Veterinary Toxicology

Veterinary Toxicology

Basic and Clinical Principles

Third Edition

Edited by

Ramesh C. Gupta, DVM, MVSc, PhD, DABT, FACT, FACN, FATS

Professor and Head, Toxicology Department, Breathitt Veterinary Center,
Murray State University, Hopkinsville, KY, United States

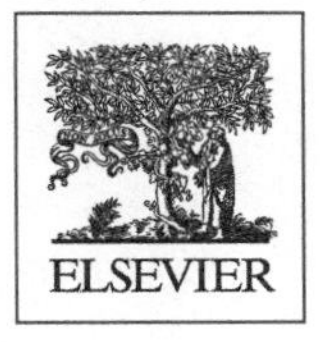

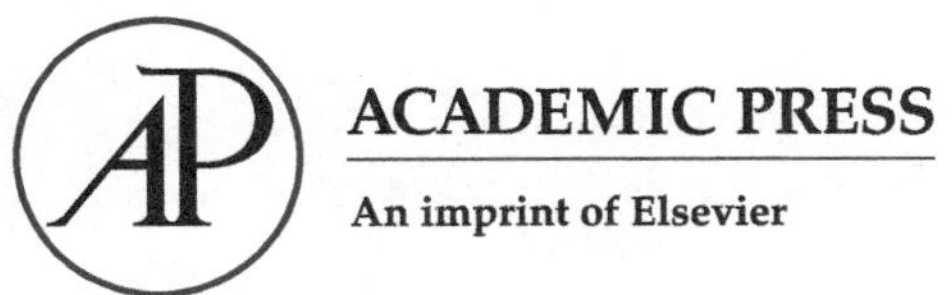

Academic Press is an imprint of Elsevier
125 London Wall, London EC2Y 5AS, United Kingdom
525 B Street, Suite 1800, San Diego, CA 92101-4495, United States
50 Hampshire Street, 5th Floor, Cambridge, MA 02139, United States
The Boulevard, Langford Lane, Kidlington, Oxford OX5 1GB, United Kingdom

Notices
Knowledge and best practice in this field are constantly changing. As new research and experience broaden our understanding, changes in research methods, professional practices, or medical treatment may become necessary.

Practitioners and researchers must always rely on their own experience and knowledge in evaluating and using any information, methods, compounds, or experiments described herein. In using such information or methods they should be mindful of their own safety and the safety of others, including parties for whom they have a professional responsibility.

To the fullest extent of the law, neither the Publisher nor the authors, contributors, or editors, assume any liability for any injury and/or damage to persons or property as a matter of products liability, negligence or otherwise, or from any use or operation of any methods, products, instructions, or ideas contained in the material herein.

British Library Cataloguing-in-Publication Data
A catalogue record for this book is available from the British Library

Library of Congress Cataloging-in-Publication Data
A catalog record for this book is available from the Library of Congress

ISBN: 978-0-12-811410-0

For Information on all Academic Press publications
visit our website at https://www.elsevier.com/books-and-journals

Publisher: Mica Haley
Acquisition Editor: Erin Hill-Parks/Kattie Washington
Editorial Project Manager: Kathy Padilla
Production Project Manager: Kiruthika Govindaraju
Cover Designer: Christian Bilbow

Typeset by MPS Limited, Chennai, India

Last digit is the print number: 9 8 7 6 5 4 3 2

Dedication

**This book is dedicated to my daughter Rekha,
my wife Denise, and to my parents,
the late Chandra and Triveni Gupta.**

Contents

7. Regulatory Aspects for the Drugs and Chemicals Used in Food-Producing Animals in the European Union

Arturo Anadón, María R. Martínez-Larrañaga, Irma Ares and María A. Martínez

8. Toxicokinetics in Veterinary Toxicology

Deon van der Merwe, Ronette Gehring and Jennifer L. Buur

9. Toxicological Testing: In Vivo and In Vitro Models

Magda Sachana and Alan J. Hargreaves

Section III
Nanoparticles, Radiation and Carcinogens

18. Toxicity of Nanomaterials

Deon van der Merwe and John A. Pickrell

19. Ionizing Radiation in Veterinary Medicine

Lisa Murphy

20. Carcinogenesis: Mechanisms and Models

Supratim Choudhuri, Ronald Chanderbhan and Antonia Mattia

Section IV
Drugs of Use and Abuse

Section V
Metals and Micronutrients

42. Fipronil

Ramesh C. Gupta and Arturo Anadón

43. Macrocyclic Lactone Endectocides

Sharon M. Gwaltney-Brant, Camille DeClementi and Ramesh C. Gupta

Section VII **Herbicides and Fungicides**

44. Toxicity of Herbicides

Pawan K. Gupta

45. Toxicity of Fungicides

Pawan K. Gupta

Section VIII **Rodenticides**

46. Anticoagulant Rodenticides

Michael J. Murphy

Section XIV
Poisonous Plants

61. Poisonous Plants of the United States

Kip E. Panter, Kevin D. Welch, Dale R. Gardner, Steven T. Lee, Ben T. Green, James A. Pfister, Daniel Cook, Thomas Z. Davis and Bryan L. Stegelmeier

62. Poisonous Plants of the Europe

Arturo Anadón, María R. Martínez-Larrañaga, Irma Ares and Maria A. Martínez

63. Poisonous Plants of Australia and New Zealand

Rhian Cope and Selina Ossedryver

64. Cyanogenic Glycoside–Containing Plants

Kip E. Panter

65. Nitrate- and Nitrite-Accumulating Plants

Jeffery O. Hall

List of Contributors

Arturo Anadón, DVM, PhD, DipECVPT, Department of Toxicology and Pharmacology, Faculty of Veterinary Medicine, Universidad Complutense de Madrid, Madrid, Spain

Irma Ares, DPharm, PhD, Department of Toxicology and Pharmacology, Faculty of Veterinary Medicine, Universidad Complutense de Madrid Madrid, Spain, Madrid, Spain

Philippe Berny, DVM, PhD, Ecole Nationale Vétérinaire de Lyon, Pharmacie-Toxicologie, Marcy l'Étoile, France

Karyn Bischoff, DVM, MS, DABVT, Assistant Professor, Animal Health Diagnostic Center, Population Medicine and Diagnostic Sciences, Cornell University, Ithaca, NY, USA; Diagnostic Toxicologist, New York State Animal Health Diagnostic Center, Cornell University, Ithaca, NY, USA

Susan J. Bright-Ponte, DVM, MPH, Division of Veterinary Product Safety, Center for Veterinary Medicine, US Food & Drug Administration, Rockville, MD, USA

Jennifer L. Buur, DVM, PhD, DACVCP, College of Veterinary Medicine, Western University of Health Sciences, Pomona, CA, USA

Francesca Caloni, DVM, PhD, Department of Veterinary Medicine (DIMEVET), Università degli Studi di Milano, Milan, Italy

Michael P. Carlson, PhD, School of Veterinary Medicine & Biomedical Sciences, University of Nebraska-Lincoln, Lincoln, NE, USA

Ronald Chanderbhan, PhD, Division of Biotechnology and GRAS Notice Review, Office of Food Additive Safety, Center for Food Safety and Applied Nutrition, US Food and Drug Administration, College Park, MD, USA

Supratim Choudhuri, PhD, Division of Biotechnology and GRAS Notice Review, Office of Food Additive Safety, Center for Food Safety and Applied Nutrition, US Food and Drug Administration, College Park, MD, USA

Ralph G. Christian, DVM, Diplomate ACVP, President, Ralph Christian Consulting Inc., Edmonton, AB, Canada

Daniel Cook, PhD, USDA-ARS Poisonous Plant Research Laboratory, Logan, UT, USA

Rhian B. Cope, BVSc, PhD, cGLPCP, DABT, DABVT, FACTRA, Senior Toxicologist, Toxicology Section, Scientific Evaluation Branch, Health Product Regulation Group, Therapeutic Goods Administration, Department of Health, Woden, ACT, Australia; Senior Advisor, Hazardous Substances, Environmental Risk Management Authority, Wellington, New Zealand; Pathobiology Section, Institute of Veterinary, Animal and Biomedical Sciences, Massey University, Palmerston North, New Zealand

Robert W. Coppock, DVM, PhD, DABVT, DABT, President and CEO, Toxicologist and Associates Ltd., Vegreville, AB, Canada; Adjunct Professor, School of Public Health and Faculty of Medicine, University of Alberta, Edmonton, AB, Canada; Adjunct Professor, Environmental Health, Concordia University College, Edmonton, AB, Canada

Siska Croubels, Pharm, PhD, Professor in Veterinary Toxicology, Ghent University, Ghent, Belgium; Faculty of Veterinary Medicine, Department of Pharmacology, Toxicology and Biochemistry, Laboratory of Pharmacology and Toxicology, Merelbeke, Belgium

Margarita Curras-Collazo, PhD, Department of Cell Biology and Neuroscience, University of California at Riverside, Riverside, CA, USA

Thomas Z. Davis, PhD, USDA-ARS Poisonous Plant Research Laboratory, Logan, UT, USA

Camille DeClementi, VMD, DABT, DABVT, Senior Director, Animal Health Services, ASPCA Animal Poison Control Center, Urbana, IL, USA

Robin B. Doss, BS, LVT, Murray State University, Hopkinsville, KY, USA

Eric Dunayer, VMD, MS, DABT, DABVT, St. Matthews University, Grand Cayman, Cayman Islands

Steve M. Ensley, BS, DVM, MS, PhD, College of Veterinary Medicine, Iowa State University, Ames, IA, USA

Tim J. Evans, DVM, MS, PhD, Veterinary Medical Diagnostic Laboratory, University of Missouri, Columbia, MO, USA

Ayhan Filazi, DVM, PhD, Department of Pharmacology and Toxicology, Faculty of Veterinary Medicine, Ankara University, Ankara, Turkey

Michael Filigenzi, PhD, California Animal Health and Food Safety Laboratory, Davis, CA, USA

Dale R. Gardner, PhD, USDA-ARS Poisonous Plant Research Laboratory, Logan, UT, USA

Tam Garland, DVM, PhD, Garland, Bailey and Associates, College Station, TX, USA

Ronette Gehring, BVSc, MMedVet, DACVCP, Department of Anatomy and Physiology, College of Veterinary Medicine, Kansas State University Manhattan, KS, USA

Ben T. Green, PhD, USDA-ARS Poisonous Plant Research Laboratory, Logan, UT, USA

Raimon Guitart, MSc, PhD, Faculty of Veterinary Sciences, Department of Pharmacology Therapeutics and Toxicology, Laboratory of Toxicology, Universitat Autònoma de Barcelona, Bellaterra, Spain

Pawan K. Gupta, BVSc, MSc VM & AH, PhD, PGDCA, FNA, VSc, FASc AW, FST, FAEB, FACVT (USA), President, Academy of Sciences for Animal Welfare, Bareilly, Uttar Pradesh, India; Former Professor and Head, Division of Pharmacology and Toxicology, Indian Veterinary Research Institute, Bareilly, Uttar Pradesh, India

Ramesh C. Gupta, DVM, MVSc, PhD, DABT, FACT, FACN, FATS, Professor and Head, Toxicology Department, Breathitt Veterinary Center, Murray State University, Hopkinsville, KY, USA

Sharon M. Gwaltney-Brant, DVM, PhD, DABVT, DABT, Veterinary Information Network, Mahomet, IL, USA

Jeffery O. Hall, DVM, PhD, DABVT, Department of Animal Dairy and Veterinary Sciences, Utah Veterinary Diagnostic Laboratory, Utah State University, Logan, UT, USA

Dwayne W. Hamar, PhD, Colorado State University, Fort Collins, CO, USA

Alan J. Hargreaves, BSc, PhD, Reader, Interdisciplinary Biomedical Research Centre, School of Science and Technology, Nottingham Trent University, Nottingham, UK

Stephen B. Hooser, DVM, PhD, DABVT, Indiana Animal Disease Diagnostic Laboratory, Purdue University, West Lafayette, IN, USA

Barry J. Jacobsen, PhD, Professor of Plant Pathology, Department of Plant Sciences and Plant Pathology, College of Agriculture, Montana State University, Bozeman, MT, USA

Un Ho Jin, PhD, Department of Veterinary Physiology and Pharmacology, Texas A&M University, College Station, TX, USA

Prasada Rao S. Kodavanti, PhD, Neurotoxicology Branch, National Health and Environmental Effects Research Laboratory, Office of Research and Development, US Environmental Protection Agency, Research Triangle Park, NC, USA

Rajiv Lall, MS, CEO and Founder, Vets Plus Inc., Menomonie, WI, USA

Steven T. Lee, PhD, USDA-ARS Poisonous Plant Research Laboratory, Logan, UT, USA

Xi Li, PhD, Department of Veterinary Physiology and Pharmacology, Texas A&M University, College Station, TX, USA

Jitendra K. Malik, BVSc & AH, MVSc, PhD, Former Joint Director (Research), and Head of the Division of Pharmacology and Toxicology, Indian Veterinary Research Institute Dehradun, Uttarakhand, India

María A. Martínez, DPharm, PhD, Department of Toxicology and Pharmacology, Faculty of Veterinary Medicine, Universidad Complutense de Madrid, Madrid, Spain

María R. Martínez-Larrañaga, DSc, DPharm, PhD, Department of Toxicology and Pharmacology, Faculty of Veterinary Medicine, Universidad Complutense de Madrid, Madrid, Spain

Antonia Mattia, PhD, Division of Biotechnology and GRAS Notice Review, Office of Food Additive Safety, Center for Food Safety and Applied Nutrition, US Food and Drug Administration, College Park, MD, USA

Roger O. McClellan, DVM, MMS, DSc (Honorary), Dipl-ABVT, Dipl-ABT, Fellow-ATS, Fellow-SRA, Fellow-AAAR, Advisor, Toxicology and Human Health Risk Analysis, Albuquerque, NM, USA

Donna Mensching, DVM, MS, DABVT, DABT, Emergency Veterinarian, Animal Emergency Clinic of Champaign County, Champaign, IL, USA

Deon van der Merwe, BVSc, MS, PhD, Department of Diagnostic Medicine/Pathobiology, Kansas State Veterinary Diagnostic Laboratory, Kansas State University, Manhattan, KS, USA

Dejan Milatovic, PhD, Independent Researcher, Charlottesville, VA, USA

Michelle S. Mostrom, DVM, MS, PhD, Diplomate ABVT and ABT, North Dakota State University, Fargo, ND, USA

Motoko Mukai, DVM, PhD, DABT, Department of Population Medicine and Diagnostic Sciences, Animal Health Diagnostic Center, College of Veterinary Medicine, Cornell University, Ithaca, NY, USA

Ida M. Mukherjee, PhD, Institute of Psychiatry and Human Behavior, Bambolim, Goa, India

Lisa Murphy, VMD, DABT, Associate Professor of Toxicology, School of Veterinary Medicine, University of Pennsylvania, Philadelphia, PA, USA; Resident Director, PADLS New Bolton Center, Kennett Square, PA, USA

Michael J. Murphy, DVM, JD, PhD, DABT, DABVT, RAC, Professor Emeritus, University of Minnesota, St. Croix Trail N, Stillwater, MN, USA

Steven S. Nicholson, DVM, DABVT, Veterinary Science Department, Louisiana State University, Baton Rouge, LA, USA

P. Nick Nation, DVM, PhD, DACVP, Laboratory Medicine and Pathology, University of Alberta, Edmonton, AB, Canada

Meliton N. Novilla, DVM, MS, PhD, Diplomate ACVP, Fellow IATP, Shin Nippon Biomedical Laboratories USA, Ltd., Everett, WA, USA

Selina Ossedryver, BVSc, MVSt, Senior Veterinary Pathologist and Curator, Natural Toxicants Database, Biosecurity Sciences Laboratory, Department of Agriculture and Fisheries Brisbane, QLD, Australia

Kip E. Panter, PhD, USDA-ARS Poisonous Plant Research Laboratory, USDA-Agricultural Research Service, Poisonous Plant Research Laboratory, Logan, UT, USA

James A. Pfister, PhD, USDA-ARS Poisonous Plant Research Laboratory, Logan, UT, USA

John A. Pickrell, DVM, MS, PhD, DABT, Department of Diagnostic Medicine/Pathobiology, Kansas State University, Manhattan, KS, USA

Robert H. Poppenga, DVM, PhD, DABVT, Professor of Clinical Veterinary Toxicology, CAHFS Toxicology Laboratory, School of Veterinary Medicine, University of California at Davis, Davis, CA, USA

Birgit Puschner, DVM, PhD, DABVT, Professor of Veterinary Toxicology, Department of Molecular Biosciences, School of Veterinary Medicine, University of California at Davis, Davis, CA, USA

Shashi K. Ramaiah, DVM, PhD, DACVP, DABT, Head-Biomarker Lab, Pfizer Inc., Cambridge, MA, USA

Magda Sachana, DVM, MSc, PhD, Faculty of Veterinary Medicine, Laboratory of Biochemistry and Toxicology, Aristotle University of Thessaloniki, Thessaloniki, Greece

Stephen H. Safe, DPhil, Distinguished Professor of Toxicology, Department of Veterinary Physiology and Pharmacology, Texas A&M University, College Station, TX, USA

Geof W. Smith, DVM, PhD, Department of Population Health and Pathobiology, North Carolina State University, Raleigh, NC, USA

Arya Sobhakumari, DVM, PhD, California Animal Health and Food Safety Laboratory, Davis, CA, USA

Ajay Srivastava, DVM, MS, PhD, Chief Scientific Officer, Vets Plus Inc., Menomonie, WI, USA

Bryan L. Stegelmeier, DVM, PhD, Diplomat ACVP, USDA-ARS Poisonous Plant Research Laboratory, Logan, UT, USA

Szabina Stice, PhD, Division of Biotechnology and GRAS Notice Review, FDA College Park, MD, USA

Snehal Tawde, BVSc & AH, MVSc, University of California at Davis, Davis, CA, USA

Larry J. Thompson, DVM, PhD, DABVT, Nestlé Purina PetCare, St. Louis, MO, USA

Mary A. Thrall, DVM, MS, DACVP, Colorado State University, Fort Collins, CO, USA

Matthew C. Valdez, PhD, Neurotoxicology Branch, Toxicity Assessment Division, National Health and Environmental Effects Research Laboratory, Office of Research and Development, US Environmental Protection Agency, Research Triangle Park, NC, USA; Oak Ridge Institute for Science and Education, US Department of Energy, Oak Ridge, TN, USA

Kevin D. Welch, PhD, DABT, USDA-ARS Poisonous Plant Research Laboratory, Logan, UT, USA

Christina R. Wilson, PhD, Department of Comparative Pathobiology, Indiana Animal Disease Diagnostic Laboratory, Purdue University, West Lafayette, IN, USA

Tina Wismer, DVM, DABVT, DABT, ASPCA Animal Poison Control Center, Urbana, IL, USA

Nobuyoshi Yamashita, PhD, National Institute of Advanced Industrial Science and Technology (AIST), Tsukuba, Ibaraki, Japan

Jae-Ho Yang, PhD, Department of Pharmacology, School of Medicine, Catholic University of Daegu, Gyeongsan, South Korea

Hany Youssef, DVM, MS, Hoopeston Pet Clinic, Hoopeston, IL, USA

Begum Yurdakok-Dikmen, DVM, PhD, Department of Pharmacology and Toxicology, Faculty of Veterinary Medicine, Ankara University, Ankara, Turkey

Tong Zhou, MS, PhD, DABT, Division of Veterinary Product Safety, Center for Veterinary Medicine, US Food & Drug Administration, Rockville, MD, USA

Csaba K. Zoltani, PhD, Emeritus US Army Research Lab, Aberdeen Proving Ground, MD, USA

Preface

Veterinary toxicology is a very complex, yet fascinating subject, as it deals with a wide variety of poisons of chemical, plant, and animal origins, as well as drugs of use and abuse. Presently, synthetic compounds constitute the largest number of chemicals that are frequently encountered in animal poisonings. The subject of veterinary toxicology is complicated greatly by the wide variations in responses of domestic, companion, aquatic, wild, and zoo species to toxicants. Of course, environmental and many other factors may be involved in the overall toxicity of a chemical. In the last few decades, veterinary toxicologists have faced the enormous task of dealing with a flood of new farm chemicals and household products. Understanding the complete profile (especially mechanisms of toxicity) of each toxicant is the biggest challenge for today's veterinary toxicologists. Highly sensitive analytical techniques for residue detection, toxicokinetics, and physiologically based pharmacokinetic modeling, biomarkers of exposure, effects and susceptibility, and the concept of adverse outcome pathway comes into play when resolving many toxicological issues, such as delineating underlying mechanisms, prompt and accurate diagnosis, and development of antidotal treatment.

By the turn of the 21st century, we began to face new problems. For example, on September 11, 2001, a large number of pets died from the collapse of the World Trade Center in New York City, while those that survived suffered from a variety of illnesses (Ground Zero illnesses) caused by the dust, debris, and toxic chemicals. In 2005, two major hurricanes (Katrina and Rita) devastated the lives of many animals in the Gulf Coast states of Louisiana and Mississippi. Thousands of animals died, while a large number of others suffered from intoxication with high levels of metals, pesticides, algal toxins, and many other unidentified toxic substances. Again, in 2017, multiple hurricanes have affected the lives of thousands of animals in the US.

In early 2007, melamine became a household name for pet owners in the United States because many dogs and cats died from renal failure, while hundreds were sickened due to the consumption of food imported from China tainted with melamine and other co-contaminants. Regulatory action of the U.S. Food and Drug Administration led to the recall of more than 150 brands of pet food. Similar recalls occurred in Asia and South Africa. In 2008, just prior to an international polo event in Florida, 21 horses from a Brazilian team died acutely due to an overdose of selenium. In 2010, the Deepwater Horizon oil rig explosion killed 11 workers. The subsequent oil spill in the Gulf of Mexico caused death, or affected the lives, of millions of birds, fish, and other species, including dolphins, costing billions of dollars. On March 11, 2011, a severe earthquake and subsequent tsunami that struck Japan led to the deaths of thousands of humans and animals. As a result of the tsunami and aftershocks, the Fukushima Daiichi Nuclear Power Plant was severely damaged. The deaths of many companion animals occurred within a few days from excess radiation exposure. A large number of surviving abandoned livestock, horses, and companion animals in the danger zone continue to suffer from cancer and other radiation-related complications. Currently, due to ongoing political unrest in Syria, thousands of humans and animals have died from chemical warfare agent (chlorine, sarin, and possibly others) exposure, and the chemical attacks are still taking place on a regular basis.

Evidently, from time to time, unusual toxicological problems are encountered on a small or large scale, and that trend will most likely continue in the future. Toxicological problems are often exacerbated by harsh weather conditions, especially in livestock species. Around the world, animals and humans are living in a more polluted environment today than ever before. Many of the toxicological problems are global, while others are regional. Unfortunately, the availability of antidotes for common poisons is still obscure and often delayed. Thus, veterinary toxicologists have a tremendous task ahead to face the new challenges of the 21st century.

The first edition of *Veterinary Toxicology: Basic and Clinical Principles* was prepared to offer a comprehensive resource to veterinary toxicologists, students, teachers, clinicians, nutritionists, animal health scientists, and environmentalists. In 2012, the 2nd edition was prepared to maintain the same temper, yet was more student-teacher-friendly and targeted primarily for the classroom. Many new chapters were added, identifying unique problems pertinent to Europe, Asia, and Africa. During the last 5 years, the book has captured its image as a Gold

Standard for veterinarians and veterinary toxicologists serving academia, government, industry, environment, and other sectors. Currently, the book is heavily used by practicing veterinarians, as it offers comprehensive information on sample submission, diagnosis and prevention, and treatment of poisonings in both small and large animals, as well as avian and aquatic species. Attorneys for legal cases and county extension agents for plant and farm chemical poisoning cases are using this book, as it offers easy access to a plethora of toxicological knowledge.

In recent years, veterinarians and veterinary toxicologists from many parts of the world have expressed the need for a 3rd edition of this book, as the field of veterinary toxicology is rapidly changing with so many emerging issues. In light of the valuable suggestions and the current world situation, the book is revised accordingly. It addresses both global as well as regional toxicological problems, adequately covers mechanistic aspects, and offers differential diagnosis and practical solutions. The entire book is organized in 18 sections, with a total of 82 chapters, to offer a stand-alone chapter on as many topics as possible; however, many of the chapters on related topics are consolidated to avoid redundancy. The book is focused heavily on target organ toxicity and poisons of various types and classes. Several chapters provide the latest information on problems related to metals, pesticides, industrial and environmental toxicants, as well as aquatic, marine, and zoo toxins. This volume extensively covers chapters on poisonous plants, mycotoxins, and feed and water contaminants. A significant portion of the book is devoted to diagnostic toxicology that entails sample submission and analytical toxicology. Finally, the book concludes with an emphasis on prevention and therapeutic measures of common poisonings.

The chapters of this book are contributed by the most qualified and well-experienced authors from academia, government, industry, environment, and the private sector, who are considered authorities in veterinary toxicology. As of today, this book remains a unique text/reference source of veterinary toxicology that is unparalleled.

Finally, the editor is deeply indebted to all authors for their sincere and dedicated contributions to this book. The editor would like to recognize Drs. Roger O. McClellan and Frederick W. Oehme, who made not only enormous contributions but also shaped the field of veterinary toxicology. A special thanks to Robin B. Doss and Denise M. Gupta for their technical assistance in preparation of this book. The editor and the authors offer their sincere thanks to the publishing editors (Erin Hill-Parks, Kathy Padilla, Molly McLaughlin, Kiruthika Govindaraju, and Kattie Washington) at Academic Press/Elsevier for their vital input in the preparation of this book.

Ramesh C. Gupta

Section I

General

Chapter 1

Concepts in Veterinary Toxicology

Roger O. McClellan

INTRODUCTION

Toxicology, from the Greek words toxicon for poison and logos for scientific study, is the study of poisons. Veterinary medicine is that branch of medical science concerned with the diagnosis, treatment, and prevention of diseases of animals. The adjective veterinary is derived from Latin: veterinae, beasts of burden. Obviously, the modern field of veterinary medicine extends beyond the "beasts of burden" to include all the domesticated animal species, both livestock and companion animals, as well as nondomesticated species. Indeed, it has expanded to include nonmammalian species. The focus of toxicology is on chemicals, including chemicals in plants. However, it is generally acknowledged that the study of effects of ionizing radiation is a part of the field or is at least a closely related specialty. Pharmacology, from the Greek words pharma for drugs and logos for scientific study, is a closely related field concerned with the science of drugs: their preparation, properties, effects and uses in the diagnosis, treatment, and prevention of disease.

The field of toxicology is very broad and includes the identification and characterization of poisons, their physical and chemical properties, their fate in the body and their biological effects. In addition, toxicology is concerned with the treatment of disease conditions caused by poisons. The terms toxicant and poison are used interchangeably. A toxicant is a material that, when it contacts or enters the body in sufficient quantity via ingestion, inhalation, dermal contact, or injection, interferes with the normal biological processes and causes adverse health effects. The term toxin is used to describe poisons originating from biological processes. The term toxic is used to describe the effects of a poison on biological systems. Toxicosis is the term used to describe the syndrome of adverse health effects that result from exposure to a toxicant. During the last several decades, increased concern has developed for the effects of long-term low-level exposures to toxicants. With these exposures, adverse health effects, if they occur, may be manifest in a nonspecific manner as an increase in the incidence of common diseases, such as cancer," in a population.

Wide ranges of materials are capable of producing toxic effects when exposure occurs at sufficiently high levels. Indeed, with extreme levels of exposure most agents can produce adverse effects. For example, while both water and oxygen are required to sustain life they are toxic when the level of intake is excessive. The nature of the toxic responses depends not only on the toxicant but also the route of exposure, the duration and intensity of the exposure, and the characteristics of the exposed individual, i.e., species, gender, age, preexisting disease states, nutritional status, and prior exposure to the agent or related compounds. The exposure may be brief or prolonged. The response may appear to be acute or chronic and occur soon after exposure or much later and only after prolonged exposure. The response may be relatively unique to the toxicant, i.e., a specific toxicosis, or distinguishable from common diseases caused by natural processes or exposure to other agents. In many cases, sophisticated statistical methods are required to associate some excess health risk, such as cancer, over and above that caused by other factors, with a particular toxicant exposure. This is especially true today after much progress has been made in controlling exposure to toxic materials.

In this chapter, I first provide a brief historical perspective on the development of veterinary toxicology as a subspecialty of the veterinary medical profession and as a specialized area within the general field of toxicology. This is followed by a section on the evolution of veterinary toxicology from an observation-based profession to one that places increasing reliance on science developed through experimentation. This includes a discussion of the risk paradigm that has become an integral part of toxicology in recent decades. In the next section, I offer several related paradigms for acquiring, organizing, and using knowledge in veterinary toxicology so as to

Veterinary Toxicology. DOI: http://dx.doi.org/10.1016/B978-0-12-811410-0.00001-5

maximize its potential impact. Next, there is a section on the sources of information that may be obtained either through observation or experimentation. These sources may include studies on the species of interest, i.e., people or some other specific animal species, controlled exposure studies in the species of interest, studies in other species, investigations using tissues and cells and structure-activity analyses. This is followed by a section discussing the design of experimental studies to optimize the interpretation and use of the results. The chapter concludes with a discussion of key toxicologic descriptors and a brief conclusions section.

HISTORICAL PERSPECTIVE

Historical Events

The father of modern toxicology is generally acknowledged to be Aureolus Philippus Theophrastus Bombastus von Hohenheim (1493–1541), who referred to himself as Paracelsus, from his belief that his work was beyond the work of Celsus, a first century Roman physician (Pagel, 1958). Paracelsus is credited with the well-known statement, "All substances are poisons; there is none which is not a poison. The right dose differentiates a poison from a remedy." Paracelsus advanced many views that were revolutionary for his time that are now accepted as fundamental concepts for the field of toxicology. In contrast to earlier emphasis on mixtures, he focused on the toxicon as a specific primary chemical entity that was toxic. Paracelsus advanced four fundamental concepts.

1. Experimentation is required for examining responses to chemicals.
2. A distinction should be made between the therapeutic and toxic properties of chemicals.
3. The therapeutic and toxic properties are something closely related and distinguishable by dose.
4. It is possible to ascertain a degree of specificity for chemicals and their therapeutic or toxic effects.

It is obvious from the foregoing that toxicology and pharmacology are closely related fields of scientific endeavor. Pharmacology is focused on drugs, including both their effectiveness and safety. Pharmaceutical agents are drugs used to diagnose, cure, treat, or prevent disease. Toxicology is concerned with all kinds of chemicals, including pharmaceutical agents, and other agents that may, at some level of exposure, cause adverse health effects. As will be noted at several places in this chapter, toxicology is increasingly concerned with low-level exposures for which the adverse effects, if any are observed or estimated to occur, may not be specific to a particular chemical and indistinguishable from those occurring naturally or from a variety of other causes.

Toxicology, in a sense, dates back to the earliest activities of humans. By observation, people came to learn that which could be ingested without harm and, by contrast, the foodstuffs to be avoided because of their harmful properties. They also came to know which animal venoms, plant extracts, and other materials could be used for hunting, warfare, and assassination. No doubt as animals were domesticated, it became apparent that the human observations and practices could be extended to domestic animals. Unfortunately, domestic animals are not always as astute as people in learning to avoid poisonous plants and other harmful situations. Thus, veterinary practitioners still encounter toxicoses involving animals ingesting poisonous plants.

The history of toxicology has been well documented by several contemporary authors (Milles, 1999; Gallo, 2013; Lane, 2014). The history of veterinary toxicology has not been as well documented, although it is apparent that veterinary toxicology has been an integral part of veterinary medicine since the earliest time of the profession. Veterinary medicine is a specialized branch of medical science with formal programs of study leading to a professional degree. The history of veterinary medicine has been reviewed by several authors (Smithcors, 1957; Stahlheim, 1994; Swabe, 1999; Wilkinson, 2005). The role of veterinary toxicology in the veterinary curriculum is well documented for one of the earliest veterinary medical colleges, that at the Free University of Berlin. Wilsdorf and Graf (1998) provide an account of the development of veterinary toxicology at that university from 1790 to 1945. Oehme (1970) has briefly reviewed the development of veterinary toxicology as a discipline in the United States.

Textbooks

In the English language, the earliest veterinary toxicology publication I am aware of is a *Synopsis of Veterinary Materia Medica, Therapeutics and Toxicology* (Quitman, 1905) apparently used at my alma mater, Washington State University College of Veterinary Medicine, in the early part of the 20th century. I am uncertain of the extent to which this synopsis may be based on a French text by Kaufmann (1901). The earliest English language veterinary toxicology textbook I was able to locate was that authored by an Englishman, Lander (1912). This book was also prepared in a second edition (1926) and a third edition was prepared by an Irishman, Nicholson (1945). I am uncertain as to how widely it was used in the United States. The text included four sections: a brief introduction to toxicology followed by sections on classes of toxicants, mineral or inorganic poisons, organic poisons and drugs, and poisonous plants. This last section represented half of the book indicating the importance of poisonous plants in that era of veterinary medicine.

Many early students in veterinary medicine in the United States used textbooks prepared for physicians such as Kobert (1897), *Practical Toxicology for Physicians and Students.* It was also common to use either textbooks in pharmacology or veterinary pharmacology that contained a brief coverage of toxicology. Indeed, few veterinary medical colleges prior to the 1950s had full-time veterinary toxicologists on their faculty. Lectures on toxicology were usually included in courses in pharmacology, pathology, and clinical medicine.

The first veterinary toxicology text I personally used was authored by R. John Garner (1957) who was then a Senior Lecturer in Chemical Pathology (Veterinary) at the University of Bristol in the United Kingdom and later Head of the Radiobiology Department at the Agricultural Research Council Field Station, Compton, Berks, United Kingdom. At the Compton Station he conducted pioneering research on the fate of important radionuclides in domestic animals. The text by Garner (1957) was intended as a successor to the third edition of *Lander's Veterinary Toxicology* (Nicholson, 1945). A second edition was prepared by Garner (1961) after he became head of the Public Health Section, Radiological Protection Division, UK Atomic Energy Authority, Harwell, Berks, United Kingdom. I visited Garner in 1962 and discussed with him the release of I^{131} in the 1957 Windscale reactor accident. This accident emphasized the importance of the dairy cow milk pathway for human exposures. Later, Garner came to the United States where he was initially associated with Colorado State University directing studies of the long-term effects of external radiation on Beagles. I recall asking Garner in the early 1970s about the possibility of preparing a third edition of his veterinary toxicology text. He responded that the field of veterinary toxicology had become so broad that it was not readily feasible for a single individual to author a text in veterinary toxicology and he was not interested in "shepherding a herd of individual chapter authors" with specialized knowledge of various aspects of veterinary toxicology. With this textbook, Gupta has responded to the challenge offered by Garner.

Radeleff (1964) authored one of the first veterinary toxicology texts published in the United States. A second edition appeared in 1970. This was followed by a text prepared by Osweiler et al. (1985). Several books published in the 1960s became classics on the effects of poisonous plants (Kingsbury, 1954, 1964; Hulbert and Oehme, 1968). Recent books on poisonous plants have been authored by Garland and Barr (1998), Burrows and Tyrl (2006), and Knight and Walter (2001). Murphy (1996) has authored a field guide to common animal poisons. It is organized by the organ system affected and then by toxicant.

Osweiler (1996) has authored a text focused on toxicology as part of the National Veterinary Medical Series for Independent Study. It has been widely used by individuals preparing for the National Board Examinations for Veterinary Medical Licensing. Roder (2001) has prepared a text, *Veterinary Toxicology*, as part of a series, *The Practical Veterinarian.* This was followed by a version edited by Chapman and Campbell, 2011. More recently, two updates have been released: *Blackwell's Five-Minute Veterinary Consult Clinics Companion: Small Animal Toxicology* (Hovda et al., 2016) and *Canine and Feline* (Tilley and Smith, 2015). Plumlee (2004) has edited *Clinical Veterinary Toxicology*, and Peterson and Talcott have edited three editions of *Small Animal Toxicology*, the most recent edited of which was published in 2012 (Peterson and Talcott, 2012). *Small Animal Toxicology Essentials*, first edition, by Poppenga and Gwaltney-Brant (2011) is also a valuable reference. In my opinion, the present multiauthored text edited by Ramesh Gupta is the most comprehensive text on veterinary toxicology published to date. It is encouraging that it is now appearing in a third edition.

There are a number of comprehensive general toxicology texts available today. I will note five that the serious student of toxicology will find useful to have in their reference library. *Casarett and Doull's Toxicology: The Basic Science of Poisons* edited most recently by Klaassen (2013) was first published in 1975 and is now in its eighth edition. As an aside, I had the opportunity to observe first hand Louis Casarett and John Doull planning the first edition of this new textbook as I served with them on the Toxicology Study Section of the National Institute of Health. Unfortunately, Louis Casarett died of cancer before the first edition (Casarett and Doull, 1975) was completed. I was pleased when John Doull asked me to prepare the chapter that Louis had intended to write on radiation toxicology, which I did with my colleague, Charles Hobbs (Hobbs and McClellan, 1975). *Hayes' Principles and Methods in Toxicology* is now in its sixth edition (Hayes and Kruger, 2014). *Toxicology*, edited by Marquardt et al. (1999) is built on an earlier German text by Marquardt and Schafer (1994, 2004). *Biological Concepts and Techniques in Toxicology: An Integrated Approach* edited by Riviere (2006) is a concise textbook. Another pioneer in toxicology, Ernest Hodgeson, has edited a textbook that is now in its fourth edition (Hodgeson, 2010). Serious students will also want to be aware of a multivolume comprehensive set of toxicology textbooks. The first edition was edited by Sipes and colleagues (1997) a 14-volume second edition edited by McQueen (2010). Moreover, there are numerous text and reference books available now covering various subspecialty areas such as inhalation toxicology, reproductive and developmental toxicology, and dermal toxicology.

Some readers of this text will also be interested in the related field of environmental medicine, which has largely developed with a focus on the influence of the environment environment, including pollutants in air, water and food, on human health.on human health. Without question, there is a need to integrate veterinary medicine, and specifically, veterinary toxicology into environmental medicine. *Environmental Medicine* (Ayres et al., 2010a) includes a lead chapter that I coauthored providing context for environmental medicine (Ayres et al., 2010b). That chapter reviews important information on causes of death in low and middle income versus high income populations (Lopez et al., 2006) and the role of environmental versus nonenvironmental factors as contributors to the global burden of disease (Kung et al., 2008). Recognizing that this text edited by Gupta is intended for international readers, the lead chapter in Ayres et al. (2010b) serves as a reminder of the wide range of environmental conditions experienced by people around the world. Veterinarians have an important role to play in promoting human health around the world in multiple ways such as by facilitating the production and availability of safe food products of animal origin and aiding in the control of infectious agents and communicating with clients and others about health issues. Indeed, over the past decade the "One Health" concept has gained increased momentum. This concept, viewed as the collaborative effort of multiple disciplines working locally, nationally, and globally to attain optimum health for people, animals, and the environment, is traceable to an initiative of the American Veterinary Medical Association (AVMA) when Roger Mahr served as president of that organization (AVMA, 2008).

In addition to text and reference books, there are numerous journals published in the field of toxicology that regularly contain articles that relate recent findings in veterinary toxicology. Many clinically oriented Veterinary Medical journals contain articles on veterinary toxicology. The on-line search capabilities serving the medical sciences, including toxicology and veterinary toxicology, are expanding at an exponential rate. Of special note are those maintained under the auspices of the US National Library of Medicine, MEDLINE and TOXLINE.

Organizations

A number of professional scientific organizations have been created as the field of toxicology, including veterinary toxicology, has matured. The most noteworthy include the American College of Veterinary Toxicology (ACVT), American Board of Veterinary Toxicology (ABVT), Society of Toxicology (SOT), American Board of Toxicology (ABT), and Academy of Toxicological Sciences (ATS). The ACVT was one of the earliest scientific societies in the field, having been founded in 1958; I joined it soon after I graduated from Washington State University in 1960. It later became the American Academy of Veterinary and Comparative Toxicology. A 1964 conference on veterinary toxicology, organized under the auspices of the New York Academy of Science (Gabriel, 1964), helped the field of veterinary toxicology gain momentum. The ACVT was instrumental in fostering the creation of the ABVT and its recognition by the AVMA as the approved certifying specialty organization for veterinary toxicology. Dorman et al. (2017) have prepared a brief commentary on the occasion of the 50th anniversary of the ABVT. The ACVT initially proposed that it would serve as the certifying body for veterinary toxicology and all of the ACVT Fellows would be "grandfathered" in as Diplomates. Ultimately, it was decided to create a new entity, the ABVT. Three well-known veterinary toxicologists, W. Binns, J.W. Dollahite, and R. Radeleff, were accepted by the AVMA as Charter Members of the ABVT. They prepared the first certifying ABVT examination, which was given in 1967 (see www.abvt.org). I was pleased to be one of five individuals (William Buck, Roger McClellan, Fred Oehme, Robert Singer and VK Singh) in the first class certified, based on examination, as Diplomates of the ABVT, with the first examination given at the 1967 AVMA meeting in Dallas, Texas, United States.

The SOT, with the world's largest membership of toxicologists, was organized in 1961 (see www.sot.org). Many of the organizers of the SOT were members of the American Society for Pharmacology and Experimental Therapeutics (ASPET) who felt toxicologists needed a "home" of their own. I recall attending the organizational meeting of the SOT held in 1961 in conjunction with an ASPET meeting at the University of Rochester and the excitement and enthusiasm of the attendees for creating the SOT. The meeting was chaired by the late Harold Hodge of the University of Rochester who would be elected as the first president of the SOT. As an aside, it would be a few years before I felt my credentials were sufficient that I could apply for membership in the SOT. The SOT now has a number of specialty sections including the Comparative and Veterinary Specialty Section and Toxicologic and Exploratory Pathology Specialty Section with veterinarians being a majority of the membership of these sections. Veterinarians have played a major role in the SOT from its founding with many serving in leadership roles. Four veterinarians (Perry Gehring, Frederick Oehme, Roger McClellan, and James Popp) have served as president of the SOT.

The SOT fostered the creation of the ABT, which held its first certifying examination in 1980 (see www.abtox.org). I was pleased to be one of the first class of individuals certified, based on examination, as Diplomates of the ABT. The ABT has become the world's largest entity certifying toxicologists from around the world, including many Veterinarians, as Diplomates.

A third certifying entity, the ATS, which accepts individuals as Fellows based on a review of credentials, was created in 1981 (see www.acadtoxsci.org). Many veterinary toxicologists belong to all of the organizations noted above and some have been certified by one or more of the certifying organizations: the ABVT, ABT, and ATS. Of special note, four veterinary toxicologists (Roger McClellan, Charles Capen, Jim Riviere, and Bernard Schwetz) have been recognized for their contributions to human health by election to the National Academy of Medicine. Veterinary toxicology has made major contributions to both animal and human health sciences as it has continued to evolve over the past decades along with the general field of toxicology.

EVOLUTION OF VETERINARY TOXICOLOGY

Roots in Veterinary Medicine and Toxicology

The evolution of veterinary toxicology occurred concurrently with evolution of its two roots: the profession of veterinary medicine and the science of toxicology. The veterinary medicine profession was initially focused on domestic animals, particularly those used for food, fiber, transportation, and to provide power for agricultural endeavors and transportation. With the growth of more specialized agriculture and production practices, the profession, with its linkage to domestic livestock, stimulated growth of veterinary toxicology. Veterinary toxicology in its earliest years had a major focus on poisonous plants and then on antidotes for various toxins. The early part of the 20th century presented a special challenge for veterinary medicine as the use of horses and mules in agriculture decreased in favor of the use of equipment powered by internal combustion engines. During this period, there must have been considerable uncertainty as to the future of the veterinary medical profession. Indeed, many individuals thought the profession would not survive, and a number of proprietary schools teaching veterinary medicine closed.

By the mid-20th century three movements transformed veterinary medicine. The first related to the traditional roots of the profession in animal agriculture and related to the increasing emphasis given to large-scale highly specialized domestic livestock endeavors. This movement was a major factor in the growth of Colleges of Veterinary Medicine at Land Grant Universities in the United States. The second related to the increased attention given to providing veterinary medical services to a growing population of companion animals, a population that included horses, dogs, and cats. In both areas the science of veterinary medicine was strengthened as observation-based medical practice was complemented and, ultimately, supplemented by science-based medicine. During this period, veterinary toxicologists began to play an important role in veterinary medical diagnostic laboratories, both in veterinary medical colleges and in state and federal agencies. With the strengthening of the science base of veterinary medicine, including the quality of the science in the veterinary medical curriculum, the third movement, the emergence of the comparative medicine character of veterinary medicine, became more apparent and was enhanced (Wilkinson, 2005). These changes in the profession were accompanied by increased involvement of veterinarians in research on the species of traditional concern to the profession, domestic and companion animals (Stahlheim, 1994), and to the participation in a broader range of biomedical research activities, involving the use of traditional laboratory animal species, driven largely by concern for human health (Wilkinson, 2005).

Emergence of Science-Based Toxicology

Toxicology, like veterinary medicine, was also rapidly changing and evolving in the mid-20th century. The previous strong emphasis on field observations was first complemented and then supplemented by experimentation. This, in turn, led to the current strong mechanistic orientation of toxicology. With this shift in toxicology came an increased awareness of the utility of a comparative medicine orientation in research directed primarily toward improving human health (Wilkinson, 2005). With this comparative medicine orientation came increased opportunities for individuals educated in veterinary medicine, including veterinary toxicology, to contribute to general toxicology and biomedical science.

These changes in the veterinary medical profession and the emergence of toxicology as a science came during a period when the public was giving increased attention to the health risks, and its counterpoint—safety, of new technologies and products. World War II resulted in the creation of the Manhattan Project in 1942 in the United States to develop nuclear weapons. Following the war, the Manhattan Project became the Atomic Energy Commission (AEC), with a broad mission that included peaceful applications of nuclear energy. A series of national and specialized laboratories were created with several having a mandate to understand the effects of external radiation and internally deposited radionuclide. Veterinarians had a key role in many of these laboratories. My career began at one of the major AEC laboratories, the Hanford Laboratories in Richland, Washington, where research was conducted on a range of topics including effects of radioactive materials on domestic animals, a research program initially led by the late Leo K. Bustad, who later served on the faculty of the College of Veterinary Medicine at the University of California-Davis and then as Dean of the College of Veterinary Medicine at Washington State University. The Hanford

Laboratories continues today as the Pacific Northwest Laboratories operated by Battelle Memorial Institute. Later I would lead one of the specialized AEC laboratories, the Lovelace Inhalation Toxicology Research Institute (ITRI) in Albuquerque, New Mexico, which continues today as part of the Lovelace Respiratory Research Institute. The initial mission of ITRI, when it was created in 1960, was to study the health consequences of exposure to airborne radioactive materials such as might occur with a catastrophic nuclear reactor accident. Later in the 1970s the mission would be broadened to include a broad range of airborne materials including coal-fired power plant and vehicle emissions. The research conducted at Hanford, Lovelace ITRI and in numerous other laboratories with support from the AEC, which later became the Energy Research and Development Administration, and then soon became the Department of Energy, provided an enormous knowledge base on the health effects of exposure to both external radiation and radionuclides that would be deposited internally. Contrary to the impression gained from many popular media reports, our understanding of the health effects of radiation probably vastly exceeds our knowledge of any other toxicant (McClellan, 2014).

It is useful to also briefly recount the role of veterinarians in the military. A Veterinary Medical Corp was organized within the US Army in 1916. Initially, these veterinarians focused their professional talents on ensuring the health of horses and mules used by the Army. This role quickly broadened to include public health activities and research. When the US Air Force was created as a separate entity, it included an Air Force Veterinary Corp. Individuals within that unit had an important role in the conduct of research related initially to aviation medicine and then in the 1960s to aerospace medicine. Many of those individuals, after completing their military service in either the US Army or US Air Force Veterinary Corp and having gained extraordinary specialized education and research experience, found opportunities in government agencies and in the pharmaceutical field as well as in other private-sector firms where they continued to make contributions.

The post–World War II era was also a period of substantial growth of the chemical and pharmaceutical industries, especially in the United States and in Europe. This included the development of a wide array of new products, including many chemicals used in agriculture, and from the pharmaceutical industry the development of a wide array of new drugs, including many that are now widely used in veterinary medicine. The growth of these industries was intertwined with an increase in research and development. This included substantial research to ensure the safe manufacture of products and their safe use. This continued a tradition that began before World War II when the major chemical companies such as Dupont, Dow, Union Carbide, Eastman Kodak, and others created laboratories that had a strong toxicology orientation. Many veterinarians played a key role in these laboratories. Unfortunately, many of these laboratories today are much smaller or have even disappeared. This, in turn, has fostered the development of many contract research organizations (CROs). Many veterinarians are employed in CROs.

The substantial knowledge base was eventually used to guide the safe use of chemicals regarding the potential impact on human health and the environment. This concern was the focus of Rachel Carson's book, *Silent Spring* (Carson, 1962). She focused on both human health and impacts on the total ecosystem of which people were just a part. Her book was certainly one of the key stimuli to a tidal wave of legislative actions in the United States that focused broadly on the environment with concern for clean air and water, safe food, pharmaceuticals, pesticides, fungicides, rodenticides, and consumer products, and a safe working environment.

Legislative actions and related administrative actions in the 1970s created the US Environmental Protection Agency (USEPA), the Consumer Product Safety Commission, the National Institute for Occupational Safety and Health (NIOSH), the National Center for Toxicological Research, the National Institute of Environmental Health Sciences, and the Cancer Bioassay Program within the National Cancer Institute (NCI), which evolved into the National Toxicology Program (NTP) now administered by the National Institute for Environmental Health Sciences. This was also a period of rapid expansion of research activities in the pharmaceutical, food, chemical, and petroleum industries. The major chemical companies started the not-for-profit Chemical Industry Institute of Toxicology (CIIT) in 1976, based on a proposal advanced by Perry Gehring, then a Veterinarian at Dow. CIIT was initially funded by the chemical industry but was later transformed into The Hamner Institutes Health Sciences. The initial mission of CIIT was to (1) test commodity chemicals, (2) investigate the mechanisms of chemical toxicity, and (3) train additional toxicologists. A senior chemical industry official in the 1970s characterized CIIT as the "crown jewel" of the industry. I concur. It was this reputation that attracted me to serve as the third President of CIIT (1988–99) following Leon Goldberg and Robert Neal. I would be followed by William Greenlee. In the early 2000s, the chemical industry changed its strategy, centralizing funding decisions in the industry's trade association and spreading its funding across many organizations in addition to CIIT. The Institute was closed in December 2016.

During its four decades of operation CIIT had a huge impact on the field of toxicology and risk assessment. All of the Institute's research findings were published in the peer-reviewed literature without prior review by the funders. Hundreds of scientists who gained valuable experience as students, postdoctoral fellows, or staff members at the Institute became leaders in the field. This included dozens of veterinarians.

In the late 20th century, the Food and Drug Administration (FDA) continued its traditional dual emphasis of ensuring both the efficacy and the safety of drugs and medical devices continued. Increased emphasis has been given by the FDA in recent decades to veterinary drugs and to the potential for veterinary drugs to contaminate meat and milk.

Increasing public concern for safety/risk and the resulting legislation led to the development of increasingly formalized approaches to both safety and risk analysis. This included more clearly defined roles for using the results of toxicological studies, including studies with laboratory animals, to assess the safety, or conversely risk, to humans of the use of pharmaceuticals, other products in commerce, and existing and new technologies. In my opinion, the same scientific knowledge base can be used to address concerns for safety and risk. Scientific information can be used to inform regulatory and other societal actions that maximize safety and minimize risk, both are relative not absolute.

Toxicology Joined to the Risk Paradigm

As noted earlier, federal legislation passed in the 1970s focused on health impacts of environmental and occupational exposures and led to more formalized approaches to evaluating the risks and safety of various exposures. The risk paradigm built on the long-standing paradigm of linking sources of dose exposure to adverse health outcomes that had guided toxicology from its earliest days (Fig. 1.1). I have reviewed elsewhere the development of the risk analysis paradigm and the use of scientific knowledge to inform regulatory actions (McClellan, 1999, 2010, 2014; McClellan et al., 2012). The development of risk analysis as a specialized area of interdisciplinary science led to the founding of the Society for Risk Analysis in 1981 of which I was a charter member and later named a Fellow. The risk analysis paradigm originally proposed by the National Research Council (1983) and used by the USEPA is shown in Fig. 1.2. A later report, *Science and Judgment in Risk Assessment* (NRC, 1994; McClellan, 1994), and reports from the Risk Commission (1997), reaffirmed use of the risk paradigm that continues to be a cornerstone of activities not just at the EPA but in other national and international agencies and in the private sector concerned with human health.

The original key elements of the risk paradigm were (1) hazard identification, (2) exposure–response assessment, (3) exposure assessment, and (4) risk assessment. The NRC (1994) report emphasized the importance of a fifth element: using the results of the risk analysis to guide future research and, thus, reduce uncertainty in future risk estimates. In addition, I have added a sixth over-arching element: risk communication. The hazard identification element has been a source of contention and confusion both with the public and in the scientific community, especially with regard to cancer, as I will discuss later.

Hazard is defined as the potential for an agent under some conditions of exposure to cause an adverse effect (NRC, 1983, 1994; McClellan, 1999, 2010, 2014). With this definition the level of exposure or dose required to produce an adverse health effect is not considered. An agent may be classified as a hazard irrespective of whether or not the exposure conditions required to elicit adverse health effects under experimental conditions are

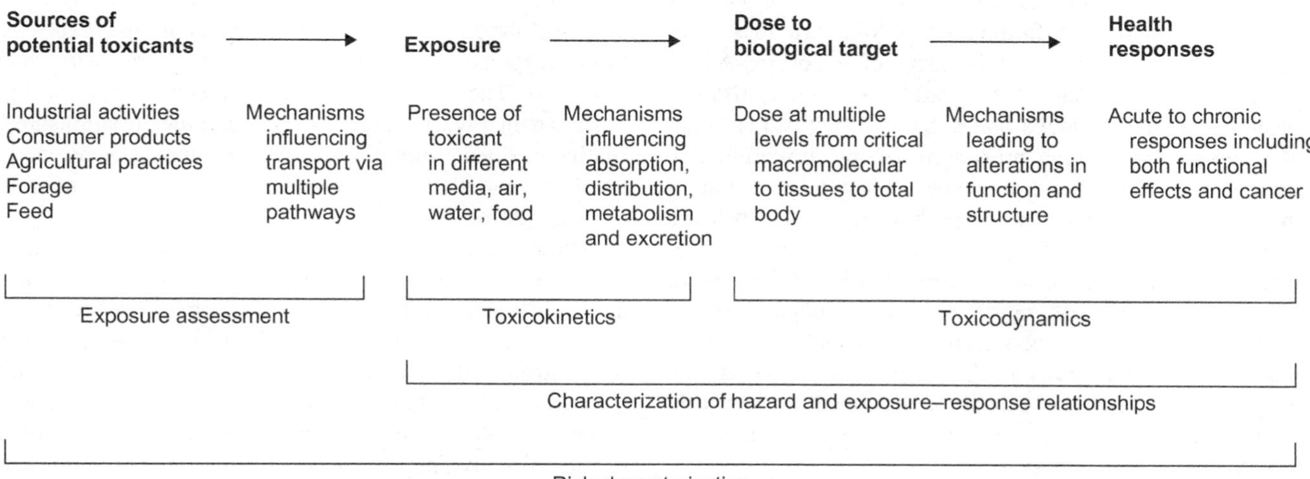

FIGURE 1.1 Critical linkages for integrating information from sources of toxicants to the development of adverse health effects.

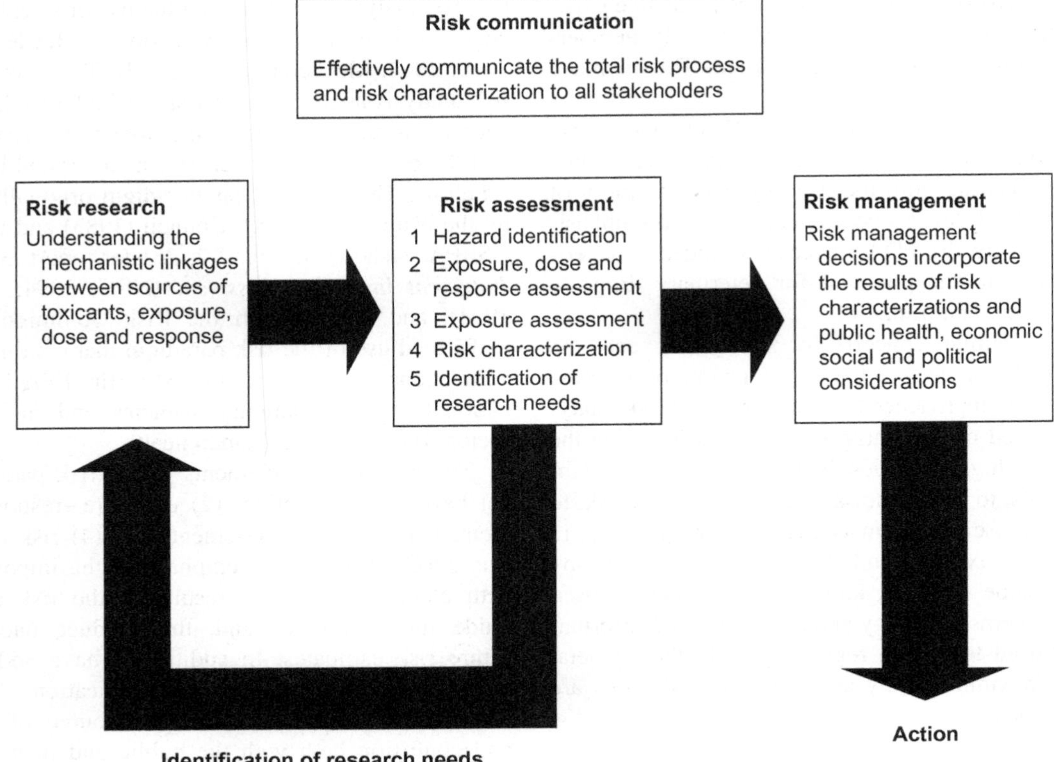

FIGURE 1.2 Risk paradigm for evaluating potential health impacts of a toxicant.

relevant to human situations. The exposure–response assessment involves characterization of this relationship as it may pertain to likely levels of human exposure. The exposure assessment quantifies, either retrospectively or prospectively, the likely duration and intensity of human exposure to the hazardous agent. The risk assessment element brings together information from the other three elements in an integrated manner to characterize risk, as illustrated in Fig. 1.1. Risk is defined as the probability of occurrence of an adverse health effect from exposure to a hazardous agent at a specified duration and intensity of exposure. As an aside, especially in Europe, the word hazard used as risk has been defined in the United States. Safety is defined as being a condition with a high probability of freedom from any increase in adverse health outcome when the agent is used in a specified manner. Obviously, both safety and risk are relative in recognizing that it is not possible to ensure absolute freedom from some small level of risk. As the control of hazards and risks has improved, in part through more and more stringent regulations, scientists and society at large are increasingly faced with the challenge of how low is low enough. Such decisions should be informed by scientific knowledge. However, it is important to recognize other factors that need to be considered.

The more formalized risk analysis approaches that were developed starting in the 1970s built on approaches developed earlier for providing guidance for controlling occupational exposures, the intake of contaminants in food, and the safety of pharmaceutical agents. Prior to World War II, the primary focus was on adverse health outcomes that caused functional impairment such as decreased respiratory function. As will be discussed later, the issue of carcinogenic responses received limited attention prior to World War II. The approach to developing guidance for the control of toxicants was based on the assumption that a threshold exists in the exposure (dose)-response relationship—just as Paracelsus had discussed. The threshold exposure–response relationship is shown in Fig. 1.3 along with four other relationships: sublinear, linear, supralinear, and a U-shaped or hormetic function. Note that both scales in this schematic rendering are logarithmic.

There is an on-going debate in the scientific community over the merits of threshold versus linear, no-threshold models for describing exposure-(dose)-response relationships, especially for carcinogenic hazards. I was first introduced to this debate in 1965 by one of my colleagues at the AEC, the late Paul Henshaw, a pioneer in cancer biology and radiation effects research. He called my attention to a paper (Henshaw, 1941) he had published on the use of tolerance dose in radiation protection. During the last decade, there has been increased

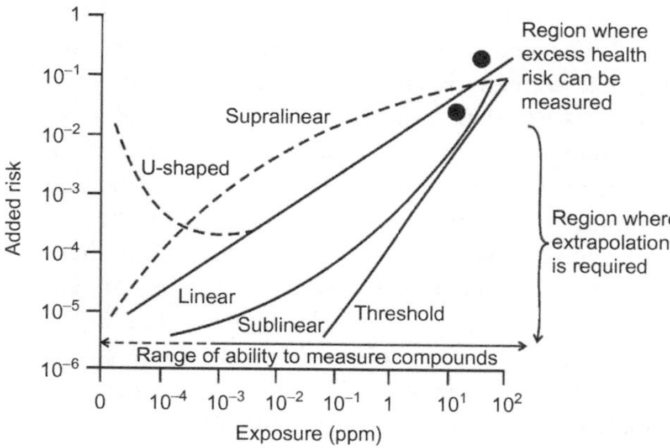

FIGURE 1.3 Schematic rendering of exposure–response relationships for various toxicants.

discussion of the concept of hormesis in which very low-level exposures have positive effects with negative effects observed only at higher exposure levels (Calabrese and Baldwin, 2003; Calabrese and Blain, 2005; Calabrese et al., 2007). Technically, in hormesis there is a beneficial effect at some low level of exposure, which decreases with increasing exposure/dose and at yet higher levels adverse effects become apparent. The concept of hormesis has been well known for decades to veterinarians who are aware that certain agents, such as vitamins and minerals, are essential for life at low concentrations and can produce toxicity with excess intake.

As an aside, there has been an on-going debate for decades as to whether linear exposure–response relationships, especially for cancer, are realistic, i.e., an added level of exposure, regardless of how small, results in a calculable monotonic increase in cancer risk. It has been argued by some that the linear exposure–response model is appropriate for regulatory purposes for assessing cancer risks because every dose of a new agent is added to a background of genetic and other damage in somatic cells arising from multiple agents and endogenous factors. I have discussed these issues in a recent book chapter on radiation toxicity (McClellan, 2014). That discussion draws on the extensive epidemiological data available on human populations exposed to radiation.

In recent years the debate over the nature of the exposure–response relationship has been extended from cancer as an endpoint to noncancer endpoints. Arguments for the use of linear nonthreshold exposure–response relationships for noncancer endpoints have been advanced by White et al. (2009). An alternative view has been advanced by Rhomberg et al. (2011a,b), namely, that linear low-dose extrapolation for noncancer health effects is the exception, not the rule. Extension of the debate over the nature of the exposure–response relationship to noncancer endpoints, such as respiratory or cardiovascular morbidity and mortality has important implications for assessing risks such as from air pollutants like particulate matter and ozone. For example, the Clean Air Act (CAA, 1970) requires the EPA administrator to set National Ambient Air Quality Standards (NAAQS) for these pollutants at levels that are protective of public health with an adequate margin of safety. If the exposure–response relationship for the pollutant in question has a threshold, then the setting of the standard is relatively straightforward, thereby identifying the threshold concentration and setting the NAAQS at a lower concentration for a given average time and statistical form. If a linear, no-threshold, exposure–response relationship is apparent, the question arises as how to determine when the NAAQS is set low enough. McClellan (2011) has addressed that topic in a paper drawing on the guidance of Supreme Court Justice Stephen Breyer in the legal case of Whitman v. American Trucking Associations (2001). McClellan (2011) has emphasized the importance of "distinguishing between (a) the science that informs the setting of the standard and (b) the policy judgments inherent in selecting the standard." This discussion is extended in a recent commentary (McClellan, 2016a) on estimates of attributable risk for ambient particulate matter.

The early development of Threshold Limit Values (TLVs) for control of occupational exposures by The American Conference of Governmental Industrial Hygienists (ACGIH), organized in 1938, assumed the existence of thresholds in exposure–response relationships. The initial data used in establishing TLVs were provided primarily by opportunistic studies of occupationally exposed human populations. In the absence of human data, data from controlled exposure studies in laboratory animals were used. This necessitated the use of safety factors to account for (1) interindividual variability, (2) interspecies extrapolation, and (3) duration of the study, as will be discussed later. The original safety factors were formally proposed by Lehman and Fitzhugh (1954) of the FDA. In 1970, the newly formed USEPA began using the same factors. However, the EPA identifies them as uncertainty factors apparently out of a desire to avoid use of a potentially contentious word: safety.

After World War II an increased public concern about the occurrence of cancer emerged. This was stimulated by multiple factors. Extensive research conducted during and after the war on the effects of both external ionizing radiation and internally deposited radionuclides emphasized the importance of cancer as a radiation-induced disease. Concern for radiation-induced cancer was further heightened when the intensive follow-up of Japanese A-bomb survivors revealed an increase, first in hematopoietic neoplasms, and, later in solid cancers. These findings soon led to abandoning a threshold approach to evaluating radiation risks in favor of using a probabilistic or stochastic approach to assess the health risks of using radiation devices in space and commercial nuclear power. The probabilistic approach using the linear no threshold exposure–response model discussed earlier was convenient to use because it could be readily applied to assessing the risks to both individuals and populations. My first experience with probabilistic risk assessment came in 1965 when I was on a temporary assignment with what was then the US AEC. I worked with a joint AEC-National Aeronautics and Space Administration Committee assessing potential human cancer risks of accidents involved with the launch of space craft containing plutonium-238–fueled thermal electric power systems.

Another factor influencing public concern was the increasing incidence of total cancers being observed in all of the economically developed countries, including the United States, that were driven largely by lung cancer. It is now well known that the increase in lung cancer, first observed in men and later in women, was largely related to cigarette smoking. The different pattern in men and women relates to a large increase in men smoking earlier than women. Many women began smoking during World War II. Rachel Carson's book also created concern for exposure to man-made chemicals contributing to the increasing incidence of cancer and encouraged the view that somehow man-made chemicals were different than chemicals of natural origin. It is now known that this is not the case (Gold et al., 2003). Ironically, some major commodity chemicals such as formaldehyde are normal constituents of mammals were related to the one-carbon metabolic cycle (Golden, 2011).

The experience with radiation soon resulted in its use as a proto-typical carcinogen in developing approaches to risk analysis and risk regulation. Albert (1994) documented the development of the USEPA's approach to assessing cancer risks. Key assumptions in the approach were: (1) cancer-causing chemical agents acted like radiation in causing cancer; (2) there was a linear relationship between exposure (dose) and increased risk of cancer extending to the lowest levels of exposure; (3) agents causing cancer in laboratory animals could be viewed as also causing cancer in people; and (4) exposure–response relationships could be extrapolated between species by considering differences in body weight and surface area, i.e., metabolic activity. These assumptions were viewed as default options to be used in the absence of specific scientific data to the contrary (McClellan, 1994, 1999, 2003; NRC, 1994).

In response to public concern for chemicals causing cancer, the International Agency for Research on Cancer (IARC), a part of the World Health Organization, was organized in Lyon, France, in 1965 under the leadership of John Higginson to develop an international research program to study cancer. Higginson's deputy, Lorenzo Tomatis, provided leadership for creating a program to classify agents or occupations as to their carcinogenic potential with the results published in a series of monographs (IARC, 1972); hence it is frequently referred to as the monograph program. The view was that if cancer-causing chemicals or other agents, such as radiation, or workplace conditions involving exposure to chemicals or other agents causing cancer could be identified, then these could be controlled, perhaps even eliminated, and the occurrence of cancer in people reduced. The IARC carcinogen classification scheme considers human, laboratory animal, and supporting data to classify agents or workplace conditions as (1) carcinogenic to humans, (2) probably carcinogenic to humans, (3) possibly carcinogenic to humans, (4) not likely to be carcinogenic to humans, or (5) not classified as to carcinogenicity. It is important to recognize that the IARC classification is strictly hazard-oriented. It does not formally evaluate the potency of these agents for causing cancer at a specific level of exposure.

The USEPA, the NTP, and other organizations have developed similar carcinogen classification schemes (EPA, 1986, 2005a,b; NTP, 2005). The EPA cancer hazard scheme is virtually identical to that of IARC. However the NTP scheme differs in that it classifies agents as (1) human carcinogens or (2) reasonably anticipated to be human carcinogens. In recent years, IARC (1991) has made provision for increased use of mechanistic data in classifying chemicals as human carcinogens. Both the EPA and NTP now also give increased emphasis to the use of mechanistic data in classifying chemicals as carcinogens (EPA, 2005a,b) unlike IARC and the NTP, the EPA does develop estimates of cancer-causing potency for some agents classified as having cancer-causing potential. This, in turn, using measurements or estimates of exposure, provides the basis for calculating lifetime cancer risks for individuals or populations.

It should be apparent that the classification of a given chemical or agent as to its cancer-causing potential is insufficient for characterizing cancer risk since the hazard-based classification does not include an estimate of the agent's potency. The USEPA has estimated the carcinogenic potency for a number of chemicals. The results are usually related as the concentration of a chemical in water or air that will result in a calculated one in a million probability of cancer occurring above the background incidence (EPA/IRIS, 2011). In viewing such estimates it is useful to recall that in developed countries of the world with long-lived populations, about one-third of the population will be diagnosed with cancer during their lifetime and one-fourth will die with a cancer. Cancers are a large family of related diseases that do occur frequently, especially in aged populations. To estimate the cancer risk for any agent and exposure situation, it is also necessary to estimate the exposure to the agent, both as to intensity, i.e., concentration and duration. In short, risk is a product of exposure *and* the potency of the agent for causing the effect. Paustenbach (2001) provides an excellent review of the practice of exposure assessment.

There has been a tendency for regulatory agencies, such as the USEPA, to use their experience with classifying chemicals as to their carcinogenic potential as a template for also classifying chemicals as to their potential for producing other noncancer hazards. Thus, there has been a trend toward classifying chemicals as to their potential hazard for causing different health outcomes and labeling them as such, i.e., neurotoxins, reproductive toxins, hepatic toxins, etc. Indeed, some even broader classifications have emerged, i.e., endocrine-disrupting chemicals. In my view, this shorthand approach to identifying and classifying hazardous agents as to their potential to cause cancer or other effects is often confusing to the public. In my opinion, the labeling approach has contributed to both radiation phobia and chemical phobia and sometimes irrational actions. It certainly flies in the face of the fact that for many chemicals the admonishment of Paracelsus that "the dose makes the poison" remains true. For numerous chemicals, even when toxic effects are apparent at high doses, these same adverse effects are no longer manifest at sufficiently low doses. Gold et al. (2003) has discussed the challenge of using high-exposure (dose) animal studies to identify either man-made or natural chemicals as human carcinogens.

In recent years increasing attention has been given to developing safer products and technologies, especially when concerns have been raised with regard to the hazards of an existing product or technology. In some cases, the focus has been on developing products that do not have carcinogenic properties to replace products that have been classified as human carcinogens or probable or possible human carcinogens by IARC or as known or reasonably anticipated to be human carcinogens in the Report on Carcinogens periodically prepared by the NTP. Endpoints other than cancer have increasingly drawn attention for chemicals such as Bisphenol A, which has been under attack as an endocrine-disrupting chemical. A committee of the National Academies of Science, Engineering and Medicine chaired by a Veterinary Toxicologist, David Dorman, has recently released a report (NASEM, 2017) that will guide future assessments of what it calls endocrine active chemicals. In general, chemicals that persist in the environment and have a long residence time in animals and humans, even when shown to have low hazard potential, have become targets for replacement. In yet other cases, the approach has been to identify replacements for chemicals that are persistent in the environment and have long residence time in animals and humans. In other cases, the approach has been to find ways to minimize the use of the chemical viewed as being unsafe. These activities have given rise to a field of science sometimes referred to as "green chemistry" (Anastas and Warner, 1998).

Controversy continues over the carcinogen hazard classification scheme used by IARC. One area of controversy concerns evaluating cancer hazards related to technologies, especially to technologies whose emissions may change over time. A specific chemical such as benzene remains constant over time with a continual increase in the knowledge that will inform the cancer hazard classification process. Benzene studied in 2017 is the same molecule as was studied at earlier times. The situation may be for different specific technologies that are constantly changing, sometimes with changes to reduce emissions.

An excellent example is the diesel engine, the compression ignition engine using liquid hydrocarbon fuel invented by Rudolph Diesel in the 1890s (McClellan et al., 2012). The utility and efficiency of diesel engines resulted in their rapid deployment and use in many applications. A pre–World War II concern for diesel exhaust emissions focused on their odor and impact on visibility. Demonstrations in the 1970s that extract of diesel exhaust particles painted on mouse skin caused cancer and were mutagenic in the newly developed Ames assay raised concern for inhalation exposure of diesel exhaust potentially causing lung cancer. These concerns stimulated research using multiple approaches. A number of epidemiological studies yielded results suggesting that exposure to exhaust from diesel engines in use in the 1950s and 1960s caused an increase in lung cancer. Four different laboratories in the United States, Germany, Switzerland, and Japan reported that long-term exposure to high concentrations of diesel exhaust particulate material caused an increase in lung cancer in rats (Hesterberg et al., 2005, 2011; McClellan et al., 2012). Mauderly et al. (1987) is an example of one of those studies of traditional diesel exhaust. An IARC (1989) panel on which I served evaluated the evidence and classified exposure to diesel exhaust as a probable human carcinogen. Soon new research provided evidence that the increase in lung cancer in rats to high concentrations of exhaust particles for long periods of time involved a nonspecific overload phenomena suggesting that the effects observed in rats were not relevant for evaluating human hazards/risks at low levels of exposure (Wolff et al., 1987; Nikula et al., 1995). Nikula et al. (1995) showed that chronic exposure of rats to high concentrations of carbon black particles free of hydrocarbons produced an increase in lung cancer.

In response to the 1988 IARC hazard classification, a related evaluation by the NTP, and an independent hazard evaluation by the USEPA, the EPA issued stringent emission standards for particulate matter and NO_2 emissions from diesel engines and mandated the use of ultra-low sulfur fuel (less than 15 ppm) for on-road vehicles. Industry responded with advances in engine technology, exhaust after-treatment, and electronic control systems that, along with use of ultra-low sulfur fuel, met the stringent particulate matter emission standards in 2007 and also stringent NO_2 emission standards in 2010 (McClellan et al., 2012).

The Health Effects Institute sponsored a study at the Lovelace Institute with rats exposed to low dilutions (as low as 20 to 1) of exhaust from a 2007 EPA-compliant engine fueled with ultra-low sulfur fuel. The highest exposures were less than 1% of the particle matter concentrations studied earlier using traditional diesel technology engines. In contrast to the findings observed earlier with the traditional diesel engines, an excess of lung cancer was not observed (Mauderly et al., 1987; McDonald et al., 2015).

Almost concurrently, results were published by NIOSH and NCI investigators on a large Diesel Exhaust in Miners Study (DEMS) (Attfield et al., 2012; Silverman et al., 2012). The DEMS involved 12,315 workers from eight nonmetal mines (three potash, three trona, one salt, and one limestone) whose exposures and vital data were assessed through 1997. Thus, these exposures were from emissions from traditional technology diesel engines. The initial reports by the NIOSH/NCI investigators revealed a positive association between respirable elemental carbon exposure (extrapolated from CO measurements) and excess lung cancer. These findings were instrumental in an IARC (2012) panel upgrading the classification of diesel exhaust exposure from a probable human carcinogen to a human carcinogen. Later, the HEI evaluated the most recent epidemiological findings, including the DEMS results and concluded that the findings could be used for quantitative risk assessment in addition to their use in cancer hazard classification (HEI, 2015).

More recently, a team I have been associated with gained access to the DEMS data, replicated the original analyses and then extended the analyses. The use of alternative exposure assessments, which were viewed as being equal to or superior to the original DEMS estimates, yielded substantially reduced lung cancer hazard estimates. When radon was included in the analyses the hazard estimates were further reduced and generally no longer statistically significant (Moolgavkar et al., 2015; Crump et al., 2015, 2016). These findings emphasize that a high degree of caution should be exercised in extrapolating the DEMS findings selectively or in toto to other populations or in using them for quantitative risk assessment. This body of work emphasizes the importance of important epidemiological data sets being made available for analysis by multiple investigators, especially when the results have public policy impact. The same applies to large data sets assembled in studies by veterinary toxicologists of animal populations. Such use should be part of the planning process when the study is designed.

A recent IARC monograph program decision of special interest to those of us interested in agricultural and food production issues concerns the widely used herbicide, glyphosate, frequently marketed as Roundup. IARC (2015) evaluated the epidemiological, animal, and supporting evidence on glyphosate and classified it as a probable human carcinogen. This action prompted an independent evaluation of the evidence, which concluded there were serious shortcomings in the IARC evaluation. The results of the independent evaluations have been published in a special Supplement to Critical Reviews in Toxicology with a commentary I prepared as editor of the journal (McClellan, 2016a,b; Williams et al., 2016a,b; Solomon, 2016; Brusick et al., 2016; Acquavella et al., 2016). I encourage individuals to read both the original IARC report and the reports prepared by the reevaluation team to gain an appreciation of the complexities of the IARC cancer hazard classification process and the uncertainties associated with evaluating the carcinogenic hazard of a single, well-studied chemical such as glyphosate. This will also give the reader an appreciation of the role of both epidemiological and animal evidence in the cancer-hazard classification process.

Increasingly, the "precautionary principle" has dominated approaches to regulation of products and technologies. The concept took hold first within Europe and was codified by the European Commission (2002), more recently its use has been advocated in the United States. In its most simple form it argues that if the product or technology has not or cannot be viewed as safe then the product or technology should be replaced or not used. It is obvious that the "devil is in the details" with regard to the basis for characterizing what is safe or not safe. There is a continuum from safe products or technologies to highly hazardous products and technologies. Indeed, some highly hazardous products may be used in a controlled manner so they do not pose a significant health risk. Some advocates of the "precautionary principle" point to thousands of untested chemicals and argue they should be tested or banned. I would argue that a critical review of past experience with many of these chemicals or closely related chemicals provides a sound basis for their continued use. Quite frankly, additional extensive testing using laboratory animals may not be warranted. Moreover, I am concerned that many of the in vitro cellular and molecular assays have not yet been appropriately validated as predictors of the presence or absence of adverse health effects in humans.

The "precautionary principle" is a core element of the Registration, Evaluation, Authorization, and Restriction of Chemicals (REACH) program established by the European Commission (2006). More details are available at REACH (2011). Thoughtful reviews of the REACH program have been written by deAvila and Sandberg (2006) and Williams et al. (2009).

Potential changes in how chemicals are regulated in the United States have been debated for decades. That debate resulted in passage in 2016 of the Frank R. Lautenberg Chemical Safety for the 21st century Act amendments to the Toxic Substances Control Act signed by the President of the United States on June 22, 2016 (TSCA, 2016). These amendments establish mandatory requirements for the USEPA to evaluate existing chemicals, have all new chemicals evaluated before commercial use, require the development of new risk-based safety standards, and provide increased public transparency for chemical hazard/risk information. During the first year after passage of the Lautenberg amendment, over 300 chemical reviews were completed by the USEPA, more than in any comparable period in the past. It will be of interest to see if the Lautenberg amendments accelerate the validation and use of in vitro (nonanimal systems) to evaluate the toxicity hazards and risks of new chemicals entering commerce.

A FRAMEWORK FOR ACQUIRING INFORMATION

Linkages From Sources to Health Impacts

The purpose of this section is to provide a conceptual framework for using information to evaluate specific cases of actual or alleged toxicosis and to facilitate the acquisition of new knowledge that will have an impact in understanding potential toxic effects. Earlier, in Fig. 1.1, a conceptual framework was provided for evaluating the linkages extending from a source of a toxic material to manifestation of an adverse health outcome in an individual or a population. The conceptual framework is equally applicable to humans or other animal species.

The source to exposure linkage has been expanded in Fig. 1.4 (Paustenbach, 2001). In this example, an industrial plant is illustrated as the source. The figure serves to illustrate the complex nature of the exposure pathways that may be encountered including the role of livestock. The focus in the figure is on the multiple pathways by which a potential toxicant may reach a human population: inhalation, drinking water, dermal absorption, ingestion of soil, and ingestion of a variety of foodstuffs including milk and meat from domestic animals. All of these pathways might also serve to expose the cow in the figure to the toxicant. Obviously, the quantities of the toxicant taken in by the single cow could also cause toxicity in a herd of cows if the combination of exposure intensity and duration were sufficient. Equally as important is the role of the cow as a pathway for the toxicant to reach people. For example, the figure illustrates that a toxicant could be present in cow's milk and the milk could be consumed by people. The cow could also be slaughtered and the meat ultimately consumed by people. Thus, it is important to recognize that the cow, or any other food animal species, can both manifest toxic effects and serve as a pathway for toxicants to reach people via the food supply.

It is readily apparent that the schematic rendering shown in Fig. 1.4 can be expanded or contracted. In natural ecosystems, multiple species might be involved as a toxicant moves from a source or multiple sources via various pathways. In some cases, various species in the

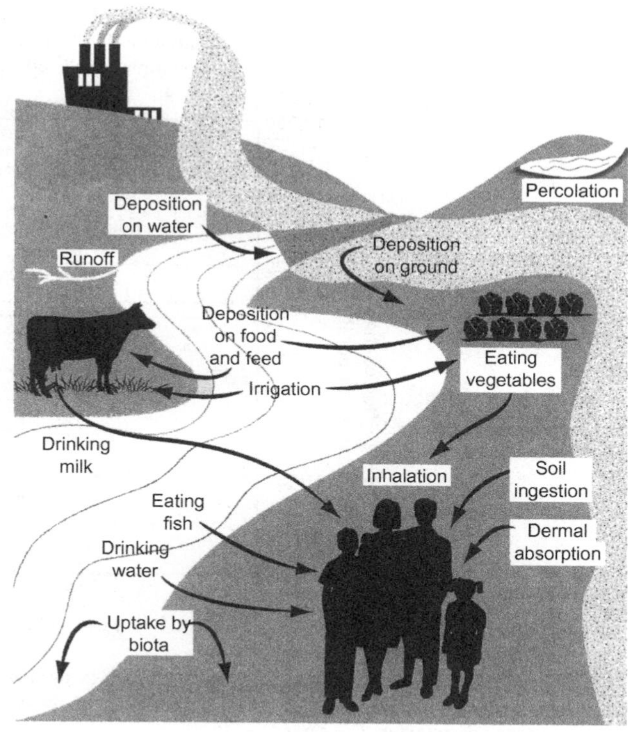

FIGURE 1.4 Schematic rendering illustrating exposure pathways extending from a source of toxicants to exposure of livestock and people. *From Paustenbach (2008).*

ecosystem may be impacted as individuals. Moreover, natural populations may be impacted. In addition, these pathways may ultimately result in the toxicant reaching people. An example is mercury in fish. In practice, veterinarians may encounter situations where poisonous plants in the pasture or in harvested forage may be the source of the toxicant. Feed may be contaminated at a mill or processing plant and serve as the pathway by which a toxicant reaches the livestock. A recent case in Europe involves contamination of eggs by a pesticide used to control lice in chicken houses. In other cases, the potential human toxicant may be a pharmaceutical agent purposefully given to the cow with the pharmaceutical appearing in the milk or in the tissues of the cow if it were slaughtered and, thus, available for human consumption. Likewise, the "contaminated" materials may be used to produce products intended for consumption by other animals such as pet food.

The utility of using the conceptual approach in Fig. 1.4 can be illustrated using the transfer of a specific radionuclide, I^{131}, from the diet of cows to the cow's milk to intake by humans and thyroid uptake. This situation was of concern when nuclear weapons were being tested in the atmosphere resulting in world-wide fallout and for releases from reactor accidents in England (Windscale), Ukraine (Chernobyl), and Japan (Fukushima). Fig. 1.5

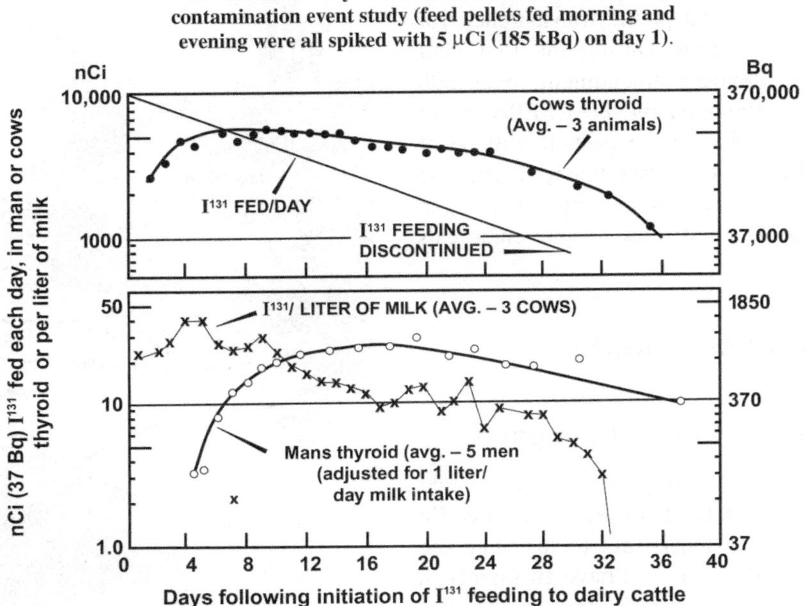

FIGURE 1.5 Interrelationships for radioiodine (I^{131}): Intake by cows, cows thyroid and milk and human thyroid. *Adapted from Bustad, L.K., McClellan, R.O., Garner R.J., 1965. The significance of radionuclide contamination in ruminants. In: Physiology of Digestion in the Ruminant. Butterworth Inc., Washington, DC, pp. 131–146.*

illustrates the results of a controlled study conducted at the Hanford Laboratories, Richland, Washington, in the early 1960s with I^{131} administered to dairy cows (Bustad et al., 1965). The "old" radiation units of microcuries for quantifying the amount of radioactive material are used in the scale on the left and the "new" International units of Becquerls are used in the scale on the right. Rather than contaminate a large quantity of feed, instead the cows were given two feed pellets each day, the feed pellets all contained 5 μCi/L (185 Bq) of I^{131} on the first day of the study. The I^{131} decayed with a physical half-life of 8.06 days so the cows ingested less I^{131} each day (the straight line in the figure). The cows' thyroids and milk were monitored for I^{131} content. Aliquots of the I^{131} contaminated milk were ingested by five volunteers, and their thyroids were monitored for I^{131}. As an aside, the calculated radiation dose to the thyroids of the volunteers was less than what would have been received from a I^{131} thyroid uptake study conducted for diagnostic purposes. Let me hasten to note that the control limits for radionuclides in milk intended for human consumption would be sufficiently stringent that the radiation dose to the cows would be much lower than required to produce toxicity in the cows. These results have been used to estimate allowable intakes from I^{131} contaminated milk and to develop guidance for monitoring pasture and hay to control milk contamination. Data such as presented in Fig. 1.5 were useful input to the control of radiation exposure of European populations from ingestion of milk following the Chernobyl accident in 1986 and the Japanese population following the Fukushima, Japan accident in 2011.

Toxicokinetics

The simple schematic rendering shown in Fig. 1.1 can be used to illustrate several important concepts. First, it is important to recognize that contrary to common usage, exposure and dose are not the same. The exposure environment is characterized by the concentration of the toxicant in the media, be it water, air or feed, the quantities taken in and the time course of the intake. Dose is the concentration, over time, of the toxicant and/or its metabolites in the various tissues of the subject, whether it be a cow, a human, or a laboratory rat.

For example, in Fig. 1.5 the exposure of the cows would be the quantity of I^{131} ingested. An example of dose would be the measured quantity of I^{131} in the thyroids of the cows and human volunteers that were ingesting aliquots of the contaminated milk. A more precise estimate of dose would be the calculated radiation dose in rem (old radiation unit) or Sievert (new radiation unit).

The information presented in Fig. 1.5 may be viewed as being a limited toxicokinetic study. The key data acquired were the intake of I^{131} and the changing concentration of I^{131} in the cow's thyroid and milk. The information on the relationship between I^{131} intake and milk content are sufficient to provide input for estimating limits of daily intake of I^{131} in forage by the cows in order to limit the I^{131} content of milk to some prescribed limit such as an Intervention Level as will be discussed later. Because the physical half-life of I^{131} is quite short, 8.06 days, and the I^{131} is concentrated in the thyroid and milk concern does not develop for the I^{131} content of the rest of the carcass. If the radionuclide or specific chemical were found in edible portions of the carcass, then information on the radionuclide, chemical, or metabolite of the chemical in the edible tissues such as muscle would be of interest. For example, cesium behaves like potassium and, thus, concern exists for radiocesium concentrations in muscle as well as milk. Strontium behaves like calcium, thus, concern exists for radiostrontium in milk and in skeleton.

The characterization of the kinetics linking exposure with dose is referred to as toxicokinetics (for a toxic agent) or pharmacokinetics (for a pharmaceutical). In actual practice, the term pharmacokinetics is frequently used when it would be more appropriate to use the term toxicokinetics. Several chapters in the book deal specifically with kinetics of toxicants and pharmaceuticals.

Toxicokinetics (see Fig. 1.1) are used to describe the movement and disposition of the toxicant in the organism. This includes consideration of the route of entry: ingestion, inhalation, dermal, or purposeful administration by injection. A complete description of the toxicokinetics of a toxicant will take into account (1) the intensity and duration of the exposure; (2) the rate and amount of absorption of the toxicant from the site of entry; (3) the distribution of the toxicant within the body; (4) potential biotransformation to less, equal or more toxic form; and (5) the rate of excretion by route (urine, feces, or exhalation). All of these aspects of toxicokinetics may be influenced by species differences in physiological and biochemical characteristics. Modern approaches to modeling toxicokinetics attempt to take account of both species differences and similarities in influencing the fate in the body of toxicants. It is also important to recognize that the exposure or dose level may influence the kinetics of a toxicant and its metabolite(s). This is an especially important consideration in extrapolating from laboratory studies that may be conducted at high exposures and doses to lower more environmentally relevant exposures/doses.

Toxicodynamics

The linkage between dose and adverse health outcome shown in Fig. 1.1 involves multiple mechanisms, as various toxicants may potentially impact all the cells and organ systems of the body. Increasingly, scientists have attempted to model these relationships that, in parallel to the nomenclature for the kinetic phase, are called toxicodynamic or pharmacodynamic models. It is obvious that multiple pathways and interactions may be involved in a toxicant producing disease and that knowledge of the individual steps and interactions will increase as knowledge of basic biological mechanisms increase. For example, the explosion of knowledge of basic biology at the level of the genome (genomics), proteins (proteomics), and metabolism (metabolomics) has provided a basis for exploring the mechanistic basis of toxicant-induced disease with a degree of refinement that could not even be envisioned even a few years ago. In recent years, the picture has become even more complicated, as it has become apparent that mammalian organisms contain large and diverse populations of microbes that may influence normal function and disease process; hence concern for the "microbome."

Later chapters review the basic mechanisms of toxicity. In addition, many of the chapters on organ toxicity and specific toxicants contain detailed information on mechanisms of toxicity. As the reader reviews this material, and especially the detailed discussion of biochemical mechanisms of action, it will be important to place those in the context of processes at the cellular and tissue level: i.e., inflammation, cell death, cell proliferation, hypertrophy, hyperplasia, metaplasia, and neoplasia. A strength of the veterinary medical curriculum, as with the human medical curriculum, is the emphasis given to understanding both normal body processes and disease processes extending from the molecular level to cells to tissues to organs and, ultimately, to the integrated mammalian organism and populations. A special opportunity exists for medically trained personnel, both veterinarians and physicians, to put the expanding knowledge of molecular and cellular processes into the context of overt disease. And vice versa, there is a need for molecular and cellular biologists to become more knowledgeable of disease processes. After years of emphasis on a reductionist approach to basic biomedical science, it has become recognized that this approach needs to be complemented by an integrative approach. This has recently been termed "systems biology." In my view, this is not really a new concept. It is more a rediscovery and refinement of the concepts of integrated biology and pathobiology used in veterinary medicine for decades.

There has been great enthusiasm for the use of mechanistic information in safety/risk evaluations as will be discussed later. Recognition of the difficulty of characterizing all of the individual mechanistic steps by which a chemical may cause disease has given rise to the term "mode of action," which has been defined as the dominant step(s) involved in producing a given toxic endpoint. An example is the role of cell killing as the mode of action for large intakes of chloroform (Butterworth et al., 1995) or formaldehyde (Conolly et al., 2004) over extended periods of time causing tumors in rodents. The exposure–response relationship for cell killing may likely have a threshold that must be considered in extrapolating the findings from high-exposure level studies in rodents to humans exposed to low concentrations of these chemicals. Readers interested in a contemporary view of the use of mode of action information to improve regulatory decision-making will be interested in a summary paper by Carmichael et al. (2011). The NRC (2011) has also addressed this issue in offering advice on the US Environmental Protection Agency draft IRIS assessment of formaldehyde. Rhomberg et al. (2011b,c) also addressed issues involving the EPA's formaldehyde assessment.

More recently, enthusiasm has developed for the concept of "Adverse Outcome Pathway" (AOP) analysis. The AOP approach focuses on developing information on the pathobiological pathway by which a critical adverse effect is observed with a particular chemical. Information obtained on detailed investigation of this pathway can then be used to inform regulatory decisions on the nature of the exposure-dose-response relationships to be considered in limiting human exposures.

It is my contention that understanding the basic concepts conveyed in Figs. 1.1, 1.2, and 1.4 can be very useful in investigating a range of situations where the objective is to establish or refute a causal association between a given source and toxic agent and an increased incidence of an adverse health outcome. The term, increased incidence, is used advisably recognizing in most situations involving domestic animals, either as commercial herds or as companion animals, the situation is one of presence or absence of a given disease and the "ruling out" of other differential diagnoses. However, in situations involving human populations and in experimental studies in animals, the issue frequently encountered is whether a given toxicant exposure has caused an increase in a disease recognizing that most diseases may have multiple etiologies, e.g., cancer, hypertension, and diabetes. This is especially the case in evaluating diseases that typically occur late in life, such as cancer and chronic diseases, and with exposure to toxicants that may occur at low levels over long periods of time. In some cases, such as lung cancer and cardiorespiratory disease in humans, a risk factor such as cigarette smoking may cause effects that are so substantial it is a challenge to determine if any concurrent low-level exposure to other toxicants, such as air pollutants, are having chronic effects at low exposure concentrations.

Veterinary Toxicology Is Multifaceted

It will be apparent to the reader of this book that veterinary toxicology is multifaceted. Thus, there are many ways to organize and synthesize the knowledge base that we call veterinary toxicology. One dimension is the various classes of toxicants. Another dimension of the field relates to the media that contains the toxicant: air, water, soil, and feed. Another dimension considers the various routes of exposure of toxicants: inhalation, ingestion, dermal, or purposeful injection. It is also convenient to consider the various organ systems and processes that may be affected by toxicants. This is the basis for organization of a major section in this book. It is also important to consider the individual toxicants or classes of toxicants. This approach is used in organizing another major section of this book. Finally, veterinary toxicologists recognize the necessity of considering the various species of concern. Increasing veterinary medical practitioners have become more specialized with many focusing their clinical skills on a single species. This book does not include a section addressing the toxicology of individual species. To have done so would have substantially increased the size of this text. However, chapter authors have endeavored to discuss species variations in responses to toxic agents. It is noteworthy that several textbooks, that of Peterson and Talcott (2012) and Poppenga and Gwaltney-Brant (2011), focus on small animals. Some of the major comprehensive veterinary medicine texts, such as the Current Veterinary Therapy series, that focus on other species include chapters on toxicology related to that species.

SOURCES OF INFORMATION

Case Observations in the Species of Interest

There are multiple sources of scientific information for characterizing the relationship between exposure to a toxicant and toxicant-induced response. Fig. 1.6 is a schematic rendering of the multiple sources of information that may be used to understand the toxicity of a given agent.

As discussed earlier, the origins of veterinary toxicology and toxicology in general are both rooted in observations. An adverse health effect, either a pattern of morbidity or mortality in an individual or population, is observed and the disease linked to exposure to a toxicant. In many instances, the time interval between exposure and the adverse health outcome was brief, which aided in deducing an association. Because the causal association was identified in the species of interest, whether it be a person, a horse, a cow, or a dog, it was not necessary to extrapolate between species. Nor was it necessary to explore in-depth the mechanistic basis for the causal association to either diagnose a particular case or prevent future cases. Action to prevent exposures and, thus, prevent disease, could be based on empirical observations.

As you read many of the chapters in this book, you will note that details of the mechanism by which

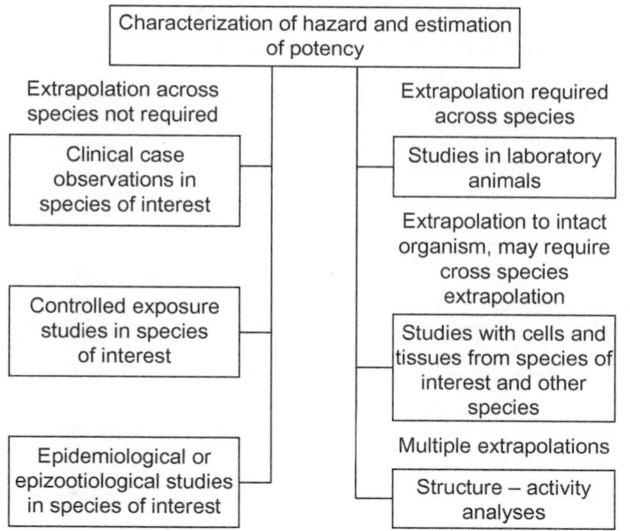

FIGURE 1.6 Sources of information for evaluating potential toxicants.

a particular toxicant causes disease have been elucidated to a variable extent. When the toxicant is exclusively of concern in veterinary medicine and has no implications for human health, there has frequently been limited impetus for developing a detailed mechanistic understanding of how a toxicant causes disease. Concern for human health has been a major driver of the biomedical research agenda. An obvious exception is when the toxicoses observed in veterinary medicine have large economic impact or toxicants can reach people via animal products.

There are many circumstances where observational knowledge is not adequate and it is necessary to conduct experiments to characterize the toxicology of an agent. It is obvious that if concern for the potential toxic response is in a nonhuman species, controlled experiments can be conducted using the species of interest. This is obviously the case for domestic livestock as well as companion animals.

A much more common situation is when concern focuses on potential toxicity of a newly developed agent for use in people or animals. For example, it is necessary to establish the safety of a potential new pharmaceutical or consumer product before it is introduced into commerce. In these instances studies in laboratory animals are conducted to provide "first approximation" of the safety of the new compounds to humans prior to administration of the agent to humans. In the case of products intended for use in animals, studies on both efficacy and safety can be conducted in the species of interest. This remains an imperative step in the safety evaluation of new products. There are also circumstances in which it is desirable to extend limited observations from opportunistic studies on people or animals that have been inadvertently exposed. When a new product is developed and marketed, either a pharmaceutical or a consumer product, various postmarketing surveillance systems should be put in place in an attempt to detecting any unexpected adverse outcomes.

Epidemiological/Epizootiological Studies

If a particular chemical has been used for an extended period of time, and human exposure has occurred previously either in the workplace or from the environment, it may be feasible to conduct epidemiological studies. Epidemiology is the study of how disease is distributed in a population and the factors that influence or determine this distribution. The design of a particular epidemiological study will be guided by the hypothesis being tested and the nature of the population(s) available for study. As an aside, the term epidemiology (epi for across, dem for people, and ology for scientific study) is applicable to people while the more appropriate related term for studies on animals would be epizootiology (epa for across, zoo for animal, and ology for scientific study). However, in common practice studies of the occurrence of disease in populations of species other than humans are frequently referred to as epidemiological studies. The details of conducting epidemiological or epizootiological studies are beyond the scope of this chapter. A relevant reference for basic concepts in epidemiology can be found in the text by Gordis (2008).

A classic paper by Austin Bradford Hill (1965), a British medical statistician, provides guidance on the interpretation of epidemiological evidence for a given agent or factor causing a health effect (Table 1.1). Although developed for interpreting epidemiological data, i.e., data acquired on human populations, the guidance is also highly relevant to interpreting data acquired on animal populations. The framework needs to be used intelligently rather than slavishly: it is a guide and not a checklist.

Retrospective epidemiological studies may be feasible for previously introduced agents for which prior exposure has occurred or prospectively for a newly introduced agent. If the agent is new it is obvious that it is not feasible to conduct epidemiological studies to retrospectively evaluate the potential safety/hazard of the agent. If the ultimate interest is in the effects on people, it may be feasible to conduct controlled exposure studies with human volunteers. It is advisable for the planning of such studies to be based on a solid database on the potential toxicity of the agent acquired from studies in laboratory animals. The design and conduct of such human studies must be guided first and foremost by ethical considerations (NRC, 2004). If a nonhuman species is the target species of concern, then it is obvious that the most relevant information is the information acquired from studies conducted in that species.

TABLE 1.1 Bradford Hill (1965): Guidance for Interpreting Epidemiological Evidence for a Given Agent or Factor Causing a Specific Disease

Strength: If there is a large effect size (a strong effect), this makes a true causal relationship more likely. There is no fundamental reason why a strong association should be more likely to be causal than a weak association. However, Bradford Hill was thinking of possible confounding factors and argued that if a strong association is not causal, an association with some other factor that varies closely with the factor originally suggested must exist. If the association is strong, this covariable will be easier to recognize than if the association is weak.
Consistency: Is there evidence for the same findings from more than one study, preferably from different settings?
Specificity: Is the effect specific to the exposure? In reality this rarely occurs, and some regard this as the "icing on the cake" when considering causal evidence. However, the specificity of a particular mechanism, if seen across a range of health endpoints, would meet the requirements of this component.
Temporality: This is the only absolute. Exposure must precede outcome.
Biological gradient: Is there a dose–response relationship? In addition (although explicit in Bradford Hill's original paper), is there a threshold of exposure below which an effect is not seen?
Plausibility: Does this exposure-effect relationship make biological sense? Is there mechanistic evidence to support the likelihood that this might occur given current knowledge? Bradford Hill pointed out that this feature should not be demanded: what is implausible today may be entirely plausible tomorrow.
Coherence: Does the proposed causal association cohere with other findings? For instance, if we were concerned that a specific exposure might be related to a health effect that was based on an inflammatory response, has a similar effect been seen with other inflammatory conditions, or is an apparent effect on mortality accompanied by effects on morbidity?
Experiment: Is there evidence from experiments (involving either animals or humans, whether individually or as populations) that removal of the exposure reduces the effect?
Analogy: Are there analogous situations that would tend to support the likelihood of a causal relationship? For instance, when considering a possible teratogen, consideration of the effects of thalidomide on the developing fetus would come to mind.

Experimentation

An additional option for acquiring information is to conduct toxicological studies with controlled exposures in typical laboratory animal species. Such studies are the cornerstone of research conducted to evaluate the safety/risk of newly synthesized agents whether they are a potential new pharmaceutical, pesticide or herbicide, a significant consumer product, or a new chemical or intermediate chemical to be used in commerce. It is well recognized, certainly by veterinarians, that no single laboratory animal species is a miniature version of the human species, i.e., 15 cm in height, weighing 180 g, and sharing all of the common biological traits and diseases of humans. However, it is fortunate that humans and laboratory animals do share many common biological traits and diseases. Knowledge of the extent to which there are similarities and differences between humans and a given laboratory animal species can be used to guide the selection of a species to serve as a surrogate for humans in developing data for safety/risk evaluations for humans. It is encouraging that some veterinary medical schools are recognizing the importance of extending the range of species studied in the core curriculum from the usual companion animal and domestic livestock species to include common laboratory animal species.

At this juncture, it is appropriate to note the importance of animal welfare issues. The Animal Welfare Act (AWA), initially enacted in 1966 and amended in 1970, 1976, 1985, 1990, and 2002, is the principal federal statute in the United States governing the sale, handling, transport, and use of animals. The AWA applies to all species of warm-blooded vertebrate animals used for research, testing, or teaching excluding animals used for agricultural research. The US Department of Agriculture's Animal and Plant Health Inspection Service (APHIS) has responsibility for implementing the AWA. The 1985 Amendments to the AWA clarified the importance of humane care, minimization of pain and distress, consideration of alternatives, the role of institutional animal care and use committees, the psychological well being of primates, and exercise for dogs. The primary reference on animal care and use is the "Guide for the Care and Use of Laboratory Animals" prepared and periodically updated under the auspices of the Institute of Laboratory Animal Resources of the National Academy of Sciences/National Research Council (ILAR, 2010). All toxicologists involved with laboratory investigations should be familiar with the contents of the Guide irrespective of the species they use for their research.

An additional matter the experimentalist should be aware of is the need for use of Good Laboratory Practices

(GLPs) in the conduct of research intended to be used for regulatory decisions. Both the FDA (2001) and the EPA (TSCA, 1985; FIFRA, 1991) have requirements for the use of GLPs. The FDA GLP requirements do not extend to exploratory, mechanism of action or efficacy studies. The basic elements of GLPs are (1) the appointment by the institution of a study director, (2) the use of an independent quality assurance unit, (3) the use of documented standard operating procedures, (4) a written protocol for each study, and (5) preparation of a final report containing a GLP compliance statement for each study. The use of GLPs is not required by FDA for studies with domestic livestock. However, investigators conducting studies using domestic livestock would be well advised to attempt to adhere to the basic principles that undergird GLPs to help ensure the quality and reproducibility of the data being generated.

In my opinion, scientists conducting exploratory or basic research studies would be well advised to use the basic concepts of GLPs in their research. I make this recommendation noting that time spent, at the beginning of a new research study, developing and documenting a protocol may be a sound investment in that it will suggest ways to improve the protocol and make it more efficient for addressing the hypothesis posed. Time invested in ensuring that the research process and records are well documented may be crucial in providing documentation for filing a patent application.

Another option for acquiring useful toxicity data beyond conducting epidemiological or whole animal studies is to conduct investigations in in vitro using tissues or cells from mammalian species, both humans and laboratory animals, and using bacteria and yeasts. An additional option is to conduct structure-activity analyses on the new agent using the large data bank of structure-activity information already available on other related chemicals.

All of the options outlined, to some extent, create extrapolation issues. Even if studies are conducted in the species of interest, it is typically necessary to extrapolate from the high levels of exposure or administered doses studied experimentally to lower exposures or doses anticipated to be representative of intended use. It may also be necessary to extrapolate from a relatively short period of study, say, days or a few weeks, to the intended period of use, over months or years. If the studies are not conducted in the species of ultimate interest, there is need to extrapolate between species. It may also be necessary to extrapolate observations made in a population of healthy individuals to a population that includes individuals with preexisting disease or altered susceptibility to development of disease. Some aspects of the extrapolation between species and across exposure/dose levels may be facilitated by physiologically based toxicokinetic and toxicodynamic modeling. However, toxicodynamic modeling is still in its relative infancy.

It is important to recognize that even with today's level of knowledge of these extrapolation issues, it is not possible to estimate, with absolute certainty, the precise numerical level of human exposure to a given agent that may be without any risk of potential harm or the level and duration of exposure that is estimated to produce a specific level of harm. This is generally recognized in contemporary safety/risk evaluation methodology such that conservative approaches are used in estimating safe levels of human intake of chemicals. By taking a conservative approach to setting standards or providing guidance to limit exposures, there can be a high degree of confidence that an agent can be used safely if used as intended. Ultimately, all processes that develop guidance or standards to limit exposures and thus, limit disease require judgments to be exercised. In short, scientific information can inform the standard or guidance development process; however, it cannot prescribe or dictate specific standards. The establishment of an adequate margin of safety or an acceptable level of risk involves value judgments that go beyond the science.

Schematic Experimental Designs

The experimental design for testing of any specific hypothesis must be matched to the hypothesis, the desired statistical power, and the resources available. Inevitably, decisions on an experimental design involve making difficult choices among options because of resource constraints. It is important to seek statistical advice during the design of a study to ensure the statistical design is matched to the hypothesis being tested. In this section, two schematic experimental designs will be discussed to illustrate some of the key issues that must be addressed in planning toxicological studies. The discussion in both cases will assume that the species to be used in the study has already been selected.

Acquiring Toxicokinetic Data

The first conceptual design, Fig. 1.7, illustrates an approach to acquiring data for understanding the link between exposure and internal dose, the kind of data that can be used for toxicokinetic modeling. Recall the toxicokinetic linkage in Fig. 1.1. The design shown is based on a single brief intake of the test agent. However, the design can be modified for studying chronic intake of an agent. A critical decision is the choice of the route of administration or intake of the test material. Obviously, such studies are most readily carried out with parenteral administration of the agent. This may be the most appropriate route for a pharmaceutical agent that is to be parentally administered.

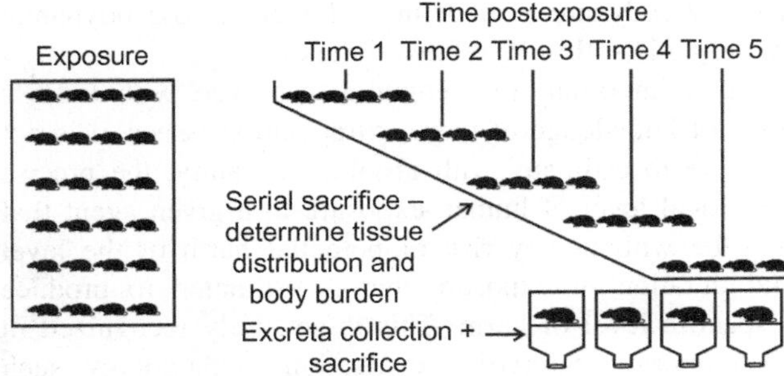

FIGURE 1.7 Schematic rendering of an experimental design for evaluating the kinetics of an administered toxicant.

However, the resulting data may be of limited relevance to other routes of intake. For example, it may not appropriately mimic oral intake since only a small fraction of some toxicants may be absorbed from the gastrointestinal tract. In short, the route of administration should be matched to the route of concern for real-world exposure to the agent.

With inhalation, the particle size distribution of the airborne toxicant will influence what portion of the inhaled material will be deposited and where it is deposited in the various regions of the respiratory tract, i.e., the oropharynx, tracheobronchial, or pulmonary regions. The pattern of deposition, retention and subsequent translocation of the deposited material will depend on the size, chemical composition and dissolution properties of the deposited material. Differences among the various species are of paramount concern. Individuals interested in details on the conduct of inhalation toxicity studies will find the book edited by McClellan and Henderson (1995) of interest as well as a summary chapter by McClellan et al. (2006). Recall also the studies of Wolff et al. (1987) on the fate of inhaled diesel exhaust particles.

Another key decision is whether conduct of the toxicokinetic studies may be facilitated by using a test agent labeled with radioactive or stable element tracers. Analytical considerations for the initial toxicant as well as any metabolites are of major importance in the conduct of toxicokinetic studies.

The schematic design (Fig. 1.7) shows a group of animals maintained for collection of excreta and, perhaps, even sampling of expired air. Data from these analyses can be used along with tissue analyses to obtain a mass-balance between the quantity administered and the quantity recovered. The schematic design shows multiple times at which animals will be euthanized and tissues collected for analysis. This allows the development of a dynamic profile of how the body handles the administered material. For organic compounds, provision needs to be made for analyzing for both the parent compound and potential metabolites.

The selection of the sacrifice times will be guided by the anticipated kinetic profile of the agent and its metabolites. It may be useful to obtain preliminary information on retention kinetics from pilot studies. Some organic compounds may be rapidly metabolized leading to the need to schedule all of the sacrifices over a few hours. On the other hand, certain inhaled relatively inherent materials may have long-term retention in the lungs extending over hundreds of days. It is important to recognize that the quantity of material administered may influence the kinetics of the material. Hence, it is desirable to use multiple administered exposure/dose levels as an experimental variable. Without question, the design of any particular toxicokinetic study requires the exercise of considerable professional judgment. Toxicological research is not a "cookie cutter" or "check the box" science.

Acquiring Exposure (Dose)-Response Data

A schematic experimental design for a study to evaluate exposure (dose)-response relationships for toxicants is shown in Fig. 1.8. Recall the exposure–response linkage shown in Fig. 1.1. The design shown is typical of that which might be used in the conduct of a 2-year bioassay, typically used to evaluate carcinogenicity, in rats and mice. Recall the studies of Mauderly et al. (1987) and McDonald et al. (2015) with exhaust from diesel engines. The same design, and indeed the same experiment, can be used to evaluate other endpoints and to conduct shorter-term studies. The study should involve administration of the material by a route matched to likely exposure conditions to be encountered with the agent. Administration of an agent by gavage may be acceptable as a surrogate for ingestion, especially when it is desirable to administer specific quantities of material. However, I am not enthusiastic about the repeated use of gavage as a substitute for ingestion of an agent in feed. The use of intratracheal instillation as a surrogate for conducting inhalation exposures to an agent remains controversial. It is my professional opinion that intratracheal administration is a nonphysiological mode for delivery of materials to the respiratory tract. It may result in exaggerated quantities of

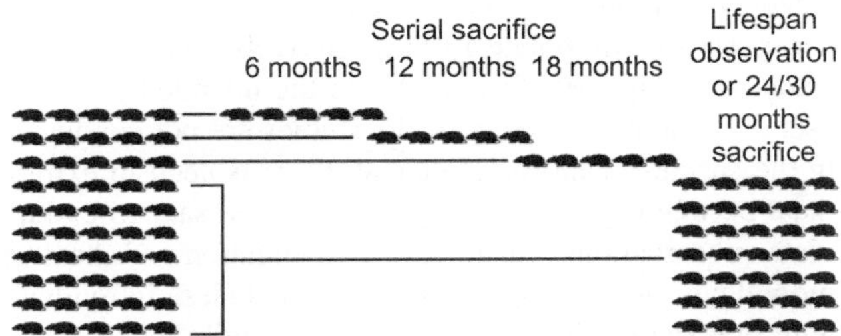

FIGURE 1.8 Schematic rendering of an experimental design for evaluating exposure (dose)-response relationships for a toxicant.

material being deposited in some regions of the respiratory tract while other regions are spared any exposure. This unusual pattern of distribution of the agent is very likely to influence the toxic responses of the airways and alveoli. Thus, I am hesitant to even recommend intratracheal instillation for mechanistic studies, the mechanistic information acquired may be irrelevant to the inhalation exposure situations that are of concern for people or other species.

It is critical that exposure-dose-response studies utilize multiple exposure levels, perhaps three or four exposure levels. The choice of the specific exposure levels is one of the most important decisions to be made in planning such studies. One consideration relates to the potential level(s) of exposure to be encountered with intended use. Higher additional levels can be selected above this base level. Selection of exposure/dose levels can also be informed by the results of the kinetic studies. For example, it would not be desirable to use only exposure levels above a level at which metabolic processes are saturated. Another consideration emphasized by the EPA and NTP, especially when cancer is an endpoint, is to select a maximum tolerated (MTD) dose level as the highest exposure/dose level and establish lower levels by some fraction of the MTD level, perhaps 1/2 and 1/4 or 1/3 and 1/9. The use of an MTD has been justified on the grounds that it is necessary to maximize exposure to potentially observe carcinogenic responses recognizing the blunt experimental approach (NRC, 1993). A useful review on the history of the use of animal bioassays to predict carcinogenicity has been authored by Beyer et al. (2011).

The extent to which animal bioassays are a blunt approach to detecting the carcinogenic potential of agents is illustrated in Fig. 1.9. It can be noted that for a species and strains of animals with a background incidence of 1%, a study of 50 animals will require a 20% response to detect a statistically significant effect. As an aside, a population of nonsmoking people will experience about a 1%

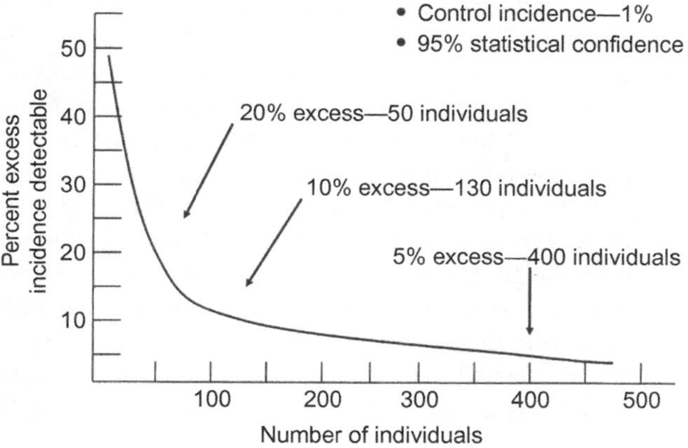

FIGURE 1.9 Relationships between number of subjects required to detect excess risk and the level of detectable excess risk.

lifetime incidence of lung cancer whereas a population of a two-pack-a-day cigarette smokers will experience about a 20% lifetime incidence of lung cancer. Consideration of statistical information such as the above emphasizes the importance of using care in interpreting the results of cancer bioassays using the typical 100 animals (50 of each sex) per exposure level. The interpretation of the relevance of the results of animal studies for estimating human hazards will be greatly enhanced by knowledge of the mechanisms involved in the toxicant causing disease in the animals.

A key feature of the exposure–response experimental design illustrated in Fig. 1.8 is the use of multiple sacrifice times for all exposure levels. In some cases it may be possible to evaluate the functional status of organs at these times, i.e., pulmonary function. In animals with inhalation exposure, when a respiratory tract response is of concern, it may be feasible to collect bronchoalveolar lavage fluid samples for analysis of biochemical and cellular parameters. Most importantly, tissue samples can be collected at the multiple time periods for histopathological evaluation. The information obtained from the serially sacrificed animals, combined with that obtained from the terminal sacrifice animals, can provide valuable insight into the progression of disease processes over the course of the study. Without question, insight into the pathogenesis of toxicant-induced disease processes will be much more complete when serial sacrifices are conducted than that obtained only from an evaluation of the terminal sacrifice animals. Another option in the design of exposure–response studies is to include a group of animals at each level that are removed from further exposure at one or more times postinhalation of exposure for maintenance without further exposure. These animals may be euthanized at later times and evaluated for evidence of recovery or reversibility of earlier toxicant-induced changes.

The basic guidance for using multiple exposure (dose) levels and making experimental observations at multiple times is as applicable to the conduct of studies examining hypotheses on the mechanisms of action of toxicants as it is to studies developing information for regulatory decisions. I remain disappointed that many published papers on mechanisms of action of specific toxicants fail to use multiple exposure (dose) levels and multiple observation times. It is only when exposure (dose) level and duration of exposure are included as experimental variables that a true understanding of the mechanisms of toxicity mode of action or AOP for an agent can be elucidated. Mechanisms, modes of action, and AOPs are frequently exposure (dose) level and exposure-duration dependent. It is important to recognize that the use of ultra-sophisticated assessment methods is not a substitute for a flawed experimental design.

As the science of toxicology has advanced, increasing attention has been given to developing specialized approaches for evaluating toxicity induced in different organ systems. The various guidelines developed by the USEPA, FDA, and NTP are useful references for these specialized approaches. For example, the EPA has published guidelines for evaluating carcinogenicity (EPA, 1996a), gene mutation (EPA, 1996b), reproductive toxicity (EPA, 1996c), developmental toxicity (EPA, 1991) and neurotoxicity (EPA, 1995). The EPA is continually reviewing and updating its guidelines for toxicity testing. Forty-nine harmonized health effects test guidelines used in the testing of pesticides and toxic substances have been developed and can be found on the EPA Office of Prevention, Pesticides and Toxic Substances website (EPA/OPPTS, 2006).

The FDA has provided specific guidance for evaluating the safety of compounds used in food-producing animals (FDA, 1994) and principles for evaluating the safety of food ingredients (FDA, 2011). The EPA has provided guidelines for evaluating the safety of products intended for use with cats and dogs (EPA, 1998) and domestic livestock (EPA, 1996d).

A special issue of concern with pharmaceutical products is the presence of trace contaminants and whether these trace contaminants should be tested individually. One approach to addressing this issue is the use of a "threshold of toxicological concern" concept championed by Kroes et al. (2005). Kroes, now deceased, was a Dutch veterinarian who developed an excellent reputation in safety and risk assessment. The concept of "safety qualification thresholds" (Ball et al., 2007, 2012) developed out of the "threshold of toxicological concern" concept. It is a promising approach to minimizing the use of laboratory animals in exhaustive testing while still assuring the safety of pharmaceuticals. The European Medicines Evaluation Agency (EMEA, 2004) has provided detailed guidelines for addressing genotoxic impurities.

The various guidelines are useful for planning safety evaluation studies. However, the guidelines should not be used as a substitute for the use of professional judgment in planning, conducting and interpreting toxicological investigations. As noted earlier, toxicology is not a "cookie cutter" or "check the box" science.

TOXICOLOGIC DESCRIPTORS

Toxicology Rooted in Observations

The results of toxicological investigations, either from clinical case observations or planned experimentation, involve describing the exposure, the dose, the response, and interrelationships among these parameters. Exquisite knowledge of exposure or dose or response is not sufficient. Ultimately, it is necessary to understand their interrelationships. With clinical case observations, the initial emphasis is on the clinical findings: what is the response and the need, on the basis of a differential diagnosis, to establish that a toxicant is or is not involved. The evidence for a specific toxicant may be based initially on clinical findings complemented by gross necropsy findings potentially buttressed by histopathological findings. The differential diagnosis of a toxicosis may be strengthened by evidence of a marker of dose, i.e., urine, blood, or tissue levels of suspected toxicant. The diagnosis may be further strengthened with evidence of exposure, i.e., the presence of the toxicant in the feed or identification of a poisonous plant or in the tissues of an exposed subject. At each step, the qualitative evidence of a toxicosis and a specific toxicant is enhanced as qualitative findings are supplemented by quantitative findings. The analysis is not completed there, though. Other reasonable differential causes of the same or similar clinical signs must also be "ruled out" if the animals or humans are in a real world or field setting.

Quantifying Exposure

Quantitation is paramount in evaluating exposure. In the experimental setting, quantitation is considered beginning with the design of the study and continued through all aspects of the experimentation. To the extent feasible, exposure to the toxicant should be rigorously characterized. This starts with physical and chemical characterization of the test material, be it an alleged pure compound or a mixture, including identification of any contaminants. The exposure circumstances need to be rigorously characterized. This, of course, is easiest to do when the test material is administered by injection. Even with injection, care must be taken to ascertain that the desired quantity of toxicant was actually injected. The quantity administered is typically related to the body weight of the subjects.

With administration by routes other than injection, the situation becomes more complicated. This may involve providing the experimental subjects' feed to which the toxicant has been added. If this approach is used, samples of the contaminated feed should be collected periodically for analysis of the test agent. In some cases, the concentration of the test agent in the feed will be used as a measure of the exposure. To accurately quantify exposure, it will be necessary to know the concentration of the test agent in the feed and also determine the quantity of the contaminated feed containing the test agent that has been ingested. For dermal administration, it is necessary to know the concentration of the test agent in the liquid media applied to the skin and the quantity of the media applied to the skin.

The situation is much more complex for a test agent in the air, whether it is a diluted gas or airborne particulate material. In both cases, it will be necessary to sample and measure the concentration of the test agent in the air at a location as close as possible to the breathing zone of the experimental subjects. For both particulate material and reactive gases, there may be substantial loss of the test agent in the delivery system between the generator used to create the test atmosphere and the breathing zone of the subject(s). Care needs to be taken to minimize such losses. For a toxic agent in a particulate matter form, it is essential to know not only the concentration of the test agent, but the size distribution of the particulate matter since the aerodynamic particle size distribution will influence the fraction of the inhaled material that will be deposited and where it deposits in the respiratory tract. In some experiments, it may be possible to use a plethysmograph to measure respiration of individual subjects during inhalation exposure. This is most readily accomplished when the exposure period is relatively brief as in a study of the toxicokinetics of the agent. The total quantity of test agent inhaled can be estimated from knowledge of the air volume inspired and the concentration of the test agent in the air. In many studies the air concentration of the test agent may be used as a surrogate measure of exposure. As indicated earlier, exposure and dose are not synonymous. However, in many studies it may be necessary to use the concentration of the test agent in the feed, water or air as a surrogate measure of dose.

Describing Absorption, Distribution, Metabolism, and Excretion

A number of different parameters may be evaluated in assessing the kinetics of a test agent (recall Fig. 1.7). Some of the common parameters and terms used are shown in Table 1.2. The four key events involved are absorption, distribution, metabolism, and excretion. It is important to recognize that species differences may exist for each of these events. Absorption is the amount of the material that enters the body. As already discussed, the

TABLE 1.2 Common Terms Used to Describe the ADME Characteristics of Chemicals

Term	Abbreviation	Definition
Concentration	C_p	Concentration of a chemical in plasma (p) at a specific time (*t*)
Time	t	Chronological measurement of a biological function
Half-life	$t_{1/2}$	Time required for exactly 50% of a drug to undergo some defined function (i.e., absorbed, distributed, metabolized, or excreted)
Volume of distribution	V_d	Unitless proportionality constant that relates plasma concentration of a chemical to the total amount of that chemical in the body at any time after some pseudo equilibrium has been attained
Volume of distribution (steady state)	$V_{d(ss)}$	Same as *V*, except measured when the chemical has reached a steady state in the body
Area under the curve	AUC	Total area under the plasma chemical concentration curve from $t=0$ to $t=\infty$ after the animal receives one dose of the chemical
Body clearance of a chemical	Cl_B	The sum of all types of clearance from the body
Renal clearance of a chemical	Cl_R	Volume of chemical that is completely cleared by the kidneys per unit of time (ml/min/kg)
Nonrenal clearance of a chemical	Cl_{NR}	Volume of chemical that is completely cleared by organs other than the kidneys per unit of time (ml/min/kg)
Dose	D	The amount of chemical that is administered to an animal; can be further defined as the total dose, that total dose the animal was exposed to, or the absorbed (effective) dose, that being the fraction of the total dose that was actually absorbed by the animal
Bioavailability	F	Also known as systemic availability of a chemical. The quantity of percentage portion of the total chemical that was absorbed and available to be processed (CME) by the animal, in the case of intravenous administration, $F=100\%$

ADME: absorption, distribution, metabolism and excretion; CME: chemical metabolism and excretion.
Adapted from Spoo, W. (2004). Toxicokinetics. In: Plumlee, K.H. (Ed.), Clinical Veterinary Toxicology. Elsevier, pp. 8–12 (Spoo, 2004).

concept is simple. However, in reality it becomes complex as one moves from parenteral administration to oral intake, to dermal uptake, or inhalation exposure. Distribution of the material will be influenced by the route of entry and the physicochemical properties of the test agent. Metabolism for compounds varies dependent on the physicochemical properties of the material. In some cases, the material may be very inert and simply be transferred mechanically within the body with some portion excreted over time. In other cases, especially with organic compounds, the metabolism may be quite complex and result in metabolites that are either more toxic, less toxic, or have toxicity similar to the parent compound.

Excretion or elimination of the material and its metabolites, if metabolized, may occur via the kidney (urine), gastrointestinal tract (feces), or the lungs (exhalation of volatile compounds). In addition, the agent or metabolites may appear in tears, sweat, or exfoliated skin. Some species, such as the rat, may engage in coprophagy, ingestion of feces, such that the test material in the feces is ingested and some portion may pass through the body multiple times. Animals may be euthanized at various times during the course of the study and samples of various tissues collected and analyzed for the test agent or metabolites. With small experimental subjects, it may be possible to analyze all the tissues and obtain an estimate of the total body burden of the test agent and metabolites.

In some short-term studies it may be possible to collect and analyze excreta and expired air, if the compound is metabolized to a form that will be present in expired air. This information, along with the results of tissue analyses, can provide an estimate of the total quantity in the body, excreta, and expired air for comparison with an estimate of the quantity administered. This kind of mass balance approach is obviously most feasible when radioactive or stable isotope tracers are used. One should not be surprised to find the estimated quantity recovered varying from 75% to 125%; there will be a high degree of experimental variability when multiple samples are being collected and analyzed. Obviously, one should view with suspicion data tables showing recovery of exactly 100% of the administered dose. Such values are typically the result of an over zealous investigator normalizing the data to 100% recovery. For chronic exposure studies, it may be possible to use kinetic modeling to estimate the quantity of the test agent or metabolites present in the experimental subjects at each exposure concentrations at various times after initiation of exposure.

Toxicant-Induced Responses

The types of studies typically used by toxicologists to investigate exposure–response relationships can be placed in four categories related to the duration of the studies; acute, subacute, subchronic and chronic (recall Fig. 1.8). Acute studies are usually of a day or less and may involve intraperitoneal, intravenous, or subcutaneous injection, gavage, dermal application or inhalation. Injections may be given once or several times in the 24-h period. Acute inhalation exposures are typically 4–6 h in duration. In all cases, the observations are made over a 24-h period. Subacute studies typically involve repeated exposures made on a daily, or 5 days per week, basis for 2–4 weeks with observations over the same period of time. Subchronic studies are usually conducted over a period of 1–3 months. In the case of inhalation exposures, these are typically conducted for 4–6 h per day, 5 days per week. Chronic studies are usually conducted for more than 3 months and, most typically, for 2 years. I personally view the use of the terms—acute, subacute, subchronic and chronic—as jargon and prefer to communicate the duration of studies in a specific manner, i.e., number of days or months, or as short or long term. I prefer to use the terms acute, subacute, or chronic as descriptors of a medical condition.

The kinds of toxicant-induced responses that may be encountered are broad, essentially mirroring the range of disease processes that may occur in humans and other animal species. In any well-conducted toxicity study, the investigator should use as broad an array of observational techniques as are reasonably available to characterize the pattern of morbidity and mortality that may develop. Inevitably, cost constraints will influence the choice of endpoints evaluated. It will be useful to prioritize the potential endpoints as to their likely value in terms of the information gained. It is crucial that detailed necropsies be conducted on subjects euthanized at prescribed times and at termination of the study. Tissues should be collected from any gross lesions and tissues identified in the protocol as likely target tissues and processed for histopathological evaluation. It is now routine to establish a defined set of criteria for evaluating the various tissues and characterizing lesions. This approach allows the quantitative evaluation of any pathological findings on a group basis rather than restricting the evaluation to qualitative descriptions of responses in individual subjects.

Toxicity studies to evaluate exposure (dose)-response relationships may extend from minutes to hours when biochemical and physiological responses are being evaluated, to hours to days when acute morbidity and mortality are being assessed, to weeks to months and finally to a significant portion of the lifespan of the species, e.g., 2 years for mice and rats when chronic effects, including cancer induction, are being evaluated. With increased attention given to animal welfare considerations, emphasis is being given to using as few animals as possible to define the acute morbidity and mortality of test materials. Rather than use a traditional approach to attempt to precisely define a lethal dose 50% (LD_{50}), it has become customary to use approaches with many fewer animals to define an approximate LD_{50}. In some cases, it may be desirable to determine the concentration of a test agent in water or air that produces 50% lethality over a defined period of time, a lethal concentration, LC_{50}. This approach remains in common use when studying aquatic organisms.

In modern toxicology, increasing attention is given to conducting studies with exposures that are defined by the anticipated conditions of use of the test material. This may involve initially conducting a study of 2 weeks duration, perhaps with up to five exposure levels anchored by a level related to anticipated use. The results of this study are then used to select exposure levels, perhaps three or four, and to sharpen the focus of a 90-day study. The results of the 90-day study, in turn, are used to select the exposure levels and sharpen the focus of a study of 2-years duration. Although it has become customary to conduct chronic exposure or 2-year studies with three exposure levels, it should be recognized that use of a control group and three exposure levels spanning a range of concentrations differing by a factor of 2, i.e., 1, 1/2 and 1/4 or a factor of 3, i.e., 1, 1/3rd, and 1/9th, does not provide a robust data set for characterizing the shape of the exposure (dose)-response relationship. On the other hand, the use of exposure levels differing by a factor of 10, i.e., 1, 1/10th, and 1/100th may provide an excessively broad range of exposure levels for identifying a lowest observed adverse effect level (LOAEL) or no observed adverse effect level (NOAEL) as will be discussed later.

In chronic studies with rodent species, major attention is directed to evaluating any toxicant-induced changes in animals at the several exposure levels compared to controls over a 2-year period or until a defined mortality level is reached, such as 20% surviving. Any changes in various indices of morbidity or pathological alterations will be evaluated compared to controls as well as tested for trends across the exposure levels. In many cases, the primary endpoint of concern will be cancer, which should include evaluation of all stages of tumor development up to sarcomas and carcinomas. It has become customary to use life table statistical methods such as that of Kaplan and Meier (1958) to evaluate the incidence of key changes. This approach allows for the use of data not only from the survivors at the end of the study, but also animals that have died or been euthanized at interim times. This situation is analogous to that encountered in human epidemiological studies when subjects may be lost to follow-up.

It has become customary when the results of chronic studies will be used for regulatory purposes to convene a pathology peer review panel of expert veterinary pathologists, typically Diplomates of the American College of Veterinary Pathology (ACVP), to evaluate histological specimens from representative cases and the diagnoses of the original pathologist to verify that the diagnoses are appropriate and consistent with the scientific norm. As an aside, I encourage veterinary toxicologists to personally review the pathology findings in studies with the study pathologist so as to be familiar with the nature of the pathology findings. However, I discourage veterinary toxicologists from taking on a dual role of toxicologist and pathologist for a study. Indeed, this approach would be unacceptable for a study to be submitted for regulatory purposes unless the toxicologist was also an ACVP Diplomate.

Describing Exposure–Response Relationships for Noncancer Endpoints

It is now appropriate to consider how the data generated from toxicological investigations can be used. Let us first examine a threshold exposure–response relationship as shown in Fig. 1.3 and shown now in an expanded form in Fig. 1.10. The first step is to examine the data set from critical exposure–response studies to identify key parameters to be used to describe the results. Key determinations are the No Observed Effect Level, the highest exposure level for which no effects are observed and the NOAEL, the highest exposure level that produces no adverse effects. Obviously, characterization of an effect as adverse or not adverse is a matter of professional judgment. For example, in a cholinesterase inhibitor study, is a reduction in blood cholinesterase in the absence of salivation or other clinical signs an adverse effect or merely an effect?

In the absence of the identification of a NOAEL, there is a need to identify the LOAEL, the highest exposure level at which an adverse effect is observed. The specific NOAEL and LOAEL that can be identified are a function

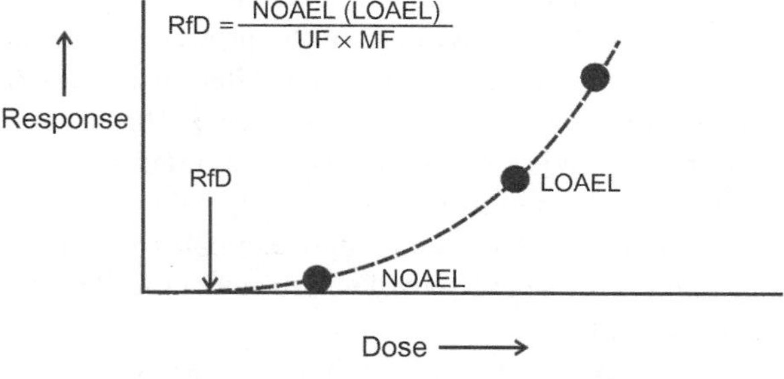

$UF = UF_H \cdot UF_A \cdot UF_S \cdot UF_L$
UF_H = Human variability (10×)
UF_A = Animal to human (10×)
UF_S = Subchronic to chronic (10×)
UF_L = LOAEL to NOAEL (10×)
MF = Modifying factor for completeness of data (1–10×)
RfD = Reference dose

FIGURE 1.10 Schematic rendering of a threshold–exposure response relationship.

of the exposure levels originally selected for studies. To state the obvious, observations can only be made at the exposure levels studied. For example, if the exposure levels studied did not extend to a sufficiently low level, the lowest level might produce an effect thereby precluding observation of a NOAEL. Alternatively, the study might be designed with three exposure levels separated by a factor of 10 with the lowest exposure level identified as a NOAEL and the next higher exposure level identified as producing some modest adverse effects and, thus, identified as the LOAEL. In retrospect, in such a study it is not known whether the "true" LOAEL might have been a factor of three or five above the NOAEL since these levels were not investigated.

Another consideration is the nature of the effects identified at the NOAEL. Was there evidence of enzyme induction or hyperplasia, hypertrophy, or atrophy with no evidence of a change in organ weight? Likewise, at the LOAEL were hyperplasia, hypertrophy, or atrophy present resulting in modest or substantial changes in organ and body weight? Were histological changes observed that were reversible? Were the changes sufficiently profound that the level would be identified as a functional effect level? These questions serve to emphasize the extent to which professional judgment is involved in interpreting the results of all toxicological investigations.

For noncancer effects a reference dose (RfD) for oral intake or a inhalation reference concentration (RfC) for airborne materials is calculated using the NOAEL or LOAEL as a starting point (Jarabek et al., 1990; Jarabek, 1994). An RfD or RfC may be defined as an estimate (with uncertainty spanning perhaps an order of magnitude) of a continuous oral or inhalation exposure to the human population (including sensitive subgroups) that is likely to be without appreciable risk of deleterious noncancer effects during a lifetime. The RfD and RfC values are developed from the experimentally determined NOAEL or LOAEL values as shown in Fig. 1.10 (Jarabek, 1994) and normalized to continuous exposure. For a more complete description of the process, the reader is referred to a book chapter by McClellan et al. (2006). The EPA maintains an Integrated Risk Information System that includes comprehensive summaries of the toxicological information available on specific chemicals including RfD and RfC values and estimates of cancer-causing potency. These profiles are available on line (EPA/IRIS, 2011).

A somewhat similar approach for noncancer effects has been used by the ACGIH to develop TLVs (ACGIH, 2011). A TLV is defined as airborne concentrations of substances that represent conditions under which it is believed that nearly all workers may be repeatedly exposed day after day without adverse health effects. Since the ACGIH TLVs apply to healthy workers they may not always incorporate a SF or UF of 10 for human variability. The exposure duration for TLVs is based on a 40-h work week and, thus, the results of animal studies will be normalized to 40 h per week.

The Agency for Toxic Substances and Disease Registry (ATSDR) develops Minimal Risk Levels (MRLs) using a similar methodology. A MRL is an estimate of the daily human exposure to hazardous substance that is likely to be without appreciable risk of adverse noncancer effects over a specified duration of exposure. For example, MRLs are derived for acute (1–14 days), intermediate (14–365 days), and chronic (365 days and longer) exposure durations. The MRLs are intended to serve as a screening tool to help public health professionals decide to look more closely at particular exposure situations. The ATSDR has prepared toxicological profiles on many chemicals including their MRLs. More than 200 profiles are available on line (ATSDR, 2006).

The NIOSH has in the past developed Recommended Exposure Levels (RELs). RELs are set at levels such that virtually all persons in the working population (with the possible exception of hypersensitive individuals) would experience no adverse effects. In late 2016, the NIOSH issued an updated cancer policy (NIOSH, 2016). This policy stated that NIOSH will no longer use the term REL for occupational carcinogens. Instead, NIOSH will provide a Risk Management Limit for a Carcinogen, which is to be identified as an RML-CA. NIOSH made this change to acknowledge there is no known safe level for exposure to carcinogens and that an RML-CA is a reasonable starting point for controlling exposures. The new policy states the RML-CA will be set for occupational carcinogens at the concentration corresponding to the 95% lower confidence limit of the 1 in 10,000 (10^{-4}) risk estimate. NIOSH intends to set RML-CA values for agents classified by IARC, EPA, or the NTP as possible, probable, or human carcinogens. The Occupational Safety and Health Administration sets Permissible Exposure Levels (PELs) based on consideration of the NIOSH RELs. Presumably in the future it will set PELs based on the RML-CA value. It is important to recognize the OSHA values are legally enforceable limits unlike the NIOSH RELs or RML-CA values, which are guidance.

The International Programme on Chemical Safety (IPCS) prepares authoritative reviews on the environmental health impact of various chemicals. The reports are available on line (IPCS, 2011). The exposure limiting values developed by the IPCS are guidance values and not legally enforceable limits. The United States makes extensive use of legal enforceable exposure limits. Many other countries emphasize the use of guidance values. This distinction is important when comparing standards versus guidance originating from different countries.

In considering all of the foregoing guidance or regulatory levels, it is important to recognize that they are set to control exposures for workers or the general public. In each case, they are set to be health protective and, thus, are set at levels below where human effects have been observed or are expected to occur. These values should not be interpreted as being equivalent to levels producing adverse effects in humans.

Cancer as an Endpoint

For cancer as an endpoint, animal exposure–response studies may provide two kinds of input. First, the results may be used in Carcinogen Classification Processes such as those of the IARC, the EPA or NTP. As discussed earlier, these are hazard-based classification schemes—a given agent capable of causing human cancer without consideration of the potency of the agent. These schemes have been described elsewhere (McClellan, 1999, 2010; McClellan et al., 2006).

If a positive cancer outcome is observed in animal studies, the quantitative exposure-cancer response data may be used in a second way: to develop a risk coefficient, lifetime cancer risk per unit of exposure, describing the potency of the agent for causing human cancer. Such extrapolations typically involve linear statistical extrapolations from high levels of exposure used in the animal studies to potential human exposure levels several orders of magnitude lower (recall Fig. 1.3). In addition, they may purposefully be calculated based on upper 95% confidence limit on some level of risk, e.g., with a probability of a one in one million occurrence for environmental exposures or 1 in 10,000 for occupational exposures as discussed earlier. In my opinion, these extrapolated values are highly uncertain. It is quite possible that for some agents classified as possibly or probably carcinogenic to humans in the absence of a positive association with cancer from epidemiological studies and, thus, based on high exposure level animal study results, there is no added cancer risk at very low levels of exposure (Gold et al., 2003). The EPA (2005a) has issued guidance for alternative approaches to estimate cancer risks when information is available on the mode of action of the agent, e.g., if the cancer arises as a result of the toxicity and secondary cell proliferation rather than a direct effect of the chemical or metabolite on DNA. For example, chloroform has been shown to cause cancer by this mode of action (Butterworth et al., 1995). The EPA (2005b) has also provided guidance for considering the impact of susceptibility of early life exposures for causing cancer.

Information on the cancer-causing potential of various chemicals is included in the material summarized in the USEPA's Integrated Risk Information System (EPA/IRIS, 2011). The IARC monographs on the evaluation of carcinogenic risks to humans are all available on line (IARC, 2011). The monographs cover the carcinogen classification reviews of nearly 1000 agents. It is ironic that over the decades IARC has only classified one chemical, caprolactan, used in the manufacture of nylon, as "unlikely to cause cancer in humans." It has clearly been easier for scientists on IARC panels to address hazards in contrast to safety. This dichotomy needs to be addressed since the public is interested in both. The NTP publishes, on an irregular schedule, a Report on Carcinogens. The 14th Report was released in November 2016 (NTP, 2016). The total number of agents listed as "human carcinogens" or "reasonably anticipated to be human carcinogens" to date is less than 300. The potency of the various agents for causing cancer is quite varied. When examining this literature, many in the public, including some scientists, are surprised to learn how few agents (less than 100) have been conclusively identified as "human carcinogens." These facts stand in sharp contrast to the view conveyed in the popular media and some scientific publications that people live in a "world of carcinogens."

New Potential Endpoints

In recent years, the expansion of knowledge at the molecular and cellular level has provided the opportunity for considering the addition of a myriad of new endpoints to toxicological evaluations. This includes an array of new molecular biomarkers that have received substantial attention. Although biomarkers are frequently discussed as new approaches, it is well known to veterinary clinicians, toxicologists, and to physicians that biomarkers have been used in both human and veterinary medicine for centuries.

In some cases, measurement of the biomarkers present in body fluids, urine, or exhaled breath, serve as an indicator of exposure or, even, dose of a toxicant. Recall the report of the individual arrested for "driving while intoxicated" based on a breathalyzer test for exhaled alcohol that has been converted to a blood alcohol level. In other cases, the biomarker is an indicator of a disease process. Recall individuals being evaluated for prostate cancer based on an elevated level of prostate specific antigen in serum samples.

New biomarkers of exposure will continue to be proposed. For each potential biomarker of exposure, it will be necessary to conduct experiments to validate the utility of the biomarker. A special challenge relates to recognizing the dynamics of the toxicokinetics of various toxicants and establishment of quantitative relationships between exposure and dose at any particular time over the course of the intoxication.

The potential list of biomarkers for toxic responses is seemingly endless. In all fields of medicine, from different kinds of cancer to various functional diseases of every organ system, new molecular markers are being identified on a regular basis (Gupta, 2014). The challenge for toxicologists is to consider from among this array of opportunities which biomarkers are sufficiently well validated with regard to their linkage to diseases and sufficiently reasonable in cost to warrant their use in exposure–response studies. This includes consideration of the new and highly sophisticated genomic tools. There is a special challenge in designing validation studies to make certain that the experimental design is directed toward identifying specific disease-related endpoints or toxicant related effects rather than merely being another, albeit more sophisticated, marker of nonspecific toxic effects. A serious issue in many previous validation studies has been the use of a single high exposure level and a few short-term observation times. Such studies are unable to evaluate exposure-related changes in biomarkers and may not be able to identify toxicant specific changes (Gupta, 2014).

Three reports prepared by Committees of the National Research Council provide insight into how some individuals envision the future of toxicity testing. The first NRC Report (2007a) addresses the application of toxicogenomic technologies in predictive toxicology and risk assessment. The second NRC Report (2007b) provides a strategy and vision for toxicity testing in the 21st century. The third and most recent NRC report (2017) provides a discussion of the multiple ways in which information acquired using new technologies can influence evaluation of health risks. I encourage veterinary toxicologists, whether they are in training or experienced, to carefully read these reports. I view both of the reports as aspirational. In my opinion, both committees would have benefitted from more participation from veterinarians and human medical doctors who understand the complexity of disease processes and toxicoses to counter-balance the views of molecular and cell biologists who are used to focusing on the microlevel and some mathematically oriented scientists who may overstate the role of mathematical models in predicting disease outcomes related to exposure to toxic agents. The concept of systems biology has come to the forefront in recent years. In my view, the concept of a systems approach to normal biology and disease processes has been a fundamental concept undergirding both veterinary medicine and human medicine for more than a century.

To illustrate the extent to which our current knowledge of biological systems and diseases processes has advanced, I will cite a single recent reference, Huttlin et al. (2017). This paper with 25 coauthors describes BioPlex 2.0 (Biophysical Interactions of ORFeome-derived complexes). BioPlex 2.0 is grounded in recognition that the physiology of a cell can be viewed as the product of thousands of proteins existing in concert to shape the cellular response. It describes more than 56,000 candidates that protein-protein interactions will contain more than 29,000 previously unknown coassociation. They identified 442 protein communities associated with more than 2000 disease connotations placing numerous candidate disease given with a cellular framework. The fundamental biology reported in this paper should serve as both a cautionary message that disease processes are extraordinarily complex and as a challenge for future scientists to build bridges from this world of basic biology to the observations of spontaneously occurring disease and toxicant-induced diseases in individuals and populations.

A related message is the increasing need for all scientists, including veterinary toxicologists to develop their communication skills. These communication skills are needed for multiple kinds of interactions, between scientists in diverse disciplines, between basic scientists and clinicians, and between medical and other scientists and the general public. The development of improved communications will require that the traditional discipline based silos of most scientific disciplines and academic institutions will need to come down. Ultimately, students who desire to become true professionals rather than mere trade persons will demand it. Moreover, many members of the public are already becoming better informed on scientific and medical matters and are developing high expectations of professionals who provide services to them or, on a broader scale, to society at large.

In closing, let me comment briefly on the role of electronic media as a source of information on toxicity and health issues, indeed, on essentially any matter in which you want to find information. It is important to recognize that a Google search will yield an astonishing amount of information. In some cases this will include original peer-reviewed papers published on-line in highly reputable journals. In other cases, careful examination will reveal the paper was published on-line in a journal with a deceptively similar title to one of the highly respected journals. In some cases material presented in a highly authoritative manner will not have a clearly related authorship, indeed, it could have been prepared as a new form of advertising. My bottom line recommendation is for users of the electronic media to carefully screen all of the material and give the highest degree of credibility to peer-reviewed material such as this text edited by Gupta.

CONCLUDING REMARKS AND FUTURE DIRECTIONS

Veterinary toxicology is a multifaceted hybrid that draws on and contributes to the veterinary medical profession, the scientific field of toxicology, and, broadly, to medical science and society at large. Some have characterized toxicology as a distinct scientific discipline. I view toxicology as an applied area of science addressing important societal issues by drawing on multiple scientific disciplines and professions. Veterinary toxicology, as a subspecialty in veterinary medicine, has a specific origin: the diagnosis and treatment of toxicoses in domestic animals and companion animals. That important role continues today. However, the field has broadened to include concern for contaminants in human food products originating from animals and for contributing to the conduct and interpretation of safety/risk evaluations for pharmaceuticals, food additives, consumer products, and specific chemicals. Veterinary toxicologists who understand both normal and disease processes extending from the molecular level to the integrated mammalian organism and, indeed, populations, have an array of opportunities for making significant contributions to medical science and to society. The prospects for the future of veterinary toxicology and the opportunities for well-educated veterinary toxicologists with broad experience have never been brighter.

DEDICATION

It is my pleasure to dedicate this chapter to a celebration of the 50th anniversary of the American Board of Veterinary Toxicology (ABVT) and my four colleagues (William Buck, Fred Oehme, Robert Singer and V.K. Singh) who passed the first ABVT examination with me in 1967 (Dorman et al, 2017).

It has been over 50 years since I filed my application to take the first examination of the ABVT. I filed the application to take the ABVT examination recognizing I had not completed a formal residency or PhD training program in veterinary toxicology. However, I was confident in my knowledge of the field acquired working a the Hanford Atomic Products Operations Biology Laboratory for 5 years with an extraordinarily talented and thoughtful mentor, the late Leo K. Bustad and the laboratory's multidisciplinary staff. I owe him a great debt of gratitude for helping shape the foundation for my career. I had a long wait for a response letter from ABVT. When it arrived I was not surprised that the letter, obviously written and reviewed by an attorney, noted that I had not completed a "formal training" program in veterinary toxicology; the examination would be very comprehensive and with my "limited training" I was unlikely to pass the examination. However, it went on to note there was no legal basis for the ABVT precluding my taking the examination. I accepted the challenge and have never regretted it. On different occasions some individuals have questioned whether I was really a veterinary toxicologist. I have always been proud to refer them to my credentials and to note, based on rigorous examinations, that I am a Diplomate of both the ABVT and the American Board of Toxicology (ABT). In my opinion, education, experience, and credentials are important. Over my career, I have recruited more than 500 students and 100 professionals. If the individuals did not already have Board or other certification, I strongly encouraged them at the first opportunity to take the appropriate examinations. I have been repaid many times over by following their successful careers and contributions to society. My career has involved working with many individuals with quite varied backgrounds in multiple disciplines and has been remarkably varied, highly productive, and enjoyable. I hope it will serve as encouragement to others to recognize that the career opportunities for veterinary toxicologists well-grounded in comparative medicine are without bounds.

I also dedicate this chapter to the memory of my longtime friend, Charles C. Capen (1936–2008), an internationally recognized comparative pathologist and endocrine toxicologist. A complete obituary was published in *Toxicologic Pathology* (Anonymous, 2008). Chuck and I were classmates in the College of Veterinary Medicine at Washington State University receiving our Doctor of Veterinary Medicine degrees in 1960. Chuck immediately entered the residency and graduate program in Veterinary Pathology at The Ohio State University (OSU). He received his PhD from OSU in 1965 and soon passed the certifying examination of the American College of Veterinary Pathologists (ACVP) and became an ACVP Diplomate. He progressed rapidly through the academic ranks, becoming a full Professor and, ultimately, a Distinguished University Professor. He provided outstanding leadership as Chairperson from 1981 to 2002 of the OSU Department of Veterinary Biosciences. He was an outstanding teacher and researcher. One of his major contributions was in the interpretation of endocrine system effects observed in laboratory animal species as to their significance as predictors of human disease for various chemicals, including candidate pharmaceuticals. His special expertise resulted in his being asked to serve on numerous advisory committees and as a consultant to many companies around the globe. He was an elected member of the National Academy of Medicine and a recipient of many other honors and a professional colleague and friend to many individuals.

ACKNOWLEDGMENTS

Many of the concepts presented in the chapter are based on my experience working with talented scientists at four institutions: the Hanford Biology Laboratory (1957–64) at Richland, Washington; the Medical Research Branch (1965–66); Division of Biology and Medicine, of what was then the US Atomic Energy Commission, Washington, DC; the Lovelace Inhalation Toxicology Research

Institute (1966–88) (now a part of the Lovelace Respiratory Research Institute) in Albuquerque, New Mexico; and the Chemical Industry Institute of Toxicology (1988–99) (in later years the Hamner Institutes Health Sciences) in Research Triangle Park, North Carolina. Moreover, my insights and their role in informing important societal decisions on human and animal health and environmental impacts have been sharpened by my experience serving as an advisor on toxicology and human health risk issues to public agencies and private clients and the opportunities I have had for working with many outstanding toxicologists and other scientists.

The excellent assistance of my long-time associate, Mildred Morgan, in preparing this chapter and the useful review comments of Drs. Ramesh C. Gupta, Fred W. Oehme, and Mike Murphy on drafts of earlier chapters are gratefully acknowledged.

POSTSCRIPT

Over the decades, I have come to appreciate that every sector of society (academic, government, industry, and private consulting firms) includes many highly qualified individuals. What one learns from experience is that what is important is the personal knowledge and integrity that each of these individuals brings to the forum, not who they are employed by at the time. It is especially gratifying when many of these professional associates over time become friends. One of those special friends was John Doull (1922–2017) who passed away on March 24, 2017 as I was finishing revision of this chapter. My primary mentor, Leo Bustad, arranged for me to visit John Doull and his colleagues at the University of Chicago in the fall of 1960. Out of that initial meeting developed a friendship that would extend for 57 years. I knew I could always call on John for advice and counsel. On many occasions in the past I would ask John to review drafts of a chapter such as this one to tell if my writing made sense or if I had missed some important concepts. That was not to be the case with this chapter. I am pleased that I was asked to author–"A Tribute to John Doull, BS, PhD, MD: Scientist, Physician, Educator, Advisor and Above All, a Gentleman and Friend to Many (McClellan, 2017)." John recognized the unique education of veterinarians in comparative medicine and their potential for contributing to veterinary toxicology, toxicology in general and, more broadly, to medical science and the well being of human kind. We will all miss this giant in the field of toxicology and medical science.

REFERENCES

ACGIH, American Conference of Governmental Industrial Hygienists, 2011. Threshold Limit Values and Biological Exposure Indices for Chemical Substances and Physical Agents. Cincinnati, OH.

Acquavella, J., Garabrant, D., Marsh, G., et al., 2016. Glyphosate epidemiology expert panel review: a weight of evidence systematic review of the relationship between glyphosate exposure and nonHodgkins's lymphoma or multiple myeloma. Crit. Rev. Toxicol. 46 (S1), 28–43.

Albert, R.E., 1994. Carcinogen risk assessment in the U.S. Environmental Protection Agency. Crit. Rev. Toxicol. 24, 70–85.

Anastas, P.T., Warner, J.C., 1998. Green Chemistry: Theory and Practice. Oxford University Press, Oxford.

Anonymous, 2008. Obituary for Charles C. Capen. Toxicol. Pathol. 36, 373–374.

ATSDR, Agency for Toxic Substances and Disease Registry, 2006. Toxicological Profiles and Minimal Risk Levels for Hazardous Substances <http://www.atsdr.cdc.gov/mrls.html>.

Attfield, M.D., Schleiff, P.L., lubin, J.H., et al., 2012. The diesel exhaust in miners study: a cohort mortality study with emphasis on lung cancer. J. Natl. Cancer Inst. 104, 1–15.

AVMA (American Veterinary Medical Association), One Health Initiative Task Force: Final Report, July 15, 2008.

Ayres, J.G., Harrison, R.M., Maynard, R., et al., 2010a. Textbook of Environmental Medicine, first ed. Hodder Arnold, London.

Ayres, J.G., Harrison, R.M., Maynard, R., McClellan, R.O., et al., 2010b. Chapter 1, Environmental Medicine. In: Ayres, J.G., Harrison, R.M., Nichols, G.L., Maynard, R. (Eds.), Textbook of Environmental Medicine, first ed. Hodder Arnold (Publisher), London, pp. 3–21.

Ball, D.J., Blanchard, J., Jacobson-Kram, D., McClellan, R.O., et al., 2007. Development of safety qualification thresholds and their use in drug product evaluation. Toxicol. Sci. 97 (2), 226–236.

Ball, D.J., Norwood, D.L., Stults, C.L.M., Nagao, L.M. (Eds.), 2012. Leachables and Extractables Handbook: Safety Evaluation, Qualification and Best Practices Applied to Inhalation Drug Products. John Wiley and Sons, Hoboken, NJ.

Beyer, L.A., Beck, B.D., Lewandowski, T.A., 2011. Historical perspective on the use of animal bioassays to predict carcinogenicity: evolution in design and recognition of utility. Crit. Rev. Toxicol. 41, 321–338.

Brusick, D., Aardema, M., Kier, L., et al., 2016. Genotoxicity expert panel review: weight of evidence evaluation of the genotoxicity of glyphosate, glyphosate-based formulations, and aminomethylphosphonic acid. Crit. Rev. Toxicol. 46 (Suppl. 1), 56–74.

Burrows, G.E., Tyrl, R.S., 2006. Handbook of Toxic Plants of North America. Blackwell Publishing, Ames, IA.

Bustad, L.K., McClellan, R.O., Garner, R.J., 1965. The significance of radionuclide contamination in ruminants. Physiology of Digestion in the Ruminant. Butterworth Inc, Washington, DC, pp. 131–146.

Butterworth, B.E., Conolly, R.B., Morgan, K.T., 1995. A strategy for establishing mode of action of chemical carcinogens as a guide for approaches to risk assessments. Cancer Lett. 93, 129–146.

CAA, 1970. The Clean Air Act Amendments of 1970-P.L. 91-04 (December 31, 1970), Plus Technical Amendments Made by P.L. 92–157 (November 18, 1971).

Calabrese, E.J., Baldwin, L.A., 2003. The hormesis model is more frequent that the threshold model in toxicology. Toxicol. Sci. 61, 246–250.

Calabrese, E.J., Blain, R., 2005. The occurrence of hormetic dose responses in the toxicological literature, the hormesis database: an overview. Toxicol. Appl. Pharmacol. 202, 289–301.

Calabrese, E.J., et al. (57 co-authors including R.O. McClellan), 2007. Biological stress response terminology: integrating the concepts of adaptive response and preconditioning stress within a hormetic dose-response framework. Toxicol. Appl. Pharmacol. 222, 122–128.

Carmichael, N., Bausen, M., Boobis, A.R., et al., 2011. Using mode of action information to improve regulatory decision-making: an ECETOX/ILSI/RF/HESI Workshop overview. Crit. Rev. Toxcol. 41, 175–186.

Carson, R., 1962. Silent Spring. Houghton Mifflin, Boston, MA.

Casarett, L.J., Doull, J. (Eds.), 1975. Toxicology: The Basic Science of Poisons. MacMillan Publishing Co., Inc.

Chapman, M., Campbell, A., 2011. Veterinary Toxicology. Blackwell Publishing, Ames, IA.

Conolly, R.B., Kimbell, J.S., Janszen, D., et al., 2004. Human respiratory tract cancer risks of inhaled formaldehyde: dose-response predictions derived from biologically-motivated computational modeling of a combined rodent and human dataset. Toxicol. Sci. 82, 279−296.

Crump, K.S., Van Landingham, C., Moolgavkar, S.H., McClellan, R., 2015. Reanalysis of the DEMS nested casecontrol study of lung cancer and diesel exhaust: suitability for quantitative risk assessment. Risk Anal. 35 (4), 676−700.

Crump, K.S., Van Landingham, C., McClellan, R.O., 2016. Influence of alternative exposure estimates in the diesel exhaust miners study: diesel exhaust and lung cancer. Risk Anal. 36 (9), 1803−1812.

deAvila, C., Sandberg, E.C., 2006. REACH: better knowledge and better use of chemicals in the European Union. Chimia. 60, 645−650.

Dorman, D.C., Beasley, V.R., McClellan, R.O., 2017. Commentary: Fifty years of contributions by the American Board of Veterinary Toxicology. JAVMA. 251, 268−270.

EC, European Commission, 2002. Communication for the Commission on the Precautionary Principle, Brussels.

EC, European Commission, 2006. Regulation No. 1907/2006 of the European Parliament and of the Council of 18 December 2006 concerning the Registration, Evaluation, Authorisation and Restriction of Chemical Substances (REACH) establishing a European Chemicals Agency, amending Directive 1999/45/EC and repealing Council Regulation (EEC) No. 793/93 and Commission Regulation (EC) No. 1488/94 as well as Council Directive 76/769/EEC and Commission Directives 91/15/EC, 93/67/EEC 93/105/EC and 20601/21/EC E.P.a.t.e. Commission. Off. J. Eur Union 30, 12.

EMEA, European Medicines Evaluation Agency, 2004. Committee for Medicinal Products for Human Use (CHMP). Guideline on the Limits of Genotoxic Impurities. CPMP/SWP/5199/02, London, 23. Available at: <http://www.emea.eu.int/pdfa/human/swp/5199902en.pdf>.

EPA, U.S. Environmental Protection Agency, 1986. Guidelines for carcinogen risk assessment. Fed. Reg. 51, 33992−34003.

EPA, U.S. Environmental Protection Agency, 1991. Guidelines for developmental toxicity risk assessment. Fed. Reg. 56, 63798−63826.

EPA, U.S. Environmental Protection Agency, 1995. Proposed guidelines for neurotoxicity risk assessment. Fed. Reg. 60, 52032−52056.

EPA, U.S. Environmental Protection Agency, 1996a. Health Effects Test Guidelines Carcinogenicity. OPPTS 870.4200, EPA 712-C-96-211, Public Draft.

EPA, U.S. Environmental Protection Agency, 1996b. Health Effects Test Guidelines. OPPTS 870.5300, Detection of Gene Mutations in Somatic Cells in Culture, EPA 712-C-96-221.

EPA, U.S. Environmental Protection Agency, 1996c. Proposed Guidelines for Reproductive Toxicity Risk Assessment. EPA-630-R-96-009.

EPA, U.S. Environmental Protection Agency, 1996d. Health Effects Test Guidelines. OPPTS 870.7200, Domestic Animal Safety. June 1996. <http://www.epa.gov/opptsfrs/publications/OPPTS_Harmonized/870_Health_Effects_Test_Guidelines/Drafts/870-7200.pc>.

EPA, U.S. Environmental Protection Agency, 1998. Health Effects Test Guidelines, OPPTS 870. 7200, Companion Animal Safety Prevention, Pesticides, and Toxic Substances, August 5, 1998. <http://www.epa.gov/OPPTSHarmonized/870>.

EPA, U.S. Environmental Protection Agency, 2005a. Guidelines for Carcinogen Risk Assessment. Risk Assessment Forum. U.S. Environmental Protection Agency.

EPA, U.S. Environmental Protection Agency, 2005b. Supplemental Guidance for Assessing Susceptibility for Early-Life Exposure to Carcinogens. Risk Assessment Form, USEPA.

EPA, U.S. Environmental Protection Agency, EPA/OPPTS, Office of Prevention, Pesticides and Toxic Substances, 2006. OPPTS Harmonized Test Guidelines. <http://www.epa.gov/opptsfrs/publications/OPPTS_Harmonized/870_Health_Effects_Test Guidelines>.

EPA, U.S. Environmental Protection Agency, Integrated Risk Information System (EPA/IRIS), 2011. <http://www.epa.gov/iris/subst/index.html>.

F.D.A., Food and Drug Administration, 1994. General Principles for Evaluating the Safety of Compounds Used in Food-Producing Animals Guidelines. <http://www.fda.gov/cvm/fda/TOCs/guideline3toc.html> (accessed 01.08.06).

F.D.A., Food and Drug Administration, 2001. Good Laboratory Practices for Non-Clinical Laboratory Studies. Code of Federal Regulations, Title 21, Part 58. <http://www.access.gpo/gov/nara/cfr/waisidx_o1/21cfr58_01.html> (accessed 01.08.06).

F.D.A., Food and Drug Administration, 2011. Toxicologic Principles for the Safety of Food Ingredients (Redbook 2000). <www.cfsan.gov/redbook/red.toct.html> (accessed 01.06.11).

FIFRA, Federal Insecticide, Fungicide and Rodenticide Act, 1991. Enforcement Response Policy for the Federal Insecticide, Fungicide and Rodenticide Act Good Laboratory Practice (GLP) Regulations.

Gabriel, K.L., 1964. Veterinary Toxicology. Ann. N.Y. Acad. Sci. III, Art. 2, 559−812.

Gallo, M.A., 2013. History and scope of toxicology. In: Klaassen, C.D. (Ed.), Casarett and Doull's "Toxicology: The Basic Science of Poisons", eighth ed. McGraw-Hill, New York, NY, pp. 3−11.

Garland, T., Barr, A.C. (Eds.), 1998. Toxic Plants and Other Natural Toxicants. CAB International, New York, NY.

Garner, R.J., 1957. Veterinary Toxicology. The Williams and Wilkins Company, Baltimore, MD.

Garner, R.J., 1961. Veterinary Toxicology, second ed. The Williams and Wilkins Company, Baltimore, MD.

Gold, L.S., Slone, T.H., Monley, N.B., Ames, B.N., 2003. Misconceptions About the Causes of Cancer. Fraser Institute, Vancouver, BC.

Golden, R., 2011. Identifying an indoor air exposure limit for formaldehyde considering both irritation and cancer hazards. Crit. Rev. Toxicol. 1−50 (Early Online Online − http://informahealthcare.com/toc/txc/0/0).

Gordis, L., 2008. Epidemiology. third ed. Saunders Elsevier, Philadelphia, PA.

Gupta, R.C. (Ed.), 2014. Biomarkers in Toxicology. Academic Press/Elsevier, Amsterdam, 1128 pp.

Hayes, A.W., Kruger, C.L., 2014. Principles and Methods of Toxicology, sixth ed. CRC Press, Boca Raton, FL.

Henshaw, P.S., 1941. Biologic significance of the tolerance dose in X-ray and radium protection. J. Natl. Cancer Inst. 1, 789−805.

Hesterberg, T.W., Bunn, W.B., McClellan, R.O., et al., 2005. Carcinogenicity studies of diesel engine exhausts in laboratory animals: a review of past studies and a discussion of future research needs. Crit. Rev. Toxicol. 35, 379–411.

Hesterberg, T.W., Long, C.M., Sax, S.N., Lapin, C.A., McClellan, R.O., et al., 2011. Particulate matter in new technology diesel exhaust (NTDE) is quantitatively and qualitatively very different from that found in traditional diesel exhaust (TDE). J. Air Waste Manage. Assn. 61, 894–913.

HEI Diesel Epidemiology Panel, 2015. Diesel Emissions and Lung Cancer: An Evaluation of Recent Epidemiological Evidence for Quantitative Risk Assessment, Special Report 19. Health Effects Institute, Boston, MA.

Hobbs, C.H., McClellan, R.O., 1975. Radiation and radioactive materials. In: Casarett, L.J., Doull, J. (Eds.), Toxicology: The Basic Science of Poisons. MacMillan Publishing Co., Inc, pp. 379–407 (Chapter 16).

Hodgson, E. (Ed.), 2010. A Textbook of Modern Toxicology, fourth ed. John Wiley, Somerset, NJ.

Hovda, L., Brutlag, A., Poppenga, R., Peterson, K. (Eds.), 2016. Blackwell's Five Minute Veterinary Consult Clinical companion: Small Animal Toxicology, second ed. Wiley Blackwell, Oxford.

Hulbert, L.E., Oehme, F.W., 1968. Plants Poisonous to Livestock. Kansas State University, Manhattan, KS.

Huttlin, E.L., Bruckner, R.J., Paulo, J.A., et al., 2017. Architecture of the human interactome defines protein communities and disease networks. Nature. 545, 505–509 (with supplemental material).

IARC, International Agency for Research on Cancer, 1972. IARC Monographs on the Evaluation of Carcinogenic Risks of Chemicals to Man, vol. 1. Lyon.

IARC, International Agency for Reseach on Cancer, 1989. Volume 45. Diesel and Gasoline Exhaust and Some Nitroarenes. IARC, Lyon.

IARC, International Agency for Research on Cancer, 1991. A Consensus Report of an IARC Monographs Working Group on the Use of Mechanisms of Carcinogenesis in Risk Identification. IARC Internal Technical Report No. 91/002, Lyon.

IARC, International Agency for Research on Cancer, 2011. IARC Monographs on Carcinogenic Risks to Humans. <http://www.iarcfr/IARCPress/general/mono.pdf>.

IARC, International Agency for Research on Cancer, 2012. Volume 105, Diesel and Gasoline Engine Exhaust and Some Nitroarenes. IARC, Lyon.

IARC, International Agency for Research on Cancer, 2015. Volume 122: Evaluation of Five Organophosphate Insecticides and Herbicides. IARC, Lyon.

ILAR, 2010. Institute of Laboratory Animal Resources. Guide for the Care and Use of Laboratory Animals. eighth ed. Committee for the Update of the Guide for the Care and Use of Laboratory Animals. National Research Council of the National Academies. National Academic Press, Washington, DC.

International Programs on Chemical Safety, 2011. Environmental Health Criteria Monographs. <http://www.inchem.org/pages/ehc.html>.

Jarabek, A.M., 1994. Inhalation RfC methodology. Dosimetry adjustments and dose-response estimation of noncancer toxicity in the upper respiratory tract. Inhal. Toxicol. 6, 301–325.

Jarabek, A.M., Menache, M.G., Overton, J.H., Jr., et al., 1990. The U.S. Environmental Protection Agency's inhalation RFD methodology: risk assessment for air toxics. Toxicol. Ind. Health 6, 279–301.

Kaplan, E.L., Meier, P., 1958. Non-parametric estimates from incomplete observations. J. Am. Stat. Assn. 53, 457–481.

Kaufmann, M., 1901. Thérapeutique et Matiére Médicale Vétérinaire, third ed. Asselin et Houzeau, Paris.

Kingsbury, J.M., 1954. Poisonous Plants of the United States and Canada. Prentice-Hall, Englewood, NJ.

Kingsbury, J.M., 1964. Poisonous Plants of the United States and Canada. Prentice-Hall, Englewood, NJ.

Klaassen, C.D., 2013. Casarett and Doull's Toxicology: The Basic Science of Poisons, eighth ed. McGraw-Hill.

Knight, A.P., Walter, R.G., 2001. A Guide to Plant Poisoning of Animals in North America. Teton New Media, Jackson Hole, WY.

Kobert, R., 1897. Practical Toxicology for Physicians and Students (L.H. Friedburg, Trans.). W.R. Jenkins, New York, 201 pp.

Kroes, R., Kleiner, J., Renwick, A., 2005. The threshold of toxicological concern concept in risk assessment. Toxicol. Sci. 86, 226–230.

Kung, H.C., Hoyert, D.L., Xu, J., Murphy, S., 2008. Final data for 2005. Natl. Vital Stat. Report. 56, 1–120.

Lander, G.D., 1912. Veterinary Toxicology. A. Eger, Chicago, IL, 312 pp.

Lane, R.W., 2014. The wissenschaften of toxicology, harming and helping through time: the history of toxicology. In: Hayes, A.W. (Ed.), Principles and Methods of Toxicology, fifth ed. Taylor & Francis, Philadelphia, PA, pp. 3–44.

Lehman, A.J., Fitzhugh, O.G., 1954. 100-Fold margin of safety. Q. Bull. Assoc. Food Drug Officials. XVIII, 33–35.

Lopez, A.D., Mathers, C.D., Ezzati, M., et al., 2006. Measuring the global burden of disease and risk factors, 1990–2001. In: Lopez, A. D., et al., (Eds.), Global Burden of Disease and Risk Factors. Oxford University Press, Oxford.

Marquardt, H., Schäfer, S.G., 1994. Lehrbuch der Toxicologie. Wissenschaftsver/ag, Mannheim.

Marquardt, H., Schäfer, S.G., 2004. Lehrbuch der Toxicologie. Wissenschaftliche Verlaggesellschaft mbh, Suttgart.

Marquardt, H., Schäfer, S.G., McClellan, R.O., Welsch, F. (Eds.), 1999. Toxicology. Academic Press, New York, NY.

Mauderly, J.L., Jones, R.K., Griffith, W.C., Henderson, R.F., McClellan, R.O., 1987. Diesel exhaust is a pulmonary carcinogen in rats exposed chronically by inhalation. Fundam. Appl. Toxicol. 9, 208–221.

McClellan, R.O., 1994. A commentary on the NRC report "Science and Judgment in Risk Assessment. Regul. Toxicol. Pharmacol. 20, S142–S168.

McClellan, R.O., 1999. Human health risk assessment: a historical overview and alternative paths forward. Inhal. Toxicol. 11, 477–518.

McClellan, R.O., 2003. Risk assessment: replacing default options with specific science. Hum. Ecol. Risk Assess. 9, 421–438.

McClellan, R.O., 2010. Hazard and risk: assessment and management. In: Ayres, J.G., Harrison, R.M., Maynard, R., Nichols, G.L. (Eds.), Textbook of Environmental Medicine, first ed. Hodder Arnold, London, pp. 59–88 (Chapter 4).

McClellan, R.O., 2011. Role of science and judgment in setting national ambient air quality standards: how low is low enough? Air Qual. Atmos. Health J. 5, 243–258.

McClellan, R.O., 2014. Radiation toxicity, Chapter 18. In: Wallace Hayes, A., Kruger, C.L. (Eds.), Principles and Methods of Toxicology, sixth ed. Taylor and Francis, Boca Raton, FL, pp. 883–955.

McClellan, R.O., 2016a. Invited commentary: Providing context for ambient particulate matter and estimates of attributable mortality. Risk Anal. 36 (9), 1755–1765.

McClellan, R.O., 2016b. Evaluating the potential carcinogenic hazard of glyphosate. Crit. Rev. Toxicol. 46 (S1), 1–2.

McClellan, R.O., 2017. A tribute to John Doull, BS, PhD, MD: scientist, physician, educator, communicator, advisor, and above all, a gentleman and friend to many. Int. J. Toxicol. in press.

McClellan, R.O., Henderson, R.F. (Eds.), 1995. Concepts in Inhalation Toxicology, second ed. Taylor & Francis.

McClellan, R.O., Hesterberg, T.W., Wall, J.C., 2012. Evaluation of carcinogenic hazard of diesel engine exhaust needs to consider revolutionary changes in diesel technology. Reg. Toxicol. Harmacol. 63, 225–258.

McClellan, R.O., Medinsky, M.A., Snipes, M.B., 2006. Inhalation toxicology. In: Riviere, J.E. (Ed.), Biological Concepts and Techniques in Toxicology. Taylor & Francis, New York, NY, pp. 295–361 (Chapter 16).

McDonald, J.D., Doyle-Eisele, M., Seagrave, J., et al., 2015. Part 1. Assessment of carcinogenicity and biologic responses I rats after lifetime inhalation of new-technology diesel exhaust in the ACES bioassay. Res. Rep. Health Effects Inst. 184, 9–44, discussion 141–171.

McQueen C.A., (Ed), *Comprehensive Toxicology* 14 volumes, 2010, second ed. Elsevier Science and Technology, Oxford, United Kingdom.

Milles, D., 1999. History of toxicology. In: Marquadt, H., Schafer, S.G., McClellan, R.O., Welsch, F. (Eds.), Toxicology. Academic Press, San Diego, CA, pp. 11–24.

Moolgavkar, S.H., Chang, E.T., Luebeck, G., et al., 2015. Diesel engine exhaust and lung cancer mortality: time-related factors in exposure and risk. Risk Anal. 35 (4), 663–675.

Murphy, M., 1996. A Field Guide to Common Animal Poisons. Iowa State University Press, Ames, IA.

National Academies of Sciences, Engineering and Medicine, 2017. Application of Systemic Review Methods in an Overall Strategy for Evaluating Low-Dose Toxicity from Endocrine Active Chemicals. The National Academies Press, Washington, DC. Available from: <http://dx.doi.org/10.17226/24758>.

Nicholson, J.A., 1945. Lander's Veterinary Toxicology. Bailliere, Tindall & Cox, London.

Nikula, K.J., Snipes, M.B., Barr, E.B., et al., 1995. Comparative pulmonary toxicities and carcinogenicities of chronically inhaled diesel exhaust and carbon black in F344 rats. Fundam. Appl. Toxicol. 25, 80–94.

NIOSH, National Institute of Occupational Safety and Health, 2016. Current Intelligence Bulletin 60. NIOSH Chemical Carcinogen Policy, December 2016, Cincinnati, OH: US Department of Health and Human Services, Centers for Disease Control and prevention, NIOSH, DHHS (NIOSH), Publication No. 2017-100.

NRC, National Research Council, 1983. Risk Assessment in the Federal Government: Managing the Process. National Academy Press, Washington, DC.

NRC, National Research Council, 1993. Issues in Risk Assessment. I. Use of the Maximum Tolerated Dose in Animal Bioassays for Carcinogenicity. National Academy Press, Washington, DC.

NRC, National Research Council, 1994. Science and Judgment in Risk Assessment. National Academy Press, Washington, DC.

NRC, National Research Council, 2004. Intentional Human Dosing Studies for EPA Regulatory Purposes: Scientific and Ethical Issues. The National Academies Press, Washington, DC.

NRC, National Research Council, 2007a. Application of Toxicogenomic Technologies to Predictive Toxicology and Risk Assessment. National Academy Press, Washington, DC.

NRC, National Research Council, 2007b. Toxicity Testing in the 21st Century: A Vision and a Strategy. National Academy Press, Washington, DC.

NRC, National Research Council, 2011. Review of the U.S. Environmental Protection Agency's Draft IRIS Assessment on Formaldehyde. Prepared by a Committee to Review EPA's Draft IRIS Assessment of Formaldehyde. National Academy Press, Washington, DC.

NRC, National Research Council, 2017. Using 21st Century Science to Improve Risk-Related Evaluations. National Academy Press, Washington, DC.

NTP, National Toxicology Program, 2005. Report on Carcinogens, 11th ed. U.S. Department of Health and Human Services, Public Health Service, National Toxicology Program, Washington, DC.

NTP, National Toxicology Program, 2016. 14th Report on Carcinogens (Released November 3, 2016. US Department of health and Human Services, Public Health Service, National Toxicology Program, Washington, DC.

Oehme, F.W., 1970. The development of toxicology as a veterinary discipline in the United States. Clin. Toxicol. 3, 211–220.

Osweiler, G.B., 1996. Toxicology. Williams and Wilkins, Philadelphia, PA.

Osweiler, G.D., Carson, T.L., Buck, W.B., Van Gelder, G.A., 1985. Clinical and Diagnostic Veterinary Toxicology, third ed. Kendall Hunt, Dubuque, IA.

Pagel, W., 1958. Paracelsus: An Introduction to Philosophical Medicine in the Era of the Renaissance. Karger, New York, NY.

Paustenbach, D.J., 2008. The practice of exposure assessment. In: Hayes, A.W. (Ed.), Principles and Methods of Toxicology. Taylor and Francis, Philadelphia, PA, pp. 475–548.

Peterson, M.E., Talcott, P.A. (Eds.), 2012. Small Animal Toxicology. third ed. Elsevier Saunders, St. Louis, MO.

Plumlee, K.H., 2004. Clinical Veterinary Toxicology. Mosby, St. Louis, MO.

Poppenga, R.H., Gwaltney-Brant, S.M., 2011. Small Animal Toxicology Essentials. Wiley-Blackwell, Hoboken, NJ.

Quitman, E.L., 1905. Synopsis of Veterinary Materia Medica, Therapeutics and Toxicology. A. Eger, Chicago, IL, 277 pp.

Radeleff, R.D., 1964. Veterinary Toxicology. Lea and Febiger, Philadelphia, PA.

REACH, Regulation, Evaluation, Authorization and Restriction of Chemical Substances, 2011. REACH Guidance. Available from: <http://guidance.echa.europa.eu/guidance_en.htm>.

Rhomberg, L.R., Bailey, L.A., Goodman, J.E., et al., 2011a. Is exposure to formaldehyde in air causally associated with leukemia?—a hypothesis-based weight-of-evidence analysis. Crit. Rev. Toxicol. 41 (7), 555–621.

Rhomberg, L.R., Chandalla, J.K., Long, C.M., Goodman, J.E., 2011b. Measurement error in environmental epidemiology and the shape of exposure-response curves. Crit. Rev. Toxicol. 41 (8), 651–671.

Rhomberg, L.R., Goodman, J.E., Haber, L.T., et al., 2011c. Linear low-dose extrapolation for non-cancer health effects is the exception, not the rule. Crit. Rev. Toxicol. 41 (1), 1–19.

Risk Commission, Presidential/Congressional Commission on Risk Assessment and Risk Management, vol. 1, 1997. A Framework for Environmental Health Risk Management, vol. 2. Risk Assessment and Risk Management in Regulatory Decision-Making, Government Printing Office, Washington, DC.

Riviere, J.E. (Ed.), 2006. Biological Concepts and Techniques in Toxicology. Taylor and Francis, New York, NY.

Roder, J.D., 2001. Veterinary Toxicology. Butterworth-Heinemann, Boston, MA.

Silverman, D.T., Samanic, C.M., Lubin, J.H., et al., 2012. The diesel exhaust in miners study: a nested case-control study of lung cancer and diesel exhaust. J. Natl. Cancer Inst. 104, 855–868.

Sipes, I.G., McQueen, C.A., Gandolph, A.J., 1997. Comprehensive Toxicology, 13 volumes. Pergamon Press, Oxford.

Smithcors, J.F., 1957. Evolution of the Veterinary Art. Veterinary Medicine Publishing, Kansas City, MO.

Solomon, K.R., 2016. Glyphosate in the general population and in applicators: a critical review of studies on exposures. Crit. Rev. Toxicol. 46 (Suppl. 1), 21–27.

Spoo W., Toxicokinetics, In: Plumlee K.H., (Ed), Clinical Veterinary Toxicology, 2004, Mosby, an Affiliate of Elsevier, St. Louis, MO, 8–12.

Stahlheim, O.H.V., 1994. The Winning of Animal Health: 100 Years of Veterinary Medicine. Iowa State University Press, Ames, IA.

Swabe, J., 1999. Animal, Disease, and Human Society: Human-Animal Relations and the Rise of Veterinary Medicine. Routledge, London/New York, NY.

Tilley, L.P., Smith, F.W.K. (Eds.), 2015. Blackwell's Five Minute Veterinary Consult Clinical Companion; 1 Canine and Feline. sixth ed. Wiley Blackwell, Oxford, England.

TSCA, Toxic Substance Control Act, 1985. Good Laboratory Practices Regulations Enforcement Response Policy.

TSCA, Toxic Substances Control Act, 2016. Frank R. Lautenberg Chemical Safety for the 21st Century Revised TSCA passed in 1976. Public Law 114-182, 130 STAT.448 (signed into law June 22, 2016).

White, R.H., Cote, I., Zeise, L., et al., 2009. State-of-the-Science Workshop Report: Issues and Approaches in Low Dose-Response Extrapolation for Environmental Health Risk Assessment. Available at: <http://www.ehponline.org/members/2008/1150211502.pdf>. Environ. Health Perspect. 117 (2), doi:10.1289/ehp.11502.

Whitman vs American Trucking Associations, 2001. 531 U.S. 457, 121 S. Ct. 903149 L. Ed. 2d1.

Wilkinson, L., 2005. Animals and Disease: An Introduction to the History of Comparative Medicine. Cambridge University Press, New York, NY.

Williams, G.M., Aardema, M., Acquavella, J., et al., 2016a. A review of the carcinogenic potential of glyphosate by four independent expert panels and comparison to the IARC assessment. Crit. Rev. Toxicol. 46 (Suppl. 1), 3–20.

Williams, G.M., Berry, C., Burns, M., et al., 2016b. Glyphosate rodent carcinogenicity bioassay expert panel review. Crit. Rev. Toxicol. 46 (Suppl. 1), 44–55.

Williams, E.S., Panko, J., Paustenbach, D.J., 2009. The European Union's REACH regulation: a review of its history and requirements. Crit. Rev. Toxicol. 39 (7), 553–575.

Wilsdorf, G., Graf, C., 1998. Historical review of development of veterinary toxicology in Berlin from 1790-1945 (in German). Berl. Munch. Tierarztl. Wochenschr. 111, 21–26

Wolff, R.K., Henderson, R.F., Snipes, M.B., et al., 1987. Alterations in particle accumulation and clearance in lungs of rat chronically exposed to diesel exhaust. Fundam. Appl. Toxicol. 9, 154–166.

Chapter 2

Epidemiology of Animal Poisonings in the United States

Sharon M. Gwaltney-Brant

INTRODUCTION

Although animals are exposed to potentially toxic agents on a daily basis, actual poisoning cases are uncommon when compared to other conditions of veterinary concern (infectious disease, trauma, metabolic disease, neoplasia, etc.). Clients will often present their animal with a suspicion of poisoning, only for the veterinarian to determine that the animal is experiencing an unrelated ailment. When evaluating information regarding suspected poisoning cases, it is important to consider the full exposure and patient history before determining whether a particular exposure is related to a clinical syndrome, as temporal coincidence does not necessarily equal causality.

The fundamental rule of toxicology as stated by Paracelsus, considered to be the "father" of toxicology, is "the dose makes the poison." Obviously, the dose required to induce toxicosis will depend on a variety of factors, including the agent in question, species of animal exposed, and route of exposure. Based on information from poison control centers (PCC), the majority of animal exposures to potentially toxic agents result in no signs developing (Hornfeldt and Murphy, 1992; Forrester and Stanley, 2004). However, clinically significant animal poisonings do occasionally occur from exposures to natural or man-made hazards. Knowledge of the most common features of animal poisonings can aid in instituting measures that may help to minimize exposures of animals to toxicants.

BACKGROUND

The lack of a central reporting agency for animal poisonings makes epidemiological study difficult. With no mandated reporting, many suspected poisoning cases are managed by the attending veterinarian and forgotten. Confirmatory testing at veterinary diagnostic laboratories is not common, and no central mechanism exists for these laboratories to report their findings for epidemiological analysis. Most published information on animal poisonings has largely come from human or animal poison control centers (APCC) that animal owners have contacted regarding potential exposures to toxic agents (Haliburton and Buck, 1983; Hornfeldt and Borys, 1985; Hornfeldt and Murphy, 1992, 1997, 1998; Forrester and Stanley, 2004) or from surveys of veterinary emergency centers or teaching hospitals (Osweiler, 1975; Cope et al., 2006). Data from these sources can be helpful in determining trends and identifying emerging toxicants, but because of the frequent lack of complete historical information and confirmatory testing, care must be taken in the interpretation of each case of suspected poisoning.

Forrester and Stanley (2004) reported that exposures of animals to toxicants occurred more commonly in the summer months, and this is consistent with data from the American Society for the Prevention of Cruelty to Animals (ASPCA) APCC AnTox database (Fig. 2.1), although a peak in December, associated with the holiday season, is also present in the APCC data (ASPCA Animal Poison Control Center, unpublished data, 2010). The uptick in cases in the spring with peak cases during the summer is likely due to a variety of factors. Domestic animals tend to be more confined during the winter, particularly indoors, limiting their access to potentially toxic agents. Toxic plants and animals are not frequently encountered during the winter months in many areas, making exposures to these potentially poisonous entities unlikely. With the advent of warmer spring weather, domesticated animals have more access to outdoors and the plants, insects and other animals that reside there. The use of agents such as fertilizers, insecticides, and herbicides also increases during these months, thereby increasing the risk of animal exposures to these agents. Cool, wet spring weather favors the rapid appearance of potentially toxic mushrooms, while hot summer weather can trigger

Veterinary Toxicology. DOI: http://dx.doi.org/10.1016/B978-0-12-811410-0.00002-7

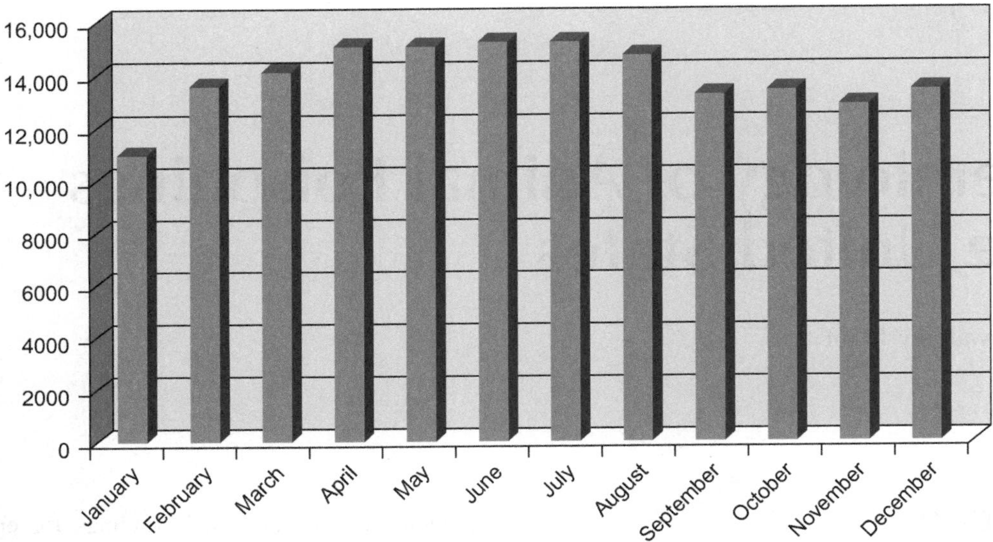

FIGURE 2.1 Monthly distribution of cases managed by ASPCA Animal Poison Control Center in 2010 (unpublished data).

growth of toxic blue-green algae in ponds, lakes, and other water sources. Other seasonal influences on the incidence of animal exposures to toxicants include increased presence of rodenticides in late fall as rodents begin to move indoors in response to cooling temperatures, increased use of psoriasis medication (e.g., calcipotriene) during winter months, increased use of ice-melting agents in winter, increased presence of lilies in the spring (Easter, Mother's Day), and increased presence of chocolate around the holidays of Valentine's Day, Easter, Halloween, and the November–December holidays (Hautekeete, 2000; Gwaltney-Brant, 2001; Volmer, 2001; Merola, 2002).

The majority (>90%) of animal poisonings are accidental, acute in nature, and occur near or at the animal owner's home (Hornfeldt and Murphy, 1992, 1998; Khan et al., 1999). Malicious intent comprises less than 1% of all exposures to potentially toxic agents. The majority (70%–95%) of exposures are due to acute ingestion, followed by acute dermal exposures (Hornfeldt and Murphy, 1992; Forrester and Stanley, 2004). Inhalation, envenomation, bites, ocular, and parenteral routes of exposure account for less than 1% of cases, and chronic exposures comprise approximately 1% of all reported cases. In 97% of exposures, a single agent is involved (Hornfeldt and Murphy, 1992, 1998).

DEMOGRAPHICS

Based on data from human and APCCs, dogs and cats are the species for which owners most frequently seek assistance with potential poisonings, accounting for 90%–98% of all reported animal cases (Hornfeldt and Murphy, 1998; Xavier et al., 2002; Forrester and Stanley, 2004; Giuliano Albo and Nebbia, 2004; McLean and Hansen, 2010). Approximately 2%–10% of reported animal poisoning cases involved other species of domesticated animals, exotic animals and wildlife, with horses and birds following dogs and cats as the third and fourth most common species. The distribution of species involved in poisonings has changed considerably since 1983, when dogs and cats accounted for 44% of calls to an APCC, with production animals (bovine, porcine, ovine) and equines making up 35% of calls (Trammel et al., 1985).

Dogs

Perhaps at least partly because of their inquisitive natures and willingness to investigate everything with their mouths, dogs far outrank other species when it comes to owners seeking aid for potential poisonings, making up 70%–80% of all animal cases reported (Hornfeldt and Murphy, 1992, 1998; Xavier et al., 2002; Forrester and Stanley, 2004; Berny et al., 2009; McLean and Hansen, 2010). There is a tendency in the veterinary community to consider certain breeds, such as Labrador Retrievers (Labradors), to be more prone to exposure to potentially toxic agents. However, to verify such an impression, one must consider the relative popularity of a particular breed. In other words: Are there more poisoning cases with Labradors because this breed is really more predisposed to misadventure, or is it just that there are more Labradors in the population?

A survey of the APCC database (2016) evaluated over 90,000 exposures of nonmixed breed dogs and compared the relative breed incidence to the 2005 Registration Statistics reported by the American Kennel Club, the oldest and largest purebred dog registry in the United States

(American Kennel Club (AKC), 2017). In 2016, Labradors accounted for approximately 15% of AKC registered breeds, with almost three times more registered than the next most popular breed, the German shepherd. During that same year, Labradors accounted for ~17% of canine exposures in APCC cases, which was also three times more than the next most popular breed (the Golden Retriever), and which was not significantly different from the AKC statistics. Rounding out the top 10 breeds for 2016 poisoning calls, in descending order, are Chihuahua, American Pit Bull Terrier, German Shepherd, Yorkshire Terrier, Beagle, Shih Tzu, Boxer, and Maltese. Table 2.1 compares the rankings of the top dog breeds in animal poisoning cases with their overall popularity according to AKC breed registration statistics. Some breeds do appear to be overrepresented in regards to exposures to potentially toxic agents. For instance, the Chihuahua ranked 30th in AKC registrations yet ranked third in cases called in to the APCC data, while Maltese were 10th in APCC cases compared to 33rd in AKC ranking, and Shih Tzus ranked eighth in poison center cases, yet 20th in AKC registrations. Parson Russell terriers appear to be markedly overrepresented in APCC data compared to AKC registrations, ranking 109th with AKC but 16th in APCC cases. However, many individuals of this breed are registered with an independent breed registry rather than the AKC, which may at least partially explain why the Parson Russell appears overrepresented in APCC data.

Reports of poisoning cases in dogs have indicated no gender predisposition, and dogs 1 year of age and under make up the largest age group of exposures to potentially toxic agents (McLean and Hansen, 2010). This is consistent with reports of canine poisonings in Europe, which indicate that dogs 2 years of age and under are the largest group of poisoning cases (Berny et al., 2009; McFarland et al., 2017).

TABLE 2.1 Comparison of Top Purebred Dog Breeds in Relation to Frequency of Exposures to Potentially Toxic Agents Reported to the ASPCA Animal Poison Control Center with the Relative Popularity of those Breed Based on Registration Statistics From the American Kennel Club in 2016 (American Society for the Prevention of Cruelty to Animals (ASPCA). Top pet toxins of 2016. http://www.aspca.org/news/announcing-top-pet-toxins-2016; accessed March 1, 2017; AKC, 2017)

Breed	APCC Ranking	AKC Ranking
Labrador Retriever	1	1
Golden Retriever	2	3
Chihuahua	3	30
American Pit Bull Terrier	4	NR
German Shepherd	5	2
Yorkshire Terrier	6	9
Beagle	7	5
Shih Tzu	8	20
Boxer	9	10
Maltese	10	33
Cocker Spaniel	11	29
Australian Shepherd	12	16
Siberian Husky	13	12
Miniature Dachshund	14	13
Pug	15	32
Parson Russell Terrier	16	109
Cavalier King Charles Spaniel	17	19
Miniature Schnauzer	18	17
Border Collie	19	38

NR, not an AKC recognized breed (ASPCA Animal Poison Control Center, unpublished data, 2016; AKC, 2017).

Cats

Due, perhaps, to their more discriminating habits and appetites, cats account for only 11%–20% of reported animal exposures to potential toxicants, which is three times less frequent than dogs (Hornfeldt and Murphy, 1992, 1998; Xavier et al., 2002; Forrester and Stanley, 2004; Berny et al., 2009; McLean and Hansen, 2010). In 2010, 71% of cats exposed to potential toxicants were identified as domestic (or American) shorthairs, 8% as domestic longhairs and 6% as domestic medium hairs (ASPCA Animal Poison Control Center, unpublished data, 2010). Excluding these types of cats due to the generic nature of their classification, the top 10 purebred cats were Siamese (24%), Main Coon (15%), Persian (10%), Himalayan (8%), Ragdoll (6%), Bengal (6%), Russian Blue (3%), Abyssinian (3%), Manx (2%), and Siberian (2%). Of these, the Persian, Maine Coon, Siamese, Abyssinian, and Ragdoll are listed in the 10 most popular breeds registered by the Cat Fancier's Association in 2010 (CFA, 2010). As with dogs, no gender differences in incidence of exposure have been noted, and cats 1 year and under comprise the largest age group (McLean and Hansen, 2010). Cats may, due to their grooming habits, be more susceptible to toxicants that come into contact with their fur; this is especially problematic with agents to which cats are extremely sensitive, such as ethylene glycol.

Other Species

Demographic information on potential poisonings in animal species other than dogs and cats in North America is largely lacking. Production animals are generally kept in large groups, meaning that when a toxicosis occurs, there is potential for multiple animals of varying age and genders to be exposed. Most production animals are kept in some form of confinement, which limits the potential for exposure to toxic agents. However, mistakes in management, such as feed mixing errors or improper ventilation, may result in acute or chronic toxicosis in large numbers of animals. A study of livestock poisonings in Greece indicated that sheep were the commonly poisoned species, attributed primarily to their ingestion of potentially contaminated soil (Guitart et al., 2010a).

Wildlife is almost continuously exposed to potentially toxic agents in the environment, but specific demographic information is not available in most cases. In France, birds are reported to be more commonly poisoned than mammals (Guitart et al., 2010b). Seasonality of poisoning incidences in wildlife would vary with the agent involved. For instance, avian botulism in waterfowl tends to be seasonal, with most cases occurring between the months of July and September (Locke and Friend, 1989). In addition to naturally occurring toxicants, exposures to man-made hazards (e.g., oil spills, industrial effluents) can result in significant wildlife morbidity and mortality.

AGENTS INVOLVED

There is an unlimited number of agents by which exposed animals may become poisoned, and for the most part the specific agents involved in animal poisonings will be dependent upon what is available in the animals' environment, the potential or inclination for the animal to be exposed to the agent, the amount of agent to which the animal is exposed, and the individual sensitivity of the animal to the effects of the agent. The potential for exposure to specific agents may be uniform throughout the year or may be seasonal, depending on the agent and the species involved. For instance, exposures to lawn care products, such as herbicides and insecticides, would be expected to be more common during the seasons when these products are most in use (i.e., spring and summer).

Table 2.2 summarizes the most common agents involved in animal exposures reported to veterinary emergency referral centers (VEC) and human or animal PCC in the United States. These exposures predominantly involve companion animals, particularly dogs and cats, and are consistent with the types of animal exposures reported by PCC in other countries (Xavier et al., 2002; Giuliano Albo and Nebbia, 2004; McFarland et al., 2017).

Rodenticides, pharmaceuticals, and chocolate make up the majority of agents involving canine poisonings presenting to VEC (Fig. 2.2) (Cope et al., 2006). Rodenticides and chocolate each accounted for approximately one quarter of all presentations to VEC, yet these agents comprised <10% of calls to PCC. This discrepancy may largely be because PCC receive calls regarding a large range of agents, many of which would not pose a toxic hazard, while VEC are most likely to see only those exposures that have potential to cause clinical problems. Pharmaceutical agents, because they are designed to have a pharmacologic effect and thereby can cause clinical effects if veterinary patients are exposed, appear to be more closely represented between VEC and PCC cases.

Pharmaceuticals exposures have increased since first reports in 1983 (Beasley and Trammel, 1994), likely due to the increased use of these agents in veterinary and human medicine over the past 30 years. The most common pharmaceutical agents associated with animal exposures are analgesics, primarily nonsteroidal antiinflammatory drugs (Hornfeldt and Murphy, 1992, 1998; McLean and Hansen, 2010). Pesticides have historically been responsible for large numbers of exposures and toxicoses in domestic animals (Beasley and Trammel, 1994), but the incidence is declining (Fig. 2.3). This may be due in part to the development of newer herbicides and insecticides

TABLE 2.2 Incidence of Exposures of Animals to Various Toxic Agents Reported by Veterinary Clinics (V) and Poison Control Centers (P), 1975–2016

	1975	1978–1981	1990	1993	2006	2011	2016
	V	P	P	P	V	P	P
Chocolate	NR	NR	NR	NR	26%	5%	8%
Glycols	1%	NR	10%	NR	4%	0.3%	NR
Metals	2%	7%	1%	NR	0%	NR	<0.5%
Miscellaneous^{+}	47%	56%	17%	34%	3%	15%	21%
Pesticides^{++}	23%	20%	21%	21%	13%	11%	7%
Pharmaceuticals^{+++}	NR	10%	25%	24%	22%	32%	43%
Plants	1%	12%	12%	10%	5%	4%	5%
Rodenticides	27%	7%	14%	7%	26%	4%	6%

NR, not reported separately; $^{+}$, foodstuffs, household items, yard/garden products; $^{++}$, combined insecticide and herbicide exposures; $^{+++}$, includes human and veterinary prescription & over-the-counter products (Osweiler, 1975; Haliburton and Buck, 1983; Hornfeldt and Murphy, 1992, 1998; Cope et al., 2006; ASPCA Animal Poison Control Center, unpublished data, 2011, 2016).

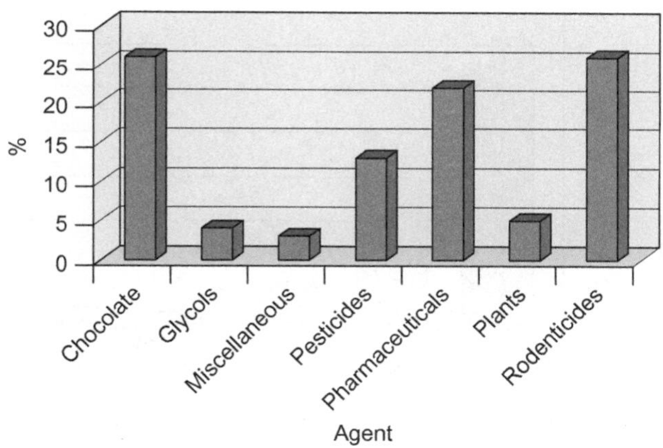

FIGURE 2.2 Most common agents involved in canine exposures presenting to a veterinary emergency center in 2006 (Cope et al., 2006).

that have a much higher margin of safety in mammals than those used in the past, as well as perhaps better public awareness of the potential hazards of these agents to pets. However, some pesticides do pose hazards to veterinary patients when used inappropriately; for instance, exposure of cats to concentrated permethrins is still a common cause of poisoning in that species (McLean and Hansen, 2010).

APCC data have revealed an increasing trend in exposures of pets to cholecalciferol, thought to be due to a combination of increased use in humans of high-dose (>5000 IU) vitamin D supplements and the increased use of cholecalciferol rodenticides in light of new EPA guidelines limiting use of second-generation anticoagulant rodenticides (McLean and Hansen, 2010). Other increasing trends noted in pet poisonings include cases of ingestion of dark chocolate and exposure of pets to synthetic cannabinoids such as "K2." A decreasing trend was noted between 2002 and 2010 in exposures of pets to the molluscicide metaldehyde, most likely due to the introduction of ferric phosphate–based molluscicides, which have a lower acute toxicity in mammals.

Less information is available regarding exposure of noncanine and nonfeline animals to potential toxicants. For livestock, plant poisoning causes tremendous economic losses to producers, estimated to exceed $350 million per year and affect 3%–5% of livestock in the United States, particularly in the western ranges (Galey, 1996; USDA, 2011). Losses from poisonous plants are due to deaths as well as loss of productivity. Other agents reported to be responsible for significant livestock loss include mycotoxins, organophosphate, and carbamate insecticides, nitrate, and lead, although lead poisoning appears to be on the decline in livestock. For waterfowl, avian botulism is a concern, resulting in the loss of thousands to millions of birds each year (Locke and Friend, 1989). Lead toxicosis was once a significant cause of loss of waterfowl in the United States due to ingestion of lead shot left by hunters, but the incidence of lead toxicosis has decreased following an enforced ban on the use of lead shot on waterfowl (Gwaltney-Brant, 2004). However, lead intoxication still occurs in raptors that ingest upland prey that have shot embedded in their tissues. Wild animals ingesting the tissues of animals that have been euthanized with barbiturates are at risk of toxicosis (Hayes, 1988), and toxicosis has been reported in a

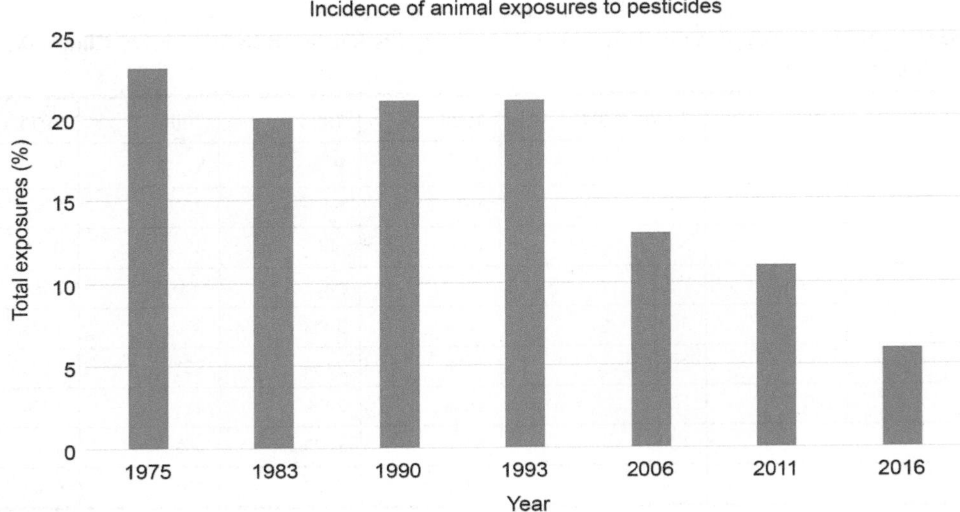

FIGURE 2.3 Comparison of incidence of animal exposures to pesticides reported to human poison control centers and veterinary clinics (Osweiler, 1975; Haliburton and Buck, 1983; Trammel et al., 1985; Hornfeldt and Murphy, 1992).

variety of species feeding on animals intentionally poisoned with pesticides (Stroud, 1998; Wobeser et al., 2004). The use of nonsteroidal antiinflammatory drugs in livestock has been linked to the marked decline in vultures and other scavenging birds in India, Asia, and Africa (Naidoo et al., 2009, 2010). Intentional poisoning of wildlife with pesticides is most commonly accomplished using carbofuran and aldicarb, while accidental or secondary poisoning of wildlife by pesticides most often involves strychnine, famphur, fenthion, and avitrol (Stroud, 1998). Oil spills near sea shores have resulted in significant loss of life of animals living in or around these areas, and industrial pollution from agricultural or industrial effluents has similarly caused deaths in a variety of wildlife species.

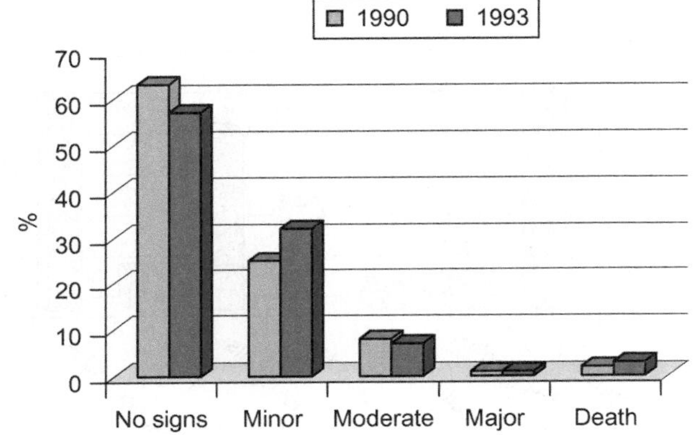

FIGURE 2.4 Degree of illness in animals following exposure to potentially toxic agents (Hornfeldt and Murphy, 1992, 1998).

SIGNS AND OUTCOMES

Based on PCC statistics, the majority (57%–63%) of animal exposures to potential toxicants result in no signs for the patient, due either to insufficient level of exposure or successful intervention (e.g., gastrointestinal decontamination) by animal caretakers (Fig. 2.4). Mild signs developed in 25%–27% of animal exposures to suspected toxicants, moderate signs developed in 7%–8%, major signs developed in approximately 1%, and death occurred in 2%–3% of cases where outcomes were known (Hornfeldt and Murphy, 1992, 1998). Mild signs are those in which some clinical signs developed but are expected to be mild and self-limiting and not in need of treatment (e.g., hypersalivation, mild vomiting, etc.). Moderate signs are those in which signs that develop are more pronounced, prolonged or of a systemic nature and merit some form of treatment, although the signs would not be expected to be life-threatening (e.g., protracted vomiting, severe diarrhea, mild to moderate hypotension). No residual effects would be expected following recovery. Major signs are those in which life-threatening conditions exist or there is potential for significant residual disability or disfigurement following recovery from the acute episode (e.g., seizures, renal injury, etc.).

Agents most frequently reported to be associated with mild to moderate signs in animals are pharmaceuticals (19%), pesticides (insecticides and herbicides, 14%), plants (10%), cleaning products (8%), and mushrooms (3%) (Hornfeldt and Murphy, 1998). Agents associated with major signs included pesticides (45%), pharmaceuticals (25%), plants (15%), rodenticides (9%), and cleaning products (8%). Deaths were most commonly associated with exposures to pesticides (24%), pharmaceuticals

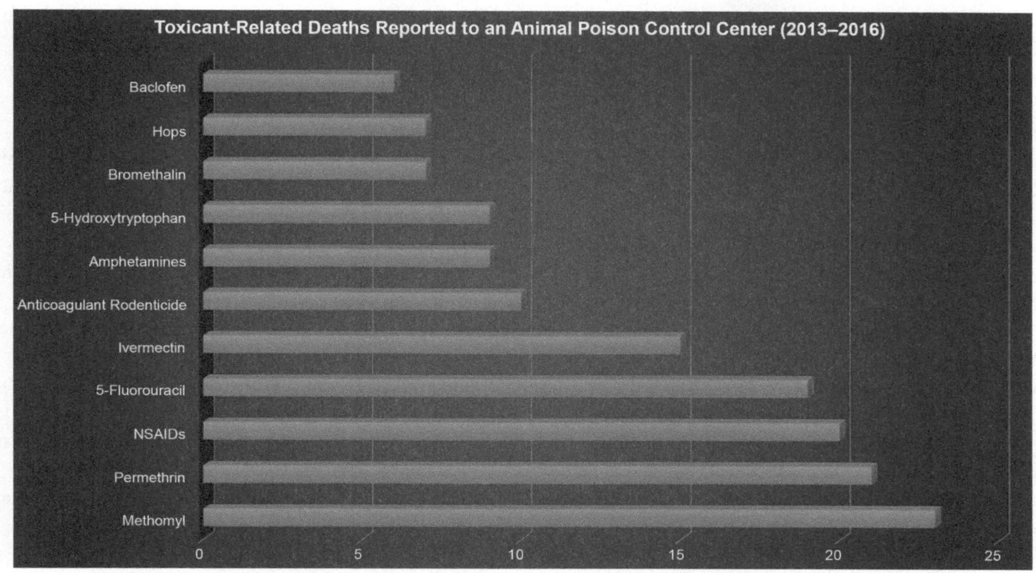

FIGURE 2.5 Most common toxicants associated with poisoning deaths reported to an animal poison control center from 2013 to 2016 (ASPCA Animal Poison Control Center, unpublished data, 2016).

(17%), rodenticides (16%), plants (9%), automotive products (predominantly ethylene glycol, 9%), and cleaning products (8%). Organophosphate insecticides, ethylene glycol and long-acting anticoagulant rodenticides were the top three agents responsible for deaths in animals in 1998, whereas between 2002 and 2010 the three most common agents associated with deaths were all insecticides: pyrethroids (permethrin), carbamates, and organophosphates (Hornfeldt and Murphy, 1998; McLean and Hansen, 2010). As shown in Fig. 2.5, between 2013 and 2016, the most common causes of animal deaths reported to one APCC were pesticides, pharmaceuticals, and rodenticides.

CONCLUSIONS

Poisonings are a serious cause of morbidity and mortality in animals, particularly in dogs and cats. Based on information obtained by veterinary clinics and human and APCC, the incidence of animal poisoning does not appear to be waning, although the agents to which animals are exposed do change with time. While significant pesticide exposures may be on the decline due to the development of newer and less toxic pesticides, exposures to other agents, such as chocolate and pharmaceutical agents, may be on the rise. Knowing what agents have the potential to be involved in serious toxicoses should allow veterinarians to better educate their clients on means of preventing animal poisonings through the appropriate use of household products and the removal of potential hazards from the animals' environments.

REFERENCES

American Society for the Prevention of Cruelty to Animals (ASPCA). Top pet toxins of 2016. <http://www.aspca.org/news/announcing-top-pet-toxins-2016> (accessed 1.03.17.).

American Kennel Club (2017) Dog Registration Statistics, 2015–2016, 2005. (http://www.akc.org/content/news/articles/most-popular-dog-breeds-full-ranking-list/?button).

ASPCA Animal Poison Control Center, unpublished data, 2010.

Beasley, V.R., Trammel, H.L., 1994. Incidence of poisonings in small animals. In: Kirk, R.W. (Ed.), Current Veterinary Therapy X. Saunders, Philadelphia, PA, pp. 97–113.

Berny, P., Caloni, F., Croubels, S., Sachana, M., Vendenbroucke, V., Davanzo, F., et al., 2009. Animal poisoning in Europe. Part 2: companion animals. Vet. J. 183, 255–259.

Cat Fancier's Association (CFA), 2010. Top 10 breeds. <http://www.cfa.org/ezine/features.html#top10>.

Cope, R.B., White, K.S., More, E., Holmes, K., Nair, A., Chauvin, P., et al., 2006. Exposure-to-treatment interval and clinical severity in canine poisoning: a retrospective analysis at a Portland Veterinary Emergency Center. J. Vet. Pharmacol. Therap. 29, 233–236.

Forrester, M.B., Stanley, S.K., 2004. Patterns of animal poisonings reported to the Texas Poison Center Network: 1998–2002. Vet. Hum. Toxicol. 46, 96–99.

Galey, F.D., 1996. Disorders caused by toxicants. In: Smith, B.P. (Ed.), Large Animal Internal Medicine, second ed. Mosby, St. Louis, MO, pp. 1974–1991.

Giuliano Albo, A., Nebbia, C., 2004. Incidence of poisonings in domestic carnivores in Italy. Vet. Res. Commun. 1, 83–88.

Guitart, R., Croubels, S., Caloni, F., Sachana, M., Davanzo, F., Vandenbroucke, V., et al., 2010a. Animal poisoning in Europe. Part 1. Farm livestock and poultry. Vet. J. 183, 249–254.

Guitart, R., Sachana, M., Caloni, F., Croubels, S., Vandenbroucke, V., Berny, P., 2010b. Animal poisoning in Europe. Part 3.Wildlife. Vet. J. 183, 260–265.

Gwaltney-Brant, S.M., 2001. Chocolate intoxication. Vet. Med. 96, 108–110.

Gwaltney-Brant, S.M., 2004. Lead. In: Peterson, M.E., Talcott, P.A. (Eds.), Small Animal Toxicology, second ed. Saunders Elsevier, St. Louis, MO, pp. 204–210.

Haliburton, J.C., Buck, W.B., 1983. Animal poison control center: summary of telephone inquiries during the first three years of service. J. Am. Vet. Med. Assoc. 182, 514–515.

Hautekeete, L.A., 2000. Ice melts are health hazards. Vet. Med. 95, 110–112.

Hayes, B., 1988. Deaths caused by barbiturate poisoning in bald eagles and other wildlife. Can. Vet. J. 29, 173–174.

Hornfeldt, C.S., Borys, D.J., 1985. Review of veterinary cases received by the Henepin Poison Center in 1984. Vet. Hum. Toxicol. 27, 525–528.

Hornfeldt, C.S., Murphy, M.J., 1992. 1990 Report of the American Association of Poison Control Centers: poisonings in animals. J. Am. Vet. Med. Assoc. 200, 1077–1080.

Hornfeldt, C.S., Murphy, M.J., 1997. Poisonings in animals: the 1993–1994 report of the American Association of Poison Control Centers. Vet. Hum. Toxicol. 39, 361–365.

Hornfeldt, C.S., Murphy, M.J., 1998. American Association of Poison Control Centers report on poisonings of animals, 1993–1994. J. Am. Vet. Med. Assoc. 212, 358–361.

Khan, S.A., Schell, M.M., Trammel, H.L., Hansen, S.K., Knight, M.W., 1999. Ethylene glycol exposures managed by the ASPCA National Animal Poison Control Center from July 1995 to December 1997. Vet. Hum. Toxicol. 41, 403–406.

Locke, L.N., Friend, M., 1989. Avian botulism: geographic expansion of a historic disease. US Fish & Wildlife Leaflet 13.2.4: 1–6.

McFarland, S.E., Msichke, R.H., Hopster-Iversen, C., von Krueger, X., Ammer, H., Potschka, H., et al., 2017. Systematic account of animal poisonings in Germany, 2012–2015. Vet. Rec. Available from: http://dx.doi.org/10.1136/vr.103973.

McLean, M.K., Hansen, S.R., 2010. An overview of trends in animal poisoning cases in the united states: 2002–2010. Vet. Clin. North Amer. Small Anim. Pract. 43, 219–228.

Merola, V.M., 2002. Anticoagulant rodenticides: deadly for pests, dangerous for pets. Vet. Med. 97, 716–722.

Naidoo, V., Wolter, K., Cuthbert, R., Duncan, N., 2009. Veterinary diclofenac treatens Africa's endangered vulture species. Regul. Toxicol. Pharmacol. 53, 205–208.

Naidoo, V., Wolter, K., Cromarty, D., Diekmann, M., Duncan, N., Meharg, A.A., et al., 2010. Toxicity of non-steroidal anti-inflammatory drugs to Gyps vultures: a new threat from ketoprofen. Bio. Lett. 6, 339–341.

Osweiler, G.D., 1975. Sources and incidence of small animal poisoning. Vet. Clin. Small Anim. 5, 589–604.

Stroud, R.K., 1998. Wildlife forensics and the veterinary practitioner. Sem. Avian. Exotic. Pet. Med. 7, 182–192.

Trammel, H.L., Buck, W.B., Beasley, V.R., 1985. National Animal Poison Control Center: seven years of service. In 29th Annual Proceedings of the American Association of Veterinary Laboratory Diagnosticians, pp. 183–191.

US Department of Agriculture, 2011. Bulletin 415: plants poisonous to livestock in the western states. Agricultural Research Service. <https://www.ars.usda.gov/ARSUserFiles/oc/np/PoisonousPlants/PoisonousPlants.pdf> (accessed 15.02.17.).

Volmer, P.A., 2001. How dangerous are winter and spring holiday plants to pets? Vet. Med. 97, 879–884.

Wobeser, G., Bollinger, T., Leighton, F.A., Blakley, B., Mineau, P., 2004. Secondary poisoning of eagles following intentional poisoning of coyotes with anticholinesterase pesticides in western Canada. J. Wildl. Dis. 40, 163–172.

Xavier, F.G., Kogika, M.M., de Sousa Spinosa, H., 2002. Common causes of poisoning in dogs and cats in a Brazilian veterinary teaching hospital from 1998 to 2000. Vet. Hum. Toxicol. 44, 115–116.

FURTHER READING

American Kennel Club, 2010. Dog Registration Statistics, 2015–2016, 2010. <http://www.akc.org/content/news/articles/most-popular-dog-breeds-full-ranking-list/?button>.

Chapter 3

Epidemiology of Animal Poisonings in Europe

Francesca Caloni, Philippe Berny, Siska Croubels, Magda Sachana and Raimon Guitart

INTRODUCTION

A centralized veterinary poison control/information center does not exist in the European Union. In many European countries information about epidemiology of animal poisonings is unavailable or inadequate, and refers only to isolated case reports. However, some epidemiological data gathered by universities, research institutes, government institutions, or independent laboratories have been published in the last decade in Austria, Belgium, Germany, Greece, Spain, Italy, and Portugal (see Table 3.1 for country abbreviations).

In certain countries such as Belgium, the Czech Republic, Greece, Spain, Finland, France, Italy, The Netherlands, Poland, and Sweden, human poison control centers also collect data on animals. In Belgium, the Belgian National Poison Center in Brussels (BPC) holds a 24/7 hotline for suspected human and animal poisoning. The Laboratory of Toxicology of Ghent University (LTGU) and the Centre d'Informations Vétérinaires en Pharmaco-toxicologie, Université de Liège, are specialized in analytical confirmation of animal poisoning for the northern and southern parts of Belgium, respectively (Vandenbroucke et al., 2010). Similarly, in Spain's National Institute of Toxicology and Forensic Sciences (INTCF) offers a 24/7 telephonic service for cases of suspected poisonings, and in recent years the Institute for Game and Wildlife Research (IREC) in Ciudad Real has been very active in the analytical confirmation of poisonings in wildlife and domestic animals.

In Italy, the Assistenza Tossicologica Veterinaria (ATV) provides telephone assistance in cases of suspected poisonings in small animals. In France, the College of Veterinary Medicine of Lyon (CNITV) offers 24-h specialized assistance for suspected cases of animal poisoning and receives between 12,000 and 14,000 calls each year, while the corresponding toxicology laboratory (ToxLab) analyses between 1500 and 2000 samples. A second center is located at the College of Veterinary Medicine of Nantes (CAPAE-*Ouest*), which is open during regular business hours (Berny, 2007; Berny et al., 2010a). In the United Kingdom, the Veterinary Poisons Information Service (VPIS) provides services only to veterinarians (Bates et al., 2012), whereas the Royal Society for the Prevention of Cruelty to Animals (RSPCA) records suspected cases of deliberate acts reported by pet owners. In cases where there is hard evidence of pesticide poisoning including sporadic incidents involving livestock and pets, surveillance is conducted by the Veterinary Laboratories Agency (VLA) for production animals and by the Wildlife Incident Investigation Scheme (WIIS) for wildlife.

SPECIES INVOLVED

In numerous EU countries such as Belgium, Denmark, Spain, France, Italy, Poland, Portugal, Sweden, and the United Kingdom, the species most commonly involved in poisoning incidents is the dog followed by the cat (Amorena et al., 2004; Giuliano Albo and Nebbia, 2004; Berny et al., 2010a; Vandenbroucke et al., 2010; Caloni et al., 2012; Novoa et al., 2012; Garcia-Cardoso, 2016). With respect to analytical investigations at the CNITV/ToxLab and LTGU laboratories (Fig. 3.1), the resulting numbers are slightly different due to the significant number of wildlife disease surveillance plans, resulting in a substantial number of baits being included in the analyses (12% of cases submitted annually at LTGU, 15% in France).

Among farm animals, most of the poisoning incidents involve cattle (Guitart et al., 2010a; Vandenbroucke et al., 2010; VIDA, 2011; Novoa et al., 2012; García-Arroyo

Veterinary Toxicology. DOI: http://dx.doi.org/10.1016/B978-0-12-811410-0.00003-9

TABLE 3.1 Abbreviations for Countries Used in Table 3.2

AT	Austria
BE	Belgium
CZ	Czech Republic
DE	Germany
DK	Denmark
EL	Greece
ES	Spain
FI	Finland
FR	France
IE	Ireland
IT	Italy
NL	Netherlands
PL	Poland
PT	Portugal
SE	Sweden
UK	United Kingdom

et al., 2015), usually followed by sheep and goats. The last two are also the most common species implicated in poisoning incidents in Greece (Roubies et al., 2008; Guitart et al., 2010a). Generally, poultry and pigs are rarely involved in poisoning episodes, and minor percentages are also reported for exotic animals and rabbits (often included in the group "other species"), although these species are becoming more present in daily calls.

As far as wildlife, birds, especially waterfowl and raptors, are more commonly reported than mammals as victims of poisoning (Samouris et al., 2007; Guitart et al., 2010b; Delahay and Spray, 2015). Apart from specific toxic environmental disasters, deliberate primary or secondary poisoning incidents are of concern in all European countries and mainly involve birds of prey such as common buzzards and red kites (Guitart et al., 2010b; Vandenbroucke et al., 2010; Berny et al., 2015). Indeed, the proportion of wildlife cases at the ToxLab diagnostic laboratory, a part of the national wildlife disease surveillance network (SAGIR), is very high (Berny, 2007; Berny et al., 2015). As this network is supported financially by hunters, it mostly deals with game species, but an increasing number of cases regarding protected and endangered species has also been recorded (Berny and Gaillet, 2008). A Spanish national program (*Programa Antídoto*) reported several cases of deliberate poisoning of wild

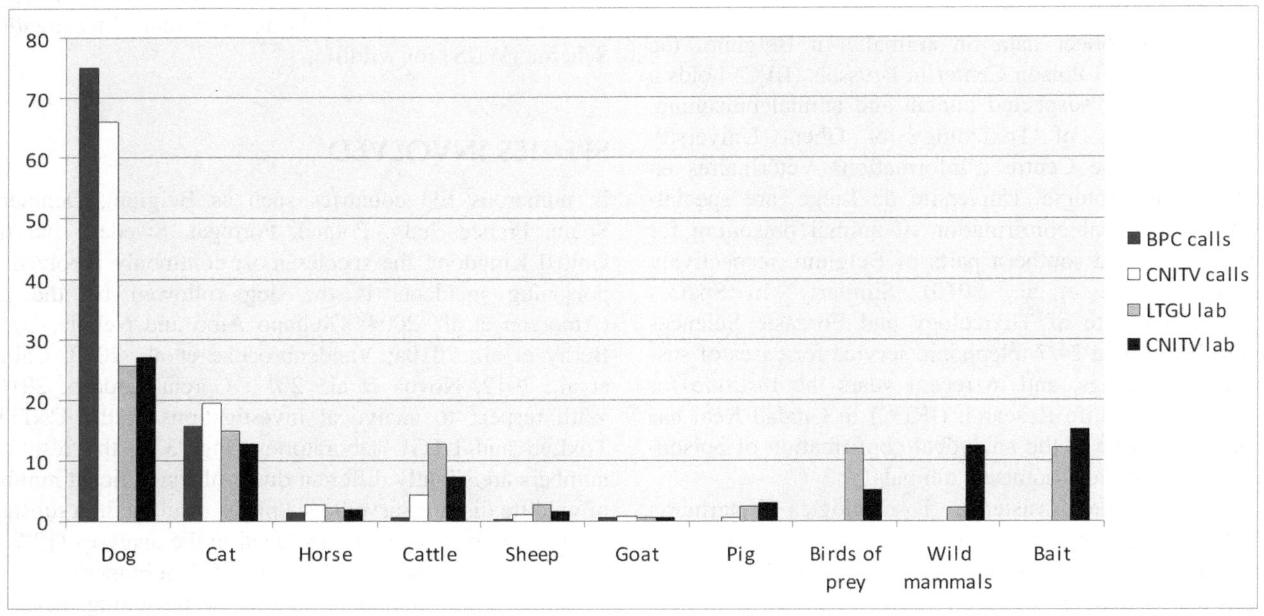

FIGURE 3.1 Distribution of species (including bait) in poisoning cases at the Belgian Poison Center (BPC calls, $n = 21{,}120$ from 2010 to 2016), the French Animal Poison Control Center (CNITV calls, $n = 115{,}502$ from 2010 to 2016), the Belgian Laboratory of Toxicology of the Faculty of Veterinary Medicine from Ghent University (LTGU lab, $n = 1155$ cases from 2010 to 2016), and the French College of Veterinary Medicine Diagnostic Toxicology Laboratory in Lyon (CNITV lab, $n = 7278$ cases from 2010 to 2016).

birds from 2006 to 2009. During this period, 243 griffon vultures, 42 red kites and 21 cinereous vultures were found dead, among other wild birds. Official data from the Ministry of the Environment in 2008 indicated that in Spain some 7000 members of protected wild species had been poisoned in the previous 15 years. Similarly, in Belgium, the Flemish government established several reporting centers in 2006, in an effort to monitor the pursuit of birds of prey in Flanders. A retrospective study conducted for the period 2011–15, dealing with 201 cases, revealed that in over 50% of the cases, an illegal cause of death was found. Poisoning was demonstrated in 38% of the cases and involved primarily cholinesterase inhibitors mostly including compounds which use is also prohibited in Belgium. But in general, a decline in the number of cases could be noticed, possibly due to the enhanced attention.

TOXIC CLASSES

In most species, pesticides are one of the main causes of poisoning (Guitart, 2012; Ruiz-Suárez et al., 2015) and statistical data from CNITV (2010–16) confirms this (Fig. 3.2).

Among pets, insecticides, rodenticides, herbicides, fungicides, and other pest control substances, used either for plant protection or for indoor pest control, are frequently involved in deliberate or accidental poisoning episodes (Berny et al., 2010a; Caloni et al., 2012; Guitart, 2012; Novoa et al., 2012). Drugs are a common source of poisoning for companion animals (Caloni et al., 2014), caused by the owner's negligence and off-label use of drugs (Modra and Svobodova, 2009; Berny et al., 2010a; Novoa et al., 2012). Other poisons include household products, plants, fuels, ethylene glycol, zootoxins, cosmetics and drugs of abuse (cocaine or cannabis) (Berny et al., 2010a). For horses, plant poisoning is most frequently reported (Berny et al., 2010a; Cortinovis and Caloni, 2013).

In food-producing animals, pesticides are again the most common class of suspected toxicants (Guitart et al., 2010a). In France, the most common culprits are mainly insecticides and seed-coated products followed by drugs, plants, and nutritional disorders resulting from the improper use of foods and feeds and unbalanced diets

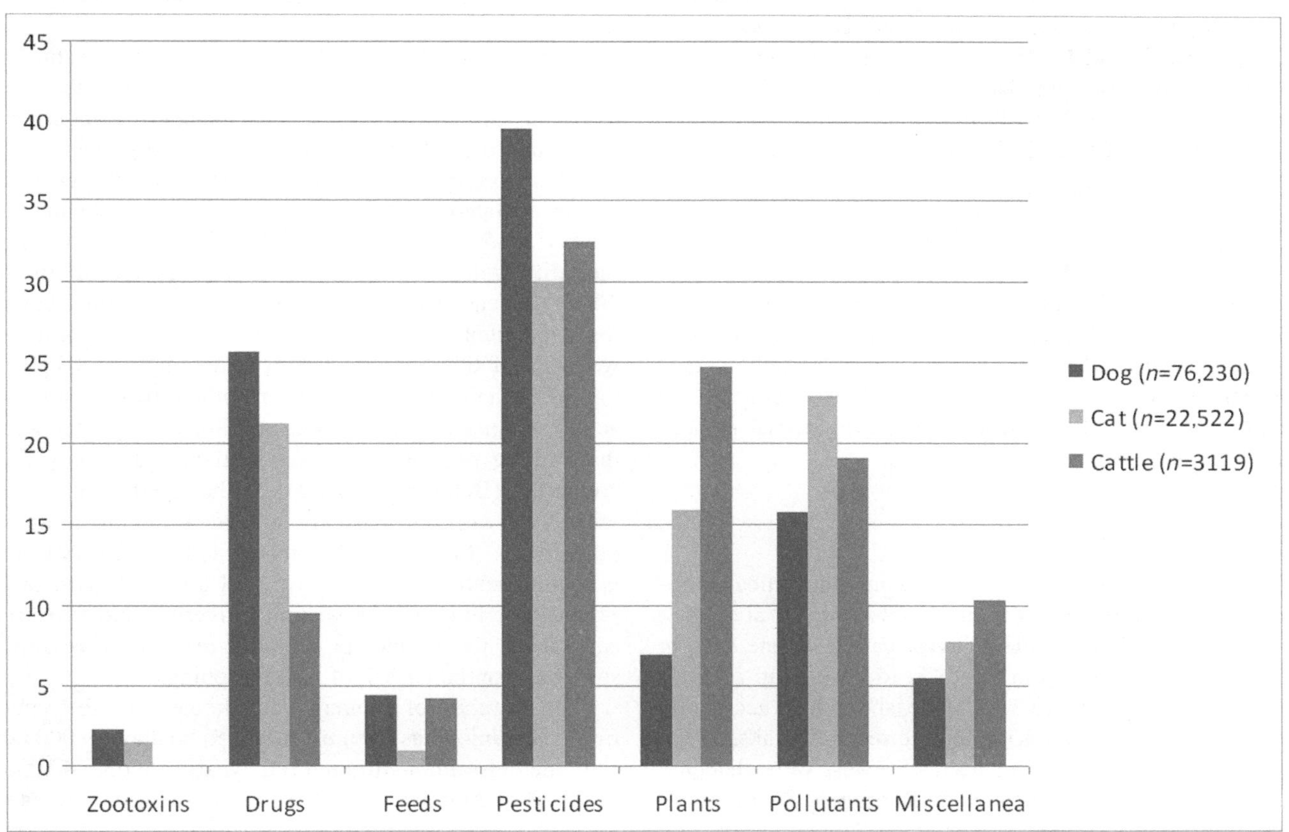

FIGURE 3.2 Toxic classes involved in suspected poisoning cases at the French College of Veterinary Medicine CNITV in Lyon (% in dogs, cats, and cattle, from 2010 to 2016).

(e.g., urea poisoning, grain overload). Other common toxicoses involving cattle and pigs result from plants and metals in ruminants and mycotoxins (Guitart et al., 2010a; García-Arroyo et al., 2015). In Greece, chronic Cu poisoning appears to be a rather common problem mainly in sheep husbandry (Roubies et al., 2008).

For wildlife, pesticides (mainly anticholinesterase and anticoagulant agents) and metals (particularly Pb from spent ammunition) are common causes of poisoning (Samouris et al., 2007; Mateo, 2009; Modra and Svobodova, 2009; Guitart et al., 2010b; Guitart, 2012; Berny et al., 2015; Ruiz-Suárez et al., 2015). Cyanobacteria toxicoses and botulism involving waterfowl have also been reported (Modra and Svobodova, 2009; Guitart et al., 2010b).

NONMETALS AND METALLOIDS

Fluorosis in the European Union has been observed following the intake of borehole water with high levels of fluorosis in region-specific deep-lying clay layers, as reported, e.g., in the case of turkeys (Berny et al., 2010a). A particular incident was reported in Belgium involving cattle, following the use of calcium sulfate ($CaSO_4$) as a binder agent in beet pulp resulting in a higher than normal level of fluorosis (Vandenbroucke et al., 2010). Poisoning with arsenic predominantly involved cattle, but rarely sheep (Sharpe and Livesey, 2005; Vandenbroucke et al., 2010). Se toxicoses are also rare but two cases have been reported involving sheep in the United Kingdom (Sharpe and Livesey, 2005) and pigs in Spain (Casteignau et al., 2006).

METALS

Telephone calls to European poison centers, however, do not give us the full picture of animal poisoning. Probably more than any other single toxic agent, certain metals, especially Pb in the case of wild birds, still continue to cause numerous suspected and confirmed animal poisoning cases in Europe.

Copper (Cu)

Chronic Cu poisoning is a fairly common clinical problem in the Greek sheep industry (Roubies et al., 2008; Guitart et al., 2010a). Field investigation of one case in Greece revealed the source of Cu to be a heap of litter from a broiler farm to which the sheep had accidental access. In the United Kingdom, three outbreaks of Cu poisoning, which killed at least 55 ewes, were detected in 2005 and 2006, associated with organic farming and the consumption of red clover (*Trifolium pratense*) and white clover (*Trifolium repens*). In Belgium, excessive amounts of Cu in commercially prepared milk replacers caused chronic toxicity in veal calves in two different farms (Vandenbroucke et al., 2010).

Lead (Pb)

In a Spanish farmland property located only several meters from a battery-recycling site that had been in operation for 20 years, the death of seven horses and one donkey was documented due to Pb poisoning. Unusual findings have been reported involving horses: a 13-year-old 700 kg Irish Draught cross gelding presenting abnormal respiratory noise during exercise caused by bilateral recurrent laryngeal nerve dysfunction, was diagnosed in the United Kingdom subsequent to Pb toxicosis (Allen, 2010).

Pb poisoning is very common for large animals, especially for cattle and sheep. In the United Kingdom, more than 450 Pb incidents were investigated by the VLA between 1998 and 2008, mostly related to discarded batteries, old paint, and geochemical sources (Payne and Livesey, 2010). In Austria, Belgium, Spain, and France, lethal cases involving cattle have also been reported due to the ingestion of fragments of discarded batteries or the contamination of pastures with ash residue from illegal bonfires (Krametter-Froetscher et al., 2007; Guitart et al., 2010a).

In the case of birds, there is extensive literature in Europe documenting poisoning episodes due to the accidental ingestion of small Pb objects, namely spent ammunition and lost fishing weights. This kind of poisoning has long been recognized as a major cause of death in several species (Mateo, 2009; Pain et al., 2009; Delahay and Spray, 2015; Berny et al., 2015). In Spain, waterfowl mortality rates were conservatively estimated to be 50,000 a year at the end of the last century, just before the implementation of a ban on the use of Pb shot in the wetlands of this country. Up to now, only about half of the European countries had taken some type of restrictive action against the introduction of Pb, mostly regulating the hunting of waterfowl over wetlands, and only four countries (Belgium, Denmark, The Netherlands and Sweden) totally or partially extended this measure to other zones (Mateo, 2009; Thomas and Guitart, 2010). It is worth mentioning that substantial amounts of metallic Pb continue to remain in wetlands, riverine, and terrestrial ecosystems for decades or centuries and this represents a source of continued risk of bird poisoning.

The number of hunters and shooters in the entire European Union has been estimated to be about 9,000,000 and the Pb ammunition fired yearly about 40,000 t (Thomas and Guitart, 2010). Very high concentrations of Pb shot (>150 per m^2 in the first 10–20 cm of depth) have been reported in some EU wetlands. Consequently a high prevalence of Pb shot ingestion was found, although the intensity varied among bird species and among regions across the European Union. Remarkably, Mateo (2009) detected a clear negative relationship between the prevalence of Pb shot ingestion and the wintering population trend in Europe of 15 waterfowl species. However, a study conducted in two wetland areas in northern Greece involving lesser and greater white-fronted goose (*Anser erythropus* and *Anser albifrons*, respectively), showed that exposure to Pb was very mild and the measured levels of Pb were well below the proposed thresholds for lethal effects of Pb poisoning (Aloupi et al., 2015). Poisoning of swans after ingestion of Pb split-shot or sinkers also occurs in Belgium, Ireland, and the United Kingdom (Perrins et al., 2003; Tavernier et al., 2004). Nonraptor upland birds are also victims, and a prevalence of 1.4% and 7.8% for red-legged partridges was found in the United Kingdom and Sweden, respectively.

There have been several reports over the last 10 years of Pb poisoning or high levels of exposure to Pb (compatible with subclinical or clinical signs) involving birds of prey (Table 3.2), both predators and scavengers (Mateo, 2009; Pain et al., 2009; Guitart et al., 2010b; Berny et al., 2015; Delahay and Spray, 2015). Raptors are at risk both from prey killed with shotguns, such as wildfowl, upland game birds and rabbits, and with rifles, such as deer and other large game. Recent radiographic studies have shown that many small bullet fragments remain inside prey shot with Pb-based bullets, posing a risk not only to raptors but also to human consumers of this hunted game (Delahay and Spray, 2015). Up to 2009, Pb poisoning had been reported in 17 species of birds of prey in Europe, some of which are near-threatened such as the white-tailed eagle or are vulnerable such as the Spanish imperial eagle (Mateo, 2009).

Last but not the least, a case of Pb poisoning involving zoo dolphins was reported in The Netherlands in 2008. Apparently, the animals had ingested metal from a damaged diving belt.

TABLE 3.2 Poisonings Reported in the Last 10–15 Years in Europe for Wildlife Species

Species	Poison	Country
American mink (*Mustela vison*)	Pesticides (anticoagulants)	FR
Atlantic puffin (*Fratercula artica*)	Oil	ES, FR, PT
Barn owl (*Tyto alba*)	Metals (Cd)	ES
	Pesticides (anticoagulants)	UK
Bearded vulture (*Gypaetus barbatus*)	Metals (Pb)	ES, FR
Beech marten (*Martes foina*)	Pesticides (anticoagulants)	BE
Cinereous vulture (*Aegypius monachus*)	Metals (Pb)	ES
	Pesticides (strychnine, carbamates)	EL, ES
Common buzzard (*Buteo buteo*)	Metals (Pb)	ES
	Oil	ES
	Pesticides (carbamates)	BE, CZ, ES
Common guillemot (*Uria aalgae*)	Oil	ES, FR, PT
Common kestrel (*Falco tinnunculus*)	Oil	ES
	Pesticides (carbamates)	ES
Common raven (*Corvus corax*)	Pesticides (carbamates)	CZ, ES
Common scoter (*Melanitta nigra*)	Oil	FR
Common vole (*Microtus arvalis*)	Pesticides (carbamates)	CZ
Common wood pigeon (*Columba palumbus*)	Pesticides (carbamates)	FR
Dolphin	Metals (Pb)	NL
Egyptian vulture (*Neophron percnopterus*)	Metals (Pb)	ES
	Pesticides (carbamates)	ES

(*Continued*)

TABLE 3.2 (Continued)

Species	Poison	Country
Eleonora's falcon (*Falco eleonorae*)	Pesticides (anticholinesterases)	EL
Eurasian eagle-owl (*Bubo bubo*)	Metals (Pb)	ES
European hare (*Lepus europaeus*)	Pesticides (anticoagulants)	FR
European hedgehog (*Erinaceus europaeus*)	Pesticides (carbamates)	ES
European rabbit (*Oryctolagus cuniculus*)	Pesticides (anticoagulants)	FR
Fallow deer (*Dama dama*)	Pesticides (carbamates)	CZ
Ferret (*Mustela putorius furo*)	Drugs of abuse (cannabis, hashish)	NL
Greater flamingo (*Phoenicopterus ruber*)	Metals (Pb)	ES, IT
	Toxins (cyanobacteria)	ES
Greylag goose (*Anser anser*)	Metals (Pb)	ES
Golden eagle (*Aquila chrysaetos*)	Metals (Pb)	AT, DE
Griffon vulture (*Gyps fulvus*)	Pesticides (anticholinesterases)	ES, EL
	Metals (Pb)	ES, PT
Herring gull (*Larus argentatus*)	Toxins (botulism)	SE
Honey bee (*Apis mellifera*)	Pesticides	UK
Marsh harrier (*Circus aureoginosus*)	Metals (Hg)	IT
	Pesticides (carbamates)	CZ
Mute swan (*Cygnus olor*)	Metals (Pb)	IE, UK
Northern gannet (*Sula bassana*)	Oil	ES, FR, PT
Northern goshawk (*Accipiter gentilis*)	Metals (Pb)	DE
	Pesticides (anticholinesterases, rodenticides)	BE
Otter (*Lutra lutra*)	Pesticides (carbamates)	CZ
Peregrine falcon (*Falco peregrinus*)	Oil (polycyclic aromatic hydrocarbons)	ES
Polecat (*Mustela putorius*)	Pesticides (anticoagulants)	BE, FR
	Oil	ES, FR, PT
Razorbill (*Alca torda*)		
Red kite (*Milvus milvus*)	Metals (Pb)	ES, FR, UK
	Pesticides (anticholinesterases, rodenticides)	BE, FR
Rock pigeon (*Columba livia*)	Metals (Pb)	BE
Rough-legged buzzard (*Buteo lagopus*)	Pesticides (carbamates)	CZ
Spanish imperial eagle (*Aquila adalberti*)	Metals (Pb)	ES
Waterbirds (several species)	Metals (Pb)	BE, ES, FR, IT, PT
	Toxins (cyanobacteria)	ES
White-tailed sea eagle (*Haliaeetus albicilla*)	Metals (Pb)	AT, DE, FI, SE
	Pesticides (carbamates)	DE, CZ
Wild boar (*Sus scrofa*)	Pesticides (carbamates, rodenticides)	CZ, FR

Other Metals and Inorganic Compounds

Mercury (Hg) poisoning is uncommon in domestic animals but should be taken into account as a potential cause of renal failure. In Germany, a 4-month-old male German shepherd dog presented with a 2-day history of vomiting, bloody diarrhea, and severe renal function impairment. After euthanasia, due to the poor prognosis, the owner admitted that a barometer containing Hg had broken in the bedroom about a week before the dog had developed clinical signs. The route of exposure to Hg was presumed to be digestive and respiratory (Hansmann et al., 2009).

In Italy, Hg exposure following the accidental ingestion of thermometers showed a clear downward trend over time in dog (Caloni et al., 2012). Also, in Italy, a marsh harrier was found dead in a wetland in the northeast, and a postmortem diagnosis of Hg poisoning was established, based on levels of 20 $\mu g\ g^{-1}$ in both liver and kidney. Hg still appears as a major threat for fish-eating predators such as otters or cormorants (Alomar et al., 2016). Zinc (Zn) toxicity is rarely observed in Europe. Two cases involving dogs were reported in the United Kingdom when both animals ingested a badly designed tag distributed by an international animal health laboratory to identify that the dogs had been microchipped (Adam et al., 2011). Unusual clinicopathological findings have also been reported, as in the case of a 6-year-old female Labrador Retriever that had ingested a Zn toy; hematological findings revealed a large number of Heinz bodies and marked anemia (Bexfield et al., 2007). Zn poisoning is regularly suspected and confirmed in cage birds (zinc cages) by the ToxLab in France.

In NL, an accident took place when a veterinarian advised the owner of a 4.5 kg Schipperke dog to give it table salt to induce vomiting after ingestion of one tablet of digoxin. Apparently, the dose administered was too large and the dog presented neurological signs of salt poisoning and died a few hours later. A similar case occurred in France with a 5-year-old female Doberman Pinscher (Pouzot et al., 2007), but this time it was treated successfully and survived.

PESTICIDES

Pesticides are common culprits in animal poisoning cases as a result of inappropriate or careless use. For companion animals, most of the suspected poisoning cases in Belgium, Greece, Spain, France, and Italy involved anticholinesterase insecticides (Berny et al., 2010a; Vandenbroucke et al., 2010; Caloni et al., 2012; Ruiz-Suárez et al., 2015). In Spain, rodenticides are as much to blame as insecticides (Berny et al., 2010a). A 6-year retrospective study in Austria investigated pesticide poisoning and revealed 123 positive cases; out of 225, 47.2% involved dogs and 34.1% cats (Wang et al., 2007). The highest percentage of incidents was associated with carbamates (50.3%), followed by herbicides and molluscicides (22.3%), anticoagulant rodenticides (18.9%), organophosphates (5.1%), and nonanticoagulant rodenticides (3.4%) (Wang et al., 2007).

Grazing animals are more exposed to pesticides than livestock kept in the barn. Nevertheless, application or storage of pesticides in barns occasionally leads to accidental animal toxicosis. In certain EU countries such as Greece and France, pesticide poisoning is, by far, the most common cause of livestock toxicosis in comparison to other countries such as Belgium, Spain, and Italy (Guitart et al., 2010a; García-Arroyo et al., 2015).

Pesticides and more specific anticholinesterase insecticides and rodenticides followed by molluscicides and avicides are among the most frequently reported causes of wildlife poisoning in Europe (Berny, 2007; Berny and Gaillet, 2008; Guitart et al., 2010b; Sharp et al., 2013). The investigation of pesticide poisoning of the cinereous vulture in Spain revealed that carbofuran, aldicarb, and strychnine account for up to 88% of all cases (Hernández and Margalida, 2008). Between 1998 and 2004, 70 animals of the wild fauna (38 birds and 32 mammals) of northern Greece were subjected to analysis and 52.63% of birds and 43.75% of mammals tested positive for toxic substances responsible for their death (Samouris et al., 2007). In Greece, it appears that anticholinesterase agents are the main cause of wildlife poisoning followed by sporadic incidents due to warfarin and cyanide salts (Samouris et al., 2007; Guitart et al., 2010b). A recent report in France shows that aldicarb and carbofuran represented 11%–33% of the identified causes of death of birds of prey (Egyptian vulture, griffon vulture, bearded vulturí, and red kite) collected along the Pyrenean Mountains (Berny et al., 2015).

Insecticides

Carbamates were found to be responsible for the majority of acute dog poisoning incidents in Belgium, the Czech Republic, Spain, and Italy (Giuliano Albo and Nebbia, 2004; Modra and Svobodova, 2009; Vandenbroucke et al., 2010; Ruiz-Suárez et al., 2015). Apart from being responsible for 46.9% of positive cases involving sheep and 66.7% involving goats in northern Greece (Guitart et al., 2010a), carbamates were also found to be the cause of a recent case involving the poisoning of 55 members of a dairy goat herd following the consumption of drenched carnations at a nearby greenhouse (Giadinis et al., 2009). Moreover, carbofuran and/or aldicarb has been, by far, the most common cause of wildlife toxicoses in Belgium, the Czech Republic, and Spain in the last decade (Modra and Svobodova, 2009; Vandenbroucke et al., 2010; Ruiz-Suárez et al., 2015).

In Italy, a retrospective study based on calls of suspected poisonings also detected several cases of pyrethrins-pyrethoids, organophosphates and neonicotinoids (imidacloprid and acetamiprid) potential exposures (Caloni et al., 2016).

Organochlorine insecticides such as DDT were banned many years ago due to their persistency in the environment and accumulation in the fatty tissues of organisms (Guitart, 2012). However, failure to meet handling regulations of toxic substances and/or waste materials led to cattle poisoning by DDT (Modra and Svobodova, 2009).

Rodenticides

The presence of rodenticides and more specific second-generation anticoagulants was analytically confirmed in the majority of suspected companion animal poisoning cases in Italy and to a lesser extent in Belgium, Spain, and France (Berny et al., 2010a). Indeed, a study in France between 2004 and 2007 showed that dogs were involved in cases of anticoagulant poisoning (over 60%) more than other domestic species (Berny et al., 2010b). Similarly, in Austria and the Czech Republic, anticoagulant rodenticides were recorded as a significant cause of acute poisoning in dogs after deliberate abuse or misuse (Wang et al., 2007; Modra and Svobodova, 2009). Additionally, anticoagulant rodenticides rank among the rare but nevertheless reportable causes of hemorrhage and epistaxis in cats and dogs (Kohn et al., 2003; Mylonakis et al., 2008). Strychnine, although banned in the majority of EU countries, is still reported as the most common form of rodenticide toxicity in Greece, Spain, France, and certain regions of Italy (Amorena et al., 2004; Berny et al., 2010a).

Hares and rabbits were also found to be significantly present in cases of anticoagulant exposure and account for almost 50% of the submitted cases in France, followed by scavengers and predators of poisoned rats (Berny et al., 2010b). In the same country, two polecats and an American mink were also reported poisoned by bromadiolone during a screening process aimed at identifying the reason behind the decline in the endangered European mink population (Fournier-Chambrillon et al., 2004). The IREC in Spain, and the Predatory Bird Monitoring Scheme (PBMS) and the WIIS in the United Kingdom, have also identified anticoagulant rodenticides as a common contaminant of wildlife and a cause of mortality (Sánchez-Barbudo et al., 2012b; Sharp et al., 2013).

Other Pesticides

Metaldehyde is usually found in pellets used for molluscicide treatment and that are palatable and easily digested by animals. Dog and cat poisoning by metaldehyde is a big issue in the Czech Republic and the United Kingdom and has alarmingly increased in other European countries such as Belgium, France, and Italy where slug pellets are used extensively, not only in farmland but also in home gardens (Modra and Svobodova, 2009; Berny et al., 2010a; Bates et al., 2012). Cases of metaldehyde poisoning involving cattle and pigs having access to stored bags of slug pellets have been recorded in the United Kingdom (Sharpe and Livesey, 2005). At least one case of iron poisoning has been diagnosed in France in a dog that ingested over 250 g of iron-phosphate–based molluscicide. The dog displayed very severe gastroenteritis, followed by neurological disorders leading eventually to death.

Occasionally, the herbicides paraquat and glyphosate have been involved in cases of companion and farm animal poisonings in Greece, Spain, France, and Italy (Berny et al., 2010a; Cortinovis et al., 2015a; Caloni et al., 2016). Other herbicides and fungicides have been more infrequently associated in the poisoning of companion animals in the European Union.

OIL

The two most recent major oil spills in Europe occurred on the Atlantic coast: the Erika (France) and the Prestige (Spain, France, and Portugal) accidents, in December 1999 and in November 2002, respectively. The Erika oil spill resulted in over 63,000 birds being stranded on beaches, while the Prestige oil spill affected between 115,000 and 230,000 birds, of which only 23,181 could be collected (Guitart et al., 2010b). Interestingly, March 2017 marks the 50th anniversary of the world's first major supertanker disaster, the Torrey Canyon, which affected and heavily polluted the coasts of southern United Kingdom, northwestern France, and the Channel Islands. It is remembered because the use of dispersants, detergents and other chemicals, exacerbated the ecological damage of the oil spill.

FEED-ASSOCIATED TOXICANTS

As far as companion animals are concerned, feed-related poisoning incidents reported in the last decade involve the accidental intake of chocolate, grapes, raisins, onions, cannabis products, and ethanol by dogs (Guitart et al., 2008; Sutton et al., 2009; Berny et al., 2010a; Gunning et al., 2010; Fitzgerald et al., 2013; Kuhne and Meisinger, 2014; Bates et al., 2015). Dogs may also be prone to the ingestion of theobromine from garden mulch made of cacao bean shells.

Current trends in feed-related livestock poisoning are related to the accidental presence of industrial chemicals/contaminants or to cross-contamination of feed batches with drugs/additives resulting in the exposure of nontarget animals. An example of the former is the Belgian dioxin incident in 1999 in which a tank of recycled fats used to produce animal feeds was accidentally contaminated with approximately 100 liters of polychlorinated biphenyl oil (Vandenbroucke et al., 2010). Another example is a melamine contaminated feed crisis in the pig industry in ES. Between 2003 and 2006, 300–400 Iberian piglets developed nephrotoxicosis subsequent to exposure to melamine and derivatives. Morbidity was 40%–60% and mortality 20%–40% in the total population of postweaning piglets (González et al., 2009).

The phenomenon of cross-contamination of feed is well known where ionophores such as monensin, lasalocid, narasin, and salinomycin are concerned. They are frequently used as feed additives and coccidiostats for cattle, sheep, and poultry. Acute monensin or other ionophores toxicosis in equids is well documented (Decloedt et al., 2012). Although ionophores are considered to be relatively safe for target animals, a number of ionophore poisoning cases in poultry were recently reported and reviewed in Markiewicz et al. (2014). A special case of acute tiamulin-salinomycin toxicosis in pigs due to a pharmacokinetic interaction between both compounds was reported in Belgium (Vandenbroucke et al., 2010).

Other feed-related poisoning incidents observed during the last years in Europe involve well-known toxicants such as nitrate, nitrite, and ammonia. Sharpe and Livesey (2005) reported three nitrate poisoning incidents involving cattle and one involving sheep in the United Kingdom between 1990 and 2002. Several cases of acute mortality in pigs in Belgium have been described in which still, standing water was identified as the nitrite source (Vandenbroucke et al., 2010). In the case of cattle, there have been occasional incidents of overconsumption of soybean meal causing acute carbohydrate fermentation and excessive ammonia release leading to nervous symptoms or of ingestion of cultivated and wild onions (*Allium* spp.) resulting in hemolytic anemia and acute death (Vandenbroucke et al., 2010).

DRUGS AND RELATED COMPOUNDS

Among the many different therapeutic classes of human drugs, nonsteroidal antiinflammatory drugs, benzodiazepines, and barbiturates are the most common contributors to animal poisoning (Berny et al., 2010a). In the United States several studies dealing with the ingestion of the nonbenzodiazepine hypnotic drug zolpidem by dogs have been reported, which are now also increasing in Europe (Caloni et al., 2014; Cortinovis et al., 2015b). In the United Kingdom, ingestion of hydroxycarbamide (hydroxyurea) tablets by a dog was associated with methemoglobinemia (Wray, 2008). Another well-known accidental ingestion of drugs involves the intake of equine deworming medication by dogs. Collies are especially known for their breed-dependent adverse reaction to ivermectin (Berny et al., 2010a).

Livestock poisoning cases related to human and veterinary drugs has seldom been reported in Europe in the last decade. Cases include the poisoning of calves by doxycycline in BE after receiving high doses as treatment for respiratory disorders (Vandenbroucke et al., 2010) and sheep and cattle in the United Kingdom due to the misuse of unlabeled or out-of-date diazinon products (Sharpe et al., 2006). A presumably deliberate oral ivermectin intoxication has been described on a veal farm in BE (Vermeulen et al., 2016). All 330 calves, aged between 2 and 4 weeks, showed severe depression, sternal to lateral recumbency, tremor, and headshaking, and 13.6% died.

HOUSEHOLD PRODUCTS

Since dogs and cats share our domestic environment, they are highly exposed to household products (e.g., 720 cases in France in 2003) (Berny et al., 2010a). Among them, hydrocarbons account for nearly 40% of poisoning incidents, especially in the case of cats exposed to domestic fuel, xylene, and other common solvents used in paint and paint solvents. Exposure to these substances usually results in very severe cases with a high mortality rate.

Other common household toxicants include detergents and caustics (bleach, strong acids and bases), accounting for almost another 40% of the 720 cases. In 2004, 69 calls related to fertilizer poisoning were registered in France and most of them (65%) resulted in moderately severe cases with digestive disorders. Similarly in Italy, bleach and detergents are often involved in the poisoning of both cats and dogs, whereas petroleum distillate poisoning was reported mainly in cats (Amorena et al., 2004; Giuliano Albo and Nebbia, 2004). In Italy and Spain, ethylene glycol poisoning involving dogs has been recorded (Berny et al., 2010a), and some recent cases involving cats have been analytically confirmed in Catalonia, Spain. Birds appear to be very sensitive to polytetrafluoroethylene (PTFE), a synthetic fluoropolymer best known as Teflon, and poisoning mostly results in sudden death. The main source of PTFE intoxication in pet birds is the overheating of nonstick cookware in the kitchen (Caekebeke et al., 2016).

TOXINS

Suspected toxin poisoning has been reported in companion animals (phytotoxins and zootoxins), in food-producing animals (phytotoxins and mycotoxins) and in wild birds (botulism and cyanobacteria).

Plants

Poisoning or suspected poisoning of companion animals as a result of ingestion of plants is a relatively common occurrence and cats appear to be more sensitive and more at risk than dogs, presumably because they tend to chew on plant leaves (Berny et al., 2010a). Often the cases are related to accidental ingestion of ornamental plants rather than wild plants, particularly at certain times of the year. Cats are generally more likely to be poisoned by household/ornamental plants and dogs are more at risk from wild plants (Giuliano Albo and Nebbia, 2004; Berny et al., 2010a).

Liliaceae and *Araceae* are the two major plant families involved in the poisoning of companion animals in France; oleander (*Nerium oleander*), castor bean (*Ricinus communis*), and Jimson weed (*Datura stramonium*) cases are also frequently observed (Berny et al., 2010a).

In Italy, ornamental plants such as dumbcane (*Dieffenbachia* spp.), ficus (*Ficus benjamina*), pittosporo (*Pittosporum tobira*), poinsettia (*Euphorbia pulcherrima*), rhododendron (*Rhododendrum hirsutum*), sago palma (*Cycas revoluta*), tiger lily (*Lilium lancifolium*), and jessamine (*Jasminum officinale*) have been involved in dog poisonings (Amorena et al., 2004; Giuliano Albo and Nebbia, 2004; Berny et al., 2010a; Cortinovis and Caloni, 2013). In Belgium, the Czech Republic, and Italy black locust (*Robinia pseudoacacia*), tansy ragwort (*Senecio jacobaea*), and oleander have been responsible for horse poisoning outbreaks (Modra and Svobodova, 2009; Berny et al., 2010a; Vandenbroucke et al., 2010). In addition, horse poisoning resulting from European yew (*Taxus baccata*) exposure is very common in Belgium and France (Berny et al., 2010a; Vandenbroucke et al., 2010). Outbreaks of atypical myopathy in horses, a fatal pasture myopathy linked to maple seed (*Acer pseudoplatanus* and *Acer negundo*) ingestion (Paulussen et al., 2015) have been recorded frequently in Europe (Votion et al., 2014).

Although livestock poisoning by toxic plants is frequent, these cases often remain only suspected, unconfirmed by analytical diagnoses. Livestock are commonly poisoned by bracken fern (*Pteridium aquilinum*), European yew, oak trees (*Quercus* spp.), and ragwort (*Senecio* spp.) in many European countries (Guitart et al., 2010a; Vandenbroucke et al., 2010; Plessers et al., 2013).

Other Toxins

In the European Union, a number of different aquatic bird species have been involved in outbreaks of botulism (Guitart et al., 2010b). Botulism outbreaks in poultry, sheep, and cattle are fairly common too (Sharpe and Livesey, 2005; Modra and Svobodova, 2009). Cyanobacteria toxic blooms are the cause of mass mortality of wild birds in inland water systems worldwide and two recent episodes have been reported in Spain in the Doñana National Park (López-Rodas et al., 2008; Guitart et al., 2010b).

Although mycotoxicoses are commonly suspected, published reports of poisoning are scarce. Episodes involving different species like cattle, pigs, poultry and sheep have been recently reported in Belgium, the Czech Republic, Spain, France, Italy, Poland, and the United Kingdom (Sharpe and Livesey, 2005; Modra and Svobodova, 2009; Obremsky and Zielonka, 2009; Guitart et al., 2010a; Moyano et al., 2010; Vandenbroucke et al., 2010).

A suspected case of poisoning with cantharidin of a great bustard (*Otis tarda*) after ingestion of several blister beetles of the species *Berberomeloe majalis* was reported in Spain (Sánchez-Barbudo et al., 2012a). Cases due to venomous bites by viper (*Vipera* spp.), common toad (*Bufo bufo*), and pine caterpillar (*Thaumetopoea pityocampa*) mostly involve dogs (Amorena et al., 2004; Giuliano Albo and Nebbia, 2004; Berny et al., 2010a; Lervick et al., 2010; Caloni et al., 2012; Niza et al., 2012). Interestingly, the last insect is endemic in southern European and Mediterranean pine forests but it is now expanding northward because of global warming (Battisti et al., 2005).

CONCLUDING REMARKS AND FUTURE DIRECTIONS

European toxicoepidemiological data demonstrate that pesticides are the most common class of toxicants in all species. Poisoning in companion animals is a frequent problem and dogs are the most commonly poisoned species, followed by cats and horses. In food-producing animals information on poisoning is limited and fragmented and occurs predominantly in cattle followed by sheep and goats. A small percentage of cases have also been reported for poultry and pigs. Poisoning episodes in wildlife are widespread and present a major investigational problem for toxicology and forensic laboratories. Knowledge of the common features of animal poisoning is central to any endeavor to reduce mortality, and it is therefore essential that coordinated and integrated efforts be made between European countries for sharing information.

REFERENCES

Adam, F., Elliott, J., Dandrieux, J., et al., 2011. Zinc toxicity in two dogs associated with the ingestion of identification tags. Vet. Rec. 168, 84–85.

Allen, K.J., 2010. Laryngeal paralysis secondary to lead toxicosis, Eq. Vet. Ed. 22, 182–186.

Alomar, H., Lemarchand, C., Rosoux, R., et al., 2016. Concentrations of organochlorine compounds (pesticides and PCBs), trace elements (Pb, Cd, Cu and Hg), ^{134}Cs, and ^{137}Cs in the livers of the European otter (*Lutra lutra*), great cormorant (*Phalacrocorax carbo*), and European catfish (*Silurus glanis*) collected from the Loire river (France). Eur. J. Wildlife Res. 62, 653–661.

Aloupi, M., Kazantzidis, S., Akriotis, T., et al., 2015. Lesser White-fronted (*Anser erythropus*) and Greater White-fronted (*A. albifrons*) Geese wintering in Greek wetlands are not threatened by Pb through shot ingestion. Sci. Total Env. 527–528, 279–286.

Amorena, M., Caloni, F., Mengozzi, G., 2004. Epidemiology of intoxications in Italy. Vet. Res. Comm. 28 (Suppl. 1), 89–95.

Bates, N.S., Sutton, N.M., Campbell, A., 2012. Suspected metaldehyde slug bait poisoning in dogs: a retrospective analysis of cases reported to the Veterinary Poisons Information Service. Vet. Rec. 171, 324.

Bates, N., Rawson-Harris, P., Edwards, N., 2015. Common questions in veterinary toxicology. J. Small Anim. Pract. 56, 298–306.

Battisti, A., Stastny, M., Netherer, S., et al., 2005. Expansion of geographic range in the pine processionary moth caused by increased winter temperatures. Ecol. Appl. 15, 2084–2096.

Berny, P., 2007. Pesticides and the intoxications of wild animals. J. Vet. Pharmacol. Therap. 30, 93–100.

Berny, P., Gaillet, J.R., 2008. Acute poisoning of red kites (Milvus milvus) in France: data from the SAGIR network. J. Wildlife Dis. 44, 417–426.

Berny, P., Caloni, F., Croubels, S., Sachana, M., et al., 2010a. Animal poisoning in Europe. Part 2: companion animals. Vet. J. 183, 255–259.

Berny, P., Velardo, J., Pulce, C., et al., 2010b. Prevalence of anticoagulant rodenticide poisoning in humans and animals in France and substances involved. Clin. Toxicol. 48, 935–941.

Berny, P., Vilagines, L., Cugnasse, J.M., et al., 2015. Vigilance poison: illegal poisoning and lead intoxication are the main factors affecting avian scavenger survival in the Pyrenees (France). Ecotoxicol. Env. Safety 118, 71–82.

Bexfield, N., Archer, J., Herrtage, M., 2007. Heinz body haemolytic anaemia in a dog secondary to ingestion of a zinc toy: a case report. Vet. J. 174, 414–417.

Caekebeke, N., Antonissen, G., De Backer, P., et al., 2016. Polytetrafluoroethylene intoxication in birds. Vlaams Diergen. Tijd. 85, 3–8.

Caloni, F., Cortinovis, C., Pizzo, F., et al., 2014. Epidemiological study (2006-2012) on the poisoning of small animals by human and veterinary drugs. Vet. Rec. 174, 222.

Caloni, F., Cortinovis, C., Rivolta, M., Davanzo, F., 2012. Animal poisoning in Italy: 10 years of epidemiological data from the Poison Control Centre of Milan. Vet. Rec. 170, 415.

Caloni, F., Cortinovis, C., Rivolta, M., Davanzo, F., 2016. Suspected poisoning of domestic animals by pesticides. Sci. Total Env. 539, 331–336.

Casteignau, A., Fontana, A., Morillo, A., et al., 2006. Clinical, pathological, and toxicological findings of an iatrogenic selenium toxicosis case in feeder pigs. J. Am. Vet. Med. Assoc. 53, 323–326.

Cortinovis, C., Caloni, F., 2013. Epidemiology of intoxication of domestic animals by plants in Europe. Vet. J. 197, 163–168.

Cortinovis, C., Davanzo, M., Rivolta, M., Caloni, F., 2015a. Glyphosate-surfactant herbicide poisoning in domestic animals: an epidemiological survey. Vet. Rec. 176, 413.

Cortinovis, C., Pizzo, F., Caloni, F., 2015b. Poisoning of dogs and cats by drugs intended for human use. Vet. J. 203, 52–58.

Decloedt, A., Verheyen, T., De Clercq, D., et al., 2012. Acute and long-term cardiomyopathy and delayed neurotoxicity after accidental lasalocid poisoning in horses. J. Vet. Int. Med. 26, 1005–1011.

Proceedings of the Oxford Lead Symposium. In: Delahay, R.J., Spray, C.J. (Eds.), Lead Ammunition: Understanding and Minimising the Risks to Human and Environmental Health. The University of Oxford, Edward Grey Institute, Oxford, 152 pp.

Fitzgerald, K.T., Bronstein, A.C., Newquist, K.L., 2013. Marijuana poisoning. Topics Compan. Anim. Med. 28, 8–12.

Fournier-Chambrillon, C., Berny, P.J., Coiffier, O., et al., 2004. Evidence of secondary poisoning of free-ranging riparian mustelids by anticoagulant rodenticides in France: implications for conservation of European mink (*Mustela lutreola*). J. Wildlife Dis. 40, 688–695.

García-Arroyo, R., Míguez, M.P., Hevia, M.L., et al., 2015. Cattle mortality due to poisoning in Spain: a cross-sectional epidemiological study. Span J. Agri. Res. 13, e05–002.

Garcia-Cardoso, J.I., 2016. *Estudo sobre intoxicações em animais de companhia no concelho de Loures*. Faculdade de Medicina Veterinária, Universidade Lusófona de Humanidades e Tecnologias, Lisboa. <http://recil.ulusofona.pt/bitstream/handle/10437/7093/ JoanaCardoso.pdf?sequence=1> (accessed 15.01.17.).

Giadinis, N.D., Raikos, N., Loukopoulos, P., et al., 2009. Carbamate poisoning in a dairy goat herd: clino-pathological findings and therapeutic approach. NZ Vet. J. 57, 392–394.

Giuliano Albo, A., Nebbia, C., 2004. Incidence of poisonings in domestic carnivores in Italy. Vet. Res. Comm. 28 (Suppl. 1), 83–88.

González, J., Puschner, B., Pérez, V., et al., 2009. Nephrotoxicosis in Iberian piglets subsequent to exposure to melamine and derivatives in Spain between 2003 and 2006. J. Vet. Diagn. Inv. 21, 558–563.

Guitart, R., Mateu, C., López, I., Agulló, A., et al., 2008. Heinz body anaemia in two dogs after Catalan spring onion ("calçot") ingestion: case reports. Vet. Med. 53, 392–395.

Guitart, R., 2012. Pesticide residues in birds and mammals. In: Rathore, H.S., Nollet, M.L. (Eds.), Pesticides: Evaluation of Environmental Pollution. CRC Press, Boca Raton, FL, pp. 393–463.

Guitart, R., Croubels, S., Caloni, F., Sachana, M., et al., 2010a. Animal poisoning in Europe. Part 1: farm livestock and poultry. Vet. J. 183, 260–265.

Guitart, R., Sachana, M., Caloni, F., et al., 2010b. Animal poisoning in Europe. Part 3: wildlife. Vet. J. 183, 249–254.

Gunning, M.E., den Hertog, E., van Velsen, N.F., et al., 2010. Chocolate intoxication in dogs. Tijds. diergen. 135, 896–899.

Hansmann, F., Stephan, I., Wirtz, A., et al., 2009. Mercury poisoning in a German shepherd dog. Vet. Rec. 165, 447–448.

Hernández, M., Margalida, A., 2008. Pesticide abuse in Europe: effects on the Cinereous vulture (*Aegypius monachus*) population in Spain. Ecotoxicology 17, 264–272.

Krametter-Froetscher, R., Tataruch, F., Hauser, S., et al., 2007. Toxic effects seen in a herd of beef cattle following exposure to ash residues contaminated by lead and mercury. Vet. J. 174, 99–105.

Kohn, B., Weingart, C., Giger, U., 2003. Haemorrhage in seven cats with suspected anticoagulant rodenticide intoxication. J. Feline Med. Surg. 5, 295–304.

Kuhne, T., Meisinger, H.C., 2014. Acute ethanol poisoning in a Labrador retriever after ingestion of uncooked stollen dough. Kleintierpraxis. 59, 608–611.

Lervick, B.J., Lilliehöök, I., Frendin, J.H.M., 2010. Clinical and biochemical changes in 53 Swedish dogs bitten by the European adder – *Vipera berus*. Acta Vet. Scand. 52, 26.

López-Rodas, V., Maneiro, E., Lanzarot, M.P., et al., 2008. Mass wildlife mortality due to cyanobacteria in the Doñana National Park, Spain. Vet. Rec. 162, 317–318.

Markiewicz, W., Barski, D., Burmanczuk, A., et al., 2014. Toxicity of salinomycin and narasin in turkeys. J. Elementol. 19, 903–914.

Mateo, R., 2009. Lead poisoning in wild birds in Europe and the regulations adopted by different countries. In: Watson, R.T.M., Fuller, M., Pokras, M., Hunt, W.G. (Eds.), Ingestion of Spent Lead Ammunition: Implications for Wildlife and Humans. The Peregrine Fund, Boise, pp. 71–98.

Modra, H., Svobodova, Z., 2009. Incidence of animal poisoning cases in the Czech Republic: current situation. Interdiscip. Toxicol. 2, 48–51.

Moyano, M.R., Molina, A.M., Lora, A.J., et al., 2010. Tremorgenic mycotoxicosis caused by Paspalum paspaloides (Michx.) Scribner infected by Claviceps paspali: a case report. Vet. Med. 55, 336–338.

Mylonakis, M.E., Saridomichelakis, M.N., Lazaridis, V., et al., 2008. A retrospective study of 61 cases of spontaneous canine epistaxis (1998 to 2001). J. Small Anim. Pract. 49, 191–196.

Niza, M.E., Ferreira, R.L., Coimbra, I.V., et al., 2012. Effects of pine processionary caterpillar *Thaumetopoea pityocampa* contact in dogs: 41 cases (2002-2006). Zoon Publ. Health. 59, 35–38.

Novoa, M.C., Melgar, M.J., García, M.A., et al., 2012. Análisis de la casuística del Servicio de Atención Toxicológica Veterinaria (SATVe) en el período 2001-2007. Rev. Toxicol. 29, 29–35.

Obremsky, K., Zielonka, L., 2009. Mycotoxins – dairy cattle breeding problem. Case report. Bull. Vet. Inst. Pulawy. 53, 221–224.

Pain, D.J., Fisher, I.J., Thomas, V.G., 2009. A global update on lead poisoning in terrestrial birds from ammunition sources. In: Watson, R. T.M., Fuller, M., Pokras, M., Hunt, W.G. (Eds.), Ingestion of Spent Lead Ammunition: Implications for Wildlife and Humans. The Peregrine Fund, Boise, pp. 99–118.

Paulussen, E., Broux, B., Lefère, L., et al., 2015. Atypical myopathy in the horse. Vlaams Diergen. Tijd. 84, 48–54.

Payne, J., Livesey, C., 2010. Lead poisoning in cattle and sheep. Practice. 32, 64–69.

Perrins, C.M., Cousquer, G., Waine, J., 2003. A survey of blood lead levels in mute swans Cygnus olor. Avian Pathol. 32, 205–212.

Plessers, E., Pardon, B., Deprez, P., et al., 2013. Acute hemorrhagic syndrome by bracken poisoning in cattle in Belgium. Vlaams Diergen. Tijd. 82, 31–37.

Pouzot, C., Descone-Junot, C., Loup, J., et al., 2007. Successful treatment of severe salt intoxication in a dog. J. Vet. Emer. Crit. Care. 17, 294–298.

Roubies, N., Giadinis, N.D., Polizopoulou, Z., et al., 2008. A retrospective study of chronic copper poisoning in 79 sheep flocks in Greece (1987–2007). J. Vet. Pharmacol. Ther. 31, 181–183.

Ruiz-Suárez, N., Boada, L.D., Henríquez-Hernández, L.A., et al., 2015. Continued implication of the banned pesticides carbofuran and aldicarb in the poisoning of domestic and wild animals of the Canary Islands (Spain). Sci. Total. Env. 505, 1093–1099.

Samouris, G., Antoniou, V., Zantopoulos, N., et al., 2007. Impact of toxic substances on animals of wild fauna in northern Greece. J. Env. Prot. Ecol. 8, 287–291.

Sánchez-Barbudo, I.S., Camarero, P.R., García-Montijano, M., et al., 2012a. Possible cantharidin poisoning of a great bustard (*Otis tarda*). Toxicon. 59, 100–103.

Sánchez-Barbudo, I.S., Camarero, P.R., Mateo, R., 2012b. Primary and secondary poisoning by anticoagulant rodenticides of non-target animals in Spain. Sci. Total Env. 420, 280–288.

Sharp, E.A., Melton, L.M., Taylor, et al., 2013. Pesticide poisoning of animals in 2012: a report of investigations in Scotland. <http://www.sasa.gov.uk/document-library/pesticide-poisoning-animals-2012> (accessed 21.12.16.).

Sharpe, R.T., Livesey, C.T., 2005. Surveillance of suspect animal toxicoses with potential food safety implications in England and Wales between 1990 and 2002. Vet. Rec. 157, 465–469.

Sharpe, R.T., Livesey, C.T., Davies, et al., 2006. Diazinon toxicity in sheep and cattle arising from the misuse of unlicensed and out-of-date products. Vet. Res. 159, 16–19.

Sutton, N.M., Bates, N., Campbell, A., 2009. Factors influencing outcome of Vitis vinifera (grapes, raisins, currants and sultanas) intoxication in dogs. Vet. Rec. 164, 430–431.

Tavernier, P., Cauwerts, K., Van Caelenberg, A., et al., 2004. Lead poisoning in anseriformes diagnosed in Flanders. Vlaams Diergen. Tijd. 73, 303–306.

Thomas, V.G., Guitart, R., 2010. Limitations of European Union policy and law for regulating use of lead shot and sinkers: comparisons with North American regulation. Env. Policy Govern. 20, 57–72.

Vandenbroucke, V., Van Pelt, H., De Backer, P., et al., 2010. Animal poisonings in Belgium: a review of the past decade. Vlaams Diergen. Tijd. 79, 259–268.

Vermeulen, H., Pardon, B., Croubels, S., et al., 2016. Oral ivermectin intoxication on a veal farm. Vlaams Diergen. Tijd. 85, 94–99.

VIDA, 2011. Veterinary Investigation Surveillance Report (VIDA): 2011 and 2004–2011. <http://webarchive.nationalarchives.gov.uk/20130822084033/http://www.defra.gov.uk/ahvla-en/publication/vida11/> (accessed 20.01.17.).

Votion, D.M., van Galen, G., Sweetman, L., et al., 2014. Identification of methylenecylclopropyl acetic acid in serum of European horses with atypical myopathy. Eq. Vet. J. 46, 146–149.

Wang, Y., Kruzik, P., Helsberg, A., et al., 2007. Pesticide poisoning in domestic and livestock in Austria: a 6 years retrospective study. For. Sci. Int. 169, 157–160.

Wray, J.D., 2008. Methaemoglobinaemia caused by hydroxycarbamide (hydroxyurea) ingestion in a dog. J. Small Anim. Pract. 49, 211–215.

Chapter 4

Epidemiology of Animal Poisonings in Asia

Pawan K. Gupta

INTRODUCTION

It is well known that human, animal, and wildlife populations are continuously exposed to environmental polluting agents that are harmful to health (Gupta, 1986). Among them are natural and manmade chemicals such as metals, pesticides, organic and inorganic substances, and animal venoms and toxins, including algal growth and industrial wastes to which domestic animals and wildlife are frequently exposed (Gupta, 2010a,b). In recent years, despite the increasing level of regulation in the use and sale of such products in Asia, their commercialization has intensified. Consequently, many cases of accidental poisoning have occurred. In addition, due to the continuous use of these poisons, accidental or otherwise, these cases have drastically increased all over the world, particularly in developing countries. There is an ongoing need for careful assessment of the risks caused by exposure to these chemicals. Information on the assessment of toxicity caused by these chemicals mainly comes from human and animal studies (Smith, 2001). However, some supporting information may also be obtained from clinical and in vitro studies. There are no reliable estimates of how many animals suffer from acute poisonings or due to long-term exposure. In general, epidemiology has been particularly helpful in the evaluation of working environments or other environments where exposure concentrations are relatively high. However, several factors limit the use of epidemiological studies by regulatory agencies (Gupta, 2010a). For example, it is difficult to define the causal elements in epidemiological investigations, particularly when complex exposures are involved. Another limitation is the frequent movement of animal populations and a large number of animal species available. As such, studies on one population under controlled conditions may be difficult to apply to predict health effects on another animal population.

In some developed countries such as the United States, human poison control centers also collect data on animals. In developing countries where there is hard evidence of poisoning including sporadic incidents involving livestock and pets, surveillance is conducted by the veterinary institutions/departments or by the wildlife departments of each country. However, a centralized veterinary poison control/information center does not exist in most countries in Asia. Therefore, in many Asian countries information related to animal poisoning is either unavailable or inadequate and refers only to isolated case reports when it does exist. Occasionally, epidemiological data on animal poisoning gathered by universities, research institutes, government institutions, or independent laboratories has been published in some local journals, which at times becomes difficult to trace. It is therefore easy to conclude that available data are inadequate to provide sound estimates of the real incidence of poisonings in animal populations and are very likely to be subjected to significant under-reporting (Litchfield, 2005; Gupta, 2016). This chapter focuses on some of the most important poisonous chemicals and plants in Asia and provides an overview of the poisoning episodes that have occurred in Asian countries.

PESTICIDES (AGROCHEMICALS AND FERTILIZERS)

Evidence is accumulating that malicious poisoning by pesticides is one of the most commonly used methods of killing animals in Asia, but the magnitude of the problem and percentage of deaths in each country is unknown. Among all pesticides, organophosphate (OP) insecticides poisons the insects and other animals, including birds, amphibians, and mammals (Gupta, 1986). This is followed by other pesticides, such as carbamate insecticides, zinc phosphide, or aluminum phosphide (fumigants) and rodenticides. Dogs were involved in cases of anticoagulant poisoning (over 60%) more than other domestic species. Occasionally, other pesticides such as the herbicide

Veterinary Toxicology. DOI: http://dx.doi.org/10.1016/B978-0-12-811410-0.00004-0

(paraquat) and fungicides have been involved in cases of animal poisonings. In food-producing animals, pesticides are again the most common class of suspected toxicants (Gunnell et al., 2007). Aluminum phosphide is a large, though under-reported, problem throughout the world, particularly in the Indian subcontinent. It is the second most common poison in India as well as in other developing countries of Asia. Death results from profound shock, myocarditis, and multiorgan failure. Such types of poisonings have also been reported in Iran. Several incidents of death in travelers in Thailand and other parts of Southeast Asia may have been caused by aluminum phosphide or chlorpyrifos because these compounds are highly toxic and dangerous to life (Sudakin, 2005). One of the reports indicates that the most commonly detected toxic substances in baits were OP and carbamate pesticides (48%), anticoagulant rodenticides (18%), zinc phosphide (12%), strychnine (9%), metaldehyde (8%), and others (5%) (Giorgi and Mengozzi, 2011).

In India there are some authentic reports of poisoning deaths in wild animals but most reports of deaths due to poisoning for large endangered wild mammalian and avian species are registered based on circumstantial evidence. Rapidly acting pesticides such as, OPs (malathion, parathion, phorate, and dimacron), carbamates, warfarin, and other anticoagulants, sodium fluoroacetate, and metaldehyde when consumed by wild beasts are undoubtedly fatal to them. Large carnivores, such as tigers, leopards, and lions have a poor sense of smell, and to kill them any such chemical poison is pasted on the live bait or poison containing capsules concealed in flesh meat that is arranged at the trap (Arora, 2003). To kill rhinoceros, poachers also use scattered poisoned food baits along their frequently used tracts or during heaves. Spreading of fresh dung of unrelated rhinoceros alongside the baited food to allure rhinoceros is also a common practice to poison these animals. A large number of such cases have been reported from various national wildlife parks in India (Arora, 2003).

There are several other reports where large carnivores are often primary targets for malicious poisonings. The effects of certain poisons do not stop with the target animal but also affects other species of wildlife in the form of secondary poisoning. One review describes incidences of secondary poisoning of a tiger (*Panthera tigris*) and a black panther (melanistic *Panthera pardus*) in the Nilgiri Biosphere Reserve. Wild boars (*Sus scrofa*), which are considered pests in horticultural plantations, were the primary targets in both cases and were poisoned using phorate, a highly toxic OP insecticide. Tigers and leopards hold significant positions in the upper most trophic level of the ecological pyramid and are grouped in schedule I of the Wildlife Protection Act of India. The tiger, as a species, is currently waging a grim battle of survival in the wild (Kalaivanan et al., 2011). In Singapore seven stray dogs were found killed, poisoned, or injured in Punggol on April 3, 2013. Over the next 2 days, several stray cats were slashed and a mini bull terrier in Changi Village had a leg cut off. On April 7, two cats, suspected of being beaten to death, were found in Tanglin Halt. A day later, a cat was found with glue on its fur. The number of reports of animal cruelty rose by a fifth last year, new figures reveal, and cases are continuing to rise due to poisoning (Anon, 2013a).

METALS

Lead (Pb)

Lead is a common cause of poisoning of domestic animals throughout the world. Pb is a heavy, low-melting, bluish-gray metal that occurs naturally in the Earth's crust. Affected animals die or perform poorly after accidentally poisoned. Gradual poisoning may also occur in areas with heavy industrial pollution (Gupta, 2016). Reports from India indicate that calves are more sensitive than adults because they are curious feeders, and both milk and milk substitutes increase the amount of Pb absorbed by calves. Suckling animals can also receive Pb in the milk. Varying degrees of Pb poisoning was recorded in cows and buffaloes near a primary Pb-zinc smelter. Affected animals had a history of clinical signs characterized by head pressing, violent movement, blindness, and salivation. These animals had considerably high Pb levels in their blood and milk. Animals from other places without the history of clinical signs suggestive of Pb poisoning recorded lower blood Pb levels than the affected animals; however, their blood Pb was higher than that reported for cattle in rural and urban areas. Affected animals also carried high levels of cadmium (Cd) in blood and milk. These values were considerably higher than those for rural cattle in India. The findings indicated varying degrees of exposure of animals to Pb and Cd in the vicinity of the smelter (Dwivedi et al., 2001).

In Japan a survey carried out between 1994 and 1997 indicated fifteen (4%) of 363 birds harvested during and after hunting seasons had one Pb pellet each in the proventriculus and gizzard. In addition, 32 (34%) of 93 swans (*Cygnus* sp.) and 2 of 14 geese (*Anser* sp.) found dead from various wetlands had lesions consistent with Pb poisoning. One to nine swans suspected of having toxicosis from ingestion of Pb shot were found dead each year. Twenty-seven (84%) of the 32 swans exposed to Pb were found in Hokkaido Prefecture indicating that that Pb poisoning remains a serious threat to waterfowl in Japan (Ochiai et al., 1999).

The Steller's Sea-Eagle (*Haliaeetus pelagicus*) and the White-tailed Eagle (*Haliaeetus albicilla*) are among the largest eagles. The total population of the Steller's Sea-Eagle is estimated at 5000–6000 on the island of Hokkaido. Pb poisoning of Steller's Sea-Eagles in Japan was first confirmed in 1996. By 2007, 129 Steller's and White-tailed Eagles died from Pb poisoning. Necropsies and radiographs also revealed pieces of Pb from rifle bullets and from shotgun slugs to be present in the digestive tracts of poisoned eagles, providing evidence that a source of Pb was spent ammunition from Pb-contaminated Sika deer carcasses. Reacting to the eagle poisoning issue, Hokkaido authorities have regulated the use of Pb rifle bullets since 2000. Despite the overwhelming evidence that Pb ammunition is toxic to wildlife and people and the broad support for eliminating its use, it remains widely used by hunters (Saito, 2009). In the United States, Pb poisoning is on the decrease due to government regulations to remove Pb from house paint in 1978. However, dogs can still be exposed to Pb through roofing materials, rug padding, linoleum, and other aged household materials (https://www.vetary.com/dog/condition/lead-poisoning). It may be worth mentioning that California, in 2013, passed the first state wide phase-out of Pb ammunition for all forms of hunting (Anon, 2016).

Mercury (Hg)

Hg toxicosis has been reported in cats, pigs, calves, horses, and laboratory animals (rats, mice, mink, ferrets, and guinea pigs) but rarely in dogs. Clinical signs and lesions of Hg intoxication depend on the species affected, dose obtained, route of administration, chronicity of exposure, and the chemical form of the Hg involved (Gupta, 2010b).

A sporadic outbreak of a curious disease occurred among dairy cattle, from early February to late May 1955, in Monbetsu District, Kitami Subprefecture of Hokkaido in Japan (Katherine et al., 2010). This disease was due to poisoning by ingested linseed meal treated with mercurial fungicide, "Ceresan." The characteristic symptoms of this disease were dyspnea and depilation; out of 29 cases, eight died while two were slaughtered. The general symptoms were fever attack, salivation, diarrhea, bloody feces, depression and anorexia, lacrimation, decrease in milk production, and cramps. In addition, partial and diffusive depilation, eczema, and swelling of the skin accompanied by itchiness on the entire body surface were found. Bronchial catarrh was observed in about half of the cases, especially; it was distinct in the severe or moderate ones. Anemia on all mucous membranes and petechial hemorrhages on the nasal and vaginal mucous membranes, cardiac disturbance, and swelling of lymph-nodes were also noted in the severe cases. In some instances, epistaxis, bloody milk, and nephritis were also observed. In another incidents, renal problems have been reported in dogs (Farrar et al., 1994).

Arsenic (As)

As poisoning due to contamination of groundwater is one of the most important causes of heavy metal poisoning in domestic animals in several countries. However, other sources of intoxication include dips, sprays, powders, or vegetation contaminated by pesticides containing As (Selby et al., 1977).

Dogs and cattle are intoxicated more frequently than other animals; yet sporadic instances of poisoning have been observed in sheep, cats, horses, and pigs. Reports from industrial cattle farm in Iran indicated poisoning is either peracute, acute, or chronic in nature. Frequently the initial and only indication that a severe problem exists with peracute poisoning in a cattle herd is dead animals. Chronic intoxications are also observed in cattle (Bazargani et al., 2007). In two other incidences, acute intoxication of As poisoning has been reported in young dog and sheep. As is a severe alimentary tract irritant in domestic animals, and treatment in most instances are primarily symptom-based and supportive (Selby et al., 1977; Javad et al., 2013).

Copper (Cu)

Cu poisoning is common in various parts of Asia. Acute Cu toxicity results from ingestion of high Cu feeds, Cu salts, pesticides, poultry litter, and other high Cu intakes of 20–100 mg/kg in sheep and young calves, and 200–800 mg/kg in adult cattle. Chronic Cu toxicity occurs when high levels of Cu are ingested over a period of time but at doses below the acutely toxic level. Sheep are the most susceptible species to chronic Cu toxicity because their liver cells have a high affinity for Cu and they excrete Cu into the bile at a very low rate, leading to a build-up of liver Cu concentration over time. One of the most common causes of toxicity in sheep is the accidental feeding of feedstuffs intended for other livestock. Field investigation of one closed herd of 400 mixed-breed dairy goats from India was examined because of a decrease in milk production and increase in mortality rate. Nine animals had died within a 1-month period. Goats were found to have been fed a mineral mix containing 3050 ppm Cu for 9 months prior to the onset of Cu toxicosis. Clinical signs were evident only in lactating goats and included anorexia and recumbency. In the most severely affected goats, signs progressed to neurologic abnormalities and death (Cornish et al., 2007; Badiye et al., 2013).

NONMETALS AND METALLOIDS

Selenium (Se)

Se has chemical and physical properties intermediate between metals and nonmetals and is similar to those of sulfur, As, and tellurium (Khanal et al., 2010). It acts as a bio accumulator which means plants and animals retain the element in greater concentrations than are present in the environment and the element can be bioconcentrated by 200–6000 times (Gupta, 1988; Dhillon and Dhillon, 1991a,b). The disease is more common in southern parts of Asia, in times of drought or where less irrigation water is predisposed to high soil Se levels and a greater uptake of Se by plants (Ghosh et al., 1993; Kunli et al., 2004; Yadav et al., 2005; Tiwary et al., 2006). The disease is commonly known as Se toxicosis. The poisoning is more common in forage-eating animals such as cattle, sheep, horses, and other herbivores that may graze Se-containing plants (Dhillon and Dhillon, 1991a,b). In acute toxicosis, the blood and serum Se concentrations were $>3-4$ ppm, and in chronic toxicosis $>1-2$ ppm. Chronic selenosis was often reported in winter season with the symptoms of hair loss, cracks on skin, hooves and horns, leading to elongation and sloughing of hooves, lameness, ataxia, and recumbency (Gupta et al., 1982). In an experimental study with buffalo calves, adverse effects appeared when the whole blood Se concentrations increased above 2 μg/mL, with mortality occurring when blood levels exceeded 3.4 μg/mL (Deore et al., 2002; Deore et al., 2005).

The disease is commonly known as alkali disease in cattle and horses and exhibit weight loss, hair loss (especially obvious in the mane and tail), and lameness in all four limbs (Gupta, 1988). The coronary bands are painful to palpation and the bands may separate with excretion of necrotic tissue from the defect. In severe cases the hoof wall sloughed off. The other form of disease is known as "blind staggers" (commonly observed in cattle and sheep), animals developed a staggery gait, wandered aimlessly, and "head pressed." Other symptoms included nausea, vomiting, nail discoloration, brittleness, hair loss, fatigue, irritability, and foul breath odor (often described as "garlic breath") (Dhillon and Dhillon, 1991a,b; Ghimire, 2012).

Nitrate and Nitrite

Nitrate can accumulate in many crop and pasture plants, weeds, and forages such as berseem (*Trifolium alexandrinum*), bajra (*Pennisetum glaucum*), maize (*Zea mays*), oats (*Avena sativa*), sorghum (*Sorghum vulgare*), and toriya (*Brassica napus*). Many species are susceptible to nitrate and nitrite poisoning, but there is considerable difference in susceptibility. Ruminants are much more susceptible to nitrate poisoning than monogastric animals (Gupta, 2016). In India, there are several documented cases of nitrate poisoning in cattle but it is rare in horses. The disease is also very common in other parts of Asia. Most cases involve ingestion of nitrate/nitrite-contaminated water, nitrate fertilizer directly, or forage or hay grown in the area of a previous fertilizer spill. In one incidence 23 cases of nitrate poisoning were diagnosed in a dairy herd due to consumption of green grass, mainly alfalfa, which was irrigated with a municipally treated wastewater. Five cows were found dead and seven fetuses were aborted. Methemoglobin was increased while hemoglobin was decreased. A clinical picture included difficulty in breathing, shivering, and brown discoloration of the mucous membranes of the vulva, vagina, and conjunctiva. The postmortem findings included dark brown carcasses, nonclotted blood in the dilated vessels. Cardiac hemorrhages, pulmonary, and rumen congestion; edema and hyperemia of the mucous membranes of the abomasums and small intestine were noticed in all examined animals. The postmortem examination of aborted fetuses revealed severe ascites and hydrothorax. Affected animals responded well to the treatment with methylene blue (Al-Qudah et al., 2009). In another incidence of poisoning at Kopargaon (Maharashtra), India, fourteen crossbred animals died within 1 day and the source was detected to be fodder of Bajari. All available fodders in eight farms were tested and were found to be positive for nitrate/nitrites (Rawte, 2012).

Nitrate/nitrite poisoning in buffalo, cattle, goat and sheep has also been reported from several other southern parts of Asia (Shinozaki, 1975; Sidhu et al., 2008; Al-Qudah et al., 2009; Sidhu et al., 2011). Although poisoning in monogastric animals is rare, in India, in one form a number of poisoning cases have been reported in pigs, wherein several of them died within very short period. Young pigs are more at risk of nitrate/nitrite induced toxicity because they have microflora that can convert nitrates into nitrites. This might be the reason for the sudden death of eight young piglets within 12 h of feed intake and 12 severely affected young ones that died despite treatment (Mahajan et al., 2007; Sidhu et al., 2014; Susan, 2016). In another incidence one rare outbreak of nitrate poisoning in combination with classical swine fever in a small pig farm has also been reported (Sidhu et al., 2014). These findings do indicate nitrate poisoning in pigs is more common in India than other countries of the world (Vyt, 2006; Rathnapraba et al., 2012).

Fluorosis

Chronic exposure to fluoride in groundwater causes adverse health problems not only in humans, but also in various species of domestic animals in the form of fluorosis. The primary manifestations are mottling of teeth (dental fluorosis) and andosteosclerosis of the skeleton (skeletal fluorosis). Besides these maladies, nonskeletal fluorosis or toxic effects of chronic fluoride exposure in soft tissues, such as gastrointestinal discomforts, neurological disorders, impaired endocrine and reproductive functions, teratogenic effects, apoptosis, genotoxic effects, excitotoxicity, etc., have also been reported in man as well as in domestic animals. Acute toxicity arises by inhalation of fluorine smoke, vapors, dust from volcanic eruptions, and dust from industries that use aluminum, Cu, enamel, glass, iron, steel, superphosphate, etc. It also may be due to accidental ingestion of large amounts of fluorine (Susan, 2016). Some Asian countries, such as India, Pakistan and neighboring countries, have a very high prevalence of fluorosis. An epidemiological survey revealed the prevalence of fluorosis in bovines in Andhra Pradesh and Uttar Pradesh (Dwivedi et al., 1997), Punjab (Sharma et al., 1997), Rajasthan (Choubisa, 1999), Karnataka (Muralidhara et al., 2000), Orissa (Maiti et al., 2003), Bihar, and Madhya Pradesh in India (Ranjan et al., 2009; Choubisa et al., 2012). Most of the animals suffered with problems after consumption of water from bore well and pastures with high fluorine content (Botha et al., 1993). Different surveys of bovine population in brick kiln areas showed signs of lameness having "knee posture," reduced appetite, loss in general body condition, loss of hair with stiff rough skin coat, poor performance, anemia, mottled teeth, enlarged mandible, painful protuberances of metacarpal, and facial bones were recorded. On the basis of clinical and circumstantial evidence, and presence of high fluoride content the problem was confirmed to be fluorosis, possibly due to environmental pollution with fluorine-bearing smoke arising from the large number of brick kilns (Swarup and Singh, 1989; Singh and Swarup, 1994). There was decrease in milk yield in buffaloes and in cattle (Jagadish et al., 1998). In several northern parts of India such as Bihar and Rajasthan, dental mottling, lameness, higher respiration and heart rates, anemia, reproductive disorders (prolonged postpartum anestrus) and increased incidence of vaginal prolapse, cases of repeat breeding due to fluorosis in cattle has come to lime light (Sharma et al., 1997; Patra et al., 2000; Swarup et al., 2001). A few other surveys of fluoride in drinking water and incidence of dental fluorosis in cows and buffaloes in Madhya Pradesh and other parts of India revealed high level of fluoride concentration in adult buffaloes (Ranjan et al., 2009). About 40% of adult and 36% of young cattle were found to have dental fluorosis (Table 4.1) with light-to-deep yellowish brown teeth, with striated and horizontal lines starting from the base of teeth. Buffaloes have a greater severity of dental and skeletal fluorosis than in cows. Young calves of both cow and buffalo were more sensitive than the adult ones (Dwivedi et al., 1997; Narwaria and Saksena, 2012). At a fluoride concentration of 4.0 ppm in water, 100% of calves, 65.6% of buffaloes, and 61.0% of cows were affected with dental fluorosis to some degree. Intermittent lameness was observed in animals above 7 years of age (Choubisa, 1998; Choubisa, 1999). Recently chronic toxic effects of fluoride in the form of osteo-dental and nonskeletal fluorosis were observed in 99 domesticated cattle (*Bos taurus*) living in Chani village, in the Bikaner district of Rajasthan (India), located in the Indian Thar Desert. Affected animals with dental fluorosis also showed signs of skeletal fluorosis as intermittent lameness and snapping sound in legs, wasting of body muscles, and excessive periosteal exostoses in the mandibles, ribs, metacarpus, and metatarsus regions. In these animals, colic, intermittent diarrhea, excessive urination, irregular reproductive cycles, repeated abortions, and stillbirths were also found as signs of nonskeletal fluorosis (Choubisa et al., 2011; Choubisa et al., 2014).

TABLE 4.1 Prevalence of Dental Fluorosis in Domestic Animals in Madhya Pradesh (India)

Animals	Number of Animals	Dental Fluorosis
Adult Animals		
Buffaloes (>1 year)	75	31 (41.34%)
Cows (>1 year)	25	10 (40.00%)
Young Animals		
Buffalo (calves) (<1 year)	36	12 (36.12%)
Cow (calves) (<1 year)	14	05 (36.72%)

Source: Data from Narwaria, Y.S., Saksena, D.N., 2012. Incidence of dental fluorosis in domestic animals of Shivepuri, Madhya Pradesh, India. J. Environ. Res. Develop. 7: 426–430.

DRUGS AND RELATED COMPOUNDS

As indicated earlier, animals are exposed to potentially toxic agents on a daily basis. Drug poisonings in animals occur commonly due to off-label use of medicines, wrong dosage, negligence, accidental ingestion, and deliberate poisonings. Toxicity of veterinary drugs may become evident also in therapeutic doses when adverse effects may occur (Siroka and Svobodova, 2013).

Each year there are more than 100,000 cases of companion animals poisoning in the United States alone. Some of the most dangerous companion animal poisons are foods and therapeutic use medications we use on a daily basis. Companion animals poisoning symptoms can include gastrointestinal and neurological problems, cardiac and respiratory distress, coma, and even death. Some of the most common and harmful substances/medications that poison companion animals include: antiinflammatory and pain medications, over-the-counter medications (acetaminophen, ibuprofen, naproxen, herbal, and nutraceutical products, and drugs of abuse (cocaine, cannabis, methamphetamine) (Berny et al., 2010).

Methamphetamine abuse has undergone a dramatic worldwide increase. Because of its increasing illicit availability, together with legitimate use in human medicine, accidental or intentional, exposure to methamphetamine in dogs is becoming a more likely scenario (Pei and Zhang, 2014). In rare instances, use of Baytril (enrofloxacin) antibacterial tablets for animal use in cats has been associated with retinal toxicity. Federal law in the United States restricts this drug to use by or on the order of prescribed Baytril (enrofloxacin) antibacterial tablets. Federal law prohibits the extra label use of this drug in food-producing animals (Bayer, 2014).

Due to the lack of a central reporting agency for animal poisonings in most of the Asian countries, epidemiological studies have not been documented on poisoning cases in animals. Therefore, it becomes extremely difficult to review the full picture of animal poisonings. However, information available from personal experience and reporting of isolated cases in newspapers are cited. For example, in Pakistan, India and Nepal, diclofenac, an antiinflammatory drug commonly prescribed for arthritis and pain in human beings and a veterinary drug administered to cattle, caused a decline of almost 99% in vulture populations that fed on the contaminated carcasses. The drug pushed three species to the brink of extinction in South Asia. Unlike DDT, which devastated populations of birds of prey, diclofenac does not accumulate in the tissues of livestock or birds. But for the vultures, it is a poison. The drug, the researchers concluded, "may also be responsible for vulture declines in the rest of the Indian subcontinent wherever diclofenac is used for the treatment of livestock." The Peregrine Fund, the researchers, and other organizations said they intend to push for a ban on the drug in veterinary use in India, Nepal, and Pakistan (Gorman, 2004).

In some developing countries discerning veterinary doctors scrupulously use tranquilizers and drugs following precautions prescribed by their manufacturers. Even then a drug reaction at times in some animals, either an overdose or individual idiosyncrasy, cannot be ruled out. Secondly, there is no policy to survey and evaluate adverse drug effects (ADEs) or pharmacovigilance program for veterinary medicines. Therefore, essential information such as frequency, severity of treated animal ADEs, and reliable data about frequent ADE-producing drugs remains unknown. However, there is one report from India that does indicate the safety and efficacy of veterinary drugs and biologicals in cattle, goats, dogs, and poultry. Survey indicated that more than 37% ADEs were related to antimicrobials, antiparasitic, and antiinflammatory agents. A further 27% of ADEs were due to vitamins and feed additives. Two percent of ADEs were observed in FMD vaccination in cattle, and canine parvo vaccine in dogs. In poultry, tiamulin and salinomycin ADEs induced serious mortality (Sarathchandra et al., 2014). The ADEs in animals have been summarized in Table 4.2.

TABLE 4.2 Summary of Adverse Drug Effects in Animals

Drugs/Vaccines	Percent
Antibiotics/antimicrobials, and antiinflammatory agents	36
Antiparasitics	19
Vitamins and feed additives	26
NSAIDs	7
Antihistamines	1
Vaccines	2
Miscellaneous drugs (Atropine, triamcinolone, oxytocin, livodex)	9

In addition, there are some authentic reports of severe ADEs or poisonings in wild and zoo animals of India. The drugs with most frequently encountered problems of poisonings/ADEs include overdosage of succinylcholine, phencyclidine HCL, etorphine HCL, tetramisole, combination of xylazine with acepromazine, and ketamine (which causes photosensitization in elephants) (Arora, 2003).

MYCOTOXINS

Mycotoxins are toxic byproducts (secondary metabolites) produced by fungi. There are 400 mycotoxins produced by 350 species of fungi. Currently, some mycotoxins, namely, aflatoxins, ochratoxin A, fumonisins, certain trichothecenes, zearalenone, and one of the fungi, fusarium, are considered the most serious threats to humans, animals, and birds due to their potential of carcinogenic, hepatogenic, teratogenic, mutagenic and other serious effects (Singh, 1988). In several Asian countries, numerous outbreaks of mycotoxicosis in animals and birds indicate heavy losses. Dogs are more vulnerable to ochratoxin A. Mortality due to facial eczema in sheep may reach to 60% (Pal, 2007; Pal et al., 2015). The economy of poultry industry is heavily affected due to wide exposure to mycotoxins leading to mortalities in birds. The economic losses are primarily due to the decreased growth rate, feed conversion efficacy, carcass yield, carcass quality, and increased susceptibility to other diseases. In addition, the possible presence of toxic residues in poultry products (egg, meat) that enter into the food chain may have potential risks due to their detrimental effects on human health (Patil et al., 2014).

Raising buffaloes and cattle in Pakistan, Nepal, and India is one way of augmenting the financial resources of village people. These animals are mainly raised on rice and wheat Straw, which are of poor nutritional quality. Rice and wheat plants, when infested by fungus *Fusarium* and in association with other fungi species, are responsible for Deg nala disease in Pakistan, Nepal, and India (Ghimire, 2012). This disease not only causes severe health problems, it can cause significant economic losses as a result of decreased production exacerbated by reduced growth rate, mortality, and poor animal performance. It causes necrosis and gangrene of the dependent parts in cows and buffaloes (*Bubalus bubalis* L.). A number of cases were recorded stemming from a monsoon rain water stream in the area of Murdike (Sheikhpura District) near Nala Deg in Pakistan (Shirlow, 1939). Subsequently, widespread occurrence of the disease has been reported from rice growing areas of Indo-Pakistan border. The diseased animals were invariably weak; ulcerative wounds and gangrene developed on the limbs and other dependent parts of the body. Almost all cases showed gangrene of the tail, which was shriveled and cold to the touch. Invariably, one or both ears showed signs of dry gangrene. In some cases, the muzzle and even the tip of the tongue became gangrenous and were shed. One or more hooves showed lesions in varying stages of development, legs were swollen up to the knee; hair was denuded and inflammatory changes set in. Later, wounds appeared on the coronet, fetlock, pastern, and knee, and in the hock region. In very advanced cases the lower regions of the feet became gangrenous, hooves were shed and bones were exposed. The gangrenous portions of the tail, tips of the ears, tongue and other affected parts of the body, dropped off, although wounds healed in the course of time (Ifran, 1971; Kalra and Bhatia, 1990; Dhillon, 1973; Ifran and Maqbool, 1986; Karki et al., 2013).

Epizootiological studies carried out during the years 1968–78, involving 370 herds from 136 villages of Haryana, India, showed the incidence of the disease varied from year to year, assuming serious proportions in certain years. The morbidity and mortality rates were 61.61% and 13.93%, respectively, in buffaloes, and 13.49% and 2.41% in cattle, with no sex and age differences (Kalra and Bhatia, 1990). Several incidences of gangrenous syndrome/Deg nala disease has been recorded in a large number of buffaloes and cows in other parts of the country, such as Murshidabad district of West Bengal, India. *Fusarium* spp. had been isolated from the moldy paddy straw that was fed to the animals. There was a reduction in the incidence of the disease following withdrawal of the moldy padded straw. Histopathological examination showed necrosis and loss of architectural details in the skin (Sikdar et al., 2000; Dandapat et al., 2011). All the cattle that were showing clinical symptoms were treated with Antidegnala liquor 5 mL s/c followed by 2 mL daily for next 10 days. The animals receiving the treatment recovered promptly (Karki et al., 2013).

Several cases of systemic mycosis have been reported in Japan. A 10-year study showed that 45 of 692 cattle aged 6 months or older had systemic mycosis. Out of these, 38 had alimentary mycosis with lesions in various sites were: rumen (73.7), omasum (71.1), abomasum (34.2), reticulum (21.1), intestine (15.8), omasoabomasal orifice (7.9), and tongue (2.6). Infections in both the fore stomachs and abomasum occurred in 31.6%; mucormycosis was found in 94.7% and aspergillosis in 31.6%; 26.3% (10 cattle) had complicated infections with both Mucorales and Aspergillus, and eight of these animals had mixed lesions of both mucormycosis and aspergillosis. Macroscopically, focal hemorrhagic necrosis was seen in all 38 cattle. Histologically, thrombosis, coagulative necrosis and hyphae typical of the order Mucorales or of *Aspergillus* spp. were found. Many of the cattle were also affected by ruminal acidosis–inducing factors (ruminal atony 81.6%, mastitis 63.2%, "downer cow syndrome" 57.9%, and parturition 50.0%). The study revealed that involvement of toxigenic fungi and their associated mycotoxins are common in various parts of Asia (Chihaya et al., 1992; Antonissen et al., 2013).

HOUSEHOLD PRODUCTS

Information on potential poisonings due to household products in animal species is largely lacking. In general, companion animals share our domestic environment; they are highly exposed to household products. They are exposed to drugs, domestic chemicals, common solvents (used in paint and paint solvents), and pesticides. Exposure to these substances usually results in very severe poisoning, at least in dogs, with a high mortality rate. Other common household substances include detergents caustics (bleach, strong acids and bases), cosmetics, fuels, ethylene glycol, zootoxins, petroleum products, kerosene and fertilizer, which results in moderately severe cases with digestive disorders (Gupta, 2014).

Poisoning or suspected poisoning as a result of ingestion of toxic ornamental plant products is a relatively common occurrence, and cats appear to be more sensitive and more at risk than dogs, presumably because they tend to chew on plant leaves. A few major plant species involved in poisoning of companion animals are *Liliaceae* and *Araceae*; oleander (*Nerium oleander*), castor bean (*Ricinus communis*), and Jimson weed (*Datura stramonium*). Rarely other ornamental plants such as dumbcane (*Dieffenbachia* spp.), ficus (*Ficus benjamina*), pittosporo (*Pittosporum tobira*), poinsettia (*Euphorbia pulcherrima*), rhododendron (*Rhododendrum hirsutum*), tiger lily (*Lilium tigrinum*) jessamine (*Jasminum officinalis*) and tansy ragwort (*Senecio jacobaea*) have been reported. Oleander has been responsible for poisoning in dogs (Berny et al., 2010).

In certain Asian countries, kerosene is commonly used because solid fuels—biomass (wood, agricultural residues, and animal dung) and coal—are major household energy sources, often burned indoors without chimneys or smoke hoods. Kerosene use for cooking and lighting remains widespread. Globally, households still rely on kerosene or other liquid fuels for lighting (Mills, 2005; Fullerton et al., 2008). There seems to have been little, if any, systematic study of the exposure implications and hazards of household kerosene combustion. In the absence of any systematic survey, the extent to which these fuels cause long-term damage, including morbidity and mortality in companion animals, is currently unclear (Ritchie et al., 2003; American Petroleum Institute, 2010). The scarcity of adequate epidemiologic and exposure investigations as well as the potential for short- and long-term exposure to household products and chemicals suggest a need for agencies to collect epidemiological data on human beings and animals (Nicholas et al., 2012).

METHYL ISOCYANATE (UNION CARBIDE PLANT DISASTER IN BHOPAL)

Thirty-two years ago, on the night of December 2, 1984, at approximately 0.30, an accident at the Union Carbide pesticide plant in Bhopal, India, released at least 30 tons of a highly toxic gas called methyl isocyanate as well as a number of other poisonous gases. The pesticide plant was surrounded by shanty towns, leading to more than 600,000 people being exposed to the deadly gas cloud that night. The gases stayed low to the ground, causing victims throats and eyes to burn, inducing nausea, and many deaths. An estimated 8000 people (official figure 2500) and 4000 animals died within minutes of exposure to the gas, and a rough estimate of 15,000 animals suffered toxic effects but survived (Mehta et al., 1994). The breakup of human and animal deaths is summarized in Table 4.3 (Gupta, 2004).

Thirty-two years later, toxic material remains, and many of those who were exposed to the gas have given birth to physically and mentally disabled children. There has, however, been no long-term epidemiological survey that conclusively proves that birth defects are directly related to the drinking of the contaminated water or toxic agents of the explosion are involved (Gupta, 2004).

The acute toxicity of inhaled MIC or its reaction products was devastating: most fatalities occurred during the first week. The common acute symptoms were associated with respiratory, ophthalmic, and psychological morbidities. The cause of death was pulmonary edema and secondary respiratory infections (bronchitis and bronchial pneumonia). Epidemiological studies in humans revealed maternal-fetal deaths, gynecological disturbances and spontaneous abortion, higher incidence of abnormal uterine bleeding, evidence of chromosomal aberrations and genetic defects, and suppression of cell mediated immunity. However, there is no report available on an epidemiological survey on long-term adverse effects of MIC in animals (Gupta, 2004).

TABLE 4.3 Deaths Due to MIC and Reaction Products During the Bhopal Gas Tragedy

Deaths	Numbers
Human deaths	2500[a]
Buffalo	790
Cows	270
Goats	483
Dogs	90
Horses	23

[a]*Unofficial figure.*
Source: Data from Gupta, P.K., 2004. Pesticide exposure – Indian scene. Toxicology 198, 83–90.

FEED ASSOCIATED TOXICANTS

Cross-contamination, resulting from the carry-over of undesirable trace amounts of pharmacologically active ingredients from a medicated/supplemented feed to a nonmedicated/nonsupplemented feed, may occur at different stages of the production process, during the storage, and transport but also on the farm (Gupta, 2006; Abdulkaf et al., 2015). The consumption of a feed, containing a pharmacologically active ingredient due to cross-contamination, by a nontarget species such as the laying hen and production animals may generate unwanted residual concentrations of these substances in edible matrices.

Ionophores such as monensin, lasalocid, narasin, and salinomycin are frequently used as feed additives and coccidiostats for cattle, sheep, and poultry (Kamashi et al., 2004, 2005). Contamination of feed with antibiotics, pesticides, metals, and with other toxins is quite common (Muhammad et al., 2009; Nisha, 2008). Although comparative toxicity was difficult to estimate, most cross-comparisons within and across species indicates relative toxicities of the ionophores from lowest to highest were salinomycin < lasalocid < or = narasin < or = monensin (but lasalocid < monensin) < maduramicin (Oehme and Pickrell, 1999). There is some evidence to suggest that because of the ubiquitous presence of dioxins in the environment, the threat of dioxin contamination posed by feed ingredients may originate from many different sources. Mycotoxins can concentrate in dried distillers' grains with solubles (DDGS) during the processing of grains for ethanol production. They also concentrate in cereal bran. Cadmium is a ubiquitous contaminant that is present in many feed and feed ingredients, in particular minerals and forages grown near smelting and mining areas. As and Hg are heavy metals that are widespread in the environment and can be found in many feeds, in particular in feeds of marine origin. Pb is also a ubiquitous contaminant (Swarup et al., 2005). Veterinary drug residues may be found in food products as a result of the carryover of veterinary drugs in feed during feed production. The continued presence of organochlorine pesticides in the environment, as well as their ongoing use in some countries, can cause exposure through food as a result of accumulation in the fat tissues of animals that have been fed on contaminated feed (Gupta, 1986). Contaminated feed containing salmonella has a direct impact on transmission to humans via food of animal origin. Some endoparasites of animals, such as *Echinococcus*, *Toxoplasma gondii*, Cysticercus, and *Trichinella*, present a risk to human health, and ingestive stages can contaminate animal feeds. There are many toxic plants found in grasslands around Asia. Their toxic effects, and the potential presence of some toxic compounds in milk and meat, are well documented. However, there is a lack of information about metabolic rates, residues, maximum residue limits (MRL), and average daily intakes (ADI) for these different toxicants (NRC, 2005). One report from Bangladesh indicates that the pleuromutilin antibiotic tiamulin is known to produce a negative interaction in broilers when administered in combination with several ionophore anticoccidials, such as salinomycin (Islam et al., 2008). This risk pathway of feed associate contaminants can be controlled by following Good Agricultural Practices (OIE, 2007; FAO/WHO, 2007).

PLASTIC BAGS

The presence of plastic bags in the Bay of Biscay (in western Europe) over 120 miles from shore in waters over 4000 m in depth have been observed. A whale dies in an urban harbor and, on being autopsied, reveals a stomach full of plastics. Whale species in particular are highly susceptible to swallowing plastic bags, as they are believed to strongly resemble their target prey, squid. Other species of large whales, which take large mouthfuls of water during feeding, also take in plastic bags by accident and hence are also at risk (Anon, 2014). In developing countries such as Pakistan, Nepal, India and several other countries in Asia and other countries of the world, severe impact of garbage on man and environment is talked about quite often, but it's far more lethal brunt on animals almost always misses the headlines. A cow eats a plastic bag from the River Ganges in India; hundreds of cows die annually from choking on plastic bags containing vegetable waste. For those living on the coasts, a mere walk on the beach can give anyone insight into how staggering our addiction to plastic has become as bottles, cans, bags, lids and straws (just to name a few) are ever-present. For other areas that insight is more poignant, as the remains of animal carcasses can frequently be observed; the plastic debris that many of them ingested or became entangled in still visible long after their death. Sadly, an overwhelming amount of plastic pollution isn't even visible to the human eye, with much of the pollution occurring out at sea or on a microscopic level (Gregory, 2008).

Several countries of Asia have an open garbage system, which means open garbage bins on the roads overflowing with stinking waste. Dogs, monkeys, pigs, rats and cows eat whatever they can find to survive. The numbers of stray dogs, rats, and monkeys are equal to the amount of garbage on which they feed and multiply. In cities and towns, large numbers of cows on the roads eat from garbage bins, foraging for fruit, vegetable leftovers, anything edible and anything smelling like food. Since plastic bags have invaded our lives, almost all garbage and food waste is disposed in plastic bags. These bags spill out either on the road or from municipality dustbins. Since the plastic bags are knotted at the mouth, cows, unable to undo the knot, eat food leftovers including the plastic. Slowly, over time, they build up a huge amount of plastic inside their stomachs. It gets entangled with different materials and it becomes hard like cement inside their rumens, which is the first belly of the cow apart from the plastic completely choking the digestive system of the cow and causing excruciating pain to the animal. Consequently, plastic residues enter the human food chain through dairy and animal products.

Animals, especially cattle, ingest the plastic and develop complications, which finally result in their death. Usually there are no reports except if cattle deaths have medico-legal implications to settle compensation claims. Otherwise, there are no figures of the number of animals dying from plastic and toxic waste. A lot of cases go unreported. The rumen is one of the four compartments of the cattle's digestive system. The feed enters from the reticulum to the rumen, omasum and finally the abomasum (true stomach). But when the plastic in the reticulum blocks the feed from entering the rumen, suffocation occurs and the animal dies (Anon, 2013b). Rumenotomy, the surgical removal of plastic up to 70 kg from the cow, has been reported (Anon, 2014).

OTHER TOXINS

A number of other toxins such as botulinum, algae (cyanobacteria toxic blooms), venomous bites, strychnine, HCN, aconite, and other phytotoxins (deadly herbal poisons), zinc phosphide, chlorinated hydrocarbon insecticides, and zootoxins, such as caterpillars, have been reported to cause poisoning in wildlife (Arora, 2003). Several toxins are known to involve domestic animals, stray cattle, sheep, goats, dogs, monkeys, poultry, pigs, and wild animals. Botulism outbreaks in poultry, sheep, and cattle are fairly common. Algae are the cause of mass mortality of wild animals and birds in inland water. Venomous bites by poisonous snakes, insects, mites and scabies have been reported from time to time in almost all species of animals (Gupta, 2016). Several cases of alopecia, with active crushed dermatitis, and an accumulation of thick scales and fissuring of the skin, have been reported in monkeys and other animals. Sarcoptes (Scabies) and other mites can also affect macaques apart from domestic animals, and other wild animals such as foxes, wolfs, and gorillas (Nagarajan et al., 2004; Sudhakara Reddy et al., 2014; Sivajothi and Sudhakara Reddy, 2015).

RADIATION EFFECTS OF THE HIROSHIMA AND NAGASAKI ATOMIC BOMBS

The first operational atomic bomb Nicknamed "Little Boy" was dropped on Hiroshima, Japan, August 6, 1945. There was probably a 40% death rate (140,000) of the 350,000 people estimated to have been in Hiroshima at the time. In Nagasaki, on which the second operational atomic bomb was dropped, nicknamed "Fat Man," was dropped August 9; about 73,884 were killed and 74,909 injured. Among those who survived, the long-term effects of radiation sickness, genetic and chromosome injury, and mental trauma have been catastrophic, even unborn children having been stunted in growth and sometimes mentally retarded. The bomb not only harmed people but animals as well. The number of animals died during these operations is unlimited. The surviving animals showed severe after effects. For example, burnt hip skin was common in horses that survived during the incidents (Anon, 1981).

CONCLUDING REMARKS AND FUTURE DIRECTIONS

Animals are exposed to potentially toxic agents on a daily basis but the lack of a central reporting agency for animal poisonings makes epidemiological study difficult. With no mandated reporting, many suspected poisoning cases are managed by the attending veterinarian and forgotten. Poisonings are a serious cause of morbidity and mortality in animals, particularly in domestic animals such as cattle (including buffaloes) and dogs; farm animals such as cattle, sheep, goats, poultry; and wild animals and vultures (but rarely cats or other animals).

Drug poisonings in animals occur commonly due to off-label use of medicines, wrong dosage, negligence, accidental ingestion, and deliberate poisonings. Accidental or malicious poisonings are due to organophosphorus and carbamate insecticides, fumigants such as aluminum phosphide and zinc phosphide, rodenticides, and rarely due to other agents. Most production animals are kept in some form of confinement, which limits the potential for exposure to toxic agents. However, mistakes in management, such as feed mixing errors or improper ventilation, may result in acute or chronic toxicosis in large number of animals. The most common amongst them is due to nitrate- and nitrites, fluoride, Se, Cu (common in sheep) ingestion of plant, or paddy straw. The other common sources of poisoning include mycotoxins, botulinum, and ionophores (monensin, lasalocid, narasin, and salinomycin). Contamination of feed with antibiotics, pesticides, metals and with other toxins is quite common but their long terms effects are still unknown. For example, in the absence of any systematic survey, the extent to which household kerosene and solid fuels-biomass (wood, agricultural residues, and animal dung) and coal fuels cause long-term damage including morbidity and mortality in companion animals is currently unclear. The scarcity of adequate epidemiologic and exposure investigations in various Asian countries and the potential for short- and long-term exposure to a vast variety of agents, including household use products and chemicals, suggest a need for agencies to collect epidemiological data on human beings and animals.

REFERENCES

Abdulkaf, K., Tariku, J., Fanos, T., et al., 2015. Assessment on chemicals and drugs residue in dairy and poultry products in Bishoftu and Modjo, Central Ethiopia. J. Nutr. Food Sci. S13, 002.

Al-Qudah, K.M., Rousan, L.M., Ereifej, K.I., 2009. Nitrate/nitrite poisoning in dairy cattle associated with consumption of forages irrigated with municipally treated wastewater. Toxicol. Environ. Chem. 91, 163–170.

American Petroleum Institute, 2010. American Petroleum Institute (editor PHT Group). Kerosene/jet fuel category assessment document #201–16846A. American Petroleum Institute, Washington, DC.

Anon, 1981. Report -Committee on Damage by Atomic Bombs in Hiroshima and Nagasaki, Hiroshima and Nagasaki: The Physical, Medical and Social Effects of the Atomic Bombings, London.

Anon, 2013a. Reports of animal cruelty cases on the rise Department of the Agri-Food and Veterinary Authority, APR 17, pp. 1–3. <http://www.straitstimes.com/singapore/reports-of-animal-cruelty-cases-on-the-rise>.

Anon, 2013b. Death by plastics. The times of India TNN I Jan 3, 2013, 04.54 AM IST, Panaji, India.

Anon, 2014. The plastic cow project. Karuna Society for animals and nature, Andhra Pradesh, India. <http://www.karunasociety.org/the-plastic-cow-project>.

Anon, 2016. Pb Ammunition: Toxic to Wildlife, People and the Environment. <http://www.humanesociety.org/issues/campaigns/wildlife_abuse/toxic-Pb-ammunition-poisoning-wildlife.html>.

Antonissen, G., Van Immerseel, F., Pasmans, F., et al., 2013. Deoxynivalenol predisposes for necrotic enteritis by affecting the intestinal barrier in broilers. Proc. Int. Poultr. Sci. Forum.9–10, Atlanta, GA, USA. 28–29 Jan.

Arora, B.M., 2003. Indian wildlife diseases and disorders. Association of Indian Zoo and Wildlife Veterinarians. Bareilly, India, pp. 520–534.

Badiye, A., Kapoor, N., Khajuria, H., 2013. Cu toxicity: a comprehensive study. Res. J. Recent. Sci. 2, 58–67.

Bayer, 2014. Baytril (enrofloxacin) antibacterial tablets for animal usage. Bayer health care LLC, Animal health division, Shawnee Mission, KS, 66201-0390. <https://www.drugs.com/vet/baytril-enrofloxacin-antibacterial-tablets.html>.

Bazargani, T.T., Ashrafihelan, J.A., Salar-amoli, J., 2007. As poisoning in a dairy herd in Isfahan. Iran. Vet. J. 3, 77–83.

Berny, P., Caloni, F., Croubels, S., Sachana, M., et al., 2010. Animal poisoning in Europe. Part 2: companion animals. Vet. J. 183, 255–259.

Botha, C.J., Naude, T.W., Minnaar, P.P., et al., 1993. Two outbreaks of fluorosis in cattle and sheep. J. South Afri. Vet. Assoc. 64, 165–168.

Chihaya, Y., Matsukawa, K., Ohshima, K., et al., 1992. A pathological study of bovine alimentary mycosis. J. Comp. Pathol. 107, 195–206.

Choubisa, S.L., 1998. Fluorosis in some tribal villages of Udaipur district (Rajasthan). J. Environ. Biol. 19, 341–352.

Choubisa, S.L., 1999. Some observations on endemic fluorosis in domestic animals in Southern Rajasthan. Vet. Res. Commun. 23, 457–465.

Choubisa, S.L., Mishra, G.V., Zulfiya, S., et al., 2011. Food, fluoride, and fluorosis in domestic ruminants in the Dungarpur District of Rajasthan, India. Fluoride. 44, 70–76.

Choubisa, S.L., Modasiya, V., Bahura, C.K., Sheikh, Z., 2012. Toxicity of fluoride in cattle of the Indian thar desert, Rajasthan, India. Fluoride. 45, 371–376.

Choubisa, S.L., 2014. Bovine calves as ideal bio-indicators for fluoridated drinking water and endemic osteo-dental fluorosis. Environ. Monit. Assess. 186, 4493–4498.

Cornish, J., Angelos, J., Puschner, B., Miller, G., 2007. Cu toxicosis in a dairy goat herd. J. Am. Vet. Med. Assoc. 231, 586–589.

Dandapat, P., Nanda, P.K., Bandyopadhyay, S., et al., 2011. Prevalence of Deg Nala disease in eastern India and its reproduction in buffaloes by feeding Fusarium oxysporum infested rice straw. Asian Pacific J. Trop. Med. 4, 54–57.

Deore, M.D., Srivastava, A.K., Sharma, S.K., 2002. Blood Se levels during different stages of selenosis in buffaloes and its evaluation as a diagnostic tool. Vet. Hum. Toxicol. 44, 260–263.

Deore, M.D., Srivastava, A.K., Sharma, S.K., 2005. Effect of reduced glutathione treatment on selenosis, blood Se concentration and glutathione peroxidase activity after repeated short term Se exposure in buffalo calves. Toxicology. 213, 169–174.

Dhillon, K.S., 1973. preliminary observation on the treatment of Deg Nala disease in Buffaloes. Indian Vet. J. 50, 482–484.

Dhillon, K.S., Dhillon, S.K., 1991a. Se toxicity in soils, plants and animals in some parts of Punjab, India. Int. J. Env. Stud. 37, 15–24.

Dhillon, K.S., Dhillon, S.K., 1991b. Accumulation of Se in sugarcane (Sachharum officinarum Linn.) in seleniferous areas of Punjab, India. Env. Geochem. Health. 13, 165–170.

Dwivedi, S.K., Dey, S., Swarup, D., 1997. Hydrofluorosis in water buffalo (*Bubalus bubalis*) in India. Sci. Total Env. 207, 105–109.

Dwivedi, S.K., Swarup, D., Dey, S., Patra, R.C., 2001. Pb poisoning in cattle and buffalo near primary Pb-zinc smelter in India. Vet. Human Toxicol. 43, 93–94.

FAO/ WHO, 2007. Animal Feed Impact on Food Safety- Health hazards associated with animal feed. Report of the FAO/WHO Expert Meeting FAO Headquarters, Rome, October 8–12, 2007.

Farrar, W., John, F., Edwards, J., Willard, M., 1994. Pathology in a dog associated with elevated tissue Hg concentrations. J. Vet. Diagn. Invest. 6, 511–514.

Fullerton, D.G., Bruce, N., Gordon, S.B., 2008. Indoor air pollution from biomass fuel smoke is a major health concern in the developing world. Trans. R. Soc. Trop. Med. Hyg. 102, 843–851.

Ghimire, L., 2012. A Case Study of Deg Nala Disease in Buffalo. Intas Pharmaceuticals Ltd. Published on: 7/24/2012, Institute of Agriculture and Animal Science (IAAS), Nepal. <http://en.engormix.com/MA-dairy-cattle/health/articles/case-study-degnala-disease-t2282/165-p0.htm>.

Ghosh, A., Sarkar, S., Pramanik, A.K., et al., 1993. Se toxicosis in grazing buffaloes and its relationship with soil and plant of West Bengal. Indian J. Anim. Sci. 63 (557), 560.

Giorgi, M., Mengozzi, G., 2011. Malicious animal intoxications: poisoned baits. Vet. Med. 56, 173–179.

Gorman, J., 2004. A Drug used for cattle is said to be killing vultures. The New York Times. 29th Jan, 2004.

Gregory, M., 2008. Plastic Bags and Animals-Making the Wild Safe for Wildlife. In: Encylopedia Britannica, 8th Dec 2008.

Gunnell, D., Eddleston, M., Phillips Michael, R., Konradsen, F., 2007. The global distribution of fatal pesticide self-poisoning: systematic review. BMC Public Health. 7, 357–371.

Gupta, P.K., 1986. Pesticides in the Indian Environment. Interprint, New Delhi.

Gupta, P.K., 1988. Veterinary Toxicology. Cosmo, New Delhi, India.

Gupta, P.K., 2004. Pesticide exposure – Indian scene. Toxicology 198, 83–90.

Gupta, P.K., 2006. WHO/FAO guidelines for cholinesterase-inhibiting pesticide residues in food. In: Gupta, R.C. (Ed.), Toxicology of Organophosphate and Carbamate Compounds. Academic Press/ Elsevier, Amsterdam, pp. 643–654.

Gupta, P.K., 2010a. Epidemiological studies of anticholinesterase pesticides poisoning in India. In: Satoh, T., Gupta, R.C. (Eds.), Anticholinesterase Pesticides: Metabolism, Neurotoxicity, and Epidemiology. John Wiley and Sons, Hoboken, pp. 417–431.

Gupta, P.K., 2010b. Modern Toxicology: Adverse Effects of Xenobiotics, vol. 2. Pharma Med Press/BSP, Hyderabad, India.

Gupta, P.K., 2014. Essential Concepts in Toxicology. BSP Publications, Hyderabad, India.

Gupta, P.K., 2016. Fundamentals of Toxicology: Essential Concepts and Applications. Elsevier/ BSP, USA, p. 398.

Gupta, R.C., Kwatra, M.S., Singh, N., 1982. Chronic Se toxicity as a cause of hoof and horn deformities in buffalo cattle and goat. Indian Vet. J. 59, 738–740.

Ifran, M., 1971. The clinical picture and pathology of Deg Nala diseases in buffaloes and cattle in West Pakistan. Vet. Rec. 88, 422–424.

Ifran, M., Maqbool, A., 1986. Studies on Deg Nala disease in cattle and buffaloes. Pakistan Vet. J. 6, 87–93.

Islam, K.M., Afrin, S., Khan, M.J., et al., 2008. Compatibility of a combination of tiamulin plus chlortetracycline with salinomycin in feed during a long-term co-administration in broilers. Poult Sci. 87, 1565–1568.

Jagadish, S., Singh, L.K., Samad, A., Bhalerao, D.P., 1998. Bovine fluorosis I: clinical pathology and investigations into source of fluorine. Indian Vet. J. 75, 335–337.

Javad, A., Jamileh, S., Amoli, N., et al., 2013. As toxicosis in sheep: the first report from Iran. Interdiscip. Toxicol. 6, 93–98.

Kalaivanan, N., Venkataramanan, R., Sreekumar, C., et al., 2011. Secondary phorate poisoning of large carnivores in India. Eur. J. Wildlife Res. 57, 191–194.

Kalra, D.S., Bhatia, K.C., 1990. Deg Nala disease in buffalo and cattle: epidemiological investigation. J. Environ. Pathol. Toxicol. 10, 132–135.

Kamashi, K., Gopala Reddy, A., Reddy, K.S., Reddy, V.R., 2004. Evaluation of zinc against salinomycin toxicity in broilers. Indian J. Anim. Sci. 48, 89–95.

Kamashi, K., Gopala-Reddy, A., Reddy, K.S., Reddy, V.R., 2005. Effect of synergistic antioxidant against salinomycin toxicity in broiler chicken. Indian J. Anim. Sci. 75, 626–630.

Karki, K., Manandhar, P., Koirala, P., Manandhar, S., 2013. Moldy rice straw poisoning in dairy cattle in Kathmandu Valley Nepal. Prime J. Microbiol. Res. 3, 170-104.

Katherine, S., Kardish, R.M., Carmichael, N.G., Fowler, B.A., 2010. Metal toxicity. In: Gupta, P.K. (Ed.), Modern Toxicology: Adverse Effects of Xenobiotics, vol. 2. Pharma Med Press/BSP, Hyderabad, India, pp. 61–130.

Khanal, D.R., Anthony, P., Knight, 2010. Se: its role in livestock health and production. J. Agri. Env. 11, 101–106.

Kunli, L., Lirong, X., Jian'an, T., Lianhua, X., 2004. Se source in the selenosis area of the Daba region, South Quinling Mountain, China. Env. Geol. 45, 426–432.

Litchfield, M.H., 2005. Estimates of acute pesticide poisonings in agricultural workers in less developed countries. Toxicol. Rev. 24, 271–278.

Mahajan, H.K., Sharma, S.V., Singh, A., et al., 2007. Concurrent pasteurellosis and classical swine fever in Indian pigs. J. Swine Health Prod. 15, 279–283.

Maiti, S.K., Das, P.K., Ray, S.K., 2003. Dental fluorosis in bovine of Nayagarh district of Orissa. J. Env. Biol. 24 (4), 465–470.

Mehta, P.S., Mehta, A.C., Mehta, S.J., Makhijani, A.B., 1994. Bhopal tragedy's health effects, a review of methyl isocyanate toxicity. JAMA 264, 2781–2787.

Mills, E., 2005. The specter of fuel-based lighting. Science. 308, 1263–1264.

Muhammad, F., Akhtar, Ml, Zia-Ur-Rahman, J.I., Irfan, A.M., 2009. Role of veterinarians: in providing residue-free animal food. Pak. Vet. J. 29, 42–46.

Muralidhara, A., Sastry, K.N.V., Madhva, R.P., Krishnamoorthy, A., 2000. Fluorosis in parts of Karnatakaan epidemiological study. Indian J. Vet. Med. 20, 86–87.

Nagarajan, P., Venkatesan, R., Kumar, J.M., Majumdar, S.S., 2004. A case of sarcoptes(scabies) infection in Bonnet monkey (Macaca). <www.priory.com/vet/Sarcoptes.htm>.

Narwaria, Y.S., Saksena, D.N., 2012. Incidence of dental fluorosis in domestic animals of Shivepuri, Madhya Pradesh, India. J. Environ. Res. Develop. 7, 426–430.

Nicholas, L., Smith, K.R., Gauthier, A., Bates, M.N., 2012. Kerosene: a review of household uses and their hazards in low- and middle group-income countries. J. Toxicol. Environ. Health B Crit. Rev. 15, 396–432.

Nisha, A.R., 2008. Antibiotics residues-A global health hazard. Vet. World. 1, 375–377.

NRC, 2005. Mineral Tolerance of Animals. Washington, DC, National Research Council.

Ochiai, K., Kimura, T., Uematsu, K., et al., 1999. Pb poisoning in wild waterfowl in Japan. J. Wildlife Dis. 35, 766–769.

Oehme, F.W., Pickrell, J.A., 1999. An analysis of the chronic oral toxicity of polyether ionophore antibiotics in animals. Vet. Hum. Toxicol. 41, 251–257.

OIE, 2007. Guidelines for the responsible and prudent use of antimicrobial agents in veterinary medicine. Terrestrial Animal Health Code, Sixteenth Edition, Appendix 3.9.3. pp. 549–556.

Pal, M., 2007. Veterinary and Medical Mycology. Indian Council of Agricultural Research, New Delhi, India, pp. 266–271.

Pal, M., Gizaw, F., Abera, F., et al., 2015. Mycotoxins: a growing concern to human and animal health. Bev. Food World. 42 (42-46), 50.

Patil, R.D., Sharma, R., Asran, R.K., 2014. Mycotoxicosis and its control in poultry: a review. J. Poult. Sci. Technol. 2, 1–10.

Patra, R.C., Dwivedi, S.K., Bhardwaj, B., Swarup, D., 2000. Industrial fluorosis in cattle and buffalo around Udaipur, India. Sci. Total Env. 253, 145–150.

Pei, Z., Zhang, X., 2014. Methamphetamine intoxication in a dog: case report. BMC Vet. Res. 10, 139–151.

Ranjan, R., Swarup, D., Bhardwaj, B., 2009. Distribution of clinical signs and lesions in fluorotic cattle. Indian J. Anim. Sci. 79, 546–549.

Rathnapraba, S., Vadivoo, V.S., Manoharan, S., et al., 2012. Molecular detection of classical swine fever from a field outbreak in Tamil Nadu. Indian J. Vet. Pathol. 36, 22–27.

Rawte, H.T., 2012. Nitrate-nitrite poisoning – report by Commissioner of Animal Husbandry and Toxicology and Regional Disease Diagnostic Laboratory (Western India). Maharashtra, India. <https://ahd.maharashtra.gov.in/pdf/dis/Nitrate%20or%20Nitratrite%20Poisoning.pdf>.

Ritchie, G., Still, K., Rossi, J., et al., 2003. Biological and health effects of exposure to kerosene-based jet fuels and performance additives. J. Toxicol. Environ. Health B. 6, 357–451.

Saito,, K., 2009. Pb poisoning of Steller's Sea-Eagle (Haliaeetus pelagicus) and White-tailed Eagle (Haliaeetus albicilla) caused by the ingestion of Pb bullets and slugs. In: Watson, R.T., Fuller, M., Pokras, M., Hunt, W.G. (Eds.), Hokkaido Japan. InIngestion of Pb from Spent Ammunition: Implications for Wildlife and Humans. The Peregrine Fund, Boise, ID, DOI 10.4080/ilsa.2009.0304.

Sarathchandra, G., Suresh, V.K., Ramesh, J., 2014. Veterinary pharmacovigilance survey conducted in Tamil Nadu State of India-A status report (20011-2012). Ind. J. Vet Anim. Sci. Res. 43, 80–97.

Selby, L.A., Case, A.A., Osweiler, G.D., Hayes Jr, H.M., 1977. Epidemiology and toxicology of As poisoning in domestic animals. Env. Health Perspect. 19, 183–189.

Sharma, S.P., Randhawa, S.S., Randhawa, C.S., 1997. Clinico-epidemiological features of bovine fluorosis in Punjab. Indian J. Anim. Sci. 67, 943–945.

Shinozaki K.I. (1975) Nitrate-nitrite poisoning in dairy cattle. The Agriculture, Forestry and Fisheries Research Information Technology Center, Japan. <http://www.affrc.go.jp/en/> (Japanese).

Shirlow, J.E., 1939. Deg Nala disease of buffaloes and cattle: epidemiological investigations, an account of the lesions and essential pathology. Indian.Vet. Sci. Anim Husb. 9, 853–864.

Sidhu, P.K., Bedi, G., Verma, S., et al., 2008. Investigations and clinical management of nitrate toxicities in dairy animals. Indian Vet. J. 85, 605–607.

Sidhu, P.K., Bedi, G.K., Meenakshi, V., et al., 2011. Evaluation of factors contributing to excessive nitrate accumulation in fodder crops leading to ill-health in dairy animals. Toxicol. Int. 18, 22–26.

Sidhu, P.K., Mahajan, V., Verma, S., et al., 2014. Toxicological and pathological review of concurrent occurrence of nitrite toxicity and swine fever in pigs. Toxicol. Int. 21, 186–190.

Sikdar, A., Chakraborty, G.C., Bhattacharya, D., et al., 2000. An outbreak of gangrenous syndrome among buffaloes and cattle in West Bengal: clinicopathological studies. Trop. Anim. Health Prod. 32, 165–171.

Singh, J.L., Swarup, D., 1994. Fluorosis in buffaloes. Vet. Rec. 135, 260–261.

Singh, Y.P., 1988. Occurrence of mycotoxins in animal feedstuffs: a challenge. In: Gupta, P.K., Raviprakash, V. (Eds.), Advances in Toxicology and Environmental Health. Jagmander Book Agency, New Dehli, India, pp. 177–202.

Siroka, Z., Svobodova, Z., 2013. The toxicity and adverse effects of selected drugs in animals--overview. Pol. J. Vet. Sci. 16, 181–191.

Sivajothi, S., Sudhakara Reddy, B., 2015. Cat affected with sarcoptic mange in Y.S.R District of Andhra Pradesh, India. Comp. Clin. Pathol. 24, 1031–1032.

Smith, G.D., 2001. The uses of epidemiology. Int. J. Epidemiol. 30, 1146–1155.

Sudakin, D.L., 2005. Occupational exposure to aluminium phosphide and phosphine gas? A suspected case report and review of the literature. Hum. Exp. Toxicol. 24, 27–33.

Sudhakara, R.B., Nalini, K.K., Sivajothi, S., Venkatasivakumar, R., 2014. Dermatitis due to mixed Demodex and Sarcoptes mites in dogs. Vet. Med. Article ID 768242, 4 pages http://dx.doi.org/10.1155/2014/768242.

Susan E. (Editor-in-Chief) (2016) Nitrate and nitrite poisoning. In The Merck Veterinary Manual. 11th ed. Whitehouse Station: Merck and Co; Toxicology. pp. 3049–3052.

Swarup, D., Dey, S., Patra, R.C., et al., 2001. Clinico-epidemiological observations of industrial bovine fluorosis in India. Indian J. Anim. Sci. 71, 1111–1115.

Swarup, D., Singh, Y.P., 1989. Bovine fluorosis in a brick kiln congested zone. Indian J. Vet. Med. 9, 12–14.

Swarup, D., Patra, R.C., Naresh, R., et al., 2005. Blood Pb levels in lactating cows reared around polluted localities; transfer of Pb into milk. Sci. Total Env. 349, 67–71.

Tiwary, A.K., Stegelmeier, B.L., Panter, K.E., et al., 2006. Comparative toxicosis of sodium selenite and selenomethionine in lambs. J. Vet. Diagn. Invest. 18, 61–70.

Vyt, S., 2006. intoxication in sows. Vet. Rec. 158, 456–458.

Yadav, S.K., Singh, I., Singh, D., Han, S.D., 2005. Se status in soils of northern districts of India. J. Environ. Manage. 75, 129–132.

FURTHER READING

Chirag, M.M., Hitesh, B.P., Shailesh, K.M., 2013. Animal husbandry practices to contaminants and residues of chemical in animal origin foods and health hazard. Inter. J. Mole. Vet. Res. 3, 55–61.

Choubisa, S.L., 2008. Dental fluorosis in domestic animals. Curr. Sci. 95, 1674–1675.

Gupta, P.K., 2010. Natural laws concerning toxicology. In: Gupta, P.K. (Ed.), Modern Toxicology: Adverse Effects of Xenobiotics, vol. 2. Pharma Med Press/BSP, Hyderabad, India, pp. 27–70.

Gupta, P.K., 2017. Herbicides and fungicides. In: Gupta, R.C. (Ed.), Reproductive and Developmental Toxicology. Academic Press/Elsevier, Amsterdam, in press.

Locke, L.N., Friend, M., 1989. Avian botulism: geographic expansion of a historic disease. US Fish Wildlife Leaflet 13.2.4.1–6.

Logrieco, A., Bottalico, A., Mulé, G., et al., 2003. Epidemiology of toxigenic fungi and their associated mycotoxins for some mediterranean crops. Eur. J. Plant Pathol. 109, 645–667.

Mandakranta, B., 2000. Faces of the Feminine in Ancient, Medieval, and Modern India. Oxford University Press, p. 26. <https://en.wikipedia.org/wiki/History_of_poison> ISBN 0-19-512229-1.

Mitsuo, S., Nakamijra, R., Too, K., Matsuhashi, A., 1956. Clinical studies on Hg poisoning in cattle. J. Vet. Res. 4, 1–16.

Swarup, D., Ranjan, R.D., Bhardwaj, B., 2009. Distribution of clinical signs and lesions in fluorotic cattle. Indian J. Anim. Sci. 79, 546–549.

Chapter 5

Chemicals of Terrorism

Tina Wismer

INTRODUCTION

Chemical agents may be chosen by terrorists, as they can be dispersed over large areas and can eventually penetrate even the most well-defended positions. These agents can be deployed against specific targets, and depending on the agent used, the effects can be immediate or delayed. Chemical agents can cause incapacitation, disorientation, or death. Many of the more commonly used agents can be produced inexpensively and easily stored.

There are four basic types of military agents that can be used for chemical terrorism: choking agents (chlorine, phosgene), blister agents (mustard, Lewisite, phosgene oxime), blood agents (cyanide, hydrogen cyanide) and nerve agents (tabun, sarin, soman, VX). Chemical warfare agents can be delivered by a variety of methods: bomb, spray tanks, rockets, missiles, land mines, and artillery projectiles (USACHPPM, 2001a). Few indicators of a chemical attack may be evident at first. The initial observation of unusual signs and symptoms that correlate with nerve agents, vesicants, blood or pulmonary agents' exposures should raise the immediate suspicion of poisoning.

The history of chemical warfare dates back to the beginning of the last century. The first chemical warfare agent of modern times was chlorine. It was used by the German army at Ypres in 1915 against the Allies. Chlorine with phosgene, or phosgene alone, followed soon after. Phosgene, arsenicals, blister agents, and mustard gas were estimated to be responsible for approximately 1.3 million casualties during the war, including at least 90,000 fatalities (Raffle et al., 1994; Bingham et al., 2001; HSDB, 2005; Johnson et al., 2015; Bajgar et al., 2015). Chemical warfare agents do not need to be lethal to be disruptive. Mustard gas caused severe injuries, and due to its persistence, remained a hazard and barrier to troop movements.

Even though they are banned, chemical weapons are still being used. Phosgene was deployed by Egyptian bombers against Yemeni royalist forces in the Yemeni civil war in the 1980s (Evison et al., 2002). The Iraqi military used both mustard gas and HCN against the Kurds leading to as many as 3000 deaths (Somani and Babu, 1989; Balali-Mood, 2015). Iraq also used "yellow rain" (a mixture of mycotoxins, mustard gas, and nerve agents) against Iran in 1984. Approximately 100,000 unprotected soldiers suffered severe and long-lasting injuries. The fatality rate was 20% (Drasch et al., 1987). Syria has also been accused of manufacturing and using chemical weapons against its own people on several occasions (Paton, 2017).

Chemical weapons have also been used by groups or individuals for political purposes. Aum Shinrikyo (Supreme Truth), a Japanese doomsday cult, used both sarin gas and phosgene in the mid-1990s to bring attention to themselves and their cause. They killed 18 people and injured over 6000 people in these attacks (Kaplan and Marshall, 1996; Okumura et al., 2015). Kim Jong Nam was assassinated in a Malaysian airport in February 2017 with VX gas after it was wiped on his face (Berlinger, 2017).

Chemical agents also have their problems as agents of terror. They are most effective in confined spaces. Chemical warfare agents dissipate quickly and degrade or adhere to surfaces. Attacks need to be well coordinated for dispersal of the agent and escape from the area of deployment.

Both livestock and pet animals can be exposed to chemical agents during a terrorist attack. Treatment of animals is secondary to treating human causalities. Humane euthanasia may be the only recourse due to financial or logistical concerns. For further details on epidemiology, toxicity, treatment, and various other aspects of chemical warfare agents, readers are referred to a recently published book, *Handbook of Toxicology of Chemical Warfare Agents* (Gupta, 2015).

CHLORINE GAS

Background

Chlorine (Agent CL, Cl_2) has been used as a choking or pulmonary agent for military purposes under the name

Veterinary Toxicology. DOI: http://dx.doi.org/10.1016/B978-0-12-811410-0.00005-2

bertholite (Budavari, 2000). It is a greenish-yellow diatomic gas with an irritating, pungent, or suffocating odor (Lewis, 2000; Budavari, 2000). Chlorine gas is heavier than air and will settle in low areas.

Pharmacokinetics/Toxicokinetics

The initial effects of chlorine gas exposure can appear very rapidly, depending upon the concentration. Due to chlorine's water solubility and chemical reactivity, it can have a greater effect on the lower respiratory tract as a large percentage bypasses the upper airways. Respiratory, dermal, and ocular irritation starts immediately and acute lung injury peaks in 12–24 h.

Mechanism of Action

Chlorine gas is a strong irritant, and in concentrated amounts may be corrosive to mucous membranes when inhaled or ingested. When chlorine combines with tissue water it produces hydrochloric acid and reactive oxygen species. These free radicals are potent oxidizers, causing further tissue damage. Nitric oxide (NO) formation is disrupted causing increased inflammation (Honavar et al., 2014). The damage to the respiratory epithelium leads to alveolar capillary congestion followed by high fibrinogen edematous fluid (Noe, 1963). Hypoxemia results from development of atelectasis, emphysema, and membrane formation. Acute lung injury and development of acute respiratory distress syndrome (ARDS) can occur. Death usually occurs within 48 h from cardiac arrest secondary to hypoxia (Decker, 1988).

Toxicity

Inhalation is the main route of chlorine gas exposure. Chlorine gas is very irritating on contact and can be caustic to the eyes, skin, nose, throat, and mucous membranes. Ocular exposure can result in severe or permanent eye injury. Dermal exposure may cause erythema, pain, and irritation. Both liquid chlorine and high concentrations of gaseous chlorine can cause dermal burns (Raffle et al., 1994). Signs of exposure to chlorine gas include: rhinorrhea, ataxia, syncope, muscle weakness, dermatitis, dyspnea, tachypnea, pneumonia, bronchospasm and acute lung injury. High concentrations may cause laryngospasm, cardiovascular collapse, tachycardia, and respiratory arrest (Noe, 1963). Respiratory symptoms may be immediate or delayed up to several hours depending on the concentration (Bingham et al., 2001). Hypoxia is common and death may be rapid. See Table 5.1 for severity of signs expected after inhalation at certain ppm concentrations of chlorine gas.

Symptoms generally disappear within 6 h after mild exposures but may continue for more than 24 h with severe exposures. Moderate to severe exposures can result in chronic respiratory dysfunction (Decker, 1988).

Treatment

Move animals into fresh air and monitor for respiratory distress. If coughing or dyspnea develops, evaluate for hypoxia, acidosis, respiratory tract irritation, bronchitis or pneumonitis. Oxygen supplementation along with intubation and ventilation may be needed. Beta adrenergic

TABLE 5.1 Different Effects of Exposure Levels of Chlorine Gas

Values in ppm	Effect
0.2–3.5	Odor detection (some tolerance develops)
1–3	Mild mucous membrane irritation that can be tolerated for up to 1 h
3	Extremely irritating to the eyes and respiratory tract
5	Severe irritation of eyes, nose, and respiratory tract; intolerable after a few minutes
14–21	Immediate irritation of the throat; dangerous if exposed for 30–60 min
15	Irritation of the throat
30	Moderate irritation of the upper respiratory tract; immediate chest pain, vomiting, dyspnea, cough
35–50	Lethal in 60–90 min
40–60	Toxic pneumonitis and acute lung injury; dangerous for even short periods
430	Lethal over 30 min
1000	Fatal within a few minutes

Source: Data from Lewis, R.J., 2000. Sax's dangerous properties of industrial materials, 10th edn. Van Nostrand Reinhold Company, New York, NY, HSDB, 2005. Hazardous Substances Data Bank. (Edition expires in 2005.) National Library of Medicine, Bethesda, MD (Internet Version). Thomson MICROMEDEX, Greenwood Village, CO; Bingham, E., Chorssen, B., Powell, C.H., 5th edn., 2001. Patty's Toxicology, vol. 3. John Wiley & Sons, New York, NY.

agonists can help if bronchospasm develops (Guloglu et al., 2002).

Flush eyes with copious amounts of room temperature 0.9% saline or water for at least 15 min. Fluorescein staining should be performed to check for corneal defects (Grant and Schuman, 1993). Animals should be bathed with copious amounts of soap and water. Chlorine blood concentrations are not clinically useful as it converts directly to hydrochloric acid in the lungs and other tissues.

Animal models have suggested that corticosteroids can hasten recovery from severe chlorine gas poisoning (Traub et al., 2002); however, administration of steroids to exposed humans has not been shown to provide any significant change (Chester et al., 1977). Pigs exposed to chlorine gas responded best to a combination of aerosolized terbutaline and budesonide than to either therapy alone (Wang et al., 2004). Sheep exposed to chlorine gas and then nebulized with 4% sodium bicarbonate had decreased mortality and improved arterial blood gas values (Chisholm et al., 1989). Other suggested therapies include IV sodium nitrite to replace NO and reduce inflammation (Honavar et al., 2017) and melatonin as a free radical scavenger (Pita et al., 2013).

Concluding Remarks

Rescuers should wear self-contained breathing apparatus and have protective clothing when entering contaminated areas. Chlorine dissipates quickly in warm climates and does not leave an environmental residue (Munro et al., 1999). The potential for secondary contamination is low, as the gas is not carried on contaminated clothing.

PHOSGENE

Background

Phosgene (Agent CG, carbonyl chloride, CCl_2O) is classified as a choking agent. It is a colorless, noncombustible, and highly toxic gas. At room temperature phosgene is easily liquefied (ACGIH, 2005; Proctor and Hughes, 2004), and at high concentrations, the gas has an odor described as strong, suffocating, and pungent. Lower concentrations are described as smelling like green corn or "haylike" (Raffle et al., 1994; Budavari, 2000).

Pharmacokinetics/Toxicokinetics

Dyspnea develops 2–6 h postexposure in most patients but may be delayed up to 15 h (Borak and Diller, 2001). With high concentrations (>200 ppm), phosgene can cross the blood–air barrier in the lung and cause hemolysis and coagulopathies (Sciuto et al., 2001).

Mechanism of Action

Phosgene is a lower-respiratory-tract irritant. Due to its low water solubility and low irritancy of the upper respiratory system, phosgene is able to penetrate deeply into the lungs (Franch and Hatch, 1986). Phosgene gas interacts with water in the lungs, where it is hydrolyzed into hydrochloric acid leading to cellular injury (Murdoch, 1993). Phosgene also acylates sulfhydryl, amine, and hydroxyl groups (Borak and Diller, 2001). This results in protein and lipid denaturation, changes in membrane structure and disruption of enzymes. Phosgene increases pulmonary vascular permeability, leading to increased fluid accumulation in the lung interstitium and alveolae. This fluid accumulation results in gas diffusion abnormalities and pulmonary edema (Diller, 1985). Phosgene also decreases energy metabolism and disrupts the glutathione redox cycle. Animals exposed to phosgene have elevated levels of leukotrienes and neutrophil chemotactic agents. Neutrophils congregate in the lung releasing cytokines and other reactive mediators that contribute to pulmonary injury (Sciuto et al., 1995). Bronchiolar epithelium is damaged, resulting in local emphysema and partial atelectasis. Death is due to anoxia secondary to pulmonary edema.

Toxicity

Most exposures to phosgene are from inhalation. The odor of phosgene gas is not sufficient to warn individuals of toxic levels and with high concentrations; olfactory fatigue can occur (Borak and Diller, 2001; ACGIH, 2005). The degree of pulmonary injury relates to the concentration and length of exposure (Bingham et al., 2001), and initial symptoms are not considered to be a good indicator of prognosis (Diller, 1985).

Exposure to concentrations less than 3 ppm may not be immediately accompanied by symptoms, but delayed effects usually occur within 24 h of exposure. Concentrations as low as 3–5 ppm can cause immediate conjunctivitis, rhinitis, pharyngitis, bronchitis, lacrimation, blepharospasm, and upper respiratory tract irritation and extended (170 min) exposure was fatal (Diller, 1985; Wells, 1985; Proctor and Hughes, 2004). A dose of 50 ppm for 5 min may cause pulmonary edema and rapid death (Chemstar, 1996; Borak and Diller, 2001; RTECS, 2006).

A lag time of 1–6 h before the onset of respiratory distress and pulmonary edema is common with acute, high-dose exposures (>50 ppm/min). Signs can be delayed for up to 24 (most common) or 72 h with exposures to lower concentrations (Proctor and Hughes, 2004). Thoracic radiographs can show evidence of pulmonary edema within 1–2 h of high-dose exposure, 4–6 h after moderate exposure, and approximately 8–24 h after low-dose exposure (Diller, 1985).

Progressive dyspnea, productive cough, cyanosis, and hemoptysis are common initial signs following exposure (Wells, 1985; Borak and Diller, 2001). Hypoxemia and hypoventilation are common secondary to respiratory distress (Wells, 1985). Animals may develop secondary GI, hepatic, renal, or brain injury, due to lack of oxygenation. In a dog model, severe phosgene poisoning caused initial bradycardia followed by tachycardia and progressive hypotension (Patt et al., 1946). Cardiac failure may occur secondary to severe pulmonary edema.

Direct contact with the liquefied material can cause dermal burns (Proctor and Hughes, 2004) and severe eye irritation, corneal opacification, and frostbite (Proctor and Hughes, 2004). Corneal opacification has also been produced in cats exposed to highly concentrated phosgene gas (Grant and Schuman, 1993).

Prognosis is directly related to the extent of pulmonary injury. If the animal survives 24–48 h, the prognosis improves. Pulmonary edema begins to resolve after 2–3 days. Survivors may have suppressed natural killer cell activity and are more susceptible to infectious agents. Secondary infections may become evident 3–5 days after exposure. They may also have persistent exertional dyspnea, reduced exercise capacity and abnormal pulmonary function tests (Borak and Diller, 2001).

Treatment

If inhalation exposure occurs, remove animals to fresh air (higher ground) and monitor for respiratory distress. Exposed skin should be washed with soap and water. Exposed eyes should be flushed for 15 min with tepid water. Asymptomatic animals should be monitored for 12–24 h for development of pulmonary edema (Borak and Diller, 2001). Symptomatic animals should receive 100% oxygen. If arterial blood gases or pO_2 continues to fall, intubation and ventilation is recommended. Plasma phosgene levels are not clinically useful, and there is no specific antidotal agent. Management of patients with pulmonary edema from phosgene is the same as for an ARDS patient. Diuretics are not indicated and can worsen volume depletion. Mechanical ventilation with oxygen and positive end-expiratory pressure is the mainstay of treatment.

Intravenous fluids can help with cardiovascular support, but monitoring closely for signs of volume overload is recommended. Colloids are preferred, as they will remain in the vascular space for a longer period of time. Most arrhythmias will resolve with adequate oxygenation.

The mechanisms underlying acute lung injury are not well understood. Nebulized beta adrenergic agonists are recommended if bronchospasm occurs. In a rabbit inhalation study, animals exposed to toxic levels of phosgene were dosed with intravenous aminophylline and subcutaneous terbutaline. If given within 10 min postexposure, it prevented noncardiogenic pulmonary edema (Kennedy et al., 1989). *N*-acetylcysteine (Mucomyst) administered intratracheally to rabbits 45–60 min after inhalational exposure to phosgene (1500 ppm/min) decreased pulmonary edema, production of leukotrienes, lipid peroxidation, and maintained normal glutathione levels as compared to rabbits exposed to phosgene only (Sciuto et al., 1995). Other treatments, such as ibuprofen (Guo et al., 1990), supplemental oxygen, sodium bicarbonate, and aerosolized surfactant (Mautone et al., 1985), or corticosteroids, prostaglandin E1 and atropine (Chemstar, 1996), have been shown to have beneficial effects in laboratory animals.

Concluding Remarks

Phosgene is heavier than air and will pool in low-lying areas. This heavy vapor density, 3.4 times that of air, made phosgene practical for trench warfare. Phosgene is considered to be nonpersistent in the environment. Air concentrations are reduced by atmospheric water, such as rain or fog (Borak and Diller, 2001). Rescuers should wear proper protective clothing when treating exposed patients. Fortunately, the potential for secondary contamination of rescue personnel is low, as the gas does not persist in fabric or leather. Phosgene is used extensively in industry as a chemical precursor and this widespread availability makes it an attractive agent for terrorist use.

MUSTARD GAS

Background

Mustard gas (Agent H, $C_4H_8C_{12}S$) is a vesicant agent used in chemical warfare. It causes necrosis of the skin, eyes, and respiratory tract. It is an organic lipophilic sulfide, which is a bifunctional alkylating agent (Borak and Sidell, 1992; Lewis, 2000). Mustard agent is a clear oily liquid in its pure state. Due to impurities, however, it is normally amber to black, or yellow to brown in color (Munro et al., 1999; USACHPPM, 2001b; HSDB, 2005). The liquid becomes aerosolized when dispersed by spraying or by explosive blast from a shell or bomb (USACHPPM, 2001a). Mustard gas has an odor resembling garlic, mustard, or horseradish. Systemic poisoning occurs more easily in warm climates than in temperate ones. Mustard gas is still considered a major threat by the US military, as it is easily manufactured and is both incapacitating and lethal.

Pharmacokinetics/Toxicokinetics

Mustard gas is toxic by all routes of exposure (oral, inhaled, dermal, and ocular) (EPA, 1985a; Sidell et al., 1997; Lewis, 2000). Skin penetration of both the liquid and vapor is rapid, and mustard causes both localized cellular and systemic damage (NATO, 1973). Mustard penetrates down hair follicles and sweat glands within minutes. Dermal absorption of mustard varies by species. About 20% of a dermal dose is absorbed through human skin, while up to 75% is absorbed through the skin in rats (Smith, 1999). Ocular absorption also happens within minutes. The latent period for absorption is inversely related to the dose, temperature and humidity (NATO, 1973). Lesions develop within 2–3 h with high-level exposures, and 8–10 h after milder exposures (Requena et al., 1988).

The chemical reaction with biological tissue occurs rapidly but symptoms are typically delayed by several hours (Grant and Schuman, 1993; Sidell et al., 1997). Dog studies show that equilibrium between blood and tissues was achieved within 5 min after inhalation (IARC, 1975). Once inside the body, mustard accumulates (in descending order) in fat, skin with subcutaneous fatty tissue, brain, kidney, muscle, liver, cerebrospinal fluid, spleen, and lung (Drasch et al., 1987; Somani and Babu, 1989). Urine is the major route of excretion in rabbits, mice, and rats. After IV administration in rats and mice, the majority is excreted in 72–96 h (Maisonneuve et al., 1993). Only about 6% is eliminated in the feces (IARC, 1975). Bone marrow damage is not evident for 3 top 5 days and leukopenia usually occurs at day 7–10 following exposures (Garigan, 1996).

Mechanism of Action

The mechanism of action for cellular damage by mustard is unknown, but four theories have been proposed: alkylation of deoxyribonucleic acid, oxidative stress upon cell components, depletion of glutathione, and an inflammatory response (Smith et al., 1995). Mustard gas is a bifunctional alkylating agent. It forms covalent cross-links between the double strands of DNA which inhibits DNA synthesis. Mustard-induced blistering appears to be correlated to DNA damage in the basal cells (Cowan et al., 1998). Mustard penetrates the skin and damages the cells separating the epidermis from the dermis. Mustard disrupts the hemidesmosomes leading to blister formation between the two layers (Sidell et al., 1997). Skin biopsies from mustard gas blisters revealed a separation of the basal cells from one another and the development of multinucleated cells (Bismuth et al., 1995).

Mustard also causes oxidative stress on intracellular molecules. Mustard forms an electrophilic ethylene episulfonium intermediate in the aqueous of the cytosol (Smith, 1999). The episulfonium ion reacts with sulfhydryl groups leading to increased intracellular calcium. The increased calcium level breaks down the microfilaments needed to maintain cell integrity and induces apoptosis by activating endonucleases, proteases, and phospholipases (Smith et al., 1995). Mustard gas may also exert its toxicity via depletion of glutathione. Without glutathione, reactive oxygen species react with membrane phopholipids causing loss of membrane function, fluidity, and integrity. Inflammation and sulfur mustard-increased proteolytic activity are also implicated in contributing to mustard pathology (Cowan et al., 1998).

Toxicity

Mustard gas is a radiomimetic, as it produces lesions similar to radiation (Sidell et al., 1997). Tissues with high cell turnover are the most affected. Being a vesicant, mustard gas can produce erythema, severe pruritus, blistering, ulceration, and necrosis of exposed skin (Borak and Sidell, 1992; Budavari, 2000). With dermal exposure, the skin initially appears pale and then becomes erythematous within a few hours of exposure (Requena et al., 1988). Blistering usually starts on the second day and progresses for several more days. Erythema disappears in 3–7 days, while the ulcers take 6–8 weeks to heal (Garigan, 1996; Sidell et al., 1997). Brown or black hyperpigmentation usually occurs after resolution of the burns, especially in areas with thinner skin. Skin involvement is most severe at warm and moist sites (genitalia, perineal regions, groin, skin folds, and axillae). This is due to the high number of sweat glands in these areas.

The eyes are very sensitive to the effects of mustard gas (NATO, 1973; Borak and Sidell, 1992). Pain, lacrimation, corneal ulceration, along with photophobia, swelling, blepharospasm, and blindness can be seen (Garigan, 1996). Conjunctivitis appears early, developing 4–6 h after exposure. Eye lesions have been reported at a Ct (concentration × time) of 10 mg-min/m^3 (Sidell et al., 1997). Porcelain-white areas in the episcleral tissues adjacent to the cornea and formation of large, tortuous, sausage-shaped varicose veins are pathognomonic signs of mustard gas poisoning (Grant and Schuman, 1993). Chronic conjunctivitis and keratopathy has been reported in people (Blodi, 1971).

The main nondermal toxic effects are on the respiratory tract. Irritation or ulceration of the respiratory tract can occur (Borak and Sidell, 1992; Budavari, 2000). Cough, dyspnea, and pulmonary edema may occur up to 24 h after inhalation. One ppm in air is a lethal concentration for dogs and 0.650 ppm mustard results in a 33% mortality rate in rabbits (OHM/TADS, 2005). See Table 5.2 for LD_{50} information in various species by multiple routes of exposure. Mild pulmonary exposures produce rhinorrhea, sneezing, epistaxis and cough within 12–24 h of exposure. Large exposures can cause pulmonary damage. In severe cases, hypoxia and respiratory

TABLE 5.2 LD_{50} for Mustard Gas

Species	Route	LD_{50} (mg/kg)
Human	Oral	0.7
	Dermal	100
Mouse	Dermal	92
	SQ	20
Rat	Oral	17
	Dermal	5
	SQ	1.5

Source: Data from Lewis, R.J., 2000. Sax's dangerous properties of industrial materials, 10th edn. Van Nostrand Reinhold Company, New York, NY; RTECS, 2006. Registry of Toxic Effects of Chemical Substances. National Institute for Occupational Safety and Health. Cincinnati, OH (CD Rom Version). Edition expires 2006; provided by Thomson MICROMEDEX, Greenwood Village, CO.

acidosis are seen. Seizures appear to occur only following extremely high acute doses (Sidell et al., 1997).

Leukopenia, thrombocytopenia, pancytopenia, and anemia have all been reported due to depressed myelopoiesis from destruction of precursor cells in the bone marrow (Borak and Sidell, 1992). Bone marrow aplasia can be seen in severe cases. Secondary to bone marrow damage, overwhelming infection can result in death (Sidell et al., 1997).

Mustard gas is considered both carcinogenic and neoplastic. Mustard gas has caused carcinomas in the skin, appendages, lungs, thorax and blood (leukemia) of rats and mice via both inhalation and IV exposure (RTECS, 2006).

Treatment

Move animal into fresh air. Do not induce emesis. Activated charcoal administration after oral ingestion is controversial. It appears to have some beneficial effects if administered within 1 h of ingestion. Sodium thiosulfate has been used as a "mustard scavenger" and giving 2% sodium thiosulfate solution orally may help in cases with ingestion exposures (Borak and Sidell, 1992). If signs or symptoms of esophageal burns are present, consider endoscopy to determine the extent of injury. Perforation and stricture formation could result.

Flush eyes with tepid water for at least 15 min. After flushing, instill 2.5% sodium thiosulfate to help neutralize the mustard. Time to decontamination is very important with ocular exposures. Mustard droplets disappear from the eye very quickly, and late flushing of the eye generally provides no benefit (Sidell et al., 1997). Topical antibiotics and mydriatics should be used if corneal lesions are present. Topical doxycycline and silibinin have been shown to decrease ocular injury (Goswami et al., 2016). Corneal transplants have been performed on some human patients with good results and may be considered for some valuable animals (Blodi, 1971).

Several general dermal decontamination methods can help reduce the toxicity of mustard gas. Bathe animals with copious amounts of soap and water. Dermal decontamination needs to be implemented quickly, as once mustard has reacted with the skin, it cannot be easily removed (Sidell et al., 1997). Many therapies have been recommended to neutralize dermal mustard exposures: 2.5% sodium thiosulfate solution (Garigan, 1996), dilute (0.5%) hypochlorite solution (Borak and Sidell, 1992), clay, such as Mineral Cationic Carrier (MCC: Kodona; Zagreb, Croatia) (Vucemilovic et al., 2008), silibinin (Tewari-Singh et al., 2012), silver sulfadiazine, dexamethasone, and diclofenac (Dachir et al., 2004). Monitor for dermal effects, which are delayed and progressive. Dermal lesions behave like a chemical burn or radiomimetic effect. Healing can take weeks to months and infection is common (Borak and Sidell, 1992). Removal and debridement of closed blisters is controversial. Blisters should be left intact until they rupture spontaneously or unless they are extremely large or inhibit motion (Roberts, 1988). Tetanus toxoid should be given to all equine and ovine patients. Tetanus prophylaxis of other species should be determined on a case-to-case basis.

Monitor for coughing and respiratory distress. If respiratory abnormalities occur, monitor arterial blood gases and/or pulse oximetry, and thoracic radiographs. Thoracic radiographs may show an infiltrate within the first 2 days (Smith, 1999). Nebulization of 2.5% sodium thiosulfate may help neutralize the mustard gas. *N*-acetylcysteine (Mucomyst) is also a potential mustard gas antagonist (Garigan, 1996). Intertracheal administration of tissue plasminogen activator has been shown to improve oxygenation in rats (Veress et al., 2015). Administer oxygen and inhaled beta agonists if needed. Intubation and ventilation may be needed. Melatonin can be beneficial in acute mustard toxicosis. It is a scavenger of both oxygen- and nitrogen-based free redicals and regulates gene expression of antioxidant enzymes (e.g., SOD, GSH-Px) (Tan et al., 2007). Melatonin also decreases inflammation by blocking proinflammatory cytokines and sparing ATP production (Tan et al., 2007). Combinations of parenteral dexamethasone, promethazine, vitamin E, and heparin have shown protective effects against mustard gas poisoning in laboratory animals (Vojvodic et al., 1985; Requena et al., 1988).

Monitor CBC with platelets for 2 weeks after exposure. Leukopenia develops at 7–10 days following a severe acute exposure (Garigan, 1996). Prophylactic antibiotics are not recommended, but a broad spectrum antibiotic should be started if leukopenia develops (Sidell et al., 1997). Antibiotic choice should be based on culture and sensitivity if possible.

Mustard can be detected in air, urine and body tissues using different methods. Mustard gas or its thiodiglycol metabolite can be detected in urine up to a week after acute exposure using gas chromatography (GC)-mass spectrometry (Vycudilik, 1985). Other than for confirming the diagnosis, measuring mustard gas levels is not likely to be of value in the management of the patient.

Concluding Remarks

Due to its low volatility, mustard is persistent in the environment. It persists for shorter periods of time in a hot climate, but reaches higher vapor concentrations more rapidly. In temperate areas mustard may persist for more than 1 week, but in desert conditions, persistence is reduced to about 1 day. Mustard will bind to vegetation for days to weeks (USACHPPM, 2001b). Detection tubes can be used to monitor airborne levels of mustard gas (IARC, 1975).

The potential for secondary contamination is high. Rescue personnel must wear protective clothing, eye protection and a respirator (HSDB, 2005). Mustard gas penetrates wood, leather, rubber and paints. Medical personnel treating mustard-exposed patients have developed toxicity.

LEWISITE

Background

Lewisite ($C_2H_2AsCl_3$) is a substituted arsine. Lewisite was first synthesized in 1918 by a research team headed by US Army Captain W.L. Lewis. It is an oily vesicant (blister-causing) liquid with potential terrorist use. Lewisite smells like geraniums. Pure Lewisite is colorless, but impurities and age cause the color to darken (amber to black or violet to brown, to olive-green) (HSDB, 2005). Lewisite remains a liquid at low temperatures and is persistent in colder climates. It hydrolyzes rapidly, making it difficult to maintain a biologically active concentration on a humid day (Sidell et al., 1997; AAR, 2000; Lewis, 2000; HSDB, 2005). Lewisite can be dispersed in air as a very fine droplet spray over a large distance (Grant and Schuman, 1993; Lewis, 2000).

Pharmacokinetics/Toxicokinetics

Lewisite can cause systemic signs when ingested, inhaled or when absorbed dermally or ocularly (Sidell et al., 1997; HSDB, 2005). Inhalation of vapor causes immediate pain, and if high enough concentrations are inhaled, death can be seen within 10 min (DeRosa et al., 2002). Dermal absorption occurs within 3–5 min, especially following liquid exposures (Sidell et al., 1997). Lewisite has extensive tissue distribution (HSDB, 2005). In rabbits, the liver, lungs and kidneys had the highest concentration of arsenic after Lewisite administration (greater than seven times blood concentration). Arsenic can cross the placenta and is passed into the milk, and nursing animals may be at risk (Barlow and Sullivan, 1982).

Animal studies showed that excretion of Lewisite oxidation products into the bile caused focal necrosis of the liver and necrosis of biliary vessel mucosa with peribiliary hemorrhages (Munro et al., 1999). The same study in rabbits found that arsenic was eliminated with a half-life in blood of 55–75 h (HSDB, 2005). The excretion of oxidized Lewisite products into the bile by the liver may result in injury to the intestinal mucosa (Munro et al., 1999).

Mechanism of Action

Besides being a vesicant, Lewisite is an arsenical compound that causes systemic effects. Lewisite directly effects enzyme systems. The exact mechanism of action is unknown, but it inhibits a variety of enzymes (pyruvic oxidase, alcohol dehydrogenase, succinic oxidase, hexokinase, and succinic dehydrogenase) (DeRosa et al., 2002). Lewisite binds with thiol groups on these enzymes, resulting in decreased ATP production. Ocular injuries following Lewisite exposure are due in part to the liberation of hydrochloric acid. Deep penetration of Lewisite into the cornea and aqueous humor causes rapid necrosis (Goldfrank et al., 1998).

Lewisite causes increased capillary permeability. Systemic absorption and increased permeability can cause a significant loss of blood plasma volume and is called "Lewisite shock" since it is similar to that of shock observed in severe burns. The leakage of fluid into the extravascular space results in hypotension (Sidell et al., 1997). The exact mechanism of increased capillary permeability is not known. Theories include a capillary dilating material released from skin or tissue, or alternatively, enhanced permeability from an interference with the metabolism of capillary endothelial cells (Goldman and Dacre, 1989). Lung capillaries appear to be the most affected due to absorption via the respiratory tract and first pass through the lungs following dermal exposure. Pulmonary edema or ARDS can develop (Sidell et al., 1997).

Toxicity

Due to its method of dispersal (bursting charge of explosive), the main routes of absorption are dermal and respiratory. Lewisite first acts as a vesicant, then as a pulmonary irritant and finally as a systemic poison.

TABLE 5.3 LD_{50} for Lewisite

Species	Route	LD_{50} (mg/kg)
Mouse	Dermal	12
Rat	Dermal	15
	Subcutaneous	1
	Oral	50
Human	Dermal	30

Source: Data from RTECS, 2006. Registry of Toxic Effects of Chemical Substances. National Institute for Occupational Safety and Health. Cincinnati, OH (CD Rom Version). Edition expires 2006; provided by Thomson MICROMEDEX, Greenwood Village, CO; Sidell, F.R., Takafuji, E.T., Franz, D.R., 1997. Textbook of Military Medicine: Medical Aspects of Chemical and Biological Warfare. TMM Publications, Washington, DC; DeRosa, C.T., Holler, J.S., Allred, M., et al., 2002. Managing hazardous materials incidents. In Agency for Toxic Substances and Disease Registry. (Website: www.atsdr.cdc.gov).

Lewisite is similar to mustard gas in that it damages the skin, eyes and airways; however, it differs in that its clinical effects appear within seconds of exposure and it is about 10 times more volatile than mustard gas (Budavari, 2000). Exposure to Lewisite is very painful, in contrast to mustard. See Table 5.3 for LD_{50s} of various species by different routes of exposure.

Dermal contact results in immediate pain. Both vapor and liquid Lewisite can penetrate skin. Reddening of the skin becomes evident within 15–30 min after exposure (EPA, 1985a; Sidell et al., 1997). Evidence of tissue destruction (grayish epithelium) will be present within minutes of skin contact (Goldman and Dacre, 1989; Sidell et al., 1997). Severe blisters develop within 12 h after exposure. The blisters may rupture, usually about 48 h after occurrence, with copious amounts of fluid seeping from the site. With dermal exposure, as little as 0.5 mL may cause severe systemic effects, and 2 mL may be lethal. Severe edema can be seen due to the Lewisite's increased capillary permeability. Dermal burns are generally deeper than those with mustard gas. Healing occurs much faster than with sulfur mustard-induced lesions and is generally complete within 4 weeks.

Ocular contact causes immediate pain, lacrimation, and blepharospasm. Permanent blindness may occur if eye exposure occurs for more than 1 min without rapid decontamination (EPA, 1985a). A small droplet (1 μL) can cause perforation and loss of vision (Sidell et al., 1997).

Inhalation of the Lewisite vapor may result in irritation to nasal passages, profuse nasal discharge and violent sneezing (HSDB, 2005). Inhalation of 6 ppm can be lethal (USACHPPM, 2001c). Following inhalation of vapor, coughing and hemoptysis commonly occurs (Sidell et al., 1997; HSDB, 2005). Lesions following Lewisite inhalation are similar to the lesions produced by mustard gas exposures. Dogs that inhaled lethal doses died of necrotizing pseudomembranous laryngotracheobronchitis (Goldman and Dacre, 1989). A thick membrane was noted in the nostrils, larynx and trachea with purulent bronchitis. Edema, hemorrhage and emphysema were seen in the lungs (Goldman and Dacre, 1989). Death can occur within 10 min with high concentrations (EPA, 1985a).

Unlike arsenic or mustard gas, Lewisite does *not* cause damage to the bone marrow or immunosuppression (Sidell et al., 1997). Even though Lewisite is a substituted arsine, it also does not appear to directly cause hemolysis of the red blood cells (HSDB, 2005). Hypovolemia, secondary to fluid loss, can be severe enough to cause renal dysfunction. Arrhythmias may occur as a result of hypovolemia rather than a direct toxic effect of Lewisite on the myocardium. Lewisite was fetotoxic to rats and rabbits, but not teratogenic (Goldman and Dacre, 1989; RTECS, 2006). It is a suspected carcinogen due to its arsenic content.

Lewisite blood levels are not clinically useful, but an arsenic blood level below 7 μg/100 mL is considered normal. Urine arsenic levels may be tested and levels of <100 μg are considered normal (Proctor and Hughes, 2004). Concentrations between 0.7 and 1.0 mg/L indicate a potentially harmful exposure.

Treatment

Move animals to fresh air and monitor for coughing and respiratory distress. Monitor blood gases and SpO_2 in patients with significant exposures. If coughing or difficulty breathing develops, administer oxygen and assist ventilation as needed. Bronchospasm should be treated with inhaled beta agonists and possibly corticosteroids. Monitor electrolytes and PCV as animals can become hemoconcentrated. Crystalloids should be given with caution not to overhydrate the patient (Goldfrank et al., 1998). Consider urinary alkalinization and maintain good urine output. Monitor for liver and kidney failure and secondary infection.

Emesis is not recommended due to the irritant and vesicant nature of Lewisite. Dilute oral ingestions with milk or water. Perforation and stricture formation may occur after ingestion as severe irritation or vesication (blistering) of the esophagus or gastrointestinal tract is likely to occur. Endoscopy may be used to determine the extent of injury.

Flush eyes with copious amounts of tepid water for at least 15 min. A 5% BAL (dimercaprol, British Anti-Lewisite) compounded ophthalmic ointment applied within 2 min may prevent a significant reaction. Treatment at 30 min will lessen the ocular reaction but does not prevent permanent damage (Goldfrank et al., 1998).

Animals should be rinsed with copious amounts of water. A 5% solution of sodium hypochlorite (diluted liquid household bleach) should be used as soon as possible on contaminated skin. Topical application of a 5% BAL ointment within 15 min of an exposure has been reported to be effective in diminishing the blistering effects of Lewisite (Smith, 1999). Wash BAL ointment off after 5 min. The ointment may cause stinging, itching or urticaria. Burns should be managed as discussed previously under mustard gas. Pain control is very important.

Chelation is indicated if there is coughing, dyspnea, pulmonary edema, or skin burns larger than palm size (Goldfrank et al., 1998). BAL is an effective arsenic chelator, but requires painful deep intramuscular injections and has numerous side effects (hypertension, tachycardia, vomiting, lacrimation, sweating). BAL will increase the clearance rate of arsenic, but it is contraindicated in animals with liver damage. 2,3-Dimercaptosuccinic acid (DMSA, Succimer) appears to be a very effective arsenic chelator in animals (Graziano et al., 1978). DMSA is an oral agent and is relatively nontoxic. It may be used following BAL. 2,3-Dimercapto-1-propanesulfonic acid is related to DMSA and is used for heavy metal poisoning, especially in Europe. It has been effective in protecting rabbits from the lethal effects of Lewisite (Aposhian et al., 1982).

Concluding Remarks

Lewisite can remain in the environment for about 1 day. It reacts with water to yield a solid arsenoxide that also has vesicant properties. When in contact with strong alkalis, Lewisite is decomposed to less harmful substances. The potential for secondary contamination is high and material spilled on clothing may be transferred to rescuers or medical personnel. Lewisite is considered a terrorist threat, as it is easy to produce and has a quick onset of signs. Carcasses should be buried deeply (away from water supplies), rendered or incinerated to insure safety of the food supply.

PHOSGENE OXIME

Background

Phosgene oxime (Agent CX, "Nettle Rush," $CHCl_2NO$) is a halogenated oxime used as a blistering agent in chemical warfare. Other halogenated oximes include diiodoformoxime, dibromoformoxime and monochloroformoxime, but phosgene oxime is the most irritant of the group and the only one considered a terrorist warfare threat. Phosgene oxime can be found as a liquid or as a colorless, low-melting point crystalline solid, readily soluble in water. The solid form can produce enough vapor to cause symptoms. Phosgene oxime has an unpleasant, peppery and irritating odor. Phosgene oxime is not a true vesicant as it does not cause skin blisters but it does have a rapid dermal urticant and corrosive effect. It can be dispersed as a liquid or vapor causing almost immediate tissue damage upon contact.

Pharmacokinetics/Toxicokinetics

Absorption in both dermal and inhalational exposures is complete and rapid (within seconds) (Sidell et al., 1997). Dermal lesions form within seconds. Phosgene oxime will dissolve in sweat and move to other nonexposed areas of the body as it is soluble in water (DeRosa et al., 2002). Pulmonary edema can be evident on thoracic radiographs within 2 h of high-dose exposure, 4–6 h of moderate exposure, and approximately 8–24 h after low-dose exposure (Sidell et al., 1997).

Mechanism of Action

The exact mechanism action is unknown, but it has been proposed that phosgene oxime reacts with SH and NH_2 groups and activates mast cells (Sidell et al., 1997; Tewari-Singh et al., 2017). Phosgene oxime exerts its greatest effects in the first capillary bed it encounters.

Toxicity

Both liquid and vaporous phosgene oxime cause intense, immediate pain and local tissue destruction on contact with skin, eyes and mucous membranes (Sidell et al., 1997). Damage to the eyes, skin and airways is similar to that caused by mustard gas. Following dermal contact with either the liquid or vapor, grayish tissue damage may be seen within several minutes. The damaged areas are erythematous and extremely painful. Within 1 h, the area becomes edematous. Browning of the skin and blistering occurs the next day. In about 3 weeks, desquamation, necrosis, crust formation, and purulent exudate occur. Pain can last for several days. Skin irritation begins at 0.2 mg/min/m^3 (12 s) for humans and is intolerable 3 mg/min/m^3 (1 min) (USACHPPM, 2001d).

Phosgene oxime is very irritating to the eyes. Very low concentrations can cause lacrimation, inflammation, and temporary blindness, and high concentrations can cause permanent corneal lesions and blindness (Sidell et al., 1997; USACHPPM, 2001d). Inhalation or oral absorption may cause respiratory tract irritation, dyspnea and pulmonary edema. The noncardiogenic pulmonary edema may occur after a several hour delay. Death is due to respiratory arrest.

Treatment

There is no antidote for phosgene oxime exposure. Move animals into fresh air. Emesis is not recommended after oral ingestion because of the irritant and corrosive effects of phosgene oxime. Immediately dilute oral ingestions with milk or water. Activated charcoal is also not recommended after ingestion, since the primary toxicity is expected to be a local corrosive injury.

Flush eyes with tepid water until pH returns to neutrality and remains so for 30 min after irrigation is discontinued (Brodovsky et al., 2000). Decontamination after ocular exposure is critical since phosgene oxime is absorbed within seconds. Corneal ulcers should be treated with mydriatic cycloplegiecs to prevent synechiae development (Grant and Schuman, 1993; Brodovsky et al., 2000). For more severe corneal lesions, topical steroids, citrate, ascorbate, and tetracycline or doxycycline may be used to aid in reepithelialization.

The skin should be flushed with large volumes of water and mild soap. As phosgene oxime reacts so quickly with tissue, decontamination is not expected to be entirely effective after pain has been produced. Isotonic sodium bicarbonate or 0.5% hypochlorite may remove phosgene oxime that has not yet reacted with tissue. Ulcerated skin lesions should be treated just like a thermal burn. Topical silver sulfadiazine is recommended (Roberts, 1988). Healing of dermal lesions can take from 1 month to over a year (Sidell et al., 1997). Both sheep and horses should receive tetanus prophylaxis. Other species should be vaccinated at the veterinarian's discretion. Large amounts of opioid analgesics may be needed to help control pain.

Monitor arterial blood gases, pulse oximetry, and thoracic radiographs in patients following significant exposures. Noncardiogenic pulmonary edema may take 12–24 h to develop. If dyspnea develops, administer 100% humidified oxygen, perform endotracheal intubation, and provide assisted ventilation as required. Beta adrenergic agonists may help if bronchospasm develops. Administer IV fluids but ensure that the animal does not become overhydrated (Hoffman, 2002).

Concluding Remarks

Phosgene oxime is considered nonpersistent in the environment. It hydrolyzes rapidly in aqueous alkaline solutions. The potential for secondary contamination is high. Veterinary personnel should wear aprons, rubber gloves, and masks when treating decontaminated patients to avoid self-contamination. Phosgene oxime is of interest to terrorists, as it penetrates garments and rubber much more quickly than other chemical warfare agents. Phosgene oxime can also be mixed with other chemical warfare agents (e.g., VX). The phosgene oxime will cause skin damage which will increase the dermal absorption of the second agent.

CYANIDE AND HYDROGEN CYANIDE

Background

Cyanide and related compounds are classified as blood agents. Cyanogen and cyanogen halides (cyanogen bromide, cyanogen chloride, cyanogen iodide) have been used historically as military chemical warfare agents (ACGIH, 2005). Today cyanide is most likely to be used for a terrorist weapon in the form of hydrogen cyanide or cyanogen chloride.

Hydrogen cyanide (Agent AC, HCN, prussic acid) is a colorless gas with a faint bitter almond-like odor (ACGIH, 2005). Hydrocyanic acid is the liquefied form of hydrogen cyanide (Lewis, 2000). Cyanogen chloride (Agent CK, ClCN) is either a colorless irritant gas or liquid with a pungent odor. It was developed to be slightly heavier than air and to have greater environmental persistence. It can release hydrogen chloride and hydrogen cyanide when it contacts water, acids, or by thermal decomposition. The water soluble salt forms (calcium cyanide, sodium cyanide, and potassium cyanide) will form HCN gas when mixed with a strong acid.

Animals with cyanide poisoning may have an odor of bitter almonds in their gastric or ruminal contents or expired breath. The ability to smell the bitter almond-like odor of cyanide is genetically determined, and 20%–60% of the population cannot detect its presence (Hall and Rumack, 1986).

Pharmacokinetics/Toxicokinetics

Cyanide and hydrogen cyanide can be absorbed by inhalation, ingestion, ocularly and through intact skin (Hall and Rumack, 1986). Cyanide rapidly diffuses into tissues and irreversibily binds to its target sites. Dermal absorption of significant amounts of hydrogen cyanide gas has not been reported. There have been no reports of systemic poisoning in humans ocularly exposed to cyanide; however, rabbits have died following ocular exposure to NaCN, KCN, and HCN.

Cyanide is distributed to all organs and tissues. The concentration of cyanide in red cells is greater than that in plasma by a factor of two or three (HSDB, 2005). Cyanide accumulates in neural tissue. It preferentially accumulates in the hypothalamus, with levels about 40% higher compared to the hippocampus, cerebellum, and cortex (Borowitz et al., 1994). In acute cyanide intoxication, there are no specific pathologic changes.

Cyanide is metabolized by rhodanase in the liver to thiocyanate (Hall and Rumack, 1986). This reaction complexes cyanide with endogenous sulfur or sulfur supplied from the sodium thiosulfate antidote. Once thiocyanate is formed it is excreted mainly in the urine. Half-life for the metabolism of cyanide to thiocyanate is 20 min to 1 h (Feldstein and Klendshoj, 1954). In animals, the dose of cyanide that produces signs is very close to the lethal dose and death can occur within seconds to minutes.

Mechanism of Action

Cyanide causes its toxicity by forming a stable complex with ferric iron (Fe^{3+}) in cytochrome oxidase enzymes. Since oxygen is unable to reoxidize the reduced cytochrome a3, this inhibits cellular respiration, oxygen utilization and ATP production, resulting in deprivation of oxygen to the body at the cellular level (Way et al., 1988). In the brain cyanide decreases oxidative metabolism, increases glycolysis and inhibits brain glutamic acid decarboxylase, thereby decreasing GABA (Bingham et al., 2001). The corpus callosum, hippocampus, corpora striata, and substantia nigra are commonly damaged in cyanide poisoning (Grandas et al., 1989).

Early in cyanide toxicosis, CNS, respiratory, and myocardial depression also contribute to decreased oxygenation of the blood and decreased cardiac output (Hall and Rumack, 1986). There is also evidence of lipid peroxidation by measurement of elevated levels of conjugated dienes in mouse brain and kidneys at 15 and 30 min after cyanide exposure (Ardelt et al., 1994). Cyanide salts are irritating upon ingestion and can cause corrosion of the oral, esophageal, or gastric mucosa (HSDB, 2005).

Toxicity

Signs following acute cyanide exposure include syncope, or CNS stimulation, dizziness, dyspnea, seizures, paralysis, apnea, and coma (Hall and Rumack, 1986). Tachypnea and hyperpnea are followed rapidly by respiratory depression. Signs of severe hypoxia without cyanosis can suggest the diagnosis. Signs in birds are similar to those in mammals. Chickens will pant, have rapid eye blinking, produce excess salivation, and experience lethargy (Wiemeyer et al., 1986). Mydriasis is common in severe poisonings, and blindness may occur from cyanide-induced damage to optic nerves and retina (Grant and Schuman, 1993). Nausea, vomiting, and abdominal pain may occur, especially after ingestion of cyanide salts (Hall and Rumack, 1986). Metabolic acidosis and lactic acidosis are frequent metabolic derrangements. Blood gases show a decreased arterial–venous oxygen saturation difference due to the cellular inability to extract oxygen (Graham et al., 1977).

TABLE 5.4 LD_{50} **for Hydrogen Cyanide**

Species	Route	LD_{50} (μg/kg)
Mouse	IM	2700
	IP	2990
	Oral	3700
Rat	SQ	3700

Source: Data from ACGIH, 2005. Threshold Limit Values (TLVs(R)) for Chemical Substances and Physical Agents and Biological Exposure Indices (BEIs(R)). American Conference of Governmental Industrial Hygienists, Cincinnati, OH; Bingham, E., Chorssen, B., Powell, C.H., 5th edn., 2001. Patty's Toxicology, vol. 3. John Wiley & Sons, New York, NY; Budavari, S., 2000. The Merck Index, 12th edn. on CD-ROM. Version 12:3a. Chapman & Hall/CRCnetBASE, Whitehouse Station, NJ; HSDB, 2005. Hazardous Substances Data Bank. (Edition expires in 2005.) National Library of Medicine, Bethesda, MD (Internet Version). Thomson MICROMEDEX, Greenwood Village, CO; Lewis, R.J., 2000. Sax's dangerous properties of industrial materials, 10th edn. Van Nostrand Reinhold Company, New York, NY; OHM/TADS, 2005. Oil and Hazardous Materials Technical Assistance Data System. U.S. Environmental Protection Agency. Washington, DC (CD Rom Version). Edition expires 2005; provided by Thomson MICROMEDEX, Greenwood Village, CO; RTECS, 2006. Registry of Toxic Effects of Chemical Substances. National Institute for Occupational Safety and Health. Cincinnati, OH (CD Rom Version). Edition expires 2006; provided by Thomson MICROMEDEX, Greenwood Village, CO.

The blood, both arterial and venous, becomes cherry red from accumulated oxyhemoglobin (Lewis, 2000; Bingham et al., 2001). The skin may also be a bright pink color from the high concentration of oxyhemoglobin in the venous return (HSDB, 2005). On funduscopic exam, retinal arteries and veins will appear equally red. A reduced arterio-central venous measured oxygen saturation difference may be seen due to the same cellular inability to extract oxygen. This arterialization of venous blood gases occurs early in the process of cyanide poisoning. Tachycardia and hypertension may be seen in the initial phases of cyanide poisoning followed by bradycardia and hypotension in the late phases. Cyanide exposure can produce death within minutes. See Table 5.4 for LD_{50}s of HCN by various routes.

Cyanide can be measured in blood. No symptoms are expected at concentrations less than 0.2 mg/L, tachycardia can be seen at 0.5–1.0 mg/L, obtundation at 1.0–2.5 mg/L, coma and respiratory depression at levels greater than 2.5 mg/L and death with blood levels greater than 3 mg/L (Graham et al., 1977). Turn-around time makes these measurements not clinically useful.

Treatment

Move animals to fresh air. Emesis is not recommended due to the rapid progression of the clinical signs and potential for seizures, coma or apnea. Activated charcoal may be beneficial if administered immediately after ingestion as the absorption of cyanide is rapid. Flush eyes for at least 15–20 min with tepid water. Wash all contaminated animals thoroughly with soap and water.

Monitor blood gases and serum electrolytes. Administer 100% humidified oxygen with assisted ventilation if needed to maintain an elevated pO_2. Hyperbaric oxygen therapy is approved for cyanide poisoning, but experimental animal studies have been questionable (Way et al., 1972). For severe acidosis ($pH < 7.1$) administer sodium bicarbonate, but acidosis may be difficult to correct prior to administration of antidotes in cyanide toxicosis (Hall and Rumack, 1986). Control seizures with benzodiazepines or barbiturates.

Cyanide toxicosis usually occurs and progresses so rapidly that treatment is rarely administered soon enough to be effective. Antidotal agents should be used if the animal is in respiratory distress or a coma. There are several different antidotal agents that can be used. Hydroxocobalamin, a vitamin B_{12} precursor, is a cobalt containing chelator. Hydroxocobalamin reverses cyanide toxicosis by combining with cyanide to form cyanocobalamin (vitamin B_{12}) (Hall and Rumack, 1987). It has been shown to be effective in treating cyanide-poisoned laboratory animals and has the advantage of producing neither methemoglobinemia nor hypotension, as sodium nitrite does.

Another choice for treatment of cyanide poisoning utilizes several steps. Sodium nitrite is given IV over 15–20 min; quick administration can cause hypotension. Sodium nitrite reacts with hemoglobin in the red blood cells forming methemoglobin. The methemoglobin will combine with free cyanide to form cyanomethemoglobin. Follow sodium nitrite with IV administration of sodium thiosulfate. Sodium thiosulfate supplies sulfur for the rhodanase reaction. Thiocyanate is formed and excreted in the urine. Oxygen, combined with traditional nitrite/thiosulfate therapy, provides better results than thiosulfate alone (Way et al., 1972). It is believed that oxygen may reverse the cyanide–cytochrome oxidase complex and aid in the conversion to thiocyanate following thiosulfate administration. Other chelators such as dicobalt-EDTA (Kelocyanor) and 4-dimethylaminophenol hydrochloride (4-DMAP) may be found in Europe, Australia, and Israel (Hillman et al., 1974; van Dijk et al., 1986).

Animal studies to identify other alternate cyanide antidotes have tested alpha-ketoglutaric acid, chlorpromazine, hydroxylamine, phenoxybenzamine, centrophenoxine, naloxone hydrochloride, etomidate, para-aminopropiophenone, and calcium-ion channel blockers (Dubinsky et al., 1984; Leung et al., 1984; Bright and Marrs, 1987; Yamamoto, 1990; Budavari, 2000). These antidotes have shown some promise in the laboratory setting but have not been tried during actual poisoning situations.

Concluding Remarks

Because HCN is lighter than air, it has a long half-life in air. However, HCN rapidly disperses and is diluted to nontoxic concentrations. Cyanide does not concentrate in soil or plant material but can mix with water. Water converts HCN gas to HCN liquid. Treat contaminated water with ozone, hydrogen peroxide, or calcium or sodium hypochlorite bleach. The potential for secondary contamination of rescue personnel is high. Boots, gloves, goggles, full protective clothing, and a self-contained positive pressure breathing apparatus are needed (AAR, 2000).

As a chemical warfare agent, cyanide is not easy to disseminate; however, it is widely available which increases the chances of its use in terrorist activities (Burklow et al., 2003). Cyanide works much better as a terrorist weapon in an enclosed space.

MILITARY NERVE AGENTS

Background

Military nerve agents are probably the most poisonous of the known chemical warfare agents and are sufficiently toxic that even a brief exposure may be fatal. They were originally synthesized by the Germans during World War II in search of alternatives to the embargos against insecticidal nicotine. Military nerve agents are rapidly acting, anticholinesterase organophosphate (OP) compounds, and are more potent than OP insecticides. Military nerve agents contain a C–P bond that is unique and very resistant to hydrolysis, except in highly alkaline solutions. At ambient temperatures, nerve agents are viscous liquids, not gases.

Military nerve agents are generally divided into "G" agents and "V" agents. The "G" agents (tabun, sarin, soman) were developed during World War II and are called "G" agents because they were first synthesized in Germany. The "G" agents are very volatile and present a vapor hazard. The vapors are more dense than air, thus they stay close to the ground (Garigan, 1996).

Tabun (Agent GA, $C_5H_{11}N_2O_2P$) is the easiest of the "G" agents to manufacture. It is a fruity-smelling (like bitter almonds) combustible colorless to brownish liquid. Contact with bleaching powder generates cyanogen chloride (EPA, 1985b). It may also undergo hydrolysis in the presence of acids or water, releasing hydrogen cyanide (Munro et al., 1999; Budavari, 2000; HSDB, 2005). Sarin (GB, $C_4H_{10}FO_2P$) is a colorless liquid with almost no odor in its pure state (Budavari, 2000). Soman (GD, $C_7H_{16}FO_2P$) is a colorless liquid with a fruity or camphor odor. Soman can release hydrogen fluoride when in contact with acids.

The "V" agents ("V" for venomous) were developed in 1954 in the United Kingdom and are more stable than the "G" agents (Sidell et al., 1997). "V" agents, such as VX, contain a sulfur group and are alkylphosphonothiolates; they are more toxic and persistent on surfaces than G-series agents. VX ($C_{11}H_{26}NO_2PS$) is a nonvolatile, amber-colored, odorless liquid.

Pharmacokinetics/Toxicokinetics

Nerve agents can be absorbed following ocular exposure, oral ingestion, inhalation, and dermal contact (HSDB, 2005; RTECS, 2006). These nerve agents are absorbed without producing any irritation or other sensation on the part of the exposed person or animal. Inhalation of military nerve agents will have initial effects on the airways within seconds. Inhalation of a large amount of the vapor will result in sudden loss of consciousness, apnea, flaccid paralysis and seizures within seconds to 2–3 min (Sidell et al., 1997). Peak effects are seen within 20–30 min and death is usually due to respiratory failure (Berkenstadt et al., 1991). Dermal exposures to nerve agents have a slower onset of action. Exposure to a large drop or more will result in clinical effects within 30 min but with small drops a delay of up to 18 h can be seen. With ingestion, initial symptoms begin in 20–30 min and are usually gastrointestinal. There is no taste to solutions containing nerve gas agents (Grob, 1956).

Distribution in the body is slightly different for each of the nerve agents. Distribution of sarin is to the brain, liver, kidney, and plasma of mice (Little et al., 1986). Radiolabeled soman was evenly distributed throughout the mouse brain after IV administration, with higher levels in the hypothalamus (Wolthuis et al., 1986). Tabun was also found in high concentrations in the hypothalamus after IV administration in mice (Hoskins et al., 1986). An unusual feature of soman toxicity is its apparent storage in body "depots" and release over time. This results in eventual death in animals who survive the initial dose of soman (Wolthuis et al., 1986).

The military nerve agents differ from other OPs in the rapidity of "aging" of the OP-enzyme complex. "Aging" is thought to be due to the loss of an alkyl group, whereby the inhibitor–enzyme complex becomes resistant to reactivation (Young et al., 1999). The half-life ($T_{½}$) of aging for soman is within minutes, for sarin is about 5 h and for both tabun and VX is greater than 40 h (Garigan, 1996).

The nerve agents are hydrolyzed by plasma and tissue enzymes to their corresponding phosphoric and phosphonic acids. Oxidative enzymes are also involved in metabolism (HSDB, 2005). Sarin is hydrolyzed in the body to isopropyl-methylphosphonic acid (IMPA). IMPA in mice studies was generally present at 20-fold higher concentrations than sarin in most tissues; exceeding sarin by four times in the brain (Little et al., 1986). In mice studies, the majority of administered radioactive sarin was detoxified and excreted by the kidneys (Little et al., 1986). Mouse studies reveal that approximately 50% of injected soman is converted to free pinacolyl-methylphosphonic-acid within 1 min, and the half-life of this metabolite is less than 1 h (Reynolds et al., 1985). Soman is mainly eliminated via enzymatic hydrolysis, in competition with binding to target acetylcholinesterase (AChE) (HSDB, 2005).

Mechanism of Action

OPs competitively inhibit AChE by binding irreversibly to its esteric site (phosphorylation). Inhibition of the AChE enzyme results in accumulation of acetylcholine (ACh) and excessive stimulation at muscarinic, nicotinic and CNS cholinergic sites. Increased acetylcholine at autonomic neuro-effector junctions results in increased smooth muscle contractions and secretions, but its effect at skeletal muscle junctions is initially stimulatory (fasciculations), followed by inhibitory (muscle weakness, paralysis). The effects on the sino-atrial node of the heart is inhibitory, causing bradycardia (Namba et al., 1971). ACh accumulation in the CNS can cause ataxia, seizures, and coma. These high levels of ACh induce massive neuronal deaths in various brain areas, particularly in limbic and cortical structures. Death from nerve agents is due to paralysis of the diaphragm, airway obstruction from increased tracheobronchial secretions and depression of the CNS respiratory center (Garigan, 1996).

VX is also thought to possibly react directly with receptors of other neurotransmitters, such as norepinephrine, dopamine and GABA. VX appears to have CNS effects that are unrelated to AChE activity and these agents may produce prolonged effects following convulsive doses (Young et al., 1999).

Toxicity

Symptoms of acute exposure to OPs may include muscarinic, nicotinic, and CNS signs. The muscarinic effects include sweating, hypersalivation, bronchoconstriction, and increased bronchial secretions, miosis, bradycardia, hypotension, vomiting and diarrhea, and urinary and fecal incontinence. The nicotinic effects include fasciculations, convulsions, and weakness of muscles (including the diaphragm). The CNS effects of nerve agents include restlessness, anxiety, headaches, seizures, and coma (Garigan, 1996). Effects after inhalation begin within seconds to minutes postexposure. Death can occur within minutes from inhibition of AChE function.

The "G" nerve gases do not readily penetrate intact skin, but toxicity significantly increases if the skin becomes permeable. Dermal toxicity of VX is high, even through intact skin as the liquid does not evaporate quickly (Berkenstadt et al., 1991; Sidell et al., 1997).

TABLE 5.5 LD_{50} (mg/kg) for Various Nerve Agents

Species	Route	Sarin	Soman	Tabun	VX
Mouse	IP				0.050
	Dermal	1.08	7.8	1	
	IM		0.089		
Rat	SQ			0.162	0.012
	Oral	0.55		3.7	
	Dermal			18	
	IM		0.062		
Human	Dermal	28	5	14	0.14

Source: Data from RTECS, 2006. Registry of Toxic Effects of Chemical Substances. National Institute for Occupational Safety and Health. Cincinnati, OH (CD Rom Version). Edition expires 2006; provided by Thomson MICROMEDEX, Greenwood Village, CO; Sidell, F.R., Takafuji, E.T., Franz, D.R., 1997. Textbook of Military Medicine: Medical Aspects of Chemical and Biological Warfare. TMM Publications, Washington, DC.

With dermal exposures, a very small drop on the skin may cause sweating and fasciculations at the site, starting within 18 h of exposure. A larger drop may cause loss of consciousness, seizures, apnea and flaccid paralysis, with effects beginning within 30 min (Sidell et al., 1997). Liquid tabun in the eye can result in death nearly as quickly as an inhaled dose (EPA, 1985b).

On a per weight basis, toxicity in descending order is: VX > soman > sarin > tabun. As used, VX is the most potent of the "G" nerve agents and it is about three times more potent a respiratory agent than sarin. VX is 300 times more lethal than tabun on skin (Sidell et al., 1997). See Table 5.5 for LD_{50}s of the various nerve agents.

Plasma cholinesterase values usually recover in a few days or weeks, due to the irreversible nature of OP inhibition. RBC AChE recovers more slowly (several days to 4 months) depending on the severity of the depression (Grob, 1956). Delayed neurotoxicity has not been reported in humans following nerve agent exposure. However, delayed peripheral neurotoxicity has been reported in animal studies. Soman, at a dose of 1.5 mg/kg, produced severe delayed neuropathy in the atropinized hen assay (Willems et al., 1984). No prenatal mortality or fetal toxicity was noted in soman-poisoned rats or rabbits, even at doses producing significant maternal toxicity, but other nerve gases showed postimplantation mortality and fetotoxicity (HSDB, 2005; RTECS, 2006).

Treatment

Remove animal from the toxic environment. Administer oxygen if needed. Intubation and ventilation may be necessary if signs progress. Flush eyes with copious amounts of tepid 0.9% saline or water for at least 15 min. Reactive skin decontamination lotion (RSDL) appears to be the best available dermal decontamination agent (Hanssen et al., 2006). If RSDL is not accessible, wash all exposed animals three times with soap and water. The use of a dilute bleach solution (1:10 with water), ethanol or tincture of green soap may be more efficacious (Cancio, 1993).

Emesis is not recommended in oral ingestion due to the rapid development of signs. Activated charcoal might provide benefits even after a topical exposure. Control seizures with diazepam, methocarbamol or barbiturates as needed before proceeding with other treatments.

Atropine sulfate is a reversal agent. It is used for the treatment of muscarinic effects of nerve agent poisoning, but will not reverse nicotinic effects (muscular fasciculations and weakness). Atropine does not affect the AChE–insecticide bond, but blocks the effects of accumulated acetylcholine at the synapse. Atropinization should be continued until the nerve agent is metabolized (Midtling et al., 1985). Effects of overdosing with atropine include hyperthermia, tachycardia, inspiratory stridor, irritability, and dilated and unresponsive pupils (Meerstadt, 1982).

Pralidoxime (2-PAM) can be used to treat the nicotinic signs. Pralidoxime is probably most effective when administered in the first 1–3 h. Pralidoxime is not as effective in the treatment of soman poisoning, due to the quick "aging" (within minutes) of the compound (Sidell et al., 1997). Since VX-inhibited AChE ages slowly, administration of 2-PAM chloride is effective in reactivating the enzyme for up to 48 h after exposure (Sidell and Groff, 1974).

In Belgium, Israel, The Netherlands, Scandinavia, Portugal, and Germany, obidoxime dichloride (Toxogonin, LüH-6) is the favored oxime (Jokanović, 2015). It may be a less toxic and more efficacious alternative to pralidoxime in poisonings from OPs containing a dimethoxy or diethoxy moiety (De Kort et al., 1988). HI-6 is an alternative oxime that has excellent AChE regenerating action with VX and very good action with sarin (GB). It has a good response to soman, but needs higher doses following tabun exposures (Hoffman, 1999). HI-6 is given in conjuction with atropine and diazepam (Kusic et al., 1991). A treatment regime of HI-6, levetiracetam and procyclidine (triple therapy) works against five times the LD_{50} in all nerve agents except tabun (Myhrer et al., 2015). Adding obidoxime to the triple therapy treat tabun doses up to five times the LD_{50} Myhrer et al., 2015).

With human exposures to nerve agents, autoinjectors (AtroPen, Mark I, Combopen MC) are available for use. Most available autoinjectors combine atropine and pralidoxime. Autoinjectors are not used in veterinary medicine as they are not adaptable for different sized patients.

Diazepam and cyproheptadine have been used for seizure control with nerve agents (Winkler et al., 2017).

The "G" agents have been detected in urine and water using capillary GC and GC-MS (Kientz, 1998). Immunoassay has been used to detect VX in biological samples (Ci et al., 1995). Nerve agent detection is not as clinically relevant as the measuring of AChE inhibition level. AChE activity can be used as a diagnostic indicator or a screening test. The test can be run on plasma, serum or whole blood. AChE activity inhibition >70% of normal (100%) is generally associated with severe symptoms (Midtling et al., 1985). Blood AChE does not always correlate well with clinical signs and poisoning has been diagnosed in patients with "normal" values.

Concluding Remarks

The "G" agents evaporate and disperse over several hours and are nonpersistent in the environment (Garigan, 1996). In contrast, VX is an oily liquid that can remain in the environment for weeks or longer after being dispersed (Garigan, 1996; Sidell et al., 1997; Munro et al., 1999; Budavari, 2000; Watson et al., 2015). Environmental persistence is estimated to be 0.5–1 day for tabun, 1–2 days for soman, 5 days for sarin and several weeks for VX. Environmental cleanup of OP spills depend on changing the pH to promote hydrolysis to inactive phosphate diester compounds (EPA, 1978). Contaminated soil can be treated with either alkaline substances (sodium carbonate, sodium bicarbonate, calcium hydroxide, calcium hydroxide, and calcium carbonate) or chlorine-active compounds (sodium hypochlorite or calcium hypochlorite) (EPA, 1975).

Veterinarians and staff can be dermally exposed to contaminated animals. Rubber gowns, aprons, and gloves along with respiratory protection must be worn. Once the animals are bathed, the risk of secondary contamination is low. Leather absorbs OPs and is extremely difficult to decontaminate. Leather collars, muzzles and other items should be incinerated.

The production of nerve agents is beyond the capabilities of most terrorist groups. Production requires a significant background in chemistry and outlay of capital. The production of sarin by the Aum Shinrikyo cult was estimated to take 1 year to make, involved 80 persons led by a PhD-level scientist and cost about $30 million (Leitenberg, 1999).

REFERENCES

AAR, 2000. Emergency Handling of Hazardous Materials in Surface Transportation. Bureau of Explosives. Association of American Railroads, Washington, DC.

ACGIH, 2005. Threshold Limit Values (TLVs(R)) for Chemical Substances and Physical Agents and Biological Exposure Indices (BEIs(R)). American Conference of Governmental Industrial Hygienists, Cincinnati, OH.

Aposhian, H.V., Mershon, M.M., Brinkley, F.B., 1982. Anti-lewisite activity and stability of meso-dimercaptosuccinic acid and 2,3-dimercapto-1-propanesulfonic acid. Life Sci. 31, 2149–2156.

Ardelt, B.K., Borowitz, J.L., Maduh, E.U., 1994. Cyanide-induced lipid peroxidation in different organs: subcellular distribution and hydroperoxide generation in neuronal cells. Toxicology. 89, 127–137.

Bajgar, J., Fusek, J., Kassa, J., et al., 2015. Global impact of chemical warfare agents used before and after 1945. In: Gupta, R.C. (Ed.), Handbook of Toxicology of Chemical Warfare Agents. Academic Press/Elsevier, Amsterdam, pp. 17–25.

Balali-Mood, M., 2015. Early and delayed effects of sulfur mustard in Iranian veterans after the Iraq-Iran conflict. In: Gupta, R.C. (Ed.), Handbook of Toxicology of Chemical Warfare Agents. Academic Press/Elsevier, Amsterdam, pp. 37–46.

Barlow, S.M., Sullivan, F.M., 1982. Arsenic and Its Compounds. Reproductive Hazards of Industrial Chemicals. Academic Press, London, pp. 62–82.

Berkenstadt, H., Marganitt, B., Atsmon, J., 1991. Combined chemical and conventional injuries – pathophysiological, diagnostic and therapeutic aspects. Isr. J. Med. Sci. 27, 623–626.

Berlinger J. VX nerve agent used to kill Kim Jong Nam, police say [Internet]. CNN; 2017 February 27. Available from: http://www.cnn.com/2017/02/23/asia/kim-jong-nam-vx-nerve-agent/.

Bingham, E., Chorssen, B., Powell, C.H., 2001. 5th edn. Patty's Toxicology, vol. 3. John Wiley & Sons, New York, NY.

Bismuth, C., Blanchet-Bardon, C., Baud, F.J., 1995. Delayed admission of five soldiers intoxicated with mustard gas. Ann. Emerg. Med. 26, 715.

Blodi, F.C., 1971. Mustard gas keratopathy. Int. Opthalmol. Clin. 11 (3), 1–13.

Borak, J., Diller, W.F., 2001. Phosgene exposure: mechanisms of injury and treatment strategies. J. Occupat. Env. Med. 43 (2), 110–119.

Borak, J., Sidell, F.R., 1992. Agents of chemical warfare: sulfur mustard. Ann. Emerg. Med. 213, 303–307.

Borowitz, J.L., Rathinavelu, A., Kanthasamy, A., 1994. Accumulation of labeled cyanide in neuronal tissue. Toxicol. Appl. Pharmacol. 129, 80–85.

Bright, J.E., Marrs, T.C., 1987. Effects of p-aminopropiophenone (PAPP), a cyanide antidote, on cyanide given by intravenous infusion. Hum. Toxicol. 6, 133–137.

Brodovsky, S.C., McCarty, A.C., Snibson, G., 2000. Management of alkali burns an 11-year retrospective review. Ophthalmology. 107, 1829–1835.

Budavari, S., 2000. The Merck Index, 12th edn. on CD-ROM. Version 12:3a. Chapman & Hall/CRCnetBASE, Whitehouse Station, NJ.

Burklow, T.R., Yu, C.E., Madsen, J.M., 2003. Industrial chemicals: terrorist weapons of opportunity. Pediatr. Ann. 32 (4), 230–234.

Cancio, L.C., 1993. Chemical casualty decontamination by medical platoons in the 82D Airborne Division. Mil. Med. 158, 1–5.

Chemstar, 1996. Phosgene Pulmonary Exposure Information, second ed. Chemical Manufacturers Association, Phosgene Panel, Arlington, VA.

Chester, E.H., Kaimal, J., Payne, C.B., 1977. Pulmonary injury following exposure to chlorine gas. Possible beneficial effects of steroid treatment. Chest. 72, 247–250.

Chisholm, C.D., Singletary, E.M., Okerberg, C.V., 1989. Inhaled sodium bicarbonate therapy for chlorine inhalation injuries (Abstract). Ann. Emerg. Med. 18, 466.

Ci, Y.X., Zhou, Y.X., Guo, Z.Q., et al., 1995. Production, characterization and application of monoclonal antibodies against the organophosphorus nerve agent VX. Arch. Toxicol. 69 (8), 565–567.

Cowan, F.M., Broomfield, C.A., Smith, W.J., 1998. Sulfur mustard exposure enhances Fe receptor expression on human epidermal keratinocytes in cell culture: implications for toxicity and medical countermeasures. Cell Biol. Toxicol. 14, 261–266.

Dachir, S., Fishbeine, E., Meshulam, Y., et al., 2004. Amelioration of sulfur mustard skin injury following a topical treatment with a mixture of a steroid and a NSAID. J. Appl. Toxicol. 24, 107–113.

De Kort, W.L., Kiestra, S.H., Sangster, B., 1988. The use of atropine and oximes in organophosphate intoxications: a modified approach. Clin. Toxicol. 26, 199–208.

Decker, W.J., 1988. Reactive airways dysfunction syndrome following a single acute exposure to chlorine gas (Abstract). Vet. Human. Toxicol. 30, 344.

DeRosa, C.T., Holler, J.S., Allred, M., et al., 2002. Managing hazardous materials incidents. In Agency for Toxic Substances and Disease Registry. <www.atsdr.cdc.gov>.

Diller, W.F., 1985. Pathogenesis of phosgene poisoning. Toxicol. Ind. Health. 1 (2), 7–15.

Drasch, G., Kretschmer, E., Kauert, G., 1987. Concentrations of mustard gas (bis(2-chloroethyl)sulfide) in the tissues of a victim of a vesicant exposure. J. Forens. Sci. 32, 1788–1793.

Dubinsky, B., Sierchio, J.N., Temple, D.E., 1984. Flunarizine and verapamil: effects on central nervous system and peripheral consequences of cytotoxic hypoxia in rats. Life Sci. 34, 1299–1306.

EPA, 1975. Guidelines for the Disposal of Small Quantities of Unused Pesticides (EPA-670/2-75-057). U.S. Environmental Protection Agency, Washington, DC. pp. 315–330.

EPA, 1978. Identification and Description of Chemical Deactivation/Detoxification Methods for the Safe Disposal of Selected Pesticides (SW-156c). U.S. Environmental Protection Agency, Washington, DC. pp. 44–88.

EPA, 1985a. EPA Chemical Profile on Lewisite. U.S. Environmental Protection Agency, Washington, DC.

EPA, 1985b. EPA Chemical Profile on Sarin; Tabun. U.S. Environmental Protection Agency, Washington, DC.

Evison, D., Hinsley, D., Rice, P., 2002. Chemical weapons. BMJ. 324 (7333), 332–335.

Feldstein, M., Klendshoj, N.C., 1954. The determination of cyanide in biologic fluids by microdiffusion analysis. J. Lab. Clin. Med. 44 (1), 166–170.

Franch, S., Hatch, G.E., 1986. Pulmonary biochemical effects of inhaled phosgene in rats. J. Toxicol. Environ. Health. 19 (3), 413–423.

Garigan, T., 1996. Medical treatment of chemical warfare casualties. Uniformed Services Academy of Family Physicians. Okinawa, Japan. <http://www.usafp.org/op_med/fieldclinical/chemcascare.html> (accessed 15.05.06.).

Goldfrank, L.R., Flomenbaum, N.E., Lewis, N.A., 1998. Goldfrank's Toxicologic Emergencies. sixth ed. Appleton & Lange, Stamford, CN.

Goldman, M., Dacre, J.C., 1989. Lewisite: its chemistry, toxicology, and biological effects. Rev. Environ. Contam. Toxicol. 110, 75–115.

Goswami, D.G., Tweari-Singh, N., Agarwal, R., 2016. Corneal toxicity induced by vesicating agents and effective treatment options. Ann. NY Acad. Sci. 1374, 193–201.

Graham, D.L., Laman, D., Theodore, J., 1977. Acute cyanide poisoning complicated by lactic acidosis and pulmonary edema. Arch. Intern. Med. 137, 1051–1055.

Grandas, F., Artieda, J., Obeso, J.A., 1989. Clinical and CT scan findings in a case of cyanide intoxication. Mov. Disord. 4, 188–193.

Grant, W.M., Schuman, J.S., 1993. Toxicology of the Eye. fourth ed. Charles C Thomas, Springfield, IL.

Graziano, J.H., Cuccia, D., Friedheim, E., 1978. The pharmacology of 2,3-dimercaptosuccinic acid and its potential use in arsenic poisoning. J. Pharmacol. Exp. Ther. 207, 1051–1055.

Grob, D., 1956. The manifestations and treatment of poisoning due to nerve gas and other organic phosphate anticholinesterase compounds. Arch. Intern. Med. 98, 221–239.

Guloglu, C., Kara, I.H., Erten, P.G., 2002. Acute accidental exposure to chlorine gas in the southeast of Turkey: a study of 106 cases. Environ. Res. 88, 89–93.

Guo, Y.L., Kennedy, T.P., Michael, J.R., et al., 1990. Mechanism of phosgene-induced lung toxicity: role of arachidonate mediators. J. Appl. Physiol. 69, 1615–1622.

Gupta, R.C., 2015. In: Gupta, R.C. (Ed.), Handbook of Toxicology of Chemical Warfare Agents. Academic Press/Elsevier, Amsterdam, p. 1184.

Hall, A.H., Rumack, B.H., 1986. Clinical toxicology of cyanide. Ann. Emerg. Med. 15, 1067–1074.

Hall, A.H., Rumack, B.H., 1987. Hydroxycobalamin/sodium thiosulfate as a cyanide antidote. J. Emerg. Med. 5, 115–121.

Hanssen, K.A., Doxzon, B.F., Lumpkin, H.L., et al., 2006. Evaluation of Decontaminaion Systems Challenged with Nerve Agents. US Army Medical Research Institute of Chemical Defense, Aberdeen Proving Ground, MD. (Conference proceedings).

Hillman, B., Bardhan, K.D., Bain, J.T.B., 1974. The use of dicobalt edetate (Kelocyanor) in cyanide poisoning. Postgrad. Med. J. 50, 171–174.

Hoffman, R.S., 1999. Soman poisoning and autoinjectors and reactivators. In Proceedings, NACCT Meeting, La Jolla, CA.

Hoffman, R.S., 2002. Respiratory principles. In: Goldfrank, L.R., Flomenbaum, N.E., Lewin, N.A. (Eds.), Goldfrank's Toxicologic Emergencies, seventh ed. McGraw-Hill, New York, NY.

Honavar, J., Doran, S., Oh, J.-Y., et al., 2014. Nitrite therapy improves survival postexposure to chlorine gas. Am. J. Physiol. Lung. Cell Mol. Physiol. 307, L888–L894.

Honavar, J., Doran, S., Ricart, K., et al., 2017. Nitrite therapy prevents chlorine gas toxicity in rabbits. Toxicol. Lett. 271, 20–25.

Hoskins, B., Fernando, J.C., Dulaney, M.D., 1986. Relationship between the neurotoxicities of soman, sarin and tabun, and acetylcholinesterase inhibition. Toxicol. Lett. 30, 121–129.

HSDB, 2005. Hazardous Substances Data Bank. (Edition expires in 2005.) National Library of Medicine, Bethesda, MD (Internet Version). Thomson MICROMEDEX, Greenwood Village, CO.

IARC, 1975. IARC Monographs on the Evaluation of the Carcinogenic Risk of Chemicals to Man, 9. World Health Organization, Geneva, Switzerland, pp. 181–192.

Johnson, N.H., Larsen, J.C., Meek El, 2015. Historical perspective of chemical warfare agents. In: Gupta, R.C. (Ed.), Handbook of Toxicology of Chemical Warfare Agents. Academic Press/Elsevier, Amsterdam, pp. 7–15.

Jokanović, M., 2015. Pyridinium oximes in the treatment of poisoning with organophosphorus compounds. In: Gupta, R.C. (Ed.),

Handbook of Toxicology of Chemical Warfare Agents. Academic Press/Elsevier, Amsterdam, pp. 1057–1070.

Kaplan, D.E., Marshall, A., 1996. The Cult at the End of the World: The Terrifying Story of the Aum Doomsday Cult, from the Subways of Tokyo to the Nuclear Arsenals of Russia. Crown Publishing, New York, NY.

Kennedy, T.P., Michael, J.R., Hoidal, J.R., et al., 1989. Dibutyryl cAMP, aminophylline, and beta-adrenergic agonists protect against pulmonary edema caused by phosgene. J. Appl. Physiol. 67 (6), 2542–2552.

Kientz, C.E., 1998. Chromatography and mass spectrometry of chemical warfare agents, toxins and related compounds: state of the art and future prospects (Review). J. Chromatogr. 814, 1–23.

Kusic, R., Jovanovic, D., Randjelovic, S., 1991. HI-6 in man: efficacy of the oxime in poisoning by organophosphorus insecticides. Hum. Exp. Toxicol. 10, 113–118.

Leitenberg, M., 1999. Aum Shinrikyo's efforts to produce biological weapons: a case study in the serial propagation of misinformation. Terr. Polit. Violence. 11 (4), 149–158.

Leung, P., Sylvester, D.M., Chiou, F., 1984. Stereospecific effect of naloxone hydrochloride on cyanide intoxication. Toxicol. Appl. Pharmacol. 83, 525–530.

Lewis, R.J., 2000. Sax's Dangerous Properties of Industrial Materials. tenth ed. Van Nostrand Reinhold Company, New York, NY.

Little, P.J., Reynolds, M.L., Bowman, E.R., 1986. Tissue disposition of (3H)sarin and its metabolites in mice. Toxicol. Appl. Pharmacol. 83, 412–419.

Maisonneuve, A., Callebat, I., Debordes, L., 1993. Biological fate of sulphur mustard in rat: toxicokinetics and disposition. Xenobiotica. 23, 771–780.

Mautone, A.J., Katz, Z., Scarpelli, E.M., 1985. Acute responses to phosgene inhalation and selected corrective measures (including surfactant). Toxicol. Ind. Health. 1 (2), 37–57.

Meerstadt, P.W.D., 1982. Atropine poisoning in early infancy due to Eumydrin drops. Br. Med. J. 285, 196–197.

Midtling, J.E., Barnett, P.G., Coye, M.J., 1985. Clinical management of field worker organophosphate poisoning. West J. Med. 142, 514–518.

Munro, N.B., Talmage, S.S., Griffin, G.D., 1999. The sources, fate, and toxicity of chemical warfare agent degradation products. Environ. Health Per. 107, 933–974.

Murdoch, C.M., 1993. Toxicity of Gases. In: Stacey, N.H. (Ed.), Occupational Toxicology. Taylor and Francis, London, pp. 233–249.

Myhrer, T., Mariussen, E., Enger, S., et al., 2015. Supralethal poisoning by any of the classical nerve agents is effectively counteracted by procyclidine regimes in rats. Neurotoxicology. 50, 142–148.

Namba, T., Nolte, C.T., Jackrel, J., 1971. Poisoning due to organophosphate insecticides. Acute and chronic manifestations. Am. J. Med. 50, 475–492.

NATO, 1973. NATO Handbook on the Medical Aspects of NBC Defensive Operations. AMedP-6, Part III. North Atlantic Treaty Organization, Brussels, Belgium. pp. 1, 3, 7, 10.

Noe, J.T., 1963. Therapy for chlorine gas inhalation. Ind. Med. Surg. 32, 411–414.

OHM/TADS, 2005. Oil and Hazardous Materials Technical Assistance Data System. U.S. Environmental Protection Agency. Washington, DC (CD Rom Version). Edition expires 2005; provided by Thomson MICROMEDEX, Greenwood Village, CO.

Okumura, T., Taki, K., Suzuki, K., et al., 2015. The Tokyo subway sarin attack: acute and delayed health effects in survivors. In: Gupta, R.C. (Ed.), Handbook of Toxicology of Chemical Warfare Agents. Academic Press/Elsevier, Amsterdam, pp. 27–35.

Patt, H.M., Tobias, J.M., Swift, M.N., et al., 1946. Hemodynamics in pulmonary irritant poisoning. Am. J. Physio. 147, 329–339.

Paton, C. Assad regime is still making chemical weapons in Syria: Report [Internet]. Newsweek; 2017 May 5. Available from: http://www.newsweek.com/russia-aware-assad-regime-continues-manufacture-and-maintain-chemical-weapons-595185.

Pita, R., Marco-Contelles, J., Ramos, E., et al., 2013. Toxicity induced by chemical warfare agents: insights on the protective role of melatonin. Chem. Biol. Interact. 206, 134–142.

Proctor, N.H., Hughes, J.P., 2004. Proctor and Hughes' Chemical Hazards of the Workplace. fifth ed. John Wiley & Sons, New York, NY.

Raffle, P.A.D., Adams, P.H., Baxter, P.J., 1994. Hunter's Diseases of Occupations. Little, Brown & Co, Boston, MA.

Requena, L., Requena, C., Sanchez, M., 1988. Chemical warfare. Cutaneous lesions from mustard gas. J. Am. Acad. Dermatol. 19, 529–536.

Reynolds, M.L., Little, P.J., Thomas, B.F., 1985. Relationship between the biodisposition of (3H)soman and its pharmacological effects in mice. Toxicol. Appl. Pharmacol. 80, 409–420.

Roberts, J.R., 1988. Minor burns (Pt II). Emerg. Med. Ambulat. Care News. 10, 4–5.

RTECS, 2006. Registry of Toxic Effects of Chemical Substances. National Institute for Occupational Safety and Health. Cincinnati, OH (CD Rom Version). Edition expires 2006; provided by Thomson MICROMEDEX, Greenwood Village, CO.

Sciuto, A.M., Strickland, P.T., Kennedy, T.P., et al., 1995. Protective effects of N-acetylcysteine treatment after phosgene exposure in rabbits. Am. J. Respir. Crit. Care Med. 151, 768–772.

Sciuto, A.M., Moran, T.S., Narula, A., et al., 2001. Disruption of gas exchange in mice after exposure to the chemical agent phosgene. Mil. Med. 116 (9), 809–814.

Sidell, F.R., Groff, W.A., 1974. The reactivatibility of cholinesterase inhibited by VX and sarin in man. Toxicol. Appl. Pharmacol. 27 (2), 241–252.

Sidell, F.R., Takafuji, E.T., Franz, D.R., 1997. Textbook of Military Medicine: Medical Aspects of Chemical and Biological Warfare. TMM Publications, Washington, DC.

Smith, K.J., 1999. The prevention and treatment of cutaneous injury secondary to chemical warfare agents. Application of these finding to other dermatologic conditions and wound healing. Dermatol. Clin. 17 (1), 41–60.

Smith, K.J., Hurst, C.G., Moeller, R.B., 1995. Sulfur mustard: its continuing threat as a chemical warfare agent, the cutaneous lesions induced, progress in understanding its mechanism of action, its long-term health effects, and new developments for protection and therapy. J. Am. Acad. Dermatol. 32, 765–776.

Somani, S.M., Babu, S.R., 1989. Toxicokinetics of sulfur mustard. Int. J. Clin. Pharmacol. Ther. Toxicol. 27 (9), 419–435.

Tan, D.X., Manchester, L.C., Terron, M.P., et al., 2007. One molecule, many derivatives: a never-ending interaction of melatonin with reactive oxygen and nitrogen species? J. Pineal. Res. 42, 28–42.

Tewari-Singh, N., Jain, A.K., Inturi, S., et al., 2012. Silibinin attenuates sulfur mustard analog-induced skin injury by targeting multiple pathways connecting oxidative stress and inflammation. PLOS. 7 (9), e46149.

Tewari-Singh, N., Goswami, D.G., Kant, R., et al., 2017. Cutaneous exposure to vesicant phosgene oxime: acute effects on the skin and systemic toxicity. Tox. Appl. Pharmacol. 317, 25–32.

Traub, S.J., Hoffman, R.S., Nelson, L.S., 2002. Case report and literature review of chlorine gas toxicity. Vet. Human. Toxicol. 44 (4), 235–239.

USACHPPM, 2001a. Detailed Facts about Sulfur Mustard Agents H and HD. U.S. Army Center for Health and Promotion and Preventive Medicine. Aberdeen Proving Ground, MD. <http://chppm-www.apgea.army.mil/dts/docs/dethhd.pdf> (accessed 15.05.06.).

USACHPPM, 2001b. General Facts about Sulfur Mustard Agents H and HD. U.S. Army Center for Health and Promotion and Preventive Medicine. Aberdeen Proving Ground, MD. <http://chppm-www.apgea.army.mil/dts/docs/genhhd.pdf> (accessed 15.05.06.).

USACHPPM, 2001c. Detailed Facts about Blister Agent Lewisite 218-14-1096. U.S. Army Center for Health and Promotion and Preventive Medicine. Aberdeen Proving Ground, MD. <http://chppm-www.apgea.army.mil/dts/docs/detlew.pdf> (accessed 15.05.06.).

USACHPPM, 2001d. Detailed Facts about Blister Agent Phosgene Oxime (CX). U.S. Army Center for Health Promotion and Preventative Medicine. Aberdeen Proving Ground, MD. <http://chppm-www.apgea.army.mil/dts/docs/detcx.pdf> (accessed 15.05.06.).

van Dijk, A., Douze, J.M.C., van Heijst, A.N.P., 1986. Clinical evaluation of the cyanide antagonist 4-DMAP. (Abstract), II World Congress of the World Federation of Associations of Clinical Toxicology and Poison Control Centers, Brussels, Belgium.

Veress, L.A., Anderson, D.R., Hendry-Hofer, T.B., et al., 2015. Airway tissue plasminogen activator prevents acute mortality due to lethal sulfur mustard inhalation. Toxicol. Sci. 143 (1), 178–184.

Vojvodic, V., Milosavljevic, Z., Boskovic, B., 1985. The protective effect of different drugs in rats poisoned by sulfur and nitrogen mustards. Fundam. Appl. Toxicol. 5, S160–S168.

Vucemilovic, A., Hadzija, M., Jukic, I., 2008. Efficacy of mineral cationic carrier against sulfur mustard in skin decontamination. Arh. Hig. Rada. Toksikol. 4, 289–293.

Vycudilik, W., 1985. Detection of mustard gas bis(2-chloroethyl)-sulfide in urine. Forens. Sci. Internat. 28, 131–136.

Wang, J., Zhang, L., Walther, S.M., 2004. Administration of aerosolized terbutaline and budesonide reduces chlorine gas-induced acute lung injury. J. Trauma. 56, 850–862.

Watson, A., Opresko, D., Young, R.A., et al., 2015. Organophosphate nerve agents. In: Gupta, R.C. (Ed.), Handbook of Toxicology of Chemical Warfare Agents. Academic Press/Elsevier, Amsterdam, pp. 87–109.

Way, J.L., End, E., Sheehy, M.H., 1972. Effect of oxygen on cyanide intoxication. IV. Hyperbaric oxygen. Toxicol. Appl. Pharmacol. 22, 415–421.

Way, J.L., Leung, P., Cannon, E., et al., 1988. The mechanism of cyanide intoxication and its antagonism. Ciba Found. Symp. 140, 232–243.

Wells, B.A., 1985. Phosgene: a practitioner's viewpoint. Toxicol. Ind. Health. 1 (2), 81–92.

Wiemeyer, S.N., Hill, E.F., Carpenter, J.W., et al., 1986. Acute oral toxicity of sodium cyanide in birds. J. Wildl. Dis. 22, 538–546.

Willems, J.L., Nicaise, M., De Bisschop, H.C., 1984. Delayed neuropathy by the organophosphorous nerve agents soman and tabun. Arch. Toxicol. 55, 76–77.

Winkler, J.L., Skovira, J.W., Kan, R.K., 2017. Anticonvulsant efficacy of antihistamine cyproheptadine in rats exposed to the chemical warfare nerve agent soman. Neurotoxicology. 58, 153–160.

Wolthuis, O.L., Vanwersch, R.A., Van Helden, H.P., 1986. Residual behavioral incapacitation after therapy of soman intoxication: the effect of a soman simulator. Neurobehav. Toxicol. Teratol. 8, 127–130.

Yamamoto, H.A., 1990. Protection against cyanide-induced convulsions with alpha-ketoglutarate. Toxicology. 61, 221–228.

Young, R.A., Opresko, D.M., Watson, A.P., 1999. Deriving toxicity values for organophosphate nerve agents: a position paper in support of the procedures and rationale for deriving oral RfDs for chemical warfare nerve agents. Hum. Ecol. Risk Assess. 5, 589–634.

Chapter 6

Regulatory Considerations in Veterinary Toxicology: An FDA Perspective

Susan J. Bright-Ponte, Tong Zhou and Michael J. Murphy

INTRODUCTION

Brief History of the Food and Drug Administration

The US Food and Drug Administration (FDA) is a regulatory, science-based federal agency responsible for protecting and promoting the public health through the monitoring and regulation of many products necessary for the health and well-being of consumers. The FDA's jurisdiction includes most food products (other than meat, poultry, and some egg products), animal food, human and animal drugs, medical devices, veterinary devices, therapeutic agents of biologic origin (e.g., vaccines, blood, and blood products) for humans, radiation-emitting products for consumer, medical and occupational use, cosmetics, and tobacco products. The history of the FDA can be traced back to the latter part of the 19th century, when Harvey Washington Wiley, chief chemist of the US Department of Agriculture (USDA) Division of Chemistry (later the Bureau of Chemistry), began conducting research into the misbranding and adulteration of food and drug products in US commerce. Wiley published the Division's findings and lobbied for new federal laws to set uniform standards for food and drugs entering into interstate commerce, resulting in the passage of the Food and Drugs Act in 1906 (FDA, 2015a). The Food and Drugs Act prohibited the interstate transport of adulterated or misbranded food, drink and drugs, and was first administered by the USDA's Bureau of Chemistry (FDA, 2009a). The Bureau of Chemistry's regulatory powers were later reorganized under a new USDA body, the Food, Drug, and Insecticide Organization, which was eventually renamed the FDA. The Food and Drugs Act of 1906 was ultimately replaced by broader legislation, in light of the "Elixir Sulfanilamide" tragedy, in which over 100 people died after using a drug formulated with a toxic solvent (diethylene glycol). The new Federal Food, Drug, and Cosmetic Act (FFDCA, the Act) was signed into law by President Franklin D. Roosevelt in 1938. This law significantly increased regulatory authority over drugs by mandating a premarket review of the safety of all new drugs, as well as banning false therapeutic claims in drug labeling. The law also authorized inspections of factories and expanded enforcement powers, set new regulatory standards for foods, and brought cosmetics and therapeutic devices under federal regulatory authority. In 1940, the FDA was transferred from the USDA to a department that would ultimately become today's Department of Health and Human Services (FDA, 2012a).

In 1962, the Kefauver-Harris Amendment to the FFDCA was passed, requiring that a new drug must also demonstrate substantial evidence of efficacy for its specific indication, in addition to the requirement for premarket demonstration of safety. Drugs approved between 1938 and 1962 were also subject to an FDA review of efficacy. The 1962 amendments also placed some restrictions on drug advertising and expanded the FDA's authority to inspect drug-manufacturing facilities (FDA, 2009b).

In 1968, Congress passed legislation to strengthen provisions of the Act that pertained to regulation of animal drugs. The Animal Drugs Amendments of 1968 required that animal drugs, medicated feeds, and food additives be safe for the animal for which they were intended for use as well as for food-producing animals (that they are safe for human consumption), and safe for the environment. Effectiveness studies were also required (FDA, 2010a).

A comprehensive history of the FDA's regulatory functions can be found on the FDA's website (FDA, 2015a). A number of amendments have been made to the FFDCA related to various areas of FDA regulatory responsibility. Information about significant amendments is available on the FDA's website (FDA, 2015b).

Veterinary Toxicology. DOI: http://dx.doi.org/10.1016/B978-0-12-811410-0.00006-4
2018 Published by Elsevier Inc.

FDA Organization

The FDA's current organization consists of the Office of the Commissioner and four major directorates overseeing the core functions of the agency: Medical Products and Tobacco, Foods and Veterinary Medicine, Global Regulatory Operations and Policy, and Operations. In addition, the FDA is organized geographically into Regional Offices and component Districts, where field staff are assigned. The Office of the Commissioner provides centralized agency-wide program direction and management services to support effective administration and the FDA's consumer protection efforts within its regulatory framework, and to put available resources to the most efficient use. The Office of Medical Products and Tobacco provides high-level coordination and leadership across the centers for human drugs, biologics, medical devices, and tobacco products. The office also oversees the agency's special medical programs. This Office consists of the Center for Drug Evaluation and Research (CDER), the Center for Devices and Radiological Health (CDRH), the Center for Biologics Evaluation and Research (CBER), and the Center for Tobacco Products (CTP). The Office of Foods and Veterinary Medicine (OFVM) has a wide range of responsibilities related to protecting the safety and security of foods for humans and animals, regulating the safety and effectiveness of animal drugs, and ensuring that food labels contain useful and reliable information. Within OFVM, the Center for Food Safety and Applied Nutrition (CFSAN), the Center for Veterinary Medicine (CVM), and the Office of Regulatory Affairs (ORA) work together to carry out the FDA's food safety, nutrition, and animal health activities. The Office of Global Regulatory Operations and Policy (also known as GO) comprises the Office of Regulatory Affairs and the Office of International Programs. The GO Office provides executive oversight, strategic leadership, and policy direction to the FDA's domestic and international product quality and safety efforts, including global collaboration, global data sharing, development and harmonization of standards, field operations, compliance, and enforcement activities. The Office of Operations is responsible for various agency functions, including finance and budget, facilities engineering, information management and technology, human resources, crisis management, and emergency operations (FDA, 2016a).

The National Center for Toxicological Research (NCTR), established by executive order in 1971, is an important research component of the FDA that plays a critical role in the FDA's mission to promote and protect public health. The NCTR, in partnership with researchers from elsewhere in the FDA, other government agencies, academia and industry, provides innovative technology, methods development, vital scientific training, and unique technical expertise which is critical in supporting FDA product centers and their regulatory roles. The NCTR conducts FDA mission-critical, peer-reviewed, critical path research targeted to developing a scientifically sound basis for regulatory decisions and reducing risks associated with FDA-regulated products. Research is aimed at evaluating the biological effects of potentially toxic chemicals or microorganisms, defining the complex mechanisms that govern their toxicity, understanding critical biological events in the expression of toxicity, and developing methods to improve assessment of human exposure, susceptibility, and risk. Customized assessment of chemicals of vital interest to the FDA involves the coordination of expertise in the areas of biochemical and molecular markers of safety and toxicity, neurotoxicology, microbiology, chemistry, genetic or reproductive/developmental toxicology and systems-biology assessments for characterizing biomarkers. The NCTR has developed and is standardizing technologies, such as genomics, proteomics, metabolomics, and nanotechnology to identify and characterize early biomarkers of toxicity using quantitative risk assessment methods. The NCTR also represents the FDA on key committees of the National Toxicology Program (NTP), a program that evaluates the effects of chemicals on health (FDA, 2016b).

Throughout this chapter, reference may be made to the US Code (USC), the Code of Federal Regulations (CFR) and certain guidance documents. The USC contains all general and permanent US laws, including the FFDCA. FDA develops regulations based on the laws set forth in the FFDCA or other laws under which FDA operates. The CFR is a codification of regulations in the Federal Register by the executive departments and agencies of the federal government. Title 21 of the CFR is reserved for rules of the FDA. Each title (or volume) of the CFR is revised once each calendar year. A revised Title 21 is issued on approximately April 1 of each year and is usually available on the US Government Publishing Office Electronic CFR website (US GPO, 2017). Guidance documents represent the FDA's current thinking on a particular subject. These documents are prepared for FDA review staff and regulated industry to provide guidelines for the processing, content, and evaluation or approval of applications and also for the design, production, manufacturing, and testing of regulated products. They also establish policies intended to achieve consistency in the FDA's regulatory approach and establish inspection and enforcement procedures. Because guidance documents are not regulations or laws, they are not enforceable, either through administrative actions or through the courts. An alternative approach may be used if such approach satisfies the requirements of the applicable statute, regulations, or both.

FDA CENTER FOR VETERINARY MEDICINE

Overview

The FDA CVM protects public and animal health by ensuring that animal drugs and medicated feeds are safe and effective and that food from treated animals is safe to eat. The responsibilities of the CVM have a direct effect on the safety of the human food supply and on the safety to animals that are treated with veterinary products. Before a new animal drug can be legally marketed in the United States, it must be approved by the FDA on the basis of quality, safety, and efficacy. When the drug is to be approved for use in food-producing animals, safety to the target animal species must be demonstrated in addition to safety of food products derived from the treated animals that are intended for human consumption. Thus, part of the preapproval process for drugs intended for use in food-producing animals includes the determination of safety of drug residues in animal-derived food products. In addition, preapproval safety evaluation of certain animal drugs includes a determination of the effects of the animal drug on the environment and on human health in some cases. Once approved products are on the market, the Center monitors the use of the products through surveillance and compliance programs. The CVM's responsibilities also include ensuring that food for animals is safe, manufactured properly and under sanitary conditions, and is properly labeled. There are currently no requirements for FDA premarket approval of medical devices intended for animal use; however, FDA can take appropriate regulatory action if a veterinary device is misbranded or adulterated.

Currently, the CVM is organized into six offices: Office of the Director, Office of Management, Office of New Animal Drug Evaluation, Office of Surveillance and Compliance, Office of Research, and Office of Minor Use and Minor Species. Most of the offices are further organized into major divisions and teams. Information about each office and their roles and responsibilities can be found on the CVM website (FDA/CVM, 2015a).

This chapter focuses on FDA regulation of new animal drugs, briefly describing parts of the approval process and examples of postapproval activities conducted to monitor drug safety and effectiveness while the drug is marketed. Animal food is also briefly discussed. A comprehensive description of these topics is not in the scope of this chapter, but more information is readily available on the CVM website. Some jurisdictional considerations and definitions are provided first.

Regulation of Animal Health Products: Jurisdiction Considerations and Regulatory Definitions

Animal health products are typically regulated by one of three federal agencies: the FDA, the Environmental Protection Agency (EPA), or the USDA, depending on whether the product is determined to be an animal drug, device or food, a pesticide, or an animal/veterinary biologic. A team of individuals within the CVM interact with these agencies to establish the appropriate jurisdiction for particular products.

The CVM's jurisdiction team often works with the Center for Veterinary Biologics (CVB) at the USDA's Animal and Plant Health Inspection Service (USDA-APHIS) to determine whether a particular product meets the definition of a biological product or a new animal drug. Unlike biologics for human use, which are regulated by FDA (CBER), veterinary biologics are regulated under the Virus-Serum-Toxin Act (VSTA) by USDA-APHIS. In Title 9 of the CFR, §101.2 defines biological products as "all viruses, serums, toxins (excluding substances that are selectively toxic to microorganisms, e.g., antibiotics), or analogous products at any stage of production, shipment, distribution, or sale, which are intended for use in the treatment of animals and which act primarily through the direct stimulation, supplementation, enhancement, or modulation of the immune system or immune response. The term 'biological products' includes but is not limited to vaccines, bacterins, allergens, antibodies, antitoxins, toxoids, immunostimulants, certain cytokines, antigenic or immunizing components of live organisms, and diagnostic components, that are of natural or synthetic origin, or that are derived from synthesizing or altering various substances or components of substances such as microorganisms, genes or genetic sequences, carbohydrates, proteins, antigens, allergens, or antibodies." Additional information about veterinary biologics and their regulation can be found at the USDA's website (USDA-APHIS, 2017).

The CVM jurisdiction team also works with the EPA's Office of Pesticide Programs (OPP) to determine whether a particular product meets the definition of a new animal drug or a pesticide. Some products used in or on animals to treat or prevent parasites are regulated by the FDA under the FFDCA Act, and some are regulated by the EPA under the Federal Insecticide, Fungicide, and Rodenticide Act (FIFRA). The term "pesticide" means, in part, any substance or mixture of substances intended for preventing, destroying, repelling, or mitigating any pest, or intended for use as a plant regulator, defoliant, or dessicant, other than any article that is a new animal drug under the FFDCA, or is an animal feed under FFDCA that bears or contains a new animal drug (40 CFR §152.3). Pesticide ingredients are evaluated by EPA to ensure that they meet federal safety standards to protect human and animal health and the environment. Information about EPA's regulation of pesticides can be found on the EPA website (US EPA, 2017).

Animal drugs, devices, and foods are regulated by the FDA under the FFDCA. The CVM's jurisdiction team also works with colleagues within the CVM and the FDA to determine the appropriate classification of these products. The FFDCA definitions (in part) for these terms are provided here, but the FFDCA should be consulted for complete definitions.

Under section 201(g) of the FFDCA, the term "drug" means articles intended for use in the diagnosis, cure, mitigation, treatment, or prevention of disease in man or other animals, and articles (other than food) intended to affect the structure or any function of the body of man or other animals, and any component of such articles. Under section 201(v) of the FFDCA, the term "new animal drug" is defined, in part, as any drug intended for use in animals other than man, including any drug intended for use in animal feed, but not including the animal feed, the composition of which is such that the drug is not generally recognized as safe and effective for the use under the conditions prescribed, recommended, or suggested in the labeling of the drug. As mandated by the FFDCA, a new animal drug may not be sold in interstate commerce unless it is the subject of an approved new animal drug application (NADA), abbreviated NADA (ANADA, which is a generic new animal drug), conditionally approved new animal drug application (CNADA), or listing on the Index of Legally Marketed Unapproved New Animal Drugs for Minor Species. Conditional approval and indexing are additional ways that drugs intended for minor uses or minor species can be legally marketed. See the CVM website for a description of these and other provisions made for minor use and minor species products (FDA/CVM, 2017a).

Under section 201(h) of the FFDCA, the term "device" means an instrument, apparatus, implement, machine, contrivance, implant, in vitro reagent, or other similar or related article, including any component, part, or accessory, which is intended for use in the diagnosis of disease or other conditions, or in the cure, mitigation, treatment, or prevention of disease, in man or other animals, or intended to affect the structure or any function of the body of man or other animals, and which does not achieve its primary intended purposes through chemical action within or on the body of man or other animals and which is not dependent upon being metabolized for the achievement of its primary intended purposes. A few examples of devices commonly used in animals include suture material, certain types of bandage materials, intravenous catheters, anesthetic machines as well as radiologic imaging equipment.

Under section 201(f) of the FFDCA, the term "food" means articles used for food or drink for man or other animals, chewing gum, and articles used for components of any such article. Also, 21 CFR §507.3 defines "animal food" as food for animals other than man and includes pet food, animal feed, and raw materials and ingredients.

New Animal Drug Approval

As part of the preapproval process for new animal drugs, a drug sponsor must provide evidence that the drug is safe for the target animal and the environment, has the intended effect, can be manufactured adequately to preserve the product's identity, strength, quality, and purity, and for drugs approved for use in food-producing animals, that the edible products derived from treated animals are safe for human consumption. For the purposes of this chapter, the drug "sponsor" owns the NADA and is the entity responsible for collecting all of the information about a new animal drug and submitting it to the CVM for review, and is also responsible for continued monitoring of the drug's safety and effectiveness after approval. Requirements for NADAs are codified in 21 CFR Part 514. Sponsors systematically address each of the required components by completing seven elements (commonly referred to as technical sections). The seven technical sections are: Chemistry, Manufacturing, and Controls (CMC); Effectiveness, Target Animal Safety (TAS); Human Food Safety (HFS); Environmental Safety; All Other Information; and Labeling. The FDA has published regulations and many guidance documents describing the approval requirements and types of studies that may be necessary to obtain approval to market animal drug products. An explanation of all steps in the process required for FDA approval is beyond the scope of this chapter; however, a brief summary of the TAS and HFS evaluation process for new animal drugs is provided below. A comprehensive description of the process is also provided on the CVM website (FDA/CVM, 2017b).

Target Animal Safety Evaluation

General Considerations

The drug sponsor must show that the drug is safe to the target animal species when it is used according to the label. The target animal species is the specific animal species in which the drug will be approved for use. The TAS information needed for approval of a particular drug depends on the type of drug, species and class of animal, route of administration, indication, dose and frequency of administration, available scientific knowledge about the drug, and potentially other factors. The principles of TAS evaluation are outlined in the FDA-CVM Guidance for Industry (GFI): TAS for Veterinary Pharmaceutical Products (FDA/CVM, 2009a). This document was developed and implemented as part of the International Cooperation on Harmonization of Technical Requirements for Registration of Veterinary Medicinal Products (VICH), a program aimed at harmonizing technical requirements for veterinary product registration among its member countries, which are the United States, the countries of the European Union, and Japan (VICH, 2017).

The components of the TAS technical section are very briefly described below. For some drugs, each of these components will be necessary, while for others, for which a lot of information is already available and drug action and safety are well understood, less information may be needed. Margin of safety and other laboratory safety studies must be performed in conformity with the principles of Good Laboratory Practices (GLP), codified in 21 CFR Part 58. The GLP regulations address nonclinical laboratory studies and ensure that methods and procedures for collecting, processing, and reporting data are standardized, allowing for an adequate level of accuracy and quality control for the studies and data submitted for review. In addition, the GLP regulations assure that records are available to provide assurance that the study was actually conducted as described in the study protocol and final study report.

Pharmacologic/Toxicologic Characterization

The pharmacologic/toxicologic characterization includes any information submitted by the sponsor that may help design the pivotal TAS study. In addition, it can help to better predict and understand any potential adverse effects that may occur in the target animal. Data in the pharmacologic/toxicologic characterization package may include published literature and preliminary studies, including various target and nontarget laboratory animal studies as well as pharmacokinetic, pharmacodynamic, and toxicology studies.

Pivotal Margin of Safety Study

Margin of safety studies have historically been used to support the safety of an investigational new animal drug. These studies are generally characterized by a small sample size, relative homogeneity of study animals, limited study duration, and the use of healthy young animals. Although the use of multiple doses is commonly needed in order to extrapolate safety findings of new animal drugs to their use under various clinical conditions, the actual multiples of the 1X dose in a margin of safety study are not strictly defined. Most typically, however, the margin of safety is demonstrated in a 0X-, 1X-, 3X-, and 5X-dose study with the drug administered for 3X the intended duration. The product safety is then established by demonstrating an acceptable level of safety (above 1X dose) and identifying (if present) the toxic syndrome. Variables that are typically assessed in a margin of safety study include physical examinations and observations; various clinical pathology tests (hematology, blood chemistry, and urinalysis); necropsy; and histopathology. Other information, such as toxicokinetic data, may also be collected if deemed necessary.

Other Laboratory Safety Studies

Additional safety studies may be needed in order to answer specific safety questions in the intended target species or class of animal. Examples of such specialized studies include reproductive safety studies; specific animal class safety studies (e.g., neonatal, geriatric); injection/administration-site safety studies; and mammary gland safety studies.

Safety Information From Field Effectiveness Studies

Additional safety information needed is gathered from field (clinical) effectiveness studies. Unlike the margin of safety studies, the field studies are conducted under clinical conditions representative of the intended use of a new animal drug (e.g., client-owned diseased animals of various breeds, classes, and ages). These studies allow detection of some adverse findings that occur at a low frequency and may have been missed in small-scale margin of safety studies. More importantly, these studies provide data on drug safety in diseased animals. Good Clinical Practice (GCP) Guidance offers the FDA's current best thinking on the conduct of effectiveness studies (FDA/CVM, 2011a).

Safety Data From Foreign Approvals

If an investigational drug is already approved in other countries, the CVM will also evaluate foreign adverse reports, if available, to learn about these adverse findings under clinical conditions of use.

Human Food Safety Assessment

General Considerations

For drugs used in food-producing animals, human food safety assessment of drug residues is required to ensure that there is reasonable certainty of no harm to human consumers with respect to human exposures to potential residues in edible tissues (muscle, liver, kidney, fat, and when applicable, milk, eggs, and honey) of animals treated with the drug product. FDA is normally concerned with intermittent and chronic exposure of people to relatively low concentrations of drug residues, including the parent drug and its metabolites. Some compounds need only a minimum of testing, while others may need more studies in various toxicological testing species. The CVM has published draft revised GFI #3 to inform sponsors of the scientific data and/or information that may be required to provide an acceptable basis to determine that the residue of a new animal drug in or on food, when consumed, presents a reasonable certainty of no harm to humans (FDA/CVM, 2016a). The overall human food safety evaluation includes hazard identification, hazard characterization, exposure assessment, and exposure mitigation. The assessment is conducted from the perspectives of toxicology, residue chemistry, and microbial food safety (for antimicrobial drugs). Pivotal toxicology studies should be conducted in compliance with the GLP regulations set forth in 21 CFR Part 58, or should address the requirements for studies not conducted under these regulations.

Toxicological Studies

The purpose of toxicological studies is to define the biological effect(s) of the new animal drug and to establish the threshold dose for the effect(s). Factors considered in determining the approach to toxicological testing needed for a new animal drug and its residues include its physicochemical properties, proposed use, mechanism of action, probable amounts and patterns of human exposure under the proposed conditions of use, possible biological effects of the residues as deduced through structure-activity comparisons, and observed effects when new animal drugs are tested in toxicological and biological model systems. In addition to the information regarding the test new animal drug, separate information on the toxicology of metabolites and/or excipients may also be considered necessary to assess human food safety. Oral administration is generally the route of choice for in vivo tests, and both rodent and nonrodent toxicological testing species are included in the testing approach in order to maximize the chance of identifying and characterizing a potential adverse effect in humans.

The recommended general testing approach is outlined in the FDA GFI #149 (VICH GL33): Studies to Evaluate the Safety of Residues of Veterinary Drugs in Human Food: General Approach to Testing (FDA/CVM, 2009b). This GFI references additional human food safety toxicology guidance documents and VICH guidelines. Basic toxicity tests recommended for all new animal drugs used in food-producing animals include repeat-dose subchronic and chronic, reproduction, developmental, and genotoxicity testing. Repeat-dose subchronic and chronic toxicity testing is performed to define toxic effects based on repeated and/or cumulative exposures to the compound and its metabolites, to determine the incidence and severity of effects in relation to dose and/or duration of exposure, to determine the doses associated with toxic and biological responses, and to determine a no-observed-effect level (NOEL) or no-observed-adverse-effect-level (NOAEL). The spacing of the doses should provide an assessment of the dose–response relationship. For the repeat-dose testing, two 90-day oral toxicity studies are usually conducted (one in a rodent species and one in a nonrodent mammalian species) to inform the conduct of a chronic oral toxicity study (usually 1 year) in the most appropriate species determined from the 90-day studies. Reproduction toxicity testing (usually two generations) is performed to detect any effect of the compound on mammalian reproduction, including effects on male and female fertility, conception, implantation, ability to maintain pregnancy to term, parturition, lactation, survival, growth and development of offspring, and subsequent reproductive function of the offspring at adulthood. Developmental toxicity testing is conducted to detect any adverse effects on the pregnant female and development of the embryo and fetus subsequent to exposure to the drug; adverse effects may include embryo or fetal death, altered fetal growth, and structural changes to the fetus. A battery of genotoxicity tests is typically used to identify substances that damage the genetic information within cells. Substances considered to be genotoxic based on a weight of the evidence evaluation for the battery of genotoxicity studies and information are regarded as potential carcinogens. Examples of additional tests that may be recommended to address safety concerns such as those based on structure, class, and mode of action of the drug include testing for effects on the human intestinal flora (for antimicrobials), immunotoxicity testing to investigate the potential for the drug to elicit an immunological or allergic reaction in sensitive individuals, neurotoxicity testing if neurotoxic potential is identified in repeat-dose tests, and carcinogenicity testing, based on results of genotoxicity testing, structure activity relationship information, and results of repeat-dose and mechanistic studies. FDA may also require special tests in order to understand the mode of action of the drug and aid in the interpretation or assessment of the relevance of the data obtained in the basic and/or additional tests.

Acceptable Daily Intake, Acute Reference Dose and Safety Factors

The safety of residues in food is usually addressed through calculation of an acceptable daily intake (ADI), defined as the daily intake which, during up to an entire life of a human, appears to be without adverse effects or harm to the health of a consumer. The toxicological ADI is based on the new animal drug's toxicological or pharmacological properties as determined through the recommended toxicology studies and other applicable scientific information, and reflects uncertainties within the information. It is usually expressed in micrograms of the total residues of the drug per kilogram body weight per day (μg/kg body wt/day) or the milligrams of the total residues of the drug per kilogram body weight per day (mg/kg body wt/day).

When establishing the ADI, the toxicity of the new animal drug and its principal metabolites are considered, and the ADI is based on the most relevant toxicological end-point. The derivation of the ADI is determined by dividing an appropriate point of departure (POD) by an appropriate safety factor. The POD is typically identified as a NOEL/NOAEL (or benchmark dose lower confidence limit (BMDL)) from an appropriate toxicology study in the most sensitive species. ADIs for animal drugs established by FDA are codified under 21 CFR Part 556, and are used to derive the enforceable tolerances for marker residues in edible tissues.

For antimicrobial drugs used in food-producing animals, a microbiological ADI may be determined if residues of antimicrobial drugs reaching the human colon remain microbiologically active and affect intestinal bacteria. FDA GFI #159 (VICH GL36(R)) describes the recommended approach (FDA/CVM, 2013).

In certain cases, there may be the potential for a new animal drug to cause acute toxicity to the human consumer following consumption of a single meal or consumption of food over a single day. Some toxicological tests may suggest the need for a safe intake value in addition to the ADI to account for the possibility of acute toxicity. In these cases, the ADI is not the appropriate safe intake value for quantifying the dose above which exposure from a single meal or over a single day can produce acute adverse effects; instead, determining an acute reference dose (ARfD) is the more appropriate approach which is described in FDA Draft GFI #232 (FDA/CVM, 2015b). An ARfD is an estimate of the amount of residues, expressed on a body weight basis, which can be ingested in a period of 24 h or less without adverse effects or harm to the health of the human consumer. The ARfD, usually reported as an amount of the drug substance on a per person (mg/person) or body weight basis (mg/kg body wt), is determined by dividing an appropriate POD by an appropriate safety factor.

The safety factors used in these calculations, whether for acute or chronic effects, reflect the uncertainties associated with the extrapolation of data and information from toxicology studies to humans, including extrapolation of long-term, chronic effects from laboratory studies with shorter-term exposures, extrapolation of animal data to humans, and interindividual variability in the sensitivity to the toxicity of the new animal drug among humans. The safety factor generally consists of multiples of 10, with each factor representing a specific uncertainty inherent in the available data. The overall safety factor is dependent upon the interplay of many factors, including the type of study from which the NOEL/NOAEL or BMDL was derived, the species of animals used in the study, and the endpoint(s) observed in the study. For example, a safety factor of 100 (the default 10-fold factor for interspecies variability and the default 10-fold for human interindividual variability) is usually applied when a POD from a chronic toxicology study is used for the ADI determination. However, information on a chemical-specific adjustment factor, when available, may justify a nondefault (either reduced or increased) safety factor.

Residue Chemistry Studies

The purpose of residue chemistry studies is to assess the quantity and nature of residues in tissues derived from animals treated with new animal drugs. The CVM has published guidance documents (FDA GFI # 3, 205, 207, and 208) which inform sponsors on the conduct of total residues and metabolism studies, comparative metabolism studies, residue depletion studies, and analytical method validation (FDA/CVM, 2011b, 2015c,d, 2016a). Total residue and metabolism studies are designed to develop information on the amount, persistence, and chemical nature of the total residues, as well as the metabolic fate of the new animal drug in the treated target animals. The total residue and metabolism data are used to determine the marker residue, the target tissue, and the marker residue to total residue ratio. The marker residue is the residue for which the concentration is in a known relationship to the concentration of total residue in an edible tissue, and the target tissue refers to the edible tissue selected to monitor for residues in the target animal.

Using information from the calculated ADI, safe concentrations, and target tissue and marker residue, a tolerance is determined for the new animal drug. Tolerance is the maximum concentration of a marker residue, or other residue indicated for monitoring, that can legally remain in a specific edible tissue of a treated animal. The tolerance is determined by examining depletion data consisting of the total residue concentrations and marker residue concentrations by a proposed analytical method. Tolerances for new animal drugs approved for use in food-producing animals are listed in the USC of Federal Regulations (21 CFR Part 556). The CVM may assign the tolerance by harmonizing with previously established international safety limits (maximum residue limits, or MRLs). Tolerances and MRLs both describe the limits of residues, but are not derived in the same manner and are used for different purposes. Tolerances are used to establish withdrawal periods or milk discard times for new animal drugs. The withdrawal period or milk discard time is the interval between the time of the last administration of a new animal drug and the time when the animal can be safely slaughtered for food or the milk can be safely consumed.

Regulating Carcinogenic Compounds

Carcinogenic risk assessment is one of the most important aspects in the safe assessment of animal drug residues.

The DES (diethylstilbestrol) proviso provides an exception to the Delaney Clause of the FFDCA, which allows for the use in food-producing animals of new animal drugs, food additives, and color additives that induce cancer in animals or humans, if (1) the compound does not adversely affect the animal, and (2) analytical methods approved by FDA do not detect residues of the compound in any edible tissues from the treated animal. If FDA determines, on the basis of the results of the chronic cancer bioassays and other information, that the sponsored compound caused cancer in man or animals, then the compound is regulated as a carcinogen under the Delaney Clause DES proviso and is subject to 21 CFR Part 500, Subpart E, to meet the FDA operational definition of no residue.

The FDA will calculate the concentration of a residue of carcinogenic concern in the total human diet that represents no significant increase in the risk of cancer to the human consumer, termed S_o. The FDA assumes this S_o will correspond to the concentration of test compound in the total diet of test animals that corresponds to a maximum lifetime risk of cancer in the test animals of 1-in-1 million (21 CFR §500.82). The no-residue regulations describe not only the calculation of a concentration of the residue of carcinogenic concern that corresponds to a maximum lifetime risk to the test animal of 1-in-1 million (21 CFR §500.84), but also the possibility of a waiver of requirements, which allows alternative procedures to provide the basis for ensuring that the approval of the compound satisfies the anticancer provisions (21 CFR §500.90). Generally speaking, for a genotoxic carcinogen or in the absence of information establishing thresholdable mode of action for carcinogenesis for a particular compound, FDA assumes that a threshold for carcinogenesis cannot be determined and determines an S_o using a default 1-in-1-million linear-at-low-dose statistical extrapolation procedure (Gaylor and Kodell, 1980; Farmer et al., 1982) based on the tumor incidence in the observed species. For a nongenotoxic carcinogen, alternative approaches for deriving the acceptable tissue residue concentrations (such as a threshold for carcinogenic effects based on the mode of action for carcinogenesis) can provide a basis for ensuring that the anticancer provisions of the FFDCA are satisfied.

Approval

After all requirements for approval have been met, the product can be legally marketed and promoted as a new animal drug. As part of the preapproval process, the CVM reviews the language and formatting that will be on each part of the drug's labeling. The labeling must provide all necessary information to use the drug safely and effectively, including the risks associated with the drug. The label must include, among other things, the drug name and active ingredient, product claim(s), pharmacology, adverse effects, precautions, warnings, and contraindications. Sections of 21 CFR Parts 200 and 201 describe the various sections and requirements for animal drug labels. A Freedom of Information (FOI) summary is prepared and published on the CVM website. The FOI summary is a public document describing the safety and effectiveness information that supports the CVM's decision to approve the drug. It includes summaries of studies that were done and explains the basis for approval. After approval, the drug is monitored through periodic and special industry drug experience reports submitted to the CVM by the sponsor, including adverse drug experience (ADE) reports that may result in label changes related to product safety.

POSTAPPROVAL SURVEILLANCE ACTIVITIES

Overview of the CVM's Pharmacovigilance Program

Although the CVM has a rigorous preapproval process for animal drugs, well-conducted, randomized, controlled clinical trials may not be of sufficient size to identify every safety problem, especially ones that are rare and unexpected. Once a product is marketed, there is a substantial increase in the number of patients exposed to the drug, including animals with coexisting medical conditions and those being treated with concomitant medications and biologic agents such as vaccines. There are potential food interactions as well. Additional information about medical product safety and effectiveness is obtained after a product is marketed and used under actual field conditions in large diverse populations of animals. This information is used to complete the safety profile of a product and helps to ensure that drug product labeling is adequate and accurate. Ultimately, this information will assist practitioners in making informed decisions to minimize risks while maximizing benefits of the drugs used in animals.

Pharmacovigilance, as defined by the World Health Organization (WHO), is "the science and activities relating to the detection, assessment, understanding, and prevention of adverse effects or any other drug-related problems" (WHO, 2017a). In general, the role of a pharmacovigilance program is to identify safety signals that, upon further evaluation, may lead to the discovery of previously unidentified or unrecognized adverse drug events and associated risk factors that were not identified in the preapproval evaluation of the product. These adverse events may be related to previously unrecognized pharmacological effects of the drug, idiosyncratic effects, drug-drug interactions, drug-food interactions, drug-disease interactions, factors specific to certain patient populations, individual patient factors, medication errors, product defects, or other factors, such as the reaction being too uncommon to be identified in the small number of animals in which the drug is tested in preapproval studies (CIOMS, 2010). Spontaneous reports of ADEs, medication errors and product defects comprise the primary data source upon which the CVM's postapproval pharmacovigilance efforts depend. Also, data from postapproval clinical studies and from the scientific literature may be utilized. Limitations of utilizing spontaneous ADE reporting databases for pharmacovigilance activities include the significant underreporting of ADEs, limited detail in submitted reports, and reporting bias. Given the variability in reporting and the many factors that affect reporting, ADE reporting rates cannot be used to reliably estimate incidence rates of ADEs in the exposed population. Despite these limitations, the monitoring and evaluation of ADE reports is very important to help ensure that the overall balance of risks and benefits of a particular drug remain acceptable. Additionally, it allows for communication of essential drug safety information to veterinarians and others involved in the treatment of animals.

Adverse Drug Experience: Definition

An ADE, as currently defined by regulation in 21 CFR §514.3, is any adverse event associated with the use of a new animal drug, whether or not considered to be drug related, and whether or not the new animal drug was used in accordance with the approved labeling (i.e., used according to label directions, or used in an extra-label manner, including but not limited to different route of administration, different species, different indications, or other than labeled dosage). ADE includes, but is not limited to: an adverse event occurring in animals in the course of the use of an animal drug product by a veterinarian or by a livestock producer or other animal owner or caretaker; failure of a new animal drug to produce its expected pharmacological or clinical effect (lack of expected effectiveness); or an adverse event occurring in humans from exposure during manufacture, testing, handling or use of a new animal drug.

Adverse Drug Experience Reporting

In the United States, ADE reporting by veterinarians and consumers is voluntary. However, manufacturers and distributors of FDA-approved animal drugs may be subject to mandatory ADE reporting requirements as described by regulation (21 CFR §514.80). All unsolicited reports from veterinarians or consumers, received by the FDA via either the voluntary or mandatory route, are called spontaneous reports. The regulations that address the spontaneous reporting obligations for manufacturers and distributors of FDA-approved animal drugs are contained in 21 CFR §514.80, "Records and reports concerning experience with new animal drugs for which an approved application is in effect." ADE reports are classified into essentially four categories: (1) 3-day field alerts, (2) 15-day alert initial reports, (3) follow-up reports, and (4) periodic reports. As defined in 21 CFR §514.80(b)(1), 3-day field alert reports contain information regarding product and manufacturing defects that may result in serious ADEs. Reports of serious, unexpected ADEs are submitted as 15-day alert or "expedited" reports. As required in 21 CFR §514.80(b)(2), these reports must be submitted on Form FDA 1932 to FDA by the applicant within 15 working days of first receiving the information. Follow-up reports are submitted on Form FDA 1932 by the applicant if significant new information is revealed during their investigation of ADEs that are the subject of 15-day alert reports. Reports of ADEs that are not serious and unexpected and reports of product defects that are not expected to result in serious ADEs are submitted in the periodic drug experience report, which is submitted every 6 months for the first 2 years after approval and annually thereafter.

Most mandatory ADE reports (from manufacturers) are submitted electronically and transmitted via the Electronic Submissions System (ESS), which is integrated with the FDA Electronic Submissions Gateway (ESG) and allows for individual or batched reports. Individual reports can also be submitted by manufacturers via a Rational Questionnaire (RQ) in the Safety Reporting Portal, or SRP. At this time, the SRP is not configured to accept adverse drug event reports from veterinarians or consumers. More information about voluntary reporting of adverse events is available on the CVM website (FDA/CVM, 2016b). All reports, mandatory and voluntary, enter the CVM ADE database for analysis and archiving.

ADE reporting to the CVM has increased dramatically over the last decade. The CVM received 28,825 ADE reports for the fiscal year 2004 and 91,592 for the fiscal year 2015. Some of the reasons for the significant increase may include an increase in number of drug approvals, label information that provides contact numbers for drug companies, and the interest of the public in reporting perceived product problems. In addition, wide access to the media and Internet has increased the public's general awareness about drug safety.

Unapproved Drugs and Veterinary Devices

ADE submission is mandatory only for companies marketing FDA-approved and conditionally approved animal drugs. Currently there are no requirements for submitting ADEs for unapproved animal drugs (animal drugs which have not gone through the FDA's approval process) or human drugs used in animals. Exceptions to this are those drugs on the FDA's Index of Legally Marketed Unapproved New Animal Drugs for Minor Species (the "Index"). These drugs are legally marketed for a specific use in certain minor species (FDA/CVM, 2014). Many approved animal drugs can be identified by the presence of a NADA number on the label, or a C-NADA number in the case of conditionally approved drugs, although these identifiers on labeling are not currently required by regulation. Veterinarians and/or animal owners are encouraged to report ADEs for unapproved animal drugs, including compounded products, to the CVM.

Although no form of premarket approval is currently required for devices used in veterinary medicine, FDA does have regulatory oversight over veterinary devices and can take appropriate regulatory action if a device is misbranded, mislabeled, or adulterated. A few examples of devices commonly used in animals include suture material, certain types of bandage materials, intravenous catheters, anesthetic machines, and equipment as well as imaging equipment. It is the responsibility of the manufacturer and/or distributor of these articles to assure that animal devices are safe, effective, and properly labeled. Although not required by regulation, the CVM accepts reports from manufacturers and distributors of veterinary devices of adverse events associated with marketed devices. Most adverse event reports that the CVM receives for animal devices are reported directly by veterinarians or animal owners.

Safety Signal Detection

A safety signal is defined by the World Health Organization as "reported information on a possible causal relationship between an adverse event and a drug, the relationship being unknown or incompletely documented previously" (WHO, 2017b). With the large volume of ADE reports that the CVM receives annually, drug safety reviewers cannot always review the reports individually. Accordingly, data mining strategies that involve the use of computer algorithms to analyze data in large, complex databases are being employed at the CVM to more efficiently identify safety signals. These methods do not replace hands-on clinical review of the case reports that generated the signal and assessment of those cases to determine the medical implications of the signal. Signals that are detected are essentially hypotheses, not causal associations, and need to be confirmed by case series examination. Signal detection processes assist the CVM in detecting potential safety signals in large volumes of data, helping to focus time and resources.

If a safety signal is identified during the ADE review process, a medical review of the case reports generating the signal is completed. For more recently approved products, part of this process is to perform a summary review, which includes a list of clinical signs for a particular product in decreasing order of their reporting frequency. The clinical sign profile that is seen postapproval is compared with the labeled adverse reactions for the product, and the development of a Postapproval Experience (PAE) section may be proposed for addition to the drug labeling. The PAE section provides a listing of adverse experiences reported for the product, and the CVM considers both frequency and severity of the events to determine their inclusion in this section of labeling. This process contributes to the safe and effective use of animal drug products by updating the label and informing the end user about the potential risks associated with the product. If ADEs during the postapproval period indicate that the risks of the product outweigh its expected benefits, the FDA may take other types of regulatory action beyond label changes.

On occasion, ADE reports will help determine changes other than postapproval experience that may be needed for labeling. A well-known example is that of fluoroquinolones and retinal toxicity in cats. Enrofloxacin was approved for use in cats in 1989 for the treatment of skin infections caused by susceptible strains of *Pasteurella multocida*, *Staphylococcus aureus*, and *Staphylococcus epidermidis*, at an oral dose of 2.5 mg/kg twice daily. This dosage regimen was changed by a supplemental approval in 1997 to provide for a range of 5–20 mg/kg as a single daily dose or divided twice daily. No ocular changes had been noted in preapproval TAS studies in cats administered up to 25 mg/kg/day for 30 days, or in cats treated with up to 125 mg/kg for 5 days. Between 1992 and 1997, the CVM had received four reports of blindness in cats treated with enrofloxacin, and between 1997 and 2000, the CVM received an additional 52 feline blindness reports (Hampshire et al., 2004). Most of the reports indicated that affected cats had been treated with greater than 5 mg/kg/day. In a postapproval study completed by the drug's sponsor, no changes in vision were seen in cats treated at the 5 mg/kg dose for up to 21 days; however, at doses of 20 mg/kg and higher, mild to severe retinal degeneration was observed. In 2001, the sponsor changed the labeled dosage for cats to a maximum of 5 mg/kg/day, and a PAE section was added to the label to include the signs of blindness and retinal degeneration. In addition, a class statement was added to all fluoroquinolones approved for use in cats, indicating that the use of fluoroquinolones in cats has been reported to adversely affect the retina and advising veterinary practitioners to use these products with caution in cats (FDA/CVM, 2001). Research published in 2011 indicated that fluoroquinolones are substrates for the ABCG2 transporter, which is found in many tissues, including the blood-retina barrier. Four feline-specific amino acid changes in the

ABCG2 transporter cause a functional defect of this transport protein in cats, leading to dysfunction of the transporter at the blood-retina barrier, accumulation of photoreactive fluoroquinolones in the retina, and ultimately retinal degeneration and blindness in some cats (Ramirez et al., 2011).

Communication of Safety Information

FDA-approved animal drug product labeling is the primary source of information about a drug's safety and effectiveness, and it summarizes the essential scientific information needed for the safe and effective use of the drug. Labeling for prescription animal drug products is directed to healthcare professionals, but may include sections that are intended for animal owners and that also must be FDA-approved. Similar to medication guides for humans that are commonly distributed with human pharmacy prescriptions, Client Information Sheets may be required by the FDA as part of the approved labeling for animal drugs. These are written in "consumer-friendly" language and provide information in easily understood terms about the benefits and side effects associated with the use of certain drugs. Examples of animal drugs that include Client Information Sheets as part of the labeling are the nonsteroidal antiinflammatory drugs intended for use in companion animals.

Certain animal drug labels may be required to bear warnings or precautions as related to human exposure to the product. For example, Regu-Mate (altrenogest) Solution 0.22% is indicated to suppress estrus in mares. The drug label for this product contains specific human warnings regarding the potential effects of exposure to the drug on human female reproduction. There has been no approved human use of this specific product. The information contained in the labeling of this product is extrapolated from data available on other products of the same pharmacological class that have been used in humans. Effects anticipated are due to the progestational activity of altrenogest. Acute effects after a single exposure are possible; however, continued daily exposure has the potential for more untoward effects such as disruption of the menstrual cycle, uterine or abdominal cramping, increased or decreased uterine bleeding, prolongation of pregnancy, and headaches.

In some cases, if label revisions are made to a product during the postapproval period to update it with new safety information, the CVM may request that a drug sponsor issue a "Dear Doctor" letter, which is sent directly to veterinarians in order to notify them of the new information. Dear Doctor letters issued since 2000 are posted on the CVM's website (FDA/CVM, 2016c). The CVM also maintains a cumulative summary of ADE reports, which contain a list of clinical signs in the reports that the CVM has received from 1987 to April 2013. This report is currently in the process of development for continued posting of information.

The CVM utilizes its website to disseminate information about ADEs and important announcements regarding animal drug product safety. One section of the website, "CVM Updates," contains brief press releases issued by the CVM on developments of interest to stakeholders and the public. CVM Updates may relate to any topic, but are often used to convey information about drug safety issues. Consumer Updates may also be published on the FDA's website. For example, in July 2010, the FDA published a Consumer Updates article, warning consumers of the dangers of inadvertent exposure of children and pets to a topical estradiol spray used to treat the symptoms of menopause in women. The CVM had received several reports of pets exhibiting mammary enlargement and vulvar swelling in female dogs. Reports had also been received for children, describing premature puberty and breast enlargement in boys and girls. The CVM worked together with CDER to develop this safety communication (FDA, 2010b).

Animal Food

A safe animal food supply is essential for the health of animals and humans. Among its animal food safety responsibilities, the CVM monitors and establishes standards for animal food contaminants, approves safe animal food additives, and manages the FDA's medicated feed and pet food programs. The CVM carries out its responsibility for the regulation of animal food in cooperation with state and local partners through a variety of mechanisms: cooperative agreements, contracts, grants, memoranda of understanding, and partnerships. For instance, the FDA cooperates with the Association of American Feed Control Officials (AAFCO) and the states for the implementation of uniform policies for regulating the use of animal food products. This includes the establishment of uniform food ingredient definitions and proper labeling to assure the safe use of animal foods. The ingredient definitions are important because animal foods and ingredients must be correctly and truthfully labeled when they enter commerce. Although FDA has the responsibility for regulating the use of these products, the ultimate responsibility for the production of safe and effective animal food products lies with the manufacturers and distributors of the products.

The FFDCA requires that any substance that is added to or is expected to become a component of animal food, either directly or indirectly, must be used in accordance with a food additive regulation unless it is generally recognized as safe (GRAS) for that intended use. Typical food ingredients such as forages, grains, and most minerals and vitamins are considered GRAS, as sources of nutrients. A list of approved food additives for use in animal food is found in 21 CFR Part 573 and a partial list of GRAS substances for use in animal food is found in 21 CFR Part 582. Substances affirmed as GRAS for use in animal foods are listed under 21 CFR Part 584.

Animal foods may be adulterated with pesticides, industrial chemicals, dioxins, elements, mycotoxins, and microbes. They may present a hazard to livestock health and production, and to the public health by residues in animal-derived human food or by their ability to cause disease. Many of the more frequently identified contaminants in animal foods are toxic, carcinogenic, mutagenic, teratogenic, or otherwise deleterious to animal and human health. The CVM may prohibit any detectable amount of a contaminant or establish a regulatory limit for the contaminant. Action is based on the protection of the public health, the extent to which the presence of the contaminant cannot be avoided, and other ways in which the consumer may be affected by the contaminant. The FDA has published GFI regarding action levels for poisonous or deleterious substances in human and animal food available on the FDA website (FDA, 2016c). Under the CVM's Feed Contaminants Program, the FDA field inspection staff conducts surveillance of the animal food industry to identify potential problem areas, collect food samples for analysis, and investigate potential violative findings.

Pet Food Adverse Event and Product Problem Reporting

Reporting of pet food adverse events to the CVM can provide an early warning of emerging food borne diseases and problems. Additionally, owners and/or veterinarians are encouraged to contact the product manufacturer or distributor on the product label to report potential problems that may be associated with the product and/or packaging, although manufacturers are not required to forward those reports to the CVM. Pet food products include pet foods, treats, puppy, and kitten milk replacers, pet nutritional supplements, and pet beverages. Examples of pet food product problems include foul odors, swollen cans or pouches, leaking containers or foreign objects. Adverse event reports can include pet illnesses or clinical signs that an animal owner or veterinarian believes are associated with pet food product consumption. The CVM website provides information about how to report a pet food problem (FDA/CVM, 2016b).

The FDA receives reports related to pet food adverse events and product problems primarily through two channels: the Safety Reporting Portal (SRP) as of 2010, and the FDA District Offices. Both are components of the Pet Food Early Warning and Surveillance System (PFEWSS), which was created after the passage of the FDA Amendments Act (FDAAA) of 2007 in response to the melamine and cyanuric acid contamination of pet food that led to the largest recall in history of pet food in the United States. During the initial weeks of this crisis, the FDA received over 11,000 pet food complaints. The combination of melamine and cyanuric acid contamination led to the development of crystals within the kidneys of dogs and cats consuming the adulterated pet foods, leading to renal failure (Dobson et al., 2008). In 2014, the Livestock Food Reporting portion of the SRP opened. Consumers and veterinarians can report adverse events and product problems related to livestock foods through this section of the portal. Another route that is available for reporting of pet or livestock food adverse events or product problems by owners and veterinarians is to call the consumer complaint coordinator in the FDA District Office that serves the geographic region in which the reporter lives (FDA, 2017). Early detection of animal food problems can lead to faster intervention by the FDA and manufacturers.

REFERENCES

Council for International Organization of Medical Sciences (CIOMS), 2010. Practical Aspects of Signal Detection in Pharmacovigilance: Report of CIOMS Working Group VIII, Geneva.

Dobson, R.L., Motlagh, S., Quijano, M., et al., 2008. Identification and characterization of toxicity of contaminants in pet food leading to an outbreak of renal toxicity in cats and dogs. Toxicol. Sci. 106, 251–262.

Farmer, J.H., Kodell, R.L., Gaylor, D.W., 1982. Estimation and extrapolation of tumor probabilities from a mouse bioassay with survival/sacrifice components. Risk Anal. 2, 27–34.

FDA, 2009a. FDA History-Part I. <http://www.fda.gov/AboutFDA/WhatWeDo/History/Origin/ucm054819.htm> (accessed .30.05.17.).

FDA, 2009b. FDA History-Part III. <http://www.fda.gov/AboutFDA/WhatWeDo/History/Origin/ucm055118.htm> (accessed 30.05.17.).

FDA, 2010a. Animal Health and Consumer Protection. <https://www.fda.gov/AboutFDA/WhatWeDo/History/ProductRegulation/AnimalHealthandConsumerProtection/default.htm> (accessed 30.05.17.).

FDA, 2010b. For Consumers: Keep Kids, Pets Away from Skin Sprayed with Evamist. <https://www.fda.gov/ForConsumers/ConsumerUpdates/ucm220217.htm> (accessed 30.05.17.).

FDA, 2012a. FDA History-Part II. <http://www.fda.gov/AboutFDA/WhatWeDo/History/Origin/ucm054826.htm> (accessed 30.05.17.).

FDA, 2015a. History. <http://www.fda.gov/AboutFDA/WhatWeDo/History/default.htm> (accessed 30.05.17.).

FDA, 2015b. Selected Amendments to the FD&C Act. <https://www.fda.gov/RegulatoryInformation/LawsEnforcedbyFDA/SignificantAmendmentstotheFDCAct/default.htm> (accessed 30.05.17.).

FDA, 2016a. FDA Organization. <http://www.fda.gov/AboutFDA/CentersOffices/default.htm> (accessed 30.05.17.).

FDA, 2016b. About the National Center for Toxicological Research. <https://www.fda.gov/AboutFDA/CentersOffices/OC/OfficeofScientificandMedicalPrograms/NCTR/default.htm> (accessed 30.05.17.).

FDA, 2016c. Guidance for Industry: Action Levels for Poisonous or Deleterious Substances in Human Food and Animal Feed. <https://www.fda.gov/Food/GuidanceRegulation/GuidanceDocumentsRegulatoryInformation/ucm077969.htm#afla> (accessed 30.05.17.).

FDA, 2017. Consumer Complaint Coordinators. <https://www.fda.gov/safety/reportaproblem/consumercomplaintcoordinators/default.htm> (accessed 30.05.17.).

FDA/CVM, 2001. Freedom of Information Summary: Baytril (enrofloxacin) Antibacterial Tablets. <https://www.fda.gov/downloads/AnimalVeterinary/Products/ApprovedAnimalDrugProducts/FOIADrugSummaries/UCM326939.pdf> (accessed 30.05.17.).

FDA/CVM, 2009a. Guidance for Industry #185(VICH GL43) – Target Animal Safety for Veterinary Pharmaceutical Products. <https://www.fda.gov/downloads/AnimalVeterinary/GuidanceComplianceEnforcement/GuidanceforIndustry/ucm052464.pdf> (accessed 30.05.17.).

FDA/CVM, 2009b. Guidance For Industry #149 (VICH GL33) – Studies to Evaluate the Safety of Residues of Veterinary Drugs in Human Food: General Approach to Testing. <https://www.fda.gov/downloads/AnimalVeterinary/GuidanceComplianceEnforcement/Guidance forIndustry/UCM052521.pdf> (accessed 30.05.17.).

FDA/CVM, 2011a. Guidance for Industry #85 (VICH GL9) – Good Clinical Practice. <https://www.fda.gov/downloads/AnimalVeterinary/GuidanceComplianceEnforcement/GuidanceforIndustry/ucm052417.pdf> (accessed 30.05.17.).

FDA/CVM, 2011b. Guidance for Industry #205 (VICH GL46) – Studies to Evaluate the Safety of Residues of Veterinary Drugs in Human Food: Metabolism Study to Determine the Quantity and Identify the Nature of Residues (MRK). <https://www.fda.gov/downloads/AnimalVeterinary/GuidanceComplianceEnforcement/GuidanceforIndustry/UCM207939.pdf> (accessed 30.05.17.).

FDA/CVM, 2013. Guidance for Industry #159 (VICH GL36(R)) – Studies to Evaluate the Safety of Residues of Veterinary Drugs in Human Food: General Approach to Establish a Microbiological ADI. <https://www.fda.gov/downloads/AnimalVeterinary/GuidanceComplianceEnforcement/GuidanceforIndustry/UCM124674.pdf> (accessed 30.05.17.).

FDA/CVM, 2014. Drug Indexing. <https://www.fda.gov/AnimalVeterinary/DevelopmentApprovalProcess/MinorUseMinorSpecies/ucm070206.htm> (accessed 30.05.17.).

FDA/CVM, 2015a. What We Do. <https://www.fda.gov/AboutFDA/CentersOffices/OfficeofFoods/CVM/WhatWeDo/default.htm> (accessed 30.05.17.).

FDA/CVM, 2015b. Draft Guidance for Industry #232 (VICH GL54) – Studies to Evaluate the Safety of Residues of Veterinary Drugs in Human Food: General Approach to Establish an Acute Reference Dose (ARfD). <https://www.fda.gov/downloads/AnimalVeterinary/GuidanceComplianceEnforcement/GuidanceforIndustry/UCM448430.pdf> (accessed 30.05.17.).

FDA/CVM, 2015c. Guidance for Industry #207 (VICH GL48(R)) – Studies to Evaluate the Metabolism and Residue Kinetics of Veterinary Drugs in Food-Producing Animals: Marker Residue Depletion Studies to Establish Product Withdrawal Periods. <https://www.fda.gov/downloads/AnimalVeterinary/GuidanceComplianceEnforcement/GuidanceforIndustry/UCM207941.pdf> (accessed 30.05.17.).

FDA/CVM, 2015d. Guidance for Industry #208 (VICH GL49(R)) – Studies to Evaluate the Metabolism and Residue Kinetics of Veterinary Drugs in Food-Producing Animals: Validation of Analytical Methods Used in Residue Depletion Studies. <https://www.fda.gov/downloads/AnimalVeterinary/GuidanceComplianceEnforcement/GuidanceforIndustry/UCM207942.pdf> (accessed 30.05.17.).

FDA/CVM, 2016a. Draft Revised Guidance for Industry #3 - General Principles for Evaluating the Human Food Safety of New Animal Drugs Used In Food-Producing Animals. <https://www.fda.gov/downloads/AnimalVeterinary/GuidanceComplianceEnforcement/GuidanceforIndustry/UCM052180.pdf> (accessed 30.05.17.).

FDA/CVM, 2016b. Report A Problem. <https://www.fda.gov/AnimalVeterinary/SafetyHealth/ReportaProblem/default.htm> (accessed 30.05.17.).

FDA/CVM, 2016c. Dear Doctor Letters. <https://www.fda.gov/AnimalVeterinary/SafetyHealth/ProductSafetyInformation/ucm055433.htm> (accessed 30.05.17.).

FDA/CVM, 2017a. Minor Use/Minor Species. <https://www.fda.gov/AnimalVeterinary/DevelopmentApprovalProcess/MinorUseMinorSpecies/default.htm> (accessed 30.05.17.).

FDA/CVM, 2017b. From an Idea to the Marketplace: The Journey of an Animal Drug through the Approval Process. <https://www.fda.gov/AnimalVeterinary/ResourcesforYou/AnimalHealthLiteracy/ucm219207.htm> (accessed 30.05.17.).

Gaylor, D.W., Kodell, R.L., 1980. Linear interpolation algorithm for low dose risk assessment of toxic substances. J. Environ. Pathol. Toxicol. 4, 305–312.

Hampshire, V.A., Doddy, F.M., Post, L.O., et al., 2004. Adverse drug event reports at the United States Food and Drug Administration Center for Veterinary Medicine. JAVMA. 225 (4), 533–536.

Ramirez, C.J., Minch, J.D., Gay, J.M., et al., 2011. Molecular genetic basis for fluoroquinolone-induced retinal degeneration in cats. Pharm. Gen. 21, 66–75.

USDA-APHIS, 2017. Common Questions about Veterinary Biologics. <http://www.aphis.usda.gov/aphis/ourfocus/animalhealth/veterinary-biologics/ct_vb_pel_faqs> (accessed 30.05.17.).

US Environmental Protection Agency, 2017. Pesticides. <https://www.epa.gov/pesticides> (accessed 30.05.17.).

US Government Publishing Office, 2017. Electronic Code of Federal Regulations. <https://www.ecfr.gov/> (accessed 30.05.17.).

VICH, 2017. (International Cooperation on Harmonisation of Technical Requirements for Registration of Veterinary Medicinal Products). <http://www.vichsec.org/> (accessed 30.05.17.).

WHO, 2017b. Safety Monitoring of Medicinal Products: Guidelines for Setting Up and Running a Pharmacovigilance Centre. <http://apps.who.int/medicinedocs/en/d/Jh2934e/14.html> (accessed 30.05.17.).

World Health Organization (WHO), 2017a. Pharmacovigilance. <http://www.who.int/medicines/areas/quality_safety/safety_efficacy/pharmvigi/en/> (accessed 30.05.17.).

Chapter 7

Regulatory Aspects for the Drugs and Chemicals Used in Food-Producing Animals in the European Union

Arturo Anadón, María R. Martínez-Larrañaga, Irma Ares and María A. Martínez

INTRODUCTION

Drugs and chemicals are essential for the production of animals intended for food. They are administered orally or systemically to treat animals or prevent disease and also to promote growth and feed efficiency. The European Union (EU) has already banned antibiotics growth promoters such as avoparcin, ardacin, zinc bacitracin, virginiamycin, tylosin phosphate, spiramycin, monensin sodium, salinomycin sodium, avilamycin, and flavophospholipol from being added to animal feed due to the fact that the use of these substances could lead to the selection of antimicrobial-resistant strains of bacteria (Anadón and Martínez-Larrañaga, 1999; Anadón, 2006). Individual animals may be treated (i.e., individual injection or by oral gavage), but it is often more efficient to treat entire groups by mass application via drinking water or feed. According to the prudent use of antimicrobials in veterinary medicine, routine prophylaxis must be avoided; prophylaxis should be reserved for exceptional case-specific indications. Certain mass-medication procedures, called metaphylaxis, are employed in an attempt to treat animal disease outbreaks while medicating others in the group of clinically healthy, but presumably infected, in-contact animals to prevent disease. Antimicrobial metaphylaxis should never be used in place of good management practices. It is a continuing concern of consumers that various drugs and chemicals may be found at above maximum residue limits (MRLs) in food. The possible effect of such drugs and chemicals on human health and safety depends on the level of exposure to animals, in particular through the foods we eat. Foods containing residues of any pharmacologically active substances (drugs and biocides) or other undesired substances (pesticides or other chemicals) above the MRLs could potentially constitute a public health hazard and could create problems in international trade, in particular, those substances that have no acceptable daily intake (ADI) and no international MRLs, or their MRLs do not cover species and uses that were considered minor by the availability of the data. The establishment of the MRL represents one of several standard options for risk managers to limit the presence of unwanted substances.

The EU took major action by introducing requirements for MRLs for residues of veterinary drugs in foods of animal origin. Residues are traces of the drug and its metabolites that remain in the animal and its edible products after treatment with veterinary medicinal products. Depending on the nature of the chemical and its metabolites, they may pose hazards with concurrent risks to consumers when the concentrations are above a safe limit. For instance, certain substances having a thyrostatic, estrogenic, androgenic or gestagenic action may be dangerous for consumers and may also affect the quality of foodstuffs. The concern for hormonal residues focuses on chronic exposure to low doses rather than an acute exposure to high doses. In summary, hazards may be toxicological, pharmacological, or microbiological in nature.

The detection of low levels of residues of certain prohibited veterinary drugs in imported animal products by laboratories in the EU at the end of 2001 and during the first months of 2002 triggered a discussion within the *Codex Alimentarius* Commission (CAC) on whether and how the problems causing such events could be addressed. Several control laboratories in member countries of the EU detected trace amounts of chloramphenicol and nitrofurans in imported animal products (e.g., shrimp and chicken). These findings were triggered mainly by improved analytical methods that significantly lowered

Veterinary Toxicology. DOI: http://dx.doi.org/10.1016/B978-0-12-811410-0.00007-6

the levels of detection for residues of these drugs. The question to study is what supranational rules apply if an importing country detects residues of unauthorized veterinary drugs in a food product. The relevant international framework that needs to be studied in order to answer this question is provided by treaties and agreements of the World Trade Organization (WTO) and the texts adopted by the CAC (Lützow, 2004).

The WTO started to work in 1995, its main objective being the facilitation and promotion of international trade. The main function of the WTO is to serve as a monitoring forum for the implementation of a number of treaties that were established during the so-called Uruguay round (1986–94) and for the settling of trade disputes subject to the rules laid down in those treaties. The more specific principles applied by the WTO when developing rules and treaties for trade between its members are: (1) countries may not discriminate trade partners; (2) national and foreign companies shall be treated equally; and (3) trade restrictions are justified for the protection of human, animal, and plant health.

The control of residues of veterinary drugs in animal products intended for human consumption is an issue related to human health that falls as such under the purview of the Agreement of Sanitary and Phytosanitary Measures (SPS). Under the SPS, WTO members can adopt SPS measures that are "necessary for the protection of human and animal health" (Lützow, 2004).

There are a number of veterinary drugs for which *Codex* has not adopted an MRL. An ADI/MRL may not have been established because the veterinary drug may not have been evaluated, the toxicological data did not support an ADI, the residue data were insufficient, a suitable validated analytical method was not identified, or good agricultural practices (GAPs) would result in exceeding the MRL. In the absence of an ADI/MRL, national authorities commonly resort to zero tolerance regulatory approaches (where no detectable residue of the veterinary drug in the food is acceptable), with the prevalence of residues of concern potentially changing as analytical method detection capabilities improve.

VETERINARY MEDICINAL PRODUCTS LEGISLATION

Veterinary medicinal products legislation is regulated in the EU by Directive 2001/82/EC (EC, 2001). In the EU legislative framework for medicines, there are a large number of directives and regulations for issuing of marketing authorizations and economic regulation of the pharmaceutical market that need to be applied and implemented effectively.

The body of knowledge relating to this implementation is constantly evolving as the EU scientific committees and their working parties develop guidelines and gain experience in new therapies and new technologies.

Marketing Authorization Procedures

Marketing authorization applications, which are to be submitted in either a national or community procedure (i.e., to competent authorities of the member states and the European Medicines Agency (EMA, previously abbreviated as EMEA)), consist of administrative information and the necessary documentation to demonstrate the quality, safety, and efficacy of the veterinary medicinal product. This applies to nonimmunological and immunological veterinary medicinal products.

A veterinary medicinal product may only be placed on the market in the European Economic Area (EEA) when a marketing authorization has been issued by the competent authority of a member state (or EEA country) for its own territory (national authorization) or when an authorization has been granted in accordance with Regulation (EC) No. 726/2004 (EC, 2004a) for the entire community (a community authorization). The marketing authorization holder must be established within the EEA.

Authorization procedures have developed over the years to become very complex with four different routes of application: (1) the centralized or community procedure, (2) the decentralized (DCP), (3) the mutual recognition (MRP), and (4) the national procedure requiring a high level of bureaucracy both for industry and regulators without gain of increased quality, safety, and efficacy.

Centralized or Community Procedure

The EMA is the EU body responsible for the scientific evaluation and monitoring of medicinals within the "centralized procedure," a procedure that allows a marketing authorization (license) for a medicine to be obtained in all EU countries simultaneously, on the basis of a single application. For veterinary medicinal products that fall within the mandatory scope of the centralized procedure in accordance with the Annex to Regulation (EC) No. 726/2004 (EC, 2004a), the application is submitted to the EMA. An application shall likewise be submitted to the EMA for veterinary medicinal products that fall within the optional scope of the centralized procedure in accordance with Article 3(2) and 3(3) of Regulation (EC) No. 726/2004 (EC, 2004) where the applicant wishes to obtain a community marketing authorization. In the "centralized" procedure, the EMA-CVMP is responsible for conducting the initial assessment of veterinary medicines for which a EU-wide marketing authorization is sought. The EMA-CVMP is also responsible for several postauthorization and maintenance activities, including the assessment of any modifications or extensions to an existing marketing authorization.

Following the scientific evaluation and upon receipt of the opinion, the European Commission drafts a decision on a community marketing authorization and, after consulting the Standing Committee for Veterinary Medicinal Products, grants a marketing authorization.

Decentralized Procedure and Mutual Recognition Procedure

Evaluation of the operation of marketing authorization procedures has revealed the need to revise the mutual-recognition procedure in order to improve the opportunities for cooperation between member states. Therefore, Directive 2004/28/EC (EC, 2004b) has introduced the decentralized procedure and the coordination group, which is responsible to settle any disagreements arising from the decentralized and mutual-recognition procedures. Both the decentralized and the mutual-recognition procedures are based on the recognition by national competent authorities of a first assessment performed by the authorities of one member state. To allow operation of the system, applicants for marketing authorization are obliged to include in their applications copies of any authorization previously obtained in other member states, as well as a list of those member states in which an application for authorization is under examination (Article 12(3)(n) of Directive 2001/82/EC) (EC, 2001).

In the "mutual-recognition" and "decentralized" procedures, the CVMP arbitrates in cases where there is a disagreement among member states concerning the marketing authorization of a particular veterinary medicine ("arbitration procedure"). The CVMP also acts in referral cases, initiated when there are concerns relating to the protection of public health or where other community interests are at stake ("community referral procedure").

Decentralized Procedure

The decentralized procedure is the most common route used and takes place in two stages: licensing in one member state (national procedure) followed by approval in other member states (mutual recognition). In this national procedure, regulatory assessors will examine the product's quality, safety, and efficacy and, if satisfied, will advise the competent authority to issue an authorization. Once a marketing authorization has been given to one member state, gaining EU-wide authorization is then possible on the basis of "mutual recognition" whereby the second and subsequent countries' regulatory authorities should, subject to certain conditions, accept the first country's national procedure. The entire process is known as the decentralized procedure.

For veterinary medicinal products not falling within the mandatory scope of the centralized procedure, the applicant may request one or more concerned member state(s) to approve a draft assessment report, a summary of product characteristics, and a labeling and package leaflet as proposed by the chosen reference member state. An application is submitted to competent authorities of the reference member state and to the concerned member state(s), together with the information and particulars referred to in Articles 12–14 of Directive 2001/82/EC (EC, 2001). The applicant must give an assurance that the dossier, including the proposed summary of product characteristics, labeling and package leaflet, is identical as submitted in all member states concerned. Differences in proposed prescription status and names of the veterinary medicinal product are acceptable, in line with national rules in force.

At the end of the decentralized procedure with a positive agreement, a national marketing authorization will be issued in the reference member state and the concerned member state. Harmonization is maintained through the procedures of Regulation (EC) No. 1084/2003 (EC, 2003) for the examination of variations and use of the decentralized and mutual-recognition procedures for extensions.

Mutual Recognition Procedure

This procedure is based on the mutual recognition by concerned member state(s) of a national marketing authorization granted by the reference member state. The concerned member state refers to the reference member state that issued the national marketing authorization on which the mutual-recognition procedure is based. At the end of the mutual-recognition procedure, a national marketing authorization will be issued in the concerned member state(s). Harmonization is maintained through the procedures of Regulation (EC) No. 1084/2003 (EC, 2003) for the examination of variations and the use of the decentralized and mutual-recognition procedures for extensions and renewals.

Independent National Procedures

Independent national procedures will continue, but are strictly limited from January 1, 1998, to the initial phase of mutual recognition (granting of the marketing authorization by the reference member state) and to veterinary medicinal products that are not to be authorized in more than one member state.

In addition, as provided for in Article 34(2) of Directive 2001/82/EC (EC, 2001), harmonization of authorizations for veterinary medicinal products authorized in the community is to be promoted via a coordinated approach for referring veterinary medicinal products, for which divergent decisions have been adopted, to the EMA and the CVMP.

TABLE 7.1 Safety and Residue Tests in Respect of Testing of Veterinary Medicinal Products

3A. Safety Tests	3B. Residue Tests
Precise identification of the product and of its active substance(s); pharmacology (pharmacodynamics, pharmacokinetics); toxicology (single-dose toxicity, repeat-dose toxicity); tolerance in the target species, reproductive toxicity including developmental toxicity (study of the effects on reproduction, study of developmental toxicity), genotoxicity, carcinogenicity, exceptions; other requirements (special studies, microbiological properties of residues (potential effects on the human gut flora; potential effects on the microorganisms used for industrial food processing)), observations in humans; development of resistance; user safety; environmental risk assessment (environmental risk assessment of veterinary medicinal products not containing or consisting of genetically modified organisms; environmental risk assessment for veterinary medicinal products containing or consisting of genetically modified organisms)	Introduction; metabolism and residue kinetics (pharmacokinetics (absorption, distribution, metabolism, excretion); depletion of residues); residue analytical method

Independent national procedures can also be used for extensions of authorized veterinary medicinal products as far as no a priori harmonization has been achieved for the initial marketing authorization.

The safety evaluation for a veterinary medicinal product and its residues is based on a package listed in Part 3 of the Commission Directive 2009/9/EC (EC, 2009a) (Table 7.1).

HUMAN HEALTH RISKS FROM DRUG RESIDUES IN FOODS

Edible or target tissues containing veterinary drug residues can pose a risk to human health, including direct toxic effects, allergic reactions, and increased bacterial resistance to common antibiotics.

The toxicity of drugs is an inherent part of all uses of medication, and there are differences from one animal or human to another, especially in allergic reactions. Residues of drugs or their metabolites in food products from treated animals are major considerations in the safety of drugs approved for use in food animals. In Europe, EMA or member states approve of drug dosages, routes of administration, durations of treatment and withdrawal times, and MRLs are designed to ensure the safety of foods derived from treated animals. EU regulations have effectively prevented allergenic, toxic, and potential carcinogenic drug residues from entering the food supply. Any adverse reaction is likely to occur due to acute rather than long-term chronic effects.

Acute Toxicity Effects

For toxicology testing, the sponsor should perform acute and chronic dosing studies. For example, the acute impact of antibiotics is not directly examined in the toxicological studies required in the preapproval process for veterinary drugs, since the primary concern has focused on chronic effects (i.e., carcinogenesis). The acute studies evaluate animals for problems such as allergies. Acute effects of food-borne drug residues on human health have also been described. These acute effects are defined as those that occur or develop rapidly after a single administration of chemical substances in a period of 24 h or fewer. Approach of a short-term high residue exposure must be presented because it could give rise to acute health effects in relation to short periods of intake, to anticipate that it is probable an ARfD (acute reference dose) will also recommended in addition to the ADI. Some examples of acute toxicity effects are hypersensitivity and pharmacological and teratogenic effects.

Hypersensitivity

Meat and other dietary products from treated food animals may contain residues of many antimicrobials or haptenized macromolecules. For small molecules to become immunologic, they must be able to form covalent bonds with macromolecules (i.e., proteins, polysaccharides, and polynucleotides). Allergic reactions can be caused by beta-lactam drugs (penicillins, cephalosporins), aminoglycosides, sulfonamides and in a few cases nitrofurans, and tetracyclines. Adverse human reactions are manifested as severe swelling of the skin, serum sickness and shock; less serious reactions such as skin rashes, asthma, and fever have been described. Drug sensitization can be acquired by antimicrobial drugs, their metabolites, or degradation products. However, cases of proven allergy to such substances in food are extremely rare, based on clinical and laboratory experience of an immunological reaction, whereas there are less well-substantiated reports blaming antibiotics in up to 50% of cases of chronic urticarial vasculitis (Dayan, 1993). Reportedly, both epidemiologic and experimental data indicate that levels of penicillin as low as 5–10 IU is sufficient to produce an allergic reaction in previously sensitized individuals (Sundlof, 1994). Adverse human reactions occur at very low doses, and it is highly probable that individuals allergic to the drug previously enumerated, when exposed via the food, could suffer an allergic reaction. The reason that so few cases are documented is likely that many cases might be masked with other health conditions, especially in elderly populations, as well as problems with underestimation and underreporting.

There are two veterinary drugs that may be toxic in humans when used therapeutically. Both are used in veterinary medicine causing adverse reactions by mechanisms involving hypersensitivity and where there is no clear relationship with dose. The first one is chloramphenicol, which may produce two types of bone marrow reactions: a reversible dose-related interference with iron metabolism and an irreversible idiosyncratic form of an often fatal aplastic anemia. The mechanism for pathogenesis of aplastic anemia is known, but it may be involved in reduction of the nitro-group to produce toxic metabolites. The reversible form is likely to occur with high doses, a prolonged duration of treatment and in patients with liver disease. Irreversible idiosyncratic aplastic anemia occurs in <1 in 25,000 patients given chloramphenicol. The onset may be delayed until after therapy has been discontinued. "Gray baby syndrome," which is often fatal, occurs in newborns and is related to the inability of the immature liver to metabolize chloramphenicol and will manifest with standard doses. The second drug is levamisole, which is known to cause reversible agranulocytosis in humans; the mechanism is unknown. Levamisole is widely used as an anthelmintic in animals, and the possible occurrence of its residues in animal tissues has caused concern (Woodward, 1991).

Pharmacological Effects

Pharmacological effects may help in the understanding of toxicological phenomena, and toxicological effects may result from exaggerated pharmacological responses. These adverse pharmacological effects are generally regarded as acute. Similarly, the pharmacological effects of some drugs can be important (e.g., clenbuterol and isoxuprine). This was illustrated by incidents where the β-agonist action of the drug clenbuterol resulted in adverse effects in those who consume liver containing residues of the drug. No observable effect levels (NOELs) can be determined for pharmacological effects and then used in the calculation of the ADI. It is known that there are two major classes of adrenergic receptors, α and β, based on the relative effectiveness of several adrenergic compounds to produce a variety of actions in different body tissues. There are two β receptor subtypes, β_1 and β_2, based on the relative potency of a series of compounds with structural similarities to epinephrine and norepinephrine on physiological processes, including cardiac stimulation and bronchodilation. The β_2 receptors predominate in smooth muscles and blood vessels whereas β_1 receptors predominate on the heart. Metabolic effects such as glycogenolysis in skeletal muscle or liver and lipolysis are mediated primarily through β_2 and β_3 receptors are expressed predominantly in adipose tissue.

It is known that the β-agonist clenbuterol has been used illegally as a growth promoter in farm animals, as a nonsteroidal anabolic and metabolism accelerator. Clenbuterol was the first of the synthetic phenethanolamine compounds with demonstrated ability to increase lean and decrease fat in food animals. In addition to their therapeutic effects, β_2-agonists are effective also as "repartitioning agents." The use of clenbuterol to enhance lean tissue growth requires a dose that is 10 times higher than the normal therapeutic dose of 0.8 μg/kg body weight. Factors affecting response to β-adrenergic agonist include level of dietary protein, length of treatment, genotype, and sex. Clenbuterol, a selective β_2-agonist, is used as a bronchodilator in human and veterinary medicine and it is available as 0.01 and 0.02 mg tablets as well as a respiratory solution. In humans, it is used at the recommended oral dosage of 0.02–0.03 mg twice daily. The eye, vitreous humor, or retina have been suggested as tissues for residue screening. More recently, accumulation of clenbuterol in hair has been demonstrated and suggested as a sensitive indicator of β-adrenergic agonist residues in animals in the EU and is listed in Table I of the Annex of Commission Regulation (EU) No., and 37/2010 (EU, 2010) as an allowed substance (Table 7.2).

TABLE 7.2 Clenbuterol and Its Classification Regarding Maximum Residue Limits (MRLs)

Pharmacologically Active Substance	Marker Residue	Animal Species	MRL (μg/kg)	Target Tissues	Therapeutic Classification
Clenbuterol hydrochloride	Clenbuterol	Bovine, *Equidae*	0.1 0.5 0.5	Muscle Liver Kidney	Agents acting on the nervous system/agents acting on the autonomic nervous system
		Bovine	0.05	Milk	

According to the Directive 2008/97/EC (EC, 2008a), β-agonists can be used to induce tocolysis in bovine and equidae as well as to treat respiratory problems, navicular disease, and laminitis.

In contrast to other β_2-agonists, clenbuterol is well absorbed after ingestion (bioavailability 70%–80%). Peak serum levels occur within 3 h, and the elimination half-life is 25–39 h. At larger doses, it also shows β_1-receptor mediated cardiac effects.

The anabolic effect of clenbuterol along with other long-acting β_2-agonists appears to be mediated through the β_2-receptors in skeletal muscle. Through its thermogenic properties, clenbuterol increases energy expenditure and hence reduces muscle glycogen and body fat deposition. In farm animals, clenbuterol accumulates in the lungs, liver, and kidney, and to a lesser extent in the muscle. Residues of β-agonists in animal tissues used for food may result in serious human health risks.

Clenbuterol has been implicated in several outbreaks of food-borne poisoning following the consumption of liver, meat, and lung of bovine and lung and liver of pig. In 1990, a poisoning incident was reported in Spain when 135 people became ill after consuming beef liver containing clenbuterol residues (Martinez-Navarro, 1990). A second episode of clenbuterol food poisoning was reported 1 year later in France affecting 22 people who consumed veal liver. The patients suffered tachycardia and tremors for 2–3 days. The infective dose is calculated as 1–2 μg/kg per day (Pulse et al., 1991). In 1992, a further episode of clenbuterol poisoning appeared in Spain after ingestion of veal liver. Analysis of liver indicated concentrations of clenbuterol in the range of 160–500 μg/kg. Consumption of 100 g of liver would exceed the pharmacological effect level of clenbuterol of 5 μg/person. Clenbuterol was detected in 47 urine samples in amounts ranging from 11 to 486 ppm. Other instances occurred in Hong Kong (1997–98) after the consumption of pig lung or liver people fell ill after eating pork products contaminated with clenbuterol. The common clinical symptoms in these food-borne clenbuterol poisonings consisted of muscle tremors, heart palpitation/sinus tachycardia, nervousness, general myalgia, fever, nausea/vomiting, headache, dizziness/vertigo, and chills. The latency period varied between 10 min and 6 h, and the duration of symptoms between 90 min and 6 days (mostly lasting less than 3 days). Some patients also presented with weakness or confusion. Others developed transient, mild hypokalemia. Electrocardiograms for some patients revealed sinus tachycardia of 120–150 beats/min with ventricular and supraventricular ectopics. Patients with underlying cardiac disease are generally expected to be more susceptible to the cardiac effects of clenbuterol. There were no reported deaths.

One side-effect of animal treatment with β-adrenergic agonists is increased heart rate. This effect may be either a direct or indirect effect of treatment. The acute toxic effects observed in animals include muscle tremors, tachycardia, and nervousness. In addition, treated animals show a higher incidence and severity of hoof lesions. Furthermore, specific histological changes have been observed in treated animals, in particular the formation of vacuoles of epithelial cells in the prostate and Bartholin's gland of male and female calves, respectively. The levels of clenbuterol in the edible tissues are expected to be at the highest.

Teratogenic Effects

Another acute toxicity effect that may occur as a result of exposure to violative animal drug residues is a teratogenic effect. Teratogens are active at very low doses and even brief exposure during a critical period of development can result in a lifelong deformation. Although the hazard associated with teratogens is severe, the possibility of the event occurring is infrequent. Therefore, the chances of a woman at the critical stage of pregnancy coming in contact with a violative residue are very low (Paige et al., 1997). Other effects caused by a single exposure can be a hemotoxicity, neurotoxicity, and endocrine effects.

Long-Term Chronic Effects (Carcinogenesis)

Long-term chronic toxicity studies identify whether or not problems such a cancer are associated with a specific drug. These studies will determine a dose that does not create any health concerns. Most residues of veterinary drugs or chemicals occur in food at low concentrations, therefore they rarely pose a chronic or long-term health hazard to consumers. Furthermore those effects as a result of exposure to drug or chemical residues in food are particularly difficult to detect and are certainly under-ascertained as well as under-reported. Carcinogenic studies are a cornerstone for toxicological assessment; however, carcinogenicity studies are rarely used to establish a NOAEL. Special problems emerge where the substance in a genotoxic, carcinogen or a mutagen, due to no threshold. A substance may not have ADI and MRL for a variety of reasons, in particular when important pivotal studies are missing or are of insufficient quality and the elaboration procedure had to be discontinued because the sponsor was not prepared to conduct further work. An example can be carcinogenicity studies. No allocation of a toxicological ADI and no recommendation of MRL mean safety concerns as a result of the substance were negatively evaluated by a competent regulatory body.

Antimicrobial Effects

Antimicrobial drug residues in contaminated foodstuffs can lead to direct toxic effects. The impact may range from sensitizing reactions to drug-inducing organ damage, or both. Moreover, many trace amounts of antimicrobial drugs may have the potential to perturb the human gut flora or to disrupt the barrier effect that it exerts, thus permitting the ingress of potentially pathogenic bacteria into the gastrointestinal tract. Antimicrobial residues in food constitute a variety of health hazards to humans that depend on the frequency and degree of exposure. The two main risks related to antimicrobials are hypersensitivity reactions, which appear in allergic individuals, and the acquisition of resistance by pathogenic microorganisms to certain antibiotics. These effects may be studied using a variety of experimental models, and they can be taken into account in the calculation of the ADI value. Derivation of a microbiological ADI (mADI) is only recommended if antimicrobial drug residues reach the human colon due to incomplete absorption, enterohepatic circulation, or secretion across the intestinal epithelial mucosa and remain microbiologically active. The following formula is used to derive a mADI based on MIC or other in vitro data generated for the antimicrobial drug (see Fig. 7.1).

- *NOAEC (No Observable Adverse Effects Concentration).* It is recommended that the NOAEC derived from the lower 90% confidence limit for the mean NOAEC from the in vitro systems be used to account for the variability of the data. In this formula uncertainty factors are not generally needed to determine the mADI.
- *Mass of colon content.* The 220 g value is based on the colon content measured from accident victims (Cummings et al., 1990). This total colonic volume of 220 g is used to calculate the mADI, being a conservative value.
- *Fraction of oral dose available to microorganism (intestinal microbiota).* The fraction of oral dose available to intestinal microflora using in vitro and/or in vivo data. In the absence of data, 100% of the oral dose is assumed to reach the colon in active form. It is recommended that the fraction of an oral dose available for colonic microorganisms be based on in vivo measurements for the drug administered orally. Alternatively, if sufficient data are available, the fraction of the dose available for colonic microorganisms can be calculated as 1 minus the fraction (of an oral dose) excreted in urine. Human data are encouraged, but, in their absence, nonruminant animal data are recommended. In the absence of data to the contrary, it should be assumed that metabolites have antimicrobial activity equal to that of the parent compound. The fraction may be lowered if the applicant provides quantitative in vitro or in vivo data to show that the drug is inactivated during transit through the intestine (FDA, 2013).
- *MIC calculation (MICcalc).* Calculation of the estimated NOAEC (MICcalc) for colonization barrier disruption uses MIC values from the lower 90% confidence limit of the mean MIC_{50} for the most relevant and sensitive human colonic bacterial genera. The strains needed to determine the MICcalc were chosen according to these guidelines, which state that an intrinsically resistant bacterial genus should not be included (FDA, 2013). MIC data, obtained by standard test methods, from the following relevant genera of intestinal bacteria (*Escherichia coli*, and species of *Bacteroides, Bifidobacterium, Clostridium, Enterococcus, Eubacterium* (*Collinsella*), *Fusobacterium, Lactobacillus, Peptostreptococcus/Peptococcus*).

The standard human food safety assessment for new animal drugs accurately determines the safe concentration for traditional toxicological endpoints as mentioned above. However, the impact of low levels of antibiotics on the intestinal microflora is not directly examined in these toxicological studies. The human gastrointestinal tract ecosystem consists of complex and diverse microbial communities that have now been collectively termed the intestinal microbiome (O'Hara and Shanahan, 2006). The intestinal microbiome is an extremely complex and dynamic ecosystem with a large and diverse group of microorganisms that include bacteria, archaea, fungi, and viruses. The intestinal microbiome contains in large part bacteria that belong to the five phyla of Firmicutes, Bacteroidetes, Actinobacteria, Proteobacteria, and Verrucomicrobia. Firmicutes and Bacteroidetes constitute approximately 90% of the total community (Lagier et al., 2012). Therapeutic doses of antibiotics can cause adverse effects on the intestinal microfloral ecology (i.e., disruption of the intestinal microflora, or effects on the metabolic activity of intestinal microflora).

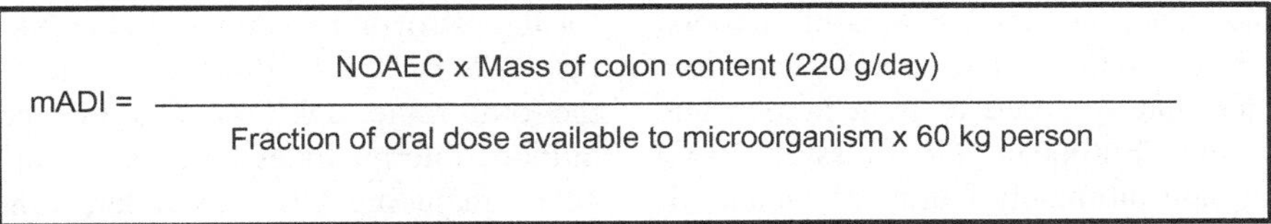

FIGURE 7.1 Derivation of a microbiological ADI from in vitro data.

The adverse effects of antimicrobials are a concern because of the important role that the intestinal microflora play in maintaining and individual's health. Also, perturbation of the intestinal microflora may compromise the effectiveness of other drug therapies and thereby adversely affect public health. Most studies of antimicrobial drugs and their effects on the human intestinal microflora were performed with therapeutic levels of antibiotics. In contrast to the well-documented negative effects of therapeutic doses of antibiotics, the effect of low levels (i.e., ppb or ppm) of antibiotics on perturbing the intestinal microflora is not well defined.

It is possible that low doses of antimicrobial agents, such as those found as residues in foods, could alter intestinal enzyme activity and have an effect on certain hormones and drugs, since in most cases the lowest doses at which the perturbations in the intestinal microflora occur have not been determined. In order to ensure human food safety the FDA's CVM considered data gathered from a large number of compounds and determined that the maximum safe concentration for antimicrobial products is 1 ppm in a total diet of 1.5 kg. This equals a maximum antibiotic dose of 1.5 mg/day from consuming residues in food. This level of an antimicrobial residue in food should produce no effects on the intestinal microflora (Paige et al., 1997).

All antimicrobial veterinary products are assessed for toxicological and pharmacological hazards as appropriate to the drug class and to the specific drug under consideration. Those animal drugs with microbiological activity are assessed for the potential hazard of ingested residues altering the intestinal microbiome and promoting emergence and selection for resistant bacteria in the gastrointestinal tract of humans. The antimicrobial substances may give rise to transfer of antimicrobial-resistant microorganisms or resistance determinant associated with animal-derived foods to humans. An ADI for chronic exposure of antimicrobial drug residues in the human diet is needed. Typically the ADI used to regulate the residues of the drug in food reflect the lowest ADI that could be established based on the endpoints evaluated. In some substances, the lowest ADI value is based on the mADI assessment of changes in the human intestinal microbiome (FDA, 2013).

Antimicrobial feed additives have been used in animal production for many decades because of their favorable economic effects in livestock production. Added in low doses to the feed of farm animals, they improve growth and performance and hence are known as antimicrobial growth promoters. Due to the emergence of microbes resistant to antibiotics that are used to treat human and animal infections, the European Commission (EC) decided to phase out, and ultimately ban as of January 1, 2006, the marketing and use of antibiotics as growth promoters in animal feed. Since then, the use of antibiotics is only allowed on veterinary prescription for direct applications or in medicated feed. These restrictions are deemed necessary, as antimicrobials may lead to the selection of resistant bacterial strains in animals that could be transferred to humans, by direct contact or via foodstuffs, and subsequently lead to an impairment of the efficacy of antibiotics used in therapy of human infectious diseases.

Hormonal Effects

Growth-promoting hormones, such as steroids and xenobiotics, have been used legally and illegally to increase live-weight gain and feed efficiency in various species, more intensively in cattle and to lesser extent in ovine, swine, poultry, and fish. Promoting steroid hormones can be divided into four groups of molecules: (1) natural steroids (oestradiol-17β, progesterone, testosterone); (2) xenobiotics (trenbolone acetate and zeranol); (3) synthetic steroids (ethinylestradiol, methyltestosterone, chlormadinone acetate, and others); and (4) diethylstilbestrol (DES) and related substances (hexestrol, dienestrol).

The endogenous steroid hormones have a wide range of actions that affect almost all systems of the body. These hormones act by binding with high affinity and high specificity to protein receptors, located in hormone-responsive tissues. The toxicity or adverse effects of the steroid hormones in humans are apparent even at physiological concentrations. A physiological level of testosterone contributes to acne, baldness, prostatic disease and prostate cancer, cardiovascular disease, and peptic ulcers. Physiological concentrations of estrogens, and to a lesser extent progesterone, have been implicated in premenstrual tension, dysmenorrhea, and some cancers of the reproductive system, including uterine and cervical, and breast (Taylor, 1983). The estrogen induction of DNA adduct formation has been described. The endogenous hormones are regulated as promoters rather than primary inducers of cancer in hormonally sensitive tissues.

The natural sex steroid hormones estradiol, testosterone, and progesterone may be in use illegally for growth promotion.

DES is perhaps the most widely known estrogenic growth–promoting agent. It is structurally different from the endogenous estrogens in that it does not possess the fused steroid ring structure but rather two phenolic hydroxyl groups, which gives DES a special orientation similar to estradiol. The relative binding affinity of DES for the estrogen receptor is 141% (vs 100% for estradiol), but DES is 10–20 times more active than estradiol via the oral route. DES is also metabolized to radical or quinone intermediates that react with cellular macromolecules, including DNA (Metzler, 1984). DES is carcinogenic in humans and in laboratory animals. DES was first used therapeutically in pregnant women in the United

States to prevent threatened abortion, and in the early 1970s a clear link was discovered between adenocarcinoma in women and their exposure to DES in utero (Herbst et al., 1971; Meyers, 1983). Furthermore, it has been shown that DES had other effects on chicken treated with DES, the most common being vaginal adenosis and other gross abnormalities of the reproductive tract (Herbst, 1976).

According to the Directive 2008/97/EC the following substances are prohibited: thyrostatic substances; stilbenes, stilbene derivatives, their salts and esters; and estradiol 17β and its ester-like derivatives (see Table 7.3).

The Opinion of the Scientific Committee on Veterinary Measures relating to Public Health (SCVPH) (EC, 2002a) concluded that there is a substantial body of recent evidence suggesting that 17β-estradiol has to be considered as a complete carcinogen, as it exerts both tumor-initiating and tumor-promoting effects, and that the data currently available do not make it possible to give a quantitative estimate of the risk to human health. The mutagenic and genotoxic potential of 17β-estradiol is a consequence of metabolic activation to reactive quinones. The report concludes that 17β-estradiol is not essential in the production of food-producing animals because the use of the available alternatives (especially prostaglandins) by practicing veterinarians is already quite common in the member states and that the complete prohibition of the use of 17β-estradiol for food-producing animals would have no, or only a negligible, impact on farming and animal welfare (EC, 2002a). Studies on the metabolism of 17β-estradiol in bovine species indicate the formation of lipoidal esters, disposed particularly in body fat. These lipoidal esters show a high oral bioavailability in rodent experiments; thus, the consequence of their consumption needs to be considered in a risk assessment (RA). It is known that experiments with heifers indicated a dose-dependent increase in residue levels of all hormones particularly at the implantation sites. Misplaced implants and repeated implanting, which seem to occur frequently, represent a considerable risk that highly contaminated meat could enter the food chain (EC, 2002a).

Zeranol and trenbolone have been tested for their mutagenic and genotoxic potential in various systems with different endpoints. Both compounds exhibited only very weak effects (EC, 2002a).

The new high-tech product bovine somatotropin, used for the enhancement of milk production in cattle, is also not authorized in the EU.

Carryover of the Feed of Coccidiostats and Other Medicated Feed

The regulatory concept of "carryover" is used specifically to designate the transfer of traces of a pharmacologically active substance contained in a medicated feed to a non-target feed, while the term "cross-contamination" is to be considered as a contamination resulting from a carryover or from the transfer in feed of any unintended substance. The best way to assess the carryover from feed to food is to determine from animal experiments the so-called "transfer factors" of chemicals from animal feed to animal products. The "transfer factor" is expressed as the concentration of the chemical in the animal food products (mg/kg wet weight) divided by the concentration of the chemical in the animal feed (mg/kg dry weight) (Leeman et al., 2007). Different studies have shown that an entire contamination-free production of premixes and compound feeds in existing multiproduct plants is not possible in practice (Strauch, 2002, 2003). Practical experience indicates that in feed mills, residual quantities of medicated feed stuffs may be retained at various points along the production line and end up at the beginning of the production of another feed product, contaminating subsequent batches of meal as they are processed. One possible

TABLE 7.3 Substances not Permitted in the European Union (EU)

1. Substances having a hormonal (stilbenes, stilbene derivatives, their salts and esters, estradiol 17β and its ester-like derivatives) or thyrostatic action, and of β-agonists (with derogations) (Council Directive 96/22/EC) (Directive 2008/97/EC)
2. Pharmacologically active substances listed in Annex, Table 7.2 of Commission Regulation (EU) No. 37/2010 (*Aristolochia* spp. and preparations thereof, chloramphenicol, chloroform, chlorpromazine, colchicine, dapsone, dimetridazole, metronidazole, nitrofurans (including furazolidone), ronidazole)
3. Antibiotic growth promoters (avoparcin, ardacin, zinc bacitracin, virginiamycin, tylosin phosphate, spiramycin, monensin sodium, salinomycin sodium, avilamycin and flavophospholipol added to animal feed due to the fact that the use of these substances could lead to the selection of resistant strains in animal and that this form of antibiotic resistance can present problems for antibiotics used in human therapy (Council Regulation (EC) No. 2821/98)) Growth factors (quinoxaline-*N*-dioxides such as carbadox and olaquindox) presented a risk to consumers (possess genotóxico and/or carcinogenic properties) to operators or to the animal itself (impairment of adrenal cortex function in pigs) (Commission Regulation (EC) No. 2788/98)
4. Pharmacologically active substances not listed in the Annex, Table 7.1 (allowed substances) of Commission Regulation (EU) No. 37/2010 (i.e., MRLs do not cover species and uses that were considered minor by the sponsors of the data)

source for contamination of nonmedicated feedstuff with medicated feed rations is the way in which it is manufactured and handled at the feed mill, where it is likely that within a short period of time, both medicated and nonmedicated batches will be milled and pelleted. The prepelleting bins, and the pelleting die, were identified as the most likely reservoirs of contamination, and feed handling at the mill was changed as a consequence. Following this, the number of feed batches containing more than 5% of the therapeutic dose of monensin dropped from 22.5% to 2.5% (Kennedy et al., 1998). Certainly, the origin of contamination of feedstuff may be located at any point along the production and distribution chain, from the point of manufacture at the feed mill to the moment of administration and use on a farm.

This unavoidable carryover may occur at all stages of production and processing of feed but also during storage and transport to feed localization (EFSA, 2007) although there are limited data on the amount and frequency of contamination of food with residues of coccidiostats resulting from feeding cross-contaminated feed stuffs to food-producing animals (Dorne et al., 2011). In conclusion, it can be either horizontal transfer and residue depletion of veterinary medicinal products in broiler chickens and horizontal transfer and residues in dairy milk following the use of medicated feeds (e.g., sulfamethazine, chlortetracycline).

In order to protect animal health, human health and the environment, maximum levels of carryover for active substances contained in medicated feed should be established, based on a scientific RA and taking into account the application of good manufacturing practice and the ALARA (As Low As Reasonably Achievable) principle. Cross-contamination of feed batches can result in the exposure of nontarget animals and induce adverse health effects in these animals due to a specific sensitivity of mammalian species as compared to poultry. Residue formation in edible tissues of nontarget species may result in unexpected human exposure through the consumption of animal products (Dorne et al., 2011). Feed additives, such as coccidiostats (polyether and nonpolyether ionophores) for poultry, are marketed as premixes, intended to be incorporated into mixed feeds during the mixing and production process. The degree of carryover depends on the technical facilities and procedures as well as on product characteristics. For example, the physicochemical characteristics of feed additives can contribute to cross-contamination. The electrostatic properties of some drugs, particularly those in powder form, aggravate the problem, making it more difficult to clean equipment between batches (Hurd, 1996). The feed additives and premixes also have an important influence on cross-contamination behavior, having the following properties of importance: adhesion strength—adhesion to walls, particle size and density (carrier, substance), and electrostatic properties. The cross-contamination decreases according to the product being less adhesive and electrostatic (EFSA, 2007).

The legal basis of this technological process is based on Regulation (EC) No. 183/2005 (EC, 2005), which replaced Council Directive No. (EC) 95/69 (EC, 1997). Article 10 of Regulation No. (EC) 183/2005 and provides that feed business operators shall ensure that establishments under their control are approved by a competent authority in case these establishments are manufacturing and/or placing on the market coccidiostats and histomonostats, or premixtures containing coccidiostats and histomonostats.

Carryover has been evaluated (Strauch, 2002, 2003; Dorne et al., 2011). Regular investigations have been performed with some coccidiostats, involving lasalocid and nicarbazin as well as sulfadiazine (McEvoy et al., 2003; Noser et al., 2006). These investigations showed the persistence of these compounds in various feed batches produced after the intentional incorporation of a polyether ionophore coccidiostat into the feed. The health risk to nontarget species resulting from the consumption of cross-contaminated feed with coccidiostats at levels of 2%, 5%, or 10% was evaluated recently by the European Food Safety Authority (EFSA) and a revision of the RAs performed can be found in the paper of Dorne et al. (2011). Overall, the toxic syndromes in nontarget animal species are related to: (1) accidental consumption of fortified feeds (in most cases intended for chickens) by other animal species; (2) feed-mixing errors or ingestion of premix concentrates with unsafe amounts of ionophores; (3) off-label (extra-label) use, either accidental or intentional, which have resulted in adverse reactions in adult poultry (laying hens), ostriches, ornamental and game birds, and humans; and (4) drug interaction with other veterinary medicinal products (target and nontarget animal species) (Dorne et al., 2011).

To avoid unintended contamination of animal feed and thereby animal products by veterinary drugs and feed additives, several measures need to be integrated. The internal control of the producers who manufacture their own medicated feed stuffs, the animal farming, the business, the slaughterhouse, and the animal processors and retailers have to maintain a documentation system providing full transparence of the food safety issues (i.e., quality and safety of their animal products). One important control point in this system is the absence of the drug in nontarget animal feed and target-animal. The key aspect in avoiding cross-contamination on nontarget animal feed by therapeutics is the introduction of reliable traceability systems, including clear labeling and the control of all feed ingredients used in the animal feed production line.

Technical improvements can reduce this cross-contamination considerably and hence limits of cross-contamination can be defined per product to exclude any health risk for human and nontarget animal species.

TABLE 7.4 Minimum Required Performance Limits (MRPLs) Established for Several Antimicrobials

Substance and/or Metabolite	Matrixes	MRPL
Chloramphenicol	Meat, eggs, milk, urine, aquaculture products and honey	0.3 μg/mL
Nitrofuran metabolites: furazolidone, furaltadone, nitrofurantoine, nitrofurazone	Poultry meat, aquaculture products	1 μg/mL for all

Recently, maximum tolerances for the presence of active substances contained in coccidiostats have been established in food of animal origin and in feed stuffs (Commission Regulation (EC) No. 124/2009 (EC, 2009b); Commission Directive 2009/8/EC (EC, 2009b)). The occurrence of unavoidable carryover and/or cross-contamination of coccidiostats in nontarget feed, even below maximum levels established, may result in the presence of residues of coccidiostats in food products of animal origin (i.e., in feed for which the use of coccidiostats or histomonostats are not authorized, such as feed intended for animal species or categories not provided for in the additive authorization). The maximum levels were set out for the coccidiostats lasalocid sodium, narasin, salinomycin sodium, monensin sodium, semduramicin, maduramicin, robenidine, decoquinate, and halofuginone. However, other antimicrobials used as premixes for medicated feed stuffs have not yet been evaluated for this purpose.

Minimum Required Performance Limits and Reference Point for Action

With the minimum required performance limits (MRPLs), the European Commission has proposed a temporary measure to address urgent problems related to prohibited or authorized substances in the EU, in particular in relation to third country trade. Commission Decision 2002/657/EC introduced MRPLs intended to ensure harmonized implementation of Directive 96/23/EC (EC, 1997) for substances for which no permitted limits have been established. MRPLs is defined as the minimum content of an analyte in a sample, which at least has to be detected and confirmed. In contrast to MRLs for substances that may be used in food-producing animals in the EU, the MRPLs would be control tools based on expert advice on feasibility of controls, and other legitimate factor in risk analysis. Consignments containing residues above the MRPLs would be rejected. If guarantees are provided, they may be returned to the sender.

The MRPLs laid down in Annex II to Commission Decision 2002/657/EC (EC, 2002b) are used as "reference points for action" irrespective of the matrix tested. The Commission Decision 2003/181/EC (EC, 2003) amended the Decision 2002/657/EC (EC, 2002b), and established MRPLs for different antimicrobials (see Table 7.4) where results of analytical tests on products: (1) are at or above the MRPLs, the consignment concerned shall be considered noncompliant with community legislation and (2) are below the MRPLs, the products will not be prohibited from entering the food chain.

On the other hand, according to Article 1 of the Regulation (EC) No. 470/2009 (EC, 2009a), the "reference point for action" is defined as the level of a residue of a pharmacologically active substance established for control reasons in the case of certain substances for which an MRL has not been laid down. The MRPL corresponds to the average limit above which the detection of a substance or its residues can be construed as methodologically meaningful. Regulation (EC) No. 470/2009 (EC, 2009c) states that the setting of reference points for action should in no way serve as a pretext for condoning the illegal use of prohibited or nonauthorized substances to treat food-producing animals. Therefore, any residues of those substances in food of animal origin should be considered undesirable. Regulation (EC) No. 470/2009 (EC, 2009c) highlighted that the reference points for action shall be reviewed regularly in light of new scientific data relating to food safety and the outcome of investigations, analytical tests, and technological progress. In conclusion, the EU would demand from its trading partners prohibition of the use of substances banned in the EU or to establish split systems and ask third countries to provide respective guarantees. As a consequence, detection of prohibited substances below the MRPL would still be documented and reported.

PESTICIDE SUBSTANCES/RESIDUES FROM CONSUMPTION OF STOCKFEED TREATED WITH AGRICULTURAL CHEMICALS

The use of agricultural chemicals can result in residues in crops and pastures that are subsequently consumed by animals and therefore pose a risk to these animals due to a single or at most a few days of exposure. Residues of pesticides are more commonly associated with foods of plant origin and it is the use of plants and plant products, such as grain, in the production of animal feed that is usually the source of residues. Organophosphates, pyrethroids, and carbamates are relatively quickly degraded and therefore less likely to be found in high concentrations if a long period of time has lapsed after application. In the EU, legislation that limits pesticide residues in feed is listed beside those for all undesirable substances. Persistent organic pollutants and, as such, residues can be found in the environment and can also be present in animal feed ingredients. Where they are used according to GAP, residues of these pesticides should not exceed MRLs, which are set on the basis of a toxicological RA and in consideration of what is achievable by best practices (i.e., correct application rates and minimum harvest intervals).

During drought conditions, the feeding of potentially contaminated crop byproducts, such as stubbles and fodder, and processed fractions, including grape marc, citrus pulp, fruit pomace, and cannery wastes, is likely to become more prevalent. In all cases, chemical residues may appear in the edible tissues, milk, or eggs derived from these animals. Some regulatory bodies also now routinely consider the need to set an ARfD for all pesticides it evaluates. The suggested numerical cut-off for setting ARfDs for pesticides is 5 mg/kg bw; consequently, if calculations indicate that an ARfD value would be greater than this value, then it would not be necessary to set an ARfD (WHO, 2015). This ARfD is not necessary for compounds with low acute toxicity value.

The approach adopted for establishing these MRLs is fundamentally different from that which applies to veterinary drug residues. Animal transfer studies, which allow for a determination of the relationship between the level of chemical in the animal diet and the concentration of residue found in edible tissues, milk, and eggs, are pivotal in determining MRL. MRL for animal tissues, milk, and eggs are established at concentrations that cover the highest residues (HRs) expected to be found from the estimated livestock dietary exposure. In animal production systems, compliance with animal commodity MRL relies on adherence to a stipulated period to allow residues in the crop to deplete prior to the commencement of animal feeding, a stipulation period to allow residues in the animal to deplete prior to slaughter, or a combination of both.

MRLs for pesticide residues and residues of veterinary drugs are the maximum concentrations of residues to be permitted in or on a food. Livestock and crop metabolism studies are the prime determinants of the residue definition in food and feed commodities. The recommended MRLs in various crops depend mainly on the data from supervised residue trials conducted in line with maximum registered uses within GAP. These trials should cover the range of conditions expected to occur in practice, including application methods, seasons, cultural practices, and crop varieties. If residue levels in the processed commodity exceed the residue levels in the raw agricultural commodity by a margin sufficient to require an MRL higher than the raw agricultural commodity MRL, it is necessary to estimate a MRL for the processed commodity. The pesticide residue dietary burden for livestock is derived from supervised residue trials for feed commodities multiplied by standard animal diets based on OECD livestock feed tables. Estimated maximum residue levels as well as HRs found in the supervised trials and supervised trial median residues (STMRs) derived from external animal treatments are compared with those derived from exposure through the feed. The recommended MRLs, HRs, and STMRs are based on whichever values are higher from this comparison. Estimates of chronic exposure are based on the STMRs from the supervised trials and food processing studies and long-term food consumption. For short-term exposure assessment, estimates of high intake of pesticide residue on a single day are based on the HRs from the supervised trials (WHO, 2015). Substances such as abamectin, cypermethrin, alpha-cypermethrin, cyfluthrin, cyhalothrin, deltamethrin, diflubenzuron, emamectin benzoate, thiabendazole, and teflubenzuron are used both as veterinary drugs and as pesticides.

BIOCIDAL SUBSTANCES USED IN ANIMAL HUSBANDRY

Biocidal substances used in animal husbandry are those used for the purposes of caring for and rearing food-producing animals, and to which food-producing animals are exposed during some stage of their life. However, biocidal substances are used in many different situations and their residues may potentially enter the food chain as a result of a number of these uses (including exposure of plants, exposure of food-producing animals, and contamination of food commodities). For instance, a pesticide is defined as a plant protection product (Regulation (EC) No. 1107/2009) (EC, 2009a), and biocidal products are defined as active substances and preparations containing one or more active substances put up in the form in which they are supplied to the user, intended to destroy, deter, render harmless, prevent the action of, or otherwise exert a controlling effect on a harmful organism by chemical or biological means (Article 1(a) of Directive 98/8/EC (EC, 1998a)). Biocidal products protect us against pests and other harmful microorganism (e.g., insect repellents, disinfectants). Biocidal product types include those intended to control vertebrates; however, the actual use of such types might give rise to concern. Where a biocidal product is identified as an insecticide, acaricide, rodenticide, avicide, or molluscicide is authorized according to the Directive 98/8/EC (EC, 1998a,b) it is also subject to classification, packaging, and labeling (CLP) according to Council Directive 78/631/EEC (EEC, 1978). The CLP introduces into the EU the globally harmonized system for classifying and labeling chemicals; this means that the same system is now used throughout the world. This will enable workers and consumers to become more familiar with the symbols and to get to know the effects of chemicals and how to use products safely. Companies need to notify European Chemicals Agency (ECHA) of the classification and labeling that they use for their chemicals.

Article 5(1)(b)(iii) of Directive 98/8/EC (EC, 1998a) specifies that for biocidal products/active substances that, as a result of their use, may lead to residues in food, member states shall ensure that products are only authorized if these residues have no adverse effects on human health.

Article 10 of Regulation (EC) No. 470/2009 (EC, 2009a) provides for the setting of MRL for pharmacologically active substances used in biocidal products used in animal husbandry and specifies that the EMA is responsible for recommending MRLs for these substances.

Under the conditions of use, the biocidal products shall pose only a low risk to humans, animals and the environment. An active substance cannot be included in Annex 1A (list of active substances with requirements agreed at the community level for inclusion in biocidal products) if it is classified as carcinogenic, mutagenic, toxic for reproduction, sensitizing, or is bioaccumulative and does not readily degrade. Inclusion of an active substance in Annexes I, IA, or IB (list of basic substances with requirements agreed at community level) shall, where appropriate, be subject to the following requirements on: (1) (a) the minimum degree of purity of the active substance; (b) the nature and maximum content of certain impurities; (c) product type in which it may be used; (d) manner and area of use; (e) designation of categories of users (e.g., industrial, professional, or nonprofessional); and (f) other particular conditions from the evaluation of the information that has been made available in the context of this directive; and (2) the establishment of the following: (a) acceptable operator exposure level, if necessary; (b) where relevant, an ADI for humans and a MRL; and (c) fate and behavior in the environment and impact on nontarget organisms.

The provisions of the last Regulation (EU) No. 528/2012 (EU, 2012) on biocidal products are underpinned by the "precautionary principle," the aim of which is to safeguard the health of humans, the health of animals, and the environment. Particular attention shall be paid to the protection of vulnerable groups. This regulation lays down rules for: (1) establishment at the union level of a list of active substances that may be used in biocidal products; (2) the authorization of biocidal products; (3) the mutual recognition of authorizations within the union; (4) market availability and the use of biocidal products within one or more member states or the union; (5) the placing on the market of treated articles.

The Regulation (EU) No. 528/2012 (EU, 2012) contains seven Annexes. Annex I: a list of active substances referred to in article 25(a) (i.e., all the active substances contained in the biocidal product appear in Annex I and satisfy any restriction specified in that Annex); Annex II: information requirements for active substances; Annex III: information requirements for biocidal products; Annex IV: general rules for the adaptation of the data; Annex V: biocidal product types and their descriptions as referred to in article 2(1); Annex VI: common principles for the evaluation of dossiers for biocidal products; and Annex VII, a correlation table.

An exhaustive list of 22 product types (PT) can be found in Annex V of Regulation (EU) No. 528/2012. Main group and product types that are relevant to substances that may be used in animal husbandry are shown in Table 7.5 and therefore a MRL should be established.

FEED ADDITIVES LEGISLATION

The Regulation (EC) No. 1831/2003 (EC, 2003) sets out rules for the authorization, use, monitoring, labeling, and packaging of feed additives. This regulation replaces Council Directive 70/524/EEC (EEC, 1970).

Directive 70/524/EEC (EEC, 1970) was fully reviewed in 2003 and Regulation (EC) No. 1831/2003 (EC, 2003) represented a major overhaul of the existing EU legislation on feed additives. All feed additives placed on the market in the EU must be authorized under Regulation (EC) No. 1831/2003 (EC, 2003). The primary scientific evaluation is conducted by the FEEDAP Panel of EFSA, assisted by the European Union Reference Laboratory for Feed Additives. The scientific evaluation may include the setting of MRLs and follow-up regulatory control if required. Authorized additives in feed stuffs containing provisional and permanent authorizations are listed in the Community Register of Feed Additives. A number of veterinary medicinals listed under EC Directive 37/2010 (EU, 2010) may be incorporated in medicated feed with a veterinary prescription. An example for a class of medication that falls into both categories (feed additives and veterinary medicinal products) is antimicrobials that are used for the prevention and therapy of coccidiosis in poultry, rabbits, calves, lambs, and piglets. A limited number of anticoccidial agents are approved for veterinary use. These are listed in the Annex of allowed substances in Commission Regulation No. 37/2010 (EU, 2010) such as amprolium, decoquinate, diclazuril, halofuginone, lasalocid, and toltrazuril. This annex contains information on

TABLE 7.5 Biocides: Main Groups and Product Types to be Used in Animal Husbandry

Main Group	Product Type	Descriptions
Group 1: Disinfectants	3: Veterinary hygiene	Products used for veterinary hygiene purposes such as disinfectants, disinfecting soaps, oral, or corporal hygiene products or with antimicrobial function
Group 1: Disinfectants	4: Food and feed area	Products used for the disinfection of equipment, containers, consumption utensils, surfaces or pipework associated with the production, transport, storage or consumption of food or feed (including drinking water) for humans and animals
Group 1: Disinfectants	5: Drinking water	Products used for the disinfection of drinking water for both humans and animals
Group 3: Pest control	18: Insecticides, acaricides and products to control other arthropods	Products used for the control of arthropods (e.g., insects, arachnids and crustaceans), by means other than repulsion or attraction
Group 3: Pest control	19: Repellents and attractants	Products used to control harmful organisms (invertebrates such as fleas, vertebrates such as birds, fish, rodents), by repelling or attracting, including those that are used for human or veterinary hygiene either directly on the skin or indirectly in the environment of human or animals
Group 4: Other biocidal products	21: Antifouling products	Products used to control the growth and settlement of fouling organisms (microbes and higher forms of plant or animal species) on vessels, aquaculture equipment, or other structures used in water

marker residues, animal species in which the substance is authorized, MRLs, target tissues, therapeutic classification and other provisions according to Article 14(7) of Regulation (EC) No. 470/2009 (EC, 2009a). In addition, Commission Directive 2009/8/EC (EC, 2009a) sets maximum content levels for 11 coccidiostats in feed including lasalocid sodium, narasin, salinomycin, monensin sodium, semduramicin sodium, maduramicin ammonium, robenidine hydrochloride, decoquinate, halofuginone hydrochloride, nicarbazin, and diclazuril. These maximum levels are set in mg/kg (ppm) relative to a feed stuff with a moisture content of 12%.

Regulations have introduced many new aspects into the preexisting legislation on feed additives, having been one of the first pieces of food safety legislation adopted following Regulation (EC) No. 178/2002 (EC, 2002b). By introducing the granting of time-limited authorizations valid for a period of 10 years and by setting up a Community Reference Laboratory for feed additives, the possibility of establishing MRLs for certain additives that may result in residues when added to feed is greatly increased and the possibility of laying down postmarketing monitoring programs at the time of authorization is enhanced as well as other provisions. The regulation also kept coccidiostats and introduced histomonostats as a new category of feed additive, while establishing the phasing out of the use (and marketing) of the existing antibiotics as feed additives from January 1, 2006, taking into account the risks of selecting bacterial strains resistant to human or veterinary medicine drugs when using antimicrobials as growth promoters.

In 1997, the European Commission introduced a requirement to monitor the occurrence of resistance in animal bacteria associated with the use of antimicrobial feed additives and related substances (EC, 1997), suspending, at the same time, the use of avoparcin as a feed additive in January 1997 and ardacin in January 1998. This obligation was reconfirmed by Council Regulation (EC) No. 2821/98 (EC, 1998a) suspending in December 1998 the use of four other antibiotics (zinc bacitracin, virginiamycin, tylosin phosphate, and spiramycin) that had been used as growth promoters in feed under the conditions that their use should be reexamined (Anadón and Martínez-Larrañaga, 1999). Subsequently, the European Commission supported a surveillance program, conducted by industry, to monitor antimicrobial resistance against feed additives in bacteria isolated from pigs and broiler chickens in the slaughterhouses in six European countries. However, as stated in the "White Paper on Food Additives" (adopted January 2000), the European Commission at that time already considered the prohibition or phase-out of antibiotics used as growth promoters within the EU, as part of a broader strategy to control and combat antibiotic resistance. With the aim of avoiding economic losses, in particular in the production of pigs and broiler chickens, and to avoid a significant increase in the use of antimicrobials under veterinary prescriptions, the EC supported the view that the phasing out of antimicrobial feed additives would be easier to pursue if other classes of growth-promoting additives could be licensed. Subsequently, several microorganisms or probiotics and an organic acid product were authorized for use as growth promoters. Moreover, enzymes preparations, such as glucanases, xylanases, proteases, and phytases as well as prebiotics (fructo-oligosaccharides and related compounds) were granted marketing authorization (Anadón et al., 2010, 2016).

The individual authorizations contain the characteristics of the products, the identification of the authorization holder, the maximum, minimum, and/or recommended dosages, the animal categories in which they can be used, MRL, and withdrawal periods where necessary as well as specific labeling provisions and further conditions where necessary.

EFSA's FEEDAP Panel evaluates safety to the target animal, the consumer, the user (farmer), and the environment in addition to the efficacy in the target species. The FEEDAP Panel carries out its work either in response to requests for scientific advice from risk managers or on its own initiative. Most commonly, and following specific authorization procedures, the European Commission asks EFSA to provide scientific advice and evaluate the safety and/or efficacy of a given substance in the context of its authorization for use in the EU. The scientific assessment performed by the panel is based on Terms of Reference provided by the European Commission or other European bodies or determined by self-tasking. This scientific assessment guides the panel approach to each question. Therefore, the authorization of an additive should be granted by the European Commission.

Article 5 of Regulation (EC) No. 1831/2003 (EC, 2003) states that a feed additive: (1) shall not have an adverse effect on animal health, human health, or the environment, (2) shall not be presented in a manner that may mislead the user, and (3) shall not harm the consumer by impairing the distinctive features of animal products, or mislead the consumer with regard to the distinctive features of animal product.

According to the Regulation (EC) No. 1831/2003 a feed additive is a substance, microorganisms, or preparations, other than feed material and premixtures that is intentionally added to feed or water in order to perform, in particular, one or more specific functions that are enumerated in Article 5(3) of the Regulation (EC) No. 1831/2003 (EC, 2003): (1) favorably affect the characteristics of feed; (2) favorably affect the characteristics of animal products; (3) favorably affect the color of ornamental fish and birds; (4) satisfy the nutritional needs of animals; (5) favorably affect the environmental consequences of animal production; (6) favorably affect animal production, performance or welfare, particularly by affecting the gastrointestinal flora or digestibility of feeding stuffs; or (7) have a coccidiostatic or histomonostatic effect; and shall be allocated to one or more of the following categories:

Technological Additives

Technological additives are defined as any substance added to feed for a technological purpose and include the following functional groups: (1) preservatives: substances or, when applicable, microorganisms which protect feed against deterioration caused by microorganisms or their metabolites; (2) antioxidants: substances prolonging the storage life of feeding stuffs and feed materials by protecting them against deterioration caused by oxidation; (3) emulsifiers: substances that make it possible to form or maintain a homogeneous mixture of two or more immiscible phases in feed stuffs; (4) stabilizers: substances which make it possible to maintain the physicochemical state of feed stuffs; (5) thickeners: substances which increase the viscosity of feed stuffs; (6) gelling agents: substances that give a feed stuff texture through the formation of a gel; (7) binders: substances that increase the tendency of particles of feed stuffs to adhere; (8) substances for control of radionuclide contamination: substances that suppress absorption of radionuclides or promote their excretion; (9) anticaking agents: substances that reduce the tendency of individual particles of a feed stuff to adhere; (10) acidity regulators: substances that adjust the pH of feed stuffs; (11) silage additives: substances, including enzymes or microorganisms, intended to be incorporated into feed to improve the production of silage; (12) denaturants: substances that, when used for the manufacture of processed feeding stuffs, allow the identification of the origin of specific food or feed materials.

Sensory Additives

Sensory additives are defined as any substance that improves or changes the organoleptic properties of the feed and/or the visual characteristics of food derived from animal, and include the following functional groups: (1) colorants: (a) substances that add or restore color in feeding stuffs; (b) substances that, when fed to animals, add color to food of animal origin; and (c) substances that favorably affect the color of ornamental fish or birds; and (2) flavoring compounds: substances, the inclusion of which in feed stuffs increases feed smell or palatability.

Nutritional Additives

Nutritional additives supply a specific nutrient required by the animal for optimal growth. The following functional groups are included: (1) vitamins, pro-vitamins, and chemically well-defined substances having similar effect;

(2) compounds of trace elements; (3) amino acids, their salts and analog; and (4) urea and its derivatives.

Zootechnical Additives

Zootechnical additives are defined as any additive used to favorably affect the performance of animals in good health or used to favorably affect the environment, and includes the following functional groups: (1) digestibility enhancers: substances that, when fed to animals, increase the digestibility of the diet, through action on target feed materials; (2) gut flora stabilizers: microorganisms or other chemically defined substances that, when fed to animals, have a positive effect on the gut flora; (3) substances that favorably affect the environment; and (4) other zootechnical additives.

Commission Regulation (EC) No. 429/2008 (EC, 2008b) on implementing rules and guidelines concerning applications for authorization of feed additives for use in animal nutrition in accordance with Regulation (EC) No. 1831/2003 is in application. This Regulation (EC) No. 429/2008 (EC, 2008b) provides specific guidelines for the authorization of feed additives. Specific guidelines have been prepared for the FEEDAP Panel of EFSA for additives that are already authorized for use in food in minor species, as nutritional additives in pets, and for other non-food producing animals as well as for sensory additives other than flavoring compounds, technological additives (silage additives), technological additives other than silage additives, zootechnical additives (enzymes, microorganisms), zootechnical additives other than enzymes and microorganisms and coccidiostats and histomonostats, among others.

COMPARATIVE SETTING TOXICOLOGICAL STANDARDS FOR FOOD SAFETY

Establishment of European Community Maximum Residue Limits for Drugs and Feed Additives

The Committee for Medicinal Products for Veterinary Use (CVMP) of the EMA and Panel on Additives and Products or Substances used in Animal Feed (FEEDAP) of the EFSA in order to protect human health, MRLs for veterinary medicinal products (EEC, 1990) and for feed additives (EC, 2003) in foodstuffs of animal origin should be established in accordance with generally recognized principles of safety assessment, taking into account toxicological risks, environmental contamination as well as unintended microbiological and pharmacological effects of residues. Council Regulation 90/2377/EEC (EEC, 1990) regulates the safety assessment for establishing the MRLs for veterinary medicinal active ingredients. From January 1992, member states were incapable to granting marketing authorization for veterinary medicines containing new pharmacologically active substances unless an MRL had been established by the EMEA-CVMP. Furthermore, the community had set MRLs for existing pharmacologically active substance in 1997. Beginning January 1, 1997, it is not possible to use any pharmacologically active substance in veterinary medicines intended for food animals for there is no community MRL.

The safety or RA of residues of veterinary drugs and feed additives is a science-based process involving the four following stages: (1) hazard identification, (2) hazard characterization, (3) exposure assessment, and (4) risk characterization. Hazard is defined as the potential of a chemical agent to cause harmful effect(s) and risk as a function of the probability that an adverse effect will occur due to the presence of a hazardous compound in food and the severity of the adverse effect (exposure × toxicity). It is not possible to completely separate the hazard identification and hazard characterization steps. For hazard identification of veterinary drugs a defined set of animal tests covering the entire range of possible adverse effects are routinely required. Information on dose-dependent toxicokinetic properties (rate and extent of absorption, distribution, metabolism, and excretion) in test animals, in the target animal species (and in humans when available), is always indispensable for hazard identification and characterization. If metabolites are formed in the target animal species that did not appear in the laboratory animal species, separate testing of those metabolites may be necessary. Other special studies may be required on a case-by-case basis. The standard approach to assessing the safety of chemical contaminants in foodstuffs intended for human consumption is the ADI defined as an estimate of the amount of a substance in food or drinking water, expressed on a body-weight basis, that can be ingested daily over a lifetime without an appreciable health risk (standard human = 60 kg) and it is expressed in units of mg per kg of body weight (FAO/WHO, 2004). For the determination of the no observable (adverse) effect level (NO(A)EL) or sometimes a lowest observed adverse effect level (LO(A)EL), a series of doses is used. In order to establish the dose—effect relationship, the dose levels are chosen in such a way that the highest dose causes an adverse effect and the lowest does not produce any adverse effect. The establishment of the ADI from the determination of a NOAEL, and application of an appropriate safety factor or uncertainty factor provide the hazard identification and characterization. The ADI approach was developed to take into account of effects based on classical toxicology and it is applied to the results of standard toxicity studies in laboratory animals. The NOAEL for the most sensitive toxicological parameter, normally in the most sensitive species of experimental animals, is used as the starting point (WHO, 1989). In order to arrive at such NOAEL, a battery of standardized toxicity tests are carried out (i.e., acute toxicity, genotoxicity studies (mutagenicity, clastogenicity), subchronic oral toxicity, chronic oral toxicity/carcinogenicity, and specific studies concerning reproduction and developmental toxicity among others) (EC, 2008b). The ADI is calculated by dividing this by a suitable safety or uncertainty factor, conventionally of 100, to account for the differences between test animals and humans (factor of 10) and possible differences in sensitivity between humans (another factor of 10). Depending on the available data set and the nature of substance under study, higher or lower safety factors may be applied (e.g., small size of the animal test group, nature of the critical effects, quality of the data). This concept cannot be applied in cases where certain genotoxic carcinogens do not show a dose-dependent threshold level.

ADIs are related to chemical substances that are deliberately added to a product or ingredient or which can be found on food following, for instance, treatment of crops with pesticide sprays or antifungal agents. A Tolerable Daily Intake (TDI) is an estimate of the quantity of a chemical contaminant to which we may be exposed through environmental contamination, and which when found in food can be ingested daily over a lifetime without posing a significant health risk. The TDI is used for contaminants, whereas the ADI is used in cases where exposure can be controlled, such as feed additives and residues of pesticides and veterinary drugs in food. Guidance values may be expressed as a TDI, provisional maximum tolerable daily intake, provisional tolerable weekly intake, or provisional tolerable monthly intake.

The ADI represents total drug residues, parent and all metabolites, that can be safely consumed daily throughout one's life. ADIs also can be developed from pharmacological or microbiological data based on no-pharmacological observed effect levels. However, the impact of low levels of antibiotics on the intestinal microflora is not examined directly in these toxicology studies. For substances with microbiological activity what is actually used is the major adverse microbiological effect arising from the effects of residues of antimicrobial drugs in food of animal origin acting on the human gastrointestinal bacteria flora, particularly those acting on the colonic flora. This approach is currently used by CVMP and JECFA (Joint FAO/WHO Expert Committee on Food Additives) but has never been used by the FEEDAP Panel as can be seen in Commission Regulation (EC) No. 429/2008 (EC, 2008b).

The use of mathematical and statistical approaches for hazard characterization appears to be valuable. One assessment approach that has been used in recent years is the use of statistical estimates based on all the available data in a dose–response series to determine the point of departure (POD) from background level response through the use of the benchmark dose (BMD) as a statistical estimate of the NOAEL. Health-based guidance values (HBGVs) (i.e., an ADI for a chronic intake or an ARfD for an acute intake) are most often established using a POD from a toxicity study in experimental animals. The most frequently used POD is either the NOAEL (mg/kg bw per day) or the BMD, which is a dose producing a low but measurable adverse response. The lower one-sided confidence limit of the BMD (the BMDL) is the POD for the derivation of a HBGV or for calculation of a margin of exposure (MOE). The MOE is derived by taking the ratio of the POD for the most relevant, sensitive end-point to an estimate of exposure by a high consumer. Where appropriate, acute dietary exposure estimates should cover a time period of food consumption over a single meal or 24 h and are intended to be used for comparison with ARfD values in a RA process. It is important to consider data of short-term or acute studies.

The HBGVs for veterinary drugs are generally established. However, when this is not possible or not appropriate, the MOE could be calculated. There are primarily two situations when this might be done: (1) when the nature of the end-point is such that derivation of a HBGV is not appropriate, and (2) when there are deficiencies in the database such that it is not possible to derive a HBGV with confidence.

The MOE approach is specially used for a number of genotoxic carcinogens using BMDL values derived by fitting a range of models to the available experimental dose–response data. The MOE approach can also be used in characterizing risks associated with certain contaminants in food for which there are deficiencies in the database and it is not possible to derive a HBGV with reliance. In general, the acceptability of an MOE is based on considerations similar to those used in the derivation of a HBGV. An MOE of at least 100 (10-fold for each of interspecies and intraspecies variability) would be considered acceptable for the effects with a biological threshold. For effects without a threshold, some regulatory bodies have suggested an MOE of greater than 10,000. This is the case with genotoxic and carcinogenic compounds, where the use of the NOAEL is not appropriate. For such compounds, where a BMDL cannot determined, a T25 (the chronic daily dose in mg/kg bw that will give 25% of the animals tumors at a specific tissue site, after correction for spontaneous incidence, within the standard lifespan of that species) is calculated (FAO/WHO, 2014).

The BMD is based on modeling all of the available dose–response data and generally estimates an excess risk of 10% over background for the response of interest. The benchmark dose lower limit (BMDL) uses the lower bound of a 95% confidence limit on the benchmark dose for an $x\%$ response (BMDLx), or a similar POD should be used. The BMD/BMDL approach is just one of a number of approaches that have been developed to refine the ability to characterize the toxicological hazard of a veterinary drug (Edler et al., 2002).

The safe concentration is the maximal allowable concentration of total residues of toxicologic concern in edible tissue and is calculated from the ADI and considers the weight of an average person and the amount of meat, milk, or eggs consumed daily by a high-consuming individual.

The identification of the residue profile and its decline in the treated animal, resulting in the setting of MRLs, enables the exposure assessment and risk characterization to be determined. Additionally the theoretical maximum daily intake (TMDI) is calculated. The TMDI is an estimate of dietary intake based on multiplying the MRL by the average food consumption for each commodity (i.e., it is assumed that a person with a body weight of 60 kg consumes every day over a lifetime 500 g of mammalian or poultry "meat" (muscle, liver, kidney, fat) or 300 g of fish plus 1500 g of milk plus 100 g of eggs plus 20 g honey) and then summing the products (Table 7.6) (EMA-CVMP and WHO, 1989). It is assumed that all the previous tissues and products contain residues at a concentration equivalent to the MRL every day.

Article 14(7) of Regulation (EC) No. 470/2009 (EC, 2009a) states "where it appears necessary for the protection of human health, the classification shall include conditions and restrictions for the use or application of a pharmacologically active substance used in veterinary medicinal products that is subject to a MRL, or for which no MRL has been set" (e.g., not for use in animals from which milk or eggs are produced for human consumption) (see Table 7.7).

The Table 7.8, "prohibited substances," includes substances considered to be unsafe on the grounds of public health (Regulation 37/2010, Table 7.2 of Annex) (EU, 2010).

Maximum Residue Level

All new pharmacologically active substances that are intended for use in food animals must have MRLs established prior to licensing. Termed tolerances in the United States, they are defined as the maximum concentration of a residue of a pharmacologically active substance that may be permitted in food of animal origin (expressed in mg/kg or μg/kg on a fresh-weight basis). It is based on the type and amount of residue considered to be without any toxicological hazard for human health as expressed by the ADI. Other relevant public risks and aspects relating to food technology, good practice in the use of veterinary drugs, and analytical methodologies are also considered when establishing MRLs. In the EU those drugs for which an MRL value should be established are governed by Regulation (EC) No. 470/2009 (EC, 2009a), repealing Council Regulation (EEC) No. 2377/90 (EEC, 1990). According to Article 6 of this regulation the scientific RA shall consider the metabolism and depletion of pharmacologically active substances in relevant animal species, the type of residues and the amount thereof that may be ingested by human beings over a lifetime without an appreciable health risk expressed in terms of ADI. Alternative approaches to ADI may also be used. The RA is concerned with the following: (1) the type and amount of residue considered not to present a safety concern for human health; (2) the risk of toxicological, pharmacological, or microbiological effects in human beings; and (3) residues that occur in food of plant origin or that come from the environment. If the metabolism and depletion of the substance cannot be assessed, the scientific RA may take into account monitoring data or exposure data.

A variety of toxicological evaluations are performed to establish the safety of veterinary drug residues in human food. The standard approach to assessing the safety of residues in foodstuffs intended for human consumption is based on the determination of the ADI on which, in turn, MRLs are based. The establishment of a

TABLE 7.6 Standard Food Basket

Mammals		Poultry		Fish		Bees	
Muscle	0.300 kg	Muscle	0.300 kg	Muscle and skin in natural proportions	0.300 kg	Honey	0.20 kg
Fat	0.050 kg[a]	Fat and skin in natural proportions	0.090 kg				
Liver	0.100 kg	Liver	0.100 kg				
Kidney	0.050 kg	Kidney	0.010 kg				
Milk	1.500 kg	Eggs	0.100 kg				

[a]*Fat and skin in natural proportions for pigs.*

TABLE 7.7 Conditions and Restrictions for the Use or Application of a Pharmacologically Active Substance Used in Veterinary Medicinal Products

Other Provisions	Pharmacologically Active Substances
Not for use in animals from which milk is produced for human consumption (according to Article 14(7) of Regulation (EC) No. 470/2009)	Abamectin (OV); acetylsalicylic acid and acetylsalicylic acid DL-lysine (all food-producing species except fin fish); aluminum salicylate (BO); apramycin (BO, OV, PO, CH, RA); bromhexine (BO); carbasalate calcium (all food-producing species except fin fish); clorsulon (BO); closantel (BO); *Cimicifugae racemosae rhizome* (all food-producing species); clodronic acid (in the form of disodium salt) (EQ); cyromazine (OV); decoquinate (BO, OV); derquantel (OV); dicyclanil (OV); difloxacin (BO, OV, CA); doramectin (all mammalian food-producing species); doxycycline (all food-producing species); florfenicol (BO, OV, CA); fluazuron (BO); flumethrin (OV); gamithromycin (all ruminants except BO); halofuginone (BO); imidocarb (OV); ivermectin (all mammalian food-producing species); levamisole (BO, OV); lasalocid (BO); mebendazol (OV, CA); monepantel (BO); oxolinic acid (all food-producing species); paromomycin (all food-producing species); phoxim (all food-producing species except fin fish); rafoxanide (BO, OV); *Ruta graveolens* (all food-producing species); sisapronil (BO, CA); sodium acetylsalicylate and salicylate (all food-producing species except fin fish); sodium salicylate (BO, PO); tildipirosin (BO, CA); toltrazuril sulfone (all mammalian food-producing species); tulathromycin (OV, CA, BO)
For milk MRL further provisions in Commission Directive 98/82/EC are to be observed	Alpha-cypermethrin (BO, OV); cypermethrin (all ruminants); permethrin (BO)
For milk MRL further provisions in Council Directive 94/29/EC are to be observed	Cyfluthrin (BO, CA); cyhalothrin (BO)
Not for use in animals from which eggs are produced for human consumption (according to Article 14(7) of Regulation (EC) No. 470/2009)	Acetylsalicylic acid and acetylsalicylic acid DL-lysine (all food-producing species except fin fish); amoxicillin (all food-producing species); ampicillin (all food-producing species except fin fish); apramycin (CH); avilamycin (POU); benzylpenicillin (all food-producing species); bromhexine (POU); carbasalate calcium (all food-producing species except fin fish); cloxacillin (all food-producing species); danofloxacin (POU); diclazuril (POU); dicloxacillin (all food-producing species); difloxacin (POU); doxycycline (POU); enrofloxacin (POU); florfenicol (POU); flumequine (POU); kanamycin (all food-producing species except fin fish); levamisol (POU); oxacillin (POU); oxolinic acid (all food-producing species); paromomycin (all food-producing species); salicylic acid (TU); sarafloxacin (CH); sodium acetylsalicylate (all food-producing species except fin fish); spectinomycin (all other food-producing species); spiramycin (CH); sulfonamides (all food-producing species); thiamphenicol (all food-producing species); tilmicosin (POU); toltrazuril (POU); trimethoprim (all other food-producing species); Virginiamycin (POU)
Not for use in fish from which eggs are produced for human consumption (according to Article 14(7) of Regulation (EC) No. 470/2009)	Azagly-nafarelin (*Salmonidae*)
Only for zootechnical use and in accordance with the provisions of Directive 96/22/EC	Altrenogest (PO, *Equidae*)
Only for intravaginal therapeutic and zootechnical use and in accordance with the provisions of Directive 96/22/EC	Progesterone (BO, OV, CA, *Equidae* (female))
For zootechnical use only	Chlormadinone (synthetic progesterone analogue) (BO)
For intravaginal use for zootechnical purposes only	Flugestone acetate (OV, CA); medroxyprogesterone acetate (OV)
For therapeutic and zootechnical purposes only	Norgestomet (bovine); 17β-oestradiol (all mammalian food-producing species)

BO, bovine; *CA*, caprine; *CH*, chicken; *EQ*, equidae; *OV*, ovine; *PO*, porcine; *POU*, poultry; *RA*, rabbit; *TU*, turkey.

TABLE 7.8 Prohibited Substances in the European Union

Substances	Toxicological End Points
Aristolochia spp. and preparations thereof	Nephrotoxicity, mutagenicity and carcinogenicity
Chloramphenicol	Aplastic anemia, carcinogenicity
Chloroform	Mutagenicity and carcinogenicity (lack of data)
Chlorpromazine	Behavioral changes
Colchicine	Genotoxicity
Dapsone	Reproductive and teratogenic effects
Dimetridazole	Reproductive and teratogenic effects
Metronidazole	Mutagenicity
Nitrofurans (including furazolidone)	Carcinogenicity
Ronidazole	Mutagenicity

toxicological ADI from the determination of a NOAEL/LOAEL and application of an appropriate safety factor provide hazard identification and characterization. The toxicological ADI approach takes into account effects based on classical toxicology. The safety factor usually chosen is 100 in the situation where a NOAEL is derived from a long-term animal study on the assumptions that humans are 10 times as sensitive as the test animals used in such studies and that a 10-fold range of sensitivity within the human population may exist. Data on human variation in the major pathways of foreign compound metabolism and pharmacological sensitivity have shown that the 10-fold factor is a reasonable default value (FAO/WHO, 2014). JECFA for certain substances has established acute reference dose (ARfD) based on pharmacological end-points.

There are very potent compounds that exert pharmacological actions through receptor pathways at very low doses; the consequences are very low ADI (or reference dose) values for human dietary consumption. The pharmacological ADI was derived for other compounds such as beta-agonists, beta-blockers, anesthetics, tranquillizers, vasodilators, and compounds that may trigger acute hypersensitivity reactions (e.g., penicillins) and for certain substances it has established ARfDs based on pharmacological end-points. The β-adrenergic agonists are an example so JECFA review of the β-adrenergic agonist ractopamine HCl resulted in a recommendation of an ADI of 0–1 μg/kg body weight/day and MRL of 10 μg/kg of muscle with higher values in liver and kidney. In contrast, this β-adrenergic agonist is not authorized in the EU because no ADI or MRL have been set.

The ADI can also be determined from microbiological data for substances with microbiological activity. An issue that needs to be addressed for veterinary antimicrobial drugs is the safety of their residues on the human intestinal flora. The objectives of this guideline are (1) to outline the steps in determining the need for establishing a mADI; (2) to recommend test systems and methods for determining NOAECs and NOAELs for the endpoints of health concern; and (3) to recommend a procedure to derive a microbiological ADI.

The mADI and the toxicological ADI calculations conservatively assume that the amount and concentration (chronic daily ingestion) of veterinary drug residue in the colon are the same daily. Recently, there have been questions regarding the applicability of the mADI calculation for purposes of assessing a single, acute residue dose exposure that is also addressed as a component of the human food safety assessment of veterinary drug use. Acute residue dose (ARD) exposure is a one-time event (e.g., ingestion would be consumption of edible tissue containing the injection site of the drug administered to the treated animal), not the chronic daily ingestion assumed in derivation of an ADI or a mADI. In such cases, an acute residue dose exposure of the intestinal microbiome to a drug is different from the chronic daily ingestion exposure assumed to establish the mADI and that the most relevant microbiological end-point for acute exposure would most likely be disruption of the colonization barrier (FDA, 2013; Cerniglia et al., 2016).

The bolus of drug contained in the ARD meal is loaded and diluted into an intestinal tract that contains no comparable high levels of ingested residue. This temporal dilution must be taken into consideration of one-time consumption of an ARD that is not taken into account in the current derivation of a mADI based on in vitro data. This is in contrast to the assumption for the chronic daily (ADI or mADI) exposure scenario that on given day, the ingested ADI is loaded into an intestinal tract that already has comparable concentrations of drug spanning the intestine due to ingestion from daily consumption of the drug at the ADI level of ingestion. What is critical in delineating this comparison of residue "loading," is the observation that the components contained within a single meal do not enter the colon as a bolus (Cerniglia et al., 2016). While this bolus approach (220 g) may be appropriate as a conservative means to derive a safe daily ingestion rate for a lifetime mADI, the 220 g bolus assumption underestimates the temporary dilution concept (i.e., ingestion of a residue in a single acute dose meal's entry into the intestinal tract). Currently, this is elaborating guidance on approaches to determine the ARD of veterinary drug from a toxicological and microbiological perspective (FDA, 2013).

To establish MRLs for a given drug requires provision of the following data: knowledge of dosage schedule (amount, dose interval, and duration) and administration route; metabolic and pharmacokinetic data in laboratory animals and each of the target food–producing species; distribution and residue depletion data for the major edible tissue (i.e., muscle, fat, liver, and kidney) in each target species using a radiolabeled drug; validated analytical methods for detection and quantitation of residues, including marker residue; and data defining the effect of residues on food processing. Under EU legislation (article 14 (2) of Regulation (EC) No. 470/2009 (EC, 2009a)) the classification of pharmacologically active substances shall also establish, in relation to each such substance, and, where appropriate, specific food stuffs or species. Substances that may be used in veterinary medicines for food-producing species or biocidal products for use in animal husbandry are listed in food stuffs Table 7.1 (allowed substances) with the following information: (1) the definitive MRL to be applied to each food commodity; (2) a provisional MRL to be applied to each food commodity (pending further data). The provisional MRL is established for a defined period and only in those cases where there are no grounds for supposing that residues of the substance at the level proposed will present a hazard to the health of the consumer but where further information is still required in order to finalize the evaluation of the substance; (3) the absence of the need to establish an MRL (i.e., no MRL is required for substances where residues at the predicted levels do not pose a hazard to the health of the consumer); and (4) a prohibition on the administration of a substance. Those substances included in Annex I, II, or III and the amount of residue are not considered to present a safety concern for human health. Those substances included in Annex I, II, or III of the Council Regulation (EEC) No 90/2377 (EEC, 1990) are listed in the Annex of Commission Regulation (EC) No. 37/2010 (EC, 2010) (Table 7.1), allowed substances, where there are listed the pharmacologically active substance, marker residue, animal species, MRL value, target tissues, other provisions (according to Article 14(7) of Regulation (EC) No. 470/2009, EC, 2009a) and therapeutic classification, and Table 7.2 (prohibited substances) (where an MRL cannot be established). These substances must not be used in veterinary medicines for food-producing animals or in biocidal products for use in animal husbandry (Table 7.9). This classification substitutes the four annexes of the Council Regulation (EEC) No. 2377/90.

Establishment of Codex Maximum Residue Limits for Drugs and Feed Additives

The JECFA is an international expert scientific committee that is administered jointly by the Food and Agricultural Organization of the United Nations (FAO) and the World Health Organization (WHO). JECFA serves as an independent scientific committee that performs RAs and provides advice to FAO, WHO, and the member countries of both organizations. Requests for scientific advice are for the main part directed through the CAC in their work to

TABLE 7.9 Active Substances Are Classified Under Four Categories

Regulation (EC) No. 470/2009	Regulation (EEC) No. 2377/90
(a) A maximum residue limit	Annex I. List of pharmacologically active substances for which maximum residue limits have been fixed
(b) A provisional maximum residue limit	Annex III. List of pharmacologically active substances used in veterinary medicinal products for which provisional maximum residue limits have been fixed
(c) The absence of the need to establish a maximum residue limit	Annex II. List of substances not subject to maximum residue limits
(d) A prohibition on the administration of a substance	Annex IV. List of pharmacologically active substances for which no maximum levels can be fixed

develop international food standards and guidelines under the Joint FAO/WHO Food Standards Program. The main purposes of this program are protecting the health of consumers and ensuring fair trade practices in the food trade industry. The advice to CAC on residues of veterinary drugs is provided by the Codex Committee on Residues of Veterinary Drugs in Food (CCRVDF). FAO and WHO have complementary functions in selecting experts to serve on the committee. For residues of veterinary drugs, the WHO panel of the Joint Expert Committee is responsible for the toxicological evaluations of the substances under consideration in order to establish ADIs (or provisional ADIs) when possible. The FAO panel develops specifications for the identity and purity of substances, assesses residue levels of veterinary drugs in food, and checks the quality of the monitoring data. It also proposes limits (MRLs or provisional MRLs) for residues of veterinary drugs in products of animal origin, based on the WHO ADIs and on information about the distribution of the residues in tissues of the target animal. In setting the MRLs, the TMDI is estimated using the exaggerated consumption package for products of animal origin. Veterinary drug residues include parent drugs as well as their metabolites. Metabolites are taken into account if they are toxicologically relevant, i.e., present in a considerable quantity or having a toxicological or pharmacological potential. The MRL is expressed in terms of parent drug levels or in terms of levels of a marker metabolite, if the percentage of the marker metabolite formed from the parent drug is known.

Changes in Calculation of MRLs

In the new JECFA approach, median residue concentration levels are used to derive an estimated daily intake rather than the MRL to better reflect estimates of chronic (lifetime) exposure (WHO, 2006). The most significant change introduced by the new approach is that the calculation of the MRL is independent of the ADI. The point at and beyond which the predicted median intake (estimated daily intake, EDI) equals the ADI is deemed an acceptable POD for the derivation of MRLs. The MRL and the median concentration are derived from the same time point of the depletion data of the marker residue. The MRL itself is a point on the curve describing the upper one-sided 95% confidence limit over the 95th percentile, and the median is the corresponding point on the regression line for the same time point. The MRL represents the upper tolerance limit for the marker residue concentration in the edible tissue at the time point when the EDI reached the level of the ADI. The JECFA concluded that the TMDI is no longer used as the most suitable estimate of chronic intake. However, where a median residue cannot be derived, the MRL may be substituted for the median residue to calculate the TMDI. JECFA's previous approach (which is still used in the EU), stated that exposure was estimated on the basis of the MRL (throughout TMDI calculation) and proposed MRLs were checked for compliance with the ADI. The new procedure uses the same formula as used previously for the calculation of the TMDI, including factors such as the ratio of marker to total residue concentrations. The only exception is that median residue level replaces the MRL as the point estimate of the residue concentration (i.e., median residue levels take place of MRLs as a starting point from which to calculate chronic exposure); therefore it is the median residue levels that are compared to the ADI rather than MRLs (WHO, 2006). The new concept is to use median residue levels in animal-derived food for the calculation of the new estimate of exposure termed the "estimated daily intake" (EDI) from a daily model food basket (i.e., the calculation of the EDI is based on the same standard figures of food basket and correction for ratios of marker to total residue concentrations as used for the calculation of the TMDI; the only exception in this procedure was the use of median residues instead of the MRLs as the point estimate of the residue concentration in animal-derived food). The EDI does not cover the scenario of a short-term/high-concentration exposure but rather is an estimate of the long-term average intake, based on long-term average consumption behavior, and long-term average residue level. Using this new approach, the MRL is calculated at the upper tolerance limit (confidence limit) in a residue study at the time point when the median residues in the food basket are below the EDI. The TMDI represents the worst case assumption of maximum permitted residue levels (i.e., at the MRL) in each food commodity consumed. This change of the model was initiated because the TMDI approach was thought to grossly overestimate the true chronic level of exposure to the population. It was recognized that, if good veterinary practice is observed, there is a relatively low statistical probability that residues in edible tissues approach the MRL.

With the current EU-MRL approach, chronic exposure is calculated on the basis of the MRL and TMDI. Summarizing, the EU throughout the EMEA should carefully consider the new MRL JECFA proposals because some impact is expected in the existing MRL assessments.

To the same extent, the modified chronic model proposed by JECFA is consistent with the approach already used by JMPR in the assessment of chronic exposure to pesticide residues. In this procedure, the TMDI concept was reviewed in 1997 and it was proposed to use results of STMR levels instead of the MRL to estimate a chronic intake (WHO, 1997). The JMPR and JECFA residue evaluation processes contribute to a better harmonization of *Codex Alimentarius* residue assessment procedures for

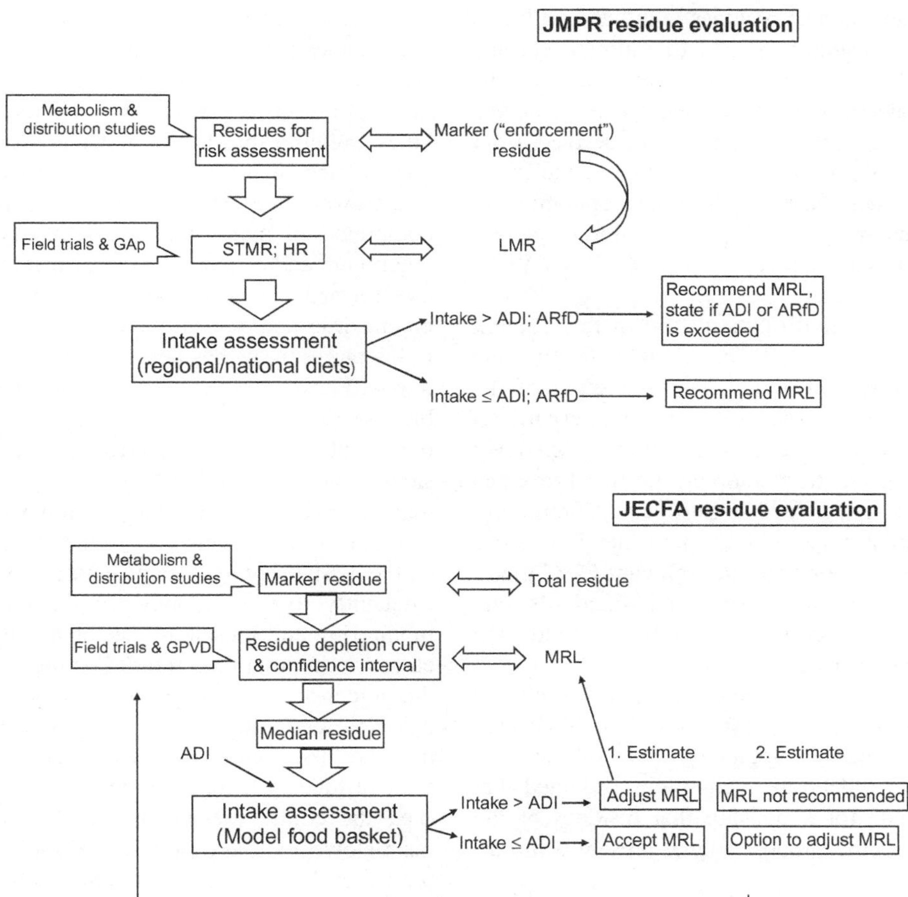

FIGURE 7.2 The JMPR and JECFA residue evaluation processes.

chemicals in food. The JMPR and new JECFA proposals are shown in Fig. 7.2.

Dietary exposure assessment plays an essential role in quantifying risk. There are methods for acute and chronic dietary exposure assessment for veterinary drug residues. The current model diet used for veterinary drug residues is intended to cover chronic high consumers of animal products. For estimating chronic dietary exposures to veterinary drug residues, JECFA uses the median of the residue depletion to derive the EDI.

The acute reference dose (ARfD) of a chemical is an estimate of the amount of the substance in food and/or drinking water, normally expressed on a body weight basis, that can be ingested in a period of 24 h or fewer, without appreciable risk to the health of the consumer. The acute dietary exposure estimates should cover a time period of food consumption over a single meal or 1 day and are intended to be used for comparison with acute reference dose (ARfD) values in a RA process. The main driver for the need to consider establishing an ARfD is the toxicological profile of the compound.

Two new methods for estimating dietary exposure are the global estimate of acute dietary exposure (GEADE) and the global estimate of chronic dietary exposure (GECDE). Both methods differ from EDI by having the capacity to estimate specific dietary exposure for additional population groups (children aged 12 months and older and infants younger than 12 months). In this approach, more detailed food consumption data are used (e.g., muscle tissue is differentiated by species, and fish are considered separately from mollusks and crustaceans) (FAO/WHO, 2014).

The current approach to estimating dietary exposure does not adequately estimate acute dietary exposure, which should be based on the highest probable exposure from a single commodity on a single day or over a single meal. This is intended to be used for comparison with ARfD values in a RA process. Therefore, an appropriate acute dietary exposure assessment method needs to be used (i.e., GEADE). The GEADE is an explicit estimate of acute dietary exposure, combining consumption at the 97.5th percentile with the 95th percentile residue concentration.

The GECDE uses median residues combined with two different types of consumption data to estimate chronic dietary exposure. Firstly, the highest exposure at the 97.5th percentile of consumption is selected from all the foods relevant to exposure. This value is derived from chronic consumers of the food, and secondly, the mean dietary exposure is derived from the total population. In addition to the general population and children, dietary exposure of infants can also be estimated (FAO/WHO, 2014).

As indicated in the modification draft of the Council Regulation (EEC) No. 2377/90 (EEC, 1990), the European Community contributes in the context of the *Codex Alimentarius* to the development of international standards on MRLs, while ensuring that the high level of human health protection adopted in the European Community is not reduced. The European Community should therefore take over, without a further RA, those codex MRLs it has supported in the relevant CAC meeting. Consistency between international standards and community legislation on residue limits in food will thereby be further enhanced.

With the modification of the Council Regulation (EEC) No. 2377/90 (EEC, 1990) a provisional MRL may be established for a pharmacologically active substance in cases where scientific data are incomplete, provided that there are no grounds for supposing that residues of the specific substance at the proposed level present a hazard for human health.

United States of America: Food and Drug Administration Tolerance Setting

The FDA does not separately regulate drugs for food-producing animals from the feed additives for animal nutrition. The toxicological assessment of a veterinary drug or a feed additive establishes the basis for identifying the most appropriates in vitro an in vivo study upon which a NOEL and, subsequently, an ADI, can be established. Based on the quantity and quality of the data and the scientific interpretation of those data, a safety factor is applied to the NOEL to establish the ADI. The second major component described in that guidance (FDA, 2003a) in regards to safety evaluation is exposure to humans from consumption of residues of toxicological concern in tissues (and milk and eggs, as appropriate). That process begins with metabolism and radiolabeled residue studies in the target animals. The three principal components of this endeavor include comparative metabolism in the toxicological species, total radiolabeled residue and metabolism studies in the food-producing animals, and residue depletion studies to establish the preslaughter withdrawal period and, when needed, the milk withdrawal and discard time. Total residue and metabolism studies provide information to establish the appropriate marker residue (i.e., the parent drug or any of its metabolites or a combination of any of these with a known relationship to the concentration of the total residue in each of the various edible tissues at the expected withdrawal time). A marker residue may be the parent compound, a major metabolite, the sum of the parent compound and/or a metabolite or metabolites, or a derivative formed during analysis by chemical reaction of the parent drug and/or metabolites. When the marker residue in the target tissue has depleted to the MRL, the total residue will have depleted to the safe concentration in all edible tissues and to determine the target tissue (represents the edible carcass from which residue depletes most slowly and is the edible tissue selected to monitor for the marker residue in the target animal). It is considered suitable for monitoring compliance with the MRL of each edible tissue from a treated animal. The target tissue is frequently liver or kidney for the purpose of domestic monitoring and muscle or fat for monitoring meat or carcasses in international trade. For the FDA, and following the guidance above when the tolerance is based on a toxicological endpoint, the concentration of the marker residue (i.e., the compound used to monitor the depletion of total residue in a food animal tissue) in the target tissue (i.e., the edible tissue from which the residue depletes most slowly) at the time the total radiolabeled residues in the target tissue have depleted to less than the target tissue in safe concentration, is the target tissue tolerance (word similar to MRLs).

When the ADI is based on a microbiological endpoint (FDA, 2013), a similar approach is used; however, only residues of microbiological concern are considered. In the FDA approach when the concentration of the marker residue in the target tissue is less than the target tissue tolerances, total residues in all the edible tissues are less than their respective safe concentrations (i.e., the entire food animal carcass is safe). Safe concentrations of residues in the animal tissues are related to the ADI and food consumption factors. The FDA uses the same food consumption factors as those used in the JECFA; however, they are applied differently (Ellis, 2004). The FDA assumes that if a person consumes 300 g of muscle tissue, he/she will not consume an allocation of liver or kidney tissue but may consume a full allocation of milk and eggs. The food allocation is 300 g for muscle, 100 g for liver, 50 g for kidney and fat, 1500 g for milk, and 100 g for eggs. Therefore, for a safe concentration in muscle for a 60 kg consumer, the ADI (in mg/kg) is multiplied by 60 kg and that value is divided by 0.3 kg. For liver, the denominator will be 0.1 kg and for kidney and fat the denominator will be 0.05 kg. The daily intake of meat products is determined to be one third of the total solid diet of 1500 g (i.e., 500 g). For milk the denominator is 1.5 kg and for eggs 0.1 kg.

Drug Withdrawal/Withholding Periods

A critical factor in the medication of all food-producing animals is the mandatory withdrawal period, defined as the time during which a drug must not be administered prior to the slaughter of the animal for consumption. The withdrawal time is the period of time between the last administration of a drug and the collection of edible tissue from a treated animal. The withdrawal period is an integral part of the regulatory authorities' approval process and is designed to ensure that no significant drug residue is present in the animal at slaughter. Drug residues in food-producing animals should comply with the MRL values for their target tissues in the animal species. The withdrawal period is intended to ensure that no harmful residues remain in edible tissues after slaughter and it is usually established at slaughter time when residue levels in all the edible tissues are below the MRL. Compliance with the preslaughter withdrawal period ensures that total residues deplete to below the safe concentration, and the marker residues deplete to below the MRL. Adherence to the withdrawal period provides assurance that food derived from treated animals will not exceed the MRL for the drug substance. Failure to keep the preslaughter withdrawal period while using veterinary drugs is the major cause of violative drug tissue residues in food animal production in the EU. Even if the withdrawal period involves only a few days or a few hours, the resulting residues can violate the national regulations against sale of adulterated foodstuffs, which can originate distortions of competition between member states of the EU. Withdrawal period, based on the MRL, is fixed by the regulatory authorities and will take into account the use of veterinary drugs in avian species. Regulatory authorities determine withdrawal periods on the basis of residue depletion data generated using healthy animals representative of those normally treated with the veterinary drug. For example, for the determination of the withdrawal period in avian species, six animals per slaughter time are needed. An appropriate withdrawal period is then established to ensure that the residues in edible tissues are depleted below the MRLs. A withdrawal period should be established for the substances with MRLs included in Annex (Table 7.1) of Regulation (EC) No. 37/2010 (EC, 2010). The EMA recommends the harmonization of withdrawal periods using linear regression analysis of log-transformed tissue concentrations determined at the time when the 95% upper one-side tolerance limit was below the MRL with 95% confidence (Anadón et al., 2008a,b, 2011, 2012). Unlike an MRL, which applies to a veterinary drug regardless of the dosage form, route of administration, or dosage regimen, the withdrawal period stated in the product labeling applies only to that particular formulation when administered via the recommended route and in accordance with the dose regime. Alteration to any of these factors affects the pharmacokinetics behavior of the drug in the animal and invalidates the withdrawal period.

In the EU a veterinary prescription is required for veterinary products for food-producing animals. If it is necessary for a VMP to be prescribed for a species for which it is not licensed or at a dosage higher than the one licensed, the veterinarian will specify an appropriate withdrawal period. In exceptional cases, where no medication is authorized, there is a possibility for the veterinarian to use, e.g., products that are authorized in other EU countries or for other animal species. This exception exists to avoid unacceptable suffering of animals. In these cases the veterinarian has to follow specific steps, the so-called "cascade," and has to make sure that there is no risk for the animal(s) concerned and for consumers of food products of animal origin. The exceptional off-label (extra-label) (cascade) use of authorized medications is allowed under specific conditions described in Directive 2001/82/EC (EC, 2001) as amended by Article 11 of Directive 2004/28/EC (EC, 2004b) (Table 7.10).

The veterinarian may administer the medicinal product personally or allow another person to do so under the veterinarian's responsibility. For food-producing animals, these provisions apply to animals on a particular holding only. The pharmacologically active substances in the medicinal products used must be listed in the Annex of the Commission Regulation (EU) No. 37/2010 (Table 7.1, allowed substances) (EC, 2010). The pharmacologically active substances in the medicinal products must have been assessed according to Regulation (EC) No. 470/2009 on the residue limits of pharmacologically active substances in foodstuffs of animal origin (EC, 2009c), and a veterinarian must specify an appropriate withdrawal period, which shall be at least 7 days for eggs, 7 days for milk, 28 days for meat from poultry and mammals (including fat and offal), and 500 days for fish.

INDUSTRIAL CHEMICALS

The area of regulations covering industrial chemicals is one of increasing harmonization within the EU. This is particularly true with regard to the need for providing adequate toxicity data on new chemicals, to allow any potential hazard to humans to be identified, and in the area of labeling of dangerous substances and preparations (i.e., mixtures of substances). A key directive is Council Directive 67/548/EEC on the approximation of the laws, regulations and administrative provisions relating to the CLP of dangerous substances, commonly referred to as

TABLE 7.10 Exceptional Off-Label (Extra-Label) Use of Authorized Medications ("Cascade" System)

No authorized veterinary medicinal product (VMP) in a member state for a specific condition (1) A VMP authorized in the member state concerned for use for another animal species, or for another condition in the same species; or	
Medicinal product (2) A medicinal product for human use authorized in the member state concerned	*Medicinal product or imported VMP* (2) If there is no such product authorized, either: (a) a medicinal product for human use authorized in the member state concerned, or (b) a VMP authorized in another member state for use in the same species or in another food-producing species for the condition in question or for another condition may be used
(3) If, however, there is no such product, a VMP prepared extemporaneously by a person authorized to do so following a veterinary prescription may be used	

the Dangerous Substances Directive (EEC, 1967) and its subsequent amendments, as well as the Council Regulation (EEC) No. 793/93 of March 23, 1993 on the evaluation and control of the risks of existing substances (EEC, 1993). On the other hand, REACH is the Regulation on Registration, Evaluation, Authorization and Restriction of Chemicals (EC, 2006). It entered into force on June 1, 2007. It streamlines and improves the former legislative framework on chemicals of the EU. The main aims of REACH are to ensure a high level of protection of human health and the environment from the risks that can be posed by chemicals, the promotion of alternative test methods, the free circulation of substances on the internal market, and enhancing competitiveness and innovation. REACH makes industry responsible for assessing and managing the risks posed by chemicals and for providing appropriate safety information to their users. Under the REACH Regulation, companies are responsible for providing information on the hazards, risks and safe use of chemical substances that they manufacture or import. REACH information requirements to be considered in the assessment embraces: (1) collecting existing data on the substance or on similar substances including information on use, exposure and risk management, and (2) data on analogous substances in a weight of evidence approach, if "read-across" or membership of a "chemical category" is possible as well as considering QSAR analyses or estimation. Data generated from in vitro test methods (validated and prevalidated) (Anadón et al., 2013) can be used either as a standalone to fill in a data gap or as part of a weight of evidence approach under REACH provided that the information for the hazard endpoint is sufficient for the purpose of classification and labeling and/or RA. In parallel, the EU can take additional measures on highly dangerous substances where there is a need for complementing action at the EU level. All manufacturers and importers of chemicals must identify and manage risks linked to the substances they manufacture and market. For substances manufactured or imported in quantities of 1 ton or more per year per company, manufacturers and importers need to demonstrate that they have appropriately done so by means of a registration dossier, which must be submitted to the ECHA. The ECHA is the driving force in implementing the EU's groundbreaking chemical legislation for the protection of human health and the environment. The ECHA work helps ensure that chemicals are used safely and that the most hazardous ones are substituted by safer alternatives. ECHA may then check that the registration dossier complies with the regulation and must evaluate testing proposals to ensure that the assessment of the chemical substances will not result in unnecessary testing, especially on animals, but also that adequate information is provided. Where appropriate, authorities may also select substances for a broader substance evaluation to further investigate substances of concern. Six substances of very high concern will be banned within the next 3–5 years unless an authorization has been granted to individual companies for their use. These substances are carcinogenic, toxic for reproduction, persist in the environment, and accumulate in living organisms. The following substances are concerned: musk xylene, 4',4'-methylenedianiline (MDA), hexabromocyclododecane (HBCDD), di-(2-ethylhexil) phthalate (DEHP), benzyl butyl phthalate (BBP) and dibutyl phthalate (DBP).

REACH also foresees an authorization system aiming to ensure that substances of very high concern are properly controlled and progressively replaced by suitable alternative substances or technologies where these are economically and technically viable. Where this is not possible, the use of substances may only be authorized where there is an overall benefit for society in using the substance. In addition, EU authorities may impose restrictions on the manufacture, use, or placing on the market of substances causing an unacceptable risk to human health or the environment. The EU member states authorities are responsible for enforcing REACH through inspections as well as penalties in case of noncompliance. From June 1, 2009, Annex XVII of the REACH Regulation replaced Directive 76/769/EEC (EEC, 1976) on the approximation of the laws, regulations and administrative provisions of the member states, relating to restrictions on the marketing and use of certain dangerous substances and preparations.

CONCLUDING REMARKS AND FUTURE DIRECTIONS

Drugs feed additives, biocides and chemicals are indispensable for the production of food animals. Complicated and extensive systems for the marketing authorization of veterinary medicinal products and other chemical compounds have existence in the EU. These systems attempt to ensure the quality, efficacy (including an objective overall assessment of the risk/benefit balance of the final product) and safety of veterinary drugs and feed additives. Safety to consumers is utmost importance and this demands a meticulous assessment of pharmacological, toxicological, microbiological, and residues data. The marketing authorization procedure for veterinary medicinal products in the EU is of great interest in terms of RA of residues. The main human health risks from drug residues in foods are the acute toxic effects (i.e., hypersensitivity, pharmacological effects, and teratogenic effects) and the long-term chronic effects (carcinogenesis).

Carryover in the feed of coccidiostats and other medicated feed can result in the exposure of nontarget animal species and induce adverse effects. The best way to assess the carryover from feed to food is to determine from animal experiments the transfer factors of chemicals from the animal feed to the animal products. The maximum levels of carryover for active substances in medicated feed should be established in order to protect animal health, human health, and the environment. MRPLs have been proposed as a temporary measure to tackle problems associated with illegal or unauthorized substances that can be used in food-producing animals in the EU.

Residues from consumption of stockfeed treated with agricultural chemicals (i.e., pesticides) should be evaluated and established the limits for pesticide residues in feed beside those for all undesirable substances.

The pharmacologically active substances contained in biocidal products or in feed additives used in animal husbandry against pests and other harmful microorganism (e.g., insect repellents, disinfectants) should be submitted to the establishment of MRL as regulated in the EU. All feed additives placed on the market in the EU must be authorized under a centralized or community procedure once it evaluates safety of the target animal, the consumer, the user and the environment besides the efficacy in the target species.

The comparative toxicological standards for food safety are very useful to raise proposed safety evaluation strategies. The HBGVs (i.e., pharmacological, toxicological, and microbiological ADI, ARfD) are most often established for veterinary drugs and chemicals used in animal food using a POD based on adversity from a toxicity study in experimental animals or for calculation of a MOE. A critical factor in the medication of all food-producing animals, with veterinary drugs and feed additive coccidiostats, is the mandatory withdrawal period. Failure to keep the preslaughter withdrawal period while using a veterinary drug is the major cause of violative drug tissue residues in food animal production in the EU. The establishment of MLRs for veterinary drugs has been submitted in the last year to change in its calculation to a better harmonization of *Codex Alimentarius* residue assessment procedures for chemicals in food.

The area of regulations covering industrial chemicals is one of increasing harmonization within the EU. The regulations and administrative provisions relating to the CLP of dangerous substances on the evaluation and control of the risk of existing substances are reviewed. Moreover, REACH came into force in 2007, addressing the production and use of chemical substances, and their potential impacts on both human health and the environment.

REFERENCES

Anadón, A., 2006. The EU ban of antibiotics as feed additives. Alternatives and consumer safety. J. Vet. Pharmacol. Ther. 29 (Suppl. 1), 41–44.

Anadón, A., Martínez-Larrañaga, M.R., 1999. Residues of antimicrobial drugs and feed additives in animal products: regulatory aspects. Livestock Prod. Sci. 59 (2–3), 183–198.

Anadón, A., Martínez, M.A., Martínez, M., de la cruz, C.O., et al., 2008a. Oral bioavailability, tissue distribution and depletion of flumequine in food producing animal, chicken for fattening. Food Chem. Toxicol. 46, 662–670.

Anadón, A., Martínez, M.A., Martinez, M., et al., 2008b. Plasma and tissue depletion of florfenicol and florfenicol-amine in chickens. J. Agric. Food Chem. 56, 11049–11056.

Anadón, A., Martínez-Larrañaga, M.R., Caballero, V., et al., 2010. Chapter 2. Assessment of prebiotics and probiotics: an overview. In: Watson, R., Preedy, V.R. (Eds.), Bioactive Foods in Promoting Health: Probiotics and Prebiotics. Elsevier Inc./Academic Press, San Diego, CA, pp. 19–41.

Anadón, A., Suarez, F.H., Martínez, M.A., et al., 2011. Plasma disposition and tissue depletion of difloxacin and its metabolite sarafloxacin in the food producing animals, chicken for fattening. Food Chem. Toxicol. 49, 441–449.

Anadón, A., Gamboa, F., Martínez, M.A., et al., 2012. Pharmacokinetics and tissue depletion of chlortetracycline after multiple oral administration to chickens for fattening. Food Chem. Toxicol. 50, 2714–2721.

Anadón, A., Martínez, M.A., Castellano, V., Martínez-Larrañaga, M.R., 2013. The role of *in vitro* methods as alternatives to animals in toxicity testing. Expert Opin. Metab. Toxicol. 10 (1), 1–13.

Anadón, A., Martínez-Larrañaga, M.R., Arés, I., et al., 2016. Prebiotics and probiotics: an assessment of their safety and health benefits.

Chapter 1. In: Watson, R., Preedy, V.R. (Eds.), Probiotics, Prebiotics, and Synbiotics. Bioactive Foods in Promoting Health: Probiotics and Prebiotics. Elsevier Inc./Academic Press, San Diego, CA, pp. 3–23. ISBN: 978-0-12-802189-7.

Cerniglia, C.E., Pineiro, S.A., Kotarski, S.F., 2016. An update discussion on the current assessment of the safety of veterinary antimicrobial drug residues in food with regard to their impact on the human intestinal microbiome. Drug Test Anal. 8 (5–6), 539–548.

Cummings, J.H., Banwell, J.G., Segal, I., et al., 1990. The amount and composition of large bowel contents in man. Gastroenterology 5, 408.

Dayan, A.D., 1993. Allergy to antimicrobial residues in food: assessment of the risk to man. Vet. Microbiol. 35, 213–226.

Dorne, J.L., Fernández-Cruz, M.L., Bertelsen, U., et al., 2011. Risk assessment of coccidostatics during feed cross-contamination: animal and human health aspects. Toxicol. Appl. Pharmacol. 8 (3), 160–171.

EC, (1997). Commission Directive 97/6/EC of 30 January Commission Directive 97/6/EC of 30 January 1997 amending Council Directive 70/524/EEC concerning additives in feedingstuffs.

EC, (1998a). Directive 98/8/EC of the European Parliament and of the Council of 16 February 1998 concerning the placing of biocidal products on the market (OJ L 123, 24.4.1998).

EC, (1998b). Council Regulation (EC) No 2821/98 of 17 December 1998 amending, as regards withdrawal of the authorisation of certain antibiotics, Directive 70/524/EEC concerning additives in feedingstuffs (OJ L 351, 29.12.1998).

EC, (2001). Directive 2001/82/EC of the European Parliament and of the Council of 6 November 2001 on the community code relating to veterinary medicinal products (OJ L 136, 30.4.2004).

EC, (2002a). Opinion of the Scientific Committee on Veterinary Measures Relating to Public Health on Review of previous SCVPH opinions of 30 April 1999 and 3 May 2000 on the potential risks to human health from hormone residues in bovine meat and meat products (adopted on 10 April 2002).

EC, (2002b). Regulation (EC) No 178/2002 of The European Parliament and of the Council of 28 January2002 laying down the general principles and requirements of food law, establishing the European Food Safety Authority and laying down procedures in matters of food safety (OJ L 31, 1.2.2002).

EC, (2003). Regulation (EC) No. 1831/2003 (EC, 2003) of the European Parliament and of the Council of 22 September on additives for use in animal nutrition (OJ No. L 268 18.10.2003).

EC, (2004a). Regulation (EC) No 726/2004 of the European Parliament and of the Council of 31 March 2004 laying down Community procedures for the authorisation and supervision of medicinal products for human and veterinary use and establishing a European Medicines Agency (OJ L 136, 30.4.2004).

EC, (2004b). Directive 2004/28/EC of the European Parliament and of the Council of 31 March 2004 amending Directive 2001/82/EC on the Community code relating to veterinary medicinal products (OJ L 136, 30/04/2004).

EC, (2005). Regulation (EC) No. 183/2005 of the European parliament and of the council of 12 January 2005 laying down requirements of feed hygiene (OJ L35, 8.2.2005).

EC, (2006). Regulation (EC) No 1907/2006 of the European Parliament and of the Council of 18 December 2006 concerning the Registration, Evaluation, Authorisation and Restriction of Chemicals (REACH), establishing a European Chemicals Agency, amending Directive 1999/45/EC and repealing Council Regulation (EEC) No 793/93 and Commission Regulation (EC) No 1488/94 as well as Council Directive 76/769/EEC and Commission Directives 91/155/EEC, 93/67/EEC, 93/105/EC and 2000/21/EC (OJ L 396, 30.12.2006).

EC, (2008a). Directive 2008/97/EC of The European Parliament and of the Council of 19 November 2008 amending Council Directive 96/22/EC concerning the prohibition on the use in stock farming of certain substances having a hormonal or thyrostatic action and of beta-agonists (OJ L 318, 28.11.2008).

EC, (2008b). Commission Regulation (EC) No 429/2008 of 25 April 2008 on detailed rules for the implementation of Regulation (EC) No 1831/2003 of the European Parliament and of the Council as regards the preparation and the presentation of applications and the assessment and the authorisation of feed additives (OJ No. L 133, 22.5.2008).

EC, (2009a). Commission Directive 2009/9/EC of 10 February 2009 amending Directive 2001/82/EC of the European Parliament and of the Council on the Community code relating to medicinal products for veterinary use (OJ L 44, 14.2.2009).

EC, (2009b). Regulation (EC) No 1107/2009 of the European Parliament and of the Council of 21 October 2009 concerning the placing of plant protection products on the market and repealing Council Directives 79/117/EEC and 91/414/EEC (OJ L 309, 24.11.2009).

EC, (2009c). Commission Regulation (EC) No 470/2009 of the European Parliament and of the Council of 6 May 2009 concerning laying down Community procedures for the establishment of residue limits of pharmacologically active substances in foodstuffs of animal origin, repealing Council Regulation (EEC) No. 2377/90 and amending Directive 2001/82/EC of the European Parliament and of the Council and Regulation (EC) No. 726/2004 of the European Parliament and of the Council (OJ L 152, 16.6.2009).

Edler, L., Poirier, K., Dourson, M., et al., 2002. Mathematical modelling and quantitative methods. Food Chem. Toxicol. 40, 283–326.

EEC, (1967). Directive 67/548/EEC on the approximation of the laws, regulations and administrative provisions relating to the classification, packaging and labelling of dangerous substances (OJ L 196, 16.8.1967).

EEC, (1970). Council Directive 70/524/EEC of 23 November 1970 concerning additives in feedingstuffs (OJ No L 270, 14.12.1970).

EEC, (1976). Council Directive of 27 July 1976 on the approximation of the laws, regulations and administrative provisions of the Member States relating to restrictions on the marketing and use of certain dangerous substances and preparations (76/769/EEC) (OJ L 262, 27.9.1976).

EEC, (1978). Council Directive 78/631/EEC of 26 June 1978 on the approximation of the laws of the Member States relating to the classification, packaging and labeling of dangerous preparations (pesticides) (OJ L 206, 29.7.1978).

EEC, (1990). Council Regulation 90/2377/EEC laying down a Community procedure for the establishment of maximum residue limits of veterinary medicinal products in foodstuffs of animal origin (OJ No L 224, 12.8.90).

EEC, (1993). Council Regulation (EEC) nº 793/93 of 23 March 1993 on the evaluation and control of the risks of existing substances (OJ L 84, 5.4.1993).

EFSA, 2007. Cross-contamination of non-target feedingstuffs by narasin authorised for use as a feed additive. EFSA J. 552, 1–35.

Ellis, R., (2004). U.S.F.D.A. Regulatory approach for control of residues of veterinary drugs. In: Technical Workshop on Residues of Veterinary Drugs Without ADI/MRL, Bangkok (Thailand), August 24–26, 2004.

EU, (2010). Commission Regulation (EU) No 37/2010 of 22 December 2009 on pharmacologically active substances and their classification regarding maximum residue limits in foodstuffs of animal origin (OJ L 15, 20.1.2010).

EU, (2012). Regulation (EU) No 528/2012 of the European Parliament and of the Council of 22 May 2012 concerning the making available on the market and use of biocidal products (OJ L 167; 27.6.2012).

FAO/WHO, (2004). Evaluation of certain veterinary drug residues in food. In: Seventy-Eighth Report of the Joint FAO/WHO Expert Committee on Food Additives. World Health Organization (Technical Report Series, 988), Geneva.

FAO/WHO (2014). Evaluation of certain veterinary drug residues in food. Seventy-eighth report of the Joint FAO/WHO Expert Committee on Food Additives. Geneva: World Healt Organization (Technical Report Series, 988).

FDA, (2003). Guidance for Industry (No.3). General Principles for Evaluating the Safety of Compounds Used in Food-Producing Animals. (http://www.fda.gov/cvm/guidance/published.htm).

FDA, (March 5, 2013). Guidance for Industry (No. 159). Studies to Evaluate the Safety of Residues of Veterinary Drugs in Human Food: General Approach to Establish a Microbiological ADI – VICH GL-36 (R).

Herbst, A.L., 1976. Summary of the changes in the human female genital tract as a consequence of maternal diethylstilbestrol therapy. J. Toxicol. Environ. Health.(Suppl. 1), 13–20.

Herbst, A.L., Ulfelder, H., Poskanzer, D.C., 1971. Adenocarcinoma of the vagina: association of maternal stilbestrol therapy with tumor appearance in young women. N. Engl. J. Med. 284, 878–881.

Hurd, D.R., 1996. Trimediazine BMP: a major advance in in-feed medication. Feed Compounder. 16, 38–39.

Kennedy, D.G., Smyth, W.G., Hewitt, A., et al., 1998. Monensin carry-over into unmedicated broiler feeds. Analyst 123, 2529–2533.

Lagier, J.C., Million, M., Hugon, P., et al., 2012. Human gut microbiota: repertoire and variations. Front. Cell. Infect. Microbiol. 2, 136.

Leeman, W.R., Van der Berg, K.J., Houben, G.F., 2007. Transfer of chemicals from feed to animal products: the use of transfer factors in risk assessment. Food Addit. Contam. 24, 1–13.

Lützow, M. (2004), Residues of veterinary drugs without ADI/MRL: what Codex and WTO rules apply? In: Technical Workshop on Residues of Veterinary Drugs Without ADI/MRL, Bangkok (Thailand), August 24–26, 2004.

Martinez-Navarro, J.F., 1990. Food poisoning related to consumption of illicit β-agonist in liver. Lancet 336, 1311.

McEvoy, J.D.G., Smyth, W.G., Kennedy, D.G., 2003. Contamination of animal feedingstuffs with nicarbazin: investigations in a feed mill. Food Addit. Contam. 20 (2), 136–140.

Metzler, M., 1984. Diethylstilbestrol. Reactive metabolites derived from a hormonally active compound. In: Greim, H., Jung, R., Kramer, M., Marquardt, H., Oesch, F. (Eds.), Biochemical Basis of Chemical Carcinogenesis. Raven Press, New York, NY, pp. 69–75.

Meyers, R., 1983. D.E.S. The Bitter Pill. Seaview/Putnam, New York, NY.

Noser, J., Wenk, P., Sutter, A., et al., 2006. Kokzidiostatika in Eiern, Geflügelfleisch und Futtermitteln: Eine Stichproben-Kontrolle über den Nordwestschweizer Markt. Mitt. Lebensmittelunters. Hyg. 97, 107–120.

O'Hara, A.M., Shanahan, F., 2006. The gut flora as a forgotten organ. EMBO Rep. 7, 688–693.

Paige, J.C., Tollefson, L., Miller, M., 1997. Public health impact on drug residues in animal tissues. Vet. Hum. Toxicol. 39 (3), 162–169.

Pulse, C., Lamaison, D., Keck, G., et al., 1991. Collective human food poisoning by clenbuterol residues in veal liver. Vet. Hum. Toxicol. 33 (5), 480–481.

Strauch, W. (2002). Causes and control of carry-over and cross-contamination. Kraftfutter/Feed Mag. 85 (4), 151–159 (Part 1); Kraftfutter/Feed Mag. 85 (6), 239–249 (Part 2).

Strauch, W., 2003. Is contamination-free feed production realistic? Feed Technol. 7 (7), 23–25.

Sundlof, S.F., 1994. Human risks associated with drug residues in animals derived foods. J. Agromed. 1, 5–22.

Taylor, W., 1983. Risk associated with the exposure of human subjects to endogenous and exogenous anabolic steroids. In: Meissonier, F., Mitchell-Vigneron, J. (Eds.), Anabolic in Animal Production. Office International des Epizooties, Paris, pp. 273–287.

WHO, 1989. Guidelines for Predicting Dietary Intake of Pesticide Residues. World Health Organization, Geneva, 24 pp.

WHO, 1997. Guidelines for Predicting Dietary Intake of Pesticides. World Health Organization, Geneva.

WHO, 2006. Evaluation of certain veterinary drug residues in food. Sixty-Sixth Report of the Joint FAO/WHO Expert Committee on Food Additives. World Health Organization, Geneva, pp. 15–16.

WHO, 2015. Pesticide Residues in Food: Guidance Document for WHO Monographers and Reviewers. World Health Organization, WHO Core Assessment Group on Pesticides Residues, Geneva.

Woodward, K.N., 1991. Hypersensitivity in humans and exposure to veterinary drugs. Vet. Hum. Toxicol. 33 (2), 160–172.

FURTHER READING

Ito, S., Alcorn, J., 2003. Xenobiotic transporter expression and function in the mammary gland. Adv. Drug Deliv. Rev. 55, 653–665.

Chapter 8

Toxicokinetics in Veterinary Toxicology

Deon van der Merwe, Ronette Gehring and Jennifer L. Buur

INTRODUCTION

The epithelial barriers that form the body's interface with the environment, and the cellular barriers that separate internal organs and tissues, have to be permeable to a wide variety of chemicals to allow nutrient absorption and waste product elimination. The permeability of these physiological barriers, however, also allows toxicants to penetrate. Exposure to toxicants through ingestion, inhalation, and dermal contact may therefore result in harmful absorption. The degree of adverse effects following exposure to a toxicant is dependent on the rate and extent of absorption into the body, distribution to susceptible organs and tissues, and specific interactions with biological targets. Living organisms are adapted to toxicant exposure through the development of transport and elimination mechanisms that prevent the build-up of harmful chemical concentrations in organs and tissues.

Toxicokinetics refers to the movement and fate, also referred to as the disposition, of toxicants. The term is most commonly used when describing the time course of absorption, distribution, and elimination (including biotransformation and excretion) of toxicants in an organism. Toxicokinetics is closely related to pharmacokinetics, and may even be viewed as the same discipline, with the only difference being the class of compound (toxicant or pharmaceutical) that is involved. Compared to typical pharmaceutical exposure, exposure to toxicants is often uncontrolled and variable, and very large doses may be involved. Toxicants are also more likely to cause lesions and abnormal physiological function that may alter the toxicant disposition, compared to exposures to pharmaceutical drugs below toxic levels. When very large doses are involved, kinetic processes that can become saturated are more likely to reach their maximum rates, resulting in altered disposition.

Predicting tissue concentrations over time is essential for the prediction of adverse effects (Andersen et al., 2006). It is also needed to prevent unwanted xenobiotic residues in animal tissues from entering the human food chain. Kinetic parameters, such as duration of internal exposure and tissue concentrations, are therefore useful metrics for assessing risk. Mathematical models are used to characterize these parameters by describing changes in toxicant concentrations over time. Models are most often used as predictive tools following exposure to toxicants, but they can also be used as an aid to understanding the underlying physiological mechanisms of chemical absorption, transport and elimination. Various types of toxicokinetic models have been developed and the appropriateness of a specific model type depends on the available data and the model's purpose (Riviere, 2011). One of the key challenges to the successful use of models is identifying the appropriate conditions for its application. Two fundamentally different types of toxicokinetic models are recognized: traditional (also called "classic") toxicokinetic models, and physiologically based toxicokinetic (PBTK) models. Traditional toxicokinetic models are mathematical descriptions of concentration/time profiles that are constructed without assuming that the compartments and functions used in the models are directly representative of physical structures or physiological processes. The selection of compartments and functions are therefore solely dependent on their ability to describe experimentally observed concentration/time profiles. PBTK models, on the other hand, are mathematical simulations of kinetic processes in organs and tissues. The mathematical constructs therefore represent actual organs, tissues, and physiological processes.

UNDERLYING PHYSIOLOGY

Absorption

Most hazardous substances must gain access to the systemic circulation to exert their toxic effects through interaction with one or more internal organs. Notable exceptions are those compounds that cause a local reaction at the site of exposure. Absorption is the process whereby toxic substances gain entrance to the body from the external

Veterinary Toxicology. DOI: http://dx.doi.org/10.1016/B978-0-12-811410-0.00008-8

environment by crossing cellular barriers. The primary routes of exposure for toxic substances are oral, respiratory, and dermal.

The gastrointestinal, respiratory, and dermal systems are lined with epithelia that present significant barriers to the entry of foreign substances due to tight junctions between their cells, or continuous lipid layers in the case of skin. The membranes of cells that form viable epithelial barriers are traversed by transporter proteins that either actively exclude xenobiotics, or facilitate the movement of specific substrates across the barrier. The onset, duration, and intensity of a substance's toxic effects are therefore dependent on the toxicant's ability to permeate lipid cell membranes directly, and its interactions with transporter proteins. Dermal penetration is unique in the sense that the outer epithelial cellular layers (corneocytes) are nonviable and do not contain transporter proteins. Absorption, in this case, is therefore dependent on the ability of toxicants to penetrate the intercellular lipid matrix found between corneocytes. There are several factors that may influence the permeability of epithelial barriers to specific xenobiotics, including the physicochemical properties of the substance, blood supply at the site of exposure, and the concentration of the substance at the site of contact. A specific compound may be categorized as relatively nontoxic by one route and highly toxic via another due to differences in absorption from these sites.

Distribution

Distribution is the process whereby toxicants move throughout the body and reach their site of action. Once absorbed, a toxicant typically enters the interstitial fluid at the site of absorption and then passes into the tissue cells or enters the blood and/or lymph. Blood is moved rapidly through the body by the cardiovascular circulatory system and this process constitutes the major mechanism whereby absorbed chemicals are distributed to the various organs and tissues of the body.

To be distributed through the body by the cardiovascular system, a toxic chemical must first cross the capillary endothelium, and then diffuse through the interstitial fluid and penetrate the cells of the target organ. The entrance of xenobiotics to some tissues is restricted by special barriers (e.g., blood–brain barrier, blood testes barrier, and blood–placenta barrier) that form continuous cellular layers with tight junctions that prevent movement of toxicants into tissues by passive diffusion through intercellular spaces. To gain entry into these protected tissues, toxicants must pass through lipid cell membranes, either by penetrating the lipid membranes directly, or by active or facilitated transport through transmembrane transporter proteins. Factors that determine a compound's rate and extent of distribution therefore include molecular size, lipophilicity, plasma protein binding and the ability to interact with transmembrane transporter proteins. Uneven distribution through the body may occur due to affinity for specific environments such as fat for highly lipophilic compounds or bone for compounds that bind to Ca^{2+}. This can lead to extremely low concentrations in the blood plasma and accumulation with prolonged storage of the compound at the depot sites.

Biotransformation

Biotransformation is a key body defense mechanism whereby chemical reactions transform xenobiotic compounds in the body. The major transformation reactions for xenobiotics are divided into two phases. Phase I reactions (oxidation, reduction, hydrolysis, and acetylation) modify the compound's structure by adding a functional group. This allows the substance to interact with Phase II enzymes, which conjugates it with a water-soluble molecule such as sulfate, glucuronide, glutathione, and amino acid. The water solubility of a compound is typically increased by this process, and it is an important step towards the excretion of lipid soluble toxicants. Water-soluble compounds that are small enough to pass through the renal glomerulus can usually be excreted relatively rapidly through the urine without biotransformation. Biotransformed toxicants will often have reduced toxicity compared to the parent compounds. In some cases, however, biotransformation increases toxicity. Biotransformation enzymes have broad substrate specificity. They are, therefore, able to transform a wide range of substrates.

Excretion

One of the primary mechanisms of protecting the body from the toxic effects of toxicants is the elimination of these compounds from the body. Compounds that are rapidly eliminated are less likely to accumulate in tissues and damage critical cells. Although the terms elimination and excretion are sometimes used synonymously, the former term encompasses all the processes that decrease the amount of parent compound in the body, including biotransformation. Excretion is the term used specifically to refer to the processes by which toxic compounds leave the body through excretory organs. The main routes of elimination are urine, feces, and exhaled air. Except for the lung, water-soluble substances are more readily excreted because they are not readily reabsorbed through cellular barriers in the excretory organs.

EMPIRICAL (COMPARTMENTAL) TOXICOKINETIC MODELS

Introduction

Empirical compartmental pharmacokinetic models describe the aggregate result of all the processes involved in determining the concentration/time curve of a compound in a reference compartment, which is most often the venous blood, and referred to as the central compartment. It uses single or multiple compartments and first-order rate equations, chosen to optimally describe experimental data, with no direct physiological relevance or fidelity to anatomical structure or physiology. The main use of these models is to predict plasma concentrations in exposure conditions that are similar to the conditions under which the data were produced from which the model was derived. Traditionally, exponential equations have been used to quantitatively describe the changes in concentrations of toxic substances in plasma and tissue over time (Riviere, 2011; Gibaldi and Perrier, 1982).

Typical biexponential equation used to describe time—concentration data of xenobiotics in plasma:

$$C(t) = Ae^{-\alpha \times t} + Be^{-\beta \times t}$$

where $C(t)$ is the xenobiotic concentration at time t, α and β are the slopes of the two phases with different disappearance rates, and A and B are their intercepts with the y-axis.

In these models, the body is viewed as comprising one or more "equilibrium compartments" from which the toxic compound disappears at the same rate. These abstract compartments are not ascribed to specific organs or regions of the body but are understood to encompass a collection of tissues with similar blood supply and affinity for the compound of interest. The number of exponential terms in these traditional compartmental kinetic models therefore reflects the number of kinetically homogenous compartments, with an additional term added to account for absorption if exposure is extravascular. These exponential equations then serve as the basis to calculate physiologically relevant pharmacokinetic parameters that reflect the various kinetic processes (V_d = apparent volume of distribution; CL = clearance). The equations are also used to predict plasma concentrations for different exposure scenarios.

The most common models used to describe plasma time—concentration profiles of xenobiotics are the one- and two-compartment open models. The one-compartment model describes the profile of a compound that distributes instantaneously and evenly in the body and is eliminated at a rate that is proportional to the amount left in the body. On a semilogarithmic scale, plasma concentrations of these compounds decline linearly over time (Fig. 8.1).

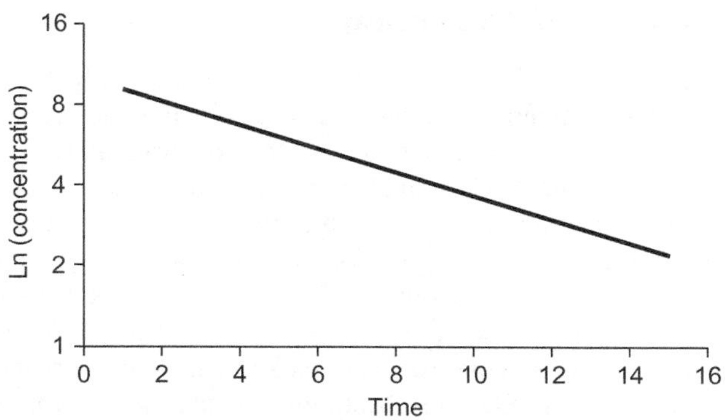

FIGURE 8.1 First-order decline in plasma concentrations on a semilogarithmic scale, according to a one-compartment model.

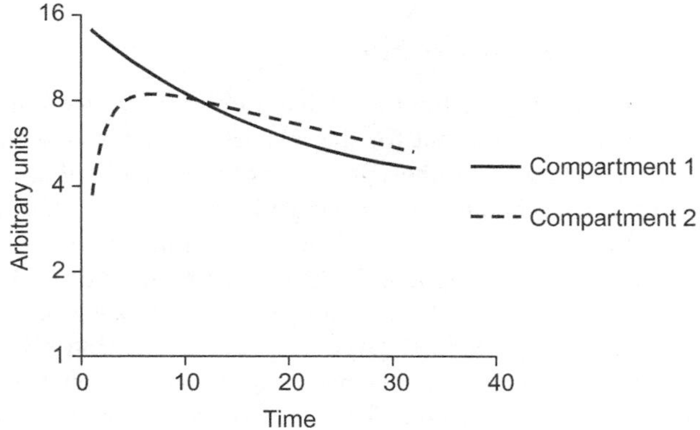

FIGURE 8.2 Plasma concentrations according to a two-compartmental model, demonstrating the separate contributions of two compartments to the rise and decline in blood concentrations.

For other compounds, an additional compartment (exponential term) must be added, because the plasma concentrations decline in two phases, with the decline during the first phase typically being more rapid than during the second phase (Fig. 8.2). Concentrations of these compounds in the second compound rise, peak, and subsequently decline over time as the substance is eliminated from the body.

This approach to toxicokinetic modeling assumes that absorption, distribution, metabolism, and excretion occur at rates that are directly proportional to the concentration of the toxicant (i.e., that they are first-order kinetic rate processes). It is important to realize that this assumption does not always apply for toxic compounds, particularly at high concentrations when the transporters and the enzymes that facilitate these processes become saturated. This means that, in the absence of evidence showing that the system maintains linear, first-order kinetics over the range of concentrations that are of interest, the values of kinetic parameters should be interpreted with caution and cannot be used to extrapolate to higher or lower doses.

Measures of Absorption

Often, only a fraction of the total dose to which an animal or human is exposed gets absorbed systemically. This fraction is referred to as the bioavailability (F) and is calculated by comparing the areas under the plasma time–concentration curves for the toxic compound administered intravenously versus the typical route of exposure. These data are not readily available for most toxic compounds, although the relative bioavailability from different routes (e.g., oral vs dermal) is often known. Other measures of the rate and extent of absorption include the absorption rate constant (k_a), maximum measured concentration in the plasma (C_{max}) and time after exposure when this concentration is measured (T_{max}).

Volume of Distribution

The total volume of fluid in which a toxic substance must be dissolved to account for the measured plasma concentrations is known as the apparent volume of distribution (V_D). If a compound is distributed only in the plasma fluid, the V_D is small and plasma concentrations are high. Conversely, if a compound is distributed to all sites in the body, or if it accumulates in a specific tissue such as fat or bone, the V_D becomes large and plasma concentrations are low. The value of this parameter is calculated from the multiexponential equation that is fit to the data using:

$$V_D = \frac{\text{Dose}}{\sum_{i=1}^{n} C_i}$$

Calculation of apparent volume of distribution from traditional pharmacokinetic parameters where C_i refers to the intercepts of the various phases of the curve with the y-axis.

Clearance

Total body clearance (CL) is the pharmacokinetic parameter that reflects the body's inherent ability to eliminate a xenobiotic through organs of elimination. The value of this parameter represents the volume of blood cleared of the toxic substance per unit time. If the total absorbed dose is known, CL can be calculated. Many times the absorbed dose in not known, in which the calculated value of this parameter reflects not only CL but also an unknown value for bioavailability (F). The lower F is, the higher the calculated value for a specific dose will be:

$$\text{CL} = \frac{\text{Dose}}{\text{AUC}_{0-\infty}}$$

Equation used to calculate total body clearance, where $\text{AUC}_{0-\infty}$ is the area under the plasma time–concentration curve extrapolated to infinity.

Half-Life

A compound's half-life in plasma ($T_{½}$) is a composite parameter that is dependent on both the body's inherent ability to eliminate the compound (CL), as well as the extent to which the compound is distributed through the body (V_D). This relationship is illustrated in the following equation:

$$T_{½} = \frac{0.693 \times V_D}{\text{CL}}$$

Widely distributed compounds have long half-lives due to their low concentrations in plasma (assuming first-order kinetics, where the rate of elimination is proportional to the amount of drug presented to the eliminating organ). Similarly, compounds with low CL values have long half-lives too.

Flip-Flop Kinetics

Flip-flop kinetics refers to a situation when the rate of absorption of a compound is significantly slower than its rate of elimination from the body. The compound's persistence in the body therefore becomes dependent on absorptive rather than elimination processes (Fig. 8.3). This sometimes occurs when the route of exposure is dermal.

Residues

An additional concern with food-producing animals is the potential for adverse effects in the human consumer if edible tissues harvested from exposed animals contain harmful residues of toxic compounds. Tolerances (also known as maximum residue levels in countries other than

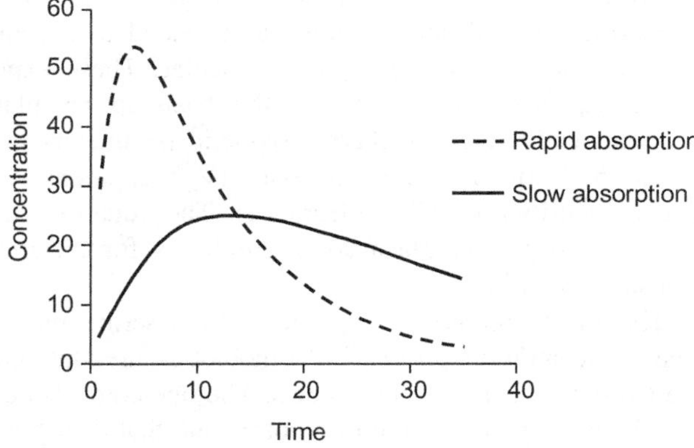

FIGURE 8.3 Plasma concentrations comparing a slow rate of absorption to a rapid rate of absorption, demonstrating "flip-flop" kinetics, where persistence of the compound is dependent on the rate of absorption, rather than the rate of elimination.

the United States) are legal limits of allowable concentrations to prevent harm in consumers from toxic compounds in foods. The length of time following exposure required for concentrations in animal tissues to deplete to levels that are below these tolerances is referred to as the withdrawal time. The length of these withdrawal times are closely related to the compounds' rates of elimination, and therefore their half-life, in the specific tissue of interest. It is important to note that the analytical technique used to measure plasma concentrations of the toxicant is unlikely to be sensitive enough to pick up the tissue depletion rate.

PHYSIOLOGICALLY BASED TOXICOKINETICS

Introduction

PBTK models are mathematical simulations of physiological processes that determine the rate and extent of xenobiotic chemical absorption, distribution, metabolism, and excretion. Such models can be used for predicting internal doses at target organs and tissues due to their conformity to actual organs, tissues, and physiological processes. Internal dose predictions are useful for dose–response analyses and risk assessment involving specific mechanisms and sites of toxicity. Successes in the application of physiologically based pharmacokinetic (PBPK) models to predict xenobiotic concentrations at target sites have led to its acceptance as a modeling technique in risk assessments. It is also used in mechanistic studies of the underlying processes that determine pharmacokinetic profiles and dose–response relationships.

In veterinary toxicology, PBPK methods can be used to improve the accuracy of predictions of toxicity across species by applying data obtained in one species to predictions in another species. It can be used to predict the effects of changes in physiological conditions, environmental conditions, activity levels, and pathological changes on xenobiotic concentrations in target tissues. This allows for more accurate assessment of risk in varied individual animals and populations. PBPK approaches can be used to study and understand the effects of mechanisms that determine the internal exposure of animals to potential toxins, such as dermal absorption and xenobiotic metabolism. PBPK models can also be used to address problems associated with the exposure of food-producing animals to drugs and chemicals that may result in potentially harmful or undesirable residues in meat, milk, and other foods of animal origin (Brocklebank et al., 1997; Craigmill, 2003; Buur et al., 2005).

PBPK models also make use of compartments, but in contrast to traditional compartmental models, the compartments are derived from mathematical descriptions of physiological body compartments or tissues. Links between the compartments simulate physiological processes of partitioning, transfer, metabolism, and excretion. If the compartments and kinetic processes are accurately described, the concentration/time curves of chemicals in specific organs and tissues can be estimated. This offers an advantage over traditional compartmental models, because differences in physiology, anatomy, environment, metabolism, and the effects of chemical-induced physiological changes and pathology can be simulated. Parameters can be scaled to reflect different dose ranges, species, breeds, genetic polymorphism and life-stages. The advantages of PBPK models are, however, difficult to achieve because the necessary anatomical and physiological parameter values are often not known, and/or the relevant pharmacokinetic processes are not well understood. The completeness of PBPK models depends entirely on the completeness of knowledge of the modeled system, and complete models are therefore not attainable in most situations. PBPK models tend, therefore, to be simplified representations of reality based on assumptions regarding the most important processes and structures that determine the pharmacokinetic profile of the chemical in question.

Typical PBPK models simplify the body and represent it as a series of well-stirred compartments representing major organs and tissues of interest, a single dose and route of exposure, and the major route of excretion. The compartments are linked by blood flow, and the movement of chemicals between compartments is determined by tissue/blood partitioning and blood flow rates. However, when enough data is available, highly detailed, multiple compartment models can be constructed that include complete dosing regimens or exposure scenarios, detailed organ structures, and physiological processes as well as specific processes of metabolism, and simulations of metabolite pharmacokinetics. Models of varying complexity focusing on specific organs and routes of absorption/elimination, such as the skin and respiratory organs, have also been developed (Andersen et al., 2002; Frederick et al., 2002; Van der Merwe et al., 2006).

Model Construction

The first step in the construction of a PBPK model is determining the purpose of the model and what internal tissue doses are needed to answer the specific scientific questions being asked. Once that is done, a schematic diagram is constructed that consists of each of the tissue compartments of interest, a plasma compartment, and a compartment or compartments that represent the rest of the physiological system. It is often necessary to include more than one compartment to represent the remaining portions of the body to reflect the differences in high and

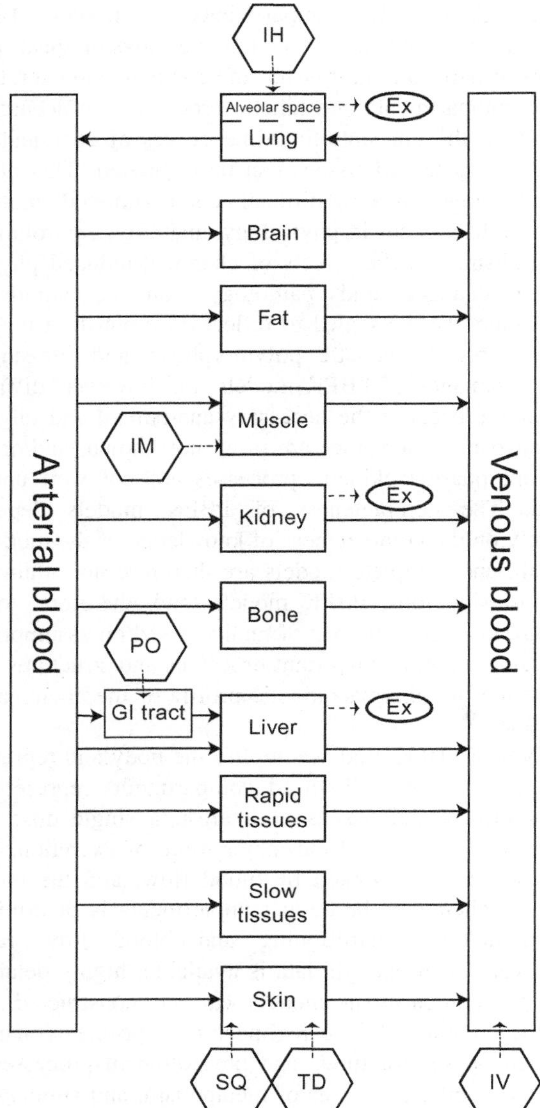

FIGURE 8.4 Schematic diagram of a generic whole body physiologically based pharmacokinetic model.

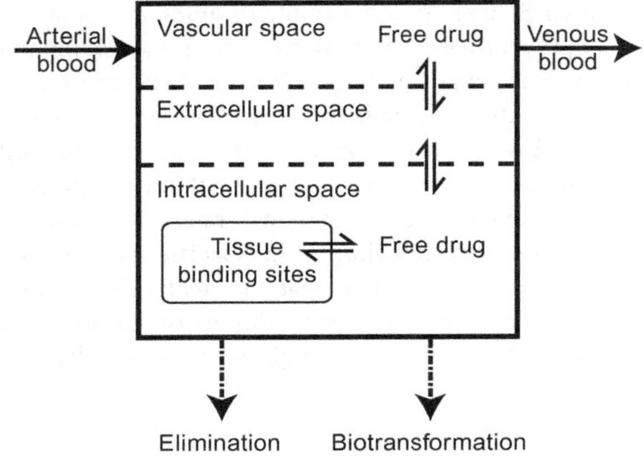

FIGURE 8.5 Schematic diagram of a generic tissue block physiologically based pharmacokinetic model, with subcompartments as well as possible binding sites and sources of elimination.

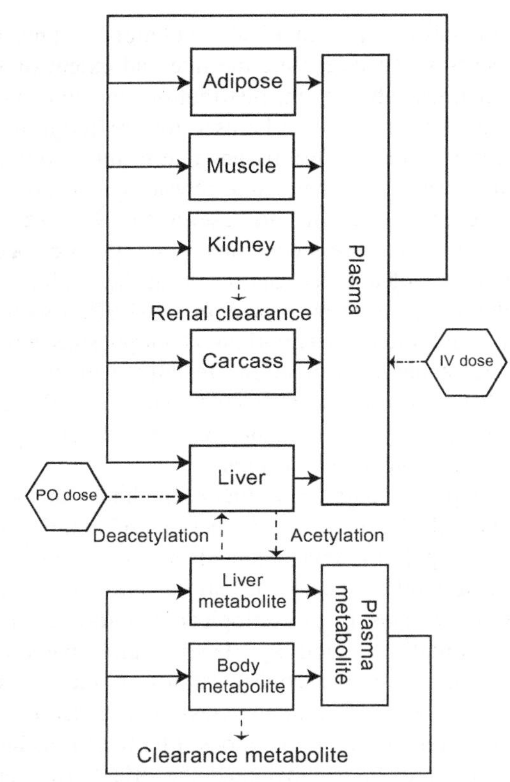

FIGURE 8.6 Schematic diagram of a physiologically based pharmacokinetic model, used in the prediction of sulfamethazine tissue residues in swine.

low blood flow tissues. The compartments can be subdivided into extracellular and intracellular spaces (Colburn, 1988). Tissue blocks and their subcompartments can be combined to make the model as simple or as complex as needed. A schematic diagram for a generic whole body model is shown in Fig. 8.4. Fig. 8.5 depicts a generic tissue block with subcompartments as well as possible binding sites and sources of elimination. In contrast to the full body model, Fig. 8.6 presents a schematic diagram used in the prediction of sulfamethazine (SMZ) tissue residues in swine (Buur et al., 2005). This model contains several simplifications, including a reduced number of tissue blocks, and the combination of tissue blocks into a single compartment. Because the model was designed to predict SMZ residues in edible swine tissues, only the edible tissues were specifically included in the model. The rest of the body was lumped into a single tissue block. Elimination occurs by renal filtration and is schematically represented using arrows that are not directed into the plasma compartment. The main metabolite is also modeled, and the two xenobiotics are linked together via the liver tissue block. This is an example of how model complexity can be optimized to achieve specific aims.

Following a schematic design of the model, the model is described using mass balance equations that represent the changes in tissue concentrations over time. The limiting factor in the exchange between compartments is an important consideration. In most models, the exchange is either limited by diffusion through a membrane barrier (diffusion-limited), or it is limited by the amount of blood flow (flow-limited). Both types of exchanges may be present in a single PBPK model. Diffusion-limited exchanges are often associated with large, polar molecules, and organs with small blood flow to mass ratios. Flow-limited exchanges are most commonly associated with small, lipophilic compounds, and organs with relatively small volume and large blood flow to mass ratios.

The basic mass balance equation for a flow-limited compartment is:

$$\frac{V_t dC_t}{d_t} = Q_t(C_a - C_v)$$

where Q_t, V_t, and C_t are the blood flow, anatomic volume, and concentration of the compound in the compartment, and C_a and C_v are the concentrations of the compound in the arterial and venous blood flowing into and out of the tissue. It is assumed in flow-limited models that the compound is in instantaneous equilibrium between the tissue and the blood, and that distribution in the compartment is homogeneous. This allows for the relationship between the venous blood concentration and the vascular space to be defined according to the partition coefficient between the tissue and blood:

$$C_v = \frac{C_t}{P_t}$$

where P_t is the tissue-to-blood partition coefficient. Therefore, the final mass balance equation is:

$$\frac{V_t dC_t}{d_t} = Q_t\left(\frac{C_a - C_t}{P_t}\right)$$

This equation can be used in models where all tissue compartments are simplified into a single compartment. In contrast, membrane-limited exchanges do not assume that tissue concentrations are in equilibrium with venous blood concentrations. Instead, it uses subcompartments representing extravascular and intracellular space. The assumption is that the vascular space is in equilibrium with the extracellular space. The mass balance equation is then defined by rate of change in the extracellular space per unit of time, and can be written as:

$$\frac{V_e dC_e}{d_t} = Q_t(C_a - C_e) - K_t(C_e - C_i)$$

$$\frac{V_i dC_i}{d_t} = K_t\left(\frac{C_e - C_t}{P_t}\right)$$

where V_e and C_e are the anatomic volume, and concentration in the extracellular space, V_i and C_i is the volume of the intracellular space, and the concentration in the intracellular space, and K_t is the membrane permeability coefficient for the membranes that separate the intracellular and extracellular spaces.

Further modifications are needed to describe metabolism or excretion. This can be done by adding a mass removal term, R_{ex}. The resulting equation for a flow-limited tissue block is:

$$\frac{V_t dC_t}{d_t} = Q_t\left(\frac{C_a - C_t}{P_t}\right) - R_{ex}$$

The mathematical definition of R_{ex} can be a simple or as complex as needed to describe the important features of the process. Commonly used functions include simple first-order exchanges, and Michaelis–Menton equations that describe processes that can become saturated. For example, if R_{ex} is defined as the clearance of a specific organ the equation would be:

$$\frac{V_t dC_t}{d_t} = Q_t\left(\frac{C_a - C_t}{P_t}\right) - C_t \mathrm{Cl}_{\mathrm{organ}}$$

where $\mathrm{Cl}_{\mathrm{organ}}$ is the clearance of the eliminating organ.

Tissue blocks can be further refined by the addition of modification terms to describe processes such as protein binding, tissue binding, active transport, biliary excretion, enterohepatic circulation, and metabolism. For example, if R_{ex} is governed by metabolism, and the appropriate parameter values of enzyme activity are known, it can described using Michaelis–Menton equations such as:

$$R_{ex} = \frac{(V_m \mathrm{f}_1)}{(K_m + \mathrm{f}_1)}$$

where V_m is the maximum rate of metabolism, K_m is the concentration at which the rate of metabolism is 50% of maximum, and f_1 is the free concentration in the metabolizing organ. The final step is to write the mass balance equation for the central (venous blood) compartment. The input into this compartment is the combined venous blood streams from the various tissue compartments. The rate of change in concentration in the central compartment is described by:

$$\frac{V_p dC_p}{d_t} = \sum Q_t C_v - Q_p C_p$$

where V_p, Q_p, and C_p are the anatomic volume, the total blood flow, and the concentration in the central compartment. C_v represents the venous blood concentration from each tissue compartment. As with other compartments, this compartment can be modified to incorporate processes such as protein binding, or partitioning into blood cells.

Parameter Estimation and Identifiability

Accurate parameter values are essential for PBPK models to achieve their full predictive potential. The relevant parameters are often physiological (blood flow, organ volume, vascular space volume, etc.), and physicochemical (partitioning coefficients, membrane permeability coefficients, rate of absorption, etc.). Some parameter values can be estimated from in vitro experiments (protein-binding rates, Michaelis–Menton constants, etc.). Many parameter values can be found in the published literature. Some parameters can be derived from in vitro and in vivo experimentation. However, there will usually be some parameters for which independent values cannot be obtained. These parameter values must be estimated using a curve fitting process against known data points (Sheiner, 1985). Several curve fitting software packages are available. Most use a function of a least likelihood ratio to estimate the parameters. It is important to emphasize that a weakness of PBPK models is their dependence upon a large number of parameters. The large numbers of parameters can also make identifiability challenging. Identifiability refers to the ability to specifically determine a unique influence on model output for each parameter, based on an ideal data set. As the number of tissue compartments increases, the ability to uniquely identify all parameters is diminished without the inclusion of additional data points. Valid inferences cannot be drawn from a model if the model contains unidentifiable parameters. To reduce the likelihood of this type of error, multiple tissue compartments may be sampled. Thus, it is not only the number of data points representing the final model output that are used, but also the number of sampled compartments that is important for accurate parameter estimation (Audoly et al., 2001). Identifiability problems can also be reduced by decreasing the number of parameters that need to be estimated. Sensitivity analysis can be used to decide which parameters can be abandoned without significantly altering model output. It compares the relative contributions of reasonable ranges of parameter values to an output of interest (Evans and Andersen, 2000). For example, in the SMZ model example, the relative contributions to plasma disposition from the parameters of renal clearance, hepatic clearance, and tissue partitioning coefficients can be compared (Fig. 8.7). The parameters of protein binding, hepatic clearance and renal clearance have the greatest effect at early time points.

The range of parameter values to use can be estimated using statistical distributions rather than fixed ranges. As with single point estimations, the accuracy of the model is directly proportional to the accuracy of the distribution. In many cases, a reasonable mean and range of parameter value distribution can be inferred from published data. Distribution patterns can also be assumed to follow a model commonly found in natural systems (normal, log-normal, beta, etc.).

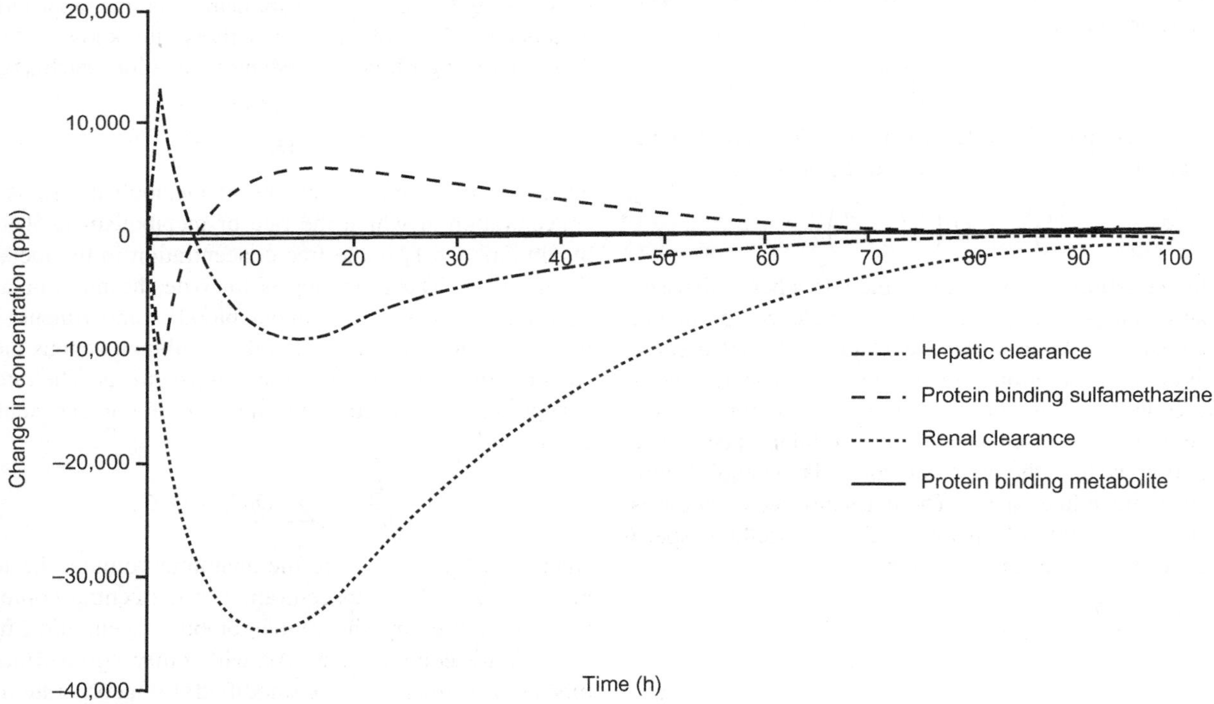

FIGURE 8.7 A comparison of the relative contributions to plasma disposition from the parameters of renal clearance, hepatic clearance, and tissue partitioning coefficients.

Model Validation

Model validation refers to the process of confirming that the model actually achieves its intended purpose. In most situations, this will involve confirmation that the model is predictive under the conditions of its intended use. This type of validation occurs by comparing model simulations to an independent experimental data set. Data used in the estimation of model parameter values cannot be included in the external data set. Simulated data derived from the model are compared to observed data points. The sets of data may be plotted side by side using simulation plots; or output values at specific times can be compared using correlation plots, and residual plots. Results are then subjected to qualitative and quantitative analysis for goodness of fit. Unlike traditional compartmental pharmacokinetic modeling approaches, there is currently no standardized method to evaluate the goodness of fit for PBPK models. Often, a combination of visual examination of residual plots and simulation plots, along with the quantification of regression correlation values (R^2 values) are used. In general, residual plots should have normal distributions around zero without any time bias. Correlation plots should have regression lines with R^2 values close to 1, and intercepts close to the starting value (in most cases, this is zero). Simulation plots are also used to detect time and concentration bias.

If a complex model was created by the incorporation of population distributions, then model validation typically becomes more qualitative in nature. In these cases, sampling methods such as Monte Carlo or bootstrapping can be used to generate specific values for the parameters in question. This parameter value assignment is repeated a large number of times, and the output becomes a set of simulations that can be plotted alongside each other. This gives a visual representation of what a population may look like (Sweeney et al., 2001). Fig. 8.8 shows a Monte Carlo analysis using the SMZ model to simulate multiple oral dosing (Buur et al., 2006). The oral absorption rate, rate of gastric emptying, protein binding, and both renal and hepatic clearances were varied. Validation of this data is performed by plotting the multiple simulations alongside independent experimental data points. However, confidence in the distributions, and in the model is determined by visual inspection, rather than correlation coefficients or residual plots, but alone. Generally, more data points covered within the spread of the output results in higher confidence in the predictive ability of the model.

Applications

PBPK models are most often used in toxicology to predict the concentrations of toxic chemicals and their metabolites in target tissues. Target tissue concentrations predict toxic effects better than exposure concentrations or concentrations in a reference compartment such as venous blood. The adaptability of PBPK models makes them suitable for extrapolations across different exposure scenarios and routes, species, breed, age, physiological state, pathological changes, and sex differences. PBPK models are also used in basic research to understand the effects and interactions between anatomical structure, tissue

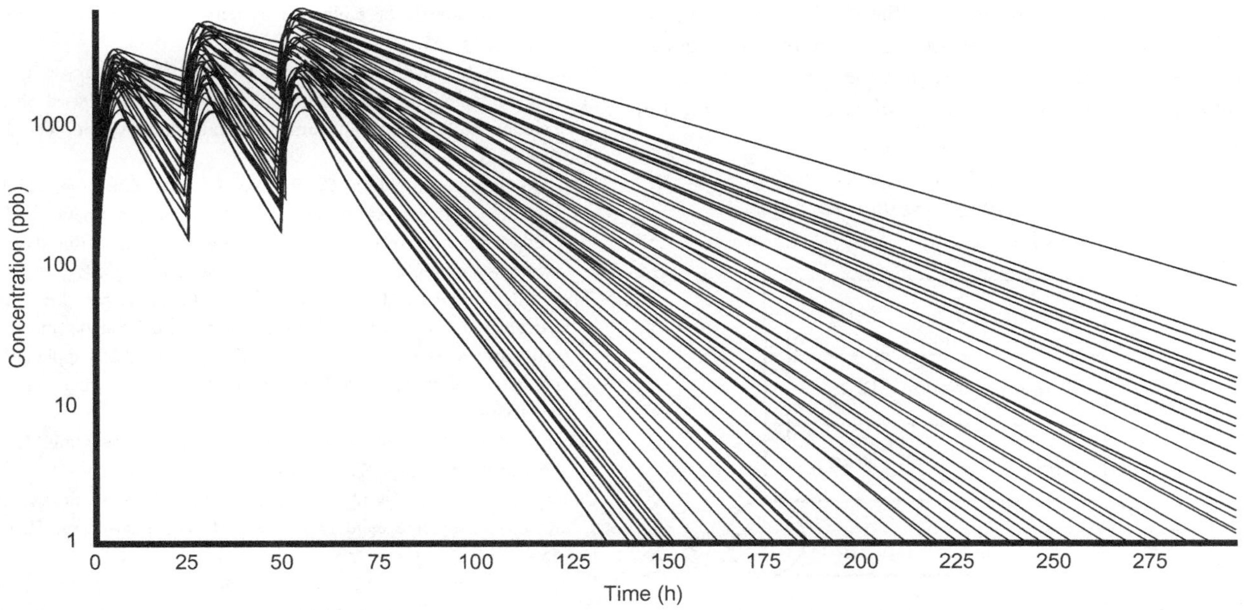

FIGURE 8.8 A Monte Carlo analysis using a physiologically based pharmacokinetic model, used in the prediction of sulfamethazine tissue residues in swine, to simulate multiple oral dosing.

composition, and physiological processes that influence the concentration/time course of xenobiotic chemicals. Toxicologists are often faced with situations where the adverse health risk from chemical exposure must be estimated without access to data obtained under the conditions of the exposure being analyzed. An advantage of well-designed, appropriately detailed, and adequately understood PBPK models is that different exposure scenarios can be simulated using the same base model by varying the mathematical descriptions of the dosing regimen. These may include single, repeated, or continuous oral ingestion, single or repeated intravenous boluses, constant intravenous infusion, single or repeated injections at various body sites, inhalation, and topical exposures under various conditions. As long as the influences of dependent parameters on the reference concentration/time curve can be reliably identified, the model can be used to simulate the effects of variations in parameter values. It can also be used to do limited hypotheses testing related to key parameters. An example of this approach is the use of a PBPK model to describe the transdermal absorption of organophosphate insecticides in flow-through diffusion cells (Fig. 8.9) (Van der Merwe et al., 2006). Detailed independent parameter estimations, in a relatively simple physiological system, reduced the dependent parameters to three—each with an identifiable influence on the concentration/time curve in the receptor chamber of the flow-through cell. Sensitivity analyses were used to identify important parameters and to generate hypotheses regarding the effects of changes in the skin related to those parameters. This approach can be used to discover important parameters in silico, which can be used to generate testable hypotheses. For example, the number of cell layers in the stratum corneum was identified as an important parameter and the effect of changing numbers of cell layers was simulated. The simulation could then be used as an hypothesis, and tested using skin with varying layers of cells in the stratum corneum in flow-through cell experiments.

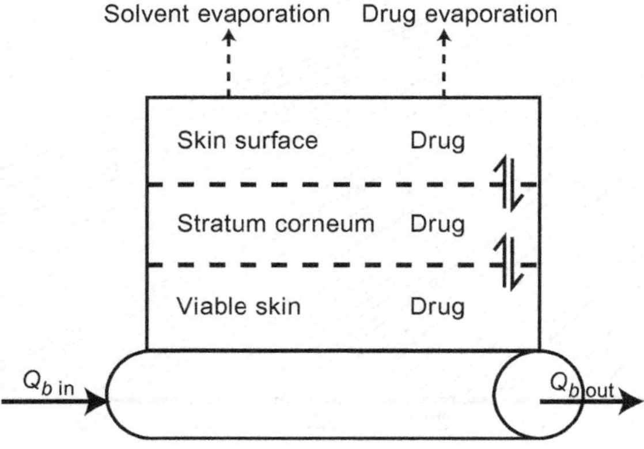

FIGURE 8.9 Schematic diagram of a physiologically based pharmacokinetic model used to describe the transdermal absorption of organophosphate insecticides in flow-through diffusion cells.

CONCLUDING REMARKS AND FUTURE DIRECTIONS

PBPK modeling is an evolving frontier in toxicokinetic modeling. As our understanding of the systems and processes involved in toxicokinetics improve and expand, so does our ability to use newly gained knowledge in models. PBPK models allow for the adaptability needed to simulate varied physiological processes and system conditions. PBPK models are therefore likely to assume an ever more important role in our efforts to understand and predict the consequences of exposure to toxicants, and its application in veterinary toxicology can be expected to expand.

REFERENCES

Andersen, M.E., Green, T., Frederick, C.B., Bogdanffy, M.S., 2002. Physiologically based pharmacokinetic (PBPK) models for nasal tissue dosimetry of organic esters: assessing the state-of-knowledge and risk assessment applications with methyl methacrylate and vinyl acetate. Reg. Toxicol. Pharmacol. 36, 234–245.

Andersen, M.E., Lutz, R.W., Liao, K.H., Lutz, W.K., 2006. Dose-incidence modeling: Consequences of linking quantal measures of response to depletion of critical tissue targets. Toxicol. Sci. 89, 331–337.

Audoly, S., Bellu, G., D'Angio, L., et al., 2001. Global identifiability of nonlinear models of biological systems. IEEE Transact. Biomed. Eng. 48, 55–65.

Brocklebank, J.R., Namdari, R., Law, F.C.P., 1997. An oxytetracycline residue depletion study to assess the physiologically based pharmokinetic (PBPK) model in farmed Atlantic salmon. Can. Vet. J. 38, 645–646.

Buur, J., Baynes, R., Smith, G., Riviere, J., 2006. Use of probabilistic modeling within a physiologically based pharmacokinetic model to predict sulfamethazine residue withdrawal times in edible tissues in swine. Antimicrob. Agents Chemother. 50, 2344–2351.

Buur, J.L., Baynes, R.E., Craigmill, A.L., Riviere, J.E., 2005. Development of a physiologic-based pharmacokinetic model for estimating sulfamethazine concentrations in swine and application to prediction of violative residues in edible tissues. Am. J. Vet. Res. 66, 1686–1693.

Colburn, W.A., 1988. Physiologic pharmacokinetic modeling. J. Clin. Pharmacol. 8, 673–677.

Craigmill, A.L., 2003. A physiologically based pharmacokinetic model for oxytetracycline residues in sheep. J. Vet. Pharmacol. Ther. 26, 55–63.

Evans, M.V., Andersen, M.E., 2000. Sensitivity analysis of a physiological model for 2,3,7,8-tetrachlorocdibenzo-p-dioxin (TCDD): assessing the impact of specific model parameters on sequestration in liver and fat in the rat. Toxicol. Sci. 54, 71–80.

Frederick, C.B., Lomax, L.G., Black, K.A., et al., 2002. Use of a hybrid computational fluid dynamics and physiologically based inhalation model for interspecies dosimetry comparisons of ester vapors. Toxicol. Appl. Pharmacol. 183, 23–40.

Gibaldi, M., Perrier, D., 1982. Pharmacokinetics. second ed. Marcel Dekker, Inc, New York, NY.

Riviere, J.E., 2011. Comparative Pharmacokinetics: Principles, Techniques, and Applications, second ed. Iowa State University Press, Ames, IA.

Sheiner, L.B., 1985. Analysis of pharmacokinetic data using parametric models 2. Point estimates of an individuals parameters. J. Pharmacokin. Biopharmaceut. 13, 515–540.

Sweeney, L.M., Tyler, T.R., Kirman, C.R., Corley, R.A., Reitz, R.H., Paustenbach, D.J., et al., 2001. Proposed occupational exposure limits for select ethylene glycol ethers using PBPK models and Monte Carlo simulations. Toxicol. Sci. 62, 124–139.

Van der Merwe, D., Brooks, J.D., Gehring, R., et al., 2006. A physiologically based pharmacokinetic model of organophosphate dermal absorption. Toxicol. Sci. 89, 188–204.

Chapter 9

Toxicological Testing: In Vivo and In Vitro Models

Magda Sachana and Alan J. Hargreaves

INTRODUCTION

The large number of new chemical entities in the human and veterinary pharmaceutical industry has led to an increased demand for safety screening to ensure successful drug development. Part of this screening process includes the determination of the toxic potential of these new compounds by applying internationally recognized in vivo or in vitro toxicological tests. The importance of toxicological testing is critical, as many pharmaceutical agents, industrial chemicals and agrochemical products must be assessed for their safety, before they become available for general use. Furthermore, in some cases, basic research can produce data that eventually leads to the ban of certain chemicals because they proved to be unsafe.

Animal studies and validated in vitro models are extensively used for screening of agents in order to identify and predict potential ill effects to humans, domestic pets, and farm animals. Although the detection of adverse health effects of xenobiotics is the main objective of toxicity testing, it can be complemented by more sophisticated biomolecular approaches aimed at the elucidation of the mechanisms of action of certain chemicals.

Another area of veterinary interest regarding toxicological testing is the evaluation of the safety of veterinary drugs for food animals as well as the safety assessment of veterinary drug residues in human food of animal origin, in order to determine the doses that cause nonobserved effect level and consequently to establish the acceptable daily intake in the human diet.

Toxicological testing laboratories now have to comply with strict official controls and inspections on animal use at any time that can be reinforced by relevant legislation. In most European countries, veterinarians play a pivotal role in toxicity testing and are required by law to be employed by designated establishments that undertake experiments on animals, including toxicological studies. More specifically, a named veterinary surgeon is responsible not only for the health and well-being of laboratory animals but also to advise on the selection of adequate in vivo models and ensure that priority is given to the use of alternative methods during the local ethical review process. Furthermore, the refinement of experimental techniques and husbandry approaches should be one of the priorities of a veterinary surgeon working in animal units, especially where regulated procedures take place, and distressed animals should be kept under very close supervision by a veterinarian. A similar approach is used in the United States, where all institutes are also obliged to establish an Institutional Animal Care and Use Committee, where the participation of a trained and experienced veterinary surgeon is essential to ensure that all aspects of the three Rs (replacement, reduction, and refinement) (Russell and Burch, 1959) have been followed before approving animal use for toxicological studies.

A veterinarian with specific professional or scientific interest in toxicology should be aware of the alternative methods in toxicity testing, advise on replacement and refinement of laboratory animals used in toxicological studies and safeguard animal welfare. The main aims of this chapter are to outline the major aspects of in vivo and in vitro models in toxicity testing and to give a brief overview of endpoint determination. The principal focus will be to highlight some of the current in vivo and in vitro models available in toxicity testing and provide information on new technologies and approaches used in this field.

IN VIVO MODELS IN TOXICITY TESTING

Introduction

With the continuous development of new chemicals and pharmaceutical products, laboratory animals have become important and well-established tools for the generation of

Veterinary Toxicology. DOI: http://dx.doi.org/10.1016/B978-0-12-811410-0.00009-X

in vivo toxicological data. Originally, in vivo experiments were aimed at the prediction of acute systemic toxicity usually in rodents. Currently, more sophisticated, targeted and multispecies approaches with well-defined endpoints and experimental protocols are applied to toxicological studies, especially for regulatory testing.

As the science of toxicology evolves, an increasing number of in vitro alternative tests have been validated or are currently under development. However, in some cases, animal models in toxicity testing are irreplaceable, especially in the tests required by the regulatory authorities to protect human and animal health. Furthermore, there is public demand to know the toxicity risks posed in everyday life, which necessitates the use of animal models comparable to humans.

Although animals are relatively expensive experimental models compared to the alternative methods discussed later, there are several important reasons for their continued use. First, there is extensive information available on their normal biochemical and physiological properties. Second, the published data from the measurement of toxicological endpoints in vivo, using models of relevance to humans and domestic/farm animals, makes animal testing a valuable tool to predict toxicity.

The animals that are most commonly used in toxicological testing are rodents and rabbits (Table 9.1). Cats and dogs are used less frequently in toxicity testing (and mostly in preclinical toxicology or phase I pharmacological studies), whereas nonhuman primates are rarely used and mainly to study metabolism of toxic compounds. Not included in this table are the studies conducted on companion animals to determine safety limits in products that are directly applied to cats or dogs (EPA, 1998a). The interested reader is referred to some more specialized books regarding animal toxicity testing (e.g., Arnold et al., 1990; Gad, 2006) and some useful websites relevant to regulatory toxicological testing (e.g., https://www.epa.gov/test-guidelines-pesticides-and-toxic-substances/series-870-health-effects-test-guidelines and http://www.oecd.org/chemicalsafety/testing/oecdguidelinesforthetestingofchemicals.htm).

Routes of Test Compound Administration

Toxicity testing in animal models is most useful if it imitates the human or domestic/farm animal route of exposure to chemical agents. Based on the medium of exposure in human and domestic animals, it is possible to decide which is the administration route of choice in animal toxicological tests (Table 9.2). Depending on the route of administration, experimental evaluation may differ because of variation in the absorption, metabolism and elimination of a compound. Oral exposure can lead to absorption by the digestive system and metabolism by the liver, whereas, following inhalation, a toxic compound is more likely to be absorbed by the respiratory system. Metabolism of xenobiotics can also occur in placenta, in the test dam and fetus. This can lead to changes in the balance of parent compound and metabolites, complicating the picture even more in developmental toxicity tests.

The metabolism of an administered chemical should be relevant to human or domestic animals and is critical for risk assessment exercises. The final toxic effect will depend on a balance between the level of toxic agent reaching the target tissue and its rate of elimination and/or bioinactivation by mixed function oxidases, serum hydrolases or binding to serum proteins. Furthermore, there are interspecies differences regarding the metabolism of xenobiotics (Nebbia, 2001). For example, cats are at high risk of developing hepatotoxicity especially after paracetamol administration. This is due to differences in bioactivation of paracetamol, which occurs only in cats through *N*-hydroxylation with the help of cytochrome P450 2E1, during the oxidative reactions in phase I transformation (Nebbia, 2001). Ruminants are less susceptible to organophosphates (OPs) such as parathion than monogastrics, because the rumen microflora play an important role by reducing the nitro group of OPs to an amino group (Nebbia, 2001).

The majority of toxicological studies commonly employ administration of the agent in animal feed or water or by stomach intubation (i.e., by gavage) in order to imitate a known or potential human or domestic animal exposure. The use of oral gavage is commonly used in administration of high doses of xenobiotics and in developmental toxicity tests, but is less practical in the case of long-duration studies. Inhalation is used when there is a need to duplicate industrial or environmental exposure to dusts, aerosols and fumes. In this case, nose, head or whole body exposure chambers are used, depending on the exposure time. For cutaneous administration, a toxic agent may be injected intradermally or simply applied topically on the skin or ears and sometimes covered with a bandage. In the case of experimental studies where the need for complete absorption of a tested compound is considered essential, parenteral routes of administration (intraperitoneal, intramuscular, intravenous, and subcutaneous) are selected. However, the solubility and bioavailability of the tested agent can also influence the degree of absorption and how much of it is directly available in a laboratory animal.

Toxicokinetic and pharmacokinetic information on tested compounds and their comparison among laboratory animals and humans are also important to determine dosing parameters and improve the toxicological data obtained. The administered dose in toxicological studies should be decided taking into account many physicochemical parameters of chemical agents, biological

TABLE 9.1 Examples of Animal Models Used in Selective Toxicity Tests

Order	Species	Toxicity Tests	References
Rodentia	Rat	Developmental toxicity	EPA (1998b, 2000), OECD (2001b, 2016a,b)
		Carcinogenicity	OECD (2009a,b)
		Cutaneous toxicity	OECD (1987)
		Genotoxicity	OECD (1984, 2013), EPA (1998c)
		Immunotoxicity	IPCS (1996), EPA (1998g)
		Neurotoxicity	OECD (1997c), EPA (1998d,e)
		Developmental neurotoxicity	EPA (1998f), OECD (2007)
		Reproductive toxicity	EPA (2000), OECD (2001a, 2012, 2016a,b)
	Mice	Carcinogenicity	OECD (2009a,b)
		Skin sensitization	EPA (2003)
		Genotoxicity	OECD (1984, 2013), EPA (1998c)
		Immunotoxicity	IPCS (1996), EPA (1998g)
		Neurotoxicity	OECD (1997c), EPA (1998d,e)
		Reproductive toxicity	OECD (2001a)
	Hamsters	Carcinogenicity	Gad (1998)
		Genotoxicity	Loomis and Hayes (1996)
	Guinea pigs	Cutaneous toxicity/skin sensitization	OECD (1987), EPA (2003)
		Developmental neurotoxicity	Kaufmann (2003)
Lagomorpha	Rabbit	Developmental toxicity	EPA (1998b), Foote and Carney (2000), OECD (2001b)
		Cutaneous toxicity	OECD (1987), Auletta (2004)
		Reproductive toxicity	Foote and Carney (2000)
Avian	Hen	Neurotoxicity	OECD (1995a,b)
Swine	Minipigs	Cutaneous toxicity	Auletta (2004)
		Developmental neurotoxicity	Kaufmann (2003)
Canine	Dog	Carcinogenicity	Loomis and Hayes (1996)
		Cutaneous toxicity	Vail et al. (1998)
		Neurotoxicity	EPA (1998e)
		Developmental neurotoxicity	Kaufmann (2003)
Nonhuman primates	Monkey	Developmental toxicity	Buse et al. (2003)
		Cutaneous toxicity	deBlois and Horlick (2001)

differences between species, previously published data and after careful planning or preliminary experimentation.

Reproductive Toxicity Tests

Reproductive toxicity testing is based on the measurement of reproductive functional and structural defects caused by toxic agents in both males and females. The toxicity endpoints most frequently studied in reproductive in vivo testing are summarized in Table 9.3. Rats and, to a lesser extent, mice are the species of choice in reproductive toxicological testing because they are considered inexpensive compared to bigger mammals (EPA, 2000; OECD, 2001a, 2012, 2016a,b). On the other hand, small rodents need to be euthanized even for simple endpoints such as collection of sperm, whereas rabbits can be sampled regularly without being sacrificed, making them an alternative in reproductive toxicological tests (Foote and Carney, 2000).

TABLE 9.2 Proposed Administration Routes of Test Compounds in Laboratory Animals Based on the Medium of Exposure

Medium of Human and Domestic/ Farm Animal Exposure to Toxicant	Administration Route
Food commodities	Oral
Water	Oral
	Inhalation
	Dermal
Air	Inhalation
Household/environmental surfaces	Oral
	Dermal

TABLE 9.3 Selective Endpoints Applied to Laboratory Animals During Reproductive Toxicity Testing

Female	Male
Reproductive tract morphology	Sperm structure/morphology
Reproductive tract receptors	Sperm motility/viability/count
Ovum properties	Sperm DNA integrity
Recovery of blastocysts	Hormonal balance/receptor interactions
Hormonal balance/receptor	Fertility testing interactions
Length and normality of estrus cycle	
Fertility testing	
Uterine condition	
Implantation	
Lactation	
Maternal behavior	

Some of the disadvantages of using rabbits are the higher cost due to greater amounts of chemical compounds administered and the increased cases of abortions because of the relatively high incidence of gastrointestinal dysfunction. For example, rabbits are poor models for veterinary residue testing and, more specifically, for antibiotics because these compounds have been found to cause diarrhea and consequently abortion (Barlow et al., 2002).

Since exposure to chemicals can occur throughout life, a multigeneration study that extends over at least two generations, using a single type of laboratory rodent, is desirable in order to reveal reproductive toxicological data (OECD, 2001a; Barlow et al., 2002; Garg et al., 2011; Estevan et al., 2011), although this approach requires large numbers of animals and is time consuming.

Developmental Toxicity Testing

Developmental toxicity testing is primarily used to determine hazard regarding the potential effects of prenatal exposure on the developing fetus. These studies focus on functional and structural changes that can be observed throughout the development from zygote to neonate. The most important developmental phase is the organogenesis period that is always taken into account in developmental toxicity testing. Based on these studies, chemical compounds can be categorized as teratogenic and/or fetotoxic by recording structural malformations, developmental retardation and/or mortality, respectively. The vast majority of teratogenic chemical agents have been identified using rodent experimental models (EPA, 1998b, 2000; OECD, 2001b, 2016a,b). However, the failure of rodents to detect teratogenic signal on some occasions and the similarities in placentation and pregnancy physiology between humans and rabbits led to the use of the rabbit as a second model for assessing the effects of toxic compounds on development (EPA, 1998b; Foote and Carney, 2000; OECD, 2001b). Furthermore, although nonhuman primates have been suggested as models for teratological testing (Buse et al., 2003; Faqi, 2011), they have several limitations such as a long gestation period, only single or twin offspring, high rates of abortion and ethical constraints.

The detection rates for veterinary pharmaceutical agents demonstrated to be teratogenic/fetotoxic were found to be 55%–79% using individual species (Hurtt et al., 2003). However, when the rat and rabbit data were both considered, there was a significant increase in detection rate to almost 100%, suggesting that in the absence of teratogenicity in rat, a second species developmental test in *lagomorpha* is required to provide high standards of public protection (Hurtt et al., 2003). The interested reader can retrieve some more information on reproductive and developmental toxicity testing by referring to a specialized textbook (Gupta, in press).

Cutaneous Toxicity Testing

The aim of in vivo assays for cutaneous toxicity is not only to assess potential acute local irritation but also to evaluate acute, subchronic and chronic systemic toxic effects. During cutaneous toxicity tests, animals are monitored for skin reactions/dermal effects, clinical, gross or microscopic pathological findings depending on the duration of a toxic compound administration and the observation period.

The albino rabbit has been until recently the animal model of choice because of the high permeability and sensitivity to toxic agents exhibited by its skin, which sometimes led to overprediction showing little relevance to human irritation (Auletta, 2004). Currently, albino rats and occasionally guinea pigs are considered preferable species to assess local irritation. Traditionally, guinea pigs and mice have been used also to perform sensitization tests (EPA, 2003; OECD, 2010). On the other hand, long-term cutaneous toxicity studies usually require the use of a rodent (albino rat and mouse) as well as a nonrodent model. Minipigs have been proven to be a reliable nonrodent species because their skin demonstrates many physiological similarities to those of humans and pigs (Auletta, 2004). Other nonrodent models are dog and nonhuman primates, commonly used to test the metabolism of toxic agents and the safety of newly designed recombinant pharmaceutical products (Vail et al., 1998; deBlois and Horlick, 2001).

Genotoxicity Testing

The aim of genotoxicity testing is to detect gene damage induced by the test compound, by measuring chromosome aberration and breakage, point mutation, and other DNA and chromosomal effects in vivo. The host-mediated assay is based on the inoculation of a microorganism into a rodent such as a mouse, rat or hamster and a subsequent assessment of the point mutations found in the microorganisms, after certain treatment of the rodents with the potential mutagen (Gabridge and Legator, 1969; Dhillon et al., 1995; Loomis and Hayes, 1996). On the other hand, to identify chromosome breakage, male rodents are treated with the test compounds and, after mating with untreated females, fetal mortality and survival are recorded (OECD, 1984; EPA, 1998c).

The mouse spot test is capable of detecting somatic gene mutations and is based on in utero exposure to the tested chemical. This in vivo mutation test works by monitoring the appearance of colored spots in the coat of the animal that may appear due to an altered or lost specific wild-type allele in a pigment precursor cell (EPA, 1998h).

A popular in vivo test to identify genetic risks is the rodent bone marrow micronucleus test, although it is not the most sensitive test and it does not improve predictivity of rodent genotoxicity when combined with in vitro tests (OECD, 1997a; Zeiger, 1998). However, this in vivo test is widely used because it is relatively easy to perform. Another in vivo test that has been validated and recommended by the Organisation for Economic Cooperation and Development (OECD, 1997b) is the rat liver unscheduled DNA synthesis test. It is worth mentioning that none of the above approaches are suggested to be used individually to predict genotoxicity. Negative or positive results should always be confirmed first by in vitro or nonmammalian mutagenicity tests.

Carcinogenicity Tests

In vivo assays of carcinogenicity examine the possibility that a tested agent might cause tumors and other chemically related effects in one or more animal species. Currently available is the rodent carcinogenicity test (OECD, 2009a). This test runs for up to 2 years and involves the use of three different concentrations, one administration route and both sexes. The results are based on clinical chemistry, gross and histopathological analysis of more than 40 tissues and organs in order to determine the site, the number and type of tumors (OECD, 2009a,b).

One serious disadvantage of using mice in carcinogenicity testing is their tendency to present high incidence of spontaneous liver or lung tumors in some strains, leading occasionally to inconclusive results (Gad, 1998). Furthermore, because of the long duration of carcinogenicity tests and therefore the old age of laboratory animals, it means that the natural occurrence of tumors increases, making it difficult to distinguish between a real treatment and a background carcinogenic effect. In addition, the most common mechanisms of tumor development in rodents may not be relevant to human carcinogenicity, posing limitations to any attempt to use in vivo data for carcinogen risk assessment.

Tumorigenic tests using dogs are limited because of the high cost and the long duration of the studies (up to 7 years). Furthermore, dogs demonstrate high susceptibility to aromatic amines and therefore care should be taken when using these animals for the evaluation of potential carcinogenic compounds of this category (Loomis and Hayes, 1996).

Neurotoxicity

The neurotoxic potential of chemical compounds can be assessed by determining relevant effects on the autonomic or central nervous system (CNS), not only in adult but also in developing animals. Clinical signs including changes in behavior (e.g., movement, motor coordination or reflexes, paralysis, tremor, learning, and memory), neurochemical (e.g., activity of enzymes associated with neuropathies, cell signaling pathways, synthesis, release and uptake of neurotransmitters), neurophysiological (e.g., electroencephalography and nerve conduction velocity) and neuroanatomical effects are commonly explored.

Rodents are the most frequently used animal models and there are a considerable number of available guidelines to examine the neurotoxicity of xenobiotics on them

(OECD, 1997c; EPA, 1998d,e). However, an important issue related to the selection of animal model in neurotoxicity testing is the delayed onset of effects manifested by toxic agents. For example, in the case of assessment of the potential of OPs to produce delayed neuropathy induced by organophosphates, as rodents are not the most sensitive models, the use of the hen model is recommended (OECD, 1995a,b). The two protocols used in the hen model involve either acute or repeated dosing for up to 28 days and determination of the enzymes acetylcholinesterase and neuropathy target esterase, clinical observation, and histopathology of the CNS (OECD, 1995a,b).

Furthermore, the need to address the specific risks of the developing nervous system has led to the application of more specific developmental neurotoxicity testing guidelines in rats (EPA, 1998f; OECD, 2007). Although rodents are the animal model of choice, the main problem using them in developmental studies is that the period of enhanced brain growth takes place during the first 10 days after birth, whereas in humans, dogs, guinea, and minipigs, this period is completed prenatally. In conclusion, for predicting developmental neurotoxicity risk in humans, the rat is the recognized model. However, due to the limitations of the rodent model, dogs, guinea, and minipigs are also widely used to test pharmaceutical compounds that target children. (Kaufmann, 2003).

Immunotoxicity

Immunotoxicity tests are designed to detect adverse effects of xenobiotics on the immune system including all the relevant cells, organs and mechanisms of immune response, whether or not there is a measurable disturbance in host resistance. Toxic substances can directly or indirectly cause immunotoxicity, either by inhibiting the enzymatic activity of esterases and serine hydrolases in the immune system or by chronic alteration in metabolism of organs in the immune and nervous system, respectively. Some of the approaches, tests, and endpoints used to assess in vivo immunotoxicity are presented in Table 9.4 (EPA, 1998g; Barlow et al., 2002; Galloway and Handy, 2003; OECD, 2008).

Laboratory rodents, especially mice, are used in toxicological tests because basic immunological studies were mainly conducted in this species. The immune elements and interactions in rodents and humans are very similar and if the toxicokinetic properties of tested chemicals are close, then the use of mice or rats is recommended (IPCS, 1996; EPA, 1998g).

Transgenic Animals in Toxicity Testing

The recent advances in genetic engineering techniques led to the development of a number of transgenic in vivo

TABLE 9.4 Immunotoxicity Endpoints, Methods and Approaches Used for In Vivo Toxicity Testing

Tests	Methods	Endpoints
Nonfunctional tests of immunotoxic response	Immunopathology	Lymphoid organ weight
		Histopathology of lymphoid tissues, including bone marrow
	Routine hematology	Immunocyte viability/differential count
		Immunoglobulin levels
Functional tests of immunotoxic response	Measurement of humoral immunity	Antibody response
		Antibody plaque forming
	Measurement of nonspecific immunity	Neutrophil and monocyte numbers
		Phagocytic activity of macrophages
	Measurement of cell mediated immunity	Mitogen-induced cell proliferation
		Natural killer cell activity
		Mixed lymphocyte reaction
		Delayed hypersensitivity
	Host resistance assays	Mortality and organ histopathology due to bacterial, virus, and parasitic infection

models that can be used in toxicity testing, mainly in carcinogenicity and mutagenicity, as well as for the study of xenobiotic metabolism. These in vivo systems permit the study of toxicological effects of tested compounds on foreign genes of human or other origin that have been genetically transferred to produce transgenic animals, by transgenesis or targeted gene modification. From the point of view of toxicity testing, it is considered that such models will lead to faster results that are more representative of human response to xenobiotics. In addition, transgenic mice can bring significant animal welfare benefits, because they are able to reduce the group size needed in experiments and replace testing in other species, including nonhuman primates. Finally, these models are also excellent experimental systems that are able to address and answer specific mechanistic questions in toxicology more efficiently (Valancius-Mangel and Doetschman, 1999). However, the use of "humanized" animal models in toxicological studies is an expensive process because it involves higher costs for their development and breeding. There is also concern that the human genome, once transferred to laboratory animals, may express the same proteins, but it does not guarantee that the protein will have similar function as that found in humans. In addition, there is limited background information on transgenic animals, making the interpretation of data in toxicological studies difficult (Valancius-Mangel and Doetschman, 1999).

The main transgenic genotoxicity systems used in toxicology to follow up in vitro genotoxicity positives are the Muta Mouse and Big Blue rat/mouse models, in which the genome is "tagged" with the markers lacZ (β-galactosidase) and lacI, respectively (Gossen et al., 1994; Winegar et al., 1994; Wahnschaffe et al., 2005a,b). Recently, these assays have been validated and approved by OECD (2013).

IN VITRO MODELS OF TOXICITY TESTING

Introduction

In vitro cellular models are relatively inexpensive and easy to maintain and manipulate compared to animal models. In vitro methods allow the study of direct cellular effects of toxins on specific cell or tissue types in a controlled environment.

However, the main disadvantage of in vitro systems over animal models is the lack of systemic effects such as an appropriate balance and supply of growth factors and a system of xenobiotic metabolism and elimination of toxins. The former can be at least partially addressed by adding appropriate growth factors and the latter can be addressed by the use of metabolic activation systems such as the introduction of nicotinamide adenine dinucleotide phosphate hydrogen-activated microsomes or a hepatic cell line in a cell culture fitted with a filter insert (Fig. 9.1). The toxin is introduced into the insert and a mixture of metabolized and nonmetabolized toxin (but not the microsomes or the hepatic cells) diffuses through the filter into the growth medium containing the target cells. Another disadvantage is that many cellular systems lack the complexity of cell–cell interactions in tissue, although this can be addressed to varying degrees using coculture systems, a three-dimensional cell culture, or a tissue slice/organ culture, which are discussed later.

Types of Cell Culture System Used in Toxicity Testing

Before discussing the assays used in the in vitro systems, it would be useful to discuss the principles, strengths and weaknesses of the main types of in vitro systems. All cell

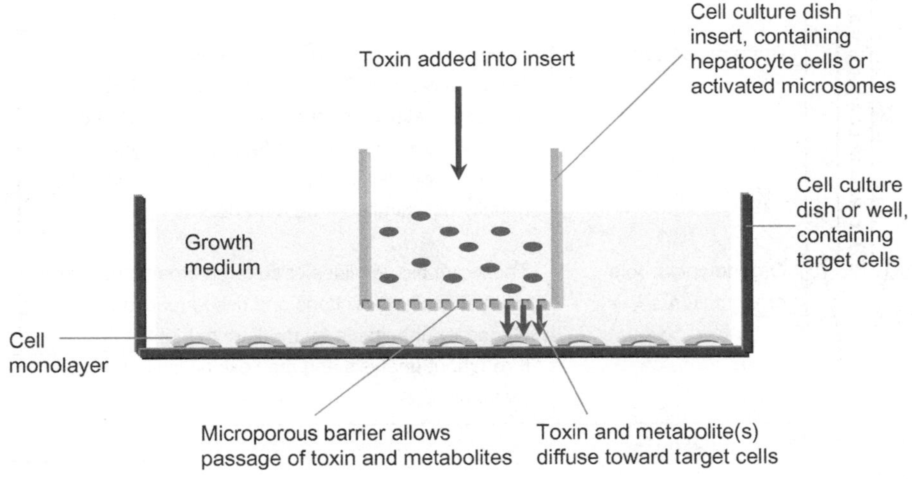

FIGURE 9.1 Metabolic activation in cell culture systems.

cultures need to be prepared and maintained under sterile conditions in order to reduce microbial contamination. Cells are maintained under defined conditions of humidity, pH, and temperature. They are grown in a specific growth medium, which may have a number of supplements, such as antibiotics, glutamine, serum, etc., which are different for each cell line. Growth conditions should be optimized prior to experimental work. Excellent reviews on practical aspects of cell culture can be found in the following sources: Cohen and Wilkin (1996), Shaw (1996), Masters (2000), Davis (2002), Gardner et al. (2004).

There are several types of cell cultures available for in vitro testing that offer various degrees of complexity and relatedness to the in vivo situation. In order of increasing complexity and genetic similarity to the tissue of origin, these include permanent cell lines, primary cultures, stem cells, and organotypic cultures (Fig. 9.2) (Noraberg, 2004; Spielmann, 2005; Sundstrom et al., 2005; Efthymiou et al., 2014; Peters et al., 2015; Van Duinan et al., 2015).

Permanent cell lines are mitotic and can be finite, established or clonal in nature. They have the advantage of being relatively easy and inexpensive to maintain compared to animals and they are amenable to cryopreservation under liquid nitrogen. However, if maintained through high numbers of divisions, there is an increasing likelihood of genetic drift that might affect phenotypic properties of relevance to toxicity testing.

Finite cell lines are normally derived from primary cultures (see below) and can survive for 40–50 divisions before finally dying (e.g., fibroblasts). Established cell lines are effectively immortal, having been transformed with a virus, a mutagen or spontaneously. These are generally tumor like in nature; some widely used examples include mouse 3T3 fibroblasts, HeLa cells, and Chinese hamster ovary cells. However, many cell lines can be induced to differentiate, making them potentially useful models of specific stages of development. For example, the use of nerve growth factor or retinoic acid to induce a neuronal phenotype in cultures of rat PC12 pheochromocytoma and human SH-SY5Y neuroblastoma cells, respectively (Fujita et al., 1989; Presgraves et al., 2004). Additionally, embryonic, progenitor, and adult stem cell lines can be immortalized and some are commercially available (Cocks et al., 2013). The advantage of such cell models is that they may replicate developmental events

Increasing complexity and similarity to in vivo systems

Culture Type	Suitability/Limitations
Mitotic cell lines	Medium to high throughput studies of basal toxicity (e.g., membrane damage, viability, etc.) and cell proliferation. If immortalized, many cell lines are tumor-like. Limited cell–cell interactions and drug metabolism.
Differentiating cell lines	Medium to high throughput screening and mechanistic studies of developmental toxicity and target cell specific toxicity. Often short-lived. Limited cell–cell interactions and drug metabolism.
Primary cell cultures	Developmental or target cell-specific toxicity. Genetically more similar to target system but generally heterogeneous and short-lived. Can be used as coculture systems (e.g., reaggregates) to simulate cell–cell interactions of target tissue but usually have limited drug metabolism.
Organotypic/whole organ cultures	These are tissue slices or cultures organs that can maintain cell interactions and tissue function. Generally unsuitable for medium to high throughput analysis and may exhibit limited drug metabolism.

FIGURE 9.2 Organization of a tiered system for in vitro toxicity testing.

more closely in models of developmental toxicity albeit at a much higher financial cost compared to the well-established tumor cell lines, such as those mentioned earlier.

Clonal cell lines are derived from the mitotic division of a single cell seeded in a sterile microtiter plate by limiting dilution as used in the cloning of hybridoma cell lines. Thus, cell lines can be cloned to exhibit a specific trait (e.g., high levels of specific receptors, drug resistance, etc.). While a homogeneous response to toxin treatment might then be expected from such a cell line, there is the risk of losing other features of a more heterogeneous population. In some cases, clones of transfected cell lines provide useful tools for mechanistic studies of cell differentiation and/or toxicity. For example, some cell cultures have been transfected with certain cytochrome P450 transgenes to make them metabolically more competent during long-term studies (Tzanakakis et al., 2002).

Primary cultures are derived by a combination of mechanical and enzymic disruption of the tissue of interest, which releases a collection of cells that most closely resembles the tissue of origin both genetically and in terms of cell heterogeneity. It is then possible to enrich specific cell types by using either selective culture media and/or cell growth inhibitors, immunomagnetic beads, or fluorescence-activated cell sorting (FACS). If a monoculture is desirable (i.e., predominantly one specific cell type), the resultant culture would then need to be screened for cell-specific markers to determine purity/enrichment of the preparation, as a pure culture is rarely achieved. Typically, this would take the form of monitoring cultures for the expression of a unique morphological or molecular trait of the desired cell type to determine the level of enrichment. For example, expression of glial fibrillary protein and aster-like morphology would be good markers for astrocytic glial cells. Cells may be cultured as monolayers or, if a system simulating cell−cell interactions of the tissue of origin is required, cells may be cultured in suspension with mild agitation or by using a rolling cell culture. Under these circumstances, cells form clusters, spheroids, or reaggregates that may continue to grow/proliferate over a period of several days or weeks, making them amenable to studies of long-term effects. For example, brain reaggregates prepared in this way have been maintained for up to several weeks and used in studies of pesticide toxicity (Sales et al., 2000). However, many primary cultures tend to be very short lived. Primary cell cultures do not necessarily exhibit identical cell−cell interaction patterns as those in the tissue of origin, and cell types that divide more rapidly could become more predominant than they would be in vivo.

A more recent development has been the use of stem cell lines as models for developmental toxicity testing (Hansen and Inselman, 2011). These cell lines are normally maintained in growth media containing mitogens, and can be induced to differentiate into different cell types (e.g., cardiomyocytes, pancreatic, and neural cells) by removal of mitogens and/or the addition of specific trophic factors (Rolletschek et al., 2004). Embryonic stem cells (ESCs) have the potential to differentiate into any cell type whereas progenitor cells are already committed to follow a specific developmental pattern. Alternatively, progenitor cell lines can be established; e.g., neural progenitor cells can be induced to differentiate into a coculture of neuronal and glial cell types, simulating the early stages and cell−cell interactions of neural development in vivo (Breier et al., 2010). However, while stem cell cultures may represent excellent in vitro models for studying developmental toxicity, they are unlikely to exhibit identical cell−cell interactions and growth patterns as those in mature adult tissue.

One way to address this issue may be to develop a postmitotic system containing predifferentiated cells prior to the addition of toxin. However, this issue may be better addressed by using organotypic cultures. In this case, tissue slices (typically 200 μm thickness) are cut from fresh tissue on a microtome, then subsequently rinsed and cultured in growth medium with agitation, as discussed above. Such slices maintain the complexity of cell−cell interactions and extracellular matrix composition of the original tissue and in some cases can survive up to several weeks (Sundstrom et al., 2005). Nevertheless, even this kind of cellular system lacks the systemic interaction with the immune and circulatory systems that would occur in vivo and is not, therefore, a complete substitute for in vivo testing. However, using cell cultures as part of a tiered system of increasing complexity from in vitro to in vivo measurements would improve throughput, decrease costs and allow drastic reduction in the use of live animals in screening compounds for potential toxic effects. Some examples of in vitro toxicity testing systems currently in use are indicated in Table 9.5.

Endpoint Determination for In Vitro Testing Systems

A good in vitro testing system should be sensitive but at the same time yield low levels of false-positive and false-negative results. It should have endpoint measurements that: (1) show dose−response relationships for a given toxin, (2) reflect and are predictive of the in vivo pattern of toxicity for a given group of agents, (3) are objective and reproducible, and (4) have internal controls. It is also useful if the testing system involves rapid assays of toxicity, allowing medium to high throughput analysis and simultaneous testing of multiple compounds and/or doses.

TABLE 9.5 Examples of Cell Culture Systems Used to Model Specific Types of Toxicity

Model	Description and Comments
Neurotoxicity	Differentiating neural cell lines (e.g., human SH-SY5Y and rat PC12 neuroblastoma). Primary cultures, whole rat brain reaggregates and organotypic brain slice cultures (Sales et al., 2000)
Hepatic toxicity	Human hepatoma HepG2 cell line and subclones expressing CYP1A1, cell lines engineered to express single human or animal P450, primary hepatocyte cultures, longer-term collagen sandwich cultures, liver slices, and isolated perfused liver (Worth and Balls, 2002)
Developmental toxicity	Whole rat embryo cultures, rat limb bud reaggregates cultures and mouse embryonic stem cell lines (Liebsch and Spielmann, 2002). Standard operating procedures available on the ECVAM–INVITTOX databases
Dermal toxicity	Keratinocyte and fibroblast cell lines. Excised rat skin models and human EPISKIN and EPIDERM skin models (Fentem et al., 2001)
Immunotoxicity	Antibody production and activation/proliferation of lymphocytes (Karol, 1998)
Genotoxicity	Mammalian cell gene mutation and chromosome aberration tests (EPA, 1998i,j)

The testing system should also be relatively inexpensive and involve technology and skills that are easily transferable to other laboratory personnel. Importantly, for a testing system to be deemed reliable for the prediction of acute in vivo human systemic toxicity, it should have been validated through a rigorous international multicenter validation program. For example, during the period 1989–96, 97 international laboratories tested the same reference chemicals (which represent different classes of chemicals with varied human toxicity) in their own in vitro systems various aspects of the overall study have been published in eight articles in *Alternatives to Laboratory Animals*. Over the past 20 years or so, recommendations governing validation of in vitro alternatives, including systems for measuring chronic effects, have been published and are regularly reviewed by international organizations, such as ECVAM (European Centre for Validation of Alternative Methods), ICCVAM (the Interagency Coordinating Committee on the Validation of Alternative Methods), and the OECD. The interested reader is referred to the following articles for publications on validated systems for toxicity testing: Liebsch and Spielmann (2002), Bhogal et al. (2005), Kandárová and Letasiová (2011).

The best way to achieve something approaching an ideal testing system is to include a battery of endpoint measurements in order to minimize the occurrence of false-negative and false-positive results. Endpoint determination should give an objective assessment of a cytostatic, cytotoxic or other functional effect. It should also be quantitative or reproducibly qualitative. The selection of endpoints chosen should enable the categorization of toxins in terms of their toxicity relative to other agents of the same or other groups, giving reproducible results in different laboratory settings.

Endpoints can take a variety of forms, including measurements of cell viability, metabolic activity, morphology, changes in protein and gene expression, and/or altered subcellular distribution of markers of interest. Some of the main endpoints are summarized below and the reader is referred to Masters (2000), and to protocols available on the following website (https://ecvam-dbalm.jrc.ec.europa.eu/) for further information and technical details about specific protocols and validated models used in toxicity testing in vitro.

Cell Viability

The traditional method of determining cell count is to determine the cell density (cells/mL) in a hemocytometer chamber. While this is a very useful method for determining cell number for seeding in cell culture experiments, it does not distinguish between viable and nonviable cells following exposure to a toxin. However, the proportion of nonviable cells can be determined in parallel by assessing the percentage of counted cells that take up the dye Trypan blue, which is excluded from viable cells. Though effective, this approach is not suited to high throughput, as measurement can be time consuming and is therefore best suited to small numbers of samples or treatments. However, relatively quick measurements can be made using automated cell counters.

An alternative approach is to use dye uptake assays. For example, neutral red accumulates on the lysosomes of viable cells, after which it can be extracted from cells with an organic solvent and determined spectrophotometrically. A variation on this is to prelabel cells with the dye prior to treatment with toxin; reduced levels of absorbance compared to untreated control cells would be indicative of dye release due to membrane damage.

Membrane Leakage

Leakage of macromolecules through the plasma membrane into the culture medium is an effective means of detecting early or late stages of membrane damage. Cells can be incubated in the presence of ^{3}H-thymidine, which is incorporated into DNA during cell proliferation. Subsequent loss of ^{3}H-labeled DNA would be indicative of cell lysis. An alternative approach is to label cells in the presence of ^{51}Cr, which binds to many cellular proteins. Loss of labeled proteins from treated cells would be indicative of membrane leakage/cell lysis. In this sense, the ^{51}Cr release assay is more sensitive than that for ^{3}H-labeled DNA as the former will detect signs of damage to the membrane at a much earlier stage.

An attractive alternative to radioisotopic methods is the release of lactate dehydrogenase (LDH) into cell culture medium, which is measured spectrophotometrically. The assay, which is commercially available in kit form, shows sensitivity comparable to the ^{51}Cr release assay and is amenable to the microtiter plate format, which would facilitate medium to high throughput analysis.

Cell Growth and Proliferation

Cell growth or proliferation can be measured in several ways. The simplest method is that of cloning efficiency. The mitotic index of cell cultures can be determined by counting the percentage of mitotic figures following staining of DNA with hematoxylin. Another approach is the measurement of cell growth in toxin-exposed cells via the incorporation of ^{3}H-thymidine into DNA (Flaskos et al., 1994). Alternatively, cell proliferation can be measured by the incorporation of 5-bromo, 2-deoxyuridine incorporated into S-phase cultured cells, and subsequent quantification is achieved by enzyme-linked immunoabsorbent assay (Lanier et al., 1989). Total DNA content can also be determined by detecting fluorescence after incubation of cells with DNA binding dyes such as Hoechst 33258, using a spectrofluorimetric microplate reader or by FACS analysis (Downs and Wilfinger, 1983).

Cell growth can also be measured by total protein content or by protein synthesis. Protein content can be estimated by a number of dye binding assays in microtiter plate format, such as the bicinchoninic acid assay (Tuszynski and Murphy, 1990).

Cell Morphology

Changes in cell morphology can be measured microscopically and are very useful in studies of mechanisms of toxicity. However, medium to high throughput analysis of toxicity would require the use of image analysis software to produce more consistent data. Specialist techniques such as Allen video-enhanced contrast differential interference contrast microscopy facilitate analysis of effects on living cells. Furthermore, high throughput assays could be developed that measure the underlying molecular changes determined from follow-up studies.

Morphological changes can take various forms, as indicated below.

Cell Volume

An increase or decrease in cell volume could indicate osmotic changes or represent the early stages of cell death by necrosis or apoptosis. Cell death or viability changes would then need to be made to confirm the type of cell death as indicated earlier.

Cell Shape

Changes in shape may occur following exposure to a toxin. These could include rounding up, flattening, spreading, or a process outgrowth in cell culture monolayers. Such changes would give an initial indication of altered cell attachment, migration, proliferation, or differentiation, indicating potential targets for follow-up molecular studies. For example, OP-induced changes in axon outgrowth in cultured neurons indicated possible changes in proteins associated with axon growth and maintenance, which were then targeted in molecular studies (Hargreaves et al., 2006).

Membrane Integrity

Changes in membrane integrity may be indicated by surface blebbing, which can occur as a result of cellular stress (e.g., oxidative stress) or during the early stages of apoptosis. These parameters could be measured further by biochemical methods to confirm the underlying molecular events associated with these morphological changes (e.g., free radical generation, lipid peroxidation, caspase activation, etc.).

Growth Patterns

Growth patterns may change as a result of exposure to toxin. Thus, the proportion of cells growing in colonies or singly would indicate changes in cell–cell interactions and potential changes in cell adhesion proteins, which could be targeted in subsequent molecular studies.

Metabolic Assay

ATP Levels

ATP is an essential requirement for many energy-dependent processes and its levels can be affected by a variety of toxins. It can be used as a marker for cell viability as it is present in all metabolically active cells and its levels decline rapidly when cells undergo apoptosis or necrosis (Kangas et al., 1984). A number of reagents and kits suitable for high throughput screening are available.

Typically, the amount of ATP in cell lysates is determined by the light released from firefly luciferase-catalyzed oxidation of D-luciferin in the presence of ATP and oxygen. ATP and its major metabolites (ADP and AMP) in cell culture extracts can also be determined using an HPLC method (Yang and Gupta, 2003).

Dehydrogenase Activity

The activity of cellular dehydrogenases can be assayed by the reduction of the yellow methyl tetrazolium dye to its blue formazan reaction product. The reduced dye forms crystals in metabolically active cells and, after removal of growth medium, can be solubilized in an organic solvent such as dimethyl sulfoxide and quantified spectrophotometrically in the microtiter plate format, e.g., in assays of in vitro toxicity of OPs (Hargreaves et al., 2006).

Although metabolic assays such as those indicated above are not direct measurements of cell viability, a significant fall in either measurement is normally taken to indicate a fall in cell viability or cell number.

Calcium Homeostasis

Many toxins have a direct or indirect effect on mechanisms involved in the control of Ca^{2+} homeostasis. Such effects could be related to a breakdown in plasma membrane integrity, which would also be detected by other methods discussed previously (e.g., leakage of LDH), or it may be the result of a selective effect on Ca^{2+} channels or Ca^{2+} ATPases that regulate Ca^{2+} movements across cellular membranes. Changes in Ca^{2+} flux can be measured using a variety of Ca^{2+} binding dyes that fluoresce when bound to Ca^{2+} (e.g., Quin 2 and Fura 2). Detection requires spectrofluorimetric analysis that is potentially applicable to high throughput analysis of average change for a given cell population. However, analysis of changes in Ca^{2+} flux in individual cells requires a system that has an integrated microscope and image analysis software package.

Cell or Tissue-Specific Markers of Toxicity

This approach is useful for targeting key proteins or enzyme activities involved in the normal function(s) of the target cells or tissues. It is particularly useful in sublethal/chronic studies of exposure to toxin, in order to determine whether a potentially reversible functional deficit occurs. The principal approaches used at the protein level are those of antibody-based detection and enzyme assays.

Proteomic Analysis

This approach can be useful in mechanistic studies of toxicity as it helps to identify novel protein markers of toxicity. Techniques of this type include the use of two-dimensional PAGE, chromatographic or protein chip fractionation of proteins from cell/tissue lysates or subcellular in order to identify changes in specific protein levels following toxin exposure. Proteins of interest are then normally digested with trypsin, and the tryptic fragments are initially identified by "peptide mass fingerprinting" in a matrix-assisted laser desorption ionization–time of flight mass spectrometer, followed by further confirmation using, e.g., tandem mass spectrometry (Steen and Mann, 2004). Identification is facilitated by the use of freely available Internet-based gene and protein sequence databases such as MASCOT, SwissProt, etc.

Genomic Analysis

Changes in the levels of specific proteins detected by proteome analysis could reflect changes in the regulation of protein turnover (i.e., how rapidly it is degraded once synthesized) or changes in gene expression. Furthermore, depending on the cell or tissue fractionation procedures adopted, changes in low abundance proteins that could be functionally important may not necessarily be detected by proteomic methods. Changes in gene expression following exposure to toxin can be determined by a number of methods including reverse transcriptase polymerase chain reaction (RT-PCR) and DNA microarray analysis (Koizimo and Yamada, 2003).

RT-PCR is a targeted approach involving the production of complementary DNA (cDNA), by treatment of cell or tissue RNA with RT. The resultant cDNA is then incubated with primers (probes) that recognize specific genes or DNA sequences of interest, followed by amplification of such sequences by the Taq polymerase reaction. Changes in the level of amplified target sequence would indicate corresponding changes in the expression of the target gene to which the primers are matched. This approach is only semiquantitative although accuracy can be improved by continuous measurement of amplicon levels using real-time quantitative RT-PCR. Levels of amplicon are normally compared to changes in household genes such as glyceraldehyde dehydrogenase or β-actin, as internal controls.

A less targeted approach that, nevertheless, could help to identify novel changes in gene expression is that of DNA microarray analysis. In this technique, up to several thousand genes are immobilized on a template and probed with labeled RNA from control and treated cells or tissues. Image analysis software is then used to determine up- or down-regulation of genes due to toxin exposure. Controls usually involve averaged changes for a series of household genes. The researcher should be aware that a change in levels of gene expression does not necessarily indicate a corresponding change in protein levels or vice versa, as there are multiple levels of control. A multidisciplinary approach is recommended to get an accurate overall picture of the chain of events following exposure to toxin.

CONCLUDING REMARKS AND FUTURE DIRECTIONS

A major issue facing toxicological science today is how to convert experimental data from in vivo and in vitro models into knowledge about molecular mechanisms of toxicity and safe levels of exposure to the agents tested. A number of animal models that have been used for many years for screening purposes have been gradually refined with increasing emphasis on improved experimental design, animal welfare, and reduced animal use. More recent developments in the area of in vitro toxicity testing have contributed significantly to the gradual reduction in animal use for toxicity screening and have helped to improve knowledge relating to mechanisms of cell- or organ-specific toxicity. Veterinarians have played an important role in the development of legislation and guidelines relating to the use and replacement of laboratory animals in toxicity assessment.

The generally accepted approach to screening compounds for toxicity is to use a multitiered system starting with simple monocultures of specific cell types, followed by cocultures that simulate metabolic effects and/or cell–cell interactions in the whole organism, before carrying out final testing on animals (Fig. 9.3). In this way,

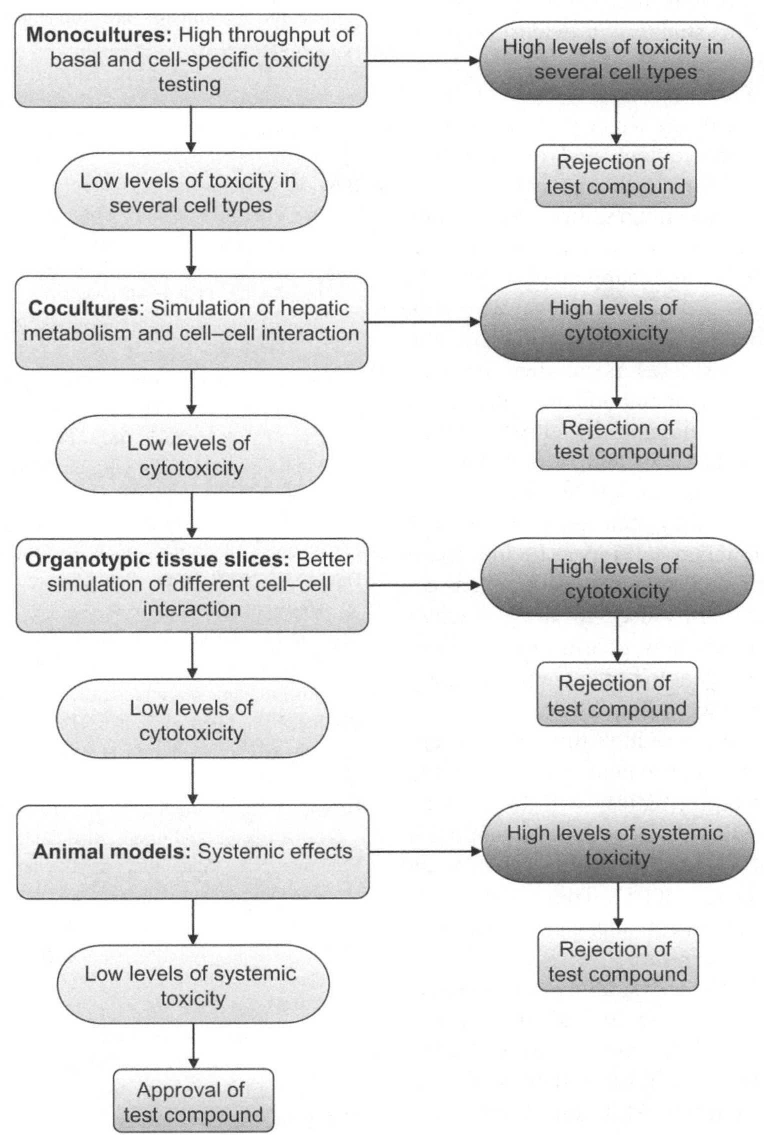

FIGURE 9.3 Flow chart showing principles of multitiered approach to toxicity testing.

it is possible to eliminate compounds that exhibit high levels of basal toxicity in several cell types and reduce unnecessary suffering in animals. In both in vitro and in vivo testing it is important to use a battery of appropriate endpoint measurements of both basal toxicity and cell/tissue-specific toxicity at each level, in order to increase the reliability and predictive potential of the data produced.

In vitro toxicology has made significant advances in the last few decades, by improving and finding solutions to its limitations. For example, cell culture systems are now being designed to be metabolically competent and viable for several weeks, making them appropriate not only for short- but also for long-term toxicity testing (Bhogal et al., 2005). Extending this approach to a wider range of cell culture systems will improve the prospect of using in vitro methods for studying a wider range of chronic toxicological phenomena. However, further development and validation of in vitro models is required if they are to be adopted on a much wider scale in order to secure further reduction, replacement, and refinement of animal models. This will require further improvements in cell culture technology and growth conditions, such as the increased use of hollow fiber systems to facilitate continuous replenishment of media and supplements (Nussler et al., 2001). The increased use of microsomal activation systems and/or established cell lines transfected with genes for mixed function oxidases is another approach that will help to increase the metabolic competence of in vitro models. Another promising in vitro approach involves the use of adult or ESCs of human or rodent origin. These cells can be either continuously cultured without being differentiated or they can generate a wide variety of functional mammalian cell types. In addition to its application in developmental toxicity testing, stem cell technology has been successfully used to study mechanisms of toxicity and to screen new pharmaceutical compounds for teratogenicity, genotoxicity, hepatotoxicity, and cardiotoxicity (Davila et al., 1998, 2004).

The development of medium to high throughput methods in proteomics, genomics, and metabolomics, together with the revolution in bioinformatics, will lead to the accumulation of vast toxicological information, helping to elucidate mechanisms of toxicity in both in vitro and in vivo models (Bhogal et al., 2005). These approaches will also help in the development and establishment of new biomarkers of effect or exposure.

In conclusion, although it is a desirable goal to replace all animal testing, animal-based toxicological testing is likely to continue for the foreseeable future. Further improvements in animal models will make them more reliable indicators of human toxicity, while the development of improved in vitro systems will eventually minimize the use of animals for toxicity studies. The veterinarian's role will therefore be to continue monitoring and improving the welfare of animals used in toxicity testing and to advise on issues relating to the development of in vitro alternatives.

REFERENCES

Arnold, D.L., Grice, H.C., Krewski, D.R., 1990. Handbook of In Vivo Toxicity Testing. Academic Press, San Diego, CA.

Auletta, C.S., 2004. Current in vivo assays for cutaneous toxicity: local and systemic toxicity testing. Pharmacol. Toxicol. 95, 201–208.

Barlow, S.M., Greig, J.B., Bridges, J.W., et al., 2002. Hazard identification by methods of animal-based toxicology. Food Chem. Toxicol. 40, 145–191.

Bhogal, N., Grindon, C., Combes, R., Balls, M., 2005. Toxicity testing: creating a revolution based on new technologies. Trends Biotechnol. 23, 299–307.

Breier, J.M., Gassmann, K., Kayser, R., et al., 2010. Neural progenitor cells as models for high-throughput screens of developmental neurotoxicity: state of the science. Neurotoxicol. Teratol. 32, 4–15.

Buse, E., Habermann, G., Ostrburg, I., et al., 2003. Reproductive/developmental toxicity and immunotoxicity assessment in the nonhuman primate model. Toxicology. 185, 221–227.

Cocks, G., Romanyuk, N., Amemori, T., et al., 2013. Conditionally immortalized stem cell lines from human spinal cord retain regional identity and generate functional interneurons and motor neurons. Stem Cell Res. Ther. 4, 69.

Cohen, J., Wilkin, G.P., 1996. Neural Cell Culture. A Practical Approach. Oxford University Press, Oxford.

Davila, J.C., Rodriguez, R.J., Melchert, R.B., Acosta Jr, D., 1998. Predictive value of in vitro model systems in toxicology. Annu. Rev. Pharmacol. Toxicol. 38, 63–96.

Davila, J.C., Cezar, G.G., Thiede, M., et al., 2004. Use and application of stem cells in toxicology. Toxicol. Sci. 79, 214–223.

Davis, J., 2002. Basic Cell Culture. A Practical Approach. Oxford University Press, Oxford.

deBlois, D., Horlick, R.A., 2001. Endotoxin sensitization to kinin B(1) receptor agonist in non-human primate model: haemodynamic and pro-inflammatory effects. Br. J. Pharmacol. 132, 327–335.

Dhillon, V.S., Singh, J., Singh, H., Kler, R.S., 1995. In vitro and in vivo genotoxicity of hormonal drugs. VI. Fluoxymesterone. Mutat. Res. 342, 103–111.

Downs, T.R., Wilfinger, W.W., 1983. Fluorometric quantification of DNA in cells and tissue. Anal. Biochem. 131, 538–547.

Efthymiou, A., Shaltouki, A., Steiner, J.P., et al., 2014. Functional screening assays with neurons generated from pluripotent stem cell-derived neural stem cells. J. Biomol. Screen. 19, 32–43.

EPA (Environmental Protection Agency), (1998a). Health Effects Test Guidelines OPPTS 870.7200 Companion Animal Safety. EPA 712-C-98-349.

EPA (Environmental Protection Agency), (1998b). Health Effects Test Guidelines OPPTS 870.3700 Prenatal Developmental Toxicity Study. EPA 712-C-98-207.

EPA (Environmental Protection Agency), (1998c). Health Effects Test Guidelines OPPTS 870.5450 Rodent Dominant Lethal Assay. EPA 712-C-98-227.

EPA (Environmental Protection Agency), (1998d). Guidelines for Neurotoxicity Risk Assessment. EPA FRL-6011-3. NTIS PB98-117831.

EPA (Environmental Protection Agency), (1998e). Health Effects Test Guidelines OPPTS 870.6200 Neurotoxicity Screening Battery. EPA 712-C-98-238.

EPA (Environmental Protection Agency), (1998f). Health Effects Test Guidelines OPPTS 870.6300 Developmental Neurotoxicity Study. EPA 712-C-98-239.

EPA (Environmental Protection Agency), (1998g). Health Effects Test Guidelines OPPTS 870.7800 Immunotoxicity. EPA 712-C-98-351.

EPA (Environmental Protection Agency), (1998h). Health Effects Test Guidelines OPPTS 870.5200 Mouse Visible Specific Locus Test. EPA 712-C-98-217.

EPA (Environmental Protection Agency), (1998i). Health Effects Test Guidelines OPPTS 870.5300 In Vitro Mammalian Cell Gene Mutation Test. EPA 712-C-98-221.

EPA (Environmental Protection Agency), (1998j). Health Effects Test Guidelines OPPTS 870.5300 In Vitro Mammalian Chromosome Aberration Test. EPA 712-C-98-223.

EPA (Environmental Protection Agency), (2000). Health Effects Test Guidelines OPPTS 870.3550 Reproduction/Developmental Toxicity Screening Test. EPA 712-C-00-367.

EPA (Environmental Protection Agency), (2003). Health Effects Test Guidelines OPPTS 870.2600 Skin Sensitization. EPA 712-C-03-197.

Estevan, C., Palmies, D., Sogorb, M.A., Vilanova, E., 2011. OECD guidelines and validated methods for in vivo testing of reproductive toxicity. In: Gupta, R.C. (Ed.), Reproductive and Developmental Toxicology. Academic Press/Elsevier, Amsterdam, pp. 121–131.

Faqi, A.S., 2011. A primate as an animal model for reproductive and developmental toxicity testing. In: Gupta, R.C. (Ed.), Reproductive and Developmental Toxicology. Academic Press/Elsevier, Amsterdam, pp. 207–218.

Fentem, J.H., Briggs, D., Chesne, C., Elliott, G.R., Harbell, J.W., Heylings, J.R., et al., 2001. A prevalidation study on in vitro tests for acute skin irritation. 2. Results and evaluation by the management team. Toxicol. In Vitro 15, 57–93.

Flaskos, J., McLean, W.G., Hargreaves, A.J., 1994. The toxicity of organophosphate compounds towards cultured PC12 cells. Toxicol. Lett. 70, 71–76.

Foote, R.H., Carney, E.W., 2000. The rabbit as a model for reproductive and developmental toxicity studies. Reprod. Toxicol. 14, 477–493.

Fujita, K., Lazarovici, P., Guroff, G., 1989. Regulation of the differentiation of PC12 pheochromocytoma cells. Environ. Health Perspect. 80, 127–142.

Gabridge, M.G., Legator, M.S., 1969. A host-mediated microbial assay for the detection of mutagenic compounds. Proc. Soc. Exp. Biol. Med. 130, 831.

Gad, S.C., 1998. Toxicity testing, carcinogenesis. In: Wexler, P. (Ed.), Encyclopedia of Toxicology, vol. 3. Academic Press, San Diego, CA, pp. 289–293.

Gad, S.C., 2006. Animal Models in Toxicology. Marcel Dekker Inc, New York, NY.

Galloway, T., Handy, R., 2003. Immunotoxicity of organophosphorus pesticides. Ecotoxicology 12, 345–363.

Gardner, D.K., Lane, M., Watson, A.J., 2004. A Laboratory Guide to the Mammalian Embryo. A Practical Approach. Oxford University Press, Oxford.

Garg, R.C., Bracken, W.M., Hoberman, A., 2011. Reproductive and developmental safety evaluation of new pharmaceutical compounds. In: Gupta, R.C. (Ed.), Reproductive and Developmental Toxicology. Academic Press/Elsevier, Amsterdam, pp. 87–107.

Gossen, J.A., de Leeuw, W.J., Vijg, J., 1994. LacZ transgenic mouse models: their application in genetic toxicology. Mutat. Res. 307, 451–459.

Gupta, R.C. Reproductive and Developmental Toxicology. Academic Press/Elsevier, Amsterdam, in press.

Hansen, D.K., Inselman, A.L., 2011. Applications of stem cells in developmental toxicology. In: Gupta, R.C. (Ed.), Reproductive and Developmental Toxicology. Academic Press/Elsevier, Amsterdam, pp. 121–131.

Hargreaves, A.J., Fowler, M.J., Sachana, M., et al., 2006. Inhibition of neurite outgrowth in differentiating mouse N2a neuroblastoma cells by phenyl saligenin phosphate: effects on MAP kinase (ERK 1/2) activation, neurofilament heavy chain phosphorylation and neuropathy target esterase. Biochem. Pharmacol. 71, 1240–1247.

Hurtt, M.E., Cappon, G.D., Browning, A., 2003. Proposal for a tiered approach to developmental toxicity testing for veterinary pharmaceutical products for food-producing animals. Food Chem. Toxicol. 41, 611–619.

IPCS (International Programme on Chemical Safety), 1996. Principles and methods for assessing direct immunotoxicity associated with exposure to chemicals. Environmental Health Criteria, International Programme on Chemical Safety, vol. 180. World Health Organization, Geneva.

Kandárová, H., Letasiová, S., 2011. Alternative methods in toxicology: pre-validated and validated methods. Interdiscip. Toxicol. 4, 107–113.

Kangas, L., Gronroos, M., Nieminen, A.L., 1984. Bioluminescence of cellular ATP: a new method for evaluating cytotoxic agents in vitro. Med. Biol. 62, 338–343.

Karol, M.H., 1998. Target organs and systems: methodologies to assess immune system function. Environ. Health Perspect. 106, 533–540.

Kaufmann, W., 2003. Current status of developmental neurotoxicity: an industry prospective. Toxicol. Lett. 140–141, 161–169.

Koizimo, S., Yamada, H., 2003. DNA microarray analysis of altered gene expression in cadmium-exposed human cells. J. Occup. Health. 45, 331–334.

Lanier, T.L., Berger, E.K., Eacho, P.I., 1989. Comparison of 5-bromo-2-deoxyuridine and [3H]thymidine for studies of hepatocellular proliferation in rodents. Carcinogenesis 10, 1341–1343.

Liebsch, M., Spielmann, H., 2002. Currently available in vitro methods used in the regulatory toxicology. Toxicol. Lett. 127, 127–134.

Loomis, T.A., Hayes, A.W., 1996. Toxicologic testing methods. In: Loomis, T.A., Hayes, A.W. (Eds.), Loomis's Essentials of Toxicology. Academic Press, San Diego, CA, pp. 205–248.

Masters, J., 2000. Animal Cell Culture. A Practical Approach. Oxford University Press, Oxford.

Nebbia, C., 2001. Biotransformation enzymes as determinants of xenobiotic toxicity in domestic animals. Vet. J. 161, 238–252.

Noraberg, J., 2004. Organotypic brain slice cultures an efficient and reliable method for neurotoxicological screening and mechanistic studies. Altern. Lab. Anim. 32, 329–337.

Nussler, A.K., Wang, A., Neuhaus, P., et al., 2001. The suitability of hepatocyte culture models to study various aspects of drug metabolism. ALTEX 18, 91–101.

OECD (Organisation for Economic Cooperation and Development), (1984). Genetic Toxicology: Rodent Dominant Lethal Test. OECD guidance 478 adopted 4-04-1984.
OECD (Organisation for Economic Cooperation and Development), (1987). Acute Dermal Toxicity. OECD guidance 402 adopted 24-02-1987.
OECD (Organisation for Economic Cooperation and Development), (1995a). Delayed Neurotoxicity of Organophosphorus Substances. Following Acute Exposure. OECD guidance 418 adopted 27-07-1995.
OECD (Organisation for Economic Cooperation and Development), (1995b). Delayed Neurotoxicity of Organophosphorus Substances: 28 Day Repeated Dose Study. OECD guidance 419 adopted 27-07-1995.
OECD (Organisation for Economic Cooperation and Development), (1997a). Mammalian Bone Marrow Chromosomal Aberration Test. OECD guidance 475 adopted 21-07-1997.
OECD (Organisation for Economic Cooperation and Development), (1997b). Unscheduled DNA synthesis (UDS) Test with Mammalian Liver Cells In Vivo. OECD guidance 486 adopted 21-07-1997.
OECD (Organisation for Economic Cooperation and Development), (1997c) Neurotoxicity Study in Rodents. OECD guidance 424 adopted 21-07-1997.
OECD (Organisation for Economic Cooperation and Development), (2001a). Two Generation Reproduction Toxicity Study. OECD guidance 416 adopted 22-01-2001.
OECD (Organisation for Economic Cooperation and Development), (2001b). Prenatal Developmental Toxicity Study. OECD guidance 414 adopted 22-01-2001.
OECD (Organisation for Economic Cooperation and Development), (2007). Developmental Neurotoxicity Study. OECD guidance 426 adopted 16-10-2007.
OECD (Organisation for Economic Cooperation and Development), (2008). Repeated Dose 28 Day Oral Toxicity Study In Rodents. OECD guidance 407 adopted 3-10-2008.
OECD (Organisation for Economic Cooperation and Development), (2009a). Carcinogenicity Studies. OECD guidance 451 adopted 7-09-2009.
OECD (Organisation for Economic Cooperation and Development), (2009b). Combined Chronic Toxicity/Carcinogenicity Studies. OECD guidance 453 adopted 7-09-2009.
OECD (Organisation for Economic Cooperation and Development), (2010). Skin Sensitisation. OECD guidance 429 adopted 23-7-2010.
OECD (Organisation for Economic Cooperation and Development), (2012). Extended One-Generation Reproductive Toxicity Study. OECD guidance 443 adopted 02-10-2012.
OECD (Organisation for Economic Cooperation and Development), (2013). Transgenic Rodent Somatic and Germ Cell Gene Mutation Assays. OECD guidance 488 adopted 26-7-2013.
OECD (Organisation for Economic Cooperation and Development), (2016a). Reproduction/Developmental Toxicity Screening Test. OECD guidance 421 adopted 29-7-2016.
OECD (Organisation for Economic Cooperation and Development), (2016b). Combined Repeated Dose Toxicity Study with the Reproduction/Developmental Toxicity Screening Test. OECD guidance 422 adopted 29-7-2016.
Peters, M.F., Lamore, S.D., Guo, L., et al., 2015. Human stem cell-derived cardiomyocytes in cellular impedance assays: bringing cardiotoxicity screening to the front line. Cardiovasc. Toxicol. 15, 127–139.
Presgraves, S.P., Ahmed, T., Borwege, S., Joyce, J.N., 2004. Terminally differentiated SH-SY5Y cells provide a model system for studying neuroprotective effects of dopamine agonists. Neurotox. Res. 5, 579–598.
Rolletschek, A., Blyszczuk, P., Wobus, A.M., 2004. Embryonic stem cell-derived cardiac, neuronal and pancreatic cells as model systems to study toxicological effects. Toxicol. Lett. 149, 361–369.
Russell, W.M., Burch, R.L., 1959. The Principles of Humane Experimental Technique. Methuen, London.
Sales, K.M., Kingston, S.T., Atterwill, C.K., Purcell, W.M., 2000. Avian whole-brain spheroid cultures: applications in pesticide toxicity. Pest Manag. Sci. 56, 825–827.
Shaw, A.J., 1996. Epithelial Cell Culture. A Practical Approach. Oxford University Press, Oxford.
Spielmann, H., 2005. Predicting the risk of developmental toxicity from in vitro assays. Toxicol. Appl. Pharmacol. 207, S375–S380.
Steen, H., Mann, M., 2004. The ABC's (and XYZ's) of peptide sequencing. Nat. Rev. Mol. Cell. Biol. 5, 699–711.
Sundstrom, L., Morrison III, B., Bradley, M., Pringle, A., 2005. Organotypic cultures as tools for functional screening in the CNS. Drug Discov. Today. 10, 993–1000.
Tuszynski, G.P., Murphy, A., 1990. Spectrophotometric quantitation of anchorage-dependent cell numbers using the bicinchoninic acid protein assay reagent. Anal. Biochem. 184, 189–191.
Tzanakakis, E.S., Waxman, D.J., Hansen, L.K., et al., 2002. Long-term enhancement of cytochrome P4502B1/2 expression in rat hepatocyte spheroids through adenovirus-mediated gene transfer. Cell. Biol. Toxicol. 18, 13–27.
Vail, D.M., Chun, R., Thamm, D.H., et al., 1998. Efficacy of pyridoxine to ameliorate the cutaneous toxicity associated with doxorubicin containing pegylated (Stealth) liposomes: a randomized, double-blind clinical trial using a canine model. Clin. Cancer Res. 4, 1567–1571.
Valancius-Mangel, V., Doetschman, T., 1999. Potential uses of transgenic and gene-targeted animals in toxicologic research. In: Puga, A., Wallace, K.B. (Eds.), Molecular Biology of the Toxic Response. Taylor and Francis, Philadelphia, PA, pp. 27–51.
Van Duinan, V., Trietsch, S.J., Joore, J., et al., 2015. Microfluidic 3D cell culture: from tools to tissue models. Curr. Opin. Biotechnol. 35, 118–126.
Wahnschaffe, U., Bitsch, A., Kielhorn, J., Mangelsdorf, I., 2005a. Mutagenicity testing with transgenic mice. Part I: Comparison with the mouse bone marrow micronucleus test. J. Carcinog. 4, 3.
Wahnschaffe, U., Bitsch, A., Kielhorn, J., Mangelsdorf, I., 2005b. Mutagenicity testing with transgenic mice. Part II: Comparison with the mouse spot test. J. Carcinog. 4, 4.
Winegar, R.A., Lutze, L.H., Hamer, J.D., et al., 1994. Radiation-induced point mutations, deletions and micronuclei in lacI transgenic mice. Mutat. Res. 307, 479–487.
Worth, A., Balls, M., 2002. Alternative (non-animal) methods for chemicals testing: current status and future prospects. Altern. Lab. Anim. 30 (Suppl. 1), 1–125.
Yang, M.S., Gupta, R.C., 2003. Determination of energy charge potential in the C6 glioma and the Hepg-2 cell culture. Toxicol. Mech. Methods 13, 97–101.

Zeiger, E., 1998. Identification of rodent carcinogens and noncarcinogens using genetic toxicity tests: premises, promises and performance. Regul. Toxicol. Pharmacol. 28, 85–95.

FURTHER READING

Amacher, D.M., Fasulo, L.M., Charuel, C., et al., 1998. In vitro toxicity of zamifenacin (UK-76,654) and metabolites in primary hepatocyte cultures. Xenobiotica 28, 895–908.

Ehrich, M., Correll, L., Veronesi, B., 1997. Acetylcholinesterase and neuropathy target esterase inhibitions in neuroblastoma cells to distinguish organophosphorus compounds causing acute and delayed neurotoxicity. Fundam. Appl. Toxicol. 38, 55–63.

Kuhn, D.M., Geddes, T.J., 2000. Molecular footprints of neurotoxic amphetamine action. Ann. N.Y. Acad. Sci. 914, 92–103.

McMorris, A.F., 1977. Norepinephrine induces glial-specific enzyme activity in cultured glioma cells. Proc. Natl. Acad. Sci. U.S.A. 74, 4501–4504.

Towbin, S., Staehelin, T., Gordon, J., 1979. Electrophoretic transfer of proteins from polyacrylamide gels to nitrocellulose sheets: procedure and some applications. Proc. Natl. Acad. Sci. U.S.A. 76, 4350–4354.

Chapter 10

Toxicoproteomics in Diagnostic Toxicology

Christina R. Wilson and Stephen B. Hooser

INTRODUCTION

During the past decade, advances in genomics research have resulted in the completion of entire genome sequences for multiple species. This abundance of genetic information, compiled in genome sequence databases, has been used to characterize changes in gene expression in response to external stimuli, such as toxicants (toxicogenomics). Because genomic data reflects changes in gene expression at the mRNA level, DNA sequence databases can be queried to predict what proteins may be present in the cell. However, this approach is problematic because there is a poor correlation between mRNA levels and protein concentrations in cells (Gygi et al., 1999a; Anderson and Seilhamer, 2005). Additionally, the biological activity of proteins is controlled by posttranslational protein modifications or protein–protein interactions, both of which cannot be predicted by the genomic data. Therefore, characterizing the entire protein complement expressed by genes (proteome) in response to external stimuli serves as a better indicator of the response of an organism, tissue, or cell to toxic insult. This has given rise to the "proteomic" approach to toxicological evaluation. Toxicoproteomics can encompass global analysis of all of the proteins expressed, called "shotgun proteomics," or can entail analyzing a subset of proteins of interest, often termed "targeted proteomics." Regardless of the approach, proteomics-based research has created an analytical challenge, requiring sophisticated, high-throughput analytical techniques, and complex computer algorithms.

ANALYTICAL TOOLS FOR PROTEOMIC ANALYSES

The Proteome and Sample Complexity

The initial step in proteome analysis typically involves the separation of intact proteins or peptides generated from proteolytic digestion of protein mixtures. Analysis of these heterogeneous components has proven to be an analytical challenge due to the large dynamic range of proteins and the microheterogeneity of protein expression in biological samples. For instance, serum albumin concentrations can range from 35 to 50×10^9 pg/mL and proteins of lower abundance, such as interleukin 6, can range in concentration from 0 to 5 pg/mL (Anderson and Anderson, 2002). This is also complicated by protein heterogeneity due to polymorphisms, alternative mRNA splicing, or variations in posttranslational modifications. When analyzing global proteolytic digests of proteins (i.e., at the peptide level), the sample complexity is compounded further. Proteolytic digests of the serum proteome, which could contain as much as 20,000 proteins, can potentially result in 200,000–600,000 peptides (Anderson and Anderson, 2002; Issaq et al., 2005). Therefore, one can appreciate the analytical challenges encountered when conducting proteomics research in complex biological systems. Attempts to overcome these drawbacks have imposed improvements in sample preparation and separation methodologies. Multidimensional levels of separation can be achieved when these techniques are combined affording increased resolution, sensitivity, and accuracy of detection.

Two-Dimensional Gel Electrophoresis

Since its inception in 1975 (O'Farrell, 1975), two-dimensional gel electrophoresis (2-DGE) has become one of the most common platforms for separating and profiling complex protein mixtures. This technique is two-dimensional in that there are two levels of protein separation. The first dimension uses immobilized pH gradient-isoelectric focusing, which separates proteins based on differences in net charge (Görg et al., 2000). In

Veterinary Toxicology. DOI: http://dx.doi.org/10.1016/B978-0-12-811410-0.00010-6

the second dimension, proteins are resolved by electrophoresis and separated based on molecular weight. Visualization of resolved protein spots is achieved using universal stains such as Coomassie blue, Coomassie brilliant blue (SeePico), silver, negative-reversible zinc, fluorescent, or radioisotope labeling dyes (Görg et al., 2000; Lopez et al., 2000; Ong and Pandey, 2001; Kuramitsu et al., 2010). If a particular subproteome is targeted for detection, more specific gel stains can be used. For example, detection of target proteins can be accomplished using stains containing antibodies for those proteins of interest or posttranslationally modified proteins can be visualized using specialized stains for phosphorylated and glycosylated proteins (Görg et al., 2004; Vlahou and Fountoulakis, 2005; Otani et al., 2011).

After staining, the gel is digitized and protein concentrations quantitated using sophisticated 2-DGE image analysis software. Comparative analysis between control samples and samples of diagnostic interest can be accomplished using these image analyzers to superimpose the digitized data from multiple gel runs. However, due to the laborious nature of this procedure and the lack of gel reproducibility, comparative analysis is often difficult. In order to circumvent these limitations, fluorescent dyes, known as Cy dyes, have been developed permitting simultaneous analysis of two samples on one gel (Ünlü et al., 1997; Hamdan and Righetti, 2002). This technique, called two-dimensional differential in-gel electrophoresis (2-D DIGE), involves labeling each sample with one of two different Cy dye fluorophores, mixing the two samples together, and analyzing them using 2-DGE and fluorescent-gel imaging.

While the gel-staining techniques used to visualize and quantitate proteins may vary, in all instances protein identification is commonly accomplished using tandem mass spectrometry (MS/MS). Excised protein spots are digested into peptides using proteolytic enzymes and subjected, offline, to MS/MS analysis. The peptide mass fingerprints generated and peptide sequence data are then compared to theoretical peptide masses in protein or genome sequence databases using specialized bioinformatics algorithms.

Despite the fact that improvements in 2-DGE technology have enabled high resolution of separated proteins and enhanced protein identification, some intrinsic problems remain. Limited throughput capabilities, inability to measure low and high molecular mass proteins, intergel variability and inefficient detection of basic and hydrophobic proteins are still inherent limitations of this proteomics platform. Regardless of these limitations, 2-DGE is still a powerful tool for the separation of intact proteins and is the most widely used technique in comparative toxicoproteomic analyses.

High Performance Liquid Chromatography

Attempts to improve protein separations have warranted the development of gel-free systems for large-scale analyses. Chromatographic strategies used to fractionate proteins and peptides have proven to be a successful alternative to 2-DGE. The chromatographic techniques commonly employed in proteomics research include affinity chromatography, capillary electrophoresis (CE), hydrophobic interaction chromatography, hydrophilic interaction chromatography, ion exchange chromatography (IEX), reversed-phase chromatography (RPC), and size exclusion chromatography (SEC) (Goheen and Gibbins, 2000; Levison, 2003; Goetz et al., 2004; Mahn and Asenjo, 2005; Mirzaei and Regnier, 2005; Babu et al., 2006; Mondal and Gupta, 2006; Wilson et al., 2008; Di Palma et al., 2011). These modes of chromatography fractionate proteins and peptides based on their adsorption and desorption on stationary phase supports through mobile phase manipulation. On the protein level, they are commonly used to prefractionate samples in order to simplify complexity prior to analysis by 2-DGE or high performance liquid chromatography (HPLC). Fractionation of proteins using these methods can also be accomplished online using high-throughput HPLC techniques. While this approach has proven to be a successful initial step in protein purification, HPLC fractionation of intact proteins is uncommon in proteomics.

HPLC is, however, the most widely used analytical tool for separating proteolytic digests of complex protein mixtures. In this approach, all of the proteins in the sample are digested into peptides using a proteolytic enzyme. After digestion, the peptides are separated using HPLC with UV detection. When interfaced with a mass spectrometer, the amino acid sequences of these peptides can be determined and their respective parent proteins identified using bioinformatics software.

Large-scale analysis of proteolytic digests can compromise the resolving power of HPLC when only one chromatographic fractionation technique is used (Davis and Giddings, 1985a,b). Therefore, orthogonal approaches using multidimensional chromatographic separations are preferred, affording greater peptide resolution and accuracy of detection. The most widely used high-throughput separation technique is the coupling of IEX and RPC with MS instrumentation. Other examples of multidimensional HPLC/MS techniques can also include RPC/CE chromatography, affinity chromatography/RP chromatography, SEC/IEX/RPC, and SEC/RPC/CE (Issaq et al., 2005; Zhang et al., 2010a).

HPLC has also been used for quantitative analysis of protein expression. Relative quantitation of proteins by HPLC is based on the theory that the concentration of the parent protein can be determined by the relative peak areas of UV-detected peptides observed from that protein (Chelius and Bondarenko, 2002). Another HPLC-based approach for relative protein quantitation involves the use of internal protein standards (Bondarenko et al., 2002). In this technique, biological samples are spiked with an internal standard protein prior to enzymatic digestion of the proteins into peptides. The chromatographic peaks observed can be normalized to the peak area of the internal standard and the relative concentrations of the proteins are inferred.

Unlike 2-DGE/MS tools, multidimensional HPLC/MS is amenable to high-throughput analyses and has the ability to resolve peptide mixtures regardless of molecular mass or hydrophobicity. This is important because resolving peptide mixtures by 2-DGE is impractical due to their narrow isoelectric points and molecular weight ranges and because 2-DGE tools cannot be directly interfaced with MS instrumentation. Even though 2-DGE is superior when separating intact proteins, methods based on pairing multidimensional HPLC and MS technology are becoming more refined and continue to advance proteomics research.

Protein and Peptide Microarrays

Protein and peptide microarray technologies offer a complimentary approach to traditional separation methodologies and mass spectrometry. This technology incorporates the use of a variety of high-throughput microarray platforms to probe protein function, abundance and to globally analyze protein expression in biological systems. The platforms commonly used in proteomics include proteome, antibody, reverse-phase protein, and lectin microarrays (Lina et al., 2011).

Protein function microarrays use immobilized capture ligands to screen for protein–drug, protein–enzyme, protein–protein interactions (Kawahashi et al., 2003; Nielsen et al., 2003; Zhu et al., 2003; Cretich et al., 2006). Analytical microarrays, such as those used in surface-enhanced laser desorption (SELDI)/TOF MS, use retentate chromatography for protein profiling and detection (Merchant and Weinberger, 2000; Cretich et al., 2006). This technique is capable of on-chip sample fractionation utilizing various chromatographic surface chemistries and can probe for chemical properties in proteins such as phosphorylation, glycosylation, hydrophobicity, or anionic–cationic properties.

Microarrays require immobilization of a capture ligand or chromatographic media onto a planar solid support, often resulting in thousands of spots per slide (MacBeath and Schreiber, 2000; Kumble, 2003). Samples of interest are added to the microarray and the entire array is scanned to detect proteins or peptides that interact with the ligand or chromatographic media.

Detection strategies for protein or peptide microarrays entail either label-free or labeled probe methods (Espina et al., 2004; Cretich et al., 2006). The label-free strategy is a direct detection method that includes MS, surface plasmon resonance, or atomic force microscopy. SELDI microarray chips commonly use MS-based detection of proteins or peptides. Labeled probe methods of detection include utilizing chromagens (similar to ELISA protocols), chemiluminescence, fluorescence, or radioactive decay-based detection techniques.

Microarray technology is progressively becoming a versatile platform for its potential use in diagnostic toxicology. Although efforts to standardize array analyses have been challenging, microarrays make it possible to simultaneously screen thousands of samples and profile large numbers of proteins from biological samples.

Mass Spectrometry

Recent developments in hybrid mass spectrometers have revolutionized the ability to analyze proteins and peptides, providing high-throughput automation combined with high sensitivity and resolving power. In general, mass spectrometers have three components, an ion source, a mass analyzer, and a detector. The ion source is the component in which protein and peptide ions are produced; the mass analyzer separates or resolves these ions based on their mass-to-charge (*m/z*); and the detector detects the selected ions from the mass analyzer. One stage mass analysis is commonly used to measure the molecular weights of intact proteins or peptides. However, in order to obtain peptide sequence information, hybrid mass spectrometers must be employed. MS/MS, or tandem mass spectrometry, detects intact peptide ions in the first mass analyzer. Once selected, the peptide ion enters the collision cell where it is fragmented into secondary ions by collision-induced dissociation (CID). These ions are then separated in the second mass analyzer, their *m/z* ratios detected, and MS/MS spectra are generated. Bioinformatics database tools use the MS/MS data to generate peptide amino acid sequence information and compare them with theoretical sequences in protein or genome databases to identify proteins.

There are two major types of hybrid mass analyzers used in proteomics research, matrix-assisted laser desorption ionization/time-of-flight (MALDI-TOF/TOF) instruments and electrospray ionization/tandem MS instruments (ESI/MS/MS) (Karas and Hillenkamp, 1988; Fenn et al., 1989; Hillenkamp et al., 1991). The MS technology chosen depends on the type of MS data that needs to be generated from toxicoproteomic experiments. For example, MALDI-TOF/TOF instruments are fast, robust mass analyzers, have a large dynamic range and do not require labor-intensive sample preparation. MALDI-TOF/TOF instruments have high resolution, making them the instruments of choice when using mass spectrometry for quantitative proteomic analyses. ESI/MS/MS instruments, including those containing hybrid combinations of quadrupole, 3-D ion trap, linear ion trap, Orbitrap, TOF, and Fourier transform-ion cyclotron resonance mass analyzers (FTICR) have approximately four times less peak capacity than MALDI-TOF/TOF; however, they have higher mass accuracy affording more accurate protein identification (Hopfgartner et al., 2004; Hu et al., 2005; O'Connor et al., 2006; Yates et al., 2006; Merchant, 2010). Additionally, they are capable of analyzing low molecular weight peptides and can be directly interfaced with HPLC instrumentation.

Innovative approaches to advance protein identification strategies have spurred the development of new MS technologies. Improvements in ion activation using electron capture dissociation (ECD) or infrared multiphoton dissociation technologies have been shown to yield more extensive peptide sequence coverage when compared to CID, resulting in significant improvements in protein identification (Wysocki et al., 2005; Bakhtiar and Guan, 2006). Although once thought to be impossible, characterization of intact, large proteins can be accomplished using ECD combined with FTICR (Sze et al., 2003; Zhang et al., 2010b). Developments in MALDI imaging mass spectrometry have paved the way to simultaneously map peptides and proteins by direct MS analysis of thin tissue sections, providing a means to correlate and monitor changes in protein patterns associated with regions of the tissue that are histologically significant (Mange et al., 2009; Stauber et al., 2010). Other significant technological advances in large biomolecule ionization and data analysis have enabled the development of miniaturized, portable mass spectrometers capable of direct analysis of complex biological samples (Laughlin et al., 2005; Cooks et al., 2006).

In addition to being essential for protein identification, MS technology is being used for quantitative proteomic profiling. Through the use of stable isotope-coded mass tags, differential quantitation of changes in peptides from control and experimental samples is possible. Quantitation of changes in global protein expression involves proteolytic or chemical labeling of peptides with isotope-coded mass tags prior to separation by HPLC. These labeling reagents are chemically identical; however, one label contains light isotope atoms and the other heavy isotope atoms. During proteolysis, enzymatic cleavage results in the incorporation of oxygen at the peptide carboxy-terminus. Exploiting this reaction, ^{18}O (heavy) and ^{16}O (light) isotopic oxygen labels can be used to differentially label two samples (Stewart et al., 2001; Ye et al., 2010). Other examples of isotope-coded reagents and their labeling strategies are listed in Table 10.1. In isotope tagging, peptides from a control sample are labeled with the light isotope and the peptides from the treated sample are labeled with the heavy isotope. After labeling, both samples are mixed together and fractionated using HPLC. When subjected to MS analysis, the mass spectrometer can distinguish between the two isotope-labeled peptide samples because a predictable mass difference will be observed between the control and experimental peptides. MS-based quantitation is then achieved by calculating the difference between the ion intensities of the light-labeled control peptide and the heavy-labeled experimental peptide samples (Fig. 10.1). From this data, differential displays of peptides that increase or decrease in response to a stimulus can be generated. These differential displays are commonly used to generate protein expression profiles or protein signature patterns that can be used in comparative toxicoproteomic investigations.

TABLE 10.1 Isotope-Coded Reagents Used for Chemical Labeling of Peptides

Reagent	Labeling Technique	Reference
ALICE	Thiol modification of cysteines	Qui et al. (2002)
AQUA	Synthetic internal standard peptide	Gerber et al. (2003)
ICAT	Iodoacetylation of cysteine	Gygi et al. (1999b)
iTRAQ	Modification of primary amines	Zieske (2006)
GIST	Acylation of primary amines	Ji et al. (2000)
MCAT	Guanidation of C-terminal lysine	Cagney and Emili (2002)
QUEST	Amidination of N-terminal lysine	Beardsley and Reilly (2003)

Bioinformatics Tools

Protein identification is accomplished by using computer search algorithms that correlate MS and MS/MS data with predicted amino acid sequences contained in protein or genome sequence databases. Even though several types of MS and MS/MS search engines have been created, databases that are used more frequently include MASCOT, SEQUEST, Spectrum Mill, X! Tandem, and Protein Prospector (Eng et al., 1994; Clauser et al., 1995; Perkins et al., 1999; Robertson and Beavis, 2004; Kapp et al., 2005). Database resources have also been created to probe

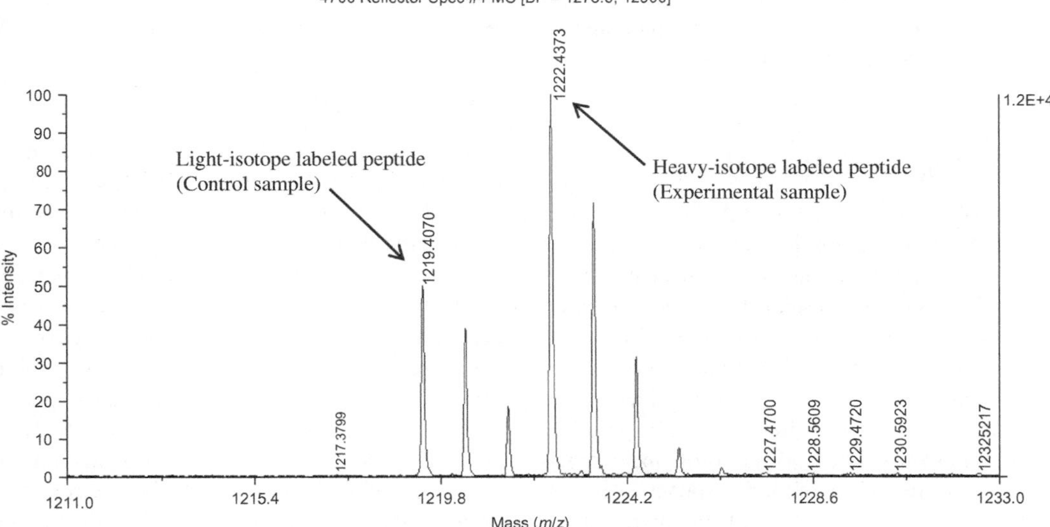

FIGURE 10.1 MALDI-TOF MS spectrum of GIST isotopically labeled peptides from control and experimental serum samples. Comparison of the relative ion intensities between the two peptides indicate that the peptide present in the experimental sample (at 1222.43 *m/z*) was present at a higher concentration when compared to the control sample (at 1219.40 *m/z*).

for posttranslational modifications on proteins and peptides. These database search engines include UniCarb-DB, for glycomics, and PHOSIDA 201, for common posttranslational modifications (Gnad et al., 2011; Hayes et al., 2011). Tox-Prot, a searchable toxin protein database, has been created that can be queried for most known animal protein toxins (Jungo and Bairoch, 2005).

Even though the computer algorithms designed for most bioinformatics databases are slightly different, their general approach to protein identification is similar. Database search engines compare the experimental precursor *m/z* ions from each MS/MS scan with hypothetical peptide *m/z* values from the database. Hypothetical peptide masses from the database that correspond with the experimental mass values are assigned probability scores. The proteins recognized with the highest scores are indicative of the best probable protein match to the experimental MS/MS data. Some bioinformatics tools assign *p*-values to the correlation scores, providing an additional means for evaluating credibility of protein matches.

Integrating MS technology with bioinformatics tools has become an indispensable tool in proteomics research. However, due to the overwhelming amounts of MS and MS/MS data generated from typical proteomics experiments, creating bioinformatics tools that adequately identify and characterize the data has been a tremendous challenge. Credible protein identification is reliant on successful interpretation of MS and MS/MS data. Unfortunately, data interpretation is often complicated by ion suppression, atypical MS/MS peptide fragmentation patterns, ill-defined universal standards for evaluating credible database matches and inability to define a single protein from one peptide spectrum (Kearney and Thibault, 2003). Additionally, variants of MS instrumentation are developing rapidly and the computer algorithms necessary to correlate the data from these next generation mass spectrometers with information contained in protein or genome sequence databases will continue to be a challenge.

PROTEOMICS APPLICATIONS IN DIAGNOSTIC TOXICOLOGY

The current objectives of toxicoproteomics in diagnostic toxicology is to define molecular mechanisms of toxicity, screen for drug toxicities and elucidate biomarkers or signature protein profiles in order to more accurately assess, predict, and diagnose toxicities (Kennedy, 2002; Guerreiro et al., 2003; Wetmore and Merrick, 2004). For decades, laboratories have relied on individual protein markers for assessing toxicity. However, some of these single biomarkers can be nonspecific and reflect protein leakage from tissues, as opposed to the direct effects of toxicants on the tissues alone (Plebani, 2005). Toxicities in biological systems are multifactorial and complex, emphasizing identification of multiple biomarkers for accurately diagnosing and classifying toxicity. This makes proteomics research in toxicologic evaluation appealing because these technologies are capable of globally profiling multiple proteins. Hence, the potential to better define molecular signatures of toxicity for clinical and diagnostic toxicology is becoming increasingly possible. Several proteomic applications have been applied to gain a better understanding of target organ toxicities, mechanisms of toxicity and biomarkers of exposure for a variety of toxicants.

Aquatic Toxicology and Pesticides

In veterinary toxicology, pesticide use and potential nontarget toxicity in aquatic organisms is always a concern. In order to gain a better understanding of the mechanisms of toxicity, changes in protein expression have been assessed in fish exposed to single or multiple pesticides. For example, proteomic analyses of proteins in brain responsive to methyl parathion in zebrafish (*Danio rerio*) have been investigated. In this study, it was found that six proteins, which were predominantly cytoplasmic proteins, significantly changed with methyl parathion exposure (Huang et al., 2011). The proteins most affected by methyl parathion are known to be involved in catalysis, binding, cell structure, and metabolic regulation. In another study in brains from male, flathead minnows (*Pimephales promelas*), protein expression was compared in fish exposed to permethrin, terbufos, or a binary mixture of both pesticides (Biales et al., 2011). In this study, 24 proteins changed with exposure to these pesticides when compared to controls. Some of the proteins identified are known to be associated with the cytoskeleton, glycolysis, hypoxia and the ubiquitin–proteasome system. The investigators also compared protein expression patterns in treated fish versus control fish. Interestingly, the permethrin protein expression pattern was distinguishable from that in the controls, enabling them to discriminate between the two treatment groups with 87.5% accuracy. When comparing the proteins identified in the aforementioned studies, the protein dihydropyrimidase-like 3 was downregulated in zebrafish exposed to methyl parathion; however, this protein was upregulated in the flathead minnows exposed to permethrin.

Since aquatic species can be affected by multiple stressors, a study was conducted in goldfish (*Carassius auratus*) in which 2-DGE was used to investigate changes in hepatic proteins after exposing the goldfish to pesticide mixtures and varying water temperatures. When compared to controls, or to goldfish exposed to one variable (pesticide mixtures or temperature changes), proteins that changed with the multiple stressors included those involved in cellular stress response, carbohydrate and lipid metabolism, and cell structure and cell death (Gandar et al., 2017). Overall, they noted that with increased temperature and pesticide exposure, there was deregulation of the cell cycle via apoptosis inhibition, a marked increase in proteins associated with oxidative stress, and a decrease in glucose formation in the liver. Therefore, the exposure to environmental cocktails of pesticides, in combination with increased water temperature, could affect the response of fish to pesticides when compared to exposure to pesticides alone.

Hepatotoxicity

Monitoring liver function is crucial in toxicologic evaluation. Hence, it is no surprise that toxicoproteomic experiments have been conducted to gain a better understanding of proteins that change with hepatotoxicity. For example, toxicoproteomics has been used to identify metabolic pathways affected by drug-induced cirrhosis in rat models. In these studies, thioacetamide and ethanol have both been shown to down-regulate proteins involved in oxidative stress and fatty acid β-oxidation pathways during early phases of cirrhosis (Low et al., 2004; Venkatraman et al., 2004). Ivermectin hepatotoxicity has been investigated in gilthead sea bream fish (*Sparus aurata*). Of the proteins that significantly changed, 30 proteins decreased and six proteins increased with exposure to ivermectin (Varo et al., 2010). The major hepatic proteins that changed were apoA-1 (lipid metabolism), β-globin, and ATP synthase subunit beta (oxidative stress response and regulation of energy).

Plasma protein biomarkers for drug-induced hepatotoxicity have also been revealed using proteomics techniques. In one study conducted to investigate plasma proteins that may correlate with acetaminophen hepatotoxicity, rats were given low (100 mg/kg) and high (1250 mg/kg) doses of acetaminophen and the liver proteins were analyzed using 2D-LC/MS/MS with $^{16}O/^{18}O$ isotope labeling (Gao et al., 2017). This study revealed 31 proteins that changed with liver toxicity; however, there was one protein that increased dramatically with liver damage, HMOX1 (heme oxygenase 1). The investigators were able to show that HMOX1 could be used as a potential plasma biomarker of liver damage.

Quantitative proteomics approaches have also been employed to study heavy metal-induced hepatotoxicity. Using 2D-DIGE, the toxic pathways by which chronic mercury hepatotoxicity occurs in aquatic organisms highlighted potential biomarkers for monitoring mercury in fish. When compared to controls, medaka fish treated with mercuric chloride (1 or 10 μg/mL) for 60 days had 45 hepatic proteins that were markedly changed. The hepatic proteins affected were related to mitochondrial function, cytoskeleton assembly, and oxidative stress (Wang et al., 2013).

Toxins

Valuable information regarding toxicological evaluation of venom ("venomics") has also been made possible through toxicoproteomic investigations. These investigations have been used to identify protein toxin components in venom, assess geographic venom variability and evaluate antivenin efficacy. In one study conducted in venom from the Asian forest scorpion (*Heterometrus petersii*), 10 families of venom peptides and proteins were identified. The proteins identified in the venom were potassium channel toxins, antimicrobial and cytolytic peptides, calcium channel toxins, La1-like peptides, phospholipase A2, serum proteases, acid phosphatases, and diuretic peptides (Ma et al., 2010). Comparative proteomic analysis of pit viper venom (*Bothrops atrox*) has been used to show geographic variation in venom phenotypes and to assess antivenin reactivity. The protein toxin phenotype in pit vipers from Colombia and Venezuela were recognized to be typical of the adult phenotype; whereas the toxin phenotype from Brazil resembled that of the juvenile snake (Calvete et al., 2011). The significance of this finding was relevant to the treatment of envenomation by this type of snake, as it was shown that the antivenins used for pit viper snake bites in these regions were more immunoreactive against the venom in the pit vipers with toxin phenotypes similar to juvenile snakes (Brazil region). Therefore, proteomics analyses of venoms have contributed to the development of improved antivenoms, termed "antivenomics," through identifying toxins that have poor or excellent immunoreactivity (Calvete et al., 2011; Utkin, 2017).

Other natural toxins examined using proteomics include mycotoxins. It is known that drought stress and high temperatures provide opportunistic conditions for fungal growth in corn and other susceptible crops (Guo et al., 2008). In an attempt to gain a better understanding of what makes certain corn crops more susceptible to aflatoxin contamination from *Aspergillus flavus*, a proteomic comparison of corn kernel proteins in resistant and susceptible crops was evaluated. Using 2-DGE and ESI/MS/MS, proteins were identified in corn kernels resistant to *A. flavus* that included proteins related to stress-tolerance (aldose reductase and glyoxalase 1 protein) and antifungal proteins T1 and PR10 (Chen et al., 2002). 2-DGE analysis of several different inbred lines of maize there were either more susceptible or resistant to *A. flavus* infection revealed that the presence of the pathogenesis-related proteins, PRm3 and chitinase in resistant maize lines (Bhatnagar-Mathur et al., 2015). These proteins are thought to be associated with higher antifungal activity in the silks in maize that is more resistant to *A. flavus* infection.

CONCLUDING REMARKS AND FUTURE DIRECTIONS

Recognition of the diagnostic accuracy of proteomics data and standardization of methodologies remain a challenge to proteomics researchers. Despite these concerns, toxicoproteomics has the potential to better define molecular mechanisms of toxicity and elucidate biomarkers or signature protein profiles for clinical and diagnostic toxicology. This technology promises to establish new guidelines for preventive and predictive toxicity, ultimately revolutionizing and redefining our future understanding of toxicology.

REFERENCES

Anderson, L., Seilhamer, J., 2005. A comparison of selected mRNA and protein abundances in human liver. Electrophoresis. 18 (3–4), 533–537.

Anderson, N.L., Anderson, N.G., 2002. The human plasma proteome. Mol. Cell Proteomics. 1, 311–326.

Babu, S., Song, E.J., Babar, S.M.E., et al., 2006. Capillary electrophoresis at the omics level: towards systems biology. Electrophoresis. 27, 97–110.

Bakhtiar, R., Guan, Z., 2006. Electron capture dissociation mass spectrometry in characterization of peptides and proteins. Biotechnol. Lett. 28, 1047–1059.

Beardsley, R.L., Reilly, J.P., 2003. Quantitation using enhanced signal tags: a technique for comparative proteomics. J. Proteome Res. 2, 15–21.

Bhatnagar-Mathur, P., Sunkara, S., Bhatnagar-Panwar, M., et al., 2015. Biotechnological advances for combating *Aspergillus flavus* and aflatoxin contamination in crops. Plant Sci. 234, 119–132.

Biales, A.D., Bencic, D.C., Flick, R.L., et al., 2011. Proteomic analysis of a model fish species exposed to individual pesticides and a binary mixture. Aquat. Toxicol. 101, 196–206.

Bondarenko, P.V., Chelius, D., Shaler, T.A., 2002. Identification and relative quantitation of protein mixtures by enzymatic digestion followed by capillary reversed-phase liquid chromatography-tandem mass spectrometry. Anal. Chem. 74, 4741–4749.

Cagney, G., Emili, A., 2002. De novo peptide sequencing and quantitative profiling of complex protein mixtures using mass-coded affinity tagging. Nat. Biotechnol. 20, 163–170.

Calvete, J.J., Sanz, L., Perez, A., et al., 2011. Snake population venomics and antivenomics of *Bothrops atrox*: paedomorphism along its transamazonian dispersal and implications of geographic venom variability on snakebite management. J. Proteomics. 74 (4), 510–527.

Chelius, D., Bondarenko, P.V., 2002. Quantitative profiling of proteins in complex mixtures using liquid chromatography and mass spectrometry. J. Proteome Res. 1, 317–323.

Chen, Z.Y., Brown, R.L., Damann, K.E., et al., 2002. Identification of unique or elevated levels of kernel proteins in aflatoxin-resistant maize genotypes through proteome analysis. Phytopathology. 92, 1084–1094.

Clauser, K.R., Hall, S.C., Smith, D.M., et al., 1995. Rapid mass spectrometric peptide sequencing and mass matching for characterization of human melanoma proteins isolated by two-dimensional PAGE. Proc. Natl. Acad. Sci. 92, 5067–5072.

Cooks, R.G., Ouyang, Z., Takats, Z., et al., 2006. Ambient mass spectrometry. Science. 311, 1566–1570.

Cretich, M., Damin, F., Pirri, G., et al., 2006. Protein and peptide arrays: recent trends and new directions. Biomol. Eng. 23, 77–88.

Davis, J.M., Giddings, J.C., 1985a. Statistical method for estimation of number of components from single complex chromatograms: theory, computer-based testing, and analysis of errors. Anal. Chem. 57, 2168–2177.

Davis, J.M., Giddings, J.C., 1985b. Statistical method for estimation of number of components from single complex chromatograms: application to experimental chromatograms. Anal. Chem. 57, 2178–2182.

Di Palma, S., Boersema, P.J., Heck, A.J., et al., 2011. Zwitterionic hydrophilic interaction liquid chromatography (ZIC-HILIC and ZIC-cHILIC) provide high resolution separation and increase sensitivity in proteome analysis. Anal. Chem. 83 (21), 8352–8356.

Eng, J.K., McCormack, A.L., Yates, J.R., 1994. An approach to correlate tandem mass spectral data of peptides with amino acid sequences in a protein database. J. Am. Soc. Mass Spectrom. 5, 976–989.

Espina, V., Woodhouse, E.C., Wulfkuhle, J., et al., 2004. Protein microarray detection strategies: focus on direct detection technologies. J. Immunol. Methods. 290, 121–133.

Fenn, J.B., Mann, M., Meng, C.K., et al., 1989. Electrospray ionization for mass spectrometry of large biomolecules. Science. 246, 64–71.

Gandar, A., Laffaille, P., Marty-Gasset, N., et al., 2017. Proteome response of fish under multiple stress exposure: Effects of pesticide mixtures and temperature increase. Aquat. Toxicol. 184, 61–77.

Gao, Y., Cao, Z., Yang, X., et al., 2017. Proteomic analysis of acetaminophen-induced hepatotoxicity and identification of heme oxygenase 1 as a potential plasma biomarker of liver injury. Proteomics Clin. Appl. 11, 1–17.

Gerber, S.A., Rush, J., Stemman, O., et al., 2003. Absolute quantification of proteins and phosphoproteins from cell lysates by tandem MS. Proc. Natl. Acad. Sci. 100 (12), 6940–6945.

Gnad, F., Gunawardena, J., Mann, M., 2011. PHOSIDA 2011: the post-translational modification database. Nucleic Acids Res. 39, D253–D260.

Goetz, H., Kuschel, M., Wulff, T., et al., 2004. Comparison of selected analytical techniques for protein sizing, quantitation and molecular weight determination. J. Biochem. Biophys. Methods. 60, 281–293.

Goheen, S.C., Gibbins, B.M., 2000. Protein losses in ion-exchange chromatography and hydrophobic interaction high-performance liquid chromatography. J. Chromatogr. A. 890, 73–80.

Görg, A., Obermaier, C., Boguth, G., et al., 2000. The current state of two-dimensional electrophoresis with immobilized pH gradients. Electrophoresis. 21, 1037–1053.

Görg, A., Weiss, W., Dunn, W.J., 2004. Current two-dimensional electrophoresis technology for proteomics. Proteomics. 4, 3665–3685.

Guerreiro, N., Staedtler, F., Grenet, O., et al., 2003. Toxicogenomics in drug development. Toxicol. Pathol. 31, 471–479.

Guo, B., Chen, Z.Y., Lee, R.D., et al., 2008. Drought stress and preharvest aflatoxin contamination in agricultural commodity: genetics, genomics and proteomics. J. Integr. Plant Biol. 50 (10), 1281–1291.

Gygi, S.P., Rochon, Y., Franza, B.R., et al., 1999a. Correlation between protein and mRNA abundance in yeast. Mol. Cell Biol. 19 (3), 1720–1730.

Gygi, S.P., Rist, B., Gerber, S.A., et al., 1999b. Quantitative analysis of complex protein mixtures using isotope-coded affinity tags. Nat. Biotechnol. 17, 994–999.

Hamdan, M., Righetti, P.G., 2002. Modern strategies for protein quantification in proteome analysis: advantages and limitations. Mass. Spectrom. Rev. 21, 287–302.

Hayes, C.A., Karlsson, N.G., Struwe, W.B., et al., 2011. UniCarb-DB: a database resource for glycomic discovery. Bioinformatics. 27 (9), 1343–1344.

Hillenkamp, F., Karas, M., Beavis, R.C., et al., 1991. Matrix-assisted laser desorption ionization mass-spectrometry of biopolymers. Anal. Chem. 63, 1139A–1202A.

Hopfgartner, G., Varesio, E., Tschäppät, V., et al., 2004. Triple quadrupole linear ion trap mass spectrometer for the analysis of small molecules and macromolecules. J. Mass Spectrom. 39, 845–855.

Hu, Q., Noll, R.J., Li, H., et al., 2005. The orbitrap: a new mass spectrometer. J. Mass Spectrom. 40, 430–433.

Huang, Q.Y., Huang, L., Huang, H.Q., 2011. Proteomic analysis of methyl parathion-responsive proteins in zebrafish (*Danio rerio*) brain. Comp. Biochem. Physiol. Part C. 153, 67–74.

Issaq, H.J., Chan, K.C., Janini, G.M., et al., 2005. Multidimensional separation of peptides for effective proteomic analysis. J. Chromatogr. B. 817, 35–47.

Ji, J., Chakraborty, A., Geng, M., et al., 2000. Strategy for qualitative and quantitative analysis in proteomics based on signature peptides. J. Chromatrogr. B. 745, 97–210.

Jungo, F., Bairoch, A., 2005. Tox-Prot, the toxin protein annotation program of the Swiss-Prot protein knowledgebase. Toxicon. 45, 293–301.

Kapp, E.A., Schütz, F., Connolly, L.M., et al., 2005. An evaluation, comparison, and accurate benchmarking of several publicly available MS/MS search algorithms: sensitivity and specificity analysis. Proteomics. 5, 3475–3490.

Karas, M., Hillenkamp, F., 1988. Laser desorption ionization of proteins with molecular masses exceeding 10,000 daltons. Anal. Chem. 60, 2299–2301.

Kawahashi, Y., Doi, N., Takashima, H., et al., 2003. In vitro protein microarrays for detecting protein-protein interactions: application of a new method for fluorescence labeling of proteins. Proteomics. 3, 1236–1243.

Kearney, P., Thibault, P., 2003. Bioinformatics meets proteomics – bridging the gap between mass spectrometry data analysis and cell biology. J. Bioinform. Comp. Biol. 1 (1), 183–200.

Kennedy, S., 2002. The role of proteomics in toxicology: identification of biomarkers of toxicity by protein expression analysis. Biomarkers. 7 (4), 269–290.

Kumble, K.D., 2003. Protein microarrays: new tools for pharmaceutical development. Anal. Bioanal. Chem. 377, 812–819.

Kuramitsu, Y., Hayashi, E., Okada, F., et al., 2010. Staining with highly sensitive Coomassie brilliant blue SeePico™ stain after Flamingo™ fluorescent gel stain is useful for cancer proteomic analysis by means of two-dimensional gel electrophoresis. Anticancer Res. 30 (10), 4001–4005.

Laughlin, B.C., Mulligan, C.C., Cooks, R.G., 2005. Atmospheric pressure ionization in a miniature mass spectrometer. Anal. Chem. 77, 2928–2939.

Levison, P.R., 2003. Large-scale ion exchange column chromatography of proteins comparison of different formats. J. Chromatogr. B. 790, 7–33.

Lina, Y., Shujuan, G., Yang, L., et al., 2011. Protein microarrays for systems biology. Acta Biochim. Biophys. Sin. 43 (3), 161–171.

Lopez, M.F., Berggren, K., Chernokalskaya, E., et al., 2000. A comparison of silver stain and SYPRO Ruby Protein Gel Stain with respect to protein detection in two-dimensional gels and identification by peptide mass profiling. Electrophoresis. 21, 3673–3683.

Low, T.Y., Leow, C.K., Salto-Tellez, M., et al., 2004. A proteomic analysis of thioacetamide-induced hepatotoxicity and cirrhosis in rat livers. Proteomics. 4, 3960–3974.

Ma, Y., Zhao, Y., Zhao, R., et al., 2010. Molecular diversity of toxic components from scorpion *Heterometrus petersii* venom revealed by proteomic and transcriptome analysis. Proteomics. 10 (13), 2471–2485.

MacBeath, G., Schreiber, S.L., 2000. Printing proteins as microarrays for high-throughput function determination. Science. 289, 1760–1763.

Mahn, A., Asenjo, J.A., 2005. Prediction of protein interaction in hydrophobic interaction chromatography. Biotechnol. Adv. 23, 359–368.

Mange, A., Chaurand, P., Perrochia, H., et al., 2009. Liquid chromatography-tandem and MALDI imaging mass spectrometry analysis of RCL2/CS100-fixed, paraffin-embedded tissues: proteomics evaluation of an alternative fixative for biomarker discovery. J. Proteome Res. 8 (12), 5619–5628.

Merchant, M., Weinberger, S.R., 2000. Recent advancements in surface-enhanced laser desorption/ionization-time of flight mass spectrometry. Electrophoresis. 21, 1164–1167.

Merchant, M.L., 2010. Mass spectrometry in chronic kidney disease research. Adv. Chronic Kidney Dis. 17 (6), 455–468.

Mirzaei, H., Regnier, F., 2005. Structure specific chromatographic selection in targeted proteomics. J. Chromatogr. B. 817, 23–34.

Mondal, K., Gupta, M.N., 2006. The affinity concept in bioseparation: evolving paradigms and expanding range of applications. Biomed. Eng. 23, 59–76.

Nielsen, U.B., Cardone, M.H., Sinskey, A.J., et al., 2003. Profiling receptor tyrosine kinase activation by using Ab microarrays. Proc. Natl. Acad. Sci. 100 (16), 9330–9335.

O'Connor, P.B., Pittman, J.L., Thomson, B.A., et al., 2006. A new hybrid electrospray Fourier transform mass spectrometer: design and performance characteristics. Rapid Commun. Mass Spectrom. 20, 259–266.

O'Farrell, P.H., 1975. High resolution two-dimensional electrophoresis of proteins. J. Biol. Chem. 250 (10), 4007–4021.

Ong, S., Pandey, A., 2001. An evaluation of the use of two-dimensional gel electrophoresis in proteomics. Biomed. Eng. 18, 195–205.

Otani, M., Taniguchi, T., Sakai, A., et al., 2011. Phosphoproteome profiling using a fluorescent phosphosensor dye in two-dimensional polyacrylamide gel electrophoresis. Appl. Biochem. Biotechnol. 164 (6), 804–818.

Perkins, D.N., Pappin, D.J., Creasy, D.M., et al., 1999. Probability-based protein identification by searching sequence databases using mass spectrometry data. Electrophoresis. 20, 3551–3567.

Plebani, M., 2005. Proteomics: the next revolution in laboratory medicine? Clin. Chim. Acta. 357, 113–122.

Qui, Y., Sousa, E.A., Hewick, R.M., et al., 2002. Acid-labile isotope-coded extractants: a class of reagents for quantitative mass spectrometric analysis of complex protein mixtures. Anal. Chem. 74, 4969–4979.

Robertson, C., Beavis, R.C., 2004. Tandem: matching proteins with mass spectra. Bioinformatics. 20, 1466–1467.

Stauber, J., MacAleese, L., Franck, J., et al., 2010. On-tissue protein identification and imaging by MALDI-ion mobility mass spectrometry. J. Am. Soc. Mass Spectrom. 21 (3), 338–347.

Stewart, I.I., Thomson, T., Figeys, D., 2001. 18O Labeling: a tool for proteomics. Rapid Commun. Mass Spectrom. 15, 2456–2465.

Sze, S.K., Ge, Y., Oh, H., et al., 2003. Plasma electron capture dissociation for the characterization of large proteins by top down mass spectrometry. Anal. Chem. 75 (7), 1599–1603.

Ünlü, M., Morgan, M.E., Minden, J.S., 1997. Difference gel electrophoresis. A single gel method for detecting changes in protein extracts. Electrophoresis. 18 (11), 2071–2077.

Utkin, Y.N., 2017. Modern trends in animal venom research – omics and nanomaterials. World J. Biol. Chem. 8 (1), 4–12.

Varo, I., Rigos, G., Navarro, J.C., et al., 2010. Effect of ivermectin on the liver of gilthead sea bream *Sparus aurata*: a proteomic approach. Chemosphere. 80 (5), 570–577.

Venkatraman, A., Landar, A., Davis, A.J., et al., 2004. Modification of the mitochondrial proteome in response to the stress of ethanol-dependent hepatotoxicity. J. Biol. Chem. 279 (21), 22092–22101.

Vlahou, A., Fountoulakis, M., 2005. Proteomic approaches in the search for disease markers. J. Chromatogr. B. 814, 11–19.

Wang, M., Wang, Y., Zhang, L., et al., 2013. Quantitative proteomic analysis reveals the mode-of-action for chronic mercury hepatotoxicity to marine medaka (*Oryzias melastigma*). Aquat. Toxicol. 130–131, 123–131.

Wetmore, B.A., Merrick, B.A., 2004. Toxicoproteomics: proteomics applied to toxicology and pathology. Toxicol. Pathol. 32, 619–624.

Wilson, C.R., Regnier, F.E., Knapp, D.W., et al., 2008. Glycoproteomic profiling of serum peptides in canine lymphoma and transitional cell carcinoma. Vet. Comp. Oncol. 6 (3), 171–181.

Wysocki, V.H., Resing, K.A., Zhang, Q., et al., 2005. Mass spectrometry of peptides and proteins. Methods. 35, 211–222.

Yates, J.R., Cociorva, D., Liao, L., et al., 2006. Performance of a linear ion trap-orbitrap hybrid for peptide analysis. Anal. Chem. 78, 493–500.

Ye, X., Luke, B.T., Johann Jr., D.J., et al., 2010. Optimized method for computing 18O/16O ratios of differentially stable-isotope labelled peptides in the context of postdigestion 18O exchange/labeling. Anal. Chem. 82 (13), 5878–5886.

Zhang, X., Fang, A., Riley, C.P., et al., 2010a. Multi-dimensional liquid chromatography in proteomics – a review. Anal. Chem. Acta. 664 (2), 101–113.

Zhang, H., Cui, W., Wen, J., et al., 2010b. Native electrospray and electron capture dissociation in FTICR mass spectrometry provide top-down sequencing of a protein complement in an intact protein assembly. J. Am. Soc. Mass Spectrom. 21 (12), 1966–1968.

Zhu, Q., Uttamchandani, M., Li, D., et al., 2003. Enzymatic profiling system in a small-molecule microarray. Organ. Lett. 5 (8), 1257–1260.

Zieske, L.R., 2006. A perspective on the use of iTRAQ™ reagent technology for protein complex and profiling studies. J. Exp. Bot. 57 (7), 1501–1508.

Chapter 11

Toxicology and the Law

Michael J. Murphy

INTRODUCTION

Much of the law of admissibility of scientific expert testimony has arisen from legal cases involving the discipline of toxicology. Consequently, toxicology has influenced the legal standards by which scientific expert testimony is admitted in a legal venue.[1] The occurrence of medical science in the courtroom has recently been reported in the introduction to the Reference Guide to Medical Testimony:[2]

> *Physicians are a common sight in today's courtroom. A survey of federal judges published in 2002 indicated that medical and mental health experts constituted more than 40% of the total number of testifying experts:*
>
> 1. *Medical evidence is a common element in product liability suits,*
> 2. *Workers' compensation disputes,*
> 3. *Medical malpractice suits, and*
> 4. *Personal injury cases.*
> 5. *Medical testimony may also be critical in certain kinds of criminal cases.*
> 6. *The goal of this reference guide is to introduce the basic concepts of diagnostic reasoning and clinical decision making, as well as the types of evidence that physicians use to make judgments as treating physicians or as experts retained by one of the parties in a case.*

Veterinarians and veterinary specialists, including toxicologists, are also called upon to provide medical evidence. Justice Breyer has stated "[w]e also need to know how best to prepare a scientist for the sometimes hostile legal environment that arises during depositions and cross-examination."[3] Hopefully this chapter can be at least partially useful preparation.

This chapter uses a hypothetical example of legal issues that may arise in an animal toxicosis case to illustrate application of the law. It is intended to introduce toxicologists and other scientists to a broad overview of some of the legal issues that may arise when a medical case becomes a "legal case." This chapter is not, and is not intended to be, a comprehensive review of the law. Neither is it intended to provide an outline of steps to take for a particular case in a particular jurisdiction or to provide any legal advice.[4]

This chapter primarily relies on the Federal Rules of Evidence, and limited case law, to identify issues[5] that may arise when the findings of a medical diagnosis are used in the courtroom. It focuses on the admissibility of expert testimony in a legal proceeding. However, the reasons for conducting toxicology analyses, jurisdiction, standard of proof, and evidence are briefly summarized to provide context for the role of expert testimony. The chapter concludes with some questions one may contemplate when analyzing a toxicology case having "legal" implications.

1. Venue. The particular county, or geographical area, in which a court with jurisdiction may hear and determine a case. Black's Law Dictionary.
2. "Reference Guide on Medical Testimony--John B. Wong, Lawrence O. Gostin, and Oscar A. Cabrera." National Research Council. 2011. Reference Manual on Scientific Evidence: Third Edition. Washington, DC: The National Academies Press. doi: 10.17226/13163.
3. "Introduction--Stephen Breyer." National Research Council. 2011. Reference Manual on Scientific Evidence: Third Edition. Washington, DC: The National Academies Press. doi: 10.17226/13163. See also Laura L. Hooper et al., Neutral Science Panels: Two Examples of Panels of Court-Appointed Experts in the Breast Implants Product Liability Litigation 93–98 (Federal Judicial Center 2001); Barbara S. Hulka et al., Experience of a Scientific Panel Formed to Advise the Federal Judiciary on Silicone Breast Implants, 342 New Eng. J. Med. 812 (2000).
4. Jurisdiction. It is the power of the court to decide a matter in controversy and presupposes the existence of a duly constituted court with control over the subject matter and the parties.
5. Issue. A single, certain, and material point, deduced by the allegations and pleadings of the parties, which is affirmed on the one side and denied on the other.

Veterinary Toxicology. DOI: http://dx.doi.org/10.1016/B978-0-12-811410-0.00011-8

REASONS FOR CONDUCTING TOXICOLOGY ANALYSES

Toxicology has been defined as "the scientific study of adverse effects of chemicals on living organisms."[Eaton] A toxicologist is one trained to examine the nature of those effects and assess the probability of their occurrence.[Ibid] Exposure, dose response, and variability of that response are fundamental principles in the science of toxicology.[Ibid] A showing that the toxicologist offered as an expert witness has applied these fundamental principles to the facts of the case at hand will likely be useful in the determination of whether toxicologist's testimony will or will not be admissible as evidence. The factors that the court uses to make this determination are discussed in the expert witness section at the end of this chapter.

A toxicologist relies on analytical toxicology analyses in many toxicology cases. In most instances, it is known at the time the sample is submitted for analytical chemistry analysis, that the results of that analysis may be used for legal purposes. Racing chemistry laboratories are one example in the veterinary profession where it is known from the outset that the results of the analytical chemistry testing performed will be used in a legal or regulatory enforcement setting. In some instances however, the purpose to which the results will be applied is not known, or perhaps that purpose changes after the testing is completed.

When the Reason for Testing the Sample Is Known

Samples are analyzed for the presence of chemical toxins for many reasons and in many settings. Analyses may take place in academic, governmental, or private laboratories. Analyses performed in these laboratories may each serve a different purpose, such as research, enforcement actions, preclinical or other regulatory testing, clinical diagnoses, or other purposes.

Toxicology analyses in academic settings are primarily conducted to support one's research or scholarly efforts. One example is the development of new analytical methods. Another example is the characterization of adverse effects of a particular dose of a particular chemical in a given species. Similarly, researchers may observe the clinical signs and adverse effects of animals exposed to chemicals, then compile these effects in retrospective or prospective case reports in the peer-reviewed literature. Such literature may be useful to support a general causation[6] argument in a legal case. However, the medical case itself, or even the analyses performed on that medical case, may not be admissible in court because of insufficient documentation supporting authenticity. Other laboratories may provide such documentation.

Veterinary diagnostic laboratories normally have some government support to assist in the clinical diagnosis of diseased animals. Such analyses are normally aimed at assisting in the determination of whether an animal may, or may not, have been exposed to a particular chemical, and if so, whether the animal has, or has not, experienced a toxicosis as a result of that exposure. These chemical analyses may give qualitative, semiquantitative, or quantitative results.

Many contemporary analytical chemistry procedures performed in each of the above-mentioned laboratory types allow detection of the presence of chemicals in biological samples that represent only "background" or "normal" exposure to that chemical. One example is micronutrients, such as vitamins A and E, copper, iron, magnesium, selenium, and zinc. Similarly, lead, and with some methods arsenic, may be detected at "background" concentrations in blood, liver, or kidney by many analytical toxicology methods available today. Consequently, the detection of the chemical is not "diagnostic" for toxicosis from that chemical, but merely indicates exposure. Information beyond the concentration of a chemical in tissues is often required to reach a toxicosis diagnosis. The distinction between "exposure to" and "toxicosis from" exposure to a chemical is fundamentally the practice of veterinary toxicology.

Samples are received from many sources. Most diagnostic laboratories accept samples from veterinarians, animal owners, animal industries, state agencies, and others. The circumstances of the collection and handling of the sample prior to submission in the diagnostic laboratory is rarely known with certainty. Similarly, routine protocols in a diagnostic laboratory may be different from those in an enforcement laboratory, particularly with respect to sample tracking, documentation, and disposal.

Some government and some private laboratories focus on performing chemical analyses in support of legal or regulatory enforcement actions. Examples of such laboratories include racing chemistry laboratories, and State or Federal Departments of Agriculture or Health. Many of these laboratories have inspectors who insure proper sample collection and transport to the laboratory. In addition, sample tracking, control, retention, and disposal are generally better documented in laboratories devoted to enforcement action, than those devoted to research or routine diagnostic testing. The analytical methods used in an enforcement setting have often have been validated by AOACI,[7] or a similar entity. This validation often

6. Causation. The fact of being the cause of something produced or of happening. The act by which an effect is produced.

7. Association of Official Analytical Chemists International

demonstrates that the method has been shown to be reliable in multiple laboratories for quantifying the concentration of an analyte, or a group of analytes, in a specific matrix.

The analytical methods useful in a diagnostic setting may be different from those that are useful in an enforcement or research setting. The analytical methods used to support a diagnostic case are often influenced by cost and turn-around-time. On the other hand, those in an enforcement setting may be more influenced by the reliability of the results reported. These factors directly and indirectly influence the collection of the original sample, tracking of the sample in the laboratory, sample retention, document retention, and sample disposal protocols. Protocols appropriate for the development of a method in a research laboratory may not be appropriate for use in an enforcement setting. These factors should be taken into account, and samples sent to the appropriate laboratory, when the reason for the analysis is known. However, the reason is not always known.

When the Reason for Testing the Sample Is Not Known or Changes After Testing

Problems are more likely to occur if the purpose for which the sample is tested is not known at the time of sample collection and testing, or changes after the testing has been completed. These problems may give rise to angst on the part of the toxicologist, counsel, and others. This angst may occur if sample collection, tracking, analysis, and interpretation, have not been documented in a way that supports proof of reliability in a legal venue. Questions of authenticity and reliability are more likely to arise in analyses performed in a research, routine clinic, or diagnostic laboratory, setting than those collected and performed by enforcement personnel. Medical samples submitted and tested for one purpose, may not be reliable if used for another purpose. In short, the lack of sample tracking or chain of custody documentation may seriously erode the admissibility of some laboratory results. A diagnosis may not be supported without laboratory results and a legal case may not succeed without the diagnosis. Put more bluntly, insufficient sample collection, retention, and chain of custody documentation may become a problem for a plaintiff or prosecutor in a legal venue. A hypothetical case may help illustrate the application of a number of the following legal concepts.

Hypothetical Case

A hypothetical individual employee of a feed additive manufacturer intentionally adds a foreign chemical to a feed premix during a step in the manufacturing process. The feed premix is distributed to many states. Many local mills purchase the premix and incorporate it into feed in appropriate amounts. The mill then delivers that feed to its customers—animal owners. These animal owners offer that finished feed to their animals in appropriate amounts. These animals ingest the feed then develop adverse effects. An adverse effect in one of the animals is death. An animal that died after ingesting this feed is submitted to a local diagnostic laboratory by the animal owner. The owner of the animal has not made any association between the new feed and the death of the animal, so the feed is not delivered when the animal is, and the new feed delivery is not part of the history provided to the diagnostic laboratory. The laboratory does a routine necropsy and case work up. A feed additive is mentioned to the animal owner as one of the possible differential diagnostic causes for the lesions seen at necropsy and associated analytical chemistry testing. The owner then takes a grab sample of feed out of the total mixed ration mixer and has her teenager drive the feed sample to the veterinary diagnostic laboratory. The chemical is detected in the feed at concentrations sufficiently high to cause the lesions observed in the dead animal.

Various types of claims[8] could arise from this case. The results of diagnostic testing may be offered as fact by the animal owner, feed manufacturer, state and federal agencies, or some combination thereof, against one or more parties. An insurance claim, and government enforcement action, are discussed very briefly before continuing with issues that may arise in civil or criminal litigation.[9]

The results of a routine diagnostic case may now be offered as fact in a claim. The animal owner will claim that the feed provided by the distributor caused the toxicosis experienced by the owner's animals. The animal owner may file a claim with the distributor of the feed for the harm done to her animals. The distributor, or the distributor's insurance company, may settle the claim with the animal owner if all agree. If all do not agree, a civil suit may be filed. The issues that arise in the civil suit are discussed in the next section.

The dispute[10] between the animal owner and the feed distributor involve private parties. The case may also give rise to an enforcement action. These actions may be on the part of one or more agencies in one or more states,

8. Claim. A cause of action. To demand as one's own or as one's right, to assert, to urge, to insist. Means by or through which claimant obtains possession or enjoyment or privilege or thing.

9. Litigation. A lawsuit. Legal action, including all proceedings therein. Contest in a court of law for the purpose of enforcing a right or seeking a remedy.

10. Dispute. A conflict or controversy, a conflict of claims or rights, an assertion of a right, claim, of demand on one side, met by contrary claims or allegations on the other.

the federal government, or any combination of state and federal government. One or more agencies of the state in which the animal was harmed may have statutory authority to protect the health of animals, humans, or both. These agencies may include the State Department of Agriculture, the State Department of Health, the State Department of Natural Resources, the State Board of Animal Health, or other similar agencies. A state agency may choose to take enforcement action against the feed distributor, premix manufacturer, or both, in order to protect the health of animals, humans, or both in its state.

The state agency may collect its own samples and perform its own analyses prior to taking enforcement action. The agency may determine that the concentration of chemical in the feed is greater than a published tolerance or action level for that chemical in that feed. This agency action may end with a fine, recall, or other administrative action, if both sides agree.

If both sides do not agree, the feed distributor and premix manufacturer may "appeal" the agency's decision. This appeal may go to an administrative law judge, or a similar official within, or outside, the agency, depending on the administrative structure of that particular agency. If the feed manufacturer or premix manufacturer agrees with the ruling of the administrative law judge, the dispute is finished. If all do not agree, the distributor or manufacturer of the feed may choose to appeal the decision of the administrative law judge to a district civil court. This may put the dispute in a venue similar to a civil suit as discussed below.

Agencies are given deference at the district court level, making this an increasingly difficult, but not insurmountable, argument to win. The specialty of administrative law is devoted to the details of administrative procedure that arises in such actions. Administrative law is beyond the scope of this chapter.

Federal agencies may also have an interest in the animal case. The Federal Food and Drug Administration (FDA) may have an interest in the case because the feed additive impacted interstate commerce when it crossed state lines, and impacted the health of the public when it caused toxicosis of a food animal. The FDA has authority to protect the public health and has authority to take administrative action against the manufacturer of the feed similar to that discussed for the state agencies above in that protection of the public's health.

Although agency decisions are normally given deference in the courtroom, regulations developed by agencies may not always address the issue of causation. Agency regulations are often promulgated to protect populations rather than individuals.[11] The affect on an individual referred to as specific causation is discussed in Section VII below. The distinction between enforcement actions taken by agencies to benefit the public as a whole and legally admissible specific causation in an individual animal is not always appreciated.

This distinction may be illustrated by a hypothetical example. A bulk tank load of milk is tested in the receiving bay and found to be positive for the presence of beta-lactam antibiotics using a test kit marketed and validated for this purpose. The entire load of milk is dumped, and the producer whose individual sample is positive is charged for the load of milk. Paying for the tanker load of milk in this situation is a contractual agreement between the milk producer and the bulk milk buyer.

The test kit is approved and validated for use in administrative action. That action is to assist in the public policy of preventing exposure of humans to beta-lactam antibiotics to prevent allergic reactions, and to reduce the likelihood of developing strains of bacteria that are pathogenic to humans and resistant to beta-lactam antibiotics. The test kit is sufficient to support the contractual agreement and perhaps administrative action of preventing these antibiotics from entering the human food supply.

The test kit result may not be sufficient, however, for litigation aimed at prosecuting one for the source of the beta-lactam. Further analytical chemistry analysis may be required to distinguish, penicillic acid, from penicillin G from, ticarcillin, as an extreme example. This distinction may be important because of the implication raised as to the potential source of the antibiotic in the bulk tank: feed, versus a treated cow, versus "spiking" the bulk tank. In short, a test that is entirely acceptable for contractual agreement or agency action may not be acceptable for a specific type of litigation. This concept is expanded upon in the section on specific causation below. See Dr. Bright's chapter on Regulatory Veterinary Medicine for a further discussion of agency issues.

The results of diagnostic testing may rarely be offered as fact in a criminal case. Animal poisoning cases have rarely risen to the level of criminal action. The addition of the chemical to the feed with the intention of causing a toxicosis may be a crime based on animal cruelty or chemical terrorism statutes. The executive branch of government may then choose to prosecute the case. The state, often through its Attorney General's office, may choose to prosecute under an animal cruelty statute. Similarly, the Department of Justice, may file criminal prosecution charges if the act is considered to be one of chemical terrorism. In these instances the state or federal government is a direct party in the case.

This discussion of legal venue is not exhaustive. The purpose of this section is merely to indicate how a routine clinical or diagnostic case could become involved in a variety of legal venues including, insurance claims,

11. See e.g. *Troy Corp* , *AFL-CIO*, and *Simpson*.

administrative action, civil, or criminal litigation at the state or federal levels.

In summary, those samples used for the purpose known at the time of submission to a laboratory can, with reasonable care, be handled, analyzed, interpreted, and stored in a manner consistent with that purpose. Angst may arise on the part of the animal owner, veterinarian, laboratory personnel, counsel, and others, in those instances where the application of results of testing are used in a venue not anticipated at the time of sample collection and analysis, particularly in those laboratories not accustomed to litigation work. This angst may rise when the documentation of laboratory results is found to not be sufficiently authentic or reliable to support a "legal" case. The importance of authenticity and reliability are discussed in the evidence section below, immediately after a brief discussion of jurisdiction and standard of "proof."

JURISDICTION: WHAT ARE THE RULES AND WHO DECIDES THE WINNER ?

The parties have met, discussed, and agreed to disagree on reaching a settlement[12] on the feed claim so they decide to take the case "to court." The owner of the animals will normally be the plaintiff,[13] and the distributor of the feed will normally be the defendant,[14] in this dispute. The manufacturer of the premix may also be named as a defendant. The animal owner may be a natural person or may have formed a legal entity[15] for example a family farm corporation. The feed manufacturer and premix manufacturer may be businesses organized as sole proprietorships, partnerships, corporations, or other legal entities.

A question arises as to "which court" will decide the dispute. The state and federal governments already have authority to rule on disputes between citizens. This authority ultimately arises from their respective constitutions. State constitutions most commonly delegate authority to the state judicial system to enforce the laws passed by the state legislature. Many state judicial systems have a three tiered structure composed of district courts, courts of appeals, and a supreme court, each with increasing authority. Similarly, the federal constitution authorizes the federal judicial system, which has district courts, courts of appeals, and the U.S. Supreme Court.

Most civil suits that are filed in the United States do not actually go to trial. A settlement is reached in the vast majority of such cases. This settlement may be reached by the parties on their own, after mediation or arbitration, or even after litigation has begun, but before a judgment is entered.

Mediation and arbitration are two forms of "alternative dispute resolution" (ADR). An outcome reached after ADR may, or may not, be disputed later "in court" depending on the final agreement of the parties in the ADR process. Judges often encourage ADR even when civil litigation is filed. Authority may be given by contract. Disputing parties may have agreed to not litigate at all but rather to use ADR. ADR is increasingly used to settle disputes between companies because it can be faster and cheaper than litigation, and because both parties have more control over the outcome of the dispute. Two parties who agree to submit themselves to ADR must grant authority to the mediator or arbitrator at the outset of the deliberation by way of contract. This authority prevails for as long as the contract between the parties is in force. Authority over citizens already exists for government.[16]

Parties with an ongoing relationship may have made a contractual agreement to argue any disputes that arise under that contract according to the laws of a particular state. For example, the manufacturer of the feed additive and the manufacturer of the final feed may have agreed to argue any dispute they may have under that contract according to the laws of X. One reason for this may be that both parties agree that the cost of arguing jurisdiction for a distributor with outlets in many states, and a manufacturer with plants in many states, is not in the economic best interest of either company.

The parties will need to decide on the state in which the dispute—lawsuit—will be litigated if they have not already made this decision by prior contract. Individuals, and particularly companies, may be citizens of more than one jurisdiction. Consequently, parties may need to decide which judicial system they choose to "sue" the case in. This decision may influence the outcome of the dispute because of differences in laws on a particular issue between states. Similarly, federal law on a particular point may be different than that of state law on arguably the same point, so one party may prefer to argue in federal court and the other in state court. The choice of venue may then become a significant part of the dispute that must be decided before the merits of the case can be

12. Settlement. Payment or satisfaction. In legal parlance, implies meeting of the minds or parties to transaction or controversy, an adjustment of differences or accounts, a coming to an agreement.

13. Plaintiff. A person who brings an action; the party who complains or sues in a civil action and is so named on the record. A person who seeks remedial relief.

14. Defendant. The person defending or denying; the party against whom relief or recovery is sought in an action or suit to the accused in a criminal case.

15. Entity. A real being. An organization or being that possesses separate existence for tax purposes.

16. See the jurisdiction discussion below.

argued. This jurisdictional decision may be made by the judge in the venue where the case was originally filed.

Each state has rules governing the procedures to be followed in conducting a civil trial and procedures to be followed in conducting a criminal trial. Although these procedural rules may have many similarities between states, they may not be uniform across all states. The federal rules are more consistent nationwide.

The federal judicial system also has rules governing civil procedure and those governing criminal procedure. These rules are the same across states, although they may be interpreted differently in different federal judicial districts in case law. In short, administrative rules guide administrative actions, state rules guide state civil and state criminal actions, and federal rules guide federal civil and criminal actions.

In our hypothetical example, the manufacturer of the premix and the manufacturer of the feed may have agreed to argue any disputes that arise under their business contract according to the laws of state X. The animal owner who chooses to sue the manufacturer of the feed may choose to sue in state court in the state in which the owner fed the feed to their animal, or perhaps in the federal court representing the same geographic area. One argument that may be used to argue that the case belongs in the federal court system is that the feed crossed state lines and therefore impacted interstate commerce. Other elements that may be required to establish federal jurisdiction are beyond the scope of this chapter.

A judgment will be entered by the judge if the dispute goes all the way through trial. Thus the animal owner may receive compensation at the insurance claim, settlement, or judgment level of this dispute if the animal owner prevails.

The point of this section is primarily to indicate that the procedures by which the dispute is handled may be different between states for an insurance claim, arbitration, mediation, or litigation. These distinctions between state court systems are beyond the scope of this chapter. On the other hand, the federal judicial system has procedures that are generally applied across the country. These procedures are more similar nationwide, so they are described below to indicate some procedural issues that may arise in toxicology cases. Although many disputes involving animal toxicoses are not tried in federal courts, the federal procedural rules provided below illustrate considerations that are likely to be similar across the country.

STANDARD OF PROOF: HOW SURE DO I NEED TO BE?

One party needs to persuade the other party once a dispute develops. This need is normally referred to as the burden of persuasion in a legal setting.[17,18,19] The burden of persuasion is colloquially referred to as a "burden of proof"—a phrase toxicologists may find familiar. This burden of persuasion is different in civil cases than it is in criminal cases. Both legal burdens may be different than that of a routine medical diagnosis. The level of medical certainty needed to treat is often illustrated by quoting the Hippocratic Oath "first do no harm." The degree of medical certainty required to treat a disease may only be that needed to give appropriate general and supportive treatment, but not that which would be required to reach an etiological diagnosis. Reaching an etiological diagnosis to any degree of medical certainty is not always done in clinical practice.

Similarly, routine cases in a diagnostic laboratory may not reach an etiological diagnosis to any degree of medical certainty either. In many instances reaching an etiological diagnosis is limited by time, cost, and the needs of the animal owner and veterinarian. This need may be merely to have guidance for providing supportive treatment. Other limits on the ability to provide an etiological diagnosis may be the available samples, the condition of the samples, the willingness of the owner to spend the money required to reach such a diagnosis, and other factors.

17. ARTICLE III. PRESUMPTIONS IN CIVIL ACTIONS AND PROCEEDINGS
Rule 301. Presumptions in General in Civil Actions and Proceedings
In all civil actions and proceedings not otherwise provided for by Act of Congress or by these rules, a presumption imposes on the party against whom it is directed the burden of going forward with evidence to rebut or meet the presumption, but does not shift to such party the burden of proof in the sense of the risk of nonpersuasion, which remains throughout the trial upon the party on whom it was originally cast.

18. Rule 302. Applicability of State Law in Civil Actions and Proceedings
In civil actions and proceedings, the effect of a presumption respecting a fact which is an element of a claim or defense as to which State law supplies the rule of decision is determined in accordance with State law.

19. Rule 1101. Applicability of Rules
(a) Courts and judges.—These rules apply to the United States district courts, the District Court of Guam, the District Court of the Virgin Islands, the District Court for the Northern Mariana Islands, the United States courts of appeals, the United States Claims Court, and to United States bankruptcy judges and United States magistrate judges, in the actions, cases, and proceedings and to the extent hereinafter set forth. The terms ''judge'' and ''court'' in these rules include United States bankruptcy judges and United States magistrate judges.
(b) Proceedings generally.—These rules apply generally to civil actions and proceedings, including admiralty and maritime cases, to criminal cases and proceedings, to contempt proceedings except those in which the court may act summarily, and to proceedings and cases under title 11, United States Code.

This distinction between a medical diagnosis and a "legal" diagnosis is appreciated by the court system. This distinction is stated for example in *Wynacht*:

> *There is a fundamental distinction between Dr. Z...'s ability to render a medical diagnosis based on clinical experience and her ability to render an opinion on causation of W.'s injuries. Beckman apparently does not dispute, and the Court does not question, that Dr. Z is an experienced physician, qualified to diagnose medical conditions and treat patients. The ability to diagnose medical conditions is not remotely the same, however, as the ability to deduce, delineate, and describe, in a scientifically reliable manner, the causes of these medical conditions.* Wynacht v. Beckman Instruments, Inc. *113 F. Supp. 2d 1205, 1209 (E.D. Tenn. 2000).*

In short, the diagnosis reached in a routine medical clinic is not always sufficient to meet a legal burden of persuasion. Similarly, a diagnosis reached in a routine veterinary clinic may not meet this burden either.

The legal burden of persuasion is different in civil and criminal cases. The burden in civil cases is often a preponderance of the evidence or clear and convincing evidence. A preponderance of the evidence is sometimes referred to as "more likely than not." Juries are sometimes instructed to consider a 51% persuasion standard. In a civil case, the plaintiff has the burden of persuading the finder of fact—judge or jury—that his or her claim is valid with a preponderance of the evidence. Similarly, the defense has the burden of persuading the finder of fact that their defense is valid with a preponderance of the evidence.

The burden of persuasion in criminal cases is much higher. Here, the burden of persuasion is often referred to as "beyond a reasonable doubt." The prosecutor has the burden of persuading the fact finder—judge or jury—beyond a reasonable doubt, that the crime was committed by the defendant. Conversely, the defendant raises "reasonable doubt" that the prosecution has met this burden. The merits of both civil and criminal cases are argued based on evidence. Some evidence will require interpretation. Interpretation of facts is one role of experts. The role and types of evidence follow.

EVIDENCE

Legal cases are decided based on an application of the law to the facts of a particular case. A dispute about facts themselves or interpretation of those facts arises in many legal cases. Disputes of fact are decided by the trier of fact. The trier of fact is the judge in a bench trial. The trier of fact is the jury in a jury trial. The trier of fact learns of these facts largely, if not entirely, through evidence.

All facts are not admissible as evidence. The judge must determine which facts are admissible as evidence and which are not admissible as evidence as a preliminary matter. Specifically, the judge must determine "the qualifications of a person to be a witness," and "the admissibility of evidence."Rule 104, (a) The weight and credibility of the evidence is not determined at this preliminary stage. Rather "evidence relevant to weight or credibility" is normally "introduce[d] before the jury." Rule 104, (e)

A major factor used to determine the admissibility of evidence is relevance. "Relevant evidence" and "material fact" are two phrases that are often used synonymously. "Relevant evidence" is "evidence having any tendency to make the existence of any fact that is of consequence to the determination of the action more probable or less probable than it would be without the evidence." Rule 401 "[A]ll relevant evidence is admissible" with few exceptions. Rule 401 "Evidence which is not relevant is not admissible." Rule 402 For example, testimony that the sky is blue may not be admitted as relevant, because the color of the sky has no tendency to indicate that the feed did, or did not, cause the toxicosis in the animals.

The judge decides which facts are admissible as evidence and which are not. The factors that influence the judge's decision on admissibility vary with the type of fact. Documents, specimens and testimony are three sources of fact that a party may desire to enter into evidence in toxicology cases.

Documents

Documents require authentication before they can be considered as evidence. Document authentication is of increasing interest in many laboratories revisiting record retention procedures. Authentication of documents is discussed in Rule 901 of the Federal Rules of Evidence.[20] Subsections of this rule specify the procedure for authenticating public[21] or ancient[22] documents. A laboratory will likely have additional influence on its record keeping. For example, veterinary diagnostic laboratories are adopting ISO standards, contract research laboratories adhere

20. Rule 901 "The requirement of authentication or identification as a condition precedent to admissibility is satisfied by evidence sufficient to support a finding that the matter in question is what its proponent claims."

21. Rule 901 (7). "Evidence that a writing authorized by law to be recorded or filed and in fact recorded or filed in a public office, or a purported public record, report, statement, or data compilation, in any form, is from the public office where items of this nature are kept."

22. Rule 901(8). "Evidence that a document or data compilation, in any form, (A) is in such condition as to create no suspicion concerning its authenticity, (B) was in a place where it, if authentic, would likely be, and © has been in existence 20 years or more at the time it is offered."

to Good Laboratory Practice standards,[23] and many state agencies have state specific data practices requirements. While the specific requirements may vary, the general purpose is to authenticate the accuracy of the document produced, such as a final report.

The case report and the documents supporting that case report may be required to authenticate that report in a legal proceeding. Authentication of case documents is one reason that many laboratories have established record retention procedures. A document and its underlying support may be retained for 7 years in some diagnostic laboratories. The specimens themselves are also important in these proceedings.

Specimens

Specimens are often relevant in toxicology cases. Toxicologists are well aware of the importance of accurate sample identification to establish the relevance of the results of testing a particular sample. Laboratories involved in racing chemistry, regulatory enforcement, GLP studies or cGMP analyses often have significant sample tracking documents to establish that the result of a test can be tracked to a specific original specimen or sample. These sample tracking or chain of custody documents are often needed to establish that the sample tested does, in fact, relate to the case report. The absence of sample tracking, or appropriate chain of custody data, may eviscerate submission of the report of that testing as evidence in a case. The federal judicial system is aware of this as well. It considers as relevant evidence "comparison by the trier of fact or by expert witnesses with specimens which have been authenticated." Rule 901, (3) Split sample testing in racing chemistry laboratories may be an example of comparison by an expert witness with authenticated samples. Such split sample testing may also be desirable in toxicology cases that reach an insurance claim, civil or criminal case level.

Toxicologists and analytical chemists are aware of the potential for different results when different analytical methods are used. This awareness has given rise over the years to recognition of the need to "validate" tests and test results. The federal judicial system is also aware of this need. It requires "[e]vidence describing a process or system used to produce a result and showing that the process or system produces an accurate result." Rule 901, (9) AOACI is an example of an entity that may validate an analytical method for a particular matrix. Normally the plaintiff has the burden of persuading the judge that the analytical results go with the correct sample, and the results of that sample's testing are on the correct report. Authenticating sample results for such proceedings is one reason for standard operating procedures, quality assurance samples, method validation, split sample testing, and other such procedures in laboratories.

Analytical toxicologists know the limits of interpretation of the results of a given test. However, some who see these reports may not. So toxicologists may take care in the wording of interpretive comments made.

Testimony

Testimony is a third means of introducing evidence. Testimony is often gathered during the discovery portion of a legal case by taking the deposition of witnesses. Testimony may also be given orally at trial. Witnesses are under oath both at the deposition and at trial. Testimony given in a deposition may be entered into evidence at trial. This is sometimes done because the witness is not available for the trial date. The same person on the same subject may give testimony in a deposition, then again at trial.

Testimony is given by both "lay" witnesses and expert witnesses. Admission of testimony from a lay witness is normally evaluated differently than that of an expert witness. A lay witness must have personal knowledge of the facts to which she or he is testifying. Specifically, "[a] witness may not testify to a matter unless evidence is introduced sufficient to support a finding that the witness has personal knowledge of the matter. Evidence to prove personal knowledge may, but need not, consist of the witness' own testimony. . . ." Rule 602

Lay witnesses must testify to their personal knowledge. This personal knowledge is their recollection of the event. For example, the animal owner in our hypothetical example may testify that she did purchase the feed, that she fed it to her animals, that she observed certain clinical signs including death in her animal(s), and that she delivered a dead animal to the veterinary diagnostic laboratory.

The animal owner may be cross examined to help verify details of the events. The animal owner's recollection may be refreshed by referring to a written document, for example, pursuant to Rule 612.[24]

23. 21 CFR 58

24. "Except as otherwise provided in criminal proceedings by section 3500 of title 18, United States Code, if a witness uses a writing to refresh memory for the purpose of testifying, either—
(1) while testifying, or
(2) before testifying, if the court in its discretion determines it is necessary in the interests of justice,
an adverse party is entitled to have the writing produced at the hearing, to inspect it, to cross-examine the witness thereon, and to introduce in evidence those portions which relate to the testimony of the witness. ... If a writing is not produced or delivered pursuant to order under this rule, the court shall make any order justice requires, except that in criminal cases when the prosecution elects not to comply, the order shall be one striking the testimony or, if the court in its discretion determines that the interests of justice so require, declaring a mistrial.Rule 612. As amended Mar. 2, 1987, eff. Oct. 1, 1987.

Examples of a writing to which the animal owner may refer are a receipt and a case report from the diagnostic facility or veterinary clinic. The receipt could be used to refresh the memory of the animal owner as to precisely when and where she purchased the feed. The case report could be used to refresh the memory of the animal owner as to when the animal died, when the diagnostic testing was performed, and the results of the testing. An expert witness may be required, however, to interpret the laboratory report.

ADMISSIBILITY OF EXPERT TESTIMONY

The lay witness is not the only source of testimony. Lay testimony is a source of facts. Some of these facts must be interpreted, which is the role of the expert. Expert testimony is the other main form of introducing testimonial evidence. Expert testimony is commonly used at trial and has become the topic of a number of evidentiary rules. Federal Rules of Evidence 701 through 706 follow in their entirety.[25,26,27,28,29,30]

Expert testimony must not only be relevant as with a lay witness, but it must also be reliable. Discussion of this reliability factor constitutes most of the remainder of this chapter. In most legal cases, the judge makes preliminary rulings that determine whether the expert may testify at all, and if so, upon which opinions. Reliability is the primary factor in the judge's determination of admissibility of expert testimony. Two approaches to determine the reliability of expert testimony have evolved, these approaches are often referred to as the "*Frye* test" and the "*Daubert* test."

Frye

The *Frye* test is the original standard of reliability for expert testimony, and it remains in several state court systems. See Table 11.1. The *Frye* test is often summarized

25. Rule 701. Opinion Testimony by Lay Witnesses
If the witness is not testifying as an expert, the witness' testimony in the form of opinions or inferences is limited to those opinions or inferences which are (a) rationally based on the perception of the witness, and (b) helpful to a clear understanding of the witness' testimony or the determination of a fact in issue, and (c) not based on scientific, technical, or other specialized knowledge within the scope of Rule 702.
(As amended Mar. 2, 1987, eff. Oct. 1, 1987; Apr. 17, 2000, eff. Dec. 1, 2000.)

26. Rule 702. Testimony by Experts
If scientific, technical, or other specialized knowledge will assist the trier of fact to understand the evidence or to determine a fact in issue, a witness qualified as an expert by knowledge, skill, experience, training, or education, may testify thereto in the form of an opinion or otherwise, if (1) the testimony is based upon sufficient facts or data, (2) the testimony is the product of reliable principles and methods, and (3) the witness has applied the principles and methods reliably to the facts of the case.
Rule 702. (As amended Apr. 17, 2000, eff. Dec. 1, 2000.)

27. Rule 703. Bases of Opinion Testimony by Experts
The facts or data in the particular case upon which an expert bases an opinion or inference may be those perceived by or made known to the expert at or before the hearing. If of a type reasonably relied upon by experts in the particular field in forming opinions or inferences upon the subject, the facts or data need not be admissible in evidence in order for the opinion or inference to be admitted. Facts or data that are otherwise inadmissible shall not be disclosed to the jury by the proponent of the opinion or inference unless the court determines that their probative value in assisting the jury to evaluate the expert's opinion substantially outweighs their prejudicial effect. Rule 703. (As amended Mar. 2, 1987, eff. Oct. 1, 1987; Apr. 17, 2000, eff. Dec. 1, 2000.)

28. Rule 704. Opinion on Ultimate Issue
(a) Except as provided in subdivision (b), testimony in the form of an opinion or inference otherwise admissible is not objectionable because it embraces an ultimate issue to be decided by the trier of fact.
(b) No expert witness testifying with respect to the mental state or condition of a defendant in a criminal case may state an opinion or inference as to whether the defendant did or did not have the mental state or condition constituting an element of the crime charged or of a defense thereto. Such ultimate issues are matters for the trier of fact alone. (As amended Oct. 12, 1984.)

29. Rule 705. Disclosure of Facts or Data Underlying Expert Opinion
The expert may testify in terms of opinion or inference and give reasons therefore without first testifying to the underlying facts or data, unless the court requires otherwise. The expert may in any event be required to disclose the underlying facts or data on cross-examination.
(As amended Mar. 2, 1987, eff. Oct. 1, 1987; Apr. 22, 1993, eff. Dec. 1, 1993.)

30. Rule 706. Court Appointed Experts
(a) Appointment.—The court may on its own motion or on the motion of any party enter an order to show cause why expert witnesses should not be appointed, and may request the parties to submit nominations. The court may appoint any expert witnesses agreed upon by the parties, and may appoint expert witnesses of its own selection. An expert witness shall not be appointed by the court unless the witness consents to act. A witness so appointed shall be informed of the witness' duties by the court in writing, a copy of which shall be filed with the clerk, or at a conference in which the parties shall have opportunity to participate. A witness so appointed shall advise the parties of the witness' findings, if any; the witness' deposition may be taken by any party; and the witness may be called to testify by the court or any party. The witness shall be subject to cross-examination by each party, including a party calling the witness. (b) Compensation.—Expert witnesses so appointed are entitled to reasonable compensation in whatever sum the court may allow. The compensation thus fixed is payable from funds which may be provided by law in criminal cases and civil actions and proceedings involving just compensation under the fifth amendment. In other civil actions and proceedings the compensation shall be paid by the parties in such proportion and at such time as the court directs, and thereafter charged in like manner as other costs. (c) Disclosure of appointment.—In the exercise of its discretion, the court may authorize disclosure to the jury of the fact that the court appointed the expert witness.(d) Parties' experts of own selection.—Nothing in this rule limits the parties in calling expert witnesses of their own selection.(As amended Mar. 2, 1987, eff. Oct. 1, 1987.)

as the "general acceptance" standard. A brief history of *Frye* may illustrate its use in a legal setting.

In 1923, a defendant was convicted of second degree murder.[Frye] The defendant appealed the trial court's ruling because the court[31] did not allow the defendant to offer expert testimony. The expert testimony would have used a precursor to the "lie detector test" known as the "systolic blood pressure deception test" ("SBPD test"). The defendant's expert claimed that the SBPD test could prove whether or not a person being examined by the SBPD was attempting to deceive the examiner or conceal his guilt with regard to the crime. The judge did not allow this testimony, and the defendant was convicted. The ruling was appealed. The court of appeals held that when "admitting expert testimony deduced from a well-recognized scientific principle or discovery, the thing from which the deduction is made must be sufficiently established to have gained general acceptance in the particular field in which it belongs."[Frye at 1013.] This holding is commonly abbreviated as the "general acceptance" test. The trial court decision was upheld, because the defendant had insufficient proof that the SBPD test had gained "general acceptance." Consequently, the defendant's expert was not allowed to testify, so this expert testimony was not entered into evidence, and this evidence was then not available to support an argument to overturn the defendant's conviction.

Frye was a federal criminal case, but the holding was later adopted in federal civil cases. Over time, *Frye* was adopted by most state courts for both civil and criminal proceedings.

However, *Frye* is no longer the standard in federal cases. The *Frye* test was superseded in federal courts by the enactment of the Federal Rules of Evidence.[Daubert at 589] The *Frye* test has also been replaced by the *Daubert* test in many state court systems. See Table 11.1. The remainder of this section is devoted to *Daubert* since it has been adopted by the federal courts and many state court systems to determine whether expert testimony is, or is not, admitted into evidence today.

Daubert

Daubert is one of three U.S. Supreme Court cases addressing the issue of admissibility of expert testimony; recently, a fourth case addresses the number of chances to select an expert. In addition, the federal court system has published a Reference Manual on Scientific Evidence[32] to assist judges in applying these rulings. This Reference Manual contains introductory material[33] and sections devoted to toxicology,[34] medical testimony,[35] admissibility of expert testimony,[36] exposure science,[37] and other sections that may be of interest to toxicologists, and other scientists. Much of the material below is summarized from these sources.

Four cases with rulings impacting expert testimony have reached the U.S. Supreme Court in recent years. The cases are *Daubert* v *Merrell Dow Pharmaceuticals, Inc.* 509 U.S. 579 (1993), *General Electric Co* v *Joiner*, 522 U.S. 136 (1997), *Kumho Tire Co v Carmichael*, 119 S. Ct. 1167 (1999), and now *Weisgram v Marley* Co, 528 U.S. 440 (2000). Both *Daubert* and *General Electric* were toxic tort cases. *General Electric, Kumho,* and *Weisgram* are briefly mentioned.

The holdings in *General Electric* and *Kumho* are of legal review and admission of testimony from nonscientists as experts, so they are summarized briefly. The holding in *General Electric* is primarily of legal interest. In *General Electric*, the Supreme Court held that the correct standard for an appellate court to apply in reviewing a district court's evidentiary ruling is an "abuse of discretion" standard. This holding most commonly has the effect of strengthening the decision made by the district court whether it is to admit, or to not admit, the expert testimony. Of potential interest to toxicologists and, other scientists, is the urging by Justice Breyer in *General Electric* that judges avail themselves of court appointed experts. [General Electric at] ... *Kumho Tire* is not directly on point for toxicologists.

The Supreme Court held in *Kumho Tire*, that the phrases "technical" and "other specialized" knowledge in the Federal Rule of Evidence 702, allows testimony from those with "skill" or "experience" based expertise and not just "science" based expertise. The Supreme Court held that an expert in tire failure analysis could testify as an expert even though his expertise was "skill" or "experience" based, rather than "science" based.[Kumho at 1171]. The holdings in *Daubert* may be of more direct interest to toxicologists, and other scientists.

In *Weisgram* the Supreme Court held that the plaintiff is entitled to only one chance to select an expert who can withstand a *Daubert* motion. Justice Ginsberg stated:[38]

> *Since* Daubert, *moreover, parties relying on expert testimony have had notice of the exacting standards of reliability such evidence must meet.... It is implausible to suggest,*

31. The judge is referred to as "the court" in legal writing.

32. Reference Manual on Scientific Evidence, Third Edition. (2011) The National Academies Press, Washington, D.C. www.nap.edu.

33. See pages 1–10.

34. See pages 633–686.

35. See pages 687–746.

36. See pages 11–36.

37. See pages 503–548.

38. 528 U.S. at 455; presented in "The Admissibility of Expert Testimony--Margaret A. Berger." National Research Council. 2011. Reference Manual on Scientific Evidence: Third Edition.

TABLE 11.1 The Status of *Daubert* in State Courts

State	Standard	References[a]
Alabama	Daubert	Ala. Code 1975, § 12-21-160 effective January 1, 2012
Alaska	Daubert	*State v. Coon*, 974 P.2d 386 (Alaska 1999)
Arizona	Daubert	2010 Legis. Bill Hist. AZ H.B. 2492
Arkansas	Daubert	Farm Bureau Mut. Ins. Co. of *Ark., Inc., v. Foote*, 14 S.W. 3d 512 (Ark. 2000)
California	Frye	*People v. Leahy*, 882 P.2d 321 (Cal. 1994)
Colorado	Daubert	*People v. Shreck*, 22 P.3d 68 (Colo. 2001)
Connecticut	Daubert	*State v. Porter*, 698 A.2d 739 (Conn. 1997)
District of Columbia	Frye	*Bahura v. S.E.W. Investors*, 754 A.2d 928 (D.C. 2000)
Delaware	Daubert	D.R.E. 702
Florida	Frye	Florida Supreme Court, 4-2 vote on Feb. 16, 2017
Georgia	Daubert	O.C.G.A. § 24-7-702
Hawaii	Daubert	*State v. Montalbo*, 828 P.2d 1274 (Haw. 1992)
Idaho	Daubert	*State v. Merwin*, 962 P.2d 1026 (Idaho 1998)
Illinois	Frye	*Donaldson v. Central Illinois Public Service Co.*, 199 Ill.2d 63, 767 N.E.2d 314 (2002)
Indiana	Daubert	*Alsheik v. Guerrero*, 956 N.E.2d 1115 (Ind. App. 2011)
Iowa	Daubert	*Ganrud v. Smith*, 206 N.W.2d 311 (Iowa 1973)
Kansas	Daubert	K.S.A. 60-456(b)
Kentucky	Daubert	Kentucky Rule of Evidence, Rule 702
Louisiana	Daubert	*State v. Foret*, 628 So. 2d 1116 (La. 1993)
Maine	Daubert	*State v. Foret*, 628 So. 2d 1116 (La. 1993)
Maryland	Frye	Md. Rule 5-702
Massachusetts	Daubert	*Commonwealth v. Lanigan*, 641 N.E.2d 1342 (Mass. 1994)
Michigan	Daubert	MRE 702
Minnesota	Frye-mack	State v. Mack, 292 N.W. 2d 764 (Minn. 1980)
Mississippi	Daubert	*Miss. Transp. Comm'n v. McLemore*, 863 So. 2d 31, 2003 Miss. LEXIS 532 (Miss. 2003)
Missouri	Daubert	House Bill 153 into law on March 28th, 2017
Montana	Daubert	*State v. Moore*, 885 P.2d 457 (Mont. 1994)
Nebraska	daubert	*Schafersman v. Agland Coop.*, 631 N.W. 2d 862 (Neb. 2001)
Nevada	Other	*Higgs v. State*, 222 P.3d 648, 126 Nev. Adv. Rep. 1, 2010 Nev. LEXIS 1 (Nev. 2010)
New hampshire	Daubert	*Baker Valley Lumber, Inc. v. Ingersoll-Rand Co.*, 813 A.2d 409 (N.H. 2002)
New Jersey	Frye	N.J. R. Evid. 702
New Mexico	Daubert	
New York	Frye	*People v. Wesley*, 633 N.E.2d 451 (N.Y.1994)
North Carolina	Daubert	*State v. McGrady*, COA13-330, 2014 WL 211962 (N.C. Ct. App. Jan. 21, 2014)
North Dakota	Other	*State v. Hernandez*, 707 N.W. 2d 449 (N.D. 2005)
Ohio	Daubert	*State v. Martens*, 629 N.E.2d 462 (3d Dist. Mercer County 1993)
Oklahoma	Daubert	Okla. Stat. tit. 12, § 2702

(*Continued*)

TABLE 11.1 (Continued)

State	Standard	References[a]
Oregon	Daubert	*State v. O'Key*, 899 P.2d 663 (Or. 1995)
Pennsylvania	Frye	Pa.R.E. 702(c)
Rhode Island	Daubert	RI R. Evid. Art. VII, Rule 702
South Carolina	daubert	
South Dakota	Daubert	*State v. Hofer*, 512 N.W.2d 482 (S.D. 1994)
Tennessee	Daubert	Tenn. R. Evid. Rule 702
Texas	Daubert	*E.I. du Pont de Nemours & Co. v. Robinson*, 923 S.W.2d 549 (Tex. 1995)
Utah	Daubert	*State v. Rinmasch*, 775 P.2d 388 (Utah 1989)
Vermont	Daubert	*State v. Brooks*, 162 Vt. 26, 30, 643 A.2d 226, 229 (1993)
Virginia	Other	Va. Code Ann. 8.01-401
Washington	Frye	*State v. Riker*, 869 P.2d 43 (Wash. 1994). Reinforced *State v. Riker*, 869 P.2d 43 (Wash. 1994)
West Virginia	Daubert	*Wilt v. Buracker*, 443 S.E.2d 196 (W. Va. 1994)
Wisconsin	Daubert	Wis. Stat. § 907.02(1)
Wyoming	Daubert	*Bunting v. Jamison*, 984 P.2d 467 (Wyo. 1999)

[a]*See https://www.theexpertinstitute.com/daubert-v-frye-a-state-by-state-comparison/ accessed April 22, 2017.*

> *post-*Daubert, *that parties will initially present less than their best expert evidence in the expectation of a second chance should their first trial fail.*[49]

Expert testimony is different from lay testimony. One difference is the possibility that "junk science" may be used to confuse, rather than assist, the trier of fact. Consequently an additional test of admissibility is applied to expert testimony. Such testimony must not only be relevant, but it must also be *reliable*. This concept is explained in the *Daubert* case. Justice Breyer, "believe[s] there is an increasingly important need for law to reflect sound science." [Justice Breyer, in the Reference Manual on Scientific Evidence, p. 5.] Justice Breyer also writes in the Manual on Scientific Evidence:

> *The judge is the evidentiary gatekeeper (*General Electric Co *v* Joiner, *522 U.S. 136 (1997);* Daubert *v* Merrel Dow Pharms Inc., *509 U.S. 579 (1993)).). "The judge, without interfering with the jury's role as trier of fact, must determine whether purported scientific evidence is "reliable" and will "assist the trier of fact" thereby keeping from juries testimony that, in Pauli's sense, isn't even good enough to be wrong." Justice Breyer, in Manual on Scientific Evidence, p. 6.*
>
> *The purpose of Daubert's gatekeeping requirement "is to make certain that an expert whether basing testimony upon professional studies or personal experience, employs in the courtroom the same level of intellectual rigor that characterizes the practice of an expert in the relevant field."* Kumho Tire Co *v* Carmichael, *119 S. Ct. 1167 (1999) at 1176. See also,* Rosen *v* Ciba-geigy Corp, *78 F.3d 316 (7th Cir) cert denied, 519 U.S. 819 (1996) at 318.*

Clearly, the U.S. Supreme Court in *Daubert* assigned the trial judge a "gatekeeping" responsibility. This responsibility is to make a "preliminary assessment of whether the reasoning or methodology underlying the testimony is scientifically valid and whether that reasoning or methodology properly can be applied to the facts in issue."[Daubert at 589] The "gatekeeper" function requires district court judges to screen proffered expert testimony.[Ibid] This screening is intended to ensure that expert testimony "is not only relevant, but reliable."[Ibid] To be relevant, the testimony "requires a valid scientific connection to the pertinent inquiry as a precondition to admissibility."[Daubert at 591–192.] Much has been written about the reliability portion of this screening.

To meet the reliability standard, the judge must determine whether testimony is "grounded in the methods and procedures of science."[Daubert, at 590.] Consequently, an expert must account for "how and why" he or she reached the expert opinion.[Kumho, at note 27.] The judge's determination is "flexible"[Daubert at 594] so the trial judge has broad latitude to determine *how* to test an expert's reliability,[Kumho, at 1176] and this determination, may be different in a criminal case than in a civil one.[Kumho at 1176] Nevertheless, guidelines for determining the reliability of expert testimony exist.

Four factors were presented in *Daubert* to assist the judge in determining whether a theory or technique has been derived by the scientific method.[*Daubert* at 593-94] These four factors are used to determine the theory's testability,[*Carmichael* at 1522] because "[w]hether [a theory or technique] can be (and has been) tested" is the "methodology [that] distinguishes science from other fields of human inquiry."[*Daubert* at 593] In short, the four factors are testability, peer review or publication, the existence of known or potential error rates, and standards controlling the techniques' operation.[*Ibid*]

In summary, the trial judge decides whether or not expert testimony is allowed. The means by which the judge makes this decision is flexible, but the judge often tests both the credentials of the expert and the opinion that expert offers. The expert's opinion must meet "the same standard of intellectual rigor" inside the court room as outside of it.[*Kumho* at 1176] This showing of intellectual rigor requires that the expert demonstrate both "how and why" the opinion was reached. This may be done by satisfying four factors, namely (1) whether the theory or technique can be tested, (2) whether it is published or peer reviewed, (3) whether it has known or potential error rates, and (4) what the control standards are.

These factors may be applied to both the analytical and interpretive portions of a toxicology case. Both *Daubert* and *General Electric* were toxic tort cases. This may be one reason that a chapter devoted to toxicology appears in the Reference Manual for Scientific Evidence. This Manual offers some questions to be asked of purported toxicology experts.

Three questions may be asked in the evaluation of a toxicology expert to determine whether the expert's testimony is reliable—and therefore admissible. These questions may be reduced to (1) is the expert qualified?, (2) has general causation been established?, and (3) has specific causation been established?

Is the Expert Qualified?[39]

The individual wanting to be allowed to testify as an expert must be "qualified as an expert by knowledge, skill, experience, training, or education, ..."[Rule 702] Toxicologists are often argued to be experts based on education, board certification, and other means. Although "... no single academic degree, research specialty, or career path qualifies an individual as an expert in toxicology. ... A number of indicia of expertise can be explored, ..."[Reference Guide on Toxicology at p. 415.]

39. See also III. Applying *Daubert* in *The Admissibility of Expert Testimony--Margaret A. Berger*. National Research Council. 2011. Reference Manual on Scientific Evidence: Third Edition.

The basis of a toxicologist's opinion is often a thorough review of the scientific literature and treatises disclosing the adverse effects of exposure to a particular chemical.[Reference Guide on toxicology, p. 415.]

HAS THE PERSON BEEN TRAINED AND EDUCATED IN THE DISCIPLINE OF TOXICOLOGY?

An advanced degree in toxicology presumptively supports the argument that the person has been trained and educated in the discipline of toxicology. One may go to the credentialing and other means portions of the analysis if the person possesses an advanced degree in toxicology. Not all toxicologists possess such a degree, however.

Many well qualified toxicologists do not have an advanced degree in toxicology, but do have an advanced degree in related disciplines such as pharmacology, biochemistry, environmental health, industrial hygiene, or other similar fields.[Reference Guide on Toxicology at 415] However, not all individuals in possession of these related degrees are toxicologists. So further evidence of training and education is often required of those who do not have an advanced degree in toxicology but do have an advanced degree in a related discipline.

This training and education is often in the form of college level course work or continuing education programs. The number of required courses in toxicology cannot be stated, but one such course is not enough. Specifically, "a single course in toxicology is unlikely to provide sufficient background for developing expertise in the field." [Reference Guide on Toxicology, p. 415.] "A physician without particular training or experience in toxicology is unlikely to have sufficient background to evaluate the strengths and weaknesses of toxicological research."[*See* Mary Sue Henifin] "[M]ost physicians have little training in chemical toxicology and lack an understanding of exposure assessment and dose-response relationships." [*Ibid.*] The same is true for veterinarians, and many other health care professionals. So, while the number of college courses, continuing education, or other training programs required to support an argument that one is a toxicologist is not established, one such course is most likely too few. Consequently, an MD or DVM without an advanced degree in toxicology may well be found to not be a toxicologist based on training and education if they have only a course in professional school to support the claim. Certification is another way to support the argument that one is a toxicologist.

HAS THE PERSON BEEN CERTIFIED AS A TOXICOLOGIST?

Some professions have a subspecialty in toxicology with a board certification. Physicians may be certified by the

American Board of Medical Toxicology.[40] Veterinarians may be certified by the American Board of Veterinary Toxicology.[41] The American Board of Toxicology (ABT) was established to provide certification of individuals trained and experienced in toxicology without consideration of whether the individual has a professional Medical or Veterinary Medical degree. [42] However, individuals with an MD, or DVM, degree may also take the ABT certifying examination. Only a few individuals are certified by more than one of these boards. Certification by other boards may be relevant for a particular legal case. A person with an advanced degree in toxicology and board certification has strong support for an argument that they are a toxicologist. This may be one reason that the American Association of Veterinary Laboratory Diagnosticians (AAVLD) has required a board certified toxicologist be on staff for an accredited laboratory. A person with an advanced degree but no board certification, or board certification but no advanced degree, may have other criteria to support a finding that they are a toxicologist.

DO OTHER CRITERIA SUPPORT AN ARGUMENT THAT THE PERSON IS A TOXICOLOGIST?

Such other criteria may be membership in one or more toxicology organizations, peer-reviewed or other publications, research grants, scientific advisory panels, university appointments and the like.[*Ibid,* p. 418.] These criteria are often documented in one's résumé or curriculum vitae.

So, a person with a professional degree, plus an advanced degree in toxicology, plus board certification in toxicology, plus membership in one or more toxicology organizations, peer reviewed toxicology literature, grants, service on scientific advisory panels, and a university appointment has very strong support for an argument that they are an expert in toxicology. On the other hand, a person with a professional degree, no advanced degree in toxicology, no board certification in toxicology, and no other publications, grants, and the like has a comparatively weaker argument, that they are an expert in toxicology. The courts recognize the distinction between a professional degree and expertise required in a legal setting. This distinction is aptly described in *Wynacht* vs *Beckman Instruments*.

> *There is a fundamental distinction between Dr. Ziem's ability to render a medical diagnosis based on clinical experience and her ability to render an opinion on causation of Wynacht's injuries. Beckman apparently does not dispute, and the Court does not question, that Dr. Ziem is an experienced physician, qualified to diagnose medical conditions and treat patients. The ability to diagnose medical conditions is not remotely the same, however, as the ability to deduce, delineate, and describe, in a scientifically reliable manner, the causes of these medical conditions.*

Many combinations of education, certification and other criteria that fall between the two above extremes are possible for toxicology experts. These would, of course, be decided by the judge in a specific case. Once found to be an expert, the toxicologist will most likely be asked to give an opinion on general causation.

GENERAL CAUSATION

"[T]he methodology prescribed by both the World Health Organization (WHO) and the National Academy of Sciences (NAS) for determining whether a person has been adversely affected by a toxin" have been described in *Mancuso* v. *Consolidated Edison Co.* as a three step procedure. Scientific validity may be argued in three steps "(1) the validity of the underlying principle, (2) the validity of the technique applying the principle, and (3) the proper application of the technique on a particular occasion." [Paul C. Giannelli].

> *First, the level of exposure of plaintiff to the toxin in question must be determined; second, from a review of the scientific literature, it must be established that the toxin is capable of producing plaintiff's illness—called "general causation"—and the dose/response relationship between the toxin and the illness—that is, the level of exposure which will produce such an illness—must be ascertained; and third, "specific causation" must be established by demonstrating the probability that the toxin caused this particular plaintiff's illness, which involves weighing the possibility of other causes of the illness—a so-called "differential diagnosis."* Mancuso *at 399*

Toxicologists may arrive at an expert opinion in a variety of ways.

> *The basis of the toxicologist's expert opinion in a specific case is a thorough review of the research literature and treatises concerning effects of exposure to the chemical at issue. To arrive at an opinion, the expert assesses the strengths and weaknesses of the research studies. The expert also bases an opinion on fundamental concepts of toxicology relevant to understanding the actions of chemicals in biological systems." Manual on Scientific Evidence at 415.*

Two key legal concepts of causation have emerged as courts have attempted to keep junk science out of the

40. A list of approved Medical subspecialties is available at: http://www.abms.org/approved.asp

41. Www.abvt.org

42. www.abtox.org

courtroom. These concepts are general causation and specific causation. The discussion of specific causation follows in the next section.

"Causation is frequently a crucial issue in toxicology cases. Establishing causation means providing scientific evidence from which an inference of cause and effect may be drawn." Reference Manual on Scientific Evidence at 32 The Manual goes on to describe the process of arriving at general causation.

> *Once the expert has been qualified, he or she is expected to offer an opinion on whether the plaintiff's disease was caused by exposure to a chemical. To do so, the expert relies on the principles of toxicology to provide a scientifically valid methodology for establishing causation and then applies the methodology to the facts of the case.*
>
> *An opinion on causation should be premised on three preliminary assessments. First, the expert should analyze whether the disease can be related to chemical exposure by a biologically plausible theory. Second, the expert should examine if the plaintiff was exposed to the chemical in a manner that can lead to absorption into the body. Third, the expert should offer an opinion as to whether the dose to which the plaintiff was exposed is sufficient to cause the disease.*

Reference Guide on Toxicology at 419

Courts define general causation as "the capacity of a product to cause injury." Siharath at xx. General causation is a scientifically established cause-and-effect relationship. To satisfy this burden, sufficient testing must be done to establish that a disease or condition can arise after exposure to a certain substance. Peer reviewed literature of epidemiology studies, case reports, in vitro, and animal studies may be used to support a general causation argument.

A toxic tort plaintiff must first show that the substance to which he was allegedly exposed is capable of causing his injury—general causation. See e.g., Raynor 7 General causation asks whether exposure to a substance causes harm to anyone. See Navigating Uncertainty

Increasingly, the discipline of epidemiology is argued as a basis for general causation. When epidemiology is used to present the incidence and distribution of disease in humans, courts have often ruled the expert opinion admissible. This has not always been the case for toxicological expert opinions because of the need to extrapolate from animal, or in vitro, studies to humans. This line of argument may be less persuasive in an animal poisoning case when such extrapolations are not needed.

Occasionally experts rely on state or federal regulations to opine that exposure to a certain amount or concentration of a chemical is associated with a particular adverse event. However, merely citing the regulation without further inquiry as to its derivation may erode the strength of such arguments. It may prove critical to the argument to know whether the regulation was established using a "reasonable certainty of no harm" standard or a "normally renders injurious to health," or other standard.

The former standard may have included various "uncertainty factors" to extrapolate below measured dose response data to obtain a safety standard. These uncertainty factors may be explored in a legal venue if one is testifying to a "reasonable degree of medical certainty" that the exposure did in fact cause harm, when the basis for the regulatory standard is a "reasonable certainty of no harm" obtained using "uncertainty factors."[43]

In short, is the alleged chemical capable of causing the disease observed at any dose or exposure ? In our hypothetical above, has the chemical that was added to the feed additive been shown to cause the clinical signs and lesions observed in the species of animal in this case ? If not, the expert's testimony may not be allowed in the case. If so, an analysis of specific causation would most likely be required.

SPECIFIC CAUSATION: THE DIFFERENTIAL DIAGNOSIS

General causation answers the question of whether the chemical in question *may* cause the disease observed. Specific causation is aimed at answering the question of whether the chemical in question *did* in fact cause the disease in the specific case at hand. This concept has been stated in a variety of ways. Specific causation is "proof that the product in question caused the injury of which the plaintiff complains"*Siharath* It is a tendency to show that the person's alleged exposure, in fact, caused his or her condition.*Siharath* at See also D.T. Ralston In other words, it is a showing that said exposure was the actual cause of the injury.See e.g., Raynor An analysis of specific causation answers the question of whether exposure to the specific chemical in question did or did not cause the disease experienced by the plaintiff, or in this chapter's hypothetical, plaintiff's animals. The specific causation analysis requires consideration of other potential causes of the disease.

Consideration of other causes of the disease is often referred to as a differential diagnosis. The differential diagnosis may not always be a common occurrence in the practice of both human and veterinary medicine. Differential diagnosis evidence is often crucial to show specific causation. See Lennon Without some evidence that the substance in question caused the specific injury to the specific plaintiff, courts are likely to grant the defendant summary judgment.

43. See Ellen K. Silbergeld. The Role of toxicology in causation: A Scientific Perspective. 1 Cts. Health Sci. & L. 374, 378 (1991).

Courts generally agree that, whenever there are different causes for the plaintiff's disease, an expert must perform a differential diagnosis before testimony will be admitted. [See Gianelli.] Courts accept the general validity of the technique of differential diagnosis.[US v Downing] An expert opinion based on a properly performed differential diagnosis analysis is not likely to be inadmissible.[Westberry at 263] More specifically, "[t]o the extent that a doctor utilizes standard diagnostic techniques in gathering this information, the more likely we are to find that the doctor's methodology is reliable."[In re Paoli, at 758.]

Put differently, "[a]n expert who opines that exposure to a compound caused a person's disease engages in deductive clinical reasoning. ... The opinion is based on an assessment of the individual's exposure, including the amount, the temporal relationship between the exposure and disease, and other disease-causing factors. This information is then compared with scientific data on the relationship between exposure and disease. The certainty of the expert's opinion depends on the strength of the research data demonstrating a relationship between exposure and the disease at the dose in question and the absence of other disease causing factors (also known as confounding factors)." [Reference guide at 422–423.] See also Joseph Sanders.

However, simply stating that a differential diagnosis was performed is not enough. This issue was discussed in *Viterbo*:

> *We do not hold, of course, that admissibility of an expert opinion depends upon the expert disproving or discrediting every possible cause other than the one espoused by him. Here, however, Dr. Johnson has admitted that Viterbo's symptoms could have numerous causes and, without support save Viterbo's oral history, simply picks the cause that is most advantageous to Viterbo's claim. Indeed, Dr. Johnson's testimony is no more than Viterbo's testimony dressed up and sanctified as the opinion of an expert. Without more than credentials and a subjective opinion, an expert's testimony that "it is so" is not admissible.* Viterbo *v* Dow Chemical

This formulation is repeated by Judge Becker in *United States* v. *Downing*.

> *The process of differential diagnosis is undoubtedly important to the question of "specific causation." If other possible causes of an injury cannot be ruled out, or at least the probability of their contribution to causation minimized, then the "more likely than not" threshold for proving causation may not be met. But, it is also important to recognize that a fundamental assumption underlying this method is that the final, suspected "cause" remaining after this process of elimination must actually be capable of causing the injury. That is, the expert must "rule in" the suspected cause as well as "rule out" other possible causes. And, of course, expert opinion on this issue of "general causation" must be derived from a scientifically valid methodology.* Cavallo *v* Star Enterprise

The order of proving causation is important. General causation should be proven first, then the specific causation differential diagnosis analysis. In virtually all cases, differential diagnosis does not provide general causation—it can only provide specific causation. [44] This may be part of the reasoning that argues that epidemiological data is rarely determinative in a specific causation analysis, and is most commonly used in the general causation argument.

To show that said exposure was the actual cause of the injury, toxic tort plaintiffs must prove the admissibility of their expert testimony in both general causation and specific causation context by a preponderance of proof.[*Daubert* at 593] A successful plaintiff must not only show that, more likely than not, the substance can cause the injury in question, but also that, more likely than not, the plaintiff's specific injury was in fact caused by the substance.[*DeLuca*, Ronald J. Allen]

A *Daubert* analysis should be performed. In fact, "a trial court that fails to justify its decision not to use *Daubert* factors risks reversal."[*Black* v *Food Lion*] *Daubert* factors may be used when assessing the admissibility of clinical medical testimony.[*Moore*] This opinion is because reliable opinions are reached using the "methods and procedures of science." Scientific validity is the foundation of "*evidentiary reliability*"[Daubert at 590] See also, Bert Black et al.

So the expert in our case, must not only rule-in the chemical added to the feed additive as the cause of the clinical signs and lesions observed, but must also rule out other diseases that cause these clinical signs or lesions in that specific animal to arrive at specific causation.

APPLICATION OF DAUBERT IN TOXICOLOGY CASES

The application of these legal rules to specific toxicology cases may be useful. Testimony may be weakened if there is no Daubert inquiry at all. [*Goebel*, 2000.]

The differential diagnosis portion of analyzing specific causation is important. Expert testimony from a forensic toxicologist has been properly excluded for insufficient proof to rule in the chemical in question and to rule out other diseases. [*Wills*, 2004.] The testimony of a toxicologist was properly excluded because the toxicologist was not a medical doctor and therefore not qualified to offer reliable differential diagnosis analysis. [*Plourde*, 2003.] On the other hand, testimony was properly allowed from two marine biologists who each performed a differential diagnosis analysis in a case involving marine animals (Clausen, 2003).

Dose is important in toxicology cases. Testimony of a treating physician, toxicologist and industrial hygienist

44. See generally, *Raynor* v. *Merrell Pharmaceuticals*, 101 F.3d 129, 138-39 (D.C. Cir. 1996). See also, *Kelly*, *Grimes*, *Rutigliano*, *Hall*, In re Breast Implant, National Bank of Commerce and Wynacht.

were excluded, and the exclusion affirmed because the literature did not support a finding of general causation at the relevant exposure (Amorgianos, 2002). Testimony of a toxicologist was properly excluded because he performed no dose assessment and showed no statistically significant link between the chemical and the type of cancer present (Burleson, 2004).

Reliance on peer reviewed literature is also important. A toxicologist's testimony was excluded, but the exclusion was reversed, because the toxicologist's testimony was supported by peer-reviewed literature (Bocanegra, 2003).

SOME QUESTIONS TO CONSIDER WHEN USING LABORATORY RESULTS

1. Was the legal aspect of the case known at the time the samples were submitted? If not, is the sample tracking or chain of custody sufficiently well documented to establish each relevant step of the analysis? Can the relevance of the documents be authenticated? Does chain-of-custody or sample tracking documentation exist?
2. What type of legal venue is the work to be used in ? Administrative enforcement, civil litigation, criminal litigation? What standard of persuasion is appropriate for this venue?
3. Can the relevance of the analytical results be authenticated? What documentation exists that the samples were collected from the appropriate animal? What documentation exists to demonstrate proper sample identification throughout the laboratory testing process? What documentation exists to demonstrate that the process used produces an accurate result—what validation processes are in place? Is the interpretation of the test results accurate for the type of analytical test performed?
4. Is the testimony to be as a lay—or fact—witness?
5. Is the testimony to be as an expert witness?
   A. Is the expert a toxicologist?
   B. Does the scientific literature support an argument of general causation?
   C. Was a differential diagnosis performed by the laboratory?
      1. Rule-in:
         a. Can the expert provide reliable testimony that the sample received by the laboratory is representative of the diseased animals?
         b. Can the expert provide reliable testimony that the animals were in fact exposed to a toxic dose of the chemical in question ? To what degree of certainty does the analytical methodology demonstrate exposure of the animal to the chemical in question?
         c. Can the expert provide reliable testimony that the animals experienced the disease expected from exposure to a toxic dose of the chemical in question? Is reliable testimony of the clinical signs and lesions available?
      2. Rule-out:
         a. Can the expert provide a differential diagnosis list?
         b. Can the expert provide reliable testimony that the diseases other than the purported one were ruled out? Can the expert explain how and why these other diseases were ruled out? Were scientifically valid methods used to rule out these diseases?

When considering exposure:[45]

1. How can we be sure that the samples taken are actually representative of the media sampled?
2. Standard methods are available to design sampling plans that have specified probabilities of being representative, but they can never provide complete assurance. Generally, when contamination is likely to be highly homogeneous, there is a greater chance of achieving a reasonably representative sample than is the case when it is highly heterogeneous. In the latter circumstance, obtaining a representative sample, even when very large numbers of samples are taken, may be unachievable.
3. How can we be sure that the analytical work was done properly?
4. What are the pathways from the source to the exposed individuals? How has it been established that those pathways exist (past? present? future?).
5. What is the concentration of the chemical in the media with which the exposed population comes into contact (past? present? future?). What is the basis for this answer: direct measurement? modeling?
6. If the concentration is based on direct measurement, what procedures were followed in obtaining that measurement? Was media sampling sufficient to ensure that it was representative? If not, why is representativeness not important? Were validated analytical methods used by an accredited laboratory? If not, how can one be assured that the analytical results are reliable?

When considering a specific causal association:[46]

45. From Reference Guide on Exposure Science--Joseph V. Rodricks. National Research Council. 2011. Reference Manual on Scientific Evidence: Third Edition. Washington, DC: The National Academies Press. doi: 10.17226/13163. See also How should the Courts Assess exposure in The Admissibility of expert Testimony – Margaret A. Berger.

46. From *Reference Guide on Toxicology--Bernard D. Goldstein and Mary Sue Henifin*.National Research Council. 2011. Reference Manual on Scientific Evidence: Third Edition. Washington, DC: The National Academies Press. doi: 10.17226/13163.

A. Was the Plaintiff Exposed to the Substance, and if So, Did the Exposure Occur in a Manner That Can Result in Absorption into the Body?
B. Were Other Factors Present That Can Affect the Distribution of the Compound Within the Body?
C. What Is Known About How Metabolism in the Human Body Alters the Toxic Effects of the Compound?
D. What Excretory Route Does the Compound Take, and How Does This Affect Its Toxicity?
E. Does the Temporal Relationship Between Exposure and the Onset of Disease Support or Contradict Causation?
F. If Exposure to the Substance Is Associated with the Disease, Is There a No Observable Effect, or Threshold, Level, and if So, Was the Individual Exposed Above the No Observable Effect Level?

When considering expert qualifications:[47]

A. Does the Proposed Expert Have an Advanced Degree in Toxicology, Pharmacology, or a Related Field? If the Expert Is a Physician, Is He or She Board Certified in a Field Such as Occupational Medicine?
B. Has the Proposed Expert Been Certified by the American Board of Toxicology, Inc., or Does He or She Belong to a Professional Organization, Such as the Academy of Toxicological Sciences or the Society of Toxicology?
C. What Other Criteria Does the Proposed Expert Meet?

CONCLUSION

The distinction between medical and legal understanding of particular terminology and statements by Justice Breyer are offered in conclusion.

Clarification of the meaning of terms, in context, is important; three examples offered in the Reference Guide are, differential diagnosis, etiology, and certainty.

Toxicologists in veterinary diagnostic laboratories and other specialists may conduct a differential diagnosis analysis more closely contemplated by the legal definition than some practitioners in other settings.

> *Differential diagnosis, for example, is an accepted method that a medical expert may employ to offer expert testimony that satisfies Daubert.*[48] *In the legal context, differential diagnosis refers to a technique "in which physician first rules in all scientifically plausible causes of plaintiff's injury, then rules out least plausible causes of injury until the most likely cause remains, thereby reaching conclusion as to whether defendant's product caused injury...."*[49] *In the medical context, by contrast, differential diagnosis*

47. From *Reference Guide on Toxicology--Bernard D. Goldstein and Mary Sue Henifin.*National Research Council. 2011. Reference Manual on Scientific Evidence: Third Edition. Washington, DC: The National Academies Press. doi: 10.17226/13163.

48. Reference guide citing Feliciano-Hill v. Principi, 439 F.3d 18, 25 (1st Cir. 2006) ("[W]hen an examining physician calls upon training and experience to offer a differential diagnosis...most courts have found no Daubert problem."); Clausen v. M/V New Carissa, 339 F.3d 1049, 1058–59 (9th Cir. 2003) (recognizing differential diagnosis as a valid methodology); Mattis v. Carlon Elec. Prods., 295 F.3d 856, 861 (8th Cir. 2002) ("A medical opinion based upon a proper differential diagnosis is sufficiently reliable to satisfy [Daubert.]"); Westberry v. Gislaved Gummi AB, 178 F.3d 257, 262 (4th Cir. 1999) (recognizing differential diagnosis as a reliable technique).

49. Reference guide citing Wilson v. Taser Int'l, Inc. 2008 WL 5215991, at *5 (11th Cir. Dec. 16, 2008) ("[N]onetheless, Dr. Meier did not perform a differential diagnosis or any tests on Wilson to rule out osteoporosis and these corresponding alternative mechanisms of injury. Although a medical expert need not rule out every possible alternative in order to form an opinion on causation, expert opinion testimony is properly excluded as unreliable if the doctor 'engaged in very few standard diagnostic techniques by which doctors normally rule out alternative causes and the doctor offered no good explanation as to why his or her conclusion remained reliable' or if 'the defendants pointed to some likely cause of the plaintiff's illness other than the defendants' action and [the doctor] offered no reasonable explanation as to why he or she still believed that the defendants' actions were a substantial factor in bringing about that illness.'"); Williams v. Allen, 542 F.3d 1326, 1333 (11th Cir. 2008) ("Williams also offered testimony from Dr. Eliot Gelwan, a psychiatrist specializing in psychopathology and differential diagnosis. Dr. Gelwan conducted a thorough investigation into Williams' background, relying on a wide range of data sources. He conducted extensive interviews with Williams and with fourteen other individuals who knew Williams at various points in his life.") (involving a capital murder defendant petitioning for habeus corpus offering supporting expert witness); Bland v. Verizon Wireless, L.L.C., 538 F.3d 893, 897 (8th Cir. 2008) ("Bland asserts Dr. Sprince conducted a differential diagnosis which supports Dr. Sprince's causation opinion. We have held, 'a medical opinion about causation, based upon a proper differential diagnosis is sufficiently reliable to satisfy Daubert.' A 'differential diagnosis [is] a technique that identifies the cause of a medical condition by eliminating the likely causes until the most probable cause is isolated.'") (stating expert's incomplete execution of differential diagnosis procedure rendered expert testimony unsatisfactory for Daubert standard) (citations omitted); Lash v. Hollis 525 F.3d 636, 640 (8th Cir. 2008) ("Further, even if the treating physician had specifically opined that the Taser discharges caused rhabdomyolysis in Lash Sr., the physician offered no explanation of a differential diagnosis or other scientific methodology tending to show that the Taser shocks were a more likely cause than the myriad other possible causes suggested by the evidence.") (finding lack of expert testimony with differential diagnosis enough to render evidence insufficient for jury to find causation in personal injury suit); Feit v. Great West Life & Annuity Ins. Co., 271 Fed. App'x. 246, 254 (3d Cir. 2008) ("However, although this Court generally recognizes differential diagnosis as a reliable methodology the differential diagnosis must be properly performed in order to be reliable. To properly perform a differential diagnosis, an expert must perform two steps: (1) 'Rule in' all possible causes of Dr. Feit's death and (2) 'Rule out' causes through a process of elimination whereby the last remaining potential cause is deemed the most likely cause of death.") (ruling that district court not in error for excluding expert medical testimony that relied on an improperly performed differential diagnosis) (citations omitted); Glastetter v. Novartis Pharms. Corp., 252 F.3d 986 (8th Cir. 2001).

refers to a set of diseases that physicians consider as possible causes for symptoms the patient is suffering or signs that the patient exhibits. [50]*By identifying the likely potential causes of the patient's disease or condition and weighing the risks and benefits of additional testing or treatment, physicians then try to determine the most appropriate approach—testing, medication, or surgery, for example.*

Veterinary diagnosticians may also be familiar with the phrase etiological diagnosis, but less so with "differential etiology."

Less commonly, courts often have used the term "differential etiology" interchangeably with differential diagnosis. [51] *In medicine, etiology refers to the study of causation in disease,* [52] *but differential etiology is a legal invention not used by physicians. In general, both differential etiology and differential diagnosis are concerned with establishing or refuting causation between an external cause and a plaintiff's condition. Depending on the type of case and the legal standard, a medical expert may testify in regard to specific causation, general causation, or both. General causation refers to whether the plaintiff's injury could have been caused by the defendant, or a product produced by the defendant, while specific causation is established only when the defendant's action or product actually caused the harm.* [53] *An opinion by a testifying physician may be offered in support of both kinds of causation.* [54]

The meaning of "certainty" may be uncertain. The reference guide states: "Courts also refer to medical certainty or probability in ways that differ from their use in medicine. The standards 'reasonable medical certainty' and 'reasonable medical probability' are also terms of art in the law that have no analog for a practicing physician."[55]

Despite uncertainty in terminology and the complexity that may occur in legal proceedings, a number of statements from Justice Breyer in the Introduction to the Reference Manual on Scientific Evidence follow as his thoughts on the current status of and future considerations for the increasing need for science in legal proceedings.

A judge is not a scientist, and a courtroom is not a scientific laboratory. But consider the remark made by the physicist Wolfgang Pauli. After a colleague asked whether a certain scientific paper was wrong, Pauli replied, "That paper isn't even good enough to be wrong!" Our objective is to avoid legal decisions that reflect that paper's so-called science. The law must seek decisions that fall within the boundaries of scientifically sound knowledge. [56]

Despite the difficulties, I believe there is an increasingly important need for law to reflect sound science. I remain optimistic about the likelihood that it will do so. . . . [57]

The judiciary, too, has begun to look for ways to improve the quality of the science on which scientifically related judicial determinations will rest. . . . [58]

Moreover, our Court has made clear that the law imposes on trial judges the duty, with respect to scientific evidence, to become evidentiary gatekeepers. [59] *The judge,*

50. Reference guide citing Steadman's Medical Dictionary 531 (28th ed. 2006) (defining differential diagnosis as "the determination of which of two or more diseases with similar symptoms is the one from which the patient is suffering, by a systematic comparison and contrasting of the clinical findings.").

51. Reference guide citing See Proctor v. Fluor Enters., Inc. 494 F.3d 1337 (11th Cir. 2007) (testifying medical expert employed differential etiology to reach a conclusion regarding the cause of plaintiff's stroke). But see McClain v. Metabolife Int'l, Inc., 401 F.3d 1233, 1252 (11th Cir. 2005) (distinguishing differential diagnosis from differential etiology, with the former closer to the medical definition and the latter employed as a technique to determine external causation).

52. Reference guide citing Steadman's Medical Dictionary 675 (28th ed. 2006) (defining etiology as "the science and study of the causes of disease and their mode of operation. . ."). For a discussion of the term "etiology" in epidemiology studies, see Michael D. Green et al., Reference Guide on Epidemiology, Section I, in this manual.

53. Reference guide citing See Amorgianos v. Nat'l R.R. Passenger Corp., 303 F.3d 256, 268 (2d Cir. 2002).

54. Reference guide citing See, e.g., Ruggiero v. Warner-Lambert Co. 424 F.3d 249 (2d Cir. 2005) (excluding testifying expert's differential diagnosis in support of a theory of general causation because it was not supported by sufficient evidence).

55. See, e.g., Dallas v. Burlington N., Inc., 689 P.2d 273, 277 (Mont. 1984) ("'[R]easonable medical certainty' standard; the term is not well understood by the medical profession. Little, if anything, is 'certain' in science. The term was adopted in law to assure that testimony received by the fact finder was not merely conjectural but rather was sufficiently probative to be reliable"). This reference guide will not probe substantive legal standards in any detail, but there are substantive differences in admissibility standards for medical evidence between federal and state courts. See Robin Dundis Craig, When Daubert Gets Erie: Medical Certainty and Medical Expert Testimony in Federal Court, 77 Denv. U. L. Rev. 69 (1999).

56. Introduction--Stephen Breyer." National Research Council. 2011. Reference Manual on Scientific Evidence: Third Edition. Washington, DC: The National Academies Press. doi: 10.17226/13163. Referencing 7. Peter W. Huber, Galileo's Revenge: Junk Science in the Courtroom 54 (1991).

57. Introduction--Stephen Breyer." National Research Council. 2011. Reference Manual on Scientific Evidence: Third Edition. Washington, DC: The National Academies Press. doi: 10.17226/13163.

58. Introduction--Stephen Breyer." National Research Council. 2011. Reference Manual on Scientific Evidence: Third Edition. Washington, DC: The National Academies Press. doi: 10.17226/13163.

59. Gen. Elec. Co. v. Joiner, 522 U.S. 136 (1997); Daubert v. Merrell Dow Pharms., Inc., 509 U.S. 579 (1993). A description of the program can be found at Committee on Science, Technology, and Law.

without interfering with the jury's role as trier of fact, must determine whether purported scientific evidence is "reliable" and will "assist the trier of fact," thereby keeping from juries testimony that, in Pauli's sense, isn't even good enough to be wrong. This requirement extends beyond scientific testimony to all forms of expert testimony.[60] *The purpose of Daubert's gatekeeping requirement "is to make certain that an expert, whether basing testimony upon professional studies or personal experience, employs in the courtroom the same level of intellectual rigor that characterizes the practice of an expert in the relevant field."* [61, 62]

Examples of courts using scientific experts include a genetic engineering patent case,[63] silicone gel breast implant,[64] environmental science,[65] "neutral science panels"[66], and others.

A number of scientific and professional organizations have come forward with proposals to aid the courts in finding skilled experts.[67] Toxicology organizations and the veterinary profession may consider such proposals.

ACKNOWLEDGMENT

My sincere appreciation to Mr. Kevin Conard, Drs. Roger McClellan, Richard Huston, Beth Thompson, Judith Kashman, and federal employees who asked to not be named, for reviewing an early draft of this chapter and providing their valuable insight.

REFERENCES

Amorgianos *v. National* R.R. Passenger Corp., 303 F.3d 256 (2d Cir. 2002). Testimony of a treating physician, toxicologist and industrial hygienist were excluded, and the exclusion affirmed because the literature did not support a finding of general causation at the relevant exposure levels when workers were exposed to xylene and developed asymmetric polyneuropathy and other neurological symptoms.

Bocanegra *v. Vicmar Services, Inc.*, 320 F.3d 581 (5th Cir.), cert. denied, 124 S. Ct. 180 (2003). A toxicologist's testimony was excluded, but the exclusion was reversed, because the toxicologist's testimony was supported by peer-reviewed literature and relied on generally accepted principles.

Burleson *v. Texas Dep't of Criminal Justice*, 393 F.3d 577 (5th Cir. 2004). Testimony of a toxicologist excluded and the exclusion was affirmed because he performed no dose assessment and offered no epidemiological studies showing a statistically significant link between thorium dioxide exposure and the type of lung and throat cancer present.

Clausen *v. M/V New Carissa*, 339 F.3d 1049 (9th Cir. 2003). Dueling marine biologist's testimony was allowed and the allowance was affirmed, because each expert performed differential diagnosis analysis in which they first "ruled in" six potential causes then both experts ruled out 4 of them. They disagreed on the remaining 2.

Daubert v. Merrell Dow Pharms., Inc., 509 U.S. 579, 1993. at 590 n. 9. See also Bert Black *et al.*, Science and the Law in the Wake of Daubert: A New Search for Scientific Knowledge, 72 TEX. L. REV. 715 (1994); Joseph Sanders, Scientific Validity, Admissibility, and Mass Torts after Daubert, 78 MINN. L. REV. 1387 (1994).

General Electric Co v. Joiner, 522 U.S. 136 (1997).

Kelley v. American Heyer-Schulte Corp., 957 F. Supp. at 882.

Kumho Tire Co v. Carmichael, 119 S. Ct. 1167, 1999. See also *Braun* v. *Lorillard Inc.*, 84 F.3d 230, 234 (7th Cir. 1996); *Rosen* v. *Ciba-Geigy Corp.*, 78 F.3d 316, 318 (7th Cir. 1996), and *Black* v. *Food Lion, Inc.*, 171 F.3d 308, 311 (5th Cir. 1999).

Mary Sue H., et al., Reference Guide on Toxicology, II, in Reference Manual on Scientific Evidence.

Rule 104, (a).

Rule 104, (e).

Rule 401.

Rule 901, (9).

Rule 402.

Rule 602.

Rule 901, (3).

Dillingham, W.O., Hagan, P.J., Salas, R.E. Blueprint for general causation analysis in toxic tort litigation†submitted by the authors on behalf of the FDCC Toxic Tort and Environmental Law Section.

FURTHER READING

AFL-CIO *v. OSHA* 965 F.2d 962, 969-70 (11th Cir. 1992).

R.J. Allen, The Nature of Judical Proof, 13 CARDOZO L. REV. 373 (1991).

Bernstein, D.E., Jackson, J.D., 2004. The Daubert Trilogy in the States, 44 Jurimetrics J. 351.

Black v. Food Lion, *Inc.*, 171 F.3d 308, 311-12 (5th Cir. 1999) "In the vast majority of cases, the district court first should decide whether the factors mentioned in *Daubert* are appropriate. Once it considers the *Daubert* factors, the court then can consider whether other factors, not mentioned in *Daubert*, are relevant to the case at hand." see also *Goebel* v. *Denver and Rio Grande W. R.R. Co.*, 215 F.3d 1083, 1087 (10th Cir. 2000).

Bonner *v. ISP Techs., Inc.*, 259 F.3d 924 (8th Cir. 2001).

Carmichael v. Samyang Tire Inc, 923 F. Supp. 1514, 1522 (S.D. Ala. 1996 at 1520-21).

60. Kumho Tire Co. v. Carmichael, 119 S. Ct. 1167 (1999).

61. Id. at 1176

62. Introduction--Stephen Breyer." National Research Council. 2011. Reference Manual on Scientific Evidence: Third Edition. Washington, DC: The National Academies Press. doi: 10.17226/13163.

63. Biogen, Inc. v. Amgen, Inc., 973 F. Supp. 39 (D. Mass. 1997). MediaCom Corp. v. Rates Tech., Inc., 4 F. Supp. 2d 17 app. B at 37 (D. Mass. 1998) (quoting the Affidavit of Engagement filed in Biogen, Inc. v. Amgen, Inc., 973 F. Supp. 39 (D. Mass. 1997) (No. 95-10496)).

64. Hall v. Baxter Healthcare Corp., 947 F. Supp. 1387 (D. Or. 1996).

65. Conservation Law Found. v. Evans, 203 F. Supp. 2d 27, 32 (D.D.C. 2002).

66. Olivia Judson, Slide-Rule Justice, Nat'l J., Oct. 9, 1999, at 2882, 2885.

67. Introduction--Stephen Breyer." National Research Council. 2011. Reference Manual on Scientific Evidence: Third Edition. Washington, DC: The National Academies Press. doi: 10.17226/13163.

Carruth, R.S., Goldstein, B.D., 2001. Relative risk greater than two in proof of causation in toxic tort litigation. Jurimetrics. 41, 195–209.

Cavallo *v. Star Enterprise*, 892 F. Supp. 756, 771 (E.D. Va. 1995), aff'd in part, rev'd in part, 100 F.3d 1150 (4th Cir. 1996). See also, *Implant Litig.*, 11 F. Supp. 2d 1217, 1230 (D. Colo. 1998); *Kelley v. American Heyer-Schulte Corp.*, 957 F. Supp. 873, 882 (W.D. Tex. 1997); *Rutigliano v. Valley Bus. Forms*, 929 F. Supp. 779, 783 (D. N.J. 1996); *Hall v. Baxter Healthcare Corp.*, 947 F. Supp. 1387, 1413 (D. Or. 1996).

Daubert I, 509 U.S. at 593 n. 10; see e.g., *Carnegie Mellon Univ. v. Hoffmann-LaRoche, Inc.*, 55 F. Supp. 2d 1024, 1030 (N.D. Cal. 1999).

DeLuca v. Merrell Dow Pharms., 911 F.2d 941, 958 (3d Cir. 1990).

Dodge v. Cotter Corp., 328 F.3d 1212 (10th Cir. 2003).

Eaton, D.L., Klaassen, C.D., 2001. Principles of toxicology. In: Klaassen, C.D. (Ed.), Casarett and Doull's Toxicology, The Basic Science of Poisons, Chapter 2, 6th edition McGraw Hill, New York, pp. 11–34.

Federal Rules of Evidence. December 31, 2004. judiciary.house.gov/media/ pdfs/printers/108th/evid2004.

Frye v. United States, 293 F. 1013 (D.C. Cir. 1923).

Giannelli, P.C., 1980. The admissibility of novel scientific evidence: *Frye v. United States*, a half-century later. 80 Colum. L. Rev. 1197, 1205.

Giannelli, P.C., 1980. , The admissibility of novel scientific evidence: *Frye v. United States*, a half–century later. 80 COLUM. L. REV. 1197, 1201.

Goeb v. Tharaldson, 615 N.W.2d 800, 816 (Minn. 2000).

Goebel v. Denver & Rio Grande Western R.R., 215 F.3d 1083 (10th Cir. 2000).

Goebel v. Denver & Rio Grande Western R.R., No. 02-1391 (10th Cir. Oct. 9, 2003).

Goldstein, B.D., 1997. Toxic substances: scientific status, modern scientific evidence. In: Faigman, Kaye, Saks, Sanders (Eds.), *The Law and Science of Expert Testimony*. West Publishing Company, St. Paul, MN, pp. 277–299.

Toxic substances: scientific status. In: Goldstein, B.D., Carruth, R.S., Faigman, Kaye, Saks, Sanders (Eds.), Modern Scientific Evidence: The Law and Science of Expert Testimony. second ed. West Publishing Company, St. Paul, MN.

Goldstein, B.D., 1993. Invited Paper "Linking scientific and technical expertise to the courts: a scientist's view of barriers and incentives". Presented at the Demonstration Project Planning Conference, Federal Judicial Center, Washington, DC. November 5, 1993.

Goldstein, B.D., 1997. Basic laws for proving causation of disease. New Jersey Lawyer. 6, 6, 72, February 10, 1997.

Goldstein, B.D., Gallo, M.A., 1995. Overview of toxicology. Shepard's Expert Sci. Evid. Quart. 3-1, 45–64.

Goldstein, B.D., Henifin, M.S., 2000. Reference guide on toxicology, Reference Manual on Scientific Evidence. second ed. Federal Judicial Center, pp. 401–437.

Grimes v. Hoffmann-LaRoche, Inc., 907 F. Supp. 33, 38 (D.N.H. 1995).

Hall v. Baxter Healthcare Corp., 947 F. Supp. 1387, 1413 (D. Or. 1996) (holding that "[t]estimony regarding specific causation in a given patient is irrelevant unless general causation is established").

In re Breast Implant Litigation, 11 F. Supp. 2d 1217, 1230 (D. Colo 1998).

In re Paoli, 35 F.3d at 758.

Lennon v. Norfolk & W. Ry. Co., 123 F. Supp. 2d 1143, 1154 (N.D. Ind. 2000).

Mancuso v. Consolidated Edison Co., 56 F. Supp. 2d 391, 403 (S.D.N.Y. 1999), rev'd on other grounds, 216 F.3d 1072 (2d Cir. 2000), at 394-95.

Moore v. Ashland Chemical, Inc. 126 F.3d 679, 5th Cir. 1997, rehearing en banc granted, opinion vacated, 151 F.3d 269 (5th Cir. 1998).

National Bank of Commerce v. Associated Milk Producers, Inc., 22 F. Supp. 2d 942, 963 (E.D. Ark. 1998), aff'd, 191 F.3d 858 (8th Cir. 1999).

Plourde v. Gladstone, No. 02-9136, 2d Cir. June 27, 2003 (unpublished): The testimony of a toxicologist was excluded, and the exclusion affirmed, because the toxicologist was not a medical doctor ans was therefore unqualified to offer a reliable differential diagnosis regarding the development of symptoms after exposure of pesticide following spraying the neighbor's farm.

Ray v. Miller Meester Advertising, Inc., Filed June 16, 2003, File No. 9817380.

Raynor v. Merrell Pharmaceuticals, 101 F.3d 129, 138-39 (D.C. Cir. 1996).

Raynor v. Merrell Pharms., Inc., 104 F.3d 1371, 1376 (D.C. Cir. 1997).

Reference Manual on Scientific Evidence. Second edition. Federal Judicial Center, 2000. The manual is available at: www.fjc.gov/public/pdf.nsf/lookup/sciman00.pdf/$file/sciman00.pdf.

Rutigliano v. Valley Business Forms, 929 F. Supp. at 783.

Sanders, J., Scientific Validity, Admissibility and Mass torts After Daubert, 78 Minn L Rev. 1387 (1994); Susan R. Poulter, Science and Toxic Torts: Is there a rational Solution to the Problem of Causation ? 7 High Tech L.J. 189 (1992).

Siharath v. Sandoz Pharms. Corp., 131 F. Supp. 2d 1347, 1352 (N.D. Ga. 2001) (citing *Wheat v. Sofamor*, S.N.C, 46 F. Supp. 2d 1351, 1357 (N.D. Ga. 1999) (product liability action excluding testimony that failed to establish (1) that Parlodel is capable of causing stroke and (2) that Palodel did in fact cause plaintiffs' strokes)).

Siharath, 131 F. Supp. 2d at 1352. See e.g. D. T. Ralston, Toxic Tort Causation – Not Just Chemical Exposure Plus Symptoms, Maely's Daubert Rep., Vol. 4, No. 5, at 15-25 (2000).

Simpson v Young, 854 f.2d 1429, 1435 (D.C. Cir, 1988).

State of Minnesota v. DeShay, June 11, 2002, MN Court of Appeals, C9-01-1128. File No. K200600502.

State v. Anderson, 379 N.W.2d 70, 79 (Minn. 1985) (Graphology "is accorded a low measure of scientific reliability in predicting character or state of mind and is not generally accepted in the scientific fields of psychology and psychiatry.").

State v. Jobe, 486 N.W.2d 407, 419-20 (Minn. 1992) (Admission of expert testimony based on DNA test results is proper because the principles underlying forensic DNA testing are generally accepted, and the laboratory complied with the appropriate standards and controls, thus rendering the results legally reliable.).

State v. Kolander, 236 Minn. 209, 221–222, 52 N.W.2d 458, 465 (1952).

State v. Mack, 292 N.W.2d 764, 768–769, 772 (Minn. 1980).

State v. Moore, 458 N.W.2d 90, 97–98 (Minn. 1990) (Admission of expert testimony on blood spatter interpretation was proper where the district court determined that the theory was generally accepted and the theory's application was legally reliable).

State v. Moore, 458 N.W.2d 90, 97–98 (Minn. 1990).

State v. Rose, 667 N.W.2d 386, 397 (Minn. 2003).

State v. Schwartz, 447 N.W.2d 422 (Minn. 1989).

Troy Corp v. Browner, 129 F.3rd 1290 (D.C. Cir 1997).

United States v. Downing, 753 F.2d 1224, 1234 (3d. Cir. 1985).

United States v. Hansen, 262 F.3d 1217 (11th Cir. 2001), cert. denied, 535 U.S. 1111 (2002).

United States v. Ledesma, No. 99-8026 (10th Cir. Feb. 14, 2000) (unpublished).

Viterbo v. Dow Chemical Co., 111. 826 F.2d 420 (5th Cir. 1987) at 424.

Westberry v. Gislaved Gummi AB, 178 F.3d 257, 263 (4th Cir. 1999).

Wills v. Amerada Hess Corp., 379 F.3d 32 (2d Cir. 2004). Testimony from a forensic toxicologist was excluded, and the exclusion was affirmed, because the toxicologist did not offer sufficient support for an oncogene theory that exposure to benzene and polycyclic hydrocarbons had caused squamous cell carcinoma, and because he had not ruled out smoking and alcohol as causes.

Wynacht v. Beckman Instruments, Inc., 113 F. Supp. 2d 1205, 1209 (E.D. Tenn. 2000).

Section II

Organ Toxicity

Chapter 12

Nervous System Toxicity

Donna Mensching and Camille DeClementi

INTRODUCTION

The nervous system is a susceptible target for toxicity because of its complex anatomy, specialized functions, high metabolic requirements, limited ability to repair itself, and the potential for life-threatening complications when disequilibrium occurs. A plethora of neurotoxicants exists including man-made pesticides, agents of chemical warfare, medications, illicit drugs, and all-natural compounds produced by a variety of organisms, such as spiders and snakes, which confer advantages to their makers such as increased predatory efficiency, avoidance of predation, or increased survivability in environmental extremes.

As is the case with any toxicant, exposure to a significant dosage of a neurotoxicant warrants appropriate decontamination in an otherwise healthy and asymptomatic patient. In the symptomatic patient, alleviation of clinical signs may be nonspecific or symptomatic (e.g., diazepam for seizures) or specifically antidotal based on the mechanism of toxicity (e.g., pralidoxime for organophosphorus (OPs) insecticides). Table 12.1 lists examples of antidotes used for select neurotoxicants. Clinical signs of nervous system toxicity (Table 12.2) can be divided roughly into stimulatory and depressant categories, although an overlap of these categories can occur with varying dosages of a given toxicant and/or class of toxicant. When severe signs are not minimized, potential complications can result including extremes of body temperature and blood pressure, hypoxia/anoxia, disseminated intravascular coagulation, rhabdomyolysis, organ failure, and trauma resulting from an inability to assess the environment and/or inability to avoid environmental hazards.

The general nature of this chapter avoids discussion of every known neurotoxicant. Instead, neurotoxicants are divided into those that affect the structural integrity of the nervous system and those that affect only its functional integrity. It is important to note, though, that the functional integrity of the nervous system can be affected by insults to its structural integrity depending on the severity and location of the insult.

STRUCTURAL TOXICOSES

Histopathological abnormalities associated with structural toxicoses can be subdivided into neuronopathy, axonopathy, or myelinopathy. The following discussion addresses each of these pathologies, providing examples relevant to veterinary toxicology.

Neuronopathy

A neurotoxicant that causes neuronopathy directly targets the neuronal cell body, resulting in cell death and secondary axonal degeneration. Gliosis, proliferation of astrocytes and/or microglial cells, is a common response to loss of neurons (Anthony et al., 2001). With few exceptions, this type of injury is irreversible. Examples of such toxicants include methyl mercury, which preferentially targets the cell bodies of the occipital cortex and the cerebellum via an unproven mechanism. Blindness and motor incoordination are common manifestations of lesions in these areas. In veterinary medicine, methyl mercury intoxication is most likely seen in animals that subsist on a diet of contaminated fish. A classic example from the 1950s involved the cats of mercury-contaminated Minamata Bay, Japan. Because of their advanced cerebellar ataxia, these cats often fell into the water of the bay and were described as "dancing" or "suicidal" (Smith and Smith, 1975; Francis, 1994). In recent years, awareness of environmental contamination with mercury has created biomonitoring programs that attempt to assess the impact of dietary mercury on piscivorous wildlife such as bald eagles (Hinck et al., 2009).

Domoic acid, the neurotoxicant responsible for amnesic shellfish poisoning in people and wildlife, is produced

Veterinary Toxicology. DOI: http://dx.doi.org/10.1016/B978-0-12-811410-0.00012-X

TABLE 12.1 Neurotoxicants and Associated Antidotes (Poppenga, 2004; Roder, 2004b,d; Plumb, 2015)

Neurotoxicant(s)	Antidote(s)
Acetaminophen	Acetylcysteine
Amitraz, brimonidine, xylazine	Atipamezole, yohimbine
Benzodiazepines	Flumazenil
Botulinum toxin	Antitoxin
Coral snake	Antivenom
Ethylene glycol	Fomepizole (4-MP), ethanol
Isoniazid	Pyridoxine/vitamin B_6
Lactrodectus spp.	Antivenin
Lead	Succimer, calcium EDTA, D-penicillamine
Metronidazole	Diazepam
Pyrethroids	Methocarbamol
Opioids	Naloxone
Organophosphorus insecticides	Pralidoxime (2-PAM), atropine
Scorpion	Antivenom
SSRIs/TCAs	Cyproheptadine
Tetanus toxin	Antitoxin

TABLE 12.2 Signs Associated With Neurotoxicoses (Podell, 2000)

Stimulatory	Depressant
Hyperactivity	Obtundation
Vocalization	Stupor
Tremors	Coma
Seizures	Ataxia
Hyperesthesia	Paresis/Paralysis
Hypermetria	Abasia
Other: Disorientation	
Paresthesia	
SLUDDE (*s*alivation, *l*acrimation, increased *u*rination, *d*iarrhea, *d*yspnea, and *e*mesis	
Cranial nerve deficits (rare)	

by the diatom *Pseudo-nitzschia* spp. The toxin is thought to exert its excitatory and cytotoxic effects on hippocampal cells because of its high affinity for binding to the kainite receptor, which is a glutamate receptor subtype. Cellular excitation ensues, resulting in an influx of Ca^{2+} ions, up-regulation of the c-Fos gene, and cell death (Jeffery et al., 2004). Domoic acid toxicity has been responsible for the considerable morbidity and mortality rate of the California sea lion (*Zalophus californianus*; Gulland et al., 2002).

A third example of neuronotoxicosis occurs in large animals, such as horses, when they ingest yellow star thistle (*Centaurea solstitialis*). This occurs typically in the dry summer and fall seasons and results in neurologic signs including involuntary lip and tongue movements, difficulty in prehending food, tremors, writhing, possible circling, persistent slow movements (dystonia), and significant weight loss. The disease is also called nigropallidal encephalomalacia because of the areas of the brain that are uniquely affected (the globus pallidus and the pars reticularis of the substantia nigra). The clinical signs manifest in these regions draw a striking similarity to Parkinson's disease in people (Burrows and Tyrl, 2013; Sanders et al., 2001), which has been associated with the selective loss of dopaminergic neurons (van den Munckhof et al., 2006). Of the guaianolide sesquiterpene lactones isolated from *Centaurea* species, cynaropicrin and an analog of solstitialin are cytotoxic in primary cultures of rat substantia nigra cells, and thus raise suspicion about their role in the toxicosis. Aspartic and glutamic acids, two excitatory amino acid neurotransmitters, are also present in *Centaurea* (Burrows and Tyrl, 2013), but their role, if any, in the mechanism of nigropallidal encephalomalacia has yet to be determined.

A final example of a neuronopathic toxicant is currently a common drug of abuse called methylenedioxyamphetamine (MDMA) or "Ecstasy." MDMA selectively targets serotonergic and dopaminergic cells depending on the species exposed, and long-term, irreversible effects may be seen (Gouzoulis-Mayfrank and Daumann, 2006). Acute physiologic effects in people include tachycardia, hypertension, euphoria, heightened sexual awareness, urinary urgency, nausea, chills, sweating, hyperthermia, among others. Signs consistent with serotonin syndrome (hyperactivity, agitation, mental confusion, hyperthermia, tachycardia and tremors) have been observed in experimentally exposed rats (Easton and Marsden, 2006). Further research is indicated to define species-specific effects, particularly the extent to which serotoninergic or dopaminergic neurons are involved. Veterinary practitioners should be aware of the potential for accidentally exposing small animals to this toxicant.

Axonopathy

The second class of structural lesions caused by neurotoxicants is axonopathy. Despite damage to the axon, the neuronal cell body remains intact, but the portion of the axon distal to the lesion degenerates, resulting in a "chemical transection" distal to the lesion that is functionally identical to a physical transection of the axon. This is also known as Wallerian or axonal degeneration. Changes in the Nissl substance, the protein synthetic material comprised of free polyribosomes and rough endoplasmic reticulum, become evident histologically in response to this degeneration. These changes include chromatolysis (dissolution of the Nissl substance) as well as margination of the Nissl and the nucleus to the periphery of the cell body. Not surprisingly, those neurons with axons of greatest length are most susceptible to axonal damage. To highlight the susceptibility of distal axons, a subclassification of axonopathy affecting these axons has been termed "central peripheral distal axonopathy." This is in contrast to "central peripheral proximal axonopathy," which involves axons proximal to the spinal cord (Anthony et al., 2001). A third subclassification of axonopathy has been termed "dying back axonopathy," which represents progressive death of the axon toward the cell body over time and continued injury. In the peripheral nervous system (PNS), the prognosis for at least partial regeneration is good, but this is less true in the central nervous system (CNS). Secondary demyelination is also possible with axonal injury (Mandella, 2002). Both sensory and motor axons can be affected.

Many agents cause axonopathies, yet just a few are particularly relevant to veterinary medicine. The first example, commonly used as an antineoplastic drug, is the vinca alkaloid vincristine, which is derived from the periwinkle plant, *Vinca rosea* or *Catharanthus rosea*. Vincristine exerts its therapeutic effect by binding to tubulin, inhibiting microtubular formation, disrupting the formation of the mitotic spindle, and arresting cell division at metaphase (Roder, 2004a). Neurotoxicity in the form of axonal degeneration can occur as a result of the disruption of fast axonal transport (rate of 400 mm/day normally), which relies on the functional integrity of the microtubules (Anthony et al., 2001). Cats are more sensitive to the neurotoxic potential of vincristine. With discontinuation of therapy and appropriate supportive care, animals exhibiting signs of peripheral neuropathy may improve over several weeks to months (Roder, 2004a). Colchicine, an antimetabolite derived from the autumn crocus (*Colchicum autumnale*) and the glory lily (*Gloriosa* spp.), also inhibits spindle formation (Burrows and Tyrl, 2013; Roder, 2004a). It is used in veterinary medicine for the treatment of amyloidosis associated with Shar Pei fever (Loeven, 1994) as well as hepatic fibrosis (Plumb, 2015). Although reported rarely in humans, no published reports of peripheral neuropathy in veterinary patients were found.

A more common, yet fortunately still rare, cause of neurotoxicosis in veterinary medicine is metronidazole. A nitroimidazole antibacterial and antiprotozoal agent used to treat *Giardia* and anaerobic intestinal bacterial overgrowth in small animals (Plumb, 2015), metronidazole can result in a sensory peripheral neuropathy manifesting as proprioceptive deficits (Gupta et al., 2000) as well as CNS effects including ataxia, nystagmus, head tilt, and seizure activity (Plumb, 2015). Myelinated fibers are most commonly affected (Anthony et al., 2001). The mechanism is unknown for both peripheral and central effects. Oral and/or IV diazepam has been associated with hastened recovery of metronidazole toxicity in dogs (Evans et al., 2003).

A final example of a class of agents that can cause axonopathy are the OPs compounds, commonly used as insecticides, which can result in signs of neuropathy 7–10 days postexposure, termed OP-induced delayed neuropathy or OPIDN. An example of historical significance was the delayed neuropathy associated with the intentional contamination of Jamaican ginger alcohol ("Jake") with tri-*ortho* cresyl phosphate (TOCP), an OPs compound, during the Prohibition Era. The TOCP was present in lindol, a substitute solvent added to the Jake to cut costs. The resulting upper motor neuron spasticity and paralysis were irreversible and affected more than 50,000 people (Woolf, 1995). In addition to humans, hens have also been shown to be very sensitive to OPIDN (Damodaran et al., 2001). The neuropathy associated with OPs is thought to involve slow axonal transport macromolecules, such as actin and tubulin, which involve movement of the neuronal cytoskeleton at a rate of 1–4 mm/day (Anthony et al., 2001).

Myelinopathy

Myelin is produced by the oligodendrocytes of the CNS and Schwann cells of the PNS. It is a lipid and forms a sheath around certain axons, namely those of the cranial and spinal nerves. It functions to increase the speed of impulse conduction by creating isolated areas of heightened electrical excitability, termed nodes of Ranvier (Spencer, 2000). Myelin gives white matter its characteristic appearance. Toxicants that result in myelinopathy may affect the myelin itself or target the cells that produce myelin. The insult may result in loss of myelin (demyelination) or edema of the myelin sheath and subsequent separation of myelin lamellae. Remyelination of segmentally demyelinated areas can occur more so in the PNS than the CNS. When peripheral nerves are remyelinated, the process involves more Schwann cells compared to the initial myelination. As a result, the nodes of Ranvier in remyelinated peripheral nerves are closer (Anthony et al., 2001).

Two examples of toxicants that result in intramyelinic edema and separation of the myelin lamellae are hexachlorophene and bromethalin. The former is an antibacterial agent frequently marketed decades ago as pHisoHex and that is still commercially available for the treatment and prevention of *Staphylococcal* infections. The latter is a rodenticide that is marketed under a variety of trade names including Assault, Sudden Death, and Vengeance. The mechanism by which hexachlorophene and bromethalin cause intramyelinic edema is due to the uncoupling of oxidative phosphorylation (Anthony et al., 2001; Dorman, 2004). This uncoupling results in decreased Na^+/K^+-ATPase activity, weakened ion gradients, and retention of water in the myelin lamellae (van Lier and Cherry, 1988). The use of mannitol or diuretics early in the course of the disease may reverse mild changes, but continued swelling of the lamellae results in a dramatic increase in intracranial and cerebrospinal fluid (CSF) pressure that is typically unresponsive to therapy. Clinical signs in an acute toxic exposure include muscle tremors, hyperthermia, generalized seizures, hyperexcitability, hyperesthesia and death within several hours of ingestion (4–18 h) for bromethalin. Cats are more sensitive to bromethalin than dogs are with a minimum lethal oral dose of 0.45 mg/kg versus 2.5 mg/kg in the dog (Dorman, 2004). At lower dosages, hind limb ataxia and paresis can develop in dogs and cats within 2–7 days of ingestion. Signs may include decreased or absent proprioception, loss of response to deep pain, upper motor neuron bladder paralysis, patellar hyperreflexia, and varying degrees of CNS depression. These sublethal effects may be spontaneously reversible with time (1–2 weeks). Histologic lesions consistent with bromethalin and hexachlorophene toxicosis include spongy degeneration (diffuse vacuolation) of the white matter of the CNS. Confirmation of a fatal bromethalin toxicosis can be accomplished by identifying the parent compound and/or its more toxic metabolite, desmethylbromethalin, in the liver. Because of their relative inability to metabolize bromethalin into desmethylbromethalin, guinea pigs are resistant to its toxic effects. Treatment of exposed susceptible species is largely aimed at initial decontamination via induction of emesis (in those species that can vomit) and administration of multiple doses of activated charcoal prior to the onset of clinical signs (Dorman, 2004).

Another toxicant that results in myelinopathy is inorganic lead. The peripheral neuropathic manifestation of lead intoxication is secondary to the segmental degeneration of myelin in distal motor fibers and is most commonly seen in veterinary medicine with chronic intoxication in horses. Sensory function is spared. Clinical signs may include dysphagia and secondary weight loss, ataxia, dysphonia, laryngeal paralysis ("roaring"), and facial nerve deficits. The CNS and other organs may be affected resulting in seizures, depression, secondary aspiration pneumonia, colic, and death (Gwaltney-Brant, 2004c).

FUNCTIONAL TOXICOSES

Most neurotoxicants exert their functional effects via the exquisitely orchestrated mechanisms involved in neurotransmission yet leave no structural footprint of their activity. This can occur at all levels within the nervous system including the CNS, PNS, and autonomic nervous system (ANS). Nervous impulses are chemically mediated across synapses by the release of neurotransmitters from the presynaptic terminal. These neurotransmitters then move across the synaptic cleft, bind to their postsynaptic target receptor, and affect either an excitatory or inhibitory response in the postsynaptic neuron or muscle (Anthony et al., 2001). Functional neurotoxicants may exert their action by preventing synthesis, storage, release, binding, reuptake or degradation of the neurotransmitter. Interference with axonal transmission via sodium, potassium, chloride or calcium channels, and the subsequent alteration of action potentials, can also result in functional toxicoses (Spencer, 2000; Hansen, 2006). Continual development of new pharmaceuticals targeting these endpoints will lead to an increased likelihood of intoxication in veterinary patients with accidental exposures, particularly in an overdose situation and/or if species differences in pharmacokinetics exist.

Examples of neurotransmitters include: acetylcholine (ACh); the catecholamine neurotransmitters (dopamine, norepinephrine and epinephrine); the amino acid derivatives serotonin (5-hydroxytryptamine; 5-HT), GABA, glycine, histamine, aspartic acid, and glutamic acid; and various neuropeptides including enkephalins, substance P (a neurokinin), orexins, endorphins, vasopressin (antidiuretic hormone), and thyroid releasing hormone (Beasley, 1999; Spencer, 2000). The complex array of neurotransmitters provides many targets for neurotoxicity. A more detailed discussion follows regarding some of the more common neurotransmitters involved in veterinary neurotoxicoses.

Acetylcholine

ACh is the neurotransmitter that mediates effects at the neuromuscular junction, at the preganglionic neurons of both the parasympathetic and sympathetic nervous systems of the ANS, and at many of the postganglionic neurons of the parasympathetic nervous system. It is the target neurotransmitter of OP and carbamate insecticides, which have been marketed since the 1970s and now are widely available commercially for home and agricultural use (Meerdink, 2004b; Gupta, 2006). Acetylcholinesterase (AChE) is the enzyme that degrades ACh to choline and acetic acid within the synaptic cleft. OP and carbamate insecticides bind to AChE—the former by phosphorylating the enzyme, the latter by carbamylating the enzyme—and prevent its degradative action on ACh. This results in an excess of ACh in the synaptic cleft and continued binding to the postsynaptic receptors. Examples of OPs include disulfoton, malathion, terbufos, phosmet, chlorpyrifos, tetrachlorvinphos, and parathion. Examples of carbamates include carbaryl, carbofuran, aldicarb, methomyl, and propoxur. The onset of action and severity of signs vary widely among these agents. OPs with a sulfur linkage need to be activated by p450 enzymes in the liver prior to exerting their toxic effects, a process which may take just minutes. Carbamates are active upon absorption but some of them are less likely to cross the blood–brain barrier than the more fat-soluble OPs. Cholinergic effects are mediated by both muscarinic and nicotinic receptors. Classic muscarinic effects include excess salivation, lacrimation, increased urination, diarrhea, dyspnea (due to increased bronchial secretions), and emesis (abbreviated as the mnemonic SLUDDE or the alternative DUMBELS, which stands for diarrhea, urination, miosis, bronchospasm, emesis, lacrimation, and salivation). Nicotinic effects include tremors, weakness, and paralysis. CNS effects can range from coma and depression to hyperactivity and seizures (Blodgett, 2006).

The main distinction between the OPs and carbamates is the reversibility of the bond between the insecticide and AChE. OPs phosphorylate affects the esteratic site of the enzyme. At variable times, depending on the type of OP bound, the carbon groups attached to the phosphorus are hydrolyzed and replaced by hydrogen. This process is classically referred to as "aging" and represents the point at which there is no possible functional recovery of that enzyme. The use of pralidoxime (2-PAM) as an antidote to preferentially bind the OP is useful only before the aging process has occurred. In contrast, the affinity of carbamates for AChE is much more labile, and aging does not occur with carbamylation of the enzyme. Therefore, the bond between AChE and carbamates is spontaneously reversible with time ($t_{½}$ = 30–40 min) and precludes the use of 2-PAM. Provided the receptor effects are not life-threatening, the prognosis for carbamate toxicoses is generally good. With potent carbamates such as methomyl, however, the signs may be severe enough and the duration of the effects long enough for the outcome to be fatal. Competitive inhibition of ACh with intravenous (IV) atropine (0.2–0.5 mg/kg, ¼ of dose IV to effect then remainder intramuscular (IM) or subcutaneous (SC)) is indicated for life-threatening bradycardia and/or dyspnea caused by bronchospasm and excess bronchial secretions (Plumb, 2015; Blodgett, 2006).

In addition to the chronic OPIDN (discussed under "Axonopathy" above) and the acute toxicosis with SLUDDE effects, there is an intermediate syndrome that is most commonly seen with more liphophilic OPs and classically with chlorpyrifos exposure in cats. It is thought to arise from a down-regulation of muscarinic receptors with sublethal, prolonged exposures. The clinical signs as a result are predominantly nicotinic in nature because those receptors are not down-regulated. Signs which typically appear within 3–10 days of exposure include generalized weakness (including ventroflexion of the neck due to the cat's lack of a nuchal ligament), anorexia, muscle tremors, seizures, depression, and/or death (Blodgett, 2006). Because of the reversibility of the bond of AChE with carbamates, the intermediate syndrome is not typically seen. However, it has been uncommonly reported with aldicarb exposures in people (Waseem et al., 2010) and has also been reported with canine aldicarb exposures (Arnot et al., 2011).

Another toxicant with muscarinic effects is the mycotoxin slaframine, produced from the fungus *Rhizoctonia leguminicola* and primarily associated with clovers (*Trifolium* species). It is a cholinergic agonist which is responsible for the clinical picture of profuse salivation or "slobbers" in affected animals (Meerdink, 2004a). Clinical signs consistent with muscarinic stimulation are also seen with ingestion of mushrooms of the genera *Inocybe* and *Clitocybe*, among others, which contain the toxic principal muscarine (Turner and Szczawinski, 1991). Anatoxin-a(s), a neurotoxin produced by the cyanobacteria *Anabaena* sp., *Aphanizomenon* sp. and *Oscillatoria* sp., inhibits AChE in the PNS. Like slaframine, the toxin does not cross the blood–brain barrier (Roder, 2004c).

Several examples of neurotoxicants exist that antagonize muscarinic effects as well. The classic poisonous plant *Atropa belladonna*, or deadly nightshade, is the source of atropine, a racemic mixture of the tropane alkaloids, D- and L-hyoscyamine (Burrows and Tyrl, 2013). Another belladonna alkaloid is scopolamine (L-hyoscine). *Datura* sp., commonly known as jimsonweed, thorn apple or devil's trumpet, contains scopolamine and hyoscyamine. Excessive anticholinergic action can result in sinus tachycardia, a dry mouth manifesting as increased thirst, dilated pupils, visual disturbances, ileus, urinary retention, restlessness, muscular twitching, incoordination, delirium (as a result of crossing the blood–brain barrier and entering the CNS), respiratory paralysis, and, uncommonly, death (Burrows and Tyrl, 2013; Pickrell et al., 2004).

Nicotinic cholinergic receptors alone can be involved with neurotoxicoses. Nature has provided several poisonous plants that stimulate these receptors including *Nicotiana* sp. (varying types of tobacco), *Conium maculatum* or poison hemlock, and *Lobelia* or Indian tobacco. The numerous alkaloids present in these plants as well as the cyanobacterial toxin anatoxin-a, most commonly produced by *Anabaena flos-aquae* (Roder, 2004c), exert their neurotoxic effects by initially stimulating nicotinic cholinergic and neuromuscular junction receptors but ultimately result in a persistent neuromuscular blocking effect. Signs include muscular weakness, tremors, nausea, vomiting, ataxia, tachypnea, tachycardia, hypertension, mydriasis, staggering, seizures, respiratory failure, and death (Panter, 2004a,b,c). Treatment is symptomatic and supportive. Prognosis is good except in cases of large overdoses.

Imidacloprid (Advantage) is a chloronicotinyl nitroguanide insecticide marketed for flea control in pets and which exerts its effects via possibly both agonist and antagonist actions at the nicotinic ACh receptor. Death of the insect is effected via the same clinical signs as previously described above, yet imidacloprid has a wide margin of safety in mammals due to its poor systemic absorption when applied dermally (as labeled) (Craig et al., 2005) and due to the higher affinity of imidacloprid for insect nicotinic receptors versus mammalian receptors. Acute oral ingestions are usually limited to nausea, salivation, and vomiting (Wismer, 2004).

Another mechanism by which ACh can be involved in toxicoses is the lack of release of the neurotransmitter from the presynaptic terminal. Botulinum toxin, produced by the anaerobic bacterium *Clostridium botulinum*, exerts its action via this mechanism. Sources of the toxin include ingestion of food contaminated with either preformed toxin or clostridial spores, contamination of a puncture wound with spores, and ingestion of spores from the environment. Exposure can be oral, inhaled, or absorbed cutaneously through devitalized skin (Bailey, 2006). The toxin consists of a 100 kDa heavy chain and a 50 kDa light chain linked by disulfide and noncovalent bonds. Upon ingestion of the toxin, its heavy chain binds synaptotagmin, a presynaptic vesicle protein. Once the toxin is internalized within the presynaptic terminal, its disulfide bonds are cleaved, releasing the light chain. The free light chain is then available to cleave proteins that are responsible for the docking and release of ACh vesicles into the synapse.

Seven different botulinum toxins (A–G) have been described. Types C and D are most commonly associated with veterinary species (type C is most common in dogs); types A, B, E and F have caused disease in humans. Although differences exist regarding which proteins are cleaved by each toxin type, the end result is the lack of ACh in the synaptic cleft of the neuromuscular junction (Roder, 2004b). The clinical result is a progressive flaccid paralysis which results in death within 3–10 days. Signs are symmetric and progress from the pelvic limbs toward the thoracic limbs. Cranial nerves may be affected, possibly resulting in megaesophagus, decreased jaw tone, facial paralysis and/or a decreased gag reflex. Autonomic functions may be affected as well (Coleman, 1998). The disease is called limber neck in affected birds. In human patients who have been supported with artificial respiration, the duration of the effect has been documented to persist for 6–8 months (Kotsonis et al., 2001).

The prognosis for severely affected animals is at best guarded, but more realistically, poor. Treatment can include debridement of wounds, penicillin therapy, and antitoxin (5 mL IV or IM) within the first 5 days of exposure. Administration of the antitoxin does not reverse the clinical signs attributed to neurons already affected by the toxin. Because of its equine source and antigenicity, an intradermal test dose is recommended prior to full administration IV or IM. For individuals already severely affected, assisted ventilation is indicated until the patient can breathe spontaneously, yet the duration of therapy required may not be practical in veterinary medicine. Extreme supportive care, including assisted or parenteral feeding, physical therapy, manual evacuation of the bladder and intermittent manipulation of body position to prevent hypostatic congestion and formation of decubital ulcers, is critical. Some laboratories can confirm the diagnosis with analysis of serum, gut contents, and/or feed for the preformed toxin (Roder, 2004b; Bailey, 2006). A mouse inoculation assay and type-specific ELISA testing may also aid in the diagnosis of botulism (Thomas, 1991).

Catecholamine Neurotransmitters

Catecholamines are "fight or flight" neurotransmitters that include norepinephrine, epinephrine and dopamine. Their synthesis begins with conversion of the amino acid L-tyrosine to L-dopa. Removal of a carboxyl group from L-dopa forms dopamine which is acted upon by dopamine β-hydroxylase to form norepinephrine (Spencer, 2000). Norepinephrine is also stored in the adrenal medulla and released into the blood with sympathetic stimulation (Capen, 2001). *N*-methylation of norepinephrine forms epinephrine, an adrenal hormone, which is only nominally present in the brain. Catecholamines are inactivated by monoamine oxidase (MAO) and catechol-*O*-methyltransferase (COMT) enzymes (Beasley, 1999; Spencer, 2000).

In addition to its role at postganglionic sympathetic neurons, norepinephrine also mediates effects in the CNS. Adrenergic receptors include α_1, α_2, β_1 and β_2 receptors. Stimulation of α_1 adrenergic receptors, present peripherally, results in vasoconstriction and mydriasis. Stimulation of α_2 adrenergic receptors, present in the CNS, mediates inhibition of norepinephrine, resulting in effects opposite those of α_1 stimulation, namely hypotension. Stimulation of β_1 receptors, located predominantly in the heart but also in the kidney, adipose, skeletal muscle, and eye, results most notably in an increase in the rate and force of cardiac contraction. The β_2 adrenergic receptors (present in skeletal muscles, the smooth muscle of the bronchi, vasculature and uterus, and the liver) mediate vasodilation, bronchodilation, uterine relaxation, and enhanced glycogenolysis in the liver (Landsberg and Young, 2001).

Examples of adrenergic toxicosis involving overstimulation of the α_2 receptors include: accidental ingestion of brimonidine, the active ingredient in Alphagan eye drops used in the treatment of glaucoma; ingestion of amitraz-containing Preventic collars; ingestion of clonidine, a human medication used for hypertension and other indications; and overdosage of the sedative/analgesic xylazine. Exposures involving Alphagan typically involve puncturing of the bottle with sparing amounts actually ingested. Clinical signs for all four toxicoses include profound hypotension and bradycardia, which can be specifically reversed with either of the α_2 antagonists, yohimbine or atipamezole (Antisedan). Patients should be closely monitored for recurrence of signs once the effect of the antagonist wears off. The half-life of atipamezole in dogs is longer than yohimbine and may require less frequent administration (Plumb, 2015; Mensching, 2011).

An example of adrenergic toxicosis involving overstimulation of the β_2 adrenergic receptors involves the accidental puncture by chewing on a pressurized albuterol inhaler. Albuterol is a β_2 adrenergic agonist used therapeutically to treat the bronchoconstriction associated with asthma. When excessive β_2 stimulation occurs, profound hypotension, a reflex tachycardia, and subsequent release of catecholamines can occur. Clinical signs usually include tachycardia with possible ventricular premature contractions, tachypnea, hyper- or hypotension (depending on the timeframe relative to exposure and the predominating neurotransmitter effect), behavioral changes including restlessness, agitation, anxiety, largely due to secondary catecholamine release, weakness later in the course, and hypokalemia, sometimes severe, because of an intracellular potassium shift. Treatment is largely supportive with fluid therapy, management of severe tachycardia with a β blocker such as propranolol, supplementation of potassium as needed, and diazepam to address behavioral changes due to secondary norepinephrine release (Mensching and Volmer, 2007).

Sympathomimetics such as amphetamines, cocaine, pseudoephedrine, phenylpropanolamine and ma huang mediate dopaminergic and norepinephrine-induced neurotoxic effects including hypertension, hyperexcitability, tachycardia, tremors, seizures, mydriasis, hyperesthesia, head-bobbing, piloerection, and death. Phenothiazine tranquilizers such as acepromazine and chlorpromazine are the mainstay of sympathomimetic overdose therapy due to their postsynaptic blocking effects of dopamine as well as inhibition of its release and increase in its turnover in the CNS. Phenothiazines also block α adrenergic and cholinergic activity and are antihistaminic (Plumb, 2015; Means, 2004).

Serotonin

Serotonin (5-hydroxytryptamine) synthesis involves the conversion of the amino acid tryptophan to 5-hydroxytryptophan (5-HTP) followed by the conversion of 5-HTP to 5-hydroxytryptamine. The various physiologic roles of serotonin include regulation of sleep, mood, cognition, appetite, and behavior (Spencer, 2000). Because of the popularity of selective serotonin reuptake inhibitors (SSRIs) in human and veterinary medicine and over-the-counter supplements containing 5-HTP for the treatment of depression in humans, accidental overdoses are common in veterinary medicine. Examples of SSRIs include fluoxetine (Prozac), fluvoxamine (Luvox), paroxetine (Paxil) and sertraline (Zoloft) (Plumb, 2015). The seeds of the West African legume *Griffonia simplicifolia* contain 5-HTP. The clinical picture of serotonin excess, termed serotonin syndrome, includes tremors, seizures, hyperthermia, depression (rarely to the point of coma), disorientation, vocalization, hyperesthesia, ataxia, tachycardia, hypertension, agitation, vomiting, and diarrhea. Treatment of the clinical patient is largely symptomatic and supportive, but the serotonin antagonist cyproheptadine specifically mediates the effects of serotonin syndrome. The drug can be given orally or crushed, mixed with water or saline, and administered rectally at a dosage of 1.1 mg/kg in dogs (Gwaltney-Brant, 2004a).

Glycine

Glycine is an inhibitory neurotransmitter that is synthesized from serine. Glycine acts predominantly in interneurons (Renshaw cells) of the brainstem and spinal cord as well as in spinal sensory, auditory, and visual pathways. Two well-known toxicants, tetanus and strychnine, act by inhibiting glycine's inhibitory effects. Tetanospasmin, a biotoxin produced by the anaerobic bacterium *Clostridium tetani*, is responsible for the prevention of glycine release (Roder, 2004b). The ubiquitous bacterial spores typically enter through a puncture or other anaerobic wound. The lack of glycine inhibition results in unchecked muscle contraction, largely of the powerful extensor muscles of the limbs and the masseter muscles. The stereotypical sawhorse stance and "lockjaw" result within 5–10 days of wound infection. Less severe signs include elevation of the nictitating membrane, which may be the earliest indication of toxicosis in the horse, the most sensitive species (Coleman, 1998). Contracture of facial muscles may result in abnormal wrinkles in the skin, erect ears or an abnormal expression, sometimes referred to as a sardonic grin. Progression of the disease results in an inability to rise and possible seizures. Severe muscular contraction or seizures may be induced by external stimuli. Death is due to an inability of the muscles of respiration to relax and subsequent hypoxia (Roder, 2004b).

Diagnosis of tetanus is based on characteristic clinical signs, history of a wound in which the organism could have proliferated, and the anaerobic culture of an infected wound. Vaccination with tetanus toxoid is recommended to prevent the disease in horses. Animals with wounds should be treated with penicillin, and the wound should be cleaned routinely to prevent proliferation of the bacteria. A tetanus antitoxin exists but is ineffective for a toxin that is already bound and will not reverse existing clinical signs. It can help to prevent progression of the disease, though. The dose for horses and cattle is 10,000–50,000 units SC or IM and 3000–15,000 units for sheep and swine and can be repeated in 7–10 days (Roder, 2004b). Contrary to popular belief, the antitoxin may be extremely cost effective. At the time of this writing, the Colorado Serum Company (Denver, CO) sells 15,000 units for $28.00 (US) (www.colorado-serum.com). Muscle spasms and seizure activity can be managed by minimization of external stimuli as well as with tranquilizers and muscle relaxants such as acepromazine, diazepam, barbiturates and methocarbamol (Coleman, 1998). The prognosis for severely affected individuals is poor.

Another antagonist of glycine is the neurotoxic bait strychnine, an alkaloid derived from the *Strychnos nux vomica* and *Strychnos ignatii* trees. It binds with high affinity to the glycine receptor and blocks its effects as a result (Patocka, 2009). Extreme muscle rigidity occurs as in the tetanus-intoxicated patient and can rapidly progress to intermittent or continuous seizures within 10–120 min of strychnine ingestion. Anxiety, apprehension, nervousness and tachypnea also may be part of the clinical presentation because of this rapid progression. Death occurs because of hypoxia as a result of contracture of the diaphragm and abdominal and intercostal muscles. The oral LD_{50} is 0.5–1.2 mg/kg for dogs; 0.5 mg/kg for horses and cows; 2 mg/kg for cats; and 0.5–1 mg/kg for pigs (Talcott, 2013). In the exposed but asymptomatic patient, aggressive decontamination is warranted. Treatment of the symptomatic patient is limited to symptomatic and supportive care. The agents used to treat muscle spasms, seizures and anxiety in the tetanic patient may also be used in the strychnine-intoxicated patient. The prognosis for symptomatic patients is grave.

GABA

GABA serves as the predominant inhibitory neurotransmitter in the brains of mammals and is synthesized from glutamic acid. Two main receptor subtypes, $GABA_A$ and $GABA_B$, exist. $GABA_A$ has at least seven subunits which combine with a chloride channel to form a receptor/ionophore complex. The complex contains binding sites not only for GABA but also for drugs such as the anticonvulsant benzodiazepines and barbiturates. Stimulation of these receptors results in CNS depression, somnolence, fatigue, lethargy, ataxia, and muscular incoordination. Paradoxical hyperactivity, excitement or aggression can also occur. In overdoses, CNS and respiratory depression may be extreme, leading to hypotension, hypoxia, hypothermia and death (Spencer, 2000; Rudolph et al., 2001).

A discussion of GABA warrants mentioning drugs of the avermectin class, commonly used in veterinary medicine for the prevention of heartworm disease (*Dirofilaria*) in dogs and cats, the treatment of endoparasitism (strongyles, ascarids, bots, threadworms, lungworms, stomach worms and summer sores (*Habronema*, *Draschia* species)), and ectoparasitism (*Sarcoptes*, *Demodex*). Examples of avermectins include ivermectin (Heartgard), selamectin (Revolution), milbemycin (Interceptor), moxidectin, and abamectin. Various mechanisms of action on target species, which lead to parasite paralysis and eventual death, have been proposed including enhanced release of GABA at presynaptic neurons (Plumb, 2015) and effects on glutamate-gated chloride channels in the CNS (Mealey, 2006). Such channels are not present in the mammalian brain, allowing for a wide margin of safety of these drugs in the host animal (Mealey, 2006). Furthermore, in genetically healthy animals, *p*-glycoprotein, part of the blood–brain barrier, is present in the apical membrane of brain capillary epithelial cells, and serves as an efflux pump to remove avermectins from the brain (Mealey, 2006).

Significant clinical signs can be seen, though, in an acute or chronic avermectin overdose, particularly with a dog that has a *p*-glycoprotein defect or MDR1 mutation. They include ataxia, CNS depression (potentially to the point of coma), recumbency, disorientation, mydriasis/apparent blindness, muscle tremors, seizures, respiratory depression, hypothermia, bradycardia, hypoxia and death. The onset of signs is expected to be more rapid and the severity of the clinical picture more extreme in the *p*-glycoprotein deficient dog. Signs may persist for weeks, but the duration of effect is often difficult to predict based on the severity of signs. Extreme supportive care is indicated for the comatose patient. Assisted ventilation may be necessary. Repeated doses of activated charcoal can be of significant benefit due to the enterohepatic recirculation of avermectin drugs. In recent years, treatment of moxidectin toxicity with an emulsion of IV lipids indicates that it may be an effective way to hasten elimination of fat-soluble toxicants (Crandell and Weinberg, 2009). If treated aggressively, with or without IV lipids, severely affected dogs can recover without long-term sequelae (Mealey, 2006; Merola et al., 2009).

A unique example of neurotoxicity in dogs relates to a species difference in metabolism. Isoniazid, an antibiotic used in the treatment of tuberculosis, is metabolized by acetylation via the enzyme *N*-acetyltransferase. Dogs are poor acetylators and, therefore, cannot effectively metabolize the drug. Isoniazid forms a complex with pyridoxine (vitamin B_6), creating a pyridoxine deficiency. Synthesis of GABA requires the cofactor pyridoxal phosphate. In the absence of sufficient cofactor, the inhibitory neurotransmitter is not made and seizures ensue. Emergency treatment involves IV administration of pyridoxine at a dose equivalent to the mg of isoniazid ingested, if known. Supportive care with fluid therapy is indicated, as may be adjunctive diazepam or other anticonvulsants, particularly if the pyridoxine is not immediately available (Villar et al., 1995).

Glutamate/Aspartate

The primary excitatory neurotransmitters of the brain are the nonessential amino acids glutamate and aspartate. Their synthesis in the brain from glucose and other molecules is tightly regulated. The blood–brain barrier excludes excesses of these excitatory neurotransmitters except in areas of the hypothalamus (arcuate nucleus) and retina where acute cellular degeneration may occur as a result. Three main receptor subtypes exist for glutamate: AMPA (DL-α-amino-3-hydroxy-5-methyl-4-isoxazole-propionic acid), kainate (KA) and NMDA (*N*-methyl-D-aspartate) receptors (Traynelis et al., 2010). As previously mentioned (see "Neuronopathy," above), domoic acid is an example of a toxicant that stimulates kainate receptors (Jeffery et al., 2004).

As discussed above, glutamate and aspartate may play a role in the pathogenesis of yellow star thistle intoxication in horses (Spencer, 2000). The plant is known to contain both excitatory amino acids in addition to several unstable guaianolide sesquiterpene lactones that may degrade to the former to exert their neurotoxic effects (Burrows and Tyrl, 2013).

A limited number of drugs used in veterinary medicine are NMDA antagonists. Ketamine, a dissociative anesthetic used commonly for induction of general anesthesia, blocks the open NMDA ion channel by binding to it. Seizures, due to elevation of CSF pressure, are a potential sequela of ketamine use at therapeutic doses. Amantadine, an antiviral drug that is an NMDA antagonist, is being used in the management of chronic pain. Particularly in the early course of treatment, stimulatory signs in dogs such as agitation may be seen. Seizures, tremors, and psychosis have been reported in relatively small overdoses in people (Plumb, 2015).

Histamine

Histamine is a physiologically active amine that is both a neurotransmitter as well as a mediator of peripheral effects relating to allergic reactions and gastric acid secretion. It is formed from the decarboxylation of L-histidine. Peripherally, histamine receptors are of two subtypes: H_1 and H_2. The former mediate allergic reactions in which histamine is released from the granules of mast cells, resulting in dilation and increased permeability of capillaries (wheal and flare reaction) and constriction of bronchial smooth muscle. The H_2 receptor stimulation increases gastric acid secretion (Gwaltney-Brant, 2004b).

Antagonists of H_1 receptors are commonly used to treat acute and chronic allergic reactions, to prevent mast cell degranulation during surgical excision as well as to minimize motion sickness in veterinary and human medicine. They are divided into first- and second-generation antagonists. The first-generation antihistamines can both stimulate and depress the CNS; while the second-generation antihistamines are considered nonsedating due to their exclusion from the brain at therapeutic dosages. At therapeutic doses and with mild overdosages, particularly with the first-generation antihistamines, CNS depression and hypotension may be seen. Epinephrine is contraindicated for management of hypotension in these patients. Paradoxical CNS excitation including restlessness, hyperactivity, tachycardia, tremors, and seizures may also occur, and the potential for it varies largely with the individual. Large overdoses of either antihistamine class can result in extreme CNS and cardiovascular stimulation to the point of seizure activity, cardiac arrhythmias, hypertension, and death. Seizures, tremors, and hyperactivity may be treated with diazepam or barbiturates (Gwaltney-Brant, 2004b).

Common H_2 blockers used in veterinary medicine to decrease gastric acidity include cimetidine, ranitidine, and famotidine. Of the H_2 blockers, cimetidine is more likely to cross the blood–brain barrier. Adverse effects are rare in veterinary patients (Plumb, 2015).

Mixed Neurotransmitter Effects

Many pharmaceuticals and toxicants exert their effects through multiple neurotransmitters. One example group is the many ergot alkaloids produced by fungi of the *Claviceps* genus. The mycotoxins can be further divided into ergopeptine and ergoline alkaloids. The alkaloids exert their toxic effects via effects on dopaminergic, serotonergic, and adrenergic pathways. Successful recovery is aimed at early diagnosis, when signs such as ataxia and confusion are reversible, and removal of the contaminated feed source is possible (Evans et al., 2004). The effects of the ergoline alkaloids, in particular, can also be seen with ingestion of the seeds of *Ipomoea* or morning glory and are very similar to those of the related street drug lysergic acid diethylamide, also known as LSD (Burrows and Tyrl, 2013).

α-Latrotoxin, the toxin in the venom of the black widow spider (*Latrodectus*), causes the release of catecholamine neurotransmitters as well as ACh, GABA and glutamate. The toxin mediates its catecholamine effects by forming a transmembrane pore through which Ca^{2+} can influx, allowing release of presynaptic vesicles containing neurotransmitters. Clinical signs associated with a bite from *Latrodectus* species include abdominal pain, ataxia, muscle fasciculations, muscle rigidity, and flaccid paralysis, which can ascend to involve the respiratory muscles. Cats are more sensitive than dogs to the effects of α-latrotoxin, but all mammalian species are susceptible. Antivenin is commercially available for black widow spider bite victims. Like all products derived from equine serum, a test dose should be administered intradermally to determine if hypersensitivity to the product exists. If none exists, the contents of the antivenin vial (2.5 mL) can be diluted 4–20 × (10–50 mL) with sterile saline and administered slowly intravenously over approximately 15 min. A slow, IV injection of 10% calcium gluconate may be given to treat the muscle fasciculations and weakness as well. Aggressive pain management with opioids or benzodiazepines is indicated (Roder, 2004d).

ION CHANNELS

The propagation of an impulse along an axon depends on an electrochemical gradient that is intricately regulated by various ion channels in an excitable membrane. Initiation of action potentials, release of neurotransmitters, axonal transport, and healthy muscle activity rely on control of ions such as sodium, potassium, chloride, and calcium (Spencer, 2000). Specific veterinary examples follow regarding the variety of natural and synthetic toxicants that target the ion channels of the nervous system.

Sodium Channels

The sodium channel of mammals is made up of three protein subunits, the largest of which is the transmembrane alpha (α) subunit, which contains the Na^+ pore and which is flanked by two smaller β subunits. The pores are voltage-gated, allowing sodium ion entrance into the cytoplasm only when charge-dependent conformational changes occur. Nature provides us with several examples of neurotoxicants which affect the sodium channel. Tetrodotoxin (TTX), present in various genera of puffer fish, in the venom of the blue-ringed octopus (*Hapalochlaena* spp.), the rough-skinned newt (*Taricha* spp.), and many other creatures, exhibits a profound binding affinity for the sodium channel peptide complex. Whereas the Na^+ ion normally reversibly binds to the peptide complex for just nanoseconds, TTX binds to the external surface of the peptide ion channel, remains bound for tens of seconds, and halts the action potential. A progression of signs occurs with TTX poisoning in people: (1) initial numbness around the mouth with or without nausea; (2) numbness of the tongue, face and skin, early motor paralysis, and incoordination manifested as slurred speech; (3) more widespread paralysis resulting in dyspnea, hypotension, an inability to speak, and fixed and dilated pupils; and (4) severe paralysis involving respiratory muscles, hypoxia, hypotension, and cardiac arrhythmias. Consciousness may be lost followed by death because of respiratory failure as early as 17 min after ingestion or as late as 24 h. No antidote currently exists. Treatment is aimed at decontamination and symptomatic and supportive care (Kaku and Meier, 1995; White, 1995).

Saxitoxin, the causative toxin for paralytic shellfish poisoning (PSP), is produced by several dinoflagellates, most notably *Alexandrium* and *Pyrodinium* species, and causes a similar clinical picture as that of TTX toxicosis also because of binding to the sodium ion channel (Smart, 1995).

Local anesthetics exert their pharmacologic effects by binding to the fast sodium channel complex when it is inactive, inhibiting its recovery after depolarization. Lidocaine, as an example, rapidly dissociates from the sodium channel complex and is also rapidly metabolized in the liver. Consequently, adverse events associated with therapeutic dosages are rare. In an overdose situation, however, CNS depression, ataxia, seizures, and circulatory collapse can occur (Welch, 2000; Plumb, 2015). Dibucaine HCl is 10 times more potent than lidocaine and much more likely to result in adverse effects as a result. Cats are especially susceptible to the methemoglobinemic potential of local anesthetics. Treatment of clinical signs is largely symptomatic and supportive, aimed at maintenance of blood pressure, addressing cardiac arrhythmias, and management of seizures (Welch, 2000). The experimental report of bupivacaine-intoxicated dogs successfully treated with IV lipid emulsion (Weinberg et al., 2003) holds promise for future use with local anesthetic toxicoses.

Several toxins affect the sodium ion channel by enhancing its activity, resulting in repetitive and prolonged neurotransmission. Brevotoxins, produced by the dinoflagellates *Karenia brevis* and *Gymnodinium breve*, prolong the opening of the sodium ion channels, perpetuating the propagation of the action potential. Bossart et al. (1998) implicated the toxin in the death of a minimum of 149 manatees along the southwest coast of Florida in 1996. Another example are ciguatoxins, which are produced by dinoflagellates and are bioaccumulated by herbivorous, and then piscivorous fish. They enhance Na^+ permeability through the ion channel (Spencer, 2000). The hallmark clinical sign of ciguatera fish poisoning in people, and presumably in affected veterinary species, is a paresthesia (tingling sensation) in the extremities as well as a perception of heat with cold stimuli ("dry-ice phenomenon") (Kaplan, 2000). The neurologic signs are attributable to edema of the adaxonal Schwann cell cytoplasm and can persist for weeks. Gastrointestinal pain and diarrhea are also typical, particularly in the early course of the disease (Glaziou et al., 1995; Spencer, 2000).

Other examples of toxicants that block inactivation of sodium channels include batrachotoxin, a steroid alkaloid isolated from the skin of *Phyllobates aurotaenia* and other species of South American poison dart frogs (Spencer, 2000); grayanotoxins, diterpene alkaloids from the plants of the *Rhododendron*, *Kalmia*, *Pieris*, *Leucothoe* and *Lyonia* genera (Puschner, 2004); aconitine, present in monkshood (*Aconitum* spp.); and veratridine from *Veratrum album* (Spencer, 2000). Both α-scorpion and β-scorpion toxins bind to Na^+ channels, albeit different sites, and enhance nerve conduction. Toxins of the Sydney funnel web spider (*Atrax robustus* and *Hadronyche* species; δ-atracotoxin, atraxotoxin, robustoxin) also block sodium channel inactivation. Persistent neuronal excitation with all of these toxins can result in a tingling sensation, muscle spasms, agitation, seizures, cardiac arrhythmias and death potentially within an hour of exposure (White et al., 1995; Spencer, 2000).

Pyrethrins, natural organic esters isolated from the flower of the *Chrysanthemum cinerariaefolium*, have natural insecticidal properties because of their ability to bind to Na^+ ion channels and slow their inactivation. These natural insecticides have a rapid knockdown effect on the insect followed by recovery. Synthetic analogs, pyrethroids, were developed to increase the insecticidal potency. Because of their relatively rapid metabolism, pyrethrins and pyrethroids are often marketed with synergists such as MGK-264 or piperonyl butoxide to inhibit enzymes which degrade them, thereby prolonging their insecticidal action. Today, pyrethroids are common ingredients in flea and tick spot-on products and sprays. Examples include permethrin, phenothrin, tetramethrin, fenvalerate, cyhalothrin, cyfluthrin, cypermethrin, cyphenothrin, and etofenprox (Volmer, 2004; Merola and Dunayer, 2006).

Fish and cats represent the most susceptible animals to pyrethroids. Fish typically die acutely when exposed to pyrethroids. Cats are most commonly presented to the veterinarian because of exposure to the highly concentrated (45%–65%) spot-on permethrin products labeled for use in dogs. Within 12–18 h of application or accidental exposure, affected cats will exhibit hyperesthesia, generalized tremors, hyperthermia, seizures, and possible death. The prognosis for complete recovery, however, is excellent with appropriate care. Seizures should be controlled with diazepam, barbiturates, inhalant anesthetics or intermittent propofol (caution regarding including Heinz body formation in cats with propofol). Tremors should be controlled with slow IV injection of methocarbamol (55–220 mg/kg) to effect. Once severe tremors and seizures have been treated, decontamination with a warm bath using a liquid dishwashing detergent is indicated. Thermoregulation is critical. Hyperthermia can arise with continued tremors and seizures and could result in life-threatening disseminated intravascular coagulation. Hypothermia can ensue following a bath and can enhance or prolong the toxicosis. Supportive care with IV fluids can help protect the kidneys from myoglobinuric damage. Other species may have dermal hypersensitivity reactions or local paresthesia effects from topical application of pyrethroids. Steady resolution with this clinical picture is expected once the dermal residue is removed post bathing (Volmer, 2004; Hansen, 2006).

Potassium Channels

Potassium channels are largely involved with repolarization of the neuron following Na^+-induced depolarization. The opening of these potassium channels is voltage dependent and allows K^+ to leave the cell, thereby restoring the resting potential of the axonal membrane. Several subtypes of potassium channels exist, the details of which exceed the scope of this text. Clinical effects of potassium channel-blocking toxicants or adverse effects of similarly acting therapeutic agents depend on the type of K^+ channel and location. A potent example of a potassium channel blocker in veterinary medicine is 4-aminopyridine (4-AP; Avitrol). Predominantly used as an avicide, 4-AP ingestion by birds results in rapid onset of seizures and death (Schell, 2004). Although its classification as a 1 A antiarrhythmic indicates it primarily blocks Na^+ channels, quinidine, derived from the *Cinchona* tree, also blocks potassium channels. Depression, confusion, and seizures are possible with quinidine overdose (Plumb, 2015). Classified as a class III (potassium channel blocker) antiarrhythmic, amiodarone also has sodium and calcium channel-blocking effects. Adverse effects include bradycardia and hypotension and potentially hepatopathy but not primary nervous system effects. Sotalol, also a class III antiarrhythmic, exerts its pharmacological effect via the blockade of cardiac potassium channels. It also has beta-blocking properties. Like amiodarone, adverse effects are primarily cardiac (bradycardia and hypotension), but nervous system effects secondary to hypoglycemia are also possible (Plumb, 2015).

Chloride Channels

As opposed to sodium and potassium channel neurotoxicants, relatively few toxicants have been identified that affect the chloride channel. Chloride ions can diffuse passively down their concentration gradient out of the neuron. Chloride ion channels regulate the entrance of chloride into the neuron and affect the membrane potential as a result. Normal resting membrane potential is 270 mV. Threshold potential, the potential at which an action potential is propagated, is roughly 250 mV. Membranes can be hyperpolarized by allowing entrance of negative chloride into the neuron and making it more difficult to reach threshold potential. Both benzodiazepines and barbiturates mediate their effects via $GABA_A$ receptors which are chloride ionophore complexes (Crystal and Schaumburg, 2000). Minute details regarding binding sites, duration, and frequency of chloride channel opening affected by barbiturates and benzodiazepines have been extensively studied (Hobbs et al., 1996; Crystal and Schaumburg, 2000; Maytal and Shinnar, 2000), yet the exact mechanism remains unclear. Ultimately, the two classes of drugs inhibit excitatory neurotransmission by increasing chloride conductance into the neuron.

The use of potassium bromide for chronic management of idiopathic epilepsy in veterinary patients is based on the competition of the bromide ion with chloride ions for transport across cell membranes. The therapeutic action relies on hyperpolarization of the neuronal membrane and a decrease in the propagation of epileptic discharges. Bromide blood levels should be monitored routinely in treated animals and particularly in those animals exhibiting signs of bromide toxicity. Neurologic signs consistent with a bromide toxicosis include ataxia, tremors and sedation to the point of stupor in veterinary species (Plumb, 2015). Headache, mood alterations, hallucinations, speech abnormalities and visual disturbances have also been reported with human bromism (Spencer, 2000). Because bromide has a longer half-life than chloride, the latter is preferentially excreted by the kidney. In animals with a deficiency of dietary salt, the half-life of bromide is prolonged, enhancing the chances of neurotoxicity. Conversely, the epileptic patient with a high dietary salt intake may have seizure activity that is poorly managed with potassium bromide treatment (Plumb, 2015).

OTHER MECHANISMS OF NEUROTOXICITY

Knowledge of the nervous system is continually expanding. Whereas the mechanisms of action of neurotoxicants discussed thus far have been simplified to affect one neurotransmitter or ion channel, the reality is likely far more complex. Additionally, clinicians should be aware of metabolic factors that can exacerbate neurotoxicoses. Examples of these factors include acidosis, hypoglycemia, and hepatic encephalopathy. Increased carbon dioxide, which readily diffuses across the blood–brain barrier, can cause narcosis by affecting neurotransmitters as well as increasing intracranial pressure. Compensation for hypercapnea with hyperventilation is the reason that metabolic acidosis is less likely to contribute to encephalopathy than respiratory acidosis (Dewey, 2008). Monitoring of acid–base status, volume restoration, correction of metabolic acidosis with sodium bicarbonate as needed (Plumb, 2015), and assisted ventilation when necessary are means by which these potential complications can be minimized.

Hypoglycemia can be a primary effect of neurotoxicoses as with sulfonylurea medication overdoses or xylitol ingestion in dogs (Meadows, 2011) or a secondary effect with increased glucose utilization in the patient with refractory seizures. Signs of neuroglycopenia occur when blood glucose goes below 45 mg/dL and include weakness, ataxia, collapse, restlessness, tremors, seizures, blindness, and potential changes in behavior (Podell, 2000; Nelson, 2009). Hypoglycemia can be corrected with administration of IV dextrose to effect (Meadows, 2011).

Finally, hepatic encephalopathy can result in neurotoxicity because of the inability of the liver to clear the body of toxins, namely ammonia, and the brain's sensitivity to it. Alterations of serotonin, GABA and glutamine, and stimulation of NMDA and benzodiazepine receptors, ensue and are responsible for potential disorientation, gait disorders, behavioral changes, and/or seizures (Watson and Bunch, 2009). Treatment with lactulose to lower blood ammonia, appropriate antibiotics, supportive care, and management of seizure activity are indicated (Webster, 2011).

CONCLUDING REMARKS AND FUTURE DIRECTIONS

The health of the nervous system, and largely that of the individual, relies on the system's structural and functional integrity. From specialized nerve cells and anatomic structures to axonal transport, myelination, neurotransmitter synthesis, storage, release, binding and degradation as well as the regulation of action potentials, maintenance of nervous system integrity is a complex task requiring significant energy expenditure. This functional complexity and structural specialization provide a plethora of targets for neurotoxicant action. The scope of this chapter precludes a detailed discussion of every known neurotoxicant. Many more mechanisms exist by which neurotoxicants exert their effects. Table 12.3 provides a

TABLE 12.3 Neurotoxicants Arranged by Mechanism of Action (Beasley, 1999; Spencer, 2000; Burrows and Tyrl, 2013; Schulze, 2002; Plumlee, 2004)

Mediation by Acetylcholine
Amanita muscaria (minute amount)
Anatoxin-a
Anatoxin-a(s)
Atropa belladonna/atropine
Botulism
Carbamate insecticides
Clitocybe mushrooms
Conium maculatum (poison hemlock)
Datura (jimsonweed)
Gymnocladus dioica (Kentucky coffee tree)
Imidacloprid
Inocybe mushrooms
Lobelia (Indian tobacco)
Nicotiana
Organophosphorus insecticides
Slaframine
Mediation by Norepinephrine
Albuterol
Atipamezole
Atomoxetine
Brimonidine
Clonidine
Doxazosin
Medetomidine
Metoprolol
Monoamine oxidase inhibitors (MAOIs)
Propranolol
Phentolamine
Phenoxybenzamine
Sotalol
Tamsulosin
Terazosin
Tricyclic antidepressants (TCAs)
Venlafaxine
Yohimbine
Xylazine

(Continued)

TABLE 12.3 (Continued)

Sympathomimetics/Catecholamines
Amphetamines
Cocaine
Ma huang (*Ephedra*)
MDMA/"Ecstasy"
Monoamine oxidase inhibitors (MAOIs)
Phenylpropanolamine
Pseudoephedrine
Tricyclic antidepressants (TCAs)
Mediation by Serotonin
Amphetamines
Griffonia/5-HTP supplements
Lysergic acid diethylamide (LSD)
MDMA/"Ecstasy"
Phalaris (Canary grass poisoning/tryptamine alkaloids)
Psilocybe mushrooms
Selective serotonin reuptake inhibitors (SSRIs)
Tricyclic antidepressants (TCAs)
Tryptophan
Venlafaxine
Mediation by Glycine
Calycanthus (bubby bush)
Strychnine
Tetanus
Tremorgenic mycotoxins (penitrem A and roquefortine)
Mediation by GABA
Avermectins
Baclofen
Barbiturates
Benzodiazepines
Bicuculline
Cicuta (water hemlock)
Cyclodiene organochlorines
Fipronil
Flumazenil
Isoniazid
Mediation by Glutamate/Aspartate
Amantadine
+/− *Centaurea solstitialis* (yellow star thistle)

(Continued)

TABLE 12.3 (Continued)

Domoic acid
Ketamine
Mediation by Histamine
Brompheniramine
Chlorpheniramine
Cetirizine
Cimetidine
Cyproheptadine
Dimenhydrinate
Diphenhydramine
Famotidine
Fexofenadine
Hydroxyzine
Loratadine
Ranitidine
Scombroid fish poisoning
Effect on Sodium Channels
Aconitine
Batrachotoxin
Brevotoxins
Ciguatoxin
Funnel web spider toxins
Grayanotoxanes
Local anesthetics
Pyrethroids
Saxitoxin
α and β scorpion toxins
Sodium intoxication
Tetrodotoxin
Veratridine
Effect on Potassium Channels
4-Aminopyridine
Amiodarone
Quinidine
Sotalol
Effect on Chloride Channel
Avermectins
Barbiturates

(Continued)

TABLE 12.3 (Continued)

Benzodiazepines
Picrotoxin
Potassium bromide
Producing Acidosis
Aspirin
Ethanol
Ethylene glycol
Metaldehyde
Methanol
Causing Hypoglycemia
Xanthium (cocklebur)
Sulfonylureas
Xylitol
Producing Hepatic Encephalopathy
Acetaminophen
Alsike clover (horses)
Blue-green algae (microcystins)
Cycas (sago palm): cycasin
Lantana
Macrozamia (cycad palms)
DL-Methionine
Nonprotein nitrogen
NSAIDs
Pyrrolizidine alkaloids:
Senecio
Crotalaria
Heliotroprium (giant hog weed)
Amsinckia (fiddle neck, tarweed)
Symphytum (comfrey)
Stimulating Cannabinoid Receptors
Cannabis sativa (marijuana)
Mediation of Opioid Receptors
Aesculus hippocastanum (horse chestnut)
Buprenorphine
Butorphanol
Codeine
Fentanyl
Heroin
Hydromorphone

(Continued)

TABLE 12.3 (Continued)

Loperamide
Meperidine
Morphine
Naloxone
Oxymorphone
Oxycodone
Tramadol
Multiple/Miscellaneous MOAs
Ageratina (white snakeroot): tremetone
Astragalus/Oxytropis (locoweed): miserotoxin
Bovine bonkers/ammoniated feed): 4-methylimidazole
Brunfelsia (yesterday, today and tomorrow plant): brunfelsamidine
Cycas (sago palm): β-methylamino-L-alanine
5-Fluorouracil/1080
Lead
Macrozamia (cycad palms): β-oxalylamino-L-alanine
Mercury
Methylxanthines, *Guarana* (adenosine receptor antagonists)
Phenothiazines (anticholinergic, antihistaminic, α-adrenergic blocking effects)
Sorghum (Sudan grass): β-cyanoalanine
Stipa (sleepy grass): ergot alkaloids
Metabolic
Carbon monoxide
Cyanide
Zinc phosphide
Thiamine Deficiency/Thiaminase Excess
Equisetum
Pteridium (bracken fern)
Raw fish diet
Excess dietary sulfur
Uncoupler of Oxidative Phosphorylation
Bromethalin
Hexachlorophene
Trialkyltin
Unknown Etiology/MOA
Desert spike
Diethyltoluamide (DEET)
Essential oils
Hydrocarbons
Indoxacarb
Macadamia nuts
Nitrofuran
Tick paralysis

comprehensive, yet certainly not exhaustive, list of neurotoxicants grouped by mechanism or site of action where known.

The extent to which a neurotoxicant exerts its effects depends on a variety of factors including dose, species, age, genetics, underlying diseases, drug therapy, diet, stress, and concurrent toxicoses. Veterinary practitioners should be aware of these underlying susceptibilities and the most common mechanisms by which neurotoxicants act so that toxicoses may be avoided or appropriately diagnosed and successfully treated when they do occur.

REFERENCES

Anthony, D.C., Montine, T.J., Valentine, W.M., Graham, D.G., 2001. Toxic responses of the nervous system. In: Klaassen, C.D. (Ed.), Casarett & Doull's Toxicology: The Basic Science of Poisons, sixth ed. McGraw-Hill, New York, pp. 535–563.

Arnot, L.F., Veale, D.J., Steyl, J.C., Myburgh, J.G., 2011. Treatment rationale for dogs poisoned with aldicarb (carbamate pesticide). J. S. Afr. Vet. Assoc. 82 (4), 232–238.

Bailey, E.M., 2006. Botulinum. In: Peterson, M.E., Talcott, P.A. (Eds.), Small Animal Toxicology, second ed. Elsevier, Inc, St. Louis, pp. 603–608.

Beasley, V.R., 1999. Veterinary Toxicology. International Veterinary Information Service. <www.ivis.org/advances/Beasley/toc.asp>.

Blodgett, D.J., 2006. Organophosphorus and carbamate insecticides. In: Peterson, M.E., Talcott, P.A. (Eds.), Small Animal Toxicology, second ed. Elsevier, Inc, St. Louis, p. 941.

Bossart, G.D., Baden, D.G., Ewing, R.Y., et al., 1998. Brevetoxicosis in manatees (Trichechus manatus latirostris) from the 1996 epizootic: gross, histologic, and immunohistochemical features. Toxicol. Pathol. 26 (2), 276–282.

Burrows, G.E., Tyrl, R.J., 2013. Toxic Plants of North America. second ed. John Wiley & Sons, Inc, Ames.

Capen, C.C., 2001. Toxic responses of the endocrine system. In: Klaassen, C.D. (Ed.), Casarett & Doull's Toxicology: The Basic Science of Poisons, sixth ed. McGraw-Hill, New York, pp. 711–759.

Coleman, E.S., 1998. Clostridial neurotoxins: tetanus and botulism. Compend. Contin. Educ. Pract. Vet. 20 (10), 1089–1097.

Craig, M.S., Gupta, R.C., Candery, T.D., Britton, D.A., 2005. Human exposure to imidacloprid from dogs treated with advantage. Toxicol. Mechan. Methods. 15, 287–291.

Crandell, D.E., Weinberg, G.L., 2009. Moxidectin toxicosis in a puppy successfully treated with intravenous lipids. J. Vet. Emerg. Crit. Care. 19 (2), 181–186.

Crystal, H.A., Schaumburg, H.H., 2000. Benzodiazepines. In: Spencer, P.S., Schaumburg, H.H. (Eds.), Experimental and Clinical Neurotoxicology, second ed. Oxford University Press, New York, pp. 231–235.

Damodaran, T.V., Abdel-Rahman, A., Abou-Donia, M.B., 2001. Altered time course of mRNA expression of alpha tubulin in the central nervous system of hens treated with diisopropyl phosphofluoridate (DFP). Neurochem. Res. 26 (1), 43–50.

Dewey, C.W., 2008. Encephalopathies: disorders of the brain. (2008), A Practical Guide to Canine & Feline Neurology. second ed. Wiley-Blackwell, Ames, IA, pp. 115–220.

Dorman, D., 2004. Bromethalin. In: Plumlee, K.H. (Ed.), Veterinary Clinical Toxicology. Mosby Inc, St. Louis, pp. 446–448.

Easton, N., Marsden, C.A., 2006. Ecstasy: are animal data consistent between species and can they translate to humans? J. Psychopharmacol. 20 (2), 194–210.

Evans, J., Levesque, D., Knowles, K., et al., 2003. Diazepam as a treatment for metronidazole toxicosis in dogs: a retrospective study of 21 cases. J. Vet. Int. Med. 17, 304–310.

Evans, T.J., Rottinghaus, G.E., Casteel, S.W., 2004. Ergot. In: Plumlee, K.H. (Ed.), Veterinary Clinical Toxicology. Mosby Inc, St. Louis, pp. 239–243.

Francis, B.M., 1994. Toxic Substances in the Environment. John Wiley & Sons, Inc, New York.

Glaziou, P., Chinain, M., Legrand, A.M., 1995. Clinical toxicology of ciguatera poisoning. In: Meier, J., White, J. (Eds.), Handbook of Clinical Toxicology of Animal Venoms and Poisons. CRC Press, Inc., Boca Raton, FL, pp. 59–74.

Gouzoulis-Mayfrank, E., Daumann, J., 2006. Neurotoxicity of methylenedioxyamphetamines (MDMA; ecstasy) in humans: how strong is the evidence for persistent brain damage? Addiction. 101 (3), 348–361.

Gulland, E.M.D., Haulena, M., Fauquier, D., et al., 2002. Domoic acid toxicity in Californian sea lions (*Zalophus californianus*): clinical signs, treatment and survival. Vet. Rec. 150, 475–480.

Gupta, B.S., Baldwa, S., Verma, S., Gupta, J.B., Singhal, A., 2000. Metronidazole induced neuropathy. Neurol. India. 48 (2), 192–193.

Gupta, R.C., 2006. Toxicology of Organophosphate and Carbamate Compounds. Academic Press/Elsevier, Amsterdam, pp. 1–763.

Gwaltney-Brant, S., 2004a. Antidepressants. In: Plumlee, K.H. (Ed.), Clinical Veterinary Toxicology. Mosby Inc, St. Louis, pp. 286–291.

Gwaltney-Brant, S., 2004b. Antihistamines. In: Plumlee, K.H. (Ed.), Veterinary Clinical Toxicology. Mosby Inc, St. Louis, pp. 204–210.

Gwaltney-Brant, S., 2004c. Lead. In: Plumlee, K.H. (Ed.), Veterinary Clinical Toxicology. Mosby Inc, St. Louis, pp. 291–293.

Hansen, S.R., 2006. Pyrethrins and pyrethroids. In: Peterson, M.E., Talcott, P.A. (Eds.), Small Animal Toxicology, second ed. Elsevier, Inc, St. Louis, pp. 1002–1010.

Hinck, J.E., Schmitt, C.J., Choinacki, K.A., Tillitt, D.E., 2009. Environmental contaminants in freshwater fish and their risk to piscivorous wildlife based on a national monitoring program. Environ. Monit. Assess. 152 (1–4), 469–494.

Hobbs, W.R., Rall, T.W., Verdoorn, T.A., 1996. Hypnotics and sedatives; ethanol. In: Hardman, J.G., Limbird, L.E. (Eds.), Goodman & Gilman's The Pharmacological Basis of Therapeutics, ninth ed. McGraw-Hill, New York, pp. 361–396.

Jeffery, B., Barlow, T., Moizer, K., Paul, S., Boyle, C., 2004. Amnesic shellfish poison. Food Chem. Toxicol. 42 (4), 545–557.

Kaku, N., Meier, J., 1995. Clinical toxicology of fugu poisoning. In: Meier, J., White, J. (Eds.), Handbook of Clinical Toxicology of Animal Venoms and Poisons. CRC Press, Inc., Boca Raton, FL, pp. 75–83.

Kaplan, J.G., 2000. Ciguatoxin. In: Spencer, P.S., Schaumburg, H.H. (Eds.), Experimental and Clinical Neurotoxicology, second ed. Oxford University Press, New York, pp. 386–390.

Kotsonis, F.N., Burdock, G.A., Flamm, W.G., 2001. Food toxicology. In: Klaassen, C.D. (Ed.), Casarett & Doull's Toxicology: The Basic Science of Poisons, sixth ed. McGraw-Hill, New York, pp. 1049–1088.

Landsberg, L., Young, J.B., 2001. Pharmacology of the sympathoadrenal system. In: Braunwald, M.D. (Ed.), Harrison's Principles of Internal Medicine, fifteenth ed. McGraw-Hill, New York, pp. 443–448.

Loeven, K.O., 1994. Hepatic amyloidosis in two Chinese Shar Pei dogs. J. Am. Vet. Med. Assoc. 204 (8), 1212–1216.

Mandella, R.C., 2002. Applied neurotoxicology. In: Derelanka, M.J., Hollinger, M.A. (Eds.), Handbook of Toxicology, second ed. CRC Press, LLC, Boca Raton, FL, pp. 371–399.

Maytal, J., Shinnar, S., 2000. Barbiturates. In: Spencer, P.S., Schaumburg, H.H. (Eds.), Experimental and Clinical Neurotoxicology, second ed. Oxford University Press, New York, pp. 219–225.

Meadows, I., 2011. Xylitol toxicosis. In: Cote, E. (Ed.), Clinical Veterinary Advisor: Dogs and Cats, second ed. Elsevier/Mosby, St. Louis, pp. 1184–1185.

Mealey, K.L., 2006. Ivermectin: macrolide antiparasitic agents. In: Peterson, M.E., Talcott, P.A. (Eds.), Small Animal Toxicology, second ed. Elsevier, Inc, St. Louis, pp. 785–794.

Means, C., 2004. Decongestants. In: Plumlee, K.H. (Ed.), Clinical Veterinary Toxicology. Mosby Inc, St. Louis, pp. 308–310.

Meerdink, G.L., 2004a. Slaframine. In: Plumlee, K.H. (Ed.), Clinical Veterinary Toxicology. Mosby Inc, St. Louis, pp. 262–264.

Meerdink, G.L., 2004b. Anticholinesterase insecticides. In: Plumlee, K. H. (Ed.), Clinical Veterinary Toxicology. Mosby Inc, St. Louis, pp. 178–180.

Mensching, D., 2011. Decongestant toxicosis. In: Cote, E. (Ed.), Clinical Veterinary Advisor: Dogs and Cats, second ed. Elsevier/Mosby, St. Louis, pp. 284–286.

Mensching, D., Volmer, P.A., 2007. Breathe with ease when managing 2-agonist inhaler toxicoses in dogs. Vet. Med. 2007, 369–373.

Merola, T., Dunayer, E., 2006. The 10 most common toxicoses in cats. Vet Med. 95, 339–342.

Merola, T., Khan, S., Gwaltney-Brant, S., 2009. Ivermectin toxicosis in dogs: a retrospective study. J. Am. An. Hosp. Assoc. 45 (3), 106–111.

Nelson, R.W., 2009. Disorders of the endocrine pancreas. In: Nelson, R. W., Couto, C.G. (Eds.), Small Animal Internal Medicine, fourth ed. Mosby/Elsevier, St. Louis, pp. 764–809.

Panter, K.E., 2004a. Piperidine alkaloids. In: Plumlee, K.H. (Ed.), Clinical Veterinary Toxicology. Mosby Inc, St. Louis, pp. 365–368.

Panter, K.E., 2004b. Pyridine alkaloids. In: Plumlee, K.H. (Ed.), Clinical Veterinary Toxicology. Mosby Inc, St. Louis, pp. 369–370.

Panter, K.E., 2004c. Quinolizidine alkaloids. In: Plumlee, K.H. (Ed.), Clinical Veterinary Toxicology. Mosby Inc, St. Louis, pp. 377–379.

Patocka, J., 2009. Strychnine. In: Gupta, R.C. (Ed.), Handbook of Toxicology of Chemical Warfare Agents. Academic Press/Elsevier, Amsterdam, pp. 199–205.

Pickrell, J.A., Oehme, F., Mannala, S.A., 2004. Tropane alkaloids. In: Plumlee, K.H. (Ed.), Clinical Veterinary Toxicology. Mosby Inc, St. Louis, pp. 381–382.

Plumb, D.C., 2015. Plumb's Veterinary Drug Handbook. eighth ed. PharmaVet Inc., Stockholm.

Plumlee, K.H., 2004. Clinical Veterinary Toxicology. Mosby Inc, St. Louis.

Podell, M., 2000. Neurologic manifestations of systemic disease. In: Ettinger, S.J., Feldman, E.C. (Eds.), Textbook of Veterinary Internal Medicine, fifth ed. WB Saunders Co., Philadelphia, pp. 548–552.

Poppenga, R., 2004. Treatment. In: Plumlee, K.H. (Ed.), Clinical Veterinary Toxicology. Mosby Inc, St. Louis, pp. 13–21.

Puschner, B., 2004. Grayanotoxins. In: Plumlee, K.H. (Ed.), Clinical Veterinary Toxicology. Mosby Inc, St. Louis, pp. 412–415.

Roder, J., 2004a. Antineoplastics. In: Plumlee, K.H. (Ed.), Clinical Veterinary Toxicology. Mosby Inc, St. Louis, pp. 299–302.

Roder, J., 2004b. Bacteria. In: Plumlee, K.H. (Ed.), Clinical Veterinary Toxicology. Mosby Inc, St. Louis, pp. 98–99.

Roder, J., 2004c. Blue-green algae. In: Plumlee, K.H. (Ed.), Clinical Veterinary Toxicology. Mosby Inc, St. Louis, pp. 100–101.

Roder, J., 2004d. Spiders. In: Plumlee, K.H. (Ed.), Clinical Veterinary Toxicology. Mosby Inc, St. Louis, pp. 111–112.

Rudolph, U., Crestani, F., Mohler, H., 2001. GABAA receptor subtypes: dissecting their pharmacologic functions. Trends Pharmacol. Sci. 22 (4), 188–194.

Sanders, S.G., Tucker, R.L., Bagley, R.S., Gavin, P.R., 2001. Magnetic resonance imaging features of equine nigropallidal encephalomalacia. Vet. Radiol. Ultrasound. 42 (4), 291–296.

Schell, M.M., 2004. 4-Aminopyridine. In: Plumlee, K.H. (Ed.), Clinical Veterinary Toxicology. Mosby Inc, St. Louis, pp. 443–444.

Schulze, G.E., 2002. Fundamental neurotoxicology. In: Derelanka, M.J., Hollinger, M.A. (Eds.), Handbook of Toxicology, second ed. CRC Press, LLC, Boca Raton, FL, pp. 353–370.

Smart, D., 1995. Clinical toxicology of shellfish poisoning. In: Meier, J., White, J. (Eds.), Handbook of Clinical Toxicology of Animal Venoms and Poisons. CRC Press, Inc., Boca Raton, FL, pp. 33–57.

Smith, W.E., Smith, A.M., 1975. Minamata. Holt, Rinehart, and Winston, New York, NY.

Spencer, P.S., 2000. Biological principles of chemical neurotoxicity. In: Spencer, P.S., Schaumburg, H.H. (Eds.), Experimental and Clinical Neurotoxicology, second ed. Oxford University Press, New York, pp. 3–54.

Talcott, P.A., 2013. Strychnine. In: Peterson, M.E., Talcott, A.A. (Eds.), Small Animal Toxicology, third ed. Elsevier, Inc, St. Louis, pp. 827–831.

Thomas, R.J., 1991. Detection of Clostridium botulinum types C and D toxin by ELISA. Aust. Vet. J. 68 (3), 111–113.

Traynelis, S., Wollmuth, L.P., McBain, C.J., et al., 2010. Glutamate receptor ion channels: structure, regulation, and function. Pharmacol. Rev. 62, 405–496.

Turner, N.J., Szczawinski, A.F., 1991. Common Poisonous Plants and Mushrooms of North America. Timber Press, Inc., Portland.

van den Munckhof, P., Gilbert, F., Chamberland, M., et al., 2006. Striatal neuroadaptation and rescue of locomotor deficit by l-dopa in aphakia mice, a model of Parkinson's disease. J. Neurochem. 96 (1), 160–170.

van Lier, R.B., Cherry, L.D., 1988. The toxicity and mechanism of action of bromethalin: a new single-feeding rodenticide. Fundam. Appl. Toxicol. 11 (4), 664–672.

Villar, D., Knight, M.K., Holding, J., et al., 1995. Treatment of acute isoniazid overdose in dogs. Vet. Human Toxicol. 37 (5), 473–477.

Volmer, P.A., 2004. Pyrethrins and pyrethroids. In: Plumlee, K.H. (Ed.), Clinical Veterinary Toxicology. Mosby Inc, St. Louis, pp. 188–190.

Waseem, M., Perry, C., Bomann, S., et al., 2010. Cholinergic crisis after rodenticide poisoning. West J. Emerg. Med. 11 (5), 524–527.

Watson, P.J., Bunch, S.E., 2009. Clinical manifestations of hepatobiliary disease. In: Nelson, R.W., Couto, C.G. (Eds.), Small Animal Internal Medicine, fourth ed. Mosby/Elsevier, St. Louis, pp. 485–495.

Webster, C.R.L., 2011. Hepatic encephalopathy. In: Cote, E. (Ed.), Clinical Veterinary Advisor: Dogs and Cats, second ed. Elsevier/Mosby, St. Louis, pp. 501–503.

Weinberg, G.L., Ripper, B.A., Feinstein, D.L., Hoffman, W., 2003. Lipid emulsion infusion rescues dogs from bupivacaine-induced cardiac toxicity. Reg. Anesth. Pain. Med. 28 (3), 198–202.

Welch, S.L., 2000. Local anesthetic toxicosis. Vet. Med. 95 (9), http://www.aspca.org/site/DocServer/toxbrief_0900.pdf?docID5122 (accessed 28.02.11.).

White, J., 1995. Clinical toxicology of blue ringed octopus bites. In: Meier, J., White, J. (Eds.), Handbook of Clinical Toxicology of Animal Venoms and Poisons. CRC Press, Inc., Boca Raton, FL, pp. 171–175.

White, J., Cardoso, J.L., Fan, H.W., 1995. Clinical toxicology of spider bites. In: Meier, J., White, J. (Eds.), Handbook of Clinical Toxicology of Animal Venoms and Poisons. CRC Press, Inc., Boca Raton, FL, pp. 259–329.

Wismer, T., 2004. Novel insecticides. In: Plumlee, K.H. (Ed.), Clinical Veterinary Toxicology. Mosby Inc, St. Louis, pp. 183–186.

Woolf, A.D., 1995. Ginger Jake and the blues: a tragic song of poisoning. Vet. Hum. Toxicol. 37 (3), 252–254.

Chapter 13

Respiratory Toxicity

Deon van der Merwe

INTRODUCTION

The respiratory system is relevant in toxicology as a target of toxic effects, and also as a major route of absorption of inhaled gases and atmospheric particles. If inhalation and subsequent absorption reach a toxic threshold, inhaled chemicals have the potential to produce lung disease. If the chemical is translocated to other organs, disease can be produced in those organs. As a highly perfused organ system, the respiratory system is also a potential target for toxic chemicals in the blood circulation, irrespective of the route of absorption. Inhalation toxicology refers to the respiratory system as a route of exposure. In contrast, respiratory toxicosis refers to respiratory organ toxicosis. The environments in which animals live are directly relevant to respiratory toxicosis (Pickrell, 1991). Different species may have anatomical features that lead to specific patterns of deposition and absorption of chemicals from the air, resulting in species variations in adverse effects (Morris et al., 1986).

To understand respiratory toxicosis we need to understand (1) the toxicant dose delivered to specific sites of the lung and (2) the effects of toxicants on respiratory system tissues under conditions of acute and chronic exposures. Many lung diseases have their beginnings with increases in oxidative lung burden. There is strong evidence that oxidative lung burden may favor development of lung diseases such as bronchitis, asthma, and interstitial lung disease (Witschi and Last, 2001).

Advances in lung toxicology are augmented by interdisciplinary collaboration between anatomists, physiologists, immunologists, pathologists, molecular biologists, epidemiologists, clinicians, and many other shared disciplines. Adaptation of pulmonary function tests to animals has led to the comparison of human and animal data, generally providing more robust conclusions compared to data from single species. Recent molecular measurements have brought home how closely tied many of these diseases are to specific protein changes. Such molecular analyses help to pinpoint specific molecular reactions to specific cell types. In addition, they help us describe the more relevant influence of each cell on the others in the near neighborhood. Tissue culture, organ minces, and in vivo animal exposure studies, such as broncho-alveolar lavage washings, further elucidate these interactions.

THE UPPER AIRWAYS

Normal Function

The nasopharynx is lined by pseudostratified columnar ciliated epithelium with goblet cells (Dungworth, 1993). Abundant lymphoid nodules are present in the submucosa. The eustachian tubes extend from the middle ear to the nasal cavity. Many animals, including horses and small laboratory rodents, are obligate nose breathers. Other animals can breathe through either their nose or mouth.

The mucous membranes of the nasal passages produce secretions from serous and mucous glands, which produce mucopolysaccharides and mucoprotein, and goblet glands, which produce similar, but sulfated, secretions. Ciliated epithelium covers a capillary net providing a rich blood supply. Mucous secretions protect the mucous membranes and can retain particulate matter and substances that dissolve in the mucous. It also allows for rapid heat transfer between the capillary net and the air (Taylor, 1974). Beating of cilia propels mucous and allergens, pathogens, and toxicants that become entrapped in the mucous towards the glottis, from where it is shunted to the digestive tract by swallowing (Dungworth, 1993). Effective mucociliary clearance depends on coordinated secretions by the goblet cells, submucous glands, and serous secretory cells to form an upper mucous layer underlying a more aqueous layer, which allows the upper mucous layer to be transported by cilia (Corcoran, 2010). Nonciliated (Clara) epithelial cells have P-450 monooxygenase systems that can metabolize xenobiotics, and they can produce inflammatory compounds such as prostaglandins.

Veterinary Toxicology. DOI: http://dx.doi.org/10.1016/B978-0-12-811410-0.00013-1

The mucociliary clearance pathway can adapt to changing environmental conditions, and forms a line of defense against a variety of airborne insults.

Upper conducting airways (bronchi, progressively smaller generations of bronchioles, and terminal bronchioles) are lined with pseudostratified columnar epithelial cells with a few goblet cells interspersed. Their support tissue contains fibrous connective tissue and cartilaginous plates (Dungworth, 1993). Animals adapted for strenuous physical activity have larger diameter airways to accommodate additional airflow. As bronchioles become progressively smaller, resistance to airflow increases. In these small conducting airways, diseases reflecting altered airflow resistance are said to be diseases of small airways or small airway resistance. As the airways narrow, the epithelium changes from pseudostratified ciliated columnar cells with goblet cells to simple columnar epithelium, reflecting the form, function, and stresses of these smaller airways. The smallest bronchioles may collapse near the end of expiration, unless there is sufficient collateral circulation to keep them open.

Upper airways (bronchi and bronchioles) have bronchial associated lymphoid tissue; this tissue is similar to gut-associated lymphoid tissue (Dungworth, 1993). Bronchial associated lymphoid tissue is responsible for local immunity in the lung.

Toxic Diseases of the Nasal Passages

Epistaxis is a typical clinical effect associated with anticoagulant pesticide toxicosis in animals (Berny, 2007). High doses of ethylene glycol (>10 mg/kg) have produced bovine epistaxis and hemoglobinuria (Crowell et al., 1979). The likelihood of equine exercise-induced pulmonary hemorrhage is increased by airborne reactive oxygen substances (ROS), which can destroy the capillary barrier and reduce vasoactive nitric oxides (Manohar et al., 1993; Mills and Higgins, 1997). Rattle snake envenomation is another toxic cause of epistaxis in horses (Dickinson et al., 1996). These horses have fever, tachycardia, cardiac arrhythmia, thrombosis, and hemorrhage. Since horses are often bitten on the nose and are obligate nose breathers, the nostril may swell and must be kept patent.

Toxic Diseases of the Conducting Airways

Allergic rhinitis that clinically resembles hay fever in humans can occur in horses, cats and dogs (Dungworth, 1993). Nasal granuloma is a chronic form of allergic rhinitis, characterized by degranulation of mast cells and infiltration by eosinophils. Horses with chronic obstructive pulmonary disease have high transpulmonary pressures (Ammann et al., 1998). Constant exposure to dust through litter use or upper respiratory tract infections were blamed as likely causes of feline upper airway inflammation. However, only certain cats become clinically ill, suggesting varying degrees of hypersensitivity to stimulating antigens in cat populations (Dye, 1992). Cattle, especially the channel island breeds, and occasionally sheep have a seasonal allergy that resembles this condition. Cattle are believed to be allergic to pollen antigens. Histologically, the epithelium is hyperplastic, eroded, and/or infiltrated with eosinophils.

A canine model of nasal congestion and allergic rhinitis has been described (Tiniakov et al., 2003). A very high prevalence of inflammatory gastrointestinal tract problems in brachycephalic dogs that presented with upper respiratory problems was observed clinically, endoscopically and histologically. Some histologically observed inflammatory lesions were not macroscopically visible at endoscopy. Respiratory and digestive signs correlated closely in French bulldog males and heavy brachycephalic dogs (Poncet et al., 2005). It is thought that systemic inflammatory disease can lead to secondary pulmonary infiltration and inflammation (Bedenice et al., 2003).

Moderate smoke inhalation injury to the upper airway is usually independent of temperature damage; after as little as 1 h, endothelin-1 in cells that line the airway increase (Cox et al., 2001). Such changes may contribute to airway inflammation, mucus secretion, pulmonary hypertension, increased airway resistance, and decreased lung compliance in an ovine model of smoke inhalation injury (Cox et al., 2001).

THE GAS EXCHANGE REGION

Normal Function

Pulmonary parenchyma is divided into units of structure and function called acini (Dungworth, 1993). An acinus is the gas exchange unit of the lung and of pulmonary parenchyma. The acinus includes all branches of respiratory bronchioles, alveolar ducts and alveoli associated with ventilation; in addition, it contains the vasculature associated with perfusion. Lobules are many acini grouped together and surrounded by connective tissue; in cattle, sheep and horses they form lobules visible at autopsy. In other species lobules are less well outlined. Cells most important to the gas exchange are epithelium (type II and type I epithelial cells). Fibroblasts provide connective tissue and structural support for the alveolus; vascular endothelial cells line the pulmonary capillaries.

Ventilation

Oxygen-rich inhaled air flows through the conducting airways to reach the acini. Oxygen and carbon dioxide are exchanged between capillary blood and air across the alveolar epithelium and vascular endothelium by diffusion along the gas concentration gradient. Carbon dioxide-enriched air is expelled upon expiration. Total lung capacity refers to the volume of air in inflated lungs. Some volume of air remains in the lungs following maximum expiration, known as the residual volume. The volume of air moved in and out during breathing is called the tidal volume (TV), while vital capacity (VC) refers to the volume of air moving in and out of the lungs during maximum inhalation and expiration. Oxygen delivery to the blood can be increased by increasing the TV, the respiratory rate, or the oxygen concentration in the inspired air. TV has a fraction in the conducting airways that does not exchange gas, known as the dead volume (West, 2000a). Anatomic dead space refers to the volume of the conducting airways to where oxygen becomes diluted (Fowler's method). Physiologic dead space refers to the portions of the airways that do not contribute to the exchange of carbon dioxide (Bohr's method; West, 2000a). As the breathing pattern becomes shallower and more rapid, the fraction of the noncontributing dead volume in each breath increases. Although we often assume that all regions of the lung are ventilated equally, positional differences are seen in humans. Such differences are minimized when humans are in the supine position. In dogs, the anterior main bronchi receive more ventilation than do the rear ones.

The water solubility of gases influences how deeply they penetrate into the airways and terminal lung structures. Highly water-soluble gases, such as SO_2, do not penetrate deeply. Less water-soluble gases, including NO_2, ozone, CO, and H_2S penetrate to the deepest lung structures.

Ozone and oxides of nitrogen and sulfur were modeled for absorption throughout the respiratory tract (Tsujino et al., 2005). All three gases had higher concentration in the airways. For example, ozone was 3–12 times higher at the 5th generation bronchus. Sensitivity analysis indicated that TV, respiratory rate, and surface area of the upper and lower airways significantly affected the results. Kinetics of inhaled gaseous substances vary substantially among animals and humans, and such variations are, at least partially, the result of anatomical and physiological differences in their airways.

Perfusion

There are two different types of blood supply to the lung: nutrient vessels that provide nutrition for the lung, and pulmonary vessels that specialize in exchanging alveolar oxygen onto the hemoglobin to be carried to the target organs (West, 2000a). The capillaries are just large enough to admit erythrocytes and they are very short. Blood flows around the alveoli as a sheet, and the network of capillaries is said to resemble a miniature underground parking garage.

Diffusion

For some gases for which the blood has a large carrying capacity, such as carbon monoxide (CO), the rate of uptake into the blood is limited by the blood–gas barrier. Thus, the gas exchange is described as diffusion limited. For certain other gases, such as nitrous oxide, which do not bind to or are taken up by the red blood cells, uptake is not limited by diffusion, but by the available blood volume provided by alveolar perfusion. These gases are described as perfusion limited. Oxygen takes the middle road so that its uptake is dependent on the blood–gas barrier characteristics (diffusion limited), as well as the blood volume (perfusion limited). If the alveolar wall becomes abnormally thick, e.g., when collagen is deposited in the interstitium or with the accumulation of interstitial fluid (edema), the oxygen uptake rate across the barrier is reduced. Alternatively, and more commonly, a failure to match ventilation with perfusion is the cause of poor gas exchange (West, 2000b). If a lung is heavily perfused with minimal ventilation because of a blocked airway, the amount of oxygen that can be exchanged is limited by the mismatch of poor ventilation with good perfusion. Alternatively, gas exchange is compromised if the lung is efficiently ventilated, but receives little or no perfusion. Both conditions are referred to as ventilation–perfusion mismatches.

Avian Respiration

There are many morphologic, physiologic, and mechanical differences between the avian and mammalian respiratory systems (Brown et al., 1997). In birds, the gas exchange unit is the parabronchus. The parabronchus has no alveoli. The walls of the narrow passageways called air capillaries serve as the gas exchange surface. Inhaled air reaches the parabronchus via the upper air passageways. Oxygen is extracted as it moves along the air capillaries. After passing through the parabronchus the air is not expelled directly, but moves on to the air sacs. From there the air is moved back through the parabronchus before it is expelled. The parabronchus does not expand and contract like mammalian lungs. Instead, air movement is controlled by expansion and compression of the air sacs. The parabronchus–air sac system provides two opportunities to extract oxygen from inhaled air. In addition, counter flow between blood and air in the parabronchus provides an effective oxygen concentration gradient over a larger fraction of the gas exchange surface area. Partially oxygenated blood comes into close proximity to the air with the highest oxygen concentration, while air with lower oxygen pressure comes into close proximity to blood with the lowest oxygen concentration. Oxygen is extracted about twice as efficiently as in mammals, which is necessary for the increased oxygen demand associated with sustained flight. Air sacs and air membrane spaces provide a reduction in density to birds; reduced density is helpful in staying afloat on water. The increased gas exchange efficiency in birds makes them more susceptible to some inhaled toxicants, such as the fumes released from overheated nonstick cookware coated with polytetrafluoroethylene (Lightfoot and Yeager, 2008). This sensitivity can also be exploited as a very sensitive monitor of air quality. An example of this is the canary in the mine that predicts toxicity to the miners (Brown et al., 1997; West et al., 2006).

GENERAL PRINCIPLES IN THE PATHOGENESIS OF LUNG DAMAGE CAUSED BY CHEMICALS

Oxidant Burden

Oxidant burden in the lung is frequently associated with airborne prooxidants such as nitrogen dioxide (NO_2), sulfur dioxide, oxidants such as ozone, free radicals, tobacco smoke, or is caused by an overzealous defense by phagocytic cells (Pickrell et al., 1987a; Pickrell and Mageed, 1995; Witschi and Last, 2001). Exposure to oxidants can lead to changes in lung structure and biochemistry (Pickrell et al., 1987b; Witschi and Last, 2001). Pivotal roles have been established for superoxide, prooxidant peroxy nitrites, and hydroxyl radicals. Responses depend on the oxidant burden in combination with the glutathione or biological antioxidant concentration. With sufficient oxidant burden and depletion of glutathione, all lung toxins have an inflammatory disease component. In the presence of significant oxidant burden, but in the presence of high levels of glutathione, lung defensive metabolic enzymes are activated. At intermediate glutathione levels, inflammation is activated using nuclear factor kappa beta. At lower levels of glutathione, mitochondrial enzymes are activated. The relation of programmed cell death (apoptosis) to mitochondrial enzyme activation is being investigated (Nel et al., 2006).

Toxic Inhalant Gases

Chlorine

Exposure to chlorine may originate from the manufacture of pulp, paper, plastics, and chlorinated chemicals (Witschi and Last, 2001). Chlorine gas is irritating to the upper airways, and can cause hemoptysis, dyspnea, tracheobronchitis, or even bronchopneumonia in animals inhaling sufficient concentrations. Peak symptoms are typically reached in 30–90 min. Patients only infrequently require more than monitoring and rudimentary support measures. Full recovery from such injuries is likely, but permanent loss of function is possible in cases of exposure to very high levels of chlorine (Winder, 2001). Humans exposed to chlorine may have a decreased VC (limited forced expiratory volume) (Mehta et al., 2005). This limitation is frequently reversible and less than that of seasonal allergic rhinitis (Shusterman et al., 2004).

Ammonia

Animals and caretakers are frequently exposed to elevated levels of ammonia (NH_3) gas in swine confinement facilities (Carson, 2004). At greater than 100 ppm, ammonia irritates eyes and respiratory membranes, increases the incidence and intensity of microbial or parasitic infections, and reduces growth rate. High levels of ammonia found in poultry houses have about the same level of toxicity to birds as they would to other animals (Brown et al., 1997). Ammonia concentrations greater than 60 ppm cause kerato-conjunctivitis in broilers; reduced bacterial clearance and enhanced sensitivities to bacterial infections (Carson, 2004).

Anhydrous Ammonia

Anhydrous ammonia (NH_3) is injected from pressurized tanks into the ground as a fertilizer nitrogen source. It can be lethal to animals and humans if pressurized tanks are breached or large containers are spilled in transit (Carson, 2004). Anhydrous ammonia reacts with air moisture to form a vapor cloud that can either remain for several hours or disperse efficiently, depending on wind velocity and humidity. In animals and man, the eyes and upper respiratory tract are prime targets. If the air ammonia concentration is higher than 5000 ppm, it can cause a fatal apnea or laryngeal edema. Survivors may be blinded by corneal lesions and sloughed epithelium. Removal of animals is important if the vapor cloud does not disperse rapidly. Supportive therapy may be curative in moderate exposures. In humans, loss of olfactory ability was associated with exposure to anhydrous ammonia, as well as a history of wheezing and asthma, and of flu-like illness (Snyder et al., 2003).

Carbon Dioxide

Carbon dioxide (CO_2) is well tolerated, even at concentrations as high as 5%. Higher concentrations stimulate the rate and depth of respiration (Carson, 2004). It is, however, being explored as a novel human stressor (Kaye et al., 2004). It is an asphyxiant at extremely high concentrations ($>40\%$). Because it is heavier than air, it collects in the lower portion of animal facilities (Carson, 2004). It is used as a euthanasia agent in some laboratory animal species.

Carbon Monoxide

CO is a product of incomplete combustion of hydrocarbon fuels. It has background levels of about 0.02 ppm in rural areas, 13 ppm in urban areas and 40 ppm in areas of high urban traffic. Improperly vented or adjusted heaters, and fires, especially those burning more coolly, are frequent sources of increased CO.

CO binds about 250 times as tightly to hemoglobin as oxygen, forming carboxyhemoglobin (COHb). Oxygen is displaced by CO, limiting the ability to take up oxygen and give off carbon dioxide in the lungs. Because of their high respiratory exchange efficiency, birds are unusually sensitive to CO (Brown et al., 1997). They often require relatively more oxygen per unit body weight because they have smaller body sizes and more active metabolisms.

Measurement of COHb is diagnostic of CO intoxication (Carson, 2004). In humans, <3% COHb is considered normal; 6%–8% causes drifting of attention; 10%–20% headaches; 20%–30% dizziness; 30%–60% tachypnea, tachycardia and confusion; and 60% fatality. Birds respond more acutely than mammals, and canaries have been used as sentinels for miners (Brown et al., 1997; Carson, 2004). Treatment requires, at a minimum, fresh circulating air; 100% oxygen may be lifesaving. Prognosis depends on the amount of COHb and the hypoxic brain damage. Pulmonary function should be monitored for at least 2 weeks, and in some cases 6 weeks.

Methane

Methane (CH_4) becomes an asphyxiant at >85%; it is an explosion hazard at 10%–15%. It is substantially lighter than air and will flow above water in a swamp (Carson, 2004).

Hydrogen Sulfide

Since hydrogen sulfide (H_2S) is insoluble in water, it may expose the deepest recesses of the lung. At 50–150 ppm level H_2S causes pulmonary edema (Carson, 2004). In vitro, H_2S induces apoptosis of aorta smooth muscle cells, regulated by mitogen-activated protein kinase (ERK MAPK) that activates caspase-3 (Yang et al., 2004). H_2S is less toxic to birds than to other animals; 2000–3000 ppm will change respiratory rate and depth, while 4000 ppm will kill them in about 15 min. The mechanism may relate to the greater gas exchange efficiency of parabronchi (Brown et al., 1997).

Hydrogen sulfide's ability to paralyze the respiratory tract is its greatest danger to animals and humans (Carson, 2004). Above 500–2000 ppm, mammals are said to take the second, but not the third, breath. Above 500 ppm, H_2S begins to cause permanent neurologic damage. Data from rats trained to run a reversed contingency maze suggested that H_2S may impair learning by increasing the animals' susceptibility to interference from irrelevant stimuli (Partlo et al., 2001).

Hydrogen sulfide is readily detectable as a rotten egg smell. Humans and presumably animals can detect hydrogen sulfide at 0.025 ppm (Carson, 2004). Above 200 ppm, however, hydrogen sulfide paralyzes the olfactory apparatus so it may not be detectable by smell. Higher concentrations seem to paralyze smell more rapidly. Thus, animals or humans may have only a very brief instant to smell hydrogen sulfide at high concentrations; it is dangerous to ignore the smell because its duration can be so brief.

Hydrogen sulfide is heavier than air and insoluble in the water of manure pits (Carson, 2004). Thus it can exist as bubbles in swine manure pits inside hog houses, ready to be released and expose animals and workers on agitation. Taking appropriate steps to protect rescuers, exposed people or animals not breathing should be dragged outside. If breathing is not reestablished spontaneously, artificial respiration should be applied until spontaneous respiration returns.

Nitrogen Dioxide and Ozone

NO_2 is considered with ozone (O_3), because NO_2 is a prooxidant and O_3 an oxidant. In agriculture, NO_2 can come from silage or relatively airtight silos, where it is usually found towards the top (Carson, 2004). Indoor air NO_2 and O_3 can come from second-hand cigarette smoke. NO_2 exposure from newly opened silage bags may modestly affect hungry cattle if exposure levels are unusually high (i.e., in large confined animal feeding operations dairies), but usually they are more likely to affect caretakers in upright silos. NO_2 has low water solubility, and can pass through the upper airway and permanently damage pulmonary parenchyma where residence times are longer. At ambient NO_2 (2–3 ppm) there is little damage or clinical signs. At higher levels, e.g., 20 ppm, it induces lung edema. Animals develop coughing, some fluid in the lungs, death of type I epithelial cells, coalescing alveoli, and an increased collagen production but no morphologic evidence of fibrosis (Gregory et al., 1983; Pickrell et al., 1987a; Mauderly et al., 1987; Carson, 2004). Animals that die at varying times after exposure have evidence of pulmonary edema and emphysema.

Birds are unusually sensitive to NO_2 and O_3, depending on exposure level. Caged pet birds may be sensitive to second-hand cigarette smoke, especially in the presence of heating/combustion sources. Newly hatched chicks die after 5 days' exposure to 1–4 ppm O_3; exposure to 0.3–0.7 ppm O_3 causes pulmonary hemorrhage in these chicks (Brown et al., 1997). Pulmonary hemorrhage in mammals is typical of acute high-level oxidant exposure of a somewhat more intense nature than that associated with pulmonary edema (Pickrell et al., 1987a).

Particle Size and Clearance

Particle Size and Deposition Mechanisms

Inhaled aerosol particles are frequently of multiple sizes (polydispersed). Particles of different aerodynamic sizes deposit in different anatomic areas of the mammalian and avian respiratory tracts. In mammalian lungs, particles with aerodynamic diameters of 5–30 μm mostly deposit by inertial impaction in the nasopharyngeal region because they do not follow curving airflow well (Witschi and Last, 2001). Inertial impaction in bird respiratory tracts is influenced by flow velocity and Reynolds numbers (Re) (trachea 100 cm/s at Re = 700; primary bronchi 130 cm/s and Re = 600; narrowed primary bronchus 200 cm/s and Re = 550). The expected sites of inertial impaction in birds are similar to those in mammals (Brown et al., 1997).

Slightly smaller particles (1–5 μm in aerodynamic diameter) mostly deposit by gravitational sedimentation in the conducting airways—the trachea, bronchi and bronchioles—as airflow speed progressively slows down towards the airway terminals. In the human lung, sedimentation is an important mechanism for deposition at sizes greater than 0.2 μm in diameter (Witschi and Last, 2001). In birds, deposition probability is a product of (residence time)(aerodynamic diameter). In parabronchi, where flows are as low as 3 cm/s (Re = 2), and residence times may be up to 1 min for complete change of air sac volume at rest, deposition probabilities can be quite high (Brown et al., 1997).

Particles <1 μm in aerodynamic diameter have a good probability to deposit by Brownian diffusion when their random movement causes them to bump into wet surfaces (Witschi and Last, 2001). Diffusion, like sedimentation, is most important where residence times are the longest. The probability of deposition by diffusion increases with decreasing particle size, so that deposition of particles with aerodynamic diameters of less than 0.5 μm is largely by diffusion. Breathing pattern can be important. During exercise particles acquire higher velocity, momentum and inertia that increase impaction deposition higher up the respiratory tract. Alternatively, breath holding causes more deposition by gravitational sedimentation and diffusion.

Particle Clearance

Particle clearance in mammals is important to defense of the lung. Rapid clearance lessens exposure time and extent of injury. Clearance of intact particles depends heavily on pulmonary alveolar macrophages and the mucociliary escalator. Alveolar macrophages phagocytose particles, then migrate to the bronchi and trachea for clearance. Ultrafine particles that enter the alveolar interstitium may be cleared at a much slower rate (Shinohara et al., 2010). Particles can leave the lung and enter the vascular system, causing a risk to organs downstream from the lung (Nemmar et al., 2001; Borm et al., 2006). Alternatively, particles may be soluble in aqueous media and can be dissolved in mucus. Fine and ultrafine (nano) particles with much of their mass in contact with the surface are especially subject to such dissolution. Factors affecting this solubility are quite complex; they include but are not limited to composition of the aqueous fluid, particle size, particle chemical composition, steepness of concentration gradient, curvature, agglomeration, and aspect ratio (Nemmar et al., 2001; Borm et al., 2006). Some ultrafine particles that are deposited in the nasal mucosa can be transported to the brain via the olfactory bulb (Oberdörster et al., 2004).

Particle solubility and chemical reactivity are influenced by the physical–chemical environment. Bicarbonate in lung simulant fluid, e.g., can enhance solubility in particles moderately soluble in aqueous media. To obtain relevant data solubility and reactivity should be measured in an environment as near to that of the lung environment as possible. This can sometimes be accomplished with in vitro conditions closely simulating biological solutions (Powers et al., 2006). Solubility is thought to be a function of chemical activity, specific surface area, radius and curvature, agglomeration, and specific chemicals that are adsorbed to the NSP (Borm et al., 2006). It is important to consider not just solubility in water, but in fluids that bear significant resemblance to that of the epithelial lining fluid (ELF). ELF is the fluid than lines the epithelial cells in the respiratory tract. A volume of 40–100 mL is predicted for mature humans. The pH varies from 6.9 at the end of inspiration to 7.5 at the end of expiration. Bicarbonate is a major buffer, and the pH variation is caused by varying CO_2 during expiration (Langmuir, 1965). Bicarbonate in lung simulant fluid increases the solubility of magnesium oxide (MgO) (Pickrell et al., 2006). Stoichiometry of the likely chemical species suggests a conversion of MgO to magnesium hydroxide ($Mg(OH)_2$) in aqueous media, and a subsequent conversion to the hydrated carbonate nesquehonite.

In chickens, small dust particles were found trapped in the respiratory epithelial cell trilaminar surfactant (Brown et al., 1997). No particles were found in the vascular system, kidneys and heart, suggesting that at least those particles did not enter the vascular system. After 1 h 54% of the particles remained, while after 36 h approximately 36% remained, suggesting that appreciable clearance took place. The mechanism of the clearance is not completely clear. However, parenchymal respiratory epithelial cells could have transported particles toward the pulmonary interstitium. Particles in the mammalian lung too small to be efficiently phagocytized were also transported into the lung's interstitium. In bird lungs, there was a virtual absence of phagocytes; the absence may have caused the epithelial cells to take on a larger role. Following experimental introduction of Sephadex or Freund's adjuvant, phagocytes with physiological features similar to macrophages can enter the bird's pulmonary spaces.

Birds living in dusty environments—kiwis near the desert with abundant sand and polydispersed loose dust, or birds living near or flying over volcanic ash—show significant pathology and signs after only short exposures to small dust particles. Confined animal feeding operations with poultry raised in high population densities often show reduced production and pathology at necropsy (Brown et al., 1997).

LUNG INJURY

Acute Responses to Lung Injury

Airway Reactivity

Large mammalian conducting airways are surrounded by bronchial smooth musculature (BSM) (Witschi and Last, 2001). The muscle tone is modulated by the autonomic nervous system. Reflex contraction occurs after stimulation by irritants. Bronchoconstriction can also be provoked by cholinergic drugs. This stimulation is used in diagnosis as a basis to assess the "twitchiness" of BSM, i.e., at how low a level the bronchi can be induced to constrict. These agents bind to receptors and trigger increased intracellular cyclic monophosphates—adenosine and guanosine, respectively (cAMP and cGMP). Histamine, prostaglandins, nitric oxide, and leukotrienes also influence bronchoconstriction.

Pulmonary Edema

Pulmonary edema is exudative, and it indicates acute lung injury (Witschi and Last, 2001). Edema is associated with leakage or interruption, as well as thickening of the alveolar capillary membrane. Edema fluid creates a thicker diffusion barrier, and contributes to a mismatch of ventilation to perfusion. The mismatch limits the rate of oxygen exchange from the air of the alveoli to the blood of the alveolar capillaries, even if the alveolar capillary unit is normal in all other respects. Frequently, very intense pulmonary edema will include some evidence of small pinpoint pulmonary hemorrhage. Even brief edema may damage or denude epithelium, or endothelium, or both.

Heart failure is often associated with cardiogenic lung edema, as demonstrated by a case of fatal *Taxus* (Japanese yew) poisoning in horses with pulmonary congestion, hemorrhage and edema (Cope et al., 2004) as well as calves given *Nerium oleander* (Oleander) clippings, which developed tachycardia and pulmonary edema (Galey et al., 1996).Very high levels of fumonisin (>100 ppm in diet) may cause fatal pulmonary edema in pigs 1–4 h after exposure (Marasas, 2001). Noncardiogenic pulmonary edema has been associated with airway obstruction, cranial trauma, seizures or electric shock (Drobatz et al., 1995). In horses, hyper hydration prior to exercise may be detrimental to respiratory function due to some degree of edema (Sosa et al., 2002). Laboratory rodents receiving very high doses of paraquat may die with pulmonary edema and hemorrhage (Witschi and Last, 2001).

Some toxic agents, such as alloxan, which denude the alveolar capillary unit, reduce the likelihood of recovery (Witschi and Last, 2001), and may lead to significant collagen deposition (Pickrell and Villegas, research communication). If the changes are intense and architecture is severely compromised, pulmonary fibrosis may result. From some insults (histamine) an uneventful recovery may result. Several other insults (e.g., paraquat) cause sufficient injury to lead to healing by secondary intent (fibrosis).

We determine the extent of pulmonary edema by relating lung wet weight to body weight (Witschi and Last, 2001). Alternatively, lungs, lobes, or slices can be weighed before and after drying. The accuracy of the second procedure is limited by the uniformity of the edema, but again this may be a useful indicator (Witschi and Last, 2001).

Acute respiratory distress, particularly acute pulmonary edema, is treated with diuretics such as furosemide, intranasal oxygen, bronchodilators, corticosteroids, and alleviation of the underlying cause (Foreman, 1999). It is especially important to address the underlying cause in many of these conditions. Furosemide was formerly used in North America as a race-day preventive for exercise-induced pulmonary hemorrhage. The difficulty with using furosemide as a preventive is that furosemide may also be a performance-enhancing agent.

Nasal and Upper Airway Reactivity

Upper airway irritant gases and particulates, especially ultrafine particulates with greatly increased surface area, stimulate nasal (trigeminal) nerve endings (Witschi and Last, 2001). They also elicit avoidance reactions. Phosphine (PH_3), e.g., is liberated after ingesting zinc phosphide rodenticide; PH_3 irritates nasal and upper airway nerve endings resulting in avoidance reactions such as breath holding and subsequent paroxysmal breathing

(Knight, 2006). Other agents, such as HCl, NH_3, NO_2, and $COCl_2$, appear to initiate serum leakage through toxic effects on epithelial cells or endothelial cells or both. Highly reactive molecules cause their reactions in a different manner. It is unlikely that ozone can penetrate fluid layers to cause direct toxicity; it is more likely that reactive molecules initiate a cascade of ROS such as aldehydes and hydroperoxides.

The lung contains most of the metabolizing P450 isoenzymes found in other tissues, but often at lower concentrations than in the rest of the body. These P450 isoenzymes are highly inducible. Activation of the enzymes is an initial defensive reaction that may contribute to healing and protecting the lung (Nel et al., 2006). Although the P450 isoenzymes are clearly activated after exposure, it is not clear whether the response is sufficiently linear and consistent to use them as a biomarker of exposure. Other metabolizing enzymes in the lung include glutathione-*S*-transferase and glutathione peroxidase. In fact, the lung has been found to contain several forms of glutathione-*S*-transferase.

Mediators of Lung Toxicosis

Cytokines (tumor necrosis factor alpha (TNFα), transforming growth factor β (TGF-β) and interleukin 1B (IL-1B)) are found in respiratory tract lavage fluid, and are associated with cultured whole lung tissue and of specific lung cells (lung epithelial cells and fibroblasts) (Witschi and Last, 2001). Cytokines can be used in studies to signal toxicant-induced lung damage. TNFα and IL-1B, e.g., signal acute lung injury. TGF-β and the cytokines signaling acute lung injury are part of the pathogenesis of pulmonary fibrosis. IL-1, IL-2, IL-5 and IL-8 are thought to be essential components of epithelial lung cell injury. Finally, IL-4, IL-5 and IL-13 are thought to be associated with allergenic responses.

Cell Proliferation

Toxicants can cause either reversible or irreversible lung changes (Witschi and Last, 2001). Toxic changes that cause major alterations in lung architecture usually cause irreversible lung injury. Severe tissue injury is followed by either tissue loss (emphysema) or healing by secondary intent (fibrosis). Although information about the typical responses associated with specific toxicants is available, it is still unclear how different responses are triggered.

When type I lung epithelial cells are injured and die following exposure to an oxidant gas, some type II lung epithelial cells proliferate, and begin to flatten and stretch to cover the denuded area. Clara cells proliferate following type II proliferation (Witschi and Last, 2001). Migration of blood monocytes to injured areas may trigger responses from other cells in the parenchymal lung unit, e.g., interstitial fibroblasts, myofibroblasts and endothelial cells. If the damage is relatively minor, the lung may heal with a relatively normal appearance, a higher total lung collagen content, and minimal, if any, alteration of pulmonary function.

Chronic Responses of the Lung to Injury

Fibrosis

Healing by secondary intent, often called pulmonary fibrosis, may be either reversible or irreversible depending on the degree of injury. When a lung injury is too severe, or persists too long to heal spontaneously, e.g., with high levels of paraquat, fibroblasts will attempt to fill the void left by type I lung epithelial cell death. Fibroblast proliferation may contribute to ventilation–perfusion mismatch, making the lung less functional than when repaired by epithelial proliferation. In addition, there would be greater alteration of pulmonary architecture and increased numbers of interstitial fibroblasts. Increased fibroblasts making normal amounts of collagen would be expected to collectively make more collagen. If minimal to moderate alterations in pulmonary architecture are present the lung will spontaneously revert back to normal (Pickrell et al., 1983). If greater alterations have been made to pulmonary architecture, the interstitial fibrosis may become irreversible and form dense fibrous scars (Pickrell et al., 1983; Witschi and Last, 2001).

There are over 10 genetically distinct collagen types in animals and humans. Types I and III are major interstitial collagens in the lung. Type III collagen is more compliant than type I. An increase in type I relative to type III collagen, which has been shown in experimental models of fibrosis caused by paraquat and asbestos, makes the lung even stiffer than if only an increased amount of collagen was present and the ratios of type I to type III collagen were unchanged (Witschi and Last, 2001).

Emphysema

Emphysema has been defined as enlarged air spaces due to tissue destruction without fibrosis (Witschi and Last, 2001). The lungs become larger, more compliant, and hyperinflated. Loss of gas exchange surfaces causes a reduction in gas exchange potential. Alveoli collapse, air spaces become distended and irregular, and air may become trapped. This makes it more difficult to expel air accumulated in distended alveoli. Patients become emaciated, have increasingly forced expirations and develop heave lines due to increasingly difficult and forceful expirations (Lowell, 1990).

Fibrosis is associated with local, heterogenic, compensatory emphysema. In areas where damage is sufficiently low, the lung heals normally. In areas where injury is more extensive, fibroblast proliferation and the excess production of collagen may result in fibrosis. In a still higher level of injury, even fibroblasts cannot effectively fill voids, healing by secondary intent fails and lung tissue is lost and emphysema forms. The extent to which this varied may be related to variations in local dose, the reserve of biological antioxidants, or the balance between proteinase–antiproteinase (Pickrell et al., 1983, 1987a,b).

Asthma

In asthma, small conducting airways constrict at lower irritant concentrations than in normal lungs. Bronchoconstriction reduces airway diameter resulting in increased small airway airflow resistance. Symptoms include coughing, wheezing, and progressive dyspnea (Witschi and Last, 2001).

Guinea pigs are highly sensitive to upper airway irritation and to subsequent development of bronchial asthma. Other animals that develop syndromes similar to human asthma include horses, dogs and cats (Padrid, 2000; Davis and Rush, 2002; McCue et al., 2003; Pirie et al., 2003; Reinero et al., 2006). In horses, an asthmatic condition known as heaves is associated with inhaled endotoxins and organic dust particulates, which are thought to be synergistic in their effects (Pirie et al., 2003). Potentially detrimental effects can be reduced by maintaining horses in "low dust" stables or at pasture, since these environments have significantly lower airborne dust and endotoxin levels (McGorum et al., 1998). Poultry farmers have significantly higher incidences of chronic bronchitis. The major risk factor for respiratory symptoms was shown to be inadequate ventilation of animal houses (Radon et al., 2002). Airborne endotoxin can cause flu like symptoms in birds; this condition must be differentiated from infectious avian influenza (Joseph and Subbarao, 2005).

Specific allergen immunotherapy is a potential therapy for feline asthma. In one study, Rush Immunotherapy (RIT) blunted eosinophilic airway inflammation in experimental feline asthma. BAL cytokine profiles favoring a Th2 response developed after giving Bermuda grass antigen. RIT shifted the response to increased IFN-γ, and IL-10 thereafter. The mechanism of RIT may involve changes in allergen-specific immunoglobulin production, induction of hyporesponsive lymphocytes or alteration of cytokine profiles (Reinero et al., 2006).

Lung Cancer

In laboratory animals, spontaneously occurring malignant pulmonary tumors are rare, except for very old animals. If lung tumors do develop in laboratory rodents, they are generally peripheral adenomas instead of the more central tumors seen in humans. Adenomas usually originate from type II pulmonary epithelial cells, or Clara cells. These adenomas rarely have sufficient time to develop into carcinomas. Occasionally, lung tissue injury causes bronchogenic adenocarcinoma, which is an unusual lung tumor in cats; it may metastasize to the digits and to the abdominal wall. Average survival time for tumors metastasizing to the digits is only ~5 weeks (Van der Linde-Sippman, 2000; Petterino et al., 2005).

Certain mouse strains (strain A and Swiss-Webster mice) with mutations in the K-ras genes similar to human carcinomas develop adenomas that increase in incidence after the inhalation of certain toxicants or carcinogens. These mice are potential models for human lung carcinogenesis (Witschi and Last, 2001).

Rat lungs occasionally contain lesions of epithelial cells surrounding material identified as keratin (Witschi and Last, 2001). The cells may compress lung parenchyma and occasionally invade it. These lesions are found more frequently in long-term tests of animals exposed to substances not considered to be carcinogens such as carbon black, titanium dioxide and certain man-made fibers. Controversy exists as to whether these are cysts filled with keratin, or can be classified as tumors.

In humans, it has been estimated that 80%–90% of all lung tumors are caused by inhaling cigarette smoke (Witschi and Last, 2001). Dogs are companion animals that live with their owners over long periods of time. Although rare, some dogs developed either nasal or lung tumors after being exposed to owner's second-hand cigarette smoke. In described cases, the tumors were carcinomas – epithelial in origin and malignant. Dogs living for protracted periods of time in a home with a smoker were more susceptible to lung cancer than those in homes of nonsmokers (odds ratio = 1.6, 95% confidence interval 0.7–3.7). No relations were found between cancer rates and increasing the number of packs of cigarettes smoked per day or the proportion of time the dog spent within the home. However, dog breeds with short- and medium-length noses had an increased tendency to develop lung cancer (odds ratio = 2.4, 95% confidence interval 0.7–7.8). Dogs with long noses (dolocephalic breeds) tend to deposit carcinogenic particles in the nasal cavity, and may develop nasal carcinomas. Alternatively, dogs with shorter noses (brachycephalic breeds) tend to allow carcinogenic particles to deposit in the upper airways and develop bronchogenic carcinomas (Reif et al., 1992). The most frequent tumors in dog lungs, however, are mammary tumors that metastasize to the lung.

Agents Known to Produce Lung Injury in Animals

Zinc Phosphide

Poultry are highly susceptible to zinc phosphide poisoning. For example, approximately 200 chickens inadvertently given zinc phosphide were found dead with no clinical signs after the flooring of a slat-and-litter house was breached (Tiwary et al., 2005). Gross necropsy revealed intense congestion of the viscera; histopathologic examination revealed severe pulmonary edema and congestion of the chickens' lungs, hearts, livers and kidneys (Tiwary et al., 2005).

Smoke

Smoke inhalation injury is common in animals when confinement does not allow them to move away from smoke-filled air. Cardiac dysfunction in sheep following combined burn and smoke injury was mostly related to hypovolemia, and was improved by aggressive fluid therapy. However, later myocardial contractile dysfunction seemed to be correlated with smoke inhalation injury (Soejima et al., 2001). In chickens, the interparabronchial septal spaces were measurably thickened and engorged as a result of hydrostatic pulmonary edema, similar to the effect of hydrostatic pulmonary edema in mammals (Weidner et al., 2002). Under similar conditions, air sacs thickened, and microvilli had increased density (Weidner, 2000).

Overheated Frying Pans

Exposure of caged birds to gases released from overheated nonstick cookware has been shown to result in a high percentage of deaths (Brown et al., 1997). Most of these birds have pulmonary edema and hemorrhages. Proximity to the source is an important risk factor. Birds in adjacent rooms may have only minimal pulmonary reactions compared to birds close to the source, even when the total exposure is similar for both (Brown et al., 1997). The mechanisms of these differences are not known at this time. It has been suggested that physical–chemical changes occur in released substances over time, making them less toxic. Alternatively, particles released from overheated surfaces in the same room are smaller in diameter, and more numerous, closer to the source, whereas those further away tend to coalesce into larger particles. Thus, birds in the same room would be exposed to more surface areas per unit mass than those in adjacent rooms.

Tryptophan and Perilla Frutescens

Tryptophan toxicity is associated with cattle consuming tryptophan in lush green forages (Pickrell and Oehme, 2004). The rumen converts tryptophan to 3-methyl indole (MI), which is metabolically activated by cytochrome P450 to a reactive compound in the lung. In a similar toxicosis, perilla ketone and 4-ipomeanol from *Perilla frutescens* (beef steak plant) damage endothelial cells and type I pulmonary epithelium (Nicholson, 2004; Pickrell and Oehme, 2004).

At high doses, MI leads to pulmonary edema, excess proteolysis, tissue destruction, emphysema, and death within 6–24 h after the onset of clinical signs (Pickrell and Oehme, 2004). Several pounds of green forage containing 4-ipomeanol may be fatal to a cow within 1–2 days (Nicholson, 2004). At lower exposure levels, animals may have respiratory signs (depression, respiratory grunt, wheeze, and froth flowing out of the nostrils) but will recover within 24–72 h with minimal to no physiological impairment. However, proliferation of type II alveolar cells may persist with no demonstrable physiological consequences. If exercised, cattle with intermediate signs can be pushed into the acute syndrome; they will worsen rapidly, develop significant lung edema and may die (Pickrell and Oehme, 2004).

REFERENCES

Ammann, V.J., Vrins, A.A., Lavoie, J.P., 1998. Effects of inhaled beclomethasonedipropionate on respiratory function in horses with chronic obstructive pulmonary disease (COPD). Equine. Vet. J. 30 (2), 152–157.

Bedenice, D., Heuwieser, W., Brawer, R., et al., 2003. Clinical and prognostic significance of radiographic pattern, distribution, and severity of thoracic radiographic changes in neonatal foals. J. Vet. Intern. Med. 17 (6), 876–886.

Berny, P., 2007. Pesticides and the intoxication of wild animals. J. Vet. Pharmacol. Ther. 30, 93–100.

Borm, P., Klaessig, F.C., Landry, T.D., et al., 2006. Research strategies for safety evaluation of nanomaterials. Part VI. Characterization of nanoscale particles for toxicological evaluation. Toxicol. Sci. 90 (2), 23–32.

Brown, R.E., Brain, J.D., Wang, N., 1997. The avian respiratory system: a unique model for studies of respiratory toxicosis and for monitoring air quality. Environ. Health Perspect. 105 (2), 188–200.

Carson, T.L., 2004. Gases. In Clinical Veterinary Toxicology, Plumlee KH (ed.), St. Louis, MO, pp. 155–161.

Cope, R.B., Camp, C., Lohr, C.V., 2004. Fatal yew (Taxus sp.) poisoning in Willamette Valley, Oregon, horses. Vet. Hum. Toxicol. 46 (5), 279–281.

Corcoran, T.E., 2010. A better picture of clearance in the nose. J. Appl. Physiol. 108, 1–2.

Cox, R.A., Soejima, K., Burke, A.S., et al., 2001. Enhanced pulmonary expression of endothelin-1 in an ovine model of smoke inhalation injury. J. Burn. Care Rehabil. 22 (6), 375–383.

Crowell, W.A., Whitlock, R.H., Stout, R.C., Tyler, D.E., 1979. Ethylene glycol toxicosis in cattle. Cornell. Vet. 69 (3), 272–279.

Davis, E., Rush, B.R., 2002. Equine recurrent airway obstruction: pathogenesis, diagnosis, and patient management. Vet. Clin. North Am. Equine. Pract. 18 (3), 453–467.

Dickinson, C.E., Traub-Dargatz, J.L., Dargatz, D.A., et al., 1996. Rattlesnake venom poisoning in horses: 32 cases (1973–1993). J. Am. Vet. Med. Assoc. 208 (11), 1866–1871.

Drobatz, K.J., Saunders, H.M., Pugh, C.R., et al., 1995. Noncardiogenic pulmonary edema in dogs and cats: 26 cases (1987–1993). J. Am. Vet. Med. Assoc. 206 (11), 1732–1736.

Dungworth, D., 1993. The respiratory system. In: Jubb, K.V.F., Kennedy, P.C., Palmer, N. (Eds.), Pathology of Domestic Animals, fourth ed. Academic Press, New York, pp. 539–699.

Dye, J.A., 1992. Feline bronchopulmonary disease. Vet. Clin. North Am. Small Anim. Pract. 22 (5), 187–201.

Foreman, J.H., 1999. Equine respiratory pharmacology. Vet. Clin. North Am. Equine. Pract. 15 (3), 665–686.

Galey, F.D., Holstege, D.M., Plumlee, K.H., et al., 1996. Diagnosis of oleander poisoning in livestock. J. Vet. Diagn. Invest. 8 (3), 358–364.

Gregory, R.E., Pickrell, J.A., Hahn, F.F., et al., 1983. Pulmonary effects of intermittent subacute exposure to low-level nitrogen dioxide. J. Toxicol. Environ. Health. 11 (3), 405–414.

Joseph, T., Subbarao, K., 2005. Human infections with avian influenza viruses. Md. Med. 6 (1), 30–32.

Kaye, J., Buchanan, F., Kendrick, A., et al., 2004. Acute carbon dioxide exposure in healthy adults: evaluation of a novel means of investigating the stress response. J. Neuroendocrinol. 16 (3), 256–264.

Knight, M., 2006. Zinc phosphide. In: Peterson, M.E., Talcott, P.A. (Eds.), Small Animal Toxicology. Elsevier-Saunders, St. Louis, MO, pp. 1103–1116.

Langmuir, D., 1965. Stability of carbonates in the system MgO-CO_2-H_2O. J. Geol. 73, 730–754.

Lightfoot, T.L., Yeager, J.M., 2008. Pet bird toxicity and related environmental concerns. Vet. Clin. N. Am.-Exotic. 11, 229–259.

Lowell, F.C., 1990. Observations on heaves. An asthma-like syndrome in the horse. Allergy Proc. 11 (3), 149–150.

Manohar, M., Hutchens, E., Coney, E., 1993. Pulmonary hemodynamics in the exercising horse and their relationship to exercise-induced pulmonary hemorrhage. Br. Vet. J. 149 (5), 419–428.

Marasas, W.F., 2001. Discovery and occurrence of the fumonisins: a historical perspective. Environ. Health Perspect. 109 (Suppl. 2), 239–243.

Mauderly, J.L., Bice, D.E., Carpenter, R.L., et al., 1987. Effects of inhaled nitrogen dioxide and diesel exhaust on developing lung. Res. Rep. Health Eff. Inst. 8, 3–37.

McCue, M.E., Davis, E.G., Rush, B.R., et al., 2003. Dexamethasone for treatment of multisystemic eosinophilic epitheliotropic disease in a horse. J. Am. Vet. Med. Assoc. 223 (9), 1320–1323.

McGorum, B.C., Ellison, J., Cullen, R.T., 1998. Total and respirable airborne dust endotoxin concentrations in three equine management systems. Equine. Vet. J. 30 (5), 430–434.

Mehta, A.J., Henneberger, P.K., Toren, K., et al., 2005. Airflow limitation and changes in pulmonary function among bleachery workers. Eur. Respir. J. 26 (1), 133–139.

Mills, P.C., Higgins, A.J., 1997. Oxidant injury, nitric oxide and pulmonary vascular function: implications for the exercising horse. Vet. J. 153 (2), 125–148.

Morris, J.B., Clay, R.J., Cavanagh, D.G., 1986. Species differences in upper respiratory tract deposition of acetone and ethanol vapors. Fund. Appl. Toxicol. 7, 671–680.

Nel, A., Xia, T., Madler, L., et al., 2006. Toxic potentials of materials at the nanolevel – review. Science. 311 (5761), 622–627.

Nemmar, A., Vanbilloen, H., Hoylaerts, M.F., et al., 2001. Passage of intratracheally instilled ultrafine particles from the lung into the systemic circulation in hamster. Am. J. Resp Crit Care. 164, 1665–1668.

Nicholson, S.J., 2004. Furans. In Plumlee, K. (Ed.), Clinical Veterinary Toxicology. St. Louis, MO, pp. 402–403.

Oberdörster, G., Sharp, Z., Atudorei, V., et al., 2004. Translocation of inhaled ultrafine particles to the brain. Inhal. Toxicol. 16, 437–445.

Padrid, P., 2000. Pulmonary diagnostics. Vet. Clin. North Am. Small Anim. Pract. 30 (6), 1187–1206.

Partlo, L.A., Sainsbury, R.S., Roth, S.H., 2001. Effects of repeated hydrogen sulphide (H_2S) exposure on learning and memory in the adult rat. Neurotoxicology. 22 (2), 177–189.

Petterino, C., Guazzi, P., Ferro, S., et al., 2005. Bronchogenic adenocarcinoma in a cat: an unusual case of metastasis to the skin. Vet. Clin. Pathol. 34 (4), 401–404.

Pickrell, J.A., 1991. Hazards in confinement housing – gases and dusts in confined animal houses for swine, poultry, horses and humans. Vet. Hum. Toxicol. 33, 32–39.

Pickrell, J.A., Mageed, A.A., 1995. Radiation in "pulmonary fibrosis". In: Phan, S., Thrall, R. (Eds.), Lung Biology in Health and Disease. Marcel Dekker, Inc, New York, pp. 363–381. Lanfant CE (series ed.).

Pickrell, J.A., Oehme, F.W., 2004. Tryptophan. In Plumlee, K. (Ed.), Clinical Veterinary Toxicology. St. Louis, MO, pp. 410–411.

Pickrell, J.A., Diel, J.H., Slauson, D.O., et al., 1983. Radiation-induced pulmonary fibrosis resolves spontaneously if dense scars are not formed. Exp. Mol. Pathol. 38 (1), 22–32.

Pickrell, J.A., Gregory, R.E., Cole, D.J., et al., 1987b. Effect of acute ozone exposure on the proteinase-antiproteinase balance in the rat lung. Exp. Mol. Pathol. 46 (2), 168–179.

Pickrell, J.A., Hahn, F.F., Rebar, A.H., et al., 1987a. Changes in collagen metabolism and proteinolysis after repeated inhalation exposure to ozone. Exper. Mol. Pathol. 46 (2), 159–167.

Pickrell, J.A., Castro, S.D., Gakhar, G., et al., 2006. Comparative solubility of nanoparticles and bulk oxides of magnesium in water and lung stimulant fluids. Toxicol. Sci. (Society of Toxicology meeting Abstract 1522).

Pirie, R.S., Collie, D.D., Dixon, P.M., McGorum, B.C., 2003. Inhaled endotoxin and organic dust particulates have synergistic proinflammatory effects in equine heaves (organic dust-induced asthma). Clin. Exp. Allergy. 33 (5), 676–683.

Poncet, C.M., Dupre, G.P., Freiche, V.G., et al., 2005. Prevalence of gastrointestinal tract lesions in 73 brachycephalic dogs with upper respiratory syndrome. J. Small Anim. Pract. 46 (6), 273–279.

Powers, K.W., Brown, S.C., Krishna, V.B., et al., 2006. Research strategies for safety evaluation of nanomaterials. Part VI. Characterization of nanoscale particles for toxicological evaluation. Toxicol. Sci. 90 (2), 296–303.

Radon, K., Monso, E., Weber, C., et al., 2002. Prevalence and risk factors for airway diseases in farmers – summary of results of the European Farmers' Project. Ann. Agric. Environ. Med. 9 (2), 207–213.

Reif, J.S., Dunn, K., Ogilvie, G.K., et al., 1992. Passive smoking and canine lung cancer risk. Am. J. Epidemiol. 135 (3), 234–239.

Reinero, C.R., Byerly, J.R., Berghaus, R.D., et al., 2006. Rush immunotherapy in an experimental model of feline allergic asthma. Vet. Immunol. Immunopathol. 110 (1–2), 141–153.

Shinohara, N., Nakazato, T., Tamura, M., et al., 2010. Clearance kinetics of fullerene C60 nanoparticles from rat lungs after intratracheal C60 instillation and inhalation C60 exposure. Toxicol. Sci. 118 (2), 564–573.

Shusterman, D., Balmes, J., Murphy, M.A., et al., 2004. Chlorine inhalation produces nasal airflow limitation in allergic rhinitic subjects without evidence of neuropeptide release. Neuropeptides. 38 (6), 351–358.

Snyder, M.C., Leopold, D.A., Chiu, B.C., et al., 2003. The relationship between agricultural environments and olfactory dysfunction. J. Agric. Saf. Health. 9 (3), 211–219.

Soejima, K., Schmalstieg, F.C., Sakurai, H., et al., 2001. Pathophysiological analysis of combined burn and smoke inhalation injuries in sheep. Am. J. Physiol. Lung. Cell Mol. Physiol. 280 (6), 1233–1241.

Sosa Leon, L., Hodgson, D.R., Evans, D.L., et al., 2002. Hyperhydration prior to moderate-intensity exercise causes arterial hypoxaemia. Equine Vet. J. Suppl. 34, 425–429.

Taylor, M., 1974. The origin and functions of nasal mucus. Laryngoscope. 84, 612–636.

Tiniakov, R.L., Tiniakova, O.P., McLeod, R.L., et al., 2003. Canine model of nasal congestion and allergic rhinitis. J. Appl. Physiol. 94 (5), 1821–1828.

Tiwary, A.K., Puschner, B., Charlton, B.R., et al., 2005. Diagnosis of zinc phosphide poisoning in chickens using a new analytical approach. Avian. Dis. 49 (2), 288–291.

Tsujino, I., Kawakami, Y., Kaneko, A., 2005. Comparative simulation of gas transport in airway models of rat, dog, and human. Inhal. Toxicol. 17 (9), 475–485.

Van der Linde-Sippman, J.S., van den Ingh, T.S., 2000. Primary and metastatic carcinomas in the digits of cats. Vet. Q. 22 (3), 141–145.

Weidner, W.J., 2000. Response of air sac mesothelium to expansion of extracellular fluid volume in Gallus domesticus. J. Comp. Pathol. 123 (2–3), 182–185.

Weidner, W.J., Kinnison, J.R., 2002. Effect of extracellular fluid volume expansion on the interparabronchial septum of the avian lung. J. Comp. Pathol. 127 (2–3), 219–222.

West, J.B., 2000a. Respiratory Physiology: The Essentials. sixth ed. Lippincott, Williams and Wilkins, Philadelphia, PA, pp. 11–61.

West, J.B., 2000b. Pulmonary Pathophysiology: The Essentials. fifth ed. Lippincott, Williams and Wilkins, Philadelphia, PA, pp. 3–35.

West, J.B., Watson, R.R., Fu, X., 2006. The honeycomb-like structure of the bird lung allows a uniquely thin blood–gas barrier. Respir. Physiol. Neurobiol. 152 (1), 115–118.

Winder, C., 2001. The toxicology of chlorine. Environ. Res. 85 (2), 105–114.

Witschi, H.P., Last, J.O., 2001. Toxic responses of the respiratory system. In: Klaassen, C.D. (Ed.), Casarett and Doull's Toxicology, The Basic Science of Poisons. McGraw Hill, New York, pp. 515–534. Chapter 15.

Yang, G., Sun, X., Wang, R., 2004. Hydrogen sulfide-induced apoptosis of human aorta smooth muscle cells via the activation of mitogen-activated protein kinases and caspase-3. FASEB J. 18 (14), 1782–1784.

Chapter 14

Cardiovascular Toxicity

Csaba K. Zoltani

INTRODUCTION

Cardiotoxicity primarily manifests itself by the dysfunction of the electrophysiology of the heart, consequently altering its mechanical functioning. With the blood unable to supply the required oxygenation to the organs, the undesirable effect of hypoxia is present. Contributing factors further include oxidative stress and the generation of reactive oxygen species (ROS) that damage cellular membranes and the energy production within the cell (Kang, 2001). The inception of the electrophysiological dysfunction in animals is primarily caused by undesirable ingested plant ingredients, envenomation, or environmental toxins (Ramachandran, 2014) including insecticides, fertilizers, herbicides, poisonous insects, vertebrates, invertebrates, or fungi of the class *Basidiomycete*.

The ingested poisonous fodder and environmental toxins may stimulate a wide variety of symptoms. In some cases, cardiotoxicity is only ancillary for the initial diagnosis, but its recognition and subsequent treatment may be of primary importance for the outcome.

Cardiotoxicity is evidenced by changes in the electrocardiogram (ECG). Initial indicators of cardiac injury include increase in the amplitude of the T-wave and ST-segment elevation. In addition, biomarkers of cardiac injury give insight into the nature of the injury. These include serum levels of the two isoforms of cardiac troponin T and I, whose levels rise after ischemia is evident and indicate myocardial necrosis. Also myoglobin, released by injured myocardial cells, is present. Levels of creatine kinase (CK), CK-MB (MB designates the isoenzyme found primarily in the myocardium), rise after the onset of infarction or even after tachycardia. LDH-1 (lactate dehydrogenase) isoenzyme is primarily found in heart tissue, while LDH-2, LDH-3, LDH-4, and LDH-5 are found in many other tissues. Tissue breakdown or cellular damage elevates LDH, the enzyme that catalyzes conversion of lactate to pyruvate and pyruvate to lactate, and its presence indicates hemolysis, the destruction of red blood cells. LDH-1 > LDH-2 indicates heart attack or injury. The FABP3 gene encodes an intracellular fatty acid–binding protein, a marker for myocardial damage. It is released into the plasma after myocardial injury.

This chapter addresses the primary cardiac problems encountered by animals as a result of unsuitable feed or the introduction of poisons into their system by alternate means.

PLANT-INDUCED CARDIOTOXICITY

The primary cause of cardiotoxicity in animals is the ingestion of plants containing phytochemicals that cause toxicity. Most plants are widely distributed, though possibly geographically contained, and toxicity depends on various factors including season, environmental conditions, particular ingredients, and part of the plant accessed.

All plants contain toxic principles that protect them and deter animals and insects from ingesting them. While these compounds may be toxic, they are essential to the plant for the formation of plant proteins and plant growth. Some grasses, such as *Phalaris* or *Festuca arundinacea,* are also poisonous. *Phalaris* species contain gramine, an indole alkaloid, that in sheep causes nervous system damage. *Phalaris* toxicity expresses itself as cardiac-sudden death (Cheeke, 1995). Initially cattle, and to a lesser extent sheep, have their tongue nerves affected causing swallowing paresis disabling the animal from normal eating.

Gossypol, a reactive polyphenolic pigment of the cotton plant, when ingested, is toxic to the heart. In livestock, lesions of the heart are observed leading to heart failure and sudden death. Pigs are similarly affected. Plant extracts containing phenolic compounds have also been implicated for their toxicity to animals.

The effect of the toxicity varies with the genus ingesting it. Excellent references and databases on plants exist (Kingsbury, 1964; Frohne and Pfander, 2005; Burrows and Tyrl, 2006; Panter et al., 2007; FDA, 2008).

Veterinary Toxicology. DOI: http://dx.doi.org/10.1016/B978-0-12-811410-0.00014-3

Additional information on plants and their effect on the cardiovascular system is found in Beasley (1999), Knight and Walter (2001) and Hoffman et al. (1975). Detailed treatment of plant toxicants are also available in Cheeke (1989).

PHYTOCHEMICALS AFFECTING THE CARDIAC SYSTEM

Plants contain on average a dozen different compounds that may cause cardiotoxicity, but two are of primary importance for inducing toxicity when consumed—glycosides and alkaloids.

Glycosides, with a digitalis-like effect, are lethal in domestic animals upon ingestion of 100–200 mg/kg of body weight (b.w.).

Mechanism of toxicity of glycosides at the cellular level involves interference with the Na^+/K^+-ATPase (Na^+/K^+-ATPase pump) resulting in decreased intracellular K^+, increase in serum K^+, and consequently decreased resting potential. At high concentrations, glycosides in the heart affect electrical conductions, resulting in increased vagal tone to the atrioventricular (AV) and the sinoatrial (SA) nodes. This may culminate in cardiac arrhythmias and asystole (cardiac arrest). Additionally, they cause hemorrhage, myocardial lesions, and myocarditis (Botha, 2013).

More than 200 cardiac glycosides are known. Digoxin, from *Digitalis purpurea* and *Digitalis lanata* (foxglove), the ingredient of digitalis, is used to enhance myocardial contractility but has a narrow therapeutic index. Overdose induces ECG changes such as ST-depression, T-wave inversion, PR-interval prolongation, and QT-interval decrease thereby leading to the signs of cardiac toxicity. Digoxin interferes with the binding sites of K^+ ions on the Na^+/K^+-ATPase pump. This increases the level of Na^+ ions in the myocytes that induces higher intercellular Ca^{2+} ion presence. Excessive Ca^{2+} increases cardiac contractions. In addition, cardiac glycosides have vagotonic effects, resulting in bradycardia and heart block (Beasley, 1999; Liu et al., 2010). Treatment for glycoside poisoning usually involves multidose activated charcoal and atropine.

Next to glycosides, alkaloids from plant ingredients play an important role in cardiac toxicity. Alkaloids are metabolites, nontoxic to the organism producing them and toxic to foreign organisms. Their function is mainly endogenous as regulators of metabolism to mimic neurotransmitters and also to influence plant growth. Alkaloids exhibit cytotoxicity against cells of foreign organisms. Among others, they can be acetylcholinesterase (AChE) inhibitors and Ca^{2+} antagonists (Aniszewski, 2007).

The alkaloids from roughly 20 botanical families are significant for their cardiac effects. The polycyclic diterpene alkaloids act as neuromuscular blocking agents, and the other two classes of steroidal alkaloids are solanum (a cholinesterase inhibitor) and veratridine (a hypotonic) (Schep et al., 2006). The glycoalkaloid solanine opens K^+ channels of mitochondria and increases Ca^{2+}, while tropane alkaloids are anticholinergic and cause arrhythmias, bradycardia, and tachycardia. Plants that harbor alkaloid toxins include Larkspur, Yew, Monkshood, Ground Hemlock, and Death Camas. The Lily family contains the alkaloid veratridine, a depolarizing agent that causes persistent opening of voltage-gated Na^+ channels and reduces channel conductance by three-quarters (Table 14.1).

GLYCOSIDE-CONTAINING PLANTS

Asclepias spp. (Milkweed) is a perennial plant indigenous to the Great Plains and from North Carolina to Maine (Kingsbury, 1964; Stevens, 2000). Most toxic is Labriform Milkweed followed by the narrow-leaf Whorled Milkweed that exudes a milky juice from its broken surfaces. *Galitoxin,* the toxic principle, is found in all vegetative parts of the plant. In addition, it contains cardenolides that may produce digitalis-like symptoms.

Horses, cattle, and sheep are all susceptible, with a dosage of Whorled Milkweed of 0.1%–0.5% b.w. of the animal being fatal. Cardiac signs include bradycardia or tachycardia, hypotension, and arrhythmia. Histological lesions and myocarditis are common (Clark, 1979). Treatment includes activated charcoal lavage and a cathartic.

Persea americana (Avocado) of the family *Lauraceae* is a tree found in Mexico and commercially grown in the United States. The toxic principle is *persin* that causes myocardial necrosis in birds and mammals. Mastitis (necrosis and hemorrhage) of mammary gland epithelium has been observed. Sheep fed 2.5 g/kg b.w. for 32 days developed cardiac insufficiency. Upon ingestion of avocado, dogs also develop cardiac insufficiency. At high doses, exceeding 100 mg/kg b.w., the myocardium is affected (Oelrichs et al., 1995) with necrosis of myocardial fibers. Goats fed fresh avocado show cardiac distress (Grant et al., 1991). Treatment is symptomatic and nonspecific.

Digitalis purpurea spp. (Foxglove) is a biennial plant found in the northeastern United States as well as California and states to the north. The poisonous constituents in Foxglove include digitoxin, digitonin, and digitalin. The LD_{50} of digitoxin for cats is 0.18 mg/kg b.w. and 60 mg/kg b.w. for guinea pigs. Poultry as well as ruminants are affected (Thomas et al., 1987). Important cardiac drugs are derived from Foxglove, including digitalis that helps to increase the force of contraction of the heart muscle. However, the effects of cardiac glycosides

TABLE 14.1 Plants Containing Cardiac Glycosides

Botanical Name	Common Designation	Cardiac Symptoms	Ancillary Cardiac Effect	Toxicity
Asclepias spp.	Milkweed	Weak, rapid pulse, arrhythmia	Hypotension, arrhythmia	Dosage of 0.5% b.w. fatal for horses, cattle
Persea americana	Avocado	Heart failure, cardiomyopathy	Necrosis of myocardial tissue, inflammation of the heart; horses, rabbits, goats, ostriches affected	Sheep fed 2.5 g/kg b.w. for 32 days developed cardiac insufficiency
Digitalis purpurea	Foxglove	Cardiac rhythm abnormality, hyperkalemia	Stronger cardiac contractions and slower contractions through stimulation of the vagus, prolonging diastole; affects cats, dogs, livestock	LD50 (cats) 0.18 mg/kg b.w., guinea pigs 60 mg/kg b.w.
Nerium spp.	Oleander	Bradycardia and/or tachycardia, ventricular fibrillation	In sheep depression of ST on ECG, hyperkalemia, serum potassium may increase twofold, second-degree AV-block	LD50 (goats) 330 mg/kg, b.w., in sheep 110 mg/kg b.w.
Convallaria majalis	Lily of the Valley	Sinus tachycardia, heart block	Cardiac signs may be delayed, heart becomes hyperirritable	LD50 (cat) 0.14 mg/kg b.w.
Rhodondendron spp.	Azalea, Rhodondendron	Arrhythmia, hypotension, weak heart rate	Contains the toxin grayanotoxin	LD50 (mice) 5.1 mg/kg b.w.
Kalmia spp.	Laurel	Bradycardia	Excitable cells remain depolarized	LD50 (rats) 2-5 mg/kg b.w.
Kalanchoe	Mother of millions	Ventricular arrhythmia	Irregular electrical activity	LD50 (rats) 560 mg/kg b.w. aqueous extract

are dose-dependent and have a tight therapeutic range. Slight overdoses induce toxicity.

Cardiac symptoms caused by steroidal glycosides of *D. purpurea* include stronger but slower cardiac contractions, prolonged diastole, also pulse and cardiac rhythm abnormalities, hyperkalemia (Lin et al., 2010), and ventricular tachycardia. Treatment includes activated charcoal lavage and cathartics.

Nerium spp. (Oleander) is an evergreen shrub of the *Apocynaceae* family that thrives principally in subtropical regions. All four Oleanders of the *Apocynaceae* family contain cardenolides that exert a positive inotropic effect on cardiac muscle. Their action is derived from inhibition of the plasmalemma (cell membrane) Na^+/K^+-ATPase.

In sheep, a dose of 110 mg/kg b.w. led to death preceded by decreased heart rate, tachyarrhythmia, and conduction defects affecting the sinus node, the AV node, and the elevated CK (Eddleston et al., 2000). ECG revealed bradycardia, AV-block, depression of the ST segment, tachycardia, and ventricular fibrillation (Aslani et al., 2004). Histopathological examination revealed myocardial degeneration. In goats, ECG showed second-degree AV-block (Barbosa et al., 2008). Digoxin immune fab treatment restores sinus rhythm and is the only proven therapy for yellow oleander poisoning (Rajapakse, 2009).

Convallaria majalis spp. (Lily of the Valley) is an herbaceous perennial woodland plant native to northern climates. The leaves contain over 30 cardiac glycosides, *Convallatoxin*, being the most important, with an LD_{50} of only 0.08 mg/kg b.w. (Fenton, 2002). *Convallatoxin* inhibits the enzyme Na^+/K^+-ATPase that increases ATP (adenosine triphosphate) found in the mitochondria and is the source of energy for cellular reactions. While useful for increasing contractility, overdose causes intoxication, sinus tachycardia, heart block, and fibrillation culminating in cardiac arrest. Cats are extremely sensitive to lilies: ingesting just two leaves will result in death (Fitzgerald, 2010). Fluid diuresis, before onset of renal failure, has been used as treatment.

Rhodonderon spp. (Azalea, Rhodondendron) is a genus of over 600 species that includes Azalea. Its toxic principle is grayanotoxin (Akera et al., 1976) compounds that affect the sodium channels on cell membranes. The grayanotoxin binds to muscarinic receptors. Bradycardia results from the peripheral vagal stimulation. Severe cases lead to cardiovascular collapse. The toxic principle interferes with cardiac muscle, and clinical effects are apparent after several hours postingestion (Sharma et al., 2009). Cardiovascular symptoms include hypotension, cardiac arrhythmias, and weak heart rate. The severity of toxicity also depends on the route of exposure. The LD_{50} in mice is 5.1 mg/kg b.w. (Barceloux, 2008). Treatment is symptomatic.

Kalmia spp. (Laurel, Lambkill) is an evergreen shrub of the family *Ericaceae,* native to North America. The plant contains the glycoside grayanotoxin that is toxic to ruminants. The LD_{50} in rats is 2–5 mg/kg b.w. (Frohne and Pfander, 2005). Minimum toxic dose in cattle is 0.4% b.w. (Beasley, 1999).

A grayanotoxin, also known as acetylandromedol, binds to Na^+ ion channel receptors involved with activation and inactivation of the cells. With inactivation blocked, the excitable cells remain depolarized. Cardiac symptoms include low blood pressure, bradycardia, and also ventricular tachycardia (Jansen et al., 2012).

Therapy includes atropine and also vasopressors to raise the blood pressure. Arrhythmias produced by grayanotoxin I can be reversed by tetrodotoxin (Akera et al., 1976; Ku et al., 1977).

Kalanchoe spp. (Mother of Millions, Chandelier Plant) are perennial plants that can be forced to bloom at any time of year. It is a genus of nearly 200 plant species native to Africa but now also found in Florida and Hawaii. Since they contain cardiac glycosides, they affect the heart by altering the electrolytic balance in the myocardium. In the wild, these plants are apt to poison sheep and cattle although household animals are also susceptible. The lethal dose for leaves of the plant for calves has been determined to be 40 g/kg b.w. The toxicity is due to the bufadienolide compounds, which are cardiac glycosides that inhibit the Na^+/K^+-ATPase pump of the myocardial cell membrane (Smith, 2012). Recommended treatment for toxicosis is symptomatic and supportive.

CYANIDE-CONTAINING PLANTS

Approximately 2500 plants contain cyanogenic glycosides (CG) (Vetter, 2000). Hydrocyanic acid/prussic acid is commonly formed in the seeds and leaves of sorghum plants and also from Cassava. Cyanide is a rapidly acting poison that inhibits the action of cytochrome oxidase that links oxygen with erythrocytes. Plants with only 20 mg of CG per 100 g (Allison and Baker, 2007) can kill livestock by asphyxia. By inhibiting cytochrome oxidase, cyanide induces cellular hypoxia. Since oxygen cannot be utilized, adenosine triphosphate is no longer formed. Cardiac symptoms include tachycardia, dysarrhythmia, and petechial hemorrhage of the heart and other organs. ECG changes include elevation or depression and shortened ST-segment, as well as fusion of the T-wave and QRS segment (Holstege et al., 2010). The amount of hydrocyanic acid formed by a plant varies, but the lethal dose for a mouse is 3.7 mg/kg b.w., and for cattle and sheep, it is 2.0 mg/kg b.w. (Speijers, 2003). Plants containing CG in excess of 20 mg/100 mg of plant material are avoided in feedstock.

Ruminant animals are more likely to be poisoned than monogastric animals (horses and pigs) because the lower pH in the stomach of monogastric animals destroys enzymes that change CG to hydrocyanic acid. Antidotes include sodium nitrate and sodium thiosulfate (Table 14.2).

ALKALOID-CONTAINING PLANTS

Delphinium spp. (Larkspur) consists of 250 species of annual and biennial flowering plants of the buttercup family *Ranunculaceae,* distributed throughout the Northern Hemisphere. Their ingestion by livestock has been responsible for extensive losses of cattle (Green et al., 2009). The plant contains numerous norditerpenoid alkaloids of the *lycoctonine* and the MDL (7,8-methylenedioxylycoctonine) and MSAL (methylsuccinyl anthranoyllycoctonine) type. Among the *lycoctonine* are three MSAL-type (potent neuromuscular poisons acting on the postsynaptic neuromuscular junction), extremely toxic neuromuscular blocking agents. MSAL-type alkaloids, the MLA (methyllycaconitine), DAN (nudicauline), and 14-DAN (14-deacetylnudicauline) cause most of the cattle poisonings from Larkspurs (Pfister et al., 1999). MSAL-type alkaloids are found to be 20 times more toxic than MDL type in mice (Panter et al., 2002; Welch et al., 2008). LD_{50} is 25–40 mg/kg b.w. depending on the type of alkaloid present.

Intoxication occurs when the nicotinic acetylcholine receptors are blocked. There are species differences in the symptoms, but the usual cardiac signs include rapid and irregular heartbeat and hypotension. The effect of Larkspur-derived MSAL alkaloids are counterbalanced by neostigmine or physostigmine. AChE inhibitors alleviate the clinical symptoms in cattle (Green et al., 2009). Physostigmine given i.v. at the rate of 0.08 mg/kg b.w. has been used under field conditions to relieve symptoms, though it may need to be repeated.

Aconitum spp. (Monkshood) is an herbaceous perennial found in elevated regions of the Northern Hemisphere. Even though, all parts of the plant are poisonous and contain polycyclic diterpene alkaloids with affinity for the open state of the voltage-sensitive sodium channel making them refractory to excitation (Chan, 2009). Aconite causes anticholinergic effects and has a positive inotropic effect by a prolonged influx of sodium. LD_{50} for mice for aconite is 130–280 mg/kg b.w. depending on the plant. Aconite causes hypotension,

TABLE 14.2 Alkaloid Metabolites Containing Plants

Botanical Name	Common Designation	Cardiac Symptoms	Ancillary Cardiac Effect	Toxicity
Delphinium spp.	Larkspur	Irregular tachycardia	Methyllycaconitine is antagonistic of nicotinic receptors; important role in poisoning of livestock	LD50 (cattle) 25–40 mg/kg b.w.
Aconitum	Monkshood	Hypotension, myocardial depression, conduction disturbance, tachycardia	Contains methyllycaconitine acts as NM blocking agent	LD50 (mice) 130–280 mg/kg b.w.
Taxus spp.	Yew	Bradycardia, acute cardiac failure	Depresses conduction of depolarization through the heart, no significant lesions	LD50 (rabbit) 8 mg/kg b.w., LD50 (mice) 15 mg/kg b.w.
Zygademus spp.	Death Camas	Weak, irregular pulse, decrease in blood pressure due to dilation of arterioles	Constricting veins, no specific lesions on autopsy, sheep especially vulnerable	Sheep lethal dose: 0.6%–6% b.w.
Cicuta maculata	Water Hemlock	Ventricular fibrillation	Change in PR of ECG	1 g/kg b.w. kills sheep
Eupatorium rugosum	White Snakeroot	Congestive heart failure	Cardiac muscle degeneration	0.5%–2.0% b.w. consumption intoxicates
Astragalus	Locoweed	Congestive right-heart failure	Accumulates selenium, heart affected	Toxin content greater than 0.001% causes poisoning
Rubiaceae	Madder	Heart failure	Galloping heart rhythm	Daily dose of 25 g/kg b.w. 4 weeks sheep cardiac failure
Cinchona officinalis	Quina	Cardiac arrhythmia	QRS duration increased	LD50 (rat) 263 mg/kg

bradycardia, superventricular tachycardia, and conduction disturbances. Treatment is symptomatic and supportive.

Taxus spp. (Yew) is an evergreen shrub found throughout North America. Ingestion of clippings from the plant causes poisoning of ruminants as well as in monogastrics. The toxic principle, taxine A and B alkaloids, causes an increase in the cytoplasmic Ca^{2+} and interferes with Na^+ and Ca^{2+} ion channel conductance that precedes bradycardia and diastolic cardiac arrest. Taxine B induces increased AV conduction times, longer QRS, and the absence of P-waves on ECG (Tiwary et al., 2005).

In ruminants, 0.5% b.w., and in monogastrics (horses) 0.1% b.w., ingestion is enough to cause clinical signs of toxicity. In mice, LD_{50} is 15 mg/kg b.w. and cardiac symptoms include arrhythmias, possibly culminating in cardiac failure (Wilson et al., 2001).

Yew has been reported to exert blockage of Na^+ and Ca^{2+} channels causing the Brugada-like syndrome (Veltmann et al., 2009). No specific treatment is known for yew poisoning except atropine and lidocaine for symptoms, and help is directed toward stabilization of the cardiovascular function.

Zygadenus spp. (*Zygadenus venenosus*, Death Camas) is an abundant perennial found in western states. It grows early in the spring but enters dormancy when soil moisture declines. It is poisonous to livestock upon ingestion, with death occurring within a few hours. The toxic principle is the cevanine steroidal alkaloid, Zigacine (Beasley, 1999). In sheep, 0.6%–6% b.w. ingestion is fatal. Zigacine causes weak, fast, irregular pulse, bradycardia, drop in blood pressure, necrosis of cardiac muscle, and cardiovascular failure. There is no known treatment for death camas poisoning.

Cicuta maculata spp. (Water Hemlock) is one of the most toxic plants found in North America (Panter et al., 1988). Water hemlock is a biennial and tall plant that grows in wet surroundings. The toxic principle is cicutoxin, which affects the central nervous system. It acts on the Gamma-aminobutyric acid (GABA) receptor, blocking the chloride channel that causes neuronal depolarization and seizures. Death occurs due to respiratory failure. Of note,

1 g/kg b.w. will kill sheep and 230 g will kill a horse or cattle. Due to its severe toxicity in cattle, it is also called "cowbane."

Cardiovascular effects include alterations in blood pressure, heart rate, a widening of the PR interval on the ECG, supraventricular tachycardia, and ventricular fibrillation (Schep et al., 2009). Degeneration and fibrosis in the heart is observed, and the blood serum shows increases in aspartate aminotransferase (AST) and lactic dehydrogenase (LDH), enzymes released upon injury to the heart or liver.

Treatment, though difficult and usually not in time due to the rapidity of the poisoning, includes intravenous administration of sodium pentobarbital to control seizure.

Eupatorium rugosum spp. (White Snakeroot) is a member of the daisy family native to the eastern United States (Kingsbury, 1964). It is an erect plant that is up to 1.5 m tall with the leaves resembling those of the nettle. Consumption of plants at 0.5%–2.0% b.w. causes poisoning in livestock (Doyle and Walkey, 1949). The plants are poisonous to horses, goats, and sheep. White snakeroot contains the toxin tremetol. Tremetol passes through the milk in cows, and thus contaminated milk causes sickness in suckling calves and humans. It is important to mention that tremetol is cumulative in that repeated exposure leads to intoxication.

The onset of clinical signs begins 2–3 weeks postingestion. In horses, it causes congestive heart failure (Maratea, 2003). The enzymes CK, alkaline phosphatase (ALP), and AST are elevated, and cardiac muscle degeneration occurs. Pale linear streaks in the myocardium as well as fluid in the pericardial sac have been observed. In horses, swelling in the neck area is also noted. Rapid heart rate, elevation of ST, and variable QRS complexes in the ECG and cardiac arrhythmias may be present. Treatment consists of supportive care.

Astragalus spp. (Locoweed) is found throughout the western United States and Canada. This perennial plant contains the toxic principle indolizidine alkaloid swainsonine (Turner et al., 2012). Animals grazing on Locoweed develop lysosomal storage disease when the lysosomal enzyme alpha mannosidase is inhibited. A toxic content of Locoweed greater than 0.001% can cause poisoning. Cytoplasmic vacuolation of cells of the CNS occurs. It increases the severity of "high mountain disease," a hypoxia-induced pulmonary hypertension and hypertrophy of the right ventricle of animals living at elevated altitudes. Sheep, cattle, and horses are affected. Some of the *Astragalus* species also accumulate large amounts of selenium complicating the effect on the heart when ingested.

Pathological effects include neurological damage and congestive right-heart failure. Treatment includes fluid therapy with potassium supplementation, dopamine, and diazepam.

Rubiaceae spp. (Madder) is the fifth-largest flowering plant family spread worldwide but found mostly in the warmer climates. An economically important member of the family is *Coffea arabica,* the source of coffee beans. Alkaloids derived from the bark of *Cinchona* yield quinine; others are antihypertensive and antiinflammatory. Gardenia (*Gardenia jasminoides*) is a garden plant of the frost-free zones planted worldwide.

On the other hand, 4–6 weeks after ingestion of plants of the *Rubiaceae* family (Kellerman, 2005), ruminants, without forewarning, drop dead with heart failure. Called gousiekte (Afrikaans name meaning quick sickness), the disease affects sheep and cattle and is characterized by myocardial necrosis consisting of a loss of myofilaments, cardiac dilations, and replacement of myocytes with collagenous tissue. In the terminal phase of the disease, the heart has a rounded, flabby appearance without an apex and has attenuated papillary muscles. In the subendocardial region of the apex and the left ventricular wall, the principal lesions are degeneration of myofibers.

The toxic principle is pavetamine from *Pavetta harborii* which inhibits myocardial protein synthesis without affecting myocardial fibers or other organs. The disease is characterized by cellular injury and is not a specific heart disease and terminates in dilated cardiomyopathy and congestive heart failure (Hay et al., 2008; Prozesky, 2008). Sheep dosed daily at 25 mg/kg b.w. after 4 weeks showed typical signs of cardiac failure with galloping heart rhythm, decrease of ejection fraction of the left ventricle (from 60% to 30%), and decrease in the pumping efficiency of the left ventricle with respect to the right ventricle (van der Walt and van Rooyen, 1977). Goats fed pavetamine showed ECG changes and tachycardia. The electrophysiology of the pacemaker cells was affected. In sheep T-wave inversion was common as was hypokalemia. In addition, calcium abnormalities were noted.

OXALATE-CONTAINING PLANTS

Many oxalate-containing plants, such as Philodendron (*Philodendron bipinnatifidum*), are kept for their ornamental beauty and are often easily accessible to pets. If ingested in large quantities, it cannot be metabolized, and the salts are absorbed into the bloodstream. Oxalic acid combines with calcium and forms the crystals. Although these crystals are primarily deposited in the kidneys, they can also be deposited in other organs, including the heart. In humans, oxalosis can lead to cardiac abnormalities correlated with decline in renal function (Mookadam et al., 2010). Oxalosis also causes heart block (Coltart and Hudson, 1971). Sheep and cattle grazing on *Rumex crispus* (Curled Dock), native to Europe and Western Asia, experienced tetany, recumbency, and death. Some grass varieties, including Buffelgrass (*Pennisetum ciliare*), which is common in southern Arizona, contain oxalates that may induce Ca^{2+} deficiency. Oxalates bind Ca^{2+} in the gastrointestinal tract, e.g., in horses, and lead to a change in the Ca^{2+} level of the blood along with a subsequent effect on the muscular system. The Ca^{2+} to oxalate ratio in the diet greater than 0.5:1 is considered safe.

The formation of calcium oxalates also leads to hypocalcemia, which interferes with electrical activity of the heart, as it inhibits the Ca^{2+} pump active in the generation of the action potential, resulting in the relaxation of the muscles. The reduced activity of the heart can culminate in cardiac arrest. The LD_{50} of oxalic acid is 375 mg/kg b.w. for rats.

Only limited data on cardiac manifestation of oxalosis in animals are available. Ingestion of sodium oxalate (VonBurg, 1994) results in weak and irregular pulse, hypotension, necrosis of the myocardium, and eventually cardiovascular collapse.

Recommended treatment includes oral dosing with calcium lactate followed by an emetic, i.e., binding the unabsorbed oxalates to calcium and then removing them.

NITRATE-CONTAINING PLANTS

Sorghum, corn, wheat, Johnson grass, pigweed, and alfalfa are a few of the plants that accumulate nitrate. The level of accumulation depends on a number of variables including the type of soil, environmental conditions, such as fertilization and climatic conditions, soil moisture, and temperature. Plants with more than 0.4% nitrate dry weight or ingestion of as little as 0.05% of the animal's weight of such plants may be lethal to livestock (Yong et al., 1990).

In the gastrointestinal tract, nitrates are converted to nitrite, which leads to the formation of methemoglobin that cannot carry oxygen to tissues. Animals thus suffocate. Clinical symptoms include rapid breathing through the mouth in livestock and an elevated heart rate. With a methemoglobin concentration greater than 35%, cardiac dysrhythmia is observed. Tissue changes are few, but hemorrhages particularly on the heart are noted. Acutely poisoned animals are usually treated with methylene blue (10 mg/kg, i.v). In view of the vasodilation caused by nitrate, vasoconstrictor drugs may also be used.

METAL-INDUCED CARDIAC TOXICITY

Arsenic

Although considerable native vegetation contains arsenic, the sources of intoxication usually are sprays or ingestion of feed contaminated by arsenic (Selby et al., 1977). Arsenic in drinking water also poses an additional risk of cardiovascular effect including hypertension, prolongation of the QT portion of the ECG, indicating a disorder of the heart's conduction system and favoring cardiac arrhythmia (Mordukhovich et al., 2009; el Bahri and Ben Romdane, 1991).

Large doses of arsenic lower blood pressure and slow down the pulse rate. In frogs the heart stops in diastole due to the paralysis of the motor ganglia. Since it is quick acting, cardiovascular collapse is to be expected. The lethal dose for arsenic trioxide for horses is 10–45 g/kg b.w. and LD_{50} of sodium arsenite in goats is 125 mg/kg b.w. (EFSA, 2005). Treatment is symptomatic and supportive.

IONOPHORES (ANTIBIOTICS)

Ionophores are carboxylic polyether antibiotics that are given as feed additives to cattle. Ionophores alter the flow of cations across cell membranes and reduce Gram-positive bacteria responsible for bloat. Since ionophores have a narrow range of safety, feed mixing errors facilitate poisoning. In horses, this leads to cardiac muscle damage; in cattle, this leads to both skeletal and cardiac muscle damage.

The cardiac signature of the poisoning in horses manifests itself by prolongation of atrial and ventricular depolarization and repolarization (Hall, 2006). Also, depression of the ST segment, absence of the P-wave, ventricular tachycardia, AV-block and atrial fibrillation are noted. Cardiac lesions and heart failure occur. In cattle, QT and QRS prolongation, first degree heart block, and T-wave amplitude increases are typical. Cardiac lesions and heart failure are also possible. Analogous effects have been noted in sheep. The LD_{50} of monensin is 2–3 mg/kg b.w. in horses; 20–34 mg/kg b.w. in cattle, and 10–12 mg/kg b.w in sheep (Doonan et al., 1989).

Beside the growth-promoting function of ionophores in ruminants, it is used as a coccidiostat in poultry. Cardiac effects of infested poultry include reduced lipid levels, reduced heart weight, low heart rates, and low blood pressure. Monensin has a narrow therapeutic window, and intoxication causes muscle necrosis and myoglobinuria. Targets include cardiac muscles. It causes inotropism, tachycardia, cardiomyopathy, and cardiac failure. Horses are especially vulnerable. There is no antidote available for monensin poisoning.

FERTILIZERS

Accidental ingestion of fertilizer can cause serious poisoning in the affected animals (Villar et al., 2003). Predominantly, though not exclusively, nitrates cause the damage. Rabbits exposed to ammonium sulfate fertilizer suffer cardiac arrest (Sato et al., 1999). In another case with fertilizer containing nitrogen, phosphoric acid, and potassium, the rabbits suffered hyperkalemia, hyperammonemia, metabolic acidosis that expressed itself on the cardiac system as ventricular tachycardia translating into ventricular fibrillation and death, though on post mortem no alterations were noted in the histopathological examination of the heart. There is no specific antidote for fertilizer poisoning.

HERBICIDES

There are a large number of herbicides (Gupta, 2012), characterized by differing chemical constituents, causing various effects on the heart. The ingestion of plants treated with herbicide can induce electrolyte abnormalities and lower blood pressure.

Paraquat is a widely used herbicide meant for killing green plants on contact although its use is restricted in the United States. Paraquat accumulates in the lungs and generates ROS (Ge et al., 2010). In rats, e.g., paraquat causes severe heart damage as seen on an ECG (Noguchi et al., 1990) including hemorrhage in the myocardium. Paraquat also elicits sinus tachycardia but no arrhythmia.

The oral LD_{50} in monkeys is 50 mg/kg b.w., and 48 mg/kg b.w. in cats. Dermal LD_{50} is 236–325 mg/kg b.w. in rabbits. An effective antidote is not available but activated charcoal, for oral ingestion, has been used.

INSECTICIDES AND OTHER PESTICIDES

Organophosphates and Carbamates

While insecticides are specifically formulated against insects, pesticides in addition work on plants, weeds and fungi. Animals by contact or ingestion may develop dangerous cardiac symptoms.

Pesticides used in agriculture and around the house contain organophosphates (OP) or carbamates. OP and carbamates differ, though their effects are similar. Their mode of action is similar, as they bind to an active site serine of AChE and inhibit its functionality, thus reducing the availability of AChE so that overstimulation of cholinergic system occurs. The inhibitory effect of carbamates on AChE is shorter than that of OPs. The function of AChE is to hydrolyze acetylcholine (ACh) to choline and acetic acid. Inhibition of AChE results in excessive ACh accumulation in synapses and at neuromuscular junctions, leading to muscarinic and nicotinic ACh receptor–associated hyper cholinergic signs. Carbamates do not age AChE, while some OPs do. Aging refers to the fact that OPs irreversibly inactivate AChE, thereby preventing its normal physiological function.

OPs are extremely toxic and cause severe electrophysiological abnormalities. Acute toxicity of OPs widely vary in different species, e.g., chlorpyrifos has an LD_{50} of 32 mg/kg b.w. in chickens, 500 mg/kg b.w. in guinea pigs, and 800 mg/kg b.w. in sheep. Similarly, among carbamates, methomyl has an LD_{50} of 17 mg/kg b.w. for dogs and 17–24 mg/kg b.w. for rats.

Animals are exposed to OPs in a large number of ways. For control of cattle grubs (*Hypoderma lineatum*), the cattle are sprayed with OPs and poisoning may occur (Khan et al., 1961; Khan, 2001). Feedstock treated with terbufos has also led to poisoning with cardiac signs in cattle. Animals that are kept indoors, e.g., marmosets, are also liable for poisoning (Brack and Rothe, 1982).

Classic signs of OP poisoning include prolonged QT interval (Abraham et al., 2001), ST–T changes, sinus tachycardia or bradycardia, and hypertension or hypotension (Saadeh et al., 1997; Karki et al., 2004).

Antidotes for OP poisoning are anticholinergics that are antagonistic to anticholinesterase activity at muscarinic receptors. Atropine, which is widely used as a muscarinic antagonist, does not bind to nicotinic receptors. Also, oximes are available to counter inhibition of AChE (Boelsterli, 2007; Kose et al., 2009).

Amitraz

Amitraz is a triazapentadiene compound used in flea collars of dogs, and is a member of the amidine chemical family. As an insecticide and acaricide, it exerts toxicity by inhibiting the activity of the enzyme monoamine oxidase and works as an alpha2-adrenergic receptor agonist. The cardiac effects of alpha2-adrenergic agonists include bradycardia, first- and second-degree AV blockage, and diminished cardiac output (Malmasi and Ghaffari, 2010). ECGs performed on an English bulldog poisoned with amitraz showed QT elongation, a precursor to ventricular arrhythmia. Amitraz apparently lengthened the QT interval by reduction of the heart rate. Thermogenesis was also affected. Hypothermia decreased the depolarization of the pacemaker cells, so that bradycardia ensued (Aslan et al., 2007). The EPA classifies it as Class III, which is slightly toxic. The oral LD_{50} of amitraz in rats is 523–800 mg/kg b.w., >1600 mg/kg for mice, and 788 mg/kg b.w., for bobwhite quail.

Metaldehyde

The molluscicide metaldehyde, used to kill slugs and snails and for the protection of crops, comes in the form of sprays and pellets. It is toxic when inhaled or ingested. Upon ingestion, mataldehyde is partially hydrolyzed by the acids in the stomach to acetaldehyde, which decreases serotonin in the brain, noradrenaline, and γ-aminobutyric acid (inhibitory neurotransmitter of the CNS). Severe muscle tremors ensue. The LD_{50} in rats is 227–690 mg/kg b.w., in rabbits 290–1250 mg/kg, and in cats 100–300 mg/kg. Cardiac symptoms (Longstreth and Pierson, 1982) include increased heart rate, increased blood pressure, and tachycardia. Autopsies on dogs revealed hemorrhage of the heart (Hayes and Laws, 1990). There is no antidote to metaldehyde poisoning. Symptomatic therapy includes gastric lavage with sodium bicarbonate and medication to control seizures.

MYCOTOXINS

Of the several thousand species of mushrooms (*Basidiomycete* fungi), less than 100 are toxic. Often mixed into feed, or ingested by pets, the toxic principle is primarily the presence of amatoxins (bicyclic octapeptides) (Berger and Guss, 2005). Amatoxin inactivates RNA polymerase II in cell nuclei and DNA transcription, thus preventing protein synthesis, curtailing cell metabolism (Duffy, 2008; Chang, 2009).

Amatoxin signature on cardiac tissue shows small hemorrhage, cloudy swelling, and degeneration. Elevation of cardiac enzymes (Unverir et al., 2007), including CK-MB isoenzyme and myoglobin, is noted. The LD_{50} is 0.1–0.3 mg/kg b.w. for most mammals. A difference in intraperitoneal and intravenous injection values is noteworthy. Also, α-amanitin LD_{50} is 0.1 mg/kg b.w. for rats, while amanullin, also an amatoxin, has an LD_{50} in mice of 20 mg/kg b.w. and is nontoxic to humans. Low calcium and phosphate levels as well as varying levels of the hormones that control their metabolism have been noted. Heart block and bradycardia have been observed. Also, sinus tachycardia and hypotension are typical cardiac clinical symptoms.

In dogs, electrolyte abnormalities and bradyarrhythmia (SA exit block and sinus arrest) symptoms reminiscent of muscarinic intoxication were noted and relieved by atropine (Lee et al., 2009). Treatment aims at minimizing amatoxin absorption, administering activated charcoal, and hydration maintenance.

ANCILLARY CAUSES OF CARDIAC TOXICITY

Anthropods

Envenomenation by arthropods (scorpions and spiders) is a serious health concern to humans and animals in many countries (Murthy et al., 1999). In dogs and rabbits, 3.5 mg/kg b.w. of scorpion venom causes an increase in LDH and CK-MB enzyme levels. ECG changes in T waves (biphasic) and ST-segment and alternans indicate myocardial damage, ancillary arrhythmias, conduction defects, and infarction-like patterns (Gueron et al., 1992; Bentur et al., 2003). Scorpion toxin includes potassium channel–blocking peptides (Kumar et al., 2011). The venom of the deathstalker scorpion (*Leiurus quinquestriatus*) includes chlorotoxin, which blocks small conductance chloride channels.

Treatment for scorpion sting is symptomatic. Hypertensive symptoms are treated with vasodilators. Scorpion antivenoms are available. Insulin administration controls effects caused by catecholamines upon scorpion envenomation.

HYMENOPTERA

Members of the order *hymenoptera* include apoidea (bees), vespoidea (wasps, hornets, and yellow jackets), and formicidae (ants). Their injected venom is poisonous. A lethal dose is approximately 20 stings/kg in most mammals (Fitzgerald and Flood, 2006). The severity of the stings is increased by anaphylactic reactions.

Stings can cause myocardial infarction and myocarditis. Increases in serum enzyme levels and necrosis in the myocardium have been reported (Levine, 1976; Ferreira et al., 1995). Mast cells in cardiac tissue may be affected by their mediators that have cardiotoxic effects, including arrythmogenesis. Wasp stings can cause Mobitz Type I heart block and myocardial infarction (Wagdi et al., 1994). ECG changes, myocardial necrosis, and arrest of cardiac beats were noted after envenomation by Africanized honeybee venom in Wistar rats. A honeybee sting can produce significant elevations of the ST-segment, CK-MB activity, and troponin I and T levels.

Treatment includes antihistamines, steroids, bronchodilators, and alpha- and beta-receptor agonists.

OPHIDIAN

The 600 known venomous snakes belong to the following four families: *Atractaspideae*, *Colubrideae*, *Elapideae,* and *Viperideae*. The *Crotalideae* is a subfamily of *Viperideae* and includes pit vipers, the moccasins, and rattlesnakes, while coral snakes belong to the *Elapideae*.

Snake venom contains biologically active ingredients with cytotoxic, neurotoxic, and coagulant effects. From the cardiac system point of view, the phosphodiestrases that lower blood pressure and phospholipase A2 that causes hemolysis are most significant.

Subcutaneous LD_{50} of cottonmouth (*Agkistrodon piscivorus*) venom is 25.8 mg/kg b.w., for *Vipera berus* the LD_{50} is 6.45 mg/kg, and for *Vipera latifii* is 4.61 mg/kg b.w.

Disruption of the normal blood clotting pathways is significant. Some prevent clot formation and induce hemorrhagic shock. Other toxins induce clotting, causing stroke and heart attacks by blocking blood flow.

Cardiotoxins bind to muscle cells causing depolarization and prevention of muscle contraction, thus interfering with the rhythmicity of the heart. Snake bites usually are noted in dogs bitten on the head or neck. In one particular study, cardiac variables were normal on auscultation postenvenomation. Twenty-four hours later, 11% had cardiac abnormalities. Muscle damage as evidenced by elevated CK values in serum biochemistry was noted in 54% of sampled dogs (Segev et al., 2008; Lervik et al., 2010). The myocardial injury was verified by ECG performed postenvenomation. Myocardial damage postenvenomation was also shown by the increase of cardiac-specific troponin I.

Polyvalent antivenoms are available for the treatment of most pit viper bites. Coral snake bites require neurotoxic antivenom.

CANTHARIDIN

Blister beetles prefer alfalfa fields where large swarms tend to congregate. When these fields are harvested, the blister beetles are crushed and incorporated into the bales of hay. They contain a poisonous substance known as cantharidin. It is an inhibitor of the serine–threonine protein phosphatase. Cantharidin blocks the adenosine A_1 receptors, regulates myocardial oxygen consumption, yielding antiadrenergic effects in ventricular cardiac myocytes (Narayan et al., 2000). Cantharidin can exert a positive inotropic effect in cardiac muscle by increasing calcium influx (Neumann et al., 1995).

In equids, the LD_{50} of cantharidin is reported to be 1 mg/kg b.w. (Guglick et al., 1996). A dose of 4 g of dried beetles is lethal to a horse and 1–1.5 mg/kg b.w. for cats and dogs. The cardiac symptoms of cantharidin poisoning include increased heart rate and myocardial dysfunction. There is no antidote for cantharidin, but symptomatic treatment is recommended with administration of fluids and maintenance of serum electrolytes.

CONCLUDING REMARKS AND FUTURE DIRECTIONS

Cardiac problems in domestic animals are primarily due to toxic plants, chemicals, and envenomation, most of which can be avoided. Genetics plays a secondary role to environmental factors (Detweiler, 1964). There is only a limited amount of published research on cases involving inadvertently affected animals. Animal cardiac responses have been extensively studied in the development of drugs. A considerable amount of work still needs to be done on cardiotoxicity in animals caused by plants, chemicals, and envenomation.

REFERENCES

Abraham, S., Oz, N., Sahar, R., Kadar, T., 2001. QTc prolongation and cardiac lesions following acute organophosphate poisoning in rats. Proc. West Pharmacol. Soc. 44, 185–186.

Akera, T., Ku, D.D., Frank, M., Brody, T.M., Iwasa, J., 1976. Effects of grayanotoxin I on cardiac Na^+ K^+ -adenosine triphosphatase activity, transmembrane potential and myocardial contractile force. J. Pharmacol. Exp. Ther. 199, 247–254.

Allison, C.D., Baker, R.D., 2007. Prussic Acid Poisoning in Livestock. Guide B-808, New Mexico State University, College of Agriculture and Home Economics, Las Cruces, NM.

Aniszewski, T., 2007. Alkaloids - Secrets of Life. Elsevier, New York.

Aslan, S., Erdem, A.F., Uzkeser, M., Cakir, Z., Cakir, M., Akoz, A., 2007. The Osborn wave in accidental hypothermia. J. Emerg. Med. 32, 271–273.

Aslani, M.R., Movassaghi, A.R., Mohri, M., Abbasian, A., Zarehpour, M., 2004. Clinical and pathological aspects of experimental oleander (*Nerium oleander*) toxicosis in sheep. Vet. Res. Commun. 28, 609–616.

Barbosa, R.R., Fontenele-Neto, J.D., Soto-Blanco, B., 2008. Toxicity in goats caused by oleander (*Nerium oleander*). Res. Vet. Sci. 85, 279–281.

Barceloux, D.G., 2008. Medical Toxicology of Natural Substances: Food, Fungi, Medicinal Herbs, Plants and Venomous Animals. Wiley, Hoboken, NJ.

Beasley, V., 1999. Other Plants that Affect the Heart. <http://www.ivis.org/advances/Beasley/Cpt14e/chapter_frm.asp?LA=1> (accessed 26.01.11.).

Bentur, Y., Taitelman, U., Aloufy, A., 2003. Evaluation of scorpion stings: the poison center perspective. Vet. Hum. Toxicol. 45, 108–111.

Berger, K., Guss, D., 2005. Mycotoxins revisited: part I. J. Emerg. Med. 28, 53–62.

Boelsterli, U.A., 2007. Mechanistic Toxicology: The Molecular Basis of How Chemicals Disrupt Biological Targets. CRC Press, Boca Raton, FL.

Botha, C., 2013. Cardiac glycoside intoxication. <http://www.afrivip.org/sites/default/files/cardiac_glycoside_intoxication_complete_2.pdf>.

Brack, M., Rothe, H., 1982. Organophosphate poisoning in marmosets. Lab Anim. 16, 186–188.

Burrows, G.E., Tyrl, R.J., 2006. Handbook of Toxic Plants of North America. Blackwell Pub, Ames, IA.

Chan, T., 2009. Aconite poisoning. Clin. Toxicol. (Phila). 47, 279–285.

Chang, C., 2009. Amatoxin Toxicity in Emergency Medicine. <http://emedicine.medscape.conv/article/820108-overview> (accessed 25.02.11.).

Cheeke, P.R., 1989. Toxicants of Plant Origin. CRC Press, Boca Raton, FL.

Cheeke, P.R., 1995. Endogenous toxins and mycotoxins in forage grasses and their effect on livestock. J. Anim. Sci. 73, 909–918.

Clark, J.G., 1979. Whorled milkweed poisoning. Vet. Hum. Toxicol. 21, 431.

Coltart, D.J., Hudson, R.E.B., 1971. Primary oxalosis of the heart: a cause of heart block. Br. Heart J. 33, 315–319.

Detweiler, D.K., 1964. Genetic aspects of cardiovascular diseases in animals. Circulation. 30, 114–127.

Doonan, G.R., Brown, C.M., Mullaney, T.P., Brooks, D.B., Ulmanis, E. G., Slanker, M.R., 1989. Monensin poisoning in horses - an international incident. Can. Vet. J. 30, 165–169.

Doyle, L.P., Walkey, F.L., 1949. *White Snakeroot (*Eupatorium urticaefolium*) Poisoning in Livestock.* Bulletin 270, Purdue University, Agricultural Experimental Station, West Lafayette, IN.

Duffy, T.J., 2008. Toxic fungi of western North America. <http://www.scribd.com/doc/45091262/Toxic-Fungi-of-Western-NA> (accessed 23.02.11.).

Eddleston, M., Ariaratnam, C.A., Sjostrom, L., Jayalath, S., Rajakanthan, K., Rajapakse, S., et al., 2000. Acute yellow oleander (*Thevetia peruviana*) poisoning: cardiac arrhythmias, electrolyte disturbances, and serum cardiac glycoside concentrations on presentation to hospital. Heart. 83, 301–306.

EFSA, 2005. Opinion of the scientific panel on contaminants in the food chain on a request from the commission related to arsenic as undesirable substance in animal feed. EFSA J. 180, 1–35.

el Bahri, L., Ben Romdane, S., 1991. Arsenic poisoning in livestock. Vet. Hum. Toxicol. 33, 259–264.

FDA, 2008. FDA Poisonous Plant Database. <http://www.accessdata.fda.gov/scripts/plantox/index.cfm> (accessed 11.02.11.).

Fenton, J.J., 2002. Toxicology: A Case-Oriented Approach. CRC Press LLC, Boca Raton, FL.

Ferreira, D.B., Costa, R.S., De Oliveira, J.A., Muccillo, G., 1995. An infarct-like myocardial lesion experimentally induced in Wistar rats with Africanized bee venom. J. Pathol. 177, 95–102.

Fitzgerald, K.T., 2010. Lily toxicity in the cat. Top. Compan. Anim. Med. 25, 213–217.

Fitzgerald, K.T., Flood, A.A., 2006. Hymenoptera stings. Clin. Tech. Small Anim. Pract. 21, 194–204.

Frohne, D., Pfander, H., 2005. Poisonous Plants: A Handbook for Doctors, Pharmacists, Toxicologists, Biologists and Veterinarians. Timber Press, Inc., Portland, OR.

Ge, W., Zhang, Y., Han, X., Ren, J., 2010. Cardiac-specific overexpression of catalase attenuates paraquat-induced myocardial geometric and contractile alteration: role of ER stress. Free Radic. Biol. Med. 49, 2068–2077.

Grant, R., Basson, P., Booker, H., Hofherr, J., Anthonissen, M., 1991. Cardiomyopathy caused by avocado (*Persea americana Mill)* leaves. J. S. Afr. Vet. Assoc. 62, 21–22.

Green, B.T., Pfister, J.A., Cook, D., Welch, K.D., Stegelmeier, B.L., Lee, S.T., et al., 2009. Effects of larkspur (*Delphinium barbeyi*) on heart rate and electrically evoked electromyographic response of the external anal sphincter in cattle. Am. J. Vet. Res. 70, 539–546.

Green, B.T., Welch, K.D., Gardner, D.R., Stegelmeier, B.L., Davis, T.Z., Cook, D., et al., 2009. Serum elimination profiles of methyllycaconitine and deltaline in cattle following oral administration of larkspur (*Delphinium barbeyi*). Am. J. Vet. Res. 70, 926–931.

Gueron, M., Ilia, R., Sofer, S., 1992. The cardiovascular system after scorpion envenomation. A review. J. Toxicol. Clin. Toxicol. 30, 245–258.

Guglick, M., MacAllister, C., Panciera, R., 1996. Equine catharidiasis. Compend. Contin. Educ. Pract. Vet. 18, 77–83.

Gupta, P.K., 2012. Toxicity of herbicides. In: Gupta, R.C. (Ed.), Veterinary Toxicology: Basic and Clinical Principles, 2nd edn. Academic Press/Elsevier, Amsterdam, pp. 631–652.

Hall, J.O., 2006. Ionophore poisoning of horses and cattle. <http://www.vin.com/proceedings/Proceedings.plx?CID = WSAVA2002&PID = 12140&Print= 1&0=Generic> (accessed 15.12.10.).

Hay, L., Schultz, R.A., Schutte, P.J., 2008. Cardiotoxic effects of pavetamine extracted from *Pavetta harborii* in the rat. Onderstepoort J. Vet. Res. 75, 249–253.

Hayes, W.J., Laws, E.R. (Eds.), 1990. Handbook of Pesticide Toxicology. Academic Press, Inc, New York.

Hoffman, B.F., Rosen, M.R., Wit, A.L., 1975. Electrophysiology and pharmacology of cardiac arrhythmias. VII. Cardiac effects of quinidine and procaine amide. Amer. Heart J. 89, 804–808.

Holstege, C.P., Forrester, J.D., Borek, H.A., Lawrence, D.T., 2010. A case of cyanide poisoning and the use of arterial blood gas analysis to direct therapy. Hosp. Pract. 38, 69–74.

Jansen, S.A., Kleerekooper, I., Hofman, Z.L.M., Kappen, I.F.P.M., Stary-Weinzinger, A., van der Heyden, M.A., 2012. Grayanatoxin poisoning: 'mad honey disease' and beyond. Cardiovasc. Toxicol. 12, 208–215.

Kang, Y.J., 2001. Molecular and cellular mechanisms of cardiotoxicity. Environ. Health Perspect. 109 (Suppl. 1), 27–34.

Karki, P., Ansari, J.A., Bhandary, S., Koirala, S., 2004. Cardiac and electrocardiographical manifestations of acute organophosphate poisoning. Singapore Med. J. 45, 385–389.

Kellerman, T.S., 2005. Plant Poisonings and Mycotoxicoses of Livestock in Southern Africa. Oxford University Press, Oxford, UK.

Khan, M.A., Kramer, T., Avery, R.J., 1961. Organophosphate poisoning in cattle with particular reference to Co-Ral. Can. Vet. J. 2, 207–211.

Khan, O., 2001. Organophosphate poisoning in a group of replacement heifers and dry cows. Can. Vet. J. 42, 561–563.

Kingsbury, J.M., 1964. Poisonous Plants of the United States and Canada. Prentice-Hall, Englewood Cliffs, NJ.

Knight, A.P., Walter, R.G., 2001. Plants affecting the cardiovascular system. <http://www.ivis.org/special_books/knight/chap2/ivis.pdf> (accessed 26.01.11.).

Kose, A., Gunay, N., Yildirim, C., Tarakcioglu, M., Sari, I., Demiryurek, A.T., 2009. Cardiac damage in acute organophosphate poisoning in rats: effects of atropine and pralidoxime. Am. J. Emerg. Med. 27, 169–175.

Ku, D.D., Akera, T., Frank, M., Brody, T.M., Iwasa, J., 1977. The effects of grayanotoxin I and alpha-dihydrograyanotoxin II on guinea-pig myocardium. J. Pharmacol. Exp. Ther. 200, 363–372.

Kumar, G.S., Upadhyay, S., Mathew, M.K., Sarma, S.P., 2011. Solution structure of BTK-2, a novel $hK_V1.1$ inhibiting scorpion toxin, from the eastern Indian scorpion *Mesobuthus tamulus*. Biochim. Biophys. Acta. 1814, 459–469.

Lee, N.S., Hyun, R.C., Hyun, C., 2009. Mushroom poisoning by *Inocybe fastiglata* in a maltese dog. J. Anim. Vet. Adv. 8, 708–710.

Lervik, J.S., Lilliehook, I., Frendin, J.H.M., 2010. Clinical and biochemical changes in 53 Swedish dogs bitten by the European adder – *Vipera berus*. Acta Vet. Scandin. 52, 26.

Levine, H.D., 1976. Acute myocardial infarction following wasp sting report of two cases and critical survey of the literature. Am. Heart J. 91, 365–374.

Lin, C.C., Yang, C.C., Phua, D.H., Deng, J.F., Lu, L.H., 2010. An outbreak of foxglove poisoning. J. Chinese Med. Assoc. 73, 97–100.

Liu, T., Brown, D.A., O'Rourke, B., 2010. Role of mitochondrial dysfunction in cardiac glycoside toxicity. J. Mol. Cell Card. 49, 728–736.

Longstreth, W.T., Pierson, D.J., 1982. Metaldehyde poisoning from slug bait ingestion. West J. Med. 137, 134–137.

Malmasi, A., Ghaffari, M.S., 2010. Electrocardiographic abnormalities in an English bulldog with amitraz toxicity. Comp. Clin. Pathol. 19, 103–105.

Maratea, K., 2003. FINAL DIAGNOSIS: white snakeroot intoxication in a calf. <http://www.addl.purdue.edu/newsletters/2004/winter/finaldx.asp> (accessed 14.02.11.).

Mookadam, F., Smith, T., Jiamsripong, P., Moustafa, S.E., Monico, C. G., Lieske, J.C., et al., 2010. Cardiac abnormalities in primary hyperoxaluria. Circ. J. 74, 2403–2409.

Mordukhovich, I., Wright, R.O., Amarasiriwardena, C., Baja, E., Baccarelli, A., Suh, H., et al., 2009. Association between low-level environmental arsenic exposure and QT interval duration in a general population study. Am. J. Epidemiol. 170, 739–746.

Murthy, K.R., Zare, M.A., Haghnazari, L., 1999. The use of serotherapy to reverse ECG and cardiac enzyme changes caused by scorpion *Mesobuthus tamulus concanesis,* Pocock envenoming. J. Venom. Anim. Toxins. 5, 154–171.

Narayan, P., Mentzer, R.M., Lasley, R.D., 2000. Phosphatase inhibitor cantharidin blocks adenosine A(1) receptor anti-adrenergic effect in rat cardiac myocytes. Am. J. Physiol. Heart Circ. Physiol. 278, H1–7.

Neumann, J., Herzig, S., Boknik, P., Apel, G., Kaspareit, G., Schmitz, W., et al., 1995. On the cardiac contractile, biochemical and electrophysiological effects of cantharidin, a phosphate inhibitor. J. Pharmacol. Exp. Ther. 274, 530–539.

Noguchi, N., Tanaka, E., Yamamoto, H., Misawa, S., 1990. Initial accumulation of paraquat in the heart leading to acute death. Nihon Hoigaku Zasshi. 44, 6–11.

Oelrichs, P.B., Ng, J.C., Seawright, A.A., Ward, A., Schaffeler, L., MacLeod, J.K., 1995. Isolation and identification of a compound from avocado (*Persea americana*) leaves which causes necrosis of the acinar epithelium of the lactating mammary gland and the myocardium. Nat. Toxins. 3, 344–349.

Panter, K.E., Gardner, D.R., Lee, J.A., Ralphs, M.H., Stegelmeier, B.L., James, L.F., 2007. Important poisonous plants of the United States. In: Gupta, R.C. (Ed.), Veterinary Toxicology Basic and Clinical Principles. Elsevier, New York, pp. 825–872.

Panter, K.E., Keeler, R.F., Baker, D.C., 1988. Toxicoses in livestock from the hemlocks (Conium and Cicuta spp.). J. Anim. Sci. 66, 2407–2413.

Panter, K.E., Manners, G.D., Stegelmeier, B.L., Lee, S., Gardner, D.R., Ralphs, M.H., et al., 2002. Larkspur poisoning: toxicology and alkaloid structure-activity relationships. Biochem. Syst. Ecol. 30, 113–128.

Pfister, J.A., Gardner, D.R., Panter, K.E., Manners, G.D., Ralphs, M.H., Stegelmeier, B.L., et al., 1999. Larkspur (*Delphinium spp.*) poisoning in livestock. J. Nat. Toxins. 8, 81–94.

Prozesky, L., 2008. A study of the pathology and pathogenesis of myocardial lesions in gousiekte, a cardiotoxicosis of ruminants. PhD thesis, University of Pretoria, Pretoria, South Africa.

Rajapakse, S., 2009. Management of yellow oleander poisoning. Clin. Toxicol. (Phila). 47, 206–212.

Ramachandran, M.S., 2014. The Heart and Toxins. Academic Press, London, GB.

Saadeh, A.M., Farsakh, N.A., Al-Ali, M.K., 1997. Cardiac manifestations of acute carbamate and organophosphate poisoning. Heart. 77, 461–464.

Sato, A., Gonmori, K., Yoshioka, N., 1999. An experimental examination of the acute toxicity of chemical fertilizers. Jap. J. Toxicol. 12, 415–421.

Schep, L.J., Schmierer, D.M., Fountain, J.S., 2006. Veratrum poisoning. Toxicol. Rev. 25, 73–78.

Schep, L.J., Slaughter, R.J., Becket, G., Beasley, D.M., 2009. Poisoning due to water hemlock. Clin. Toxicol. (Phila). 47, 270–278.

Segev, G., Ohad, D.G., Shipov, A., Kass, P.H., Aroch, I., 2008. Cardiac arrhythmias and serum cardiac troponins in Vipera palaestinae envenomation in dogs. J. Vet. Intern. Med. 22, 106–113.

Selby, L.A., Case, A.A., Osweiler, G.D., Hayes, H.M., 1977. Epidemiology and toxicology of arsenic poisoning in domestic animals. Env. Health Persp. 19, 183–189.

Sharma, U.R., Surendra, V., Jha, S.K., Nitesh, S.C., Prakash, T., Goli, D., 2009. Evaluation of anti-inflammatory activity of *Rhododendron Arboreum* herb extract on experimental animal. Arch. Pharm. Sci. Res. 1, 58–61.

Smith, G., 2012. *Kalanchoe* species poisoning in pets. <http://aspcapro.org/sites/pro/files/v-vetm1104-933_936-0.pdf>

Speijers, G., 2003. *Cyanogenic glycosides.* <http://www.inchem.org/documents/jecfa/jecmono/v30je18.htm> (accessed 15.02.11.).

Stevens, M., 2000. Common Milkweed. <http://plants.usda.gov/plantguide/pdf/cs_assy.pdf> (accessed 31.01.11.).

Thomas, D.L., Quick, M.P., Morgan, R.P., 1987. Suspected foxglove (*Digitalis purpurea*) poisoning in a dairy cow. Vet. Rec. 120, 300–301.

Tiwary, A.K., Puschner, B., Kinde, H., Tor, E.R., 2005. Diagnosis of *Taxus* (yew) poisoning in a horse. J. Vet. Diagn. Invest. 17, 252–255.

Turner, J.L., Ashcroft, N., Moore, S., 2012. Locoweed poisoning of horses. <http://aces.nmsu.edu/pubs/_b/B713/welcome.html>

Unverir, P., Soner, B.C., Dedeoglu, E., Karcioglu, O., Boztok, K., Tuncok, Y., 2007. Renal and hepatic injury with elevated cardiac enzymes in Amanita phalloides poisoning: a case report. Hum. Exp. Toxicol. 26, 757–761.

van der Walt, J.J., van Rooyen, J.M., 1977. Use of technetium-99 to determine haemodynamic changes during the development of ventricular failure with gousiekte. SA Med. J. 52, 375.

Veltmann, C., Borggrefe, M., Schimpf, R., Wolpert, C., 2009. Images in cardiovascular medicine. Yew causes Brugada ECG. Circulation. 119, 1836–1837.

Vetter, J., 2000. Plant cyanogenic glycosides. Toxicon. 38, 11–36.

Villar, D., Schwartz, K.J., Carson, T.L., Kinker, J.A., Barker, J., 2003. Acute poisoning of cattle by fertilizer-contaminated water. Vet. Hum. Toxicol. 45, 88–90.

VonBurg, R., 1994. Oxalic acid and sodium oxalate. J. App. Tox. 14, 233–237.

Wagdi, P., Mehan, V.K., Burgi, H., Salzmann, C., 1994. Acute myocardial infarction after wasp stings in a patient with normal coronary arteries. Am. Heart. J. 128, 820–823.

Welch, K.D., Panter, K.E., Gardner, D.R., Green, B.T., Pfister, J.A., Cook, D., et al., 2008. The effect of 7,8-methylenedioxylycoctonine-type diterpenoid alkaloids on the toxicity of methyllycaconitine in mice. J. Anim. Sci. 86, 2761–2770.

Wilson, C.R., Sauer, J., Hooser, S.B., 2001. Taxines: a review of the mechanism and toxicity of yew (*Taxus spp.*) alkaloids. Toxicon. 39, 175–185.

Yong, C., Brandow, R.A., Howlett, P., 1990. Brandow, R.A., Howlett, P., An unusual cause of nitrate poisoning in cattle. Can. Vet. J. 31, 118.

Chapter 15

Liver Toxicity

Karyn Bischoff, Motoko Mukai and Shashi K. Ramaiah

INTRODUCTION

The liver is a remarkable organ that usually protects the individual against injury from xenobiotic compounds. However, this organ is often the site of metabolism and it is where some chemicals concentrate and become bioactivated, leading to hepatic injury. Although its capacity for repair and regeneration (Ramaiah et al., 2004; Mehendale, 2005) makes it a quite robust organ, if the ability to regenerate is not adequate, or if injury to the liver is very severe, liver damage can progress to liver failure and death.

There is continued interest concerning the higher incidence of liver damage caused by prescription/injectable drugs, over-the-counter medications, dietary supplements, and special diets, in addition to environmental chemicals/xenobiotics (Watkins, 1999). Though alcohol consumption is not a major risk factor in most veterinary patients, other factors such as toxic pasture or house plants, cyanobacterial toxins, pollutants, pesticides, fungal toxins, and toxicants in household waste can cause hepatic injury. An incomplete list of hepatotoxins is found in Table 15.1. Complicating matters is the increasing population of geriatric veterinary patients. Preexisting liver disease must be considered in patients exposed to liver toxicants.

In humans, drug-induced liver injury (DILI) has become the most frequent cause of acute liver failure in the United States and around the world, exceeding all other causes combined. Although the incidence of idiosyncratic DILI with approved drugs at therapeutic doses is relatively low and estimated at 1−10 per 100,000 treated patients, the outcome is potentially a very grave one. Approximately 10% of those human patients will die or require liver transplantation, making idiosyncratic DILI the leading causes for urgent liver transplantation (Stirnimann et al., 2010). Toxic liver disease also remains the single major cause for regulatory actions concerning drugs. Such actions may include failure of approval, withdrawal from the market, restrictions on use and warnings to physicians.

Liver injury by xenobiotics is encountered in a variety of circumstances. Some natural toxins such as the cyclic peptides of *Amanita phalloides*, pyrrolizidine alkaloids, cycasin from cycad palms and other phytotoxins are examples of environmental hazards. They may be ingested by the curious or very hungry veterinary patient. Others, such as mycotoxins, are ingested unknowingly because of feed contamination due to climatic conditions favorable to fungal growth. A striking example of this phenomenon was the aflatoxin contamination of dog food, which resulted in dozens of canine deaths in late 2005 and early 2006 (Stenske et al., 2006; Newman et al., 2007; Dereszynski et al., 2008). Other circumstances of exposure to hepatotoxins in the home or farm have included accidental food or feed contamination with industrial chemicals or pesticides. For example, in 1955, a human outbreak of hepatic porphyria in Turkey was caused by ingestion of wheat to which hexachlorobenzene, a fungistatic agent, had been added (Can and Nigogosyan, 1963).

The goal of this chapter is to provide a basic understanding of the liver physiology and pathophysiology, and to expand on the common toxicosis inducing liver injury in veterinary medicine.

STRUCTURAL AND FUNCTIONAL ORGANIZATION OF THE LIVER

Lobule and Acinus

The structural and functional organization of the liver has been described by two concepts: the hepatic lobule and hepatic acinus models. The hepatic lobule, the classic model, is defined histologically as a hexagonal region of parenchyma surrounding the central vein. Six portal triads, composed of branches from the portal vein, hepatic artery and bile ductules, border the edge of the lobule. One-cell thick plates or cords of hepatocytes are arranged radially around the central vein, forming the blood sinusoids between them. The hepatic

Veterinary Toxicology. DOI: http://dx.doi.org/10.1016/B978-0-12-811410-0.00015-5

TABLE 15.1 Incomplete List of Hepatotoxins of Veterinary Interest

Classification of Mechanism	Toxicant	Source of Toxicant	Source Classification	Species Affected
Free radical	Carbon tetrachloride	Cleaning agents	Industrial	All
	Yellow phosphorus	Fireworks	Industrial	All
	Iron	Dietary supplement	Household	All
	Copper	Dietary supplement	Feed, industrial	Sheep, some dog breeds
Electrophile	Aflatoxins	*Aspergillus* spp.	Mycotoxin	All
	Acetaminophen	NSAID	Household	All, cats
	Phenazopyridine	Analgesic	Household	Dogs
	Sesquiterpene lactones	*Helenium* spp., *Hymenoxis* spp.	Plant	Herbivores
	Pyrrolizidine alkaloids	*Amsinkia* spp.	Plant	Herbivores
		Crotolaria spp.		
		Cynoglossum spp.		
		Echium spp.		
		Erechtites glomerulata		
		Senecio spp.		
Biliary obstruction	Sporodesmin	*Pithomyces chartarum*	Mycotoxin	Herbivores, ruminants
	Sapogenins	*Tribulus terrestris*	Plant	Herbivores, ruminants
		Panicum spp.	Plant	Herbivores, ruminants
		Agave lecegilla	Plant	Herbivores, ruminants
		Nolina texana	Plant	Herbivores, ruminants
Other	Glycosides of methylazocymethanol	*Cycas* spp.	Plant	Dogs
	Xylitol	Sugar substitute	Food, household	Dogs
	Carboxyatractyloside	*Xanthium* spp.	Plant	Swine, herbivores
	Triterpenes	*Lantana* spp.	Plant	Herbivores
	Amatoxins	*Amanita* spp.	Mushroom	All
	Microcystins	*Microcystis* spp.	Cyanobacteria	All
	Nodularins	*Nodularia* spp.	Cyanobacteria	All
	Phenolics and coal tar derivatives	Disinfectants, clay pigeons	Household	All
	Unknown	Joint supplements	Drug	Dogs
Idiosyncratic	Sulfonamides	Antimicrobial	Drug	Dogs
	Carprofen	Antiinflammatory	Drug	Dogs
	Diazepam	Sedative	Drug	Cats
	Lomustine	Chemotherapeutic	Drug	Dogs
	Zonisamide	Anticonvulsant	Drug	Dogs
	Mitotane			
	Methimizole	Antithyroid	Drug	Cats
	Carbamizole	Antithyroid	Drug	Cats

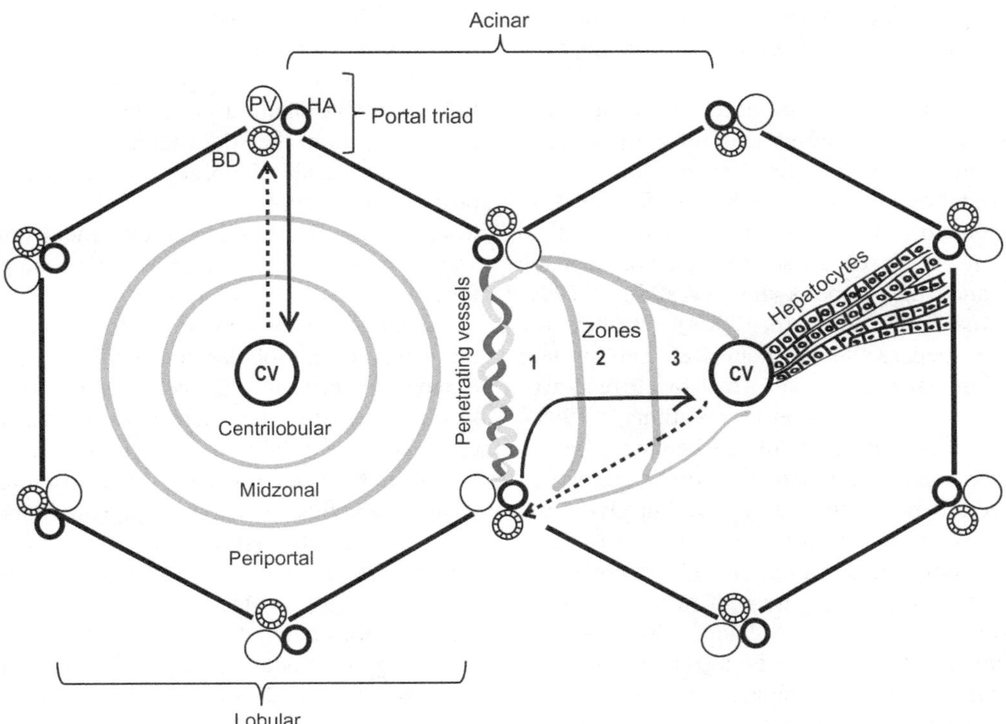

FIGURE 15.1 Lobular versus acinar concept in liver architecture. The hepatic lobule is defined histologically as a hexagonal region of parenchyma surrounding the central hepatic vein. The hepatic acinus is a functional unit based on the microcirculation of the liver, and is preferred as a concept of a functional hepatic unit. The hepatic parenchyma is divided into three sections based on proximity to the central vein in the case of lobular model (centrilobular, midzonal, periportal), and according to the sequence of the blood flow in the case of acinar model (zones 1–3). Blood flows towards the central vein (solid line) and bile blow towards to bile duct (dotted line). *CV*, hepatic central vein; *BD*, bile duct; *HA*, hepatic artery; *PV*, portal vein.

parenchyma is divided into three zones based on proximity to the central vein (Fig. 15.1, left). The area adjacent to the central vein is termed *centrilobular*, the area adjacent to the portal triad is *periportal*, and between the centrilobular and periportal parenchyma is the *midzonal* area.

The hepatic acinus, on the other hand, was defined by Rappaport as the smallest structural and functional unit in the liver based on the microcirculation, and is preferred as a concept of a functional hepatic unit (Fig. 15.1, right). The blood in the liver flows from the portal vein and hepatic artery of the portal triad, is mixed in the penetrating vessels, enters the sinusoids, and eventually exits via central hepatic vein. The cells of the acinus are arbitrarily divided into three zones according to the sequence of the blood flow: zone 1 corresponds to the periportal zone, zone 2 corresponds to the midzonal area, and zone 3 corresponds to the centrilobular zone.

Diverse Function of the Liver

The liver is a functionally diverse organ. The liver is directly involved in (1) nutrient homeostasis, including glucose regulation, cholesterol synthesis and uptake (Treinen-Moslen, 2001), storage of glycogen, lipids, minerals and vitamins (Treinen-Moslen, 2001; Pineiro-Carrero and Pineiro, 2004; Plumlee, 2004; Thawley, 2016), (2) synthesis of clotting factors, albumin, very low density lipoprotein and other proteins (Treinen-Moslen, 2001; Plumlee, 2004; Thawley, 2016) and (3) metabolism and excretion of such things as hemoglobin breakdown products, steroid hormones, and xenobiotics (Brown, 2001; Plumlee, 2004).

Blood from the gastrointestinal tract (GIT), via the portal vein, is filtered for bacterial products, such as endotoxin and ammonia, and xenobiotics (Treinen-Moslen, 2001; Plumlee, 2004). Energy-dependent transport exists for certain xenobiotics and endogenous hormones. These include a group of multiple drug resistance *p*-glycoproteins that transport lipophilic cationic drugs, estrogens and phospholipids, as well as the canalicular multiple organic anion transporters involved in movement of molecules conjugated to glutathione (GSH), glucuronide and sulfate. Metal and mineral transport functions are important for mineral homeostasis and occur through facilitated diffusion and receptor mediated endocytosis across the sinusoidal membrane. Lysosomes within hepatocytes are involved in storage and export of metals and minerals into canaliculi.

Sinusoids are located between cords of hepatocytes, which are larger than capillaries and lined by specialized endothelium. The endothelial lining is discontinuous, the sinusoidal endothelial cells having fenestrae, to allow movement of fluid and molecules less than 259 kDa into the space of Disse, located between the endothelium and the hepatocytes (Watkins, 1999; Treinen-Moslen, 2001; Plumlee, 2004). Within the space of Disse, hepatocytes contact free and protein bound molecules that may be absorbed by diffusion or aforementioned active transport (Watkins, 1999). Remarkable metabolic diversity of the hepatic zones is needed in order to accommodate the liver's numerous functions. Zone 3 hepatocytes are involved in glycolysis and lipogenesis. Zone 1 hepatocytes are involved in bile salt extraction, fatty acid oxidation, gluconeogenesis and protein synthesis and thus are rich in mitochondria for energy production (Treinen-Moslen, 2001; Pineiro-Carrero and Pineiro, 2004; Plumlee, 2004). Gradients of metabolic enzymes involved in bioactivation and detoxification have been shown along different zones of the acinus (reviewed by Jungermann and Katz, 1989). Zone 3 is particularly rich in phase I metabolic enzymes and zone 1 has the highest concentration of GSH involved in phase II metabolism (Thawley, 2016).

The blood supply of the liver is mainly from the portal vasculature: 60%–80% from branches of the portal vein, which is oxygen depleted but supplies nutrients, xenobiotics, and toxicants from the GIT, and 20%–40% from the hepatic artery, which is oxygenated (Treinen-Moslen, 2001). Oxygen is quickly consumed to meet the high metabolic demands of the parenchymal cells as the blood flows towards the terminal hepatic venule, also known as central vein. As a consequent of this structure, hepatocytes in zone 1 receive blood that is 9%–13% oxygenated but nutrient replete, whereas blood received by zone 3 is only 4%–5% oxygenated and nutrient depleted (Sturgill and Lambert, 1997; Treinen-Moslen, 2001). Therefore zone 3 or the centrilobular zone is susceptible to hypoxia (Thawley, 2016).

Another well-known gradient seen in acinar zonation is that of bile. Bile salts and bilirubin from blood enter hepatocytes via active transporters on the sinusoidal membrane, then are secreted into canalicular lumen via the canalicular membrane (Treinen-Moslen, 2001). Bile canaliculi are dynamic structures formed between hepatocytes by the hepatocyte membranes (Treinen-Moslen, 2001; Plumlee, 2004). Bile flows from hepatocytes into canaliculi, and towards the bile duct within the portal triad of the acinus, from zone 3 to 1, in the opposite direction of the blood flow. Bile salts are efficiently extracted from the blood in zone 1, and there is little uptake by the time blood reaches zone 3.

Bile secretion is a major hepatic function and essential for uptake of lipid nutrients, protection against oxidative insults in the small intestine, and for excretion of endogenous and xenobiotic compounds. Bile is composed of bile salts, bilirubin, GSH, phospholipids, cholesterol, proteins, organic anions, metals and conjugated xenobiotics (Treinen-Moslen, 2001; Pineiro-Carrero and Pineiro, 2004).

Canaliculi enter canals of Hering in the portal triad that leads to interlobular and intrahepatic bile ducts, surrounded by bile duct epithelial cells, which coalesce to form the hepatic bile duct. Most animal species have a gall bladder for bile storage but it is absent in others: horses and related species, rhinoceroses and tapirs, elephants, camelids, porcupines, pigeons, rats, deer, ratites, and many parrots. Gall bladders may or may not be present in giraffes and hippopotamuses (Oldham-Ott and Gilloteaux, 1997). Most carnivores have a gall bladder, the exceptions being dolphins and other cetaceans.

The gall bladder stores and concentrates bile, then empties into the duodenum. When the gall bladder is absent, bile empties directly into the duodenum (Ramaiah, 2007). Bile enhances nutrient uptake in the small intestine, protects enterocytes from oxidation and facilitates excretion of xenobiotics and endogenous waste in the feces (Treinen-Moslen, 2001).

Cell Types of the Liver

Seven intrinsic cell types have been identified in the liver: the parenchymal cells (or hepatocytes), the hepatocytic stem cells (oval cells) and five nonparenchymal cell types. Nonparenchymal cells include bile duct epithelium, sinusoidal endothelium, described above, as well as resident macrophages (Kupffer cells), large granular lymphocytes (pit cells), and lipid storing hepatic stellate cells (HSC or Ito cells). Hepatocytes represent about 60% of the total cell number and 80% of hepatic tissue volume in the rat liver, and the smaller nonparenchymal cells are estimated to constitute about 30% of total cellular population, but only 6%–7% of tissue volume (Dahm and Jones, 1996).

Oval cells, the hepatocytic stem cells, are located in the canals of Hering, where bile canaliculi from the hepatic cords converge with bile ductules of the portal triad. If hepatocyte replication is impaired, the oval cells proliferate and differentiate and eventually become both hepatocytes and biliary epithelial cells (Fausto and Campbell, 2003; Jaeschke, 2008). Experimental blockade of hepatocyte proliferation can potentially lead to continued oval cell proliferation, leading to neoplastic transformation and resulting in hepatocellular tumors.

New hepatocytes from zone 1 progress down hepatic cords to replace the aging zone 3 hepatocytes.

Kupffer cells represent 80% of the fixed macrophages in the body (Treinen-Moslen, 2001). These macrophages are usually located within sinusoids and are closely associated with endothelial cells, though they can migrate to areas of injury (Thawley, 2016). Kupffer cells are phagocytes, ingesting foreign material from the portal circulation (Treinen-Moslen, 2001; Plumlee, 2004; Thawley, 2016), debris from apoptotic or necrotic hepatocytes, and microbes and microbial antigens (Thawley, 2016). Kupffer cells act as antigen presenting cells and secrete various cytokines (Treinen-Moslen, 2001; Plumlee, 2004), and are involved in destruction of metastatic neoplastic cells (Plumlee, 2004). Kupffer cells may store minerals and are involved in the pathogenesis of a variety of liver diseases induced by toxicants such as ethanol (Laskin, 1990; Thurman, 1998).

Pit cells are natural killer cells with antineoplastic functions, are involved in granuloma formation, and reside within sinusoids (Treinen-Moslen, 2001; Plumlee, 2004). Pit cells can proliferate locally when stimulated to attack tumor cells together with Kupffer cells (Wisse et al., 1997).

HSCs or Ito cells are located in space of Disse and store fat and vitamin A (Treinen-Moslen, 2001; Pineiro-Carrero and Pineiro, 2004; Plumlee, 2004). When there is liver injury, HSCs are activated to myofibroblast-like cells (Plumlee, 2004; Maddrey, 2005). Activated stellate cells produce collagen and play a role in hepatic fibrosis (Treinen-Moslen, 2001; Plumlee, 2004).

FACTORS INFLUENCING TOXIC LIVER INJURY

Uptake and Concentration of Xenobiotics

The liver has a dual blood supply as noted above. The hepatic artery brings blood from the systemic circulation and the portal system brings blood directly from the gastrointestinal system. The portal system is involved in the "first pass effect," meaning that nutrients and xenobiotics absorbed by the digestive system are filtered through the liver before entering the systemic circulation (Treinen-Moslen, 2001).

The space of Disse allows close contact between circulating plasma, plasma proteins, and hepatocytes, allowing rapid diffusion of lipophilic compounds across the hepatocyte membrane (Treinen-Moslen, 2001). Some compounds are specifically taken up by sinusoidal transporters, including bile acids, phalloidin from several *Amanita* spp. of mushrooms, and microcystin produced by the cyanobacteria *Microcystis aeruginosa*. Canalicular transporters include multidrug resistance-associated (MDR) proteins. Polymorphisms in these proteins have been associated with increased susceptibility to certain xenobiotics (Shehu et al., 2016). Other xenobiotics can affect the activity of MDR and canalicular transport proteins.

Liver cells can accumulate high concentrations of metals and vitamins, leading to injury. For example, excessive storage of vitamin A in stellate cells produces engorgement, activation, and proliferation of these cells (Treinen-Moslen, 2001). Chronic high vitamin E concentrations produce hepatic fibrosis and portal hypertension in humans, precipitating continued fibrosis (Zimmerman, 1999; Pineiro-Carrero and Pineiro, 2004; Maddrey, 2005). Cadmium is sequestered by hepatic metallothioneins but produces pathology when storage capacity is exceeded.

The liver is also responsible for iron homeostasis. Iron uptake from the sinusoids is receptor mediated and sequestration occurs through binding with iron storage proteins such as ferritin. High hepatic iron concentrations produce lipid peroxidation affecting zone 1 hepatocytes (Treinen-Moslen, 2001). Certain mammals, including Egyptian fruit bats, and some fruit-eating bird species including mynahs, toucans, aracari, and birds of paradise, tend to have hemosiderosis (accumulation of iron in the liver) and are prone to hemochromatosis (disease associated with iron sequestration). Increased expression of iron transporters DMT1 and Ireg1 has been found in mynahs, and likely causes iron accumulation in this particular species (Mete et al., 2005). However, the genetic cause(s) of hemosiderosis have not been completely determined yet.

The liver also plays an important role in copper homeostasis and is the most important organ in the body for copper homeostasis and storage (Dirksen and Fieten, 2017). Inability to export copper into bile is the cause of Wilson's disease in humans. This disease is caused by a defect or lack of an autosomal recessive gene called *P*-type ATPase (ATP7B), a copper transporter (Jaeschke, 2008). Treatment involves life-long chelation therapy (Dirksen and Fieten, 2017). Copper storage disease of veterinary relevance, either mediating or as a result of chronic liver damage, is noted in certain breeds of dogs: Anatolian shepherds, Bedlington terriers, Cardigan Welsh corgies, clumber spaniels, cocker spaniels, Dalmatians, Doberman pinschers, Labrador retrievers, Pembroke Welsh corgies, poodles, Skye terriers, West Highland white terriers, and others (Rolfe and Twedt, 1995; Spee et al., 2006; Dirksen and Fieten, 2017). Copper storage disease in Labrador retrievers has been linked to the ATP7B gene, like Wilson's disease (Dirksen and Fieten, 2017). Deletion of exon 2 of the MURR1 (COMMD1) gene, important in regulation of biliary copper excretion, was found to be the genetic defect in Bedlington terriers (Klomp et al., 2003). Molecular causes in other susceptible breeds remain to be confirmed. Similar to dogs, copper storage disease has been reported in cats and ferrets (Huynh and Laloi, 2013). Sheep and some other species are susceptible to a form of copper storage disease with an acute presentation. Other causes of hepatocellular damage in sheep cause copper release and oxidative damage to surrounding hepatic parenchyma as well as erythrocytes.

The ability to excrete a toxicant into the bile duct will usually result in clearance by excretion in feces or urine. However, certain lipophilic compounds such as methylmercury and diclofenac can be reabsorbed from the intestinal lumen back into the portal circulation, a process known as *enterohepatic cycling*. This will lead to prolonged biological half-life and can increase the toxicity of the compound (Jaeschke, 2008).

Bioactivation and Metabolism

One of the major functions of the liver is the elimination of both endogenous and exogenous compounds. Some xenobiotic agents absorbed by the small intestine are highly lipophilic. Renal excretion is the primary mechanism of removal for many xenobiotics, but renal excretion of lipophilic compounds, which are frequently protein bound in the circulation, is poor (Dahm and Jones, 1996; Sturgill and Lambert, 1997; Watkins, 1999). Therefore, in order for these xenobiotics to be eliminated, biotransformation needs to occur in the liver first to increase their water solubility.

Hepatocytes contain phase I enzymes, which expose or introduce functional groups ($-OH$, $-NH_2$, $-SH$ or $-COOH$) and generate reactive electrophilic metabolites. Hepatocytes also have a wide variety of phase II enzymes that enhance the hydrophilicity by a conjugation reaction, which adds a polar group to promote excretion. The functional groups exposed or introduced by the phase I enzymes often become the site of action for the phase II reactions. Though these reactions function to detoxify compounds, if there is a mismatch between phase I and II reactions, there is potential for accumulation of toxic phase I metabolites (Zimmerman, 1999; Jaeschke, 2008).

Phase I reactions, ubiquitous in mammals, involve oxidation, reduction and hydrolysis, and sometimes produce biologically active metabolites (Brown, 2001). Phase I enzymes are predominantly located in zone 3, as mentioned previously. Many of these phase I enzymes are present in the smooth endoplasmic reticulum of the hepatocyte. When liver tissue is homogenized mechanically in a laboratory, the endoplasmic reticulum breaks down into small vesicles known as microsomes and can be retrieved by differential centrifugation. Thus these enzymes are often referred to as *microsomal enzymes*. As a rule, microsomal enzymes require oxygen and NADPH to function (Dahm and Jones, 1996; Brown, 2001).

Cytochrome P450 enzymes, a major group of the microsomal enzymes, are the most common players of phase I oxidation. All P450 enzymes contain a heme iron center and when complexed within carbon monoxide, absorb light at a wavelength of 450 nm. These enzymes were first discovered in an unknown pigment thus named cytochrome P450: P for pigment and 450 for the wavelength of absorbed light. Liver P450 enzymes involved in xenobiotic biotransformation belong to three main P450 gene families, CYP1, CYP2, and CYP3. More than 36 cytochrome P450 isoenzymes have been identified in animals (Dahm and Jones, 1996; Watkins, 1999; Jaeschke, 2008). P450s can be induced or inhibited by drugs such as phenobarbital and cimetidine, respectively. Oxidation is the major phase I reaction, and the most important enzyme system for oxidative reactions are the cytochrome P450 (Gu and Manautou, 2012). Important substrates include steroid hormones, bile acids, fat soluble vitamins, and more than 90% of drugs (Brown, 2001; Gu and Manautou, 2012). Oxidative reactions can produce highly reactive epoxides, which are usually detoxified rapidly by phase II conjugation or hydrolysis by microsomal epoxide hydrolase enzymes (Watkins, 1999; Pineiro-Carrero and Pineiro, 2004). If an individual is exposed to the xenobiotic in high enough doses that these mechanisms are overwhelmed, reactive phase I metabolites produce injury.

Noncytochrome P450 enzymes are also involved in oxidative reactions. One such enzyme is alcohol dehydrogenase, a cytosolic enzyme, whose substrates include vitamin A, ethanol, and ethylene glycol. Others such enzymes include aldehyde dehydrogenase, aldehyde oxidase, xanthine oxidase, monoamine oxidase, diamine oxidase, peroxidase, and flavin-monooxygenases (Jaeschke, 2008).

Examples of phase I reduction reactions include reduction of nitro compounds to amines, and dehalogenation of volatile anesthetics. Phase I hydrolysis reactions are required for metabolism of compounds with amide bonds or ester linkages, as in the conversion of aspirin to salicylate (Brown, 2001). Carboxylesterase, alkaline phosphatase, peptidase, and epoxide hydrolase are involved in phase I hydrolysis reactions (Jaeschke, 2008).

Most phase II enzymes are cytosolic, but others are mitochondrial or microsomal. Phase II enzymes are predominantly involved in conjugating xenobiotics at the functional groups of the parent compound or the phase I metabolites. Unlike the phase I metabolites, phase II metabolites are rarely reactive, with some exceptions such as the glucuronide product of some nonsteroidal antiinflammatory drugs and aromatic amines (Jaeschke, 2008), which will be discussed later.

Phase II enzymes conjugate a polar group to a hydroxyl-, carboxyl-, amino- or sulfhydryl-group on the substrate. These polar molecules include glucuronic acid, sulfate derived from sulfuric acid ester, acetate, GSH, methyl groups derived from methionine, and amino acids such as glycine and cysteine. These groups enhance water solubility to allow for renal or biliary excretion of the metabolite. Disruption of phase II reactions allows accumulation of reactive phase I metabolites (Sturgill and Lambert, 1997).

Glucuronidation is the most common phase II reaction in humans, though it is deficient in the neonate (Sturgill and Lambert, 1997; Brown, 2001; Pineiro-Carrero and Pineiro, 2004), and, of considerable veterinary importance, cats, which lack a functional UGA1A6 gene for glucuronyl transferase (van Beusekom et al., 2015). Substrates with a molecular weight greater than 500, such as steroid hormones, thyroxin, bilirubin, salicylates, acetaminophen and many other drugs are likely to undergo glucuronide conjugation. Glucuronyltransferases are microsomal enzymes that catalyze the transfer of glucuronide from uridine 5′-diphosphate (UDP). UDP becomes depleted in overdoses of acetaminophen or other drugs that undergo this detoxification pathway. Products of glucuronide conjugation are excreted in bile or urine. Those excreted in bile sometimes undergo hydrolysis in the intestine, leading to enterohepatic cycling. Phenobarbital is an agent that induces glucuronyltransferases.

Sulfation is the primary conjugation reaction for aliphatic alcohols and substrates with phenol groups (Sturgill and Lambert, 1997; Brown, 2001). These reactions are catalyzed by cytoplasmic sulfotransferases. Substrates for sulfate conjugation include acetaminophen, morphine, ascorbic acid and endogenous compounds like chondroitin, heparin and some steroid hormones. The pool of available sulfates may become saturated in drug overdoses.

Drugs with amine and hydrazine groups, such as sulfonamides, are often conjugated to acetate (Sturgill and Lambert, 1997; Brown, 2001). *N*-acetyltransferase is a cytoplasmic enzyme involved in acetylation reactions.

GSH and cysteine have sulfhydryl groups that readily bind many phase I metabolites (Brown, 2001). GSH, a free radical scavenger, prevents membrane damage from reactive metabolites in spontaneous reactions or with the selenium-dependent GSH peroxidases as a catalyst. Because these enzymes are cytosolic, damaged membrane phospholipids must be released by phospholipase A2 for detoxification. GSH is also involved in reduction and recycling of other antioxidants such as vitamins E and C (Dahm and Jones, 1996). When oxidized, GSH forms a dimer that must be reduced by NADPH-dependent GSH reductases. GSH becomes depleted in the fasting or overdosed patient (Dahm and Jones, 1996; Sturgill and Lambert, 1997; Pineiro-Carrero and Pineiro, 2004). *N*-acetylcysteine is used to replenish GSH.

Significant species differences exist in phase II enzymes. UDP-glucuronosyltransferase is deficient in cats, as noted above, affecting their ability to detoxify numerous compounds including acetaminophen (Court and Greenblatt, 1997; Brown, 2001). The Gunn rat, a mutant strain of the Wistar rat, is also deficient in UDP-glucuronosyltransferase enzyme. Ferrets also have less capability to glucuronidate (Court, 2001). Swine have reduced sulfate conjugation abilities (Brown, 2001). Dogs do not have the ability to acetylate aromatic groups, which may interfere with their ability to metabolize sulfonamide antimicrobials (Brown, 2001; Trepanier, 2004).

Reactive metabolites of phase I metabolism can act as free radicals, substances with unpaired electrons. Free radicals generate reactive oxygen species (ROS) such as superoxide ($O_2-\bullet$), hydroxyl radicals ($\bullet OH$), and hydrogen peroxide (H_2O_2) through interactions with other molecules. Free radicals reacting with phospholipids of the plasma membrane, endoplasmic reticulum membrane or mitochondrial membranes cause a self-propagating chain reaction leading, eventually, to cell death (Dahm and Jones, 1996; Watkins, 1999).

Epoxides and other electrophiles are molecules with electron seeking properties. These form covalent bonds with nucleophilic molecules, e.g., by binding thiol groups on proteins (Dahm and Jones, 1996; Watkins, 1999; Zimmerman, 1999). Electrophiles produced by phase I reactions cause cell death by damage to critical proteins such as membrane calcium transport proteins. Aflatoxin B_1 binds to guanine residues in the DNA, leading to defects in protein transcription, resulting in carcinogenesis or cell death.

Aromatic amines and NSAIDs can form reactive phase II metabolites, as mentioned previously. Glucuronides of aromatic amine metabolites, *N*-hydroxyaromatic amines, form highly electrophilic aromatic nitrenium ions that can bind to DNA and other macromolecules, leading to urinary bladder cancer. Several drugs, including NSAIDs, can form acyl-glucuronides, which are reactive intermediates that bind to proteins to form adducts.

In addition to phase I and II biotransformation enzymes, studies suggest drug efflux from hepatocytes using hepatic transporter systems as a means of hepatic xenobiotic excretion. These are called the phase III transporter systems. Several transporter families that mediate uptake of chemicals into liver and excretion of chemicals from liver into blood and/or bile have been identified. Generally, the organic anion transporting polypeptide family (OATPS), organic cation transporter 1 (OCT1), and organic anion transporter 2 mediate uptake of a large number of xenobiotics from the blood to the liver. Conversely, multidrug resistance proteins (MDRS), multidrug resistance-associated proteins (MRPS) and breast cancer resistance protein (BCRP) mediate efflux of xenobiotics from liver into bile or blood (Klaassen and Slitt, 2005). Similarly to phase I and II enzymes, these transporters can be induced or inhibited by drugs that are ligands of various nuclear receptors, such as aryl hydrocarbon receptor (AhR), constitutive androstane receptor (CAR), and pregnane x receptor (PXR).

The ABCB1 gene for *p*-glycprotein is of particular interest in veterinary medicine because a defect in this gene caused by a base pair deletion is common in many dog breeds (Merola and Eubig, 2014). A deletion mutation has also been described in cats (Mealey and Burke, 2015). *P*-glycoprotein is well known as an efflux mechanism that excludes certain xenobiotics, such as avermectins, from the blood-brain barrier, but *p*-glyoprotein is also involved in transport across canalicular epithelium, and thus is involved in xenobiotic excretion (Merola and Eubig, 2014).

Inflammation

Inflammatory reactions represented by activation of resident Kupffer cells, natural killer cells, and natural killer T cells, and migration of activated neutrophils, lymphocytes, and monocytes in the damaged areas of liver parenchyma are commonly seen in toxin-induced hepatopathy. Although the main role of this inflammatory response is to remove dead and damaged cells, it can also aggravate the injury by releasing or forming cytotoxic pro- and antiinflammatory mediators (Jaeschke, 2008).

Upon activation, Kupffer cells generate ROS, such as hydrogen peroxide, by the action of NADPH oxidase. These ROS will diffuse into neighboring hepatocytes, produce oxidative stress, and lead to cell injury. It has been determined that intracellular proteins, such as high-mobility group protein 1 (HMGB-1), released by cells during necrosis bind to toll-like receptors on Kupffer cells, induce synthesis and release of cytokines and chemokines (such as TNF-α, IL-1) leading to recruitment of cytotoxic neutrophils, which can directly cause apoptotic cell death or generate ROS, such as hypochlorus acid, by the actions of NAPDH oxidase and myeloperoxidase, leading to cell injury and death (Jaeschke, 2008).

The role of Kupffer cells in toxicant-induced liver injury from variety of chemicals such as ethanol, acetaminophen, CCl_4 and 1,2-dichlorobenzene has been studied. Involvement of neutrophils has been shown with hepatotoxicity associated with alpha-naphthylisothiocyanate and halothane. Although many compounds such as ethanol, allyl alcohol, aflatoxin B_1, monocrotaline, ranitidine and diclofenac are capable of causing liver injury without the involvement of neutrophils, inflammatory response initiated by endotoxin triggers a neutrophil-induced injury or aggravates the existing injury.

TYPES OF TOXICANT-INDUCED LIVER INJURY

Cell Death

Necrosis is the predominant form of cell death in most toxic insults. Microscopically visible degenerative changes to the hepatocyte may precede necrosis, including ballooning degeneration, hyaline degeneration, and the presence of Mallory bodies (Zimmerman, 1999). Cells lose osmotic homeostasis and swell, as can be seen on light microscopy. Swelling of organelles is seen only on an ultrastructural basis (Dahm and Jones, 1996; Treinen-Moslen, 2001). Energy production fails due to loss of calcium homeostasis (Dahm and Jones, 1996; Zimmerman, 1999). Eventually there is rupture of cellular membranes and leakage of cell contents, including cytosolic enzymes such as alanine transaminase and sorbitol dehydrogenase. Aspartate transaminase is a mitochondrial enzyme that can also into the circulation from necrotic hepatocytes (Chapman and Hostuler, 2013). Depending on the extent of liver necrosis, overall liver function may or may not be affected.

As noted, necrosis is often initiated by damage to membranes, either the plasma membrane of the cell or the membranes of organelles, particularly the mitochondria, such as with acetoaminophen toxicosis. Cell membrane damage can be caused by peroxidation of membrane phospholipids, such as with carbon tetrachloride (CCl_4). Damage to the plasma membrane interferes with ion regulation; damage to the membranes of the mitochondria interferes with calcium homeostasis and energy production; and damage to the smooth endoplasmic reticulum membrane diminishes the ability of that organelle to sequester calcium (Zimmerman, 1999). Inhibition of protein synthesis is an alternate mechanism of cell necrosis. Toxicants that inhibit protein synthesis include amanitin and related mushroom toxins, which inhibit the action of RNA polymerase and therefore mRNA synthesis (Pineiro-Carrero and Pineiro, 2004).

Necrotic liver injury can be focal, zonal, bridging, or massive and panlobular. Focal necrosis is randomly distributed and involves hepatocytes individually or in small clusters (Treinen-Moslen, 2001). Zonal necrosis is common and usually occurs in zone 3, the centrilobular area (Zimmerman, 1999; Treinen-Moslen, 2001; Plumlee, 2004) due to a higher concentration of phase I enzymes in this region. Grossly, the liver will have a reticulated pattern of dark red central areas separated by brown to yellow areas. Bridging necrosis describes confluent areas of necrosis extending between zones of the lobule or between lobules (Treinen-Moslen, 2001). Panlobular or massive necrosis denotes hepatocyte loss throughout the lobule and loss of lobular architecture.

The liver is grossly swollen and friable with panlobular injury.

Apoptotic cells undergo cell shrinkage, nuclear condensation and pyknosis (Dahm and Jones, 1996; Treinen-Moslen, 2001), but mitochondrial function (Pineiro-Carrero and Pineiro, 2004) is maintained and the cell membrane remains intact (Zimmerman, 1999). Phagocytes immediately remove the dead cell (Shehu et al., 2016). This type of cell death is not associated with inflammation. Although apoptosis, sometimes termed "programmed cell death," is a normal physiological process, it may be induced by xenobiotics causing oxidative stress, decreased expression of apoptotic suppressors, or enhanced expression of proapoptosis genes. Apoptotic cells are occasionally seen in the centrilobular area but are rapidly phagocytized by macrophages and other hepatocytes.

Although necrosis and apoptosis are considered separate entities, an alternate view is emerging that apoptosis and necrosis are frequently the consequence of the same initiating factors and signaling pathways. Rather than being separate entities, apoptosis and necrosis represent extremes on a continuum of cell death. Thus necrosis resulting from oncosis is termed "oncotic necrosis," and that originating from apoptosis is termed "apoptotic necrosis" (Levin et al., 1999; Jaeschke et al., 2004; Malhi et al., 2006).

The nature of the lesions can tell us something about the mechanism of injury. Several xenobiotics, such as CCl_4, acetaminophen, thioacetamide, allyl alcohol and ethanol, produce oncotic necrosis. Centrilobular necrosis is a common pattern seen with CCl_4, acetaminophen and thioacetamide. Hypoxia also causes centrilobular necrosis since zone 3, the centrilobular region, is oxygen stressed.

Less commonly, a midzonal pattern is seen in endotoxin-mediated hepatitis in the rat model (Ramaiah et al., 2004). Necrosis of periportal hepatocytes, although rare, can be observed with compounds such as allyl alcohol. Hepatocytes in this region are relatively young and necrosis can lead to portal fibrosis and bile duct proliferation. Ethanol produces multifocal, random hepatic necrosis.

Necrosis may be a primary event caused by reactive intermediates (e.g., acetaminophen, thioacetamide and CCl_4) or a secondary event following infiltration of inflammatory cells, as seen with ethanol.

Hepatic Steatosis

Hepatic steatosis/lipidosis or fatty liver is simply the accumulation of fat vacuoles within hepatocytes. Steatosis is a common response to a variety of hepatotoxins and represents a potentially reversible injury (Treinen-Moslen, 2001). Grossly, the affected liver is swollen with rounded edges, friable, and light brown to yellow. Due to the fat accumulation, sections of the affected liver will float in formalin (Plumlee, 2004). Compounds that produce prominent steatosis associated with mortality include the antiepileptic drug valproic acid and the antiviral agent fialuridine. Other toxins that cause hepatic steatosis include aflatoxin, white or yellow phosphorus, ethanol, and CCl_4.

Although steatosis has been considered a benign and reversible change, studies have determined biochemical alterations that lead to steatohepatitis, fibrosis and cirrhosis (Ramaiah et al., 2004). Nonalcoholic fatty liver disease (NAFLD), a syndrome associated with obesity in humans, often type II diabetics, has a marked inflammatory component (Diehl, 2002). Several endocrine abnormalities also result in steatosis, making it challenging to determine a cause. Serum transaminase concentrations in patients with steatosis are variable, but can be moderately to markedly increased. Cholestasis occurs with marked lipid accumulation.

Steatosis is termed microvesicular if fat vacuoles are small and do not displace the nucleus. Microvesicular steatosis is often associated with slow lipid accumulation (Bastianello et al., 1987; Plumlee, 2004). This form of steatosis may indicate deficiency in mitochondrial β-oxidation of fatty acids. This relatively severe form of steatosis and has been seen in primates and dogs with aflatoxicosis (Bastianello et al., 1987; Zimmerman, 1999) and people with valproic acid toxicosis (Sturgill and Lambert, 1997; Zimmerman, 1999).

Macrovesicular steatosis, more common in domestic animals, describes hepatocytes containing one, or occasionally a few, large fat vacuole(s) that displace the nucleus to the periphery of the cytoplasm (Plumlee, 2004). Macrovesicular steatosis indicates an imbalance between fatty acid uptake and secretion of very low density lipoproteins secondary to increased triglyceride mobilization, decreased fatty acid oxidation, decreased synthesis of very low density lipoproteins, or other metabolic anomalies (Sturgill and Lambert, 1997; Zimmerman, 1999; Treinen-Moslen, 2001; Plumlee, 2004). Macrovesicular steatosis occurs with a variety of metabolic disease in domestic animals, particularly in obese cats with anorexia and preparturient cattle due to mobilization of lipids. Macrovesicular steatosis has been reported in dogs with subacute aflatoxicosis (Bastianello et al., 1987). Zone 1 macrovesicular steatosis has been reported with yellow phosphorus toxicosis (Zimmerman, 1999).

Steatohepatitis

Steatohepatitis is usually the next stage of untreated steatosis (Lieber, 1994; Bautista, 2002; French, 2003). Steatohepatitis is the hepatocellular accumulation of lipid and inflammation of hepatic parenchyma. The inflammatory cells involved are usually neutrophils and mononuclear leukocytes. There is no specificity noted with this pathologic stage and the distribution of lipidosis and inflammation is random and multifocal. Conditions usually associated with steatohepatitis are alcoholic liver disease, NAFLD, and endotoxemia secondary to intestinal disease. Any toxic compounds that can cause steatosis can cause steatohepatitis if left untreated. Steatohepatitis in humans can progress to fibrosis/cirrhosis and hepatocellular carcinoma (Diehl, 2002). The clinical biochemistry alterations include elevated serum transaminases.

Hepatic Fibrosis

Fibrosis is a nonspecific lesion that usually results from chronic inflammation. Chronic inflammation can be the result of continuous exposure to a variety of hepatotoxic chemicals such as organic arsenicals, vinyl chloride, high doses of vitamin A (Zimmerman, 1999), chronic ethanol ingestion and nonalcoholic fatty liver disease. Fibrosis usually occurs around the portal area, in the space of Disse, and around the central veins. Hepatocytes are lost and replaced with fibrous connective tissue. Periportal fibrosis can lead to portal hypertension.

Cirrhosis

Hepatic cirrhosis is end-stage liver disease. Cirrhosis describes irreversible changes characterized by accumulation of excessive collagen deposition in the form of bridging fibrosis, disrupting hepatic architecture. Entrapped hepatocytes undergo random mitosis and growth, termed nodular regeneration. Cirrhosis is either micronodular or macronodular, depending on the amount of fibrosis and tissue regeneration. A liver with micronodular fibrosis has a grossly cobblestoned surface and is firm and difficult to cut with a knife.

Serum transaminase concentrations are low at this stage due to the lack of functional hepatocytes. Bile acids and ammonia are markedly elevated due to loss of hepatic function. Prognosis for recovery is poor. Physicians resort to liver transplantation in human patients.

Alcoholic hepatic steatosis, steatohepatitis, fibrosis and cirrhosis represent a sequential progression in alcoholic liver disease. Investigations of animals dosed with ethanol for one to several months have shown that the mechanisms of liver injury are numerous, indicating a complex, multifactorial pathogenesis for alcoholic liver disease, as seen in Fig. 15.2 (Lieber, 1994). The roles of CYP2E1, fatty acid metabolism, oxidative damage, endotoxin, Kupffer cell and neutrophil infiltration have been extensively investigated (Di Luzio, 1966; Bardag-Gorce et al., 2000; Kono et al., 2000; Hoek and Pastorino, 2002). Progression of liver disease correlates well with the dose of ethanol consumed daily and the duration of alcohol consumption. Females are more sensitive than males and experience a higher incidence of liver injury (Apte et al., 2005). Inflammation is predominantly neutrophilic within regions of necrosis and Mallory body formation. Although many of these changes have been observed in experimental models of alcoholic hepatitis, progression to cirrhosis has rarely been experimentally reproduced.

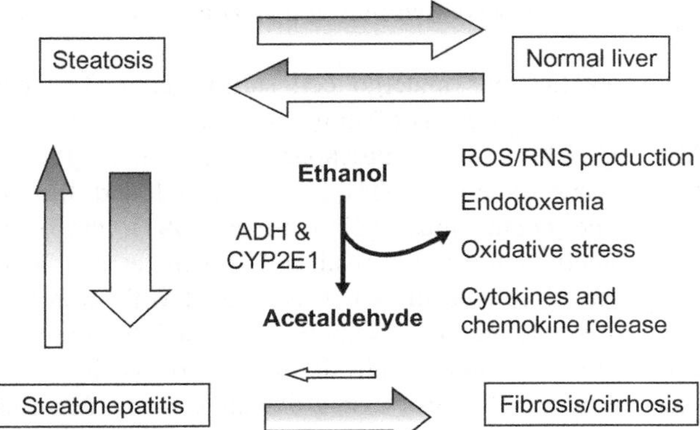

FIGURE 15.2 Progression of alcoholic liver disease. Consumption of ethanol produces hepatic pathology in a sequence ranging from steatosis (fatty liver) on one extreme to fibrosis/cirrhosis on the opposite end of the spectrum. Steatosis and steatohepatitis represent acute stages of alcoholic liver disease. *ROS*, reactive oxygen species; *RNS*, reactive nitrogen species.

Pigment Accumulation

Various substances can accumulate within hepatocytes or Kupffer cells and are often microscopically visible as pigment. Occasionally, these pigments lend a grossly visible tint to the liver. If there is cholestasis due to damage to the biliary tract or biliary obstruction, bile pigment can accumulate in canaliculi and bile ducts, producing a grossly yellow to green color (Zimmerman, 1999; Plumlee, 2004). Yellow pigment can be seen in hepatocytes and Kupffer cells in the event of canalicular rupture.

Iron in the form of hemosiderin, a yellow-brown pigment, is stored in the liver and can be better visualized using Pearl's Prussian blue (Plumlee, 2004). Copper is yellow-brown and is visualized using rhodanese. Newly regenerated hepatocytes may not have had time to accumulate copper, thus showing less pigment.

Lipofuscin can be present as a yellow-brown pigment within hepatocytic lysosomes and is a senile change, resulting from the inability of cells to break down old and damaged cytosolic organelles (Plumlee, 2004). Melanin can also be present in hepatocytes, Kupffer cells, and the portal connective tissue, particularly in reptiles, without any disease or toxic insults. Differentiation of pigments can be difficult histologically without the use of histochemistries and special stains.

Hepatic Neoplasia

Chemically induced neoplasms can originate from hepatocytes, biliary epithelium, and very rarely from sinusoidal endothelium. Neoplasms occur months or years after toxin exposure (Plumlee, 2004). If a toxin produces direct damage to DNA, a single exposure can lead eventually to neoplastic changes (Zimmerman, 1999; Pineiro-Carrero and Pineiro, 2004). Aflatoxin B_1 is an agent that acts by alkylating DNA and is associated with hepatocellular carcinoma in humans infected with hepatitis B virus. Aflatoxin B_1 has also been implicated in liver cancers in trout and laboratory animals (Newberne and Butler, 1969). Nongenotoxic agents must be given at high doses for long periods of time to induce cancer. Examples of nongenotoxic agents include phthalate esters in plasticizers, phenoxy acid herbicides and hypolipidimic drugs.

Hepatic adenomata are benign hepatocytic tumors associated with contraceptive steroid use in humans (Zimmerman, 1999). Hepatocellular carcinomata are malignant neoplasms induced by various chemicals and botanical toxins and are of more concern. These have been found in humans affected with hepatitis B virus and exposed to aflatoxin B_1, as noted above, and have been associated with anabolic steroid abuse. Other risk factors include viral hepatitis C and D, ethanol abuse, and exposure to microcystin.

Biliary carcinomata or cholangiocarcinomata are uncommonly associated with exposure to drugs/chemicals. Biochemical indicators of note include normal, elevated, or low concentrations of serum transaminases, loss of liver function, and the resulting increase in bile acid and ammonia concentrations.

Angiosarcomata or hemangiosarcomata derive from sinusoidal epithelium (Zimmerman, 1999; Treinen-Moslen, 2001; Plumlee, 2004). These neoplasms are rare but rapidly lethal and have been associated with exposure to vinyl chloride, inorganic arsenics, and Thorotrast, a form of radioactive thorium dioxide once used in radiographic contrast studies.

Megalocytosis

Hepatic megalocytosis can be observed in some aged animals, but is characteristic lesion observed in toxic insult by pyrrolizidine alkaloids and aflatoxins. Megalocytosis is caused by impaired cell division, resulting in enlarged hepatocytes with markedly enlarged nuclei (Plumlee, 2004). Pyrrolizidine alkaloids have an antimitotic effect on the hepatocytes but don't inhibit DNA synthesis. Since hepatocytes naturally proliferate to replace the damaged cells, hepatocytes are active in DNA and protein synthesis; when they cannot divide, megalocytosis results. Very often, chronic pyrrolizidine intoxication is accompanied by hepatic fibrosis as well as biliary hyperplasia and sometimes nodular regeneration of parenchyma.

MECHANISMS OF LIVER DAMAGE

Mechanisms of liver injury have been classified as either intrinsic or idiosyncratic. Intrinsic injury can produce steatosis, necrosis, cholestasis, or multiple lesions, often with minimal inflammation (Sturgill and Lambert, 1997). Intrinsic liver injury is a predictable, reproducible, dose-dependent response to a xenobiotic (Dahm and Jones, 1996; Sturgill and Lambert, 1997; Zimmerman, 1999; Pineiro-Carrero and Pineiro, 2004). A threshold dose exists for xenobiotics causing intrinsic liver injury, and there is often a predictable latent period between the time of exposure and clinical evidence of liver injury. Intrinsic liver injury accounts for the vast majority of toxic liver injury cases and is often produced by reactive products of xenobiotic metabolism, such as electrophiles or free radicals, though a few drugs cause intrinsic liver injury without bioactivation. An abbreviated summary of mechanisms of intrinsic liver injury is illustrated in Fig. 15.3.

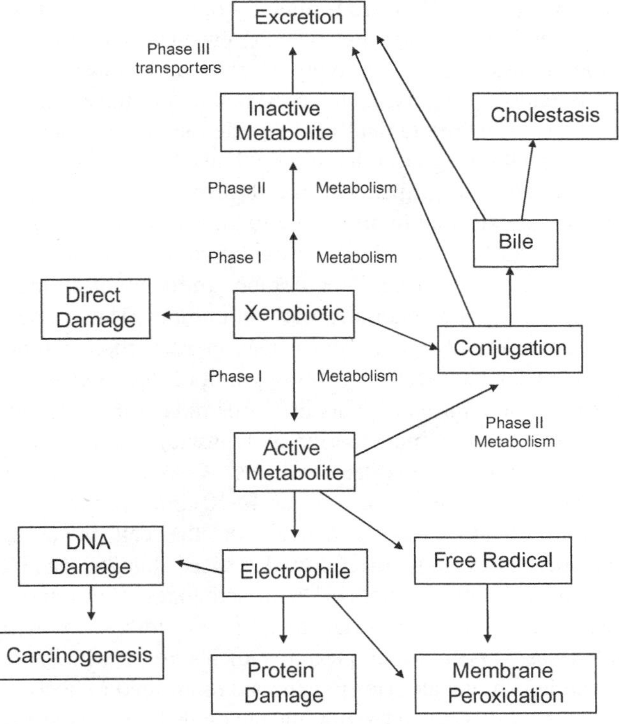

FIGURE 15.3 Basic mechanisms of hepatic injury showing the relationship between multiple pathways for metabolism and toxicity for any compound. The liver metabolizes xenobiotics (and some endogenous compounds) to form water-soluble products appropriate for urinary or biliary excretion. Some compounds are activated through these metabolic processes to free radicals, electrophiles or other toxic products that may induce hepatic injury.

Idiosyncratic reactions are, by contrast, unpredictable responses to a drug or other xenobiotic. They are rare, not dependent on dose, and can be associated with extrahepatic lesions (Sturgill and Lambert, 1997; Zimmerman, 1999; Pineiro-Carrero and Pineiro, 2004; Shenton et al., 2004). Extrahepatic clinical signs can include pyrexia, rash, and peripheral eosinophilia. Some idiosyncratic drug reactions resemble serum sickness. Hepatic lesions associated with idiosyncratic drug reactions include necrosis, cholestasis, or both, and there is often an inflammatory response involving macrophages and eosinophils.

Oxidative Stress Mediated by Free Radicals

Free radicals are generated from within hepatocytes through a variety of mechanisms: oxidative metabolism by cytochrome P450s, reduction and oxidation (redox) reactions of normal metabolism, transition metals such as iron and copper, nitric oxide generated by inflammatory cells, and ion radiation. Free radicals produce lipid peroxidation of membranes, oxidative modification of proteins, and DNA disruption (Crawford, 1999).

Free radicals have unpaired electrons, making them highly reactive. They are formed by one electron oxidation and reduction reactions, which produce cationic and anionic radicals, respectively (Dahm and Jones, 1996). Alternately, homolytic bond scission produces neutral radicals. The free radical nitric oxide (•NO), an important cell signaling agent released by leukocytes, reacts with superoxide to form peroxinitrite. Hydroxyl radicals, superoxide radicals, and hydrogen peroxide are major ROS.

Free radicals produce peroxidation of phospholipids within the cell plasma membrane, mitochondrial membrane, and the endoplasmic reticulum. The radicals remove a proton (H^+) from a methylene carbon within a polyunsaturated fatty acid, forming a lipid-free radical. This step is called *initiation*. This lipid-free radical then abstracts a proton from a neighboring polyunsaturated fatty acid, generating more lipid-free radicals. *Propagation* by this mechanism is estimated to occur 4–10 times per initiation. Effects of lipid peroxy radicals on the cell membrane include: increased permeability, decreased fluidity, inactivation of membrane proteins (Dahm and Jones, 1996) and, in the case of mitochondrial membranes, loss of polarity (Watkins, 1999). Lipid peroxy radicals react with stored metal ions in hepatocytes to generate more lipid radicals.

The most frequent initiating factor in free radical production inducing hepatocellular injury is the bioactivation of xenobiotics by the cytochrome P450 system. Phase I metabolism activates substrates to reactive intermediate molecules in preparation for phase II conjugation reactions. However, in circumstances of high exposure, phase I products accumulate (Gu and Manautou, 2012). Lesions produced by these compounds are usually centrilobular due to the location of the cytochrome P450s responsible.

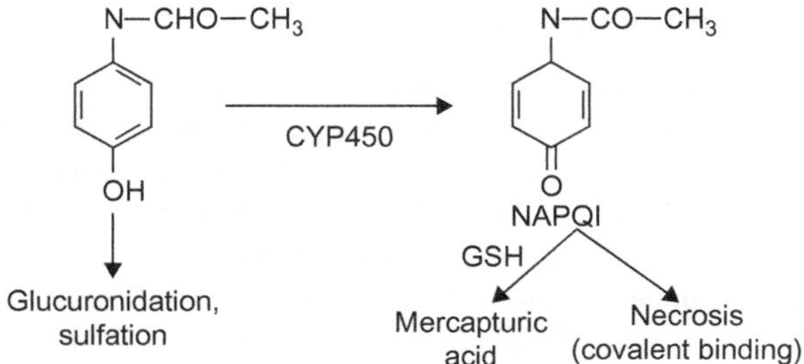

FIGURE 15.4 Metabolism and mechanism of acetaminophen toxicity. Bioactivation of acetaminophen by P450 enzymes results in the formation of the reactive intermediate (NAPQI) that forms covalent adducts with glutathione which is then converted to mercapturic acid. When the amount of the reactive metabolite formed exceeds the glutathione available for binding, the excess metabolite binds to tissue molecules, forming covalent adducts, resulting in centrilobular hepatic necrosis.

A classic example of phase I bioactivation is cell death resulting from acetaminophen (Fig. 15.4). Acetaminophen is a widely used analgesic that rarely induces clinical signs at therapeutic doses, except in the particularly susceptible feline species where metabolites of acetaminophen produce acute liver failure and oxidation of hemoglobin to methemoglobinemia. The details of acetaminophen toxicosis are described in another chapter, but one unstable intermediate metabolite, *N*-acetyl-*p*-benzoquinone imine (NAPQI), is the primary cause of hepatocyte injury.

The reaction that produces NAPQI generates superoxide anions as a by-product. NAPQI itself also acts as an electrophile, targeting mitochondria in particular, forming covalent adducts with protein thiol groups and other cellular macromolecules. Interaction of NAPQI with other cellular molecules generates more ROS, leading to oxidative stress (Dahm and Jones, 1996; Zimmerman, 1999). Adenine nucleotides and plasma membrane proteins involved in calcium homeostasis are also targeted (Dahm and Jones, 1996; Sturgill and Lambert, 1997). The role of Kupffer cell activation has been implicated as contributing to acetaminophen-induced liver injury through the production of reactive nitrogen species (Treinen-Moslen, 2001).

Another classic example of xenobiotic bioactivation, generation of free radicals, and peroxidative damage is conversion of CCl_4 into trichlorocarbon radical (•CCl_3) and then to trichloroperoxy radical (CCl_3OO•) (Fig. 15.5). The main phase I enzyme involved in bioactivation of both aforementioned acetaminophen and CCl_4 is CYP2E1, which can be induced by ethanol consumption in humans. Lipid peroxidation caused by free radicals increases the Ca^{2+} permeability of the plasma membrane, leading to disruption of calcium homeostasis and centrilobular cell necrosis. In addition, •CCl_3 directly binds to

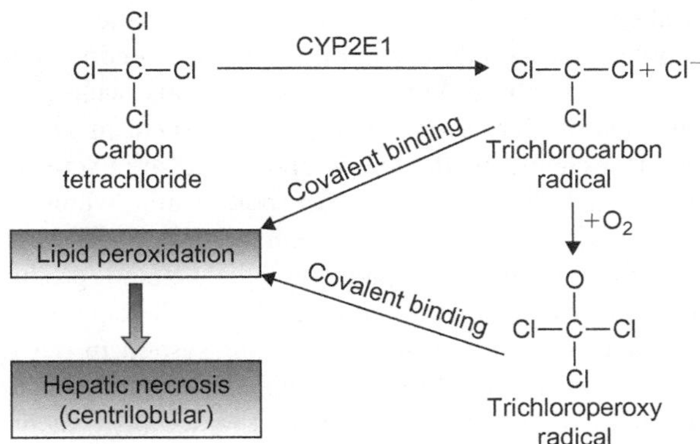

FIGURE 15.5 Metabolism and mechanism of carbon tetracholoride toxicity. Carbon tetrachloride metabolism by CYP450 leads to free radicals such as trichlorocarbon and trichloroperoxy radical that initiate lipid peroxidation. The centrilobular location of CYP2E1 enzyme is mainly responsible for carbon tetrachloride metabolism and contributes to centrilobular necrosis similar to acetaminophen toxicity.

tissue macromolecules and lipid peroxyl radicals form protein adducts (Jaeschke, 2008).

Disruption of Calcium Homeostasis and Cell Membrane Damage

Calcium ions (Ca^{2+}) are important for the mediation of hepatocellular injury. Cytosolic-free calcium is maintained at relatively low concentrations compared to extracellular concentrations. The majority of intracellular calcium is sequestered within the mitochondria and endoplasmic reticulum. Membrane-associated calcium and magnesium ATPases are responsible for maintaining this calcium gradient (Farrell et al., 1990).

Disruption or changes in permeability of the plasma membrane, mitochondrial membranes and membranes of the smooth endoplasmic reticulum lead to significant and persistent increases in the intracellular calcium. Depletion of available NADPH leads to calcium release, since calcium pumps in the mitochondrial membrane require NADPH (Cullen, 2005).

Excessive cytoplasmic calcium ions activate a variety of enzymes, including ATPases, phospholipases, proteases and endonucleases, producing further membrane damage. Thus increased calcium causes increased mitochondrial membrane permeability and induces apoptosis and necrosis. Additionally, calcium is required for cytoskeletal maintenance and function (Dahm and Jones, 1996; Delgado-Coello et al., 2006) and increased calcium can stimulate release of cytokines and eicosanoids by the Kupffer cells. Chemicals that cause liver damage by this mechanism include CCl_4, quinines, peroxides, acetaminophen, iron and cadmium.

Mitochondrial Injury

Mitochondria function in the production of energy, in the form of ATP, for cellular function by the process of oxidative phosphorylation. Hepatocytes are highly metabolically active and thus require a continuous supply of ATP. Hepatocytes active in detoxification or replication and replacement of damaged tissue have a still higher ATP requirement (Dahm and Jones, 1996). Compounds that disrupt mitochondrial oxidative phosphorylation include bile acids and amiodarone. Mitochondria are critical to modulation of cell redox status, osmotic regulation, pH control, cytosolic calcium homeostasis, and cell signaling. Mitochondrial DNA is more susceptible to oxidant damage than nuclear DNA (Stirnimann et al., 2010). Mitochondria are affected by virtually all types of injurious stimuli, including hypoxia, oxidants, electrophiles, lipophilic cations, and weak acids. Damage is often precipitated by increases in cytosolic calcium.

Hepatic injury is frequently accompanied by morphological mitochondrial changes. These structural abnormalities, such as greatly increased size and development of crystalline inclusions, are regarded as pathologic, reflecting either protective or degenerative response to injury. Mitochondrial damage results in formation of high conductance channels, the so-called mitochondrial permeability transition, in the inner mitochondrial membrane. This is an irreversible change and, because membrane potential is critical for mitochondrial oxidative phosphorylation, constitutes a deathblow to the cell.

Oxidative phosphorylation produces ROS that are deactivated within the mitochondria by antioxidants (Watkins, 1999). GSH within mitochondria functions as a scavenger for peroxides and electrophiles. Synthesis of GSH takes place within the cytosol and requires ATP. Greater than 90% depletion in the GSH reserve decreases the ability of the mitochondrion to detoxify the ROS associated with ATP production (Watkins, 1999). GSH *S*-transferase, the enzyme required for recycling of GSH, can be overwhelmed by xenobiotics and reactive metabolites (Dahm and Jones, 1996).

Xenobiotics can also cause cell death by their effects on mitochondrial DNA. Some antiviral deoxynucleoside analogs disrupt mitochondrial DNA synthesis through the inhibition of DNA polymerase gamma, thus depleting mitochondria, resulting in hepatocyte death.

Chemicals that damage mitochondrial structure, enzymes, or DNA synthesis disrupt beta oxidation of lipids and oxidative energy production within hepatocytes, which, if prolonged, leads to microvesicular steatosis, which can progress to macrovesicular steatosis. This sequence of events is seen in alcoholic and nonalcoholic steatohepatitis. The role of mitochondria has been extensively studied with nonalcoholic fatty liver disease in people. Alcoholic steatosis and other forms of hepatic steatosis have been linked to impairment of ATP homeostasis and mitochondrial abnormalities have been reported in a growing body of literature. Aspirin, valproic acid, and tetracyclines inhibit beta oxidation of fatty acids in mitochondria leading to lipid accumulation.

Disruption of Cytoskeleton

Changes in intracellular calcium homeostasis produced by active metabolites of xenobiotics can disrupt the dynamic cytoskeleton. A few toxicants cause disruption of the cytoskeleton through mechanisms independent of biotransformation. Microcystin is one example. Microcystin is produced by the cyanobacterium *M. aeruginosa* and other species of cyanobacteria. The hepatocyte is the specific target of microcystin, which enters the cell through a bile-acid transporter. Microcystin covalently binds to serine/threonine protein phosphatase, leading to the hyperphosphorylation of cytoskeletal proteins, and deformation and loss of function of the cytoskeleton (Treinen-Moslen, 2001).

Phalloidin and related toxins found in some mushrooms, including *A. phalloides*, act by binding tightly to actin filaments and preventing cytoskeletal disassembly, again causing deformation and loss of cytoskeletal function (Treinen-Moslen, 2001).

Cholestasis

Cholestasis can be transient or chronic (Treinen-Moslen, 2001). If severe, bile pigments make the liver appear grossly yellow to yellow-green (Plumlee, 2004). Cholestasis is subdivided into canalicular cholestasis and cholangiodestructive cholestasis.

Canalicular cholestasis can be produced by drugs/chemicals that damage the structure and function of bile canaliculi. A key component of bile secretion involves several ATP-dependent export pumps, such as the canalicular bile salt transporter and other transporters that export bile constituents from the hepatocyte cytoplasm to the lumen of the canaliculus. Some drugs bind these transporter molecules, arresting bile formation and movement within the canalicular lumen (Klaassen and Slitt, 2005). Secondary bile injury results if there is cholestasis due to the detergent action of bile salts on the biliary epithelium or hepatocytes in areas of cholestasis. Enzymes associated with the bile duct canaliculus include aldehyde dehydrogenase and gamma-glutamyltransferase, which can leak into the circulation during bile stasis or damage to the biliary epithelium, as can bile acids (Chapman and Hostutler, 2013).

Cholestasis can also occur simply from physical obstruction of canaliculi within the liver parenchyma (intrahepatic) or outside the liver (extrahepatic). Causes of cholestasis include hepatobiliary tumors, endotoxemia, hepatocyte swelling and intraductal crystals such as calcium salts of plant saponins, e.g., those found in *Tribulus* spp. Most chemicals that cause cholestasis are excreted in the bile, including the mycotoxin sporidesmin, which concentrates 100-fold in the bile (Treinen-Moslen, 2001).

Disruption of the hepatocyte cytoskeleton produces cholestasis by preventing the normal pulsatile contractions that move bile through the canalicular system to the bile ducts. Drugs that bind to actin filaments, such as phalloidin, those that affect cytoskeletal assembly, such as microcystin, and those that affect calcium homeostasis and cellular energy production can generate this type of injury. Cholestatic disorders typically result in elevated serum alkaline phosphatase, gamma-glutamyltransferase and serum bilirubin.

Cholangiodestructive cholestasis is caused by intrahepatic or extrahepatic bile duct obstruction. Injury of biliary epithelium leads to cell edema, sloughing into the lumen, and inflammation, contributing to obstruction (Treinen-Moslen, 2001; Plumlee, 2004). Chronic lesions of cholangiodestructive cholestasis typically include bile duct proliferation and periductular fibrosis. Vanishing bile duct syndrome, characterized by a loss of bile ducts, has been described in chronic cholestatic disease in humans (Zimmerman, 1999; Treinen-Moslen, 2001) and produced experimentally in dogs (Uchida et al., 1989).

Hepatogenous Photosensitization

Cholestatic diseases in herbivores, ruminants in particular, are associated with dermal photosensitization. The presentation of photosensitization is similar to that of sunburn, but with a more rapid onset and associated with different wavelengths of light (Rowe, 1989). Photosensitization is caused by circulation of photoactive compounds. Primary photosensitization involves ingestion or dermal absorption of a photodynamic compound that enters the circulation, such as hypericin from *Hypericum perforatum* or St. John's wort, and is described elsewhere. The second type of photosensitization is hepatogenous photosensitization.

Hepatogenous photosensitization usually occurs secondary to cholestasis. Herbivores ingest large quantities of chlorophyll. Metabolism of chlorophyll by bacteria in the GIT produces phylloerythrin, a photoactive compound that is absorbed and is predominantly excreted in the bile (Rowe, 1989; Burrows and Tyrl, 2001). Cholestasis prevents excretion of this compound and, upon exposure to light of wavelengths 320–400 nm, circulating phylloerythrin contributes to generation of singlet oxygen, causing lipid peroxidation in areas of skin unprotected by hair or melanin (Burrows and Tyrl, 2001). Not all causes of cholestasis produce photosensitization, and icterus can occur in the absence of photosensitization (Rowe, 1989).

Hepatocyte swelling can produce cholestasis. Agents that cause photosensitization through hepatocyte damage include the toxic plant *Lantana camera* that causes steatosis. Plants containing pyrrolizidine alkaloids (such as *Senecio* spp., *Crotalaria* spp., *Cynoglossum* spp., *Tetradymia* spp., *Trifolium hybridum*, *Artemisia nigra*) also cause secondary photosensitization due to portal fibrosis. Because significant hepatocyte damage must occur before the individual presents with photosensitization, damage of this type usually carries a poor prognosis (Rowe, 1989).

Other agents that damage bile ducts include the mycotoxin sporidesmin and sapongenins from the plant *Tribulus terrestris*. Sporidesmin is produced by *Pithomyces chartarum*, which grows predominantly on ryegrass pastures in Australia and New Zealand. Sporidesmin acts by directly damaging biliary epithelium, producing cell necrosis and degeneration. Bile ducts become occluded with cell debris and inspissated bile, and periductular fibrosis further occludes bile ducts (Rowe, 1989).

Several plant species cause bile stasis through precipitation of calcium salts of sapogenic glucuronides within bile ducts. The major toxic sapongenins from *T. terrestris* are diosgenin and yamogenin. These compounds are hydrolyzed in the GIT to sapogenins, which are further metabolized before glucuronidation (Burrows and Tyrl, 2001). Sapogenins directly occlude bile ducts and damage canalicular membranes. Note that while *T. terrestris* poisoning is reported with some frequency in South Africa and Australia, it is believed that the toxic sapogenins are either absent or only present in lower concentrations in *T. terrestris* growing in the United States (Burrows and Tyrl, 2001).

Inhibition of Tissue Repair Response

Tissue repair is a dynamic response, involving compensatory cell proliferation and tissue regeneration, and is stimulated to recover hepatic structure and function after injury. Extensive evidence from rodent models using structurally and mechanistically diverse hepatotoxicants such as acetaminophen, CCl_4, chloroform, thioacetamide, trichloroethylene and allyl alcohol have demonstrated that tissue repair plays a critical role in determining the final outcome of toxic insult, i.e., either recovery from injury and survival or progression of injury leading to liver failure and death (Mehendale, 2005).

Thioacetamide, originally used as a fungicide, is potently hepatotoxic after being bioactivated by cytochrome P450 and/or flavin-containing monooxygenase systems to sulfine (sulfoxide) and sulfene (sulfone) metabolites, which cause centrilobular necrosis. Thioacetamide bioactivation is primarily mediated by the cytochrome P450 enzyme CYP2E1. Studies suggest that thioacetamidesulfoxide, a relatively stable intermediate of thioacetamide metabolism, is obligatory for the hepatotoxic effects, indicating that it is the penultimate reactive metabolite. Accordingly, it has been reported that the hepatotoxic effects of thioacetamide are only expressed after metabolic conversion to thioacetamide *S*-oxide, which undergoes further metabolism to an as yet unidentified metabolite, most likely the reactive unstable thioacetamidesulfone. The reactive metabolite of thioacetamide binds to liver proteins with the formation of acetylimidolysine derivatives that are responsible for thioacetamide-induced hepatotoxic effects. Progression of thioacetamide-induced liver injury has also been attributed to inhibition of the tissue repair response in dietary restriction (Ramaiah and Mehendale, 2000).

Tissue repair is a complex process governed by the intricate cellular signaling involving chemokines, cytokines, growth factors, and nuclear receptors, leading to promitogenic gene expression and cell division. Tissue repair encompasses regeneration of hepatocytes, hepatic extracellular matrix, angiogenesis, and other processes necessary to completely restore hepatic structure and function after injury. New insights have emerged over the last quarter century indicating that tissue repair follows a dose response: at increasing doses of xenobiotics, a threshold is reached beyond which repair is delayed or impaired through inhibition of cellular signaling. Runaway secondary events then cause tissue destruction, organ failure and death. Prompt and adequate tissue repair after toxic injury is critical for recovery. Tissue repair is modulated by species, strain, age, nutrition, disease condition, and other factors, accounting for the marked differences in individual susceptibility and toxic outcome (Ramaiah et al., 1998; Mehendale, 2005).

IDIOSYNCRATIC REACTIONS

Idiosyncratic drug reactions occur when sensitization is followed by reexposure to a drug, classified as immune-mediated idiosyncratic hepatotoxicity (Dahm and Jones, 1996; Sturgill and Lambert, 1997; Zimmerman, 1999; Treinen-Moslen, 2001). A delay of 3–4 weeks after 1–2 weeks course of medication (e.g., amoxicillin-clavulanic acid) occurs before clinical signs become evident (Kaplowitz, 2001; Zimmerman, 1999), but onset is expedited with rechallenge (Dahm and Jones, 1996; Sturgill and Lambert, 1997; Watkins, 1999).

Neoantigens result from adducts formed by interaction of reactive drug metabolites with cellular proteins. These neoantigens are processed by Kupffer cells or other antigen presenting cells, transported to the cell surface, and presented to the immune system. Cell and antibody-mediated immune responses can cause severe liver damage. Various drugs believed to cause immune-mediated

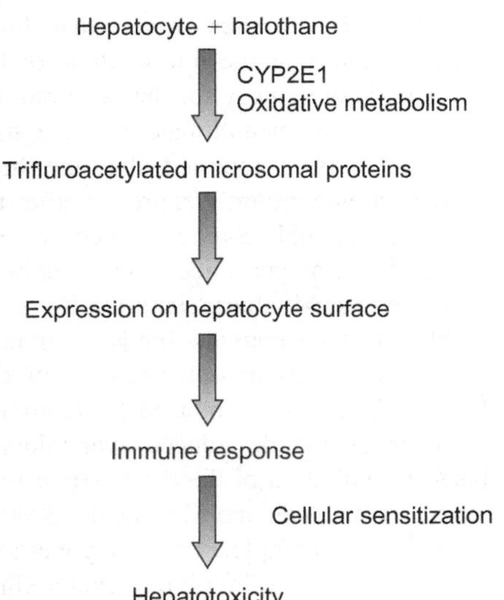

FIGURE 15.6 Postulated mechanism of immune-mediated halothane hepatotoxicity. Halothane-mediated hepatitis is the best example for immune-mediated liver damage. Oxidative pathway yields trifluoroacetylchloride, which can react with microsomal proteins to form a neoantigen which then can generate immune response leading to hepatic injury.

idiosyncratic reactions in humans include halothane, diclofenac, phenytoin, and sulfonamides (Sturgill and Lambert, 1997; Watkins, 1999; Zimmerman, 1999; Treinen-Moslen, 2001). The idiosyncratic reaction to halothane has been well studied (Fig. 15.6).

Clinical signs of the idiosyncratic reaction to carprofen, an NSAID, in dogs include anorexia, vomiting, and icterus and occur approximately 20 days following the first exposure to the drug. Signs do not correlate with drug dose. Affected dogs have elevated alanine transaminase, aspartate transaminase, alkaline phosphates and serum total bilirubin. There is mild to severe bridging hepatocyte degeneration and necrosis with evidence of apoptosis. Mild to moderate periportal inflammation is reported. Spayed female dogs are overrepresented among the affected (MacPhail et al., 1998). This idiosyncratic reaction to carprofen is most likely similar to that of diclofenac in humans. Diclofenac generates reactive metabolites and forms a hapten (Trepanier, 2013).

Methimazole is another example of agents causing idiosyncratic hepatotoxicosis affecting humans and cats. Patients usually present with icterus. The hepatic effect appears to be associated with metabolism by hepatic flavin monooxygenase to a reactive *N*-methylthiourea metabolite. GSH depletion is believed to play a role in human cases (Trepanier, 2013).

Many drugs implicated in idiosyncratic liver injury are known to affect mitochondrial function (Stirnimann et al., 2010). Part of the mechanism of injury due to diclofenac in humans could be due to mitochondrial injury (Trepanier, 2013). A proposed explanation for the delayed onset of clinical signs is that mitochondrial damage is not manifested until a threshold has been reached, then cell death occurs. Genetic polymorphisms in activation of detoxifying enzymes have been associated with increased susceptibility to idiosyncratic drug reactions in some people, further implicating the role of oxidative stress (Stirnimann et al., 2010).

Other idiosyncratic reactions of veterinary importance include diazepam in cats, which could be based on humoral or T-cell mediated immunity (Center et al., 1996; Trepanier, 2013). The clinical presentation in cats is similar to that described with carprofen in dogs. Idiosyncratic reactions to sulfonamides occur in about 0.25% of dogs and a variety of organ systems are affected, hepatopathy being the third most reported sequela. Other effects include polyarthropathy, which predominates in Doberman pinschers, thrombocytopenia, pyrexia and dermal drug eruptions. A reactive metabolite of sulfonamide binds to protein creating a hapten and may activate drug-specific T-cells, as occurs in humans (Trepanier, 2013). Methimazole and carbimazole are antithyroid drugs that have caused idiosyncratic reactions in cats and can cause hepatocellular and cholestatic liver damage, thrombocytopenia or neutropenia, or pruritis within a month of initiating therapy (Trepanier, 2013). Recently, zonisamide has been reported to cause acute liver failure after 10–20 days of dosing (Trepanier, 2013; Weingarten and Sande, 2015).

Some idiosyncratic drug reactions are associated with very long latency (up to 12 months), but are usually not associated with features of hypersensitivity and have variable response to rechallenge. These are classified as nonimmuno-mediated idiosyncratic reactions (Kaplowitz, 2001). Examples of drugs that are known to cause this type of idiosyncratic reaction include troglitazone, valproate, amiodarone, ketoconazole, disulfiram, and isoniazid. However, some involvement of allergic mechanism cannot be completely rejected in these drugs, thus this classification should still be viewed as tentative (Kaplowitz, 2005).

CONCLUDING REMARKS AND FUTURE DIRECTIONS

Research has focused on understanding the different mechanisms for chemical-induced liver injury. Researchers have attempted to understand the molecular basis for injury and the contribution of individual cell types to ultimate hepatic pathology. Recently, techniques such as microarray-based toxicogenomics, 2D gel electrophoresis, mass spectrometry-based proteomics and ^{1}H-NMR spectroscopy-based metabonomics have attempted to further design novel hypotheses to test the molecular players involved in liver damage (Craig et al., 2006; Blomme et al., 2009; Kienhuis et al., 2011).

Toxicogenomics will enable the detection of specific biomarkers used to predict adverse drug effects at low-level exposure (Kienhuis et al., 2011). Several signature biomarkers have been elucidated that may eventually be useful in the diagnosis of hepatotoxicosis: serum proteomic analysis revealed increased concentrations of vitamin D-binding protein, malate dehydrogenase, and purine nucleoside phosphorylase in several models of chemically induced hepatopathies. These enzymes were elevated in the serum before microscopic changes or conventional serum markers such as transaminase or alkaline phosphates elevations (Amacher et al., 2005). Once validated for use in humans and domestic animals, these proteins are potentially predictive of hepatotoxicity. The use of biomarkers will assist in identifying drugs that can cause serious adverse reactions, such as idiosyncratic liver injury, that could be missed in conventional preclinical or clinical drug trials. Further, research involving transgenic and knockout models provides insight into the mechanistic and molecular basis of liver injury.

Genetic predispositions to idiosyncratic drug reactions have been elucidated in humans, such as sensitivity to diclofenac and other xenobiotics in patients with a mutation in the gene for multidrug resistance-associated protein 2. Mutations in the genes for superoxide dismutase and GSH transferase also account for increased susceptibility to the toxic effects of certain drugs (Stirnimann et al., 2010). Animal models for idiosyncratic drug reactions remain elusive, but form another area requiring investigation.

REFERENCES

Amacher, D.E., Adler, R., Herath, A., Townsend, R.R., 2005. Use of proteomic methods to identify serum biomarkers associated with rat liver toxicity or hypertrophy. Clin. Chem. 51, 1796–1803.

Apte, U.M., Banerjee, A., McRee, R., et al., 2005. Role of osteopontin in hepatic neutrophil infiltration during alcoholic steatohepatitis. Toxicol. Appl. Pharmacol. 207, 25–38.

Bardag-Gorce, F., Yuan, Q.X., et al., 2000. The effect of ethanol-induced cytochrome p4502E1 on the inhibition of proteasome activity by alcohol. Biochem. Biophys. Res. Commun. 279, 23–29.

Bastianello, S.S., Nesbit, J.W., Williams, M.C., Lange, A.L., 1987. Pathological findings in a natural outbreak of aflatoxicosis in dogs. Onderstepoort J. Vet. Res. 54, 635–640.

Bautista, A.P., 2002. Neutrophilic infiltration in alcoholic hepatitis. Alcohology. 27, 17–21.

Blomme, E.A., Yang, Y., Waring, J.F., 2009. Use of toxicogenomics to understand mechanisms of drug-induced hepatotoxicity during drug discovery and development. Toxicol. Lett. 186, 22–31.

Brown, S.A., 2001. Pharmakokinetics: disposition and fate of drugs in the body. In: Adams, R. (Ed.), Veterinary Pharmacology and Therapeutics, 8th edn Iowa State University Press, Ames, IA, pp. 15–56.

Burrows, G.E., Tyrl, R.J., 2001. Toxic Plants of North America. Iowa State University Press, Ames, IA, pp. 1196–1200.

Can, C., Nigogosyan, G., 1963. Acquired toxic porphyria cutanea tarda due to hexachlorobenzene. Report of 348 cases caused by this fungicide. JAMA. 183, 88–91.

Center, S.A., Elston, T.H., Rowland, P.H., et al., 1996. Fulminant hepatic failure associated with oral administration of diazepam in 11 cats. J. Am. Vet. Med. Assoc. 209, 618–625.

Chapman, S.E., Hostutler, R.A., 2013. A laboratory diagnostic approach to hepatobiliary disease in small animals. Vet. Clin. North Amer. Small Anim. Pract. 43, 1209–1225.

Court, M.H., 2001. Acetaminophen UDP-glucuronosyltransferase in ferrets: species and gender differences, and sequence analysis of ferret UGT1A6. J. Vet. Pharmacol. Ther. 24, 415–422.

Court, M.H., Greenblatt, D.J., 1997. Molecular basis for deficient acetaminophen glucuronidation in cats. An interspecies comparison of enzyme kinetics in liver microsomes. Biochem. Pharmacol. 53, 1041–1047.

Craig, A., Sidaway, J., Holmes, E., et al., 2006. Systems toxicology: integrated genomic, proteomic and metabonomic analysis of methapyrilene induced hepatotoxicity in the rat. J. Proteome Res. 5, 1586–1601.

Crawford, J.M., 1999. The liver and the biliary tract. In: Cotran, R.S., Kumar, V., Collins, T. (Eds.), Robbins: Pathologica Basis of Disease, sixth ed. Saunders, Philadelphia, pp. 845–901.

Cullen, J.M., 2005. Mechanistic classification of liver injury. Toxicol. Pathol. 33, 6–8.

Dahm, L.J., Jones, D.P., 1996. Mechanisms of chemically induced liver disease. In: Zakim, D., Boyer, T.D. (Eds.), Hepatology, A Textbook of Liver Disease. W.B. Saunders Company, Philidelphia, pp. 875–890.

Delgado-Coello, B., Trejo, R., Mas-Oliva, J., 2006. Is there a specific role for the plasma membrane Ca^{2+}-ATPase in the hepatocyte? Mol. Cell Biochem. 285, 1–15.

Dereszynski, D.M., Center, S.A., Randolph, J.F., et al., 2008. Clinical and clinicopathologic features of dogs that consumed foodborne hepatotoxic aflatoxins: 72 cases (2005–2006). J. Am. Vet. Med. Assoc. 232, 1329–1337.

Di Luzio, N.R., 1966. A mechanism of the acute ethanol-induced fatty liver and the modification of liver injury by antioxidants. Am. J. Pharm. Sci. Support Public Health. 15, 50–63.

Diehl, A.M., 2002. Nonalcoholic steatosis and steatohepatitis. IV. Nonalcoholic fatty liver disease abnormalities in macrophage function and cytokines. Am. J. Physiol. Gastrointest Liver Physiol. 282, 1–5.

Dirksen, K., Fieten, H., 2017. Canine copper-associated hepatitis. Vet. Clin. North Amer. Small Anim. Pract. 47 (3), 631–644.

Farrell, G.C., Duddy, S.K., Kass, G.E., et al., 1990. Release of Ca^{2+} from the endoplasmic reticulum is not the mechanism for bile acid-induced cholestasis and hepatotoxicity in the intact rat liver. J. Clin. Invest. 85, 1255–1259.

Fausto, N., Campbell, J.S., 2003. The role of hepatocytes and oval cells in liver regeneration and repopulation. Mech. Dev. 120, 117–130.

French, S.W., 2003. Alcoholic liver disease. In: Zakim, D., Boyer, T.D. (Eds.), Hepatology, A Textbook of Liver Disease. W.B. Saunders Company, Philidelphia, pp. 839–922.

Gu, X., Manautou, J.E., 2012. Molecular mechanisms underlying chemical liver injury. Exp. Rev. Mol. Med. 14, e4.

Hoek, J.B., Pastorino, J.G., 2002. Ethanol, oxidative stress, and cytokine-induced liver cell injury. Alcohology. 27, 63–68.

Huynh, M., Laloi, F., 2013. Diagnosis of liver disease in domestic ferrets (*Mustela putorius*). Vet. Clin. North Amer. Exot. Anim. Pract. 16, 121–144.

Jaeschke, H., 2008. Toxic responses of the liver. In: Klaassen, C.D. (Ed.), Casarette & Doull's Toxicology: The Basic Science of Poisons, seventh ed. McGraw Hill, Columbus, OH, pp. 557–582.

Jaeschke, H., Gujral, J.S., Bajt, M.L., 2004. Apoptosis and necrosis in liver disease. Liver Int. 24, 85–89.

Jungermann, K., Katz, N., 1989. Functional specialization of different hepatocyte populations. Physiol. Rev. 69, 708–764.

Kaplowitz, N., 2001. Drug-induced liver disorders: implications for drug development and regulation. Drug Saf. 24, 483–490.

Kaplowitz, N., 2005. Idiosyncratic drug hepatotoxicity. Nat. Rev. Drug Discov. 4, 489–499.

Kienhuis, A.S., Bessems, J.G., Pennings, J.L., et al., 2011. Application of toxicogenomics in hepatic systems toxicology for risk assessment: acetaminophen as a case study. Toxicol. Appl. Pharmacol. 250, 96–107.

Klaassen, C.D., Slitt, A.L., 2005. Regulation of hepatic transporters by xenobiotic receptors. Curr. Drug Metab. 6, 309–328.

Klomp, A.E., van de Sluis, B., Klomp, L.W., Wijmenga, C., 2003. The ubiquitously expressed MURR1 protein is absent in canine copper toxicosis. J. Hepatol. 39, 703–709.

Kono, H., Rusyn, I., Bradford, B.U., et al., 2000. Allopurinol prevents early alcohol-induced liver injury in rats. J. Pharmacol. Exp. Ther. 293, 296–303.

Laskin, D.L., 1990. Nonparenchymal cells and hepatotoxicity. Semin. Liver. Dis. 10, 293–304.

Levin, S., Bucci, T.J., Cohen, S.M., et al., 1999. The nomenclature of cell death: recommendations of an ad hoc Committee of the Society of Toxicologic Pathologists. Toxicol. Pathol. 27, 484–490.

Lieber, C.S., 1994. Alcohol and the liver: 1994 update. Gastroenterology. 106, 1085–1105.

MacPhail, C.M., Lappin, M.R., Meyer, D.J., et al., 1998. Hepatocellular toxicosis associated with administration of carprofen in 21 dogs. J. Am. Vet. Med. Assoc. 212, 1895–1901.

Maddrey, W.C., 2005. Drug-induced hepatotoxicity: 2005. J. Clin. Gastroenterol. 39, S83–S89.

Malhi, H., Gores, G.J., Lemasters, J.J., 2006. Apoptosis and necrosis in the liver: a tale of two deaths? Hepatology. 43, S31–S44.

Mealey, K.L., Burke, N.S., 2015. Identification of a nonsense mutation in feline ABCB1. J. Vet. Pharmacol. Therapeut. 38 (5), 429–433.

Mehendale, H.M., 2005. Tissue repair: an important determinant of final outcome of toxicant-induced injury. Toxicol. Pathol. 33, 41–51.

Merola, V.M., Eubig, P.A., 2014. Toxicology of avermectins and milbemycins (macrolytic lactones) and the role of p-glycoproteins in dogs and cats. Vet. Clin. North Am. Small Anim. Pract. 42 (2), 313–336.

Mete, A., Jalving, R., van Oost, B.A., et al., 2005. Intestinal overexpression of iron transporters induces iron overload in birds in captivity. Blood Cells Mol. Dis. 34, 151–156.

Newberne, P.M., Butler, W.H., 1969. Acute and chronic effects of aflatoxin on the liver of domestic and laboratory animals: a review. Cancer Res. 29, 236–250.

Newman, S.J., Smith, J.R., Stenske, K.A., et al., 2007. Aflatoxicosis in nine dogs after exposure to contaminated commercial dog food. J. Vet. Diagn. Invest. 19, 168–175.

Oldham-Ott, C.K., Gilloteaux, J., 1997. Comparative morphology of the gallbladder and biliary tract in vertebrates: variation in structure, homology in function and gallstones. Microsc. Res. Tech. 38, 571–597.

Pineiro-Carrero, V.M., Pineiro, E.O., 2004. Liver. Pediatrics. 113, 1097–1106.

Plumlee, K.H., 2004. Hepatobiliary system. In: Plumlee, K.H. (Ed.), Clinical Veterinary Toxicology. Mosby, St. Louis, pp. 61–68.

Ramaiah, S., Rivera, C., Arteel, G., 2004. Early-phase alcoholic liver disease: an update on animal models, pathology, and pathogenesis. Int. J. Toxicol. 23, 217–231.

Ramaiah, S.K., 2007. A toxicologist guide to the diagnostic interpretation of hepatic biochemical parameters. Food Chem. Toxicol. 45, 1551–1557.

Ramaiah, S.K., Mehendale, H.M., 2000. Diet restriction as a protective mechanism in non cancer toxicity outcomes: a review. Int. J. Toxicol. 19, 413–424.

Ramaiah, S.K., Bucci, T.J., Warbritton, A., et al., 1998. Temporal changes in tissue repair permit survival of diet-restricted rats from an acute lethal dose of thioacetamide. Toxicol. Sci. 45, 233–241.

Rolfe, D.S., Twedt, D.C., 1995. Copper-associated hepatopathies in dogs. Vet. Clin. North Am. Small Anim. Pract. 25, 399–417.

Rowe, L.D., 1989. Photosensitization problems in livestock. Vet. Clin. North Am. Food Anim. Pract. 5, 301–323.

Shehu, A.I., Ma, X., Venkataramanan, R., 2016. Mechanisms of drug-induced hepatotoxicity. Clin. Liver Dis. 21, 35–54.

Shenton, J.M., Chen, J., Uetrecht, J.P., 2004. Animal models of idiosyncratic drug reactions. Chem. Biol. Interact. 150, 53–70.

Spee, B., Arends, B., van den Ingh, T.S., et al., 2006. Copper metabolism and oxidative stress in chronic inflammatory and cholestatic liver diseases in dogs. J. Vet. Int. Med. 20, 1085–1092.

Stenske, K.A., Smith, J.R., Newman, S.J., et al., 2006. Aflatoxicosis in dogs and dealing with suspected contaminated commercial foods. J. Am. Vet. Med. Assoc. 228, 1686–1691.

Stirnimann, G., Kessebohm, K., Lauterburg, B., 2010. Liver injury caused by drugs: an update. Swiss Med. Wkly. 140, 13080.

Sturgill, M.G., Lambert, G.H., 1997. Xenobiotic-induced hepatotoxicity: mechanisms of liver injury and methods of monitoring hepatic function. Clin. Chem. 43, 1512–1526.

Thawley, V., 2016. Acute liver injury and failure. Vet. Clin. North Am. Small Anim. Pract. 47 (3), 617–630.

Thurman, R.G., 1998. II. Alcoholic liver injury involves activation of Kupffer cells by endotoxin. Am. J. Physiol. 275, 605–611.

Treinen-Moslen, M., 2001. Toxic responses of the liver. In: Klaassen, C. D. (Ed.), Casarette & Doull's Toxicology: The Basic Science of Poisons, sixth ed. McGraw Hill, Columbus, OH, pp. 471–489.

Trepanier, L.A., 2004. Idiosyncratic toxicity associated with potentiated sulfonamides in the dog. J. Vet. Pharmacol. Ther. 27, 129–138.

Trepanier, L.A., 2013. Idiosyncratic drug toxicity affecting the liver, skin, and bone marrow in dogs and cats. Vet. Clin. North Am. Small Anim. Pract. 43, 1055–1066.

Uchida, H., Tomikawa, S., Nishimura, Y., et al., 1989. Vanishing bile duct syndrome in canine liver allotransplants. Trans. Proc. 21, 404–406.

van Beusekom, C.D., van den Heuvel, J.J.M.W., Koenderink, J.B., et al., 2015. Feline hepatic biotransformation of diazepam: differences between cats and dogs. Res. Vet. Sci. 103, 119–125.

Watkins, P.B., 1999. Mechanisms of drug induced liver disease. In: Schiff, E.R., Sorrell, M.F., Maddrey, W.F. (Eds.), Schiff's Diseases of the Liver. Lippincott-Raven Publishers, Philidelphia, pp. 1065–1080.

Weingarten, M.A., Sande, A.A., 2015. Acute liver failure in dogs and cats. J. Vet. Emerg. Crit. Care. 25 (4), 455–473.

Wisse, E., Luo, D., Vermijlen, D., et al., 1997. On the function of pit cells, the liver-specific natural killer cells. Semin. Liver Dis. 17, 265–286.

Zimmerman, H.J., 1999. Drug induced liver disease. In: Schiff, E.R., Sorrel, M.F., Maddrey, W.F. (Eds.), Schiff's Diseases of the Liver. Lippincott-Raven Publishers, Philidelphia, pp. 973–1064.

Chapter 16

Renal Toxicity

Sharon M. Gwaltney-Brant

INTRODUCTION

The kidney plays a vital role in maintaining homeostasis through the elimination of waste products, conservation of fluid and electrolyte balance, maintenance of acid–base balance, secretion of hormones and regulatory peptides, and metabolism and excretion of both endogenous compounds and xenobiotics. Although the kidney comprises roughly 0.5% of bodily mass, it receives up to 20%–25% of cardiac output, which can expose renal tissue to relatively high levels of blood-borne toxicants. The kidney may also be exposed to toxicants through the metabolic activation of xenobiotics by enzyme systems within the renal tubular epithelium, and through the process of urine concentration the kidney can be exposed to higher concentrations of toxicants than other tissues. Injury to the kidney can lead to widespread systemic derangements, and due to limited regenerative ability, long-term renal insufficiency may result from exposure to nephrotoxic agents.

FUNCTIONAL ANATOMY

Kidneys are paired organs residing ventrolaterally to the lumbar vertebrae in mammals. Mammalian kidneys are bean- to horseshoe-shaped with uniform exterior surfaces, although some species (e.g., bears, oxen, whales) have multilobulated surfaces. Kidneys can be unipyramidal (e.g., horses, dogs, cats) or multipyramidal (e.g., pigs, oxen) depending on the number of renal papillae into which renal lobes empty. Mammalian kidneys are of equal size and are roughly the equivalent of three vertebrae in length. The surface of the kidney is covered by a fibrous capsule, and is brown-red in color in most species; in the cat, normal high fat content within the tubules results in a kidney that is a pale, yellow-gray color. Viewed on sagittal section, the kidneys have medial indented hilar regions from which renal artery, renal vein, lymphatics, nerves and ureter emerge. Viewing the cut surface of the sagitally incised kidney, the renal interior can be divided into two distinct sections, the cortex and medulla. The renal cortex in mammals comprises approximately 80% of the renal mass, and the normal cortex to medulla ratio is 1:2–1:3 in most species (Maxie and Newman, 2007). The medulla is divided into ray-shaped sections known as renal pyramids, which have their bases at the corticomedullary junction and apices that empty into the renal calyx (cats, oxen) or pelvis (dogs, horses). From the hilar region, the ureter directs urine to the distal urinary bladder.

The functional unit of the kidney is the nephron, which comprises the renal corpuscle (Bowman's capsule and the glomerulus), proximal tubule, loop of Henle and distal tubule. The number of nephrons per kidney ranges from 200,000 in cats and 400,000 in dogs to 1,000,000 in humans. The ultimate number of nephrons is fixed at birth, although kidneys of altricial offspring of some species (e.g., dog, cat, pig) undergo nephrogenesis for several weeks after birth (Maxie and Newman, 2007). Renal blood flow originates from the renal arteries which are direct branches from the aorta. The kidneys receive 20%–25% of cardiac output, allowing the entire plasma volume to be filtered approximately 100 times daily. Renal arteries progressively branch to form interlobar arteries, arcuate arteries, interlobular arteries and afferent arterioles, which feed blood to the glomerulus. The high hydrostatic pressure from afferent arterioles provides the force for ultrafiltration of plasma by the glomerulus, a tuft of branching and anastomosing capillaries. The glomerular "sieve" consists of the capillary endothelium, basement membrane and epithelial *podocytes* that anchor foot processes (*pedicels*) within the lamina rara of the glomerular basement membrane (GBM). These pedicels are separated by filtration slits covered by slit diaphragms containing 6–9 nm diameter pores through which plasma is filtered, permitting filtration of compounds up to approximately 60 kDa in size. The glomerular mesangium

Veterinary Toxicology. DOI: http://dx.doi.org/10.1016/B978-0-12-811410-0.00016-7

provides the supporting framework for the glomerular capillaries, and is composed of an extracellular matrix, contractile stellate cells which respond to vasoactive hormones, and phagocytic cells which are involved in local immune reactions (Khan and Alden, 2002). The distal ends of glomerular capillaries merge to form efferent arterioles that progress further down the nephron and form the peritubular capillary network that surrounds the renal tubules and helps to drive the countercurrent absorption mechanisms responsible for concentration of the urine and regulation of electrolyte balance. The majority of renal blood flow and oxygen is expended in the cortex, making the medulla a relatively hypoxic area of the kidney.

Fluid filtered by the glomerulus enters Bowman's capsule and flows into the proximal renal tubule. The proximal tubule is divided into three segments that differ anatomically and functionally. The most proximal segment, S_1, consists of the convoluted portion of the proximal tubule and possesses epithelial cells with tall brush borders, well-developed lysosome systems, and numerous basally located mitochondria. The S_2 segment extends from the end of the convoluted segment to the beginning of the straight segment and constitutes a transition segment. S_2 segment epithelia have shorter brush borders, fewer mitochondria and fewer lysosomes than cells in the S_1 segment. The S_3 segment encompasses the remaining distal portion of the proximal tubule and extends into the outer reaches of the medulla. Oxygen consumption, Na^+/K^+ ATPase activity and gluconeogenic capacity are greatest in the first two segments, while the S_3 segment has higher transport capabilities for some compounds, such as ascorbic acid (Castro et al., 2008). The S_3 segment is also the site for metabolic activation of some toxicants.

In the proximal tubule, passive reabsorption of water and active reabsorption (via Na^+/K^+ ATPases) of sodium occurs. Other solutes reabsorbed by the proximal tubule include potassium, calcium, phosphorus, bicarbonate, glucose, amino acids and proteins, and various xenobiotics, with each segment having a different range of and capacity for reabsorption. For instance, the S_1 segment is primarily responsible for the reabsorption of bicarbonate, glucose, amino acids and low molecular weight proteins. The proximal tubule ultimately reabsorbs 60%–80% of solute and water filtered by the glomerulus. Excretory functions of the proximal tubule include the active secretion of weak organic anions and cations. The proximal tubular epithelium possesses cytochrome P450-dependent mixed function oxidases capable of metabolizing a variety of endogenous compounds and xenobiotics. Agents that are bioactivated to toxic metabolites (e.g., acetaminophen) can induce proximal renal tubular injury.

Filtrate passes from the proximal tubule into the loop of Henle, which has a thin-walled descending limb and a thick-walled ascending limb that extends to the level of the outer medullary region. Some nephrons, termed long-looped nephrons, dip deeply into the inner medulla; in these nephrons, the proximal aspect of the ascending limb is thin-walled, becoming thick-walled as the tubule reaches the level of the outer medulla. Countercurrent exchange mechanisms within the loop result in the reabsorption of approximately 20% of filtered water and 25% of filtered sodium and potassium (Schnellmann, 2008). In the thin descending limb, water and interstitial solutes such as urea and electrolytes are able to freely pass into the tubule. At the level of the thin ascending limb, the tubule becomes impermeable to water and urea, and chloride and sodium ions are actively transported via Na^+/K^+ ATPases. The loop of Henle resides largely within the poorly oxygenated renal medulla, so the high oxygen demand of the Na^+/K^+ ATPases makes this segment especially susceptible to hypoxic injury (Brezis et al., 1984).

The macula densa is composed of specialized cells located between the end of the thick ascending limb of the loop of Henle and the most proximal aspect of the distal tubule. This area is in close proximity to afferent arterioles, allowing for communication between the macula densa and afferent arteriole of the same nephron. An increase in intratubular solute concentration at the macula densa results in a feedback signal to the afferent arteriole, resulting in vasoconstriction and reduction of glomerular filtration rate (GFR). This feedback mechanism helps prevent massive loss of fluid and solute in the face of impaired renal tubular absorption. The proximal-most aspect of the renal distal tubule is responsible for reabsorption of most of the remaining intraluminal electrolytes such as sodium and potassium. The remaining segment of the distal tubule and collecting duct absorb sodium, eliminate excessive potassium and hydrogen ions, and absorb additional water (influenced by antidiuretic hormone) as needed to regulate the volume and composition of the urine. Agents that disrupt the osmotic gradient of the medullary region (e.g., by increasing medullary blood flow) can disrupt the ability of the kidney to concentrate urine. Collecting ducts progressively intersect and anastomose toward the renal papilla and ultimately empty into the renal calyx, renal pelvis, or ureter, depending on species. Peristaltic action of the ureter propels urine toward the urinary bladder for temporary storage and elimination.

In addition to its role in regulation of waste excretion and water/electrolyte balance, the kidney secretes a variety of hormones and regulatory peptides vital for normal systemic homeostasis. Secretion of erythropoietin by renal peritubular interstitial cells promotes red blood cell formation; significant chronic renal disease is often associated with anemia due to decreases in erythropoietin secretion. Renin secreted from the juxtaglomerular cells increases systemic and renal blood pressure and aldosterone release. Prostaglandins (PGs) and prostacyclin are produced by a variety of renal cells and aid in regulation of renal vascular tone, mesangial contractility and processing of water and electrolytes by the renal tubules. The kidney also plays an important role in xenobiotic clearance and/or metabolism.

TOXIC EFFECTS ON THE KIDNEY

Acute Renal Failure

Acute renal failure is defined as an abrupt decrease in renal function leading to retention of nitrogenous wastes (Langston, 2010), and is one of the most common manifestations of nephrotoxic injury (Schnellmann, 2008). The term *acute renal failure* is sometimes used interchangeably with *acute renal insufficiency* or *acute renal injury (AKI)*. The latter term has been suggested as the proper term to use in order to encompass the entire spectrum of renal injury, from minor elevations of serum chemistry values (i.e., blood urea nitrogen and creatinine) to anuric renal failure.

The primary manifestation of AKI is a decrease in GFR leading to an excess of nitrogenous wastes in the blood (azotemia). Decreases in GFR may result from prerenal, renal or postrenal causes. Prerenal causes of decreased GFR include hypovolemia, renal vasoconstriction and poor cardiac output. Postrenal factors include obstruction of the ureters, bladder or urethra (e.g., bladder stones). Primary renal factors that can result in AKI leading to decreased GFR include tubular injury, glomerular injury, interstitial disease and renal vascular compromise. In humans, prerenal factors are said to account from 20% to 80% of cases of AKI, while renal factors account for 10%–45% and postrenal factors account for 5%–15% (Langston, 2010). Of causes of primary renal injury, ischemia/reperfusion and nephrotoxicosis are considered to account for over 90% of AKI cases (Schnellmann, 2008). Nephrotoxicants damage the kidneys by a variety of different mechanisms including: (1) direct injury to renal tubular epithelium, leading to epithelial cell necrosis, sloughing and obstruction of tubules by cellular debris (tubular casts), (2) detachment of lethally injured cells from the basement membrane, resulting in back-leakage of filtrate across the exposed basement membrane and adherence of detached cells to sublethally injured cells still attached to the basement membrane causing lumen obstruction, (3) renal vasoconstriction, resulting in hypoxia and ischemic necrosis of renal structures, (4) damage to the glomerular filtration barrier, and (5) impairment of renal healing and repair (Counts et al., 1995). Most nephrotoxicants exert their damage at the level of the renal tubules, with many toxicants targeting specific segments of the tubules. For instance, aminoglycoside antibiotics cause damage primarily to the S_1 and S_2 segments of the proximal tubule, while mercuric chloride-induced injury is restricted to the S_3 segment at low doses, extending into the S_2 and S_1 segments only at higher doses (Diamond and Zalups, 1998).

The clinical signs of acute renal injury and/or failure can include polydipsia, nausea or vomiting, lethargy, anorexia, weakness, dehydration and polyuria/oliguria/anuria. More severe cases may have halitosis, oral ulceration, abdominal (renal) pain, palpably enlarged kidneys and cardiac arrhythmias. Clinical laboratory abnormalities indicative of AKI include elevations in blood urea nitrogen and serum creatinine (azotemia), hyperphosphatemia, hyper- or hypokalemia and metabolic acidosis. *Uremia* is the term used when azotemia is accompanied by typical clinical signs of AKI. Advanced cases of uremia may present with gastrointestinal ulceration, anemia, peripheral neuropathy, encephalopathy and cardiac dysfunction.

The ability of the kidney to heal following an acute toxic insult is dependent upon several factors including the dose and type of toxicant, the amount of functional kidney remaining, the presence and severity of secondary uremic conditions (e.g., soft tissue mineralization) and the degree of medical intervention and supportive care provided during the acute crisis. Mild to moderate renal tubular injury with retention of tubular basement membranes has a reasonable prognosis for tubular regeneration provided that supportive care is administered until tubules have had a chance to recover. In uncomplicated acute tubular injuries, regeneration of epithelial cells generally begins after about 7–10 days following the renal insult; in mild cases, full recovery of architecture may occur within 2–3 weeks, with longer recovery periods being required for more severe renal injury (Maxie and Newman, 2007). In situations where nephrons have been fully obstructed by cellular debris or crystals, or if basement membrane integrity is lost, regeneration may be incomplete, resulting in long-term renal insufficiency and/or progression to chronic renal failure (CRF).

Chronic Renal Failure

CRF is most commonly the result of long-term exposure to toxicants, and many of the alterations seen in CRF are related to the secondary compensatory changes triggered by the initial injury. Upon loss of nephrons (and thus decrease in overall renal GFR), hemodynamic alterations occur that increase the blood flow and pressure to surviving nephrons in an attempt to reestablish normal whole-kidney GFR. Although changes such as increased glomerular pressures can help to maintain overall GFR, these increased pressures may contribute to glomerular sclerosis, tubular atrophy and interstitial fibrosis, thus furthering the progression of renal injury (Brenner et al., 1982). Increased pressure within glomerular capillaries results in an increase in volume of the glomerular tuft, glomerular hypertrophy and intraglomerular hypertension. Consequences of these changes include hyaline accumulation within glomerular capillary walls, mesangial dysfunction associated with matrix accumulation and microaneurysm formation, and thrombosis due to endothelial injury (Polzin, 2010). As the glomerulus expands, podocytes are unable to maintain the integrity of slit diaphragms and focal denudation of GBM occurs, allowing leakage of larger proteins into the glomerular filtrate (proteinuria). In addition to hemodynamically induced progression of CRF, there is evidence to suggest that T-lymphocytes and interleukin-6 contribute to the ongoing interstitial fibrosis in dogs with chronic progressive kidney disease (Yhee et al., 2008).

Clinical effects associated with CRF include uremia, gastrointestinal disorders (uremic gastritis, uremic enterocolitis), polyuria, polydipsia, nocturia, dehydration, atrial hypertension, peripheral neuropathy, uremic encephalopathy, myopathy, anemia, platelet dysfunction, renal secondary hyperparathyroidism, cachexia and hypokalemia (especially in cats) (Polzin, 2010). Immunosuppression is a potential complication of CRF in humans, and studies of dogs with CRF have shown impaired immunological function as well (Kravola et al., 2010). Animals with CRF may show few outward signs of illness until late in the course of their disease; in some instances acute decompensation may occur during periods of physical or emotional stress (Hosseininejad and Hosseini, 2008). Lesions found in animals with CRF include kidneys that are small and irregular in shape, with uneven capsular surfaces. On cut section, pale streaks (fibrosis) may be seen within the interstitium and the parenchyma may be gritty upon cutting due to mineralization and/or crystal deposition.

PATTERNS OF TOXIC RENAL INJURY

Identification of the target site of action of nephrotoxicants can assist in determining the functional impact and potential mechanism of toxicity (Fig. 16.1). Toxicants that are directly toxic to cells may cause injury to the glomerulus or the S_1 segment of the proximal tubule as they first enter the nephron. Conversely, direct-acting toxicants may be dilute in the initial ultrafiltrate, and may not cause injury until they reach the more distant nephron, where they may reach toxic concentrations as water is gradually reabsorbed and/or the pH changes. Some toxicants require bioactivation in order to exert their toxic effects, so they may cause site-specific injury to the S_3 segment of the proximal tubule, where bioactivation processes are most active. A list of nephrotoxicants and their primary sites of action can be seen in Table 16.1.

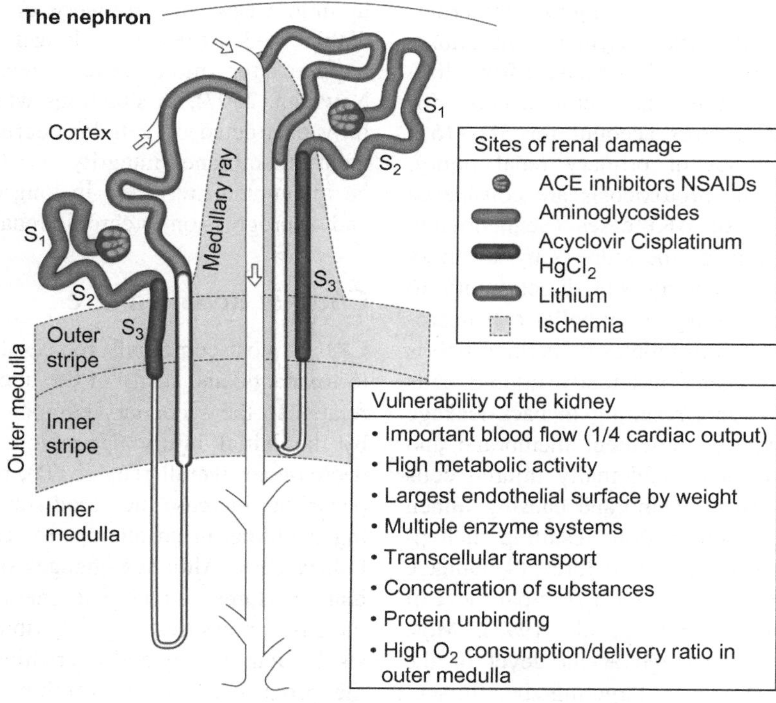

FIGURE 16.1 Sites of renal damage, including factors that contribute to the kidney's susceptibility to injury. *ACE*, angiotensin converting enzyme; *NSAIDs*, nonsteroidal antiinflammatory drugs; *$HgCl_2$*, mercuric chloride. Source: *Adapted from Berl, T., Bonaventure, J.V., 1998. Atlas of Diseases of Kidney. Schrier, R.W. (Ed.), Blackwell Publishing, Philadelphia, with permission.*

TABLE 16.1 Urinary Tract Toxicants Listed by Site of Injury

Toxicant	Species	Lesion	Comment
Glomerular Injury			
Bacterial endotoxin (hemolytic-uremia syndrome)	All	Mesangiolysis	Intravascular fibrin deposition of glomerular capillaries (Schwartzman reaction)
Crotalid snake venom	All	Mesangiolysis	Also tubular degeneration
Cyclosporine	Dogs, cats	Thrombotic microangiopathy	
Gold salts	Dogs	Membranous glomerulonephritis	Also acute tubular necrosis, vasculopathy, interstitial fibrosis
Mercury	Oxen	Membranous glomerulonephritis; proximal tubule degeneration and necrosis	Affects S_1 segment of proximal tubule
Proximal Tubular Injury			
Acer rubrum (red maple)	Horses	Acute tubular degeneration and necrosis; hemoglobin casts in tubules	
Acetaminophen	All	Acute tubular degeneration and necrosis	Metabolic activation results in damage to S_3; hepatotoxicity more common
Amaranthus spp.	Herbivores, especially pigs, calves	Acute tubular degeneration and necrosis; perirenal edema	See text for more information
Aminoglycoside antibiotics	All	Acute tubular degeneration and necrosis	Predominantly S_1 and S_2 segments; see text for more information
Amphotericin B	Dogs, cats	Acute tubular degeneration and necrosis; tubular dilatation; glomerular and interstitial mineralization	Arteriolar vasoconstriction results in decrease in GFR
Arsenic	All	Acute tubular degeneration and necrosis, cortical necrosis (dogs)	All segments
Cadmium	All	Acute tubular degeneration and necrosis	Glomerular injury reported in seals[a]
Cantharadin (blister beetle, *Epicuata* spp.)	Herbivores, especially horses	Acute tubular degeneration and necrosis; renal cortical hemorrhages; hyperemia and hemorrhage of mucosa of renal crest, ureter, bladder, urethra	Vesicant effect on mucosa of alimentary tract, cardiac lesions
Carbon tetrachloride	All	Tubular degeneration and necrosis	Hepatic injury most prominent
Cephalosporin antibiotics (and other β-lactam antibiotics)	All	Tubular degeneration and necrosis	High intracellular concentrations in S_3 segment due to action of organic ion transporter result in cell injury
Cholecalciferol (1,25-dihydroxy cholecalciferol, vitamin D_3), calcitriol, calcipotriene, *Cestrum diurnum*, *Solanum* spp., *Trisetum* spp.	All	Tubular degeneration and necrosis; mineralization	Renal ischemia due to vasoconstriction and mitochondrial calcification secondary to hypercalcemia[b]
Cisplatin	Dog	Tubular degeneration and necrosis	Primary effect on S_3 segment due to metabolic activation

(*Continued*)

TABLE 16.1 (Continued)

Toxicant	Species	Lesion	Comment
Citrinin	All species, pigs most common	Tubular degeneration and necrosis	Primary effect on S_2 segment, thick ascending limb, distal convoluted tubule and collecting ducts; see text for more information
Copper	Sheep, other ruminants less common	Tubular degeneration and necrosis; hemoglobinuric and bile nephrosis (gunmetal kidney)	Nonruminants develop liver injury without hemolysis
Ethylene glycol	All, dogs and cats most common	Tubular degeneration and necrosis; intratubular calcium oxalate crystals	Oxalate crystals may be found in vessels of meninges, heart, liver, intestinal mucosa; see text for more information
Lantana spp.	All grazing animals except horses	Tubular degeneration and necrosis	Lesions primarily in liver; secondary photosensitization; cardiac lesions
Lead	All	Tubular degeneration and necrosis; intranuclear inclusion bodies; karyomegaly of tubular epithelium	
Lilium spp., *Hemerocallis* spp.	Cats only	Tubular degeneration and necrosis; vascular fibrinoid necrosis	See text for more information
NSAIDs (see distal tubule section for phenylbutazone and flunixinmeglumine)	Dogs, cats, vultures, other species likely susceptible	Tubular degeneration and necrosis; occasionally papillary necrosis in dogs	See text for more information
OchratoxinA	All, pigs most commonly affected	Tubular degeneration and necrosis; cystic tubular dilatation; interstitial fibrosis; renal edema in chickens	Primary effect on S_3 segment due to bioactivation;[c] carcinogen; see text for more information
Oosporein	Chickens	Tubular degeneration and necrosis; interstitial pyogranulomatous inflammation and fibrosis	Periodic-acid-Schiff-positive granules in macula densa[d]
Oxalic acid, soluble oxalates (*Halogetonglomeratus*, *Sarcobatusverniculatus*, *Rheum rhaponicum*, *Rumex* spp., *Chenopodium*spp.)	All, ruminants and pigs most common	Tubular degeneration and necrosis; intratubular calcium oxalate crystals	Precipitation of soluble oxalates with serum calcium; hypocalcemic tetany possible
Paraquat	All	Tubular degeneration and necrosis	Pulmonary lesions most common effect (progressive pulmonary fibrosis); corrosive lesions in GI tract
Pine oil	Cats	Tubular degeneration and necrosis	Hepatic lesions more prominent
Pyrrolizidine alkaloids (*Amsinckia*, *Crotolaria*, *Cynoglossum*, *Echium*, *Heliotropium*, *Senecio* spp.)	All, predominantly horses, cattle, pigs	Tubular degeneration and necrosis; megalocytosis of tubular and glomerular cells	Hepatic lesions more prominent; secondary photosensitization, hepatic encephalopathy
Quercus spp. (Oaks)	Grazing animals, cattle most common	Tubular degeneration and necrosis; perirenal edema	See text for more information
Sulfonamide antibiotics	Ruminants	Tubular degeneration; grossly visible intratubular crystals	
Vitis spp. (grapes, raisins, Zante currants)	Dogs	Tubular degeneration and necrosis	See text for more information

(*Continued*)

TABLE 16.1 (Continued)

Toxicant	Species	Lesion	Comment
Zinc	All	Tubular degeneration and necrosis; hemoglobinuric nephrosis	
Distal Tubular/Collecting Duct Injury			
Fluoride	All	Distal tubular degeneration and necrosis	
Melamine:cyanuric acid	Dogs, cats, raccoon dogs, pigs, rats, fish; others likely susceptible	Distal tubular degeneration and necrosis; crystals in distal tubules and collecting ducts	See text for more information
Interstitial Injury			
Vicia spp. (vetch)	Grazing animals, primarily cattle	Eosinophilic granulomatous nephritis	Lesions can occur in any organ
Lower Urinary Tract Injury			
Cyclophosphamide	Dogs	Hemorrhage and necrosis of urinary bladder	Bioactivation and concentration of toxic metabolites in urine
Ptaquiloside (*Pteridium* spp., bracken fern)	Cattle	Necrosis and hemorrhage of urinary bladder; urinary bladder neoplasia	Enzootic hematuria
Ptaquiloside (*Sorghum* spp.)	Horses	Necrosis and hemorrhage of urinary bladder	Equine cystitis ataxia syndrome

[a]*Sonne-Hansen C, Dietz R, Lieffson PS, et al. (2002) Cadmium toxicity to ringed seals* (Phocahispida)*: an epidemiological study of possible cadmium-induced nephropathy and osteodystrophy in ringed seals* (Phocahispida) *from Qaanaaq in Northwest Greenland.* Sci Total Environ ***295:*** *167–181.*
[b]*Haschek WM, Rousseaux CG, Wallig MA (2007) Kidney and lower urinary tract. In* Fundamentals of Toxicologic Pathology, *second ed. Academic Press, San Diego, pp. 221–238.*
[c]*Boorman GA, McDonald MR, Imoto S, Persing R (1992) Renal lesions induced by ochratoxin A exposure in the F344 rat.* Toxicol Pathol ***20:*** *236–245.*
[d]*Brown TP, Fletcher OJ, Osuna O, Wyatt RD (1987) Microscopic and ultrastructural renal pathology of oosporein-induced toxicosis in broiler chicks.* Avian Dis***31:*** *868–877.*

Glomerular Injury

The glomerular capillaries are the first component of the nephron to be exposed to blood-borne toxicants. The glomerular cells, matrix and mesangium are susceptible to toxic injury by several different mechanisms including direct injury to cellular components, formation of oxygen-derived free radicals, disruption of extracellular substrates (e.g., basement membranes), immune-mediated injury and disruption of renal hemodynamics (Khan and Alden, 2002). Direct injury or injury secondary to reactive oxygen intermediates can result in endothelial loss, glomerular podocyte injury and necrosis of mesangial cells and substrate (mesangiolysis). Further damage may occur secondary to cytokines released by inflammatory cells responding to the site of injury. Alterations in the GBM subsequent to cellular injury can result in disruption of the glomerular filtration barrier, leading to proteinuria. Deposition of toxicant-immune complexes and immune-mediated reactions to various toxicants (e.g., mercurial, gold salts) can result in thickening of the GBM, disrupting the glomerular filtration barrier and leading to membranous glomerulonephropathy.

Proximal Tubular Injury

Tubular injury is the most common pattern of renal injury induced by toxicants and the proximal tubule is most frequently affected by nephrotoxicants (Schnellmann, 2008). Damage to the proximal tubule may occur from direct damage from toxicants, metabolic activation of toxicants, ischemia-reperfusion, or physical or chemical disruption of endothelium and/or basement membrane. The S_1 segment is the most vulnerable to injury from toxicants that exert direct injury as the epithelium in this area is exposed to the toxicant first. The proximal convoluted tubule epithelium is actively involved in endocytosis of various compounds that bind to the brush border, sequestering the compounds in phagolysosomes. When this process is overwhelmed by the presence of certain toxicants (e.g., aminoglycoside antibiotics), loss of phagolysosome membrane integrity occurs, resulting in lysosomal leakage and cell injury or necrosis (Khan and Alden, 2002). This type of injury is most commonly associated with the S_1 and S_2 segments of the proximal tubule. In contrast, the straight segment (S_3) is most susceptible to injury by metabolic activation, transporter-associated accumulation, and reperfusion injury.

Distal Nephron/Renal Papillary Injury

Toxic injury to the distal nephron is relatively uncommon, and injury to this area generally manifests as decreased urine concentration ability or defects in acid secretion. Injury to the renal papilla is most commonly seen with chronic consumption of nonsteroidal antiinflammatory drugs (NSAIDs), although the use of NSAIDs in hypovolemic animals or in conjunction with other nephrotoxicants (e.g., aminoglycoside antibiotics) has also been associated with the development of renal papillary necrosis (Talcott, 2006).

NEPHROTOXIC AGENTS

Mycotoxins

Ochratoxins

Ochratoxins are produced by various species of the fungi *Aspergillus* and *Penicillium* and are produced on a variety of cereal grains, cottonseed, nuts, dried beans and coffee beans (Haschek et al., 2002). Ochratoxin A (OTA) is the most common and most toxic of the ochratoxins that have been identified to date. The coproduction of penicillic acid by *Penicillium ochraeus* or citrinin by *Aspergillus* spp. or *Penicillium* spp. greatly enhances the toxicity of OTA (Haschek et al., 2002; Kumar et al., 2007). OTA is thought to be the causative factor in endemic Balkan nephropathy of humans (Maxie and Newman, 2007). Ochratoxin toxicosis has been reported in a variety of animal species including swine, ducklings, horses, chickens, rabbits, turkeys, dogs and fish (Kitchen et al., 1977; Haschek et al., 2002; Kumar et al., 2007; El-Sayed et al., 2009). Cattle are thought to be resistant due to degradation of ochratoxins within the rumen, although preruminant calves are susceptible (Haschek et al., 2002). In domestic animals, ochratoxicosis is most commonly reported in pigs and chickens as a subchronic to chronic disease affecting growth and production (Maxie and Newman, 2007; Sakthivelan and Sudhakar Rao, 2010). Pigs are considered to be the most sensitive species, with chronic toxicosis occurring following ingestion of diets containing 0.2–4 ppm OTA, while broiler chickens develop toxicosis at 2 ppm OTA (Haschek et al., 2002). The renal lesions in pigs consist of proximal tubular degeneration and atrophy with interstitial fibrosis and infiltration by mononuclear cells. Cystic dilatation of degenerated tubules occurs, which can lend a pitted, irregular appearance to the renal capsule; glomerular hyalinization may occur in severe cases. In acute cases, perirenal edema may occur (Maxie and Newman, 2007). Additional lesions of OTA toxicosis in pigs include multifocal necrotizing enteritis, fatty degeneration of the liver and lymphoid necrosis (Szczech et al., 1973). In broilers, OTA causes renal edema and renal tubular necrosis (Huff et al., 1975). OTA is teratogenic, mutagenic and carcinogenic, and it induces renal tumors in rat models (Haschek et al., 2002).

Citrinin

Citrinin is produced by toxic strains of several *Penicillium*, *Aspergillus* and *Monascus* spp. (Bennett and Klich, 2003), and has been associated with rice, wheat, oats, rye, corn, barley, vegetarian foods colored with red *Monascus* pigments, and naturally fermented sausages from Italy. Citrinin is often found in association with OTA and is less toxic than OTA (Kitabatake et al., 1993). Dogs receiving citrinin at dosages of 80 micromoles/kg intravenously or 10 mg/kg orally developed proteinuria, glucosuria, and ultrastructural changes in the epithelium of the S_2 segment, thick ascending limb, distal convoluted tubule and collecting ducts (Kitchen et al., 1977; Krejci et al., 1996). Dogs given oral 10 mg/kg citrinin twice at 24 h intervals developed similar lesions and developed glucosuria, proteinuria, and granular casts in the urine; glucosuria was the earliest abnormality noted and persisted for 5 days, as did proteinuria (Kogika et al., 1993). Cylindruria persisted from days 1 to 15, and renal values (BUN, creatinine) were elevated from days 2 to 5. Clinical signs in dogs administered 10 mg/kg citrinin per day for 14 days included anorexia, retching, tenesmus, weight loss, prostration, and death. Citrinin is teratogenic, embryotoxic, and a putative carcinogen.

Drugs

Aminoglycoside Antibiotics

Aminoglycoside antibiotics exert their nephrotoxic effects through induction of apoptosis and necrosis within the renal tubular epithelial cells of the proximal convoluted tubule as well as the distal tubules and collecting ducts (Lopez-Novoa et al., 2011). Within these cells, aminoglycosides internalized though endocytosis accumulate in lysosomes, Golgi apparatus and endoplasmic reticulum. As the aminoglycoside concentration increases beyond a threshold level, the endosomal membranes become disrupted and the drug leaks into the cytosol where it activates the intrinsic apoptotic pathway, increases production of reactive oxygen intermediates, and interacts with mitochondria to interrupt the respiratory chain. Interaction with endoplasmic reticulum and Golgi apparatus results in dysfunction of protein synthesis and packaging. In sublethally affected cells, aminoglycosides interfere with cell membrane transporter systems, altering tubular reabsorption and threatening epithelial cell viability. Cellular necrosis and apoptosis result in the accumulation of cellular residues in the tubular lumen, causing obstruction which increases the intratubular hydrostatic pressure. This back-pressure results in leakage of ultrafiltrate into the interstitium and peritubular capillaries and reduces the glomerular filtration pressure gradient, resulting in decrease in GFR. Aminoglycosides also have some direct glomerular effects including mesangial contraction, mesangial cell proliferation and alteration of filtration barrier selectivity. Toxicosis from aminoglycosides results in loss of urine concentration ability, polyuria, proteinuria, hematuria, cylindruria, azotemia and acute renal failure. In spite of the significant renal injury that may develop due to aminoglycoside exposure, the renal effects are generally considered reversible once the drug is withdrawn (Maxie and Newman, 2007). Additional adverse effects of aminoglycoside antibiotics include ototoxicity and induction of neuromuscular blockade.

NSAIDs

Nonsteroidal antiinflammatory drugs are the most widely used analgesics in veterinary medicine and are the most common drugs involved in accidental overdoses in companion animals (Sebastian et al., 2007; Gwaltney-Brant, 2007). In both therapeutic and overdose situations, the potential of most NSAIDs to have deleterious effects on the kidney must be considered. The adverse effects of NSAIDs on the kidney result from the inhibition of cyclooxygenases (COX) which results in decreased synthesis of PGs. COX has two distinct isoforms, COX-1 and COX-2. COX-1 is constitutively expressed in most tissues through the body, while COX-2 is normally expressed in tissues at low levels but can be induced in the presence of proinflammatory mediators that are expressed in sites of inflammation, pain or injury (Radi, 2009). COX-1 is the most abundant isoform expressed in the kidneys, and is located in the renal vasculature, collecting ducts and papillary interstitial cells. COX-2 is minimally expressed in the kidney and its localization within the different areas and impact on production of PGs in the kidney is species and maturation dependent. The kidney is a major site of PG synthesis, and PGs exert a variety of diverse functions within the kidney, including modulation of renal blood flow and GFR, regulation of sodium excretion and influencing renin release. PGs produced through the action of COX-1 are considered "protective," as inhibition of these PGs is associated with the majority of adverse effects from NSAIDs. NSAIDs such as ibuprofen are nonselective inhibitors of both COX isoforms, while newer NSAIDs may target COX-2, sparing COX-1 and resulting in fewer gastrointestinal and renal adverse effects (Khan and Alden, 2002). However, COX selectivity is species-dependent and can be lost in overdose situations. The primary impact of COX-induced inhibition of PG synthesis in the kidney is reduction of renal blood flow, resulting in ischemia. The medulla and renal papillae are at increased risk for NSAID-induced hypoxic injury due to their low oxygenation and relatively slow blood flow that predisposes to accumulation of toxic substances (Radi, 2009). Dogs, rats, mice, and pigs are thought to be most sensitive to NSAID-induced papillary necrosis (Khan and Alden, 2002). Clinical effects of NSAID-induced renal injury include polyuria, polydipsia, dehydration, electrolyte imbalances and azotemia. Acute renal failure, interstitial nephritis and nephrotic syndrome have also been reported. Nonrenal effects of NSAIDs include gastrointestinal ulceration.

Metals

Cadmium

The primary sources of exposure to cadmium are due to contamination of food, water and air. Cadmium in soil can be taken up by plants (Doris et al., 2002), and cadmium in water can bioaccumulate in shellfish. Inhalation exposure to cadmium can occur through exposure to industrial exhaust, fossil fuel combustion products and cigarette smoke; the latter is one of the major nonoccupational sources of inhaled cadmium in humans (Gwaltney-Brant, 2002). Acute cadmium toxicosis primarily manifests as pulmonary injury, while nephrotoxicity resulting from cadmium is most commonly due to chronic exposure. Cadmium is poorly absorbed via the gastrointestinal tract, with less than 5% of ingested cadmium being absorbed. Inhaled cadmium is more readily absorbed into the blood, where it binds to metallothionein, a 6800 Da, cysteine-rich protein. Metallothionein transports cadmium primarily to the kidney and liver, with lesser amounts accumulating in bone and testicle. The cadmium–metallothionein complex is filtered through the glomerulus and reabsorbed from the filtrate into the proximal renal tubules by endocytosis (Khan and Alden, 2002). Within the phagolysosome, metallothionein is hydrolyzed, which releases the cadmium; the free cadmium triggers the de novo synthesis of additional metallothionein. Once the level of intracellular cadmium exceeds a species-specific threshold of tolerance (10–200 μg/g wet weight), cellular injury progresses. Cadmium-injured renal epithelial cells have decreased reabsorptive capacity and decreased ability to concentrate urine (Gwaltney-Brant, 2002). Low molecular weight proteinuria (particularly β_2-microglobulinuria), amino aciduria, calciuria and glucosuria develop. Renal lesions include proximal tubular cell degeneration and necrosis, granular casts, hyaline casts, tubular atrophy, interstitial inflammation and interstitial fibrosis. Additional chronic renal lesions include nephrocalcinosis, fatty degeneration of pars recta tubular epithelium, and glomerular disease resembling immune complex glomerulonephritis. Extra-renal effects of cadmium include osteoporosis and osteopenia, hepatocellular necrosis, myocardial injury and testicular injury. Cadmium is a mutagen and putative carcinogen.

Lead

The incidence of lead toxicosis has declined in the United States since the banning of lead-based paints in residential domiciles in 1977 and leaded gasoline in 1996 (with significant reductions in use of leaded gasoline for the prior 20 years). However, lead is still present in the paint of many older homes as well as common household items such as toys, artists' paints, linoleum, lead weights, lead fishing sinkers and ornaments. Additionally, despite bans on the use of lead shot for hunting waterfowl, lead ammunition is still widely used on upland game, and lead toxicosis is still a significant cause of death among scavengers such as eagles and condors (Hunt et al., 2009; Stauber et al., 2010). Birds with lead toxicosis frequently present with emaciation and evidence of renal tubular degeneration (Pattee et al., 2006). Acute lead toxicosis is most commonly associated with neurological signs in mammals, while chronic lead toxicosis can result in dysfunction of a variety of organ systems including gastrointestinal, neuromuscular, central nervous, hematological and renal (Gwaltney-Brant, 2002). Degeneration and necrosis of proximal renal tubules results in oliguria, amino aciduria, glucosuria and altered tubular ion transport. Acute renal failure may occur following exposure to lead, but CRF is more common. Dense, homogeneous, eosinophilic intranuclear inclusion bodies may be visualized in affected renal tubular cells; although suggestive for lead toxicosis, these inclusions are not pathognomonic as they can occur following exposure to other metals such as bismuth.

Plants

Amaranthus spp.

The pigweed family includes several different species capable of producing toxicosis, but *Amaranthus retroflexus* is the species most commonly associated with disease in domestic animals (Burrows and Tyrl, 2001). Renal injury from pigweed has been reported in pigs, cattle and sheep. Other herbivorous species are likely susceptible, although the disease was not able to be reproduced in rabbits fed *A. retroflexus* (Schamber and Misek, 1985). The toxic principle is not known. Although pigweeds do contain some oxalates, the levels are low and the clinical syndrome and lesions caused by pigweed toxicosis are not consistent with those seen in oxalate nephrosis (Burrows and Tyrl, 2001). Clinical signs generally begin following several days of ingesting the plant, although renal lesions have been identified within 24 h of ingestion. Clinical signs include weakness, ataxia, knuckling of pasterns, recumbency, paralysis and coma; death occurs within 1–2 days of onset of signs. Gross lesions of pigweed toxicosis include widespread edema, most prominently around the kidneys, rectum and omentum. Kidneys are pale and normal to swollen in size. Histopathologic changes within the kidney include interstitial edema, scattered hemorrhages and proximal tubular degeneration and necrosis. Dilated tubules and tubules filled with necrotic debris are often present and interstitial fibrosis may be present in chronic cases. Extra-renal lesions include edema and ulceration of the digestive tract.

Lilium spp. and Hemerocallis spp.

Ingestion of some species of the genera *Lilium* and *Hemerocallis* by cats has resulted in potentially fatal renal dysfunction that has not been successfully reproduced in other species including dogs, rats, and rabbits (Rumbeiha et al., 2004). Although the toxic principle remains unknown, Rumbeiha et al. (2004) were able to demonstrate that the toxic effects originated from an aqueous floral extract of the Easter lily. All parts of the plant, including pollen, are toxic, and even small ingestions can result in significant renal injury (Fitzgerald, 2010). Prevention of serious renal injury can often be achieved if aggressive intravenous fluid therapy is instituted within the first 18 h following exposure. Clinical effects include vomiting, depression, polyuria, polydipsia, azotemia, glucosuria, proteinuria and isosthenuria. Serum creatinine levels tend to elevate disproportionately to blood urea nitrogen. Histopathologic lesions include proximal convoluted tubule degeneration and necrosis with denudation of basement membrane and filling of tubular lumens with cellular debris (Rumbeiha et al., 2004). Extra-renal lesions include vacuolar degeneration of pancreatic acinar cells.

Quercus spp.

Oak foliage and acorns provide forage to a variety of wildlife and livestock, but when oak is the primary source of feed for more than a few days, toxicosis can develop (Burrows and Tyrl, 2001). Oak buds, acorns and young leaves are involved in the majority of reported livestock poisonings, and most oak species have, at one time or another, been implicated in animal poisonings. Cattle are most commonly affected, and reports in other species such as horses, goats and sheep are rare. The primary toxic principles in oak are tannins, phenolic and polyphenolic compounds such as ellagic and gallic acids, and tannin metabolites such as pyrogallol. At toxic doses, oak tannins precipitate proteins in the digestive tract, causing erosions and ulcerations as well as altering mucosal absorption barriers. Increased absorption of polyphenolic tannins via injured mucosa results in damage to the liver and kidney; in rats, gallic acid was identified as the compound responsible for renal tubular necrosis (Harris et al., 1966). Clinical signs begin 2 days to a week or longer after animals have been consuming large amounts of oak. Affected cattle initially develop anorexia, depression, rumen stasis and constipation which are followed by diarrhea (+/− blood), dehydration, colic, polyuria and subcutaneous edema of ventral areas such as neck, brisket, abdomen and perineum (Panciera, 1978). Clinical pathologic evaluation of serum reveals metabolic acidosis, elevations in BUN and serum creatinine, and electrolyte abnormalities (e.g., hyperkalemia). Cattle with severe renal injury become weak and die, while less severely affected animals may survive, although many will become chronically debilitated due to persistent renal insufficiency (Burrows and Tyrl, 2001). The disease progression is similar in other species, though sheep and goats do not develop appreciable edema and horses tend to have more severe diarrhea (+/− blood), colic and tenesmus. Gross findings include fluid accumulations within body cavities, subcutaneous edema, mesenteric edema and retroperitoneal edema (especially perirenal). Kidneys are swollen, pale and may have petechiae within the cortex; chronic cases may have shrunken, irregular and fibrotic kidneys. Extra-renal lesions include edema, congestion, erosions and ulcerations of the alimentary tract mucosa and some cases may have hepatocellular degeneration.

Vitis spp.

Ingestion of members of *Vitis* spp., including grapes, raisins and Zante currants, has been associated with acute renal failure in dogs (Morrow et al., 2005) and, anecdotally, cats and ferrets (ASPCA Animal Poison Control Center, unpublished data). The toxic principle is unknown, but attempts to identify known nephrotoxins such as mycotoxins, pesticides, vitamin D_3 and heavy metals have been unsuccessful. Affected dogs generally demonstrate vomiting and/or diarrhea within 12 h of ingestion of grapes or raisins, accompanied by anorexia, lethargy and abdominal discomfort in some cases (Morrow et al., 2005). Severely affected dogs rapidly progress to anuria, and death or euthanasia occurs within 23−289 h. Histopathological changes in the kidney include renal tubular degeneration and necrosis, primarily in the proximal tubules. Extensive sloughing of proximal tubule epithelium results in extensive necrotic debris within tubular lumens. Extra-renal lesions consist of centrilobular hepatic degeneration or necrosis, myocardial necrosis, soft tissue mineralization and fibrinous arteritis in colon, myocardium and aorta.

Miscellaneous

Ethylene Glycol

The most common cause of ethylene glycol toxicosis in domestic animals is by consumption of automotive antifreeze, and dogs and cats are the most commonly affected species, although all mammals are susceptible to toxicosis. Ethylene glycol intoxication has three distinct stages: (1) initial CNS depression and derangement due to an alcohol-like effect on the brain, (2) profound metabolic acidosis with significant cardiorespiratory effects due to formation of acidic metabolites of ethylene glycol and (3) acute renal failure due to renal tubular injury (Thrall et al., 2006). Renal tubular injury is due to direct action of the nephrotoxic metabolites glycoaldehyde and glyoxylate on the renal tubules as well as mechanical injury and obstruction by calcium oxalate crystals (Thrall et al., 2006; Maxie and Newman, 2007). Calcium oxalate crystalluria is considered by some to be a hallmark of ethylene glycol, but crystalluria is present in less than half of all intoxications. Therefore, the absence of oxalate crystals does not eliminate ethylene glycol as a potential toxicant. Renal changes associated with ethylene glycol intoxication include pale, swollen kidneys which may be gritty when cut. Microscopically, proximal tubular degeneration and necrosis is associated with the deposition of birefringent, light yellow crystals arranged in sheaves, rosettes or prisms (Maxie and Newman, 2007). Oxalate crystals may also be found within tubular lumens, within renal tubular epithelial cells, and within the interstitium (Fig. 16.2). Animals surviving more than a few days may show areas of tubular regeneration and/or interstitial fibrosis. Extra-renal lesions may include deposition of oxalate crystals within small vessels of the brain, heart, liver and intestinal mucosa.

Melamine:Cyanuric Acid

In North America in 2007, the discovery of renal injury in dogs and cats ingesting commercial pet foods led to the recall of over 60 million cans and pouches of "cuts and gravy"-style pet food contaminated with melamine and cyanuric acid. The contamination was found to have originated in wheat gluten from China, where the melamine had been added to artificially inflate the apparent protein level of the product. Cyanuric acid is a hydrolysis product of melamine that may also have either been intentionally added or coincidentally present as a melamine by-product (Puschner et al., 2007). Subsequent to the pet food recall of 2007, the contamination of various food sources by melamine has been identified in several countries around the world including Italy, China, Spain, Korea, Taiwan, and other Asian countries (Brown et al., 2007; Gonzalez et al., 2009; Yhee et al., 2009; Brown and Brown, 2010; Cocch et al., 2010). Separately, melamine and cyanuric acid are of low toxicity, but in combination these compounds precipitate in acidic environments to form melamine cyanurate crystals (MCA) (Puschner et al., 2007). In animals ingesting feed containing melamine and cyanuric

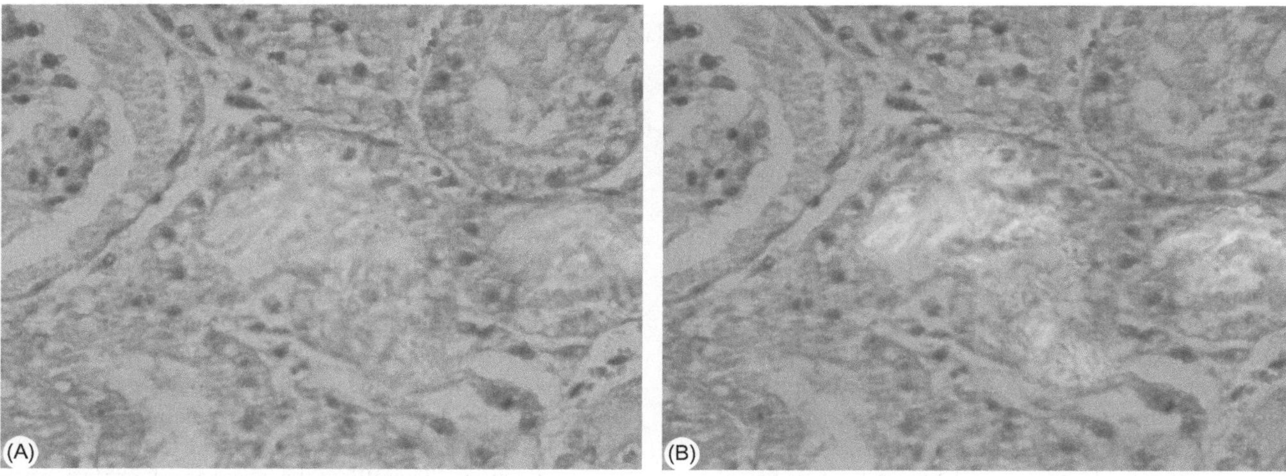

FIGURE 16.2 Ethylene glycol poisoning, canine kidney.

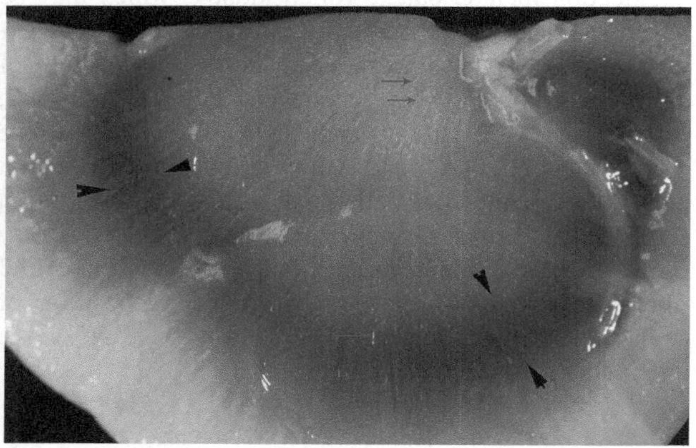

FIGURE 16.3 Melamine:cyanurate crystals, feline kidney. The corticomedullary junction is obscured by a broad, dark red band of hemorrhage (between black arrowheads). Fine dots to 0.1 cm long threads of an opaque, variably white to yellow substance (i.e., crystals) are observed (arrows). These crystals extend from the papilla of the medulla into the obscured corticomedullary junction and are in parallel with the medullary rays. They are most concentrated at the renal crest. Source: *Courtesy of Drs. Patricia Pesavento and Birgit Puschner, University of California, Davis.*

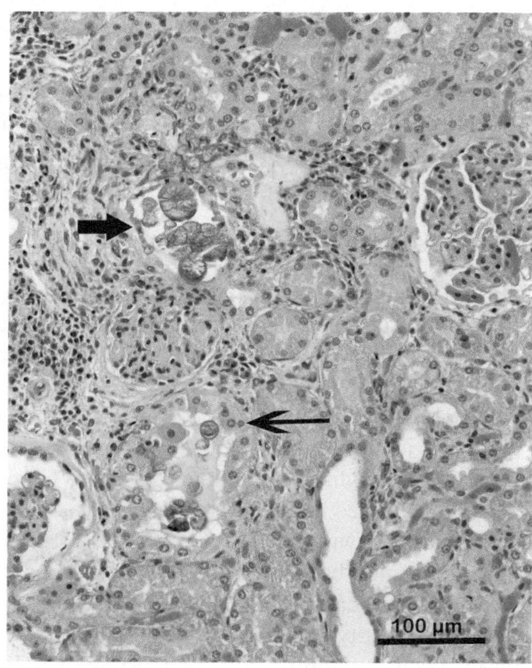

FIGURE 16.4 Melamine:cyanurate crystals, canine kidney. Renal tubular epithelium is attenuated and the lumen is expanded by variably sized, fan-shaped to starburst, gray-brown crystals (thick arrow). Another tubule has attenuated epithelium and detached and necrotic cells, proteinaceous fluid and smaller crystals within the lumen (thin arrow). Inflammatory cells are present within the adjacent interstitium. H&E, Bar = 100 μm. Source: *Courtesy of University of California, Davis Anatomic Pathology.*

acid, precipitation of MCA in the renal tubules has been associated with tubular injury, interstitial edema and renal failure. The exact mechanism of renal injury is not known, although mechanical injury from deposition of the large crystals is likely contributory. In cats, acute renal failure was induced within 48 h following oral administration of 32 mg/kg of melamine and cyanuric acid. MCA-induced nephropathy has been documented in humans, pigs, dogs, cats, fish, raccoon dogs, and rats (Reimschuessel et al., 2008; Bhalla et al., 2009; Gonzalez et al., 2009; Yhee et al., 2009; Brown and Brown, 2010), although most species are likely susceptible. Affected animals develop clinical signs typical of renal injury: vomiting, anorexia, lethargy, polyuria/oliguria and dehydration. Renal lesions include hemorrhage and edema of the interstitium, predominantly in the medullary region (Fig. 16.3). Degeneration and necrosis of the distal straight tubules is associated with the presence of large, translucent, pale yellow to brown, fan-shaped to starburst to globular crystals (Fig. 16.4) (Puschner et al., 2007). Crystals are also present in collecting ducts. The presence of these crystals in the more distal tubules, in addition to their morphology, can help to distinguish MCA from calcium oxalate crystals, which are found in the proximal tubules and tend to be smaller with variable shapes and sizes.

CONCLUDING REMARKS AND FUTURE DIRECTIONS

The vital role that the kidney plays in maintaining homeostasis makes renal injury due to nephrotoxic agents a serious and potentially life-threatening problem. In many instances, prevention of renal injury can be achieved through proper gastrointestinal decontamination and implementation of aggressive intravenous fluid therapy following exposure to nephrotoxicants. Once renal injury has developed, veterinary intervention is essential in order to support the patient through the acute crisis and to allow time for regeneration and repair of injured renal tissues. Depending on the extent of injury and degree of regeneration, the patient may fully recover, may be left with residual renal insufficiency, or may progress to CRF.

REFERENCES

Bennett, J.W., Klich, M., 2003. Mycotoxins. Clin. Microbiol. Rev. 16, 497–516.

Bhalla, V., Grimm, P.C., Chertow, G.M., Pao, A.C., 2009. Melamine nephrotoxicity: an emerging epidemic in an era of globalization. Kidney Int. 75, 774–779.

Brenner, B.M., Meyer, T.H., Hotstetter, T.H., 1982. Dietary protein intake and the progressive nature of kidney disease: the role of hemodynamically mediated glomerular injury in the pathogenesis of glomerular sclerosis in agina, renal ablation and intrinsic renal disease. N. Engl. J. Med. 307, 652–659.

Brezis, M., Rosen, S., Silva, P., 1984. Transport activity modifies thick ascending limb damage in isolate perfused kidney. Kidney Int. 25, 65–72.

Brown, C.A., Brown, S.A., 2010. Food and pharmaceuticals: lessons learned from global contaminations with melamine/cyanuric acid and diethylene glycol. Vet. Pathol. 47, 45–52.

Brown, C.A., Kyu-Shik, J., Poppenga, R.H., Puschner, B., et al., 2007. Outbreaks of renal failure associated with melamine and cyanuric acid in dogs and cats in 2004 and 2007. J. Vet. Diagn. Inv. 19, 525–531.

Burrows, G.E., Tyrl, R.J., 2001. Toxic Plants of North America. Iowa State Press, Ames IA, pp. 687–699.

Castro, T., Low, M., Salazar, K., et al., 2008. Differential distribution of the sodium-vitamin C cotransporter-1 along the proximal tubule of the mouse and human kidney. Kidney Int. 74, 1278–1286.

Cocch, M., Vascellari, M., Gallina, A., et al., 2010. Canine nephrotoxicosis induced by melamine-contaminated pet food in Italy. J. Vet. Med. Sci. 72, 103–107.

Counts, R.S., Nowak, G., Wyatt, R.D., Schnellmann, R.G., 1995. Nephrotoxicants inhibition of renal proximal tubule cell regeneration. Am. J. Physiol. 269, F274–F281.

Diamond, G.L., Zalups, R.K., 1998. Understanding renal toxicity of heavy metals. Toxicol. Pathol. 26, 92–103.

Doris, J., Atieh, B.H., Gupta, R.C., 2002. Cadmium uptake in radishes from soil contaminated with nickel-cadmium batteries: toxicity and safety considerations. Toxicol. Mech. Methods. 12, 265–276.

El-Sayed, Y.S., Khalil, R.H., Saad, T.T., 2009. Acute toxicity of ochratoxin-A in marine water-reared sea bass (Dicentrarchuslabrax L.). Chemosphere. 75, 878–882.

Fitzgerald, K.T., 2010. Lily toxicity in the cat. Top. Compan. Anim. Med. 25, 213–217.

Gonzalez, J., Puschner, B., Perez, V., et al., 2009. Nephrotoxicosis in Iberian piglets subsequent to exposure to melamine and derivatives in Spain between 2003 and 2006. J. Vet. Diagn. Inv. 21, 558–563.

Gwaltney-Brant, S.M., 2002. Heavy metals. In: second ed. Haschek, W. M., Rousseaux, C.G., Wallig, M.A. (Eds.), Handbook of Toxicologic Pathology, vol. 1. Academic Press, San Diego, CA, pp. 701–733.

Gwaltney-Brant, S.M., 2007. Epidemiology of animal poisonings. In: Gupta, R.C. (Ed.), Veterinary Toxicology: Basic and Clinical Principles. Academic Press, Elsevier, Amsterdam, pp. 67–73.

Harris, P.A., Zboralske, F.F., Rambo, O.N., et al., 1966. Toxicity studies on tannic acid administered by enema. 2. The colonic absorption and intraperitoneal toxicity of tannic acid on the colon and liver of rats. Am. J. Reontgenol. 96, 498–504.

Haschek, W.M., Voss, K.A., Beasley, V.R., 2002. Mycotoxins. In: second ed. Haschek, W.M., Rousseaux, C.G., Wallig, M.A. (Eds.), Handbook of Toxicologic Pathology, vol. 1. Academic Press, San Diego, CA, pp. 645–699.

Hosseininejad, M., Hosseini, F., 2008. Spontaneous manifestation of polycystic kidney disease following separation anxiety in a Persian cat. Pak. J. Biol. Sci. 11, 2171–2172.

Huff, W.E., Wyatt, R.D., Hamilton, P.B., 1975. Nephrotoxicity of dietary ochratoxinA in broiler chickens. Appl. Microbiol. 30, 48–51.

Hunt, W.G., Parish, C.N., Orr, K., Aquilar, R.F., 2009. Lead poisoning and the reintroduction of the California condor in northern Arizona. J. Avian. Med. Surg. B23, 145–150.

Khan, K.N.M., Alden, C.E., 2002. Kidney. In: second ed. Haschek, W. M., Rousseaux, C.G., Wallig, M.A. (Eds.), Handbook of Toxicologic Pathology, Vol. 2. Academic Press, San Diego, CA, pp. 255–336.

Kitabatake, N., Doi, E., Trivedi, A.B., 1993. Toxicity evaluation of the mycotoxins, citrinin and ochratoxin A, using several animal cell lines. Comp. Biochem. Physiol. C. 105, 429–433.

Kitchen, D.N., Carlton, W.W., Tuite, J., 1977. Ochratoxin A and citrinin induced nephrosis in beagle dogs. II. Pathology. Vet. Pathol. 14, 261–272.

Kogika, M.M., Hagiwara, M.K., Mirandola, R.M., 1993. Experimental citrinin nephrotoxicosis in dogs: renal function evaluation. Vet. Hum. Toxicol. 35, 136–140.

Kravola, S., Leva, L., Toman, M., 2010. Changes in lymphocyte function and subsets in dogs with naturally occurring chronic renal failure. Can. J. Vet. Res. 74, 124–129.

Krejci, M.E., Bretz, N.S., Koechel, D.A., 1996. Citrinin produces acute adverse changes in renal function and ultrastructure in pentobarbital-anesthetized dogs without concomitant reductions in [potassium] plasma. Toxicology. 106, 167–177.

Kumar, M., Dwivedi, P., Sharma, A.K., et al., 2007. Ochratoxin A and citrinin nephrotoxicity in New Zealand white rabbis: an ultrastructural assessment. Mycopathologia. 163, 21–30.

Langston, C., 2010. Acute uremia. In: seventh ed. Ettinger, S.J., Feldman, E.C. (Eds.), Textbook of Veterinary Internal Medicine, vol. 2. Saunders/Elsevier, St. Louis, pp. 1969–1984.

Lopez-Novoa, J.M., Quiros, Y., Vicente, L., et al., 2011. New insights into the mechanism of aminoglycoside nephrotoxicity: an integrative point of view. Kidney Int. 79, 33–45.

Maxie, M.G., Newman, S.J., 2007. Urinary system. In: fifth ed. Maxie, M.G. (Ed.), Pathology of Domestic Animals, Vol. 2. Saunders/Elsevier, Philadelphia, pp. 425–522.

Morrow, C.M.K., Valli, V.E., Volmer, P.A., Eubig, P.A., 2005. Canine renal pathology associated with grape or raisin ingestion. J. Vet. Diagn. Inv. 17, 223–231.

Panciera, R.J., 1978. Oak poisoning in cattle. In: Keeler, R.F., van Kampen, K.R., James, L.F. (Eds.), Effects of Poisonous Plants on Livestock. Academic Press, New York, pp. 499–506.

Pattee, O.H., Carpenter, J.W., Fritts, S.H., et al., 2006. Lead poisoning in captive Andean condors (Vulturgryphus). J. Wildl. Dis. 43, 566.

Polzin, D.J., 2010. Chronic kidney disease. In: seventh ed. Ettinger, S.J., Feldman, E.C. (Eds.), Textbook of Veterinary Internal Medicine, vol. 2. Saunders/Elsevier, St. Louis, pp. 1990–2021.

Puschner, B., Poppenga, R.H., Lowenstine, L.J., et al., 2007. Assessment of melamine and cyanuric acid toxicity in cats. J. Vet. Diagn. Inv. 19, 616–624.

Radi, Z.A., 2009. Pathophysiology of cyclooxygenase inhibition in animal models. Toxicol. Pathol. 37, 34–46.

Reimschuessel, R., Gieseker, C.M., Miller, R.A., et al., 2008. Evaluation of the renal effects of experimental feeding of melamine and cyanuric acid to fish and pigs. Am. J. Vet. Res. 69, 1217–1228.

Rumbeiha, W.K., Francis, J.A., Fitzgerald, S.D., et al., 2004. A comprehensive study of Easter lily poisoning in cats. J. Vet. Diagn. Inv. 16, 527–541.

Sakthivelan, S.M., Sudhakar Rao, G.V., 2010. Effect of ochratoxina on body weight, feed intake and feed conversion in broiler chickens. Vet. Med. Int. 2010, 590432.

Schamber, G.J., Misek, A.R., 1985. *Amaranthus retroflexus* (redroot pigweed): inability to cause renal toxicosis in rabbits. Am. J. Vet. Res. 46, 266–267.

Schnellmann, R.G., 2008. Toxic responses of the kidney. In: Klaassen, C. D. (Ed.), Casarett and Doul's Toxicology: The Basic Science of Poisons, seventh ed. McGraw-Hill Medical, New York, pp. 583–608.

Sebastian, M.M., Baskin, S.I., Czerwinski, S.E., 2007. Renal toxicity. In: Gupta, R.C. (Ed.), Veterinary Toxicology Basic and Clinical Principles. Academic Press/Elsevier, Amsterdam, pp. 161–176.

Stauber, E., Finch, N., Talcott, P.A., Gay, J.M., 2010. Lead poisoning of bald (Haliaeetus leucocephalus) and golden (Aquila chrysaetos) eagles I the U.S. inland Pacific northwest region – an 18-year retrospective study: 1991–2008. J. Avian. Med. Surg. 24, 279–287.

Szczech, G.M., Carlton, W.W., Tuite, J., Caldwell, R., 1973. Ocharatoxin A toxicosis in swine. Vet. Pathol. 10, 347–364.

Talcott, P.A., 2006. Nonsteroidal anti-inflammatories. In: Peterson, M. E., Talcott, P.A. (Eds.), Small Animal Toxicology, second ed. Saunders/Elsevier, St. Louis, pp. 902–933.

Thrall, M.A., Connally, H.E., Grauer, G.F., Hamar, D., 2006. Ethylene glycol. In: Peterson, M.E., Talcott, P.A. (Eds.), Small Animal Toxicology, second ed. Saunders/Elsevier, St. Louis, pp. 702–725.

Yhee, J.Y., Yu, C.H., Kim, J.H., Sur, J.H., 2008. Effects of T lymphocytes, interleukin-1 and interleukin-6 on renal fibrosis in canine end-stage renal disease. J. Vet. Diagn. Invest. 20, 585–592.

Yhee, J.Y., Brown, C.A., Yu, C.H., et al., 2009. Retrospective study of melamine/cyanuric acid-induced renal failure in dogs in Korea between 2003 and 2004. Vet. Pathol. 46, 348–354.

Chapter 17

Reproductive Toxicity and Endocrine Disruption

Tim J. Evans

INTRODUCTION

Reproduction is a critical biological process in all living systems and is required for species survival. Toxicant-induced abortions, congenital defects and infertility can have devastating effects on livestock production. Wildlife species living in environments contaminated by industrial and/or agricultural chemicals have experienced impaired fertility and declining populations. There is growing concern within the scientific community and among government regulatory agencies about the effects of occupational and environmental exposures to reproductive toxicants on human fertility.

For the purposes of this chapter, the term "reproduction" will be used primarily in reference to vertebrate species of animals (especially mammals) and will be inclusive of "development," which is sometimes treated as a separate topic in toxicology texts. This particular book chapter will emphasize the interactions between toxicants and the male and female reproductive tracts, as well as xenobiotic-induced effects on the growth, maturation and sexual differentiation of the embryo and fetus. Since "endocrine disruption" is an extremely common mechanism of action for xenobiotics associated with impaired reproductive function, reproductive toxicity and endocrine disruption will be discussed together in this chapter. Efforts will be made to clarify the current terminology related to reproductive toxicity and endocrine disruption and to introduce the reader to normal reproductive anatomy and physiology, as well as important concepts associated with embryonic and fetal development. Endocrine disruption in wildlife species and humans and the effects of xenobiotics, including endocrine disrupting chemicals (EDCs), on reproductive function in domestic animals will be discussed along with a brief description of proposed mechanisms of action and the effects of some selected reproductive toxicants.

Unfortunately, space constraints limit the amount of information which can be presented in this chapter, and many of the presented topics cannot be discussed at great length. There are a number of recently published textbooks and issues of journals which cover some of these subjects in greater detail and provide information which is complementary to what is presented in this chapter (Burrows and Tyrl, 2001; Plumlee, 2004; Naz, 2005; Golub, 2006a; Hood, 2006; Jobling and Tyler, 2006; Jørgensen et al., 2006b; Mukerjee, 2006; Gupta, 2017). The reader is directed to these publications and other references cited in this chapter in order to gain additional insight into specific areas of reproductive function and toxicology.

It is important that the reader understand that the areas of toxicology involving reproductive toxicity and endocrine disruption, in particular, are in continual flux. New data and exceptions to "classical" mechanisms of action are being reported on a regular basis, and there continues to be ongoing debate about the various aspects of normal as well as xenobiotic-induced abnormal reproductive function. Every effort has been made to accurately represent what is currently understood about the topics of discussion in this chapter. Controversial topics or those currently still subject to debate within the scientific community have been noted wherever possible.

IMPORTANT DEFINITIONS AND CONCEPTS

Reproduction

Reproduction in domestic, wild and laboratory vertebrates encompasses the wide range of physiological processes and associated behaviors and anatomical structures involved in the production of the next generation and

Veterinary Toxicology. DOI: http://dx.doi.org/10.1016/B978-0-12-811410-0.00017-9

the survival of a given species of animal (Senger, 2003). The physiological processes involved in reproduction generally include the following: (1) gametogenesis (production of sperm or ova) and the pre- and peri-pubertal changes leading up to its onset; (2) release of gametes (i.e., sperm transport and maturation, penile erection and ejaculation of sperm (mammals), copulation between a male and a female of the same species (several vertebrate classes) and ovulation of oocytes); (3) formation of the zygote (i.e., sperm storage, capacitation and other processes leading to fertilization, or union, of a single sperm with an egg); (4) embryonic and fetal development during the incubation process in egg-bearing vertebrates or, especially in the case of mammals, during pregnancy (gestation) (i.e., activities related to the initiation and progression of zygote cleavage, blastocyst formation, separation of the germ layers, placentation (mammalian species), neurulation and organogenesis (including sexual differentiation)); and finally (5) "birth" of a single or multiple offspring (hatching in oviparous vertebrates). In the conventional sense, the reproductive process culminates with birth or parturition (mammals); however, the initiation and maintenance of milk production (lactation) for the postpartum nutrition of offspring can also be considered a critical aspect of mammalian reproduction (Evans et al., 2007; Evans and Ganjam, 2017).

Reproductive Toxicity

For the purposes of this chapter, "reproductive toxicity" will refer to any manifestations of xenobiotic exposure reflecting adverse effects on the physiological processes and associated behaviors and/or anatomical structures involved in animal reproduction or development. This is a fairly broad definition which encompasses developmental toxicity, as well as any toxic effects of post-pubertal exposures to xenobiotics on either male or female reproduction. "Developmental toxicity" refers to any adverse effect on the developing organism associated with either pre-conception parental exposures to toxicants or post-conception xenobiotic exposures to the embryo, fetus or pre-pubertal offspring (Hodgson et al., 2000; Eaton and Klaassen, 2001; Foster and Gray, 2008). Adverse effects associated with developmental toxicity of xenobiotics might not necessarily be observed until after the affected individuals have reached sexual maturity (Foster and Gray, 2008; Rogers and Kavlock, 2008).

Teratogenesis

The term "teratogenesis" is derived from the Greek word for monster ("teras") and is a form of developmental toxicity (Panter, 2002; Rogers and Kavlock, 2008). "Teratogenesis" refers specifically to developmental defects induced by toxicant exposures occurring between conception and birth (Hodgson et al., 2000; Eaton and Klaassen, 2001; Rogers and Kavlock, 2008). The types of abnormalities that are typically associated with teratogenesis include embryonic or fetal death; morphological, functional and/or neurobehavioral abnormalities; and decreased growth rate and/or birth weight (Panter, 2002; Rogers and Kavlock, 2008).

Wilson's General Principles of Teratology

With respect to teratogenesis, there are six basic tenets of teratology, first defined by Wilson in 1959, which need to be kept in mind whenever gestational exposure to a teratogenic xenobiotic is suspected or when a chemical is being evaluated for its teratogenic potential. As stated by Wilson in the *Handbook of Teratology* (Wilson, 1977), the general principles of teratology are as follows:

1. Susceptibility to teratogenesis depends on the geno-type of the conceptus and the manner in which it interacts with environmental factors.
2. Susceptibility to teratogenic agents varies with the developmental stage at the time of exposure.
3. Teratogenic agents act in specific ways (mechanisms) on developing cells and tissues to initiate abnormal embryogenesis.
4. The final manifestations of abnormal development are death, malformation, growth retardation and functional disorder.
5. The access of adverse environmental influences to developing tissues depends on the nature of the influences (agent).
6. Manifestations of deviant development increase in degree as dosage increases from no effect to the totally lethal level.

Mechanisms of Reproductive Toxicity and Teratogenesis

There are a wide range of specific mechanisms of action by which xenobiotics can adversely affect reproductive function, including embryonic and fetal development. In general, many of these mechanisms are the same as those for toxicants affecting other organ systems and essentially involve some sort of toxicant-induced cellular dysregulation and alterations in cellular maintenance which, when possible, the body attempts to repair, either successfully or unsuccessfully (Gregus, 2008). Oxidative damage and interference with normal enzymatic reactions are two common mechanisms by which xenobiotics can cause the dysregulation and altered maintenance of cells within various organs and tissues.

Normal reproduction and development require, by their very nature (see review in this chapter), signaling within and between a variety of diverse organs. In sexual reproduction and mammalian pregnancy, critical communication even takes place between distinctly different organisms (i.e., male and female and mother and offspring, respectively). The dependency of reproductive function on signaling pathways inclusive of gene transcription makes this physiological process especially prone to adverse effects associated with xenobiotic-induced disruption of or interference with cell-to-cell, organ-to-organ and/or even animal-to-animal communication. Many of the mechanisms which interfere with physiological signaling activity can be classified as forms of "endocrine disruption," which will be discussed in much greater detail in this chapter.

There is a great deal of overlap between the various different mechanisms for reproductive toxicity. The level of exposure to a particular toxicant is an important determinant of what toxic effects are observed. Xenobiotics which "disrupt" endocrine pathways can do so without interactions with endogenous receptors, using mechanisms of action which can cause other forms of toxic insult at various dosages.

Reproductive Toxicants and Teratogens

Any xenobiotic associated with adverse effects on development or male or female reproductive function can be classified as a "reproductive toxicant." Xenobiotics capable of inducing teratogenesis are referred to as "teratogens." Although any chemicals adversely affecting animal well-being have the potential to have a negative impact on development and reproductive function, this chapter will attempt to focus on mechanisms of actions and toxicants which specifically target normal embryonic or fetal growth and maturation or have a direct effect upon the male and/or female reproductive tract.

Hormones and Hormone Receptors

The term "hormone" classically refers to a substance which is secreted into the circulation by a ductless gland and which alters the function of its target cells (Hodgson et al., 2000). While the traditional "endocrine" aspect of hormone action involves organ-to-organ signaling (and in the case of mammalian pregnancy animal-to-animal signaling), it is recognized that hormones can also be involved in "paracrine" (cell-to-cell) communication and signaling pathways within the same cell in which they were produced ("autocrine" function) (Evans et al., 2007; Evans and Ganjam, 2017). In vertebrates there are a wide variety of different hormones involved in reproductive function. The major reproductive hormones are generally grouped according to their basic molecular structure and include amino acid derivatives (e.g., dopamine or prolactin inhibitory factor (PIF) and melatonin); peptides (e.g., oxytocin, adrenocorticotropin hormone (ACTH), corticotropin releasing factor or hormone (CRF or CRH), gonadotropin releasing hormone (GnRH) and thyrotropin releasing hormone (TRH)); proteins (e.g., activin, inhibin, insulin-like growth factors, prolactin and relaxin); glycoproteins (e.g., follicle-stimulating hormone (FSH), luteinizing hormone (LH) and thyroid stimulating hormone (TSH or thyrotropin)); steroids (e.g., androgens, estrogens and progestagens); and eicosanoids, which include prostaglandins (Evans et al., 2007; Evans and Ganjam, 2017).

The actions of hormones on their targets are generally mediated through receptors which initiate or inhibit some sort of signal transduction pathway or are required for hormone-induced alterations in gene expression. Hormone–receptor interactions can be modulated by a number of factors including the amount of hormone present, the affinity of the hormone for the receptor, receptor density and occupancy and interaction with other hormones, receptors and hormone–receptor complexes, as well as a variety of endogenous co-activators and inhibitors (Genuth, 2004a; Bigsby et al., 2005). It should be clear by the end of this chapter that various xenobiotics are also capable, under certain exposure conditions, of modulating the interactions between endogenous hormones and their receptors.

Gonadal Steroid Hormones and their "Nuclear" Receptors

The primary gonadal steroids (i.e., androgens and estrogens (some references also include progesterone)) are also referred to as the "sex" steroids, and the imitation and/or inhibition of the actions of these hormones by xenobiotics is what was first referred to as "endocrine disruption" (Krimsky, 2000; McLachlan, 2001). The major androgens (testosterone and dihydrotestosterone (5α-reductase conversion product of testosterone in the testes and selected non-gonadal tissues)), estrogens (estradiol and estrone) and progesterone and endogenous progestagens facilitate the development and regulation of reproductive function in animal species, in large part by interacting with (i.e., functioning as ligands for) receptors which are members of the steroid/thyroid ("nuclear") receptor superfamily, the largest family of transcription factors in eukaryotic systems (Tsai and O'Malley, 1994; Genuth, 2004a). Receptors in this superfamily are large oligomeric proteins (Genuth, 2004a), which generally consist of five domains (A/B, C, D, E and F) (Tsai and O'Malley, 1994). Although specific portions of the gonadal steroid nuclear receptor molecules can interact with a variety of co-activators as well as inhibitors, the most important domains of these receptors are generally considered to be those involved in transactivation (*N*-terminal A/B domain; also C-terminus in estrogen receptors (ERs)); DNA-binding and hormone–receptor complex dimerization (middle portion containing two helical zinc fingers; C domain); and hormone (ligand) binding (C-terminus; E domain) (Genuth, 2004a; Bigsby et al., 2005). While androgen, estrogen and progesterone receptors, which are members of the steroid/thyroid superfamily, are often thought of as being exclusively nuclear in their location, these receptors can also be located in the cytoplasm of some cells (Tsai and O'Malley, 1994; Genuth, 2004a). Cytoplasmic and nuclear gonadal steroid receptors can be bound to a variety of different heat shock proteins, which interact with the receptor's hormone-binding domain. Heat shock proteins can act as "blocking" molecules and are displaced by hormones binding to the receptors (Genuth, 2004a; Bigsby et al., 2005) or as "chaperones" involved in receptor turnover and "trafficking" of these receptors between the nucleus and the cytoplasm (Pratt and Toft, 1997).

There is reportedly a single type of androgen receptor which is a member of the steroid/thyroid superfamily. In contrast, there are two types of nuclear ERs (ERα and ERβ), which are the products of distinct genes on separate chromosomes (O'Donnell et al., 2001). ERα and ERβ differ in their amino acid structure, tissue distribution, affinity for selective ER modulators (SERMs) and their role in female (Britt and Findlay, 2002) as well as, somewhat surprisingly, male fertility (O'Donnell et al., 2001; Hess, 2003). The nuclear progesterone receptor also has two isoforms, progesterone receptor A and progesterone receptor B (PRA and PRB, respectively), which differ slightly in their amino acid sequences and their interactions with co-activators. However, unlike ERα and ERβ, PRA and PRB are the products of a single gene (Brayman et al., 2006).

Genomic and Non-Genomic Mechanisms of Action of Gonadal Steroid Hormones

Traditionally, the receptor-mediated reproductive effects of gonadal steroids were thought to occur almost exclusively through interactions between homodimers of the hormone–nuclear receptor complexes and specific regions of DNA upstream from the basal promoter of a given gene, referred to as hormone-response elements (HREs) or, more specifically, androgen and estrogen-response elements (ARE and ERE, respectively) (Tsai and O'Malley, 1994; Genuth, 2004a). It is now understood that these "genomic" effects of gonadal steroids and their nuclear receptors, which involve alterations in gene transcription, can, in some instances, involve heterodimers of different nuclear steroid–receptor complexes, indirect binding of hormone–receptor complexes to DNA via proteins within a preformed transcriptional complexes and even ligand (hormone)-independent "activation" of nuclear gonadal steroid receptor molecules (O'Donnell et al., 2001; Bigsby et al., 2005; Thomas and Khan, 2005). In addition, it is also apparent that gonadal steroids can affect cellular function by non-genomic mechanisms of action involving changes in intracellular concentrations of ions, cAMP and its second messengers, and the mitogen-activated protein (MAP) kinase pathway. These non-genomic mechanisms are independent of the somewhat "time-consuming" alterations in gene expression traditionally associated with gonadal steroids and occur rapidly within seconds or minutes (O'Donnell et al., 2001; Thomas and Khan, 2005). While the rapid, non-genomic effects of gonadal steroids most likely involve receptors bound to the plasma membrane, the specific identity and classification of these receptors remain unclear and might involve a number of different receptor types (Razandi et al., 1999; O'Donnell et al., 2001; Thomas and Khan, 2005; Warner and Gustafsson, 2006).

Endocrine Disruption

"Endocrine disruption" is a developing, multidisciplinary area of research, involving aspects of both toxicology and endocrinology (McLachlan, 2001). "Endocrine disruption" is also a potential mechanism of action for many toxicants, and this term has been defined in a variety of different ways, depending on the circumstances and the intended audience. Some of these definitions can be fairly "broad," such as the one which will be used in this chapter (see below). However, "endocrine disruption" can also be defined fairly narrowly with respect to toxicant origin (synthetic versus naturally occurring); source or site of toxicant exposure (environmental contamination versus occupational exposure); xenobiotic mechanism of action (receptor agonism and/or antagonism (see definition below) versus other mechanisms independent of direct interactions between xenobiotics and receptors); and/or the timing of exposure (pre- natal versus postnatal exposures) (Krimsky, 2000, 2001). It is critically important for one to carefully define the context in which "endocrine disruption" is being used in order to clearly and accurately discuss one's research findings or opinions with toxicologists, physiologists, wildlife biologists, medical professionals, regulatory personnel, the popular press and/or the general public (McLachlan, 2001).

Although the imitation and/or inhibition of the actions of androgens and, especially, estrogens by xenobiotics is what was first referred to as "endocrine disruption," both the multidisciplinary area of study and mechanism of action generally referred to as "endocrine disruption" have evolved over the years to encompass a wide range of specific mechanisms of action which can ultimately result in adverse effects on invertebrate and/ or vertebrate animals (McLachlan, 2001). As scientists continue to investigate the effects of xenobiotics on biological systems, the paradigm of endocrine disruption will continue to "shift," and a willingness to "step out of the box" and discuss endocrine disruption in a broader context will be necessary in order to participate in scientific discussions, to design future experiments and/or to make informed, medical or policy decisions based on "good" science (McLachlan, 2001; Guillette, 2006). For the purposes of this chapter "endocrine disruption" will refer to the effects of any synthetic or naturally occurring xenobiotic which can affect the endocrine system of exposed individuals (i.e., the balance of normal hormonal functions) and, as a result of exposure, cause physiological alterations (Keith, 1997; Hodgson et al., 2000). Within the broad scope of this definition, reproduction, including prenatal and pre-pubertal development, certainly would be expected to be one of the physiological functions most profoundly affected by chemicals capable of endocrine disruption. In fact, it could be argued that the majority of reproductive toxicants interfere with endocrine function in one way or another. However, adverse effects on other, "non-reproductive" endocrine systems can also be associated with exposures to xenobiotics, and these "non-reproductive" effects need to be taken into consideration as well when describing the endocrine disruption associated with exposure to a given chemical (Guillette, 2006).

Mechanisms of Endocrine Disruption

Endocrine disruption encompasses a wide range of mechanisms of action which can ultimately result in adverse effects on animal species. The mechanisms of action involved in endocrine disruption can include effects which are mediated directly by interactions between the xenobiotic and an endogenous hormone receptor (i.e., the xenobiotic functions as a ligand for an endogenous receptor and a receptor–ligand complex is formed), as well as those adverse effects which alter hormonal functions without direct interactions between the toxicant and an endogenous receptor (Keith, 1997). In addition, it should be noted that some xenobiotics are capable of causing endocrine disruption by functioning as an endogenous hormone receptor ligand, as well as by mechanisms of action which are independent of the formation of a xenobiotic (ligand)–receptor complex.

"Classic" Receptor-Mediated Endocrine Disruption

"Classic" endocrine disruption can involve imitation or mimicry of the interactions between cellular receptors and endogenous hormones (i.e., receptor agonism) and/or a blockade or inhibition of the formation of receptor–hormone complexes (i.e., receptor antagonism) (McLachlan, 2001). With respect to gonadal steroids, both genomic and non-genomic physiological responses can be affected by this mimicry or blockade of endogenous hormone receptor-mediated activity (Thomas and Khan, 2005). Xenobiotics which mimic the actions of endogenous androgens or estrogens (i.e., gonadal steroid receptor agonists) are referred to, respectively, as being either "xenoandrogens" or "xenoestrogens." Conversely, reproductive toxicants which inhibit or block endogenous estrogens or androgens from interacting with their respective receptors (i.e., gonadal receptor antagonists) are generally classified as "antiandrogens" or "antiestrogens." Progestagens" ("progestogens" or "progestins" in some literature) is a generic term for endogenous or synthetic compounds which interact with progesterone receptors, and there is evidence of increasing environmental contamination with these types of EDCs.

Some xenobiotics can act as receptor agonists or antagonists, depending on the circumstances or tissues involved. "Selective ER modulators" or "SERMs" refer to a class of xenobiotics which, although originally classified as antiestrogens, can function as either ER agonists or antagonists, depending on the tissue in which estrogen-dependent responses are being discussed (Dutertre and Smith, 2000; Katzenellenbogen and Katzenellenbogen, 2000). SERMs are particularly relevant with respect to observed differences in their binding affinities to ERα or ERβ and their development as therapeutic agents for different types of estrogen-responsive neoplasia.

Endocrine Disruption Independent of Receptor-Mediated Interactions

Endocrine disruption which is independent of interactions between xenobiotics and endogenous hormone receptors can occur in a variety of different ways. Xenobiotic exposure can result in alterations in the number of hormone receptor sites (up- or down-regulation) or can cause direct or indirect hormone modifications which alter hormonal function (Keith, 1997). Xenobiotics can change the rate of synthesis or destruction of endogenous hormones and can alter how hormones are stored, how they are released into and/or transported within the circulation or even how they are eventually cleared from the body (Keith, 1997; Sikka et al., 2005). Any xenobiotic which is toxic to organs or tissues producing hormones (e.g., testis and ovary) has the potential to decrease hormone synthesis and thereby indirectly cause endocrine disruption (Devine and Hoyer, 2005). It should also be noted that some of these mechanisms of endocrine disruption are not necessarily exclusive of one another. A given xenobiotic can potentially disrupt the normal balance of hormonal function by more than one mechanism which is independent of direct interactions between the toxicant and an endogenous hormone receptor.

"Androgenic" and "Estrogenic" Effects of Xenobiotics

The terms "androgenic" and "estrogenic" and their antonyms "antiandrogenic" and "antiestrogenic" have been used in a number of different contexts. Some authors have used these terms to refer specifically to the agonistic and antagonistic receptor interactions of xenobiotics (Hodgson et al., 2000). Because the precise mechanism of endocrine disruption of a given toxicant might not always be known or might involve multiple mechanisms of action, these terms have also been used in a more general sense, especially in livestock and wildlife species, to refer to phenotypic changes which were similar to or the opposite of the effects which would be expected with exposure to endogenous androgens or estrogens (Guillette, 2006). This type of general usage can be helpful in some instances but can also be confusing, given that xenoandrogens and progestagens frequently have the opposite phenotypic effects as xenoestrogens. For instance, the effects of estrogenic xenobiotics can be described as antiandrogenic or anti-progestagenic in some instances, while the effects of xenoandrogens and progestagens can be referred to as being antiestrogenic in nature. Further confusion can be associated with exposures to mixtures of chemicals having different phenotypic effects, as is often the case in instances of environmental contamination, or with exposures to xenobiotics having mixed antiestrogenic and antiandrogenic effects (i.e., methoxychlor). When the terms "androgenic," "estrogenic" or their antonyms are used within this chapter, an attempt will be made to clearly denote the intended specific or general meaning of the terms in the context in which they are used. The discretionary use of the terms "feminization" and "masculinization," as well as "defeminization" and "demasculinization," can also, in some instances, help to clarify and/or describe the phenotypic effects of a chemical suspected of endocrine disruption.

Endocrine Disrupting Chemicals, Endocrine Disruptors and Hormonally Active Agents

Any reproductive toxicant capable of endocrine disruption can be considered an "EDC" or an "endocrine disruptor." Obviously, this includes a large number of xenobiotics which are used in commercially available industrial, agricultural and pharmaceutical products, as well as naturally occurring toxicants produced by plants and fungi. An effort will be made later in this chapter to discuss some of the xenobiotics most often associated with endocrine disrupting mechanisms of action.

Another term frequently used with respect to endocrine disruption, especially regarding xenobiotics which interact with endogenous hormone receptors, is "hormonally active agent" or "HAA." In most instances, "endocrine disrupting chemical," "endocrine disruptor" or "hormonally active agent" can be used interchangeably to discuss the actions of a given xenobiotic. However, whereas "endocrine disrupting chemical" and "endocrine disruptor" generally have negative connotations and imply, by virtue of the inclusion of the term "disrupt," something "dangerous" and the likelihood of adverse or toxic effects, the term "hormonally active agent" is more benign and only indicates that a given xenobiotic has the potential to affect a hormonal pathway in an animal (Krimsky, 2001). As pointed out by Krimsky (2001), a mechanism rather than a specific pathology is inferred by "hormonally active," and "hormonally active agent" is the nomenclature preferred by the National Research Council (Knobil, 1999), especially when referring to xenobiotics which interact with endogenous hormone receptors.

The circumstances and intended audience will often dictate the terms used to describe xenobiotics associated with or suspected of being having endocrine activity. "Environmental hormone" and "environmental signal" have also been used, along with "HAA," "EDC" and endocrine disruptor, to describe xenobiotics capable of interacting with endogenous hormone receptors (McLachlan, 2001; McLachlan et al., 2006). However, the context in which these two terms have been routinely used generally implies environmental contaminants with documented adverse endocrine effects on animals or humans. In some instances, the term "HAA" might be more "politically correct" (Krimsky, 2001) than "EDC," "endocrine disruptor," "environmental hormone" or "environmental signal" when discussing chemicals with a suspected hormonal activity that has not been clearly associated with adverse effects on animals in a research and/or clinical setting.

Aryl Hydrocarbon Receptor-Mediated Endocrine Disruption

Endocrine disruption mediated by the aryl hydrocarbon receptor (AhR) is a relatively complex, species- and tissue-dependent phenomenon, involving several of the previously described mechanisms of EDC action and interactions with many important, environmentally persistent compounds. Some aspects of AhR-mediated endocrine disruption are reminiscent of the ligand-induced transcription associated with gonadal steroid receptor function. However, the unique nature of the endogenous AhR and its interactions with primarily xenobiotic agonists warrants further discussion.

Aryl Hydrocarbon Receptor Agonists

The major agonists for the AhR protein belong to the class of environmental contaminants referred to collectively as "halogenated" or "polyhalogenated aromatic hydro-carbons" (HAHs or PAHs, respectively) and includes many highly stable and lipophilic organochlorine industrial chemicals (e.g., polycyclic aromatic hydrocarbons (PAHs), polychlorinated biphenyls (PCBs), polychlorinated dibenzo-*p*-dioxins (PCDDs) and polychlorinated dibenzodifurans (PCDFs)), as well as their metabolites (Safe, 2005). In addition, other organic compounds, such as polycyclic aromatic hydrocarbons (PAHs) (e.g., 3-methylcholanthrene and benzo[a]pyrene) (BaP)) and flavones (e.g., β-naphthoflavone), have also been shown to be AhR agonists (Parkinson and Ogilvie, 2008).

Mechanisms of Aryl Hydrocarbon Receptor-Mediated Endocrine Disruption

Many of the mechanisms of action mediated by AhR–ligand interactions have been elucidated using 2,3,7,8-tetrachlorodibenzo-*p*-dioxin (TCDD) as a prototypical AhR agonist (Safe, 2005; Parkinson and Ogilvie, 2008). TCDD is considered by many to be the most toxic of all of the HAHs, and it is reported to have the highest AhR-binding affinity of any of the xenobiotics in that class of chemicals (Safe, 2005). The AhR, also referred to as the "dioxin receptor," is located in the cytoplasm bound to heat shock proteins (Parkinson and Ogilvie, 2008). Following ligand (i.e., TCDD) binding and the subsequent disassociation of the heat shock proteins, the AhR is activated by phosphorylation (Parkinson and Ogilvie, 2008) and the activated ligand–AhR complex undergoes a rapid sequence of events involving interactions with the AhR nuclear translocator protein (Arnt) and relocation of the ligand–AhR–Arnt complex into the nucleus (Safe, 2005).

Within the nucleus, the liganded AhR/Arnt heterodimer can facilitate a variety of endocrine disrupting mechanisms. This activated heterodimer complex can interact with dioxin/xenobiotic-response elements (DREs/XREs), which function in much the same way as the previously discussed HREs, and with various co-activators to increase the expression of selected genes (Safe, 2005; Parkinson and Ogilvie, 2008). Depending on the animal species and the tissue, multiple-phase I drug-metabolizing enzymes (e.g., cytochrome P450 (CYP) enzymes (CYP1A1, CYP1A2 and CYP1B1)) and enzymes involved in phase II drug-biotransformation reactions (e.g., glutathione-*S*-transferase and glucuronosyl transferase), are induced by TCDD (Safe, 2005).

Although the antiandrogenic and antiestrogenic properties of TCDD have been associated with the ability of HAHs to induce enzymes involved in androgen and estrogen metabolism, TCDD can interact with androgen-, estrogen- and progestagen-modulated pathways in a number of ways, including interference with neuroendocrine development (Petersen et al., 2006). AhR-mediated effects of TCDD can interfere with the biosynthesis of testosterone by a mechanism which alters the regulation of the synthesis and release of LH (Sikka et al., 2005). It has also been shown in cell cultures that TCDD can disrupt testosterone signal transduction pathways (Jana et al., 1999). The liganded AhR/Arnt heterodimer appears to be able to interact with inhibitory DREs (iDREs) in selected tissues to suppress the expression of some genes induced by estrogens (Safe, 2005), as well as be able to actually block the ability of estrogen–ER complexes to bind to their HREs (Kharat and Saatcioglu, 1996; Thomas and Khan, 2005). It is likely that a variety of other means of crosstalk between TCDD- and estrogen-mediated signaling pathways exist, and, in fact, TCDD has actually been shown to have the potential for estrogenic activity through interactions between liganded AhR/Arnt heterodimers and unliganded ERs (both ERα and ERβ) (Ohtake et al., 2003; Bigsby et al., 2005; Thomas and Khan, 2005). Ohtake et al. (2003) have reported that these novel interactions resulted in the recruitment of unliganded ERs and p300 co-activator to gene promoters which are responsive to estrogens. Based on the results of the various experiments performed with TCDD, it is important to remember that the effects observed following exposure to HAHs and EDCs, in general, can be dependent on animal species involved, as well as the type of tissue, organ or physiological response being evaluated.

Epigenetic Mechanisms of Action of Endocrine Disrupting Chemicals

In recent years there has been increasing interest in the association between prenatal exposures to some reproductive toxicants and the postnatal development of neoplasia (cancer) involving the reproductive tract, as well as the occurrence of transgenerational or vertically transmitted adverse reproductive effects (Crews and McLachlan, 2006). These two phenomena are not mutually exclusive of one another, and, in fact, there is increasing evidence of vertically transmitted neoplasia involving reproductive organs (McLachlan et al., 2006). Both tumor formation and transgenerational reproductive abnormalities can occur because of "genetic" mutations or alterations in the genotype (i.e., DNA sequence) or as a result of "epigenetic" changes where there are heritable modifications in the properties of a cell which do not represent genetic changes (inherited phenotypic alteration without genotypic change) (Lewin, 1998; McLachlan, 2001; Crews and McLachlan, 2006).

Epigenetic changes are a normal part of development and most likely represent one means for heritable environmental adaptation (Crews and McLachlan, 2006). One of the more common mechanisms of epigenetic modification in mammals is DNA methylation of CpG nucleotides in the promoter regions of genes, which results in methylated genes being "turned off" and unmethylated or demethylated genes being "turned on" (McLachlan, 2001; Anway and Skinner, 2006). Patterns of DNA methylation are generally established during development at the gastrulation stage (i.e., lineage-specific pattern in somatic cells) and after sex determination (i.e., germ line-specific lineage pattern in the gonad) (Anway and Skinner, 2006). DNA methylation can facilitate "genomic imprinting," a form of epigenetic gene regulation resulting in the expression of the allele from only one parent (i.e., monoallelic expression) (McLachlan, 2001; Anway and Skinner, 2006). The ability of developmental exposures to xenobiotics to provide a basis for adult disease, such as neoplasia, might very likely involve epigenetic changes involving methylation or demethylation of the promoters for specific genes (Newbold et al., 2006). Epigenetic modification by alterations in DNA methylation patterns in the germ line might be one mechanism for observed xenobiotic-induced transgenerational (vertically transmitted) effects associated with infertility and tumor susceptibility in rodents (Anway and Skinner, 2006; Newbold et al., 2006).

Disruption of "Non-Reproductive" Endocrine Systems

Although it can be argued that almost all endocrine systems are "reproductive" to some extent, there are multiple systems with primary functions which are not directly related to reproduction, and several of these systems have also been identified as potential targets of EDCs. In addition, gonadal steroids and xenobiotics which mimic these endogenous hormones can have "non-reproductive" effects. The synthesis of triiodothyronine (T_3) and thyroxine (T_4) by the thyroid gland can be decreased by chemicals which inhibit the uptake of iodine (e.g., perchlorate and thiocyanate) and also by xenobiotics which inhibit thyroperoxidase (e.g., thiourea, propylthiourea (PTU), some sulfonamides, methimazole, carbimazole, aminotriazole and acetoacetamide) (Capen, 2008). Polybrominated diphenyl ethers (PBDEs) have been shown to have antithyroidal activity (Guillette, 2006), and thyroid hormone secretion can be inhibited by exposure to excessive amounts of iodine or lithium (Capen, 2008). Xenobiotics, such as the *o,p*′-DDD metabolite of dichlorodiphenyltrichloroethane (DDT), can interfere with glucocorticoid metabolism (Guillette, 2006), and there has been increasing interest in the relationship between gestational and neonatal exposures to xenoestrogens and the development of obesity (Cooke and Naz, 2005; Newbold et al., 2005, 2006). Some EDCs (e.g., organotin compounds) have recently been described as "obesogens" because of their ability to affect adipogenesis by several different mechanisms, including interactions involving the isoforms of 11β-hydroxysteroid dehydrogenase (11β-HSD) which play key roles in glucocorticoid metabolism (Grün and Blumberg, 2006). Because of increased societal concerns about obesity, there is likely to be greater future interest in organotins and other EDCs with similar "obesogenic" activities.

NORMAL ANIMAL REPRODUCTION

Reproduction is a complex and dynamic process involving precise coordination and integration of the functions of multiple organs within the body. The production of viable and functional gametes and their transport and union to form a zygote which develops into a healthy and fertile individual require that many stringent physiological and metabolic needs be met. A thorough understanding of the mechanisms involved in reproduction is absolutely essential in order to recognize which steps in the reproductive process are most susceptible to the adverse effects of potential toxicants. It is critical that one be able to understand the pathophysiological basis for reproductive abnormalities. In addition, it is necessary, from a clinical perspective, to identify what constitutes "normal" reproduction in order to recognize abnormal reproductive behaviors and morphological changes in both domestic and wild animals. Impaired reproductive function in domestic animals, which is associated with exposure to toxic amounts of xenobiotics, necessitates the use of diagnostic, prognostic and therapeutic procedures which require a thorough knowledge of normal reproductive anatomy and physiology.

Normal reproduction will be reviewed in this chapter to provide a basis for discussion concerning specific reproductive toxicants. Although the emphasis will be on mammalian reproduction, many of the principles will be applicable to other classes of vertebrates. If additional information is needed, textbooks are available which provide a comprehensive overview of animal reproduction (Hafez and Hafez, 2000; Senger, 2003), as well as general veterinary anatomy (Dyce et al., 2002). Other references can be consulted for descriptions of various aspects of normal reproduction in species of domestic or laboratory animals, which might be of particular interest to the reader (Johnston et al., 2002; Hedrich and Bullock, 2004; Suckow et al., 2006; Youngquist and Threlfall, 2007).

Neuroendocrine Control of Reproduction

In humans and animals alike, visual, olfactory, auditory and other sensory data are integrated within the brain and are reflected in endocrine events. The neuroendocrine functions of the pineal gland, hypothalamus and pituitary gland play an important role in the integration and endocrine regulation of the body's physiological processes and are potential targets for many reproductive toxicants (i.e., dioxins). These structures within the brain and proper function of the hypothalamic–pituitary–gonadal axis facilitate development of the reproductive tract and endocrine regulation of spermatogenesis in the male and the estrous or menstrual cycle in the female. The onset of puberty and sexual behavior in males and females, the ability to achieve erection and ejaculation in males, and the normal progression of gestation, parturition and lactation in females are all affected by the secretions of the hypothalamus and pituitary gland, as well as interactions between these structures and the reproductive tract (Ginther, 1992; Senger, 2003; Evans et al., 2007; Evans and Ganjam, 2017).

The hormones involved in the neuroendocrine control of reproduction are produced in several regions of the brain. Melatonin is produced in the pineal gland. The major hormones of reproductive interest which are of hypothalamic origin are dopamine, CRF, GnRH and TRH. Oxytocin is released from the posterior pituitary (neurohypophysis), and ACTH, FSH, LH, prolactin and TSH are synthesized and released from the anterior pituitary (adenohypophysis) (Ginther, 1992; Evans et al., 2007; Evans and Ganjam, 2017). The production and release of these hormones are regulated by various positive and negative feedback loops, which are potentially susceptible to the effects of hormonally active xenobiotics.

Puberty

The Onset of Puberty

Puberty in male and female offspring implies reproductive competence and corresponds to the onset of normal spermatogenesis in the male and reproductive cyclicity in the female. Puberty can be indicated in the female by the age at first estrus or ovulation or even the age at which pregnancy can be maintained safely (Senger, 2003; Evans et al., 2007; Evans and Ganjam, 2017). In the male, the age at the time of preputial separation and the acquisition of the ability to ejaculate or the age at the first appearance of spermatozoa in the ejaculate or urine, as well as the production of threshold concentrations of fertile sperm in the ejaculate, have all been used as indicators of puberty (Senger, 2003). Species, nutritional status, environmental and social factors, pheromones and photoperiod in short- or long-day breeders can all influence the age of onset of puberty in animal species (Senger, 2003; Evans et al., 2007; Evans and Ganjam, 2017).

The Endocrinology of Puberty

From an endocrine perspective, puberty is associated with the ability of the hypothalamus to release enough GnRH to induce gonadotropin production by the anterior pituitary gland (Senger, 2003). This endocrine milestone is brought about by the postnatal developmental changes which allow the hypothalamus to overcome the negative feedback of testicular androgens and estrogens in males and which facilitate the ovary's ability to produce sufficient estrogens to induce the preovulatory surge of GnRH in females (Senger, 2003; Evans et al., 2007; Evans and Ganjam, 2017). Many of the endocrine changes which come into play with the onset of puberty are also involved in the transition from anestrus to the ovulatory season in seasonally polyestrous female animals (Evans et al., 2007; Evans and Ganjam, 2017).

The Susceptibility of the Pubertal Process to Reproductive Toxicants

While puberty is often described simply in terms of a single, initial reproductive event (e.g., first estrus, ovulation or ejaculation), the attainment of reproductive competency is actually a process which is susceptible to the effects of reproductive toxicants. Xenobiotics can interfere with important physiological and morphological transformations necessary for the normal stepwise progression toward reproductive competency. Pre-pubertal follicular development, as well as the onset of the preovulatory LH surge in the female and the transition in testicular estrogen synthesis from the Sertoli cell to the Leydig cell in the males of many species, in addition to the postnatal proliferation of Sertoli cells in some mammals, are all potentially susceptible to the adverse effects of xenobiotics. Pre- or peri-pubertal exposure to hormonally active xenobiotics, such as anabolic steroids and antiandrogens, can interfere with postnatal reproductive development and function and can impair an animal's ability to reach its maximum reproductive potential (Monosson et al., 1999; Evans et al., 2007; Evans, 2011a; Evans and Ganjam, 2017).

Normal Male Reproductive Anatomy and Physiology

Reproductive Anatomy of the Male

Anatomical structures associated with reproduction in the male usually include, especially in mammals, paired testes (male gonads) positioned outside the abdominal cavity in most species; an excurrent duct system (i.e., efferent ductules, paired epididymides, vas deferens and urethra); accessory sex glands (i.e., ampullae, seminal vesicles, prostate and bulbourethral glands); a scrotum and its associated thermoregulatory functions to protect the testes from mechanical and thermal insult and some form of copulatory organ or penis with a mechanism for protrusion, erection, emission of glandular secretions and ejaculation of sperm. The primary functions of the testis (testicle) are spermatogenesis (production of male gametes (sperm or spermatozoa)) and steroidogenesis (production of androgens and estrogens). Unlike the female in which oogonia are no longer replicating and the full complement of potential oocytes are present at birth, spermatogonia are proliferating and differentiating into spermatozoa continuously, and the testis is organized in such a way as to maximize sperm production (Senger, 2003; Evans and Ganjam, 2017).

Testicular Structure

The parenchyma of the testis is divided into the tubular and interstitial compartments (Senger, 2003; Evans and Ganjam, 2017) (Figure 17.1A). The structural and functional units of the testis are the seminiferous tubules within the tubular compartment and the Leydig (interstitial cells) within the interstitial compartment. Depending on the species, it is estimated that the seminiferous tubules comprise approximately 80% of the adult testis, with the interstitium comprising most of the remaining 20% (Genuth, 2004b). Seminiferous tubules form highly convoluted loops (tubulus contortus) which begin and end with straight portions (tubulus rectus) that connect to the rete tubules (Thomas and Thomas, 2001; Genuth, 2004b; Senger, 2003; Evans and Ganjam, 2017). In some species, the rete tubules coalesce in a fibrous region of the testis referred to as the mediastinum, which joins with septal projections of the tunica albuginea, part of the testicular capsule (Senger, 2003). The rete tubules join with the efferent ductules which attach to the epididymidis.

Within the seminiferous tubules are germ cells at various stages of differentiation and Sertoli cells which provide germ cells with structural support and nutrients, as well as regulatory and paracrine factors (Thomas and Thomas, 2001) (Figure 17.1B). Tight junctions (junctional complexes) between adjacent Sertoli cells divide the seminiferous epithelium into basal and adluminal compartments, with Sertoli cells anchored to the basement membrane and surrounding the developing populations of germ cells (Thomas and Thomas, 2001; Genuth, 2004b; Senger, 2003; Evans and Ganjam, 2017). The seminiferous tubules are surrounded by peritubular myoid cells, which in combination with the junctional complexes, form the "blood–testis barrier" to prevent free exchange of large proteins and some xenobiotics between the blood and the fluid within the seminiferous tubules (Thomas and Thomas, 2001; Senger, 2003; Evans and Ganjam, 2017).

Within the interstitial compartment are the Leydig (interstitial) cells, as well as capillaries, lymphatic vessels

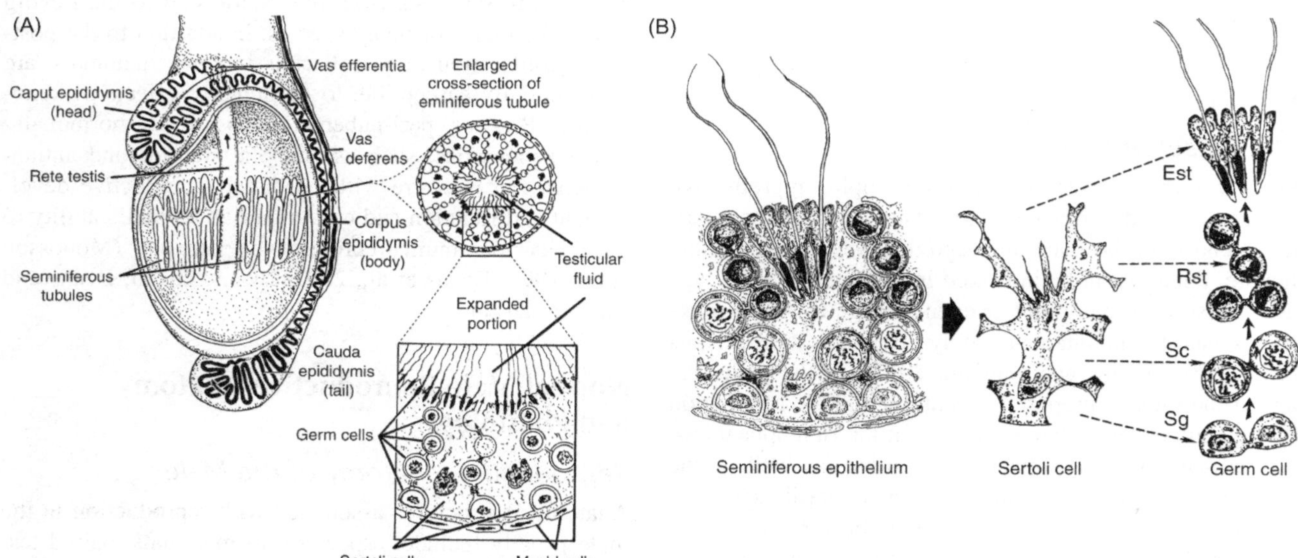

FIGURE 17.1 Loops of the seminiferous tubules, rete testis and excurrent duct system (i.e., efferent ductules (vas efferentia), epididymidis (epididymis) and ductus deferens (vas deferens)), as well as a cross-section of a seminiferous tubule showing the microanatomy of the seminiferous epithelium in a "typical" mammalian testis, are shown in (A). Mature spermatozoa follow the pathway denoted by arrows. Testicular fluid is secreted by the Sertoli cell into the lumen of the seminiferous tubule. The portion of the testicular parenchyma outside of the seminiferous tubules is the interstitium. The predominant cell type within the interstitium is the Leydig or interstitial cell. The complex nature of the association between Sertoli cells and developing germ cells within the seminiferous epithelium in a "typical" mammalian testis is shown in (B). The Sertoli cell and germ cells are shown schematically disassociated to demonstrate how spermatozoal precursors occupy spaces between adjacent Sertoli cells. Spermatogonia, spermatocytes, round spermatids and elongate spermatids are denoted by Sg, Sc, RSt and ESt, respectively. *This figure was adapted, with permission, from Garner DL, Hafez ESE (2000) (modifications and artwork courtesy of Don Connor and Howard Wilson).*

and connective tissue (Senger, 2003; Evans and Ganjam, 2017). The Leydig cells are homologous to the theca interna cells in the ovary and produce testosterone (also estrogen in some species). There are species differences with respect to the abundance of Leydig cells in the interstitium, and these differences are important to recognize when reporting Leydig or interstitial cell hyperplasia in response to toxicant exposure. It should also be noted that Leydig and, to a lesser extent, Sertoli cells contain enzymes involved in xenobiotic biotransformation, and the synthesis of toxic metabolites can actually occur within the testis, in close proximity to the target cells for a given reproductive toxicant (Thomas and Thomas, 2001; Haschek et al., 2010).

Excurrent Duct System

The excurrent duct system consists of the efferent ductules, the epididymal duct and the ductus deferens. This duct system functions to conduct spermatozoa, rete fluid and some testicular secretory products away from the testis and eventually into the pelvic urethra (Senger, 2003; Evans and Ganjam, 2017). The reabsorption of fluid by a species-variable number of efferent ductules is essential for normal testicular function (O'Donnell et al., 2001; Hess, 2003), and these tubules terminate by joining a single highly coiled epididymal duct, commonly referred to as the epididymidis or epididymis. Depending on the species, the epididymidis is generally subdivided into the initial segment, head (caput), body (corpus) and tail (cauda), with the various portions sometimes being further subdivided (França et al., 2005). The primary functions of the epididymidis are transport and sustenance of sperm, reabsorption and secretion of fluid (initial segment and head, respectively); spermatozoal acquisition of motility and fertile potential (i.e., sperm maturation); recognition and elimination of defective spermatozoa; sperm storage prior to ejaculation and secretory contributions to the seminal fluid (Sutovsky et al., 2001). The epididymal transit time varies somewhat with species, but is generally approximately 7 to 14 days in length, depending on several factors including ejaculation frequency. The ductus deferens conducts spermatozoa matured in the epididymidis to the pelvic urethra which helps to form the penis.

Accessory Sex Glands

There are a number of accessory sex glands (the complement of which varies with species) that contribute to the composition of the seminal fluid in mammals. These glands include the ampullae, seminal vesicles (vesicular glands), prostate and bulbourethral glands (Senger, 2003; Evans and Ganjam, 2017). Laboratory rodents (i.e., mice and rats) have an additional gland referred to as the preputial gland, which appears to have a role in the production of pheromone (Haschek et al., 2010). These accessory sex glands in the male are generally considered to be androgen dependent, with conversion of testosterone to DHT occurring in the prostate and seminal vesicles of many species (Senger, 2003; Haschek et al., 2010; Evans and Ganjam, 2017). The weights of the accessory sex glands can be used as an indirect measure of testosterone concentrations or exposure to antiandrogens (Thomas and Thomas, 2001; Senger, 2003; Evans and Ganjam, 2017).

External Genitalia

The external genitalia of the male consist of the copulatory organ or penis, the prepuce, which protects the penis from environmental and mechanical injury, and the scrotum for testes positioned outside of the abdominal cavity. Penile structure is extremely species variable, with some species even having a special penile bone (i.e., os penis), but the shaft of the penis generally consists of erectile tissue (corpus cavernosum and corpus spongiosum) which surrounds the pelvic urethra. The glans penis is homologous to the female clitoris, and stimulation of the glans is the primary factor involved in the initiation of ejaculation (Senger, 2003; Evans and Ganjam, 2017). The scrotum protects the testes from mechanical injury and, in conjunction with the tunica dartos, cremaster muscle and pampiniform plexus, plays a major thermoregulatory role with respect to temperature-sensitive, testicular spermatogenesis. In some species of wildlife (e.g., elephants and marine mammals), the testes are positioned intra-abdominally. Xenobiotics, which cause hyperthermia (i.e., ergopeptine alkaloids) or which induce fever, have the potential to adversely affect spermatogenesis.

Spermatogenesis

Spermatozoa are highly specialized haploid cells equipped with a self-powered flagellum to facilitate motility, as well as an acrosome to mediate penetration of the zona pellucida. Spermatogenesis takes place within the seminiferous tubules and consists of all the changes germ cells undergo in the seminiferous epithelium in order to produce adequate numbers of viable spermatozoa each day and to continuously replace spermatogonial stem cells (Thomas and Thomas, 2001; Senger, 2003; Evans and Ganjam, 2017). Spermatogenesis provides for genetic diversity and ensures that germ cells are in an immunologically favored site (Senger, 2003; Evans and Ganjam, 2017). The duration of spermatogenesis varies with species but generally ranges between 4 and 8 weeks (approximately 30–60 days) in domestic and laboratory animals and is approximately 75 days (almost 11 weeks) in humans. It is important to keep in mind the durations of spermatogenesis and epididymal sperm transport in a given species, as well as the normal, species-specific number of spermatozoa produced daily by the testes, when determining the period of toxicant exposure relative to the appearance of abnormal spermatozoa in an ejaculate and when assessing the severity and reversibility of toxicant-induced damage to sperm precursors within the testes.

Spermatogenesis can be subdivided into three phases or stages referred to as "proliferation," "meiosis" and "differentiation." During each of these phases, sperm precursors or male germ cells (spermatogonia, spermatocytes or spermatids) undergo specific, stepwise changes as they develop into spermatozoa which will eventually be released into the excurrent duct system. Each of these phases involves a different type of germ cell undergoing a different developmental process, and, as such, these phases have the potential to differ in their susceptibility to the mechanisms of action of various reproductive toxicants.

Proliferation (Mitosis or Spermatocytogenesis)

The "proliferation" phase of spermatogenesis has also been referred to as "mitosis" or "spermatocytogenesis" and occurs within the basal compartment of the seminiferous tubule. Proliferation denotes all of the mitotic divisions involving spermatogonia (Senger, 2003; Evans and Ganjam, 2017). A large number of B-spermatogonia result from the mitoses of several generations of spermatogonia (e.g., A_1, A_2, A_3, A_4 and I; some species variations in nomenclature) (Senger, 2003; Genuth, 2004b; Evans and Ganjam, 2017). Stem cell renewal is accomplished during proliferation by the reversion of some spermatogonia to more primitive germ cells (Senger, 2003; Evans and Ganjam, 2017). Germ cell mitosis during spermatogenesis ends with the transformation of B-spermatogonia into primary spermatocytes, and this process is particularly susceptible to toxicants, such as chemotherapeutic agents and radiation, which target rapidly dividing cells.

Meiosis

"Meiosis" takes place within the adluminal compartment of the seminiferous tubules and involves the participation of primary and secondary spermatocytes in a total of two meiotic divisions. The chromosomal reduplication, synapsis and crossover, as well as cellular division and separation, which occur during this phase of spermatogenesis, are extremely complex and guarantee genetic diversity (Senger, 2003; Genuth, 2004b; Evans and Ganjam, 2017). The meiosis phase of spermatogenesis is considered by some to be most susceptible to toxic insult (Thomas and Thomas, 2001) and ends with the production of haploid round spermatids (Senger, 2003; Evans and Ganjam, 2017).

Differentiation (spermiogenesis)

Spermatozoa have been aptly characterized as "sophisticated, self-propelled packages of DNA and enzymes" (Senger, 2003; Evans and Ganjam, 2017). "Differentiation" or "spermiogenesis" involves all the changes occurring within the adluminal compartment, which transform round spermatids into spermatozoa possessing an acrosome for penetration of the zona pellucida and a tail or flagellum to facilitate motility (Genuth, 2004b). Differentiation can be subdivided into the "Golgi," "cap," "acrosomal" and "maturation" phases, which correspond respectively to acrosomal vesicle formation; spreading of the acrosomal vesicle over the nucleus; elongation of the nucleus and cytoplasm and final assembly involving the formation of the post nuclear cap organization of the tail components (Senger, 2003; Evans and Ganjam, 2017). Following the nuclear and cytoplasmic reorganization which characterizes the changes to germ cells during spermiogenesis, differentiated spermatozoa are released from Sertoli cells into the lumen of the seminiferous tubules by a process referred to as "spermiation." The complex signaling pathways and genomic imprinting involved in regulating the differentiation of round spermatids into spermatozoa are potential targets for EDCs.

The Cycle of the Seminiferous Epithelium

In most sexually mature mammals, spermatozoa are produced continuously, with the entry of germ cells into the proliferation phase of spermatogenesis occurring in a coordinated cyclic manner (Genuth, 2004b). Spermatogonia A in a given region of the seminiferous tubule commit to proliferate in a synchronous manner, with cohorts of their progeny germ cells (cellular generations) connected by intercellular bridges and developing and differentiating in unison (Thomas and Thomas, 2001; Senger, 2003, Evans and Ganjam, 2017). Including spermatogonia A, four or five generations or concentric layers of sperm precursors are present in each cross-section of the seminiferous tubules (Figure 17.1) (Thomas and Thomas, 2001; Senger, 2003; Haschek et al., 2010; Evans and Ganjam, 2017). The cycle of the seminiferous epithelium in most mammals is characterized by germ cells in each spermatogenic phase associating with contiguous generations in a repeatable pattern of specific cellular associations or "stages" (Thomas and Thomas, 2001; França et al., 2005). There is generally only one stage per seminiferous tubular cross-section in subprimates (França et al., 2005), and each stage transitions into the next at predictable intervals (Senger, 2003). At any given point along a seminiferous tubule, the entire cycle of the seminiferous epithelium occurs over a set time interval closely associated with the spermatogonial turnover rate for that particular mammalian species (Thomas and Thomas, 2001;

Haschek et al., 2010). The number and duration of the various stages of the cycle of the somniferous epithelium vary with species (Senger, 2003), and various classification schemes have been used, based on the morphological characteristics of the spermatid nucleus or the development of the acrosomic system (França et al., 2005). In subprimates, sequential stages are arranged along the length of the seminiferous tubule in consecutive order, forming a "spermatogenic wave" (Senger, 2003; Haschek et al., 2010). The progeny of one spermatogonium A will progress through approximately 4.5 cycles of the seminiferous epithelium before being released into the lumen of the seminiferous tubule and progressing through the rete testis into the excurrent duct system (Thomas and Thomas, 2001). An understanding of the cycle of the seminiferous epithelium is very useful for the evaluation of the effects of xenobiotics on spermatogenesis and for the determination of populations of germ cells most susceptible to a given toxicant.

Male Reproductive Physiology

Gonadal Steroid Synthesis in the Testes

The endocrine events which regulate spermatogenesis and sexual behavior in males are very distinct from those which take place in females (see below). The primary gonadal steroids produced by the testes are androgens (testosterone and DHT (also produced from testosterone in selected non-gonadal tissues)) and estrogens (primarily estradiol in most species), which are now recognized as playing essential roles in male reproductive development and function (O'Donnell et al., 2001; Hess, 2003). Leydig cells in the interstitium synthesize pregnenolone and then progesterone from cholesterol and convert progesterone to testosterone under the influence of LH (Senger, 2003; Genuth, 2004b; Evans and Ganjam, 2017). The site of estrogen synthesis (i.e., aromatase activity) varies with the age and species of animal. In the male fetus, postnatal immature male and, in some species, the adult male, Sertoli cells within the seminiferous tubules play a major role in the aromatase-mediated conversion of testosterone to estradiol under the influence of FSH (O'Donnell et al., 2001; Senger, 2003; Evans and Ganjam, 2017). In many mammals, Leydig cells in the fetal testis and, especially, the postnatal immature testis gradually begin to synthesize estrogens, and, at sexual maturity, a major portion of the estrogens in these species is produced by aromatase activity in the Leydig cells, under the influence of LH rather than FSH (O'Donnell et al., 2001; Hess, 2003; Evans and Ganjam, 2017). More recently, germ cells have been identified as another potential source of estrogens in the testis, and it is possible that germ cell-derived estrogens play major roles in regulating male reproductive function (Hess, 2003).

Endocrine Regulation of Spermatogenesis

While the female hypothalamus has both fully developed tonic and surge centers for GnRH release (especially prior to ovulation), the hypothalamic GnRH surge center in the male is diminished, and the anterior pituitary gland of the male does not experience surges in GnRH stimulation (Senger, 2003; Evans and Ganjam, 2017). This gender-specific alteration in the hypothalamus facilitates the normal endocrine milieu which maintains continuous spermatogenesis and stimulates normal sexual behavior (Figure 17.2). The tonic pulsatile release of GnRH induces the anterior pituitary to produce pulses of LH and FSH several times during the day and facilitates adequate LH-dependent testosterone production and, depending on the species, normal FSH-dependent Sertoli function, both

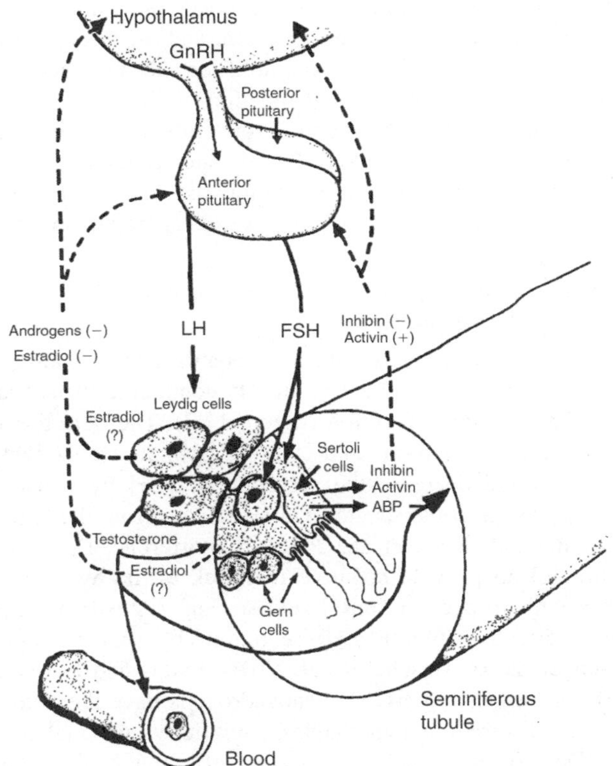

FIGURE 17.2 The relationship between the tubular and the interstitial compartments of the testicular parenchyma and the endocrine regulation of testicular function in mammalian species is shown. Solid lines indicate positive feedback mechanisms, and dashed lines denote negative feedback pathways. The question mark associated with the production of estradiol by the Sertoli cells and Leydig cells is used to indicate that this hormone, as well as other estrogens, can be produced in the testis by either primarily Sertoli or Leydig cells, depending on the species and stage of development. Although not shown, it should be kept in mind that DHT also provides negative feedback to the hypothalamus and anterior pituitary and germ cells can also aromatize testosterone and produce estradiol. *This figure was adapted, with permission, from Garner DL, Hafez ESE (2000) (modifications courtesy of Don Connor and Howard Wilson).*

of which are essential for spermatogenesis to occur continuously in the seminiferous tubules (Senger, 2003; Genuth, 2004b; Evans and Ganjam, 2017). In some species, FSH is primarily required for the onset of puberty and the initiation of spermatogenesis, with many of the functions of FSH in the immature male being taken over by testosterone in the sexually mature animal (Haschek et al., 2010).

Testosterone stimulates Sertoli cells to produce several androgen-regulated proteins (including androgen-binding protein), which are required for spermatogenesis (Senger, 2003; Haschek et al., 2010). Interference with this testosterone-mediated effect by antiandrogens (e.g., vinclozolin) which prevent interactions between testosterone and the androgen receptor or by the inhibition of testosterone synthesis by excessive glucocorticoids (e.g., chronic stress, alterations in endogenous glucocorticoid metabolism or the administration of xenobiotics with glucocorticoid-like activities) has the potential to adversely affect Sertoli cell function, and, therefore, spermatogenesis. Estrogens are required for various aspects of the normal development and function of Sertoli cells and germ cells within the seminiferous tubules (O'Donnell et al., 2001; Hess, 2003; Evans and Ganjam, 2017). Xenobiotics which mimic or inhibit the actions of estradiol within the testis can disrupt normal spermatogenesis.

Positive and Negative Feedback Loops Involved in Male Reproduction

Positive and negative feedback mechanisms help maintain an endocrine environment which is conducive to normal male reproductive function (Figure 17.2). The Sertoli cell can produce activin and inhibin which respectively increase and decrease the secretion of FSH by gonadotropes and, in some species, GnRH release from the hypothalamus (Haschek et al., 2010). Testosterone, DHT and estradiol all provide negative feedback to the hypothalamus with respect to GnRH release, and testosterone can also directly inhibit LH secretion by gonadotropes (Senger, 2003; Haschek et al., 2010; Evans and Ganjam, 2017). Xenoestrogens and xenoandrogens have the potential to disturb the hypothalamic–pituitary–gonadal axis (O'Donnell et al., 2001). It is currently thought that antiandrogens and a variety of other xenobiotics can interfere with these feedback loops and possibly other endocrine pathways, resulting in Leydig or interstitial cell hyperplasia (Thomas and Thomas, 2001; O'Connor et al., 2002; Evans, 2017).

Epididymal and Accessory Sex Gland Function

Epididymal development and function are dependent on the proper balance of androgenic and estrogenic stimulation and are required for normal male reproductive function and fertility. The accessory sex glands are considered to be primarily androgen dependent, and the secretions of these glands, as well as those of the epididymidis, are important components of seminal fluid. Conversion of testosterone to DHT can generally occur in the epididymidis, prostate and seminal vesicles. Hormonally active xenobiotics which alter the normal endocrine events associated with epididymal and accessory gland development and function can have adverse effects on male fertility.

Sexual Behavior, Erection, Emission and Ejaculation

Sexual behavior is mediated by estradiol in postnatal males and females. The conversion of the steadily produced testosterone in the male to estradiol in the brain (plus the effects of estrogens of testicular origin) results in the male being sexually receptive most of the time (Senger, 2003). Adequate libido and sexual receptivity, as well as adequate concentrations of testosterone, are necessary for erection of the penis, which is required for intromission during copulation (Sikka et al., 2005). Olfactory (detection of pheromones), auditory and visual stimuli play roles in facilitating cholinergic and NANC (non-adrenergic/non-cholinergic) parasympathetic neuron-mediated penile erection, which, depending on the species, involves various degrees of nitric oxide-associated vasodilation and vascular engorgement (Senger, 2005; Sikka et al., 2005). During copulation, the events which lead to emission of the secretions of the accessory sex glands and the ejaculation of spermatozoa generally involve tactile stimuli to the glans penis and stimulation by sympathetic neurons (Sikka et al., 2005).

Normal Female Reproductive Anatomy and Physiology

Reproductive Anatomy of the Female

Although there are some distinct morphological differences between species (e.g., simplex uterus in primates, duplex cervices in rabbits), the female reproductive tract generally consists of paired ovaries and the "tubular genitalia," which include the paired oviducts (uterine tubes) and uterine horns contiguous with a uterine body and cervix, vagina, vestibule and vulva (Senger, 2003; Evans et al., 2007; Evans and Ganjam, 2017). The organs involved in female reproductive function are physiologically and morphologically dynamic and function to produce the oocyte, facilitate its fertilization, provide an environment for embryonic and fetal development, and transport the fetus from the maternal to the external environment. Variations in size, appearance, location and function of the female reproductive organs depend on the endocrine milieu dictated by the effects of sexual maturation, stage of the estrous or menstrual cycle, gestational hormone production of maternal, fetal and/or placental origin, exposure to exogenous HAAs and seasonal influences (Ginther, 1992; Senger, 2003; Evans et al., 2007).

The primary functions of the ovary are oogenesis (production of female gametes (oocytes or ova)) and steroidogenesis (production of estrogens and progesterone). The ovaries of most domestic mammals consist of a peripheral parenchymatous zone (cortex), containing various stages of follicular and luteal gland development and a central vascular zone (medulla), comprised of collagenous connective tissue rich in blood vessels (Senger, 2003; Evans and Ganjam, 2017) (Figure 17.3). The structural and functional unit of the ovary is the follicle. Follicles are classified as primordial, primary (some become atretic), secondary and tertiary (antral) follicles based on their stage of development (Evans et al., 2007; Evans and Ganjam, 2017).

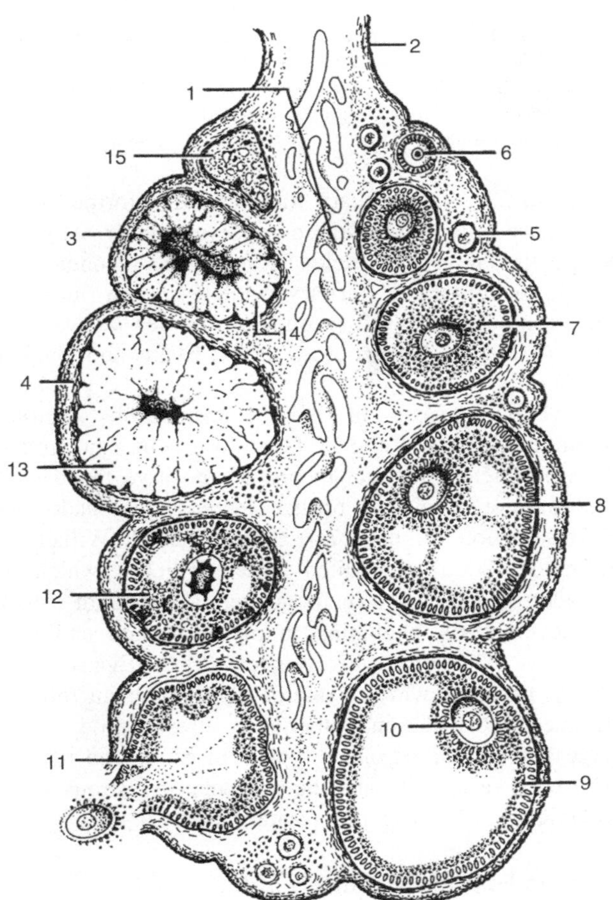

FIGURE 17.3 Although there is some interspecies variation with respect to ovarian structure, a schematic representation of a "typical" mammalian ovary is shown to demonstrate the major ovarian structures: (1) medulla; (2) mesovarium; (3) surface epithelium; (4) tunica albuginea, which is poorly developed in the ovary as compared to the testis; (5) primordial follicle; (6) primary follicle; (7) secondary follicle; (8) early tertiary or antral follicle; (9) mature antral follicle; (10) oocyte; (11) ruptured follicle and ovulated secondary oocytes (except for the dog); (12) atretic follicle; (13) CL; (14) atretic CL; (15) corpus albicans. *This figure was adapted, with permission, from Dyce et al. (2002) (modifications courtesy of Don Connor and Howard Wilson).*

A primary oocyte surrounded by a single, flattened cell layer is a primordial follicle. A basal lamina separates the single layer of what will become granulosa cells from the adjacent stromal tissue which eventually develops into the theca cells (theca interna and theca externa). The granulosa cells homologous to the Sertoli cells in the testis, and the theca interna cells are the female equivalent of the Leydig cells (Senger, 2005). Following the appropriate endocrine stimulation, primordial follicles are recruited to undergo possible further differentiation into estrogen-producing antral follicles and ultimately ovulation, which results in the release of a secondary oocyte (primary oocyte in dogs) and formation of a corpus luteum (CL) which produces progesterone (Ginther, 1992; Senger, 2003; Evans et al., 2007; Evans and Ganjam, 2017).

Female Reproductive Physiology

Females are born with a finite pool of primordial follicles (up to hundreds of thousands), and reproductive cyclicity (i.e., estrous or menstrual cycles) provides females with repeated opportunities for the establishment of pregnancy. The majority of mammalian species (subprimates) have estrous cycles, which reflect the physiological changes occurring between successive ovulations and/or periods of sexual receptivity (estrus) (Senger, 2005; Evans and Ganjam, 2017). Humans and non-human primates experience menstrual rather than estrous cycles and do not have defined periods of sexual receptivity (i.e., estrus). Unlike the estrous cycles in subprimates, the reproductive cycle in menstruating animals is divided into phases (i.e., menses, proliferative and secretory phases), which are defined based on the physiological state of the uterine endometrium, rather than on the predominant ovarian structures (Senger, 2003; Genuth, 2004b; Evans and Ganjam, 2017).

The Estrous Cycle

The follicular and luteal phases of the estrous cycle describe the predominant ovarian structures and the corresponding gonadal steroid concentrations which result from the follicular secretion of estrogens or the luteal secretion of progesterone, respectively (Ginther, 1992; Senger, 2003; Evans et al., 2007). Both the follicular and luteal phases can generally be further subdivided into two stages each, proestrus and estrus (sexual receptivity) for the follicular phase and metestrus and diestrus (sexual non-receptivity) for the luteal phase (Senger, 2003). Proestrus represents the period of transition from the diestrus dominance of progesterone to the dominance of estrogens during estrus, while metestrus represents the opposite shift in the endocrine milieu (estrogen dominance to progesterone dominance) (Senger, 2003; Evans et al., 2007).

The durations of the various stages of the estrous cycle vary with species and can, depending on the animal in question, either occur throughout the year, multiple times within an ovulatory season that is dependent on photoperiod (long-day or short-day polyestrous animals) or only once a year (Senger, 2003). The domestic bitch does not have a metestrus and, in fact, is actually most receptive to copulation when estradiol is declining and there is a unique, preovulatory surge in progesterone. This endocrine environment predisposes the bitch to cystic endometrial hyperplasia and pyometra following exposure to some xenoestrogens and progestagens. Felids, which are induced (reflex) ovulators, like ferrets, mink, camelids and rabbits, the period of time following an estrus in which copulation has not occurred has been described as post-estrus rather than metestrus because there is no increase in progesterone secretion following the end of sexual receptivity (Senger, 2003). Anestrus is the time period during which reproductive cyclicity ceases and can be seasonal (estradiol and progesterone production are at basal levels) or can be associated with various endocrine milieus related to species of animal, pregnancy, lactation, stress and/or pathological conditions, some of which can be induced by xenobiotics.

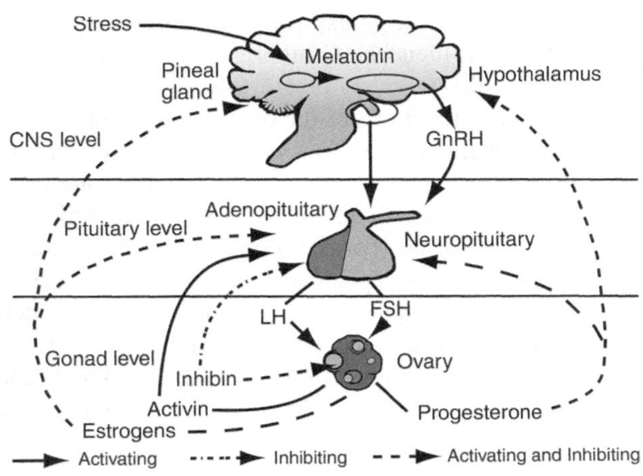

FIGURE 17.4 The endocrine regulation of ovarian function and the feedback loops for the hypothalamic–pituitary–gonadal (ovarian) axis in the female are depicted. *This figure was adapted, with permission, from Wilker and Ellington (2006) (modifications courtesy of Don Connor and Howard Wilson).*

Follicular Development

The general sequence of endocrine and morphological changes occurring during the estrous cycle involves a variety of positive and negative feedback loops affecting the hypothalamic–pituitary–gonadal axis and leads to the development of antral follicles, the primary source of estrogens, and, eventually, the formation of corpora lutea, which produce progesterone (Figures 17.3 and 17.4). During the time of year when females are exhibiting reproductive cyclicity, there are cyclic alterations in the pattern of hypothalamic GnRH secretion from the tonic and surge centers, which interact with the anterior pituitary to influence the relative amounts of FSH and LH secreted by anterior pituitary gonadotropes. Over the course of the ovulatory season, many (up to several hundred or more) primordial follicles leave the reserve pool in a cyclic fashion (under the influence of FSH) and enter the active pool of follicles (primary follicles) undergoing growth and differentiation (folliculogenesis) and eventually atresia or ovulation (Senger, 2003; Evans et al., 2007; Evans and Ganjam, 2017). The oocyte in the developing follicle grows in size, the zona pellucida is formed and the granulosa cells surrounding the oocyte undergo mitosis and further differentiation (Senger, 2003; Evans and Ganjam, 2017). A primary follicle is transformed into a secondary follicle when there are several layers of granulosa cells. Preantral follicles (primary and secondary follicles) become antral (tertiary) follicles, when fluid from the granulosa cells of secondary follicles coalesces to form an antrum (Evans et al., 2007; Evans and Ganjam, 2017).

Cyclic increases in FSH concentrations facilitate recruitment antral follicles. Granulosa cells can produce activin which is thought to provide positive feedback to the anterior pituitary, further increasing gonadotropic FSH secretion (Figure 17.4) (Senger, 2003; Wilker and Ellington, 2006). Recruited antral follicles, which are gonadotropin sensitive, undergo several waves of follicular development beginning in metestrus and ending in proestrus (Ginther, 1992; Senger, 2003; Evans et al., 2007). The final wave of one or more dominant follicles, destined for ovulation, rather than atresia, produces the large amounts of estrogens typical of estrus and required for sexual receptivity and the preovulatory estrous surges in GnRH and LH secretion (Senger, 2003).

Ovarian Follicular Synthesis of Estrogens

The production of estrogens (predominantly estradiol) by antral follicles is accomplished by a mechanism termed the "two-cell or two-gonadotropin model," which can vary somewhat between species (Senger, 2003; Evans et al., 2007; Evans and Ganjam, 2017). Cells from the theca interna and/or granulosa cells (depending on the species) produce progesterone from pregnenolone synthesized from cholesterol and, under the influence of relatively low concentrations of LH, theca interna cells convert this progesterone into androgens and, ultimately, testosterone (Evans et al., 2007; Evans and Ganjam, 2017). In granulosa cells (reportedly theca interna cells in some species), the release of FSH from the anterior pituitary induces aromatase-mediated conversion of testosterone produced in the theca cells into estradiol (Senger, 2003; Evans et al., 2007; Evans and Ganjam, 2017). Stimulation of aromatase activity by xenobiotics can have an overall estrogenic effect on exposed animals (increased production of estradiol).

The Effects of Estrogenic Feedback on the Hypothalamic–Pituitary–Gonadal Axis

Increasing concentrations of estrogens associated with estrus alter the hypothalamic GnRH secretory pattern and decrease pituitary secretion of FSH, while greatly increasing the amount of LH produced and released by the anterior pituitary gland (preovulatory LH surge) (Senger, 2003; Evans et al., 2007; Evans and Ganjam, 2017). Although inhibin produced by granulosa cells further decreases FSH secretion, dominant follicles surviving to estrus do not undergo atresia because of an enhanced sensitivity to basal FSH levels (Senger, 2003; Wilker and Ellington, 2006). Xenoestrogens have the potential to either imitate or inhibit these estradiol feedback mechanisms in sexually mature females, depending on the amount of estrogenic xenobiotic, the endocrine milieu at the time of the exposure and the relative binding affinity of the xenobiotic for ERs.

Ovulation

The granulosa cells in the one or more dominant estrous follicles (Graafian follicles) cease to divide shortly prior to ovulation and undergo further differentiation, with increased numbers (up-regulation) of LH receptors which will be responsive to the estrogen-induced preovulatory LH surge (Senger, 2003; Evans et al., 2007; Evans and Ganjam, 2017). As LH increases, granulosa cells (theca interna cells in some species) continue to convert pregnenolone to progesterone, but estradiol production decreases, resulting in a slight preovulatory decline in estradiol (Evans et al., 2007; Evans and Ganjam, 2017). The preovulatory LH surge is associated with increased follicular pressure, degeneration of theca cells and weakening of the follicular wall, completion of the first meiotic division within the oocyte (end of meiotic inhibition except in dogs and foxes) and, finally, ovulation of a secondary oocyte arrested in metaphase II (Senger, 2003; Evans et al., 2007; Evans and Ganjam, 2017). In felids, ferrets, mink, camelids and rabbits, the preovulatory LH surge is induced by copulation (intromission or vaginal stimulation in most induced ovulators; seminal fluid in camelids). Toxicants which interfere with copulation or sexual contact in these species can interfere with the ovulatory process.

Formation and Function of a CL

Following ovulation, a cascade of endocrine changes takes place in the female subprimate which facilitates the transition from sexual receptivity to non-receptivity. Once an ovulation occurs, blood concentrations of follicular estradiol and inhibin return to their basal levels, and granulosa cells continue their growth, differentiation and increased production and release of progesterone (luteinization) under the influence of LH (Evans et al., 2007). The functional ovarian structure which eventually develops from each ovulated follicle is a CL, which is comprised of large and small luteal cells derived from the granulosa and theca interna cells (granulosa cells in horses), respectively (Senger, 2003; Evans et al., 2007). In most species, luteal cells are responsive to LH and produce progesterone until, shortly before the usual end diestrus in non-pregnant animals, the CL undergoes luteolysis mediated by oxytocin-stimulated production of prostaglandins $F_{2\alpha}$ ($PGF_{2\alpha}$) (Ginther, 1992; Senger, 2003; Evans et al., 2007). While luteolysis is an intraovarian event in primates, oxytocin-stimulated endometrium produces the luteolysin ($PGF_{2\alpha}$) in subprimates (Senger, 2003; Evans and Ganjam, 2017). Xenobiotics, which can cause endometritis or mimic the actions of oxytocin or $PGF_{2\alpha}$ (e.g., endotoxin or lipopolysaccharide (LPS)) can be associated with premature luteolysis. Conversely, toxicants with the opposite oxytocin/$PGF_{2\alpha}$-related effects would be expected to disrupt normal reproductive cyclicity by prolonging the lifespan of the CL and causing a prolonged diestrus or pseudo-pregnancy (e.g., xenoestrogens in swine).

Species of animals can vary in the number of fertile ovulations and, therefore, CLs, which are characteristically associated with each estrous cycle. Monotocous mammalian species usually only ovulate a single secondary oocyte each estrous cycle. The ovaries of litter-bearing (polytocous) mammals generally develop multiple follicles which mature, ovulate and form functional CLs.

Summary of the Effects of Estrogens and Progesterone During the Female Reproductive Cycle

The endocrine changes which occur during the estrous cycle are reflected in behavior and the size, morphology, position and function of the tubular genitalia. Estrogens have multiple effects on the female reproductive tract which include: the previously discussed interactions with the hypothalamus and anterior pituitary to alter the patterns GnRH and gonadotropin secretion, which govern follicular development and ovulation; facilitation of sexual receptivity; increased blood flow, genital swelling, leukocytosis, mucosal secretion and myometrial tone; altered tissue electrical conductivity; and initiation of the growth of endometrial and mammary glands (Senger, 2003). Like estrogens, progesterone also has several effects on the reproductive tract of the female, but the effects of progesterone generally oppose those of estrogens, favoring pregnancy maintenance and sexual nonreceptivity over ovulation and appropriately timed sexual receptivity associated with estrogenic stimulation (Ginther, 1992; Senger, 2003; Evans et al., 2007). Progesterone is generally associated with negative feedback to the hypothalamus and anterior pituitary gland which limits GnRH and gonadotropin secretion (Senger, 2003; Evans et al., 2007; Evans and Ganjam, 2017). Sexual receptivity and myometrial contractility and tone are diminished in an endocrine environment dominated by progesterone, while mammary and endometrial gland development and secretion are promoted (Senger, 2003). Toxicants which disrupt the communication and coordination between the ovary and the other parts of the reproductive tract (e.g., xenoestrogens, xenoandrogens and antiestrogens) will alter the appearance and function of the reproductive organs and can interfere with survival of the oocyte, embryo and/or fetus.

Oocyte/Sperm Transport, Normal Capacitation of Sperm and Fertilization

Transport of the Ovulated Oocyte

The primary reproductive organs involved in the transport of ovulated secondary oocytes (primary oocytes in the bitch) are the oviducts or uterine tubes. Each oviduct consists of an infundibulum, isthmus and ampulla, which have some distinct differences in structure, as well as function (Evans et al., 2007; Evans and Ganjam, 2017). The ovulated ovum enters the funnel-like opening to the infundibulum and is transported through the isthmus to the ampulla or ampullary–isthmic junction for fertilization. Unlike spermatozoa which can generally survive for several days in the oviduct, secondary oocytes usually, depending on the species, are viable for 12–24 h (Genuth, 2004b). The appropriate endocrine environment is required for adequate oviductal entry and transport of ovulated oocytes to the site of fertilization. Delayed transport of oocytes within the uterine tubes can result in the death of ova before contact can be made with fertile spermatozoa.

Transport and Capacitation of Spermatozoa

Transport of Spermatozoa

During mammalian copulation, mature sperm stored in the caudae epididymidies travel through the vas deferens and penile urethra to be ejaculated into the anterior vagina, cervix or uterine body of the female reproductive tract, depending on the species. Spermatozoa can be lost from the female reproductive tract by retrograde loss and phagocytosis by leukocytes (Senger, 2003). Contractions of the smooth muscle within the tubular genitalia (muscularis), as well as interactions involving components of the seminal fluid and luminal secretions of the female reproductive tract, facilitate the transport of sperm to the oviducts (uterine tubes) where, depending on the species, fertilization takes place in the ampulla or at the junction of the ampulla and the isthmus (ampullary–isthmic junction) (Senger, 2003; Genuth, 2004b). While sperm can be rapidly transported to the ampullary–isthmic junction or ampullae of the oviducts within minutes of natural or artificial semination, the relatively slow, sustained transport of motile sperm from reservoirs of spermatozoa in the cervix and uterotubal junctions is the primary mechanism by which the viable sperm that can participate in fertilization actually enter the oviducts (Senger, 2003). Xenobiotics which interfere with the endocrine milieu required for appropriate muscularis contractility and the cervical and uterine mucosal secretions which facilitate sperm transport (e.g., phytoestrogens) can prevent spermatozoa from getting to the site of fertilization in a timely manner.

Capacitation of Spermatozoa

Spermatozoa can generally survive in the oviducts for several days following insemination. Ejaculated sperm are not competent to either bind to the zona pellucida or to undergo the acrosomal (acrosome) reaction, both of which are required for fertilization of ova by mature spermatozoa. Sperm must be capacitated in order to interact with the ovum. The capacitation process involves calcium influx and biochemical changes to the sperm plasma membrane which result in the "removal" or modification of epididymal and seminal plasma proteins and the exposure of the surface molecules required for spermatozoal binding to the zona pellucida of the ovulated secondary oocyte (Senger, 2003; Genuth, 2004b). Depending on the species and, to some extent, the site of their deposition, spermatozoa become capacitated within the cervix, uterus and/or the oviduct (Senger, 2003).

Fertilization

Fertilization of secondary oocytes by capacitated sperm is a complex process involving a cascade of events which prevents fertilization of an ovum by more than one sperm (polyspermy) and ends in the fusion of the male and female pronuclei (syngamy) (Senger, 2003; Evans and Ganjam, 2017). In the oviductal ampulla or at the ampullary–isthmic junction, the motility of capacitated sperm becomes hyperactive, facilitating the precise sequence of events which includes the following in their respective order: (1) sperm binding to the zona pellucida of the oocyte involving interactions between species-specific sperm and oocyte proteins; (2) the sperm acrosomal reaction, which results in the release of acrosomal enzymes and exposure of the equatorial segment of the sperm plasma membrane; (3) acrosomal enzyme-associated penetration of zona pellucida by a single spermatozoon; (4) fusion of the plasma membrane of the sperm at its equatorial segment with the plasma membrane of the oocyte; (5) membrane fusion-associated sperm engulfment and the oocyte cortical reaction, which prevents additional oocyte zona binding and membrane fusion (i.e., polyspermy prevention); female pronucleus formation and completion of meiosis; decondensation within the sperm nucleus and male pronucleus formation and, finally, the fusion of male and female pronuclei or syngamy which produces a zygote ready to undergo embryogenesis (Senger, 2003; Genuth, 2004b; Evans and Ganjam, 2017). From the complexity of the fertilization process, it is apparent that toxicants which result in subtle aberrations in sperm and oocyte formation and maturation can have profound effects on gamete function.

The Endocrinology of Pregnancy and Placentation

Gestational Hormones

Pregnancy begins with fertilization of the oocyte within the oviduct, followed by the first cleavage of the zygote, and terminates with parturition. Although the endocrine physiology and duration of mammalian pregnancy are very species specific and are characterized by a great deal of interspecies variation, the overall goals during the entire gestation for all pregnant mammals, their embryo(s) and, eventually, the maternal—fetal—placental unit are the same. A uterine environment conducive to embryonic and fetal development must be facilitated and the pregnancy (pregnancies in multitocous animals) must be maintained for the entire normal gestational length. The primary hormones involved in establishing the proper uterine environment and maintaining pregnancy are progesterone secreted by the maternal ovary and/or the placenta, as well as, in some species, a variety of placental progestagens. In addition, a variety of other endogenous hormones of maternal, fetal and/or placental origin (depending on the species and gender of the offspring), including androgens, estrogens, prolactin, placental lactogen, equine and human chorionic gonadotropins (eCG and hCG, respectively) and relaxin, also have important gestational functions. Normal embryonic and fetal development require that gestational hormones, especially endogenous androgens and estrogens, be synthesized and secreted in sufficient quantities and at the appropriate time during pregnancy. The proper reproductive development of the female fetus is primarily dependent on exposure to estrogens at specific times during gestation. However, the male fetus must have appropriately timed exposure to normal amounts of both androgens and estrogens for normal development of the reproductive tract and optimal adult reproductive performance (Hess, 2003). Depending on the timing of exposure, EDCs, especially those which function as gonadal steroid receptor agonists and antagonists, can potentially interfere with normal gestational signaling and sexual differentiation.

Maternal Recognition of Pregnancy

The embryo generally enters the uterus several days after fertilization. One of the first endocrine events which must occur in most mammalian species, other than those for which the timing of luteolysis and duration of pregnancy are very similar to one another (i.e., dogs and cats), is the prevention of luteolysis (i.e., entry into the next estrus or period of sexual receptivity) and the maintenance of luteal phase progesterone concentrations (Senger, 2003; Evans *et al.*, 2007). The mechanism for this embryo—endometrium interaction in subprimates (intraovarian event in primates), also referred to as "maternal recognition of pregnancy," has been elucidated in several species and involves embryonic production of species-specific interferon-τ in ovine and bovine species (o-IFN-τ and b-IFN-τ, respectively), estradiol secretion by porcine embryos, intrauterine embryonic migration in equids and placental chorionic gonadotropin (hCG) in humans (Senger, 2003; Genuth, 2004b). The timing of "maternal recognition of pregnancy" is species specific and in subprimates generally corresponds to the time period spanning the normal oxytocin-mediated synthesis and release of $PGF_{2\alpha}$ the endometrium, as well as transport of the luteolysin to the ovary. Xenobiotics which interfere with embryonic and, in the case of humans, placental development or those toxicants which mimic the actions of the luteolysin (e.g., endotoxin) can terminate early pregnancies. Some species of mammals, such as dogs, cats, camelids, goats, swine and rabbits, depend solely on luteal progesterone secretion for the maintenance of pregnancy (Senger, 2003). The placenta takes over progesterone-associated pregnancy maintenance in sheep at approximately 50 days post-conception and between the 6th and 8th month of gestation in cattle (Senger, 2003). The uterofetoplacental unit of the mare begins to produce a unique assortment of progestagens classified as 5α-pregnanes, beginning at about day 70 of pregnancy (Ginther, 1992; Evans et al., 2007; Evans, 2011b). A number of toxicants (e.g., ergopeptine alkaloids) have been found to interfere with normal progestagen metabolism in the mare (Evans, 2011b).

Placentation

Most mammalian species are "eutherian" and, during pregnancy, form a placenta comprised of both fetal and maternal components, which acts as an attachment between the fetal and the maternal systems, functions as a transient endocrine organ and plays essential roles in the exchange of gases, nutrients and metabolic wastes between the maternal and the fetal circulations (Ginther, 1992; Senger, 2003). The yolk sac, chorion, amnion and allantois are the extraembryonic membranes formed by the pre-attachment mammalian embryo (Senger, 2003). While the yolk sac in most mammalian species normally undergoes regression, the allantois and chorion generally fuse to form the allantochorion, and the fluid-filled amnion provides a shock absorbing, aquatic environment to facilitate fetal development and transport (Ginther, 1992; Senger, 2003). The allantochorionic membrane is the fetal contribution to the placenta and the chorionic villi are the structures which interdigitate with the maternal endometrium (Senger, 2003).

Types of Placentas

Mammalian placentation can be classified according to the degree of intimacy between the maternal and the fetal circulations (i.e., the number of tissue layers separating maternal and fetal blood) and by the pattern of distribution of the chorionic villi on the surface of the placenta facing the maternal endometrium (Senger, 2003). Epitheliochorial placentas (placentae) have a total of six layers separating the maternal and fetal circulations and are observed in a variety of species, including equids and swine. Ruminant placentation is described as syndesmochorial because of the transient erosion and regrowth of the maternal epithelium, which results in the intermittent exposure of maternal endothelium (capillaries) to chorionic epithelium (Senger, 2003). Canine and feline placentas are classified as endotheliochorial, and the hemochorial placentation observed in rodents and primates has essentially only chorionic epithelium separating the maternal blood from that of the fetus. The placenta of each species is associated with a typical distribution of the chorionic villi, classified as being either diffuse (e.g., equids and swine), cotyledonary (e.g., ruminants), zonary (e.g., dogs and cats) or discoid (e.g., rodents and primates). Some species, such as the rabbit, have variations in their placentation over the course of gestation, and what begins as an epitheliochorial placenta has transformed into a hemoendothelial type of placentation by the end of pregnancy (Lehman-McKeeman, 2008).

Placental Function

In multitocous species, each fetus has its own placenta, with the previously described endocrine functions, which "attaches" the fetus to the endometrium and facilitates the exchange of gases, nutrients, metabolic wastes and xenobiotics between the fetal and the maternal circulations. Although the term "implantation" is frequently used to describe the appropriately timed attachment of the placental membranes to the endometrium, only the conceptuses of rodent and primate species undergo true implantation (Senger, 2003). Placental exchange involves the processes of simple (passive) diffusion, facilitated diffusion and active transport, as well as pinocytosis and phagocytosis of some nutrients (Senger, 2003).

The passage of materials across the placenta has been traditionally thought of as primarily a function of the intimacy (i.e., number of tissues layers) between the maternal and the fetal circulations, especially with respect to maternal immunoglobulins which cross hemo- and endotheliochorial placentas but not those types of placentae having more layers. However, since most xenobiotics cross the placenta by simple diffusion, it is currently thought that molecular size and solubility are the most important determinants of the ability of potential teratogens in the maternal circulation to cross the placenta into the fetal circulation (Senger, 2003; Lehman-McKeeman, 2008). Some toxic xenobiotics can be actively transported by mechanisms intended for structurally similar endogenous molecules (Lehman-McKeeman, 2008), and it is thought that transplacental transport of lead can mimic that of calcium (Evans et al., 2003).

The "Placental Barrier"

Because the placenta "blocks" the ability of very large molecules to cross from the maternal circulation into the fetal circulation, the term "placental barrier" has been used to describe this protective function of the placenta. Given that a large number of potential toxicants diffuse across the placenta and reach the fetus, the term "barrier" might be somewhat of a misnomer. However, multidrug resistance protein and enzymes involved in biotransformation of xenobiotics have been found in the placenta (Lehman-McKeeman, 2008), The placenta is multifunctional, and regardless of its relative inefficacy as a "barrier" between the maternal and fetal circulations, with respect to at least some xenobiotics, the nutritional and endocrine functions of the placenta are essential for successful completion of the mammalian pregnancies. Placental toxicity has been discussed in much greater detail elsewhere (Gupta and Gupta, 2017).

Normal Embryonic and Fetal Development

Blastocyst Formation and Differentiation of the Germ Cell Layers

In order for a zygote to develop into a viable offspring, multiple steps involving cellular division, migration, differentiation and organization must take place. Embryonic and fetal survival requires that these various steps take place in a precise order and at set times during the gestation of each species. Within 24 h following fertilization, the zygote located in the oviduct begins to divide, within the confines of the zona pellucida, into multiple blastomeres, which ultimately form a ball of cells referred to as the morula (Ginther, 1992; Senger, 2003). A fluid-filled cavity (blastocoele) develops, and the newly formed blastocyst, which is divided into cells forming either the inner cell mass (future embryo proper) or the trophoblast (future chorion), enters the uterus (Senger, 2003). The blastocyst undergoes rapid growth and "hatches" from the zona pellucida. The subsequent cellular division and differentiation results in the formation of the three germ layers (i.e., endoderm, mesoderm and ectoderm), which are destined to develop into the embryonic tissues forming the various organs and body systems, as well as the extraembryonic membranes involved in placental formation and attachment (Ginther, 1992; Senger, 2003). Germ layer differentiation leads to organogenesis and the transformation of an embryo into the fetus which continues to grow and develop for the remainder of pregnancy. With respect to reproductive toxicity in non-rodent mammals, the organogenic and other developmental processes occurring during the first trimester of pregnancy are especially susceptible to the teratogenic effects of xenobiotics. The abnormalities induced by a teratogen are dependent on the specific developmental processes or signaling pathways targeted by that toxicant and the timing of the exposure.

Sex Determination and Sexual Differentiation of Reproductive Function

Genotypic Sex and Development of the Primitive Sex Cords

The genotypic sex of a mammalian conceptus is determined at fertilization by the sex chromosome (X or Y) contributed by the sperm, which, in combination with the X chromosome in the ovum, denotes either a genotypically female (XX) or a male (XY) zygote. During early gestation in most species, the primordial germ cells arise from the epithelium of the embryonic yolk sac and migrate through the developing mesentery to the gonadal (genital) ridge (testicular or ovarian anlage) in its position contiguous with the mesonephros (Senger, 2003; Evans et al., 2007). Germ cells and stimulated somatic cells proliferate and organize into primitive sex cords within undifferentiated (bipotential) gonads, which have the potential to develop into either ovaries or testes (Senger, 2003; Basrur, 2006).

Gonadal Sex Determination and Phenotypic Sexual Differentiation

Development of a phenotypically male or female mammalian fetus occurs during the first trimester of pregnancy in most species and consists of the determination of gonadal sex followed by the further development and differentiation of either the mesonephric or the paramesonephric ducts and regression of the other duct system. The selection of the mesonephric or paramesonephric ducts for retention and further differentiation results in the formation of genitalia (phenotypic sex) appropriate for either the male or female gonads, respectively (Genuth, 2004b). Gonadal sex determination and phenotypic sexual differentiation are dependent on complex and carefully timed signaling events and are extremely susceptible to disruption by xenobiotics. Toxicants which alter epigenetic programming or mimic or inhibit endogenous hormones can have potentially deleterious effects on sexual development (Basrur, 2006). Xenobiotic-induced abnormalities in phenotypic sexual differentiation can arise from defects in testicular formation, defects in androgen production and defects in androgenic action (Basrur, 2006; Hughes et al., 2006). While some toxicant-induced abnormalities in sexual differentiation can be very obvious (e.g., hermaphroditism (presence of ovotestes), pseudohermaphroditism (differences in gonadal and phenotypic sex), hypospadias (feminized external genitalia; failure of urethral fold fusion) and cryptorchidism (failure of testicular descent)), other more subtle effects can be related to functional rather than structural abnormalities. In order to identify the steps in gonadal sex determination and phenotypic sexual differentiation most likely to be targeted by the effects of EDCs and other reproductive toxicants, it is important to understand how these processes are initiated within the fetus and how they impact subsequent fetal development.

For the last several decades, the model for gonadal sex determination and phenotypic sexual differentiation has been based on the premise that a "testis determining factor" (TDF) on the Y chromosome dictates that a gonad differentiates into a testis and initiates the cascade of endocrine changes (Figure 17.5) which results in a pheno-typically male fetus (developed mesonephric duct system; regressed paramesonephric ducts) (Senger, 2003; Genuth, 2004b; Basrur, 2006; Evans and Ganjam, 2017). Without the determination that the gonads will develop into testes, the "default" or "constitutive" pathway is followed and ovarian gonads are formed in association with a developed paramesonephric duct system and regressed mesonephric ducts (Senger, 2003; Genuth, 2004b; Basrur, 2006). While this model is useful to explain rather complex developmental processes, it should be kept in mind that other toxicant-susceptible mechanisms

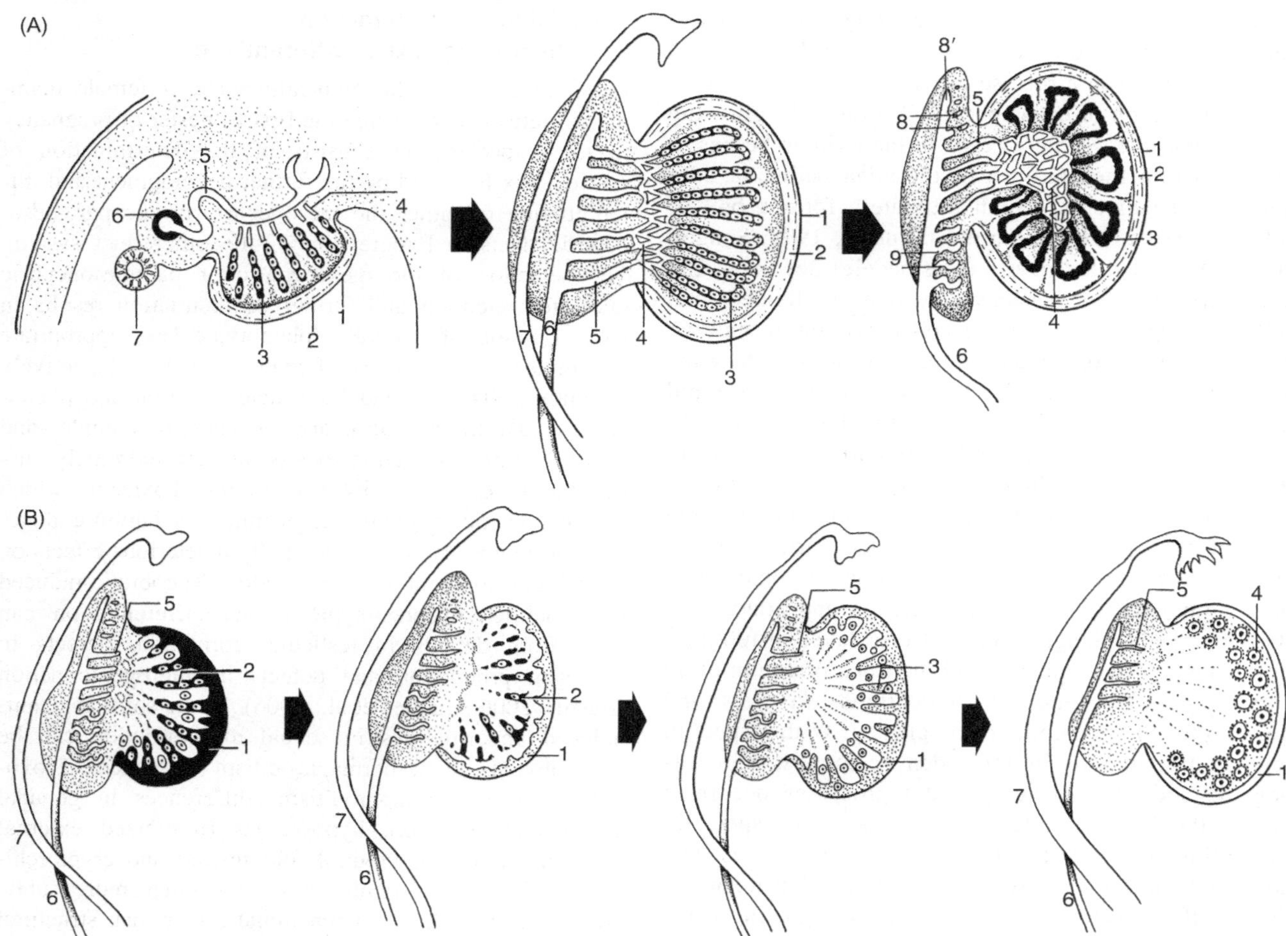

FIGURE 17.5 The initial stages in the development of the testis and the formation of the excurrent duct system are shown in (A). The initial formation of the tunica albuginea isolates the epithelial cords from the surface epithelium, and the epithelial cords, rete testis and mesonephric tubules (also referred to as the mesonephric ductules or mesonephric duct system) subsequently interconnect. The epithelial cords (sex cords) will eventually become the seminiferous tubules, and the mesonephric ductules will be incorporated into the formation of the excurrent duct system. (1) Celomic epithelium; (2) tunica albuginea; (3) epithelial cords (future seminiferous tubules); (4) rete testis; (5) mesonephric tubules (later efferent ductules); (6) mesonephric duct (future epididymis (proximal portion contiguous with mesonephric tubules and ductus deferens (distal portion)); (7) paramesonephric duct; (8) cranial remnant of mesonephric duct system (aberrant ductules); (8′) remnant of mesonephric duct (appendix of epididymis); and (9) caudal remnant of mesonephric duct (paradidymis). The initial stages in the development of the ovary and the formation of paramesonephric ducts are shown in (B). The epithelial cords (sex cords) penetrate and then regress within the developing ovary, eventually fragmenting and organizing into cell clusters which consist of a single oocyte surrounded by a layer of granulosa cells (primordial follicles). The paramesonephric ducts undergo further development and differentiation, and the mesonephric duct system begins to regress: (1) celomic epithelium; (2) epithelial cords which initially penetrate then regress and fragment; (3) early formation of future cortical region; (4) primordial follicles; (5) regressing mesonephric tubules; (6) mesonephric duct which will eventually regress; and (7) paramesonephric duct which will undergo further development and differentiation into the major female tubular genitalia. *This figure was adapted, with permission, from Dyce et al. (2002) (modifications courtesy of Don Connor and Howard Wilson).*

might also play a role in gonadal sex determination and sexual differentiation. It is apparent that very precise, sex-specific patterns of germ line epigenetic programming and interactions with somatic cells take place during the early stages of sexual differentiation (Anway and Skinner, 2006). Recent data have suggested that these signaling pathways are susceptible to epigenetic modifications induced by some antiandrogens (Anway et al., 2005; Anway and Skinner, 2006). It has also been suggested that gonadal sex determination involves other genes on both sex and autosomal chromosomes that might be targeted by reproductive toxicants (Genuth, 2004b; Basrur, 2006).

Development of the Male Phenotype

Once previously undifferentiated gonads commit to testes development (TDF present), a coordinated series of endocrine-induced morphological changes take place, resulting in both a genotypically and a phenotypically male fetus (Figure 17.5a). The sequence of signaling and developmental changes, which result in male sexual differentiation, include the following: (1) Sertoli cell development and secretion of anti-Müllerian hormone (AMH) or Müllerian inhibiting substance (MIS); (2) AMH-induced regression of the paramesonephric (Müllerian) ducts and differentiation of Leydig cells capable of producing testosterone; (3) testosterone-facilitated development of the mesonephric or Wolffian ducts; (4) differentiation of the mesonephric ducts into the rete testes, efferent ductules, epididymidies and ducti deferens; (5) development of primordial accessory sex glands and the formation of external genitalia from primordia and, finally, in most species (some exceptions in wildlife species); (6) testicular descent of the intra-abdominal testes into their extra-abdominal position in the scrotum, prior to or very shortly after birth (some species) (Senger, 2003; Genuth, 2004b; Basrur, 2006; Edwards et al., 2006).

Development of the Female Phenotype

If the previously undifferentiated gonads do not commit to testes development (TDF absent), ovaries are formed and a cascade of morphological changes occurs in the absence of AMH and testosterone stimulation, resulting in a genotypically and phenotypically female fetus (Figure 17.5b). This sequence of "default" or "constitutive" morphological and endocrine alterations results in the following sequence of developmental events: (1) regression of mesonephric (Wolffian ducts); (2) differentiation of the paramesonephric (Müllerian) ducts into the oviducts, uterine horns, uterine body, cervix and anterior vagina; (3) remodeling of the ovary into its typical parenchymal and cortical structure; (4) cortical development of primordial follicles, with primary oocytes arrested in meiosis and surrounded by future granulosa and theca interna cells; and (5) development of the caudal vagina and vulva from the urogenital sinus (external genitalia primordia) (Senger, 2003; Genuth, 2004b; Basrur, 2006; Edwards et al., 2006; Evans et al., 2007).

Sexual Differentiation of the Brain

Sex-specific endocrine patterns and the resulting gender appropriate sexual behaviors in animals are necessary for fertile copulations to occur and require that the brain also undergo prenatal (postnatal in some species) sexual differentiation. Although large amounts of estradiol defeminize the brain, alpha-fetoprotein prevents most of the endogenous estrogens in the female fetus from crossing the blood–brain barrier (Senger, 2003). The brain remains inherently female under the influence of minimal amounts of estradiol, and both the GnRH tonic and surge centers are maintained within the hypothalamus of the female fetus in this low-estradiol environment (Ford and D'Occhio, 1989; Senger, 2003). Testosterone produced by the fetal testes crosses the blood–brain barrier and is converted to estradiol within the brain, and, as a result of this estradiol synthesis, the hypothalamic GnRH surge center in the male fetus is minimized (Senger, 2003).

While the differentiation of male sexual behavior in large domestic animals generally involves prenatal defeminization, especially in species having longer gestations, it should be noted that postnatal defeminization of the brain is occurs in male swine and rodents (Ford and D'Occhio, 1989). There is also evidence to suggest that the males of some species with prenatal defeminization of the brain might also require postnatal exposure to androgens for maximum masculinization of the brain (Senger, 2003). Depending on the timing of exposure, xenoestrogens and exogenously administered testosterone and, possibly, some xenoandrogens, which cross the placenta and the blood–brain barrier have the potential to have profound effects on sexual differentiation of the brain and future reproductive function.

Parturition and Lactation

Physiology of Parturition

Parturition constitutes transport of the fetus and its associated membranes from the maternal to the external environment, and represents transition of the fetus to a neonate. Maturation of the fetal hypothalamic–pituitary–adrenal axis plays an important role in the cascade of neural and endocrine events which lead to parturition in most mammals (Senger, 2003; Evans et al., 2007). As most clearly demonstrated in ruminants, fetal CRF stimulates the release of ACTH from the fetal pituitary, and ACTH, in turn, stimulates fetal secretion of cortisol by the adrenal glands (Senger, 2003). Elevations in fetal cortisol (fetal LH may be involved as well) activate placental steroidogenic enzyme systems, resulting in decreased progestagens and elevated estrogens prior to parturition (Ginther, 1992; Evans et al., 2007). The resulting increase in the estrogen:progestagen ratio facilitates several important processes (e.g., cervical softening, up-regulation of myometrial oxytocin receptors, uterine synthesis of $PGF_{2\alpha}$ and increased blood flow to the gravid uterus and placenta) which prepare the uterus for parturition (Evans et al., 2007). Teratogen-induced congenital defects in the fetal pituitary gland can result in prolonged gestation (e.g., *Veratrum californicum*), and any xenobiotic exposure causing maternal and/or fetal stress can be associated with abortion or premature parturition (e.g., nitrates and pine needle abortion).

Normal parturition approaches as neural signals caused by fetal movements and myometrial contractions, along with elevated basal levels of oxytocin and increased secretion of $PGF_{2\alpha}$, bring about the first stage of labor. A rapid increase in oxytocin and $PGF_{2\alpha}$ secretion leads to rupture of the allantochorionic membrane and the commencement of the second stage of labor. Strong myometrial contractions result in the delivery of offspring, as well as the expulsion of the fetal membranes during the third stage of labor (Senger, 2003; Evans et al., 2007).

Physiology of Lactation

Lactogenesis

Appropriately timed lactogenesis is critical for survival of mammalian offspring. Lactogenesis is a two-stage process involving: (1) the enzymatic and cytological differentiation of the alveolar cells within the mammary gland and (2) the copious secretion of milk, which is distinct from the colostral sequestration of antibodies (Tucker, 1994). Growth hormone, aldosterone, prostaglandins, insulin, estrogens, progestagens and prolactin are required for the first stage of lactogenesis, which generally occurs during the last trimester of pregnancy (McCue, 1993; Tucker, 1994). Large increases in pulsatile prolactin secretion by lactotropes in the anterior pituitary are necessary for the initiation of the second stage of lactogenesis, which generally occurs in close temporal association with the endocrine milieu of parturition (Evans, 1996). In many species, circulating concentrations of prolactin are elevated above basal levels for a month or two after parturition (McCue, 1993). In some species of animals, a placental lactogen performs many of the same endocrine functions as prolactin.

Control of Prolactin Secretion

Lactotropic prolactin secretion is tonically inhibited by dopamine secreted by hypothalamic neurons belonging to either the tuberoinfundibular or tuberohypophysial dopaminergic systems (TIDA and THDA, respectively) (Neill and Nagy, 1994; Evans et al., 2007; Evans and Ganjam, 2017). Vasoactive intestinal peptide (VIP) and TRH are thought to act as prolactin releasing factors and can interfere with the dopamine-associated tonic inhibition of prolactin release (Evans, 1996). Oxytocin, in conjunction with the suckling reflex, will increase pituitary lactotropic production and secretion of prolactin (Neill and Nagy, 1994). In species strictly dependent on prolactin for lactogenesis (e.g., equids and swine), toxicants which mimic dopamine and tonically inhibit prolactin secretion (e.g., ergopeptine alkaloids) pose a risk to fetal survival (Evans, 2011b; see Chapter 72 in this book).

THE MECHANISMS AND EFFECTS OF REPRODUCTIVE TOXICANTS

The Effects of EDCs on Wildlife Species, Humans and Domestic Animals

It should be evident from the previous discussion that maximum reproductive efficiency, including normal embryonic and fetal development, is dependent on the structural and functional integrity of multiple organs and tissues, as well as various signaling pathways (Figure 17.6). Within the broad definition for "endocrine disruption" used in this chapter, without any restrictions as to whether the xenobiotics involved are synthetic or naturally occurring or by which specific mechanism they exert their endocrine effects, no doubt should remain in even the harshest skeptic's mind that "endocrine disruption" is a real phenomenon. The current debate should not focus on "whether" endocrine disruption occurs, but, rather, "when" it occurs and under what circumstances. There is increasing concern within the scientific and regulatory communities regarding the effects of prenatal and early postnatal exposures to EDCs on wildlife species and humans (Evans, 2017). Domestic animals have been known to be susceptible to the effects of several naturally occurring reproductive toxicants in clinical settings, and it is possible that low-level environmental exposures to

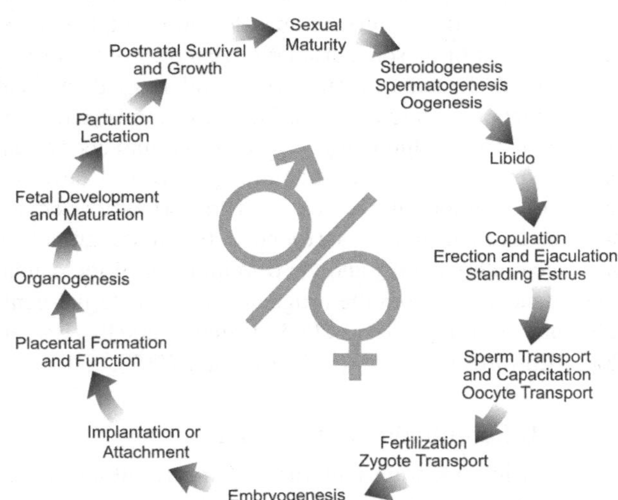

FIGURE 17.6 The multiple steps involved in reproductive development and function in both males and females are shown schematically to illustrate the complexity of reproduction in mammalian species and to demonstrate the various stages in the reproductive process which can be targeted for toxic insult. With respect to embryonic, fetal and placental development, it should be understood that these events are species dependent and interrelated, with many of them taking place concurrently. *This figure was adapted, with permission, from Ellington and Wilker (2006) (modifications and artwork courtesy of Don Connor and Howard Wilson).*

EDCs can also hinder reproductive function in these species (Evans, 2011a).

Endocrine Disruption in Wildlife Species

There have been many, well-documented instances of reproductive abnormalities in species of wildlife living in environments contaminated by industrial and/ or agricultural chemicals (McLachlan, 2001; Hess and Iguchi, 2002; Jobling and Tyler, 2006; McLachlan et al., 2006). The deleterious reproductive effects of DDT on birds reported in Rachel Carson's *Silent Spring* have been shown to be the result of eggshell thinning related to abnormalities in prostaglandin synthesis induced by the *p,p*-DDE metabolite of DDT (Lundholm, 1997; Guillette, 2006). Wildlife populations are very likely sentinels for endocrine disruption because of the contamination of the aquatic habitats in which many of them live and the likelihood that predatory animals will have relatively high exposures to chemicals which bioaccumulate within the environment (Hess and Iguchi, 2002). Lessons learned from instances of endocrine disruption in wildlife species can be applied to EDC exposures involving humans and domestic animals (Evans, 2017).

"Androgenic" and "Estrogenic" Effects of EDCs on Wildlife Species

Prenatal and postnatal exposures to androgenic and estrogenic environmental contaminants, as well as chemicals classified as having the opposite phenotypic effects, have been associated with various reproductive abnormalities in wildlife. Effluents from pulp and paper mills, as well as runoff from cattle feedlots where the synthetic androgen trenbolone was used for growth promotion, have been shown to be androgenic and capable of masculinizing female fish (Orlando et al., 2004; Gray et al., 2006). "Androgenization" or a state of indeterminate sexual development encompassing both feminization and demasculinization in males has been observed in populations of fish, amphibians, reptiles, birds and mammals and is thought to be similar to the testicular dysgenesis syndrome described in humans (Edwards et al., 2006). Adult and immature amphibians exposed to the herbicide atrazine, which has been associated with increased aromatase activity in a number of species, have been reported to exhibit various manifestations of feminization (Hayes et al., 2006). Hatchling, juvenile and adult male alligators (*Alligator mississippiensis*), originating from a Florida lake previously contaminated with DDT and other persistent, bioaccumulated pesticides, as well as ethylene dibromide and DBCP, have demonstrated varying patterns of androgynization, including phallic malformations, which are thought to result from ovo exposure of maternal origin, as well as post-embryonic modifications and/or continuing environmental exposures to EDCs (Milnes et al., 2006).

Endocrine Disruption in Humans

Based, in part, on the observations of endocrine disruption in wildlife and ongoing concerns about reproductive dysgenesis, as well as the effects of embryonic and/or fetal exposure to diethylstilbestrol (DES), the emphasis with respect to endocrine disruption in humans and one of the bases for the "Theory of Hormone Disrupting Chemicals" (THDC) or the "Environmental Endocrine Hypothesis" (Krimsky, 2000, 2001) has been the enhanced effects of prenatal, as compared to postnatal, exposures to suspected endocrine disruptors. The embryo and fetus, without a developed blood–brain barrier and with only rudimentary DNA repair mechanisms and hepatic detoxifying and metabolizing capabilities, are especially susceptible, as compared to adults, to the adverse effects of low-level exposures to xenobiotics (Newbold et al., 2006). In addition, previous discussions in this chapter and other testbooks have described the important organizational events taking place during gonadal and phenotypic sexual differentiation, which are potentially very sensitive to alterations in the normal endocrine milieu (Evans, 2017).

Although still controversial, there is a growing body of evidence to support the observation that sperm counts in men within some industrialized regions of the world have been decreasing over the last several decades (Swan et al., 2000; Skakkebæk et al., 2006; Jørgensen et al., 2006a). In conjunction with these alterations in sperm numbers within ejaculates, there appears to have been a concurrent increase in developmental abnormalities within the male reproductive tract consistent with TDS (Skakkebæk et al., 2001). Similar to what has been observed in xenobiotic-exposed wildlife, reproductive dysgenesis in human males (i.e., TDS) is associated with a suite of clinical abnormalities which include reduced semen quality, cryptorchidism, hypospadias, decreased anogenital distance and testicular cancer (Skakkebæk et al., 2001; Edwards et al., 2006). Failure of Sertoli cell proliferation and functional maturation within the seminiferous tubules has been one mechanism proposed for the pathogenesis of TDS (Sharpe et al., 2003). The findings of a recently completely epidemiological study have suggested a relationship between decreased anogenital distance and prenatal phthalate exposure in male infants (Swan et al., 2005), and a possible rodent model for human TDS has been developed using prenatal exposure to dibutyl phthalate [di (*n*-butyl) phthalate] (Fisher et al., 2003; Mahood et al., 2005, 2006).

In addition to phthalates, which are used as plasticizers, a number of other widely used agricultural and industrial chemicals have been associated with adverse reproductive effects in humans and/or rodent models. In epidemiological studies a correlation has been shown between reduced semen quality in men within certain regions of the United States and the metabolites of several economically important herbicides (Swan et al., 2003a, b). Metabolites of the commercially available fungicide vinclozolin have been demonstrated to interfere with interactions between androgens and their nuclear receptor, resulting in antiandrogenic effects on exposed rodents (Wong et al., 1995; Monosson et al., 1999; O'Connor et al., 2002; Kubota et al., 2003; Gray et al., 2006). It has been reported that, at concentrations well below those routinely found in humans, bisphenol A, which is widely used in the plastics industry and other manufacturing processes, can initiate nongenomic estrogenic responses with plasma membrane receptors and interact with the nuclear estrogen receptor as a SERM (Welshons et al., 2006). It has also recently been reported that, as might be expected, more bisphenol A is absorbed if included in the diet similar to what would be observed in actual environmental exposures, as opposed to administered as an oral bolus, which is normally what occurs in an experimental setting (Sieli et al., 2011). Concerns have also been raised about the antiandrogenic activity of pyrethroid insecticides (Zhang et al., 2008), which are commonly used without the awareness that these compounds have the potential to affect reproductive function at levels of exposures less than those associated with neurotoxicity. With the increased societal awareness of the possible effects of hormonally active xenobiotics on human reproduction, further research is required to make educated decisions, based on "good science," with respect to label instructions and precautions for continued use and/or regulation of economically important chemicals associated with the potential for reproductive abnormalities in humans and/or documented impairment of reproductive function in laboratory animals.

The Effects of Reproductive Toxicants on Domestic Animals

Abortion, Teratogenesis and Impaired Fertility in Domestic Animals

Animal-based agriculture is dependent on the efficient production of viable and reproductively functional offspring. Toxicant-induced abortions, congenital defects and male or female infertility can have devastating effects on livestock production. Cattle are commonly at increased risk, especially under drought conditions, for adult mortality and abortions in pregnant cows related to the consumption of nitrate-accumulating forages (e.g., *Sorghum* spp., oat hay (*Avena sativa*), cornstalks (*Zea mays*), and many others), which cause nitrite-induced fetal methemoglobinemia, hypoxia and, consequently, fetal stress and, potentially, even death (Casteel and Evans, 2004). Multiple congenital contractures (MCC) ("crooked calf disease") associated with the ingestion of lupines (*Lupinus* spp.) have resulted in the loss of large numbers of calves in the western United States (Panter, 2002), and multiple species of livestock exposed to swainsonine-containing plants (e.g., species of *Astragalus* and *Oxytropis* in North America species of *Swainsona* in Australia) have experienced congenital defects, abortions and/or ovarian and testicular abnormalities (Cheeke, 1998). Cleft palate, cyclops lambs, prolonged gestation and various tracheal and limb deformities have resulted from different periods of exposure of pregnant ewes to *Veratrum californicum* (false hellebore) (Burrows and Tyrl, 2001). Ergot alkaloids produced by the tall fescue endophyte *Neotyphodium coenophialum* are responsible for suboptimal reproductive performance in large numbers of cattle and horses, with late-gestational mares being particularly susceptible to endophyte-related prolonged gestation and agalactia (Evans et al., 2004; see Chapter 72 of this book).

Endocrine Disruption in Domestic Animals

With respect to the adverse reproductive effects of endocrine disruption on domestic animals, there have been many instances of impaired reproductive function involving naturally occurring EDCs of plant and fungal origin. However, there is still much to be learned about the potential adverse effects of pre- as well as postnatal environmental exposures to EDCs in these species where selection of breeding animals is often based on reproductive soundness. Postnatal exposures to phytoestrogens in some leguminous plants, including soybeans, have resulted in reproductive abnormalities and subfertility in multiple species (Cheeke, 1998; Ford et al., 2006). The adverse effects of postnatal exposures to the estrogenic mycotoxin zearalenone on swine fertility have also been well documented (Cheeke, 1998). Many of the reproductive effects of the common forage-related disease syndrome referred to as "fescue toxicosis" clearly involve the endocrine disruptive effects of ergot alkaloids on prolactin secretion. In experimental studies, female swine appear to be more sensitive than rodents to the effects of the synthetic herbicide atrazine on the hypothalamic–pituitary–gonadal axis (Gojmerac et al., 2004), and it is possible that companion and agricultural animals are also more susceptible than laboratory species to other EDCs. As many hormonally active xenobiotics also have important agricultural and industrial uses, it is important to continue research which attempts to accurately predict the effects of environmental exposures to EDCs, as well as other reproductive toxicants, on domestic animals.

Toxicants Affecting the Male Reproductive Function

There have been relatively few documented reports regarding the adverse effects of reproductive toxicants on male fertility in the major animal species of veterinary interest. Realistically the lack of examples is more likely a reflection of the limited number of controlled studies performed using non-rodent mammalian species and/or the number of toxicant-associated reproductive abnormalities which remain undiagnosed, rather than an accurate indication of the scope of the problem (Schrader, 2002). A large number of chemicals are currently thought to have the potential for causing abnormalities in male reproductive function in domestic animals. Based on extrapolations from effects observed in a various mammalian species and the limited scientific and anecdotal reports, a partial listing of these compounds is presented in Table 17.1 (Ellington and Wilker, 2006). In the following section a few selected male reproductive toxicants and their proposed mechanisms of action will be described in order to familiarize the reader with the various different ways that male fertility can be affected by reproductive toxicants.

Selected Male Reproductive Toxicants and Mechanisms of Action

Cell-Specific Reproductive Toxicants

Some reproductive toxicants adversely affect specific cells within the testes. Ethane dimethane sulfonate is specifically cytotoxic to the Leydig cells, and excessive exposure to this compound results in complete loss of this population of cells within the interstitium, and, consequently, the ability of the testes to synthesize testosterone and, in some species, estrogens (Haschek et al., 2010). Tri-*o*-cresyl phosphate (TOCP) is an industrial chemical used in lacquers and varnishes, which inhibits LH-induced steroidogenesis in the Leydig cells and, after Leydig cell-mediated conversion to its active metabolite, morphological abnormalities in Sertoli cells (Thomas and Thomas, 2001; Haschek et al., 2010).

Sertoli cells are specifically targeted by several toxicants, including diethylhexyl phthalate (DEHP), 1,3-dinitrobenzene (DNB) and 2,5-hexanedione (metabolite of *n*-hexane) (Haschek et al., 2010) and the effects of these xenobiotics are age and species specific (Thomas and Thomas, 2001). With respect to DNB, the parent compound is converted to its toxic metabolites, nitosonitrobenzene and nitroaniline, within the target Sertoli cells, and, similar to other Sertoli cell-specific toxicants, germ cell death and exfoliation occur secondary to toxic insult to the Sertoli cells (Haschek et al., 2010). Sertoli cell microtubules appear to be the intracellular targets of 2,5-hexanedione (Thomas and Thomas, 2001; Haschek et al., 2010). The fungicide dibromochloropropane (DBCP) appears to affect the Sertoli cell (Thomas and Thomas, 2001), but its metabolites epichlorhydrin and α-chlorhydrin induce capillary permeability and vascular damage within the epididymis (Haschek et al., 2010).

There are a number of reproductive toxicants which target-specific populations of germ cells. Spermatogonia, spermatocytes, round spermatids and elongate spermatids are specifically targeted by busulfan, 2-methoxyethanol, ethylmethane sulfonate and dibromacetic acid, respectively (Haschek et al., 2010). Ionizing radiation and a variety of chemotherapeutic agents, including cyclophophamide, nitrogen mustard, vincristine and vinblastine, generally target rapidly dividing mitotic or meiotic germ cells in the testes, and TCDD appears to adversely affect several populations of spermatozoal precursors (Thomas and Thomas, 2001). The compound 7,12-dimethylbenz[*a*]anthracene (DMBA) is toxic to spermatogonia but must undergo a stepwise biotransformation in the Leydig cell and, subsequently, the Sertoli cell to produce the ultimately toxic metabolite (Haschek et al., 2010).

Heavy Metals

Lead and cadmium are ubiquitous heavy metals and have both been associated with testicular toxicity and impaired fertility in a number of species. Excessive cobalt can potentially interfere with normal spermatogenesis, and severe cobalt intoxications have actually resulted in generalized hypoxia related to increased blood viscosity which affects the testes (Thomas, 1995). Chromium and vanadium have also been associated with adverse reproductive effects (Thomas and Thomas, 2001), and cis-platinum exposure has been associated with the death of spermatocytes and spermatids, as well as disruption of Sertoli cell tight junctions (Thomas, 1995). Although testicular toxicity is generally not observed with excessive parenteral exposure to zinc (other than possibly secondary to hemolytic anemia-related hypoxia) (Thomas, 1995), intratesticular injections with zinc gluconate have been successfully used for chemical castration in several species.

Divalent lead is known to interact with physiological processes involving calcium and generally has an affinity for sulfhydryl groups. Lead is reported to be directly toxic to germ cells and Leydig cells and can suppress anterior pituitary secretion of LH and FSH (Thomas and Thomas, 2001). Lead also appears to be able to adversely affect the ability of spermatozoa to fertilize ova, but this effect, like others associated with lead exposure, appears to be dependent on age and individual variations in susceptibility, adaptation and reversibility (Sokol, 2006).

TABLE 17.1 Xenobiotics/Environmental and Physiological Factors that Affect Male Fertility

Xenobiotic	Observed Effect(s) on Male
Antimicrobials	
Metronidazole	High doses: ↓ sperm number; ↑ abnormal morphology
Nitrofurantoin	High doses: ↓ sperm number
Tetracycline	Very high doses: ↓ sperm number; ↓ sperm capacitation; testis atrophy
Trimethoprim	1-month course: ↓ sperm number by 7–88%
Antifungals	
Ketaconazole	Decreased testosterone and libido; ↓ sperm number and motility
Miconazole	Interferes with testosterone in male fetus
Immunosuppressants	
Cyclophosphamide	Decreased sperm number; birth defects in offspring
Hormones	
Testosterone	Decreased sperm number; testicular degeneration
Anabolic steroids	Decreased sperm number, motility and morphology
Trenbolone	Increased sperm abnormalities
Estrogens	Decreased sperm number; behavioral feminization
Phytoestrogens	Bioaccumulation in cats on soy diets can cause poor fertility
Zearanol	Decreased spermatogenesis
Antivirals	
Acyclovir	Dose- and age-dependent testicular degeneration
Ganciclovir	Decreased sperm number and quality
Carbonic anhydrase inhibitors	
Acetazolamide	Decreased libido and impotence
Psychoactive drugs	
Buspirone	Decreased libido and impotence
Benzodiazepine tranquilizers	Impotence and possible ejaculatory dysfunction
Tricyclic antidepressants	Decreased libido and erectile dysfunction
Antihistamines	
Chlorpheniramine	In vitro experiments: ↓ sperm motility
Antineoplastics	
Adrimycin	Dose- and age-dependent testicular toxicity
Cisplatin	Decreased sperm number; ↓growth in offspring; pregnancy loss
Vincristine	Decreased sperm number; possible reversibility
Antimetabolite	
Cytarabine	Decreased sperm number
Gastrointestinal tract drugs	
Cimetidine	Decreased sperm number
Metaclopramide	Impotence

(Continued)

TABLE 17.1 (Continued)

Xenobiotic	Observed Effect(s) on Male
Non-steroidal antiinflammatories	
Naproxen	Decreased seminal prostaglandins; ↓ sperm motility
Phenylbutazone	Inhibition of sperm acrosome reaction; unknown effect on fertility
Sulfasalazine	Decreased sperm number and motility
Glucocorticoids	
Prednisone	Decreased sperm number and motility; ↓ testosterone
Herbicides	
2,4-D (dichlorophenoxyacetic acid)	Abnormal sperm quality; testicular degeneration; ↓ fertility
Diquat and paraquat	Altered sexual differentiation in the male
Solvents	
Nitrobenzene	Decreased sperm number and motility; testicular degeneration
Naphtha	Decreased fertility
Phthalic acid esters	
Diethylhexaphthalate (DEHP)	Testicular atrophy
Gasoline additives	
Ethylene dibromide	Testicular degeneration and poor sperm quality
Insecticides	
Carbamates	Decreased sperm quality
Chlorinated hydrocarbons	Testicular degeneration and atrophy
Methoxychlor	Testicular degeneration associated with estrogenic activity
Kepone	Decreased sperm number
Lindane	High doses: testicular toxicant
	In utero exposure: ↓ sperm number and ↓ testosterone in offspring
Organophosphates	No information
Pyrethrins	In vitro: 40–60% ↓ in testosterone binding to androgen receptor
Fungicides/nematocides	
DBCP (dibromochloropropane)	Decreased sperm number; testicular toxicant
Fungicide	
Vinclozolin	Antiandrogen: disruption of male phenotypic sexual differentiation
Heavy metals	
Cadmium	High doses: ischemic necrosis of the testis
Chromium	Decreased testosterone; ↓ sperm number
Lead	Decreased testosterone; ↓ sperm number; ↓ fertilization rates
Mercury	Decreased sperm quality
Miscellaneous xenobiotics	
Dioxin	Decreased libido; abnormal sperm morphology; ↓ response to GnRH
DBP (dibutyl phthalate)	Altered sexual differentiation
PCBs	Decreased sperm number; altered hypothalamic–pituitary–adrenal axis
Gossypol	Decreased sperm number

(*Continued*)

TABLE 17.1 (Continued)

Xenobiotic	Observed Effect(s) on Male
Ethylene glycol	Decreased sperm number and motility
Environmental factors	
Heat	Damaged sperm chromatin and quality
Microwaves	Decreased sperm number
Radiation	High doses: death of stem cells and permanent azoospermia
Stray voltage (AC and DC)	Decreased sperm number
Physiological factors	
Stress	Decreased sperm motility
Fever (hyperthermia)	Damaged sperm chromatin and quality

This table was adapted, with permission, from Ellington and Wilker (2006).

Like lead, cadmium is thought to adversely affect male reproduction by several different mechanisms. With respect to spermatogenesis, the stage of the seminiferous epithelium associated with spermiation appears to be specifically inhibited by cadmium (Thomas, 1995). Cadmium has also been shown to have possible interactions with the hypothalamic–pituitary–gonadal axis (Akinloye et al., 2006). The endothelium of the testicular and epididymal vasculature is extremely susceptible to toxic insult by cadmium, potentially resulting in reduced vascular perfusion and testicular necrosis (Haschek et al., 2010). Cadmium can also alter the actin filaments in the junctional complexes between adjacent Sertoli cells, thereby disrupting the integrity of the blood–testis barrier (Thomas and Thomas, 2001). Cadmium can interfere with the cellular metabolism of zinc, an essential trace element necessary for normal reproductive function, and diets deficient in zinc can predispose individuals to the toxic effects of cadmium (Akinloye et al., 2006). Pre-treatment with zinc has been reported to reduce the incidence of cadmium-induced Leydig cell cytotoxicity and neoplasia (Thomas, 1995).

Gossypol

Gossypol is a yellow, polyphenolic pigment, which is contained in most of the parts of plants belonging to the *Gossypium* genus and is concentrated in pigment glands within the seeds (Morgan, 2004; Casteel, 2007). Gossypol exists as two isomers (enantiomers) within plants (+ and the more toxic −), and these isomeric forms can be non-toxic and bound to plant proteins or toxic and "free" or unbound (Cheeke, 1998). The concentrations of the toxic free form of gossypol vary widely in whole seeds and meals, with the gossypol in direct solvent-extracted cottonseed meal being much more readily bioavailable than the gossypol contained in whole seeds (Cheeke, 1998; Casteel, 2007).

Gossypol can cause systemic and reproductive disease syndromes, depending on the species of exposed animal and the dosage of free gossypol consumed (Randel et al., 1992). The toxic effects of gossypol are cumulative, and systemic disease, characterized by hepatic, renal, cardiovascular and pulmonary abnormalities, is generally observed in monogastric animals (Cheeke, 1998). Mature ruminants are considered to be relatively resistant to the severe systemic effects of free gossypol because of the propensity of this form of the pigment to become bound to proteins in ruminal fluid and, therefore, "detoxified" (Casteel, 2007). Gossypol-induced male subfertility has been observed in monogastrics and, especially, ruminant species and is dependent on the dosage of free gossypol and the duration of gossypol exposure (Randel et al., 1992; Cheeke, 1998).

Exposure of peri-pubertal or sexually mature males to sufficient dosages of free gossypol adversely affects the seminiferous epithelium and disrupts normal spermiogenesis, resulting in spermatozoa with aplastic midpieces (i.e., segmental aplasia of the mitochondrial sheath) (Randel et al., 1992; Chenoweth et al., 2000). Additional sperm abnormalities, possibly associated with gossypol-induced oxidative damage (Velasquez-Pereira et al., 1998), can potentially develop as stressors related to the acquisition of motility in the epididymidis, and alter the structural integrity of already weakened spermatozoa (Chenoweth et al., 2000). The spermatozoal abnormalities induced by exposure of immature bulls to free gossypol are most likely reversible (Hassan et al., 2004) and can be ameliorated by concurrent treatment with vitamin E (Velasquez-Pereira et al., 1998). Total dietary concentrations of free gossypol supplied as cottonseed meal or whole cottonseed should not exceed 150 and 600 ppm, respectively, in young developing bulls, or, similarly, 200 and 900 ppm in sexually mature animals (Morgan, 2004).

Xenoestrogens and Antiestrogens

Reproductive function in sexually mature males can potentially be adversely affected by exposures to nuclear ER agonists or antagonists, as well as by estrogenic or antiestrogenic EDCs acting independently of receptor-mediated interactions (Evans, 2017). However, it is clear from the feminizing effects of prenatal exposures to DES (McLachlan, 2001; Newbold et al., 2006) and observations of androgynization in wildlife species (Edwards et al., 2006) that the male fetus is much more sensitive to the adverse effects of endocrine disruptors than male animals during the postnatal period (Hess and Iguchi, 2002). It is also important to remember that, even in males, xenobiotics which interfere with estrogenic signaling pathways can adversely affect normal reproductive development and function (O'Donnell et al., 2001; Hess, 2003).

Xenoandrogens and Antiandrogens

Normal phenotypic sexual differentiation of the male fetus, as well as all of the postnatal events which result in the delivery of fertile spermatozoa to the female reproductive tract, is dependent on appropriately timed androgenic stimulation of the male. It has been well recognized for quite some time that xenoandrogens (e.g., anabolic steroids and exogenous testosterone and DHT) can interfere with hypothalamic–pituitary–gonadal feedback mechanisms (Figure 17.2), resulting in decreased LH release, sperm abnormalities and testicular atrophy (Ellington and Wilker, 2006). In recent years, there has been increasing interest in xenobiotics which can interfere with interactions between androgens and their receptors or, in some other way, disrupt androgen-dependent signaling pathways. The dicarboximide fungicides vinclozolin and procymidone and/or their metabolites inhibit the binding of androgens to nuclear androgen receptors and can demasculinize and feminize the prenatally exposed male fetus or induce important alterations in pre- or peripubertally exposed offspring (Monosson et al., 1999; Gray et al., 2006). Vinclozolin has also recently been shown to be capable, in some experimental settings, of inducing epigenetic modifications which facilitate the occurrence of transgenerational or vertically transmitted reproductive abnormalities (Anway et al., 2005; Anway and Skinner, 2006). Other potential EDCs, including linuron, *p,p′*-DDE (another metabolite of DDT), prochloraz and, more recently, pyrethroid insecticides can also function as androgen receptor antagonists, with PBDEs acting as competitive inhibitors of the androgen receptor as well as androgen-induced gene expression (Gray et al., 2006; Zhang, 2008: Evans, 2017). The AhR-mediated effects of TCDD can interfere with the biosynthesis of testosterone and disrupt testosterone signal transduction pathways (Jana et al., 1999; Sikka et al., 2005).

Phthalates

It is recognized that phthalates, which are used as plasticizers and which are abundant within the environment, share a unique antiandrogenic mechanism, which can result in reproductive dysgenesis in male offspring. Unlike vinclozolin, phthalates are not androgen receptor antagonists, but it is also clear that they are not uterotropic nor are they capable of inducing a persistent estrus, as would be expected with estrogenic EDCs (Gray et al., 2006). Phthalates actually alter fetal Leydig cell function, resulting in decreased testosterone synthesis and down-regulated expression of insulin-like peptide-3, which is required for gubernacular cords formation (Foster, 2006; Gray et al., 2006; Foster and Gray, 2008). Appropriately timed fetal exposure to di (*n*-butyl) phthalate can result in an abnormal aggregation of Leydig cells in the fetal rat testis, resulting in a failure of Sertoli cell proliferation and functional maturation, similar to what has been proposed as a possible mechanism the development of TDS in humans (Sharpe et al., 2003; Mahood et al., 2005, 2006).

Toxicants Affecting the Female Reproductive Function

There have been many documented reports of female reproductive abnormalities associated with exposures of domestic animal species to naturally occurring EDCs (i.e., phytoestrogens and zearalenone) (Evans, 2011a). Likewise, the adverse endocrine disruptive effects of the ergot alkaloids produced by the tall fescue endophyte *Neotyphodium coenophialum* are also very well understood (Evans et al., 2004; see Chapter 72 in this book). Unfortunately, however, there are still instances of toxicant-induced subfertility which very likely go unrecognized. An effort will be made to review some of the major mechanisms of action for toxic insult to the female reproductive tract in domestic animals, in the hope that the reader might better understand the potential scope of xenobiotic-induced reproductive effects.

Selected Female Reproductive Toxicants and Mechanisms of Action

Cell-Specific Reproductive Toxicants

In general, the effects of toxicants on specific cell types within the female reproductive tract, and especially the ovaries, are not as well understood as they are in the testes (Thomas and Thomas, 2001). Many female reproductive toxicants do not target particular cell lines *per se*, but, rather, disrupt the endocrine milieu of the tubular genitalia or cause changes in ovarian structures secondary to alterations in the hypothalamic–pituitary–gonadal axis (Haschek et al., 2010). There are, however, a number of xenobiotics considered to be "ovotoxic." Phthalates and TCDD can delay or decrease ovulations (Devine and Hoyer, 2005). Ionizing radiation and some of the same chemotherapeutic agents reported to adversely affect rapidly dividing germ cells within the testes (e.g., cyclophosphamide, nitrogen mustard and vinblastine) can also adversely affect primordial follicles within the ovary (Thomas and Thomas, 2001; Devine and Hoyer, 2005). Several PAHs (i.e., BaP, 3-methylcholanthrene (3-MC) and DMBA) and 1,3-butadiene appear to target oocytes in preantral follicles, and DMBA, BaP and 1- and 2-bromopropane, as well as 1,2-dibromopropane, can adversely affect antral follicular development (Devine and Hoyer, 2005). Exposure to free gossypol has been associated with increased numbers of degenerating embryos in heifers (Casteel, 2007).

Like the testes, the ovaries also have some xenobiotic biotransformation capabilities (Thomas and Thomas, 2001; Haschek et al., 2010). As in other organs, oxidative damage can adversely affect ovarian structure and function. In the case of 1,3-butadiene and 4-vinylcyclohexene, the adverse effects of these toxicants on small and growing follicles are due, in part, to the toxic actions of the epoxidated metabolites of these xenobiotics (Devine and Hoyer, 2005).

Heavy Metals

The ovaries do not appear to be as sensitive to the toxic effects of heavy metals as do the testes, and those adverse effects which are observed are more subject to variation between species than what was observed in the male gonads (Thomas, 1995). Anterior pituitary release of FSH and LH and ovarian steroidogenesis appear to be inhibited by cadmium in the female (Hoyer, 2006). With respect to lead, the neuroendocrine function of the hypothalamic–pituitary–gonadal axis appears to be targeted by lead in the female, as well as in the male (Thomas, 1995; Hoyer, 2006).

Phytoestrogens

Several genera of leguminous plants produce estrogenic compounds collectively referred to as "phytoestrogens," which can be associated with clinically relevant effects in livestock species and companion animals. Species of clover, including subterranean clover (*Trifolium subterraneum*), red clover (*Trifolium pratense*), white clover (*Trifolium repens*) and alsike clover (*Trifolium hybridum*), contain phytoestrogens classified as isoflavones (Cheeke, 1998; Burrows and Tyrl, 2001; Mostrom and Evans, 2011; Evans, 2011a). It should also be noted that other leguminous plants, such as soybean (*Glycine max*), which is commonly used as a feed source for agricultural animals, can contain varying amounts of isoflavones. Alfalfa (*Medicago sativa*) contains another class of phytoestrogenic compounds referred to as coumestans (Cheeke, 1998; Mostrom and Evans, 2011).

The relatively inactive, "parent" glycosides for the most clinically relevant isoflavones in clover are formononetin, biochanin A and genestin, and the total concentration of these phytoestrogens can be as high as 2 to 4% (20,000–40,000 ppm) in clover (Burrows and Tyrl, 2001). Primarily within the gastrointestinal tract and, especially, the rumen, formononetin is converted into an intermediate metabolite, daidzein, and, then subsequently into the more estrogenically active phytoestrogen, equol (Cheeke, 1998; Burrows and Tyrl, 2001). Conversely, biochanin A and genestin are initially converted into genestein and then subsequently into estrogenically inactive phenolic compounds (i.e., phenolic acid and *p*-ethylphenol).

Coumestrol is the primary phytoestrogen in alfalfa. This compound has significantly greater estrogenic activity than many of the isoflavones present in other legumes, and this activity generally decreases during the drying process involved in hay production (Cheeke, 1998; Burrows and Tyrl, 2001). Coumestrol is usually only present at very low concentrations (10 to 20 ppm) in the vegetative stages of alfalfa growth, but its estrogenic activity can vary with plant maturity and from year to year (Burrows and Tyrl, 2001; Mostrom and Evans, 2011; Evans, 2011a).

A number of clinical syndromes have been associated with phytoestrogen exposure in domestic animals. Precocious mammary development has been reported in several instances of phytoestrogen exposure and can be especially evident in dairy breeds of cattle and goats (Evans, 2011a). "Clover disease" in sheep and, to a lesser extent, cattle is associated with the consumption of the isoflavones in clover, resulting in infertility associated with abnormal estrous cycles and structural and functional changes in the cervix (Cheeke, 1998; Burrows and Tyrl, 2001). Phytoestrogen-induced alterations in ovine cervical mucus interfere with the slow, sustained transport of motile spermatozoa from their cervical reservoirs (Cheeke, 1998). Genestein can induce structural changes and, possibly, irreversible organizational abnormalities in the cervix and uterus of exposed gilts (Ford et al., 2006). Coumestan exposure in cattle can be associated with various and, sometimes, seemingly conflicting clinical presentations (e.g., hyperestrogenism, nymphomania, swelling of the external genitalia, estrus suppression, inhibition of ovulation and cystic ovarian disease) (Cheeke, 1998; Casteel, 2007). It is important to remember, particularly when clinical signs are very different from what was anticipated, that phytoestrogens, like other xenoestrogens, can function also as antiestrogens through the inhibition of LH and FSH release from the anterior pituitary and by competing with endogenous estrogens for receptor sites within the tubular genitalia (Cheeke, 1998; Evans, 2017).

Zearalenone

The estrogenic mycotoxin zearalenone is produced by *Fusarium graminearum* (formerly *Fusarium roseum*), under certain environmental and storage conditions and, sometimes, in conjunction with vomitoxin or deoxynivalenol (DON). Cereal grains associated with zearalenone production include corn, wheat, barley and oats, and some grasses in New Zealand have also been reported to have been contaminated with zearalenone (Cheeke, 1998). Swine have been shown to be particularly susceptible to the adverse effects of zearalenone, with pre-pubertal gilts being affected by concentrations of zearalenone in the feed as low as 1 to 3 ppm (Cheeke, 1998; Casteel, 2007). The increased sensitivity of pigs to the estrogenic effects of zearalenone is most likely related to the slow metabolism and enhanced enterohepatic recirculation of zearalenone noted in this particular species (Cheeke, 1998). Cattle and other ruminants can be affected by zearalenone but only at dietary concentrations much higher than those associated with clinical signs in swine (Casteel, 2007). Hyperestrogenism in pre-pubertal gilts is characterized by swelling of the vulva and mammary glands, uterine enlargement and ovarian atrophy, and testicular atrophy and preputial swelling have been observed in immature male swine (Cheeke, 1998). As with other xenoestrogens, interference with estrogenic feedback mechanisms and various ovarian abnormalities, including follicular cysts, have been observed with excessive exposure to zearalenone. Since estrogens are luteotrophic in swine, zearalenone can be associated with prolonged luteal phases (pseudopregnancy), as well as nymphomania in cycling gilts and sows, depending on the phase of the estrous cycle at the time of exposure.

Synthetic Xenoestrogens and Antiestrogens

A wide range of agricultural and industrial chemicals, as well as pharmaceuticals used in birth control preparations, have estrogenic and/or antiestrogenic activities, depending on the endocrine environment, presence of endogenous estrogens and stage of development at the time of exposure. The type of tissue and physiological response being discussed, as well as the relative distribution of ERα and ERβ receptors, will also affect the types of endocrine effects observed in a given circumstance. As has been emphasized previously, the developing fetus is particularly susceptible to the adverse effects of estrogenic and antiestrogenic endocrine disruptors (Hess and Iguchi, 2002).

Some of the synthetic xenobiotics most commonly discussed with respect to their estrogenic and/or, in some instances, their antiestrogenic activity include DES, DDT, PCBs, bisphenol A, nonylphenol, kepone and TCDD (MacLachlan, 2001). While the overall adverse effects of xenoestrogens have already been discussed in this chapter with respect to reproductive development and endocrine disruption, there are several unique clinical aspects of exposures to these types of xenobiotics which should be addressed for completeness. Prenatal human exposures to the synthetic, non-steroidal xenoestrogen DES have been associated with feminization of the male fetus, as well the increased occurrence of clear cell adenocarcinoma of the vagina in young women (McLachlan 2001; McLachlan et al., 2006; Newbold et al., 2006; Rogers and Kavlock, 2008). The use of DES for mismating or pregnancy prevention in dogs has been, in some instances, associated with an increased incidence of cystic endometrial hyperplasia and pyometra. The apparent ability of the widely distributed xenoestrogen bisphenol A to cause adverse developmental effects at very low environmental concentrations and in a manner characterized by a non-monotonic (inverted U- or U-shaped) dose response has been difficult for some researchers to reproduce and remains controversial (Welshons et al., 2006). However, this particular issue is worthy of further, detailed discussions regarding appropriate reproductive endpoints and necessary experimental controls, given the topic's scientific ramifications, societal relevance and potential applications to other EDCs (Evans, 2017).

Xenoandrogens

While the emphasis in the area of endocrine disruption has traditionally been on the adverse effects of xenoestrogen reproductive development and function, there is increasing evidence that there are also instances of endocrine disruptors having androgenic activity. The effluents from pulp and paper mills have recently been shown to be able to masculinize female fish (Gray et al., 2006). In addition, the runoff from cattle feedlots, where the synthetic androgen trenbolone was used for the promotion of growth, has also been shown to have androgenic activity and is also suspected of being associated with masculinization of females in wildlife species (Orlando et al., 2004).

Teratogenesis and Abortion

Mechanisms of Actions of Teratogenesis and Abortion

A large number of xenobiotics have been classified with respect to their teratogenic potential, and these are listed in Table 17.2. The ability of EDCs to interfere with phenotypic sexual differentiation in the fetus has already

TABLE 17.2 Safety of Drugs in Pregnancy

Drug	Recommendation	Comments
Antimicrobial drugs		
Amikacin	C	Aminoglycoside antibiotics easily cross the placenta and may cause 8th nerve toxicity or nephrotoxicity.
Ampicillin	A	Crosses the placenta but has not been shown to be harmful to fetus.
Amoxicillin	A	Crosses the placenta but has not been shown to be harmful to fetus.
Carbenicillin	A	Crosses the placenta but has not been shown to be harmful to fetus.
Cephalosporins	A	Crosses the placenta but has not been shown to be harmful to fetus.
Chloramphenicol	C	May decrease protein synthesis in fetus, particularly in bone marrow.
Ciprofloxacin	D	Do not use during pregnancy; quinolones have been associated with articular cartilage defects.
Clavulanic acid–amoxicillin (Clavamox, Beecham)	A	Crosses the placenta but has not been shown to be harmful to fetus.
Clindamycin	A	Crosses the placenta but has not been shown to be harmful to fetus.
Cloxacillin	A	Crosses the placenta but has not been shown to be harmful to fetus.
Dicloxacillin	A	Crosses the placenta but has not been shown to be harmful to fetus.
Doxycycline	D	Tetracyclines can cause bone and teeth malformations in fetus and may cause toxicity in mother.
Enrofloxacin	D	See ciprofloxacin.
Erythromycin	A	Appears to be safe except for erythromycin estolate, which has been shown to increase the risk of hepatotoxicity in women.
Gentamicin	C	Aminoglycoside antibiotics easily cross the placenta and may cause 8th nerve toxicity or nephrotoxicity. However, specific toxicities from gentamicin have not been reported, and it may be used for a serious infection in place of a suitable alternative.
Hetacillin	A	Crosses the placenta but has not been shown to be harmful to fetus.
Kanamycin	C	Aminoglycoside antibiotics easily cross the placenta and may cause 8th nerve toxicity of nephrotoxicity.
Lincomycin	A	Crosses the placenta but has not been shown to cause problems in fetus.
Metronidazole	C	Teratogenic in laboratory animals, but there is no information for dogs and cats. It should be avoided during the first 3 weeks of pregnancy.
Neomycin	A	Not absorbed sufficiently to cause systemic effects after oral administration.
Oxacillin	A	Crosses the placenta but has not been shown to be harmful to fetus.
Oxytetracycline	D	Toxic to fetus and may increase risk of hepatitis in mother (see tetracycline).
Penicillin G (benzyl penicillin)	A	Crosses the placenta but has not been shown to be harmful to fetus.
Streptomycin	D	See gentamicin. Streptomycin is associated with higher incidence of 8th nerve toxicity than other aminoglycosides.
Sulfonamides	B	Sulfonamides cross the placenta and have produced congenital malformations in rats and mice, but problems have not been reported in dogs or cats; in people, they have caused neonatal icterus when administered near term. Avoid long-acting sulfonamides.
Tetracycline	D	Tetracyclines can cause bone and teeth malformations in fetus and may cause toxicity in mother.

(*Continued*)

TABLE 17.2 (Continued)

Drug	Recommendation	Comments
Trimethoprim–sulfadiazine (Tribrissen, Coopers)	B	Manufacturer states that it is safe during pregnancy in dogs; see also trimethoprim and sulfonamides.
Trimethoprim	B	Teratogenic in rats but probably safe in other species. Folate antagonism and bone marrow depression are possible with prolonged use.
Ticarcillin	A	Crosses the placenta but has not been shown to be harmful to fetus.
Tobramycin	C	Aminoglycoside antibiotics easily cross the placenta and may cause 8th nerve toxicity or nephrotoxicity.
Tylosin	B	No information is available.
Antifungal drugs		
Amphotericin-B	C	There are no known teratogenic effects, but amphotericin is extremely toxic. Use only if the disease is life threatening, in absence of a suitable alternative.
Griseofulvin	D	Teratogenic in rats; causes multiple skeletal and brain malformations in cats.
Ketoconazole	B	Teratogenic and embryotoxic in rats; antiandrogenic; stillbirths have been reported in dogs.
Miconazole	A	Apparently safe if applied topically.
Antiparasitic drugs		
Amitraz	C	Manufacturer states that reproduction studies have not been done; no information available.
Diethylcarbamazine	A	Manufacturer states that the drug may be given to dogs throughout gestation.
Dithiazanine iodide (Dizan, TechAmerica)	B	No information is available; iodide salts may cause congenital goiter if administered for prolonged periods during pregnancy.
Fenbendazole	A	Safe. Has been administered to pregnant bitches without producing adverse effects.
Dichlorvos (Task, Solvay)	B	Caution is advised when administering cholinesterase inhibitors to pregnant animals; it should not be administered to puppies or kittens, but studies in pregnant dogs and cats suggest that there are no adverse effects during pregnancy.
Ivermectin	A	Safe. Reproduction studies in dogs, cattle, horses and pigs have not shown adverse effects.
Levamisole	C	No information available.
Mebendazole	A	Safe. In reproduction studies in dogs, it was not teratogenic or embryotoxic.
Piperazine	A	Safe. No known contraindications for the use of piperazine.
Praziquantel	A	Safe. No adverse effects were seen when tested in pregnant dogs and cats.
Thiacetarsamide (Caparsolate sodium, CEVA)	C	No specific information regarding toxicity to fetus is available. It can be hepatotoxic and nephrotoxic, and heartworm adulticide should be postponed until after parturition.
Bunamidine	A	Has been administered to pregnant bitches without problems and is safe in pregnant cats. Slight interference with spermatogenesis has been seen in male dogs.
Pyrantel	A	Safe. Toxicity studies have not shown any adverse effects.
Thenium	A	Safe. Manufacturer states that except in young puppies, there are no known contraindications.
Thiabendazole	B	Thiabendazole is not teratogenic in laboratory animals, but high doses have produced toxemia in ewes.

(Continued)

TABLE 17.2 (Continued)

Drug	Recommendation	Comments
Trichlorfon	C	Caution is advised when administering organophosphates to pregnant animals. Congenital toxicoses have been reported following administration to pregnant sows. Manufacturer states that trichlorfon should not be administered to pregnant mares, but there are no recommendations for dogs and cats.
Anticancer drugs		
Doxorubicin hydrochloride (Adriamycin, Adria)	C	May produce malformations in newborn or embryotoxicity.
Azathioprine	C	May produce congenital malformations but has been used in pregnant women safely. It may be a suitable alternative to other drugs when immunosuppressive therapy is required.
Chlorambucil	C	May produce malformations in newborn or embryotoxicity.
Cisplatin	C	May produce congenital malformations, embryotoxicity or nephrotoxicity.
Cyclophosphamide	C	May produce malformations in newborn or embryotoxicity.
Methotrexate	C	May produce malformations in newborn or embryotoxicity.
Vincristine	C	May produce malformations in newborn or embryotoxicity.
Analgesic drugs		
Acetaminophen	C	Safety not established in dogs; toxic in cats.
Aspirin	C	Embryotoxicity has been seen in laboratory animals but not in other species. Late in pregnancy, it may produce pulmonary hypertension and bleeding problems (see text).
Flunixin meglumine	C	Safety in pregnancy has not been determined.
Gold (aurothioglucose)	D	Laboratory animal studies clearly show increased congenital malformations.
Ibuprofen	C	Safety in dogs and cats not established.
Indomethacin	C	Can be toxic in adult dogs; can cause premature closure of ductus arteriosus if administered near term.
Phenylbutazone	C	Safety has not been established. Long-term use can depress bone marrow.
Salicylates		Embryotoxicity has been seen in laboratory animals but not in other species. Late in pregnancy, it may produce pulmonary hypertension and bleeding disorders.
Anesthetic and preanesthetic drugs		
Acepromazine	B	Phenothiazines should be avoided near term; they may produce neonatal CNS depression.
Atropine	B	Crosses the placenta and has been used safely but may cause fetal tachycardia.
Butorphanol	B	Safe for short-term use. Neonatal depression can be treated with naloxone.
Codeine	B	Safe for short-term use. Neonatal depression can be treated with naloxone.
Diazepam	C	See anticonvulsants.
Fentanyl	B	Safe for short-term use. Neonatal depression can be treated with naloxone.
Glycopyrrolate	B	Safe. Does not cross placenta as readily as astropine. Studies in rats and rabbits have not revealed teratogenic effects.
Halothane	C	Decreased learning ability has been reported in rats after *in utero* exposure; depression may be seen in neonates after cesarean section; excessive uterine bleeding may be seen when administered during cesarean section.
Isoflurane	B	Probably safe. Depression may be seen in neonates after cesarean section.

(*Continued*)

TABLE 17.2 (Continued)

Drug	Recommendation	Comments
Ketamine	B	Probably safe. Depression may be seen in puppies delivered by cesarean section; may increase intrauterine pressure and induce premature labor.
Lidocaine	A	All local anesthetics appear to be safe when used for a local nerve block or epidural anesthesia.
Meperidine	B	Opiates can produce neonatal sedation and respiratory depression, but the effects can be reversed with the administration of naloxone.
Methoxyflurane	C	Neonatal depression is seen when used for cesarean section.
Morphine	B	Opiates can produce neonatal sedation and respiratory depression, but the effects can be reversed with the administration of naloxone.
Naloxone	A	Has been shown to be safe when administered to newborns within a few minutes after birth.
Nitrous oxide	B	Probably safe. Used frequently for cesarean section without adverse effects.
Oxymorphone	B	Opiates can produce neonatal sedation and respiratory depression, but the effects can be reversed with the administration of naloxone.
Pentobarbital	D	Associated with high incidence of neonatal mortality.
Thiamylal	C	Easily crosses the placenta; all barbiturates produce respiratory depression in fetus; however, thiobarbiturates are not as toxic as pentobarbital.
Thiopental	C	Easily crosses the placenta. All barbiturates produce respiratory depression in fetus; however, thiobarbiturates are not as toxic as pentobarbital.
Gastrointestinal drugs		
Antacids	A	Safe. Not absorbed systemically.
Antiemetics	B	Probably safe if administered short term.
Cimetidine	B	Safety has not been established, but no reports of toxicity in humans.
Dimenhydrinate	B	Safe if used short term.
Diphenhydramine	B	Safe if used short term.
Diphenoxylate	C	Studies have reported adverse effects in laboratory animals, but no adverse effects havebeen reported in pregnant dogs, cats and humans.
Laxatives	B	All laxatives, except castor oil (Squibb), are considered safe if they are used short term. Castor oil causes premature uterine contractions.
Loperamide	C	Same comment as diphenoxylate.
Metoclopramide	B	Safe in laboratory animals, but no studies available for cats or dogs.
Methscopolamine	C	Safety not established.
Misoprostol	D	Synthetic prostaglandin, causes a termination of pregnancy.
Prochlorperazine	B	No reports of toxicity when administered short term.
Ranitidine	B	Safety has not been established, but no reports of toxicity were reported in humans.
Sucralfate	A	Probably safe. Not absorbed systemically.
Sulfasalazine	B	Salicylate component is not absorbed enough to produce adverse effects; sulfonamide may produce neonatal icterus when used near term (see text).
Cardiovascular drugs		
Atropine	B	Probably safe but may produce fetal tachycardia.
Captopril	C	Has been shown to be embryotoxic in laboratory animals and goats.

(Continued)

TABLE 17.2 (Continued)

Drug	Recommendation	Comments
Digitalis	A	Probably safe. No adverse effects seen in humans and laboratory animals (see text).
Furosemide	B	No adverse effects have been reported.
Dopamine	B	Probably safe at therapeutic doses.
Heparin	B	Does not appear to cross placenta.
Hydralazine	B	Probably safe. There have been reports of minor toxicity in rats, but it has been administered safely to pregnant women.
Isoproterenol	C	May cause fetal tachycardia; beta-adrenergic drugs inhibit uterine contractions.
Lidocaine	B	Probably safe. May cause fetal bradycardia.
Nitroglycerin	C	No information available.
Nitroprusside	C	There is a risk of fetal cyanide toxicity with prolonged use.
Procainamide	B	Probably safe. May cause fetal bradycardia.
Propranolol	C	May cause fetal bradycardia, respiratory depression and neonatal hypoglycemia; avoid use near term.
Quinidine	B	Probably safe. May cause fetal bradycardia.
Theophylline	B	No reports of adverse effects.
Thiazide diuretics	C	May cause increased incidence of perinatal mortality.
Warfarin	D	Causes embryotoxicity and congenital malformations, neural tube defects in laboratory animals and humans.
Anticonvulsant drugs		
Diazepam	C	Has been associated with congenital defects in mice, rats and people.
Phenobarbital	B	Has been associated with rare congenital defects and bleeding tendencies in newborn but may be safer than other anticonvulsants (see text).
Phenytoin	C	Teratogenic in rats, mice and people.
Primidone	C	Same risks as phenobarbital and has been associated with increased incidence of hepatitis in adult dogs.
Valproic acid	C	May cause congenital malformations.
Muscle relaxants		
Dantrolene	C	Safety not established.
Dimethyltubocurarine	B	Quarternary base with negligible placental transfer; it does not affect the fetus unless administered in large doses.
Gallamine	B	Quarternary base with negligible placental transfer; it does not affect the fetus unless administered in large doses.
Methocarbamol	C	Safety not established; manufacturer states that it should not be administered during pregnancy.
Pancuronium	B	Quarternary base with negligible placental transfer; it does not affect the fetus unless administered in large doses.
Succinylcholine	B	Quarternary base with negligible placental transfer; it does not affect the fetus unless administered in large doses.
Endocrine drugs		
Betamethasone	C	Corticosteroids have been associated with increased incidence of cleft palate and other congenital malformations, and they may induce premature labor and abortion in dogs (see text).

(*Continued*)

TABLE 17.2 (Continued)

Drug	Recommendation	Comments
Cortisone	C	Corticosteroids have been associated with increased incidence of cleft palate and other congenital malformations, and they may induce premature labor and abortion in dogs (see text).
Dexamethasone	C	Corticosteroids have been associated with increased incidence of cleft palate and other congenital malformations, and they may induce premature labor (see text). Dexamethasone has caused abortion and fetal death in dogs.
Diethylstilberstrol (DES)	D	Malformation of male and female genitourinary systems.
Estradiolcypionate (ECP)	D	Malformation of male and female genital tracts and bone marrow depression.
Flumethasone	C	Corticosteroids have been associated with increased incidence of cleft palate and other congenital malformations, and they may induce premature labor and abortion in dogs (see text).
Mitotane (*o,p*-DDD)	D	Adrenocortical necrosis.
Prednisolone	C	Although prednisolone has been administered to pregnant women without adverse effects, caution is advised (see dexamethasone). Prednisolone may be used in serious diseases in absence of a suitable alternative.
Stanozolol	D	Manufacturer states that it should not be administered to pregnant dogs and cats.
Testosterone	D	Causes masculinization of female fetus.
Thyroxine	B	Does not cross placenta easily and has not been associated with any problems.
Miscellaneous drugs		
Ammonium chloride	B	May cause fetal acidosis; discontinue use during pregnancy.
Aspartame (Nutra Sweet)	A	No risk.
Dimethylsulfoxide (DMSO)	C	Teratogenic in laboratory animals; manufacturers state that it should not be applied to breeding animals.

A: Probably safe. Although specific studies may not have proved the safety of all drugs in dogs and cats, ther are no reports of adverse effects in laboratory animals or in women.
B: Safe for use if used cautiously. Studies in laboratory animals may have uncovered some risk, but these drugs appear to be safe in dogs and cats or these drugs are safe if they are not administered when the animal is near term.
C: These drugs may have potential risks. Studies in people or laboratory animals have uncovered risks, and these drugs should be used cautiously, as a last resort when the benefit of therapy clearly outweighs the risks.
D: Contraindicated. These drugs have been shown to cause congenital malformations or embryotoxicity.

been extensively reviewed in this chapter. Teratogenesis can be associated with each of the following mechanisms of action: (1) excessive cell death; (2) interference with apoptosis; (3) reduced cellular proliferation rate; (4) failed interactions between cells; (5) impaired morphogenetic movements; (6) reduced synthesis of components essential for growth and development; (7) mechanical disruption; (8) and alterations in pH (Hood et al., 2002; Hood, 2006). Some teratogens are capable of more than one mechanism of action. Premature parturition or abortion can be induced by any xenobiotics which cause fetal or, potentially, maternal stress and initiate the cascade of endocrine and neural signaling events which would normally lead to parturition. Any intoxication in a pregnant animal has the potential to threaten fetal survival. Toxicants which cause sudden fetal death or complete cessation of placental function or disruption of the gestational source of progestagens can also induce abortion in animals.

Heavy Metals

Several heavy metals have been identified as teratogens and possible abortifacients in humans and animals. The adverse effects of *in utero* lead exposure, on the developing nervous systems of both humans and laboratory animal species, have been well documented (Evans et al., 2003; Rogers and Kavlock, 2008). Prenatal exposure to organotins has been associated with pregnancy loss and impaired ossification in rodents (Ema and Hirose, 2006), and organic mercury is a known developmental neurotoxicant (Golub, 2006b). Other heavy metals, including cadmium and mercury, have been associated with placental toxicity, and this topic is covered in greater detail in Chapter 20 of this book.

Selected Plant-Associated Teratogens and Abortifacients

Many potentially toxic plants have been found to induce teratogenesis and/or abortion in mammals, including swainsonine-containing species of *Astragalus* and *Oxytropis* and plants associated with nitrate/nitrite intoxication. While it is not possible to extensively review all of these plants in this chapter, there are several well-documented examples of plant-induced birth defects and abortion which clearly illustrate the basic principles regarding the pathogenesis of teratogenesis and abortion in domestic animals. There are a number of references which review the adverse effects of specific plants and/or toxicants on reproduction in some detail (Burrows and Tyrl, 2001; Evans, 2011a; Panter and Stegelmeier, 2011; Panter et al., 2017).

Veratrum Californicum

Jervanine alkaloids (e.g., cyclopamine, cycloposine and jervine) in *Veratrum californicum* (false hellebore) and, potentially, some closely related plants have been associated with the occurrence of cyclops lambs and other developmental abnormalities in sheep, as well as, less commonly, cattle and goats (Burrows and Tyrl, 2001; Panter and Stegelmeier, 2011; Panter et al., 2017). The mechanism of action of the teratogenic alkaloids in species of *Veratrum* involves interference with the *sonic hedgehog* (SHH) signal transduction pathway and the inhibition of neuroepithelial cell mitosis and migration during neurulation and decreased proliferation of chondrocytes (Cheeke, 1998; Burrows and Tyrl, 2001; Panter and Stegelmeier, 2011). The specific developmental abnormalities and the precise timing of maternal exposure to *Veratrum californicum*, which results in these defects is as follows: cyclops lambs and prolonged gestation (associated with the absence of pituitary gland) from maternal exposure on days 12 to, particularly, day 14 of gestation; embryonic death from maternal exposure on gestational days 19 to 21; cleft palate from maternal exposure on gestational days 24 to 30, metacarpal and metatarsal defects (limb reductions) and tracheal cartilage defects (tracheal stenosis) from maternal exposure on gestational days 28 to 31 and 31 to 33, respectively (Burrows and Tyrl, 2001). No abnormal effects were observed with maternal exposure to *Veratrum californicum* before day 10 or after day 35 of pregnancy, and *Veratrum*-associated birth defects can generally be prevented by avoiding exposure until at least 5 weeks after breeding.

Multiple Congenital Contractures

Species of tobacco (*Nicotiana* spp.), poison hemlock (*Conium maculatum*) and lupines (*Lupinus* spp.) have all been shown to be able to induce MCC or "crooked calf disease" in cattle and, potentially, other species exposed to their toxic principles at the appropriate stage of gestation. The condition is characterized by cleft palate and limb and spinal contractures. Pyridine alkaloids (e.g., anabasine) in tobacco, piperidine alkaloids in poison hemlock (e.g., coniine and γ-coniceine) and piperidine-derived and quinolizidine alkaloids in lupines (e.g., ammodendrine and anagyrine, respectively) cause stimulation then depression (depolarizing neuromuscular blockade) of nicotinic receptors in the fetus (Cheeke, 1998; Burrows and Tyrl, 2001; Panter, 2002). This stimulation followed by neuromuscular blockade of fetal nicotinic receptors during the critical period of palate and joint development (i.e., gestational days 40 to 100 in cattle; days 30 to 60 in sheep; days 30 to 60 in swine) results in decreased fetal movement and the failure of the palate and joints to form in a normal fashion (Panter, 2002; Panter and Stegelmeier, 2011).

Pine Needle Abortion

Ingestion by cattle of pine needles (*Pinus ponderosa*) containing isocupressic acid (also possibly present in the vegetation of some junipers and cypresses) results in late-term abortion (Cheeke, 1998). Inhibition of the catechol estrogen-induced blockade of potential-sensitive $Ca2+$ channels by isocupressic acid leads to enhanced entry of divalent calcium into arterial smooth muscle cells supplying the gravid uterus and results in profound vasoconstriction (Casteel, 1997; Cheeke, 1998; Burrows and Tyrl, 2001; Panter and Stegelmeier, 2011; Panter et al., 2017). This isocupressic acid-induced vasoconstriction can lead to at least a 50% reduction in the blood flow reaching the fetal circulation and causes fetal stress, leading to the induction of premature parturition or abortion (Cheeke, 1998; Burrows and Tyrl, 2001). Late-term abortion occurs 2–14 days following heavy consumption of green or dry pine needles and results in up to 75% of exposed cows aborting or delivering dead or weak calves (Cheeke, 1998; Burrows and Tyrl, 2001; Casteel, 2007; Panter and Stegelmeier, 2011). Dams are frequently dull and depressed, with weak uterine contractions, incomplete cervical dilation, retained placenta and frequent postpartum metritis (Cheeke, 1998).

CONCLUDING REMARKS

Reproduction is a critical biological process, required for financially viable livestock production, as well as species survival. Toxicant-induced abortions, congenital defects and subfertility can have devastating effects on both domestic animals and wildlife species. There is growing concern within the scientific and government regulatory communities, and especially the general public, about the potential for these toxicant-induced effects in humans. The information presented in this chapter was intended to familiarize the reader with terminology and concepts pertinent to reproductive toxicity and endocrine disruption, as well as to provide an overview of reproductive development, anatomy and physiology and aspects of these processes susceptible to toxic insult by naturally occurring and synthetic xenobiotics. The information and references provided should assist readers in making informed decisions in the course of their future clinical investigations, experimental designs and interpretations of scientific literature and/or regulatory policies.

REFERENCES

Akinloye, O., Arowojulu, A.O., Shittu, O.B., Anetor, J.I., 2006. Cadmium toxicity: a possible cause of male infertility in Nigeria. Reprod Biol. 6 (1), 17–30.

Anway, M.D., Skinner, M.K., 2006. Epigenetic transgenerational actions of endocrine disruptors. Endocrinology 147 (6 Suppl.), S43–S49.

Anway, M.D., Cupp, A.S., Uzumcu, M., Skinner, M.K., 2005. Epigenetic transgenerational actions of endocrine disruptor and male fertilitys. Science 308, 1466–1469.

Basrur, P.K., 2006. Disrupted sex differentiation and feminization of man and domestic animals. Environ Res. 100 (1), 18–38.

Bigsby, R.M., Mercado-Feliciano, M., Mubiru, J., 2005. Molecular mechanisms of estrogen dependent processes. In: Naz, R.K. (Ed.), Endocrine Disruptors: Effects on Male and Female Reproductive Systems, second edn. CRC Press and Taylor and Francis Group, LLC, Boca Raton, FL, pp. 217–247.

Brayman, M.J., Julian, J., BiserkaMulac-Jericevic, B., Conneely, O.M., Edwards, D.P., Carson, D.D., 2006. Progesterone receptor isoforms A and B differentially regulate MUC1 expression in uterine epithelial cells. Mol. Endocrinol. 20, 2278–2291.

Britt, K.L., Findlay, J.K., 2002. Estrogen actions in the ovary revisited. J. Endocrinol. 175, 269–276.

Burrows, G.E., Tyrl, R.J., 2001. Toxic Plants of North America. Iowa State University Press, Ames, IA, pp. 1–1342.

Capen, C.C., 2008. Toxic responses of the endocrine system. In: Klaassen, C.D. (Ed.), Casarett and Doull's Toxicology: The Basic Science of Poisons, seventh edn. McGraw-Hill, New York, pp. 807–877.

Casteel, S.W., 2007. Reproductive toxicants. In: Youngquist, R.S. (Ed.), Current Therapy in Large Animal Theriogenology, second edn. Saunders Elsevier, St. Louis, pp. 420–427.

Casteel, S.W., Evans, T.J., 2004. Nitrate. In: Plumlee, K.H. (Ed.), Clinical Veterinary Toxicology. Mosby, Inc, St. Louis, MO, pp. 127–130.

Cheeke, P.R., 1998. Natural Toxicants in Feeds, second edn. Interstate Publishers, Inc, Danville, IL, pp. 1–479.

Chenoweth, P.J., Chase, C.C., Risco, C.A., Larsen, R.E., 2000. Characterization of gossypol-induced sperm abnormalities in bulls. Theriogenology 53, 1193–1203.

Cooke, P.S., Naz, A., 2005. Effects of estrogens and the phytoestrogen genistein on adipogenesis and lipogenesis in males and females. Birth Defects Res. A Clin. Mol. Teratol. 73, 472–473.

Crews, C., McLachlan, J.A., 2006. Epigenetics, evolution, endocrine disruption, health and disease. Endocrinology 147 (6 Suppl.), S4–S10.

Devine, P.J., Hoyer, P.B., 2005. Ovotoxic environmental chemicals: indirect endocrine disruptors. In: Naz, R.K. (Ed.), Endocrine Disruptors: Effects on Male and Female Reproductive Systems, second edn. CRC Press and Taylor and Francis Group, LLC, Boca Raton, FL, pp. 67–100.

Dutertre, M., Smith, C.L., 2000. Molecular mechanisms of selective estrogen receptor modulator (SERM) action. J Pharmacol. Exper. Ther. 295 (2), 431–437.

Dyce, K.M., Sack, W.O., Wensing, C.J.G., 2002. Textbook of Veterinary Anatomy, third edn. Saunders, Philadelphia, PA, pp. 1–840.

Eaton, D.L., Klaassen, C.D., 2001. Principles of toxicology. In: Klaassen, C.D. (Ed.), Casarett and Doull's Toxicology: The Basic Science of Poisons, sixth edn. McGraw-Hill, New York, pp. 11–34.

Edwards, T.M., Moore, B.C., Guillette Jr, L.J., 2006. Reproductive dysgenesis in wildlife: a comparative view. Environment, reproductive health and fertility. Internat J Androl. 29 (1), 109–119.

Ellington, J.E., Wilker, C.E., 2006. Reproductive toxicology in the male companion animal. In: Peterson, M.E., Talcott, P.A. (Eds.), Small Animal Toxicology, second edn. Elsevier Saunders, St. Louis, MO, pp. 500–518.

Ema, M., Hirose, A., 2006. Reproductive and developmental toxicity of organotin compounds. Metals, Fertility and Reproductive Toxicity. CRC Press and Taylor and Francis Group, LLC, Boca Raton, FL, pp. 23–64.

Evans TJ (1996) The effects of bromocriptine, domperidone, and reserpine on circulating, maternal levels of progestins, estrogens, and prolactin in pregnant pony mares. Masters Thesis, University of Missouri-Columbia, MO.

Evans, T.J., 2011a. Diminished reproductive performance and selected toxicants in forages and grains. Vet. Clin. North Am. Food Anim. Pract. 27, 345–371.

Evans, T.J., 2011b. The endocrine disruptive effects of ergopeptine alkaloids on pregnant mares. Vet. Clin. North Am. Equine. Pract. 27, 165–173.

Evans, T.J., 2017. Endocrine disruptors. In: Gupta, R.C. (Ed.), Reproductive and Developmental Toxicology, 2nd edn. Academic Press, San Diego, CA, pp. 1091–1110.

Evans, T.J., Ganjam, V.K., 2017. Reproductive anatomy and physiology. In: Gupta, R.C. (Ed.), Reproductive and Developmental Toxicology, 2nd edn. Academic Press, San Diego, CA, pp. 7–37.

Evans, T.J., James-Kracke, M.R., Kleiboeker, S.B., Casteel, S.W., 2003. Lead enters Rcho-1 trophoblastic cells by calcium transport mechanisms and complexes with calcium-binding proteins. Toxicol. Appl. Pharmacol. 186, 77–89.

Evans, T.J., Rottinghaus, G.E., Casteel, S.W., 2004. Fescue. In: Plumlee, K.H. (Ed.), Clinical Veterinary Toxicology. Mosby, Inc, St. Louis, MO, pp. 243–250.

Evans, T.J., Constantinescu, G.M., Ganjam, V.K., 2007. Clinical reproductive anatomy and physiology of the mare. In: Younquist, R.S., Threlfall, W.R. (Eds.), Current Therapy in Large Animal Theriogenology, second edn. Saunders Elsevier, St. Louis, pp. 47–67.

Fisher, J.S., MacPherson, S., Marchetti, N., Sharpe, R.M., 2003. Human "testicular dysgenesis syndrome": a possible model using in-utero exposure to dibutyl phthalate. Hum. Reprod. 18 (7), 1383–1394.

Ford, J.J., D'Occhio, 1989. Differentiation of sexual behavior in cattle, sheep and swine. J. Anim. Sci. 67 (7), 1816–1823.

Ford Jr, J.A., Clark, S.G., Walters, E.M., Wheeler, M.B., Hurley, W.L., 2006. Estrogenic effects of genestein on reproductive tissues of ovariectomized gilts. J. Anim. Sci. 84, 834–842.

Foster, P.M.D., 2006. Disruption of reproductive development in male rat offspring following in utero exposure to phthalate esters. Internat. J. Androl. 29 (1), 140–147.

Foster, P.M.D., Gray Jr, L.E., 2008. Toxic responses of the reproductive system. In: Klaassen, C.D. (Ed.), Casarett and Doull's Toxicology: The Basic Science of Poisons, seventh edn. McGraw-Hill, New York, pp. 761–806.

França, L.R., Avelar, G.F., Almeida, F.F.L., 2005. Spermatogenesis and sperm transit through the epididymis in mammals with emphasis on pigs. Theriogenology 63, 300–318.

Genuth, S.M., 2004a. General principles of endocrine physiology. In: Berne, R.M., Levy, M.N., Koeppen, B.M., Stanton, B.A. (Eds.), Physiology, fifth edn. Mosby, Inc, St. Louis, MO, pp. 719–742.

Genuth, S.M., 2004b. The reproductive glands. In: Berne, R.M., Levy, M.N., Koeppen, B.M., Stanton, B.A. (Eds.), Physiology, fifth edn. Mosby, Inc, St. Louis, MO, pp. 920–978.

Ginther, O.J., 1992. Reproductive Biology of the Mare: Basic and Applied Aspects. second edn. Equiservices, Cross Plains, WI.

Gojmerac, T., Pleadin, J., Zuric, M., Rajkovic-Janje, R., Korsic, M., 2004. Serum luteinizing hormone response to administration of gonadotropin-releasing hormones to atrazine-treated gilts. Vet. Hum. Toxicol. 46 (5), 245–247.

Golub, M.S. (Ed.), 2006a. Metals, Fertility and Reproductive Toxicity. CRC Press and Taylor and Francis Group, LLC, Boca Raton, FL.

Golub, M.S., 2006b. Reproductive toxicity of mercury, arsenic and cadmium. Metals, Fertility and Reproductive Toxicity. CRC Press and Taylor and Francis Group, LLC, Boca Raton, FL, pp. 6–22.

Gray Jr, L.E., Wilson, V.S., Stoker, T., Lambright, C., Furr, J., Noriega, N., et al., 2006. Adverse effects of environmental antiandrogens and androgens on reproductive development in mammals. Environment, reproductive health and fertility. Internat. J. Androl. 29 (1), 96–104.

Gregus, Z., 2008. Mechanisms of toxicity. In: Klaassen, C.D. (Ed.), Casarett and Doull's Toxicology: The Basic Science of Poisons, seventh edn. McGraw-Hill, New York, pp. 45–106.

Grün, F., Blumberg, B., 2006. Environmental obesogens: organotins and endocrine disruption nuclear receptor signaling. Endocrinology 147 (6 Suppl.), S50–S55.

Guillette Jr, L.J., 2006. Environmental disrupting contaminants – beyond the dogma. Environ Health Perspect. 114 (S-1), 9–12.

Gupta, R.C. (Ed.), 2017. Reproductive and Developmental Toxicology, 2nd edn. Academic Press, Amsterdam.

Gupta, R.K., Gupta, R.C., 2017. Placental toxicity. In: Gupta, R.C. (Ed.), Reproductive and Developmental Toxicology, 2nd ed Academic Press/Elsevier, Amsterdam, pp. 1301–1325.

Hafez, B., Hafez, E.S.E. (Eds.), 2000. Reproduction in Farm Animals. seventh edn. Lipincott Williams & Wilkins, Philadelphia, PA.

Haschek, W., Rousseaux, C.G., Wallig, M.A., 2010. Fundamentals of Toxicologic Pathology. 2nd edn Academic Press, San Diego, CA, pp. 1–691.

Hassan, M.E., Smith, G.W., Ott, R.S., Faulkner, D.B., Firkins, L.D., Ehrhardt, E.J., et al., 2004. Reversibility of the reproductive toxicity of gossypol in peripubertal bulls. Theriogenology 16 (6), 1171–1179.

Hayes, T.B., Stuart, A.A., Mendoza, M., Collins, A., Noriega, N., Vonk, A., et al., 2006. Characterization of atrazine-induced gonadal malformations in African clawed frogs (*Xenopus laevis*) and comparisons with effects of an androgen antagonist (cypterone acetate) and exogenous estrogen (17-estradiol): support for the demasculinization/feminization hypothesis. Environ. Health Perspect. 114 (S-1), 134–141.

Hood, R.D., Rousseaux, C.G., Blakely, P.M., 2002. Embryo and fetus. In: Haschek, W.M., Rousseaux, C.G., Wallig, M.A. (Eds.), Handbook of Toxicologic Pathology, Vol. 2. Academic Press, San Diego, CA, pp. 895–936.

Hedrich, H.J., Bullock, G. (Eds.), 2004. Elsevier Academic Press, Boston, MA.

Hess, R.A., 2003. Estrogen in the adult male reproductive tract: a review. Reprod. Biol. Endocrinol. 1, 52–65.

Hess, R.A., Iguchi, T., 2002. Role of herbicides and pesticides on endocrine disruption. Proceedings of Annual Conference of the Society for Theriogenology and American College of Theriogenologists. Colorado Springs, CO, pp. 443–452.

Hodgson, E., Mailman, R.B., Chambers, J.E., Dow, R.E., 2000 second edn. Grove's Dictionaries Inc., New York. pp. 1–504.

Hood, R.D. (Ed.), 2006. Developmental and Reproductive Toxicology: A Practical Approach, second edn. CRC Press and Taylor and Francis Group, LLC, Boca Raton, FL.

Hoyer, P.B., 2006. Impact of metals on ovarian function. In: Golub, M.S. (Ed.), Metals, Fertility and Reproductive Toxicity. CRC Press and Taylor and Francis Group, LLC, Boca Raton, FL, pp. 155–173.

Hughes, I.A., Martin, H., Jääskeläinen, J., 2006. Genetic mechanisms of fetal male undermasculinization: a background to the role of endocrine disruptors. Environ. Res. 100, 44–49.

Jana, N.R., Sarkar, S., Ishizuka, M., Yonemoto, J., Tohyama, C., Stone, H., 1999. Cross-talk between 2,3,7,8-tetrachlorodibenzo-*p*-dioxin and testosterone signal transduction pathways in LNCaP prostate cancer cells. Biochem. Biophys. Res. Commun. 256, 462–466.

Jobling, S., Tyler, C.R., 2006. The ecological relevance of chemically induced endocrine disruption in wildlife. Environ. Health. Perspect. 114 (S-1), 1–160.

Johnston, S.D., Root, M.V., Olson, P.N.S. (Eds.), 2002. Canine and Feline Theriogenology. W.B. Saunders, Philadelphia, PA.

Jørgensen, N., Asklund, C., Carlsen, E., Skakkebæk, N.E., 2006a. Coordinated European investigations of semen quality: results from studies of Scandinavian young men is a matter of concern. Internat. J. Androl. 29 (1), 51–59.

Jørgensen, N., McGrigor, K., Toppari, J., Skakkebæk, N.E. (Eds.), 2006b. Environment, reproductive health and fertility. Internat. J. Androl 29 (1), 1–312.

Katzenellenbogen, B.S., Katzenellenbogen, J.A., 2000. Estrogen receptor transcription and transactivation: estrogen receptor alpha and estrogen receptor beta: regulation by selective estrogen receptor modulators and importance in breast cancer. Breast Cancer Res. 2, 335–344.

Keith, L.H., 1997. Environmental Endocrine Disruptors: A Handbook of Property Data. John Wiley & Sons, Inc, New York, pp. 1–1232.

Kharat, I., Saatcioglu, F., 1996. Antiestrogenic effects of 2,3,7,8-tetrachlorodibenzo-*p*-dioxin are mediated by direct transcriptional interference with the liganded estrogen receptor. J. Biol. Chem. 271 (18), 10533–10537.

Knobil, E., 1999. Chair, Committee on Hormonally Active Agents in the Environment. Hormonally Active Agents in the Environment. National Academy Press, Washington, DC, pp. 1–430.

Krimsky, S., 2000. Hormonal Chaos: The Scientific and Social Origins of the Environmental Endocrine Hypothesis. Johns Hopkins University Press, Baltimore, MD, pp. 1–284.

Krimsky S (2001) An epistemological inquiry into the endocrine disruptor thesis. In Environmental Hormones: The Scientific Basis of Endocrine Disruption, McLachlan JA, Guillette LJ, Iguchi T, Toscano Jr WA (eds). Annals NY Acad Sci 948: 130–142.

Kubota, K., Ohsako, S., Kurosawa, S., Takeda, K., Qing, W., Sakaue, M., et al., 2003. Effects of vinclozolin administration on sperm production and testosterone biosynthetic pathway in adult male rat. J. Reprod. Develop. 49, 403–412.

Lehman-McKeeman, L.D., 2008. Absorption, distribution, and excretion of toxicants. In: Klaassen, C.D. (Ed.), Casarett and Doull's Toxicology: The Basic Science of Poisons, seventh edn. McGraw-Hill, New York, pp. 131–159.

Lewin, B., 1998. Genes. sixth edn. Oxford University Press, New York, pp. 1–1260.

Lundholm, C.D., 1997. DDE-induced eggshell thinning in birds; effects of p,p-DDE on the calcium and prostaglandin metabolism of the eggshell gland. Comp. Biochem. Physiol. C Pharmacol. Toxicol. Endocrinol. 118 (2), 113–128.

Mahood, I.K., Hallmark, N., McKinnell, C., Walker, M., Fisher, J.S., Sharpe, R.M., 2005. Abnormal Leydig cell aggregation in the fetal testis of rats exposed to di (*n*-butyl) phthalate and its possible role in testicular dysgenesis. Endocrinology 146 (2), 613–623.

Mahood, I.K., McKinnell, C., Walker, M., Hallmark, N., Scott, H., Fisher, J.S., et al., 2006. Cellular origins of testicular dysgenesis in rats exposed in utero to di(*n*-butyl) phthalate. Internat. J. Androl. 29 (1), 148–154.

McCue, P.M., 1993. Lactation. In: McKinnon, A.O., Voss, J.L. (Eds.), Equine Reproduction. Lea & Febiger, Philadelphia, pp. 588–595.

McLachlan, J.A., 2001. Environmental signaling: what embryos and evolution teach us about endocrine disrupting chemicals. Endocrine Rev. 22 (3), 319–341.

McLachlan, J.A., Simpson, E., Martin, M., 2006. Endocrine disrupters and female reproductive health. Best Pract. Res. Clin. Endocrinol. Metab. 20 (1), 63–75.

Milnes, M.R., Bermudez, D.S., Bryan, T.A., Edwards, T.M., Gunderson, M.P., Larkin, I.L.V., et al., 2006. Contaminant-induced feminization and demasculinization of nonmammalian vertebrate males in aquatic environments. Environ Res. 100 (1), 3–17.

Monosson, E., Kelce, W.R., Lambright, C., Ostby, J., Gray Jr, L.E., 1999. Peripubertal exposure to the antoandrogenic fungicide, vinclozolin, delays puberty, inhibits the development of androgen-dependent tissues, and alters androgen receptor function in the male rat. Toxicol. Ind. Health. 15, 65–79.

Morgan, S., 2004. Gossypol. In: Plumlee, K.H. (Ed.), Clinical Veterinary Toxicology. Mosby, Inc, St. Louis, MO, pp. 119–120.

Mostrom, M., Evans, T.J., 2011. Phytoestrogens. In: Gupta, R.C. (Ed.), Reproductive and Developmental Toxicology. Academic Press, San Diego, CA, pp. 707–722.

Mukerjee, D. (Ed.), 2006. Endocrine disruptors. Environ. Res. 100 (1), 1–99.

Naz, R.K. (Ed.), 2005. Endocrine Disruptors: Effects on Male and Female Reproductive Systems, second edn. CRC Press and Taylor and Francis Group, LLC, Boca Raton, FL.

Neill, J.D., Nagy, G.M., 1994. Prolactin secretion and its control. In: Knobil, E., Neill, J.D. (Eds.), The Physiology of Reproduction, second edn. Raven Press, New York, pp. 1833–1860.

Newbold, R.R., Padilla-Banks, E., Snyder, R.J., Jefferson, W.N., 2005. Developmental exposure to estrogenic compounds and obesity. Birth Defects Res. A Clin. Mol. Teratol. 73, 478–480.

Newbold, R.R., Padilla-Banks, E., Jefferson, W.N., 2006. Adverse effects of the model environmental estrogen diethylstilbestrol are transmitted to subsequent generations. Endocrinology 147 (6 Suppl.), S11–S17.

O'Connor, J.C., Frame, S.R., Ladics, G.S., 2002. Evaluation of a 15-day screening assay using intact male rats for identifying antiandrogens. Toxicol. Sci. 69 (1), 92–108.

O'Donnell, L., Robertson, K.M., Jones, M.E., Simpson, E.R., 2001. Estrogen and spermatogenesis. Endocrine Rev. 22 (3), 229–318.

Ohtake, F., Takeyama, K., Matsumoto, T., Kitagawa, H., Yamamoto, Y., Nohara, K., et al., 2003. Modulation of oestrogen receptor signalling by association with the activated dioxin receptor. Nature 423, 545–550.

Orlando, E.F., Kolok, A., Binzcik, G.A., Gates, J.L., Horton, M.K., Lambright, C.S., et al., 2004. Endocrine-disrupting effects of cattle feedlot effluent on an aquatic sentinel species, the fathead minnow. Environ Health Perspect. 112, 353–358.

Panter, K.E., 2002. Plant and chemical teratogens. Proceedings of Annual Conference of the Society for Theriogenology and American College of Theriogenologists. Colorado Springs, CO, pp. 463–472.

Panter, K.E., Stegelmeier, B.E., 2011. Effects of xenobiotics and phytotoxins on reproduction in food animals. Vet. Clin. North Am. Food Anim. Pract. 27, 430–446.

Panter, K.E., Welch, K.D., Gardner, D.R., 2017. Toxic plants. In: Gupta, R.C. (Ed.), Reproductive and Developmental Toxicology, 2nd edn. Academic Press/Elsevier, Amsterdam, pp. 903–923.

Parkinson, A., Ogilvie, B.W., 2008. Biotransformation of xenobiotics. In: Klaassen, C.D. (Ed.), Casarett and Doull's Toxicology: The Basic Science of Poisons, seventh edn. McGraw-Hill, New York, pp. 161–304.

Petersen, S.L., Krishnan, S., Hudgens, E.D., 2006. The aryl hydrocarbon receptor pathway and sexual differentiation of neuroendocrine functions. Endocrinology 147 (6 Suppl.), S33–S42.

Plumlee, K.H. (Ed.), 2004. Clinical Veterinary Toxicology. Mosby, Inc, St. Louis, MO.

Pratt, W.B., Toft, D.O., 1997. Steroid receptor interactions with heat shock proteins and immunophilin chaperones. Endocrine Rev. 18 (3), 306–360.

Randel, R.D., Chase, C.C., JrWyse, S.J., 1992. Effects of gossypol and cottonseed products on reproduction of mammals. J. Anim. Sci. 70 (5), 1628–1638.

Razandi, M., Pedram, A., Greene, G.L., Levin, E.R., 1999. Cell membrane and nuclear estrogen receptors (ERs) originate from a single transcript: studies of ERα and ERβ expressed in Chinese hamster ovary cells. Mol. Endocrinol. 13 (2), 307–319.

Rogers, J.M., Kavlock, R.J., 2008. Developmental toxicology. In: Klaassen, C.D. (Ed.), Casarett and Doull's Toxicology: The Basic Science of Poisons, seventh edn. McGraw-Hill, New York, pp. 415–449.

Safe, S., 2005. 2,3,7,8-Tetrachlorodibenzo-*p*-dioxin (TCDD) and related environmental antiandrogens: characterization and mechanism of action. In: Naz, R.K. (Ed.), Endocrine Disruptors: Effects on Male and Female Reproductive Systems, second edn. CRC Press and Taylor and Francis Group, LLC, Boca Raton, FL, pp. 249–287.

Schrader, S.M., 2002. Sites of toxicant action of male reproductive toxicants. Proceedings of Annual Conference of the Society for Theriogenology and American College of Theriogenologists. Colorado Springs, CO, pp. 437–442.

Senger, P.L., 2003. Pathways to Pregnancy and Parturition, second edn. Current Conceptions, Inc., Moscow, ID, pp. 1–368.

Sharpe, R.M., McKinnell, C., Kivlin, C., Fisher, J.S., 2003. Proliferation and functional maturation of sertoli cells, and their relevance to disorders of testis function in adulthood. Reproduction 125, 769–784.

Sieli, P.T., Jašarevi, E., Warzak, D.A., Mao, J., Ellersieck, M.R., Liao, C., et al., 2011. Comparison of serum bisphenol A concentrations in mice exposed to bisphenol A through the diet versus oral bolus exposure. Environ Health Perspect. Available from: http://dx.doi.org/10.1289/ehp.1003385.

Sikka, S.C., Kendirci, M., Naz, R., 2005. Endoctine disruptors and male infertility. In: Naz, R.K. (Ed.), Endocrine Disruptors: Effects on Male and Female Reproductive Systems, second edn. CRC Press and Taylor and Francis Group, LLC, Boca Raton, FL, pp. 291–312.

Skakkebæk, N.E., Rajpert-de Meyts, E., Main, K.M., 2001. Testicular dysgenesis syndrome: an increasingly common developmental disorder with environmental aspects. Hum. Reprod. 16 (5), 972–978.

Skakkebæk, N.E., Jørgensen, N., Main, K.M., Rajpert-de Meyts, E., Leffers, H., Andersson, A.-M., et al., 2006. Is human fecundity declining? Internat. J. Androl. 29 (1), 2–11.

Sokol, R.Z., 2006. Lead exposure and its effects on the reproductive system. In: Golub, M.S. (Ed.), Metals, Fertility and Reproductive Toxicity. CRC Press and Taylor and Francis Group, LLC, Boca Raton, FL, pp. 117–154.

Suckow, M.A., Weisbroth, S.H., Frankin, C.L. (Eds.), 2006. The Laboratory Rat. second edn. Elsevier Academic Press, Burlington, MA.

Sutovsky, P., Moreno, R., Ramahlho-Santos, J., Dominko, T., Thompson, W., 2001. A putative, ubiquitin-dependent mechanism for the recognition and elimination of defective spermatozoa in the mammalian epididymis. J. Cell Sci. 114 (9), 1665–1675.

Swan, S.H., Elkin, E.P., Fenster, L., 2000. The question of declining sperm density revisited: an analysis of 101 studies published 1934–1996. Environ. Health Perspect. 108 (10), 961–966.

Swan, S.H., Brazil, C., Drobnis, E.Z., Liu, F., Kruse, R.L., Hatch, M., et al., 2003a. Geographical differences in semen quality of fertile U.S. males. Environ. Health Perspect. 111 (4), 414–420.

Swan, S.H., Kruse, R.L., Liu, F., Barr, D.B., Drobnis, E.Z., Redmon, J.B., et al., 2003b. Semen quality in relation to biomarkers of pesticide exposure. Environ. Health Perspect. 111 (12), 1478–1484.

Swan, S.H., Main, K.M., Liu, F., Stewart, S.L., Kruse, R.L., Calafat, A. M., et al., 2005. Decrease in anogenital distance among male infants with prenatal phthalate exposure. Environ. Health Perspect. 113 (8), 1056–1061.

Thomas, J.A., 1995. Gonadal-specific metal toxicology. In: Goyer, R.A., Klaassen, C.D., Waalkes, M.P. (Eds.), Metal Toxicology. Academic Press, Inc, San Diego, CA, pp. 413–436.

Thomas, M.J., Thomas, J.A., 2001. Toxic responses of the reproductive system. In: Klaassen, C.D. (Ed.), Casarett and Doull's Toxicology: The Basic Science of Poisons, sixth edn. McGraw-Hill, New York, pp. 673–709.

Thomas, P., Khan, I.A., 2005. Disruption of nongenomic steroid actions on gametes and serotonergic pathways controlling reproductive neuroendocrine function by environmental chemicals. In: Naz, R.K. (Ed.), Endocrine Disruptors: Effects on Male and Female Reproductive Systems, second edn. CRC Press and Taylor and Francis Group, LLC, Boca Raton, FL, pp. 3–45.

Tsai, M.-J., O'Malley, B.W., 1994. Molecular mechanisms of action of steroid/thyroid receptor superfamily members. Annu. Rev. Biochem. 63, 451–486.

Tucker, A., 1994. Lactation and its hormonal control. In: Knobil, E., Neill, J.D. (Eds.), The Physiology of Reproduction, second edn. Raven Press, New York, pp. 1065–1098.

Velasquez-Pereira, J., Chenoweth, P.J., McDowell, L.R., Risco, C.A., Williams, S.N., Wilkinson, N.S., 1998. Reproductive effects of feeding gossypol and vitamin E to bulls. J. Anim. Sci. 76, 2894–2904.

Warner, M., Gustafsson, J.-A., 2006. Nongenomic effects of estrogen: why all the uncertainty? Steroids 71, 91–95.

Welshons, W.V., Nagel, S.C., vom Saal, F.S., 2006. Large effects from small exposures. III. Endocrine mechanisms mediating effects of bisphenol A at levels of human exposure. Endocrinology 147 (6 Suppl), S56–S69.

Wilker, C.E., Ellington, J.E., 2006. Reproductive toxicology in the female companion animal. In: Peterson, M.E., Talcott, P.A. (Eds.), Small Animal Toxicology, second edn. Elsevier Saunders, St. Louis, MO, pp. 475–499.

Wilson, J.G., 1977. Current status of teratology: general principles and mechanisms derived from animal studies. In: Wilson, J.G., Clarke Foster, F. (Eds.), Handbook of Teratology, Vol. 1. Plenum Press, New York, pp. 47–74.

Wong, C., Kelce, W.R., Sar, M., Wilson, E.M., 1995. Androgen receptor antagonist versus agonist activities of the fungicide vinclozolin relative to hydroxyflutamide. J. Biol. Chem. 270, 19998–20003.

Youngquist, R.S., Threlfall, 2007. Current Therapy in Large Animal Theriogenology, second edn. Saunders Elsevier, St. Louis, MO, pp. 1–1061.

Zhang, J., Zhu, W., Zheng, Y., Yang, J., Zhu, X., 2008. The antiandrogenic activity of pyrethroid pesticides cyfluthrin and βcyfluthrin. Reprod. Toxicol. 25, 491–496.

FURTHER READING

Garner, D.L., Hafez, E.S.E., Hafez, B. (Eds), 2000. Lipincott Williams & Wilkins, Philadelphia, PA.

Section III

Nanoparticles, Radiation and Carcinogens

Chapter 18

Toxicity of Nanomaterials

Deon van der Merwe and John A. Pickrell

INTRODUCTION

The toxicology of nanomaterials has emerged as a challenging field of investigation because the widely applied toxicological paradigm, "the dose makes the poison," appears to break down when the toxicological effects of materials are investigated at the nanometer scale. At this scale, the physical–chemical characteristics of materials are highly dependent on unit size and shape, and their interactions with biological systems may differ markedly from chemicals in solution, and from larger particles. The mass of nanomaterial to which susceptible tissues are exposed therefore becomes relatively less important as a determinant of the degree of biological impact compared to the size and form of the material. Particles, fibers, rods, or tubes with one or more dimensions <100 nm are generally referred to as nanomaterials, or more specifically as nanoparticles (also known as ultrafine particles), nanofibers, nanorods, or nanotubes. Nanomaterials are formed in nature during combustion, geological processes, and biological processes. They are also commonly produced unintentionally by man in processes such as power generation from coal, the combustion of fuels in automobiles, and by many other industrial, engineering, and domestic activities. Additionally, and at a rate that is rapidly accelerating, nanomaterials are manufactured intentionally through molecular-level engineering to obtain materials with unique mechanical, optical, electrical, magnetic, and chemical properties (Tsuji et al., 2006; Richards, 2009). These materials can be referred to as engineered nanomaterials (ENMs). They form the core of a rapidly growing industry where ENMs are incorporated into a wide variety of manufactured products. The increasing use of ENMs, and the uncertainties associated with their unusual and often poorly understood biological effects, creates concern regarding their potential for causing unanticipated adverse health effects (Fig. 18.1).

Investigators continue to discover unique properties of materials at the nanometer scale (Hoet et al., 2004). Commercialization of products that exploit these unique properties is increasing, and have already found commercial application in sporting goods, tires, sunscreens, sanitary ware coatings, stain resistant textiles and clothing, food products, and electronics (Hoet et al., 2004; Nel et al., 2006 Tsuji et al., 2006). The list of products incorporating nanotechnology is expected to continue to expand indefinitely. By some estimates, growth of nanotechnologies and use of ENMs will far exceed the impact of the industrial revolution; they were predicted to become a one-trillion-dollar market by 2015 (Nel et al., 2006). However, in spite of the seemingly unstoppable success of this technology, the unique properties of ENMs also present considerable new challenges to understanding, predicting, and managing potential adverse health effects following exposure. Technological development and applications are outpacing research for safe use and documentation of health and environmental risk (Hoet et al., 2004; Tsuji et al., 2006). Although exposure to ENMs is often intentional and controlled, widespread use of increasing quantities of ENMs increases the likelihood of uncontrolled human and animal exposure to nanomaterials in quantities that may result in biological effects. The future success of nanotechnology will be influenced by the level of public acceptance of the risks from exposure to ENMs, relative to the benefits. The increased demands for development to obtain the promised benefits from nanomaterials is balanced by an increasing need for a proactive approach in estimating the environmental and health costs (Ngo et al., 2008).

Concerns regarding the suitability of traditional toxicological assessment methods for evaluating ENMs gave birth to a relatively new discipline, named nanotoxicology. The discipline can be defined as: "the study of the adverse effects of ENMs on living organisms and ecosystems, including the prevention and amelioration of such adverse effects" (Oberdörster, 2010). As with conventional chemicals, risk assessment will be the basis of assessing and regulating exposure to nanomaterials to protect human, animal, and environmental health. Many applications will likely have limited, or at least

Veterinary Toxicology. DOI: http://dx.doi.org/10.1016/B978-0-12-811410-0.00018-0

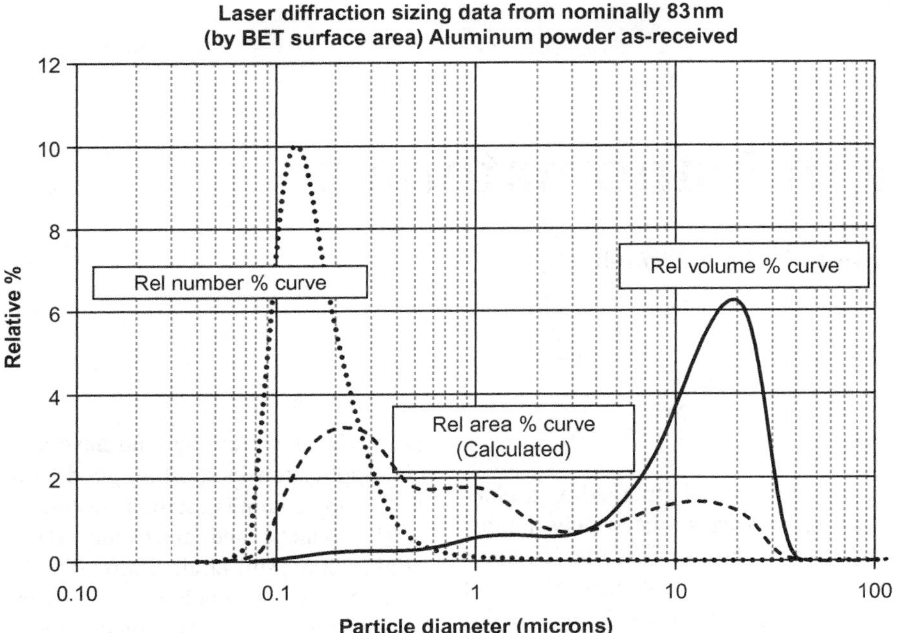

FIGURE 18.1 An example of relative abundance of particulate sizes in a sample.

manageable, exposures and effects, and are therefore expected to cause insignificant adverse health effects; however, these assumptions may be difficult to substantiate based on traditional assessment methods because the effects of ENMs may be unique, product-specific, and unpredictable from data derived from larger particles or from chemicals in solution (Hoet et al., 2004; Tsuji et al., 2006). Studies have shown that some ENMs are not inherently benign and that they may distribute throughout the body, inducing inflammation, oxidative stress, and other adverse effects (Nel et al., 2006). The results of studies demonstrating ENM adverse effects should, however, be interpreted with caution, especially when very high experimental doses are used that may not represent realistic exposure scenarios. Meaningful risk assessments should address questions related to the identification of hazards, exposure assessment, and toxicokinetics including persistence in cells and subcellular structures (Oberdörster, 2010). Assuming public acceptance, a toxicologist's experience with past "miracle" materials advises us that caution in using novel substances without fully evaluating potential health risks may be ill advised (Hoet et al., 2004; Tsuji et al., 2006). The discovery of serious adverse health effects, such as asbestos-like effects associated with multiwalled carbon nanotubes, has prompted nanotoxicologists to recommend heightened caution in the release of ENMs until more adequate information becomes available (Oberdörster, 2010). Moving forward, the field of nanotoxicology is faced with many challenges, including the need to modify our understanding of the concept of "dose," which, at the nanoscale level, is dependent on multiple physical–chemical factors other than the familiar mass or concentration used in traditional toxicology. Another significant challenge is the dynamic nature of the physicochemical characteristics of materials at the nanoscale, which often change over time, and as a consequence of interaction with biological systems. (Maynard et al., 2011). The specific changes that occur and their implications for biological interaction depends on the specific nanomaterial. Metal oxide nanoparticles, e.g., may aggregate and agglomerate without significant reduction of the total surface area of the agglomerate, but it may limit interaction with internal surfaces of the agglomerate to substances that are small enough to penetrate the agglomerate (Pickrell et al., 2010). Thus, unique effects, associated with repeated and combined exposures, are expected to emerge. The formation of reactive oxygen species and resulting oxidative stress has emerged as an important mechanism of toxicity of nanomaterials. The specific mechanisms of free radical formation and oxidative stress effects are, however, difficult to study in detail in vivo, and much of the current knowledge are derived from cell culture studies. Factors that appear to influence free radical formation include particle size, shape, aggregation and surface chemistry, particle dissolution rate, release of metal ions and oxides, UV light activation, and cellular environment factors such as pH and inflammatory responses (Fu et al., 2014). The complexity and multidimensional nature of nanomaterial toxicity makes it necessary to follow a comprehensive approach when performing nanotoxicity assessments, including physical characterization of nanomaterials, and studies to determine nanomaterial behavior at cellular and organismal levels (Caballero-Diaz and Cases, 2016).

NANOMATERIALS CHARACTERIZATION

The unusual physicochemical properties of ENMs are attributable to their morphology, composition, and surface characteristics. In an effort to standardize the description of nanomaterials in a way that will reduce uncertainty in data interpretation and facilitate cross-comparison between studies, the Minimum Information on Nanoparticle Characterization (MINChar) initiative (MINChar Initiative, 2008) identified a list of parameters that should ideally be characterized during studies. The parameters include particle size and size distribution, agglomeration state and aggregation, particle shape, chemical composition, crystal structure, surface composition, purity and levels of impurities, surface area, surface chemistry (including reactivity and hydrophobicity), and surface charge. It was also recognized that the characteristics of ENMs may not be stable during storage, handling, preparation, and delivery into biological systems. Since the media used for delivery may change ENM properties, particular emphasis should be placed on characterization of ENMs "as administered." It was also recommended that responses should be interpreted against a range of dose metrics, including mass, surface area, and number concentration.

Particles or particle agglomerates are usually not perfect spheres and are almost never singly dispersed. However, particle size is most often defined as the diameter of a sphere that is equivalent in the selected property to the particle measured; this makes it possible to conveniently plot size distributions of irregularly shaped particles or particle-agglomerates using a single value (diameter) along a single axis. The properties most often described are volume or mass; i.e., the diameter of a sphere of equal volume or mass to the particle(s) in question (volume or mass diameter).

The changes in ENM surface characteristics following delivery into a biological system are of particular importance when biological interactions are assessed. Proteins attach selectively to nanoparticle surfaces to form nanoparticle-protein coronas. This process, which depends on the adsorption properties of nanomaterial surfaces (Xia et al., 2010), can dramatically change particle surface characteristics and, consequently, interactions with biological systems. Combination with biological macromolecules may both detoxify nanomaterials, and promote uptake into cells that can reduce clearance and lead to chronic, degenerative changes.

Solubility can be an important determinant of biological response. Solubility is a function of chemical activity, specific surface area, radius and curvature, agglomeration and specific chemicals that are adsorbed to the ENM (Borm et al., 2006). Larger, more densely aggregated particles will dissolve more slowly. Adsorbed organic chemicals will slow solvation (Powers et al., 2006). Solubility of ENMs is inversely correlated with their biopersistence. Since solubility and chemical reactivity are strongly dependent on the physical–chemical environment, they should be measured in an environment as near to that of the target biological environment as possible. This can sometimes be accomplished with in vitro conditions closely simulating biological solutions (Powers et al., 2006). Specific interactions may be present in biological fluids that are absent in simple solvents. For example, when determining solubility and reactivity in the lung, it is important to consider not just solubility in water, but in fluids that bear significant resemblance to that of the epithelial lining fluid (ELF). A minimal ELF volume is predicted at 40–100 mL for mature humans. The pH varies from 6.9 at the end of inspiration, to 7.5 at the end of expiration. Bicarbonate acts as a buffer, and the change in pH is caused by removing CO_2 of expiration (Langmuir, 1965). Bicarbonate concentration in lung simulant fluid increases the solubility of MgO (Pickrell et al., 2009). Surprisingly, macrocrystalline (bulk) MgO is dissolved as extensively as nanosized MgO in lung stimulant fluids in about 10–20 min (Pickrell et al., 2009). This paradoxical result suggests that bicarbonate chemical activity may have a direct relation to the rapid dissolution of MgO in lung simulant fluid related to its modest solubility in distilled water. Stoichiometry of the likely chemical species suggests a conversion of MgO to $Mg(OH)_2$ in aqueous media and a subsequent conversion to the hydrated carbonate (Langmuir, 1965; Pickrell et al., 2010). These phenomena serve to illustrate the potential error associated with studies conducted in simple solutions when attempting to predict activity in complex biological systems.

ANIMAL OR TISSUE EXPOSURES

In Vitro Exposures to Nanomaterials

Early indicators for ENP-derived adverse health effects were needed for an adequate assessment cytotoxicity of different types of well characterized ENPs; cytotoxicity was used to infer relative risk (Brunner et al., 2006). For this purpose, the authors chose a mesothelioma and a fibroblast cell line. Two assays were performed. The first was mean culture activity, indicated by mitochondrial activity in converting a formazan type of dye from its leukoform to an active dye. In addition, DNA content, indicating cell number was measured (Brunner et al., 2006). Other than the positive asbestos control, none had >20% of the particles larger than 200 nm. Specific surface area was also higher than the asbestos positive control (90–190 m^2/g vs the 8.5 m^2/g of the asbestos). Mass median sizes were 20–50 nm and surface area median sizes were 6–21 nm, although they differed in terms of the shape and degree of agglomeration (Brunner et al., 2006). Soluble amorphous silicate, a negative control caused minimal response in either cell line, consistent with its anticipated lack of toxicity (Brunner et al., 2006). Crocidolite asbestos had a significant reduction in both cell activity and cell number (DNA) in both cell lines. The mesothelioma cell line was more severely affected, perhaps reflecting its metabolic activity. This toxicity was consistent with expectations from a positive control (Brunner et al., 2006). Calcium phosphate had no significant cytotoxicity at 3 days; these data are consistent with it having no toxicity like the negative control particle, amorphous silica (Brunner et al., 2006). Insoluble metal oxides (TiO_2, ZrO_2 and CeO_2) had modest toxicity at 3 days of exposure that was most prominent in mesothelioma cells. By 6 days of exposure, these cells had returned to normal (Brunner et al., 2006). Morphologically, the high dose of zirconium oxide caused the appearance of decreased cell number and function, even after 6 days incubation. These data are consistent with only a modest health effect relative to the positive control (Brunner et al., 2006). Zinc and ferric oxide were slightly soluble and quite toxic to both cell lines after 3 days incubation (Brunner et al., 2006). The authors advance no specific explanation for zinc toxicity beyond chemical toxicity, but experimental conditions suggest considerable local particle concentrations. For iron, the toxicity resulted from free radical production from the Haber–Weiss reaction. Because this reaction occurred at 40-fold less than the chemical toxicity of iron, it is said to be specific for the nanoparticle (Brunner et al., 2006).

In vitro analysis of particle size-related effects on alveolar macrophages, epithelial cells, and neutrophils, demonstrates size- and oxidant-dependent responses. Increased interleukin 6 (IL-6) in cultured lung cells suggested a proinflammatory, oxidant response. Reduced cell numbers, especially with Mn-containing nanoparticles, suggested cytotoxicity at high doses, probably from local concentration of particles (Pickrell et al., 2010). These effects were observed after in vitro exposure to concentrated PM (2.5) ambient particles collected in real time. Oxidative stress, mediated by ROS, is an important mechanism of particle-induced lung inflammation (Tao et al., 2003).

INTRATRACHEAL INSTILLATION–PHARYNGEAL ASPIRATION

Ultrafine Particles

Exposure to ambient air pollution particles caused increased cardiopulmonary morbidity and mortality, particularly with preexisting disease (Tao et al., 2003). Exacerbation of pulmonary inflammation in susceptible people (e.g., asthmatics, chronic obstructive pulmonary disease (COPD) patients) is a central mechanism by which particles cause lung disease, primarily from organic dusts (Pickrell et al., 2009, 2010). Metal oxide nanoparticles may also have direct cytotoxic effects in lung cells (Pickrell et al., 2010). After intratracheal instillation, ultrafine colloidal silica (UFCS) particles had greater ability to induce tissue damage and inflammation compared to fine colloidal silica (FCS) particles. Electron microscopy demonstrated UFCS and FCS particles on both bronchiolar and alveolar wall surfaces; type I epithelial cell necrosis and basement membrane damage was greater in UFCS than in FCS particles (Kaemawatawong et al., 2005).

Inhalation of highly insoluble ultrafine particles (diameter 20 nm) of low intrinsic toxicity (TiO_2) resulted in pulmonary inflammatory responses. However, these effects were not acute and occurred only after prolonged inhalation exposure of the aggregated ultrafine particles at high levels $> 1\ mg/m^3$ (Oberdörster et al., 1995). Ultrafine carbon particles are more toxic on an equal mass basis than fine carbon particles, but this is not true if they are examined on a total surface area basis (Oberdörster et al., 2010).

Carbon Nanotubes

Pharyngeal aspiration of single-walled carbon nanotubes (SCWNT) elicited an acute pulmonary inflammation in C57BL/6 mice that progressed to fibrosis and granulomas (Shvedova et al., 2005). SWCNT caused a dose-dependent release of protein, LDH, and gamma-glutamyl transferase activities into bronchoalveolar lung washings (lavage). In addition, elevated 4-hydroxynonenal (oxidative biomarker), depleted glutathione in lungs, leukocyte accumulations, and cytokines were present in lavage fluids on days 1–7. This was followed by fibrogenic transforming growth factor (TGF-β1) that peaked on day 7. The progressive fibrosis found in mice exhibited two distinct morphologies: SWCNT-induced granulomas, and diffuse interstitial fibrosis and alveolar wall thickening. Functional respiratory deficiencies and decreased bacterial clearance (*Listeria monocytogenes*) were found in mice treated with SWCNT (Shvedova et al., 2005). In vitro exposures of multiwalled carbon nanotubes to fibroblasts at high doses induces a similar inflammation (Ding et al., 2005). Equal doses of ultrafine carbon black particles or fine crystalline silica (SiO_2) did not cause either granulomas or alveolar wall thickening. Instead, they caused weaker pulmonary inflammation and damage (Shvedova et al., 2005). Inhalation of multiwalled carbon nanotubes induced no lung changes, but marginal pulmonary and systemic immunosuppression was observed (Mitchell et al., 2007).

INTRANASAL EXPOSURE

High doses of carbon black, given intranasally, showed adjuvant activity as indicated by enlargement of peribronchial lymph nodes and ovalbumin specific production of thymocyte (Th) 2 specific IL4, IL5, and IL10. Local cytokine production after carbon black exposure is predictive of allergic airway inflammation (De Haar et al., 2005).

INHALATION EXPOSURE

Both particle size and solubility are important determinants of biological response after lung exposure. If cleared rapidly they will be less injurious; if not they will remain as a chronic irritating source (Pickrell et al., 2004, 2009). Particles must be small enough to be inhaled into deep lung—usually taken to be $< 4\ \mu m$ (4000 nm). Particles between 4000 and 500 nm will be phagocytized and cleared rapidly. Particles < 500 nm aggregate size will be less efficiently phagocytized by phagocytes and may translocate to the pulmonary interstitium and remain there for relatively long periods of time. For example, in a recent study of fullerene particles with a geometric mean diameter of 96 nm (based on number) in rat lungs, it was estimated that $>99\%$ of particles remaining in the lung 6 months after exposure were in the interstitium, while particles that did not enter the interstitium were cleared by alveolar macrophages relatively rapidly with a half-life of 15–24 days (Shinohara et al., 2010).

Thermodegradation products of polytetrafluoroethylene (PTFE) contain singlet ultrafine particles (median diameter 26 nm); the fumes are toxic to rats at inhaled concentrations of $0.7-1.0 \times 10^6$ particles/cm^3. Inhalation studies with ultrafine particles (≤ 100 nm; NP) in rats suggest that particles ≤ 50 nm in diameter, may contribute to increased mortality and morbidity. Inhalation exposure rats caused an acute hemorrhagic pulmonary inflammation and death after 10–30 min (Oberdörster et al., 1995). These results confirmed reports from other laboratories that the toxicity of PTFE fumes should not be attributed only to gas-phase components of these fumes. Aging of PTFE fumes with concomitant aggregation of the ultrafine particles greatly decreases their toxicity (Oberdörster et al., 1995).

Fumes from overheated Teflon (PTFE)-coated frying pans cause a fatal hemorrhagic pneumonitis in caged birds directly adjacent in both time and space to the overheating (Blandford et al., 1975). Birds appear to be more sensitive than rats and humans to direct inhalation of Teflon fumes from overheated skillets; this sensitivity probably reflects their physiologically more efficient respiratory system. When birds are removed from the overheating event by a short period of time, or when birds are in an adjacent room, there is a comparatively minimal reaction. Current understanding implies that the small particles released from heated PTFE rapidly condense into larger and less biologically potent particles (Lee and Seidel, 1991). Aged particles collected as agglomerates were not toxic when given intratracheally to rats, but the particles became toxic when rats were given inhalation exposure to fumes evolved from the reheated agglomerate. Rats died with pulmonary edema and hemorrhage reflecting Type I pneumocyte damage (Lee and Seidel, 1991).

EPIDEMIOLOGICAL DATA

Epidemiological studies show an association between particulate air pollution and acute mortality and morbidity down to ambient particle concentrations below 100 μg/m^3. Whether this association also indicates causality between acute health effects and particle exposure at these low levels is still unclear, but several examples of associations between particulate air pollution and adverse health effects are available, and it suggests a high probability that a cause and effect relationship exists.

Sulfur Dioxide (Oxides of Sulfur Particles)

Sulfur dioxide (oxide of sulfur particles) comes mainly from burning sulfur containing fuels (Sullivan et al., 2006), causing both indoor and outdoor pollution. For example, poorly ventilated kerosene space heaters are sources of indoor sulfur dioxide. Sulfur dioxide particles are hygroscopic and tend to grow larger with increasing hydration of the atmosphere (Sullivan et al., 2006).

Nasal breathing filters out much of the inhaled sulfur dioxide; it is water-soluble and is often absorbed in the upper portion of the respiratory tract (Sullivan et al., 2006). Sulfur dioxide is irritating to the eyes, nose and airways, and its odor is detected at concentrations as low as 0.5 ppm. At >6 ppm, companion animals often show acute clinical signs including tearing, runny nose, cough, bronchospasm, and shortness of breath. Additional chronic signs that come from prolonged exposure at lower exposure concentrations include cough, mucus hypersecretion, and frequent clearing of the throat; these reflect airway inflammation and chronic bronchitis. Massive exposure is capable of inducing severe, permanent pulmonary damage (Sullivan et al., 2006). Low level prolonged human exposures correlate well with bronchial asthma.

Swine Barn Dust Exposure

Gases and/or ultrafine particles in swine barns can be important factors in the development of increased bronchial responsiveness both in animals and their human caretakers. For example, healthy human volunteers weighing pigs for 3 h developed a neutrophilic pneumonitis, and they had an increased bronchial responsiveness to methacholine. Wearing a mask reduced, but did not abolish, the inflammatory response (Larsson et al., 2002). In vitro data suggest that airway epithelial cell swine dust extract exposure enhances subsequent lymphocyte adhesion to epithelial cells by a modulation of the expression of intracellular adhesion molecule 1, and protein kinase C α (Mathiesen et al., 2004). The associated inflammation is characterized by increased numbers of neutrophils, macrophages, and lymphocytes to a lesser degree, in pigs and their caretakers. The inflammation is associated with increased IL-6 in cultured cells, suggesting an asthma-like reaction (Pickrell et al., 2010). Interestingly, this inflammation is most pronounced in caretakers with no prior exposure to this environment, which suggests a tolerance to endotoxin or other substances in this environment associated with repeated exposures (Von Essen and Romberger, 2003).

Nanoparticle Exposure in the Home

Environmental tobacco smoke (ETS) is a health risk for companion animals. It is a major source of indoor particles, and can release more than 4000 potential toxicants into the air (Sullivan et al., 2006). While the effects of smoke inhalation may be mostly due to toxic gases (e.g., carbon monoxide), ETS particles, such as acrolein, are capable of producing pulmonary damage (Fitzgerald and Vera, 2006). Frequently observed signs include wheezing, chronic cough, chronic hyper reactive airways, and chronic bronchitis. Water soluble toxins are absorbed and injure mostly the upper respiratory tract, while less soluble materials go deeper into the lungs and injure the pulmonary parenchyma (Fitzgerald and Vera, 2006). The EPA has classified ETS a group A carcinogen, meaning that there is sufficient evidence to indicate that it will produce cancer in humans (Sullivan et al., 2006). Epidemiological evidence in humans demonstrates a strong relationship between ETS and cancer. Mice exposed to ETS experimentally at high doses developed increased incidences of cancer (Hecht, 2005). Although most investigators continue to compare experimental results in animals with human data in humans, most animals appear to be less sensitive than man (Coggins, 2002). Beta-carotene supplementation attenuated cardiac remodeling induced by 1-month of tobacco smoke exposure in rats (Zornoff et al., 2006). After 1-month's exposure to ETS cardiac remodeling was present as indicated by disorganization or loss of myofilaments, infolding of plasma membrane, dilatation of the sarcoplasmic reticulum, and polymorphic mitochondria with swollen or decreased cristae. Rats given beta-carotene during cigarette smoke exposure had minimal or no significant cardiac remodeling. These data suggest beta carotene attenuates, reduces, or minimizes cardiac remodeling induced by cigarette smoke (Zornoff et al., 2006). These data are probably most relevant to obese cardiac-compromised companion animals. Differential diagnoses or conditions that must be adequately distinguished from smoke inhalation include asthma, heart disease, allergic pulmonary disease, inhalation of toxic solvents or sprays, pneumonia, neoplasia, trauma, COPD, and pneumothorax (Fitzgerald and Vera, 2006).

Household use of metal oxide ENMs in sunscreens (mostly zinc oxide or titanium dioxide), or as cosmetics, has not led to reports of toxicities in humans (Nel et al., 2006). Other metal oxide ENMs such as ferric oxide, however, are cytotoxic to mesothelioma cells and fibroblasts in vitro (Brunner et al., 2006). In comparison, zinc oxide fumes at high doses (500 $\mu g/m^3$), in an occupational setting, cause fume fever (fatigue, chills, fever, myalgia, cough and leukocytosis) (Nel et al., 2006).

Dog Exposures to Automobile Exhaust Aerosols

Repeated, high exposures to the complex pollutant mixtures in automobile exhaust aerosols cause lung structural changes induced by sustained inflammatory processes resulting in airway and vascular remodeling and altered repair. These exposures are complicated by a heavy load of oxidant gases. Bronchoalveolar lavage from dogs in heavily exhaust-polluted environments show increased numbers of activated alveolar macrophages in association with ultrafine particles in alveolar type I and II cells. Cytokines released from both circulating inflammatory cells and resident lung cells, in response to endothelial and epithelial injury, are thought to play important roles. The lung changes are typically associated with myocardial and endothelial pathology (Calderon-Garciduenas et al., 2001a,b).

EMERGING CHALLENGES

A question that received recent scientific scrutiny is the potential indirect impact that ENMs may have as contaminant carriers. For example, the uptake of phenanthrene by daphnids is increased by C_{60} nanoparticles, and it increases phenanthrene toxicity to algae. Effects on uptake and toxicity are, however, variable depending on the organism and the toxicant (Baun et al., 2008). The significance of these observations is still unclear, but it indicates that the possibility of ENMs affecting the potency and/or kinetics of toxicant coexposures should be considered. On the other hand, ENMs can be used to reduce the impacts of environmental contaminants. Iron (0 valence/charge) particles, e.g., may be used to remove chromium and lead in drinking water (Iseli et al., 2009).

Evidence of ecotoxicological effects associated with nanomaterials is emerging. For example, leachates from low-purity fullerenes were shown to be toxic to aquatic organisms (Hull et al., 2009). Nanotechnology may lead to novel types of pollutant effects. Organisms may not have the ability to metabolize and detoxify ENMs, using pathways evolved to prevent poisoning from chemicals in solution. The diversity of environmental conditions and possible ecological impacts pose additional challenges to ecotoxicological risk assessment. Data from diverse test organisms are needed, and a general scarcity of data is still a major concern (Cattaneo et al., 2009).

REFERENCES

Baun, A., Sorensen, S.N., Rasmussen, R.F., et al., 2008. Toxicity and bioaccumulation of xenobiotic organic compounds in the presence of aqueous suspensions of aggregates of nano-C_{60}. Aquat. Toxicol. 86 (3), 379–387.

Blandford, T.B., Seamon, P.J., Hughes, R., et al., 1975. A case of polytetrafluoroethylene poisoning in cockatiels accompanied by polymer fume fever in the owner. Vet. Rec. 96 (8), 175–178.

Borm, P., Klaessig, F.C., Landry, T.D., et al., 2006. Research strategies for safety evaluation of nanomaterials. Part VI. Characterization of nanoscale particles for toxicological evaluation. Toxicol. Sci. 90 (2), 23–32.

Brunner, T.I., Wick, P., Manser, P., et al., 2006. In vitro cytotoxicity of oxide nanoparticles: comparison to asbestos, silica and the effect of particle solubility. Environ. Sci. Technol. 40 (14), 4374–4381.

Caballero-Diaz, E., Cases, M.V., 2016. Analytical methodologies for nanotoxicity assessment. Trends Anal. Chem. 84 (A), 160–171.

Calderon-Garciduenas, L., Gambling, T.M., Acuna, H., et al., 2001a. Canines as a sentinel species for assessing chronic exposures to air pollutants: part 2. Cardiac pathology. Toxicol. Sci. 61 (2), 356–367.

Calderon-Garciduenas, L., Mora Tiscareno, A., Fordham, L.A., et al., 2001b. Canines as sentinel species for assessing chronic exposures to air pollutants: part 1. Respiratory pathology. Toxicol. Sci. 61 (2), 342–355.

Cattaneo, A.G., Gornati, R., Chriva-Internati, M., et al., 2009. Ecotoxicology of nanomaterials: the role of invertebrate testing. ISJ. 6 (1), 78–97.

Coggins, C.R., 2002. A minireview of chronic animal inhalation studies with mainstream cigarette smoke. Inhal. Toxicol. 14 (10), 991–1002.

De Haar, C., Hassing, I., Bol, M., et al., 2005. Ultrafine carbon black particles cause early airway inflammation and have adjuvant activity in a mouse allergic airway disease model. Toxicol. Sci. 87 (2), 409–418.

Ding, L., Stilwell, J., Zhang, T., et al., 2005. Molecular characterization of the cytotoxic mechanism of multiwall carbon nanotubes and nano-onions on human skin fibroblast. Nano Lett. 5 (12), 2448–2464.

Fitzgerald, K.T., Vera, R., 2006. Smoke inhalation. In: Peterson, M.E., Talcott, P.A. (Eds.), Small Animal Toxicology. Elsevier-Saunders, St Louis, MO, pp. 439–458.

Fu, P.F., Xia, Q., Hwang, H., et al., 2014. Mechanisms of nanotoxicity: generation of reactive oxygen species. J. Food Drug Anal. 22 (1), 64–75.

Hecht, S.S., 2005. Carcinogenicity studies of inhaled cigarette smoke in laboratory animals: old and new. Carcinogenesis. 26 (9), 1488–1492.

Hoet, P.H.M., Bruski-Hohlfeld, I., Salata, O.V., 2004. Nanoparticles – known and unknown health risks. J. Nanobiotechnol. 2 (12), 1–15.

Hull, M.S., Kennedy, A.J., Steevens, J.A., et al., 2009. Release of metal impurities from carbon nanomaterials influences aquatic toxicity. Environ. Sci. Technol. 43 (11), 4169–4174.

Iseli, A., Kwen, H., Rajagopalan, S., 2009. Nanomaterials for Environmental Remediation. In: Klabunde, K.J., Richards, R.M. (Eds.), Nanoscale Materials in Chemistry, second ed. John Wiley & Sons, Inc, Hoboken.

Kamawatawong, T., Kawamura, N., Okajima, M., et al., 2005. Acute pulmonary toxicity caused by exposure to colloidal silica: particle size dependent pathological changes in mice. Toxicol. Pathol. 33 (7), 745–751.

Langmuir, D., 1965. Stability of carbonates in the system MgO-CO_2-H_2O. J. Geol. 73, 730–754.

Larsson, B.M., Larsson, K., Malmberg, P., et al., 2002. Airways inflammation after exposure in a swine confinement building during cleaning procedure. Am. J. Ind. Med. 41 (4), 250–258.

Lee, K.P., Seidel, W.C., 1991. Pulmonary response to perfluoropolymer fume and particles generated under various exposure conditions. Fundam. Appl. Toxicol. 17 (2), 254–269.

Mathisen, T., Von Essen, S.G., Wyatt, T.A., et al., 2004. Hog barn dust extract augments lymphocyte adhesion to human airway epithelial cells. J. Appl. Physiol. 96 (5), 1738–1744.

Maynard, A.D., Warheit, D.B., Philbert, M.A., 2011. The new toxicology of sophisticated materials: nanotoxicology and beyond. Toxicol. Sci. 120 (Suppl. 1), 109–129.

MINChar Initiative, 2008. Recommended Minimum Physical and Chemical Parameters for Characterizing Nanomaterials on Toxicology Studies. Available: <http://characterizationmatters.org/parameters/>.

Mitchell, L.A., Gao, J., Wal, R.V., et al., 2007. Pulmonary and systemic immune response to inhaled multiwalled carbon nanotubes. Toxicol. Sci. 100 (1), 203–214.

Nel, A., Xia, T., Madler, L., et al., 2006. Toxic potentials of materials at the nanolevel – review. Science. 311 (5761), 622–627.

Ngo, M.A., Smiley-Jewell, S., Aldous, P., et al., 2008. Nanomaterials and the environment. In: Grassian, V.H. (Ed.), Nanoscience and Nanotechnology: Environmental and Health Impacts. John Wiley and Sons Ltd., Hoboken, pp. 3–18.

Oberdörster, G., 2010. Safety assessment for nanotechnology and nanomedicine: concepts of nanotoxicology. J. Int. Med. 267 (1), 89–105.

Oberdorster, G., Gelein, R.M., Ferin, J., et al., 1995. Association of particulate air pollution and acute mortality: involvement of ultrafine particles? Inhal. Toxicol. 7 (1), 111–124.

Pickrell, J.A., Erickson, L.E., Klabunde, K.J., 2009. Toxicity of Inhaled Nanomaterials. In: Klabunde, K.J., Richards, R.M. (Eds.), Nanoscale Materials in Chemistry, second ed. John Wiley & Sons, Inc, Hoboken, NJ.

Pickrell, J.A., Gakhar, G., Mulukutla, R.S., et al., 2004. Safety of glycol, diesel fuel or combustion smokes in the presence of magnesium of titanium dioxide clearing agents. Progr. 39th Midwest Reg. Meet. (MWRM) Am. Chem. Soc.183.

Pickrell, J.A., Van der Merwe, D., Erickson, L.E., et al., 2010. Comparative pulmonary toxicity of metal oxide nanoparticles.

Nanoscale Mater. Chem. Environ. Appl. ACS Symp Series. 1045, 225–233.

Powers, K.W., Brown, S.C., Krishna, V.B., et al., 2006. Research strategies for safety evaluation of nanomaterials. Part VI. Characterization of nanoscale particles for toxicological evaluation. Toxicol. Sci. 90 (2), 296–303.

Richards, R.M., 2009. Introduction to nanoscale materials in chemistry. In: Klabunde, K.J., Richards, R.M. (Eds.), Nanoscale Materials in Chemistry, second ed. John Wiley & Sons, Inc, Hoboken, NJ.

Shinohara, N., Nakazato, T., Tamura, M., et al., 2010. Clearance kinetics of fullerene C60 nanoparticles from rat lungs after intratracheal C60 instillation and inhalation C60 exposure. Toxicol. Sci. 118 (2), 564–573.

Shvedova, A.A., Kisin, E.R., Mercer, R., et al., 2005. Unusual inflammatory and fibrogenic pulmonary responses to single-walled carbon nanotubes in mice. Am. J. Physiol. Lung. Cell Mol. Physiol. 289 (5), 698–708.

Sullivan, J.B., Van Ert, M.D., Krieger, G.R., et al., 2006. Indoor environmental quality and health. In: Peterson, M.E., Talcott, P.A. (Eds.), Small Animal Toxicology. Elsevier-Saunders, St Louis, MO, pp. 244–272.

Tao, F., Gonzalez-Flecha, B., Kobzik, L., 2003. Reactive oxygen species in pulmonary inflammation by ambient particulates. Free Radic. Biol. Med. 35 (4), 327–340.

Tsuji, J.S., Maynard, A.D., Howard, P.C./, et al., 2006. Research strategies for safety evaluation of nanomaterials, Part IV, Risk assessment of nanoparticles. Toxicol. Sci. 89 (1), 42–50.

Von Essen, S., Romberger, D., 2003. The respiratory inflammatory response to the swine confinement building environment: the adaptation to respiratory exposures in the chronically exposed worker. J. Agric. Saf. Health. 9 (3), 185–196.

Xia, X., Monteiro-Riviere, N.A., Riviere, J.E., 2010. An index for characterization of nanomaterials in biological systems. Nat. Nanotechnol. 5, 671–675.

Zornoff, L.A.M., Matsubara, L.S., Matsubara, B.B., et al., 2006. Beta-Carotene supplementation attenuates cardiac remodeling induced by one-month tobacco-smoke exposure in rats. Toxicol. Sci. 90 (1), 259–266.

Chapter 19

Ionizing Radiation in Veterinary Medicine

Lisa Murphy

INTRODUCTION TO IONIZING RADIATION

Atoms are made up of protons, neutrons, and electrons. An element is defined by the number of protons in its nucleus. When the number of protons and neutrons are balanced, the atom is referred to as a stable isotope. Too few or too many neutrons make the atom an unstable radioisotope or radionuclide. Radionuclides release ionizing radiation as electromagnetic waves or atomic particles as they decay to form new (daughter) radioisotopes or stable elements. These emissions are able to strike an electron with enough force to strip it away from its atom, creating an ion (Rebois and Ray, 2012). Ionizing radiation can also generate highly reactive nonionic free radicals. Hydroxyl-free radicals (OH•), formed by the ionization of water, are responsible for the biochemical abnormalities associated with radiation toxicity. Radiation damage either kills cells or causes damage to molecules that increases cancer risk, particularly when DNA is involved. Other health concerns include cardiovascular effects, cataracts, shortened lifespan, and effects on the immune and gastrointestinal systems and reproduction.

As radioactive emissions travel through cells and deposit a concentrated amount of energy, DNA breakage and other biological damage occur. Cells can repair much but not all of this damage; this unrepaired damage can lead to an increased risk of cancer or adverse genetic effects in offspring. Any dose of radiation could potentially cause cancer. Other authors have previously covered ionizing radiation extensively (Henriksen and Maillie, 2003; McClellan, 2014), mainly as it pertains to human exposures and experimental animal data. Information regarding unintentional exposures of animals to ionizing radiation is more limited.

Nonionizing radiation has lower energy and frequencies and higher wavelengths than ionizing radiation. Common forms of nonionizing radiation that are not covered in this chapter include ultraviolet, visible light, infrared, microwave, and radio frequency radiation.

Alpha and Beta Particles

Alpha particles are ionized helium atoms consisting of two protons and two neutrons with an electrical charge of +2. The large size of alpha particles lowers their penetration capacity and makes it possible to stop them with skin, clothing, or a sheet of paper, but they can densely transfer their energy along a very short track. External exposures are unable to penetrate skin. However, internal exposures to alpha particles can be extremely harmful. Damage from alpha particles is less easily repaired compared to that from beta particles and gamma rays. Radon gas that occurs in homes emits alpha particles.

Beta particles are high-energy, negatively-charged electrons that are less densely-ionizing than alpha particles though able to penetrate more deeply due to their lighter weight. Beta particles are stopped by thin barriers such as wood or metal. Radium 228 (^{228}Ra), one of two isotopes of radium used in luminescent paints, and Iodine 131 (^{131}I) emit beta particles.

Gamma Rays and X-rays

Gamma rays and X-rays are highly-penetrating forms of electromagnetic radiation with unionization density that varies inversely with their energy (Nussbaum and Köhnlein, 2003) and are distinguishable by their source (Rella, 2015). Gamma rays are emitted by unstable nuclei via radioactive decay with a fixed wavelength. X-rays originate outside of the nuclei. For instance, an X-ray machine that accelerates electrons through a large voltage collides them into a metal target. Both require thick layers of heavy material, such as lead or concrete for shielding. The cosmic radiation that astronauts and airline personnel are exposed to consists mainly of gamma rays and neutrons.

Veterinary Toxicology. DOI: http://dx.doi.org/10.1016/B978-0-12-811410-0.00019-2

MEASURING IONIZING RADIATION

The number of radioactive disintegrations per second (radioactive decay) is measured in becquerels (Bq) or curies (Ci). Curies compares the number of disintegrations per second to that of roughly 1 g of Radium-226 (Rella, 2015). One Bq is equal to one atomic disintegration per second.

$$1 \text{ Ci} = 3.7 \times 10^{10} \text{ Bq}$$

Radiation that simply passes through the body causes no harm. Biological injury results from the deposition of radioactive energy in a tissue or organ, quantified as the absorbed dose. Linear energy transfer (LET) for a charged particle refers to its average energy lost due to interactions per unit length of its trajectory (Hoel, 2013). X-rays, gamma rays, and beta particles are classified as low-LET radiation because they produce sparse ionization tracks. Neutrons and alpha particles dissipate large amounts of energy over very short distances.

Calculating an effective dose, using a relative biologic effectiveness (RBE) multiplying factor, makes it possible to compare biologic effects from different types of radiation exposures. RBE is defined as the biological potency of one radiation exposure compared with another to produce the same biological endpoint (National Research Council, 1990). RBE varies with the type and energy of the radiation, the selected biologic endpoint, and with dose and dose rate (Nussbaum and Köhnlein, 2003; Hoel, 2013).

$$\text{Effective dose} = \text{RBE} \times \text{Absorbed dose}$$

The units for effective dose are Sieverts (Sv) or rems.

$$1 \text{ Sv} = 100 \text{ rem}$$

Absorbed dose is expressed as grays (Gy) or radiation absorbed dose (rads).

$$1 \text{ Gy} = 100 \text{ rad}$$

One gray is defined as one joule of energy released in one kilogram of tissue.

Gas-filled tubes are used in ionization survey meters and Geiger-Mueller survey meters to accurately detect gamma radiation associated with nuclear incidents (Berger et al., 1987). A typical Geiger-Mueller survey meter reads dose rate as mrem per hour (mR/h) with a range switch that indicates how to multiply the dial reading. For example, when the needle is pointing to 10 and the range switch is set at X100, the dose rate is 1000 mrem (or 10 Sv) per hour.

SOURCES OF RADIATION

While radiation is ubiquitous, some natural exposures and accidental or intentional exposures related to incidents involving nuclear or medical uses of radiation and transportation accidents involving associated materials can result in harmful impacts on humans, animals, and the environment.

Natural Sources

Among the human population of the United States, approximately 52% of natural background radiation exposures are due to radon, 16% from cosmic radiation, 20% from terrestrial sources, and 12% from internal exposures (National Research Council, 2006). These natural exposures account for 82% of annual human radiation exposure. Radon (Rn) is a natural decay product of uranium and thorium. Daughter isotopes of ^{222}Rn decay to emit alpha particles and are associated with increased incidences of lung cancer in humans (Rella, 2015).

Nuclear Weapons

Two atomic bomb blasts at the end of World War II in Japan were estimated to have killed or injured more the 200,000 people. Most people died as a result of the bomb blast, though many others eventually succumbed to either acute radiation syndrome (ARS) or radiation-induced cancers.

In the United States, radioactivity released into the Columbia River by the nuclear weapons plant in Hanford, Washington resulted in radioisotope contamination of fish and shellfish hundreds of miles downriver to levels greater than 100,000 times what was detectable in the river water (Stenehjem, 1990). Radioactive waste is still stored at Hanford. Global fallout from atmospheric nuclear weapons testing carried out primarily in the 1950s and early 1960s is the main source of anthropogenic radionuclides, including Cesium 137 (^{137}Cs), in the environment (Povinec et al., 2013).

Nuclear Power

Uranium (U) ore as mined is approximately 99% ^{238}U and 1% ^{235}U (Rella, 2015). Uranium enrichment separates these so the ^{235}U can be used as nuclear fuel. The leftover ^{238}U, also known as depleted uranium (DU), is approximately 40% less radioactive than natural uranium ore and can be used in munitions. A nuclear power plant (NPP) generating 1000 MW of electricity requires about 30 tons of enriched uranium fuel rods each year (Nussbaum and Köhnlein, 2003). The resulting waste must be isolated from people and water supplies. Due to high levels of heat output, these spent fuel rods are stored, at least temporarily, in on-site storage pools, potentially vulnerable to natural disasters such as earthquakes.

The two most notable NPP incidents in recent history are the 1986 Chernobyl NPP accident that released large quantities of radionuclides over Belarus, Ukraine, and the Russian Federation, and the 2011 Fukushima Daiichi NPP accident. At Chernobyl, radioactive material dispersed into the atmosphere eventually settled back to the ground as influenced by local wind and rainfall conditions, spreading the contamination throughout a wide area and prompting human evacuations from a roughly 4300-km^2 area. Similar to nuclear warhead detonations, NPP accidents release ^{131}I, ^{137}Cs, strontium 90 (^{90}Sr), uranium, and plutonium. The estimated releases for Fukushima are 150–160 petabecquerel (PBq) ^{131}I and 10–15 PBq ^{137}Cs into the atmosphere, and 4–27 PBq ^{137}Cs and 0.1–1 PBq ^{90}Sr into water (Povinec et al., 2013). Large volumes of fresh water were used during emergency cooling of the reactor and some of this was unintentionally discharged into coastal waters. Other released radionuclides included ^{134}Cs, tellurium 132 (^{132}Te), ^{132}I, ^{136}Cs, and the radioactive noble gases xenon 133 (^{133}Xe) and ^{135}Xe. Radiation dispersion devices or "dirty bombs" will probably involve a single radionuclide, most likely ^{137}Cs, but potentially also cobalt 60 (^{60}Co) or ^{90}Sr (Yamamoto, 2013).

As of December 2015, there were 441 operational nuclear reactors worldwide (IAEA, 2016). Increased leukemia clusters have been reported near civilian NPPs in the United States, United Kingdom, and Germany (Nussbaum and Köhnlein, 2003).

Sterilization of Food

An irradiated object or living organism does not become radioactive, meaning they pose no risk to others or to the environment. Irradiation of food is accepted by the AMA, CDC, and WHO as a method of safely and effectively controlling *Escherichia coli*, *Salmonella*, and *Campylobacter* in food without decreasing its nutritional quality.

Medical Uses of Radiation in Human and Veterinary Medicine

In the United States, medical X-rays and nuclear medicine make up about 79% of man-made radiation exposures (National Research Council, 2006). Multiple computed tomography (CT) scans are associated with a small but measureable increase in certain childhood cancers. Radionuclides such as ^{60}Co and ^{137}Cs have medical applications, and unintended exposures have occurred following accidental releases. Other examples include diagnostic bone scans (technetium 99 m [^{99m}Tc]) or positron emission tomography (PET) scans (Fludeoxyglucose 18 [^{18}F]) and the use of radioactive iodine (^{131}I), a gamma and beta emitter, to treat thyroid disease in people and cats.

Radiation is currently used in veterinary medicine to cure oncology patients or provide palliative care, most commonly as a localized treatment either with or without chemotherapy (Kent, 2017). The forms most commonly used for malignancies are teletherapy, usually delivered using a linear accelerator, and plesiotherapy, which places a radioactive source such as strontium 90 (^{90}Sr) directly on the tumor. Total delivered dose and the number of treatment sessions (fractionation) will vary on a case-by-case basis.

Radiation burns to the skin can occur with X-rays or gamma rays used for teletherapy and interventional radiology (Waghmare, 2013). Chemotherapy, other medical treatments, and individual susceptibility may increase this risk, though full epidermal recovery can be complete within 6 weeks unless permanent damage has occurred (ICRP, 1992).

ABSORPTION, DISTRIBUTION, AND ACCUMULATION OF RADIOACTIVE CONTAMINANTS IN ANIMALS

Shielding and distance greatly decrease exposures and health hazards associated with external sources of radiation. For people in the United States, the U.S. Nuclear Regulatory Commission (NRC) regulates radiation exposures by setting exposure limits for individuals through a system of practices that keeps all exposures as low as reasonably achievable.

External contamination occurs when radioactive particles are deposited on an object or a living organism, such as what would be expected following the detonation of a radiological dispersal device ("dirty bomb") or accidental spill in a medical, laboratory, or industrial setting. Risk can be relatively low with evacuation, appropriate decontamination, and controlling further access to the source of the contamination. Unless decontamination of the ground and surrounding environment is possible, affected areas may need to be abandoned for an extended period of time.

Internal contamination is when a radionuclide enters the body, usually by ingestion or inhalation. Incorporation occurs when the radionuclide is then taken up by tissue, such as what happens with diagnostic bone scans (^{99m}Tc) or PET scans (^{18}F) and the use of radioactive iodine (^{131}I) to treat thyroid disease in cats. Incorporation can also lead to tissue damage. Internal exposures only diminish as a result of radioactive decay or physiologic elimination. Determining the degree of internal versus external exposure can be difficult. However, following a release of radioisotopes, it is reasonable to expect that increased levels of internal contamination may occur in animals compared to people in the same affected area. In addition to being more likely to ingest contaminated food and water than people, animals may also internally contaminate themselves through normal grooming behaviors.

The physical half-life of a radioisotope is the time required for its initial rate of emissions to decrease by

TABLE 19.1 Target Tissues and Physical and Biological Half-Lives for Selected Radionuclides Commonly Associated With Radiological Incidents

Radionuclide	Target Tissue(s)	Physical Half-Life	Biological Half-Life
Cesium-134 (^{134}Cs)	Muscle and whole body	2 years	70 days
Cesium-137 (^{137}Cs)	Muscle and whole body	31 years	70–140 days
Iodine-131 (^{131}I)	Thyroid and breast	8 days	12–138 days
Strontium-90 (^{90}Sr)	Bone and lung	28 years	18–50 years

Source: Adapted from Nussbaum, R.H., Köhnlein, W., 2003. Ionizing radiation. In Greenberg, M.I., Hamilton, R.J., Phillips, S.D., McCluskey, G.J. (Eds.), Occupational, Industrial, and Environmental Toxicology (2nd ed.). Mosby. Philadelphia, (pp. 702-715).

50% and is specific to the radioisotope. Biologic half-life is determined by physical half-life and also the body's ability to excrete the radioisotope. Excretion varies among the different tissue types in the body and also between animal species and individuals. Both physical and biological half-lives vary from hours to years (Table 19.1).

Like stable or nonradioactive elements, radioisotopes can accumulate in plant and animal tissues, and exposures to multiple radioisotopes are additive. Radioisotopes accumulate in tissues using the same pathways as their stable analogs. This is why ^{137}Cs accumulates in muscle, ^{90}Sr in bone, and ^{131}I in the thyroid. Animal food products would be expected to be most commonly contaminated with ^{131}I (mainly milk) and ^{134}Cs and ^{137}Cs (mainly meat) (Beresford and Howard, 2011). The International Atomic Energy Agency published a handbook of parameter values that predict transfer of radionuclides to animal products (IAEA, 2010).

Iodine is completely absorbed from the gastrointestinal tract, concentrates in the thyroid, and transfers to milk and eggs (Crout et al., 2000). High concentrations of ^{131}I and radiocesium were detected in raw milk sampled in Ibaraki prefecture following the Fukushima accident (Povinec et al., 2013). Because of the relatively short physical half-life of ^{131}I, contaminated milk could be processed into food products that are then held until the ^{131}I has decayed to acceptable levels (Beresford and Howard, 2011).

Cesium absorption varies with the form involved and is distributed throughout soft tissues (Beresford et al., 2000). Its rate of loss from meat is faster for smaller animals, such as 1–2 days for chickens (Pöschl et al., 1997), compared to 60 days for a larger animal like a beef cow (Voight et al., 1989). In wild boar collected around the site of the Chernobyl accident, highest concentrations of ^{137}Cs were detected in muscle and kidneys, sometimes at levels >660 kBq/kg, and ^{90}Sr concentrated mainly in the bone (Gulakov, 2014). Wild boar hunted in Fukushima and its neighboring prefectures had detectable levels of ^{134}Cs and ^{137}Cs in their muscle (Ishida, 2013). More than 50% of Fukushima prefecture's boars, animals that forage through ground litter and in the soil for animals and plants, had radiocesium levels >500 Bq/kg. Muscle radiocesium levels in wild Japanese monkeys were significantly related to levels of soil contamination (Hayama et al., 2013). Cattle fed contaminated rice straw also resulted in radiocesium concentrations >500 Bq/kg (Povinec et al., 2013). In March 2011, the Japanese Ministry of Health, Labor, and Welfare adopted a provisional regulation level of radioactive substances in foods of <5 mSv/year (Hosono et al., 2013). Under this regulation the upper radiocesium limits were set at 200 Bq/kg for drinking water and dairy products, and 500 Bq/kg for meat, vegetables, and grains. In April 2012 a new standard of 1 mSv/year was established, along with new upper limits of radiocesium of 100 Bq/kg for general food products and 50 Bq/kg for milk. Studies on the distribution of radiocesium in cattle suggest that when suspicious levels of 50–100 Bq/kg are detected in the neck tissues, where radioactivity inspection is generally conducted at slaughter, another portion of muscle should be reinspected (Okada et al., 2013).

ACUTE EFFECTS OF RADIATION EXPOSURE IN ANIMALS

Acute radiation syndrome (ARS) was first described in human victims of Hiroshima and Nagasaki. Whole-body irradiation doses associated with ARS in people generally exceed 1 Gy, or about 160 times an average annual exposure (Rella, 2015). The sequence of events observed with ARS varies with the severity of the exposure (Waselenko et al., 2004). The effects of radiation exposure, including time until death occurs following whole-body irradiation, vary among animal species and are determined by the exposure duration and the radioisotope(s) involved (Sample and Irvine, 2011; von Zallinger and Tempel, 1998). Survival times for lethally exposed animals vary from minutes for an absorbed dose of 1000 Gy to 3–5 days for 10–100 Gy and up to 30–60 days for 2–10 Gy (Coggle, 1983). $LD_{50/30}$ is defined as the radiation dose that is lethal to 50% of the population within 30 days. $LD_{50/30}$ values for six domestic mammal species are summarized in Table 19.2. Similar data has been published for effective radiation doses (Berger et al., 1987). Acute whole-body exposures of >20 Sv are fatal within minutes to hours, 5−20 Sv produces symptoms within minutes to hours and death within approximately 1 week, and <5 Sv results in hematopoietic effects developing over days to weeks with death more probably at doses >3 Sv. Mild symptoms may occur with 0.5−1 Sv and <0.5 Sv is not expected to produce any early effects. An estimated LD_{50} for humans and several animal species is 3.5 Sv.

In general, as the severity of exposure increases, so does the severity of clinical signs and the time of onset decreases, with some differences among animal species (von Zallinger and Tempel, 1998). Burros are relatively resistant to total-body radiation doses that are lethal for other mammals, and cattle have a delayed hematopoietic response. The main feature of ARS in swine is severe hemorrhage. Breed differences have been documented in pigs, with Hampshires surviving 57 days of daily 1 Gy doses of ^{60}Co, compared to 19 days for Yorkshires (Brown et al., 1964). ARS in dogs most similarly resembles what occurs in humans (Tempel, 1983). Minipigs have been developed as a highly sensitive model for studying ARS and potential countermeasures (Elliott et al., 2014). Gamma radiation doses <2 Gy are lethal due to hematopoietic ARS (H-ARS). 2−5 Gy are associated with an accelerated hematopoietic syndrome. 5−12 Gy produces the classic signs of gastrointestinal ARS (GI-ARS): vomiting, diarrhea, abdominal cramping, bacterial translocation, and decreased plasma citrulline levels, a routine biomarker for gastrointestinal syndrome (Kaore and Kaore, 2014).

Previous stresses such as high levels of production or extreme climates at the time of the exposure may reduce survival times in animals even further than initially expected. Even surviving animals may have late effects that impact their meat, milk, and egg production. While animals will not be permanently sterilized by radioactive contamination (Berger et al., 1987), fertility may be decreased, even in recovered individuals.

The four classical clinical stages of ARS are described in Table 19.3. Lethally exposed patients may rapidly progress through the first three stages within a few hours before succumbing (Rella, 2015). The various body systems exhibit their own clinical pictures during the manifest illness stage as listed in Table 19.3 and outlined in

TABLE 19.2 $LD_{50/30}$ **Values for Selected Domestic Mammals**

Species	Dose
Burros	1.8−2.8 Gy
Cattle	1.6−2.75 Gy, 1.5 Gy for calves
Goats	2.37 Gy
Pigs	2.18−2.47 Gy
Dogs	2.55−3.35 Gy

Source: Adapted from von Zallinger, C., Tempel, K., 1998. The physiologic response of domestic animals to ionizing radiation: a review. Vet. Radiol. Ultras 39(6), 495−503.

TABLE 19.3 Clinical Stages of Acute Radiation Syndrome (ARS)

Stage	Time of Onset Postexposure	Clinical Features	Duration
Early prodromal stage	Hours to days, inversely proportional to dose received	Nausea and vomiting	Directly proportional to dose except when death occurs rapidly
Latent period	Hours to days	Apparent clinical improvement	Days to weeks, inversely related to dose
Manifest illness	3−5 weeks	Cerebrovascular injury	Variable, until death or recovery
		Pulmonary disease	
		Gastrointestinal syndrome	
		Hematopoietic syndrome	
		Cutaneous syndrome	
Recovery	Variable	Clinical improvement and eventual recovery	Weeks to months

Source: Adapted from Rella, J.G., 2015. Radiation. In Hoffman, R.S., Howland, M.A., Lewin, N.A., Nelson, L.S., Goldfrank, L.R. (Eds.), Goldfrank's Toxicologic Emergencies (10th ed.) (pp. 1703-1712). McGraw-Hill Education, New York.

TABLE 19.4 Body System-Specific Manifestations Associated With Acute Radiation Syndrome (ARS)

Syndrome	Associated Exposure Dose	Clinical Manifestations
Cerebrovascular	≥15–20 Gy (humans) >80–100 Gy (lethal dose in animals)	Hyperthermia, ataxia, loss of motor control, apathy, lethargy, cardiovascular shock, seizures, coma
Pulmonary	6–10 Gy (humans)	Pneumonitis within 1–3 months of exposure followed by respiratory failure, pulmonary fibrosis, or cor pulmonale months to years later
Gastrointestinal	≥6 Gy (humans) 10–100 Gy (lethal dose for animals)	Anorexia, nausea, vomiting, diarrhea with or without blood, loss of peristalsis, abdominal distension, dehydration, sepsis
Hematopoietic	≥1 Gy (humans) 2–10 Gy (lethal dose for animals)	Pancytopenia, hemorrhage, sepsis
Cutaneous	3–50^{+} Gy (humans)	Bullae, blisters, hair loss, pruritis, ulceration, onycholysis

Source: Adapted from Rella, J.G., 2015. Radiation. In Hoffman, R.S., Howland, M.A., Lewin, N.A., Nelson, L.S., Goldfrank, L.R. (Eds.), Goldfrank's Toxicologic Emergencies (10th ed.) (pp. 1703–1712). McGraw-Hill Education, New York; von Zallinger, C., Tempel, K., 1998. The physiologic response of domestic animals to ionizing radiation: a review. Vet. Radiol. Ultras 39(6), 495–503.

more detail in Table 19.4. Time to onset of vomiting and kinetics of lymphocyte depletion have been used as the basis of triaging human radiation exposures. The gold standard is analyzing the number of dicentric chromosomes in lymphocytes, which can be correlated to a whole-body radiation dose (Rella, 2015).

The generalization that young, rapidly growing tissues are most radiosensitive was postulated by Bergonie and Tribondeau (1906). In mammals this includes reproductive germ cells, dermal and gastrointestinal stem cells, and erythroblasts (Sample and Irvine, 2011). Cattle studied after the first atomic bomb test in 1945 were estimated to have received 1.5 Gy of penetrating whole-body radiation and 370 Gy of beta radiation to the skin over the dorsum (Brown et al., 1966). The animals developed epilation and blistering 3–4 weeks later that healed with scarring after several months. Three years later, hyperkeratosis, epilation, depigmented hair, and other abnormalities were still evident, and cows surviving ≥15 years developed squamous cell carcinomas in the previously-affected areas. Compared to adult cattle, calves with ARS develop more severe respiratory infections, diarrhea, and hemorrhage (von Zallinger and Tempel, 1998).

The $LD_{50/30}$ for birds ranges from 5 to 20 Gy for most species (Woodhead, 1998), making them about as sensitive to acute radiation exposures as mammals. A gradual decline and subsequent recovery was observed in newly hatched white leghorn chicks exposed to 2.25 Gy of gamma source radiation (Malhotra et al., 1990). In the same study, single exposures of 15 day old chicks to 6.6 Gy of gamma radiation was 100% lethal within 7 days.

In domestic and exotic vertebrate animals receiving radiation therapy, side effects are generally categorized as acute effects and late effects (Kent, 2017). Acute effects reported near the end of therapy or soon after include mucositis and desquamation, usually resolving within weeks. Examples of late effects seen after months or years are fibrosis, necrosis, and new tumor formation.

Acute radiation doses that are lethal to vertebrates are generally lower than lethal doses in invertebrates. In a similar fashion, reproductive success in mammals is more radiosensitive than in invertebrates, with fish falling somewhere in between. Various databases of radiation exposure and effects, exposure estimation and risk evaluation models, and effects thresholds have been developed and are reviewed in detail elsewhere (Sample and Irvine, 2011). Most recently, the International Commission of Radiological Protection (ICRP) introduced a system of Reference Animals and Plants (ICRP, 2009). By providing radioisotope effects data for 39 elements in 12 species found in a variety of habitats (deer, rat, duck, frog, trout, flatfish, bee, crab, earthworm, pine tree, wild grass, and brown seaweed), exposures and effects in other animals can be estimated.

LONG-TERM IMPACTS OF RADIATION EXPOSURE IN ANIMALS

Based on observations among human survivors of Hiroshima and Nagasaki and Chernobyl cleanup workers, other adverse effects besides cancer can be associated with radiation exposure such as heart disease

(Darby et al., 2010) and cataracts (Worgul et al., 2007). More than 30 years after the 1986 Chernobyl NPP accident in Ukraine, very little is known about the current health status of mammalian species within the Chernobyl Exclusion Zone (CEZ). Following the Chernobyl accident, reproductive effects were noted in carp from a fish farm established in the power plant's cooling pond (Belova et al., 1993; Makeeva et al., 1994). Genetic effects have been seen in barn swallows breeding near Chernobyl, along with an increased frequency of albinism (Ellegren et al., 1997; Moller et al., 2007; Bonisoli-Alquati et al., 2009). Additional studies document negative impacts on plant and animal life (Geras'kin et al., 2008) and substantial accumulations of radionuclides in wildlife (Chester et al., 2001). Recent data suggest that wildlife populations are not depleted within even the most ^{137}Cs-contaminated areas of the 4300 km^2 CEZ (Webster et al., 2016). However, further studies are needed. In animals that appear to be the least sensitive to radiation, insects and soil invertebrates, levels of chronic exposure producing effects vary from 2 to 1000 mGy per day (Wood et al., 2005). Chronic exposures of up to 192 mGy per day of gamma radiation produced no adverse effects in terrestrial isopods (Hingston et al., 2005).

MITIGATING ACUTE RADIATION EXPOSURES IN ANIMALS

Minimizing Exposure

Following the Chernobyl disaster, the maximum exposures to animals and plants occurred within the first 10–20 days, with the main contributors being the short-lived radionuclides (Alexakhin and Geras'kin, 2011). For people responding to radiological incidents, exposures are minimized by isolating them from potential sources using personal protective equipment (PPE), including respirators and goggles. Strategies to consider for animals postincident should include confining either the source or the animals, preventing or minimizing uptake, reducing uptake, or increasing excretion.

Animals left outside should be washed before bringing them inside. Any structure will provide some shielding against sources of radiation outside. Controlling access to contaminated food and water and providing clean or at least less-contaminated sources to confined animals may be an important first step that can be accomplished by either first responders on scene, owners, or caretakers who are sheltered in place or returned following the incident, though depending on the scope of the incident and the number of animals involved this may be difficult to accomplish in a timely manner or at all. Water from wells and covered tanks are least likely to be contaminated following an incident compared to water in ponds and open tanks (Berger et al., 1987). If a water source appears to be grossly contaminated, which is common following any natural or man-made disaster, boiling or chlorination may be helpful but will not remove all contaminants, including radiation.

Use of uncontaminated animal feed is best. However, when this is not possible, at least initially, potentially contaminated outer layers of hay bales and feed piles should be carefully removed and set aside to allow time for radioactive decay. To reduce the possibility of radioiodine contamination of milk, this retention time should be at least 40 days for dairy cattle (Berger et al., 1987). Closed bags or barrels of feed should be carefully handled and decontaminated when necessary to prevent contamination of the feed inside.

Prophylaxis

Internal contamination with radionuclides persists until they either decay or are eliminated. This, and therefore the management of internally contaminated patients, is isotope dependent. Interventions can be useful, however are only available for a few specific isotopes. For beta emitter ^{131}I that was associated with increased risk of childhood thyroid cancers following Chernobyl, the half-life of only 8 days is relatively short compared to those for ^{134}Cs and ^{137}Cs, which are instead 2 years and 31 years, respectively. Potassium iodide (KI) can be used prophylactically to reduce thyroid uptake of ^{131}I if taken within 4 hours of the incident. Oral potassium iodide has been used in veterinary medicine as an extra-label treatment for sporotrichosis (Plumb, 2015). It should be noted that iodides are excreted in milk.

Clay minerals (bentonites, vermiculites, zeolites) can be used to reduce animals' absorption of radiocesium and its subsequent transfer to food products (Howard et al., 2001). Prussian blue (ferric hexacyanoferrate) enhances fecal cesium excretion (Yamamoto, 2013). Oral Prussian blue has been shown to be relatively nontoxic in dogs, though it is most effective when given within 1 day of cesium intake (Melo et al., 2014). Several forms of ferrocyn were used after the Chernobyl accident to reduce radiocesium transfer to meat and milk (Ratnikov et al., 1998).

Calcium and zinc DTPA (diethylenetriamine pentaacetic acid) form stable, urine-excretable complexes with plutonium, americium, and curium (Yamamoto, 2013). While treatment typically involves intravenous infusions (Singh et al., 2015), studies using an oral form of zinc DTPA dogs and rats have demonstrated low toxicity, with a no-observed-adverse-effect level of approximately 1325 mg/kg/day in dogs and $>$1000 mg/kg/day in rats (Shankar et al., 2014).

Triage and Screening

In human medicine, being irradiated or contaminated with radiation is not generally considered a medical emergency (Rella, 2015). However, animals are much more likely to internally contaminate themselves if triage and external decontamination is delayed. Animal patients will need to be evaluated for burns or injuries following a radiological incident in addition to being screened for radiation exposure. Personnel can likely accomplish this wearing dosimeters and Level C PPE. Animal recovery and decontamination plans that will require animal handling and contact should incorporate the basic radiation safety principles of time, distance, and shielding. Can a team approach be used to decrease the total exposure for any one individual? Can animals be removed from heavily contaminated environments to decrease their exposure but also limit the proximity of personnel to these areas? Can shielding be practically employed?

When personnel initially encounter animals involved in a radiological incident they should be considered potentially contaminated in one or both of the following ways (Berger et al., 1987). First, animals may have had radioactive particles deposited directly on their skin or on the ground around them. Second, animals may ingest radioactive particles from contaminated food, water, or other environmental sources. The likelihood of both scenarios may be increased because animals may not be initially accessed or evacuated as quickly as people following a radiological incident. This delay may also further complicate the ability to accurately estimate doses received by animals compared to estimates for people in the same geographic area, particularly when large flocks or herds are involved that make assessment of individuals less practical. When dose estimates are not available, the following procedure has been suggested: 80%–100% of animals will survive if no or mild signs are apparent within 21 days of the incident, 50%–75% will survive if signs of illness develop on or after 14 days postincident, and <5% will survive if severe signs begin within 10 days of the incident (Berger et al., 1987). This may be a useful tool for assessing groups of animals and to direct segregation of animals based on their likelihood of survival.

Decontamination

Ideally, decontamination should occur before transporting animals away from the incident scene or receiving area to minimize cross-contamination of vehicles, equipment, facilities, personnel, and other animals. A minimum of Level C PPE, consisting of a respirator, chemical-resistant clothing and gloves, boots, and eye protection, should be used to protect personnel working with animals from solid, liquid, and aerosolized forms of contamination. Depending on the nature of the incident, animals may have also been exposed to chemical and biological hazards that are beyond the scope of this chapter (Gwaltney-Brant et al., 2003; Soric et al., 2008).

Prior to decontaminating animals, any collars, halters, or other items should be removed, labeled, and retained in a designated location. Documentation of all such items may be critical to reuniting an animal and its owner, even if the items cannot be returned. When possible, radiologic assessment should occur prior to decontamination. Depending on the type of incident involved, it is probably prudent to fully decontaminate all stable animal patients whether or not radiologic contamination is evident to facilitate the removal of other chemical or biological hazards that may be present on the animal.

The most common decontamination method for people and animals is using soap and water. Ideally the wash water should be uncontaminated. However, using slightly-contaminated water when necessary is preferable to no decontamination at all. Washing must be thorough enough to penetrate through hair or feathers to reach and clean skin, without producing abrasions or excessive skin irritation. Eyes, nares, and ears should all be flushed. Skin folds, such as those between toes and where limbs meet the torso, may inadvertently trap contamination and will require additional inspection and cleaning. Fully fleeced sheep are more protected from radioactive particles than shorn animals (Berger et al., 1987), so shearing may be a decontamination approach to consider for sheep. Wash water and other waste generated during animal decontamination should be contained as much as possible. Animals determined to be "clean" by the use of a radiation survey meter can either be returned to their owners or transferred to an animal housing or sheltering facility for continued care.

Animals with urgent but potentially treatable medical problems that are not necessarily directly related to radiation exposure, such as traumatic injuries, may require expedited external decontamination so they can receive immediate care. An isolation area will be needed for treating and at least temporarily housing these animals. After patients are stabilized a more thorough decontamination should take place, followed by a radiologic assessment.

Additional Treatments and Monitoring

A more thorough physical examination and baseline laboratory testing should occur after initial triage and decontamination. These activities may need to occur in an isolated environment if there are any concerns about residual external contamination or any internal contamination, especially for patients that are injured or already exhibiting clinical signs consistent with ARS. Strategies for managing internally contaminated animals are limited. However, providing good quality food and water in sufficient quantities may be helpful. It will then be necessary to remove the radiologically contaminated urine, manure, and fecal material as soon as possible. A major challenge to consider should be whether or not there are enough trained animal caretakers and veterinary personnel available who are willing to work in proximity to internally contaminated animals and their waste products for weeks or months depending on the radionuclides involved.

Based on human recommendations (Rella, 2015) and if feasible, initial laboratory testing should include a complete blood count (CBC), urinalysis, baseline radiologic assessment of the urine, and initiation of a 24-hour urine collection. Nasal swabs, vomitus, and feces can also be collected for radiologic assessment. In people, decreased monocyte counts are associated with internal exposures to radioisotopes that localize in bone, making monocyte count a potential tool in estimating exposure levels to these particular radioisotopes (Ogunranti, 1989). Hematopoietic-based algorithms, using standard CBCs and serum chemistry results, have been developed to estimate the severity of H-ARS using minipigs and Rhesus macaques as part of the triage process rather than waiting for peak hematological abnormalities to develop (Bolduc et al., 2016).

Medical management of patients with ARS is primarily symptomatic and supportive, aimed at managing gastrointestinal signs and fluid losses, pain, and risk of infection (Rella, 2015). Granisetron has been effectively used to alleviate nausea and vomiting association with radiation and chemotherapeutic treatments for cancer (Singh et al., 2015). Based on experimental animal evidence and limited human use after Chernobyl, administration of probiotics may be beneficial (Ciorba et al., 2012; Urbancsek et al., 2001). Vitamin E analogs are being developed as a safe and effective radioprotectant and radiomitigant (Compadre et al., 2014). Alpha-tocopherol is the most widely studied form of vitamin E. However, tocoflexols promise to be more potent. Studies in mice have shown that ciprofloxacin enhances stress erythropoiesis in the spleen, potentially increasing survival following whole-body irradiation (Fukumoto et al., 2014).

CONCLUDING REMARKS AND FUTURE DIRECTIONS

Compared to other toxicants, ionizing radiation is especially challenging because contaminated animals cannot be definitively identified without the use of specialized detection equipment. The principles of time, shielding, and distance can be used to protect both humans and animals from ongoing exposures to sources of radioactivity. However, animal patients are much more likely to become both externally and internally contaminated because of their natural grooming behaviors, increased likelihood of consuming contaminated food and water, and the probable delay of addressing animal issues in a timely manner following a radiological event because people will have also been affected. Early effects of ARS are somewhat nonspecific and more specific illness can manifest slowly over several weeks. Recovery of surviving animals may be prolonged and can result in increased risk of chronic diseases, decreased fertility, and cancer. Food-producing animals may never return to previous levels of production and at least temporarily their meat, milk, and eggs may not be safe for consumption. If time and resources allow without compromising human safety, animals potentially exposed to radioactive contaminants can be triaged, decontaminated, and treated by properly trained personnel equipped with appropriate PPE and screening equipment.

REFERENCES

Alexakhin, R.M., Geras'kin, S.A., 2011. 25 years after the accident at the Chernobyl nuclear power plant: radioecological lessons. Radioprotection. 46, S595–S600.

Belova, N.V., Verigin, B.V., Emelianova, N.G., et al., 1993. Radiobiological analysis of silver carp *Hypophthalmichthys molitrix* in the Chernobyl NPP cooling pond in the post-accident period. I. The reproductive system status in the survived fish. J. Ichthyol. 33, 814–828.

Beresford, N.A., Howard, B.J., 2011. An overview of the transfer of radionuclides to farm animals and potential countermeasures of relevance to Fukushima releases. Integr. Env. Assess. Manag. 7 (3), 382–384.

Beresford, N.A., Mayes, R.W., Cooke, A.I., et al., 2000. The importance of source dependent bioavailability in determining the transfer of ingested radionuclides to ruminant derived food products. Environ. Sci. Technol. 34, 4455–4462.

Berger, C.D., Frazier, J.R., Greene, R.T., et al., 1987. Radiological emergency manual for livestock, poultry, and animal products. IT Corporation/Radiological Sciences Laboratory Publication 87 168. IT RSL, Oak Ridge.

Bergonie, J., Tribondeau, L., 1906. De quelques résultats de la radiotherapie et essai de fixation d'une technique rationnelle. Comptes-Rendue des Séances de l'Acad des Sci. 143, 983–985.

Bolduc, D.L., Bünger, R., Moroni, M., et al., 2016. Modeling H-ARS using hematological parameters: a comparison between the non-human primate and minipig. Rad. Prot. Dosim. 172, 161–173.

Bonisoli-Alquati, A., Voris, A., Mousseau, T.A., et al., 2009. DNA damage in barn swallows (*Hirundo rustica*) from the Chernobyl region detected by use of the comet assay. Comp. Biochem. Physiol. Part C Toxicol. Pharmacol. 151 (3), 271–277.

Brown, D.G., Gramly, W.A., Cross, F.H., 1964. Response of three breeds of swine exposed to whole-body cobalt-60 gamma radiation in daily doses of 100 roentgens. Am. J. Vet. Res. 25, 1347–1353.

Brown, D.G., Reynolds, R.A., Johnson, D.F., 1966. Late effects in cattle exposed to radioactive fallout. Am. J. Vet. Res. 27, 1509–1514.

Chester, R.,K., Rodger, B.E., Wickliffe, J.K., et al., 2001. Accumulation of ^{137}cesium and ^{90}strontium from abiotic and biotic sources in rodents at Chornobyl, Ukraine. Environ. Toxicol. Chem. 20 (9), 1927–1935.

Ciorba, M.A., Riehl, T.E., Rao, M.S., et al., 2012. Lactobacillus probiotic protects intestinal epithelium from radiation injury in a TLR-2/cyclo-oxygenase-2-dependent manner. Gut. 61 (6), 829–838.

Coggle, J.E., 1983. Biological Effects of Radiation. second ed. Taylor & Francis Ltd, London.

Compadre, C.M., Singh, A., Thakkar, S., et al., 2014. Molecular dynamics guided design of tocoflexol: a new radioprotectant tocotrienol with enhanced bioavailability. Drug Dev. Res. 75, 10–22.

Crout, N.M.J., Beresford, N.A., Mayes, R.W., et al., 2000. A model of radioiodine transfer to goat milk incorporating the influence of stable iodine. Rad. Environ. Biophys. 39, 59–65.

Darby, S.C., Cutter, D.J., Boerma, M., et al., 2010. Radiation-related heart disease: current knowledge and future prospects. Int. J. Rad. Oncol. Biol. Phys. 76 (3), 656–665.

Ellegren, H., Lindgren, G., Primmer, C.R., et al., 1997. Fitness loss and germline mutations in barn swallows breeding in Chernobyl. Nature. 389, 593–596.

Elliott, T.B., Deutz, N.E., Gulani, J., et al., 2014. Gastrointestinal acute radiation syndrome in Göttingen minipigs (*Sus scrofa domestica*). Comp. Med. 64 (6), 456–463.

Fukumoto, R., Burns, T.M., Kiang, J.G., 2014. Ciprofloxacin enhances stress erythropoiesis in spleen and increases survival after whole-body irradiation combined with skin-wound trauma. PLoS One. 9 (2), e90448.

Geras'kin, S.A., Fesenko, S.V., Alexakhin, R.M., 2008. Effects of non-human species irradiation after the Chernobyl NPP accident. Environ. Int. 34, 880–897.

Gulakov, A.V., 2014. Accumulation and distribution of ^{137}Cs and ^{90}Sr in the body of the wild boar (*Sus scrofa*) found on the territory with radioactive contamination. J. Env. Rad. 127, 171–175.

Gwaltney-Brant, S.M., Murphy, L.A., Wismer, T.A., et al., 2003. General toxicologic hazards and risks for search-and-rescue dogs responding to urban disasters. J. Am. Vet. Med. Assoc. 222 (3), 292–295.

Hayama, S., Nakiri, S., Nakanishi, S., et al., 2013. Concentration of radiocesium in the wild Japanese monkey (*Macaca fuscata*) over the first 15 months after the Fukushima Daiichi nuclear disaster. PLoS One. 8 (7), e68530.

Henriksen, T., Maillie, H.D., 2003. Radiation and Health. Taylor & Francis, New York.

Hingston, J.L., Wood, M.D., Copplestone, D., et al., 2005. Impact of chronic low-level ionising radiation exposure on terrestrial invertebrates. Radioprotection. 40 (S1), S145–S150.

Hoel, D.G., 2013. Toxic effects of radiation and radioactive materials. In: Klaassen, C.D. (Ed.), Casarett & Doull's Toxicology: The Basic Science of Poisons, eighth ed. McGraw-Hill Education, New York, pp. 1113–1129.

Hosono, H., Kumagai, Y., Sekizaki, T., 2013. Development of an information package of radiation risk in beef after the Fukushima Daiichi Nuclear Power Plant accident. In: Nakanishi, T.M., Tanoi, K. (Eds.), Agricultural Implications of the Fukushima Nuclear Accident. Springer, Tokyo, pp. 187–204. Chapter 17.

Howard, B.J., Beresford, N.A., Voight, G., 2001. Countermeasures for animal products: a review of effectiveness and potential usefulness after an accident. J. Environ. Rad. 56, 115–137.

IAEA (Internal Atomic Energy Agency), 2010. Handbook of Parameter Values for the Prediction of Radionuclide Transfer in Terrestrial and Freshwater Environments. International Atomic Energy Agency, Vienna.

IAEA (International Atomic Energy Agency), 2016. Nuclear Power Reactors in the World. IAEA, Vienna.

ICRP (International Commission on Radiological Protection), 1992. The Biological Basis for Dose Limitation in the Skin. ICRP Publication 59. Pergumon, Oxford.

ICRP, 2009. Environmental protection: transfer parameters for reference animals and plants. ICRP Publication 114. Ann. ICRP. 39, 6.

Ishida, K., 2013. Contamination of wild animals: effects on wildlife in high radioactivity areas of the agricultural and forest landscape. In: Nakanishi, T.M., Tanoi, K. (Eds.), Agricultural Implications of the Fukushima Nuclear Accident. Springer, Tokyo, pp. 119–129. Chapter 12.

Kaore, S.N., Kaore, N.M., 2014. Citrulline: pharmacological perspectives and role as a biomarker in diseases and toxicities. In: Gupta, R.C. (Ed.), Biomarkers in Toxicology. Academic Press/Elsevier, Amsterdam, pp. 883–905.

Kent, M.S., 2017. Principles and applications of radiation therapy in exotic animals. Vet. Clin. North Am. Exotic. Anim. Pract. 20 (1), 255–270.

Makeeva, A.P., Emelianova, N.G., Belova, N.V., et al., 1994. Radiobiological analysis of silver carp *Hypophthalmichthys molitrix* in the Chernobyl NPP cooling pond in the post-accident period. II. Development of the reproductive system in offsprings of the first generation. J. Ichthyol. 34, 681–696.

Malhotra, N., Rani, N., Rana, K., et al., 1990. Radiation induced blood pathology in chick erythrocytes and related parameters. Exp. Pathol. 38 (4), 241–248.

McClellan, R.O., 2014. Radiation toxicity. In: Hayes, A.W., Kruger, C. L. (Eds.), Hayes' Principles And Methods of Toxicology, sixth ed. CRC Press, Boca Raton, FL, pp. 883–955.

Melo, D.R., Lipsztein, J.L., Leggett, R., et al., 2014. Efficacy of Prussian blue on ^{137}Cs decorporation therapy. Health Phys. 106 (5), 592–597.

Moller, A.P., Mousseau, T.A., de Lope, F., et al., 2007. Elevated frequency of abnormalities in barn swallows from Chernobyl. Biol. Lett. 3 (4), 414–417.

National Research Council, 1990. Health Risks From Exposure to Low Levels of Ionizing Radiation: BEIR V. The National Academies Press, Washington, DC.

National Research Council, 2006. Health Risks From Exposure to Low Levels of Ionizing Radiation: BEIR VII, Phase 2. The National Academies Press, Washington, DC.

Nussbaum, R.H., Köhnlein, W., 2003. Ionizing radiation. In: Greenberg, M.I., Hamilton, R.J., Phillips, S.D., McCluskey, G.J. (Eds.), Occupational, Industrial, and Environmental Toxicology, second ed. Mosby, Philadelphia, pp. 702–715.

Ogunranti, J.O., 1989. Haematological indices in Nigerians exposed to radioactive waste. Lancet. 334 (8664), 667–668.

Okada, K., Sato, I., Deguchi, Y., et al., 2013. Distribution of radioactive cesium in edible parts of cattle. An. Sci. J. 84, 798–801.

Plumb, D.C., 2015. Plumb's Veterinary Drug Handbook. eighth ed. Wiley-Blackwell, Ames, pp. 561–563.

Pöschl, M., Borkovec, V., Zelenka, J., 1997. Dynamics and distribution of radiocaesium in broiler chicken. Rad. Env. Biophys. 36, 169–174.

Povinec, P.P., Hirose, K., Aoyama, M., 2013. Fukushima Accident: Radioactivity Impact on the Environment. Elsevier, Waltham.

Ratnikov, A.N., Vasiliev, A.V., Alexakhin, R.M., et al., 1998. The use of hexacyanoferrates in different forms to reduce radiocaesium contamination of animal products in Russia. Sci. Total Env. 223, 167–176.

Rebois, R.V., Ray, K., 2012. Ionizing radiation and radioactive materials in health and disease. In: Gupta, R.C. (Ed.), Veterinary Toxicology, second ed. Academic Press/Elsevier, Amsterdam, pp. 391–405.

Rella, J.G., 2015. Radiation. In: Hoffman, R.S., Howland, M.A., Lewin, N.A., Nelson, L.S., Goldfrank, L.R. (Eds.), Goldfrank's Toxicologic Emergencies, tenth ed. McGraw-Hill Education, New York, pp. 1703–1712.

Sample, B.E., Irvine, C., 2011. Radionuclides in biota. In: Nelson, W.N., Meador, J.P. (Eds.), Environmental Contaminants in Biota: Interpreting Tissue Concentrations, second ed. CRC Press, Boca Raton, FL, pp. 703–732.

Shankar, G.N., Potharaju, S., Green, C.E., 2014. Evaluating the toxicity of novel Zn-DTPA tablet formulation in dogs and rats. Drug Dev. Res. 75, 37–46.

Singh, V.K., Romaine, P.L.P., Seed, T.M., 2015. Medical countermeasures for radiation exposure and related injuries: characterization of medicines, FDA-approval status and inclusion into the Strategic National Stockpile. Health Phys. 108 (6), 607–630.

Soric, S., Belanger, M.P., Wittnich, C., 2008. A method for the decontamination of animals involved in floodwater disasters. J. Am. Vet. Med. Assoc. 232 (3), 364–370.

Stenehjem, M., 1990. Indecent exposure. Nat. History. 9 (90), 6–14.

Tempel, K., 1983. Radiologie für veterinärmediziner (Radiology for veterinarians). Enke Verlag, Stuttgart.

Urbancsek, H., Kazar, T., Mezes, I., et al., 2001. Results of a double-blind, randomized study to evaluate the efficacy and safety of Antibiophilus® in patients with radiation-induced diarrhea. Eur. J. Gastroenterol. Hepatol. 13 (4), 391–396.

Voight, G., Pröhl, G., Müller, H., et al., 1989. Determination of the transfer of cesium and iodine from feed into domestic animals. Sci. Total Environ. 85, 329–338.

Waghmare, C.M., 2013. Radiation burn – from mechanism to management. Burns. 39, 212–219.

Waselenko, J.K., MacVittie, T.J., Blakely, W.F., et al., 2004. Medical management of the acute radiation syndrome: recommendations of the Strategic National Stockpile Radiation Working Group. Ann. Int. Med. 140 (12), 1037–1051.

Webster, S.C., Byrne, M.E., Lance, S.L., et al., 2016. Where the wild things are: influence of radiation on the distribution of four mammalian species within Chernobyl Exclusion Zone. Front Ecol. Environ. 14 (4), 185–190.

Wood, M.D., Hingston, J.L., Copplestone, D., et al., 2005. Development of experimental protocols for chronic irradiation studies: the application of a good practice guide framework. Radioprotection. 40 (S1), S229–S234.

Woodhead, D.S., 1998. The Impact of Radioactive Discharges on Native British Wild-Life and the Implications for Environmental Protection. R&D Technical Report P135. Environment Agency, Bristol.

Worgul, B.V., Kundiyev, Y.I., Sergiyenko, N.M., et al., 2007. Cataracts among Chernobyl clean-up workers: implications regarding permissible eye exposures. Rad. Res. 167 (2), 233–243.

Yamamoto, L.G., 2013. Risks and management of radiation exposure. Ped. Emer. Care. 29 (9), 1016–1026.

von Zallinger, C., Tempel, K., 1998. The physiologic response of domestic animals to ionizing radiation: a review. Vet. Radiol. Ultras. 39 (6), 495–503.

Chapter 20

Carcinogenesis: Mechanisms and Models*

Supratim Choudhuri, Ronald Chanderbhan and Antonia Mattia

INTRODUCTION

Cancer is a general term used to refer to a pathological condition that is characterized by aberrant cell growth and proliferation. Carcinogenesis is the process of cancer development. Animals, like humans, have always been exposed to thousands of man-made and naturally occurring chemical substances in their daily lives. This exposure may come from the food they eat, the water they drink, and the air they breathe. Both the level of exposure and duration of exposure are factors that impact whether chemicals cause cancer in humans and animals. In 1915, Katsusaburo Yamagiwa and Koichi Ichikawa at Tokyo University pioneered the field of experimental cancer research when they produced tumors by repeated application of coal tars on the skin of rabbits. Over the last 50 years or so, remarkable progress has been made in understanding the mechanism of carcinogenesis, which has both a genetic and an environmental component. The present chapter primarily focuses on the mechanism and models of chemical carcinogenesis.

TERMINOLOGY

Tumors or neoplasms (new growth of tissue) can be benign or malignant (cancerous). In the parlance of cancer biology, the suffix "oma" means tumor—whether benign or malignant. For example, adenoma, fibroma, and lipoma are benign tumors of glandular, fibrous (connective), and adipose tissues, respectively, while melanoma, hepatoma, and seminoma are malignant tumors of skin, liver, and germ cells, respectively. Cancer arising in the epithelial tissues lining the outer or inner surfaces of the body is called carcinoma. Carcinomas are classified according to histological type, and include adenocarcinoma (glandular carcinoma), squamous cell carcinoma, small cell carcinoma, large cell carcinoma, etc. The most common types of cancers in humans are carcinomas. Cancers of embryonic tissues are denoted with the suffix "blastoma," such as neuroblastoma and retinoblastoma. Similarly, cancers of connective tissue, such as bone, cartilage, fat, muscle, and blood vessels are denoted with the suffix "sarcoma," such as fibrosarcoma, liposarcoma, and rhabdomyosarcoma.

Sometimes nonneoplastic lesions end with the "oma" suffix, such as hematoma and granuloma. A hematoma is a localized collection of blood outside the blood vessels that occurs when blood escapes into the surrounding tissue because of damage to the blood vessels. A granuloma is a small patch of inflamed tissue that results from infection or inflammation. The terms used to describe these noncancer tissue alterations are a reminder that the terminology surrounding cancer and carcinogenesis is not simple. Tumor typing and cancer diagnosis require the expertise of trained pathologists.

AGENTS CAUSING CARCINOGENESIS

Three main types of agents that can lead to the development of cancer are chemicals, viruses and radiation. Chemical carcinogenesis is an important topic in toxicology and will be the primary focus of this chapter. The genetic basis of carcinogenesis including virus-induced carcinogenesis and radiation-induced carcinogenesis will be discussed briefly.

Chemical Carcinogenesis

Chemical Carcinogens Occur in Nature and Can Also Be Formed by Nonindustrial and Industrial Processes

Chemical carcinogens are extremely diverse in structure and they belong to very different chemical classes,

* The opinions expressed in this chapter are the authors' personal opinion and they do not necessarily reflect those of FDA, DHHS, or the federal government.

Veterinary Toxicology. DOI: http://dx.doi.org/10.1016/B978-0-12-811410-0.00020-9

TABLE 20.1 Some Examples of Chemical Carcinogens

Carcinogens occurring naturally	• Aflatoxin (from the fungus *Aspergillus flavus*) • Aristolochic acid (in plant family Aristolochiaceae) • Toxic metals (e.g., As, Ni) • Safrole (from the root-bark or the fruit of sassafras plants) • Ionizing radiation
Carcinogens produced by industrial and nonindustrial processes	• Benzo[a]pyrene formed by incomplete combustion (e.g., vehicle emissions, tar and asphalt fumes, meat barbeque) • Acrylamide formed during cooking French fries and potato chips • Tobacco smoke • Coal tar that is produced by the carbonization of coal, i.e., heating of coal in the absence of air at very high temperatures • Benzene • Dyes (aromatic amines, such as 2-Naphthylamine)

such as inorganic, organic, fibers, plastic, hormones, etc. Table 20.1 shows some chemical carcinogens.

Chemical Carcinogens Can Be Genotoxic or Nongenotoxic

Based on their biological activities, chemical carcinogens can be classified as genotoxic carcinogens that are DNA-reactive, and nongenotoxic carcinogens that are not DNA-reactive.

Genotoxic (DNA-Reactive) Carcinogens Interact With DNA

Most genotoxic carcinogens act as tumor initiators. Genotoxic carcinogens interact directly with DNA through the formation of covalent bonds, resulting in DNA-carcinogen complexes (DNA adducts). These complexes lead to various types of DNA damage, such as point mutations, chromosome breakage, fusion, missegregation and nondisjunction, all of which result in modifications to the information stored in DNA as well as genomic instability. Some of the mechanisms underlying structural alterations include the formation of cross-links between the two helices, chemical bonds between adjacent bases, removal of DNA bases (hydration) and cleavage of the DNA strands. Such mutations are typically fixed by DNA repair mechanisms; however, if DNA replication occurs prior to the action of a repair mechanism, mutations can become permanent (Lee et al., 2013). In addition, DNA repair process is not devoid of errors; therefore, mutations can be induced by the very repair processes cells use to rid themselves of DNA damage. An affected cell first tries to reverse the damage by DNA repair. If DNA repair and removal of the damage fails the cell often undergoes programmed cell death (apoptosis). If the cell fails to undergo apoptosis, the result is a permanent fixation of the damage in the DNA, which provides the first trigger of tumor development.

A genotoxic carcinogen can be a direct genotoxic carcinogen or an indirect genotoxic carcinogen (procarcinogen). A direct genotoxic carcinogen is DNA-reactive without metabolic activation, whereas an indirect genotoxic carcinogen (procarcinogen) becomes DNA-reactive following metabolic activation. Metabolic activation of the indirect genotoxic carcinogen (procarcinogen) generates the ultimate carcinogen, which is DNA-reactive (Table 20.2). The majority of genotoxic carcinogens are indirect carcinogens because they need metabolic activation to form an electrophile that reacts with nucleophilic DNA (Marquardt, 1999).

Nongenotoxic (Non DNA-Reactive) Carcinogens Do Not Directly Interact With DNA

Most nongenotoxic carcinogens act as tumor promoters (Table 20.2). Nongenotoxic carcinogens do not directly induce DNA damage. They can act through a number of different mechanisms, such as specific protein binding, receptor interactions, hormonal and endocrine modifier effects, epigenetic changes in the DNA, etc. (Benigni et al., 2013). Thus, any genotoxic event in response to challenge by nongenotoxic carcinogen is secondary to other biologic activity. For example, oxidative stress produced by a nongenotoxic carcinogen as a primary effect can cause DNA damage as a secondary effect, but this secondary effect of DNA damage does not make the oxidative stress causing chemical a genotoxic carcinogen (Trosko and Upham, 2005). Nongenotoxic carcinogens usually exhibit tissue and species specificity.

Increasing evidence suggests that the demarcation between genotoxic and nongenotoxic carcinogens may not be as distinct as initially thought. For example, epigenetic changes may play a causative role in carcinogenic process induced by genotoxic agents as well (Pogribny et al., 2008). Tumor initiators can both initiate and promote

TABLE 20.2 Examples of Genotoxic and Nongenotoxic Carcinogens

Type	Subtype and Mechanism of Action	Some Examples
Genotoxic carcinogen (DNA-reactive) Linear dose-response used for risk assessment	Direct genotoxic carcinogen (No metabolic activation needed) Many compounds in this class are used as chemotherapeutic agents because they are cytotoxic	• Nitrogen mustards (e.g., mechlorethamine, also known as mustargen and mustine): Alkylate DNA • Nitrosoureas (the simplest one is *N*-nitrosourea that has an H-atom for the R_1, R_2 and R_3 groups. The H can be substituted to give rise to more complex nitrosoureas, such as *N*-methyl-*N*-nitrosourea or MNU; *N,N'*-bis (2-chloroethyl) nitrosourea or BCNU): Alkylate DNA • β-propiolactone: Alkylates DNA (used as antiviral)
	Indirect genotoxic carcinogen (metabolic activation needed) The carcinogenic metabolite is called the ultimate carcinogen	• Polycyclic aromatic hydrocarbons, such as benzo[a] pyrene (B[a]P-7,8-dihydrodiol-9,10-epoxide is the ultimate carcinogen produced from the metabolism of benzo[a]pyrene) • Aromatic amines (The key reaction producing the ultimate carcinogen is the *N*-oxidation to aryl-*N*-hydroxylamines that form esters. An example is *N*-acetoxyarylamine produced from 2-naphthylamine. In acidic pH, such as in urine these metabolites produce aryl nitrenium ion which is DNA-reactive; hence aromatic amines often induce bladder tumor) • Aflatoxin B1 (AFB_1-*exo*-8,9-epoxide is the ultimate carcinogen produced from the metabolism of aflatoxin B1)
Nongenotoxic carcinogen (non DNA-reactive) Nonlinear dose-response possible	Protein binding	• D-limonene (binds $\alpha_{2u}G$ in the kidney of male rats; $\alpha_{2u}G$ is not degraded, hence accumulates in the proximal tubular cells, becomes cytotoxic and causes cell death by necrosis. A sustained compensatory cell proliferation results in malignancy)
	Receptor activation	• PCBs, Dioxins: AhR activation (causes dysregulation of cellular physiology, growth and proliferation) • Fibrates, such as Clofibrate, Ciprofibrate: PPARα activation (induces oxidative stress and DNA damage as a 2° effect of oxidative stress; alters hepatocyte growth control)
	Endocrine modifier	• Diethylstilbesterol and other phytoestrogens
	DNA methylation (epigenetic)	• Wy-14643, Trichloroethylene (can also cause peroxisome proliferation) (cause promoter hypomethylation of oncogenes, such as *c-Jun*, *c-Myc*, and dysregulation of cell proliferation)

tumor development and also cause progression to malignancy, if applied repetitively (Tennant, 1999). There are relatively few DNA reactive complete carcinogens that can induce cancers following single exposures (e.g., X-rays, urethane, and ethyl nitrosourea). For most other carcinogens, repetitive or prolonged exposures are necessary. Additionally, new chemicals introduced into commerce or the environment are rarely traditional genotoxic carcinogens (Tennant, 1999). Thus, the study of nongenotoxic carcinogens (tumor promoters) is an important aspect of the study of chemical carcinogenesis.

Carcinogens and Dose-Response

In cancer risk assessment, the dose-response to genotoxic carcinogens is assumed to be linear, i.e., a straight line approaching zero. In other words, there is no safe level of exposure; any exposure to a genotoxic carcinogen is assumed to have a risk and the higher the exposure the greater the risk. In contrast, nongenotoxic carcinogens are assumed to produce nonlinear dose-response curve. Therefore, nongenotoxic carcinogens are assumed to have a threshold of exposure below which tumor development is not expected.

Carcinogenesis Is a Multistep Biological Process That Involves Three Major Events: Initiation, Promotion, and Progression

The three distinct steps of chemical carcinogenesis are initiation, promotion, and progression (Foulds, 1954). Based on the experimental data, Isaac Berenblum and Philippe Shubik (1947) first proposed the two-stage "initiation–promotion model" of carcinogenesis. The term "progression" was later added as a distinct step by Leslie Foulds, although the concept of progression of cancer had already been articulated by Peyton Rous and others (Foulds, 1954).

Tumor Initiation Is an Irreversible Genetic Event That Produces Preneoplastic Cells

The chemical causing initiation is called an initiator. In the initiation phase, the chemical or its reactive metabolite causes a permanent change in the DNA of the target cell(s), such as a mutation, a distortion of the DNA structure with further consequences, deletion of a component of DNA (bases or sugars), or errors in DNA repair (Pitot, 2002). Thus, initiation is a genetic event. If the DNA damage is not repaired or the cell containing the damage does not undergo apoptosis, the damage is fixed in the cellular genome and the target cell is initiated. From this point on initiation is irreversible. An initiated cell is preneoplastic and by itself is not a cancer cell because it has not acquired the property of uncontrolled growth. In order for an initiated cell to transform into a cancer cell and eventually produce a detectable tumor, promotion is necessary.

In 1971 Alfred Knudson proposed the two-hit hypothesis of cancer initiation, which postulates that cancer results from more than a single mutation in the DNA. Statistical analysis of the data revealed that dominantly inherited predisposition to retinoblastoma needs a germline mutation (the inherited "first hit"), while tumor development requires a second mutation, which is somatic. Nonhereditary retinoblastoma also requires two hits, but both are somatic. The two-hit hypothesis is the simplest form of the multiple hit hypothesis of carcinogenesis first proposed by Nordling (1953) and postulating that cancer results from multiple genetic mutations (hits). In the two-hit hypothesis, the first hit required for tumor development is part of the initiation step discussed above. DNA adduct formation, (i.e., covalent bonding of the initiator with the DNA) is an important mechanism of tumor initiation because adducts have the potential to induce mutations.

TABLE 20.3 Examples on the Mechanism of Action of Two Tumor Initiators

- DMBA forms DNA adduct by covalently binding through its 12-methyl group to the N-7 position of adenine (major adduct) or guanine (minor adduct). Removal of the N-7 purine adducts leads to depurination and mutation. If the mutation involves an oncogene or a tumor suppressor gene, such as A→T transversion in *ras* oncogene, the result could be disastrous
- *N*-methyl-*N*-nitrosourea (MNU) forms DNA adduct by modifying guanine to O^6-methylguanine in the target tissue. The 'suicide enzyme' O^6-methylguanine-DNA methyltransferase (MGMT) repairs this lesion. It is called suicide enzyme because following repair the enzyme is inactivated because Cys145 residue in the active site of MGMT binds the methyl group removed by the O^6-methylguanine. Unrepaired O^6-methylguanine lesion leads to G→A transition. Transgenic mice overexpressing MGMT are less sensitive to tumor development in the tissue overexpressing the enzyme. Methyl group is the preferred substrate of MGMT, but it can remove larger and complex alkyl groups, which makes MGMT an alkyltransferase

TABLE 20.4 Examples of Tumor Initiators, Promoters, and Progression Agents

Tumor initiators	• Benzo[a]pyrene • 7,12-dimethylbenz[a]anthracene (DMBA) • *N*-methyl-*N*-nitrosourea (MNU) • 3-methylcholanthrene • 2-acetylaminofluorene • Dimethylnitrosamine • Diethylnitrosamine
Tumor promoters	• TPA (12-*O*-tetradecanoylphorbol-13-acetate, a phorbol ester isolated from croton oil) is skin-specific • Chlordane, DDT (dichlorodiphenyltrichloroethane), TCDD (2,3,7,8-tetrachlorodibenzo-*p*-dioxin), phenobarbital, β-naphthoflavone, peroxisome proliferators and polybrominated biphenyls are hepatic tumor promoters • Mirex (an organochlorine) is a promoter in both skin and liver • Saccharin is a bladder tumor promoter
Tumor progression agents(no initiator activity)	• Benzene • Benzoyl peroxide • 2,5,2′5′-tetrachlorobiphenyl

Table 20.3 describes the mechanisms of action of two representative tumor initiators, DMBA and MNU; Table 20.4 lists some common tumor initiators.

Tumor Promotion Is a Nongenetic Process That Affects the Growth Kinetics of the Initiated Cells and It Can Be Reversible

Tumor promoters alter the expression of genetic information of the cell and in many cases inhibit programmed cell death (Pitot, 2002). Tumor promoters are involved in mitogenic signaling to trigger increased cell proliferation, thereby influencing the proliferation of initiated cells as well. Irigaray and Belpomme (2010) defined tumor promoters as nongenotoxic carcinogens capable of causing clonal expansion of initiated cells, i.e., able to induce proliferation of mutated cells and to prevent these cells from apoptotic loss, so the possibility of additional genetic and/or epigenetic changes is preserved.

The proliferation of preneoplastic cells leads to the formation of benign focal lesions, such as enzyme-altered foci in the liver, nodules in the mammary gland, polyps in the colon, papillomas in the skin. Because tumor promoters alter the expression of genetic information without changing the DNA sequence, tumor promotion is an epigenetic process. In addition to causing cell proliferation, tumor promoters appear to block apoptosis, thus leading to the accumulation of preneoplastic cells within a tissue. Some of the lesions that develop due to promotion may regress, but others acquire additional mutations and progress to malignant neoplasm. Tumor promotion is a reversible process up to a certain stage if the promoter is withdrawn.

In order for the tumors to develop, the target tissue must be exposed to an initiator first and then repeatedly exposed to promoters. If the time gap between the exposure to initiator and promoter varies from a week to a year, tumors will still develop. However, if the exposure to promoter is first and is followed by exposure to initiator, tumors will not develop. Fig. 20.1 shows the importance of the sequence of exposure to tumor initiator and tumor promoter in tumor development. Table 20.4 shows some common tumor promoters.

Tumor Progression Is a Genetic Process That Involves Transformation of a Benign Tumor Into a Malignant Tumor and Metastasis of the Malignant Neoplasm

The term tumor progression, coined by Leslie Foulds, refers to the stepwise transformation of a benign tumor into a malignant tumor and involves autonomous growth and metastasis of the malignant neoplasm. Irigaray and Belpomme (2010) defined tumor progressors as carcinogens that advance mutated cells from promotion to progression, i.e., that allow premalignant mutated cells to irreversibly acquire the phenotype of fully malignant

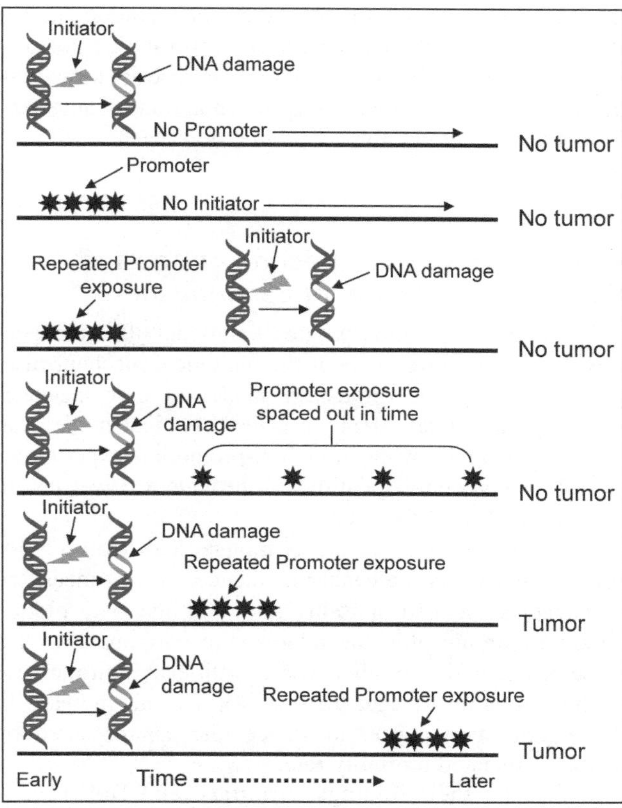

FIGURE 20.1 The target tissue must be exposed to an initiator first followed by repeated exposure to promoters in order for the tumors to develop. If the time gap between the exposure to initiator and promoter varies from a week to a year, tumors will still develop. However, if the exposure to promoter is first and is followed by exposure to initiator, tumors will not develop. Also, if the exposure to promoter is not repeated and spaced over time, tumors is not likely to develop even if the exposure to promoter occurs after exposure to initiator.

cells. At the cytogenetic level, progression is associated with additional mutations and a karyotypic change because virtually all tumors are aneuploid (have the wrong number of chromosomes). Additionally, chromosomal abnormalities, such as deletion, duplication, or translocation of chromosomal fragments are hallmarks of tumor progression. Additional mutations in the oncogenes and tumor suppressor genes also accumulate during this phase. Because tumor progression is a genetic process that involves the accumulation of additional mutations (beyond the initiating mutation), tumor initiators can also cause tumor progression (Qin et al., 2000; Becker et al., 2003).

Karyotypic instability and accumulation of additional mutations reflect an ongoing selection of cells suitable for neoplastic growth and metastasis (Okey et al., 1998). Such increased fitness of a subset of cells for neoplastic growth and metastasis is thought to be conferred by specific mutation(s) called driver mutations. The rest of the mutations that outnumber the driver mutations do not confer any survival advantage to the cells and do not contribute to the overall process of carcinogenesis; these neutral mutations are called passenger mutations. Table 20.4 lists some common tumor progression agents with no initiator activity.

Carcinogenesis as a Function of Age and the Multistage Model of Carcinogenesis

The initiation-promotion-progression model of carcinogenesis discussed above is about the biological mechanism of carcinogenesis. The multistage model of carcinogenesis (Armitage and Doll, 1954) is a mathematical model that integrates data from the initiation-promotion experiments as well as epidemiological data to provide a power law to the age incidence of cancer.

In their original paper, Armitage and Doll (1954) showed that when the cancer incidence rate (as measured by cancer-associated mortality rate) and age were plotted on a logarithmic plot, the relationship was linear with a slope of about six. In other words, with each unit increase in the logarithm of age, there was a six-unit increase in the logarithm of cancer incidence rate, as measured by cancer-associated mortality rate.

Based on their findings, Armitage and Doll (1954) proposed what is commonly known as the multistage model of carcinogenesis. They inferred that six or seven independent, sequential, and stable events are needed to occur in the cancer lineage before malignancy could be observed. Therefore, according to this model, cancer is the end-result of a series of discrete cellular changes with a long latency period before cancer is manifest. Armitage and Doll's original model has been subsequently refined by many authors. The multistage model does not hold particularly true for hormonal carcinogenesis, nor for cancers in people above the age of 75 because at this age cancer incidence significantly drops.

Before Armitage and Doll proposed their multistage model of carcinogenesis, Nordling (1953) hypothesized that cancer development requires mutations in multiple genes. As mentioned above, Knudson's two-hit hypothesis is the simplest form of this multiple hit hypothesis. Based on the current state of understanding of carcinogenesis, the inferred six or seven independent events that Armitage and Doll hypothesized as needed for cancer development, may be all genetic events or a combination of genetic and epigenetic events.

Mode of Action of Chemical Carcinogens

As discussed above, the majority of genotoxic carcinogens are indirect genotoxic carcinogens because the parent compound needs to be metabolized into a carcinogenic metabolite, which is called the ultimate carcinogen. The carcinogens form DNA adducts that are often, but not always, properly repaired. The biological activity of the carcinogens depends on a balance between their activation and detoxification in the target tissue.

The Majority of Genotoxic Carcinogens Interact With DNA Through Three Different Types of Chemical Reactions: Alkylation, Arylamination, and Aralkylation

The DNA-reactive groups are generated through specific reaction chemistries, such as oxidation at carbon-carbon double bonds yielding alkylating or aralkylating agents; oxidation or reduction at nitrogen producing arylaminating agents; conjugations of hydroxy compounds producing aralkylating or arylaminating agents and conjugation between glutathione with dihaloalkanes producing alkylating agents. There are some carcinogens that do not fit these categories, such as acylating agents, α,β-unsaturated aldehydes, chloroethylene oxide, etc. (Dipple, 1995).

Alkylation Involves the Addition of an Alkyl Carbocation to DNA

Alkylating carcinogenic agents add an electrophilic (electron-poor) alkyl carbocation to nucleophilic (electron-rich) sites in DNA. Carbocations, formerly known as carbonium ions, carry a positive charge on a carbon atom. The reactivity of alkyl carbocations from higher to lower is as follows: methyl carbocation (also known as methyl carbonium ion; CH_3^+) > primary alkyl carbocation ($R_1CH_2^+$; R_1 = single alkyl group) > secondary alkyl carbocation (R_2CH^+; R_2 = two alkyl groups) > tertiary alkyl carbocation (R_3C^+; R_3 = three alkyl groups). Examples of alkylating agents include nitrosamines, aliphatic epoxides, aflatoxins, lactones, nitrosoureas, nitrogen mustards, haloalkanes, aryl triazenes, and sultones (Dipple, 1995). The sites of substitution in DNA bases by alkylating agents are many (see Figure 26.2 in Choudhuri et al., 2012). Alkylating agents are produced by enzymatic reactions, such as P450-mediated microsomal oxidation in the liver.

An example of alkyl carbocation alkylating agent is methyl carbonium ion (CH_3^+) produced by P450 2E1 (CYP2E1)-mediated metabolism of dimethylnitrosamine. Methyl carbonium ion is a highly reactive alkylating agent that methylates DNA and proteins (Fig. 20.2A). Another example is the aflatoxin B1 (AFB_1)-*exo*-8,9-epoxide produced by the metabolism of AFB_1. The AFB1-*exo*-8,9-epoxide forms DNA adducts almost exclusively at the N-7 position of guanine (Fig. 20.2B) that ultimately results in a GC → TA transversion. These mutations are thought to be the major mechanism of

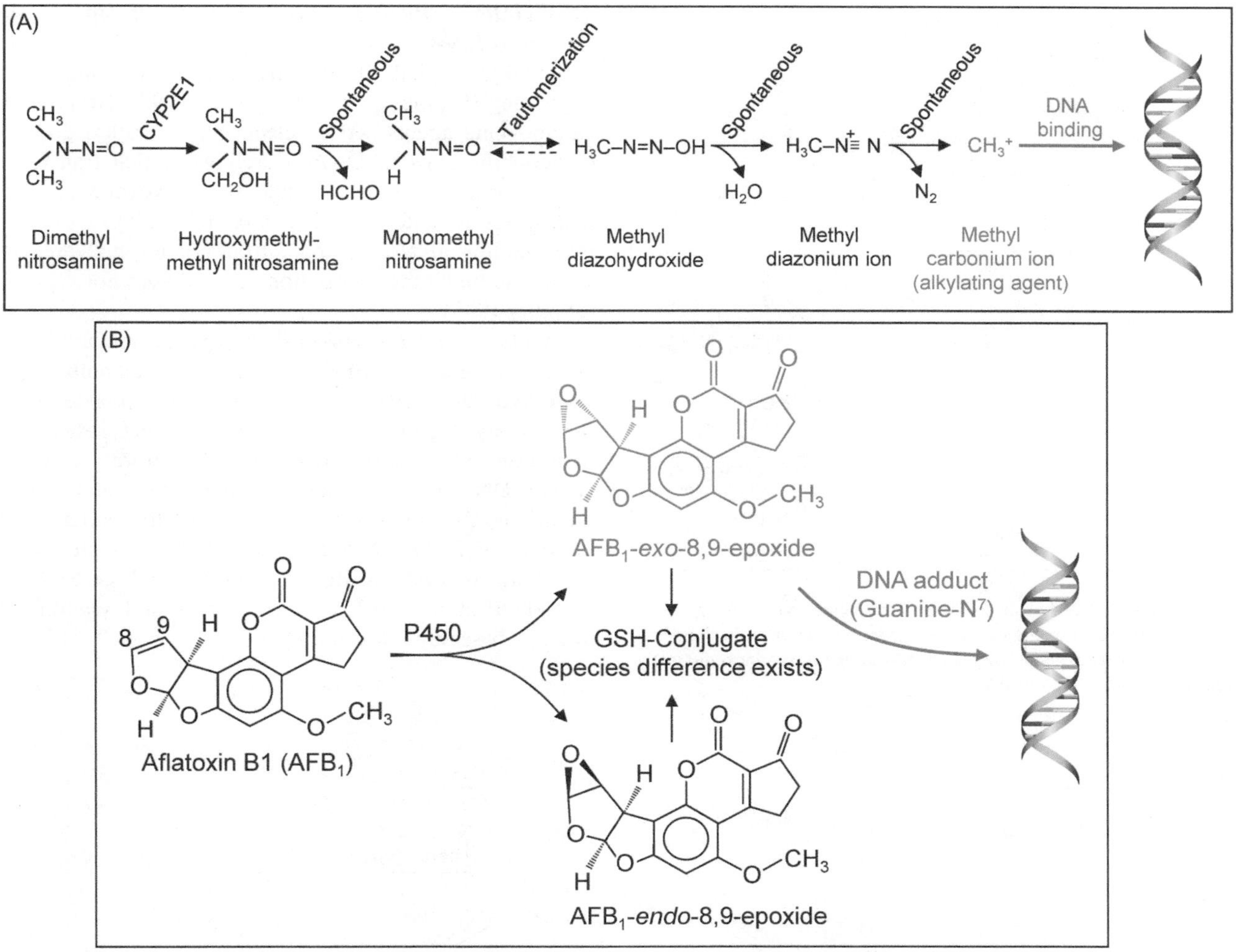

FIGURE 20.2 (A) Metabolism of dimethylnitrosamine produces methyl carbonium ion (CH_3^+), which is a highly reactive alkyl carbocation that methylates nucleophilic sites on DNA and proteins. (B) Metabolism of aflatoxin B1 (AFB_1) results in the formation of the reactive AFB_1-*exo*-8,9-epoxide intermediate, which forms DNA adducts almost exclusively at the N-7 position of guanine. This results in a GC→TA transversion mutation.

aflatoxin-induced carcinogenesis. Most of the hepatocellular carcinomas observed in an aflatoxin-exposed population have the GC→TA transversion at codon 249 of the *p53* gene (Smela et al., 2001; Okey et al., 1998).

Arylamination Involves the Addition of an Electrophilic Aryl Nitrenium Ion to DNA

An arylamine contains an amine-substituted aromatic ring (Dipple, 1995; Okey et al., 1998). Arylaminating carcinogenic agents add an electrophilic aryl nitrenium ion ($Ar\text{-}NH^+$) to nucleophilic sites in DNA. The nitrenium ion is the *N*-analogue of carbocation; it has a positive charge on the nitrogen atom. Metabolism of aromatic amines (arylamines), amides, aminoazo dyes, heterocyclic amines, and similar compounds forms electrophilic aryl nitrenium ions. The major sites of substitution in DNA by arylaminating agents appear to be the C-8 position and the amino group of the purine nucleotides (Dipple, 1995). See Figure 26.2 in Choudhuri et al. (2012) for the potential arylamination sites in DNA bases by arylaminating agents.

A prototypical example is DNA arylamination following the metabolic activation of 2-naphthylamine. *N*-oxidation by CYP1A2 forms the corresponding *N*-hydroxyarylamine (e.g., *N*-hydroxynaphthylamine), which can undergo a number of conjugation reactions forming sulfate, acetate or glucuronide conjugates. These conjugates can be excreted in the urine. In the acidic pH of urine, the conjugate dissociates and the *N*-hydroxynaphthyl moiety is protonated to form the nitrenium ion (Fig. 20.3). The site-specific formation of the nitrenium ion, is the ultimate carcinogen, explains why 2-naphthylamine is carcinogenic in the urinary tract and urinary bladder.

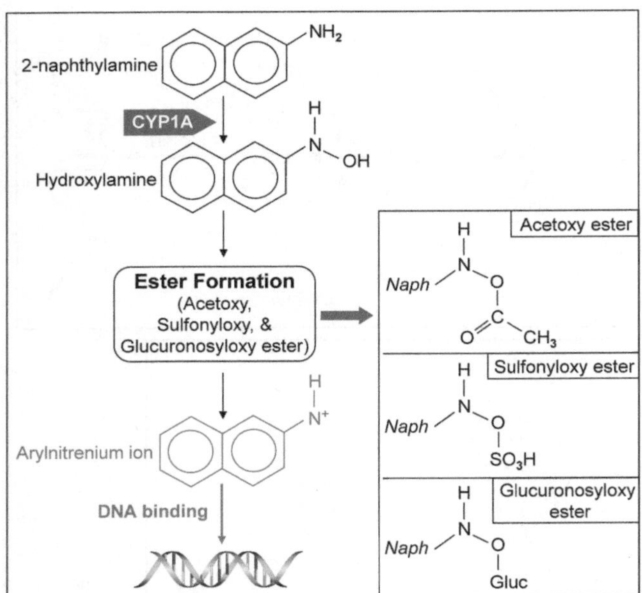

FIGURE 20.3 Metabolism of 2-naphthylamine produces the arylnitrenium ion, the ultimate carcinogen, from its conjugate in the acidic pH of urine. This explains why 2-naphthylamine is carcinogenic in the urinary tract and urinary bladder.

Aralkylation Involves the Addition of an Aralkyl Group to DNA

An aralkyl (arylalkyl) contains an alkyl-substituted aromatic ring (Dipple, 1995; Okey et al., 1998). Aralkylating carcinogenic agents add an electrophilic aralkyl group to nucleophilic sites in DNA. Carcinogens that transfer an aralkyl group to DNA include the polycyclic aromatic hydrocarbons and related compounds, alkyl benzenes, pyrrolizidine alkaloids, and nitroaromatics that are activated through the formation of dihydrodiol epoxide (Dipple, 1995).

A classic example of this class is the metabolism of benzo[a]pyrene (B[a]P) (Fig. 20.4). The metabolite B[a]P 7,8 dihydrodiol-9,10 epoxide has the 9,10 epoxide as part of the bay region; it is electrophilic, and resistant to hydration by epoxide hydrolase. Therefore, it readily attacks DNA bases, covalently binds DNA and induces mutations. B[a]P is known to cause initiating mutations in the cellular *H-ras* oncogene; these mutations are associated with tumors of different organs. See Figure 26.2 in Choudhuri et al. (2012) for the potential aralkylation sites in DNA bases by aralkylating agents.

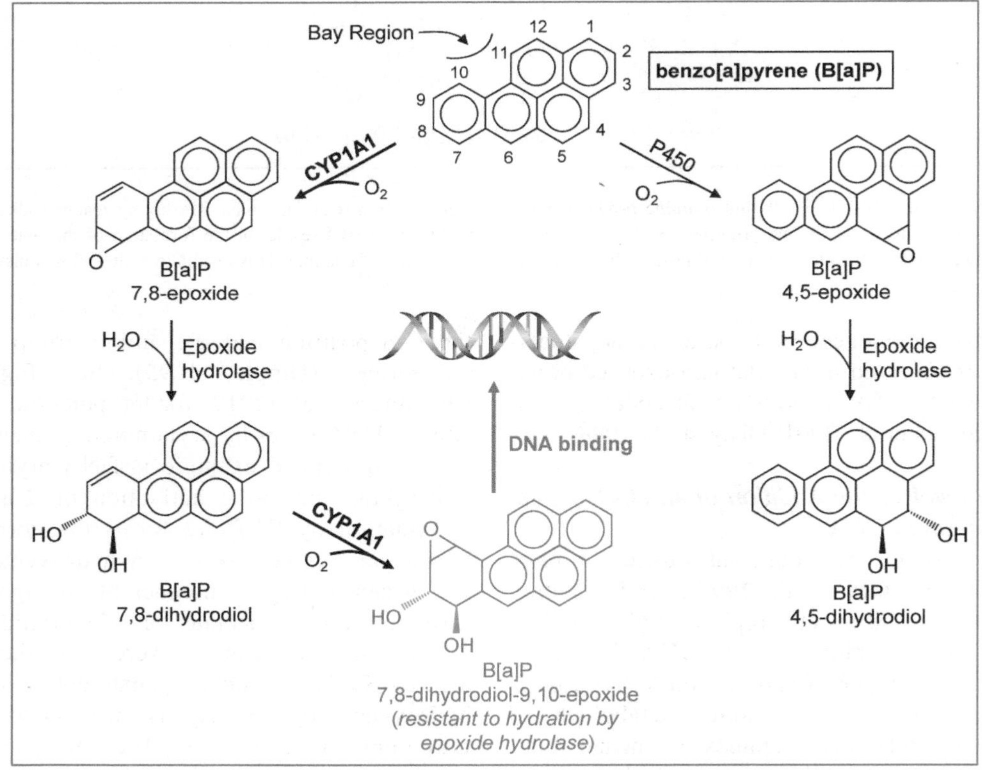

FIGURE 20.4 Metabolism of benzo[a]pyrene produces 7,8 dihydrodiol-9,10 epoxide, which is resistant to hydration by epoxide hydrolase because of the position of the epoxide close to the bay region; therefore it readily attacks DNA bases, covalently binds DNA and induces mutation.

Cellular Defense Against DNA Damage: DNA Repair and Removal of DNA Adducts

There are a number of mechanisms to repair DNA damage, including the removal of DNA adducts: (1) direct repair, (2) base excision repair (BER), (3) nucleotide excision repair (NER), (4) mismatch repair (MMR), and (5) single and double strand break repair. The common steps in DNA repair involve recognition of the lesion by specific protein complex, removal of bases around and including the lesion using specific nucleases, repair synthesis by DNA polymerase and gap sealing by ligase. Some of the relevant repair mechanisms are discussed below.

In direct repair, the bond between the nucleotide and adduct is broken restoring the original conformation. An example is MGMT-mediated O^6-methylguanine repair by direct demethylation of the methylguanine (Fig. 20.5A). In animals that have photolyase, thymine dimers are also repaired by the direct repair mechanism that involves breaking of the bond causing the dimer (Fig. 20.5B).

The BER works mainly on nonbulky base modifications, such as those produced by methylation in positions where it does not interfere with H-bonding, such as N3- or N7-methyladenine, N7-methylguanine or 8-hydroxyguanine. For example, *N*-methyl-*N*-nitrosourea produces these types of methylation patterns. The BER involves the following steps: (1) removal of the inappropriate base by a specific DNA glycosylase that cleaves the *N*-glycosidic bond between the deoxyribose sugar and the base, thereby creating an apurinic or apyrimidinic (AP) site, (2) AP endonuclase-mediated nick in the sugar-phosphate backbone 5′ to the AP site, (3) deoxyribophosphodiesterase (an excision endonuclease)-mediated nick in the sugar-phosphate backbone 3′ to the AP site, thereby creating a one nucleotide gap, (4) recruitment of the appropriate base (nucleotide) by DNA polymerase followed by sealing of the gaps by ligase (Fig. 20.5C). Many DNA glycosylases have been discovered so far; specific DNA glycosylases excise specific types of damaged bases, such as those spontaneously formed (e.g., hypoxanthine), oxidized (e.g., 8-oxo-7, 8-dihydroguanine), alkylated (e.g., 3-methyladenine), or mismatched (e.g., T:G) bases.

The NER is a versatile mechanism that can eliminate a wide range of structurally unrelated lesions from the DNA, including bulky base modifications, such as B[a]P-guanine adducts caused by smoking, cisplatin-guanine adducts and psoralen-thymine adducts resulting from chemotherapy, and UV-induced multiple thymine dimers. In humans, thymine dimers are repaired by NER because humans do not have photolyase. The steps of NER involves (1) damage recognition by DNA damage-binding

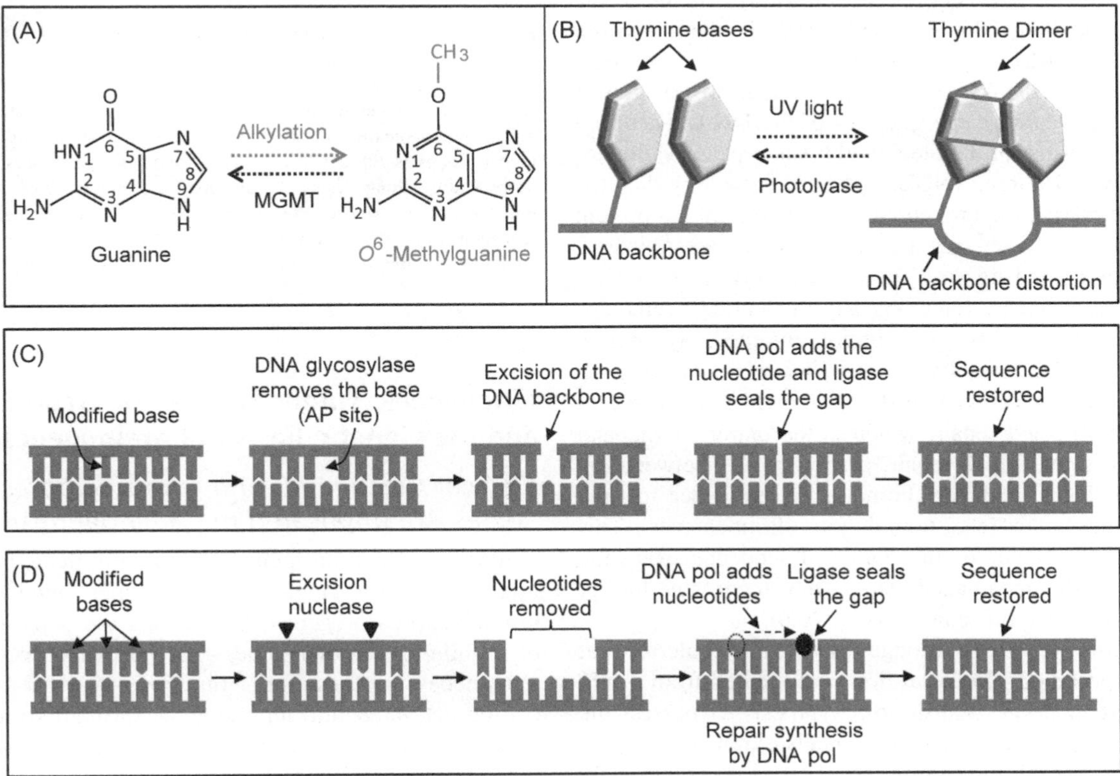

FIGURE 20.5 Three DNA repair mechanisms shown in the figure are: (A) direct repair, (B) base excision repair, and (C) nucleotide excision repair (see text for details). In humans, thymine dimers cannot be directly repaired because humans do not have photolyase.

protein complex, (2) unwinding of the DNA duplex around the damage, (3) dual incision of the damaged DNA strand to remove 30 or more nucleotides creating a gap, (4) gap repair synthesis by DNA polymerase, and (5) sealing of the gaps by ligase. The damage recognition in transcriptionally silent region versus transcriptionally active region requires different sets of proteins, but the subsequent steps are essentially identical (Fig. 20.5D).

The MMR mechanism repairs bases that violate Watson-Crick base pairing rules. The classic example is that of *Escherichia coli*. The sequence 5′-GATC-3′ in *E. coli* DNA is methylated at adenine, and the sequences 5′-CCAGG-3′ and 5′-CCTGG-3′ are methylated at cytosine. When DNA replicates, the daughter strand methylation is delayed. As a result, the newly synthesized daughter strand remains undermethylated for some time compared to the parental strand. If there is a base misincorporation, the MMR machinery (MutS-MutL-MutH protein complex) identifies the misincorporated base by scanning the methylation status of both strands. The mismatched base is excised from the undermethylated daughter strand.

DNA strand breaks are frequently caused by ionizing radiation and chemicals that generate free radicals. Single strand breaks do not disrupt the integrity of the DNA. The intact single strand is coated by Poly(ADP-ribose) polymerase-1 (PARP 1) protein near the lesion site of the other strand. The single strand break is then repaired using the excision repair mechanisms already described. Double strand breaks, on the other hand, are dangerous because they damage the integrity of the DNA. There are two mechanisms for double strand break repair; (1) nonhomologous end joining (NHEJ), and (2) homology-directed repair. In NHEJ, the broken ends are bound by Ku protein that recruits the necessary nucleases, polymerases, kinases, phosphatases, and ligases. The broken ends are enzymatically blunt-ended by removing any nucleotide overhangs, and the blunt ends are simply rejoined by ligase. Therefore, NHEJ results in the loss of some original sequence and may even lead to frameshift mutation. In homology-directed repair, which is the major mechanism of double strand break repair, pairing occurs between the damaged DNA and the homologous sequence of the undamaged duplex (e.g., homologous chromosomes). This results in the repair of the damaged sequence using the template of the undamaged DNA. Thus, there is no loss of original sequence information (Fig. 20.6).

Sometimes, a DNA damage lesion can be tolerated, at least temporarily, in order to first save the cell from death. During replication, translesion synthesis bypasses the damage and does not repair it; it is also known as bypass synthesis. The bypass can be error-free or error-prone. In the absence of translesion synthesis, a replication fork that is stalled for long would cause cell death.

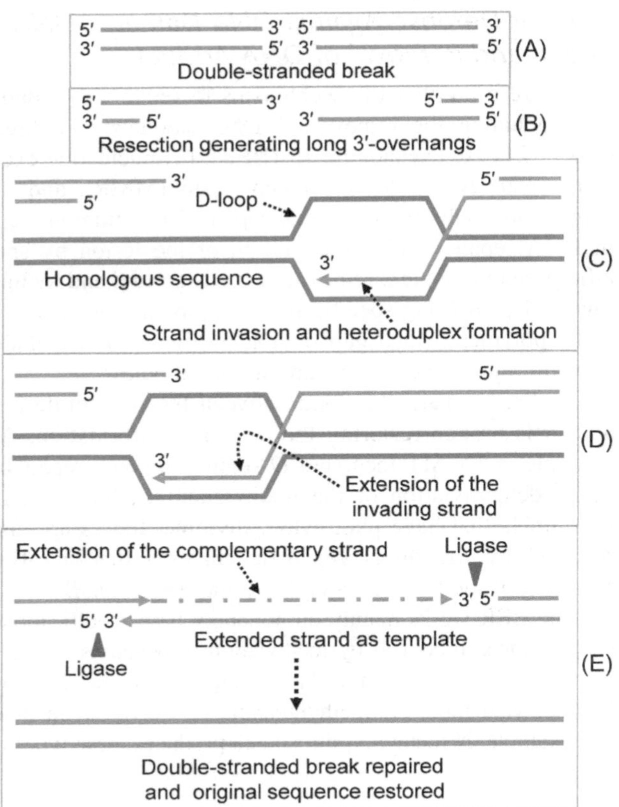

FIGURE 20.6 In homology-directed DNA repair using homologous chromosome, the 5′-end of each duplex fragment is resected to create a long single-stranded 3′-overhang (tail). This is followed by strand invasion to form a heteroduplex. In the heteroduplex one strand of the undamaged duplex becomes displaced and a three-stranded displacement loop (D-loop) is formed. As the DNA synthesis progresses the D-loop keeps sliding along. Using the undamaged template, DNA synthesis is initiated at the 3′-end of the invading strand. Newly synthesized DNA regenerates one strand, which is then used as a template to regenerate the complementary strand. As always, the gaps are sealed by ligase.

Oncogenes, Tumor Suppressor Genes, and the Genetic Basis of Carcinogenesis

Cellular Oncogenes and Tumor Suppressor Genes Are Implicated in Carcinogenesis

A number of cellular genes are now implicated in carcinogenesis. These genes are of two types; oncogenes and tumor suppressor genes. Oncogenes are activated form of cellular proto-oncogenes that normally encode proteins necessary for cellular functions. A proto-oncogene can be activated into an oncogene through structural or functional alterations. Broadly speaking, activation of oncogenes and inactivation of tumor suppressor genes may have similar consequences in terms of tumor development.

Activation of Oncogenes and Inactivation of Tumor Suppressor Genes are Intimately Associated With Tumor Development

Proto-oncogenes may be activated by mutation, chromosomal rearrangement (e.g., translocations and inversions), or gene amplification to become a cellular oncogene (*c-onc*). An example of cellular oncogenic activation through gene amplification is *Myc*, which codes for a transcription factor that plays a role in cell division. Generation of high amounts of *Myc* oncogene product can also be due to high levels of transcription without gene amplification. This has been reported in Burkitt's lymphoma where translocation of the *Myc* proto-oncogene from its normal location in chromosome 8 to chromosome 14 brings it close to the immunoglobulin heavy chain gene promoter. As a result, *c-Myc* now finds itself in a region of vigorous transcriptional activity, with a consequent overproduction of its product.

Another example of chromosomal translocation and cellular oncogenic activation is found in chronic myelogenous leukemia (CML). In CML, a reciprocal translocation occurs between chromosomes 9 and 22 [*t*(9;22)]. A portion on the long arm of chromosome 9 (9q) containing the *Abl* gene is translocated next to the *Bcr* gene on the long arm of chromosome 22 (22q). The altered chromosome 22 is called the Philadelphia chromosome (Ph′). The *Bcr-Abl* fusion gene produces higher levels of a fusion protein Bcr-Abl. The Abl portion of the fusion protein has constitutive protein tyrosine kinase activity, whereas the Bcr portion of the fusion protein can bind to many proteins. Binding of the Bcr-Abl fusion proteins with proteins involved in the mitogenic signaling pathway can cause activation of mitogenic signaling and increased cell proliferation.

Tumor suppressor genes, which also participate in the regulation of normal cell growth, are usually inactivated by point mutations or truncation of their protein sequence coupled with the loss of the normal allele. The first mutation may be inherited or somatic. The second mutation will often be a gross event leading to loss of heterozygosity and tumor suppressor function. This mechanism provides support to the two-hit hypothesis of Alfred Knudson, discussed earlier in the chapter. Frequent loss of heterozygosity in the tumor cells provides support to Knudson's hypothesis.

Oncogenes and Tumor Suppressor Genes Encode Protein Products That Are Involved in the Regulation of Growth and Survival of Cells as Well as Programmed Cell Death

Proto-oncogenes encode proteins that are involved in the regulation of cell growth as well as division and differentiation, such as growth factors, growth factor receptor-associated tyrosine kinases, membrane-associated nonreceptor tyrosine kinases, G-protein-coupled receptors, membrane-associated G-proteins, serine-threnine kinases, transcription factors, and regulators of programmed cell death. For example, *Sis*, *Int-2* encode growth factors; *Src*, *Abl*, *erbB* encode protein tyrosine kinases; Ras is a GTP-binding GTPase; and *Fos*, *Jun*, *Myc*, and *Myb* encode transcription factors. There are many other such examples. These proteins, when encoded by oncogenes, are called oncoproteins, which are either mutated or with unregulated expressions. In most cases, the oncogenes encode mutant forms of the proteins so that they are not subject to the on-off regulation in response to mitogenic signals. In other words, the mitogenic signal is perpetually "on," resulting in uncontrolled cell proliferation.

The cell growth and division suppressor effects are also lost in the mutant p53 gene; p53 is a tumor suppressor gene that encodes a transcription factor (p53 protein). The amino acids that are involved in DNA binding show the highest mutation rate in various cancers. This demonstrates how mutations in tumor suppressor genes can abrogate their tumor suppressor function by disrupting the transcriptional regulation of their target genes. Another role of p53 is to regulate apoptosis or programmed cell death by upregulating the proapoptotic gene Bax. Mutant p53 cannot mediate apoptosis; thus cells with unrepaired DNA damage are prevented from undergoing apoptosis. Survival of these cells and their subsequent division may lead to the development of tumor.

Viral Carcinogenesis

Viruses are implicated in approximately 15% of all cancers, such as nasopharyngeal carcinoma, T-cell leukemias, hepatocellular carcinoma, and Kaposi's sarcoma. Only a small proportion of people infected with any of the human tumor viruses develop tumors, and those that are infected rarely (if ever) serve as sources for ongoing transmission. Instead, most human tumor virus transmissions are asymptomatic or mildly symptomatic but do not lead to neoplasia (Butel, 2000; Moore and Chang, 2010). Oncogenes are found in both cancer-causing DNA viruses and RNA viruses. DNA viruses with oncogenic potential are from six distinct viral families: hepatitis B viruses, simian virus 40 (SV40) and polyomavirus, papillomaviruses, adenoviruses, herpesviruses, and poxviruses. In contrast, members of only one family of RNA viruses, the retroviruses, are capable of inducing oncogenic potential (Cooper, 1995). Papillomavirus, hepatitis B virus and Kaposi's sarcoma-associated herpes virus are the main DNA tumor viruses relevant in human cancer development. Like the tumorigenic DNA viruses, there are tumorigenic retroviruses. Whereas DNA tumor viruses encode oncogenes of viral origin that are essential for viral replication and cell transformation, transforming retroviruses carry oncogenes derived from cellular proto-oncogenes that are involved in mitogenic signaling and growth control (Butel, 2000).

The model for the acquisition of oncogenes by retroviruses from cellular proto-oncogenes was first provided by Takeya and Hanafusa (1983) from their work on the *c-Src* proto-oncogene. Cellular proto-oncogenes contain introns while the corresponding viral oncogenes lack introns. The retroviral oncogene capture model postulates that the *c-onc* sequence was captured by virus through recombination that occurred at the level of proviral DNA. Retroviruses replicate inside the cell through a DNA intermediate, called provirus, which is integrated into the chromosomal DNA of the infected cell. Chance integration of provirus next to the cellular proto-oncogene creates a viral-cellular fusion gene. Read-through transcription of this fusion gene creates a hybrid (viral + cellular) RNA. Processing of this read-through transcript removes the introns. When this hybrid RNA sequence undergoes recombination with the viral RNA during reverse-transcription, the cellular oncogene (without the introns) is captured by the viral genome. Fig. 20.7 shows how a cellular proto-oncogene (*c-onc*) could be acquired by the viral genome. The function of the *v-onc* products is similar or identical to that of the *c-onc* products, and the expression is generally unregulated.

Radiation Carcinogenesis

The Risk of Radiation-Induced Carcinogenesis Is Directly Related to the Amount of Energy Deposited Into the Tissue by Radiation

In the following discussion, radiation will refer only to ionizing radiation. A radiation dose to tissue is expressed as absorbed energy per unit tissue mass. The Gray (Gy) is the unit of radiation dose and is quantified as 1 joule/kg tissue. The older unit rad is still used and 1 rad = 0.01 Gy. Carcinogenic potential of radiation depends upon the absorbed dose (energy).

LET (linear energy transfer; L) is a measure of the rate at which energy (E) is deposited to the absorbing medium per unit distance (l) traversed by the radiation ($L = dE/dl$; if the distance traversed is measured in mm, then $L = \text{keV/mm}$). Consequently, high-LET radiations (e.g., α-particles; neutrons; heavy ions; pions, also known pi mesons) will deposit greater amounts of energy in the absorbing media than low-LET radiations (e.g., γ-rays;

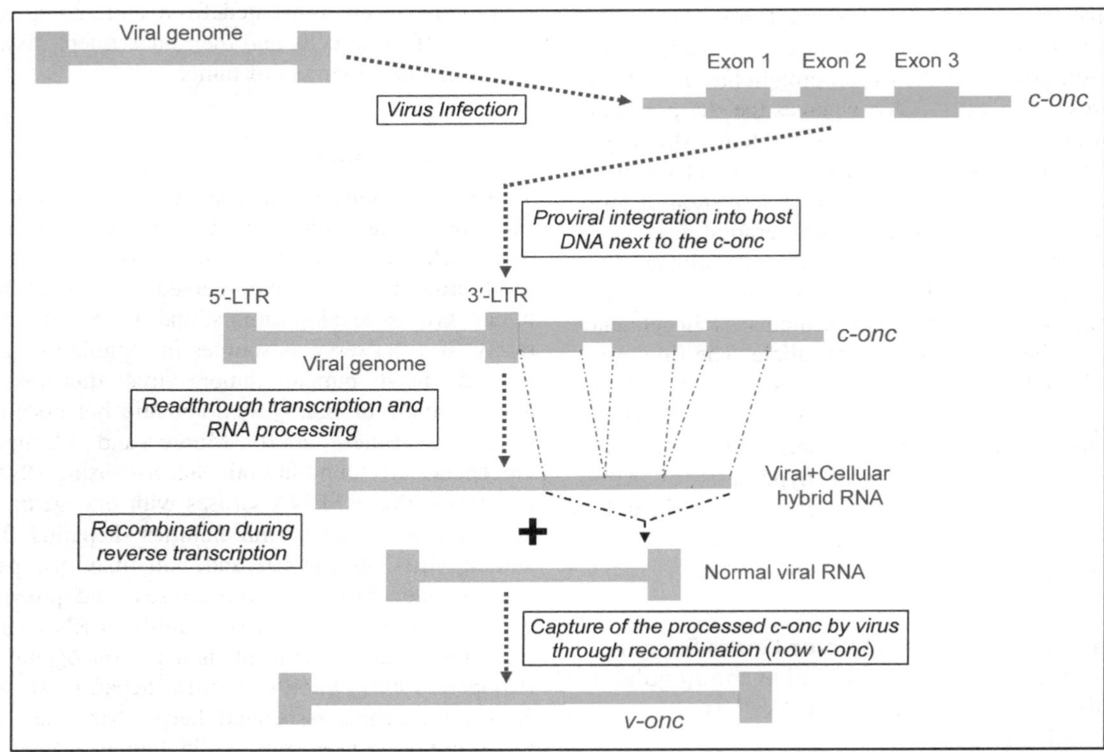

FIGURE 20.7 Mechanism by which a cellular proto-oncogene (*c-onc*) is captured by retrovirus to give rise to a viral oncogene (*v-onc*). It is triggered by proviral integration next to the cellular proto-oncogene creating a viral-cellular fusion gene. RNA processing following read-through transcription removes the introns from this hybrid (viral + cellular) RNA sequence. When this hybrid RNA sequence undergoes recombination with the viral RNA during reverse-transcription, the cellular oncogene is captured by the viral genome without the introns.

X-rays; electrons). Human skin can stop α-particles from penetrating and reaching the internal organs. This is because α-particles deposit most of their energy onto the skin and may damage the skin in that process, but are unable to penetrate any further. Both α- and β-particles penetrate cell membranes more easily than they penetrate human skin. Therefore, ingesting or inhaling radioactive chemicals that can emit α- or β-particles can pose serious threats to human health.

In the case of tissue exposure, the energy deposited by the radiation causes ionizations and the generation of free radicals, which cause macromolecular damage. Thus, high-LET radiations are more destructive to biological materials than low-LET radiations. At the same dose, low-LET radiations induce the same number of radicals more sparsely within a cell, whereas high-LET radiations transfer most of their energy to a small region of the cell. The localized DNA damage caused by dense ionizations from high-LET radiations is more difficult to repair than the diffuse DNA damage caused by the sparse ionizations from low-LET radiations.

Experimental studies with animals as well as epidemiological studies indicate that higher or continual radiation exposure increases the incidence of specific cancers, such as (1) increased incidence of lung cancer among uranium miners, fluorspar miners, zinc and iron ore miners (Adams and Cox, 1997); (2) increased occurrence of osteosarcoma among workers in luminous dial watch factories (workers licked the paint brush to maintain sharp edges and in the process consumed radium-226 and radium-228; the ingested radium deposited in the bone was the source of short range α-particles); (3) increased incidence of thyroid cancer after the Chernobyl incident (those who continued to live in the contaminated region and consumed locally produced milk for the 3 months after the accident, had about 85% of the radiation dose to their thyroid from iodine-131) (Stsjazhko et al., 1995). Following the Chernobyl incident, the incidence of thyroid cancer among children under 15 was 30.6 per million during 1991–94 as compared to 0.3 during 1981–85. Another source of human data on carcinogenesis by ionizing radiation is from the A-bomb survivors from Hiroshima and Nagasaki. Data show that in the first 5–10 years after the exposure, the risk of leukemia increased rapidly but declined thereafter. The risk of solid tumors in many organs also increased significantly (Okey et al., 1998).

The Mechanism of Radiation-Induced Carcinogenesis Involves Severe Macromolecular Damage and Genomic Instability

An absorbed dose of 1 Gy generates about 2×10^5 ionizations within the mammalian cell. Approximately 1% of these ionizations occur in the DNA itself (Adams and Cox, 1997). Ionizing radiation and oxidative stress are closely associated. Irradiated cells produce damaging reactive oxygen species (ROS), which can cause severe damage to cellular macromolecules including nuclear DNA (Spitz et al., 2004; Wu et al., 1999). A cell's oxidative status plays an important role not only at the time of radiation exposure, but also long after exposure. Irradiation may produce ROS for several minutes or even hours after exposure (Spitz et al., 2004).

At the cytological level, the extension of radiation-induced DNA damage is chromosome breakage, nondisjunction of homologous chromosomes, aberrant intrachromosomal crossing over, and scrambling of DNA sequences (Adams and Cox, 1997). Therefore, radiation can cause increased genomic instability and the extent of damage is dependent on the energy of the radiation. If an oncogene or a tumor suppressor gene is mutated or severely damaged by radiation, then radiation-induced damage may have serious consequences.

EPIGENETIC BASIS OF CARCINOGENESIS

The mechanisms of carcinogenesis discussed above mostly involve changes in DNA sequence and/or integrity. However, carcinogenesis has an important epigenetic component as well. As indicated above, nongenotoxic mechanism of carcinogenesis is epigenetic.

Epigenetic Changes During Carcinogenesis Have Been Widely Studied and Well Documented

Epigenetic regulation involves heritable changes in gene expression that are not accompanied by changes in DNA sequence. Three main mechanisms of epigenetic regulation of gene expression are mediated by: (1) DNA methylation, (2) histone modifications, and (3) RNA interference by small noncoding RNA, such as microRNA (miRNA). Epigenetic changes can collaborate with genetic changes to cause the evolution of a cancer because they are mitotically heritable (Jones and Baylin, 2007).

Studies over the last 30 years or so have confirmed that the genome in a cancer cell is characterized by genome-wide hypomethylation and site-specific promoter hypermethylation. Many of these epigenetic changes probably occur very early in cancer development and may contribute to cancer initiation (Jones and Baylin, 2007; Sharma et al., 2010).

Global DNA hypomethylation basically has two effects: it increases genomic instability and activates genes including growth promoting genes. Hypomethylation affects repeat sequences, leading to increased genomic instability by promoting chromosomal rearrangements. Additionally, hypomethylation of retrotransposons can result in their activation and translocation to other genomic regions, thus increasing genomic instability. DNA hypomethylation can activate growth promoting genes (proto-oncogenes), thereby inappropriately turning on mitogenic signals. DNA hypomethylation can also lead to the loss of genomic imprinting. In contrast, site-specific hypermethylation can contribute to tumorigenesis by silencing tumor suppressor genes (Sharma et al., 2010).

Silencing of gene expression in carcinogenesis also involves global loss of transcription-activating histone modifications, such as acetylation and activating methylation. All known histone acetylations are transcription-activating. In contrast, certain histone methylations are transcription-activating, such as histone H4 lysine 20 methylation, whereas others are transcription-repressing, such as histone H3 lysine 9 and lysine 27 methylation. Loss of histone acetylation is carried out by histone deacetylase (HDAC), which is often overexpressed in various types of cancer (Sharma et al., 2010). In addition to the loss of transcription-activating modifications, cancer cells also have active transcriptional silencing modifications as well, such as histone H3 lysine 9 and lysine 27 methylation.

The third arm of epigenetic regulation, the RNA interference caused by miRNA, also shows widespread dysregulation of expression in carcinogenesis. Because miRNAs are involved in transcriptional regulation, cell proliferation and apoptosis, dysregulation in their expression can promote tumorigenesis. Oncogenic miRNAs (oncomirs) target tumor suppressors and growth inhibitory pathways and are often up-regulated in various types of cancer. Examples of oncomirs are miR-21 (targets the tumor suppressor "phosphatase and tensin homolog deleted on chromosome 10" (PTEN)), which is upregulated in human glioblastoma; miR-155, which is upregulated in breast, lung and several hematopoietic malignancies; miR-17-92 cluster, which targets the proapoptotic gene *Bim* and is overexpressed in many different types of cancers. In contrast to oncomirs, tumor suppressor miRNAs target oncogenes and growth promoting pathways, and are often down-regulated in cancers. For example, miR-15 and miR-16 target the antiapoptotic gene *BCL2* and are down-regulated in chronic lymphocytic leukemia; miR-127 targets BCL6 and is down-regulated in prostate and bladder tumors (Sharma et al., 2010).

Clearly, the normal cellular epigenetic landscape is significantly altered in cancer. The underlying mechanisms that initiate these global changes are not fully understood, and neither are the causative versus correlative nature of the changes observed. Nevertheless, recent studies indicate that some changes occur very early in cancer development and may contribute to cancer initiation (Jones and Baylin, 2007; Sharma et al., 2010).

CLASSIFICATION OF CARCINOGENS

The most widely used system for classifying carcinogens comes from the International Agency for Research on Cancer (IARC). The US Environmental Protection Agency (EPA) has also developed a very similar classification scheme. In the past 30 years, IARC has evaluated nearly 1000 chemicals for their cancer-causing potential in humans. Most of the chemicals that IARC evaluated are classified as probably or possibly carcinogenic or not classifiable. About 12% are classified as carcinogenic to humans. The IARC classification scheme is described in Table 20.5.

ASSAYS FOR CARCINOGENS

Tests most frequently used to determine the carcinogenic potential include (1) long term rodent cancer bioassays and (2) short term assays.

TABLE 20.5 IARC Classification of Human Carcinogens

Carcinogen Classification	Explanation
Group 1 *Known* human carcinogen	Sufficient evidence of carcinogenicity in humans
Group 2A *Probable* human carcinogen	Limited evidence of carcinogenicity in humans; sufficient evidence in experimental animals, and strong evidence that carcinogenesis in experimental animals is mediated by a mechanism that also operates in humans
Group 2B *Possible* human carcinogen	Limited evidence of carcinogenicity in humans, and less than sufficient evidence of carcinogenicity in experimental animals
Group 3 *Not classifiable* for human carcinogenicity	The evidence of carcinogenicity is inadequate or limited in experimental animals
Group 4 *Not likely* to be a human carcinogen	Not carcinogenic to humans

TABLE 20.6 Genotoxicity, Mutagenicity, and Carcinogenicity Tests

Test	In Vitro/In Vivo	Endpoint/Brief Description
Bacterial reverse mutation assay (Ames assay)	In vitro mutagenicity	Gene mutation detection
Mammalian cell gene mutation assay (mouse lymphoma assay)	In vitro mutagenicity	Gene mutation detection
Mammalian chromosome aberration test	In vitro genotoxicity	Chromosome aberration detection
Sister chromatid exchange assay in mammalian cells	In vitro genotoxicity	Mammalian DNA damage detection
Unscheduled DNA synthesis in mammalian cells	In vitro *genotoxicity*	Mammalian DNA damage detection
Comet assay	In vitro *genotoxicity*	Eukaryotic cell DNA damage detection
Mammalian cell micronucleus assay	In vitro genotoxicity	Detection of damage to chromosomes or mitotic apparatus
Bone marrow micronucleus assay	In vivo genotoxicity	Detection of damage to chromosomes or mitotic apparatus
Structure-activity relationship	In silico prediction	Predicts the mutagenic, genotoxic and carcinogenic potential of a compound based on its structural similarity with other compounds that are known to be mutagenic, genotoxic or carcinogenic
Bioassay in rats and mice	In vivo carcinogenicity	• Long term (2 years) • Highest dose: MTD (maximum tolerated dose) or MFD (maximum feasible dose) • Route: Depending on the route of exposure in humans • Expensive
Bioassay in transgenic mice	In vivo carcinogenicity	• Can be short term (6 months) • Some models are: Tg.rasH2, p53$^{+/-}$, Tg.AC, XPA$^{-/-}$, K6/ODC
Cell transformation assay	In vitro carcinogenicity	• Induction of phenotypic changes in cultured cells, usually Syrian hamster embryo (SHE) cells or BALBc/3T3 cells • Changes are characteristic of tumor cells (from "normal" to neoplastic state), such as morphologically transformed colonies that are characterized by aberrant growth patterns, compared to controls

The long term (2-year) rodent bioassay is still the accepted standard in evaluating the carcinogenic potential of a compound, despite some shortcomings of the assay. For example, these assays are expensive and the dose range includes the maximum tolerated dose, which is high enough to potentially cause cellular injury. Compensatory and repetitive cell proliferation in response to the injury could trigger uncontrolled cell proliferation. One alternative to the 2-year bioassay is the 6-month study in transgenic mice. The short term assays represent alternatives to major animal testing and are used to determine a chemical's ability to cause mutational events, chromosomal aberrations, or DNA damage in vitro or in vivo. Positive results in one or more of these short term tests may suggest the carcinogenic potential. Table 20.6 lists some of these assays.

CONCLUDING REMARKS AND FUTURE DIRECTIONS

After more than four decades since President Nixon declared the "War on Cancer" with the enactment of the National Cancer Act in 1971, the war continues. Routine checkups have been effective in the early diagnosis and cure of certain forms of cancer, such as colon cancer, and breast cancer. Inventions in modern medicine have further added to better prognosis. Nevertheless, cancer largely remains an incurable disease unless it is detected early.

In spite of significant advances in our knowledge of the molecular mechanisms of carcinogenesis, scientists still have a long way to go before all these advances in knowledge could be translated into effective and curative therapy. In the meantime, more work is needed to understand the biological and molecular underpinnings of carcinogenesis. Nevertheless, the accumulated knowledge on various aspects of carcinogenesis has definitely helped scientists conduct appropriate risk assessment that lead to health policy recommendations. One arena of risk assessment that is still under development is the extent to which a threshold can be determined for a genotoxic carcinogen. Finally, recent progress in the science of genomics has provided scientists and clinicians alike with renewed hope that further breakthroughs in understanding carcinogenesis and cancer detection will lead to new therapies that will allow us to effectively control the disease.

REFERENCES

Adams, G.E., Cox, R., 1997. Radiation carcinogenesis. In: Franks, L.M., Teich, N.M. (Eds.), Cellular and Molecular Biology of Cancer, third ed. Oxford University Press, Oxford, pp. 130–150.

Armitage, P., Doll, R., 1954. The age distribution of cancer and a multi-stage theory of carcinogenesis. Br. J. Cancer. 8, 1–12.

Becker, K., Gregel, C., Fricke, C., Komitowski, D., Dosch, J., Kaina, B., 2003. DNA repair protein MGMT protects against *N*-methyl-*N*-nitrosourea-induced conversion of benign into malignant tumors. Carcinogenesis. 24, 541–546.

Benigni, R., Bossa, C., Tcheremenskaia, O., 2013. Nongenotoxic carcinogenicity of chemicals: mechanisms of action and early recognition through a new set of structural alerts. Chem. Rev. 113, 2940–2957.

Berenblum, I., Shubik, P., 1947. A new, quantitative, approach to the study of the stages of chemical carcinogenesis in the mouse's skin. Br. J. Cancer. 1, 383–391.

Butel, J.S., 2000. Viral carcinogenesis: revelation of molecular mechanisms and etiology of human disease. Carcinogenesis. 21, 405–426.

Choudhuri, S., Arvidson, K., Chanderbhan, R., 2012. Carcinogenesis: mechanisms and models. In: Gupta, R.C. (Ed.), Veterinary Toxicology, second ed. Academic Press, Oxford, pp. 406–425.

Cooper, G.M., 1995. Oncogenes. second ed. Jones and Bartlett, Boston, MA.

Dipple, A., 1995. DNA adducts of chemical carcinogens. Carcinogenesis. 16, 437–441.

Foulds, L., 1954. The experimental study of tumor progression: a review. Cancer Res. 14, 327–339.

Irigaray, P., Belpomme, D., 2010. Basic properties and molecular mechanisms of exogenous chemical carcinogens. Carcinogenesis. 31, 135–148.

Jones, P.A., Baylin, S.B., 2007. The epigenomics of cancer. Cell. 128, 683–692.

Knudson Jr., A.G., 1971. Mutation and cancer: statistical study of retinoblastoma. Proc. Natl. Acad. Sci. USA. 68, 820–823.

Lee, S.J., Yum, Y.N., Kim, S.C., Kim, Y., Lim, J., et al., 2013. Distinguishing between genotoxic and non-genotoxic hepatocarcinogens by gene expression profiling and bioinformatic pathway analysis. Sci. Rep. 3, 2783.

Marquardt, H., 1999. Chemical carcinogenesis. In: Marquardt, H., Schäfer, S.G., McClellan, R.O., Welsch, F. (Eds.), Toxicology. Academic Press, San Diego, CA, pp. 151–178.

Moore, P.S., Chang, Y., 2010. Why do viruses cause cancer? Highlights of the first century of human tumor virology. Nat. Rev. Cancer. 10, 878–889.

Nordling, C.O., 1953. A new theory on cancer-inducing mechanism. Br. J. Cancer. 7, 68–72.

Okey, A.B., Harper, P.A., Grant, D.M., Hill, R.P., 1998. Chemical and radiation carcinogenesis. In: Tannock, I.F., Hill, R.P. (Eds.), The Basic Science of Oncology, third ed. McGraw-Hill, New York, pp. 166–196.

Pitot, H.C., 2002. Fundamentals of Oncology. fourth ed. Marcel and Dekker, Inc., New York.

Pogribny, I.P., Rusyn, I., Beland, F.A., 2008. Epigenetic aspects of genotoxic and non-genotoxic hepatocarcinogenesis: studies in rodents. Environ. Mol. Mutagen. 49, 9–15.

Qin, X., Zhang, S., Matsukuma, S., Zarkovic, M., Shimizu, S., Ishikawa, T., et al., 2000. Protection against malignant progression of spontaneously developing liver tumors in transgenic mice expressing O^6-methylguanine-DNA methyltransferase. Jpn. J. Cancer Res. 91, 1085–1089.

Sharma, S., Kelly, T.K., Jones, P.A., 2010. Epigenetics in cancer. Carcinogenesis. 31, 27–36.

Smela, M.E., Currier, S.S., Bailey, E.A., Essigmann, J.M., 2001. The chemistry and biology of aflatoxin B(1): from mutational spectrometry to carcinogenesis. Carcinogenesis. 22, 535–545.

Spitz, D.R., Azzam, E.I., Li, J.J., Gius, D., 2004. Metabolic oxidation/reduction reactions and cellular responses to ionizing radiation: a unifying concept in stress response biology. Cancer Metas. Rev. 23, 311–322.

Stsjazhko, V.A., Tsyb, A.F., Tronko, N.D., Souchkevitch, G., Baverstock, K.F., 1995. Childhood thyroid cancer since accident at Chernobyl. Br.Med. J. 310, 801.

Takeya, T., Hanafusa, H., 1983. Structure and sequence of the cellular gene homologous to the RSV *src* gene and the mechanism for generating the transforming virus. Cell. 32, 881–890.

Tennant, R., 1999. What is a tumor promoter? Environ. Hlth. Perspec. 107, A390–A391.

Trosko, J.E., Upham, B.L., 2005. The emperor wears no clothes in the field of carcinogen risk assessment: ignored concepts in cancer risk assessment. Mutagenesis. 20, 81–92.

Wu, L.J., Randers-Pehrson, G., Xu, A., Waldren, C.A., Geard, C.R., Yu, Z., et al., 1999. Targeted Cytoplasmic Irradiation with Alpha Particles Induces Mutations in Mammalian Cells. Proc. Natl. Acad. Sci. USA. 96, 4959–4964.

Section IV

Drugs of Use and Abuse

Chapter 21

Toxicity of Over-the-Counter Drugs

Karyn Bischoff

INTRODUCTION

The topic of over-the-counter (OTC) drugs is complicated, encompassing a large number of products, many containing multiple active ingredients. Products are available for oral, topical, intraocular, intranasal, and intrarectal administration, although most veterinary exposures are through ingestion. These products are readily available in many homes. Toxicosis can result when animals are medicated by well-intentioned animal owners or even veterinarians, or accidental exposure, in which case, the amount of medication ingested may not be known. Response to a given drug may be species-specific or different between individuals of the same species. Idiosyncratic and allergic reactions to drugs must also be considered, although reports in domestic animals are rare (Papich, 1990; Brumbaugh, 2001; Meani and Nixon, 2015; Stewart et al., 2016).

Approximately one-quarter of the calls to human poison control centers in 1990 dealt with OTC drugs (Murphy, 1994; Villar et al., 1998). More than 16% of calls to the American Society for the Prevention of Cruelty to Animals' Animal Poison Control Center (ASPCA-NAPCC) in 2016 were for OTC medications (http://aspcapro.org/resource/shelter-health-poison-control/top-10-toxins-2016). It is estimated that there are more than 300,000 OTC drug formulations available, with approximately 700 active ingredients in various combinations (Papich, 1990); only a small fraction will be addressed in this chapter.

Important classes of drugs that will be addressed include analgesics, cold, flu, and allergy medications, and drugs used to treat gastrointestinal symptoms. Nutritional supplements, for the most part, will not be addressed here, although a few herbal preparations (ma huang and guarana) are discussed. Supplements containing cyanobacteria (blue-green algae) have been associated with microcystin toxicosis in dogs, which is addressed elsewhere in this text (Bautista et al., 2015). There have been several reports of joint supplement overdose associated with acute liver failure in dogs, likely due to the hypermanganesemia (Khan et al., 2010; Borchers et al., 2014). Toxicologically important minerals, such as iron, and important vitamins, such as vitamin D, are addressed in other chapters. Stimulants and diet pills often contain methylxanthines, such as caffeine, which are also addressed in appropriate chapters, or sympathomimetic amines, which are discussed later with decongestants.

SUSPECTED OTC DRUG REACTIONS

Obtaining a thorough history is of great importance when dealing with suspect OTC drug-related problems (Talcott, 2006). Animal owners do not always volunteer critical information. Well-intentioned pet owners sometimes administer OTC drugs to treat perceived symptoms in their pets (Papich, 1990; Jones et al., 1992; Villar et al., 1998; Roder, 2004a; Sellon, 2006). Veterinarians sometimes share the blame for inappropriate dosing. Chronic analgesic administration to treat orthopedic problems is a particular hazard in many species of domestic animals.

Accidental ingestions can occur when drugs are improperly stored. Careful assessment of the history can be challenging, but is critical, and unexpected circumstances can arise. For example, severe clinical signs prompted euthanasia in a kitten that was later discovered to have been playing with an empty acetaminophen tablet container (Allen, 2003). In another example, appropriate treatment was delayed when an owner failed to report ingestion of analgesics containing acetaminophen and codeine upon presenting their puppy to the veterinarian for anxious behavior and cyanosis (Stewart et al., 2016).

If an adverse reaction to an OTC drug is suspected, administration of the drug should be immediately discontinued. The owner should be instructed to bring the drug container to the veterinarian as a source of information on the active ingredients, indications for use, and manufacturer identification, telephone number, and address. Many manufacturers have information on treatment and prognosis, and, in the United States, will use the

Veterinary Toxicology. DOI: http://dx.doi.org/10.1016/B978-0-12-811410-0.00021-0

information you provide for adverse events reporting to the Food and Drug Administration (FDA). More information on adverse event reporting can be found at the FDA website: http://www.fda.gov/cvm/adetoc.htm. Any material remaining in the container can be analyzed to verify that the contents are as expected (Brumbaugh, 2001). Serum, urine, vomitus, and gastric lavage (liver, kidney, and GI content for postmortem) should also be saved for analysis if it is unclear what the animal has ingested. Early gastrointestinal decontamination is sometimes helpful in the asymptomatic animal, and can involve emetics or gastric lavage and instillation of activated charcoal and cathartics depending on the situation. If drugs are used topically, removal with a mild detergent bath is usually beneficial. Careful monitoring and maintenance of body temperature is required after bathing, and bath towels may be warmed by tumbling in a heated clothes dryer to help prevent hypothermia.

ANALGESICS

According to Jones et al. (1992), about 5% of dog- and cat-related calls to one poison control center were in response to analgesic ingestion; nearly 80% involved dogs. Analgesics are listed every year on the ASPCA Animal Poison Control Center and the Pet Poison Helpline's websites among the most common causes of poisonings in domestic animals. Commonly used OTC analgesics include acetaminophen and nonsteroidal antiinflammatory drugs (NSAIDs), such as aspirin, ibuprofen, naproxen, and ketoprofen. Aspirin shares many properties with other NSAIDs, but will be addressed separately due to some of its unique features.

Acetaminophen

Acetaminophen is an analgesic and antipyretic, although it does not have the antiinflammatory properties of NSAIDS (Hjelle and Grauer, 1986). Acetaminophen is a metabolite of the historic drug phenacetin. Acetaminophen is found in a variety of OTC pain relievers, and is often combined with other drugs in cold, flu, and allergy medications (Roder, 2004a). Common brand names in the United States include Tylenol and Anacin-3. Acetaminophen is sold under the name Paracetamol in Australia and Great Britain. Overdose is a common cause of morbidity in humans, with almost 80,000 hospital emergency room visits per year due to acetaminophen hepatotoxicosis. Acetaminophen toxicosis in domestic animals is most commonly reported in cats (Rumbeiha et al., 1995). Clinical acetaminophen toxicosis is usually associated with a single exposure, although adverse effects as a result of multiple dosing have been reported (Hjelle and Grauer, 1986; Villar et al., 1998). The most common clinical situation results from the owner medicating their animal without the benefit of a veterinarian's advice and supervision (Hjelle and Grauer, 1986; Aronson and Drobatz, 1996). One report documents severe poisoning in a kitten that had played with an empty acetaminophen tablet container (Allen, 2003). Although the hepatotoxic effects of acetaminophen have been described in many species, the hematotoxic effects have only been documented in cats and dogs (McConkey et al., 2009).

Toxicity

Individual differences in sensitivity are reported within and across species (Webb et al., 2003), but the use of acetaminophen is always contraindicated in cats due to their extreme sensitivity (Jones et al., 1992; Roder, 2004a; Villar et al., 1998; Wallace et al., 2002). Clinical signs of acetaminophen toxicosis, up to and including death, have been reported in cats at doses of 10 mg/kg (Aronson and Drobatz, 1996); however, most poisonings are associated with doses of 50 mg/kg and greater (Murphy, 1994; Allen, 2003; MacNaughton, 2003; Roder, 2004a; Sellon, 2006). Villar et al. (1998) reported 50% methemoglobinemia within 4 h in cats dosed with 120–140 mg/kg acetaminophen. One of four cats dosed with 143 mg/kg died. One regular acetaminophen tablet contains 352 mg of the active ingredient, and an extra-strength tablet contains 500 mg.

The recommended oral dose for acetaminophen in dogs is 15 mg/kg every 8 h, or 10 mg/kg every 12 h for long-term dosing (Plumb, 2015). Toxicosis has been reported at a dose of 46 mg/kg (Sellon, 2006), although doses of 100 mg/kg or greater are more likely to be associated with clinical signs (Jones et al., 1992; Boothe, 2001; Roder, 2004a). Most dogs dosed with less than 460 mg/kg will recover (Villar et al., 1998). Doses over 460 mg/kg in dogs are associated with methemoglobinemia, and deaths have occurred (Schlesinger, 1995; Villar et al., 1998; Wallace et al., 2002); a dose of 900 mg/kg caused "fulminant liver failure" (Boothe, 2001). Doses greater than 1 g/kg (1000 mg/kg) are reported to cause unconsciousness and cyanosis within hours and death within 12 h (Villar et al., 1998).

Toxicokinetics

After ingestion, acetaminophen is rapidly absorbed in the stomach and small intestine (Schlesinger, 1995; Wallace et al., 2002). Peak plasma concentrations occur 4 h after ingestion in cats (Rumbeiha et al., 1995). Circulating acetaminophen is minimally bound to plasma protein and widely distributed. The therapeutic plasma concentration of acetaminophen in a dog is near 30 μg/mL, and toxicosis is associated with concentrations of 300 μg/mL and greater.

Metabolism of acetaminophen occurs primarily in the liver. There are three major pathways: direct glucuronide conjugation, direct sulfate conjugation, and oxidation mediated by cytochrome P450 enzymes (Hjelle and Grauer, 1986; Wallace et al., 2002). Acetaminophen has an available hydroxyl group. Immediate phase II conjugation is the primary route of metabolism in most species, and involves glucuronide and sulfate (Dahm and Jones, 1996). Due to limitations of cat physiology, they have only about one-tenth the acetaminophen biotransformation ability of dogs (Hjelle and Grauer, 1986; Sellon, 2006). Glucuronide conjugation is the fate of 50%–60% of a dose of acetaminophen given to either a human or dog (Aronson and Drobatz, 1996); this pathway is deficient in cats due to decreased microsomal UDP-glucuronosyltransferase enzyme activity (Wallace et al., 2002).

The amount of acetaminophen that is conjugated to glucuronide in cats is dependent upon dose, but is always a relatively small proportion. After an oral dose of 20, 60, and 120 mg/kg acetaminophen, only 1%, 5%, and 16% undergo glucuronide conjugation, respectively (Hjelle and Grauer, 1986). Sulfate conjugation is less important than glucuronide conjugation in the disposition of acetaminophen in most species aside from cats (Aronson and Drobatz, 1996; Boothe, 2001; Allen, 2003). Dogs metabolize only about 10%–20% of a given dose of acetaminophen via sulfate conjugation. Again, use of this pathway is dependent upon the dose of acetaminophen. After cats were dosed with 20 mg, 60 mg, and 120 mg acetaminophen/kg, 92%, 78%, and 57% of the acetaminophen underwent sulfate conjugation, respectively. The sulfate conjugation pathway can be saturated due to the limited availability of inorganic sulfates (Hjelle and Grauer, 1986).

Metabolism of acetaminophen by phase I processes is relatively minimal in most species, but is very important to the mechanism of toxicity of this drug, as will be described later. Cytochrome P450 oxidation increases as phase II pathways become saturated (MacNaughton, 2003; Sellon, 2006). Approximately 5% of a dose of acetaminophen undergoes oxidation by cytochrome P450s in dogs. When cats are dosed with 20 mg/kg acetaminophen, 5% undergoes oxidation, but this number increased to 10% at doses of 60–120 mg/kg (Hjelle and Grauer, 1986). The product of the oxidation pathway is *N*-acetyl benzoquinoneimine (NAPQI). NAPQI is conjugated to reduced glutathione (GSH), forming an inactive product. A second byproduct of acetaminophen metabolism, via phase I deacetylation, is para-aminophenol (PAP), which is of importance to the mechanism of toxicity in dogs and cats. PAP is rapidly conjugated to GSH or acetate in laboratory rodents, but cats have reduced capacity for *N*-acetylation and dogs lack the hepatic *N*-acetyltransferase enzyme (McConkey et al., 2009).

The byproducts of acetaminophen metabolism are excreted predominantly through the urine (MacNaughton, 2003; Sellon, 2006; Sturgill and Lambert, 1997). Less than 5% of a dose is excreted as the parent compound in humans (Wallace et al., 2002), and some conjugates are eliminated in the bile (Sturgill and Lambert, 1997; Maddrey, 2005). The rate of elimination is dependent upon the species and the dose. The elimination half-life of a 100–200 mg/kg dose of acetaminophen is 72 min in dogs, and increases to 210 min when the dose is increased to 500 mg/kg. The elimination half-life in cats for a 20 mg/kg, dose is 36 min, but increases to 144 min and 288 min for a 60 mg/kg and a 120 mg/kg dose, respectively (Hjelle and Grauer, 1986). The half-life is longer in male cats compared to females (Rumbeiha et al., 1995).

Mechanism of Action

Unlike NSAIDs, the therapeutic effects of acetaminophen are independent of cyclooxygenase (COX), and are based on interference with endoperoxidase (Boothe, 2001). A new isoenzyme of COX, however, COX3, has been identified in dogs, and is reported to be a target of acetaminophen. COX3 could be responsible for decreased tear production in acetaminophen-induced keratoconjunctivitis sicca (Stewart et al., 2016). The main target organ for acetaminophen in most species is the liver. The hepatotoxic effects of acetaminophen are due primarily to the metabolite NAPQI. Large doses of acetaminophen overwhelm the sulfide and glucuronide conjugation pathways and lead to increased formation of active metabolite (Hjelle and Grauer, 1986; Dahm and Jones, 1996; Sturgill and Lambert, 1997; MacNaughton, 2003; Roder, 2004a). NAPQI is usually conjugated with GSH, as noted above. GSH stores become depleted 16–24 h after exposure to acetaminophen.

Hepatotoxic effects predominate in dogs, mice, rats, and humans, and occur in dogs and cats (Wallace et al., 2002; Sellon, 2006). Oxidative damage to hepatocytes leads to zone 3 (centrilobular) hepatocyte degeneration and necrosis (Hjelle and Grauer, 1986; Dahm and Jones, 1996; Treinen-Moslen, 2001; Wallace et al., 2002). NAPQI acts as an electrophile, causing tissue damage through formation of covalent adducts with biological macromolecules (Savides and Oehme, 1985; Hjelle and Grauer, 1986; Jones et al., 1992; Dahm and Jones, 1996; Sturgill and Lambert, 1997; Villar et al., 1998; Zimmerman, 1999; Treinen-Moslen, 2001). NAPQI interacts with cysteine residues on mitochondrial proteins, leading to mitochondrial dysfunction and adenosine triphosphate (ATP) depletion (Khayyat et al., 2016). NAPQI is also believed to bind to membrane proteins that regulate calcium homeostasis, thus increasing intracellular calcium concentrations. Cytoskeletal damage/activation of endonucleases and DNA fragmentation are proposed causes of cell death. Production of superoxide anions causing peroxidative injury occur during phase I metabolism of acetaminophen, causing oxidative stress in the cell, especially once glutathione has been depleted. Endothelial damage is the likely cause of clinical signs such as edema of the face and extremities and hemorrhage.

PAP, another reactive metabolite, is implicated in the hematotoxic effect seen in cats and dogs (McConkey et al., 2009). Unlike most species, erythrocyte injury is a major adverse effect associated with acetaminophen ingestion in cats. It is also observed in dogs at high doses, although hepatotoxic effects predominate at relatively low doses in dogs. Oxidative injury to the erythrocyte takes the form of methemoglobin production or Heinz body production (Rumbeiha et al., 1995; Webb et al., 2003; McConkey et al., 2009). GSH becomes depleted in erythrocytes, and hemoglobin is oxidized to methemoglobin, which cannot carry oxygen (Hjelle and Grauer, 1986; Aronson and Drobatz, 1996). Animals with 30% of their hemoglobin converted to methemoglobin show clinical signs and cyanosis (Rumbeiha et al., 1995). Methemoglobinemia is reversible through conversion back to hemoglobin by methemoglobin reductase (Schlesinger, 1995). Cats have less methemoglobin reductase activity than other domestic species (MacNaughton, 2003). Acetaminophen can produce methemoglobinemia in dogs as well, but this change has not been reported in other species (Hjelle and Grauer, 1986; McConkey et al., 2009).

Heinz body formation is an irreversible change caused by the precipitation of hemoglobin (Schlesinger, 1995; Aronson and Drobatz, 1996). Heinz bodies increase red cell fragility and decrease survival time of erythrocytes, and thus, may cause hemolysis and anemia. Until recently, it was believed that NAPQI bound to the sulfhydryl groups and oxidized hemoglobin (Allen, 2003). However, erythrocytes lack the enzymes to metabolize acetaminophen to NAPQI, and circulating NAPQI is unlikely to be bioavailable to erythrocytes. Another reactive metabolite, PAP, was found to oxidize hemoglobin in vitro, and thus, has recently been proposed as the cause of methemoglobinemia in cats and dogs (McConkey et al., 2009). There are eight sulfhydryl groups on feline hemoglobin, but only four on the hemoglobin of other domestic species and two on the human molecule, making cat erythrocytes much more prone to oxidative injury (Hjelle and Grauer, 1986; Rumbeiha et al., 1995; Aronson and Drobatz, 1996; Allen, 2003; Sellon, 2006).

Factors that enhance the toxic effects of acetaminophen include glutathione depletion due to fasting (Treinen-Moslen, 2001) and induction of P4502E1, as occurs with barbiturate exposure (Sturgill and Lambert, 1997). Cimetidine inhibits cytochrome P450s, and has been used therapeutically for acetaminophen toxicosis. Young animals are sometimes less sensitive to acetaminophen toxicosis than mature animals. This is the case in children and neonatal mice, and is believed to be due to the immaturity of the mixed-function oxidase system and more rapid glutathione synthesis in these youngsters (MacNaughton, 2003).

Clinical Signs

Clinical signs of acetaminophen toxicosis in cats and dogs are attributable to its toxic effects on erythrocytes and hepatocytes. Clinical methemoglobinemia is the most common problem in cats, and can also occur in dogs. Centrilobular hepatic necrosis is most common in dogs, also occurring in other species, including cats, humans, rats, and hamsters (Hjelle and Grauer, 1986).

Clinical signs in cats usually occur within a couple of hours of exposure. Anorexia and vomiting are reported in 35% of cats presenting for acetaminophen exposure, and hypersalivation is reported in 24% (Aronson and Drobatz, 1996), and commonly occurs within 2 h of exposure (Savides and Oehme, 1985). Diarrhea occurred in 18% of cats. Mental depression is reported in 76%, and usually takes place within 3 h.

Methemoglobinemia occurs within the 4 h of acetaminophen ingestion in cats, and is dose-dependent. Cats given a dose of 60 mg/kg acetaminophen had 21.7% of their hemoglobin converted to methemoglobin, and the methemoglobin concentration in cats dosed with 120 mg/kg acetaminophen was 45.5% (Hjelle and Grauer, 1986). Clinically evident cyanosis occurs at about 30% methemoglobinemia. Fifty-nine percent of the cats in the Aronson and Drobatz (1996) study had pale or dark mucous membranes and respiratory distress, and the blood was brown in 12%. Affected cats were weak and depressed (Hjelle and Grauer, 1986; Jones et al., 1992; Allen, 2003), 12% presented comatose, and 18% tachycardic (Aronson and Drobatz, 1996). Hemolysis, anemia, icterus, and pigmenturia have been described, and are seen within 48 h of exposure. In addition to characteristic methemoglobinemia, edema of the face and forelimbs or front paws is commonly described in affected cats. Death in cats is usually due to methemoglobinemia, but fatal liver failure can also occur. Hepatic necrosis is most commonly associated with high-dose exposures, particularly in male cats.

Dogs often vomit soon after ingesting a high dose of acetaminophen, which can serve a protective function (Schlesinger, 1995). Severe clinical signs in dogs are usually attributable to hepatic necrosis (Hjelle and Grauer, 1986; Schlesinger, 1995; Sellon, 2006). Signs commence within 36 h of ingestion, and include nausea and vomiting, anorexia, abdominal pain, and depression;

tachycardia and tachypnea have also been reported (Roder, 2004a; Sellon, 2006; Stewart et al., 2016). Mild cases usually recover in another 2–3 days, but severe cases progress to icterus and death, usually within 4 days (Murphy, 1994; Sellon, 2006).

Methemoglobinemia also occurs in dogs after ingesting high doses of acetaminophen, and is more likely to cause death than is liver failure. Methemoglobinemia usually occurs within 12 h of ingestion, but some dogs present after 48 h. Doses of 200 mg/kg acetaminophen PO converted 18.8% of hemoglobin to methemoglobin in dogs; 500 mg/kg produced 51.5% methemoglobinemia (Hjelle and Grauer, 1986). Signs reported included cyanosis, brown blood, brown urine, tachypnea, tachycardia, lethargy, and recumbence (Schlesinger, 1995; Wallace et al., 2002; MacNaughton, 2003; Stewart et al., 2016). Hemolysis, anemia, icterus, and shock have been described. Several authors report pigmenturia. Occasionally, signs of methemoglobinemia occur in acetaminophen-intoxicated dogs in the absence of clinically evident liver damage. Facial edema, keratoconjunctivitis sicca, and edema of the forelimbs or paws have been observed in dogs (Stewart et al., 2016).

Clinical Chemistry

Methemoglobinemia and hemolysis are noted, especially in cats. Whole blood exposed to air appears brown. Heinz bodies in cats and dogs are evident on blood smears stained with new methylene blue. Heinz bodies occur within 3 days of dosing (Webb et al., 2003), and were evident in 12% of accidentally exposed cats (Aronson and Drobatz, 1996). Anemia occurred in 75% of cats (Aronson and Drobatz, 1996), and has been reported in dogs (Schlesinger, 1995; Wallace et al., 2002; MacNaughton, 2003). In addition to Heinz bodies, ghost cells, nucleated erythrocytes, eccentrocytes, and reticulocytes have been reported in affected dogs (Stewart et al., 2016). Hyperbilirubinemia occurred within 48 h of acetaminophen ingestion in cats, and has been reported in dogs with hemolysis (Schlesinger, 1995; Sellon, 2006). Evidence of regeneration has been reported in dogs 2–11 days after acetaminophen ingestion.

Hypoglycemia, mild hyperbilirubinemia, elevated ALT, ALP, blood urea nitrogen (BUN), creatinine, and CK were the changes reported in a dog that had ingested acetaminophen (Rumbeiha et al., 1995; Webb et al., 2003; Sellon, 2006). This change was reported by Aronson and Drobatz (1996) in 35% of exposed cats. Increased ALT in dogs is a direct result of toxic hepatic injury, though hypoxic injury may contribute, and occurs within 24 h of acetaminophen ingestion. Increased aspartate transaminase (AST) and alkaline phosphatase (ALP) activities are reported. Evidence of severe liver damage includes elevated prothrombin time (PT), partial thromboplastin time (PTT), and progressively decreased serum cholesterol albumin concentrations (Sellon, 2006). Forty-one percent of cats presenting for acetaminophen toxicosis had hypocholesterolemia and 12% had hypoalbuminemia (Aronson and Drobatz, 1996). Hemoglobinuria and hematuria have been observed in dogs and cats with acetaminophen toxicosis.

Diagnosis and Management

Diagnosis of acetaminophen poisoning is usually based on a history of clinical exposure and appropriate clinical signs. Plasma, serum, and urine can be tested for acetaminophen at human hospitals and some veterinary laboratories to confirm the diagnosis. However, test results are usually not available for hours or days, and acetaminophen toxicosis presents as an emergency, thus treatment should be initiated immediately.

If the animal presents within 6 h of ingestion, decontamination measures can be instituted to prevent further absorption. Emetics can be used in the alert animal within a couple of hours of ingestion. However, if large doses were ingested, gastric lavage of the anesthetized, intubated animal is more likely to be appropriate. Activated charcoal and a cathartic such as sorbitol are given to prevent further absorption.

Antidotal therapy must be initiated as soon as possible in animals suspected of ingesting a toxic dose of acetaminophen. Antidotal therapy involves use of sulfate sources to bind the active metabolites and enhance glutathione production. Several sulfur donors are available, and include *N*-acetylcysteine, *S*-adenosyl methionine (SAMe), and sodium sulfate. *N-acetylcysteine therapy is the most accepted treatment for acetaminophen toxicosis.* Additionally, antioxidants can be used to reduce methemoglobin.

N-acetylcysteine is a glutathione precursor. *N*-acetylcysteine acts as source of sulfhydryl groups to be used for phase II sulfate conjugation or for glutathione production (Hjelle and Grauer, 1986; Savides and Oehme, 1985; Villar et al., 1998). *N*-acetylcysteine is hydrolyzed to L-cysteine by deacetylase enzymes. Use of *N*-acetylcysteine promotes conjugation of acetaminophen metabolites in cats. Rumbeiha et al. (1995) reported a 50% decrease in the plasma half-life of acetaminophen in cats treated with *N*-acetylcysteine, and Savides and Oehme (1985) reported an increase in the total fraction excreted as a sulfate conjugate. Cats treated with *N*-acetylcysteine have a more rapid recovery of blood GSH concentrations than untreated cats. *N*-acetylcysteine decreased the half-life of methemoglobin in the blood of cats from more than 10 to 5 h and prevented anemia.

N-acetylcysteine therapy should be initiated in any suspected case of acetaminophen toxicosis, even if treatment is delayed or exposure is unconfirmed. This treatment is most effective within 8 h of exposure; however, treatment within 24 h decreases mortality from liver failure. *N*-acetylcysteine is sold in 10% and 20% solutions. Twenty percent solutions are diluted 1:1 in normal saline or a 5%–10% dextrose solution (MacNaughton, 2003; Plumb, 2015; Sellon, 2006). An initial dose of 140 mg/kg is given intravenously (IV) slowly. Alternately, the dose can be given orally if no vomiting is evident and activated charcoal has not been given recently. Doses of 70 mg/kg *N*-acetylcysteine should be given IV or PO every 6 h thereafter for 48 h. A new drug, *N*-acetylcysteine amide, with greater bioavailability, has shown promise in experimental studies of acetaminophen toxicosis (Khayyat et al., 2016).

SAMe is another possible sulfate source used to treat acetaminophen toxicosis in dogs and cats. Decreased hemolysis and overall improvement were reported in treated dogs (Wallace et al., 2002). Prevention of methemoglobin production in cats by SAMe has been inconsistent. The number of Heinz bodies was lower and the packed cell volume (PCV) remained higher in treated versus untreated experimental cats (Webb et al., 2003; Sellon, 2006). Dogs are given 40 mg/kg PO as their first dose and 20 mg/kg daily for 7–9 days thereafter. Protocols recommended for cats include 180 mg/kg SAMe PO every 12 h for 3 days and 90 mg/kg SAMe PO every 12 h for 14 days.

There are reports of sodium sulfate as a treatment for acetaminophen toxicosis. This protocol decreased the plasma half-life of acetaminophen in cats and increased the amount excreted as a sulfate conjugate, similar to *N*-acetylcysteine (Savides and Oehme, 1985). Severity and duration of clinical signs and methemoglobin concentrations were decreased in treated animals, and glutathione concentrations rebounded faster than in untreated cats (Villar et al., 1998). Sodium sulfate was given as a 1.6% solution at a dose of 50 mg/kg IV every 4 h for six treatments.

Ascorbic acid and methylene blue are commonly used to reduce methemoglobin to hemoglobin. Ascorbic acid causes nonenzymatic reduction of methemoglobin, but is slow-acting. Ascorbic acid is given at a dose of 30 mg/kg PO every 6 h for six or seven treatments. Methylene blue has a rapid onset, but can induce hemolytic anemia in cats, making it a risky choice; still, methylene blue has been used successfully for short-term management of feline methemoglobinemia. Use of methylene blue concurrently with *N*-acetylcysteine in cats should be avoided.

Supportive and symptomatic therapy for acetaminophen toxicosis includes administration of oxygen to animals with methemoglobinemia. Transfusion or hemoglobin replacement is needed in cases of severe anemia (Murphy, 1994; Sellon, 2006). Fluid therapy is aimed at improving hydration, electrolyte balance, and pH.

Cimetidine has been recommended for use in dogs and cats to inhibit acetaminophen metabolism through inhibition of cytochrome P450 enzymes; however, the doses required for enzyme inhibition are higher than doses used routinely (Sellon, 2006).

The time that elapses between exposure and treatment seems to be as, if not more, important in estimating the prognosis for survival. Most cats that survived were treated within 14 h of exposure, although one cat was not treated for 24 h. Most of the cats for which treatment was delayed 17 or more hours postexposure died. There were no differences in exposure–dose between the group of cats that died and those that survived. Cats with underlying disease most likely have a worse outcome than otherwise healthy cats. The survival rate in dogs decreases if treatment is delayed more than 72 h (Sellon, 2006). Animals that were treated and survived usually recovered within 48 h, and were hospitalized for 3 days (Aronson and Drobatz, 1996).

Postmortem Findings

Icterus is a common finding secondary to acute hemolysis or chronic cholestasis. Centrilobular necrosis occurs commonly in dogs, and has been described in cats, although necrosis is likely to be more diffuse in cats. Bile duct proliferation, vacuolar hepatocyte degeneration, and mononuclear cholangitis are reported in dogs with chronic liver injury. Subcutaneous edema extends from the head along the fascial planes of the neck and thorax in some affected cats and dogs, and can affect the conjunctiva (Allen, 2003).

Nonsteroidal Antiinflammatory Drugs

NSAIDs are defined as "compounds that are not steroidal and that suppress inflammation" (Boothe, 2001). These drugs have antithrombotic actions when taken at low doses, relieve minor pain and pyrexia at moderate doses, and have antiinflammatory effects at higher doses (Rubin and Papich, 1990; Boothe, 2001). NSAIDs are commonly used to treat orthopedic problems in dogs (Wallace et al., 1990). About 8% of all human- and veterinary-related calls to the Illinois Poison Control Center were reported to involve NSAIDs, most commonly aspirin, ibuprofen, naproxen, piroxicam, indomethacin, and phenylbutazone. Out of those calls, 70% of the nonhuman animal calls were for dogs and 25% for cats (Kore, 1990). NSAID toxicosis can be caused by a single large dose or multiple smaller doses (Albretsen, 2002).

There are more than 30 commercially available NSAIDs (Mazué et al., 1982). They are classified based on their structure into the carboxylic acid group, which includes salicylic acid derivatives, acetic acid derivatives, fenamates,

TABLE 21.1 An Incomplete List of Nonsteroidal Antiinflammatory Drugs

Carboxylic Acid Group	Enolic Group
Salicylic Acid Derivatives	**Pyrazolone Derivatives**
Aspirin	Azapropazone
Diflunisal	Dipyrone
Salicylates	Isopyrin
	Oxyphenbutazone
	Phenylbutazone
Acetic Acid Derivatives	**Oxicam Derivatives**
Etodolac	Lornoxicam
Indomethacin	Meloxicam
Sulindac	Piroxicam
Tolmetin	Tenoxicam
Diclofenac	
Fenamates/Anthranilic Acid Derivatives	**Coxibs**
Flufenamic acid	Celecoxib
Meclofenamic acid	Deracoxib
Mefenamic acid	Firocoxib
Tolfenamic acid	Robenacoxib
Propionic Acid Derivatives	
Carprofen	
Ibuprofen	
Fenoprofen	
Flurbiprofen	
Ketoprofen	
Naproxen	
Suprofen	
Tiaprofenic acid	
Flurbiprofen	
Aminonicotinic Acid Derivatives	
Flunixin meglumine	

or anthranilic acid and propionic acid derivatives, as well as the enolic acid groups. An incomplete list of NSAIDs is provided in Table 21.1.

The mechanism of action is similar for all drugs in this classification. However, toxicity and pharmacokinetic data vary markedly between the different compounds and species. Cats, e.g., are more susceptible to salicylate toxicosis than other species (Roder, 2004a), and dogs are very sensitive to ibuprofen (Rubin and Papich, 1990). Attempts should not be made to extrapolate the therapeutic dose from one species to another (Lees et al., 1991).

Individual factors also affect susceptibility to NSAIDs. Young and aged animals do not have the same metabolic capacity as mature animals. Drug excretion can be delayed in animals with poor hepatic or renal function (Lees et al., 1991; Isaacs, 1996; Roder, 2004a). Dehydration and cardiac disease decrease renal circulation, slowing drug excretion and promoting renal damage. Preexisting gastrointestinal disease could predispose to ulceration when NSAIDs are used.

Various drugs interact with NSAIDs. Changes in bioavailability are by inhibition of absorption, displacement from plasma- and tissue-binding proteins, and competition for active renal secretion. Some drugs enhance or diminish metabolism of other drugs by hepatic cytochrome P450 enzymes. An incomplete list of possible interactions is provided in Table 21.2. NSAIDs also affect the bioavailability of other drugs. There have been reports of deaths in people using NSAIDs with methotrexate, and ibuprofen decreases renal clearance of digoxin and lithium. The diuretic effects of furosemide and bumetanide, which are mediated by prostaglandins (PGs), are inhibited by NSAIDs. NSAIDs do not influence response to thiazide diuretics in this way, but decrease the hypotensive response. NSAIDs can decrease the effectiveness of angiotensin-converting enzyme (ACE) inhibitors such as captopril. NSAIDs have additive effects when used together, with decreased rates of metabolism and clearance for each (Lees et al., 1991; Verbeeck, 1990). NSAIDs also have additive effects when used with corticosteroids, and such mixing should be avoided.

Toxicity

There are species differences in NSAID tolerance, as noted above. Dogs are more susceptible to ibuprofen and naproxen toxicosis than many other species (Kore, 1990; McKellar et al., 1991; Isaacs, 1996). Use of these drugs in dogs should be avoided. Ibuprofen doses greater than 5 mg/kg have been associated with adverse reactions in dogs (Villar et al., 1998). Gastric lesions occurred in dogs when 8 mg/kg/day ibuprofen was given over a 30-day period, either PO or parenterally, although clinical signs were not evident (McKellar et al., 1991; Godshalk et al., 1992; Boothe, 2001; Talcott, 2006). Clinical signs were evident in dogs dosed with 16 mg/kg/day for 8 weeks. Single doses of 50–125 mg/kg have been associated with gastrointestinal signs (Jackson et al., 1991; Murphy, 1994; Talcott, 2006), and a perforating gastric ulcer was reported in a dog given a cumulative dose of 110 mg/kg ibuprofen over a period of 48 h (Godshalk et al., 1992).

TABLE 21.2 Some NSAID–Drug Interactions

Drugs that Decrease Absorption of Some NSAIDs
Aluminum hydroxide
Drugs that Compete for Protein Binding with NSAIDs
Acetazolamide
Corticosteroids
Coumarin
Digitoxin
Hydantoin
Methotrexate
Phenylbutazone
Phenytoin
Salicylates
Sulfonamides
Tolbutamide
Valproic acid
Drugs that Increase Metabolism Rate of Some NSAIDs
Antihistamines
Phenobarbital
Phenytoin
Rifampicin
Drugs that Decrease Metabolism Rate of Some NSAIDs
Anabolic steroids
Chloramphenicol
Drugs that Increase Excretion Rate of Some NSAIDs
Aluminum hydroxide
Magnesium hydroxide
Drugs that Decrease Excretion Rate of Some NSAIDs
Probenecid
Methotrexate

An incomplete list of NSAID-drug interactions. For more detailed information, consult Verbeeck (1990).

Doses of 175–250 mg/kg have been associated with acute renal failure. Serum ibuprofen concentrations less than 31 μg/mL have not been associated with clinical signs in dogs, but melena was noted with serum concentrations of 138 μg/mL.

Less information on ibuprofen in cats is available, though they are considered very susceptible. Cats dosed with 50 mg/kg ibuprofen had gastrointestinal hemorrhage and irritation (Kore, 1990). Doses of 200 mg/kg were associated with renal failure, and doses over 600 mg/kg caused death. A ferret that ingested at least 347 mg/kg ibuprofen died from respiratory failure and asystole approximately 12 h postexposure (Cathers et al., 2000). Ketoprofen given as a subcutaneous dose of 2 mg/kg to 3-month-old kittens and mature cats produced lesions in the small intestine that were more severe in adult cats (Takata et al., 2012).

Naproxen induced toxicosis in dogs at a dose of 5 mg/kg/day, and plasma concentrations were >50 μg/mL (Daehler, 1986; Rubin and Papich, 1990; Boothe, 2001). Severe toxicosis was produced in a Samoyed dosed with 5.6 mg/kg naproxen, presumably once per day, over a week. Common clinical signs are anemia, melena, and renal and hepatic dysfunction. A perforating ulcer was described in a dog given 10–20 mg/kg/day naproxen for several weeks (Daehler, 1986). Doses of 15 mg/kg/day have been lethal in some dogs (Daehler, 1986; Gfeller and Sandon, 1991). Horses do not appear to be sensitive to naproxen toxicosis. Horses given three times the recommended dose of naproxen for 6 weeks did not have adverse clinical signs (Boothe, 2001).

Phenylbutazone is commonly used in horses. The recommended oral dose is 4 mg/kg/day (Plumb, 2015). A dose of 4.4 mg/kg every 12 h over a 2-week period was associated with changes of mineralization patterns in cortical bone in growing horses 18–30 months of age, an effect that was reversible (Brumbaugh, 2001). The same dose has been associated with other clinical signs, including CNS depression and protein-losing enteropathy. Shock was reported in one of nine horses after 5 days of dosing (Collins and Tyler, 1985). Therapeutic plasma concentrations for phenylbutazone in a horse range from 10 to 30 μg/mL. The therapeutic range in humans, 100–150 μg/mL, would be lethal in a horse (Lees et al., 1991). Phenylbutazone doses of 100 mg/kg/day did not cause gastrointestinal ulcers in dogs (Mazué et al., 1982).

Vultures are exquisitely sensitive to some NSAIDS, which has led to their near extinction in parts of Asia after diclofenac entered their food chain. Diclofenac and ketoprofen are known to cause renal failure in Old World vultures, and carprofen, flunixin, and phenylbutazone produced clinical toxicosis in experimental vultures (Fourie et al., 2015).

Toxicokinetics

NSAIDs are small, weakly acidic molecules with pK_a values less than 4.5, and thus, are well-absorbed in the stomach (Mazué et al., 1982; Kore, 1990; Rubin and Papich, 1990; Verbeeck, 1990; Isaacs, 1996; Boothe, 2001). Peak plasma concentrations for most NSAIDs occur within 3 h of oral dosing. Some absorption probably occurs in the proximal small intestine.

Ibuprofen and naproxen are 60%–80% and 68%–100% bioavailable, respectively, in dogs (McKellar et al., 1991; Boothe, 2001), and blood concentrations are almost identical whether dosing is PO or IV (Runkel et al., 1972). Naproxen is 50% bioavailable in horses (Boothe, 2001) and nearly 100% bioavailable in pigs (Runkel et al., 1972).

NSAID distribution is variable between individual drugs and animal species. Because they are highly protein-bound in the circulation, mostly to albumin, NSAIDs generally have a low volume of distribution (Brater, 1988; Verbeeck, 1990; Boothe, 2001; Talcott, 2006). Protein binding in humans is 99% for ibuprofen (Brater, 1988), >99% for naproxen (Runkel et al., 1972; Rubin and Papich, 1990), and 98.7% for ketoprofen (Brater, 1988). The remaining unbound fraction becomes distributed in the extracellular fluid and is responsible for the clinical effects (Brater, 1988; Kore, 1990; Boothe, 2001; Talcott, 2006). Hypoalbuminemia or displacement from protein-binding sites by other drugs leads to a transient increase in the unbound fraction. Although this unbound drug is normally rapidly excreted, clinical effects can be evident. NSAIDs can partition into lipid, allowing them to cross cell membranes.

Metabolism of NSAIDs takes place primarily in the liver. Most undergo cytochrome P450-mediated oxidation to increase water solubility. Phenylbutazone is converted to oxyphenbutazone, which is similarly potent, via phase I hepatic metabolism (Lees et al., 1991). Phase I metabolites and, in the case of carboxylic acid-group NSAIDs, the parent compound can undergo phase II reactions such as glucuronide conjugation, sulfate conjugation, and glutathione conjugation, which further increase water solubility and usually inactivate the drug. Acyl-glucuronide conjugation of propionic acid NSAIDs such as ibuprofen and naproxen is reversible, and these drugs deconjugate if excretion is delayed.

Drug elimination is dependent upon compound and animal species. Animals younger than 6 weeks old, as well as geriatric animals, usually metabolize drugs slower; hepatic or renal failure further delays elimination. High plasma protein binding also slows excretion. Plasma clearance is biphasic, with a rapid initial decline as the drug is distributed to the tissues, and then a slower decline as it is metabolized and excreted, terminating drug activity (Lees et al., 1991). Less than 1% of a dose of naproxen or ketoprofen is eliminated unchanged, and approximately 1% of a given dose of ibuprofen is excreted in the urine as the parent compound (Brater, 1988). Urinary excretion is pH-dependent, and tends to be more rapid in alkali urine due to ion trapping.

Fecal elimination through biliary excretion is important for ibuprofen, naproxen, and carprofen in dogs (Runkel et al., 1972; Gfeller and Sandon, 1991; Isaacs, 1996; Talcott, 2006; Koenigschof et al., 2015). Half of a given dose of naproxen is eliminated in the bile of dogs (Runkel et al., 1972). Drugs eliminated in the bile, such as ibuprofen and naproxen, as well as carprofen, indomethacin, piroxicam, flunixin, tolfenamic acid, meclofenamic acid, and diclofenac, undergo enterohepatic circulation in dogs. This prolongs the plasma half-life, and is likely the cause of increased susceptibility of dogs to these compounds.

The plasma half-life of ibuprofen is 2.5–6 h in dogs and cats and 1 h in rats (Mazué et al., 1982; Lees et al., 1991; Boothe, 2001). The half-life for naproxen in plasma is 35 h in beagles (Runkel et al., 1972), 74 h in mixed-breed dogs (Isaacs, 1996), 5 h in h (Lees et al., 1991; Isaacs, 1996), 4.8 h in cows (Lees et al., 1991), 4.8 h in minipigs, 1.9 h in rhesus monkeys, and 8.7 h in guinea pigs. Elimination of phenylbutazone in dogs appears to follow zero-order kinetics (Lees et al., 1991). The plasma half-life for phenylbutazone is between 5 and 8 h in horses, 37 h in cattle, and 4 h in swine.

Mechanism of Action

The basic mechanism of action of NSAIDs is inhibition of COX enzymes. These enzymes are found in all cells except mature erythrocytes (Kore, 1990; Boothe, 2001). Arachidonic acid, a 20-carbon unsaturated fatty acid, is released from the cell membrane by phospholipase A_2 and phospholipase C when a cell is damaged. Carprofen causes moderate inhibition of these phospholipases (Lees et al., 1991; McKellar et al., 1991). Although arachidonic acid itself has little activity, it can enter two pathways: the COX pathway, which produces eicosanoids, or the lipoxygenase pathway, which produces leukotrienes (LTs). Oxidation of arachidonic acid by COX, and further metabolism by other enzymes, leads to the production of various PGs and the release of oxygen-free radicals (Lees et al., 1991; Boynton et al., 1998). These PGs include PGH_2, PGE_2, and PGI_2. With the addition of prostacyclin synthase, $PGF_2\alpha$ is formed; thromboxane synthase is needed for production of thromboxane A_2.

PGE_2 and PGI_2 have similar actions, although the effects of PGI_2 tend to be of shorter duration. PGE_2, which is secreted by the gastrointestinal mucosa and at other sites, causes smooth muscle relaxation and vasodilation, which enhances blood flow to the kidneys and gastric mucosa and increases vascular permeability. It inhibits gastric acid production, inhibits pepsin production, increases gastric mucus synthesis, and is believed to mediate repair and turnover of gastric epithelium (Collins and Tyler, 1985; Boynton et al., 1988; Wallace et al., 1990). PGE_2 is also found in inflammatory exudate and enhances pain response due to bradykinin and histamine. PGI_2 also inhibits platelet aggregation.

NSAIDs bind the active site of COX, usually through competitive inhibition, although aspirin binds platelet COX irreversibly (Rubin and Papich, 1990). There are three isoforms of COX; designated COX_1, COX_2, and COX_3. COX_1 is found in almost all tissues, including the gastrointestinal tract, platelets, endothelium, and kidneys, is continuously produced, and functions in tissue homeostasis. Most of the adverse effects associated with NSAID use are due to inhibition of COX_1. Inhibition of PGE_2 promotes production of gastric acid and pepsin, and decreases the ability of the mucosa to secrete mucus glycoproteins and bicarbonate and respond to injury. Impairments to mucosal circulation due to loss of PG activity produce mucosal hypoxia and thrombosis.

Loss of the vasodilative actions of PGE_2 and PGI_2 in the kidneys through inhibition of COX_1 leads to hypoxic renal injury (Isaacs, 1996; Rubin and Papich, 1990). Production of PG by the kidneys is relatively low. With the possible exception of vultures, renal pathology is most often associated with chronic NSAID use (Fourie et al., 2015). Reversible urinary incontinence and isosthenuria was reported in a dog exposed to an unknown dose of carprofen (Hutchins et al., 2013). Renal papillary necrosis is frequently seen in horses, and is often associated with chronic phenylbutazone use (Gunson, 1983; Rubin and Papich, 1990). This lesion is also reported in cats, dogs, mice, rats, gerbils, hamsters, rabbits, desert mice, primates, and pigs (Brix, 2002). Renal failure in cats administered meloxicam first parenterally and then orally has been reported, and oral exposure to flurbiprofen was recently reported to cause death in cats (Dyer et al., 2009).

Evidence suggests that low doses of NSAIDs cause degeneration of medullary interstitial cells and, later, damage to vascular endothelium, leading to microvascular thrombosis and hypoxia. Higher doses produce more rapid endothelial damage (Brix, 2002). Dehydration is a major predisposing factor for renal papillary necrosis. Dehydration commonly occurs with gastrointestinal disease, diuretic use, anesthesia, surgical stress, hemorrhagic shock, or sepsis. Other risk factors described for dogs include advancing age, congestive heart failure, hepatic cirrhosis, preexisting renal problems, hypotension, and concurrent administration of nephrotoxic drugs such as gentamicin or amphotericin.

COX_2 is produced by macrophages, fibroblasts, chondrocytes, endothelial cells, and some other cell types (Roder, 2004a). This isoform only functions intermittently, and is induced by cytokines in areas of inflammation (Isaacs, 1996; Roder, 2004a; Talcott, 2006). Inhibition of this enzyme produces antipyretic, analgesic, and antiinflammatory effects of NSAIDs. Little is yet known about the function of COX_3, which is present in dogs but not functional in humans.

Most NSAIDs inhibit both COX_1 and COX_2, but a new class of COX_2-specific NSAIDs was developed as a safer alternative. These drugs include celecoxib, deracoxib, rofecoxib, diclofenac, etodolac, firocoxib, flosulide, and meloxicam. However, rofecoxib (Vioxx) was voluntarily withdrawn from the market in 2004 due to increased risk of adverse cardiovascular events in humans, and controversies still exist whether other compounds of this class pose a similar risk. Selectivity is species-specific, and thus, these new drugs sometimes cause COX_1 inhibition in domestic species (Talcott, 2006). Dogs treated with deracoxib and firocoxib did have fewer clinical signs and gastric lesions than dogs treated with other NSAIDs in one study (Sennello and Leib, 2006). Interestingly, carprofen is COX_2-specific in dogs but not in humans (Talcott, 2006).

LTs are also produced from arachidonic acid via the lipoxygenase pathway. 5-Lipoxygenase produces LTA4, which is converted to LTB4, LTC4, LTD4, LTE4, and others. LTB4 is an important chemoattractant for neutrophils. Various LTs cause vasoconstriction, bronchospasm, and increased vascular permeability (Boynton et al., 1988; Strøm and Thomsen, 1990; Lees et al., 1991). Some NSAIDs inhibit lipoxygenase. It has been found that in dogs, flunixin is a more potent inhibitor of LTB4-mediated neutrophil migration than phenylbutazone, which is more potent than indomethacin. Alternately, some NSAIDs actually increase LT production due to increased availability of arachidonic acid not entering the COX pathway.

NSAIDs can also inhibit phosphodiesterase. Phosphodiesterase breaks down cyclic AMP (cAMP). Increased intracellular cAMP can stabilize lysosomal membranes in polymorphonuclear leukocytes, inhibiting release of inflammatory products (Kore, 1990). Other effects of NSAIDs include inhibition of phosphatidylinositol 3′-kinase Akt signaling, important in cytokine pathways and cell regulation, mitogen-activated protein kinases involved in cell regulation, peroxisome proliferator-activated receptors, NFκB, and heat shock proteins involved in transcription. NSAIDs also uncouple oxidative phosphorylation and, thus, inhibit cellular energy production (Little et al., 2007).

Some NSAIDs have topical irritant properties. As weak acids, they partition to the gastric mucosa, leading to decreased hydrophobicity of mucus and thinning of the mucus barrier, allowing gastric acid to penetrate to the epithelial layer. NSAIDs frequently cause mild and transient liver damage associated with cholestasis and increased liver enzymes (Boynton et al., 1988; Isaacs, 1996; Roder, 2004a). More severe problems, such as hepatic necrosis, are rare. Hepatotoxicity is uncommon with ibuprofen in dogs. More commonly reported in dogs is idiosyncratic hepatotoxicosis due to carprofen

(Albretsen, 2002; Roder, 2004a; Talcott, 2006); approximately one-third of these cases were in Labrador retrievers.

Cartilage degeneration has been reported in mice given aspirin, phenylbutazone, indomethacin, ibuprofen, and naproxen (Isaacs, 1996). Anaphylactic reactions have been reported, but hypersensitivity to NSAIDs is rare. This problem is has been documented in dogs due to phenylbutazone administration (Rubin and Papich, 1990; Lees et al., 1991; Isaacs, 1996).

Clinical Signs

The most commonly reported clinical signs associated with NSAIDS in dogs and cats are gastrointestinal disturbance, renal insufficiency, lethargy, and death; gastrointestinal disturbance, particularly vomiting and diarrhea, but also including melena, colitis, abdominal pain, and icterus, are far more frequent than the others and most likely underreported (Hunt et al., 2015; Montiero-Steagall et al., 2013). Use of NSAIDs is the most common predisposing factor to gastrointestinal ulceration in dogs requiring emergency intervention (Montiero-Steagall et al., 2013). Clinical signs do not always correlate well with the severity of the lesion, probably due to the analgesic effect of NSAIDs. The asymptomatic ulcer rate among NSAID users is estimated at 50% (Isaacs, 1996). Animals with gastric perforations usually present with a distended abdomen due to effusion, dehydration, pyrexia, collapse, pallor, and abdominal pain (Godshalk et al., 1992; Talcott, 2006).

Lower gastrointestinal tract effects can include protein-losing enteropathy, most common in horses, and stricture formation; horses with hypoproteinemia often have secondary edema (Collins and Tyler, 1984, 1985). Endotoxemia and shock have been noted in horses secondary to gastrointestinal ulceration.

Analgesic nephropathy occurs in humans, has been reported in dogs given naproxen and, more recently, in cats given meloxicam or accidentally exposed to flurbiprofen (Isaacs, 1996; Boothe, 2001; Dyer et al., 2009; Anonymous 2015). Chronic use of NSAIDs in high doses appears to be a predisposing factor, except with flurbiprofen. It is likely that preexisting kidney disease in cats predisposes them to NSAID-associated renal insufficiency, making it critical to assess hydration status before prescribing NSAIDS (Hunt et al., 2015). Clinical signs are evident 2 weeks or many months after chronic dosing or, sometimes, after single, very high doses. Acute onset of oliguric renal failure has been described (Kore, 1990; Villar et al., 1998; Roder, 2004a). Animals may present with polyuria and polydipsia, dehydration, oral ulceration, and uremic coma (Mazué et al., 1982). Renal failure and visceral gout has been associated with low-dose NSAID exposure in Old World vultures (Fourie et al., 2015).

Transient increases in liver enzymes are frequently seen in NSAID overdose in small animals. Severe hepatotoxicosis is not common in NSAID-intoxicated small animals, although it has been reported in a dog given naproxen (Kore, 1990; Lees et al., 1991; Isaacs, 1996) and as an idiosyncratic reaction to carprofen (Albretsen, 2002). Clinical signs include anorexia and weight loss, vomiting, lethargy, icterus, ascites, and coagulopathy. Increased bleeding times are rarely reported in domestic animals (Murphy, 1994). Prolonged gestation and teratogenesis have been seen experimentally (Lees et al., 1991).

Clinical Chemistry

Approximately one-quarter of gastroduodenal ulceration cases in dogs present with microcytic hypochromic anemia due to chronic blood loss (Stanton and Bright, 1989); acute blood loss is uncommon. Individuals with acute blood loss present with rapid deterioration, normocytic and normochromic anemia, a normal albumin to globulin ratio, and evidence of regeneration (Stanton and Bright, 1989; Wallace et al., 1990). Peracute hemorrhage is rare, and occurs when a mesenteric blood vessel becomes eroded in the area of ulceration. Such a complication would be rapidly lethal and not allow time for a regenerative response. Increased PCV has been seen in horses with dehydration secondary to diarrhea (Collins and Tyler, 1985).

Fecal occult blood is unreliable. It can be negative for low-level blood loss or positive if red meat was fed within 72 h of testing (Talcott, 2006). Hypoalbuminemia has been observed with gastrointestinal ulcers and protein-losing enteropathy secondary to NSAID use. Both albumin and globulin concentrations are decreased. Coagulation profiles reveal poor platelet aggregation, thrombocytopenia, and increased bleeding times.

Serum chemistry reveals increased ALT, AST, ALP, and bilirubin (Albretsen, 2002; Roder, 2004a). A mild, transient rise in liver enzymes often occurs during the first week of NSAID administration. Elevated BUN indicates nephropathy. Phosphorus, calcium, and potassium are usually also elevated. Animals with renal damage due to NSAIDs present with isosthenuria, hematuria, and proteinuria. Ketonuria and pyuria have also been reported. Horses on chronic, high-dose phenylbutazone therapy had normal lymphocyte counts, with a left shift due to neutrophil loss into the gastrointestinal tract. Increased serum glucose concentrations were attributed to endotoxemia. Hypokalemia and hyponatremia are commonly seen in horses with diarrhea (Collins and Tyler, 1985).

Diagnosis and Management

Diagnosis of NSAID toxicosis is often based on history and clinical signs. Serum or plasma testing for NSAID drugs is available at many veterinary laboratories and human hospitals. Serum drug concentrations are unlikely to be useful in management, but some reference values are listed in the toxicokinetics portion of this section.

Endoscopy is the most sensitive test for gastric ulceration, although occasionally the ulcer will not be visible. Anesthesia is required, thus the patient must be stabilized. Survey radiographs are not usually useful. If there is gastrointestinal perforation, then poor visualization of serosal surfaces, peritoneal effusion, free gas in the peritoneal cavity, and intestinal ileus are often noted (Godshalk et al., 1992; Talcott, 2006). Large ulcers have been identified on contrast radiographs; however, if perforation is present, barium sulfate will complicate peritonitis, thus a water soluble agent is preferred. Ulcers can be detected using ultrasound in an animal given water by stomach tube. The gastric wall is thickened with a loss of the normal five-layer structure, disruption of the mucosa, and gas bubble formation. Increased fluid in the abdomen is seen in the case of peritonitis due to perforation.

Renal papillary damage can be diagnosed in humans, horses, and foals using ultrasound (Brix, 2002; Roder, 2004a). Computed tomography has been used to diagnose renal papillary necrosis in humans, and magnetic resonance imaging has been used experimentally (Brix, 2002).

Animals on NSAID therapy should be closely monitored for adverse effects: attitude, appetite, hydration, electrolyte status, urine concentrating ability, urine protein concentrations, BUN, creatinine, and liver enzymes can be monitored (Villar et al., 1998; Roder, 2004a).

When animals present with adverse effects attributable to NSAIDs, administration of the drug should be discontinued. Gastric emptying is appropriate for animals that have ingested large quantities of NSAIDs but are not yet showing clinical signs (Kore, 1990). Emetics are sometimes used for large single ingestions, although they are contraindicated in animals with severe CNS suppression. Gastric lavage can be performed in the anesthetized, intubated animal (Cathers et al., 2000). Activated charcoal and cathartics are given after gastric emptying or if the animal presents later. Repeated activated charcoal administration has been recommended for various reasons. Some tablets are sustained-release, and regular tablets can form concretions in the stomach and have delayed absorption. Furthermore, activated charcoal prevents enterohepatic cycling, which is the cause of a prolonged half-life of ibuprofen and other NSAIDs in dogs. However, a report looked at the effect of activated charcoal, activated charcoal plus sorbitol as a cathartic, or multiple doses of activated charcoal on a moderate overdose of carprofen in dogs (Koenigschof et al., 2015), and determined that a single dose of activated charcoal was as effective as multiple doses and produced fewer adverse effects. Sorbitol plus activated charcoal increased rate of elimination but did not change the maximum circulating concentration compared to activated charcoal alone, but the addition of sorbitol did not cause clinically evident adverse effects.

Intravenous lipid infusion has been used to treat ibuprofen and naproxen overdoses in dogs by providing a lipid compartment and enhancing elimination (Bolfer et al., 2014; Herring et al., 2015). Lipid emulsion therapy was used in a dog that ingested a high dose of ibuprofen (>1800 mg/kg) and became comatose within 30 min of arrival to the veterinary clinic (Bolfer et al., 2014). The patient showed slight improvement within 3 h, and was alert and responsive 13 h after lipid administration, but had evidence of coagulopathy. The dog survived and was discharged after 5 days of hospitalization, and appeared to be completely recovered on examination 1 week later. Three dogs that ingested between 60 and 200 mg/kg of naproxen were given intravenous lipid infusion (Herring et al., 2015); circulating naproxen concentrations declined quickly. After treatment, dogs developed relatively mild clinical signs, including azotemia in one and melena in another, and all were discharged without further complications.

Animals should be monitored for hydration, electrolyte imbalances, acid–base imbalances, blood glucose, liver enzymes, BUN, creatinine, body temperature, and blood pressure. Deviations from expected values can be corrected as needed. Fluid therapy is needed to correct dehydration, hypotension, electrolyte imbalances, and improve renal perfusion. It has been suggested that fluids be given at twice the maintenance rates. Villar et al. (1998) recommended 0.9% saline, or 0.45% saline plus 2.5% dextrose, in hypoglycemic animals, given at a rate of 120 mL/kg/day plus estimated fluid losses over a 48- to 72-h period. Lactated Ringers solution can contribute to electrolyte imbalances and, thus, should be used with caution. Dopamine at a dose of 2.5 μg/kg/min, or dobutamine at 2.5 mg/kg/min, can be given to increase renal perfusion (Kore, 1990). Diuretics can predispose animals to dehydration and subsequent renal hypoperfusion and, thus, should be avoided (Albretsen, 2002). Sodium bicarbonate is used cautiously to treat acidosis and for ion trapping (Murphy, 1994; Roder, 2004a). Urine alkalization for ion trapping is sometimes useful with salicylates, aspirin, and ibuprofen, but urinary pH must exceed 7.5–8 to increase naproxen secretion.

Gastric lavage with iced saline or water has been recommended for severe and continued gastric bleeding, but the efficacy of this treatment is questionable, and surgical correction is often required (Wallace et al., 1997). Severe anemia is treated with transfusions or blood substitutes (Murphy, 1994; Sellon, 2006). Acute loss of greater than 30% of the blood volume, a PCV less than 20%, plasma protein less than 3.5 g/dL, or continued blood loss are possible indications for transfusion (Talcott, 2006); vitamin K_1 is given to aid coagulation (Kore, 1990). Perforating ulcers are a surgical emergency.

Gastrointestinal protectants are typically used in NSAID overdose cases to prevent or heal gastric ulcerations. Gastric pH must be maintained above 3 for 18–20 h a day for effective healing, and above 4 in critically ill patients. Gastric pH above 4 inhibits fibrinolysis and the activity of pepsin. Gastric pH must be above 6 to promote platelet aggregation and prevent clot dissolution, therefore allowing hemostasis. Gastric secretion is variable in beagles, which can have a pH of pH of 1.30 under normal conditions and 4.44 if fasted (Bersenas et al., 2005). Therefore, simply withholding food benefits the patient by decreasing gastric acid secretion and minimizing emesis.

Treatment with antacids such as magnesium hydroxide (milk of magnesia) or aluminum hydroxide is probably adequate for animals exposed to low NSAID doses. Antacids require dosing every 2–4 h, and sometimes produce changes in fecal consistency (Wallace et al., 1990). Products containing bismuth subsalicylate (Pepto Bismol and Kaopectate) should be avoided because salicylate acts as an NSAID.

Misoprostol is a long-lasting synthetic analog of PGE_1. It is the only agent that consistently prevents and treats NSAID-induced gastric and duodenal ulcers (Isaacs, 1996). When given concurrently with aspirin, misoprostol prevented gastric ulcers in dogs (Villar et al., 1998). Dogs given NSAIDs and misoprostol had less gastrointestinal hemorrhage, less vomiting, and less mucosal ulceration on endoscopy than dogs given NSAIDs only (Talcott, 2006). Misoprostol is believed to protect renal function in domestic animals and be chondroprotective in pigs (Isaacs, 1996). At high doses, misoprostol can cause diarrhea, and use of this synthetic PG is contraindicated in pregnant animals (Villar et al., 1998). Dogs can be given 1–5 μg/kg misoprostol PO every 8 h (Plumb, 2015).

Proton pump inhibitors suppress gastric acid secretion by inhibiting the H^+/K^+-ATPase pump in gastric parietal cells (Walan et al., 1989; Villar et al., 1998). Omeprazole and pantoprazole are proton pump inhibitors (Bersenas et al., 2005). Omeprazole has been used successfully in humans and dogs to treat gastric ulcer. Bersenas et al. (2005) found that 2 mg/kg omeprazole PO given to dogs twice per day kept their gastric pH from going below 3 for 90.9% of the day, and kept the gastric pH above 4 for 78.3% of the day, although one in six dogs vomited. Omeprazole remains biologically active for nearly 24 h and only need be given once daily. Plumb (2015) lists the canine daily dose as 0.5–1.0 mg/kg PO, and the feline dose as 0.7 mg/kg. Villar et al. (1998) recommend a 3- to 4-week treatment protocol. Rebound acid secretion has been reported at discontinuation of omeprazole therapy (Driman et al., 1995).

Sucralfate is an aluminum salt of sucrose sulfate. This drug complexes with exposed proteins on the surface of gastric ulcers, specifically fibrinogen and albumin, and acts as a direct mucosal protectant. Sucralfate has five times as much affinity for damaged mucosa as it does for normal mucosa (Villar et al., 1998). Sucralfate also adsorbs pepsin and bile acids. This drug is believed to promote bicarbonate and mucus secretion by the gastric mucosa. Sucralfate is equally as effective as cimetidine at reducing discomfort and promoting ulcer healing. Dogs given sucralfate to treat gastric ulcers, with and without concurrent cimetidine treatment, had completed healing of the gastric mucosa within 9 days. Sucralfate can be used alone if gastric hyperacidity is not suspected (Wallace et al., 1990). If used with cimetidine, dosing should be staggered or cimetidine should be given by a parenteral route because sucralfate interferes with gastrointestinal absorption of cimetidine (Wallace et al., 1990). Cimetidine should be given 1 h before a meal. Dogs are dosed every 8 h. Dogs weighing >20 kg are given 1 g per dose, and smaller dogs are dosed with 0.5 g (Murphy, 1994; Albretsen, 2002; Plumb, 2015). Cats are given a total of 0.25–0.5 g every 8–12 h, and ferrets are given 75 mg/kg four to six times a day, preferably 10 min before feeding. Foals are given 1–2 g PO two to three times daily.

H_2 histamine receptor antagonists, including cimetidine, ranitidine, and famotidine, are routinely used to treat NSAID-induced gastric ulcers. Histamine stimulates gastric parietal cells to secrete hydrogen ions through an H^+/K^+-ATPase pump. Acetylcholine, gastrin, and histamine stimulate this proton pump. H_2 inhibitors only block the histaminic effect on parietal cells, but cause significant inhibition of gastric acid secretion nonetheless (Bersenas et al., 2005). H_2 inhibitors are likely to suppress clinical signs associated with unhealed ulcers (Talcott, 2006).

Cimetidine has been commonly used to treat and prevent NSAID-induced ulcers. Cimetidine is believed to decrease gastrointestinal discomfort, and does decrease gastric acid secretion (Boulay et al., 1986; Isaacs, 1996). Cimetidine has not been proven to be effective with continued NSAID use, and did not prevent gastric ulcer formation when used concurrently with aspirin. Cimetidine is more useful when NSAID administration has ended and, possibly, after a single large dose (Kore, 1990). Gastric acid production is dependent on local circulation, which provides oxygen and energy. Cimetidine decreases gastric blood flow, which contributes to decreased mucosal alkalinity (Cheung and Sonnenscheine, 1983). Reduced circulation also contributes to tissue hypoxia. Cimetidine is known to inhibit hepatic cytochrome P450 enzymes and, therefore, could decrease the rate of

NSAID metabolism (Talcott, 2006; Wallace et al., 1990; Verbeeck, 1990). Cimetidine given at a dose of 6 mg/kg every 6 h caused decreased basal acid output in dogs by 30%–50%, and food induced output by 63%–71%. When 12 mg/kg was used every 6 h, there was a 70%–80% decrease in basal acid output and complete suppression of food-induced output (Boulay et al., 1986). Cimetidine is given to dogs at a dose of 5–10 mg/kg PO, SC, or slow IV every 6–8 h (Villar et al., 1998; Plumb, 2015). Similar dosing protocols are used in cats and ferrets.

Ranitidine does not inhibit microsomal enzymes like cimetidine. However, Bersenas et al. (2005) found no significant effect on gastric acid secretion in dogs dosed with ranitidine. Ranitidine also decreases gastric blood flow. It is given at a dose of 0.5–2.0 mg/kg PO, IV, or IM every 8–12 h in dogs, and 2.5 mg/kg IV or 3.5 mg/kg PO in cats every 12 h (Plumb, 2015). Villar et al. (1998) recommend continuous treatment for 3–6 weeks.

Famotidine increases intragastric pH in dogs better than ranitidine. However, a 0.5 mg/kg dose of famotidine given two to three times a day did not result in a prolonged gastric pH increase (pH > 4) in dogs (Bersenas et al., 2005). Famotidine was found protective against gastric hypoxia from reduced perfusion when used at a dose of 0.5 mg/kg IV in dogs given diclofenac (Hata et al., 2005). Dogs are given 0.5–1 mg/kg famotidine PO or slow IV every 12 h. The dose for cats is 0.5 mg/kg, and 0.25–0.5 mg/kg is the dose for ferrets. Horses are given 0.23 mg/kg IV or 1.88 mg/kg PO every 8 h or 0.35 mg/kg IV or 2.8 mg/kg PO every 12 h.

The prognosis for NSAID toxicosis is dependent on chronicity, dose, and clinical signs (Talcott, 2006). A study by Wallace et al. (1990) found that seven out of seven dogs treated for chronic NSAID toxicosis recovered after 2–9 days of hospitalization. The mean hospital stay was 6 days. Gastrointestinal irritation and ulceration are reversible, but perforation and peritonitis require immediate surgical intervention plus intensive medical management and have a guarded prognosis. Renal effects, such as nephropathy, are often reversible. Papillary necrosis is a permanent change, but well-tolerated. Loss of the long loops of Henle decreases urine concentrating ability, but horses with renal papillary necrosis usually appear clinically normal (Gunson, 1983; Roder, 2004a). Severe, acute cortical necrosis is associated with irreversible renal failure. NSAID-induced coagulopathies are reversible once the NSAID has been eliminated. Dogs with idiosyncratic hepatic injury usually recover within 4 weeks (Albretsen, 2002).

Postmortem Findings

NSAID toxicosis is most commonly associated with gastrointestinal lesions in domestic animals. Mild lesions include mucosal edema, irritation, and petechiation, which progress to erosive and, then, ulcerative lesions. The location for gastric ulceration in the canine stomach is variable; lesions can be near the pylorus, lesser curvature of the fundus or diffuse. Duodenal ulcers and perforations have been reported in dogs, but can be influenced by predisposing factors. Perforations are reported to occur in the stomach, small intestine, or colon. Ulcers that erode mesenteric vasculature are rapidly lethal.

Gastric ulcerations in the horse usually occur in the glandular mucosa adjacent to the margo plicatus (Collins and Tyler, 1984, 1985; Roder, 2004a). Linear-to-circular erosions were reported in the duodenums of horses dosed with phenylbutazone, and ulcers and erosions were found throughout the small intestines. Ulcerative colitis of the right dorsal colon is commonly seen in horses with NSAID toxicosis. Fibrinonecrotic typhlocolitis was reported by Collins and Tyler (1985).

Papillary necrosis occurs with long-term NSAID administration (Mazué et al., 1982). The lesion is bilateral and the papillae are cavitated, yellow-green to orange, and demarcated from the medulla by hemorrhage. The lesion is most severe at the poles. Microscopically, the papilla has undergone coagulative necrosis, with dilation of the collecting ducts and loops of Henle. Interstitial fibrosis extends through the medulla and cortex in chronic cases (Gunson, 1983). This lesion has been reported in horses, dogs, cats, mice, rats, gerbils, hamsters, rabbits, desert mice, primates, and pigs (Brix, 2002). The lesion is common in horses given phenylbutazone, but has also been reported with flunixin, aspirin, and dipyrone (Gunson, 1983). Papillary necrosis occurred in two of five dogs dosed with piroxicam (Talcott, 2006).

Interstitial nephritis, with multifocal or diffuse infiltrates of lymphocytes, has been reported, as has vacuolar degeneration of proximal and distal convoluted tubules (Kore, 1990). Tubular nephritis with epithelial necrosis and regeneration has also been described (Mazué et al., 1982). Acute cortical necrosis due to NSAID toxicosis has been documented in small animals (Jones et al., 1992).

Lymphoid necrosis has been noted in dogs and a ferret. Mild necrosis in the white pulp of the spleen was described in the ferret (Cathers et al., 2000). Depletion and necrosis of germinal centers was discovered in a dog, although circulating lymphocytes were within the reference range.

Aspirin and Other Salicylates

This group, which constitutes the most extensively used OTC drugs, includes acetylsalicylic acid, or aspirin, sodium salicylate, bismuth subsalicylate, and diflunisal. Aspirin and salicylates are NSAIDs with many characteristics similar to those of other NSAIDs, as described previously. Aspirin and salicylate also have certain unique properties. Clinical toxicosis of products containing bismuth subsalicylate, an OTC drug commonly used for gastrointestinal distress, are similar to those associated with other sources of salicylate, thus these products will be further discussed in this section. However, lesions unique to bismuth subsalicylate are described under gastroprotectants.

Salicylates have been used since ancient times by Greek and Roman physicians, Hippocrates and Galen, by South African tribes, and by North American Indians. Reverend Edmund Stone wrote of the use of *Salix alba* bark in the journal of the Royal Philosophical Society in London in 1763. Salicylic acid was first isolated from the bark of willows (*Salix* spp.) and beech trees (*Fagus* spp.) in the early 19th century (Lees et al., 1991). Bayer Pharmaceutical Company synthesized acetylsalicylic acid in 1893, and aspirin has been marketed since 1899.

Contraindications for aspirin use include coagulation disorders, recent (within 1 week) surgery, and concurrent use with certain drugs. See Table 21.2 for a list of drugs that may interact with aspirin and other NSAIDs. Aspirin inhibits the diuretic effects of spironolactone (Verbeeck, 1990).

Toxicity

The efficacy of aspirin is dose-dependent. Aspirin is used in dogs at doses of 10–25 mg/kg every 8–12 h for analgesia. Dogs dosed with 25 mg/kg aspirin every 8 h for up to 3 weeks had no serious adverse effects, and peak plasma concentrations were >50 μg/mL in mature dogs (Lees et al., 1991). The half-life is likely to be increased in pups less than 30 days old due to limited metabolic capability (Waters et al., 1993). A study of dogs dosed with 25–35 mg/kg aspirin every 8 h found increased fecal hemoglobin, and gastric ulcerations were visualized on endoscopy (McKellar et al., 1991). Seizures were reported in a dog given 37 mg/kg aspirin every 12 h for 2 weeks (Schubert, 1984). Clinical signs in dogs dosed with 50 mg/kg aspirin every 12 h included emesis, and similar daily doses were associated with perforating gastric ulcers within 4 weeks (Kore, 1990). One dose of 400 mg/kg caused hemorrhage, and daily dosing caused pyloric ulcers within 2 weeks (Mazué et al., 1982).

Cats are more susceptible to the toxic effects of aspirin than dogs and humans (Papich, 1990; Roder, 2004a). Doses of 25 mg/kg every 2–3 days are recommended to control thromboembolic disease, and 10 mg/kg every other day can be used for analgesia and antipyresis (Plumb, 2015). A dose of 10.5 mg/kg aspirin every 52 h produced plasma concentrations ranging from 50 to 20 μg/mL. No clinical signs were seen in cats dosed with 25 mg/kg aspirin every 48 h, and no severe signs were seen in cats dosed with 25 mg/kg aspirin every 24 h for 2–3 weeks (Lees et al., 1991; Boothe, 2001). Daily aspirin doses between 100 and 110 mg/kg in cats have caused death within 7 days (McKellar et al., 1991). Young cats, old cats, or cats with renal or hepatic disease are believed to be particularly sensitive (Kore, 1990).

Aspirin can be used in cattle and goats, but they require larger oral doses to reach appropriate plasma concentrations. A dose of 100 mg/kg PO given every 12 h in cattle maintains a therapeutic concentration of 30 μg/mL (Davis, 1980; Boothe, 2001). IV dosing with 6.5 mg/kg hourly is associated with plasma concentrations of 50–20 μg/mL, 26 mg every 1.6 h yields plasma concentrations of 200–50 μg/mL, and 39 mg every 2 h yields concentrations of 300–50 μg/mL in the plasma. Horses can be given 35 mg/kg aspirin IV, according to Davis (1980). However, a single oral dose of 20 mg/kg was associated with prolonged bleeding times (Boothe, 2001).

Toxicokinetics

Aspirin is lipophilic at acid pH, thus it is readily absorbed from the stomach and duodenum in dogs and cats (Rubin and Papich, 1990; Talcott, 2006). Aspirin is 68%–76% bioavailable in dogs, with some variation based on the formulation (Boothe, 2001). Enteric-coated and buffered products are used in humans and dogs (McKellar et al., 1991; Murtaugh et al., 1993; Boothe, 2001). Buffered aspirin is more soluble and less ionized, thus slowing absorption and decreasing gastric irritation. Acid-resistant forms are more readily absorbed at the relatively alkaline pH range of the duodenum, and absorption is delayed up to 12 h (Verbeeck, 1990). Ingestion of a fatty meal can reduce aspirin bioavailability by 30% (Mazué et al., 1982). Aspirin is 70% bioavailable in cattle, but absorption is relatively slow. Salicylates in bismuth subsalicylate are 97.5% absorbed in dogs and 85.4% absorbed in cats (Papich et al., 1987).

Peak serum concentrations occur 4 h after oral dosing with buffered aspirin. Peak serum concentrations are lower in immature dogs than in mature dogs after PO or IV dosing. Circulating salicylate is 72% protein-bound in humans and 45% protein-bound in dogs. There is more free and, therefore, bioavailable salicylate in the hypoalbuminemic animal, but the excess is rapidly eliminated (Boothe, 2001). Aspirin is rapidly distributed to most tissues, including synovial fluid, peritoneal fluid, saliva, and milk. Aspirin has a lower volume of distribution in cattle compared to other domestic species (Davis, 1980).

Aspirin is rapidly hydrolyzed to salicylate by esterases in the gastrointestinal tract, liver, and erythrocytes. These enzymes are less efficient in immature dogs (Waters et al., 1993). Most of the metabolism takes place in the liver. Salicylate is bioactive, and responsible for most of the clinical effects of aspirin. Salicylate is conjugated to glucuronide or glycine. The glucuronide pathway is deficient in cats, limiting their elimination of salicylate. Bismuth subsalicylate is metabolized to bismuth and salicylate in the gastrointestinal tract (Boothe, 2001).

The kidneys eliminate salicylate and its glycine conjugate (Boothe, 2001). Two to thirty percent of a dose of aspirin is excreted as unconjugated salicylate (Verbeeck, 1990). The rate of elimination for aspirin varies with species and age (McKellar et al., 1991). The elimination half-life in dogs is dependent upon the dose form. The half-life for enteric-coated products ranges from 7.5 to 12.2 h. The elimination half-life for aspirin given IV is 2.2–8.7 h (Boothe, 2001). The elimination half-life in cats is long, and increases with dose. If low doses of 5–12 mg/kg are given, the elimination half-life is 22–27 h, but the half-life for the much higher dose of 25 mg/kg is 45 h. Salicylate is considered to have zero-order kinetics in cats (Lees et al., 1991). The elimination half-life in horses is about an hour due to ion trapping in alkaline urine. Salicylates are normal components of equine urine (Boothe, 2001). The elimination half-life of salicylates in cattle is about 30 min (Lees et al., 1991; Boothe, 2001). Young animals metabolize aspirin more slowly, and the elimination half-life may be prolonged in puppies less than 30 days old, piglets, kids, and foals.

Mechanism of Action

The effects attributed to aspirin are mostly caused by the active metabolite salicylate (McKellar et al., 1991). Salicylate inhibits COX to block PG synthesis, as described for NSAIDs. Other NSAIDs competitively inhibit COX, but salicylates permanently inactivate the enzyme by acetylating a serine residue (Kore, 1990; Rubin and Papich, 1990; Boothe, 2001; Talcott, 2006). Platelets are unable to synthesize COX. Unlike other NSAIDs, where coagulopathy resolves once the drug is eliminated, it takes about 1 week to resolve aspirin-induced coagulopathy.

Aspirin has a direct irritant effect on the gastric mucosa. Aspirin is an acidic drug, and is taken up by the mucosal epithelium, where it becomes concentrated (Carson and Strom, 1988; Rubin and Papich, 1990; Isaacs, 1996). Aspirin inhibits oxidative phosphorylation of the gastric mucosal epithelium, thus decreasing ATP production and Na^+/K^+ movement across the cell membrane and producing cell swelling and necrosis (Rubin and Papich, 1990). Disruption of ion transport allows increased H^+ ion back-diffusion into the mucosa. Injury can extend into submucosal capillaries, leading to hemorrhage, inflammation, and ulceration. IV dosing of cats produced gastric erosions and ulcers, confirming that there is also a role for COX inhibition and reduced PG synthesis in the pathophysiology of gastric mucosal damage (Villar et al., 1998).

Aspirin uncouples oxidative phosphorylation, as noted above. Aspirin allows penetration of H^+ across the mitochondrial membrane, thus disrupting the proton gradient. The result is inhibition of the enzyme ATP synthetase. Energy that would go into ATP production is dissipated as heat. When oxidative phosphorylation is uncoupled systemically, the result is elevated body temperature (Roder, 2004a).

Salicylates can produce acidosis and increase the anion gap. Salicylate and metabolites thereof increase the anion gap directly (Schubert, 1984; Kore, 1990). Anaerobic metabolism compensates for the reduced ATP production when oxidative phosphorylation is inhibited, producing metabolites such as lactic acid, pyruvic acid, and ketones, thus contributing to acidosis. Aspirin is also believed to directly stimulate respiratory centers in the CNS, causing hyperventilation and respiratory alkalosis and promoting renal secretion of bicarbonate (Kore, 1990; Boothe, 2001). Later in the progression of the toxicosis, CNS suppression can decrease the respiratory rate, also contributing to acidosis.

Clinical Signs

Similar to other NSAIDs, gastric irritation is the most common side effect of aspirin. Vomiting, gastric ulceration, and hemorrhage are often observed. Depression is also reported in aspirin toxicosis in dogs and cats (Kore, 1990; Jones et al., 1992). Profound depression has been reported in dogs given high doses of aspirin. Affected dogs have sometimes collapsed or appeared too weak to stand. Restlessness progressing to tremors, seizures and, eventually, coma has been observed in dogs (Kore, 1990). One dog had a progressive increase in seizure duration from 5 to 45 min (Schubert, 1984). Seizures and coma have also been observed in cats (Jones et al., 1992; Isaacs, 1996). Seizures have been attributed to hypoventilation, acidosis, and hypoglycemia. Aspirin toxicosis can cause hyperthermia in children and cats. There can be an initial hyperpnea in acute aspirin toxicosis due to stimulation of respiratory centers.

Clinical Chemistry and Postmortem Findings

Metabolic acidosis and increased anion gap have been noted in acute aspirin toxicosis (Roder, 2004a). Bone marrow suppression can cause anemia in cats (Kore, 1990; McKellar et al., 1991). Other changes are similar to those described with other NSAIDs. Lesions similar to other NSAIDs are expected on necropsy. Gastric mucosal lesions have been documented in the pyloric antrum, body, and cardiac region of the stomach of dogs (Boulay et al., 1986).

Management

Diagnosis and treatment of salicylate toxicosis is similar to that described above for NSAIDs. Urine and plasma testing is available at many veterinary and hospital laboratories, but there is a poor correlation between plasma salicylate concentrations and clinical signs (Talcott, 2006). The presence of salicylate in horse urine is expected, even in horses not given aspirin, and is, therefore, not a significant finding (Boothe, 2001).

Salicylates can inhibit gastric emptying, and gastrointestinal absorption is prolonged with enteric-coated tablets; therefore, gastric lavage is sometimes useful up to 12 h after exposure. Activated charcoal is most useful within 2 h of aspirin ingestion. Cathartic use does not appear to decrease absorption.

Forced alkaline diuresis is more useful for aspirin than for other NSAIDs, and is frequently used by physicians. High urinary pH promotes salicylate elimination by trapping the ionic form in the urine. Alkaline peritoneal dialysis has been recommended for large overdoses (Davis, 1980; Kore, 1990). Acetazolamide, a carbonic anhydrase inhibitor, can be used to alkalinize urine, but will exacerbate metabolic acidosis. Acid–base status must be closely monitored in any animal undergoing alkaline diuresis. Monitoring and supportive care for changes in hydration, electrolyte balance, and body temperature are warranted. Clearly, use of NSAIDs to treat hyperthermia must be avoided. Diazepam can be used for seizure management.

COLD, COUGH AND ALLERGY MEDICATIONS

Medications for the symptomatic relief of cold, flu, and allergies are common, and can contain multiple active ingredients, including analgesics, decongestants, antihistamines, antitussives, and expectorants. Other possible ingredients include ethanol, caffeine, xylitol, and benzocaine. These medications can come in a variety of forms, including oral tablets, extended-release tablets, dissolving granules/tablets, lozenges, and as syrup (liquid).

Dextromethorphan is a centrally active antitussive. Structurally similar to opioids, it acts on the medullary cough center and directly suppresses its activity. Due to its dissociative effects at high doses, illicit use of dextromethorphan as a recreational drug has been reported (Romanelli, 2009). This effect is similar to those of ketamine and phencyclidine, which are both controlled substances discussed in an upcoming chapter. However, dextromethorphan toxicoses are rare in small animals, sedation being the most common effect, and respiratory suppression is unlikely. If an animal is overdosed with dextromethorphan, activated charcoal can be given early. Treatment consists of observation and supportive and symptomatic care as needed.

Guaifenesin, or glyceryl guaiacolate, is the most common expectorant or mucolytic agent. It is used in veterinary medicine as a sedative and muscle relaxant at high parental doses as an adjunct to anesthesia or for seizure controlling. Mild decreases in blood pressure, increases in heart rate, and thrombophlebitis are possible side effects of parental exposures (Plumb, 2015). However, guaifenesin is present in relatively small concentrations in OTC products, and oral exposure will most likely cause only minimal effects such as vomiting and gastritis. Treatment for guaifenesin overdose would include early routine detoxification (emesis is likely to be contraindicated), and symptomatic and supportive care (Papich, 1990).

Decongestants

Decongestants can be largely divided into sympathomimetic amines such as pseudoephedrine, ephedrine, phenylephrine, and phenylpropanolamine (PPA), and imidazolines such as oxymetazoline, xylometazoline, and tetrahydrozoline. Sympathomimetic amines and imidazolines are used as decongestants because of their vasoconstriction effects.

Among these, pseudoephedrine is the most common decongestant associated with toxicosis in small animals, more often dogs than cats (Papich, 1990). Pseudoephedrine has been commonly used in cold and allergy preparations, but due to its illicit use in the manufacture of methamphetamine, many US states now regulate its sale. Pseudoephedrine is a stereoisomer of the plant alkaloid ephedrine. Ephedrine is found in *Ephedra* spp. and *Sida cordifolia*. *Ephedra* spp. are used to produce ma huang, an herbal drug used in asthma, allergy, and cold formulations, diet pills, and in various supplements (Means, 1999, 2005; Ooms and Khan, 2001). Phenylephrine is found in nasal sprays and hemorrhoid creams.

PPA was commonly available, both OTC and by prescription, in diet pills, cold and allergy products, and, currently, to treat urinary incontinence in dogs (Papich, 1990; Means, 2005). FDA issued a public health advisory in November 2000 due to increased risk of hemorrhagic stroke associated with the use of PPA in humans (Cantu, 2003). Following the advisory, it was voluntarily withdrawn from the market for human use in the United States. Although cardiotoxic effects have been reported in dogs by accidental ingestion (Crandell and Ware, 2005), PPA is still available as a veterinary prescription drug for the control of urinary incontinence in dogs.

Imidazolines are commonly used in OTC eye drops and nasal sprays. Oxymetazoline is found in nasal sprays as a topical decongestant as treatment for allergic rhinitis and epistaxis, as well as in eye drops (marketed as Visine LR).

Sympathomimetic amines can interact with digoxin, MAO inhibitors, halothane, and methylxanthines (Means, 1999, 2005; Ooms and Khan, 2001). Certain conditions are known to predispose animals to adverse reactions when given sympathomimetic amines. These include diabetes, hypothyroidism, hyperthyroidism, cardiac disease, hypertension, seizure disorders, renal disease, and glaucoma.

Toxicity

Pseudoephedrine is used as a treatment for urinary incontinence in dogs because it improves urethral sphincter. The dose is usually 1–2 mg every 12 h (Means, 2005). Clinical toxicosis has been reported in dogs given 5–6 mg/kg, and death was documented in dogs given 10–12 mg/kg (Means, 1999, 2005; Ooms and Khan, 2001).

Drugs containing ephedrine, in the form of ma huang, are often combined with caffeine, in the form of guarana. This combination of drugs acts synergistically, enhancing the toxicity of this product. Doses of 1.3–88.9 mg/kg ma huang given concurrently with 4.4–296.2 mg/kg guarana have been associated with clinical toxicosis in dogs. One dog given a dose of 5.8 mg/kg ma huang and 19.1 mg/kg guarana died. There seems to be great individual difference in sensitivity to this combination of drugs, and prognosis is also dependent on the time that elapses between exposure and treatment (Ooms and Khan, 2001).

The therapeutic dose of PPA for urinary incontinence in dogs is 1.1 mg/kg (Crandell and Ware, 2005; Means, 2005). Clinical signs of irritability, tachycardia, hypertension, and urinary retention have been observed at the therapeutic dose (Ginn et al., 2013). Elevated blood pressure was seen in beagles given 3.1 mg/kg PO every 8 h, and myocardial damage was noted in a dog given 48 mg/kg.

Pharmacokinetics

Decongestants are rapidly absorbed by the gastrointestinal tract (Papich, 1990; Means, 2005). Ephedrine is absorbed within 2 h of ingestion (Ooms and Khan, 2001). The onset of action is usually within 30 min, although it is delayed up to 8 h with extended-release products. Sympathomimetic amines are believed to cross the blood–brain barrier (BBB) and the placenta, and are known to be secreted into milk. Metabolism occurs primarily in the liver. Most of a dose of ephedrine is excreted unchanged in the urine, and other decongestants are excreted 55%–75% as the parent compound. The elimination half-life of pseudoephedrine is 2–21 h; 2–4 h for PPA. Urinary excretion is accelerated with low urine pH (Ooms and Khan, 2001; Means, 2005).

Mechanism of Action

Adrenergic stimulation is responsible for the effects produced by decongestants (Papich, 1990; Means, 1999, 2005; Ooms and Khan, 2001; Crandell and Ware, 2005). Stimulation of α-1 receptors causes vasoconstriction and subsequent drying of the mucous membranes of the nasal mucosa and sinuses. Ophthalmic solutions decrease eye redness by constriction of conjunctival and scleral vasculature. Peripheral vasoconstriction leads to increased systemic vascular resistance and hypertension. Stimulation of the α-1 receptor can cause vasospasm of the coronary artery and myocardial necrosis. Other α-adrenergic effects may include appetite suppression, CNS stimulation, and mydriasis. The effects of phenylephrine and oxymetazoline are α-receptor-specific. Stimulation of α-receptors by PPA causes release of endogenous catecholamines in the brain and heart, and can inhibit MAO at high doses. Stimulation of β-receptors is the cause of some of the cardiac effects attributed to decongestants, which include increased contractility and output, increased heart rate, and tachyarrhythmia. Reflex bradycardia is possible. Bronchodilation is also mediated through β-receptors.

Clinical Signs

CNS stimulation is the common presentation for animals with decongestant overdose. Hyperactivity, restlessness, agitation, pacing, and vocalization are reported (Papich, 1990; Means, 1999, 2005). Hallucinatory behaviors in dogs include staring into a corner or at unseen objects, perhaps even biting at them. Tremors, seizures, and head-bobbing can be observed. Hyperthermia can be secondary to increased activity, and DIC or rhabdomyolysis with associated renal failure are possible outcomes. Cardiovascular changes include tachycardia, reflex bradycardia, and hypertension. Blood pressure can remain elevated in dogs for 6 h. Animals can die from cardiovascular collapse. Vomiting, diarrhea, dehydration, and anorexia were reported in one dog with PPA toxicosis, along with ataxia, lethargy, tachycardia, and tachypnea. Pupils were bilaterally dilated with loss of pupillary light reflex and vertical nystagmus. This dog was not hypertensive at presentation to the veterinarian 12 h after ingestion (Crandell and Ware, 2005). Another dog was treated for hypertension and tachycardia after ingesting a dose of PPA greater than 50 mg/kg (Ginn et al., 2013). The dog had a markedly elevated creatinine kinase indicating muscle damage, and cardiac troponin 1 indicating myocardial damage, hypertensive retinopathy, retinal detachment, and developed oral mucosal ulcers during hospitalization, which resolved after recovery.

Ooms and Khan (2001) studied dogs accidentally overdosed with a combination of ma huang and guarana herbal preparations, and found that the onset of clinical signs could be as early as 30 min after ingestion, and was usually within 8 h. Duration of signs ranged from 10 to 48 h. Vomiting was seen in 47% of dogs, 5% were anorexic, 30% were tachycardic, 6% were tachypneic, 21% had mydriasis, 27% had tremors, 6% had behavioral changes such as snapping, pacing, and head shaking, 6% had seizures, 5% had depression, 5% were weak, and 5% were apprehensive. Hyperthermia was reported in 28% of these dogs.

Clinical Chemistry

Hypokalemia, hyperglycemia, and hyperinsulinemia are usually reported in dogs with decongestant toxicosis (Means, 1999, 2005). Changes reported in a dog that had ingested PPA included hypoglycemia, mild hyperbilirubiemia, and elevated ALT, ALP, BUN, creatinine, and CK. Blood pH and calcium concentrations were elevated. Polycythemia and thrombocytopenia were noted. A urine sample contained blood, hemoglobin or myoglobin, and protein. Elevated serum cardiac troponin concentrations indicate myocardial damage (Crandell and Ware, 2005; Ginn et al., 2013).

Diagnosis and Management

Diagnosis of decongestant toxicosis is usually based on history and clinical signs. Some laboratories are able to test for pseudoephedrine, ephedrine, and PPA in plasma or urine to confirm exposure, but it takes hours or days for results to be available. Treatment must be initiated in the poisoning case before analytical results are available.

Treatment consists of detoxification, symptomatic, and supportive care. Emetics use is contraindicated in dogs with central nervous system signs due to the potential for aspiration. Gastric lavage can be performed in the stabilized, anesthetized, and intubated patient after a large ingestion. Activated charcoal and cathartic have been recommended. Blood pressure, ECG, and body temperature should be monitored closely, and CBC, serum chemistry, and acid–base status should be monitored every day or so. Cardiac troponin can be measured to diagnose myocardial damage.

Tachycardia is treated with β-blockers. Propranolol can be administered at a dose of 0.02–0.06 mg/kg slowly by IV (Means, 1999, 2005; Ooms and Khan, 2001). Propranolol therapy will help to stabilize hypokalemia. Alternately, lidocaine has been used at a dose of 2 mg/kg IV by intermittent bolus or by continuous infusion at a rate of 80 μg/kg/min (Crandell and Ware, 2005). Crandell and Ware (2005) recommend atenolol at 0.2 mg/kg every 12 h and enalapril 0.5 mg/kg every 12 h, both given orally, to support myocardial function for PPA toxicosis. Ginn et al. (2013) used a combination of drugs, including esmolol, via bolus (2 μg/kg IV) and continuous rate infusion (30 μg/kg/min), in addition to aggressive supportive care in a dog that ingested a large dose of PPA. Papich (1990) recommend atropine at a dose of 0.04 mg/kg SC or IV. High peripheral vascular resistance and hypertension are relieved with α-adrenergic receptor-blocking agents. Prazosin can be given at 1–2 mg every 8 h or phentolamine can be given at 0.1 mg/kg IV as needed (Papich, 1990; Ooms and Khan, 2001).

Severe CNS stimulation sometimes requires treatment with more than one anticonvulsant. Acepromazine can be used to treat pseudoephedrine, ephedrine, or PPA toxicosis. Acepromazine is given at a dose of 0.05–1.0 mg/kg IM, IV or SC, starting with a low dose and adding more as needed. Alternately, chlorpromazine is given IM or IV at a dose of 0.5–1.0 mg/kg, starting with a low dose and increasing as needed. If needed, phenobarbital can be given for refractory seizures at a starting dose of 3 mg/kg to effect (Means, 1999, 2005). Isoflurane anesthesia has been recommended to control severe clinical signs (Ooms and Khan, 2001). Use of benzodiazepines is considered contraindicated because the dissociative effects of this drug class can exacerbate clinical signs of sympathomimetic amines.

Fluid therapy and cautious urinary acidification helps promote excretion (Ooms and Khan, 2001; Means, 2005). Urinary acidifiers enhance excretion of pseudoephedrine in humans, and may be used in dogs, but acid–base status must be monitored closely. The dose for ascorbic acid is 20–30 mg/kg IM or IV every 8 h. Ammonium chloride is given 50 mg/kg PO every 6 h. Glucose is added to intravenous fluids to treat hypoglycemia. Overhydration must be avoided to prevent pulmonary edema in the hypertensive patient.

Adverse clinical signs associated with decongestants can last for 72 h or more (Means, 2005). One dog with severe clinical signs after PPA ingestion required 6 days of hospitalization (Crandell and Ware, 2005); most animals respond to treatment more rapidly. Clinical signs that have been associated with an unfavorable outcome include uncontrollable seizures, DIC, myoglobinuria, and head-bobbing. Ooms and Khan (2001) report that 26 out of 34 dogs recovered with treatment, usually within 10–48 h after ingestion of a ma huang and guarana combination drug. The remaining eight dogs died or were euthanized.

Antihistamines

Antihistamines act by competitive inhibition of histamine at histamine receptors. Compounds referred to as antihistamines in this section are the H_1 histamine receptor antagonists. H_2 histamine receptor antagonists are also sold over the counter, and are covered later, with drugs affecting the gastrointestinal system. They will be referred to as H_2 histamine receptor antagonists (or H_2-blockers).

Many antihistamines, including brompheniramine, chlorpheniramine, clemastine, diphenhydramine, loratadine, and triprolidine, are found in allergy, cold, and flu formulations. Others, such as dimenhydrinate and meclizine, are used as antiemetics to treat motion sickness. Doxylamine is used as a sedative in sleep aids. Hydroxyzine is used by veterinarians to treat canine atopy (Tegzes et al., 2002). Malicious poisoning with diphenhydramine has been reported in a dog (Buchweitz et al., 2014).

Toxicity

An incomplete list of antihistamines is provided in Table 21.3. Chlorpheniramine is the antihistamine most commonly associated with adverse effects in dogs (Papich, 1990; Gwaltney-Brant, 2004). The IV LD_{50} for diphenhydramine is 24–30 mg/kg in dogs, and the human minimum oral lethal dose is about 10 mg/kg. The oral LD_{50} for clemastine in dogs is 175 mg/kg. The therapeutic dose for hydroxyzine is 2.2 mg/kg, and 111 mg/kg is reported as toxic in dogs (Tegzes et al., 2002). Terfenadine, which is no longer sold in the United States, caused clinical signs of toxicosis in a dog at a dose of 6.6 mg/kg (Otto and Greentree, 1994; Gwaltney-Brant, 2004). Electroencephalogram changes were noted in dogs dosed with 30 mg terfenadine/kg, clinical signs were noted in dogs given in 100 mg/kg/day for 2–3 weeks, and vomiting was a consistent finding in dogs dosed with 150 mg/kg.

Pharmacokinetics

Antihistamines are well-absorbed by the monogastric gastrointestinal tract, but oral doses are poorly absorbed in ruminants (Adams, 2001; Gwaltney-Brant, 2004). The anticholinergic effects of antihistamines can slow absorption by delaying gastric emptying. Peak plasma concentrations usually occur within 2–4 h of ingestion, and the onset of clinical effects tends to be 20–45 min after ingestion. Therapeutic effects usually last from 3 to 12 h. Antihistamines are highly protein-bound. First-generation antihistamines freely cross the BBB, and are more likely to cause CNS effects than second-generation products, which do not normally enter the CNS, unless given at very high doses. Terfenadine has been detected in cerebrospinal fluid in overdose situations (Otto and Greentree, 1994).

Metabolism of antihistamines takes place predominantly in the liver, and there can be significant first-pass effect. Only 40%–60% of diphenhydramine enters the general circulation from the portal circulation in humans. Hydroxyzine is metabolized to the active product cetirizine, which does not cross the BBB. The elimination half-life of antihistamines is dependent upon the individual compound. Most metabolites are excreted in the urine, although there is some biliary excretion of terfenadine. Antihistamines excreted into the bile can undergo enterohepatic cycling.

TABLE 21.3 Antihistamines (H_1 Histamine Receptor Inhibitors) See Gwaltney-Brant (2006) for more detailed information

First Generation	Second Generation
Alkylamines	**Piperadines**
Brompheniramine	Terfenadine
Chlorpheniramine	Astemizole
Dexbrompheniramine	Levocabastine
Dexchlorpheniramine	Loratadine
Dimetindene	
Pheniramine	**Third Generation**
Triprolidine	Desloratadine
Ethanolamines	Fexofenadine
Clemastine	Levocetirizine
Dimenhydrinate	
Diphenhydramine	
Bromodiphenhydramine	
Carbinoxamine	
Doxylamine	
Phenyltoloxamine	
Ethylenediamines	
Antazoline	
Pyrilamine	
Tripelennamine	
Phenothiazines	
Methdilazine	
Trimeprazine	
Piperazines	
Hydroxyzine	
Cyproheptadine	
Meclozine	
Cyclizine	
Buclizine	
Chlorcyclizine	
Niaprazine	
Certirizine	
Tricyclics	
Promethazine	

Mechanism of Action

Antihistamines act by competitive inhibition of histamine at H_1 receptors (Papich, 1990; Gwaltney-Brant, 2004). Binding is reversible, but can become irreversible or slow to dissociate at high doses, as with terfenadine (Otto and Greentree, 1994; Gwaltney-Brant, 2004). H_1 receptors are found in a variety of tissues, including the mast cells of the skin, the smooth muscle of airways, gastrointestinal tract, urogenital tract, and cardiovascular system, the endothelial cells and lymphocytes, and the mammalian CNS. Histamine produces dermal itching and allergic responses in the skin and contraction of smooth muscle in the bronchial tree and intestine. Low doses of histamine produce a rapid onset of vascular dilation. The wheal-and-flair reaction associated with histamine release is due to increased vascular permeability. Histamine in the CNS modulates sleep/wake cycles.

Antihistamines are used to block allergic response and reduce itching. Antihistamines block smooth muscle contraction, reducing bronchoconstriction, and affecting vascular and uterine smooth muscle. Effects on intestinal smooth muscle can cause gastrointestinal disturbances. Antihistamines also prevent increased vascular permeability associated with histamine release. CNS effects produced by antihistamines can include sedation or excitement.

Muscarinic stimulation is believed to be involved in motion sickness-induced vomiting. The antimuscarinic actions of antihistamines decrease nausea and vomiting (Papich, 1990). Gastrointestinal motility is decreased, and respiratory suppression is sometimes seen with antihistamines. Phenothiazine-type antihistamines also block α-adrenergic receptors. Allergic reactions to antihistamines have been noted.

Clinical Signs

Clinical signs of antihistamine overdose are usually evident within 30 min of dosing. Signs of CNS depression can occur with therapeutic doses of first-generation antihistamines, and include sedation, ataxia, and drowsiness. More severe clinical signs, such as profound depression, coma, respiratory suppression, convulsions, and myocardial depression, can lead to death (Buchweitz et al., 2014). A dog with hydroxyzine toxicosis presented with tachycardia and weakness progressing to stupor, coma, loss of gag reflex, and apnea (Tegzes et al., 2002). Higher doses of antihistamines can have a stimulatory effect on the CNS, particularly in children and young animals. These effects are less common in adults. Overdosed young individuals appear to experience hallucinations, lack of coordination, disorientation, irritability, anxiety, aggression, seizures, and pyrexia.

Salivation, vomiting, and diarrhea have been associated with first-generation antihistamines. Anticholinergic effects include dry mucous membranes, fixed and dilated pupils, tachycardia, and arrhythmia, and animals can be either hypertensive or hypotensive. Cardiac abnormalities were documented in humans and dogs that ingested terfenadine (Otto and Greentree, 1994; Gwaltney-Brant, 2004). Animals can have allergic reactions to topical or oral antihistamines. A list of associated clinical signs includes dermatitis, pyrexia, and photosensitization (Gwaltney-Brant, 2004). Teratogenic effects have been detected in experimental animals treated with piperazine.

Metabolic acidosis and electrolyte abnormalities have been documented based on serum chemistry of antihistamine-overdosed animals, but overall changes are nonspecific. Changes reported on postmortem examination also tend to be nonspecific. Rhabdomyolysis, and associated renal lesions, or DIC are possible complications of antihistamine toxicosis.

Management

Diagnosis of antihistamine toxicosis is usually based on history and clinical signs. Laboratory testing of urine or plasma can be helpful to confirm exposure, but results will be delayed for hours or days, and quantitation is unlikely to be of value.

Emetics are appropriate to promote gastric emptying in asymptomatic animals after large, recent ingestions of antihistamines, but caution is advised because onset of clinical signs can be rapid. Gastric lavage of the anesthetized, intubated animal is more appropriate in symptomatic patients. Activated charcoal and a cathartic can be instilled after lavage, or given to the stable patient. Multiple doses of activated charcoal have been recommended to interrupt enterohepatic cycling.

Drugs such as penicillin G and NSAIDs have been recommended to reduce protein binding and enhance excretion (Tegzes et al., 2002). However, in the short term, this can worsen clinical signs.

Serum chemistry should be assessed and monitored for hydration, electrolyte balance, acid–base status, and liver and kidney function. Animals with poor hepatic or renal function can eliminate antihistamine more slowly (Gwaltney-Brant, 2004). Cardiac function, blood pressure, and body temperature should be monitored, and respiratory function should be closely monitored, because intubation is sometimes required to support the comatose patient.

Fluid therapy is useful to maintain hydration for cardiac support, diuresis, and correction of pH and electrolyte imbalances. Animals rarely require treatment for hypotension or mild-to-moderate cardiac arrhythmias, which usually respond to fluid therapy. Epinephrine should not be used in promethazine overdose (Staley and Staley, 1995). Promethazine inhibits adrenergic receptors, and addition of epinephrine can lead to further decrease in blood pressure. Atropine can potentiate the anticholinergic effects of antihistamines, and is best avoided.

Seizures can be treated cautiously with benzodiazepines or short-acting barbiturates. The depressive effects of antihistamines are additive with these sedatives, and can produce "rebound depression." Although cholinergic signs are sometimes present, treatment with physostigmine potentiates cardiovascular dysfunction and seizures, and is contraindicated.

Animals overdosed with antihistamines usually improve within 24 h, although signs sometimes persist for up to 3 days. Prognosis is dependent on the severity of signs, and is guarded in animals presenting with seizures or coma (Gwaltney-Brant, 2004). Tegzes et al. (2002) report recovery of a comatose dog due to hydroxyzine overdose, though the authors note that supportive care can be required for up to 2 weeks.

DRUGS USED TO TREAT GASTROINTESTINAL SYMPTOMS

This classification includes antacids, laxatives, and antidiarrheal drugs.

Antacids

H_2 histamine receptor antagonists and mineral antacids are used to increase gastric pH and reduce discomfort. Use of these products to aide in healing of gastroduodenal ulcers secondary to NSAID use is noted in a previous section. Few adverse effects have been reported with these drugs, although contact dermatitis in a horse trainer associated with ranitidine has been reported (Meani and Nixon, 2015).

H_2 Histamine Receptor Antagonists

H_2 histamine receptor antagonists include cimetidine, famotidine, nizatidine, and ranitidine. Cimetidine impairs gastrointestinal absorption of some drugs and prolongs the effects of others by inhibiting their metabolism by microsomal enzymes.

Pharmacokinetics

Cimetidine is rapidly absorbed, and 70% of a given dose is bioavailable. Absorption can be slowed by the presence of food in the stomach. The mean absorption time for ranitidine was reported as approximately 1 h, and absorption was not impaired by the presence of food in the stomach. Ranitidine is 73% bioavailable in dogs and 27% available in horses after oral dosing. Famotidine is poorly absorbed and only 37% bioavailable. Nizatidine is rapidly and almost completely absorbed (Boothe, 2001). H_2 receptor antagonists (or H_2-blockers) are less lipid soluble than H_1 receptor antagonists (or H_1-blockers) and less likely to cross the BBB. Ranitidine is about 15% protein-bound.

Cimetidine and ranitidine are metabolized predominantly in the liver. Seventy-three percent of an oral dose of ranitidine undergoes hepatic metabolism in people, compared to 40% in dogs. Unchanged cimetidine, famotidine, and nizatidine are excreted in the urine. The plasma half-life for cimetidine is about 1 h, but can be prolonged in individuals with renal or hepatic insufficiency. The elimination half-life of ranitidine is 2.5 h in humans and 4 h in beagles (Boothe, 2001).

Mechanism of Action

H_2 receptor antagonists specifically bind to and block the actions of H_2 receptors by competitive inhibition. H_2 receptors are present in the enterochromaffin cells of the gastric mucosa. Histamine stimulates acid secretion and, to a limited extent, pepsin secretion (Adams, 2001; Tegzes et al., 2002). High doses of histamine produce a slow-onset, prolonged vasodilatory response. H_2 receptor inhibitors decrease acid and pepsin secretion. They also block some of the cardiovascular effects of histamine (Adams, 2001). Famotidine is nine times more potent as an H_2-blocker than ranitidine, which is 5–12 times more potent than cimetidine. Famotidine also has the longest duration of clinical effects (Boothe, 2001). Cimetidine reduces hepatic blood flow by around 20% and inhibits microsomal cytochrome P450 enzymes, thus it interferes with metabolism of other drugs.

Clinical Signs

There are no reports of adverse effects in domestic animals associated with these H_2 receptor antagonists.

Mineral Antacids

An incomplete list of active ingredients in mineral antacids can be found in Table 21.4. Products may contain more than one active ingredient. These products are common in many households, and may be accidentally ingested by pets or administered by pet owners. They are used in veterinary medicine to decrease gastric hyperacidity and treat peptic ulcers, uremic ulcers, reflux esophagitis, and rumen acidosis secondary to grain overload (Boothe, 2001). Few adverse effects are associated with mineral antacids (Papich, 1990). Mineral antacids increase gastric pH. Rebound acid secretion can occur when dosing is discontinued.

Sodium bicarbonate is present in baking soda and in effervescent antacid products. Sodium bicarbonate and calcium carbonate are absorbed after ingestion. Transcutaneous absorption of sodium bicarbonate across damaged skin can occur (Gonzalez and Hogg, 1981). Carbon dioxide is produced rapidly when sodium bicarbonate is introduced to an

TABLE 21.4 An Incomplete List of Mineral Antacids

Aluminum Salts
Aluminum hydroxide
Aluminum magnesium silicate
Aluminum phosphate
Magnesium Salts
Magnesium hydroxide
Magnesium oxide
Magnesium silicate
Others
Calcium carbonate
Sodium bicarbonate

TABLE 21.5 Irritant Cathartics

Diphenylmethanes
Phenolphthalein
Bisacodyl
Vegetable Oils
Castor oil
Raw linseed oil
Olive oil
Anthraquinones
Cascara sagrada
Senna
Aloin

acid, and this reaction may cause gastric distension (Boothe, 2001). Chronic use of calcium carbonate antacids can produce metabolic acidosis, hypercalcemia, hypophosphatemia, and calciuria with urolithiasis and metastatic calcification (Fitzgibbons and Snoey, 1999; Boothe, 2001).

Some of the magnesium in magnesium salt-containing antacids are absorbed, and hypermagnesemia has been reported with repeated dosing (Boothe, 2001). Magnesium-containing salts have a laxative effect, and aluminum-containing salts have a constipating effect, and these active ingredients are often used in combination. Aluminum complexes phosphate in the intestine and aluminum hydroxide has been used to decrease phosphate absorption in patients with renal disease (Segev et al., 2008).

Laxatives, Cathartics and Enemas

Drugs in this category are designated as bulk-forming laxatives, lubricant laxatives, irritant laxatives, hyperosmotic cathartics, or enemas.

Bulk-Forming Laxatives

Nonabsorbable polysaccharide cellulose derivatives are used as bulk-forming laxatives. Natural sources include psyllium or plantago seed, wheat bran, and fruits such as prunes. Synthetic forms include methylcellulose and carboxymethylcellulose. These products act by absorbing water in the gastrointestinal tract, swelling, and softening fecal mass, resulting in intestinal distension and reflex peristaltic contractions. Intestinal bacteria act on cellulose and hemicellulose, and produce volatile fatty acids, enhancing the osmotic effect; fluid feces and tympany can result (Boothe, 2001). No serious adverse effects have been reported in companion animals, although these products cause fluid and electrolyte loss secondary to diarrhea. Papich (1990) suggests that subsequent dehydration can lead to intestinal impaction. Animals treated with bulk-forming laxatives should have fresh water available. If diarrhea occurs, monitor hydration and electrolyte status and correct as needed.

Lubricant Laxatives

Lubricant laxatives, including mineral oil and white petrolatum, are hydrocarbon mixtures derived from petroleum. Mineral oil is frequently used in large animals, and white petrolatum products are used to treat trichobezoars in cats (Papich, 1990). These large hydrocarbons are minimally absorbed, and act by coating feces with a film that entraps moisture and lubricates the passage. Hydrocarbon laxatives reduce absorption of fat-soluble vitamins and possibly other nutrients; thus, chronic use can produce deficiencies. The small amount of absorbed hydrocarbons can provide a nidus for granuloma formation in the intestinal mucosa, mesenteric lymph nodes, or liver. Adverse effects, however, are rarely reported with lubricant laxatives.

Irritant Laxatives

Table 21.5 lists common types of irritant laxative. Phenolphthalein laxatives are often chocolate flavored to increase palatability, but are reportedly only effective in primates and swine (Boothe, 2001). Bisacodyl is structurally similar to phenolphthalein. Some vegetable oil products contain irritant fatty acids such as ricinoleic acid in castor oil, linoleates in linseed oil, and oliveates in olive oil. Common anthraquinone-type cathartics are derived from plants: cascara sagrada from *Rhamnus* spp., senna from *Senna* spp., and aloin from *Aloe* spp. Danthron

(1,8-dihydroxyanthroquinone) is a synthetic anthraquinone drug.

Five percent of an oral dose of bisacodyl is absorbed. There is some absorption of anthraquinone glycosides, and delayed transit through the small intestine decreases effectiveness. Anthraquinones are secreted in the milk, causing clinical effects in the nursing young (Boothe, 2001).

As suggested by the term "irritant laxative," these compounds cause contact irritation of gastrointestinal mucosa and increase fluid secretion into the lumen. Diarrhea occurs 6–8 h after diphenylmethane cathartics are administered, and can be severe after large doses (Boothe, 2001). Pink discoloration of alkaline urine can be used to confirm phenolphthalein ingestion. Acidic urine will turn pink with addition of sodium hydroxide or sodium bicarbonate (Papich, 1990).

Vegetable oil laxatives are hydrolyzed by lipase in the small intestine and form sodium and potassium salts, which act as soaps, producing irritation (Boothe, 2001). Ricinoleic acid is the most potent of these compounds, and initiates rapid and complete colonic emptying. This clinical effect is seen 4–8 h after administration of castor oil in small animals and 12–18 h postdosing in large animals. Animals treated with castor oil should be fed moist, bulky material afterward.

Anthraquinones are hydrolyzed by bacteria in the large intestine to emodins, which stimulate the myenteric plexus. Anthraquinones produce catharsis after 6–12 h in small animals and 12–36 h in large animals (Boothe, 2001). Catharsis is accompanied by reduced hydration and electrolyte loss. Abdominal pain or colic is produced by large doses. Changes in urine color have been reported with anthraquinones. With chronic use of these laxatives, the myenteric plexus degenerates, causing a loss in intestinal motility.

Hyperosmotic Cathartics

Magnesium sulfate, or Epsom salt, is commonly used as an osmotic cathartic in 6% isotonic solution. Other magnesium-containing cathartics include magnesium hydroxide (milk of magnesia), magnesium oxide, and magnesium citrate. Sodium sulfate (Glauber's salt), sodium phosphate, potassium sodium tartrate, and sodium tartrate (Rochelle salt) are used as cathartics, and ingestion of large quantities of sodium chloride also produces catharsis. The sugar alcohols mannitol and sorbitol, and synthetic disaccharides such as lactulose, are also used as cathartics. Polyethylene glycol 3350 (PEG), once available only with prescription for whole-bowel irrigation before colonoscopy procedures and to treat body-packer patients (Farmer and Chan, 2003), is currently available over the counter (MiraLAX).

Osmotic cathartic use should be avoided in dehydrated animals, and water must be freely available. Other contraindications for use include congestive heart failure, gastrointestinal stasis, and hepatic or renal impairment (Henninger and Horst, 1997; Ezri et al., 2006). Hyperosmotic cathartics draw water into the intestinal tract via osmosis. Intestinal distension promotes motility. Effects are usually evident 3–12 h after dosing in monogastrics and within 18 h in ruminants.

There is minimal slow absorption of most cathartics, but up to 20% of the magnesium in a dose of magnesium sulfate is absorbed in the small intestine (Henninger and Horst, 1997; Boothe, 2001). Renal failure enhances systemic magnesium accumulation, leading eventually to hypermagnesemia. Magnesium ions promote the release of cholecystokinin, which promotes peristalsis. Systemic effects of magnesium include inhibition of calcium ion release at neuromuscular junctions, inhibition of acetylcholine release, decreased sensitivity of motor endplates, and decreased excitability of myocyte membranes, leading to paralysis. Clinical signs of hypermagnesemia secondary to magnesium sulfate administration in the horse occurred within 6 h of magnesium sulfate administration and included perspiration, progressive tremors, recumbence, severe tachycardia, tachypnea, pale mucous membranes, prolonged capillary refill times, flaccid paralysis of the head and neck, and loss of flexor and perineal reflexes, but horses remained alert.

Absorbed phosphate from phosphate-containing cathartics can deplete intracellular potassium ions and induce hypokalemia. Dehydration and electrolyte imbalances are the most common changes associated with cathartics (Papich, 1990). Management is aimed at correcting these imbalances. Calcium is used to treat hypermagnesemia. Calcium ions displace magnesium ions from cell membranes. Response to therapy is rapid, but repeated dosing with calcium gluconate is sometimes needed. Diuresis with IV fluids and furosemide promote renal excretion. Henninger and Horst (1997) reported that horses treated for hypermagnesemia had serum magnesium concentrations within reference ranges the next day. Electrolyte changes in asymptomatic patients given oral sodium phosphate for presurgical catharsis returned to normal within 24 h (Ezri et al., 2006).

Enemas

An enema is a material given intrarectally to induce defecation. Commonly used enemas include soft anionic soap in water, isotonic or hypertonic sodium chloride, sorbitol, glycerol, sodium lauryl sulfate, sulfoacetate, mineral oil, olive oil, and phosphate salts (Boothe, 2001).

Toxicosis has been reported in people and small animals administered hypertonic sodium phosphate solutions, or fleet enemas. Debilitated cats are commonly affected (Papich, 1990). Predisposing factors include administration of a full-strength fleet enema (intended for human use) to a small animal, dehydration, preexisting electrolyte abnormalities, renal or hepatic dysfunction, colonic dilatation, and colonic ulceration. A 60 mL hypertonic phosphate enema can cause toxicosis in a cat (Roder, 2004b). Toxicosis has also been reported in alpaca crias that were inadvertently given sodium phosphate enemas intravaginally (Bragg et al., 2010).

Sodium and phosphate are absorbed in the colon, and absorption is increased with disruption of the mucosa or in animals with chronic constipation (Jorgensen et al., 1985). Uptake of phosphate promotes cellular uptake of calcium, and phosphate can directly bind serum calcium, both contributing to hypocalcemia. Adverse effects associated with sodium phosphate enemas usually occur within 1 h of dosing. Vomiting and bloody diarrhea have been observed. Nervous signs that have been reported include depression, ataxia, anxiety, neuromuscular irritability, tremors, opisthotonus, and convulsions. Dehydration, weak pulses, tachycardia, hypothermia, shock, and death have also been observed. Serum chemistry in these patients often reveals hyperphosphatemia, hypernatremia, hypocalcemia, metabolic acidosis, and hyperglycemia. Hyperkalemia or hypokalemia can occur.

Intensive fluid therapy is required in acute sodium phosphate enema overdose situations. The purpose is to correct dehydration, electrolyte imbalances, acid–base imbalances, and hypoglycemia and to treat circulatory shock. Isotonic saline solution can increase renal calcium loss and, thus, should be avoided. Saline solutions containing 0.45% sodium chloride and 2.5% dextrose, or 2.5%–5.0% dextrose solutions, have been recommended for hypoglycemic patients. Lactated Ringers solution can be used in hyperglycemic patients. Fluid therapy may be required for up to 4 days. Jorgensen et al. (1985) suggested instillation of aluminum carbonate or aluminum hydroxide to bind phosphate in the intestine and maintain body temperature. Prophylactic antibiotics are given for compromise of the colonic mucosa. Intoxicated cats showed improvement within 6 h of initiation of therapy, and electrolyte imbalances resolved within 2 days.

Antidiarrheal Drugs

Active ingredients in products used to treat diarrhea include bismuth subsalicylate, kaolin–pectin, and opioid receptor agonists. Most of the toxic effects associated with bismuth subsalicylate are due to the salicylate component; therefore, this formulation is discussed in more detail with aspirin and salicylates. Bismuth is believed to adsorb bacterial endotoxin and have a direct antimicrobial effect. Bismuth does react with hydrogen sulfide to produce black crystals, and though minimally absorbed, chronic dosing was associated with discoloration of the kidneys in a rhesus monkey due to accumulation of black crystals in the renal tubular epithelium (Johnson et al., 2016).

Kaolin and pectin were previously the active ingredients in the popular OTC product Kaopectate, but bismuth subsalicylate is now used. Kaolin is hydrated aluminum silicate, and acts as an adsorbent. Pectin is a carbohydrate extracted from citrus fruit that acts as an adsorbent and intestinal protectant. Toxicosis attributed to kaolin–pectin preparations has not been observed, though these products are likely to decrease absorption of other drugs.

The OTC drug Imodium, and the prescription drug Lomotil, contain the opioid receptor agonists loperamide and diphenoxylate, respectively. Loperamide is sold in 2 mg capsules and 0.20 mg/mL liquid formulations. The effective dose for loperamide is 0.08 mL/kg PO every 12 h in small dogs and cats. These products are poorly absorbed, and function to decrease gastrointestinal secretion and motility. Side effects include constipation, abdominal pain, vomiting, and drowsiness. Collies and other dog breeds with a mutation in the *ABCB1* gene are believed to have increased susceptibility to loperamide (Sartor et al., 2004). Clinical signs in collies include salivation, weakness, ataxia, and disorientation. Management consists of monitoring and supportive and symptomatic care. Activated charcoal can be given to decrease intestinal absorption in the case of a large ingestion. Neuromuscular signs in one collie resolved about 1 day after the drug was discontinued (Sartor et al., 2004). The opioid antagonist naloxone can be used to manage severe clinical signs, but is usually unnecessary. Naloxone has a short half-life, requiring repeated dosing as needed (Papich, 1990).

TOPICAL DRUGS

Toxicosis secondary to topical preparations can occur through dermal absorption or ingestion. Cats, in particular, are fastidious groomers, thus any product that is used *on* a cat is likely to end up *in* the cat. Some animals, dogs in particular, have been known to chew through tubes containing topical drugs (Papich, 1990).

Like other OTC drugs, topical products frequently contain more than one active ingredient. Antibiotic preparations can contain bacitracin, neomycin, and polymyxin. These antimicrobials are poorly absorbed from the normal gastrointestinal tract, limiting their systemic effects (Papich, 1990). However, if large quantities are ingested, damage to the resident gastrointestinal microflora can lead to diarrhea and discomfort. Use of these products in hamsters or guinea pigs, which are predisposed to develop antibiotic-induced enterocolitis, should probably be avoided.

Benzoyl peroxide is present in some topical antiseptics and acne medications. It acts by releasing hydrogen peroxide, which has antibacterial and keratinolytic effects and promotes epithelial cell turnover. Hyperemia and blistering have been reported with overuse of benzoyl peroxide-containing products. Ingestion can lead to intragastrointestinal gas production and distension. Emetics are contraindicated if this should happen. Gastric decompression requires use of a stomach tube.

CONCLUDING REMARKS AND FUTURE DIRECTIONS

OTC drugs, which are widely available to consumers, encompass a large number of products, often contain multiple active ingredients, and have been developed for oral, topical, intraocular, intranasal, and intrarectal administration. Of the thousands of OTC drugs available, only a fraction were addressed in this chapter, including some analgesics, cold, flu, and allergy medications, and drugs used to treat gastrointestinal symptoms. Obtaining a thorough history is of great importance when dealing with suspect OTC drug-related problems. It is often helpful if the owner brings the drug container to the veterinarian as a source of information on the active ingredients, indications for use, and manufacturer identification, telephone number, or address. Treatment for most OTC drugs includes decontamination, stabilization, and symptomatic and supportive care with careful monitoring.

REFERENCES

Adams, R.H., 2001. Autocoids and anti-inflammatory drugs. In: Adams, R. (Ed.), Veterinary Pharmacology and Therapeutics, eighth ed. Iowa State University Press, Ames, IA, pp. 403–412.

Albretsen, J.C., 2002. Oral medications. Vet. Clin. N. Amer. Small Anim. 32, 421–442.

Allen, A.L., 2003. The diagnosis of acetaminophen toxicosis in a cat. Can. Vet. J. 44, 509–510.

Anonymous, F.D.A. Center for Veterinary Medicine, 2015. FDA warns of illnesses and deaths in pets exposed to prescription topical pain medications containing Flurbiprofen. <https://www.fda.gov/animal-veterinary/newsevents/cvmupdates/ucm443333.htm> (accessed 22.05.17.).

Aronson, L.R., Drobatz, K., 1996. Acetaminophen toxicosis in 17 cats. J. Vet. Emerg. Cri. Care. 6, 65–69.

Bautista, A.C., Moore, C.E., Lin, Y., et al., 2015. Hepatopathy following consumption of a commercially available blue-green algae dietary supplement in a dog. BMC Vet. Res. 11, 136.

Bersenas, A.M.E., Mathews, K.A., Allen, D.G., et al., 2005. Effects of ranitidine, famotidine, pantoprazoline, and omeprazole on intragastric pH in dogs. Am. J. Vet. Res. 66, 425.

Bolfer, L., McMichael, M., Ngwenyama, T.R., et al., 2014. Treatment of ibuprofen toxicosis in a dog with IV Lipid Emulsion. J. Am. Anim. Hosp. Assoc. 50, 136–140.

Boothe, D.M., 2001. The analgesic, antipyretic, anti-inflammatory drugs. In: Adams, R. (Ed.), In Veterinary Pharmacology and Therapeutics, eighth ed. Iowa State University Press, Ames, IA, pp. 433–451.

Borchers, A., Epstein, S.E., Gindiciosi, B., et al., 2014. Acute enteral manganese intoxication with hepatic failure due to ingestion of a joint supplement overdose. J. Vet. Diag. Invest. 26 (5), 658–663.

Boulay, J.P., Lipowitz, A.J., Klausner, J.S., 1986. Effects of cimetidine on aspirin-induced gastric hemorrhage in dogs. Am. J. Vet. Res. 47, 1744–1746.

Boynton, C.S., Dick, C.F., Mayor, G.F., 1988. NSAIDs: an overview. J. Clin. Pharmacol. 28, 512–517.

Bragg, R., Hackett, E.S., Callan, R.J., et al., 2010. Inadvertent transvaginal administration of sodium phosphate enemas in 2 alpaca crias. J. Vet. Emerg. Crit. Care. 60 (6), 623–627.

Brater, D.C., 1988. Clinical pharmacology of NSAIDs. J. Clin. Pharmacol. 28, 518–523.

Brix, A.E., 2002. Renal papillary necrosis. Toxicol. Pathol. 30, 672–674.

Brumbaugh, G.W., 2001. Adverse drug reactions and interactions in the horse. Vet. Clin. North Am. Equine Pract. 17, 445–453.

Buchweitz, J.P., Raverty, S.A., Johnson, M.B., et al., 2014. Fatal diphenhydramine poisoning in a dog. Can. Vet. J. 55, 1089–1092.

Cantu, C., Arauz, A., Murillo-Bonilla, L.M., et al., 2003. Stroke associated with sympathomimetics contained in over-the-counter cough and cold drugs. Stroke. 34, 1667–1672.

Carson, J.L., Strom, B.L., 1988. The gastrointestinal side effects of the nonsteroidal anti-inflammatory drugs. J. Clin. Pharmacol. 28, 554–559.

Cathers, A.T.E., Isaza, R., Oehme, F., 2000. Acute ibuprofen toxicosis in a ferret. J. Am. Vet. Med. Assoc. 216, 1246–1248.

Cheung, L.Y., Sonnenschein, L.A., 1983. Effect of cimetidine on canine gastric mucosal pH and blood flow. Am. J. Surg. 145, 24–28.

Collins, L.G., Tyler, D.E., 1984. Phenylbutazone toxicosis in a horse: a clinical study. J. Am. Vet. Med. Assoc. 184, 699–703.

Collins, L.G., Tyler, D.E., 1985. Experimentally induced phenylbutazone toxicosis in ponies: description of the syndrome and its prevention with synthetic prostaglandin E2. Am. J. Vet. Res. 46, 1605.

Crandell, J.M., Ware, W.A., 2005. Cardiac toxicity from phenylpropanolamine overdose in a dog. J. Am. Anim. Hosp. Assoc. 41, 413–420.

Daehler, M.H., 1986. Transmural pyloric perforation associated with naproxen administration in a dog. J. Am. Vet. Med. Assoc. 189, 694–695.

Dahm, L.J., Jones, D.P., 1996. Mechanisms of chemically induced liver disease. In: Zakim, D., Boyer, T.D. (Eds.), Hepatology A Textbook of Liver Disease. W.B. Saunders Company, Philadelphia, pp. 875–890.

Davis, L.E., 1980. Clinical pharmacology of salicylates. J. Am. Vet. Med. Assoc. 176, 65–66.

Driman, D., Wright, C., Tougas, G., et al., 1995. Omeprazole produces parietal cell hypertrophy and hyperplasia in humans. Gastroenterology. 108, A87.

Dyer, F., Diesel, G., Cooles, S., Tait, A., 2009. Suspected adverse reactions. Vet. Rec. 167, 118–121.

Ezri, T., Lerner, E., Muggia-Sullam, M., et al., 2006. Phosphate salt bowel preparation regimens alter perioperative acid–base and electrolyte balance. Can. J. Anesth. 53, 153–158.

Farmer, J.W., Chan, S.B., 2003. Whole body irrigation for contraband bodypackers. J. Clin. Gastroenterol. 37, 147–150.

Fitzgibbons, L.J., Snoey, E.R., 1999. Severe metabolic acidosis due to baking soda ingestion: case reports of two patients with unsuspected antacid overdose. J. Emerg. Med. 17, 57–61.

Fourie, T., Cromarty, D., Duncan, N., et al., 2015. The safety and pharmacokinetics of carprofen, flunixin, and phenylbutazone in the cap vulture (*Gyps coprotheres*) following oral exposure. PLoS One. 10 (10), e0141419.

Gfeller, R.W., Sandon, A.D., 1991. Naproxen-associated duodenal ulcer complicated by perforation and bacteria- and barium sulfate-induced peritonitis in a dog. J. Am. Vet. Med. Assoc. 198, 644–646.

Ginn, J.A., Bentley, E., Stepien, R.L., 2013. Systemic hypertension and hypertensive retinopathy following PPA overdose in a dog. J. Am. Anim. Hosp. Assoc. 49, 46–53.

Godshalk, C.P., Roush, J.K., Fingland, R.B., et al., 1992. Gastric perforation associated with administration of ibuprofen in a dog. J. Am. Vet. Med. Assoc. 201, 1734–1736.

Gonzolez, J., Hogg, R.J., 1981. Metabolic Alkalosis secondary to baking soda treatment of a diaper rash. Pediatrics. 67 (6), 820–822.

Gunson, D.E., 1983. Renal papillary necrosis in horses. J. Am. Vet. Med. Assoc. 182, 263–266.

Gwaltney-Brant, S., 2004. Antihistamines. In: Plumlee, K. (Ed.), Clinical Veterinary Toxicology. Mosby, St. Louis, pp. 291–293.

Hata, J., Kamada, T., Manabe, N., et al., 2005. Famotidine prevents canine gastric blood flow reduction by NSAIDs. Alim. Pharm. Ther. 21, 55–59.

Henninger, R.W., Horst, J., 1997. Magnesium toxicosis in two horses. J. Am. Vet. Med. Assoc. 211, 82–85.

Herring, J.M., McMichael, M.A., Corsi, R., et al., 2015. Intravneous lipid emulsion therapy in three cases of canine naproxen overdose. J. Vet. Emerg. Crit. Care. 25 (5), 672–678.

Hjelle, J.J., Grauer, G.F., 1986. Acetaminophen-induced toxicosis in dogs and cats. J. Am. Vet. Med. Assoc. 188, 742–746.

Hunt, J.R., Dean, R.S., Davis, G.N.D., et al., 2015. An analysis of the relative frequencies of reported adverse events associated with NSAID administration in dogs and cats in the United Kingdom. Vet. J. 206, 183–193.

Hutchins, R.G., Messenger, K.M., Vaden, S.L., 2013. Suspected carprofen toxicosis caused by coprophagia in a dog. J. Am. Vet. Med. Assoc. 243 (4), 709–711.

Isaacs, J.P., 1996. Adverse effects of non-steroidal anti-inflammatory drugs in the dog and cat. Aust. Vet. Practit. 26, 180–186.

Jackson, T.W., Costin, C., Link, K., et al., 1991. Correlation of serum ibuprofen concentration with clinical signs of toxicity in three canine exposures. Vet. Hum. Toxicol. 33, 486–488.

Johnson, A.L., Blaine, E.T., Lewis, A.D., 2016. Renal pigmentation due to chronic bismuth administration in a rhesus macaque (*Macaca mulatta*). Vet. Pathol. 52 (3), 576–579.

Jones, R.D., Baynes, R.E., Nimitz, C.T., 1992. Nonsteroidal anti-inflammatory drug toxicosis in dogs and cats: 240 cases (1989–1990). J. Am. Vet. Med. Assoc. 201, 475–477.

Jorgensen, L.S., Center, S.A., Randolph, J.F., et al., 1985. Electrolyte abnormalities induced by hypertonic phosphate enemas in two cats. J. Am. Vet. Med. Assoc. 187, 136–137.

Khan, S.A., McLean, M.K., Gwaltney-Brandt, S., 2010. Accidental overdose of joint supplements in dogs. JAVMA. 236 (5), 509–510.

Khayyat, A., Tobwala, S., Hart, M., et al., 2016. *N*-acetylcysteine amide, a promising antidote for acetaminophen toxicity. Toxicol. Lett. 241, 133–142.

Koengshof, A.M., Beal, M.W., Poppenga, R.H., et al., 2015. Effects of sorbitol, single, and mutlidose activated charcoal administration on carprofen absorption following experimental overdose in dogs. J. Vet. Emerg. Crit. Care. 25 (5), 606–610.

Kore, A.M., 1990. Toxicology of nonsteroidal anti-inflammatory drugs. Vet. Clin. North Am. Small Anim. Pract. 20, 419–430.

Lees, R., May, S.A., McKellar, Q.A., 1991. Pharmacology and therapeutics of non-steroidal anti-inflammatory drugs in the dog and cat: general pharmacology. J. Small Anim. Pract. 32, 183–193.

Little, D., Jones, S.L., Blikslager, A.T., 2007. Cyclooxygenase (COX) inhibitors and the intestine. J. Vet. Int. Med. 21, 367–377.

MacNaughton, S.M., 2003. Acetaminophen toxicosis in a Dalmatian. Can. Vet. J. 44, 142–144.

Maddrey, W.C., 2005. Drug-induced hepatotoxicity. J. Clin. Gastroenterol. 39, S83–S89.

Mazué, G., Richez, P., Berthe, J., 1982. Pharmacology and comparative toxicology of non-steroidal anti-inflammatory agents. In: Ruckebush, Y., Toutain, P., Koritz, G.D. (Eds.), Veterinary Pharmacology and Toxicology. AVI Roslyn, pp. 321–331.

McConkey, S.E., Grant, D.M., Cribb, A.E., 2009. The role of para-aminophenol in acetaminophen-induced methemoglobinemia in dogs and cats. J. Vet. Pharmacol. Therap. 32, 585–595.

McKellar, Q.A., May, S.A., Lees, P., 1991. Pharmacology and therapeutics of non-steroidal anti-inflammatory drugs in the dog and cat: 2 individual agents. J. Small Anim. Pract. 32, 225–235.

Meani, R., Nixon, R., 2015. Allergic contact dermatitis caused by ranitidine hydrochloride in a veterinary product. Contact Dermatitis. 73, 125–126.

Means, C., 1999. Ma huang: all natural but not always innocuous, Vet. Med., 94. pp. 511–512.

Means, C., 2005. Decongestants. In: Plumlee, K. (Ed.), Clinical Veterinary Toxicology. Mosby, St. Louis, pp. 309–311.

Montiero-Steagall, B.P., Steagall, P.V.M., Laschelles, B.D.X., 2013. Systematic review of nonsteroidal anti-inflammatory drug-induced adverse effects in dogs. J. Vet. Int. Med. 27, 1011–1019.

Murphy, M.J., 1994. Toxin exposures in dogs and cats: drugs and household products. J. Am. Vet. Med. Assoc. 205, 557–560.

Murtaugh, R.J., Matz, M.E., Labato, M.A., et al., 1993. Use of synthetic prostaglandin E1 (misoprostol) for prevention of aspirin-induced gastroduodenal ulceration in arthritic dogs. J. Am. Vet. Med. Assoc. 202, 251–256.

Ooms, T.G., Khan, S., 2001. Suspected caffeine and ephedrine toxicosis resulting from ingestion of an herbal supplement containing guarana and ma huang in dogs: 47 cases (1997–1999). J. Am. Vet. Med. Assoc. 218, 225–229.

Otto, C.M., Greentree, W.F., 1994. Terfenadine toxicosis in dogs. J. Am. Vet. Med. Assoc. 205, 1004–1006.

Papich, M.G., 1990. Toxicosis from over-the-counter human drugs. Vet. Clin. North Am. Small Anim. Pract. 20, 431–451.

Papich, M.G., Davis, C.A., Davis, L.E., 1987. Absorption of salicylate from an antidiarrheal preparation in dogs and cats. J. Am. Anim. Hosp. Assoc. 23, 221–226.

Plumb, D.C., 2015. Plumb's Veterinary Drug Handbook. eighth ed. Blackwell Publ, Stockholm, WI.

Roder, J.D., 2004a. Nonsteroidal anti-inflammatory agents. In: Plumlee, K. (Ed.), Clinical Veterinary Toxicology. Mosby, St. Louis, pp. 282–284.

Roder, J.D., 2004b. Hypertonic phosphate enema. In: Plumlee, K. (Ed.), Clinical Veterinary Toxicology. Mosby, St. Louis, p. 319.

Romanelli, 2009. Dextromethorphan abuse: clinical effects and management. J. Am. Pharm. Assoc. 49, e20–e25.

Rubin, S.L., Papich, M.G., 1990. Clinical uses of nonsteroidal anti-inflammatory drugs in companion animal practice – Part II: drugs, therapeutic uses and adverse effects. Canine Pract. 15, 27–32.

Rumbeiha, W.K., Lin, Y., Oehme, F.W., 1995. Comparison of N-acetylcysteine and methylene blue, alone or in combination, for treatment of acetaminophen toxicosis in cats. Am. J. Vet. Res. 56, 1533–1592.

Runkel, R., Chaplin, M., Boost, G., Segre, E., et al., 1972. Absorption, distribution, metabolism, and excretion of naproxen in various laboratory animal and human subjects. J. Pharmaceut. Sci. 61, 703–708.

Sartor, L.L., Bentjen, S.A., Trepanier, L., et al., 2004. Loperamide toxicity in a collie with the MDR1 mutation associated with ivermectin sensitivity. J. Vet. Int. Med. 18, 117–118.

Savides, M.C., Oehme, F.W., 1985. Effects of various antidotal treatments on acetaminophen toxicosis and biotransformation in cats. Am. J. Vet. Res. 46, 1485–1489.

Schlesinger, D.P., 1995. Methemoglobinemia in a dog with acetaminophen toxicity. Can. Vet. J. 36, 515–517.

Schubert, T.A., 1984. Salicylate-induced seizure in a dog. J. Am. Vet. Med. Assoc. 185, 1000–1001.

Segev, G., Bandt, C., Francey, T., et al., 2008. Aluminum toxicity following administration of aluminum-based phosphate binders in 2 dogs with renal failure. J. Vet. Int. Med. 22, 1432–1435.

Sellon, R.K., 2006. Acetaminophen. In: Petersen, M.E., Talcott, P.A. (Eds.), Small Animal Toxicology, second ed. Saunders, St. Louis, pp. 550–558.

Sennello, K.A., Leib, M.S., 2006. Effects of deracoxib or buffered aspirin on the gastric mucosa of healthy dogs. J. Vet. Int. Med. 20, 1291–1296.

Staley, E.C., Staley, E.E., 1995. Promethazine toxicity in a seven-month-old Doberman pinscher. Vet. Hum. Toxicol. 37, 243–244.

Stanton, M.E., Bright, R.M., 1989. Gastroduodenal ulceration in dogs retrospective study of 43 cases and literature review. J. Vet. Int. Med. 3, 238–244.

Stewart, J.E., Haslam, A.K., Puig, J., 2016. Pathology in practice. JAVMA. 248 (9), 1009–1010.

Strøm, H., Thomsen, M.K., 1990. Effects of non-steroidal anti-inflammatory drugs on canine neutrophil chemotaxis. J. Vet. Pharmacol. Therap. 13, 186–191.

Sturgill, M.G., Lambert, G.H., 1997. Xenobiotic-induced hepatotoxicity: mechanisms of liver injury and methods of monitoring hepatic function. Clin. Chem. 43, 1512–1526.

Takata, K., Hikasa, Y., Satoh, H., 2012. Comparison of gastrointestinal adverse effects of ketoprofen between adult and young cats. J. Vet. Med. Sci. 74 (12), 1545–1550.

Talcott, P.A., 2006. Nonsteroidal antiinflammatories. In: Petersen, M.E., Talcott, P.A. (Eds.), Small Animal Toxicology, second ed. Saunders, St. Louis, pp. 902–933.

Tegzes, J.H., Smarick, S.D., Puschner, B., 2002. Coma and apnea in a dog with hydroxyzine toxicosis. Vet. Hum. Toxicol. 44, 24–26.

Treinen-Moslen, M., 2001. Toxic responses of the liver. In: Klaassen, C. D. (Ed.), Casarette and Doull's Toxicology: The Basic Science of Poisons. McGraw Hill, New York, pp. 471–489.

Verbeek, R.K., 1990. Pharmacokinetic drug interactions with nonsteroidal anti-inflammatory drugs. Clin. Pharm. 19, 44–66.

Villar, D., Buck, W.B., Gonzalez, J.M., 1998. Ibuprofen, aspirin, acetaminophen toxicosis and treatment in dogs and cats. Vet. Hum. Toxicol. 40, 156–161.

Walan, A., Bader, J., Classen, M., et al., 1989. Effect of omeprazole and ranitidine on ulcer healing and relapse rates in patients with benign gastric ulcer. N. Engl. J. Med. 320, 69–75.

Wallace, K.B., Eells, J.T., Madeira, V.M., 1997. Mitochondria-mediated cell injury. Symposium overview. Fundam. Appl. Toxicol. 38, 23–37.

Wallace, K.P., Center, S.A., Hickford, F.H., et al., 2002. S-adenosyl-L-methionine (SAMe) for treatment of acetaminophen toxicity in a dog. J. Am. Anim. Hosp. Assoc. 38, 254–256.

Wallace, M.S., Zawie, D.A., Garvey, M.S., 1990. Gastric ulceration in the dog secondary to use of nonsteroidal anti-inflammatory drugs. J. Am. Anim. Hosp. Assoc. 26, 467–472.

Waters, D.J., Bowers, L.D., Cipolle, R.J., et al., 1993. Plasma salicylate concentrations in immature dogs following aspirin administration: comparison with adult dogs. J. Vet. Pharmacol. Therapeut. 16, 275–282.

Webb, C.B., Twedt, D.C., Fettman, M.J., et al., 2003. S-adenosylmethionione (SAMe) in a feline acetaminophen model of oxidative injury. J. Feline Med. Surg. 5, 69–75.

Zimmerman, H.J., 1999. Drug induced liver disease. In: Schiff, E.F., Sorrell, M.F., Maddrey, W.F. (Eds.), Schiff's Diseases of the Liver. Lippincott-Raven Publishers, Philadelphia, pp. 973–1064.

FURTHER READING

Vander Werf, K.A., Davis, E.G., Kukanich, B., 2012. Pharmacokinetics and adverse effects of oral meloxicam tablets in healthy adult horses. Vet. Pharmacol. Therap. 36, 376–381.

Chapter 22

Toxicity of Drugs of Abuse

Karyn Bischoff

INTRODUCTION

Potential for exposure to illegal drugs exists for many companion animals, horses, and even other livestock on occasion. Forty-seven percent of graduating American high-school students surveyed had used illegal drugs in some form (Latimer and Zur, 2010). The illegal drug trade in the United States peaked in the late 1970s, declined in the 1980s and early 1990s, and increased again through the late 1990s only to stabilize by 2000 (Compton et al., 2005). Morbidity and mortality related to drug use began to rise after 2000, in a large part because of increased abuse of prescription opioids and heroin (Martins et al., 2015).

Marijuana is one of the most prevalent recreational drugs in the world and is legal as either a medical therapy or for recreational use in a little more than half of US states as of this writing. Ethanol and nicotine, legal throughout the United States, are even more prevalent (Janczyk et al., 2004; Compton et al., 2005; Johnson et al., 2005; Vitale and van de Mheen, 2005; Latimer and Zur, 2010). Cocaine was, for a long time, second to marijuana in popularity in some areas of the United States and Europe (Kisseberth and Trammel, 1990; Dumonceaux, 1995; Queiroz-Neto et al., 2002; Vitale and van de Mheen, 2005). Since the 1980s, the term "club drugs" has come into use, representing drugs frequently found at nightclubs and all-night "rave" parties. Club drugs are a continuing trend (Smith et al., 2002; Banken, 2004). Many are stimulants, though depressants may be used to counter the effects of the stimulants or given covertly to sedate a victim prior to theft or assault. Hallucinogens are also used. Some of the most common club drugs include ketamine, 3,4-methylene-dioxymethamphetamine (MDMA), commonly called "ecstasy," flunitrazepam (Rohypnol), the "date rape drug," and γ-hydroxybutanoic acid (GHB). Beginning in late 2010, the abuse of the substances mephedrone, methylenedioxypyrovalerone, and others, which were legal at that time and marketed as "bath salts," has come into vogue, prompting an emergency order to remove them from the market in Louisiana. Around the same time, a variety of synthetic cannabinoids became popular.

Illicit Drugs and Small Animals

Among companion animals, dogs are the most susceptible to poisoning with illicit substances, though toxicoses occasionally arise in cats, ferrets, birds, or other household pets. Exposure may be through voluntary ingestion, malicious poisoning, or other forms of animal abuse (Kisseberth and Trammel, 1990). There are reports of adolescents entertaining themselves by intoxicating dogs, cats, and birds with second-hand marijuana smoke (Schwartz and Riddle, 1985; Buchta, 1988). Legalization of marijuana in some states has led some to take a more cavalier attitude towards the substance, and carelessness has allowed more access to this drug to companion animals.

Police dogs are at particular risk for ingestion of illegal drugs. They can contact large quantities of the high-purity chemicals in the line of duty (Dumonceaux and Beasley, 1990; Kisseberth and Trammel, 1990). They sometimes ingest whole bags of drugs, which must be removed surgically or via endoscopy with extreme caution to prevent rupture and massive exposure. Police dogs are also likely to be at increased risk for malicious poisonings. A news report in the early 2000s documented the use of dogs as "drug mules" to move bags of heroin, which were surgically implanted. Deaths of several of the dogs were attributed to secondary infections.

Illegal drug ingestion in small animals presents a diagnostic challenge, and often an ethical challenge, to the clinician. Pet owners may not be aware of what the animal was exposed to, as in the case of animal intoxication by adolescents (Schwartz and Riddle, 1985; Buchta, 1988). Jones (1978) reports that a dog ingested illicit substances from a neighbor's garbage can. Violence is intrinsic to the drug culture in poor neighborhoods (Johnson and Myron, 1995). It can take the form of

Veterinary Toxicology. DOI: http://dx.doi.org/10.1016/B978-0-12-811410-0.00022-2

malicious poisoning or other forms of animal abuse. Suspected malicious poisoning with illicit drugs has been reported (Bischoff et al., 1998).

The pet owner who is aware that the animal ingested an illegal substance may be reluctant to admit it (Godbold et al., 1979; Kisseberth and Trammel, 1990; Dumonceaux, 1995; Welshman, 1986; Frazier et al., 1998; Janczyk et al., 2004; Volmer, 2005). Veterinarians are tasked with balancing client confidentiality with legal obligation. The client bringing the pet to a veterinary clinic is aware that the pet requires medical attention, but may be unwilling to disclose critical information under the threat of legal action. It is prudent for the veterinarian to be aware of the local laws concerning animal abuse, drug possession, and their responsibility towards reporting illegal activities. Sadly, animals have been euthanized in part because of an incomplete history (Smith, 1988). The owner must be made aware that a proper history is required if appropriate treatment is to be administered.

Diagnostic laboratories have screens available to detect the presence of many illegal drugs, but testing can be costly and results are usually not available right away (Janczyk et al., 2004). Over-the-counter testing kits have been developed for rapid analysis of human urine and are available at pharmacies. One study has found these kits useful in detection of barbiturates, some opioids, benzodiazepines, and amphetamines in canine urine, but less accurate in the detection of other opioids and marijuana (Teitler, 2009). Based on the author's experience, false negatives for marijuana are common with over-the-counter test kits. Awareness of the animal's home situation, including the neighborhood or the presence of adolescent children, can be helpful in determining the potential for exposure to illegal substances and can give the client or owner the opportunity to explain the exposure while diverting blame from themselves. The astute clinician might ask if there was a party in the home when the pet became ill (Kisseberth and Trammel, 1990). Pet owners who do admit that their pet ingested illegal drugs are not always fully aware of what was ingested or know only the street name of the drug. Drug dealers often combine drugs or make substitutions, and many drugs are very similar in appearance. The results of marijuana legalization in US states have been mixed—clients and owners will be more likely to report exposures, but exposures have already become more common.

Illicit Drugs and Large Animals

Horses may be "doped" to improve athletic performance or to hide soundness or temperament problems. The first laws regarding equine doping were put in place in England in 1666, though the practice certainly predates the law. Cocaine has been detected in urine samples from horses at athletic events (Queiroz-Neto et al., 2002; Kollias-Baker et al., 2003). It is expected that such drugs would be given in relatively small doses, but dose miscalculations can occur. Illicit use of anabolic steroids was reported in 1941 and involved testosterone use, drugging with such compounds as stonozolol and androstenedione, as well as numerous new "designer" anabolic steroids. This continues to be reported in equine athletes (Waller and Mcleod, 2016). Exposure to plants grown for illicit drug manufacture has occurred in herbivores. There are reports of lethal marijuana exposure in cattle fed marijuana hay and horses on pasture (Cardassis, 1951; Driemeier, 1997). Impaction from the fibrous nature of the plant and underlying illnesses probably contributed to the deaths in those cases.

Anhydrous ammonia is an ingredient in illegal methamphetamine production. It is also used to instill nitrogen into the soil for fertilization, and tanks are sometimes stored near animal facilities. Unscrupulous manufacturers of the drug steal anhydrous ammonia from farm tanks and have been known to fail to close the tank valves before leaving the premises. The death of 64 out of 260 dairy cattle in Michigan resulted from anhydrous ammonia theft (Fitzgerald et al., 2006).

The Veterinarian and the Drug Enforcement Administration

Title 21 of the US Code of Federal Regulations establishes the Drug Enforcement Administration (DEA), which classifies drugs into five categories as listed in Table 22.1. Because some veterinary drugs, such as ketamine and some opioids, are coveted on the illegal drug market, failure of the veterinarian to prescribe drugs appropriately has led to the loss of licenses and the risk of imprisonment (Gloyd, 1982). A veterinarian was fined and lost his license in 2000 for selling steroids illegally (AVMA News, October 15, 2000), and a few years later, an Internet pharmacy was fined more than $40,000 for contracting veterinarians to write prescriptions without examining animals and for dispensing drugs not approved by the FDA (AVMA News, April 19, 2002).

DEPRESSANTS

Substances that have a depressant effect on the central nervous system (CNS) include marijuana, barbiturates, opioids, and the club drugs flunitrazepam (Rohypnol) and GHB. Ketamine, a sedative-hypnotic, will be discussed with the related compound phencyclidine under the category of hallucinogens. Depressants act at a variety of receptor sites within the CNS. Some receptors are named

TABLE 22.1 DEA Drug Schedules

Classification	Description	Examples
Schedule I	1. High potential for abuse	Heroin
	2. No accepted medical use in United States	LSD
	3. Lack of accepted safety for use under medical supervision	Marijuana
		MDMA
		Mescaline
		Psilocybin
Schedule II	1. High potential for abuse	Amphetamine
	2. Currently accepted medical uses; may have restrictions	Cocaine
	3. Severe physical or psychological dependence potential with abuse	Methamphetamine
		Morphine
		Opium
		Pentobarbital
		Phencyclidine
Schedule III	1. Less potential for abuse than Schedule I or II drugs	Ketamine
	2. Currently accepted medical uses	Testosterone
	3. Moderate or low potential for physical or psychological dependence with abuse	Thiopental
Schedule IV	1. Low potential for abuse relative to Schedule III	Butorphanol
	2. Currently accepted medical use	Diazepam
	3. Limited physical or psychological dependence potential with abuse	Midazolam
Schedule V	1. Low potential for abuse compared to Schedule IV	Low-dose codeine preparations
	2. Currently accepted medical use	Low-dose opium preparations
	3. Limited potential for physical or psychological dependence with abuse compared to Schedule IV	Pregablin

for the drugs that bind to them, including opioid receptors and cannabinoid receptors.

Marijuana

Cannabis sativa has been used for over 4000 years for its psychotropic effects (Di Marzo and De Petrocellis, 2006). Surveys of US students found that approximately 33%–37% had used marijuana by the last year of high school and 11% had used it in eighth grade (Eaton et al., 2010; Latimer and Zur, 2010). Common names include marijuana, hemp or Indian hemp, pot, ganja, dagga, hashish, and kief (Burrows and Tyrl, 2001). The crude product, usually called marijuana in the United States, is produced from dried chopped leaves and the female inflorescences (Kisseberth and Trammel, 1990; Frohne and Pfänder, 2004; Volmer, 2005). Sinsemilla, Spanish for "without seeds," accounts for approximately 85% of US marijuana production because of the absence of seeds and the very high content of the active ingredient. Hashish is a dried and compressed resin made from the *C. sativa* and is often formed into balls, sheets, and cakes to be used for smoking. Hashish oil, even more concentrated, may be mixed with tobacco or marijuana and smoked.

Cannabinoids are a variety of related compounds found in *C. sativa*. More than 60 are known, the most important being Δ^9-tetrahydrocannabinol (THC). THC is a lipid soluble monoterpene present in all parts of the plant, with the highest concentrations in the flowers and leaves (Ashton, 2001; Burrows and Tyrl, 2001). The THC content of marijuana can range from 0.4% to 20% (Fitzgerald et al., 2013). Common cultivars grown in 1974 contained approximately 1% THC; whereas a more recent average THC concentration in seized marijuana samples was recent average THC concentration in seized marijuana samples was 10.1% (Anonymous, 2011). Hashish can contain more than 10% THC; hashish oil can contain more than 20% THC and may be added to a marijuana cigarette to double the potency.

There are a variety of accepted and controversial medical uses for marijuana and its active compound. Though still illegal under federal law, some states allow possession and use of marijuana, often under certain conditions and for medical treatment. Though laws change frequently, as of this writing more than half of the states in the US allow some form of marijuana use. Prescription products include dronabinol (Marinol) capsules, which contain THC in sesame oil and remain classified as a Schedule I drug by the DEA, and Nabilone (Cesamet), a synthetic form of THC classified as Schedule II. These drugs are used to treat nausea in cancer patients and may be superior in efficacy to other antiemetic drugs. They improve weight gain among patients with AIDS, cancer, or Alzheimer's disease and have been considered for use in the treatment of glaucoma, multiple sclerosis, chronic pain, epilepsy and various psychiatric disorders (Di Marzo and De Petrocellis, 2006).

Illegal marijuana is most commonly used in the form of marijuana cigarettes called "joints" or "reefers." Alternately, marijuana may be rolled in a tobacco leaf and called a "blunt" or smoked using a water pipe ("bong") or other type of pipe. Marijuana may be brewed into a tea, or more commonly baked into brownies, cookies, or cakes (Ashton, 2001; Volmer, 2005). Many veterinary exposures come from the ingestion of tainted baked goods.

Marijuana cigarettes are sometimes dipped in a mixture of phencyclidine, methanol, and formaldehyde. Ketamine, opium, cocaine, and heroin may be added to a marijuana cigarette or used with marijuana. Street names for marijuana include "grass," "hemp," "Mary Jane" or "MJ," "pot," "puff," and "weed."

Dogs less than 1 year of age are the most likely companion animal to ingest marijuana (Kisseberth and Trammel, 1990; Janczyk et al., 2004). Marijuana leaves or marijuana cigarettes were recovered from 203 of 213 canine ingestions. Fresh plants and refined resins are also occasionally available to companion animals. Intentional intoxication of small animals using second-hand smoke has been reported (Schwartz and Riddle, 1985; Buchta, 1988; Frohne and Pfänder, 2004). THC is highly fat-soluble. Marijuana can be processed with a source of fat, such as butter, allowing the THC to partition into the lipid matrix, which can be used in cooking. This "pot butter" is now frequently used to make baked goods containing high concentrations of THC (Fitzgerald et al., 2013). These baked goods are attractive to dogs and possibly other companion animals and are a common source of exposure.

New synthetic cannabinoids, which aren't structurally related to THC but can have exponentially higher potency, have been developed since the 1960s, but have only become popular in the United States since around 2008. There are currently hundreds of these compounds available on the market (Rech et al., 2015). One is 1-penthyl-3-(1-naphthoyl) indole, or JWH-018, which is mixed with leafy herbs and sold as "spice" or "K2" to be smoked as an alternative to marijuana. These products are readily available, frequently as "incense" and typically marked "not for human consumption," but are intentionally smoked, ingested, or taken parenterally. Laws concerning these products vary by country, state, and city and are made more complicated by the difficulty in identifying and testing for new compounds entering the market. Adverse effects in dogs that have been exposed to synthetic cannabinoids have been reported.

Large animals have been exposed through grazing marijuana or ingesting dry baled marijuana as hay (Cardassis, 1951; Driemeier, 1997). Horses have been bedded on hemp fiber, which presents an impaction risk (Green, 1996; Smith and Papworth, 1996).

Toxicity

Few veterinary deaths have been reported from marijuana intoxications. Marijuana has a very wide safety margin in that the lethal dose is approximately 1000 times the effective dose (Volmer, 2005). No deaths were reported in dogs and monkeys ingesting 3–9 g of marijuana per kg of body weight (Burrows and Tyrl, 2001). Janczyk et al. (2004) documented the survival of a dog that ingested 26.8 g marijuana/kg body weight. The LD_{50} for oral marijuana exposure in rats is 666–1000 mg/kg (Kisseberth and Trammel, 1990; Burrows and Tyrl, 2001). Driemeier (1997) reports that four out of five debilitated cattle died after the group ingested 35 kg of dried marijuana. Horses and mules have died after ingesting large quantities of fresh marijuana of the species *Cannabis indica* (Cardassis, 1951).

Toxicokinetics

Absorption of inhaled THC approaches 50% and clinical signs occur in 6–12 min (Burrows and Tyrl, 2001; Janczyk et al., 2004). Gastrointestinal absorption is erratic in humans and dogs. Blood concentrations obtained by ingestion are 25%–30% of those obtained by smoking in humans (Ashton, 2001). Onset of clinical signs is usually delayed at least 30 min after ingestion.

Circulating THC is up to 99% protein bound in humans (Volmer, 2005). Plasma concentrations peak within 2–3 h. This lipid soluble compound is rapidly distributed to the brain and other tissues. Within the brain, THC accumulates in the neocortical, limbic, sensory, and motor areas. Distribution is blood flow dependent, and peak accumulation in adipose tissue occurs in 4 or 5 days in humans (Ashton, 2001). The plasma half-life of THC is short because of the rapid tissue distribution.

THC is rapidly metabolized by the mixed-function oxidase system of the liver (Burrows and Tyrl, 2001). The significant first-pass effect likely accounts for the lower blood concentrations associated with ingestion versus inhalation (Ashton, 2001; Janczyk et al., 2004). 11-Hydroxy-Δ^9-THC is the physiologically active major metabolite of THC (Volmer, 2005). There are more than 20 other known metabolites (Ashton, 2001).

Between 65% and 90% of a dose of THC is excreted as the parent compound or conjugated metabolites through the feces, and there can be significant enterohepatic cycling (Kisseberth and Trammel, 1990; Ashton, 2001; Volmer, 2005). Ten to twenty-five percent of THC is excreted as the parent compound, metabolites, and conjugates in the urine in humans, and renal excretion is unlikely to be a major elimination pathway in dogs.

Mechanism of Action

CB1 and CB2 are the cannabinoid receptors that have been identified in rats, guinea pigs, dogs, monkeys, pigs, and humans (Ashton, 2005). CB1 is widely distributed in certain areas of the brain: receptors in the cerebral cortex regulate cognitive function; receptors in the hippocampus and amygdala are important in emotional status; cerebellar receptors influence dopaminergic signaling, movement and postural reflexes; and receptors in the basal ganglia, brainstem and autonomic nervous system (ANS) regulate pain perception and cardiovascular and gastrointestinal function (Ashton, 2005; Di Marzo and De Petrocellis, 2006). CB1 receptors are located within lipid membranes of presynaptic neurons and coupled to G-proteins. They inhibit cAMP and stimulate mitogen-activated protein kinases to modulate control of ion channels, particularly voltage-activated calcium ion channels and potassium channels (Ashton, 2005; Di Marzo and De Petrocellis, 2006; Janczyk et al., 2004). The end result is inhibition of neurotransmitter release, both excitatory and inhibitory. CB1 receptors also activate phospholipase C and PI-3-kinase. The endogenous ligand for cannabinoid receptors, known as endocannabinoids, are derived from arachidonic acids and closely related to prostaglandins. CB2 receptors are absent in the CNS but found in the peripheral nervous system (PNS) and immune system where they play a part in inflammation and pain regulation (Di Marzo and De Petrocellis, 2005; Volmer, 2005). CB2 receptors regulate ceramide biosynthesis (Di Marzo and De Petrocellis, 2006).

Clinical Signs

Clinical signs of marijuana intoxication reported in dogs are similar to those in humans (Dumonceaux and Beasley, 1990; Dumonceaux, 1995). Symptoms are evident 30–60 min after ingestion and attributable to the CNS effects: depression, ataxia, mydriasis, disorientation, behavioral disturbances, hyperesthesia, recumbence, tachycardia, hypotension, or less commonly, stupor, tremors, or seizures. Urinary incontinence is reported in exposed dogs about half the time. Ingestion exposures can also cause mild gastrointestinal irritation and vomiting. Other symptoms that have been reported include hypothermia, or less commonly, hyperthermia as well as bradycardia, vocalization, and compulsive eating. Severe clinical signs described in a ferret included ataxia with rapid onset of coma, muscle twitching, hypotension, and hypothermia (Smith, 1988). A case of atopic dermatitis was reported in a dog living in a home where *C. sativa* had been cultivated (Evans, 1989).

Synthetic cannabinoids can have a higher potency than THC, and clinical signs of anxiety, hallucinations, seizures, psychosis, and tachycardia are reported in people and most recover within several hours (Rech et al., 2015). One case report describes a dog and its owner. The dog presented with anxiety and hyper responsiveness; the owner had a tonic-clonic seizure while the dog was being examined, which progressed until the owner was unresponsive. The dog was placed in a low-stimulus environment and treated with supportive care. Dog and owner recovered, though the dog remained agitated at the time of discharge.

Onset of clinical signs in cattle began 20 h after ingesting dried plant material and included muscle tremors, hypersalivation, and mydriasis. Animals were reluctant to move and lacked coordination. Four of the five exposed animals died within 3 days; one recovered with no treatment. These cattle were already debilitated at the time of exposure (Driemeier, 1997). Rapid onset of clinical signs was described in eight horses and seven mules ingesting fresh plant material, including dyspnea, tremors, hypothermia, hypersalivation, sweating, recumbence, and death within 30 min (Cardassis, 1951).

Treatment

The prognosis for full recovery in small animals exposed to marijuana is usually excellent with proper treatment. Janczyk et al. (2004) describe 213 cases with 100% survival. Rate of recovery is dependent on dose and route of exposure. Most animals exposed to second-hand smoke recover within a few hours. Dogs who ingest a small dose of plant material usually recover within 24 h, but those ingesting large doses can have clinical signs for several days (Kisseberth and Trammel, 1990; Dumonceaux, 1995; Burrows and Tyrl, 2001; Volmer, 2005). More severe clinical effects have been recently reported and may be due to the increased use of medical-grade marijuana products and baked goods that use "pot butter" and contain other compounds such as methylxanthines.

Treatment for THC exposure includes decontamination with supportive and symptomatic care. Mild intoxication only requires observation most of the time. Gastrointestinal decontamination to decrease THC absorption can be used in animals that have ingested large quantities of marijuana or more concentrated marijuana products. Emesis can be attempted with great caution in animals believed to have ingested a high dose of THC within the past hour if they remain asymptomatic but must be avoided in animals with clinical signs such as CNS depression or remarkable agitation (Dumonceaux and Beasley, 1990; Dumonceaux, 1995). Repeated dosing with activated charcoal and cathartics can prevent absorption and enterohepatic cycling and thus decreases the duration of clinical signs, but this too must be used judiciously (Fitzgerald et al., 2013). Keeping the patient in an area with minimal external stimulation (low light, activity, and noise) and appropriate symptomatic care will be adequate treatment most of the time. Recovery can take several days. THC is highly lipid soluble, and, in the author's experience, intravenous (IV) lipid infusion can be used to diminish clinical signs of the THC toxicosis in dogs (unpublished information).

Observation of the patient includes monitoring cardiac function, body temperature and respiration. Stuporous or comatose dogs are at risk for respiratory suppression or hypothermia and must be treated appropriately. Marked central nervous stimulation can be treated with diazepam.

Treatment of large animals was not attempted in the few cases presented in the literature. The rapid onset and progression of clinical signs in the horses did not allow time for veterinary intervention. Basic treatment procedures in large animals parallel those used in small animals. Gastrointestinal decontamination for large ingestions can involve gastric lavage or, in cattle, rumenotomy, and intragastric or intraruminal instillation of mineral oil or activated charcoal and cathartics. Monitoring and symptomatic and supportive care should proceed as above.

Two dog deaths were recently reported in dogs that ingested baked goods made with marijuana butter (Meola et al., 2012). One dog presented minimally responsive and was treated with IV lipid infusion but died with coagulopathy on the second day of treatment. The second presented unresponsive and underwent aggressive decontamination measures but developed respiratory difficulty and died, possibly because of aspiration pneumonia.

Veterinary laboratories test blood or plasma for THC using gas chromatography/mass spectrometry (GC/MS) or immunoassays. Drug testing kits are available over the counter from pharmacies but are unlikely to be useful in dogs.

Pathology

There is little information on lesions associated with marijuana overdose in small animals because so few have died. Pulmonary edema was noted in a cow (Driemeier, 1997). *C. indica* was identified in the stomach of the horses with edema as well as petechiation of the gastric wall and myocardial hemorrhage (Cardassis, 1951).

Barbiturates

Barbiturates are derived from the nonsedative barbituric acid. They are a bitter tasting white powder in the pure form and are most frequently available as a sodium salt in a weakly acidic aqueous solution. Barbiturates have been used in anesthesia, sedation, and seizure control, and though still commonly used by veterinarians, are becoming more uncommon in human medicine (Kisseberth and Trammel, 1990). The four classifications of barbiturates are based on the duration of their activities. The expected duration of an ultrashort-acting barbiturate in general is approximately 20 min with a duration of approximately 3 h. These drugs are given IV to effect for anesthesia. Examples include thiamylal sodium and thiopental sodium, both Schedule III, and methohexital sodium, which is Schedule IV. The duration of short-acting barbiturates, which are given IV for anesthesia, is approximately 3 h. Common examples of these are pentobarbital sodium and secobarbital sodium, both Schedule II drugs. The duration of intermediate-acting barbiturates, such as butobarbital or amobarbital, both Schedule III, is 3–6 h. Long-acting barbiturates can produce clinical effects for 12 h and these drugs have use in sedation and anticonvulsant therapy. Phenobarbital, methylphenobarbital, and barbital sodium are examples of long-acting barbiturates and are Schedule IV drugs (Kisseberth and Trammel, 1990; Branson, 2001; Volmer, 2005). Barbiturates are known as downers, reds, Christmas trees, and dolls on the illegal market.

Barbiturate overdose in companion animals is usually iatrogenic or due to accidental ingestion of prescription or illicit drugs. A common problem in veterinary medicine is exposure to carcasses of animals that were euthanized with barbiturates. This problem has been diagnosed by the author and reported in dogs and in wildlife in the literature (Humphreys et al., 1980; Branson, 2001; Volmer, 2005). According to the AVMA News, in 2003, at least 34 bald eagles have died from pentobarbital poisoning. Veterinarians and animal owners are responsible for proper carcass disposal and may be liable for wildlife poisonings (Volmer, 2005).

Toxicity

The LD_{50} for pentobarbital in dogs is 40–60 mg/kg by the IV route or 85 mg/kg per os. The oral LD_{50} for cats is

125 mg/kg. The margin of safety for barbiturates is low; the therapeutic dose may be 50%–70% of the LD_{50} (Kisseberth and Trammel, 1990; Branson, 2001).

Toxicokinetics

Gastrointestinal absorption of barbiturates is variable, with rapid absorption of short-acting compounds and slower absorption of long-acting barbiturates. Barbiturates are rapidly distributed throughout the body and readily cross the blood–brain barrier (Kisseberth and Trammel, 1990; Branson, 2001; Volmer, 2005). Short-acting thiobarbiturates are highly lipid soluble and enter the brain rapidly, resulting in rapid onset of CNS depression. This is followed by rapid redistribution to tissues with less perfusion and thus rapid clinical recovery. Longer-acting barbiturates are less lipophilic; therefore, they enter and leave the brain more slowly and have a more gradual onset and longer duration of action. Barbiturates cross the placenta and fetal concentrations equilibrate with those of the dam within minutes.

There is significant variation in barbiturate metabolism and excretion based on the barbituric acid derivative, the species of animal, and the individual. Barbiturates are metabolized by microsomal P450 enzymes in the liver. Barbiturates interfere with metabolism of other compounds either through competitive inhibition of the P450 enzymes or, in chronic exposures, by inducing P450 enzymes and thus increasing the rate of metabolism of xenobiotics and endogenous substances, including steroids (Volmer, 2005). Some barbiturates, in particular the short-acting thiobarbiturates, undergo significant oxidation in the tissue. Phenobarbital is metabolized very rapidly in ruminants and horses, relatively rapidly in dogs, more slowly in humans, and slower still in cats (Branson, 2001).

Barbiturates are excreted as both parent compound and metabolites in the urine. Excretion of some barbiturates is dependent on urine pH and is increased 5–10 times in alkaline urine through ion trapping. Ion trapping is less effective with short-acting barbiturates, which are highly metabolized, highly protein bound drugs, and have high pK_as (Kisseberth and Trammel, 1990; Volmer, 2005). Barbital is excreted very slowly in birds (Branson, 2001).

Mechanism of Action

Barbiturates bind to the γ-aminobutyric acid (GABA) receptor complex and decrease the rate of GABA dissociation (Branson, 2001). These actions increase permeability of the postsynaptic membrane to chloride, causing membrane hyperpolarization and reduced excitability. GABA receptors are found in motor and sensory areas of the cerebral cortex and possibly in the thalamus, where barbiturates act to control seizures and induce anesthesia. Barbiturates also act to inhibit glutamate receptors and decrease norepinephrine (NE) release (Volmer, 2005). Actions on the PNS include inhibition of acetylcholine sensitive nerve depolarization at postsynaptic junctions and motor end plates. Respiratory depression is caused by chemoreceptor suppression by barbiturates. This effect is more marked in cats where the reticular formation governs medullary control of respiration. Control of respiratory activity is believed to be more complex in other species.

Barbiturates can cause hypotension and secondary anuria (Branson, 2001; Volmer, 2005). Increased heart rate is believed to be governed by arterial pressoreceptors. The effects of barbiturates on concentrations of sodium, potassium, and calcium in cardiac myocytes produce a change in cardiac contractility. Hypothermic animals are predisposed to ventricular fibrillation with barbiturates. Fibrillation is reported in 100% of hypothermic animals given pentobarbital and 50% of those given thiopental.

Clinical Signs

Onset of clinical signs depends on the route of exposure, the barbiturate involved, and the presence or absence of food in the stomach. Animals that have ingested short-acting barbiturates usually have clinical signs within 30 min. If long-acting barbiturates were ingested, the first effects might not be observed for an hour (Kisseberth and Trammel, 1990). The time to onset of clinical anesthesia is doubled if phenobarbital is given to an animal with food in its stomach versus an empty stomach or if contaminated carrion is ingested. Duration of effects is also variable, as alluded to previously, and dependent on the agent involved, species of animal, nutritional status, age, sex, and weight. The duration of a given barbiturate is expected to be prolonged in greyhounds, which have less adipose tissue for the drug deposition.

The predominant symptoms of barbiturate intoxication are profound CNS depression and anesthesia (Humphreys et al., 1980; Kisseberth and Trammel, 1990; Volmer, 2005). Animals usually present with severe ataxia, weakness, disorientation, and loss of deep tendon reflexes. Hypothermia is common and is associated with cardiac dysrhythmia in humans and dogs as noted previously. Rapid, weak pulse and severe respiratory depression can lead to cyanosis and death.

Certain preexisting conditions enhance the effects of barbiturates, such as renal failure, uremia, and decreased rate of excretion. Barbiturates can accelerate liver damage in an individual with preexisting liver disease. Allergic and idiosyncratic reactions to barbiturates have been reported, including necrolytic dermatitis and Stevens-Johnson syndrome (Cornelis et al., 2016).

Treatment

Decontamination for recent exposures, monitoring, and symptomatic and supportive therapy are the basis of treatment for barbiturate overdose. Respiratory function, cardiac function, and body temperature are closely monitored (Kisseberth and Trammel, 1990; Branson, 2001; Volmer, 2005). Emetics are given only to the *asymptomatic* animal if it is soon after ingestion. Gastric lavage after intubation is more appropriate when possible in animals with CNS depression. Repeated doses of activated charcoal function to decrease the biological half-life of barbiturates. A cathartic such as sorbitol can be added, but magnesium-containing cathartics such as magnesium sulfate (Epsom salt) should be avoided because they can enhance CNS depression. IV lipid emulsion has been used for lipid soluble barbiturates to decrease the bioavailability and minimize clinical signs (Bischoff et al., 2011).

Monitoring and control of body temperature is essential to prevent ventricular fibrillation and decrease the duration of the clinical signs. Intubation and assisted ventilation are required when marked respiratory suppression is noted. Fluid therapy is necessary in some cases to maintain cardiac and renal function. Alkaline diuresis has been used to increase the rate of excretion of some barbiturates but is ineffective with short-acting barbiturates. Because tissue partitioning attenuates the effects of barbiturates, it is possible for the patient to relapse as the drug repartitions from the tissues back into plasma. Certain drugs are contraindicated in the barbiturate overdose patient. Dextrose, fructose, lactate, pyruvate and glutamate can increase partitioning of barbiturates into the CNS. Epinephrine and isoproterenol cause reanesthetization after thiopental exposure. Sulfonamides, salicylates, and doxycycline increase bioavailability of barbiturates by displacing them from plasma proteins.

Many laboratories can analyze samples such as urine, blood products, or tissues for barbiturates. Common techniques include TLC and GC/MS. In one study, over-the-counter drug testing kits for urine were successful in barbiturate detection in canine urine, though these kits are not always reliable (Teitler, 2009).

Opioids

Opium is produced from *Papaver somniferum*, a poppy, and its use was recorded in the Ebers Papyrus, one of the oldest known medical texts, dated around 1500 BC. The unripe seed capsule is incised after the petals have fallen. Material that exudes from the capsule is dried, collected, and dried further to produce opium. Powdered opium is 75% inert ingredients, about 10% morphine, which is the major active alkaloid, 0.5% codeine, and dimethyl-morphine or thebaine, which acts as a convulsant (Branson and Gross, 2001). Laudanum is deodorized tincture of opium and paregoric is camphorated tincture of opium.

Morphine sulfate is a Schedule II drug commonly used medicinally for pain control and sedation. Oxymorphone is a Schedule II morphine derivative approved for use in dogs and cats in the United States. Oxymorphone is approximately 10 times more potent than morphine (Branson and Gross, 2001). Other morphine derivatives include codeine and the more potent hydromorphone, both Schedule II drugs. Heroin is a Schedule I morphine derivative.

Synthetic opioids include butorphanol and tramadol, which are Schedule VI drugs, and methadone, propoxyphene, meperidine, and pentazocine, all Schedule III drugs. Oxycodone and hydrocodone are prescription synthetic opioids classified as Schedule II. Fentanyl is formulated into injectable solutions, slow-dissolving sticks for oral transmucosal absorption, and patches that release doses of 25, 50, 75 or 100 μg/h for transdermal absorption. Fentanyl is about 80 times more potent than morphine (Branson and Gross, 2001). Other potent synthetic opioids are alfentanil, sufentanil citrate, and etorphine HCl, which is 10,000 times as potent as morphine and used in wildlife capture. These potent drugs are classified in Schedule II. Desomorphine is a schedule I drug.

The morphine derivative heroin is one of the most abused opioids, and use is increasing because of increased availability and relatively low cost (Dumonceaux, 1995; Anonymous, 2011). A survey of US high-school students found that 2.5% had used heroin, though another survey stated that only about 1% had used heroin in the past year, and up to 25% said it was accessible to them (Latimer and Zur, 2010). A white to dark brown powder, heroin often contains additives such as sugar, starch, powdered milk, quinine, or strychnine. Heroin was traditionally injected, but insufflation (snorting) and smoking are becoming more popular. Heroin is also available as a black sticky substance termed "black tar heroin," which is dissolved, diluted, and injected.

Oxycodone, sold as OxyContin, Percocet, and in a generic form, is commonly used recreationally. A recent survey found that 9% of US high-school seniors had used prescription opioids recreationally (Latimer and Zur, 2010). Pills are time-released but may be crushed and insufflated or injected in solution. Hydrocodone, sold under various trade names and in formulations with acetaminophen (Vicodin) is also commonly sold on the illegal drug market. Fentanyl can be produced in clandestine laboratories and is used intravenously.

Desomorphine is a synthetic morphine derivative that is easily manufactured and considered 10 times as potent as heroin (Rech et al., 2015). More common in Russia than the United States, desomorphine, also known as krokodil, is usually injected and has gained notoriety because of the necrotizing skin lesions caused by contaminants. It has been estimated that the survival time for krokodil users is 2 years.

Small animal exposure to opioids may be because of accidental ingestion of pharmaceuticals, illegal drugs, or occasionally by oral or parenteral dosing with malicious intent (Kisseberth and Trammel, 1990; Volmer, 2005). There have been several reports in the US news media of small animals that accidentally ingested or were intentionally injected with heroin. Ingestion of therapeutic fentanyl patches has been reported in children, dogs, and monkeys (Deschamps et al., 2012).

Toxicity

With such a wide variety of opioids, there is much variation in toxicity. The lethal parenteral dose of morphine in dogs is between 110 and 210 mg/kg (Kisseberth and Trammel, 1990; Branson, 2001; Volmer, 2005). The minimum lethal dose for subcutaneous (SC) injection of morphine in cats is 40 mg/kg. The minimum lethal dose of heroin for dogs is 25 mg/kg given subcutaneously. Approximately 0.20 mg/kg heroin causes clinical signs in dogs, including sedation and respiratory depression; whereas, a dose of 0.58 mg/kg causes increased duration of effects, respiratory difficulty, and aggressive behavior with clinical signs lasting up to 8 h (Garrett and Gürkan, 1980). The minimum oral lethal dose of heroin for cats is 20 mg/kg. Meperidine causes clonic convulsions in cats at a dose of 30 mg/kg (Branson and Gross, 2001).

Toxicokinetics

Opioids are weakly acidic, and absorption after oral dosing is predominantly in the small intestine. There is rapid absorption from the subcutis after SC injection (Branson and Gross, 2001). Distribution is variable. Heroin is more lipophilic than morphine and more readily crosses the blood–brain barrier (Garrett and Gürkan, 1980). Opioids are also distributed to skeletal muscle, kidney, liver, intestine, lungs, spleen, brain, and placenta (Kisseberth and Trammel, 1990). Opioids are readily metabolized in the liver with a significant first pass effect after ingestion. Phase I metabolism includes hydrolysis, oxidation, and *N*-dealkylation. Approximately 50% of a dose of morphine is conjugated to glucuronide in most species. A notable exception is cats, accounting in part for the increased sensitivity of this species. The primary glucuronide conjugate is morphine-3 glucuronide, though the metabolically active morphine-6-glucuronide is also produced. Heroin is metabolized in the liver and other tissues and is cleared more rapidly than morphine. Deacetylation produces 6-*o*-acetylmorphine and morphine, which appear in the plasma of dogs within minutes (Garrett and Gürkan, 1980).

Opioids are excreted predominantly as metabolites in the urine. Metabolites may be detected in horse urine for up to 6 days (Branson and Gross, 2001). There is some biliary excretion and enterohepatic cycling. The biological half-life of morphine in cats is about 3 h. The initial plasma half-life of heroin in dogs is 8 min, but the terminal half-life is 80 min due to repartitioning from the tissues (Garrett and Gürkan, 1980).

Mechanism of Action

Major opioid receptors are designated μ, δ, and κ and are believed to be stimulated by endogenous endorphins (Branson and Gross, 2001; Volmer, 2005). The μ receptors are activated by endogenous enkephalins, and are further differentiated into μ_1 and μ_2. Activation of the μ_1 receptor induces supraspinal analgesia, and μ_2 receptor activation causes spinal analgesia, suppression of respiration, and inhibition of gastrointestinal motility. The δ receptors are more selective for enkephalins than the μ opioid receptors and are also involved in spinal analgesia. Activation of κ receptors produces spinal and supraspinal analgesia, sedation, and dysphoria. The σ receptor, previously classified as an opioid receptor, does not appear to mediate analgesia.

Opioid receptors are found in the CNS, ANS, gastrointestinal tract, heart, kidney, pancreas, adrenal glands, vas deferens, lymphocytes, and adipocyte (Volmer, 2005). Opioid receptors in the CNS are concentrated in the amygdala and frontal cortex in dogs, monkeys, and humans where stimulation is associated with CNS depression (Branson and Gross, 2001; Kisseberth and Trammel, 1990). Activation in cats, swine, goats, sheep, horses, or oxen alters dopaminergic or noradrenergic function, leading to excitation. Activation of opioid centers in the chemoreceptor trigger zone in the fourth ventricle of the brain produces emesis. Opioid receptors are present in the brain stem, including the cough centers where they suppress the cough reflex, and the respiratory centers, though initial increases in respiration are followed by respiratory suppression because of generalized CNS depression. Stimulation of gastrointestinal opioid receptors decrease motility, leading to delayed passage of ingesta, increased water absorption and constipation.

Opioid drugs act as agonists, partial agonists, or antagonists. Morphine and related drugs are agonists at μ receptors. Naloxone is an antagonist with a high affinity for the μ receptors and a low affinity for δ receptors (Volmer, 2005). An opioid is classified as a partial agonist if it acts as an agonist at one receptor but an antagonist at another.

Tramadol is a special case, in that it acts as a weak μ receptor agonist but also acts as a serotonin reuptake inhibitor (Indrawirawan and McAlees, 2014).

Clinical Signs

The clinical effects of opioid drugs are dependent on age (as neonates have an incomplete blood–brain barrier), species, and the drug involved. Clinical signs in dogs are similar to those described in humans. Early clinical signs can include transient excitation and rapid respiration, drowsiness and ataxia, decreased pain perception, hypersalivation, vomiting, defecation, and urination. Dogs progress to stupor or coma with hypothermia, hypotension, respiratory depression, and death (Kisseberth and Trammel, 1990; Dumonceaux, 1995; Branson and Gross, 2001; Volmer, 2005). Other symptoms include decreased urination and constipation. Symptoms in dogs given low doses of heroin included early aggressive behavior, brief unconsciousness, weakness, hypersalivation, and respiratory difficulty, and last up to 8 h (Garrett and Gürkan, 1980). Propoxyphene can induce tremors and convulsions in dogs. Cats present with excitation, aggression, insomnia, and hyperthermia as well as increased pain threshold. Tramadol overdose in a cat was associated with constipation and sedation, but other clinical signs were attributed to serotonin syndrome (Indrawirawan and McAlees, 2014). Cats are highly resistant to the emetic effects of opioids. Horses, ruminants, and swine also exhibit CNS stimulation. Clinical signs in rabbits depend on the drug used: morphine induces hypothermia; whereas, apomorphine induces hyperthermia.

Treatment

The basis of treatment for opioid exposure is early decontamination, symptomatic and supportive care, and the judicious use of opioid antagonists. Fentanyl patches have been discovered in the check pouches of monkeys that overdosed; thus, checking the oral cavity can be warranted (Deschamps et al., 2012). Vomiting can be induced in animals presenting immediately after ingestion of narcotics if they have not already vomited and no contraindications exist. If large doses are ingested and contraindications against emetic use are present, enterogastric lavage on the intubated animal can be performed to evacuate the stomach and instill activated charcoal and cathartics. Decontamination is likely to be effective for several hours after ingestion because of decreased gastrointestinal motility. Animals must be monitored closely for respiratory depression, the most common cause of death in opioid overdoses. Assisted ventilation is often necessary. Body temperature is maintained and seizures treated with diazepam.

The opioid antagonist Naloxone is used to treat severe CNS or respiratory depression. Naloxone can be given parenterally at a dose of 0.01–0.02 mg/kg and repeated as necessary since it has a very short half-life. Patients that fail to respond to a 10 mg dose of Naloxone are unlikely to respond to a higher dose.

Testing of urine or plasma for opioids is available at some diagnostic laboratories. Over-the-counter drug tests kits have been used with variable success to detect opioids in canine urine (Teitler, 2009).

Other CNS Depressants

Other drugs may have depressant activities on the CNS. Two commonly used "club drugs" are discussed below: flunitrazepam and GHB. Both are often used by assailants to sedate potential victims; thus, there is potential for their use on guard dogs.

Flunitrazepam

Flunitrazepam is not sold in the United States but is available in more than 60 countries, including many in Europe and Latin America, as Rohypnol, Narcozep, and under other trade names, as a sedative. Rohypnol has gained notoriety as the "date rape drug" and is sold as tablets imprinted "Roche 1" and "Roche 2," designating their manufacturer and milligram dosage. Tablets are crushed and insufflated or dissolved in a drink intended for an unsuspecting victim (Smith et al., 2002; Anonymous, 2011). Blue coloring has been added to these pills to reduce the potential for this use (Smith et al., 2002; Rimsza and Moses, 2005). Street names include "roofies" or "rophies," "Roche" or "la rocha," "Mexican valium," "forget me pills," "Rope," and "R2." Injectable forms of flunitrazepam are also available.

Animals that have ingested flunitrazepam should be monitored closely for respiratory and CNS depression, changes in heart rate, and body temperature fluctuations. If ingestion was recent and CNS depression is not yet evident, emetics can be given followed by activated charcoal and cathartics to help minimize absorption. Gastric lavage can be performed on the intubated patient who has ingested a large dose and presents with severe CNS depression. Analysis is available at some laboratories for flunitrazepam, but doses are often quite low and urine must be collected soon after ingestion.

GHB

Another popular "club drug" that has been associated with date rape is GHB. This compound is a derivative of GABA and is present in the body under normal conditions. Synthetic GHB can be produced in clandestine laboratories. It was sold as a nutritional supplement for body builders at one time, and is currently used to treat narcolepsy. Industrial solvents γ-butyrolactone (GBL) and 1,4-butanediol (BD) are metabolized to GHB. BD is available in printer ink cartridges and has been sold as a supplement at health food stores (Smith et al., 2002; McDonough et al., 2004; Anonymous, 2011). BD was also used as a substitute for 1,5-pentanediol in the production of a children's craft product called "Aqua Dots" in the United States and "Bindeez" in Australia (Suchard et al., 2009). The substitution was made in 2007 and resulted in clinically affected children. GHB is most commonly sold as a clear liquid in small vials and added to bottled water (Smith et al., 2002; Rimsza and Moses, 2005). Street names include "Liquid X" or "liquid ecstasy," "soap" or "salty water" because of the flavor of the product, "easy lay," "Georgia homeboy," "grievous bodily harm," "G," "goop," "gib," or "scoop."

GHB receptors are present in the hippocampus, cortex, and other areas of the brain (McDonough et al., 2004). GHB is involved in regulation of sleep cycles, body temperature, memory, glucose metabolism, and dopamine levels (Smith et al., 2002). GHB can also be converted back to GABA. Human death has been reported at an oral GHB dose of 5.4 g, but some patients have survived doses of 29 g. The LD_{50} for rodents and rabbits is approximately 2 g/kg. GHB is rapidly absorbed from the gastrointestinal tract, and, because it is highly lipophilic, it readily crosses the blood–brain barrier. GHB is rapidly metabolized to carbon dioxide, though 2%–4% of a given dose can be excreted in the urine (Smith et al., 2002; Gable, 2004). Half-life is dose dependent.

Clinical signs attributed to GHB usually occur within half an hour of ingestion and include euphoria, reduced anxiety, and drowsiness. CNS depression sometimes progresses to loss of motor control, unconsciousness, and respiratory depression (Smith et al., 2002; McDonough et al., 2004; Rimsza and Moses, 2005). Clinical signs reported in children ingesting "Aqua Dots" were vomiting, ataxia, and coma (Suchard et al., 2009). Seizures have been reported, and bradycardia and hypothermia are reported in nearly a third of overdose patients.

Treatment consists of decontamination of the intubated patient with either gastric lavage, after large ingestion, or activated charcoal—*emetics are contraindicated* because of the rapid onset of CNS depression—and close monitoring of respiratory, cardiovascular, CNS function, and body temperature. Supportive care is instituted based on clinical signs. Seizures have been treated with benzodiazepines. Patients who appear stable should be monitored for at least 8 h (Smith et al., 2002). GHB is difficult to analyze for, and results are difficult to interpret because this compound is rapidly metabolized and normally present in the body.

STIMULANTS

The major illicit drugs classified as stimulants are cocaine and the amphetamines. Cocaine is a plant alkaloid, and amphetamines are a large group of compounds, including prescription drugs such as methylphenidate, sold as Ritalin, and methamphetamine, which is produced in clandestine laboratories. Stimulants in general act on the ANS, usually on adrenergic receptors. Popular "club drug" MDMA, or "ecstasy," also has significant action on serotonin receptors. Related to amphetamines are cathinones. Naturally occurring cathinone is found in the plant *Catha edulis*, known as Khat, but synthetic forms, often sold as "bath salts," have become popular in the United States since 2010. Various legally available compounds act as stimulants through various mechanisms. These include nicotine, caffeine, and related compounds, and are discussed elsewhere in the text. Areca alkaloids, described below, are commonly used as stimulants across much of Asia and are available in some parts of the United States and Europe.

Cocaine

Cocaine is the natural alkaloid of the shrubs *Erythroxylun coca* and *Erythroxylun monogynum*, originally from the Andes Mountains in South America and most commonly grown in Bolivia, Peru, and Columbia (Queiroz-Neto et al., 2002; Volmer, 2005; Anonymous, 2011). Traditionally, *E. coca* leaves are brewed into tea by those native to the Andes Mountains, who share this delightful beverage with unsuspecting tourists in order to counter the effects of the high altitude. Cocaine is a Schedule II drug used for topical anesthesia and vasoconstriction of mucous membranes (Kisseberth and Trammel, 1990). At times, it has been second only to marijuana in illegal consumption in the United States (Dumonceaux, 1995; Queiro-Neto et al., 2002; Vitale and van de Mheen, 2005). Based on surveys in the 1980s, approximately 15% of the US population had tried cocaine (Kabas et al., 1990). More recent surveys of high-school students in the US found that 5%–6.4% had used cocaine (Eaton et al., 2010; Latimer and Zur, 2010).

Cocaine is sold as a powdered white salt, cocaine HCl, ranging in purity from 12% to >60% (Kisseberth and Trammel, 1990). It is usually diluted or "cut" with inert ingredients such as lactose, inositol, mannitol, corn starch, or sucrose, or with active compounds including procaine, lidocaine, tetracaine, caffeine, amphetamine, or quinine. Cocaine cut with levamisole has been associated with severe adverse effects in users, including agranulocytosis and vasculitis (Buchanan et al., 2010; Wiegand, 2010). The water soluble salt can be injected, ingested, or insufflated (Rimsza and Moses, 2005; Anonymous, 2011).

Common street names for cocaine HCl include "bernies," "blow," "C" or "big c," "coke," "girl" or "white girl," "gold dust" or "star dust," "her," "lady" or "white lady," "nose candy," "snow," or "toot."

Cocaine HCl is converted to the free alkaloid by dissolving it in a basic solution, which is then boiled to precipitate the alkaloid. The dry precipitate is broken into "rocks" which are 75%–90% pure, and often subsequently diluted with inert ingredients or active compounds such as procaine, lidocaine, amphetamines, heroin, caffeine, phencyclidine, ergot alkaloids, and strychnine. The free base readily vaporizes with heat and the smoke is inhaled, though it may be taken orally. This form of cocaine is termed "crack" because of the sound produced when it is heated, but it is sometimes called "bedrock," "beamers," "BJ's," "bolo," "crank," "crystal," "flake," "ice," "jelly beans," "rock," "rooster," "space," "tornado," or "24/7."

Exposure to illicit cocaine is most likely to affect dogs, particularly police dogs, but it's also been used in racing greyhounds. Athletic horses are also sometimes dosed with cocaine to improve performance (Dumonceaux and Beasley, 1990; Kisseberth and Trammel, 1990; Frazier et al., 1998; Queiroz-Neto et al., 2002; Kollias-Baker et al., 2003; Volmer, 2005). A clinical study found that 8 of 19 dogs that presented for cocaine toxicosis were also exposed to THC (Thomas et al., 2014).

Toxicity

The LD_{50} for cocaine in dogs is 3 mg/kg IV, and the LD_{99} is 20 mg/kg IV. Dogs can tolerate two to four times the above doses if it is given PO. The minimum lethal dose in cats is approximately 7.5 mg/kg IV or 16 mg/kg SC. Horses given 50 mg of cocaine IV showed no clinical signs, but performance was enhanced at 200 mg (Kollias-Baker et al., 2003).

Toxicokinetics

Cocaine is highly lipophilic and readily absorbed from all mucosal surfaces, including those of the nose, oral cavity, gastrointestinal tract, and alveoli. Approximately 20% of an ingested dose is absorbed. Peak plasma concentrations appear between 15 min and 2 h after ingestion and cocaine readily crosses the blood–brain barrier. The neurological effects of cocaine and crack last for 15–20 min after insufflation or 5–10 min after smoking recreational doses.

Cocaine undergoes hydrolysis by plasma esterases to water soluble metabolites benzoylecgonine, ecgonine methyl ester, and others (Queiroz-Neto et al., 2002). Hepatic esterases and demethylating enzymes play a role in cocaine metabolism (Kisseberth and Trammel, 1990; Volmer, 2005). Up to 20% of a dose of cocaine is excreted unchanged in the urine. Benzoylecgonine and ecgonine methyl ester are the primary metabolites excreted in the urine of most mammals in both conjugated and unconjugated forms (Kollias-Baker et al., 2003). Other metabolites include norcocaine, benzoylecgonine, norecgonine, and ecgonine. Kollias-Baker et al. (2003) found cocaine in the urine for up to 24 h when horses were dosed sublingually with 2.5 mg. Larger doses are detectable for a few days.

Mechanism of Action

Cocaine increases release of catecholamines and blocks reuptake of NE, serotonin, and dopamine, leading to increased neurotransmitter concentrations at synaptic junctions (Kisseberth and Trammel, 1990; Volmer, 1995; Queiroz-Neto et al., 2002; Vroegop et al., 2009). NE regulates thalamic effects on appetite, body temperature, and sleep. Cocaine also influences the endogenous opiate system. Local anesthetic actions occur through inhibition of membrane sodium ion channels.

Cardiac effects are often associated with IV dosing of cocaine (Kabas et al., 1990; Kisseberth and Trammel, 1990). Cocaine acts directly on myocardium by blocking sodium ion channels, thus causing conduction disturbances and prolonged R waves. Cocaine increases calcium concentrations within cardiac myocytes and can promote depolarization during the diastolic interval leading to ventricular fibrillation. Cocaine slows conductance at the bundle of His. Oxygen demand is increased within the myocardium but constriction of the coronary vasculature leads to hypoxia and infarction (Kabas et al., 1990; Volmer, 2005; Vroegop et al., 2009).

Clinical Signs

Clinical signs of cocaine toxicosis are associated with CNS stimulation, sometimes followed by depression (Kisseberth and Trammel, 1990). Clinical signs described in dogs admitted to an emergency clinic for cocaine toxicosis include muscle tremors (7/19), ataxia (4/19), and hyperesthesia or hyperexcitability (3/19). Other complaints included altered mentation, seizures, licking, vocalization, hypersalivation, vomiting, and nystagmus. Mydriasis (11/19), tachcardia (10/19), obtundation (6/19), hypertension (4/19), seizures (2/19), anisocoria, ptosis, and blindness were noted on physical examination or during hospitalization of affected dogs (Thomas et al., 2014). Cardiac changes are consistently reported. Dogs dosed IV with cocaine had increased heart rate, cardiac output, and mean arterial pressure (Catravas and Waters, 1981). Electrocardiographic changes were absent in the clinical study but have been described to include increased duration of QRS complexes and P-wave abnormalities (Llera and Volmer, 2006; Thomas et al., 2014). Death was attributed to hyperthermia, secondary to increased muscular activity and peripheral vasoconstriction (Catravas and Waters, 1981; Dumonceaux and Beasley, 1990; Dumonceaux, 1995; Frazier et al., 1998; Vroegop et al., 2009). Frazier et al. (1998) report a body temperature of 105°F (40.56°C) in one dog. Respiratory and cardiac arrest, the latter attributed to coronary vasospasm, have also been implicated as cause of death.

Hyperglycemia (4/19), increased serum lactate or lactic acidosis (12/19),and hypernatremia (9/19), were reported clinically, with occasional respiratory alkalosis, hyponatremia, and hypochloremia (Thomas et al., 2014).

Queiroz-Neto et al. (2002) report mild clinical signs in horses given low IV doses of cocaine: increased alertness, irritability, muscle tremors, vocalization, and stereotypical behaviors like head-bobbing and pawing at the ground. Cribbing was reported at higher doses. Most horses defecated within 10 min of dosing and recovered within 20 min.

Lesions reported in dogs include subendocardial and epicardial hemorrhage, degeneration of cardiac myofibers, coronary vasoconstriction, pericardial effusion, and pulmonary hemorrhage.

Treatment

Early decontamination of dogs that have recently ingested cocaine has been recommended, but is likely to have limited effects because the drug is absorbed extremely rapidly (Dumonceaux and Beasley, 1990; Dumonceaux, 1995). Furthermore, emesis is likely to induce seizures (Volmer, 2005; Llera and Volmer, 2006). Sedation and gastric lavage in the patient who has ingested a large quantity of cocaine is a safer method of decontamination. Activated charcoal and a cathartic can be given orally. Police dogs that have ingested bags of cocaine require cautious endoscopic or surgical retrieval to prevent bags from rupturing or causing obstruction. Surgically implanted bags must be removed with equal caution and secondary infection treated as necessary. Because cocaine is highly lipophilic, IV infusion of lipid emulsion is likely to decrease the bioavailability and clinical effects of cocaine.

Symptomatic and supportive care includes maintaining body temperature, acid–base and electrolyte status, and monitoring cardiac and respiratory function. Body temperature can be maintained by use of a cool environment, cool fluids, cool bath, wet towels, fans or cool water enemas, but avoid inducing shivering, which will increase body temperature. Decreased stress also prevents hyperthermia.

Seizure control also prevents hyperthermia. Diazepam and midazolam have been used to control hyperexcitability and seizure activity; however, two out of six animals with an apparently favorable response to diazepam died within 72 h according to one study (Catravas et al., 1977). A clinical study found that two of three dogs had seizures that were refractory to benzodiazepines (Thomas et al., 2014). Barbiturates or propofol CRI have been recommended to treat refractory seizures. Chlorpromazine given before cocaine dosing was effective experimentally to reduce severity of seizures, maintain blood pH, maintain body temperature, decrease heart rate and blood pressure, and prevent arrhythmias (Catravas and Waters, 1981). Clinically, acepromazine and chlorpromazine have been used to control hyperexcitability refractory to benzodiazepine, but multiple doses of acepromazine were sometimes required (Thomas et al., 2014). Affected animals with severe, prolonged respiratory depression require respiratory support, including intubation and mechanical ventilation. Cardiac symptoms such as tachycardia are usually short-lived and respond to sedation (Thomas et al., 2014). IV fluids with sodium bicarbonate are likely to effectively decrease electrocardiogram changes and risk of ventricular arrhythmia development. Treatment of *life-threatening* cardiac arrhythmia with beta-blockers such as propranolol has been recommended, but pretreatment of dogs with propranolol before cocaine injection did not increase survival. Beta-blockers are known to produce systemic hypertension (Vroegop et al., 2009).

Urine and plasma are routinely tested for cocaine at many laboratories. Thin-layer chromatography and immunoassays are used as a screening method with confirmation by GC/MS. Over-the-counter test kits are available to test for cocaine in urine and have proved useful clinically (Thomas et al., 2014).

The prognosis is guarded to good with aggressive medical treatment, and in a clinical study 19/19 dogs survived with medical treatment, though some neurologic and cardiovascular symptoms remained after discharge (Thomas et al., 2014).

Amphetamines

The term "amphetamine" refers specifically to α-methylphenylethylamine, a Schedule II drug, but the term is often used to describe various derivatives. The term "amphetamines" (plural) is used here to describe a group of related compounds unless specified otherwise. Common amphetamines include the Schedule II drug methamphetamine and Schedule I drugs 2,5-dimethyoxy-4-methylamphetamine ("DOM," "STP"), 2,5-dimethoxy-4-bromoamphetamine ("DOB"), methylphenidate, 4-methylaminorex (4MA), and 3,4-methylenedioxy-*N*-ethylamphetamine (MDEA). The "designer drug" MDMA ("ecstasy") has some unique characteristics and is discussed separately below.

Historically, amphetamines were used by veterinarians for the stimulation of medullary respiratory centers in order to increase respiratory rate and depth in animals (Adams, 2001). These drugs are not currently used in veterinary medicine. Physicians have used amphetamines to control appetite in obese patients, to treat narcolepsy, depression, alcoholism and, counter-intuitively, to control hyperkinetic behavior in children. Most are sold as tablets or capsules, which may be sustained release (Kisseberth and Tremmel, 1990). One study found that 5% of eighth grade students in the United States and 7% of high school students surveyed had used amphetamines over a 1 year period (Latimer and Zur, 2010).

Amphetamines on the illegal market are sold as "bennies," "dex" or "dexies," "speed," or "uppers." Prescription products may find their way to the illegal market, but many "designer" amphetamines such as methamphetamine are created in clandestine laboratories. Crystal methamphetamine, called "ice" or "glass," may be smoked; powdered methamphetamine, termed "crank" or "meth," may be dosed intravenously, orally, or insufflated (Rimsza and Moses, 2005; Anonymous, 2011). "Yaba" contains methamphetamine and caffeine. A survey found that about 4% of US high-school students have used methamphetamine (Eaton et al., 2010). Other "designer" amphetamines include 4-methylaminorex, sold as "euphoria," "U4EUH," or "ice," MDEA, sold as "Eve," methylcathinone (see Khat) and MDMA. Drug dealers may combine amphetamine with inert or other active ingredients or may substitute other drugs such as heroin, cocaine, or phenylethylamine.

Accidental ingestion of prescription amphetamines is the most likely exposure risk for companion animals, but potential exists for exposure of companion animals to illegal drugs. Illegal doping is a possible exposure risk for equine and canine athletes.

Toxicity

Catravas et al. (1977) found that 10 mg/kg IV amphetamine killed dogs within 3 h. LD_{50}s for orally administered amphetamine sulfate and methamphetamine in dogs are 20–27 mg/kg and 9–100 mg/kg, respectively (Diniz et al., 2003; Volmer, 2005).

Toxicokinetics

Absorption of amphetamines through the gastrointestinal system is usually rapid, though it is slower with sustained release products (Dumonceaux and Beasley, 1990; Kisseberth and Trammel, 1990; Dumonceaux, 1995; Volmer, 2005). Methamphetamine absorption is more rapid by insufflation, with onset of clinical signs in 2–5 min; whereas, the onset after PO dosing is 15–20 min (Anonymous, 2011).

Peak plasma concentrations of amphetamine occur 1–3 h after ingestion, unless a sustained release product was ingested. Amphetamines are highly lipid soluble and readily cross the blood–brain barrier (Volmer, 2005). Concentrations in the cerebral spinal fluid can be 80% of those found in the plasma (Kisseberth and Trammel, 1990). Methamphetamine has increased partitioning to the CNS compared to other amphetamines (Rimsza and Moses, 2005). Amphetamine is also distributed to the kidneys, liver and lungs, with negligible storage in the adipose tissue (Baggot and Davis, 1972).

There is significant hepatic metabolism of amphetamines. The two major pathways are hydroxylation and deamination. Deaminated products can be oxidized and conjugated to glycine (Baggot and Davis, 1972). Active metabolites are produced. Amphetamine and its metabolites are excreted primarily in the urine and minimally in the bile. About 8% of an amphetamine sulfate dose is excreted unchanged in the urine in swine and 30% in dogs. The rate of excretion is significantly increased as urine pH declines (Baggot and Davis, 1972; Kisseberth and Trammel, 1990; Volmer, 2005). Amphetamine is almost completely eliminated within about 6 h in dogs with an average urinary pH of 7.5, and in 3.3 h if the urinary pH averages around 6.0.

Mechanism of Action

Questions remain concerning the mechanism of action of amphetamines. Sympathetic central and peripheral effects are because of direct actions on α and β adrenergic receptors, increased release of catecholamines, particularly NE, inhibition of monoamine oxidase (MAO), and inhibition of catecholamine reuptake (Kisseberth and Trammel, 1990; Adams, 2001; Diniz et al., 2003; Volmer, 2005; Llera and Volmer, 2006). Amphetamines also promote serotonin and dopamine release and act directly on dopamine receptors.

Clinical Signs

Common clinical signs of amphetamine toxicosis in animals include mydriasis, hyperactivity, restlessness, tremors and seizures, circling and other stereotypic repetitive behaviors, and occasionally ataxia and depression. Hyperthermia can be secondary to seizures and peripheral vasoconstriction. Tachycardia and ventricular premature contractions, hypertension, or occasionally hypotension, have all been observed. Other reported symptoms are mydriasis, hypersalivation, vocalization, bloody diarrhea, and petechiation of the abdominal skin (Fitzgerald and Bronstein, 2013).

Reported causes of death in amphetamine overdosed dogs include disseminated intravascular coagulation (DIC) secondary to hyperthermia and respiratory failure

(Davis et al., 1978; Diniz et al., 2003). Cerebrovascular hemorrhages due to hypertension, hypoglycemia, lactic acidosis and cardiac failure have all been implicated in amphetamine overdose deaths (Catravas et al., 1977).

Serum chemistry abnormalities in addition to lactic acidosis and hypoglycemia have been reported to include hyperkalemia, hyperphosphatemia and elevated liver enzymes such as alanine transaminase, alkaline phosphatase, and aspartate transaminase (Catravas et al., 1977; Diniz et al., 2003; Llera and Volmer, 2006). Rhabdomyolysis is evident in the presence of increased creatine kinase, myoglobinuria, and there is evidence of renal failure (Kisseberth and Trammel, 1990; Diniz et al., 2003). DIC was suspected in a dog that presented with bloody diarrhea, petechia of the skin, thrombocytopenia, and increased prothrombin time and activated partial thromboplastin time subsequent to methamphetamine ingestion. Lesions in experimental dogs dosed with amphetamines included subendocardial and epicardial hemorrhage and myocardial necrosis.

Low doses of amphetamine given to horses caused increases in heart rate during rest and exercise, increased blood pressure, second degree AV block, and premature ventricular contractions (Smetzer et al., 1972).

Treatment

The prognosis for animals that have ingested amphetamines depends on the dose, time between exposure and presentation, and severity of clinical signs. Gastrointestinal decontamination should be initiated in animals that present within 2 h of ingestion (Kisseberth and Trammel, 1990; Dumonceaux, 1995). Rapid onset of clinical signs usually precludes the use of emetics. Gastric lavage of the sedated animal can be considered if large doses were ingested. Activated charcoal and a cathartic can help prevent absorption, but repeated dosing is necessary for sustained release products.

Animals should be monitored closely for neurologic symptoms, hyperthermia, cardiac arrhythmias, or respiratory insufficiency. Baseline serum chemistries should be taken to monitor for hypoglycemia, electrolyte abnormalities, lactic acidosis, myoglobinuria, liver and kidney damage, etc.

Minimal external stimulation helps to prevent seizure activity. Diazepam may paradoxically exacerbate the clinical signs of many amphetamines (a possible exception is MDMA, see below), and is thus contraindicated (Volmer, 2005). Chlorpromazine given at 10–18 mg/kg IV was determined by Catravas et al. (1977) to prevent death in experiment dogs dosed with amphetamine when given early in the progression of clinical signs. Treatment decreased hyperthermia, convulsions, hypertension, and heart rate. Normal respiration was maintained. Haloperidol at 1 mg/kg IV also decreased the clinical effects of amphetamines on body temperature, blood pressure, heart rate, respiration, and decreased convulsions in experiment dogs. Chlorpromazine and haloperidol block α-adrenergic and dopaminergic receptors. Propofol at continuous rate infusion or short-acting barbiturates have also been recommended for treatment of amphetamine-induced seizures. Methocarbamol has been used to control tremors. Because of the lipophilic nature of many amphetamines, IV lipid infusion could be a useful treatment (Fitzgerald and Bronstein, 2013).

Cool IV fluids, ice packs, fans, cool water baths or cool moist towels, or gastric lavage with cool water can be used to treat hyperthermia. However, the shivering response increases body temperature (Smith et al., 2002).

Cardiac arrhythmias in the amphetamine overdose patient often resolve with treatment of central nervous symptoms (Smith et al., 2002; Diniz et al., 2003). Propranolol decreased the heart rate and blood pressure in experiment dogs given amphetamines, but did not improve survival (Catravas et al., 1977). The use of β-blockers may lead to α-receptor-mediated vasoconstriction and spasms of the coronary artery. Lidocaine, procainamide or amiodarone have been recommended to treat ventricular arrhythmias.

Urinary acidification with ascorbic acid or ammonium chloride increases amphetamine excretion but should not be attempted in the presence of acidosis or rhabdomyolysis or if acid–base status cannot be monitored. Treatment for acidosis and rhabdomyolysis involves fluid diuresis and alkalinization. Respiratory support is sometimes required (Liechti et al., 2005). Treatment of hepatic damage with *N-acetylcysteine* has been recommended but the effectiveness is not known.

Based on the literature, dogs presenting with severe toxicosis because of exposure to amphetamines have survived with aggressive therapy, but there is inadequate information to formulate a prognosis.

Urine or plasma samples can be tested for amphetamines at many diagnostic laboratories. Thin-layer chromatography is commonly used, and immunologic assays are available for some compounds. GC and MS may be used for confirmation. There has been some success using over-the-counter drug test kits to detect amphetamines in canine urine (Teitler, 2009).

Other Stimulants

MDMA, sold as "ecstasy," is a common illegal club drug and will be discussed in some detail. Laws vary between countries and states as to the legality of the herbal stimulant Khat and the related synthetic compounds mephedrone and methylenedioxypyrovalerone, which have become common in the United States where they are sold in certain products with innocuous sounding names like "bath salts" and "plant food." Many legally available compounds are commonly used as stimulants and sometimes incorporated into illegal drugs. These include nicotine from tobacco products, methylxanthines such as caffeine, theobromine and theophylline, found in common food and drink products, and alkaloids of the areca nut, present in betel quid. The latter compounds will be addressed briefly.

MDMA

MDMA, more frequently known as "ecstasy," is a Schedule I drug. MDMA was used as an appetite suppressant and in psychotherapy (Smith et al., 2002). The drug has shown some promise in the treatment of Parkinson's disease and posttraumatic stress disorder, but there are no accepted medical uses at this time (Morton, 2005). Currently, MDMA is one of the most popular club drugs in the United States and use increased 70% worldwide between 1995 and 2001 (Anonymous, 2011). Surveys of US students found that 5%–6.7% of students had used MDMA in high school and 2% of 8th graders had used it (Eaton et al., 2010; Latimer and Zur, 2010).

MDMA has been sold under numerous different names, a short list of which includes "Adam," "Batman," "bibs," "blue kisses," blue Nile," "charity," "clarity," "Debs," "decadence," "E," "Eve," "go," "happy pill," "hug drug," "lover's speed," "M," "roll" or "rolling," "Scooby snacks," "X" and "XTC." Tablets containing 50–150 mg MDMA are often brightly colored with pressed images such as product logos, butterflies, smiley faces, numbers, or letters. Less commonly encountered are the powdered or capsule forms. "Ecstasy" tablets tested in Europe during the 1990s only contained 50% MDMA on average (Libiseller et al., 2005). Those tested in the US averaged 83% MDMA (Anonymous, 2011). Other common ingredients included ketamine, methamphetamine, MDA, and MDEA.

The LD_{50} of MDMA in rats is between 160 and 325 mg/kg PO. Dogs given 15 mg/kg MDMA showed severe clinical signs, and one of six of the dogs died (Frith et al., 1987). MDMA is metabolized in the liver by *N*-demethylation to the active metabolite MDA (Smith et al., 2002).

MDMA is structurally similar to amphetamines and mescaline, which likely explains some of the clinical effects (Lyles and Cadet, 2003). MDMA increases neurotransmitter release, including serotonin, dopamine, and NE (Smith et al., 2002; Morton, 2005; Rimsza and Moses, 2005). Hallucinogenic effects have been attributed to serotonin release and inhibition of reuptake. This drug also inhibits MAO. MDMA directly binds to certain receptors, including 5-HT_2 receptors, α_2-adrenergic receptors, M_1 muscarinic receptors, and H_1 histamine receptors, with less affinity for 5-HT_1, dopamine, α_1, and β receptors.

Frith et al. (1987) described the effects of MDMA given to dogs in increasing oral doses, and they were similar to those described for other amphetamines. Clinical signs began after about 45 min and continued for 6–8 h. Dogs given low doses (3 mg/kg) most frequently showed symptoms of hyperactivity and mydriasis. Dogs given 9 mg/kg also became tachypneic with hypersalivation and circling behavior. One of six dogs given 15 mg/kg MDMA died after showing clinical sings that included vocalization, aggression, convulsions, and front limb paralysis.

Onset and duration of clinical signs are similar in humans, though onset is more rapid with insufflation (Smith et al., 2002; Rimsza and Moses, 2005). Mydriasis, delirium confusion, agitation, bruxism, tremors, seizures, and loss of consciousness have been reported in MDMA users, as have hyperthermia and rhabdomyolysis (Kisseberth and Trammel, 1990; Smith et al., 2002; Liechti et al., 2005; Rimsza and Moses, 2005). Cardiovascular changes can include tachycardia, or less commonly bradycardia, AV block, and hypertension. A few deaths have been attributed to cardiopulmonary arrest (Liechti et al., 2005) and liver failure (Andreu et al., 1998; Gable, 2004; Rimsza and Moses, 2005; Liechti et al., 2005). Onset of liver failure occurs days to weeks after exposure, and the mechanism is not understood, though a hypersensitivity reaction has been suggested in some cases.

Treatment of MDMA exposure consists of appropriate gastrointestinal detoxification, as with amphetamines, and symptomatic and supportive care.

Khat, Mephedrone and Methylenedioxypyrovalerone

Khat (*C. edulis*) is a plant found in East Africa and the Arabian Peninsula. Traditionally, leaves of this shrub have been chewed or consumed as a stimulant, but they are sometimes smoked. The leaves contain cathinone, a DEA Schedule I substance, which breaks down after about 36 h, and the more stable compound cathine, which is a Schedule IV substance (Anonymous, 2011). Clinical signs associated with khat use include reduced appetite, tachycardia, hypertension, and insomnia.

Bupropion is a synthetic cathinone prescribed for smoking cessation and depression, and diethylpropion is used for appetite suppression (Rech et al., 2015). Mephedrone (4-methylmethcathinone) and methylenedioxypyrovalerone (MDPV) are compounds related to cathinone that have increased exponentially in popularity as recreational drugs over the past couple of decades. Mephedrone became illegal in the United Kingdom in April 2010 where it sold for approximately 20% of the cost of cocaine and was that nation's fourth most popular drug, after marijuana, cocaine and MDMA (Elwell, 2010). Mephedrone and MDPV are sold in the United States as "bath salts" and "plant food" under brand names such as "Ivory Snow," "Red Dove," and "Vanilla Sky."

Mephedrone and MDPV are snorted or ingested. Clinical signs usually last a few hours, but can linger for days (Elwell, 2010). Users report euphoria, increased energy, and talkativeness. Poison centers report agitation, confusion, tachycardia, hypertension, mydriasis, tremors, fever, rhabdomyolysis, electrolyte abnormalities, renal failure, seizures, psychosis, hypertension, and violent behavior (Rech et al., 2015). Other reported adverse effects have included epistaxis, mydriasis, and cardiac arrhythmias. Later, users experience fatigue, dizziness, and depression.

Betel quid

Though not common in most areas of the United States, alkaloids of the areca nut are believed to be one of the most commonly used psychoactive substances in the world after caffeine, ethanol, and nicotine. It is estimated that 10%–20% of the world's population have access to "betel quid" containing these alkaloids, mostly in South and Southeast Asia and the Asia Pacific regions. These products can also be purchased in US cities with large populations of Asian immigrants.

Palm trees of the genus *Areca* are cultivated in tropical and subtropical areas of the world to produce betel quid (Deng et al., 2001). The nut of this palm tree may be ingested green, ripe, raw, baked, roasted, boiled, fermented, or processed with various sweeteners. It is most commonly processed with leaves from the betel shrub, *Piper betle*, and calcium hydroxide. Tobacco and various spices are sometimes added. The betel quid industry is worth hundreds of millions of dollars. Betel quid is produced both regionally and under trade names such as Supari, Mainpuri tobacco, mawa, pan masala and Gutka. Gutka is illegal in some parts of India.

Alkaloids present in areca nut include arecoline, arecaidine, guvacine and guvacoline. These alkaloids bind with muscarinic receptors, induce coronary vasospasms, and have weak activity on nicotinic receptors in the ganglia.

Oral submucosal fibrosis is a preneoplastic lesion common in young people who use betel quid. Clinical signs seen in inexperienced users and overdoses are more likely to be of interest to the veterinarian and include mucosal irritation, nausea and vomiting, bronchoconstriction, hypersalivation, lacrimation, urinary incontinence, diarrhea, hypertension or hypotension, tachycardia, acute myocardial infarction, and extrapyramidal symptoms. Most patients given supportive care recover within 24 h. Atropine has not been found effective as a treatment in humans (Deng et al., 2001).

HALLUCINOGENS AND DISSOCIATIVE DRUGS

The clinical effects of hallucinogenic and dissociative drugs are unpredictable and dependent very much on the individual and his or her environment (Nichols, 2004). Many compounds that alter consciousness have been termed "hallucinogens," though some, like marijuana and MDMA, only induce hallucinations under specific circumstances or at very high doses. "Psychomimetic" is a term used to describe drugs that cause behavioral changes mimicking psychosis, but this terminology is of limited usefulness in veterinary medicine. "Psychedelic" is a term commonly used by the media and translates from the Greek, more or less, as "mind revealing," but again, this term is unlikely to be useful in veterinary medicine.

Lysergic acid diethylamide (LSD), a synthetic product similar to natural ergot alkaloids, is a common hallucinogen that acts on serotonin receptors. Hallucinogens with a similar mechanism of action include mescaline and *N,N*-dimethyltryptamine (DMT), described below. *Psilocybe* spp. and related mushroom species contain the hallucinogen psilocybin. Vomiting was reported after *Psilocybe* spp. mushroom ingestion in a dog (Spoerk, 2005). Behavioral changes in a horse suspected of ingesting *Psilocybe* spp. included fear and extreme aggression with recovery in 48 h (Hyde, 1990). Symptoms of severe toxicosis in a colt included hyperexcitability, tremors, mydriasis, and bruxism. The colt was eventually euthanized because of traumatic injuries and weakness (Jones, 1990). Symptoms of psilocybin in cats are similar to those described below with LSD (Jacobs et al., 1977). DMT is produced by several plants including *Psychotria viridis*, used to produce a tea known as Ayahuasca in the traditional practices of the indigenous people of the Amazon, *Anadenanthera peregrina* seeds, called yopo by native people of the Amazon rain forest, and *Phalaris* spp. of grass, which grows around the world. 5-methoxy-*N*, *N*-dimethyltryptamine and/or *N*, *N*- (bufotenin) are serotonergic compounds produced in the parotid glands of various species of toads, along with bufodienolide glycosides, which are potent cardiac glycosides.

Leaves of the plant *Salvia divinorum* are illegal to possess in some states of the United States and some European countries. *S. divinorum* preparations are commonly used to produce hallucinogenic effects, though by a unique mechanism described below.

Dissociative anesthetics are so-called because they uncouple functions of the brain such as sensory/motor activity and emotion/consciousness, sometimes producing a cataleptic-type state (Branson, 2001). Affected individuals become disconnected from their environment, and there is an absence of response to nociceptive stimuli. The synthetic drug phencyclidine is an example of a dissociative agent. Ketamine, a familiar therapeutic drug to most veterinarians, is a dissociative anesthetic and popular as a "club drug."

Several naturally occurring substances other than those mentioned above have been used to produce hallucinogenic effects by various mechanisms. Certain species of mushrooms in the genus *Amanita*, specifically *A. muscaria* and *A. pantherina*, are sometimes intentionally ingested. These mushrooms contain ibotenic acid and muscimol, which bind glutamate receptors. Various plants containing atropine and scopolamine, including *Datura stramonium*, *Atropa belladonna*, *Mandragora officinarum* and *Hyoscyamus niger*, are routinely smoked or ingested as recreational drugs (Halpern, 2004). The drug dextromethorphan has been used recreationally for its dissociative effects.

LSD and LSA

LSD is the most powerful known hallucinogen (Nichols, 2004; O'Shea and Fagan, 2006). The D-isomer of LSD is responsible for the molecule's effect on the CNS. The story of Albert Hoffman's synthesis and subsequent exposure to LSD is well documented elsewhere. LSD was marketed under the trade name Delysid and used in psychotherapy and for experimental purposes. Though there are no currently accepted medical uses for this drug, it has shown some promise for use in the treatment of alcoholism, drug addiction, and obsessive-compulsive disorder. After becoming a popular recreational drug, LSD use was banned by the US government in 1966, and it is currently a Schedule I drug (Nichols, 2004; Volmer, 2005).

LSD is a colorless, odorless, and flavorless white powder that is usually dissolved in water and then applied to other substances such as blotter paper, microdots, tiny tablets, gelatin squares (termed "window pane" or "window glass"), stamps, gummy bears and other candies, and sugar cubes (Rimsza and Moses, 2005; Volmer, 2005; O'Shea and Fagan, 2006; Anonymous, 2011). Street names for LSD reflect these applications and include "acid," as in "spiked with acid," "blotter" or "blotter acid," "cubes," "dots" or "microdot," "L," "sugar" or "sugar cubes," "trip," or "wedding bells." Use of LSD is declining in the United States (Banken, 2004; Nichols, 2004). Still, a survey found that 3% of US high-school seniors had used LSD over a period of 12 months (Latimer and Zur, 2011).

The seeds of *Ipomoea violacea*, the morning glory, contain lysergic acid amide (LSA), which is approximately 1/10th as potent as LSD, at a concentration of 0.02% dry matter (Halpern, 2004). Ingestion of 150–300 seeds causes clinical effects in humans (Frohne and Pfänder, 2004; Halpern, 2004; Volmer, 2005). The seed coat is protective, thus seeds must be crushed, germinated, or soaked in water for ingestion to be effective. A word of caution to the adventurous: emetics are sometimes added to commercial morning glory seeds. Other sources of LSA include seeds of the Hawaiian baby woodrose, *Argyreia nervosa*, at a concentration of 0.14% dry matter, and endophyte-infected sleepy grass, *Stipa robusta*. *S. robusta*, is present in the southwestern United States.

Toxicity

The effective dose of LSD for humans is between 0.05 and 0.20 mg. Products sold currently usually contain 0.04–0.06 mg and are less likely to cause an adverse reaction than the pills sold in the 1960s, which could contain up to 0.25 mg LSD. Increasing the dose produces both quantitative and qualitative differences in the response (Nichols, 2004). Some cats given intraperitoneal (IP) injections of 2.5 μg LSD/kg body weight showed mild clinical signs, and a dose of 50 μg/kg produced significant clinical signs in all cats tested (Jacobs et al., 1977). The IV LD_{50} for rats is 16 mg/kg (Volmer, 2005).

Toxicokinetics

LSD is rapidly absorbed after ingestion in humans (Riordan et al., 2002; Volmer, 2005). Peak plasma concentrations occur within 6 h and LSD is approximately 80% protein bound. Metabolism occurs primarily in the liver by hydroxylation and glucuronide conjugation to an inactive metabolite. A dose of LSD is 89% excreted in the feces, and the elimination half-life is between 2 and 5 h. Clinical effects can persist for 12 h (Nichols, 2004).

Mechanism of Action

Like many "recreational" hallucinogens, LSD acts primarily as an antagonist at serotonin receptors (Volmer, 2005; O'Shea and Fagan, 2006). LSD is structurally similar to serotonin. Actions at the 5-HT_{2A} receptor are believed to be responsible for the hallucinogenic effects, though the signaling pathways involved have not been completely elucidated. The 5-HT_{2A} receptors are located in the pyramidal cells of the prefrontal cortex, the reticular nucleus of the thalamus, and possibly the locus coeruleus, where they are involved in sensory processing. LSD and some other hallucinogens also have a strong affinity for the 5-HT_{1A}, 5-HT_{2C} and other serotonin receptors, but the significance of this is not understood (Nichols, 2004). LSD causes increased release of glutamate in the prefrontal cortex, has a high affinity for dopamine receptors D_1 and

D_2, and shows some affinity for α_1 and α_2 adrenergic receptors (Nichols, 2004; Volmer, 2005).

Clinical Signs

General symptoms reported in nonhuman animals include disorientation, mydriasis, depression or excitation, and vocalization (Volmer, 2005). Behavioral changes reported in cats given IP injections of LSD included paw flicking, head and body shaking, yawning, chops licking, bizarre sitting and standing positions, falling from their perch, "leaping about," compulsive scratching at the litter, pawing at the water, biting objects in the cage, play behaviors including pawing and sniffing objects, tail chasing, "hallucinatory behavior," described as tracking, staring at, batting at, or pouncing on objects that were not apparent to the observer, frequent defecation and occasionally emesis. Grooming behaviors included rubbing the head with paws, licking, biting and scratching, and were sometimes "incomplete"—the cat would lick or bite the air or stick her tongue out. Rage behavior and vocalization were not seen in these cats (Jacobs et al., 1977). Based on this study, one can only imagine the presenting complaint in a companion animal exposed to LSD.

Treatment

Treatment is based on close observation with supportive and symptomatic care. Because absorption of LSD is relatively rapid and effects are self-limiting, gastrointestinal decontamination is unlikely to be beneficial (Riordan et al., 2002; Volmer, 2005). Clinical signs sometimes persist for up to 12 h after ingestion of a large dose. Animals should be kept in a quiet, dark room to minimize sensory stimulation and restraint should be minimized to prevent hyperthermia. Laboratory techniques that have been employed in the detection of LSD include immunoassays, thin-layer chromatography, HPLC, and LC/MS.

Phencyclidine and Ketamine

Phencyclidine, 1-(1-phenylcyclohexyl) piperidine, is a Schedule II synthetic drug with more than 80 known analogs. One such analog, ketamine or 2((-*o*-chlorophenyl)-2-methylamino)-cyclohexanone HCl, has less than 1/10th the potency of phencyclidine and is a Schedule III drug. Phencyclidine was originally used as an anesthetic under the trade names Sernyl for human patients and later Sernylan for veterinary patients. Sernyl, given IV, produces decreased response to nociceptive stimuli with insignificant respiratory and cardiac depression and no loss of corneal, papillary, or other reflexes (Branson, 2001). However, Sernyl was associated with postoperative psychosis, dysphoria, delirium, violent behavior, and hallucinations (Kisseberth and Trammel, 1990; Pestaner and Southall, 2003; Volmer, 2005; Anonymous, 2011). Sernylan was used in dogs and nonhuman primates and was the preferred anesthetic for crocodilians (Ortega, 1967; Stunkard and Miller, 1974). Phencyclidine was last used commercially in the United States in 1978.

Phencyclidine is easily synthesized in clandestine laboratories. It is available in powdered or crystal form, which is dissolved in liquids such as water or "embalming fluid" containing formaldehyde and methanol, or it can be sold as tablets or capsules. Street products range from 5% to 90% purity, and phencyclidine is sometimes substituted for THC, mescaline, LSD, amphetamines, or cocaine. Phencyclidine is said to have a distinctive odor (Anonymous, 2011). This drug is frequently sold under the name "PCP," but other terms include "angel dust" or "angel hair," "boat" or "love boat," "dummy dust," "CJ," "hog" or "hog dust," "PeaCe Pill," "rocket fuel," "stardust," "whack," and "zombie dust." "Embalming fluid" is added to cigarettes containing tobacco, marijuana or other leafy material such as parsley, mint, or oregano. Names for this type of product include "supergrass," "amp," "happy sticks," "sherm," and "wet sticks."

Ketamine is not as readily produced by the amateur chemist but is used in veterinary and, less commonly, human medicine. Ketamine is a racemic mixture of R-ketamine and S-ketamine. Ketamine is labeled for use in cats and nonhuman primates. It is still used by physicians in pediatrics and in emergency and critical care situations where maintaining blood pressure and respiration are challenging. Ketamine is an odorless, flavorless liquid, which is often dried and crystallized, then powdered for illicit use. Ketamine can be ingested, injected, insufflated, or placed into tobacco or marijuana cigarettes and smoked and has been used to "spike" drinks. Street names for ketamine include "cat valium," "green," "jet," "K," "special K," or "vitamin K," "keets," "kit-kat," "super acid," and "super C."

Toxicity

Phencyclidine given orally at doses of 2.5–10 mg/kg produces clinical effects in dogs and doses of 25 mg/kg were lethal in all of six dogs treated (Kisseberth and Trammel, 1990; Volmer, 2005). Given via intramuscular (IM) injection, 2 mg/kg caused muscular incoordination, 5 mg/kg caused immobilization and convulsions in 1/5 of dogs, and 15 mg/kg caused convulsions in 2/2 dogs treated (Ortega, 1967).

Ketamine has a high therapeutic index in domestic mammals. The sedative dose in cats is 20 mg/kg IM. Doses of 5–10 mg/kg IM have produced convulsive seizures in dogs. IV injections of 2 mg/kg produce ataxia in sheep and dissociative analgesia in cattle. Doses of 5–15 mg/kg IV caused struggling and vocalization in goats (Branson, 2001). The approximate LD_{50} for ketamine in rodents is 600 mg/kg PO (Gable, 2004). Large doses of ketamine do not appear to produce analgesia in chickens or pigeons, but a dose of 0.11 mg/kg was reportedly associated with respiratory failure in pigeons. A dose of 0.05–0.1 mg/kg produced anesthesia in parakeets, but 0.5 mg/kg IM was lethal (Branson, 2001).

Toxicokinetics

Phencyclidine is ionized at gastric pH, thus little is absorbed in the stomach, but there is significant intestinal absorption (Kisseberth and Trammel, 1990; Volmer, 2005). Inhaled phencyclidine is well absorbed. The drug is lipophilic, with a wide tissue distribution that includes the CNS, adipose tissue, and gastric secretions. The latter leads to recycling and increases the biological half-life. Metabolism is variable between species. In the dog, approximately 68% of a given dose undergoes hepatic metabolism to a monohydroxyl form which is then conjugated for excretion. The remaining 32% is excreted unchanged in the urine. Approximately 88% of a dose of phencyclidine is excreted unchanged in the urine in cats.

Peak plasma concentrations in cats occur 10 min after IM injection of ketamine (Branson, 2001; Volmer, 2005). Ketamine is about 50% bound to plasma proteins in horses. It is distributed to the brain, adipose tissue, liver, lung, and other tissues. Ketamine undergoes hepatic metabolism via *N*-demethylation or hydroxylation and glucuronide conjugation to a water soluble metabolite for excretion in the urine. The elimination half-life is approximately 67 min in the cat after parenteral dosing, 60 min in the calf, 42 min in the horse after IV dosing, and 2–3 h in the human (Branson, 2001).

Mechanism of Action

How compounds like phencyclidine and ketamine produce their dissociative effects is not entirely understood. It is known that these drugs act on sites in the cerebral cortex, thalamus, and limbic system (Branson, 2001; Pal et al., 2002; Volmer, 2005). The effects on behavior and cognition in humans can mimic schizophrenia. Phencyclidine and ketamine bind to *N*-methyl-D-aspartate (NMDA) receptors at a different site than glutamate, the excitatory neurotransmitter, and therefore, act as noncompetitive inhibitors. Reuptake of NE, dopamine, and serotonin is decreased through inhibition of the biogenic amine reuptake complex. The sympathomimetic effects are associated with changes in heart rate, blood pressure, and cardiac output, and increased myocardial oxygen consumption. Phencyclidine inhibits γ-aminobutyric acid. Cardiovascular effects are more prominent with ketamine than phencyclidine.

Ketamine induces stage I and stage II anesthesia but not stage III. Ketamine acts on non-NMDA glutamate receptors, dopaminergic receptors, nicotinic receptors, muscarinic receptors, and opioid receptors. Analgesic properties are most likely attributable to the actions of ketamine on opioid receptors.

Ketamine is usually sold as a racemic mixture, but the S-enantiomer is the active portion. S-ketamine is being studied for therapeutic use by physicians treating major depressive disorder and by veterinarians for use in anesthesia.

Clinical Signs

Dogs dosed with phencyclidine appear depressed at low doses and stimulated at high doses, with the potential for convulsive seizures (Branson, 2001). Onset of clinical effects is within 2 min of IV dosing (Ortega, 1967). Symptoms reported in dogs include muscular rigidity, risus sardonicus-like facial expression, increased motor activity, head weaving, stereotyped sniffing behavior, blank staring, incoordination, hypersalivation, nystagmus, opisthotonos, ascending loss of motor function, coma, tonic–clonic convulsions, and hyperthermia (Ortega, 1967; Kisseberth and Trammel, 1990; Volmer, 2005). Cardiovascular effects include tachycardia, hypertension, and cardiac arrhythmia. Deaths have been attributed to respiratory failure. Symptoms associated with phencyclidine in swine include muscle tremors and hypersalivation (Jones, 1972). Behavioral changes have been noted in neonates that were exposed during gestation (Branson, 2001). Reported changes in clinical chemistry parameters include acidosis, hypoglycemia, electrolyte imbalances, and increased creatine phosphokinase and aspartate transaminase. Postmortem lesions associated with phencyclidine include epicardial and subendocardial hemorrhage and pulmonary congestion and hemorrhage (Kisseberth and Trammel, 1990; Volmer, 2005).

Pineal, pedal, photic, corneal, papillary, laryngeal, pharyngeal, and other reflexes are maintained during ketamine anesthesia (Branson, 2001; Volmer, 2005). There are significant species differences in the effects of ketamine. Ketamine increases muscle tone in cats, sometimes causing forelimb extensor rigidity or opisthotonos. Other symptoms in cats include mydriasis and fixed staring. Hypersalivation and chops licking are associated with oral dosing. Most cats can sit upright within 2 h and recover completely within 10 h. Ketamine causes excitation in dogs and can produce tonic–clonic seizures. Tonic-clonic seizures have been described in dogs undergoing an anesthesia protocol that utilized S-ketamine (Adami et al., 2013). Pulmonary edema was reported in a dog 2 days after anesthesia with ketamine and xylazine. Hypersalivation, apneustic breathing, and increased pulse are reported in sheep. Goats salivate, struggle, and vocalize but usually recover within 20 min of dosing.

Nonhuman primates have increased heart and respiratory rates, hypertension, and tonic-clonic seizures (Christie et al., 2013).

Treatment

Prognosis for an animal overdosed with phencyclidine or ketamine is generally good with early intervention, but self-induced trauma and rhabdomyolysis are possible complications. Cats that have undergone ketamine anesthesia usually recover rapidly and are able to sit up within 2 h (Branson, 2001). Dogs injected with low doses of phencyclidine (1 mg/kg IM) recovered almost completely in a little over an hour, and at higher doses (5 mg/kg) were able to sit up within 2 h (Ortega, 1967).

Treatment of phencyclidine or ketamine overdose is generally symptomatic and supportive. Animals must be kept in a dark, quiet room and restraint is to be avoided.

Inducing emesis is of limited use because of the rapid absorption of phencyclidine, but may be attempted in very recent ingestions of large doses if no contraindications exist (Kisseberth and Trammel, 1990). Activated charcoal binds phencyclidine, prevents recycling, and is reported to reduce mortality in dogs and rats. Repeated dosing of activated charcoal is recommended because of enterohepatic cycling. Forced diuresis with mannitol or furosemide will increase the rate of clearance. Urinary acidification enhances excretion but is contraindicated in the presence of acidosis or rhabdomyolysis. Electrolyte abnormalities and hypoglycemia should be corrected as necessary.

Cardiorespiratory abnormalities have been reported in some species. Muscle rigidity, hyperactivity, and seizures associated with ketamine have been treated successfully with diazepam. Severe seizures require barbiturates or general anesthesia. The body temperature of the patient must be closely monitored.

Other Compounds

Mescaline, the active compound in peyote, is a well-studied hallucinogen because of its significance both culturally and in the illicit drug trade. Salvinorin-A is an agent with hallucinogenic potential that is found in the legal herb *S. divinorum*.

Mescaline

Use of mescaline (3,4,5-trimethoxyphenethylamine) dates back to approximately 8500 BC (Bruhn et al., 2002). It is derived from several species of cactus including *Lophophora williamsii*, the peyote *Echinopsis pachanoi*, the San Pedro cactus, and *E. peruvianus*, the Peruvian torch cactus. The latter two cacti are native to South America and are common ornamental plants. Both can be boiled into a soup for ingestion. Peyote grows in the southwestern United States and Mexico and is used legally by indigenous people. A tuberous root grows into the ground and is capped by crowns or "buttons" which are removed. The buttons may contain 1.5% mescaline on a dry matter basis. Buttons can be eaten fresh but are often dried. Dried buttons are chewed, powdered, reconstituted, or steeped into a tea. Pickled buttons have caused botulism (Halpern, 2004). Though traditional uses are permitted, mescaline is a Schedule I drug.

Mescaline is well absorbed by oral and parenteral routes in the dog, with maximum plasma concentrations detected within an hour of ingestion. Mescaline concentrations detected in the brain reflect blood concentrations. Renal, hepatic, and splenic concentrations are three to six times blood concentrations. Mescaline can be detected in the urine within 30 min of exposure and remains detectable for up to 24 h. Between 28% and 46% of a given dose is excreted unchanged in the urine (Cochin et al., 1950). The mescaline molecule is structurally similar to serotonin and acts on the 5-HT_{2A} receptor (Nichols, 2004).

Clinical signs of mescaline intoxication in dogs include vomiting, mydriasis, injection of the conjunctiva, hyperreflexia, chewing motions of the jaw, excitation and disorientation, or sometimes profound depression. Dogs are reported to recover from severe depression within 10 h (Cochin et al., 1950). Symptoms in humans are fairly similar and may include emesis, especially after ingestion of *Echinopsis* spp. (Halpern, 2004). Other symptoms that have been reported are mydriasis, sweating, hallucinations, synesthesia, disorientation, incoordination, increased heart rate and blood pressure, and hyperthermia.

Salvia divinorum

S. divinorum, known as salvia, is a perennial sage closely related to mint. The plant is native to Mexico and grows in humid, semitropical climates. It is cultivated in California and Hawaii (Anonymous, 2011). The plant is of cultural significance to the Mazatec Indians of Oaxaca, Mexico, where it is used to treat diarrhea, headaches, rheumatism, and semimagical diseases (Prisinzano, 2005). These indigenous Mexicans either chew the fresh leaves or extract the juice. Salvia is also smoked (Frohne and Pfänder, 2005; Prisinzano, 2005). Salvia is a controlled substance in parts of Europe and the United States.

Salvia contains various diterpenes, including salvinorins A through F and divinatorins A through C. Similar compounds are present in plants of the genus *Coleus*. Biological effects are attributed to salvinorin-A. Salvinorin-A is absorbed through the oral mucosa (Halpern, 2004). Little is known about the metabolism of this compound, but the elimination half-life in nonhuman primates averages 55.6 min (Prisinzano, 2005). Unlike other traditional hallucinogens, salvinorin-A is an agonist at the κ receptor and has no known effect on the 5-HT_{2A} receptor. There is evidence that salvinorin-A also acts at the CB1 receptor. Clinical signs reported in humans have included disorientation, tachycardia, and acute psychosis (Rech et al., 2014). No toxic effects were seen in mice given high doses of salvia. No poisonings have been reported in domestic animals.

CONCLUDING REMARKS AND FUTURE DIRECTIONS

Toxicoses due to ingestion of illegal substances are infrequently reported in veterinary literature but are anecdotally common. With the high incidence of "recreational" drug use in the United States, occasional companion animal exposures are expected. Exposures are through accidental ingestion of the owner or neighbor's private "stash" or intentional exposure, either in attempting to get the pet "stoned" or with lethal intent. Though companion animals are far more likely to ingest "recreational" drugs, there are documented exposures of cattle and horses to illegally cultivated marijuana, and illegal drugs have been used to alter the performance of horses and other animal athletes.

There are numerous drugs used for recreational purposes, and their actions vary mechanistically, producing a broad range of clinical signs. Treatment requires detoxification and symptomatic and supportive therapy. Rarely are specific antidotes available, though antagonists are available for opioid drugs. The quantity of the drug ingested and the severity of clinical signs are important factors for determining the treatment regimen and prognosis. Some drugs, however, such as marijuana, can cause severe CNS symptoms in animals and yet have an excellent prognosis with early and appropriate intervention.

REFERENCES

Adami, C., Spadavecchia, C., Casoni, D., 2013. Seizure activity occurring in two dogs after S-ketamine induction. Schweiz Arch Tierheilkd. 155 (10), 569–572.

Adams, H.R., 2001. Adrenergic agonists and antagonists. In: Adams, R. (Ed.), Veterinary Pharmacology and Therapeutics, eighth ed. Iowa State University Press, Ames, IA, pp. 91–116.

Andreu, V., Mas, A., Bruguera, M., et al., 1998. Ecstasy: a common cause of severe acute hepatotoxicity. J Hepatol. 29, 394–397.

Anonymous, 2011. Street Drugs: A Drug Identification Guide. Publishers Group, LLC, Long Lake, MN.

Ashton, C.H., 2001. Pharmacology and effects of cannabis: a brief review. Brit. J. Psychatr. 178, 101–186.

Baggot, J.D., Davis, L.E., 1972. Pharmacokinetic study of amphetamine elimination in dogs and swine. Biochem. Pharmacol. 21, 1967–1976.

Banken, J.A., 2004. Drug abuse trends among youth in the United States. Ann. NY Acad. Sci. 1025, 465–471.

Bischoff, K., Beier, E., Edwards, W.C., 1998. Methamphetamine poisoning in three Oklahoma dogs. Vet. Hum. Toxicol. 40, 19–20.

Bischoff, K., Jaeger, R., Ebel, J.G., 2011. An unusual case of relay pentobarbital toxicosis in a dog. J. Med. Toxicol. 7 (3), 236–239.

Branson, K.R., 2001. Injectable anesthetics. In: Adams, R. (Ed.), Veterinary Pharmacology and Therapeutics, eighth ed. Iowa State University Press, Ames, IA, pp. 213–267.

Branson, K.R., Gross, M.E., 2001. Opioid agonists and antagonists. In: Adams, R. (Ed.), Veterinary Pharmacology and Therapeutics, eighth ed. Iowa State University Press, Ames, IA, pp. 213–267.

Bruhn, J.G., De Smet, P.A.G.M., El-Seedi, H.R., et al., 2002. Mescaline use for 5700 years. Lancet 359: 1866.

Buchanan, J.A., Vogel, J.A., Eberhardt, A.M., 2010. Levamisole-induced occlusive necrotizing vasculitis of the ears after use of cocaine contaminated with levamisole. J. Med. Toxicol. Online First Accessed February 19, 2011.

Buchta, R., 1988. Deliberate intoxication of young children and pets with drugs: a survey of an adolescent population in a private practice. Am. J. D. C. 142, 701–702.

Burrows, G.E., Tyrl, R.J., 2001. Toxic Plants of North America. Iowa State University Press, Ames, IA, pp. 316–319.

Cardassis, J., 1951. Intoxication des équidés par *Cannabis indica*. Rec. Méd. Vét. 127, 971–973.

Catravas, J.D., Waters, I.W., 1981. Acute cocaine intoxication in the conscious dog: studies on the mechanism of lethality. J. Pharmacol. Exp. Thet. 217, 350–356.

Catravas, J.D., Waters, I.W., Hickenbottom, J.P., et al., 1977. The effects of haloperidol, chlorpromazine, and propranolol on acute amphetamine poisoning in the conscious dog. J. Pharmacol. Exp. Ther. 202, 230–243.

Christie, K.L., Lee, U.J., Lemoy, J.-J., et al., 2013. Generalized seizure activity in an adult Rhesus macaque (*Macaca mulatta*) during ketamine anesthesia and urodynamic studies. Comp. Med. 63 (5), 445–447.

Cochin, J., Woods, L.A., Seevers, M.H., 1950. The absorption, distribution, and urinary excretion of mescaline in the dog. J. Pharmacol. Exp. Ther. 101, 205–209.

Compton, W.M., Thomas, Y.F., Conway, K.P., et al., 2005. Developments in the epidemiology of drug use and drug use disorders. Am. J. Psychiatr. 162, 1492–1502.

Cornelis, I., Vandenbeele, S., Dunon, D., et al., 2016. Presumed phenobarbital-inducedd Stevens-Johnson syndrome in a 4-year-old female Great Dane. Vet. Quart. 36 (4), 242–246.

Davis, W.M., Bedford, J.A., Buelke, J.L., et al., 1978. Acute toxicity and gross behavioral effects of amphetamine, 4-methoxyamphetamines, and mescaline in rodents, dogs, and monkeys. Toxicol. Appl. Pharmacol. 45, 49–62.

Deng, J.F., Ger, J., Tsai, W.J., et al., 2001. Acute toxicities of betel nut: rare but probably overlooked events. Clin. Toxicol. 39, 355–360.

Deschamps, J.-Y., Gualier, J.-M., Podvin, G., et al., 2012. Fatal overdose after ingestion of a transdermal fentanyl patch in two non-human primates. Vet. Anaesth. Analg. 39, 653–656.

Di Marzo, V., De Petrocellis, L., 2006. Plant, synthetic, and endogenous cannabinoids in medicine. Ann. Rev. Med. 57, 17.1–17.22.

Diniz, P.P., Sousa, M.G., Gerardi, D.G., et al., 2003. Amphetamine poisoning in a dog: case report, literature review, and veterinary medical perspectives. Vet. Hum. Toxicol. 45, 315–317.

Driemeier, D., 1997. Marijuana (*Cannabis sativa*) toxicosis in cattle. Vet. Human. Toxicol. 39, 351–352.

Dumonceaux, G.A., 1995. Illicit drug intoxication in dogs. In: Kirk, R.W. (Ed.), Current Veterinary Therapy XII: Small Animal Practice. W.B. Saunders Co, Philadelphia, pp. 250–252.

Dumonceaux, G.A., Beasley, V.R., 1990. Emergency treatment for police dogs used for illicit drug detection. J. Am. Vet. Med. Assoc. 197, 185–187.

Eaton, D.K., Kann, L., Kinchen, S., et al., 2010. Youth risk behavior surveillance – United States, 2009. Morbid Mortal Weekly Rept. 59 (SS5), 1–142.

Elwell, A., 2010. Britain moves to curtail new drug craze. Can. Med. Assoc. J. 182, E393–E394.

Evans, A.G., 1989. Allergic inhalant dermatitis attributed to marijuana exposure in a dog. J. Am. Vet. Med. Assoc. 195, 1588–1590.

Fitzgerald, K.T., Bronstein, A.C., 2013. Adderall® (amphetamine-dextroamphetaime) toxicity. Topics Compan. Anim. Med. 28, 2–7.

Fitzgerald, K.T., Bronstein, A.C., Newquist, K.L., 2013. Marijuana poisoning. Topics Compan. Anim. Med. 28, 8–12.

Fitzgerald, S.D., Grooms, D.L., Scott, M.A., et al., 2006. Acute anhydrous ammonia intoxication in cattle. J. Vet. Diag. Invest. 18, 485–489.

Frazier, K., Colvin, B., Hullinger, G., 1998. Postmortem diagnosis of accidental cocaine intoxication in a dog. Vet. Human. Toxicol. 40, 154–155.

Frith, C.H., Chang, L.W., Lattin, D.L., et al., 1987. Toxicity of methylenedioxymethamphetamine (MDMA) in the dog and rat. Fund. Appl. Toxicol. 9, 110–119.

Frohne, D., Pfänder, H.J., 2004. Poisonous Plants. second ed. Timber Press Inc, Portland, pp. 118–119., 239–241.

Gable, R.S., 2004. Acute toxic effects of club drugs. J. Psychoact. Drugs. 36, 303–313.

Garrett, E.R., Gürkan, T., 1980. Pharmacokinetics of morphine and its surrogates IV: pharmacokinetics of heroin and its derived metabolites in dogs. J. Pharmaceut. Sci. 69, 1116–1134.

Gloyd, J.S., 1982. Abused drugs, street drugs, and drug misuse. J. Am. Vet. Med. Assoc. 181, 880–881.

Godbold, J.C., Hawkins, J., Woodward, M.G., 1979. Acute oral marijuana poisoning in the dog. JAVMA. 175, 1101–1102.

Green, P., 1996. Intestinal obstruction with hemp bedding. Vet. Rec. 138, 71–72.

Halpern, J.H., 2004. Hallucinogens and dissociative agents naturally growing in the United States. Pharmacol. Therapeut. 102, 131–138.

Humphreys, D.J., Longstaffe, J.A., Stodulski, J.B., et al., 1980. Barbiturate poisoning from pet shop meant: possible associated with perivascular injection. Vet. Rec. 107, 517.

Hyde, P.N., 1990. High horse? Vet. Rec. 22, 554.

Indrawirawan, Y., McAlees, T., 2014. Tramadol toxicity in a cat: case report and literature review of serotonin syndrome. J. Fel. Med. Surg. 16, 572–578.

Jacobs, B.L., Trulson, M.E., Stern, W.C., 1977. Behavioral effects of LSD in the cat: proposal of an animal behavior model for studying the actions of hallucinogenic drugs. Brain Res. 132, 301–314.

Janczyk, P., Donaldson, C.W., Gwaltney, S., 2004. Two hundred and thirteen cases of marijuana toxicosis in dogs. Vet. Hum. Toxicol. 46, 19–21.

Johnson, E.M., Myron, L.B., 1995. Substance abuse and violence: cause and consequence. J. Health Care Poor. Underserved. 6, 113–121.

Johnson, L.D., O'Malley, P.M., Bachman, J.G., et al., 2005. Teen Drug Use Down But Progress Halts Among Youngest Teens. University of Michigan News and Information Service, Ann Arbor, MI.

Jones, D.L., 1978. A case of canine cannabis ingestion. New Zealand Vet. J. 26, 135–136.

Jones, J., 1990. "Magic mushroom" poisoning in a colt. Vet. Rec. 24, 603.

Jones, R.S., 1972. A review of tranquilisation and sedation in large animals. Vet. Rec. 90, 613–617.

Kabas, J.S., Blancahrd, S.M., Matsuyama, Y., et al., 1990. Cocaine-mediated impairment of cardiac conduction in the dog: a potential mechanism for sudden death after cocaine. J. Pharmacol. Exper. Therapeut. 252, 185–191.

Kisseberth, W.C., Trammel, H.L., 1990. Illicit and abused drugs. Vet. Clin. N Am. Small Anim. Pract. 20, 405–418.

Kollias-Baker, C., Maxewell, L., Stanley, S., et al., 2003. Detection and quantification of cocaine metabolites in urine samples from horses administered cocaine. J. Vet. Pharmacol. Ther. 26, 429–434.

Latimer, W., Zur, J., 2010. Epidemiologic trends of adolescent use of alcohol, tobacco, and other drugs. Child Adolesc. Pshyciatr. Clin. N Am. 19, 451–646.

Libiseller, K., Pavlic, M., Rabl, W., et al., 2005. An announced suicide with ecstasy. Int. J. Leg. Med. 21, 1–4.

Liechti, M.E., Kunz, I., Kupferschmidt, H., 2005. Acute medical problems because of ecstasy use. Swiss Med. Wkly. 135, 652–657.

Llera, R.M., Volmer, P.A., 2006. Toxicologic hazards for police dogs involved in drug detection. J. Am. Vet. Med. Assoc. 228, 1028–1032.

Lyles, J., Cadet, J.L., 2003. Methylenedioxymethamphetamine (MDMA, Ecstasy) neurotoxicity: cellular and molecular mechanisms. Bran. Res. Rev. 42, 155–168.

Martins, S.S., Sampson, S., Cerdá, M., et al., 2015. Worldwide prevalence and trends in unintentional drug overdose: a systematic review of the literature. Am. J. Publ. Health. 105 (11), e29.

McDonough, M., Kennedy, N., Glasper, A., et al., 2004. Clinical features and management of gamma-hydroxybutyrate (GHB) withdrawal: a review. Drug Alcohol. Depend. 75, 3–9.

Meola, S.D., Tearney, C.C., Haas, S.A., et al., 2012. Evaluation of trends in marijuana toxicosis in dogs living in a state with legalized medical marijuana: 125 dogs (2005-2010). J. Vet. Emer. Crit. Care. 22, 690–696.

Morton, J., 2005. Ecstasy: pharmacology and neurotoxicity. Curr. Opin. Pharmacol. 5, 79–86.

Nichols, D.E., 2004. Hallucinogens. Pharmacol. Ther. 101, 131–181.

Ortega, J.J.Z., 1967. Phencyclidine for capture of stray dogs. J. Am. Vet. Med. Assoc. 150, 772–776.

O'Shea, B., Fagan, J., 2006. Lysergic acid diethylamide. Irish Med. J. 94, 217.

Pal, H.R., Berry, N., Kumar, R., et al., 2002. Ketamine dependence. Anaesth. Intens. Care. 30, 382–384.

Pestaner, J.P., Southall, P.E., 2003. Sudden death during arrest and phencyclidine intoxication. Am. J. Foren. Med. Pathol. 24, 119–122.

Prisinzano, T.E., 2005. Psychopharmacology of the hallucinogenic sage Salvia divinorum. Life Sci. 78, 527–531.

Queiroz-Neto, A., Zamur, G., Lacerda-Neto, J.C., et al., 2002. Determination of the highest no-effect dose (HNED) and of the elimination pattern for cocaine in horses. J. Appl. Toxicol. 22, 117–121.

Rech, M.A., Donahey, E., Cappiello Dziedzic, J.M., et al., 2015. New drugs of abuse. Pharmacotherapy. 35 (2), 189–197.

Rimsza, M.E., Moses, K.S., 2005. Substance abuse on the college campus. Pediatr. Clin. North Am. 52, 307–319.

Riordan, M., Rylance, G., Berry, K., 2002. Poisoning in children 5: rare and dangerous poisons. Arh. Dis. Child. 87, 407–410.

Schwartz, R.H., Riddle, M., 1985. Marijuana intoxication in pets. J. Am. Vet. Med. Assoc. 187, 206.

Smetzer, D.L., Senta, T., Hensel, J.D., 1972. Cardiovascular effects of amphetamine in the horse. Can. J. Comp. Med. 36, 185–194.

Smith, K.M., Karvube, K.L., Romanelli, F., 2002. Club drugs: methylenedioxymethamphetamine, flunitrazepam, ketamine HCl, and ©-hydroxybutyrate. Am. J. Health-Syst. Pharm. 59, 1067–1076.

Smith, R.A., 1988. Coma in a ferret after ingestion of cannabis. Vet. Hum. Toxicol. 31, 262.

Smith, R.K., Papworth, S., 1996. Intestinal obstruction with hemp bedding. Vet. Rec. 138, 71–72.

Spoerk, D., 2005. Mushrooms. In: Peterson, M.E., Talcott, P.A. (Eds.), Small Animal Toxicology, second ed. Saunders, Philadelphia, pp. 273–311.

Stunkard, J.A., Miller, J.C., 1974. An outline guide to general anesthesia in exotic species. Vet. Med. Sm. Anim. Clin. 69, 1181–1186.

Suchard, J.R., Nizkorodov, S.A., Wilkinson, S., 2009. 1,4-Butandiol content of aqua dots in children's craft toy beads. J. Med. Toxicol. 5, 120–124.

Teitler, J.B., 2009. Evaluation of a human on-site urine multidrug test for emergency use with dogs. J. Am. Anim. Hosp. Assoc. 45, 59–66.

Thomas, E.K., Drobatz, K.J., Mandell, D.C., 2014. Presumptive cocaine toxicosis in 19 dogs: 2004-2012. J. Vet. Emerg. Crit. Care. 24 (2), 201–207.

Vitale, S., van de Mheen, D., 2005. Illicit drug use and injuries: a review of emergency room studies. Drug Alcohol. Dependen. 82, 1–9.

Volmer, P.A., 2005. "Recreational" drugs. In: Peterson, M.E., Talcott, P.A. (Eds.), Small Animal Toxicology, second ed. Saunders, Philadelphia, pp. 273–311.

Vroegop, M.P., Franssen, E.J., van der Voort, P.H.J., et al., 2009. The emergency care of cocaine intoxications. J. Med. 67, 122–126.

Waller, C.C., McLeod, M.D., 2016. A review of designer anabolic steroids in equine sports. Drug Testing Anal. Available from: http://dx.doi.org/10.1002/dta.2112.

Weigand, T.J., 2010. Adulterated cocaine and lessons learned from the Jake Walk Blues. J. Med. Toxicol. 6, 63–66.

Welshman, M.D., 1986. Doped doberman. Vet. Rec. 119, 512.

Section V

Metals and Micronutrients

Chapter 23

Arsenic

Tam Garland

INTRODUCTION

Arsenic is a ubiquitous element with several different forms. The toxicity of arsenic is determined by its form (Vahter, 1983). The prevalent valences are the +3 and the +5 form. Arsenic is found in both an organic form and an inorganic form with valence numbers ranging from +3 to +5. As^{+3}, or arsenite, is more toxic than arsenate, or As^{+5}.

It is found as different ores and rocks, which are mined, then smelted resulting in elemental arsenic and arsenic trioxide. In the environment, arsenic usually exists in the pentavalent form and soil microorganisms may methylate it. Since it is ubiquitous in many forms, complete avoidance is nearly impossible.

Arsenic's sources and uses have a long and varied history. A partial list is available in Table 23.1.

BACKGROUND

The ubiquitous element arsenic (As) is a nonmetal or metalloid in group V of the period chart. Frequently it is referred to as arsenic metal and is classified for many toxicological purposes as a metal. It exists in several forms with a long history of various uses. It has been used in preparations from insecticides, wood preservatives, herbicides, and medicinal uses. It is responsible for many poisonings in people and animals, both large and small.

PHARMACOKINETICS/TOXICOKINETICS

Different toxic disease syndromes are caused by the different forms of arsenic. Inorganic arsenicals and trivalent organics cause disease syndromes characterized by an effect on the gastrointestinal (GI) tract and the capillaries. In extremely low doses, it is possible the body will develop a tolerance to the arsenic. Pentavalent organic arsenicals produce a neurological syndrome.

There are many factors influencing the absorption of arsenicals. Among those variables are the form of the metal, the particle size, the purity, the solubility, the species affected, and the physical condition of the animal exposed. Susceptibility to inorganic arsenicals varies among species and is highest in humans, followed by dogs, rats, and mice (Harrison et al., 1958; Hays, 1982). Clearly there are many variables affecting the absorption and toxicity of this metal, which increases the difficulty of making accurate predictions of lethal amounts.

Pentavalent organic arsenicals are more easily absorbed than are the trivalent arsenicals, especially through the GI tract. Small amounts of either form may be absorbed via the intact skin, but it usually remains locally within the skin. However, absorption is limited by the size of the arsenical particle size. If the particle size is too large, it is not absorbed. Hence, a more toxic arsenical that is not absorbed because of large particle size may effectively be less toxic.

Once arsenicals are absorbed, the distribution is through the blood to all the organs of the body. Arsenic accumulates in the liver and is slowly distributed to the other tissues. The spleen, kidneys, and lungs are able to accumulate large amounts of arsenic. Arsenic has been shown to cross into the placental barrier, particularly in monkeys, hamsters, and gerbils (Flora and Agrawal, 2017). Chronic doses are stored in the bone, the skin, and other keratinized tissues, such as skin, hair, hooves, and nails (Agency for Toxic Substances and Disease Registry, 2007).

The biotransformation of the arsenicals is poorly understood. There is some conversion from the +5 state to the +3 state, but the redox equilibrium favors the +3.

Methylation occurs by microorganism in the soil, but inorganic arsenicals are also methylated in vivo. The in vivo process may aid in the detoxification process. The kidneys may reduce a small amount of pentavalent arsenic to the more toxic trivalent form.

Arsenicals are excreted through many processes. In most species, between 40% and 70% of the absorbed amount of pentavalent arsenicals are excreted through the urine within 48 h (Vahter, 1983), while smaller quantities may be excreted through the sweat. Trivalent forms of

Veterinary Toxicology. DOI: http://dx.doi.org/10.1016/B978-0-12-811410-0.00023-4

TABLE 23.1 Sources and Uses of Arsenic

Sources	Valence/Form	Uses
Commercial uses and products	Inorganic arsenic trioxide (+3)	Insecticide, cattle dip (0.18%)
	Inorganic sodium arsenite (+3)	Defoliant (highly toxic)
	Inorganic copper acetoarsenite (+3)	Paris green—insecticide (emerald green)
	Inorganic arsenic trioxide (+3)	Smelters
	Inorganic sodium arsenate (+5)	Herbicide
	Inorganic chromated copper arsenate (+5)	Wood preservative
	Inorganic lead arsenate (+5)	Insecticide and medicinal
	Organic pentavalent (+5)	Monosodium methylarsenate (MSMA) and disodium methylarsenate (DSMA) (highly toxic to cattle)
		Ant bait
		Leaded gasoline
Natural sources		Ores, minerals, volcanoes
		Ground water and soil
Medicinals	Potassium arsenite (+3)	Fowler's solution tonic/conditioner
	Organic trivalent arsenical	Thiacetarsamide—heartworm treatment in dogs
	Organic pentavalent arsenical	Tryparsamide—trypanosomiasis—old
	Organic trivalent arsenical	Melarsoprol—trypanocidal
	Organic pentavalent arsenical	Arsenical feed additives (arsanilic acid, sodium arsanilate, 3-nitro, 4-hydroxyphenylarsonic acid)

arsenic are excreted more slowly and through the bile into the feces.

MECHANISM OF ACTION

Arsenite (+3) reacts with sulfhydryl groups (−SH) of proteins and inhibits the enzymes by blocking the active groups. The arsenite inhibits alpha-keto oxidases which contain dithiol groups and are involved in oxidation of pyruvate. Lipoic acid, an essential coenzyme for pyruvic acid oxidase, and alpha-oxyglutaric acid oxidase are inhibited by the arsenite. These play an essential role in the tricarboxylic acid cycle. Actively dividing cells having a high oxidative energy requirement are most susceptible to the effects of arsenicals.

Arsenites induce vasodilation and can cause capillary damage. The cellular integrity of the capillary is affected by an unknown mechanism. Evidence of vascular instability is seen by the presence of congestion, edema, and hemorrhage in most of the visceral organs of animals with acute poisoning. This same mechanism of action occurs with inorganic arsenicals and with organic trivalent arsenicals, and they may be considered as "vascular poisons" (Hann and McHugo, 1960; Jubb and Huxtable, 1993; Agency for Toxic Substances and Disease Registry, 2007).

Arsenates (+5) are a little different. They are uncouplers of oxidative phosphorylation. The inorganic pentavalents may substitute phosphate in this reaction. The result is an increase in body temperature. Organic pentavalents have an unknown mechanism of action. There is some thought that they may interfere with vitamins B_6 and B_1, which may allow for the demyelination and subsequent axonal degeneration that occurs.

From experimental and clinical studies, evidence suggests that arsenic exposure is associated with various cardiopathologic effects, including ischemia, arrhythmia and heart failure. Possible mechanisms of cardiotoxicity include oxidative stress, DNA fragmentation, apoptosis and functional changes of ion channels (Alamolhodaei et al., 2015). Evidence also suggests that ROS mediated mitochondrial disruption, caspase activation, MAPK, and P^{53} are the pathways for arsenic induced apoptosis (Chen et al., 1998).

Although arsenicals have been classified as carcinogens in people, this has not been the case in animals. Experimentally, there have been attempts to document arsenic-related cancer in animals, but the experiments have been unsuccessful (Chan and Huff, 1997; Agency for Toxic Substances and Disease Registry, 2007; Hughes et al., 2011).

TOXICITY

Inorganic arsenicals are up to ten times more toxic than pentavalent arsenicals. The order of toxicity from greatest to least follows this schematic: inorganic As^{+3} (arsenite) > inorganic As^{+5} (arsenate) > trivalent organics > pentavalent organics (I As^{+3} > I As^{+5} > O As^{+3} > O As^{+5}). In other metal toxicities, the organics are more toxic, but with arsenicals the inorganics are the more toxic.

Toxicity is also influenced by many factors, including particle size. The more finely ground, the more surface area there is for reactions. Solutions, such as dips and defoliants, are the most dangerous. However, the causes of the poisonings are varied. Debilitated animals are more sensitive. Since arsenic is not biodegradable, the soil and the old corrals around old dipping vats are still sources for arsenic poisoning. The area around smelters is also a source of poisoning, similar to that of dipping vats. Human mistakes and carelessness are the largest contributing factors to toxic events. For example, feeding a product known as gin trash instead of cotton seed hulls has resulted in numerous animals being poisoned.

Clinical signs caused by either inorganic or trivalent aliphatic arsenicals are similar. Peracute toxicities often result in sudden death within minutes to a few hours if the dose of dissolved arsenic ingestion is high. Acute poisonings have more clinical signs: abdominal pain or colic, vomiting (in those animals capable of vomiting), a staggering gait and weakness, incoordination, rapid weak pulse and shock, diarrhea, followed by collapse and death. If the acute poisoning is through dermal contact, then the arsenic will also be systemic. The skin will have blisters and edema and may be cracked and bleeding, leaving the skin susceptible to secondary infection (National Academy of Science, 1977; Evinger and Blakemaore, 1984). Those receiving a lower dose over a period of time may have subacute poisonings and will likely live several days, developing depression and anorexia. Movements may be difficult, stiff, and uncoordinated. Diarrhea is dark and possibly hemorrhagic and very fluid. Hematuria may be present, or the urine may contain protein and casts (National Academy of Science, 1977; Osweiler et al., 1985). However, those suffering chronic poisoning are easily fatigued and have dyspnea when they are moved. These animals display intense thirst and have a rough dry hair coat as well as dry, brick-red mucous membranes. Cattle are described as having enlarged joints.

Clinical signs of phenylarsenic poisoning occur within 3 days of a high dose or after chronic exposure. Most noticeable are the neurological signs. The animal is generally bright and alert but uncoordinated. The animal may or may not be blind, and these animals may have erythema in the skin. Some of the neurological damage may be reversible unless the nerves are damaged.

Lesions are often dependent upon the dose and survival times. There may be no lesions at all in animals dying from peracute poisoning. However, even these animals have some degree of GI irritation. With the exception of peracute deaths, most of the other animals dying from some form of arsenic poisoning may have excess fluid in the GI tract. In cattle, there is hyperemia of the abomasum, and this may be the only finding. This "paint brush" hyperemic lesion is characteristic of arsenic poisoning. If there are other lesions in cattle, it is often necrosis of the rumen mucosal epithelium. Ruminants have gelatinous serosal edema in the rumen, reticulum, omasum, and abomasum. The GI tract may have indications of irritation and be hemorrhagic. Lesions are indicative of capillary damage, and the liver is usually soft and yellow.

The phenylarsonics (+5) were previously used in feed additives, and lesions would be expected to be associated with overdoses in the feed mixture. A "downer pig" would have severe abrasions with muscle atrophy. Microscopic lesions indicate there was demyelination in the optic nerve and the posterior cord. The FDA announced in 2013 the voluntary withdrawal of roxarson, arsanilic acid, and carbarsone by Zoetis and Fleming Laboratories, leaving only nitarsone approvals in place (CFSAN).

TREATMENT

A diagnosis of arsenic poisoning is important and is based upon clinical history and clinical signs. If more than one animal is involved, then lesions may also be important. Diagnostic arsenic levels in the kidney and liver are usually more than 8–10 parts per million (ppm) unless several days have lapsed since exposure, in which case it would likely be 2–4 ppm. Diagnostic levels of arsenic in the urine and feces are greater, between 10 and 20 ppm. Arsenic should not be found in phenylarsonic acid intoxications.

Removal of the source of arsenic from the animal is critical. Treatment must be directed toward the clinical signs of the patient. There are no specific treatments for organic arsenicals. However, the neurotoxic effects are usually reversible. This involves removing any offending feed early in the process, within 2–3 days of the onset of ataxia. If there is paralysis and nerve damage, then the damage is irreversible. A blind animal usually does not regain sight, but appetite and weight gain will continue if the offending arsenic containing food is removed. The more prolonged the exposure or slow the onset of toxicity, the less likely there will be of recovery.

Inorganic arsenicals can be treated. In small animals, if no clinical sigs are evident in a recent exposure, the animal should have its stomach emptied with warm water or a 1% solution of sodium bicarbonate solution for gastric lavage. Emetics and strong cathartics and parasympathomimetic drugs are not recommended as they may cause rupture of the walls of a weakened GI system (Neiger, 2001). Emesis, cathartics, and charcoal have been used when very early in the process and when there are no clinical signs, but are used with caution if at all. However, in arsenic intoxication, the efficacy of charcoal is undetermined. Following gastric emptying, provide GI protectants, such as kaolin-pectin. If charcoal has been used, then protectants should follow approximately 1–2 h later in small animals. Fluid therapy is appropriate. If the patient is showing clinical signs, then aggressive fluid therapy and if needed, a blood transfusion should be instituted. In cases with clinical signs, British antilewisite (BAL, dimercaprol, or 2,3-dimercaptopropanol), at 2.5–5 mg/kg, IM as a 10% solution in oil is administered every 4 h for 2 days, then every 8 h for the third day and only bid for the next 10 days or until recovery (Neiger, 2001). Recall IM solutions with oil can be painful.

In large animals, the efficacy of BAL alone is questionable. Thioctic acid (lipoic acid or α-lipoic acid) (50 mg/kg, IM, tid, as a 20% solution) is usually combined with BAL (3 mg/kg, IM as a 10% solution in oil, every 4 h for the first 2 days then qid for the third day, then bid treatment for 10 days or until recovery). Thioctic acid may be used alone at the same rate with a reasonable expectation of recovery.

Treatment of large and small animals should include sodium thiosulfate at 0.5–3 g PO, or as a 20% solution, IV, at 30–40 mg/kg, bid-tid for 3–4 days or until recovery. In horses and cattle, sodium thiosulfate has been used, PO, at 20–30 g in 300 mL of water. In goats and sheep, one-fourth of this dose should be used. More recently, it has been shown in cattle that doses of sodium thiosulfate at higher dosages (40 mg/kg IV q8h and 80 mg/kg PO q24h instead of 20–40 mg/kg IV q8h) have achieved better results (Bertin et al., 2013).

The water-soluble analogues of dimercaprol, 2,3-dimercaptopropane-1-sulfonate (DMPS) and dimercapto-succinic acid (DMSA) are considered less toxic (Neiger, 2001), more effective, and may be given orally. In people, D-penicillamine is reportedly an effective chelator, having a wide margin of safety and could be used at 10–50 mg/kg, PO, tid-qid for 3–4 days in animals.

Include specific therapy with supportive therapy. Supportive therapy may be of even greater value, particularly when cardiovascular collapse is imminent, and should involve IV fluids to restore blood volume and correct dehydration. Amino acids and B-complex vitamins should also be included. Kidney and liver function should be monitored during treatment.

CONCLUDING REMARKS AND FUTURE DIRECTIONS

Determining the diagnosis and initiating treatment early will determine the prognosis. Acutely poisoned animals have a poor prognosis without early intervention. Understanding the differentials is important to institute the appropriate treatment for the appropriate condition. Arsenic produces signs of severe gastroenteritis, similar to those of pancreatitis, viral or bacterial gastroenteritis, irritating plants, caustic agents, and zinc phosphide poisoning. Likewise, other heavy metals will produce similar clinical signs. However, poisoning with phenylarsonics, used most frequently in feed additives, has a high morbidity rate but is associated with a low mortality rate. Recovery generally requires 2–4 weeks.

REFERENCES

Agency for Toxic Substances and Disease Registry (ATSDR), 2007. Arsenic Toxicity, Case Studies in Environmental Medicine. US Department of Health and Human Services, Washington, DC.

Alamolhodaei, N.S., Shirani, K., Karimi, G., 2015. Arsenic cardiotoxicity: an overview. Env. Toxicol. Pharmacol. 40, 1005–1014.

Bertin, F.R., Baseler, L.J., Wilson, C.R., et al., 2013. Arsenic toxicosis in Cattle: meta-analysis of 156 cases. J. Vet. Int. Med. 27, 977–981.

Chan, P.C., Huff, J., 1997. Arsenic carcinogenesis in animals and in humans: mechanistic, experimental, and epidemiological evidence. Evniron. Carcino. Ecotox. Rev. 15 (2), 83–122.

Chen, Y.C., Lin-Shiau, S.Y., Lin, J.K., 1998. Involvement of reactive oxygen species and caspase 3 activation in arsenite-induced apoptosis. J. Cell Physiol. 177, 324–333.

Evinger, J.F., Blakemaore, J.C., 1984. Dermatitis in a dog associated with exposure to an arsenic compound. J. Am. Vet. Med. Assoc. 184, 1281–1282.

Flora, S.J.S., Agrawal, S., 2017. Arsenic, cadmium and lead. In: Gupta, R.C. (Ed.), Reproductive and Developmental Toxicology, second ed. Academic Press/Elsevier, Amsterdam, pp. 537–566.

Hann, C., McHugo, P.B., 1960. Studies on the capillary and cardiovascular actions of intravenous sodium arsenate and arsenite. Toxicol. Appl. Pharmacol. 2, 674–682.

Harrison, W.E., Packman, E.W., Abbott, D.D., 1958. Acute oral toxicity and chemical and physical properties of arsenic trioxides. AMA Arch. Ind. Health. 17, 118–123.

Hays, W.J., 1982. Pesticides Studied in Man. Williams & Wilkins, Baltimore.

Hughes, M.F., Beck, B.D., Chen, Y., et al., 2011. Arsenic exposure and Toxicology: a historical perspective. Toxicol. Sci. 123, 305–332.

Jubb, K.V.F., Huxtable, C.R., 1993. The nervous system. In: Jubb, K.V.F., Kennedy, P.C., Palmer, N. (Eds.), Pathology of Domestic Animals, vol. 1. fouth ed. Academic Press, New York.

National Academy of Science (NAS), 1977. Arsenic. National Academy of Science, Washington, DC.

Neiger, R.D., 2001. Arsenic. In: Peterson, M., Talcott, P.A. (Eds.), Small Animal Toxicology. W.B.Saunders Co, New York.

Osweiler, G.D., Carson, T.L., Buck, W.B., Van Gelder, G.A., 1985. Clinical and Diagnostic Veterinary Toxicology. Kendall/Hunt, Dubuque, IA.

Vahter, M., 1983. Metabolism of arsenic. In: Fowler, B.A. (Ed.), Biological and Environmental Effects of Arsenic. Elsevier, New York, NY.

FURTHER READING

Center for Food Safety (CFSAN)Press Release. FDA to Withdraw Approvals of Arsenic in Animal Feed. October 1, 2013. at <http://www.centerforfoodsafety.org/press-releases/2620/fda-to-withdraw-approvals-of-arsenic-in-animal-feed#>.

Chapter 24

Cadmium

Stephen B. Hooser

INTRODUCTION

Cadmium accumulation in plants and animals from several sources of environmental exposure is increasing. The application of rock phosphate (which contains varying amounts of cadmium depending on the source) and sewage sludge fertilizers results in cadmium deposition in the soil of pastures (Piscator, 1985; ATSDR, 2009). In addition to direct ingestion of soil containing cadmium, some forage plants extract cadmium from the soil. Although cadmium accumulation in the soft tissues of livestock has been demonstrated and there is ample experimental documentation of the toxicity of cadmium in animals, under natural conditions, documented cases of direct toxic or carcinogenic effects of cadmium in domestic livestock have been very uncommon (Dorn, 1979); no clinical cases have been reported in farmed ruminants (Lane et al., 2015).

BACKGROUND

Pure cadmium is a soft, silver-white metal with an atomic number of 48 and a molecular weight of 112.41. It is a divalent transition metal with chemical properties that are similar to zinc, and is usually found as a mineral in combination with other elements to form cadmium oxide, cadmium chloride, or cadmium sulfate (ATSDR, 2009). Since numerous compounds are formed from cadmium, it is used in batteries, solders, semiconductors, solar cells, plastics stabilizers, and to plate iron and steel. All soil and rocks contain some cadmium. It can enter the environment from zinc smelting and refining, coal combustion, mine wastes, iron and steel production, and from the use of rock phosphate and sewage sludge as fertilizers (Klasing, 2005).

Cadmium accumulation in plants and animals from a variety of sources is increasing, the most severe being in the vicinity of zinc smelters. The use of cadmium-containing mineral supplements in feed (e.g., from calcium phosphate), the application on pastures and hay fields of phosphate fertilizers (which contain varying amounts of cadmium depending on the source), and sewage sludge results in cadmium deposition in the soil (Piscator, 1985; Lane et al., 2015). Some plants readily extract cadmium from the soil, making it available for consumption. For example, cadmium concentrations in clover grown in soil fertilized with high cadmium rock phosphate were significantly higher than the concentrations in clover grown in soils treated with low cadmium phosphate fertilizer (McLaughlin et al., 1997). A New Zealand national survey of soils and plants, and random testing of kidneys from grazing animals revealed that there was an approximately twofold increase in soil cadmium, while over a 3-year period, 14%–20% of cattle kidneys exceeded the New Zealand maximum residue level of 1 μg Cd/g (Roberts et al., 1994). In a study in which cattle were allowed to graze pastures treated with anaerobically digested sewage sludge for up to 8 years, cadmium was the only metal to accumulate consistently in increased amounts in the tissues of the cattle (Fitzgerald et al., 1985). It has been reported that cattle grazing on sewage sludge-treated pastures consumed significantly more (up to three times) cadmium than cattle on control pastures (Reddy and Dorn, 1985). In addition, a Swedish study has found a direct correlation between cadmium in feed and pig kidneys (Grawe et al., 1997). A study reporting the analysis of Wisconsin dairy feeds for heavy metals found that cadmium concentrations in complete dairy feed rations were the closest of the heavy metals to United States maximum acceptable concentrations, suggesting that cadmium has the greatest potential to exceed those maximum standards if the amounts of cadmium in feeds increase in the future (Li et al., 2005). However, several studies have failed to demonstrate any adverse clinical manifestations related to increased cadmium concentrations in the animals examined, and naturally occurring cadmium toxicity in farmed ruminants has not been reported (Lane et al., 2015). In one study, although cattle on pasture fertilized with sewage sludge consumed increased amounts of cadmium and had

Veterinary Toxicology. DOI: http://dx.doi.org/10.1016/B978-0-12-811410-0.00024-6

increased fecal excretion and kidney accumulation of cadmium (Reddy et al., 1985), there were no adverse health effects noted in these cattle (Dorn et al., 1985). Similarly, when corn silage or corn that was grown on sewage sludge fertilized fields were fed to sheep or pigs, respectively, significant increases in kidney cadmium concentrations were measured, but no other adverse treatment-related effects were noted (Lisk et al., 1982; Telford et al., 1982). Although cadmium is of concern in the environment, and cattle grazing on cadmium-contaminated pastures have increased tissue concentrations of cadmium, two additional studies conclude that accumulation of cadmium in the liver and kidneys of cattle may be a moderately effective screen for the entry of cadmium into the human food chain, as long as liver and especially kidneys are not consumed (Sharma and Street, 1980; Johnson et al., 1981). It has been reported that regardless of the concentrations of cadmium fed to livestock, the amount in meat, milk, and eggs is always lower than that in the diet that the animal was eating. Thus, foods derived from those products decrease human exposure (Klasing, 2005). This is fortunate, as chronic cadmium poisoning has been documented in humans. In these cases, it has been associated with osteoporosis, renal lesions, tissue mineral imbalances, and death. In addition, the Department of Health and Human Services has determined that cadmium and cadmium compounds may be reasonably anticipated to be carcinogens.

PHARMACOKINETICS/TOXICOKINETICS

In animals, cadmium exposure is primarily through oral ingestion. Compared to other divalent cations such as zinc and iron, intestinal absorption of cadmium is relatively low, ranging from approximately 1%–5% in most species, with up to as much as 16% in cattle, dependent on the dose (Klasing, 2005). Interestingly, cadmium bound to metallothionein in foods of animal origin is absorbed less efficiently than cadmium salts; therefore, it may be less available for uptake (Groten et al., 1990). After absorption, cadmium is transported in the plasma bound to albumin and, in lesser amounts, other serum proteins. It distributes throughout the body, with the highest concentrations in the liver and kidneys, which account for approximately one-half of the total cadmium in the body. Muscle and bone do not accumulate high concentrations of cadmium. Blood cadmium concentrations are indicators of recent exposure, while urine cadmium is a better indicator of the body burden. Cadmium is not transported well into milk or eggs, or across the placental barrier (Klasing, 2005). In pregnant and lactating livestock, the toxicokinetics of cadmium have been compared. In this study, the kinetics of cadmium were measured in lactating versus nonlactating ewes after a single intravenous or oral administration of cadmium chloride. The nonlactating ewes exhibited a low cadmium bioavailability (0.12%–0.22%), a large steady-state volume of distribution (23.8 ± 5.4 L/kg), and a low blood clearance (0.20 ± 0.03 L/kg/day) with a mean residence time of 113 ± 28 days. The lactating ewes had a higher bioavailability (0.33%–1.7%), and the mean residence time was close to that of the nonlactating ewes, despite a greater blood clearance (0.46 ± 0.013 L/kg/day), because the volume of distribution of cadmium in the body was larger. The cadmium clearance in milk remained low in the lactating ewes (Houpert et al., 1997).

In the body, cadmium is excreted very slowly, with daily losses of approximately 0.009% via the urine and 0.007% in the feces via the bile. Cadmium–protein complexes are excreted in the kidneys and then resorbed from the filtrate in the proximal tubules. This area of the renal cortex accumulates cadmium, and is susceptible to damage and necrosis. Depending on the species, the biological half-life of cadmium can vary from months to years, which results in cadmium accumulating in animals as they age (Klasing, 2005). For example, several studies have documented age-related increases in cadmium in the kidneys of horses (Elinder et al., 1981a; Anke et al., 1989).

In mammals and birds, cadmium accumulates in the liver and kidneys at concentrations of 0.1–2.0 and 1–10 mg/kg wet weight, respectively. It has been discovered that animals with long life spans, such as horses, can accumulate large amounts of cadmium in their organs, particularly in their kidneys. In samples of renal cortex from old horses, concentrations of up to 200 mg/kg have been reported (Elinder, 1992).

MECHANISM OF ACTION

Experimentally, acute exposure to high doses of inorganic cadmium leads to its accumulation in many organs, eliciting liver and, in some cases, testicular damage (Dixit et al., 1975; Habeebu et al., 1998; Klasing, 2005). Once inside the cell, free cadmium binds to protein sulfhydryl groups, disrupting the cellular redox cycle, depleting glutathione, and eliciting intracellular oxidant damage. In addition, its similarity to other divalent cations such as calcium interferes with their normal functioning (Klasing, 2005). Cadmium ions can displace zinc and other divalent metals from their binding sites on metalloproteins. For example, in the testis, cadmium can interfere with zinc proteins, leading to widespread apoptosis and necrosis (Marettova et al., 2015; Xu et al., 1999). In the liver, acute cadmium toxicity results in widespread hepatocyte apoptosis, followed by varying degrees of necrosis, depending on the dose (Habeebu et al., 1998). This is related, in part, to the effects of resident liver macrophages (Kupffer cells) to potentiate and increase the initial liver damage caused by cadmium alone. This has been demonstrated in several systems in which inhibition of Kupffer cells significantly decreases liver damage caused by a toxic dose of cadmium (Sauer et al., 1997a,b).

Cadmium readily binds to, and induces, the production of metallothionein, a cysteine-rich, metal-binding protein. Binding to metallothionein does not have a major effect on the uptake of cadmium, but is, in part, responsible for retention of cadmium within cells and its long half-life (greater than 10 years in humans). Metallothionein does this by decreasing cadmium elimination, especially in bile. Within hepatocytes, metallothionein binds to cadmium, decreasing its hepatotoxicity. Experimentally, rats that have greater induction of metallothionein in the liver are somewhat protected from cadmium hepatotoxicity (Kuester et al., 2002). However, in the kidneys the cadmium–metallothionein complex is nephrotoxic, and has been theorized that it may play a role in chronic poisoning in humans (Klaassen and Liu, 1997).

TOXICITY

Increased exposure to cadmium in combination with zinc, lead, and/or other metals continues to occur in the vicinity of nonferrous metal smelters and processing facilities. These exposures have resulted in toxicoses, although it can be difficult to separate the effects of cadmium from those of lead, zinc, and other metals. In one such case in the Netherlands, kidney cadmium concentrations were found to be twice those of cattle in control areas. However, although hemoglobin, blood iron concentrations, and iron-binding capacity were lower in the cadmium-exposed cattle compared to controls, no adverse clinical effects were observed (Wentink et al., 1992). In an additional study in the Netherlands, bulls fed diets containing increased concentrations of cadmium, lead, mercury, and arsenic had increased concentrations of cadmium in the kidney and liver, but did not exhibit histological lesions related to the intake of heavy metals (Vreman et al., 1988). However, more recently, deaths in horses exposed to cadmium, lead, and zinc from a nonferrous metal processing plant in Eastern Europe were attributed to ingestion of these metals in their feed. Analysis of tissues from a number of these horses revealed extremely high concentrations of cadmium (40–100 times normal) and three to six times the normal concentrations of lead (Bianu and Nica, 2004). Toxicoses have also been reported in sheep and horses in the vicinity of nonferrous metal smelters in China. Analysis of the tissues from these animals revealed lead and cadmium concentrations significantly higher than those of controls (Liu, 2003).

A survey of cadmium concentrations in tissues from healthy swine, cattle, dogs, and horses in the Midwestern United States was conducted in the mid-1970s. While the median cadmium concentration was low, at or below 0.6 ppm in the kidneys of cattle, swine, and dogs, the median concentration in the kidneys was four times greater in horses (Penumarthy et al., 1980). One study has indicated that horses may be more at risk for cadmium toxicity than other species. In this Swedish study, the cadmium concentrations in the kidney cortices of 69 otherwise normal horses were measured and correlated to any histological lesions that were noted. In that study, renal cadmium concentrations ranged from 11 to 186 μg Cd/g wet weight, with an average of 60 μg Cd/g. This study found a correlation between increased chronic interstitial nephritis and increasing cadmium concentrations in the renal cortex. There was no obvious relationship between the age and the frequency of renal lesions (Elinder et al., 1981a). These same authors also found that cadmium concentrations in the kidney cortices were approximately 15 times greater than those in the liver of the same animals (Elinder et al., 1981b). Age-dependent increases in kidney metallothionein and cadmium have also been reported in horses (Elinder et al., 1981a; Jeffrey et al., 1989; Plumlee et al., 1996). However, these later studies and others (Holterman et al., 1984) have not reported renal lesions similar to those reported by Elinder et al. (1981a). One diagnostic investigation has reported lameness and swollen joints (i.e., lesions of osteochondrosis) in addition to osteoporosis and nephrocalcinosis in horses near a zinc smelter in Pennsylvania. In the horses examined, kidney zinc and cadmium concentrations were elevated. It this case, it was postulated that the osteoporosis that was observed in one foal and the nephrocalcinosis seen in the foal and its dam were related to the elevated renal cadmium (Gunson et al., 1982). When ponies were raised near a similar zinc smelter for periods of time up to 18.5 months, there were significant elevations in tissue zinc and cadmium concentrations. Increases in tissue cadmium concentrations were correlated with increasing age, although increases in tissue zinc concentrations were not. Generalized osteochondrosis was present in joints of the limbs and cervical vertebrae, as well as lymphoid hyperplasia. From this study, it was concluded that the development of osteochondrosis was associated with increased exposure to zinc and, possibly, cadmium. However, other lesions of cadmium toxicosis, such as renal damage or osteomalacia, were not present (Kowalczyk et al., 1986).

In wildlife, white-tailed deer (*Odocoileus virginianius*) harvested within 20 km of zinc smelters in Pennsylvania had very high kidney concentrations of cadmium and zinc. These deer were also reported to have had joint lesions similar to zinc-poisoned horses from the same area (Sileo and Beyer, 1985).

In humans, occupational exposure to cadmium has been associated with renal dysfunction and osteomalacia with osteoporosis. One of the earliest effects of chronic cadmium exposure is renal tubular damage with proteinuria (Bernard et al., 1992). Other chronic effects can include liver damage, emphysema (through inhalation), osteomalacia, neurological impairment, testicular, pancreatic and adrenal damage, and anemia. Reproductive, developmental, and tumorigenic effects have been reported in experimental animals (Lee and White, 1980; Thompson and Bannigan, 2008; Siu et al., 2009; Flora and Agrawal, 2017). Historically in the 1940s, high environmental exposure in one area of Japan from eating cadmium-contaminated rice resulted in itai-itai (ouch-ouch) disease. This was manifested by intense bone pains and pathological bone fractures, mainly in elderly women, with osteoporosis and renal dysfunction (Kobayashi, 1978). In addition, studies in Europe and China have demonstrated that low-to-moderate exposure to cadmium from zinc smelters resulted in a decrease in bone density and an increase in fractures in women. In one of these studies, cadmium concentrations in the blood and urine were taken as biomarkers of exposure (Katzantzis, 2004). Experimental studies in animals have confirmed the adverse effects of cadmium on bones. Six mechanisms have been theorized to explain these effects: (1) interference with parathyroid hormone stimulation of vitamin D production in the kidney, (2) reduced renal vitamin D activation, (3) increased urinary excretion of calcium, (4) reduced intestinal calcium absorption, (5) interference with calcium deposition in bones, and (6) interference with bone collagen production (Kjellstrom, 1992).

TREATMENT

In animals, cadmium toxicosis is prevented by minimizing exposure in the environment and in feedstuffs.

CONCLUDING REMARKS AND FUTURE DIRECTIONS

Although toxicoses in domestic animals are very uncommon, exposure is gradually increasing, especially in grazing animals. Since chronic cadmium toxicity is of concern to humans, continued close observation and analysis of cadmium in animals is indicated to provide a system for environmental cadmium surveillance.

REFERENCES

Anke, M., Kosla, T., Groppel, B., 1989. The cadmium status of horses from central Europe depending on breed, sex, age, and living area. Arch. Tierernahrung. 39, 657–683.

ATSDR, 2009. Toxicological Profile for Cadmium. Agency for Toxic Substances and Disease Registry. Department of Health and Human Services, Public Health Service, Atlanta, GA.

Bernard, A., Roels, H., Buchet, J.P., et al., 1992. Cadmium and Health, the Belgian Experience, vol. 118. IARC Scientific Publications, Lyon, pp. 15–33.

Bianu, E., Nica, D., 2004. Chronic intoxication with cadmium in the horses at Copsa Mica area. Rev. Rom. Med. Vet. 14, 99–106.

Dixit, V.P., Lohiya, N.K., Agrawal, M., 1975. Effect of cadmium chloride on testis and epididymis of dog. A biochemical study. Acta Biol. 26, 97–103.

Dorn, C.R., 1979. Cadmium and the food chain. Cornell. Vet. 69, 323–344.

Dorn, C.R., Reddy, C.S., Lamphere, D.N., et al., 1985. Municipal sewage sludge application on Ohio farms: health effects. Environ. Res. 38, 332–359.

Elinder, C.G., 1992. Cadmium as an Environmental Hazard, vol. 118. IARC Scientific Publications, Lyon, pp. 123–132.

Elinder, C.G., Jonsson, L., Piscator, M., et al., 1981a. Histopathological changes in relation to cadmium concentration in horse kidneys. Environ. Res. 26, 1–21.

Elinder, C.G., Nordberg, M., Palm, B., et al., 1981b. Cadmium, zinc, and copper in horse liver and in horse liver metallothionein: comparisons with kidney cortex. Environ. Res. 26, 22–32.

Fitzgerald, P.R., Peterson, J., Lue-Hing, C., 1985. Heavy metals in tissues of cattle exposed to sludge-treated pastures for eight years. Am. J. Vet. Res. 46, 703–707.

Flora, S.J.S., Agrawal, S., 2017. Arsenic, cadmium and lead. In: Gupta, R.C. (Ed.), Reproductive and Developmental Toxicology, Second edn. Academic Press/Elsevier, Amsterdam, pp. 537–566.

Grawe, K.P., Thierfelder, T., Jorhem, L., et al., 1997. Cadmium levels in kidneys from Swedish pigs in relation to environmental factors – temporal and spatial trends. Sci. Total Environ. 208, 111–122.

Groten, J.P., Sinkeldam, E.J., Luten, J.B., et al., 1990. Comparison of the toxicity of inorganic and liver-incorporated cadmium: a 4-wk feeding study in rats. Food Chem. Toxicol. 28, 435–441.

Gunson, D.E., Kowalczyk, D.F., Shoop, C.R., et al., 1982. Environmental zinc and cadmium pollution associated with generalized osteochondrosis, osteoporosis, and nephrocalcinosis in horses. J. Am. Vet. Med. Assoc. 180, 295–299.

Habeebu, S.S.M., Liu, J., Klaassen, C.D., 1998. Cadmium-induced apoptosis in mouse liver. Toxicol. Appl. Pharmacol. 149, 203–209.

Holterman, W.F., de Voogt, P., Peereboom-Stegeman, J.H., 1984. Cadmium/zinc relationships in kidney cortex and metallothionein of horse and red deer: histopathological observations on horse kidneys. Environ. Res. 35, 466–481.

Houpert, P., Federspiel, B., Milhaud, G., 1997. Toxicokinetics of cadmium in lactating and nonlactating ewes after oral and intravenous administration. Environ. Res. 72, 140–150.

Jeffrey, E.H., Noseworthy, R., Cherian, M.G., 1989. Age dependent changes in metallothionein and accumulation of cadmium in horses. Comp. Biochem. Physiol. C Comp. Pharm. Toxicol. 93, 327–332.

Johnson, D.E., Kienholz, E.W., Baxter, J.C., et al., 1981. Heavy metal retention in tissues of cattle fed high cadmium sewage sludge. J. Anim. Sci. 52, 108–114.

Katzantzis, G., 2004. Cadmium, osteoporosis, and calcium metabolism. Biometals. 17, 493–498.

Kjellstrom, T., 1992. Mechanism and Epidemiology of Bone Effects of Cadmium. IARC Scientific Publications, Lyon, pp. 301–310.

Klaassen, C.D., Liu, J., 1997. Role of metallothionein in cadmium-induced hepatotoxicity and nephrotoxicity. Drug Metab. Rev. 29, 79–102.

Klasing, K.C., 2005. Cadmium. Mineral Tolerances of Animals. National Research Council. The National Academies Press, Washington, DC.

Kobayashi, J., 1978. Pollution by cadmium and the itai-itai disease in Japan. In: Oehme, F. (Ed.), Toxicity of Heavy Metals in the Environment. Marcel Dekker, Inc, New York, NY, pp. 199–259.

Kowalczyk, D.F., Gunson, D.E., Shoop, C.R., et al., 1986. The effects of natural exposure to high levels of zinc and cadmium in the immature pony as a function of age. Environ. Res. 40, 285–300.

Kuester, R.K., Waalkes, M.P., Goering, P.L., et al., 2002. Differential hepatotoxicity induced by cadmium in Fischer 344 and Sprague-Dawley rats. Toxicol. Sci. 65, 151–159.

Lane, E.A., Canty, M.J., More, S.J., 2015. Cadmium exposure and consequence for the health and productivity of farmed ruminants. Res. Vet. Sci. 101, 132–139.

Lee, J.S., White, K.L., 1980. A review of the health effects of cadmium. Am. J. Ind. Med. 1, 307–317.

Li, Y., McCrory, D.F., Powell, J.M., et al., 2005. A survey of selected heavy metal concentrations in Wisconsin dairy feeds. J. Dairy Sci. 88, 2911–2922.

Lisk, D.J., Boyd, R.D., Telford, J.N., et al., 1982. Toxicologic studies with swine fed corn grown on municipal sewage sludge-amended soil. J. Anim. Sci. 55, 613–619.

Liu, Z.P., 2003. Lead poisoning combined with cadmium in sheep and horses in the vicinity of non-ferrous metal smelters. Sci. Total Environ. 309, 117–126.

Marretova, E., Maretta, M., Legath, J., 2015. Toxic effects of cadmium on testis of birds and mammals: a review. Anim. Reprod. Sci. 155, 1–10.

McLaughlin, M.J., Simpson, P.G., Fleming, N., et al., 1997. Effect of fertilizer type on cadmium and fluorine concentrations in clover herbage. Aust. J. Exp. Agric. 37, 1019–1026.

Penumarthy, L., Oehme, F.W., Hayes, R.H., 1980. Lead, cadmium, and mercury tissue residues in healthy swine, cattle, dogs, and horses from the midwestern United States. Arch. Environ. Contam. Toxicol. 9, 193–206.

Piscator, M., 1985. Dietary exposure to cadmium and health effects: impact of environmental change. Environ. Health Perspect. 63, 127–132.

Plumlee, K.H., Johnson, B., Gardner, I.A., 1996. Heavy metal concentrations in injured racehorses. Vet. Hum. Toxicol. 38, 204–206.

Reddy, C.S., Dorn, C.R., 1985. Municipal sewage sludge application on Ohio farms: estimation of cadmium intake. Environ. Res. 38, 377–388.

Reddy, C.S., Dorn, C.R., Lamphere, D.N., et al., 1985. Municipal sewage sludge application on Ohio farms: tissue metal residues and infections. Environ. Res. 38, 360–376.

Roberts, A.H.C., Longhurst, R.D., Brown, M.W., 1994. Cadmium status of soils, plants and grazing animals in New Zealand. New Zeal. J. Agric. Res. 37, 119–129.

Sauer, J.-M., Waalkes, M.P., Hooser, S.B., et al., 1997a. Suppression of Kupffer cell function prevents cadmium induced hepatocellular necrosis in the male Sprague-Dawley rat. Toxicology. 121, 155–164.

Sauer, J.-M., Waalkes, M.P., Hooser, S.B., et al., 1997b. Tolerance induced by all-trans-retinol to the hepatotoxic effects of cadmium in rats: role of metallothionein expression. Toxicol. Appl. Pharmacol. 143, 110–119.

Sharma, R.P., Street, J.C., 1980. Public health aspects of toxic heavy metals in animal feeds. J. Am. Vet. Med. Assoc. 177, 149–153.

Sileo, L., Beyer, W.N., 1985. Heavy metals in white-tailed deer living near a zinc smelter in Pennsylvania. J. Wildl. Dis. 21, 289–296.

Siu, E.R., Mruk, D.D., Porto, C.S., et al., 2009. Cadmium-induced testicular injury. Toxicol. Appl. Pharmacol. 238, 240–249.

Te lford, J.N., Thonney, M.L., Hogue, D.E., et al., 1982. Toxicologic studies in growing sheep fed silage corn cultured on municipal sludge-amended acid subsoil. J. Toxicol. Environ. Health. 10, 73–85.

Thompson, J., Bannigan, J., 2008. Cadmium: toxic effects on the reproductive system and the embryo. Reprod. Toxicol. 25, 304–315.

Vreman, K., van der Veen, N.G., van der Molen, E.J., et al., 1988. Transfer of cadmium, lead, mercury and arsenic from feed into tissues of fattening bulls: chemical and pathological data. Neth. J. Agric. Sci. 36, 327–338.

Wentink, G.H., Wensing, T., Kessels, B.G., 1992. Toxicity of cadmium in cattle. Tijdschrift Diergeneeskunde. 117, 548–550.

Xu, G., Zhou, G., Jin, T., et al., 1999. Apoptosis and p53 gene expression in male reproductive tissues of cadmium exposed rats. Biometals. 12, 131–139.

Chapter 25

Chromium, Iodine, and Phosphorus

Larry J. Thompson

CHROMIUM

Chromium is a metallic element that can exist in six valence states, with the trivalent chromium form most commonly found in nature as ferrochromite ores. Both trivalent (+3) and hexavalent (+6) chromium are widely used in various industrial and manufacturing processes. Chromium is an essential trace element, and functions in a number of metabolic processes, including glucose, lipid, and amino acid metabolism (NRC, 2005a). Hexavalent chromium is considered to be more toxic than the trivalent form, which may be a direct result of its increased systemic availability.

While hexavalent chromium is considered to be a human carcinogen, acute chromium toxicosis in animals is probably of minimal concern in all but the most unusual circumstances. Both hexavalent chromium and dichromate are easily converted to trivalent chromium in mammalian systems, but the burning of chromium-treated lumber does not produce enough heat to convert the dichromate to the trivalent chromium form. Oil field contamination with hexavalent chromium has been associated with cases of cattle death (Thompson et al., 1991), and a solution of strong, oxidizing chromium was responsible for dairy cattle deaths when the solution dripped on cattle and was absorbed dermally (Talcott et al., 2005). Acute chromium toxicosis is associated with severe congestion and inflammation of the digestive tract, kidney damage, and liver damage.

Dogs were given potassium chromate in drinking water for 4 years with hexavalent chromium concentrations up to 11.2 ppm (Anwar et al., 1961). The calculated dose was up to 0.30 mg/kg BW/day of hexavalent chromium (Grevatt, 1998), with no significant adverse effects reported in the dogs. No adverse effects were reported in cats fed diets containing chromium oxycarbonate for 80 days, which delivered up to approximately 100 mg/kg BW/day trivalent chromium (Akatsuka, 1934). Maximum tolerated levels of trivalent chromium were set at 100 ppm for mammalian species and 500 ppm for poultry, with allowances for insoluble chromic oxide up to 3000 ppm (NRC, 2005a). However, using a safety factor of 10 for cross-species extrapolation, a maximum tolerated dose of 10 ppm total chromium in dog and cat food products was determined by the FDA-CVM in response to confusion concerning the misinterpretation of chromium analytical results in pet food products (FDA-CVM, 2011).

IODINE

Iodine is a non-metallic element of the halogen group that occurs as a purple-black crystalline solid, but has several common other forms, including iodide (I^{-1}) and iodate (IO^{-3}). Iodine is widely distributed in nature in both organic and inorganic forms, but only in low concentrations, with rare exceptions. Iodine is essential for the normal synthesis of thyroid hormones and a deficiency of iodine can result in thyroid enlargement or goiter. Deficiencies may occur from eating feeds grown on iodine-deficient soils or from the presence of goitrogenic substances (NRC, 2005b). High dietary iodine for a prolonged period of time can reduce the iodine uptake by the thyroid, thus causing a clinical syndrome of iodine deficiency, especially when normal levels are subsequently fed.

Common dietary sources of iodine include iodized salt, ethylenediamine dihydroiodide (EDDI), calcium iodate, as well as naturally high iodine sources such as kelp and certain seaweeds. Iodized salt can contain 0.01% iodine (100 ppm), and has not been associated with excess iodine exposure. EDDI has been used to prevent and treat foot rot in cattle, although its efficacy is unclear (Morgan, 2004). Toxic effects of iodine excess have been reported in cattle consuming iodine-containing feed additives (Thompson et al., 1991). Clinical signs include decreased feed intake, decreased milk production, rapid breathing, nasal and ocular discharge, dry hair coat, and non-responsive hock lesions. Affected cattle were on high intakes of iodine (68–600 mg/head/day and above) for several weeks before obvious clinical signs appeared. Young calves exhibited chronic coughing and profuse nasal discharge at

Veterinary Toxicology. DOI: http://dx.doi.org/10.1016/B978-0-12-811410-0.00025-8

100–200 ppm dietary iodine. Puppies have been reported to have depressed thyroid gland function and bone abnormalities when fed diets high in iodine (Castillo et al., 2001, 2003). Removal of the excess iodine from the diet, as well as supportive care, usually result in rapid return to normal.

Maximum tolerated levels of iodine in the diet vary widely, including swine (400 ppm), chicken and turkey (300 ppm), cattle and sheep (50 ppm), horses (5 ppm) (NRC, 2005b), dogs (11 ppm), and cats (9 ppm) (AAFCO, 2017).

PHOSPHORUS

Most phosphorus in nature exists in combination with oxygen in the form of phosphates, primarily in igneous and sedimentary rocks. Inorganic phosphates are commonly used as chemical fertilizers and food and feed supplements, and have many industrial uses. Phosphorus is abundant in the animal body, primarily as a structural component of crystalline hydroxyapatite in bone and teeth, but also as required components of phospholipids, nucleic acids, nucleotides, and enzyme cofactors. Phosphate ions also function in acid–base balance and other essential body functions. Phosphorus is an essential macroelement in nutrition, and is an important consideration in the formulation of animal diets. The largest dietary source of phosphate will be in the form of inorganic phosphate supplements, and other dietary sources may include plant-origin feeds, as well as bone, meat, poultry, and fish meals. Normal phosphorus nutrition and metabolism requires adequate calcium in the diet with an appropriate calcium-to-phosphorus ratio (Ca:P). While adverse effects of excess phosphorus are rare, they can occur with either excess dietary phosphates or deficient dietary calcium. If the Ca:P ratio is balanced, usually no wider than 2:1, animals can tolerate a wide range of dietary phosphorus levels (NRC, 2005c).

Excess phosphorus in the diet of ruminants, especially sheep, can result in the formation of urinary calculi in the kidney or bladder. This formation of stones can obstruct or completely block urine flow, especially in males, resulting in the bladder filling with urine and eventually rupturing into the abdominal cavity, causing death. The problem can be prevented by correctly balancing calcium and phosphorus in the diet. Excess phosphorus in the diet of horses has resulted in nutritional secondary hyperparathyroidism, a condition usually associated with a high grain diet without appropriate calcium supplementation. The high dietary phosphate will depress the intestinal absorption of calcium, with a decrease in plasma calcium and an increase in plasma phosphate levels. Low plasma calcium will stimulate the secretion of parathyroid hormone, which will increase bone mineral resorption activity. The skeletal bones will lose calcium, and the demineralized bone will be replaced by fibrous connective tissue, with the facial bones often becoming enlarged (Joyce et al., 1971), leading to the common term of big head disease in horses. It is also known as bran disease, since feeding high dietary levels of bran, which is high in phosphate and low in calcium, has historically been a cause of the disease. In all animals, optimum animal performance will be closely associated with optimum dietary calcium and phosphorus balance.

Phosphorus, white or yellow, has historically been used as a rodenticide, which is uncommon today. Initial clinical signs following ingestion would include gastroenteritis with vomiting and diarrhea. If the animal survived several days, it would often develop a secondary phase of severe liver damage, with renal insult also occurring.

REFERENCES

AAFCO, 2017. Association of American Feed Control Officials. 2017 Official Publication. Champaign, IL.

Akatsuka, K., Fairhall, L.T., 1934. The toxicology of chromium. J. Ind. Hyg. 16, 1–28.

Anwar, R.A., Langham, R.F., Hoppert, C.A., et al., 1961. Chronic toxicity studies III. Chronic toxicity of cadmium and chromium in dogs. Arch. Environ. Health. 3, 456–460.

Castillo, V.A., Lalia, J.C., Junco, M., et al., 2001. Changes in thyroid function in puppies fed a high iodine commercial diet. Vet. J. 161, 80–84.

Castillo, V.A., Rodriguez, M.S., Lalia, J.C., et al., 2003. Morphologic changes in the thyroid glands of puppies fed a high-iodine commercial diet. J. App. Res. Vet. Med. 1, 45–50.

FDA-CVM, 2011. Target animal safety review memorandum. <https://www.fda.gov/downloads/aboutfda/centersoffices/officeoffoods/cvm/cvmfoiaelectronicreadingroom/ucm274327.pdf> (accessed 01.03.17.).

Grevatt, P.C., 1998. Toxicological Review of Hexavalent Chromium. Support of Summary Information on the Integrated Risk Information System (IRIS). US Environmental Protection Agency, Washington, DC.

Joyce, J.R., Pierce, K.R., Romane, W.M., et al., 1971. Clinical study of nutritional secondary hyperparathyroidism in horses. J. Am. Vet. Med. Assoc. 158, 2033.

Morgan, S.E., 2004. Iodine. In: Plumlee, K.H. (Ed.), Clinical Veterinary Toxicology. Mosby, St. Louis, MO, pp. 200–202.

National Research Council (NRC), 2005a. Chromium, Mineral Tolerance of Animals. second revised ed. The National Academies Press, Washington, DC, pp. 115–123.

National Research Council (NRC), 2005b. Iodine, Mineral Tolerance of Animals. second revised ed. The National Academies Press, Washington, DC, pp. 182–198.

National Research Council (NRC), 2005c. Phosphorus, Mineral Tolerance of Animals. second revised ed. The National Academies Press, Washington, DC, pp. 290–299.

Talcott, P.A., Haldorson, G.J., Sathre, P., 2005. Chromium poisoning in a group of dairy cows. Proceedings of the AAVLD 48th Annual Conference. Hershey, PA, p. 45.

Thompson, L.J., Hall, J.O., Meerdink, G.L., 1991. Toxic effects of trace element excess. Vet. Clin. North Am. Food Anim. Pract. 7, 277–306.

Chapter 26

Copper

Larry J. Thompson

INTRODUCTION

Copper is a transition group metal with high electrical and thermal conductivity. The chemical abbreviation for copper is Cu, which comes from the Latin word *cuprum*, which refers to the island of Cyprus, known in the ancient times for large deposits of copper ore. The Bronze Age followed the discovery that adding tin (and other metals) to copper made the resulting metal alloy much more durable. Copper has been shown to be an essential element for both animals and plants but can be toxic under certain conditions. This chapter describes the toxicity and deficiency of copper in animals.

BACKGROUND

Toxic insults from copper occur in two main categories, acute and chronic. The acute overexposure of animals to copper can occur by both oral and parenteral routes (Galey et al., 1991) but is relatively uncommon. Sheep are very susceptible to chronic copper poisoning, where even a slight excess of copper in the diet can build up over weeks or months to cause problems. Cattle and other ruminants are less likely to suffer from chronic mild to moderate copper excesses in the diet but can be affected by relatively high levels (Gummow, 1996; Engle, 2014). Monogastric animals seem to tolerate excess dietary copper much better than ruminants and high dietary copper additions (up to 250 ppm) have been used for growth promotant effects, such as in pigs and poultry. Finally, certain breeds of dogs (e.g., Bedlington terriers) have a genetic predisposition for liver copper accumulation similar to Wilson's disease in humans (Taboada and Thompson, 1997). Genetic characterization of Labrador Retrievers has shown other genes and expression patterns may represent a new model for copper metabolism disorders (Fieten et al., 2016; Wu et al., 2016; Dirksen et al., 2017).

Each of these may have a different clinical presentation, with the main target organs for acute copper exposure generally being the gastrointestinal (GI) tract, liver, and kidney, with the target organs for chronic problems being the liver, red blood cells, and kidney.

Dietary sources of copper include normal plant concentrations of copper, with forages and cereal grains usually containing less than 10 ppm copper on a dry matter (DM) basis. Some oilseed meals can contain up to 35 ppm copper in DM. By far the largest source of copper in the diet will be feed additives such as copper sulfate, copper chloride, and copper oxide. Additional sources of copper for the animal may be chelated copper sources in the diet or the administration of boluses containing copper metal wires or other solid forms of copper that remain in the rumen/reticulum and slowly dissolve over time. Misformulation of rations or errors in the mixing of feed can result in high concentrations of copper. Problems can arise from the use of feed formulated for a copper-tolerant species when used for a copper-sensitive species such as sheep, or the use of trace mineralized salt in sheep diets. Other sources for large acute oral copper exposures would include copper sulfate foot baths and copper algaecides or fungicides. Most water sources have low copper concentrations but the use of copper piping with slightly acidic water can result in additional copper being dissolved.

PHARMACOKINETICS

Copper is primarily absorbed in the small intestine and transported in the blood by transcuprein and albumin, which serve to reduce the oxidative effects of divalent copper. In the liver, copper can be stored in the lysosomes, excreted in the bile or incorporated into ceruloplasmin for use and transport to cells in other parts of the body. Biliary excretion is the major mechanism responsible for copper homeostasis and identified genetic disorders of copper accumulation are due to impaired biliary

Veterinary Toxicology. DOI: http://dx.doi.org/10.1016/B978-0-12-811410-0.00026-X

excretion. Copper is utilized by essentially every cell in the body, and there are several important copper-dependent enzymes including cytochrome C oxidase, superoxide dismutase, lysyl oxidase, and dopamine beta hydroxylase (Gaetke et al., 2014).

In the ruminant, copper has a complex interrelationship with dietary molybdenum and sulfur which, when present in excess, will both decrease copper absorption and inhibit copper utilization. In the reducing environment of the rumen, excess sulfur favors the formation of sulfides, which can inhibit copper absorption from the GI tract. Additionally, the formation of tri- and tetrathiomolybdates can also inhibit the absorption of copper or, if in high amounts, can cause systemic effects by holding copper in a nonbiologically available form (NRC, 2005).

MECHANISM OF ACTION

Acute exposure to excess copper causes GI irritation and can cause erosions of the mucosa as well as a blue-green discoloration of the contents and wall. Normally, the free copper concentration in cells is kept very low by copper-binding proteins such as metallothionein, glutathione, and copper chaperone proteins. An excess of copper can overwhelm these binding proteins and allow free copper ions to exist in the cell, which can directly bind proteins and nucleic acids. Additionally, the free copper can form reactive oxygen species and hydroxyl radicals, causing lipid peroxidation of membranes and damage to nucleic acids and cellular proteins (NRC, 2005; Gaetke et al., 2014). In a recent experimental study, Keswani et al. (2013) demonstrated copper-induced immunotoxicity involving cell cycle arrest and apoptosis in the liver.

Chronic copper toxicosis in sheep is caused by the inability of the sheep to increase the biliary excretion of copper in response to dietary increases. Copper will then accumulate in the liver but during this accumulation phase there will be little or no evidence of negative effects (Bremner, 1998). If accumulation continues, the liver can suffer direct damage from the high concentrations of copper. When damage is severe, hepatic necrosis develops and copper is released into the bloodstream. Additionally, stress to the animal can also accentuate this mobilization of copper from the liver and into the bloodstream. Increasing copper concentrations in the bloodstream will overwhelm the protective transport actions of transcuprein and albumin, which can then result in the lysis of red blood cells due to the oxidation of the red blood cell membrane by ionic copper. As copper is mobilized from the liver, it can accumulate in the kidney. The kidney can be damaged both from the accumulation of copper as well as the direct toxic effects of hemoglobin following the hemolytic event. Cattle can also be affected by chronic copper toxicosis, with a strong suspicion of breed differences (Du et al., 1996) but with hemolysis occurring with less frequency than in sheep.

Chronic copper toxicosis in dogs is primarily seen in the Bedlington Terrier where genetic studies have shown it to be an autosomal recessive disorder (Forman et al., 2005). Other breeds including West Highland White Terriers, Skye Terriers, and Doberman Pinschers (Speeti et al., 1998) have breed-related hepatic copper accumulation, the origin of which is less defined. Chronic copper toxicosis in dogs will also have a period of copper accumulation without clinical signs or detectable damage to the liver. As copper concentrations increase, the animal develops a chronic active hepatitis with necrosis and inflammation. As with sheep, excess free copper damages many cellular components of the liver, including the lipid peroxidation of mitochondrial membranes. A sudden release of copper with the resulting hemolytic crisis is much less likely to occur in dogs. The disease usually appears at 2–6 years of age, with animals often showing no problems before this time.

TOXICITY

There is a paucity of information on the amount of copper needed for acute poisoning in various species, but the general range is given as 25–50 mg/kg of body weight. Copper sulfate is most often implicated in clinical cases as the copper source. The toxic dose of copper sulfate in cattle is 200–800 mg/kg, with sheep more sensitive at 20–100 mg/kg. Affected animals show clinical signs of salivation, gastroenteritis, and abdominal pain, which may rapidly develop to dehydration, shock, and death. Animals that survive longer than 24–48 h develop liver and kidney damage and the animal may have an acute hemolytic crisis. Postmortem findings include gastroenteritis and a blue-green discoloration to the GI tract and contents. Varying degrees of liver and kidney lesions are present, with milder lesions in acute deaths and more dramatic lesions developing after 48 h. Diagnostic testing of the intestinal tract contents shows a high level of copper. In acute deaths, there are normal levels of copper in the liver and kidney. If the animal survives over 24 h, elevated copper levels are found in liver and kidney.

In sheep, even normal levels of copper in feeds (10–20 ppm) can cause hepatic copper accumulation when the molybdenum level in feed is low (less than 1 ppm). As the copper-to-molybdenum ratio (Cu:Mo) increases above 6:1, the risk of copper accumulation increases, with those diets whose ratio is above 20:1 being very dangerous for sheep. At the higher Cu:Mo ratios, toxic accumulation of copper in the liver can occur over a matter of weeks. In affected animals, there may be an acute hemolytic crisis and the animals show clinical signs of weakness, anorexia, icterus, dyspnea and pale mucous membranes. There may be hemoglobinuria, and death is common among severely affected animals. Postmortem findings include icterus, swollen liver, enlarged spleen, and the kidneys appear dark, often referred to as gunmetal blue or black kidneys. Antemortem testing of serum copper often shows an elevation above normal, but this decreases over time with a rapid decrease following fluid therapy. Postmortem diagnostic testing for copper should be performed on both liver and kidney. Mobilization of copper from the liver may reduce copper concentrations to normal levels but the mobilized copper is then accumulated in the kidney. The ratio should be tested for both copper and molybdenum. The close environment of the sheep should be inspected for extraneous sources of copper.

Young dogs with genetic susceptibility to chronic copper toxicosis may develop an acute syndrome of weakness, vomiting, and anorexia. Older dogs may present with a more chronic syndrome of weight loss and anorexia, which may progress to ascites and neurological signs related to a developing hepatic encephalopathy. If untreated, the animal may succumb to liver dysfunction, and postmortem findings may include a cirrhotic liver. Antemortem diagnostics would include an evaluation of liver enzymes. In suspect cases, a liver biopsy should be used to confirm elevated copper content (Taboada and Thompson, 1997).

TREATMENT

Treatment of animals acutely poisoned with copper mainly consists of supportive treatment directed at the shock, dehydration, and damage to the GI tract.

Treatment of sheep with severe clinical signs following hemolytic crisis is often unrewarding. Supportive care should include fluid therapy and the consideration of a blood transfusion. Ammonium or sodium molybdate (50–500 mg) and sodium thiosulfate (0.3–1 g) should be used daily as a drench for up to 3 weeks not only in affected animals but also in other animals that have received the same diet. Ammonium tetrathiomolybdate has been suggested as a treatment but is difficult to obtain. It can be administered IV or SQ at 1.7–3.4 mg/kg on alternate days for three treatments. Molybdenum in the diet can be increased to 5 ppm and zinc can be supplemented at 100 ppm to reduce copper absorption.

Dogs affected with chronic copper toxicosis should be fed a low copper diet, e.g., avoiding organ meats that are usually higher in copper. The use of oral chelating agents is suggested to enhance urinary excretion of copper. The use of D-penicillamine at 10–15 mg/kg PO twice daily or the use of trientine hydrochloride at 10–15 mg/kg PO twice daily have been suggested. Liver enzymes should be monitored every 6 months and consideration be given to liver biopsy to assess liver copper concentrations. The addition of elemental zinc to the diet (100–200 mg/day as the acetate) should be considered to reduce copper absorption.

CONCLUDING REMARKS AND FUTURE DIRECTIONS

In trace amounts, copper is an essential element, but in excess it is a toxicant. In general, sheep and certain breeds of dogs are more susceptible to copper poisoning. Copper produces toxicity by multiple mechanisms. Poisoned animals are usually treated with ammonium molybdate and sodium thiosulfate. In addition, supportive care including fluid therapy and blood transfusion are beneficial.

REFERENCES

Bremner, I., 1998. Manifestations of copper excess. Am. J. Clin. Nutr. 67 (Suppl), 1069S–1073S.

Dirksen, K., Spee, B., Penning, L.C., et al., 2017. Gene expression patterns in the progression of canine copper-associated chronic hepatitis. PLoS One. 12 (5), 1–19.

Du, Z., Hemken, R.W., Harmon, R.J., 1996. Copper metabolism of Holstein and Jersey cows and heifers fed diets high in cupric sulfate or copper proteinate. J. Dairy Sci. 79, 1873–1880.

Engle, T.E., 2014. Copper and lipid metabolism in beef cattle: a review. J. Anim. Sci. 89, 591–596.

Fieten, H., Gill, Y., Martin, A.J., et al., 2016. The Menkes and Wilson disease genes counteract in copper toxicosis in Labrador retrievers: a new canine model for copper-metabolism disorders. Dis. Model Mech. 9, 25–38.

Forman, O.P., Boursnell, M.E.G., Dunmore, B.J., et al., 2005. Characterization of the COMMD1 (MURR1) mutation causing copper toxicosis in Bedlington terriers. Anim. Genet. 36, 497–501.

Gaetke, L.M., Chow-Johnson, H.S., Chow, C.K., 2014. Copper: toxicological relevance and mechanisms. Arch. Toxicol. 88, 1929–1938.

Galey, F.D., Maas, J., Tronstad, R.J., et al., 1991. Copper toxicosis in two herds of beef calves following injection with copper disodium edetate. J. Vet. Diagn. Invest. 3, 260–263.

Gummow, B., 1996. Experimentally induced chronic copper toxicity in cattle. Onderstepoort J. Vet. Res. 63, 277–288.

Keswani, T., Mitra, S., Bhattacharyya, A., 2013. Copper-induced immunotoxicity involves cell cycle arrest and cell death in the liver. Environ. Toxicol. 30, 411–421.

National Research Council (NRC), 2005. Copper. Mineral Tolerance of Animals. second revised ed. The National Academies Press, Washington, DC, pp. 134–153.

Speeti, M., Eriksson, J., Saari, S., et al., 1998. Lesions of subclinical Doberman hepatitis. Vet. Pathol. 35, 361–369.

Taboada, J., Thompson, L.J., 1997. Copper hepatopathy. In: Tilley, L.P., Smith, F.W.K., MacMurray, A.C. (Eds.), The 5 Minute Veterinary Consult: Canine and Feline. Williams and Wilkins, Baltimore, MD, pp. 478–479.

Wu, X., Leegwater, P.A., Fieten, H., 2016. Canine models for copper homeostasis disorders. Int. J. Mol. Sci. 17, 196–209.

Chapter 27

Fluoride

Larry J. Thompson

INTRODUCTION

Fluorine is a member of the halogen group on the periodic table and is rarely found in elemental form in nature but instead exists as fluoride, the monovalent anion, combined with other elements. The most common mineral containing fluoride is fluorspar, also known as fluorite (CaF_2), and soils generally contain calcium fluoride (CaF_2). Although now rare, sodium fluoride and sodium fluorosilicate (Na_2SiF_6) have been used as insecticides and anthelminthics. Sodium fluoroacetate (compound 1080) is another formerly used rodenticide that is rarely seen in the United States today but may be found in other parts of the world (e.g., Australia). Fluoroacetate can also be found naturally in several species of plants (*Gastrolobium* spp., *Oxylobium* spp. and others). Sodium fluoride, sodium fluorosilicate, and fluorosilicic acid have been used in the United States for the fluoridation of drinking water for humans to prevent the development of dental caries (CDC, 2001). When the gas hydrogen fluoride is dissolved in water it forms hydrofluoric acid, a very hazardous chemical that has industrial and laboratory uses such as purifying metals, etching glass and cleaning semiconductors due to its ability to dissolve silicates and metal oxides. This chapter will stress the chronic effects of fluoride excess, also called fluorosis or fluoride toxicosis, in large animals.

BACKGROUND

Fluoride is present at low levels in virtually all feed and water sources, thus animals will have continuing exposure throughout their lifetime. While a small amount of fluoride in the diet has been shown to improve bone and teeth development, a chronic excess of fluoride can have adverse effects on teeth, bone, and other body systems. Large animals have been exposed to excess fluorides through the ingestion of high-fluoride rock phosphates used as nutritional supplements, by the ingestion of forages contaminated with excess fluorides from industrial pollutants or volcanic emissions, or through water containing excess fluorides from industrial pollution or dissolved from natural sources (Shupe and Olson, 1971, 1983). Rock phosphates destined for animal diets must be defluorinated before use or have a phosphorus to fluorine ratio (P:F) of more than 100:1 in order to avoid exposing the animal to excess fluoride (Osweiler, 2004). Following a long history of problems, industrial contamination of forages and water with excess fluoride has decreased due to recognition of the problems caused by excess fluoride and increased regulatory controls on fluoride-emitting industries. Historical point sources for fluoride emissions have included the smelting industries (e.g., aluminum, copper, and steel), brick or ceramic product factories, coal-fired power plants, and the phosphate-processing industries. Plant uptake of fluoride by translocation from the soil is usually not an important source of fluoride for grazing animals. Much more significant sources include airborne fluoride that settles on plant surfaces and fluoride from soil that is ingested directly or contaminates the plant (NRC, 2005). Acute fluoride poisoning in large animals is rare but can occur following exposure to fluoride-containing commercial products (Bischoff et al., 1999) or to ash and tephra following volcanic eruptions (Shanks, 1997).

PHARMACOKINETICS AND MECHANISM OF ACTION

Sodium fluoride is readily absorbed from the digestive tract and is several times more biologically available than fluoride compounds from feed or environmental sources. Fluoride is distributed to all parts of the body, with approximately 50% of absorbed fluoride being excreted by the kidneys. The remainder will be incorporated into bone and teeth with very little accumulation in the soft tissue. Fluoride concentrations in the blood, urine, and soft tissues may reflect recent ingestions but will also increase slowly over time with continuing excess fluoride

Veterinary Toxicology. DOI: http://dx.doi.org/10.1016/B978-0-12-811410-0.00027-1

exposure and accumulation in the bone. Greater than 95% of the body burden of fluoride will be contained in the bones with bone levels dependent upon the amount of fluoride ingested, duration of exposure, bioavailability, species, age, and diet of the animal involved. If dietary fluoride exposure decreases, bone fluoride levels will decrease slowly over a long period of time. In cattle there appears to be a partial placental barrier to the movement of fluoride to the fetus as even high levels of fluoride in the diet of the dam did not adversely affect the health of the calves, even though higher fetal blood and bone fluoride concentrations resulted (NRC, 2005). Fluoride is excreted in the milk but this does not appear to be a significant source for the neonate.

The major adverse effects of chronic excess fluoride ingestion concern the teeth and bones of affected animals. Fluoride substitutes for hydroxyl groups in the hydroxyapatite of the bone matrix, which alters the mineralization and crystal structure of the bone. Bone changes induced by excess fluoride ingestion, termed skeletal fluorosis or osteofluorosis, include the interference of the normal sequences of osteogenesis and bone remodeling with the resulting production of abnormal bone or the resorption of normal bone. The fluoride content of bone can increase over a period of time without other noticeable changes in the bone structure or function. Once lesions start to develop, they are usually bilateral and symmetric. The most consistent gross changes are abnormal bone formation on the periosteal surface with thickening of the cortex. In cattle, earliest clinical changes usually occur on the ribs and mandible as well as the medial surfaces of the metatarsal and metacarpal bones. Histologically, bones will have abnormal remodeling and mineralization with irregular collagenous fibers and excess osteoid tissues. While an excess of ingested fluorides can adversely affect the bones at any time in the animal's life, the bones in younger animals are more responsive to the excess fluoride.

Dental fluorosis develops when the period of excess fluoride intake occurs during the period of tooth development; in cattle this will generally be before 30–36 months of age. Teeth are affected during development with damage to ameloblasts and odontoblasts and the resulting abnormal matrix unable to mineralize normally (Shearer et al., 1978). Both enamel and dentine are adversely affected. Affected teeth may erupt with mottling (alternating white opaque horizontal areas or striations in the enamel), hypoplasia, dysplasia (abnormal soft dull white chalky enamel or horizontal zones of constriction), erosion or pitting of enamel and affected teeth are prone to excessive abrasion and discoloration.

Acute fluoride toxicosis occurs when soluble forms of fluoride (e.g., sodium fluoride) are ingested in large doses. Absorption is rapid and clinical signs can appear within 30–60 min following ingestion. Although the exact mechanism of action is not known with certainty, fluoride concentrations in blood and soft tissues rapidly increase, which leads to hypocalcemia. Sudden death from acute fluoride exposure is thought to involve the development of hyperkalemia or diminished Na/K-ATPase activity and the inhibition of glycolysis (NRC, 2005). Fluoride can induce oxidative stress and modulate intracellular redox homeostasis, lipid peroxidation and protein carbonyl content (Ranjan et al., 2009; Dubey et al., 2013). Fluoride is thought to inhibit the activity of antioxidant enzymes, such as superoxide dismutase, glutathione peroxidase and catalase. Depletion of glutathione results in excessive production of reactive oxygen species at the mitochondrial level, leading to the damage of cellular components. In an experimental study, Agalakova and Gusev (2013) demonstrated that excessive chronic fluoride consumption leads to accelerated death of erythrocytes and anemia in rats. Fluoride can also alter gene expression and cause apoptosis (Barbier et al., 2010). Genes modulated by fluoride include those related to the stress response, metabolic enzymes, the cell cycle, cell–cell communication and signal transduction.

TOXICITY

There are a number of factors that influence the amount of fluoride required to produce specific lesions and clinical signs including the amount of fluoride ingested, duration of exposure, bioavailability, species, age and diet of the animal involved. The point where fluoride ingestion becomes detrimental to the animal also varies from animal to animal. Clinical signs develop slowly and can be confused with other chronic problems. Animals often show nonspecific intermittent stiffness and lameness, which appear to be associated with periosteal overgrowth leading to spurring and bridging near joints as well as ossification of ligaments, tendon sheaths and tendons. The clinical presentation may easily be confused with other conditions, such as degenerative arthritis, but the lesions associated with fluorosis are not primarily associated with articular surfaces. In severe cases, affected cattle may become progressively lamer and eventually may refuse to stand or may stand with rear legs upright and be on their knees to graze (Shupe and Olson, 1983). Lameness in cattle leads to abnormal hoof wear with elongated toes, especially in the rear legs. In long-term studies with cattle on varying levels of fluoride intake, skeletal neoplasms were not seen even in cattle with severe osteofluoritic lesions (Shupe et al., 1992).

A great deal of effort has gone into the classification of dental lesions in cattle produced by excess fluoride ingestion. The incisor teeth are evaluated for enamel defects and abrasion pattern. The usual classification system ranges from a value of 0 for normal teeth to a value of 5 for severe fluoride effects (Shearer et al., 1978;

Shupe et al., 1992). Because of the nature and complexity of the disease these dental lesions should not be the sole criterion for diagnosis. In general, severely affected teeth appear with brown or black discoloration, may have enamel defects and show increased wear including exposure of the pulp cavity, which causes pain while chewing roughage or swallowing extremely cold water. There will be a correlation between lesions on incisor teeth and those cheek teeth that form and mineralize at the same time. Cheek teeth that are abnormally worn cause improper mastication with roughage being difficult for the animal to utilize. The animal will have variable and decreased intake and the decreased production, slowed growth, and general poor health associated with poor nutritional status. Animals with chronic exposure to excess fluorides have dry skin and hair coat.

Acute fluoride poisoning of cattle can result in clinical signs of depression, weakness and ataxia with postmortem findings of gastroenteritis (Bischoff et al., 1999) and degenerative changes in the renal tubular epithelium.

TREATMENT

Diagnosis of chronic fluoride toxicosis is based upon clinical signs, exposure history, dental lesions, evaluation of lameness and bony lesions and elevated urinary fluoride concentrations. Normal cattle urine contains less than 6 ppm fluoride. Animals having recent exposure or continuing release from fluorotic bone will have 15–20 ppm urinary fluoride (Osweiler, 2004). The biopsy of a rib or coccygeal vertebrae for fluoride analysis, as well as radiographic examination of teeth or bones, may also be helpful. A full postmortem examination should be performed, with attention to bone and teeth for both gross and histopathologic examination. Various bone samples should be submitted for fluoride analysis including metatarsal, metacarpal, rib, pelvis and mandible. Normal values for cattle are 400–1200 ppm fluoride on a dry, fat-free basis. Animals affected with chronic fluorosis can contain 3000–5000 ppm fluoride on a dry, fat-free basis. Analysis of feed, water or suspect material should also be included.

There is no specific antidote or treatment for chronic fluoride toxicosis. Sources of excess fluoride should be identified and removed from the diet. With reduction of dietary fluoride to background levels, mild to moderate bone changes may be reduced and normal bone laid down. Extensive bone lesions will not be remodeled to normal and teeth lesions are irreversible. Symptomatic and supportive care for animals with bone and teeth changes include providing high-quality easily masticated feeds, limited grazing area, and provisions to avoid cold or frozen water. For mild fluorotic changes, improving the diet and grazing may avoid excess wear on the teeth and reduce mastication problems.

CONCLUDING REMARKS AND FUTURE DIRECTIONS

Animals can be intoxicated with fluoride from its higher concentrations in supplemented feed or drinking water. The level of fluoride contamination in drinking water is dependent on the nature of the rocks and the occurrence of fluoride-bearing minerals in ground water. While in small amounts fluoride is necessary for teeth and bone development, in higher concentrations fluoride is toxic. Fluoride causes toxicity through multiple mechanisms. In addition to inhibition of Na/K-ATPase, fluoride can induce oxidative stress and modulate intracellular redox homeostasis, lipid peroxidation and protein carbonyl content, as well as alter gene expression and cause apoptosis. A chronic excess to fluoride can have adverse effects on teeth, bones and other body systems. Diagnosis is based on analysis of feed, water, and bones. There is no specific treatment for fluoride toxicosis.

REFERENCES

Agalakova, N.I., Gusev, G.P., 2013. Excessive fluoride consumption leads to accelerated death of erythrocytes and anemia in rats. Biol. Trace Elem. Res. Available from: http://dx.doi.org/10.1007/s12011-013-9691-y.

Barbier, O., Arreola-Mendoza, L., Razo, L.M.D., 2010. Molecular mechanisms of fluoride toxicity. Chemico-Biol. Interact. 188, 319–333.

Bischoff, K.L., Edwards, W.C., Fearer, J., 1999. Acute fluoride toxicosis in beef cattle. Bovine Pract. 33, 1–3.

Centers for Disease Control and Prevention (CDC), 2001. Recommendations for using fluoride to prevent and control dental caries in the United States. MMWR Recomm Rep 50 (RR-14): 1–42.

Dubey, N., Khan, A.M., Raina, R., 2013. Sub-acute deltamethrin and fluoride toxicity induced hepatic oxidative stress and biochemical alterations in rats. Bull. Environ. Contam. Toxicol. 91, 334–338.

National Research Council (NRC), 2005. Fluorine. Mineral Tolerance of Animals. second revised ed. The National Academies Press, Washington, DC, pp. 154–181.

Osweiler, G.D., 2004. Fluoride. In: Plumlee, K.H. (Ed.), Clinical Veterinary Toxicology. Mosby, St. Louis, MO, pp. 197–200.

Ranjan, R., Swarup, D., Patra, R.C., 2009. Oxidative stress indices in erythrocytes, liver, kidneys of fluoride-exposed rabbits. Fluoride. 42, 88–93.

Shanks, D.F., 1997 Clinical implications of volcanic eruptions on livestock – case studies following the 1995 and 1996 eruptions of Mt. Ruapehu. Proc of the Society of Sheep and Beef Cattle Veterinarians of the New Zealand Veterinary Association. Massey University, Palmerston North, New Zealand, 27(1): 1–13.

Shearer, T.R., Kolstad, D.L., Suttie, J.W., 1978. Bovine dental fluorosis: histologic and physical characteristics. Am. J. Vet. Res. 39, 597–602.

Shupe, J.L., Olson, A.E., 1971. Clinical aspects of fluorosis in horses. J. Am. Vet. Med. Assoc. 158, 167–174.

Shupe, J.L., Olson, A.E., 1983. Clinical and pathological aspects of fluoride toxicosis in animals. In: Shupe, J.L., Peterson, H.B., Leone, N.C. (Eds.), Fluorides: Effects on Vegetation, Animals and Humans. Paragon Press, Inc, Salt Lake City, UT, pp. 319–338.

Shupe, J.L., Bruner, R.H., Seymour, J.L., et al., 1992. The pathology of chronic bovine fluorosis: a review. Toxicol. Pathol. 20, 274–285.

Chapter 28

Iron

Stephen B. Hooser

INTRODUCTION

Iron is an essential element for animal and plant life. It works as an oxygen (O_2) carrier in hemoglobin/myoglobin and is involved in numerous biological oxidation–reduction reactions, including photosynthesis. Iron is present in cytochrome P450 and is crucial for the metabolism of many chemicals in the liver, kidney, and other organs. Deficiencies in iron can result in anemia. Excess iron can cause iron overload and organ damage, while oxidation of ferrous to ferric iron in hemoglobin results in methemoglobinemia and an inability of red blood cells (RBCs) to carry O_2. Consequently, because of its importance, the uptake, distribution, storage, and excretion of iron is very tightly regulated in animals under normal conditions. Because of their reactivity, free iron compounds are sequestered with proteins to ensure that they do not initiate intracellular oxidative damage through electron donation and the formation of reactive oxygen species (ROS) such as hydroxyl radical. In this chapter, we will deal primarily with clinical animal exposures to excess iron through ingestion, parenteral administration, or genetic iron storage abnormalities. Nutritional deficiencies or exposure to chemicals causing methemoglobin formation such as nitrates in ruminants, or nitrites and chlorates in all species, are discussed elsewhere.

BACKGROUND

Iron is abundant in the universe and is the fourth most abundant element on earth. Its atomic number is 26 and its atomic weight is 55.847. It has been recognized to be an essential nutrient for more than 100 years and is present in all the cells of the body. The largest amount of iron is incorporated into proteins, hemoglobin, and myoglobin. Within RBCs (erythrocytes), hemoglobin transports O_2 from the lungs to cells throughout the body, while myoglobin binds O_2 for use in muscle cells (Klasing, 2005). Iron present in the serum is bound to the protein transferrin and in milk is bound to lactoferrin. Iron-containing proteins in the mitochondrial electron transport chain are essential for oxidative phosphorylation and energy production. Iron is also contained in enzymes of the Krebs cycle and in cytochromes P450, which are necessary for the metabolism of chemicals (Fairbanks, 1994).

The iron content of feedstuffs can be highly variable depending on the components. Iron in plants is subject to wide variation depending on the type of plant and the amount of iron in the soil, while many animal-based feed components are often rich in usable iron. The iron content of water can also vary greatly (Klasing, 2005). Large amounts of iron in water give the water a rusty color and a metallic taste, but upper limits of iron in drinking water for livestock and poultry have not been established since experimental data are not sufficient to make definite recommendations (NRC, 1974).

Worldwide, iron-deficiency anemias affect large numbers of people, but nutritional iron deficiencies are much less of a problem in animals. However, there are groups of animals that are vulnerable to iron deficiency including newborn piglets, veal calves, and those animals with parasitic infestations (Underwood, 1977). For instance, newborn piglets have very low concentrations of liver iron (29 mg/kg) compared to newborn rabbits whose liver iron stores average 135 mg/kg.

There is accumulating experimental evidence in laboratory animals that excessive iron deposits in the brain and abnormal iron homeostasis play an important role in neurodegenerative diseases such as Alzheimer's disease and Parkinson's disease (Connor et al., 1995; Lan and Jiang, 1997; Fredriksson et al., 1999; Dal-Pizzol et al., 2001; Qian and Shen, 2001; Arosio and Levi, 2002; Jomova et al., 2010; Singh et al., 2013; Ward et al., 2014; Zecca et al., 2004).

PHARMACOKINETICS/TOXICOKINETICS

The homeostatic regulation of iron in the body is complex and involves uptake, transport, utilization, storage, and

Veterinary Toxicology. DOI: http://dx.doi.org/10.1016/B978-0-12-811410-0.00028-3

loss. Under normal conditions, iron is poorly absorbed from most diets with approximately 5%–15% absorbed from the gastrointestinal (GI) tract. This uptake can double in iron deficiency. The body has a very limited ability to excrete iron; therefore, iron homeostasis is maintained by adjusting iron absorption to the body's needs. The amount of dietary iron that is absorbed through the GI tract is determined by the needs of the individual animal and is inversely related to serum ferritin concentrations (Bothwell et al., 1979). There are four main factors influencing iron absorption in the GI tract: (1) individual factors including the animal's age, iron status, and health; (2) conditions in the GI tract; (3) the chemical form and amount of iron ingested; and (4) other components of the diet which can enhance or reduce intestinal absorption. Iron is absorbed by enterocytes of the small intestine in ferrous (Fe^{2+}) form and transferred to the serum where it is converted to the ferric (Fe^{3+}) form and bound to transferrin (Goyer and Clarkson, 2001). In normal animals, most of fecal iron comes from ingested iron, which is not absorbed. Once absorbed, the body vigorously retains ingested iron unless bleeding occurs with daily iron loss limited to about 0.01% (of the body total) per day (Goyer and Clarkson, 2001). It has been found that even in the face of hemolytic anemia with destruction of erythrocytes, less than 1% of the iron is excreted in the urine and feces (Underwood, 1977).

In the bloodstream, serum iron is primarily bound to transferrin with lesser amounts bound to ferritin. Iron in the serum forms a pool from which it enters, is transported, leaves and reenters at a variable rate for the synthesis of hemoglobin, ferritin, cytochromes, and other iron-containing proteins. Of the total iron in the body, approximately two-thirds is bound to hemoglobin and 10% to myoglobin and iron-containing enzymes, with the remainder bound to the storage proteins ferritin and hemosiderin (Goyer and Clarkson, 2001). Ferritin and hemosiderin are found throughout the body with the main concentrations being in the liver, spleen, and bone marrow. They are protective in that they keep cellular iron in a bound form. Ferritin contains up to 20% iron, while hemosiderin is up to 35% iron. In the normal animal, nonviable RBCs are removed from the circulation by cells of the reticuloendothelial system in the liver, spleen, and bone marrow. There, heme is broken down, and the iron recycled for further use. In aged animals, when large amounts of iron are injected and rapidly cleared from the serum, or during chronic iron storage disease, the iron is preferentially deposited as hemosiderin, thereby increasing intracellular concentrations and giving rise to the hemosiderosis that can be seen histologically (Underwood, 1977; Goyer and Clarkson, 2001).

MECHANISM OF ACTION

For many functions, the body utilizes ferrous (Fe^{2+}) iron to bind molecular O_2. In this way, O_2 is transported by hemoglobin to cells in the peripheral tissues; myocytes bind O_2 for intracellular utilization; mitochondrial proteins of the electron transport chain bind O_2 for energy production; and P450 enzymes bind O_2 for its use in phase I metabolism of endogenous and xenobiotic chemicals. However, because of its reactivity, iron in its ferrous state must be carefully sequestered away to prevent the formation of highly ROS which can elicit severe cellular damage. Ferrous iron (Fe^{2+}) and other transition metal ions, Cu^+, Cr^{5+}, Ni^{2+} or Mn^{2+}, can catalyze the formation of hydroxyl ion (HO^-) and the extremely reactive and dangerous hydroxyl radical ($HO^•$) from the reduction of endogenous hydrogen peroxide (HOOH) via the *Fenton reaction*:

$$HOOH + Fe^{2+} \rightarrow Fe^{3+} + HO^- + HO \tag{28.1}$$

The Fenton reaction causes site-specific accumulation of free radicals and initiates biomolecular damage. Free radicals are molecules or molecular fragments that contain one or more unpaired electrons in their outer orbital shell. If produced in great enough quantities to overwhelm the cellular antioxidant and radical-quenching protective mechanisms, hydroxyl radicals promote the formation of more hydroxyl radicals and other ROS such as superoxide. Superoxide combines with nitric oxide and forms peroxynitrite, which is as detrimental as hydroxyl radical. These ROS and reactive nitrogen species (RNS) damage and destroy proteins and DNA by causing cross-linking, which inhibits their normal functions, or by initiating extensive damage and spontaneous degeneration of molecules such as lipids (Avery, 2011). ROS/RNS not only cause DNA damage but also inhibit repair activities. ROS induce lipid peroxidation, which if not quenched, can initiate a chain reaction of lipid destruction and ROS formation destroying vital cell membranes in mitochondria, nuclei and the cell periphery. Together, these effects can be of great enough magnitude to cause cell death, organ dysfunction, and death. However, it is also of interest to note that iron is necessary for the normal functioning of macrophages and other leukocytes during the respiratory burst in inflammation to catalyze the formation of bactericidal hydroxyl radical (Gregus and Klaassen, 2001).

TOXICITY

General

Iron poisoning is not common in animals, although potentially it could occur in any species. Clinical cases of acute iron toxicosis have been reported in dogs, pigs, horses, cattle and goats (Greentree and Hall, 1983; Ruhr et al., 1983; Osweiler et al., 1985; Holter et al., 1990). Toxicity can occur through ingestion or parenteral administration. Because of their indiscriminate eating habits and close proximity to people and their nutritional supplements, dogs are the species most likely to ingest large quantities of iron-containing vitamins or molluscicide applied to rid gardens of snails and slugs. Baby pigs are iron deficient at birth and require iron supplementation, which can result in peracute or acute toxicity. Limited cases of iron poisoning have occurred in horses and cattle through the use of iron supplements. In general, toxicity occurs in the GI mucosa (oral exposure), liver, myocardium, and other tissues when the iron-binding capacity of the body is overwhelmed, and free iron causes oxidative damage. Genetic iron storage diseases are uncommon, but have been reported in mynah birds, blackbirds (and other members of the Turdidae family), toucans, Saler cattle, Egyptian fruit bats, and rarely in horses.

Acute Toxicity in Dogs, Cattle, Pigs and Adult Horses

Acute iron toxicity has been reported in dogs (Greentree and Hall, 1983), cattle (Ruhr et al., 1983), pigs (Velasquez and Aranzazu, 2004), horses (Arnbjerg, 1981), and humans. In dogs, toxicosis primarily occurs through the accidental ingestion of large amounts of iron-containing vitamins or other iron supplements. In addition, acute toxicity can occur in dogs as the result of ingestion of molluscicide containing iron phosphate and/or iron EDTA (Buhl et al., 2013; Haldane and Davis, 2009) In cattle, horses, and pigs, it has occurred through accidental administration of excess amounts of iron supplements by oral or parenteral routes. Diagnosis is based on history, appropriate clinical signs, and radiography in small animals as iron-containing pills are radiodense. In general, if the animals remain asymptomatic for greater than 8 h following a single exposure, it is reported that they are unlikely to develop iron toxicity. In all species, ingestion of a toxic dose (roughly greater than 20 mg/kg in dogs) initially results in necrosis of the GI mucosal cells. This is followed by fluid loss, direct cardiotoxicity, and widespread organ damage through the mechanisms described above. Fluid loss and decreased cardiac output can lead to circulatory shock. Iron toxicity has been described as occurring in four stages. Stage I occurs 0–6 h postingestion and is characterized by vomiting, diarrhea, abdominal pain, and depression. Stage II occurs from 6 to 24 h postingestion and is characterized by apparent recovery. Stage III begins at 12–96 h with commencement of additional vomiting, diarrhea, abdominal pain, GI hemorrhage, weakness, shock, and possibly death. Stage IV, if it occurs, begins 2–6 weeks after ingestion and is characterized by GI fibrosis and obstruction (Greentree and Hall, 1983).

Neonatal Pigs

Paradoxically, iron toxicity in piglets resulting from oral supplementation or parenteral injection occurs because of the very low liver iron stores in newborn pigs, the low expression of duodenal iron transporters in the first few days postpartum (Lipinski et al., 2010), and the need to supplement the small amounts of iron that they receive in sow's milk. Because of their low iron stores at birth, iron-deficiency anemia can occur in nonsupplemented baby pigs within 2–4 weeks after birth. This is manifested clinically in the pigs as dyspnea, anorexia, increased infections, and poor growth, with some deaths. It is prevented by oral or parenteral injection of iron-containing compounds (Underwood, 1977; Osweiler et al., 1985). When comparing routes of administration of the same iron compound, the potential for toxicity is the greatest after intravenous injection followed by intramuscular injection with oral administration being the least toxic. In acute iron toxicosis of pigs, two syndromes are recognized. The first is a peracute syndrome which is characterized by sudden death minutes to a few hours after iron injection. In some ways, this resembles an anaphylactic reaction in its rapidity of onset, vascular collapse and death, but the exact mechanism is not known. This peracute syndrome has also been reported in horses following administration of iron compounds (Lannek and Persson, 1972; Bergsjoe, 1974). The second syndrome described in pigs is a subacute to acute syndrome characterized by GI necrosis, severe depression, coma and death, which can occur in the four stages described above. Pigs born to sows deficient in vitamin E and selenium are reported to be more susceptible to iron toxicosis (Osweiler et al., 1985; Velasquez and Aranzazu, 2004).

Neonatal Horses

Although reports of iron toxicosis in horses and ponies are rare, several cases in the 1980s are of note. Newborn foals, 2–5 days old, were given an oral nutritional supplement containing ferrous fumarate. They became ill, icteric, weak, and died of liver failure within 1–5 days following administration. The histologic lesions in the livers of these foals were remarkable in that they had the appearance of longer-term chronic lesions even though they were as little as 24 h old. These hepatic lesions consisted of prominent bile ductule proliferation, hepatic cell necrosis, and periportal fibrosis (Divers et al., 1983; Acland et al., 1984). Through experimental administration, it was determined that ferrous fumarate, administered orally to foals within the first few days after birth, caused the liver failure seen in the earlier clinical cases (Mullaney and Brown, 1988). The increased sensitivity of the neonatal foals is thought to be from increased absorption in the GI tract and lower systemic iron-binding capacity (Poppenga, 2002). The iron overload in these foals, resulting from oral administration of ferrous fumarate, caused hepatic necrosis with bile ductule proliferation and fibrosis. It is speculated that what was histologically interpreted as proliferation of bile ductules was, in fact, proliferation of hepatic stem cells (oval cells) in response to the severe hepatic damage (personal observation). Experimentally, adult ponies have been administered iron as ferrous sulfate at 50 mg/kg/day orally for up to 8 weeks. Through the study and for 20 weeks after the end of dosing, no adverse clinical signs or hepatic damage were reported (Pearson and Andreasen, 2001).

Iron Storage Disease

Iron storage disease, resulting in hemosiderosis and hemochromatosis, has been reported in several different species of animals. Hemochromatosis is the pathologic accumulation of iron in tissues, while hemosiderosis is the non-pathologic accumulation of iron. In birds, iron storage disease has been reported in mynah birds, toucans, birds of paradise, quetzals, and birds of the Turdidae family (blackbirds, song thrushes, fieldfares, and redwings, Pavone et al., 2014). The clinical signs are dyspnea, hepatic damage/insufficiency, and death in mynah birds. Sudden death has been reported in toucans. It has been shown that the cause in mynah birds is due to maintenance of iron uptake from the GI tract, despite excess hepatic iron accumulation (Mete et al., 2003). The treatment in birds can consist of a low iron diet with phlebotomy or the use of iron chelators (Rodenbusch et al., 2004). A genetic, inheritable defect resulting in hemochromatosis, clinical wasting, and skeletal defects can occur in Salers cattle beginning at 9–22 months of age (O'Toole et al., 2001; Norrdin et al., 2004). Egyptian fruit bats (*Rousettus aegyptiacus*) are also known to have genetic iron storage disease. In these bats, it was found that if the sum of transferrin saturation and serum iron was greater than 51, the individual bat had a high probability of having iron overload. When the sum was greater than 90, there was a high probability of having hemochromatosis (Farina et al., 2005). In addition, although rarely reported, hemochromatosis with liver damage has also been reported in horses (Pearson et al., 1994) and captive northern fur seals (Mazzaro et al., 2004). Finally, one case of hemochromatosis secondary to repeated blood transfusions every 6–8 weeks for 3 years for the treatment of red cell aplasia has been reported in an aged miniature schnauzer (Sprague et al., 2003).

TREATMENT

Treatment of iron toxicity varies with the inciting cause, dose, and duration of the disease. General therapy is to limit absorption (although activated charcoal is ineffective at binding iron), provide symptomatic and supportive care, remove gastric bezoars of sticky iron-containing pills (surgically if necessary), and increase excretion. Because the body has limited ability to excrete excess iron (other than through bleeding), urinary excretion can be enhanced through the use of a chelating agent. A specific chelator of iron, deferoxamine, has been used in the treatment of iron toxicity. Deferoxamine has a strong affinity for iron and a low affinity for calcium and competes effectively for iron in ferritin and hemosiderin but not in transferrin, hemoglobin or heme-containing enzymes. It is poorly absorbed orally and so is given parenterally by slow intravenous drip. Since it is excreted primarily by the kidneys, it should be given carefully to patients with renal insufficiency (Osweiler et al., 1985; Goyer and Clarkson, 2001; Poppenga, 2002).

CONCLUDING REMARKS AND FUTURE DIRECTIONS

Iron is essential for normal physiological functioning. Iron-deficiency anemia is common in humans and also occurs in piglets, veal calves and parasitized animals. Therefore, iron supplements are readily available and widely used. In addition, some species have a propensity for genetic iron storage diseases. Fortunately, both acute and chronic iron toxicoses are rare in animals. When toxicosis does occur, cellular damage is caused by the presence of free iron in excess of the body's capacity to bind and sequester it. The free iron then initiates the generation of ROS in excess of cellular oxidant defenses resulting in lipid peroxidation of membranes, protein and DNA cross-linking, and cell death.

REFERENCES

Acland, H.M., Mann, P.C., Robertson, J.L., et al., 1984. Toxic hepatopathy in neonatal foals. Vet. Pathol. 21, 3–9.

Arnbjerg, J., 1981. Poisoning in animals due to oral application of iron. With description of a case in a horse. Nordisk Vet. 33, 71–76.

Arosio, P., Levi, S., 2002. Ferritin, homeostasis, and oxidative damage. Free Rad. Biol. Med. 33, 457–463.

Avery, S., 2011. Molecular targets of oxidative stress. Biochem. J. 434, 201–210.

Bergsjoe, T., 1974. Death in association with parenteral administration of iron in horses. Also a short comparison with similar events in other species. Norsk Veterinaer-Tidsskrift. 85, 346–349.

Bothwell, T.H., Charlton, R.W., Cook, J.D., et al., 1979. Iron Metabolism in Man. Blackwell Scientific Publications, Oxford.

Buhl, K.J., Berman, F.W., Stone, D.L., 2013. Reports of metaldehyde and iron phosphate exposures in animals and characterization of suspected iron toxicosis in dogs. J. Am. Vet. Med. Assoc. 242, 1244–1248.

Connor, J.R., Pavlick, G., Karli, D., et al., 1995. A histochemical study of iron-positive cells in the developing rat brain. J. Comp. Neurol. 355, 111–123.

Dal-Pizzol, F., Klamt, F., Frota Jr, M.L.C., et al., 2001. Neonatal iron exposure induces oxidative stress in adult Wistar rat. Develop. Brain Res. 130, 109–114.

Divers, T.J., Warner, A., Vaala, W.E., et al., 1983. Toxic hepatic failure in newborn foals. J. Am. Vet. Med. Assoc. 183, 1407–1413.

Fairbanks, V.F., 1994. Iron in medicine and nutrition. In: Shils, M., Olson, J., Shike, M. (Eds.), Modern Nutrition in Health and Disease. Lea & Febiger, Philadelphia, pp. 185–213.

Farina, L.L., Heard, D.J., LeBlanc, D.M., et al., 2005. Iron storage disease in captive Egyptian fruit bats (*Rousettus aegyptiacus*): relationship of blood iron parameters to hepatic iron concentrations and hepatic histopathology. J. Zoo Wild. Med. 36, 212–221.

Fredriksson, A., Schröder, N., Eriksson, P., et al., 1999. Neonatal iron exposure induces neurobehavioural dysfunction in mice. Toxicol. Appl. Pharmacol. 155, 25–30.

Goyer, R.A., Clarkson, T.W., 2001. Toxic effects of metals. In: Klaassen, C.D. (Ed.), Toxicology, the Basic Science of Poisons. McGraw-Hill Co, New York, pp. 811–867.

Greentree, W.F., Hall, J.O., 1983. Iron toxicosis. In: Bonagura, J.D. (Ed.), Kirk's Current Veterinary Therapy XII. W.B. Saunders Co, London, pp. 240–242.

Gregus, Z., Klaassen, C.D., 2001. Mechanisms of toxicity. In: Klaassen, C.D. (Ed.), Toxicology, the Basic Science of Poisons. McGraw-Hill Co, New York, pp. 35–81.

Haldane, S.L., Davis, R.M., 2009. Acute toxicity in five dogs after ingestion of a commercial snail and slug bait containing iron EDTA. Austr. Vet. J. 87, 284–286.

Holter, J.A., Carson, T.L., Witte, S.T., 1990. Acute iron intoxication in a herd of young bulls. J. Vet. Diag. Invest. 2, 229–230.

Jomova, K., Vondrakova, D., Lawson, M., et al., 2010. Metals, oxidative stress and neurodegenerative disorders. Mol. Cell Biochem. 345, 91–104.

Klasing, K.C., 2005. Iron. Mineral Tolerances of Animals. National Research Council. The National Academies Press, Washington, DC.

Lan, J., Jiang, D.H., 1997. Excessive iron accumulation in the brain: a possible potential risk of neurodegeneration in Parkinson's disease. J. Neural. Transm. 104, 649–660.

Lannek, N., Persson, S., 1972. Shock following parenteral iron injections in horses. Svensk Veterinartidning. 24, 341–343.

Lipinski, P., Starzynski, R.R., Canonne-Hergaux, F., et al., 2010. Benefits and risks of iron supplementation in anemic neonatal pigs. Am. J. Pathol. 177, 1233–1243.

Mazzaro, L.M., Dunn St., J.L., Aubin, D.J., et al., 2004. Serum indices of body stores of iron in northern fur seals (Callorhinus ursinus) and their relationship to hemochromatosis. Zoo Biol. 23, 205–218.

Mete, A., Hendriks, H.G., Klaren, P.H.M., et al., 2003. Iron metabolism in mynah birds (Gracula religiosa) resembles human hereditary haemochromatosis. Avian Pathol. 32, 625–632.

Mullaney, T.P., Brown, C.M., 1988. Iron toxicity in neonatal foals. Eq. Vet. J. 20, 119–124.

Norrdin, R.W., Hoopes, K.J., O'Toole, D., 2004. Skeletal changes in hemochromatosis of Salers cattle. Vet. Pathol. 41, 612–623.

NRC (National Research Council), 1974. Nutrients and Toxic Substances in Water for Livestock and Poultry. National Academy Press, Washington, DC.

Osweiler, G.D., Carson, T.L., Buck, W.B., van Gelder, G.A., 1985. Iron. Clinical and Diagnostic Veterinary Toxicology. Kendall/Hunt Publishing Co, Dubuque, pp. 104–106.

O'Toole, D., Kelly, E.J., McAllister, M.M., et al., 2001. Hepatic failure and hemochromatosis of Salers and Salers-cross cattle. Vet. Pathol. 38, 372–389.

Pavone, S., Salamida, S., Pecorelli, I., et al., 2014. Deadly outbreak of iron storage disease (ISD) in Italian birds of the family Turdidae. J. Vet. Med. Sci. 76, 1209–1212.

Pearson, E.G., Andreasen, C.B., 2001. Effect of oral administration of excessive iron in adult ponies. J. Am. Vet. Med. Assoc. 218, 400–404.

Pearson, E.G., Hedstrom, O.R., Poppenga, R.H., 1994. Hepatic cirrhosis and hemochromatosis in three horses. J. Am. Vet. Med. Assoc. 204, 1053–1056.

Poppenga, R.H., 2002. Iron toxicosis. In: Brown, C., Bertone, J. (Eds.), The 5-Minute Veterinary Consult – Equine. Lippincott, Williams & Wilkins, Baltimore, pp. 590–591.

Qian, Z.M., Shen, X., 2001. Brain iron transport and neurodegeneration. Trends Mol. Med. 7, 103–108.

Rodenbusch, C.R., Canal, C.W., dos Santos, E.O., 2004. Hemosiderosis and hemochromatosis in wild birds – a review. Clin. Vet. 9, 44–50.

Ruhr, L.P., Nicholson, S.S., Confer, A.W., et al., 1983. Acute intoxication from a hematinic in calves. J. Am. Vet. Med. Assoc. 182, 616–618.

Singh, B., Haldar, S., Tripathi, A.K., et al., 2013. Brain iron homeostasis: from molecular mechanisms to clinical significance and therapeutic opportunities. Antioxid. Redox Signal. 20, 1324–1363.

Sprague, W.S., Hackett, T.B., Johnson, J.S., et al., 2003. Hemochromatosis secondary to repeated blood transfusions in a dog. Vet. Pathol. 40, 334–337.

Underwood, E.J., 1977. Iron. In: Underwood, E.J. (Ed.), Trace Elements in Human and Animal Nutrition. Academic Press, New York, pp. 13–55.

Velasquez, J.I., Aranzazu, D.A., 2004. An acute case of iron toxicity in newborn piglets from vitamin E/Se deficient sows. Rev. Col. Cien. Pecuarias. 17, 60–62.

Ward, R.J., Zucca, F.A., Duyn, J.H., et al., 2014. The role of iron in brain ageing and neurodegenerative disorders. Lancet Neurol. 13, 1045–1060.

Zecca, L., Youdim, M.B.H., Riederer, P., et al., 2004. Iron, brain ageing and neurodegenerative disorders. Nat. Rev. Neurosci. 5, 863–873.

Chapter 29

Lead

Larry J. Thompson

INTRODUCTION

Lead is a bluish white to gray heavy metal that was probably the first toxic element recognized by man and still has great relevance today. The chemical symbol for lead, Pb, is short for the Latin word *plumbum*, meaning liquid silver. The main source of lead is the ore named galena, which contains lead sulfide. The main use of lead today is in lead-acid storage batteries, but historically it has had widespread usage in paints (white, yellow and red pigments) and as a gasoline additive (tetraethyl lead), although these latter uses have essentially been phased out. A debate still continues as to the role lead played in the fall of the Roman Empire. Although lead was indeed used in some Roman water pipes (the word *plumbum* leading to our modern word plumber), the main source of lead for the Romans was probably sapa, a syrup used to sweeten wine and preserve fruit, which was made by boiling grape juice in lead pots thereby adding lead acetate to the liquid. The use of lead continues in our modern world with lead-containing solder in our electronics as well as lead-containing glass, from cathode ray tube monitors to fine crystal. Among all the metals, lead poisoning is encountered with greatest frequency in certain species of animals and poses a serious concern to animal health. This chapter describes the toxicity of lead in mammalian and avian species.

BACKGROUND

Lead is a toxic element and has not been shown to be an essential trace element for nutrition. The historical use of lead in gasoline, paint, construction materials, and many other products has resulted in lead being one of the most significant environmental contaminants in the world. Additional sources of lead have included lead weights (e.g., for fishing or curtains), small lead trinkets and toys, lead shot and bullets for weapons, lead arsenate pesticides, and many other products as well as single source environmental contamination from mining, smelting, and recycling operations. As a result of increased regulation of lead and the decreasing use of lead-containing products, the overall incidence of lead poisoning (also called plumbism) in animals and humans has been decreasing. While environmental contamination with lead does not resolve readily, the overt poisoning of domestic animals from environmental sources (e.g., from contaminated forages, plants, water, or other food sources) has been decreasing in number. Still, lead poisoning in animals is encountered with greatest frequency compared to any other metal.

TOXICOKINETICS

The main route of entry of lead into the body is the digestive tract with absorption dependent upon the chemical form of lead and the physiological state of the animal. Organic lead compounds are, in general, more readily absorbed than either inorganic lead salts or the metallic form of lead. Dermal absorption of organolead compounds can be significant, but the salt or metallic forms of lead are not absorbed dermally. The fumes from heated lead or very fine particles (<0.5 μm) of lead can enter the lung alveoli and be absorbed with the larger particles lodging in the ciliated portion of the bronchial tree. These larger particles can be transported up by mucociliary action and then swallowed with absorption through the gastrointestinal (GI) tract. Fine particles of lead and lead salts can be solubilized in the acid environment of the stomach, and the small intestine is the site of most lead absorption. Absorption of lead from the alimentary tract is usually influenced by dietary factors and by the size of lead particles. High dietary fat and mineral deficiency can increase lead absorption by seven and 20-fold, respectively. In an experimental study, dogs maintained on a high-fat, low-calcium diet absorbed significantly more lead than those kept on a balanced diet (Hamir et al., 1988). Young animals absorb a larger portion of the lead

Veterinary Toxicology. DOI: http://dx.doi.org/10.1016/B978-0-12-811410-0.00029-5

from the GI tract than do adults. Animals with a calcium deficiency have increased absorption of lead. Pregnancy or lactation as well as deficiencies of iron, zinc, or vitamin D can also enhance lead absorption. Lead crosses the placental barrier, and the residue can be detected in significant amounts in fetal blood and organs. Among the fetal organs, the highest concentrations are found in the blood and liver (Kelman and Walter, 1980; O'Hara et al., 1995; Flora and Agrawal, 2017). Lead also passes through the milk.

Adult monogastric animals absorb approximately 10% of dietary lead, and adult ruminants absorb less than 3%. Young animals can absorb up to 90% of the ingested lead. Following absorption, a large proportion of lead is carried on erythrocyte membranes (60%–90%, species dependent) with most of the remainder of lead bound to protein or sulfhydryl compounds, with only a very small proportion found free in the serum. Lead is widely distributed in the body, including crossing the blood–brain barrier (BBB) (Seimiya et al., 1991). In the soft tissues, lead binds to various proteins as well as metallothionein but accumulates in the active bone matrix (about 90%) serving as a relatively inert reservoir of lead in the body. This reservoir can be mobilized by lactation, pregnancy, or the action of certain chelating agents. Otherwise, lead has a very slow turnover rate from the bone. Lead is normally very slowly excreted via the bile with very little in the urine. Chelation therapy greatly increases the urinary output of lead.

MECHANISM OF ACTION

Lead interferes with several biochemical processes in the body by binding to sulfhydryl and other nucleophilic functional groups causing inhibition of several enzymes and changes in calcium/vitamin D metabolism. Lead also contributes to oxidative stress within the body. Lead inhibits the body's ability to make hemoglobin by interfering with several enzymatic steps in the heme pathway. Specifically, lead decreases heme biosynthesis by inhibiting delta-aminolevulinic acid dehydratase and ferrochelatase activity. These changes contribute to the anemia that develops in chronic lead poisoning. An increased fragility of red blood cells also contributes to the anemia.

From various experimental studies, biochemical and pathological evidence demonstrates that lead is a neurotoxicant, as it significantly disrupts certain brain structures and functions. High-dose exposure to lead (i.e., blood levels in excess of $4\ \mu M = 0.83$ ppm) disrupts the BBB. Molecules such as albumin that normally are excluded will freely enter the brain of immature animals exposed to these concentrations of lead (Clasen et al., 1973; Goldstein et al., 1974; Bressler and Goldstein, 1991). Ions and water follow, and edema is produced. Intracranial pressure rises as edema accumulates in the brain because of the physical restraint of the skull. When the intracranial pressure approaches the systemic pressure, cerebral perfusion decreases, and brain ischemia occurs.

Many of the neurotoxic effects of lead appear related to the ability of lead to mimic, or in some cases, inhibit the action of calcium as a regulator of cell function (Bressler and Goldstein, 1991). At a neuronal level, exposure to lead alters the release of neurotransmitters (dopamine, acetylcholine and γ-aminobutyric acid) from nerve endings. Spontaneous release is enhanced and evoked release is inhibited. The former may be due to activation of protein kinases in the nerve endings and the latter to blockade of voltage-dependent calcium channels. Lead also inhibits *N*-methyl-D-aspartate receptors containing NR2A, NR2C and NR2D subunits, thereby causing decreased calcium influx and reduced brain derived neurotrophic factor, leading to neuroinflammation and neuronal injury and death.

Brain homeostatic mechanisms are disrupted by exposure to higher levels of lead. The final pathway appears to be a breakdown in the BBB. Again, the ability of lead to mimic or mobilize calcium and activate protein kinases may alter the properties of endothelial cells, especially in an immature brain, and disrupt the barrier. In addition to a direct toxic effect upon the endothelial cells, lead may alter indirectly the microvasculature by damaging the astrocytes that provide signals for the maintenance of BBB integrity, and necrosis in neurons with shrunken cytoplasm, pyknotic nuclei and increased perineuronal space.

Recent studies provide evidence of increased production of reactive oxygen species following lead exposure. Lead induces oxidative damage in several tissues by enhancing lipid peroxidation through Fenton reaction or by direct participation in free radical-mediated reactions, such as inhibition of δ-aminolevulinic acid dehydratase (ALAD) activity or accumulation of ALA, a metabolite that can release Fe^{2+} from ferritin and induce oxidative damage.

TOXICITY

Mammals, birds and reptiles have all been found to develop lead poisoning. The toxic dose of lead has been determined for several species but is difficult to apply to clinical cases where the exposure history is unclear (Gwaltney-Brant, 2004). In general, young animals are more susceptible to lead toxicosis because they are more prone to lead pica and have a higher rate of absorption (about 90%) from the intestinal tract. Cattle have been most widely reported with lead toxicosis, probably because of their propensity to ingest discarded lead–acid batteries and construction materials including paints. Dogs are also commonly reported with lead toxicosis, probably because of their chewing habits and ingestion of small lead objects around the house. Both cats and dogs have been exposed to lead by the renovations of older homes containing leaded paints. The main route seems to be the ingestion of fine dust by the grooming habits of indoor pets and their tendency to ingest small objects. A proximal renal tubulopathy has been described in a dog diagnosed with lead intoxication (King, 2016).

Clinical signs of lead toxicosis vary with the species involved, duration of exposure, and amount of lead absorbed. The major systems affected by lead poisoning are the GI system, central nervous system, and hematological system. Abdominal pain and diarrhea can be common clinical signs in animals exposed to excess lead. Anorexia is common as well as vomiting in those species that are able to. Neurological signs including depression, weakness and ataxia can progress to more severe clinical signs of muscle tremors or fasciculations, head pressing (especially in ruminants), blindness, seizure-like activity, and death. Many animals with chronic lead poisoning will show subtle and nonspecific clinical signs such as abdominal discomfort, vague GI upsets, anorexia, lethargy, weight loss, and behavior changes. Horses develop acute lead toxicosis and show clinical signs of laryngeal paralysis and "roaring," in addition to colic and seizure-like activity. Evidence suggests that horses may be more susceptible to chronic lead toxicosis than cattle. Horses exposed to a daily intake as low as 1.7 mg/kg body weight (approximately 80 ppm Pb in forage dry matter) were poisoned (Aronson, 1972). A maximum tolerated dose of 10 ppm lead in dog and cat food products was determined by the FDA-CVM in response to confusion concerning the misinterpretation of lead analytical results in pet food products (FDA-CVM, 2011). Clinical signs of lead toxicosis in avians vary with waterfowl and raptors mainly displaying a chronic wasting disorder with apparent peripheral neuropathy. Psittacines are more likely to display GI problems and neurological abnormalities.

Gross lesions in animals dying of lead poisoning are often minimal and nonspecific, although lead-containing objects may be visible in the GI tract. Histologically, there may be degeneration and necrosis of the renal tubular epithelium or the presence of acid-fast inclusion bodies (Hamir et al., 1988; O'Hara et al., 1995). Brain lesions in a calf poisoned with lead included multiple focal or laminar lesions of neuronal necrosis in the cerebral cortex, caudatum, and medial nuclei of thalamus, predominantly at the tips of gyri in the occipital and parietal lobes. The lesions spread occasionally to the deeper region of the gyri along the sulci (Seimiya et al., 1991). The affected neurons were shrunken and angular, sometimes triangular in outline with pale eosinophilic cytoplasm. The nuclei showed pyknosis and rhexis. Edematous dilation of perivascular and perineuronal spaces with spongiotic state of neuropil was observed from the molecular layer to outer zone of the white matter. Astrocytic proliferation was also observed. Blood capillaries were congested with enlarged and increased endothelial cells. Meningeal blood vessels were prominently congested with mild lymphocytic infiltration. Edema of Purkinje cell layer in the cerebellum and mild neuronal degeneration in the nucleus of mesencephalon were seen.

Lead is also a reproductive and developmental toxicant and details can be found in other publications (Flora and Agrawal, 2017).

Diagnosis of lead poisoning in animals should be made with a combination of history, clinical or necropsy findings, and lead analysis of tissue. Basophilic stippling of erythrocytes and inhibition of hemoglobin synthesis are characteristic hematological features of lead poisoning. From a living animal, whole blood is the best sample for laboratory determination of lead. The normal background concentration of lead in the blood of mammals is below 0.1 ppm. Whole blood lead concentrations above 0.35 ppm, when combined with indicative clinical signs in the suspect animal, are compatible with a diagnosis of lead toxicosis. Many authors use a blood lead concentration of 0.6 ppm and above as diagnostic for lead toxicosis. Postmortem samples of choice are kidney and liver with lead concentrations above 10 ppm on a wet weight basis being diagnostic for lead toxicosis in domestic species.

TREATMENT

Acute lead poisoning in animals is usually fatal if the animals are not treated promptly. The treatment approach for lead poisoning in animals includes stabilizing and supporting the animal, especially if severe clinical signs are present, preventing additional exposure to lead, and chelation therapy to quickly reduce the body burden of lead. The exposure history of the animal should be reviewed for potential sources of lead and the need for GI decontamination. The use of chelating agents when large amounts of lead are present in the GI tract may actually enhance the absorption of lead into the body. Physical removal of lead-containing objects by surgical means may be necessary with larger objects. The parenteral use of calcium disodium ethylenediaminetetraacetic acid (CaEDTA) has been commonly used for several decades as a chelation agent in domestic animals (Kowalczyk, 1984).

Although other chelators may be superior, CaEDTA is still widely used in veterinary medicine, especially in large animals. CaEDTA is given intravenously (IV) or subcutaneously (SQ) and chelates and mobilizes the lead from bone resulting in a transient increase in blood lead levels. This increase in blood lead can increase soft tissue lead levels leading to an exacerbation of clinical signs. Preceding CaEDTA usage with a chelator that specifically targets lead in the soft tissue (e.g., British Anti-Lewisite or BAL) has been recommended but is difficult to accomplish in most practice settings. CaEDTA can be nephrotoxic, especially in situations where the animal is dehydrated. Recommended treatment with CaEDTA for large animals is 73 mg/kg/day, divided into two or three doses given over the course of a day by slow IV. For example, a 6.6% solution of CaEDTA (in normal saline or 5% dextrose) can be given IV at a rate of 1 mL per 2 pounds (0.9 kg) of body weight per day in divided doses. Treatment should continue for 3–5 days. If additional treatment is needed, a rest period of 2 days with continued supported care is suggested before the additional 3–5-day second treatment period. An alternative treatment regimen is to administer CaEDTA at 110 mg/kg IV twice daily for 2 days. If additional treatment is needed, first apply the 2-day rest period of supportive care before initiating the second treatment period of 2 days at 110 mg/kg twice daily. Thiamine has been shown to be a valuable adjunct to the treatment of lead poisoning in ruminants (Bratton et al., 1981) and is recommended for other species as well. A dose of 2 mg/kg/day for calves and 250–2000 mg/day for adult cattle has been recommended. A 2-day withdrawal period for both meat and milk is recommended (Haskell et al., 2005).

If commercial CaEDTA is unavailable, a stock solution can be formulated for emergency antidotal usage. A 10% stock solution can be made by dissolving 101.1 g of tetrasodium EDTA (Na_4EDTA) plus 30 g of anhydrous calcium chloride ($CaCl_2$) in distilled water to a final volume of 1000 mL. From the stock solution, a working 2.22% solution can be made by mixing 220 mL of the 10% stock solution with 780 mL distilled water. Using the 2.22% solution, the daily dosage of 73 mg/kg/day is equal to approximately 3.5 mL/kg of body weight. This should be divided into two or three separate administrations (Thompson, 1992). Tetrasodium EDTA should never be administered by itself as it may cause hypocalcemia.

Recommended treatment with CaEDTA for dogs is 100 mg/kg/day in four divided doses. Treatment should continue for 2–5 days, and a second round of treatment is rarely needed. A 5-day rest period is recommended before applying additional treatment. CaEDTA concentration should be 10 mg/mL and may be administered by slow IV or by SQ route. Cats can be treated with 27.5 mg in 15 mL normal saline or 5% dextrose SQ every 6 h for 5 days or the same dose as a slow IV infusion.

Succimer (meso-2,3-dimercaptosuccinic or DMSA) is an orally administered chelating agent that is less likely to have adverse side effects associated with CaEDTA. The recommended treatment in dogs is an oral dose of succimer at 10 mg/kg, repeated three times daily for 10 days (Ramsey et al., 1996). Succimer has also been used orally in caged birds at a dose of 25–35 mg/kg twice daily for 5 days. Several weeks of therapy may be needed in avians. In initial experimental work, succimer given to experimentally lead-poisoned calves IV at 25 mg/kg/day for 4 days was more effective than CaEDTA at decreasing lead concentrations in the liver and kidney (Meldrum and Ko, 2003).

In an recent experimental study, Pachauri et al. (2009) provide evidence of the efficacy of combinational therapy using an antioxidant with a thiol chelator in reversing neurological dystrophy caused by chronic lead exposure in rats.

CONCLUDING REMARKS AND FUTURE DIRECTIONS

While cases of lead toxicosis in animals have been decreasing, it should remain on the clinician's list of rule-outs for seizure-like activity, blindness, and vague neurological and GI disorders. At a minimum, the environment of the animal should be reviewed for possible lead sources.

REFERENCES

Aronson, A.L., 1972. Lead poisoning in cattle and horses following long-term exposure to lead. Am. J. Vet. Res. 33, 627.

Bratton, G.R., Zmudzki, J., Kincaid, N., et al., 1981. Thiamine as treatment of lead poisoning in ruminants. Mod. Vet. Pract. 62, 441–446.

Bressler, J.P., Goldstein, G.W., 1991. Mechanisms of lead neurotoxicity. Biochem. Pharmacol. 41, 479–484.

Clasen, R.A., Hartmann, J.F., Starr, A.J., et al., 1973. Electron microscopic and chemical studies of the vascular changes and edema of lead encephalopathy. Am. J. Pathol. 74, 215–240.

FDA-CVM, 2011. Target animal safety review memorandum. https://www.fda.gov/downloads/aboutfda/centersoffices/officeoffoods/cvm/cvmfoiaelectronicreadingroom/ucm274327.pdf. (accessed 01.03.17.).

Flora, S.J.S., Agrawal, S., 2017. Arsenic, cadmium and lead. In: Gupta, R.C. (Ed.), Reproductive and Developmental Toxicology, second ed. Academic Press/Elsevier, Amsterdam, pp. 537–566.

Goldstein, G.W., Asbury, A.K., Diamond, I., 1974. Pathogenesis of lead encephalopathy. Uptake of lead and reaction of brain capillaries. Arch. Neurol. 31, 382–389.

Gwaltney-Brant, S., 2004. Lead. In: Plumlee, K.H. (Ed.), Clinical Veterinary Toxicology. Mosby, St. Louis, MO, pp. 204–210.

Hamir, A.N., Sullivan, N.D., Handson, P.D., 1988. Tissue lead distribution and pathological findings in lead exposed dogs maintained on fat and calcium modified diets. Br. Vet. J. 144, 240–245.

Haskell, S.R., Payne, M., Webb, A., et al., 2005. Antidotes in food animal practice. J. Am. Vet. Med. Assoc. 226 (6), 884–887.

Kelman, B.J., Walter, B.K., 1980. Transplacental movements of inorganic lead from mother to fetus. Proc. Soc. Exp. Biol. Med. 163, 278–282.

King, J.B., 2016. Proximal tubular nephropathy in two dogs diagnosed with lead toxicity. Aust. Vet. J. 94, 280–284.

Kowalczyk, D.F., 1984. Clinical management of lead poisoning. J. Am. Vet. Med. Assoc. 184, 858–860.

Meldrum, J.B., Ko, K.W., 2003. Effects of calcium disodium EDTA and meso-2,3-dimercaptosuccinic acid on tissue concentrations of lead for use in treatment of calves with experimentally induced lead toxicosis. Am. J. Vet. Res. 64, 672–676.

O'Hara, T.M., Bennett, L., McCoy, P.C., et al., 1995. Lead poisoning and toxicokinetics in a heifer and fetus treated with $CaNa_2EDTA$ and thiamine. J. Vet. Diag. Investig. 7, 531–537.

Pachauri, V., Saxena, G., Mehta, A., et al., 2009. Combinational therapy abrogates lead-induced neurodegeneration in rats. Toxicol. Appl. Pharmacol. 240, 255–264.

Ramsey, D.T., Casteel, S.W., Faggella, A.M., et al., 1996. Use of orally administered succimer (meso-2,3-dimercaptosuccinic acid) for treatment of lead poisoning in dogs. J. Am. Vet. Med. Assoc. 208, 371–375.

Seimiya, Y., Itoh, H., Ohshima, K.-I., 1991. Brain lesions of lead poisoning in a calf. J. Vet. Med. Sci. 53, 117–119.

Thompson, L.J., 1992. Heavy metal toxicosis. In: Robinson, N.E. (Ed.), Current Therapy in Equine Medicine, vol. 3. W.B. Saunders Co, Philadelphia, PA, pp. 363–366.

Chapter 30

Manganese

Dejan Milatovic and Ramesh C. Gupta

INTRODUCTION AND BACKGROUND

Manganese (Mn) is a naturally occurring trace metal commonly found in the environment. It is the twelfth most abundant element in the earth's crust, present in rocks, soil, water, and food. It does not occur naturally in a pure state and the most important Mn-containing minerals are oxides, carbonates, and silicates (Post, 1999). As a transition metal, Mn exists in more than five valence states, with a majority as Mn^{2+} or Mn^{3+}. Mn is abundantly found in the environment, including rocks, soil, water, and food, with the highest concentrations typically in nuts, cereals, grains, fruits, vegetables, and tea. Mn is a component of certain aluminum alloys, particularly those used in the manufacture of soft drink cans. Inorganic Mn is also used in dry cell batteries, animal feed, brick coloring, and fertilizers (Aschner et al., 1999; ATSDR, 2000; Corathers, 2001; O'Neal and Zheng, 2015). Organic Mn is used as a fuel additive and in fungicides, such as mancozeb and maneb (ATSDR, 2000; Kaiser, 2003).

Mn is an essential element for maintaining the proper function and regulation of many biochemical and cellular reactions (Takeda, 2003) that are critical for humans, animals, and plants (Takeda, 2003; Tarale et al., 2016). It is required for growth and development and plays a role in immune response, blood sugar homeostasis, adenosine triphosphate (ATP) regulation, digestion, bone growth, reproduction, and lactation. It is a necessary component of numerous metalloenzymes, such as Mn superoxide dismutase, arginase, phosphoenol-pyruvate carboxylase, and glutamine synthase (Aschner and Aschner, 2005). As a result, dietary deficiency of Mn is known to affect several enzymes, including glycosyltransferases, xylosyltransferases, arginase, and mitochondrial superoxide dismutase (NRC, 2005). The dietary requirement of Mn is 10 ppm in rats and mice, 40 ppm in guinea pigs, 20 ppm in pigs, 28–30 ppm in chickens, 20 ppm in beef cattle and 40 ppm in dairy cattle. Practically, Mn deficiency occurs more frequently in cattle, pigs, and poultry. In ruminants, Mn deficiency can be linked to silent heat, reduced conception, abortions, reduced birth weight, an increased percentage of male calves, paralysis and skeletal damage in calves. Mn deficiency can cause delayed estrus, reduced fertility, and spontaneous abortions in mares. Foals are born with skeletal deformities and muscle contractures, such as asymmetry of the skull, curvature of the vertebral column, shortened limb bones, enlarged joints, and contracture of neck muscles. In dogs, Mn deficiency can cause crooked and shortened soft bones (Puls, 1994).

Despite its essentiality, Mn overexposure can cause a variety of toxic effects in humans and animals. Mn has been linked to a peculiar extrapyramidal syndrome in occupational workers since 1837. Since then, incidences of Mn poisoning, especially in mines and steel factories, have been reported in many countries (Wang et al., 1989; Lucchini et al., 2009; Racette et al., 2012; Chen et al., 2014). Fortunately, in the last three decades there has been a declining trend even in developing countries. Mn poisoning can occur in animals or humans if the exposure level of Mn exceeds the normal levels in the environment. Toxicity can also occur if either the dietary concentration exceeds the maximal tolerable levels or if dietary intake of other minerals is marginal (Hartman et al., 1955; Ivan and Hidiroglou, 1980; Southern and Baker, 1983; Baker and Halpin, 1991; Hauser et al., 1994). The brain, in particular, is highly susceptible to Mn toxicity. Excessive accumulation of Mn in specific brain areas, such as the substantia nigra, the globus pallidus and the striatum, produce neurotoxicity leading to a degenerative brain disorder, referred to as manganism. In addition to neurological effects, Mn accumulation is also associated with reproductive and developmental effects. High-dose exposure to Mn has been associated with increased fetal brain Mn concentrations (Kontur and Fechter, 1985) although several studies have reported an ability of the placenta to reduce systemic delivery of Mn to the fetal brain. Moreover, Mn plays a role in the modulation of the immune system, and in protein, lipid and carbohydrate metabolism (Addess et al.,

Veterinary Toxicology. DOI: http://dx.doi.org/10.1016/B978-0-12-811410-0.00030-1

1997; Malecki et al., 1999; Aschner et al., 2002; Fitsanakis and Aschner, 2005). This chapter describes deficiency and toxicity of Mn in animals.

PHARMACOKINETICS/TOXICOKINETICS

Absorption of Mn is via oral and inhalation routes. Absorption of Mn through the skin is negligible. Apparent absorption of orally administered ^{54}Mn has been estimated to range from 1% to 5% in rats, humans and livestock (Hurley and Keen, 1987; Davis et al., 1993). In young rats, Mn absorption has been reported to be 8%. Absorption of Mn appears to occur by a low-capacity saturable process and by diffusion (Garcia-Aranda et al., 1983; ATSDR, 2000). Uptake and retention of dietary Mn was found to be greater in suckling than postweaning rats (Keen et al., 1986). In cattle, using $MnSO_4$ as 100% available, MnO is 58%, MnO_2 is 33% and $MnCO_2$ is 28% available (Puls, 1994). Mn is more available from hay to cattle than from silage. It is important to note that newborn calves absorb and retain more dietary Mn than adults.

Absorption of Mn can be influenced by various dietary factors such as iron, calcium, phosphorus, phytate, and amino acids. Henry (1995) estimated the relative bioavailability of Mn to poultry was 0.55 from manganese carbonate, 0.3 from manganese dioxide and 0.75 from manganese monoxide, when the bioavailability of manganese from manganese sulfate and manganese chloride was considered to be 1. Manganese from manganese carbonate, dioxide and monoxide (relative bioavailabilities were 0.3, 0.35 and 0.6, respectively) was even less available to sheep than manganese sulfate (relative bioavailability was 1).

Following absorption, Mn can be distributed to many organs. The average adult human has about 12 mg of Mn, of which about 43% resides in the skeletal system and the rest in soft tissues including the liver, pancreas, kidneys, and central nervous system (CNS). Such information about Mn is not available for animals. It is interesting to note that in dogs, the pancreas accumulates 3–60 times more Mn than other soft tissues. Furthermore, colored hair has higher Mn levels than noncolored hair.

After absorption from the gut, Mn is transported to the liver by α2-macroglobulins and albumin (Andersen et al., 1999). This protein-bound Mn is efficiently cleared in the liver and is bound to transferrin. Transferrin is believed to be the primary transporter of Mn across the blood–brain barrier (BBB) and Mn is taken up into astrocytes and neurons in the brain. Astocytes serve as the major homeostatic regulator and storage site for Mn in the brain (Aschner et al., 1992; Sidoryk-Wegrzynowicz and Aschner, 2013). Increased accumulation of Mn in astrocytes may alter release of glutamate and elicit excitatory neurotoxicity (Erikson and Aschner, 2003). Neuronal uptake of Mn involves transferrin (Suarez and Eriksson, 1993) and utilization of specific transporter systems, such as the dopamine transporter (Chen et al., 2006a; Anderson et al., 2007). At the subcellular level, Mn preferentially accumulates in mitochondria, where it disrupts oxidative phosphorylation and increases the generation of reactive oxygen species (ROS) (Gunter et al., 2006).

Rodent studies of enhanced CNS uptake during development have been contradictory. While one study indicates that the amount of Mn that crosses the placenta was not increased by enhanced maternal exposure via diet (Jarvinen and Ahlstrom, 1975), another study indicated increased neonatal brain Mn following chronic high-level exposure of the dam to Mn in drinking water throughout gestation (Kontur and Fechter, 1985). Other studies also showed that, when compared with adults, neonatal rodents attained higher brain Mn levels following similar oral exposures (Kontur and Fechter, 1985; Dorman et al., 2000). This tendency of neonates to attain higher brain Mn concentrations may reflect a less than optimal BBB, markedly reduced biliary Mn excretion rates, and/or increased placental Mn concentration (Aschner and Aschner, 2005; Austinc et al., 2016). However, an increase in the placental concentrations does not necessarily mean higher placental transfer of Mn to the fetus or higher fetal exposure (Dorman et al., 2005; Yoon et al., 2009a). Furthermore, brain Mn concentrations are higher in developing animals, suggesting that high amounts of Mn are required for normal brain development in infants (Keen et al., 1986; Takeda et al., 1999). Therefore, whether the relatively higher net increase in brain Mn observed in neonates compared to adults would pose an increased risk for neurotoxicity requires further understanding of the Mn requirements for normal brain development (Yoon et al., 2009b).

The absorbed Mn can be excreted via urine and bile. Excretion of Mn through urine is minor. Bile is the major excretory route of injected or ingested Mn. Rats excreted 15%–40% (Ballatori et al., 1987) and calves excreted 21% (Abrams et al., 1977) of injected doses of Mn in bile. In humans, Mn is eliminated almost entirely with feces, and only 0.1%–1.3% of daily intake through urine. Klaassen (1974) observed that rats excreted proportionately more Mn into bile than rabbits and dogs. Following ingestion, effectiveness of the gut in preventing excess absorption blunts the effect of biliary excretion (Abrams et al., 1977; Davis et al., 1993; Malecki et al., 1996). Calves excreted 0.2% of a duodenal dose of Mn into bile in one study (Abrams et al., 1977), and 2.1%–3.6% of high levels of Mn infused intraduodenally in another study (Symonds and Hall, 1983).

MECHANISM OF ACTION

Mn is generally described as a neurotoxicant, selectively affecting basal ganglia structures. Although it is known that Mn is a cellular toxicant which can impair the transport system, enzyme activity and receptors function, the principal mechanism by which Mn neurotoxicity occurs has not yet been clearly established (Aschner and Aschner, 1991; Aschner et al., 2007; Martinez-Finley et al., 2013; O'Neal and Zheng, 2015). Since mitochondria are the principal intracellular repository for metals (Cotzias and Greenough, 1958), binding of Mn to inner mitochondrial membrane or matrix proteins (Gavin et al., 1990) directly interacts with proteins involved in oxidative phosphorylation. Mn directly inhibits complex II (Singh et al., 1974) and complexes I–IV (Zhang et al., 2003) in brain mitochondria, and suppresses ATP-dependent calcium waves in astrocytes, suggesting that Mn promotes potentially disruptive mitochondrial sequestration of calcium (Tjalkens et al., 2006). Elevated matrix calcium increases the formation of ROS by the electron transport chain (ETC) (Kowaltowski et al., 1995) and results in inhibition of aerobic respiration (Kruman and Mattson, 1999). Recent studies with primary astrocytes and neurons have shown that Mn exposure induces an increase in the biomarkers of oxidative stress (Milatovic et al., 2007, 2009). Measurement of F_2-isoprostanes (F_2-IsoPs) (Morrow and Roberts, 1999; Milatovic and Aschner, 2009), a group of arachidonic acid-derived prostanoid isomers generated by free radical damage due to arachidonic acid, revealed that astrocytes exposed to Mn at a neurotoxic level (100 μM, 500 μM or 1 mM) induced significant elevations in F_2-IsoPs (Fig. 30.1). Thus, increases in ROS, which are generated by electron leak

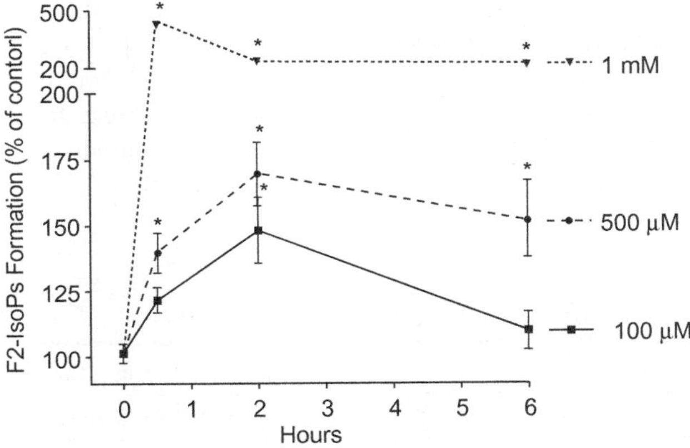

FIGURE 30.1 Effects of $MnCl_2$ on F_2-IsoPs formation in cultured astrocytes. Rat primary astrocyte cultures were incubated at 37°C in the presence or absence on $MnCl_2$ (100 μM, 500 μM or 1 mM), and F_2-IsoPs levels were quantified at 30 min, 2 h and 6 h. Data represent the mean ± S.E.M. from three independent experiments. * Significant difference between values from control and Mn-treated astrocytes ($*p < .05$).

from the ETC (Turrens and Boveris, 1980), potentially damage mitochondria directly or through the effects of secondary oxidants like superoxide, H_2O_2 or peroxynitrite ($ONOO^-$), mediate Mn-induced oxidative damage. Moreover, superoxide produced in the mitochondrial ETC may catalyze the transition shift of Mn^{2+} to Mn^{3+} through a set of reactions similar to those mediated by superoxide dismutase and thus lead to the increased oxidant capacity of this metal (Gunter et al., 2006). Consequent oxidative damage produces an array of deleterious effects: it may cause structural and functional derangement of the phospholipids bilayer of membranes, disrupt energy metabolism, metabolite biosynthesis, calcium and iron homeostasis and initiate apoptosis (Attardi and Schatz, 1988; Yang et al., 1997; Uchida, 2003).

Consistent and preceding the Mn-induced increased in biomarkers of oxidative damage (F_2-IsoPs) (Fig. 30.1), Milatovic et al. (2007) demonstrated an early decrease in astrocytic ATP levels. As a consequence, ATP depletion or a perturbation in energy metabolism might diminish the ATP-requiring neuroprotective action of astrocytes, such as glutamate and glutamine uptake and free radical scavenging (Rao et al., 2001). In addition, depletion of high-energy phosphates may affect intracellular Ca^{2+} in astrocytes through mechanisms involving the disruption of mitochondrial Ca^{2+} signaling. This assertion is supported by data showing that Mn inhibits Na^+-dependent Ca^{2+} efflux (Gavin et al., 1990) and respiration in brain mitochondria (Zhang et al., 2004), both critical for maintaining normal ATP levels and ensuring adequate intermitochondrial signaling. Decrease in ATP following Mn exposure is also associated with excitotoxicity, suggesting a direct effect on astrocytes with subsequent impairment of neuronal function. Mn down-regulates the L-glutamate/L-aspartate transporter in astrocytes (Erikson and Aschner, 2002) and decreases levels of glutamine synthase in exposed primates (Erikson et al., 2008). Studies with a neonatal rat model indicated that both pinacidil, a K^+ channel agonist, and nimodipine, a Ca^{2+}channel antagonist, reversed Mn neurotoxicity and loss of glutamine synthase activity, further indicating excitotoxicity in the mechanism of Mn-induced neurotoxicity. Excessive Mn may lead to excitotoxic neuronal injury both by decreased astrocytic glutamate uptake and by loss of ATP-mediated inhibition of glutamatergic synapses.

Another consequence of Mn-associated increased oxidative stress and mitochondrial energy failure is the induction of the mitochondrial permeability transition (MPT), a Ca^{2+}-dependent process characterized by the opening of the permeability transition pore in the inner mitochondrial membrane. This process results in increased permeability to protons, ions and other solutes (Zoratti and Szabo, 1995), which subsequently leads to a collapse of the mitochondrial inner membrane potential ($\Delta\Psi_m$). Loss of the $\Delta\Psi_m$ results in colloid osmotic swelling of the mitochondria matrix, movement of metabolites across the inner membrane, defective oxidative phosphorylation, cessation of ATP synthesis and further generation of ROS. Researchers have shown a concentration-dependent effect of Mn on the mitochondrial inner membrane potential in cultured astrocytes (Rao and Norenberg, 2004; Milatovic et al., 2007). Zhang et al. (2004) revealed that high levels of Mn chloride (1 mM) cause a significant dissipation of the $\Delta\Psi_m$ in isolated rat brain mitochondria, consistent with induction of the MPT.

Oxidative stress as an important mechanism in Mn-induced neurotoxicity has also been confirmed in the in vivo model. Analyses of cerebral biomarkers of oxidative damage revealed that a one-time challenge of mice with Mn (100 mg/kg) was sufficient to produce significant increases in F_2-IsoPs (Table 30.1) 24 h following the last injection. Increased striatal concentrations of ascorbic acid and glutathione (GSH), antioxidants that when increased signal the presence of an elevated burden from ROS, as well as other markers of oxidative stress, have been previously reported (Desole et al., 1994; Dobson et al., 2004; Erikson et al., 2007). Mn-induced decrease in GSH and increased metallothionein was reported in rats (Dobson et al., 2003) and nonhuman primate studies (Erikson et al., 2007). ROS may act in concert with reactive nitrogen species derived from astroglia and microglia to facilitate the Mn-induced degeneration of dopaminergic (DAergic) neurons. DAergic neurons possess reduced antioxidant capacity, as evidenced by low intracellular GSH, which renders these neurons more vulnerable to oxidative stress and glial activation relative to other cell types (Sloot et al., 1994; Greenamyre et al., 1999). Therefore, the overactivation of glia and release of additional neurotoxic factors may represent a crucial component associated with the degenerative process of DAergic neurons.

Mn-induced ROS generation is also associated with inflammatory responses and release of inflammatory mediators, including prostaglandins. Recent studies confirmed that in parallel with an increase in biomarkers of oxidative damage, Mn exposure also induced an increase in biomarkers of inflammation, prostaglandin E_2 (PGE_2), in vitro and in vivo (Milatovic et al., 2007, 2009). Results from an in vivo study showed that Mn exposure induced a time-dependent increase in PGE_2 (Table 30.1). Recent studies have also shown an inflammatory response of glial cells following Mn exposure (Chen et al., 2006b; Zhang et al., 2009; Zhao et al., 2009). Mn potentiates lipopolysaccharide-induced increases in proinflammatory cytokines in glial cultures (Filipov et al., 2005) and increases in nitric oxide production (Chang and Liu, 1999). An increase in proinflammatory genes, such as tumor necrosis factor-α, iNOS and activated inflammatory proteins such as P-p38, P-ERK and P-JNK have been measured in primary rat glial cells after Mn exposure (Chen et al., 2006b). However, data from a recent study indicate that release of proinflammatory mediators following Mn exposure is not only associated with glial response, but neurons as well, and suggests that these two events are mechanistically related, with neuroinflammation either alone or in combination with activated glial response contributing to oxidative damage and consequent cell injury.

Dysregulation of excitatory glutamatergic neurotransmission by Mn is also associated with DAergic and GABAergic neuronal dysfunction. It is known that in vitro Mn can promote autooxidation of dopamine, which leads to the creation of reactive quinones (Miller et al., 1990; Shen and Dryhurst, 1998). However, rodent and nonhuman primate data offer conflicting evidence on the influence of Mn exposure on catecholamine concentrations (Olanow et al., 1996; Struve et al., 2007). Additional evidence from nonhuman primate data suggests an Mn-induced postsynaptic decrease of D2-like dopamine receptor levels (Eriksson et al., 1992). Several rodent studies support an association between Mn exposure and increased brain GABA concentration (Gwiazda et al., 2002; Reaney et al., 2006). However, other rodent studies suggested that Mn decreases striatal and frontal cortex GABA levels (Seth et al., 1981; Brouillet et al., 1993) or has no effect on GABA levels (Bonilla et al.,

TABLE 30.1 Cerebral F2-IsoPs and PGE2 Levels in Saline (control) or MnCl2 (100 mg/kg, s.c.) Exposed Mice

Exposure	F_2-IsoPs (ng/g tissue)	PGE_2 (ng/g tissue)
Control (saline)	3.013 + 0.03939	9.488 + 0.3091
Single Mn	4.302 + 0.3900[a]	12.03 + 0.4987[a]
Multiple Mn	4.211 + 0.4013[a]	14.22 + 1.019[a]

Brains from mice exposed once or three times (day 1, 4 and 7) to MnCl2 were collected 24 h post last injection. Values of F_2-IsoPs represent mean ± SEM ($n = 4-6$).
[a]*Significant difference between values from control and Mn-treated mice (*P < .05).*

1994). Additional findings also suggest that in the absence of extracellular Ca^{2+}, Mn induces a long-lasting potentiation of acetylcholine (ACh) release from cardiac parasympathetic nerve terminals following tetanic nerve stimulation (Kita et al., 1981). In combination with glutamate-gated cation channel activation, e.g., *N*-methyl-D-aspartate receptor, secondary excitotoxicity mechanisms play an important role in the development of Mn-induced neurodegeneration.

Neurotoxicity of Mn reflects alterations in the integrity of DAergic striatal neurons and DA neurochemistry, including decreased DA transport function and/or striatal DA levels. The striatum is a major recipient structure of neuronal afferents in the basal ganglia. It receives excitatory input from the cortex and DAergic input from substantia nigra and projects to the internal segment of the globus pallidus (Dimova et al., 1993; Saka et al., 2002). Nigrostriatal DAergic neurons appear to be particularly sensitive to Mn-induced toxicity (Sloot and Gramsbergen, 1994; Sloot et al., 1994; Defazio et al., 1996). Intense or prolonged Mn exposure in adulthood causes long-term reductions in striatal DA levels and induces a loss of autoreceptor control over DA release (Autissier et al., 1982; Komura and Sakamoto, 1992). Nigrostriatal DA axons synapse onto striatal medium spiny neurons (MSNs), and these neurons have radially projecting dendrites that are densely studded with spines (Wilson and Groves, 1980). Recent data show the effects of Mn on degeneration of striatal neurons. Representative images of Golgi-impregnated striatal sections with their traced MSNs from control and Mn-exposed animals are presented in Fig. 30.2. Images of neurons with Neurolucida-assisted morphometry show that Mn-induced oxidative damage and neuroinflammation targeted the dendritic system with profound dendrite regression of striatal MSNs. While a single Mn exposure altered the integrity of the dendritic system and induced significant decrease in spine numbers and total dendritic lengths of MSNs, prolonged Mn exposure led to further reduction in spine numbers and dendritic lengths (Milatovic et al., 2009). In essence, MSNs neurodegeneration could result from loss of spines, removing the pharmacological target for DA-replacement therapy, without overt MSNs death (Stephens et al., 2005; Zaja-Milatovic et al., 2005).

TOXICITY

Mn is considered to be one of the least toxic of the essential elements (NRC, 2005). There are no reports of acute toxicity of Mn in animals. Therefore, all toxicity studies described here are chronic in nature. A diet can be consumed without any adverse effect when the Mn level is 2000 ppm for calves, 3000 ppm for sheep, 3000 ppm for chickens, 4000 ppm for turkeys and 7000 ppm for rats. However, decreased growth is observed at 500–3000 ppm in swine. These data indicate that pigs are more sensitive to excess Mn than other livestock (NRC, 2005). Mn at a 5000 ppm dietary level is lethal to preruminant calves (Puls, 1994). Clinical signs of toxicity include reduced appetite and growth rate, anemia and abdominal discomfort. Excess Mn may be associated with abortions and cystic ovaries. In all domestic animals and poultry, excess dietary Mn is known to cause reduced feed intake, growth rate, and lethargy. In dogs, a

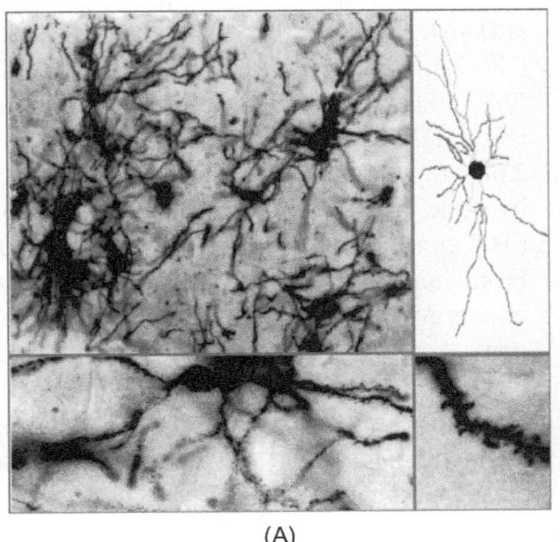

(A)

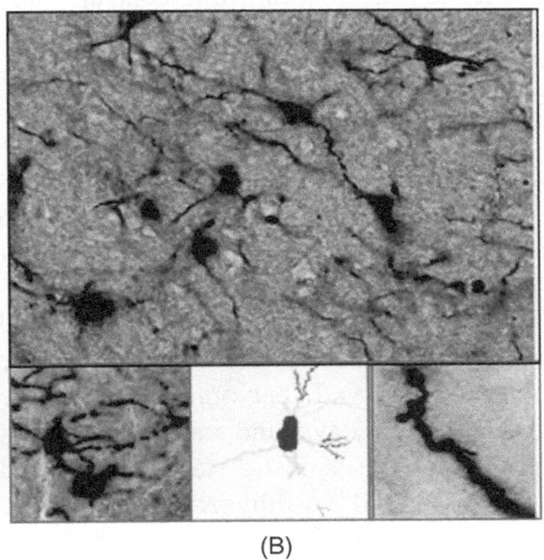

(B)

FIGURE 30.2 Photomicrographs of mouse striatal sections with representative tracings of medium spiny neurons (MSNs) from mice treated with saline (control) (A) or $MnCl_2$ (100 mg/kg, s.c.) (B). Brain from mouse exposed three times (day 1, 4 and 7) to $MnCl_2$ was collected 24 h post last injection. Treatment with Mn-induced degeneration of striatal dendritic system, decrease in total number of spines and length of dendrites of MSNs. Tracing and counting are done using a Neurolucida system at 100 × under oil immersion (MicroBrightField, VT). Colors indicate the degree of dendritic branching (yellow = 1 degree, red = 2 degrees, purple = 3 degrees, green = 4 degrees, turquoise = 5 degrees).

neurological syndrome of gait disorders is common and indicative of Mn-induced injury to the extrapyramidal motor system in the brain.

Mn can have a damaging effect on many body organs, including the brain, liver, pancreas and reproductive system. In addition to these well-established neurotoxic effects, Mn has been extensively studied for its reproductive and developmental effects. Evidence obtained from laboratory animals indicates that exposure to high levels of Mn may adversely affect sperm quality (Elbetieha et al., 2001; Ponnapakkam et al., 2003a,b), cause decreased testicular weights (Laskey et al., 1982) and impair development of the male reproductive tract. Impaired fertility was observed in male mice exposed to Mn in drinking water for 12 weeks at a daily dose level of 309 mg/kg/day, but not at doses ≤ 154 mg/kg/day (Elbetieha et al., 2001). Decreased sperm motility and sperm counts were observed in male CD-1 mice after 43 days of exposure to manganese acetate (4.6–9.6 mg/kg/day). But these doses did not impair the ability of these males to impregnate unexposed females (Ponnapakkam et al., 2003a,b). Szakmary et al. (1995) reported that Mn did not result in any reproductive effect in the rabbit when exposed to 11, 22 or 33 mg/kg/day on gestation days 6–20. In 13-week dietary studies, no gross or histopathological lesions or organ weight changes were observed in reproductive organs of rats fed up to 618 mg Mn/kg/day or mice fed up to 1950 mg Mn/kg/day.

Many developmental toxicity studies in animals exposed to Mn have focused on possible effects on reproductive and neurological functions. Animal studies have shown that Mn exposure decreased the growth of reproductive organs (preputial gland, seminal vesicle and testes) (Gray and Laskey, 1980). Testes weights in males were significantly decreased from controls only when Mn was administered in conjunction with an iron-poor diet (Laskey et al., 1982). Studies in neonatal animals have detected structural and neurochemical changes at doses of Mn similar to or slightly above dietary levels (1–10 mg Mn/kg/day) (Chandra and Shukla, 1978; Deskin et al., 1980), suggesting that young animals might be more susceptible to Mn than adults. Another study by Dorman et al. (2000) also suggested that neonatal rats are at greater risk than adults for Mn-induced neurotoxicity when compared under similar exposure conditions. Their study showed that oral Mn exposure (11 or 22 mg/kg/day for 21 days) induced a significant increase in amplitude of the acoustic startle reflex and an increase in striatal DA and 3,4-dihydroxyphenylacetic acid concentrations in neonates treated with high doses. In a similar study, neonatal rats exposed to Mn (0.31 mg Mn/kg/day for 60 days in water) suffered neuronal degeneration and increased brain monoamine oxidase on day 15 and 30 of the study, but did not show any clinical or behavioral signs of neurotoxicity (Chandra and Shukla, 1978). Developmental studies involving the use of laboratory animals have also detected subtle changes in growth (decreased body weight in animals provided with relatively high doses of Mn). These changes were observed both when the animals were exposed while in utero or postpartum. In a developmental rat model of chronic Mn toxicity, administration of Mn in drinking water was associated with increased levels of iron, copper, selenium, and calcium in various brain regions. The biochemical mechanisms underlying the interaction between Mn and other minerals are unclear. For further details on Mn-induced reproductive and developmental effects, readers are referred to a recent publication (Milatovic et al., 2017).

Several studies have also addressed gene expression changes in Mn-treated cells and animals and the complex interaction of Mn with other minerals (Baek et al., 2004; HaMai et al., 2006). Mn-induced expression changes were noted in genes involved in inflammation, DNA replication and repair. Recent work in nonhuman primates (Guilarte et al., 2008) detected Mn-induced brain gene expression changes associated mainly with genes affecting apoptosis, protein folding and degradation, inflammation and axonal/vesicular transport. Cumulative evidence has established that Mn exposure induces signs and symptoms similar but not identical to Parkinson's disease (Tuschl et al., 2013; Rutchik et al., 2012; O'Neal and Zheng, 2015; Kwakye et al., 2015; Guilarte and Gonzales, 2015).

DIAGNOSIS

Diagnosis of Mn deficiency and toxicity is based on quantitative determination of Mn in biological specimens (body tissue or fluid). Normal values of Mn in liver and kidney are reported in cattle (2.5–6.0 ppm and 1.2–2.0 ppm), horses (1.0–6.0 ppm and 0.5–2.4 ppm), sheep (2.0–4.4 ppm and 0.8–2.5 ppm), goats (2.0–6.0 ppm and 1.0–3.0 ppm), pigs (2.30–4.00 ppm and 1.30–2.0 ppm), dogs (3.0–5.0 ppm and 1.2–1.8 ppm) and rabbits (1.0–2.0 ppm and 2.0–3.0 ppm). Mn levels are also reported for blood in cattle (0.07–0.09 ppm), sheep (0.02–0.025 ppm), dogs (0.02 ppm), pigs (0.04 ppm) and poultry (0.085–0.091 ppm). From human studies it is indicated that neither blood nor urinary Mn levels correlates with any neurological manifestations. Analysis is performed by Flame Atomic Absorption or Furnace Atomic Absorption Spectrometer or Inductively Coupled Plasma (ICP)/ICP-Mass Spectrometer. It is worth mentioning that none of the methods distinguish between different oxidation states of Mn.

TREATMENT

The very first step in the treatment of Mn poisoning should be to remove the animals from any further exposure by avoiding contaminated feed, water or any other source. Some studies investigating Mn poisoning suggest that chelation therapy may be considered to reduce the body burden of Mn and to alleviate toxicity symptoms. Chelators bind metal ions in a stable form and the compound chelator plus metal are then excreted by the urinary and/or biliary routes. Ethylene diaminetetraacetic acid (EDTA) is a polyaminocarboxylic acid that chelates many divalent metals, a property that finds commercial application as a metal sequestrant in food additives. Several studies suggested that EDTA successfully increased Mn excretion in urine and decreased Mn concentration in blood. However, EDTA cannot effectively chelate and remove Mn ions from brain and damaged neurons, and it appears to be of limited therapeutic value for more advanced cases of Mn intoxication.

Since Mn has been shown to catalyze the oxidation of dopamine in vitro and the production of dopamine quinine and hydrogen peroxide, it was also suggested that antioxidants may be effective in suppressing Mn toxicity. In addition, interference with oxidation of Mn may affect cellular uptake, elimination of Mn^{3+} and neurotoxicity. Further investigation of the inhibition of Mn oxidation as a possible mitigation method should be preceded by additional studies to elucidate the role of Mn in its various oxidation states in normal cell metabolism, and to determine whether oxidative stress is a primary mechanism for neurotoxicity by Mn exposure.

CONCLUDING REMARKS AND FUTURE DIRECTIONS

Acute Mn poisoning is rare in animals, but chronic toxicosis can occur as a result of excess dietary exposure. Mn-induced toxicity can affect several body organs involving multiple mechanisms of actions. Several studies suggest that oxidative stress, mitochondrial dysfunction and neuroinflammation are underlying mechanisms in Mn-induced vulnerability of dopaminergic (DAergic) neurons. Mediation of any of these mechanisms and control of alterations in biomarkers of oxidative injury, neuroinflammation and synaptodendritic degeneration may provide a therapeutic strategy for the suppression of dysfunctional DAergic transmission and slowing of the neurodegenerative process. In addition, multiple mechanisms of Mn action are not sufficiently known and may vary with environmental factors and susceptibilities, including single nucleotide polymorphisms that may alter Mn homeostasis, Mn transport and metabolism. Therefore, further research is required to investigate the direct link between Mn uptake, distribution, accumulation and its downstream target(s), as well as associated clinical manifestations. Importantly, more conclusive studies on mechanisms associated with the extracellular transport on Mn, mechanistic effects of Mn at the molecular level and its effects on signal transduction pathways, as well as studies on effective diagnosis and treatment, are needed.

ACKNOWLEDGMENTS

The authors gratefully acknowledge support by a grant from the Department of Defense W81XWH-05-1-0239 (DM). The authors would like to thank Mrs. Robin B. Doss for her technical assistance in the preparation of this chapter.

REFERENCES

Abrams, E., Lassiter, J.W., Miller, W.J., et al., 1977. Effect of normal and high manganese diets on the role of bile in manganese metabolism of calves. J. Aim. Sci. 45, 1108–1113.

Addess, K.J., Basilion, J.P., Klausner, R.D., et al., 1997. Structure and dynamics of the iron responsive element RNA: implications for binding of the RNA by iron regulatory binding proteins. J. Mol. Biol. 274, 72–83.

Andersen, M.E., Gearhart, J.M., Clewell III, H.J., 1999. Pharmacokinetic data needs to support risk assessment for inhaled and ingested manganese. Neurotoxicology. 20, 161–172.

Anderson, J.G., Cooney, P.T., Erikson, K.M., 2007. Inhibition of DAT function attenuates manganese accumulation in the globus pallidus. Environ. Toxicol. Pharmacol. 23, 179–184.

Aschner, J.L., Aschner, M., 2005. Nutritional aspects of manganese homeostasis. Mol. Aspects Med. 26, 353–362.

Aschner, M., Aschner, J.L., 1991. Manganese neurotoxicity: cellular affects and blood–brain barrier transport. Neurosci. Biobehav. Rev. 15, 333–340.

Aschner, M., Gannon, M., Kimelberg, H.K., 1992. Manganese uptake and efflux in cultured rat astrocytes. J. Neurochem. 58, 730–735.

Aschner, M., Shanker, G., Erikson, K., et al., 2002. The uptake of manganese in brain endothelial cultures. Neurotoxicology. 23, 165–168.

Aschner, M., Guilarte, T.R., Schneider, J.S., et al., 2007. Manganese: recent advances in understanding its transport and neurotoxicity. Toxicol. Appl. Pharmacol. 35, 1–32.

Aschner, M., Vrana, K.E., Zheng, W., 1999. Manganese uptake and distribution in the central nervous system (CNS). Neurotoxicology. 20, 173–189.

ATSDR (Agency for Toxic Substances and Disease Registry), 2000. Toxicological Profile for Manganese. Atlanta, GA.

Attardi, G., Schatz, G., 1988. Biogenesis of mitochondria. Annu. Rev. Cell Biol. 4, 289–333.

Austinc, C., Niedzwiecki, M., Arora, M., 2016. Multi-elemental bio-imaging of tissues in children's environmental health research. Curr. Opin. Pediatr. 28, 216–220.

Autissier, N., Rochette, L., Dumas, P., et al., 1982. Dopamine and norepinephrine turnover in various regions of the rat brain after chronic manganese chloride administration. Toxicology. 24, 175–182.

Baek, S.Y., Cho, J.H., Kim, E.S., et al., 2004. cDNA array analysis of gene expression profiles in brain of mice exposed to manganese. Industr. Health. 42, 315–320.

Baker, D.H., Halpin, K.M., 1991. Manganese and iron interrelationship in the chick. Poult. Sci. 70, 146–152.

Ballatori, N., Miles, E., Clarkson, T.W., 1987. Homeostatic controls of manganese excretion in the neonatal rat. Am. J. Physiol. 252, R842–R847.

Bonilla, E., Arrieta, A., Castro, F., et al., 1994. Manganese toxicity: free amino acids in the striatum and olfactory bulb of the mouse. Invest. Clin. 35, 175–181.

Brouillet, E.P., Shinobu, L., McGarvey, U., et al., 1993. Manganese injection into the rat striatum produces excitotoxic lesions by impairing energy metabolism. Exp. Neurol. 120, 89–94.

Chandra, S.V., Shukla, G.S., 1978. Manganese encephalophathy in growing rats. Environ. Res. 15, 28–37.

Chang, J.Y., Liu, L.Z., 1999. Manganese potentiates nitric oxide production by microglia. Brain Res. Mol. Brain Res. 68, 22–28.

Chen, C.J., Ou, Y.C., Lin, S.Y., et al., 2006a. Manganese modulates proinflammatory gene expression in activated glia. Neurochem. Int. 49, 62–71.

Chen, M.K., Lee, J.S., McGlothan, J.L., et al., 2006b. Acute manganese administration alters dopamine transporter levels in the non-human primate striatum. Neurotoxicology. 27, 229–236.

Chen, P., Parmalee, N., Aschner, M., 2014. Genetic factors and manganese-induced neurotoxicity. Front. Genet. 5, 265.

Corathers, L.A., 2001. *Manganese*. US Geological Survey Mineral Yearbook, Available at http://mineral.usgs/mineral/pubs/community/manganese.

Cotzias, G.C., Greenough, J.J., 1958. The high specificity of the manganese pathway through the body. J. Clin. Invest. 37, 1298–1305.

Davis, C.D., Zech, L., Greger, J.L., 1993. Manganese metabolism in rats: an improved methodology for assessing gut endogenous losses. Proc. Soc. Exp. Biol. Med. 202, 103–108.

Defazio, G., Soleo, L., Zefferino, R., et al., 1996. Manganese toxicity in serumless dissociated mesencephalic and striatal primary culture. Brain Res. Bull. 40, 257–262.

Deskin, R., Bursian, S.J., Edens, F.W., 1980. Neurochemical alterations induced by manganese chloride in neonatal rats. Neurotoxicology. 2, 65–73.

Desole, M.S., Miele, M., Esposito, G., et al., 1994. Dopaminergic system activity and cellular defense mechanisms in the striatum and striatal synaptosomes of the rat subchronically exposed to manganese. Arch. Toxicol. 68, 566–570.

Dimova, R., Vuillet, J., Nieoullon, A., et al., 1993. Ultrastructural features of the choline acetyltransferase-containing neurons and relationships with nigral dopaminergic and cortical afferent pathways in the rat striatum. Neuroscience. 53, 1059–1071.

Dobson, A.W., Weber, S., Dorman, D.C., et al., 2003. Oxidative stress is induced in the rat brain following repeated inhalation exposure to manganese sulfate. Biol.Trace Elem. Res. 93, 113–126.

Dobson, A.W., Erikson, K.M., Aschner, M., 2004. Manganese neurotoxicity. Ann. NY Acad. Sci. 1012, 115–128.

Dorman, D.C., Struve, M.F., Vitarella, D., et al., 2000. Neurotoxicity of manganese chloride in neonatal and adult CD rats following subchronic (21-day) high-dose oral exposure. J. Appl. Toxicol. 20, 179–187.

Dorman, D.C., McElveen, A.M., Marshall, M.W., et al., 2005. Maternal–fetal distribution of manganese in the rat following inhalation exposure to manganese sulfate. Neurotoxicology. 26, 625–632.

Elbetieha, A., Bataineh, H., Darmani, H., et al., 2001. Effects of long-term exposure to manganese chloride on fertility of male and female mice. Toxicol. Lett. 119, 193–201.

Erikson, K., Aschner, M., 2002. Manganese causes differential regulation of glutamate transporter (GLAST) taurine transporter and metallothionein in cultured rat astrocytes. Neurotoxicology. 23, 595–602.

Erikson, K.M., Aschner, M., 2003. Manganese neurotoxicity and glutamate–GABA interaction. Neurochem. Int. 43, 475–480.

Erikson, K.M., Dorman, D.C., Lash, L.H., et al., 2007. Manganese inhalation by rhesus monkeys is associated with brain regional changes in biomarkers of neurotoxicity. Toxicol. Sci. 97, 459–466.

Erikson, K.M., Dorman, D.C., Lash, L.H., et al., 2008. Duration of airborne-manganese exposure in rhesus monkeys is associated with brain regional changes in biomarkers of neurotoxicity. Neurotoxicology. 29, 377–385.

Eriksson, H., Gillberg, P.G., Aquilonius, S.M., et al., 1992. Receptor alterations in manganese intoxicated monkeys. Arch. Toxicol. 66, 359–364.

Filipov, N.M., Seegal, R.F., Lawrence, D.A., 2005. Manganese potentiates in vitro production of proinflammatory cytokines and nitric oxide by microglia through a nuclear factor kappa B-dependent mechanism. Toxicol. Sci. 84, 139–148.

Fitsanakis, V.A., Aschner, M., 2005. The importance of glutamate, glycine, and gamma-aminobutyric acid transport and regulation in manganese, mercury and lead neurotoxicity. Toxicol. Appl. Pharmacol. 204, 343–354.

Garcia-Aranda, J.A., Lifhitz, A.F., Wapnir, R.A., 1983. In vivo intestinal absorption of manganese in the rat. J. Nutr. 113, 2601–2607.

Gavin, C.E., Gunter, K.K., Gunter, T.E., 1990. Manganese and calcium efflux kinetics in brain mitochondria. Relevance to manganese toxicity. Biochem. J. 266, 329–334.

Gray, L.E., Laskey, J.W., 1980. Multivariate analysis of the toxic effects of manganese on the reproductive physiology and behavior of the male house mouse. J. Toxicol. Environ. Health. 6, 861–867.

Greenamyre, J.T., MacKenzie, G., Peng, T.I., et al., 1999. Mitochondrial dysfunction in Parkinson's disease. Biochem. Soc. Symp. 66, 85–97.

Guilarte, T.R., Gonzales, K.K., 2015. Manganese-induced parkinsonism is not idiopathic Parkinson's disease: environmental and genetic evidence. Toxicol. Sci. 146, 204–212.

Guilarte, T.R., Burton, N.C., McGlothan, J.L., et al., 2008. Impairment of nigrostriatal dopamine neurotransmission by manganese is mediated by pre-synaptic mechanism(s): implications to manganese-induced Parkinsonism. J. Neurochem. 107, 1236–1247.

Gunter, T.E., Gavin, C.E., Aschner, M., et al., 2006. Speciation of manganese in cells and mitochondria: a search for the proximal cause of manganese neurotoxicity. Neurotoxicology. 27, 765–776.

Gwiazda, R.H., Lee, D., Sheridan, J., et al., 2002. Low cumulative manganese exposure affects striatal GABA but not dopamine. Neurotoxicology. 23, 69–76.

HaMai, D., Rinderknecht, A.L., Guo-Sharman, K., et al., 2006. Decreased expression of inflammation-related genes following inhalation exposure to manganese. Neurotoxicology. 27, 395–401.

Hartman, R.H., Matrone, G., Wise, G.H., 1955. Effect of high dietary manganese on hemoglobin formation. J. Nutr. 57, 429–439.

Hauser, R.A., Zesiewicz, T.A., Rosemurgy, A.S., et al., 1994. Manganese intoxication and chronic liver failure. Ann. Neurol. 36 (6), 871–875.

Henry, P.R., 1995. Manganese bioavailability. In: Ammerman, C.B., Baker, D.H., Lewis, A.J. (Eds.), Bioavailability of Nutrients for Animals: Amino Acids, Minerals, and Vitamins. Academic Press, Orlando, FL, pp. 239–256. http://mineral.usgs/mineral/pubs/community/manganese. (accessed 29.12.03.).

Hurley, L.S., Keen, C.L., 1987. Manganese. In: fifth ed. Mertz, W. (Ed.), Trace Elements in Human and Animal Nutrition, vol. 1. Academic Press, Orlando, FL, pp. 185–232.

Ivan, M., Hidiroglou, M., 1980. Effect of dietary manganese on growth and manganese metabolism in sheep. J. Dairy Sci. 63, 385–390.

Jarvinen, R., Ahlstrom, A., 1975. Effect of the dietary manganese level on tissue manganese, iron, copper and zinc concentrations in female rats and their fetuses. Med. Biol. 53, 93–99.

Kaiser, J., 2003. Manganese: a high-octane dispute. Science. 300, 926–928.

Keen, C.L., Bell, J.G., Lonnerdal, B., 1986. The effect of age on manganese uptake and retention from milk and infant formulas in rats. J. Nutr. 116, 395–402.

Kita, H., Narira, K., Van der Kloot, W., 1981. Tetanic stimulation increases frequency of miniature end-plate potentials at the frog neuromuscular junction in Mn-, Ni-saline solution. Brain Res. 205, 121–122.

Klaassen, C.D., 1974. Biliary excretion of manganese in rats, rabbits, and dogs. Toxicol. Appl. Pharmacol. 29, 458–468.

Komura, J., Sakamoto, M., 1992. Effects of manganese forms on biogenic amines in the brain and behavioral alterations in the mouse: long-term oral administration of several manganese compounds. Environ. Res. 57, 34–44.

Kontur, P.J., Fechter, L.D., 1985. Brain manganese, catecholamine turnover, and the development of startle in rats prenatally exposed to manganese. Teratology. 32, 1–11.

Kowaltowski, A.J., Castilho, R.F., Vercesi, A.E., 1995. Ca^{2+}-induced mitochondrial membrane permeabilization: role of coenzyme Q redox state. Am. J. Physiol. 269, 141–147.

Kruman, I.I., Mattson, M.P., 1999. Pivotal role of mitochondrial calcium uptake in neural cell apoptosis and necrosis. J. Neurochem. 72, 529–540.

Kwakye, G.F., Paoliello, M.B., Mukhopadhyay, S., et al., 2015. Manganese-induced parkinsonism and Parkinson's disease: shared and distinguishable features. Int. J. Environ. Res. Public Health. 12, 7519–7540.

Laskey, J.W., Rehnberg, G.L., Hein, J.F., 1982. Effects of chronic manganese ($M_{n3}O_4$) exposure selected reproductive parameters in rats. J. Toxicol. Environ. Health. 9, 677–687.

Lucchini, R.G., Martin, C.J., Doney, B.C., 2009. From manganism to manganese-induced Parkinsonism: a conceptual model based on the evaluation of exposure. Neuromol. Med. 11, 311–321.

Malecki, E.A., Radzanowski, G.M., Radzanowski, T.J., et al., 1996. Biliary manganese excretion in conscious rats is affected by acute and chronic manganese intake but not by dietary fat. J. Nutr. 126, 489–498.

Malecki, E.A., Devenyi, A.G., Beard, J.L., et al., 1999. Existing and emerging mechanisms for transport of iron and manganese to the brain. J. Neurosci. Res. 56, 113–122.

Martinez-Finley, E.J., Gavin, C., Aschner, M., et al., 2013. Manganese neurotoxicity and the role of reactive oxygen species. Free Radic. Biol. Med. 62, 65–75.

Milatovic, D., Aschner, M., 2009. Measurement of isoprostanes as markers of oxidative stress in neuronal tissue. Curr. Prot. Toxicol. 12 (14), 1–12, unit.

Milatovic, D., Yin, Z., Gupta, R.C., et al., 2007. Manganese induces oxidative impairment in cultured rat astrocytes. Toxicol. Sci. 98, 198–205.

Milatovic, D., Zaja-Milatovic, S., Gupta, R.C., et al., 2009. Oxidative damage and neurodegeneration in manganese-induced neurotoxicity. Toxicol. Appl. Pharmacol. 240, 219–225.

Milatovic, D., Gupta, R.C., Yin, Z., Zaja-Milatovic, S., et al., 2017. Manganese. In: Gupta, R.C. (Ed.), Reproductive and Developmental Toxicology, 2nd Edn. Academic Press/Elsevier, Amsterdam, pp. 567–582.

Miller, D.M., Buettner, G.R., Aust, S.D., 1990. Transition metals as catalysts of "autoxidation" reactions. Free Radic. Biol. Med. 8, 95–108.

Morrow, J.D., Roberts, L.J., 2nd, 1999. Mass spectrometric quantification of F_2-isoprostanes in biological fluids and tissues as measure of oxidant stress. Methods Enzymol. 300, 3–12.

NRC (National Research Council), 2005. Manganese, Mineral Tolerance of Animals. second edn The National Academies Press, Washington, DC, pp. 235–247.

Olanow, C.W., Good, P.F., Shinotoh, H., et al., 1996. Manganese intoxication in the rhesus monkey: a clinical, imaging, pathologic, and biochemical study. Neurology. 46, 492–498.

O'Neal, S.L., Zheng, W., 2015. Manganese toxicity upon overexposure: a decade in review. Curr. Environ. Health Rep. 2, 315–328.

Ponnapakkam, T.P., Bailey, K.S., Graves, K.A., et al., 2003a. Assessment of male reproductive system in CD-1 mice following oral manganese exposure. Reprod. Toxicol. 17, 547–551.

Ponnapakkam, T.P., Sam, G.H., Iszard, M.B., 2003b. Histopathological changes in the testes of the Sprague Dawley rat following orally administered manganese. Bull. Environ. Contam. Toxicol. 71, 1151–1157.

Post, J.E., 1999. Manganese oxide minerals: crystal structures and economic and environmental significance. Proc. Natl. Acad. Sci. USA. 96, 3447–3454.

Puls, R., 1994. Mineral Levels in Animal Health. second ed. Sherpa Intl, Clearbook, BC, pp. 173–182.

Racette, B.A., Criswell, S.R., Lundin, J.I., et al., 2012. Increased risk of parkinsonism associated with welding exposure. Neurotoxicology. 33, 1356–1361.

Rao, K.V., Norenberg, M.D., 2004. Manganese induces the mitochondrial permeability transition in cultured astrocytes. J. Biol. Chem. 279, 32333–32338.

Rao, V.L., Dogan, A., Todd, K.G., et al., 2001. Antisense knockdown of the glial glutamate transporter GLT-1, but not the neuronal glutamate transporter EAAC1, excerbates transient focal cerebral ischemia-induced neuronal damage in rat brain. J. Neurosci. 21, 1876–1883.

Reaney, S.H., Bench, G., Smith, D.R., 2006. Brain accumulation and toxicity of Mn(II) and Mn(III) exposures. Toxicol. Sci. 93, 114–124.

Rutchik, J.S., Zheng, W., Jiang, Y.M., et al., 2012. How does an occupational neurologist assess welders and steelworkers for a manganese-induced movement disorder? An international team's experiences in Guangxi, China, part I. J. Occup. Environ. Med. 54, 1432–1434.

Saka, E., Iadarola, M., Fitzgerald, D.J., et al., 2002. Local circuit neurons in the striatum regulate neural and behavioral responses to dopaminergic stimulation. Proc. Natl. Acad. Sci. USA. 99, 9004–9009.

Seth, P.K., Hong, J.S., Kilts, C.D., et al., 1981. Alteration of cerebral neurotransmitter receptor function by exposure of rats to manganese. Toxicol. Lett. 9, 247–254.

Shen, X.M., Dryhurst, G., 1998. Iron- and manganese-catalyzed autoxidation of dopamine in the presence of l-cysteine: possible insights into iron- and manganese-mediated dopaminergic neurotoxicity. Chem. Res. Toxicol. 11, 824–837.

Sidoryk-Wegrzynowicz, M., Aschner, M., 2013. Role of astrocytes in manganese mediated neurotoxicity. BMC Pharmacol. Toxicol. 14, 23.

Singh, J., Husain, R., Tandon, S.K., et al., 1974. Biochemical and histopathological alterations in early manganese toxicity in rats. Environ. Physiol. Biochem. 4, 16–23.

Sloot, W.N., Gramsbergen, J.B.P., 1994. Axonal transport of manganese and its relevance to selective neurotoxicity in the rat basal ganglia. Brain Res. 657, 124–132.

Sloot, W.N., van der Sluijs-Gelling, A.J., Gramsbergen, J.B.P., 1994. Selective lesions by manganese and extensive damage by iron after injection into rat striatum or hippocampus. J. Neurochem. 62, 205–216.

Southern, L.L., Baker, H., 1983. Excess manganese ingestion in the chick. Poult. Sci. 62 (4), 642–646.

Stephens, B., Mueller, A.J., Shering, A.F., et al., 2005. Evidence of a breakdown of corticostriatal connections in Parkinson's disease. Neuroscience. 132, 741–754.

Struve, M.F., McManus, B.E., Wong, B.A., et al., 2007. Basal ganglia neurotransmitter concentrations in rhesus monkeys following subchronic manganese sulfate inhalation. Am. J. Ind. Med. 50, 772–778.

Suarez, N., Eriksson, H., 1993. Receptor-mediated endocytosis of a manganese complex of transferrin into neuroblastoma (SHSY5Y) cells in culture. J. Neurochem. 61, 127–131.

Symonds, H.W., Hall, E.D., 1983. Acute manganese toxicity and the absorption and biliary excretion of manganese in cattle. Res. Vet. Sci. 35, 5–13.

Szakmary, E., Ungvary, G., Hudak, A., et al., 1995. Developmental effect of manganese in rat and rabbit. Cent. Eur. J. Occup. Environ. Med. 1, 149–159.

Takeda, A., 2003. Manganese action in brain function. Brain Res. Rev. 41, 79–87.

Takeda, A., Ishiwatari, S., Okada, S., 1999. Manganese uptake into rat brain during development and aging. J. Neurosci. Res. 56, 93–98.

Tarale, P., Chakrabarti, T., Sivanesan, S., et al., 2016. Potential role of epigenetic mechanism in manganese induced neurotoxicity. Biomed. Res. Int. 2016, 1–18.

Tjalkens, R.B., Zoran, M.J., Mohl, B., et al., 2006. Manganese suppresses ATP-dependent intercellular calcium waves in astrocyte networks through alteration of mitochondrial and endoplasmic reticulum calcium dynamics. Brain Res. 1113, 210–219.

Turrens, J.F., Boveris, A., 1980. Generation of superoxide anion by the NADH dehydrogenase of bovine heart mitochondria. Biochem. J. 191, 421–427.

Tuschl, K., Mills, P.B., Clayton, P.T., 2013. Manganese and the brain. Int. Rev. Neurobiol. 110, 277–312.

Uchida, K., 2003. 4-Hyroxy-2-nonenal: a product and mediator of oxidative stress. Prog. Lipid. Res. 42, 318–343.

Wang, J.D., Huang, C.C., Hwang, Y.H., et al., 1989. Manganese induced Parkinsonism: an outbreak due to an unrepaired ventilation control system in a ferromanganese smelter. Br. J. Ind. Med. 46, 856–859.

Wilson, P., Groves, P.M., 1980. Fine structure and synaptic connections of the common spiny neuron of the rat neostriatum: a study employing intracellular inject of horseradish peroxidase. J. Comp. Neurol. 194, 599–615.

Yang, J., Liu, X., Bhalla, K., et al., 1997. Prevention of apoptosis by Bcl-2 release of cytochrome c from mitochondria blocked. Science. 275, 1129–1132.

Yoon, M., Nong, A., Clewell 3rd, H.J., et al., 2009a. Evaluating placental transfer and tissue concentrations of manganese in the pregnant rat and fetuses after inhalation exposures with a PBPK model. Toxicol. Sci. 112, 44–58.

Yoon, M., Nong, A., Clewell 3rd, H.J., et al., 2009b. Lactational transfer of manganese in rats: predicting manganese tissue concentration in the dam and pups from inhalation exposure with a pharmacokinetic model. Toxicol. Sci. 112, 23–43.

Zaja-Milatovic, S., Milatovic, D., Schantz, A., et al., 2005. Dendritic degeneration in neostriatal medium spiny neurons in late-stage Parkinson disease. Neurology. 64, 545–547.

Zhang, P., Wong, T.A., Lokuta, K.M., et al., 2009. Microglia enhance manganese chloride-induced dopaminergic neurodegeneration: role of free radical generation. Exp. Neurol. 217, 219–230.

Zhang, S., Zhou, Z., Fu, J., 2003. Effect of manganese chloride exposure on liver and brain mitochondria function in rats. Environ. Res. 93, 149–157.

Zhang, S., Fu, J., Zhou, Z., 2004. In vitro effect of manganese chloride exposure on reactive oxygen species generation and respiratory chain complexes activities of mitochondria isolated from rat brain. Toxicol. Vitro. 18, 71–77.

Zhao, F., Cai, T., Liu, M., et al., 2009. Manganese induces dopaminergic neurodegeneration via microglial activation in a rat model of manganism. Toxicol. Sci. 107, 156–164.

Zoratti, M., Szabo, I., 1995. The mitochondrial permeability transition. Biochim. Biophys. Acta. 1241, 139–176.

Chapter 31

Mercury

Ramesh C. Gupta, Dejan Milatovic, Rajiv Lall and Ajay Srivastava

INTRODUCTION

Mercury (Hg) is a naturally occurring element that exists in several forms, such as elemental (metallic), inorganic and organic. About 80% of the mercury released into the environment is metallic mercury; it comes from human activities, such as fossil fuel combustion, mining, smelting and from solid waste incineration, as well as from volcanoes and forest fires. Human activities can lead to mercury levels in the soil as much as 200,000 times higher than natural levels. Metallic mercury in a pure form looks like a shiny-white liquid substance at room temperature. It is commonly used in thermometers, barometers, blood pressure measuring devices, button-cell batteries, electric switches, dental fillings (amalgams), etc. Inorganic mercury compounds, or mercury salts, occur when Hg combines with other elements, such as chlorine, sulfur, and oxygen. Most of these compounds are white, except mercuric sulfide or cinnabar ore (i.e., red, which turns black after exposure to light). Some mercury compounds are used as fungicides, while others are used for medicinal purposes, e.g., laxatives, deworming agents, antiseptics, and disinfectants. When mercury combines with carbon, it is called organic mercury (organomercurials). Methylmercury, ethylmercury, and phenylmercury are a few examples. In the environment and mammalian systems, various forms of mercury are interchangeable. For example, inorganic mercury can be methylated to methylmercury and methylmercury can change to inorganic or elemental mercury. Animals at the top of the food chain tend to bioaccumulate methylmercury in their bodies. Therefore, poisoning by mercury is due to consumption of meat or grain contaminated with mercury. Poisoning can also result from excessive exposure to inorganic and organic mercury compounds from misuse of mercury-containing products. Much of the information presented in this chapter is from experimental studies conducted in laboratory animals and poisoning incidents in humans, animals and wildlife.

BACKGROUND

Mercury exists naturally in the environment (soil, water, and air), and as a result everyone is exposed to very low levels. Aristotle named it "quicksilver," because it is a silver-colored liquid. Animal poisoning by mercury is rare because of strict federal, state, and local regulations. The most common natural forms of mercury found in the environment are metallic mercury, mercury sulfide, mercuric chloride, and methylmercury. Methylmercury is of particular concern because it is bioaccumulated and biomagnified in certain edible freshwater and saltwater fish and marine mammals to levels that are many times greater than levels in the surrounding water. As a result, older and predatory fish living in contaminated water build up levels of mercury in their bodies (especially in the liver, kidneys, brain, and muscle). Inorganic mercury does not bioaccumulate in the food chain to any extent. Cultivation of edible mushrooms, where waste as compost material with unsafe levels of mercury is used, can also accumulate high levels of mercury (Bressa et al., 1988). The release of methylmercury into an ocean bay (Minamata) in Japan in the 1950s led to a massive health disaster, and the clinical syndrome was named Minamata disease (Tsubaki and Krukuyama, 1977; Tsubaki and Takahashi, 1986). Thousands of people were poisoned, and hundreds developed severe brain damage.

Currently, Hg is ranked third by the US Agency for Toxic Substances and Disease Registry (ATSDR, 2011) Substance Priority List and is listed as one of the WHO's top 10 chemicals of major public health concern (Ray et al., 2014). The Food and Drug Administration (FDA) estimates that, on average, most people are exposed to about 50 ng mercury/kg body weight/day in the food they eat. This level is not enough to cause any harmful effects. A large part of this mercury is in the form of methylmercury and the majority of that comes from eating fish. Fish for food consumption is not allowed to have more than 1 ppm mercury. This level is below a level that can be

Veterinary Toxicology. DOI: http://dx.doi.org/10.1016/B978-0-12-811410-0.00031-3

associated with adverse effects. Foods other than fish that may contain higher levels of mercury include wild animals, birds, and mammals (bears) that eat large amounts of contaminated fish (ATSDR, 1999). Meat and/or fat from fish, marine mammals, fish-eating wildlife and birds, and mercury-based fungicide-treated grains have the highest mercury levels. Certain species of commercially available saltwater fish, such as shark, swordfish, kingfish and tilefish, can contain high levels of methylmercury. These are all potential sources of mercury poisoning. In horses, mercury toxicity occurs from wound dressings (blisters) when dimethyl sulfoxide (DMSO) is applied simultaneously, because DMSO enhances the absorption of mercury (Schuh et al., 1988).

TOXICOKINETICS

Absorption of mercury from oral ingestion depends upon the form of mercury. Metallic mercury is maximally absorbed (about 80%) from the lungs, while very little is absorbed from the gastrointestinal (GI) tract. Once mercury enters the circulation, it is rapidly distributed to other tissues, but more so in the kidneys, where it accumulates. Metallic mercury can stay in the body for weeks to months. Due to its high lipophilicity, metallic mercury can readily cross the blood–brain barrier (BBB) and placental barrier. When metallic mercury enters the brain, it is readily converted to an inorganic divalent mercury (oxidized by the hydrogen peroxidase–catalase pathway), and it gets trapped there for an extended period. The inorganic divalent cation can, in turn, be reduced to metallic mercury. Most of the absorbed metallic mercury excretes in the urine and feces, some amount passes in the milk, and very little in the exhaled air.

Inorganic mercury compounds (e.g., mercurous chloride and mercuric chloride) are absorbed 10%–40% from the GI tract upon ingestion, distributed to different organs and mainly accumulate in the kidneys. In an experimental study, female Sprague-Dawley rats given a single dose of mercuric chloride (7.4 or 9.2 mg Hg/kg, po) showed 12.6 and 18.9 ppm mercury, respectively, in the kidneys when sacrificed 14 days postexposure (Lecavalier et al., 1994). Trace amounts were also detected in the liver, brain, and serum. These compounds do not readily cross the BBB or placental barrier. Inorganic mercury excretes in the urine and feces, and only detectable levels pass through the milk.

Organic mercury, such as methylmercury, is readily absorbed from the GI tract (about 90%–95%) and has a long retention time (half-life of ~70 days). After ingestion, the distribution to the blood compartment is complete within 30 h, and the blood level accounts for about 7% of the ingested dose. Methylmercury distributes to all vital organs (Fig. 31.1). Circulating methylmercury accumulates predominantly in the red cells where it binds to cysteinyl residues (–SH) on the hemoglobin beta-chain, and is then slowly distributed to other tissues, reaching equilibrium with other tissues at ~4 days. The distribution of methylmercury is similar to that of metallic mercury, i.e., a relatively large amount of mercury can accumulate in the brain and fetus (compared to inorganic mercury) because of its ability to penetrate the BBB and placental barrier and its conversion in the brain and fetus to the inorganic divalent cation mercury. Organic mercury excretes in the form of inorganic mercury in the feces over a period of several months. Some organic mercury also excretes in the urine and milk.

Depending upon the route of exposure, dose, and single versus repeat exposure, toxicokinetics of mercury can

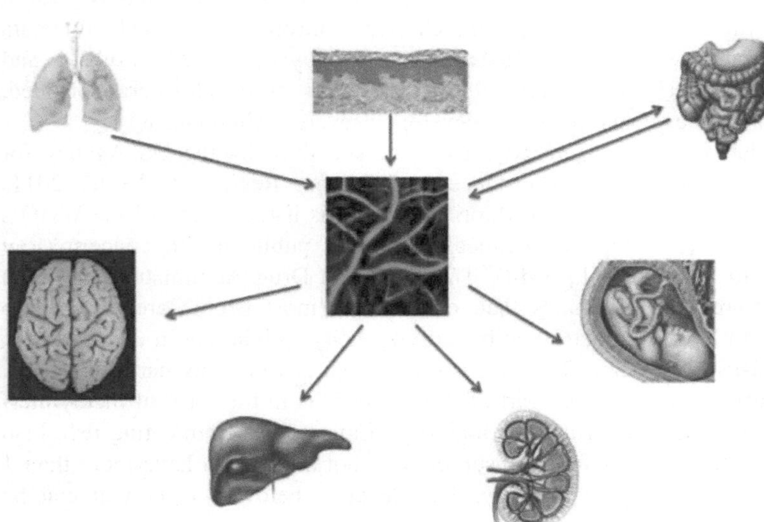

FIGURE 31.1 The distribution of MeHg in the human body. MeHg is readily absorbed by the lung, skin, and gastrointestinal tract and distributed to the CNS, kidneys, and liver. MeHg can cross the placental–blood barrier and it accumulates in the fetus at higher concentrations compared to the mother.

follow a one-compartment or two-compartment model. Studies have shown that repeat or continuous exposure to any form of mercury can result in the accumulation of mercury in the body. In vertebrates, mercury tends to accumulate in the liver and kidney, but it also has a high-affinity for the brain and endocrine system. Mercury in the brain may persist long after cessation of short- and long-term exposures. Blood levels of mercury are closely related to its levels in the whole body during the first 3 days following administration. Thereafter, the amount of mercury in the blood declines more rapidly than the whole-body burden. Animal studies show disparity in mercury body burden in terms of gender. In general, females are believed to have higher body burdens of methylmercury at given doses than males. Furthermore, in rodents, females accumulate more mercury in the brain, while males accumulate higher levels of mercury in the kidneys.

Evidence suggests that the metabolism of all forms of mercury is similar for humans and animals. Mercury is metabolized through the oxidation–reduction cycle that takes place in intestinal microflora, and after absorption in many tissues and in the red blood cells. Elimination rates for methylmercury appear to vary with species, dose, sex, and strain. The elimination half-life in the blood of monkeys receiving inorganic and organic mercury was found to be 26 days (Vahter et al., 1994). In a study of organs from sled dogs fed methylmercury-laden meat and organs from predatory marine animals, the highest concentration of total mercury was found in the mesenterial lymph nodes, followed by liver and kidneys, indicating that the lymphatic system may play an important role in the transport of mercury to target organs (Hansen and Danscher, 1995). The tissue concentrations of mercury observed in this study were found to be age related, and the results suggest that demethylation takes place in all organs, except the skeletal muscles. Demethylation of methylmercury was found to be lower in the brain than in other organs. For further details on toxicokinetics of mercury refer to Bernhoft (2012).

MECHANISM OF ACTION

Toxicities of the different forms of mercury are related, in part, to its differential accumulation in sensitive tissues. This theory is supported by the observation that mercury rapidly accumulates in the kidneys and specific areas of the brain (Yilmaz et al., 2014; Pletz et al., 2016; Ni et al., 2017). High-affinity binding of the divalent cationic mercury to thiol or sulfhydryl groups of proteins is believed to be a major mechanism involved in the toxicity of mercury. As a result, mercury can cause inactivation of various enzymes, structural proteins, transport proteins and alteration of cell membrane permeability by the formation of mercaptides. In addition, mercury may induce one or more of the following effects: increased oxidative stress, mitochondrial dysfunction, changes in heme metabolism, glutathione depletion, increased permeability of the BBB and disruption of microtubule formation, protein synthesis, DNA replication, DNA polymerase activity, calcium homeostasis, synaptic transmission and immune response (Farina et al., 2011a,b; Sharma et al., 2014; Ni et al., 2017).

The nervous system is especially sensitive to mercury. The degree of damage depends upon the form of mercury and its dose. The effects of Hg on the developing central nervous system (CNS) are more severe than those in the mature CNS (Taber and Hurley, 2008; Eriksson et al., 2010; Sokolowski et al., 2011; Bernhoft, 2012; Ni et al., 2017). Metallic mercury at high doses causes irreparable damage to the brain. In many poisoning incidents, permanent damage to the brain occurred by methylmercury. Since inorganic mercury does not readily cross the BBB, it is highly unlikely that inorganic mercury may cause any damage to the brain or nerves. Most of the information concerning neurotoxicity in humans following oral exposure to organic mercury comes from reports describing the effects of ingesting contaminated fish or fungicide-treated grains, or meat from animals fed such grains. Studies conducted in experimental animals strongly indicate that organic mercury is a potent neurotoxicant (Kaur et al., 2007; Ceccatelli et al., 2010; Farina et al., 2011a,b; Ni et al., 2017).

Evidence suggests that a single dose of mercuric chloride (0.74 mg/kg) caused disruption of the BBB barrier in rats (Chang and Hartman, 1972). These investigators also administered mercuric chloride to rats at the same dose daily for 11 weeks. Within 2 weeks, there were coagulative or lucid changes in cerebellar granule cells and fragmentation, vacuolation and cytoplasmic lesions in the neurons of dorsal root ganglia. Neurological disturbances consisted of severe ataxia and sensory loss.

Neurotoxic effects seen in the Minamata (Japan) and Iraqi poisonings were associated with neuronal degeneration and glial proliferation in the cortical and cerebellar gray matter and basal ganglia (Al-Saleem, 1976). Derangement of basic developmental processes, such as neuronal migration (Matsumoto et al., 1965; Choi et al., 1978) and neuronal cell division (Sager et al., 1983) were also observed. In the brain, Purkinje, basket, stellate and granule cells are severely affected by methylmercury.

Methylmercury selectively inhibits protein synthesis in the brain (reversibly in neurons from the cerebrum and Purkinje cells; and irreversibly in granule cells of the cerebellum), and this effect usually precedes the appearance of clinical signs. This selective action on the brain may be due to the fact that certain cells are susceptible because they cannot repair damage from methylmercury. Cheung and Verity (1985) identified the most sensitive step in the protein synthesis, i.e., peptide elongation can be affected by the high concentrations of mercury, but the first stage of synthesis associated with tRNA may be the most sensitive. Methylmercury inhibits one or more of the amino acyl tRNA synthetase enzymes. Microtubules are essential for cell division (main component of the mitotic spindle), and methylmercury reacts with the SH groups on tubulin monomers, and thereby disrupts the assembly process. The dissociation process continues, and this leads to depolymerization of the tubule. Excess generation of reactive oxygen species and inhibition of antioxidant enzyme appear to be the major mechanisms in methylmercury-induced neurotoxicity (Franco et al., 2009; Farina et al., 2009, 2011a,b; Hwang, 2012; Kirkpatrick et al., 2015). The most recent findings suggest that methylmercury triggers multiple pathways, which may be activated concomitantly, and ensuing cell death by apoptosis (Ceccatelli et al., 2010; Farina et al., 2011a,b; Sokolowski et al., 2011).

In all forms, mercury accumulates in the kidneys, and thereby causes greater damage to this organ. The kidney damage appears to be dose dependent, and that means recovery can occur if exposure is at low-level. Following entry of the mercuric or methylmercuric ion into the proximal tubular epithelial cells via transport across the brush-border or basolateral membrane, mercury interacts with thiol-containing compounds, such as glutathione and metallothionein. This interaction initially produces alterations in membrane permeability to calcium ions and inhibition of mitochondrial function. Subsequently, by unknown signaling mechanisms, mercury induces the synthesis of glutathione, glutathione-dependent enzymes, metallothionein and several stress proteins. Finally, epithelial cell damage occurs in the kidney as a result of excess free radical formation and lipid peroxidation, and inhibition of antioxidant enzymes.

TOXICITY

In general, the toxic effects of mercury depend upon the form of mercury, the dose, duration and route of exposure. Mercury, in all forms, has been found to be toxic to both man and animals. There are many similarities in the toxic effects of the various forms of mercury, but there are also differences. Practically, it is organic mercury, which is more toxic and often encountered in poisonings following oral ingestion. The major targets of toxicity to inorganic and organic mercury are the kidneys and the CNS, respectively.

Signs and symptoms associated with short-term exposure to metallic mercury may include nausea, vomiting, diarrhea, increase in blood pressure or heart rate, skin rashes, and eye irritation.

Inorganic mercury, if swallowed in large quantities, may cause damage to the kidney, and also in the stomach and intestine, including nausea, diarrhea and ulcers. Animal studies revealed that long-term oral exposure to inorganic mercury salts causes kidney damage, an increase in blood pressure and heart rate, and effects on the stomach. Studies also show that nervous system damage occurs after long-term exposure to high levels of inorganic mercury. Short-term, high-level exposure of laboratory animals to inorganic mercury has been shown to affect the developing fetus and may cause termination of the pregnancy.

Laboratory animals exposed to long-term, high levels of methylmercury or phenylmercury showed damage to the kidneys, stomach and large intestine, changes in blood pressure and heart rate, and adverse effects on the developing fetus, sperm and male reproductive organs, as well as increases in the number of spontaneous abortions and stillbirths.

In livestock animals, clinical signs of mercury poisoning vary greatly. In cattle, toxicity signs include ataxia, neuromuscular incoordination and renal failure, followed by convulsions and a moribund state. Average time from ingestion to death is reported to be about 20 days. Ingestion of phenylmercuric acetate may cause sudden death with massive internal hemorrhage, without other signs of toxicity (Puls, 1994). In horses, signs of acute toxicity include severe gastroenteritis and nephritis. In chronic cases, signs may include neurological dysfunction, laminitis, in addition to renal disease, which is characterized by glycosuria, proteinuria, phosphaturia, reduced urine osmolarity, reduced glomerular filtration rate, azotemia and elevated creatinine and blood urea nitrogen. In sheep, the poisoning is characterized by severe neurological symptoms and tetraplegia. Pigs show incoordination, unstable gait, lameness, recumbency and death.

Some of the toxic effects are described below in detail for each organ/system affected by mercury exposure.

Nervous System

Adverse effects on the nervous system of animals occur at lower doses than do harmful effects to most other systems of the body. This difference indicates that the nervous system is more sensitive to mercury than are other organs in the body. Animal studies also provide evidence of damage to the nervous system from exposure to methylmercury during development, and findings suggest that the effects worsen with age, even after the exposure stops. The reason for this greater susceptibility is that mercury affects processes unique to the developing nervous system, namely cell migration and cell division (Clarkson, 1987; Ni et al., 2017).

Both human epidemiology and experimental animal studies indicate that organic mercury is a potent neurotoxicant (Ni et al., 2017). Studies suggest that cats and monkeys are more sensitive than rodents to the neurotoxic effects of mercury (especially methylmercury). In several animal species, the major effects that are seen across the studies include motor disturbances, such as ataxia and tremors, as well as signs of sensory dysfunction, such as impaired vision. The predominant pathological feature is degenerative changes in the cerebellum, which is likely to be the mechanism involved in many of the motor dysfunctions. In a chronic study, cats fed tuna contaminated with methylmercury showed degenerative changes in the cerebellum and the cortex (Chang et al., 1974). Neonatal monkeys exposed to methylmercuric chloride at 0.5 mg Hg/kg/day for 28–29 days exhibited stumbling, falling, blindness, crying, temper tantrums and coma. Histopathological analysis revealed diffuse degeneration in the cerebral cortex, cerebellum basal ganglia, thalamus, amygdala and lateral geniculate nuclei (Willes et al., 1978).

Rats acutely intoxicated with methylmercury (19.9 mg Hg/kg, oral gavage) showed signs of lethargy and ataxia, which was not accompanied by histopathological changes. Symptoms disappeared within 2–3 h. Administration of a single dose of methylmercuric chloride (0.8 mg Hg/kg) produced BBB dysfunction in rats (Chang and Hartman, 1972) similar to that described for inorganic mercury. Neurotoxic signs observed in rats exposed to methylmercury (4 mg Hg/kg/day for 8 days) include muscle spasms, gait disturbances, flailing and hind limb crossing (Inouye and Murakami, 1975; Fuyuta et al., 1978; Magos et al., 1980, 1985). Histopathological examination of the nervous system of affected rats has shown degeneration of cerebellar granular cells and dorsal root ganglia (Magos et al., 1980, 1985) and degenerative changes in peripheral nerves (Fehling et al., 1975; Miyakawa et al., 1976).

Mice exposed to 1.9 or 9.5 mg Hg/kg/day as methylmercury in the drinking water for 28 weeks exhibited degeneration of Purkinje cells and loss of granular cells in the cerebellum (MacDonald and Harbison, 1977). At higher doses, hind limb paralysis was observed. Neuronal degeneration and microgliosis were observed in the corpus striatum, cerebral cortex, thalamus and hypothalamus, accompanied by hind leg weakness, in mice given 1 or 4 mg Hg/kg/day as methylmercuric chloride by gavage for 60 days (Berthoud et al., 1976). In rabbits given 5.5 mg Hg/kg as methylmercuric acetate for 1–4 days, widespread neuronal degenerative changes in cervical ganglia cells, cerebellum and cerebral cortex have been observed without accompanying behavioral changes (Jacobs et al., 1977).

Following inhalation exposure to metallic mercury vapors, the CNS has been found to be the most sensitive organ in guinea pigs, rats and mice. With increasing concentrations of mercury, damage to CNS becomes irreversible. Rabbits appear to be less sensitive to mercury following inhalation exposure.

Renal System

Mercury, in all forms, has been shown to cause renal toxicity (structural and functional damage) in humans and animal species that are tested. Renal toxicity has been observed in rats (Fisher 344) and mice ($B6C3F_1$) following acute, intermediate and chronic exposures to mercuric chloride (Dieter et al., 1992; NTP, 1993). In a 14-day study, male and female rats were exposed by gavage to 0.93–14.8 mg Hg/kg/day as mercuric chloride for 5 days a week. There was a significant increase in the absolute and relative kidney weights of males beginning at the 1.9 mg Hg/kg/day dose level. An increased incidence of tubular necrosis was observed in rats exposed to at least 3.7 mg Hg/kg/day. Severity was dose dependent. In chronic studies, mercuric chloride produced a variety of pathological changes in kidneys (Carmignani et al., 1992; Hultman and Enestrom, 1992; NTP, 1993). Degenerative effects have been found in the kidneys of animals exposed to moderate to high levels of metallic mercury vapors following acute or subacute exposures (Ashe, 1953). Effects ranging from marked cellular degeneration to tissue destruction and widespread necrosis were observed in rabbits exposed to mercury vapor at a concentration of 28.8 mg/m^3 for 2–3 h. In rats, slight degenerative changes (i.e., dense deposits in tubule cells and lysosomal inclusions) in the renal tubular epithelium were evident following exposure to 3 mg/m^3 mercury vapor for 3 h/day/5 days a week, for 12–42 weeks (Kishi et al., 1978). Low-level, long-term exposure to mercury (0.1 mg/m^3) has not been found toxic to the kidneys of rats, rabbits, and dogs (Ashe, 1953).

Cardiovascular System

Mercury has been shown to produce adverse effects on the cardiovascular system. A decrease in heart rate was observed in male rats given two gavage doses of 2 mg Hg/kg as methylmercuric chloride (Arito and Takahashi, 1991). An increase in systolic blood pressure was observed in male rats after daily oral gavage doses of 0.4 mg Hg/kg/day as methylmercuric chloride for 3–4 weeks (Wakita, 1987). This effect began approximately 60 days after initiation of exposure and persisted for at least 9 months.

GI Tract

Ingestion of mercuric chloride is highly irritating to the tissues of the GI tract. Inflammation and necrosis of the glandular stomach were observed in mice that were given oral doses of 59 mg/kg as mercuric chloride 5 days a week for 2 weeks (NTP, 1993). In a 2-year gavage study, an increased incidence of forestomach hyperplasia was observed in male rats exposed to 1.9 or 3.7 mg Hg/kg/day as mercuric chloride compared to the control group. Mice showed ulceration of the glandular stomach after 2 years of dietary exposure to methylmercuric chloride at 0.69 mg Hg/kg/day (Mitsumori et al., 1981, 1990).

Hematopoietic System

In general, acute mercury toxicity does not produce any characteristic hematological changes. In a chronic study conducted in rats, phenylmercuric acetate given in water at a dose of 4.2 mg Hg/kg/day caused decreases in hemoglobin, hematocrit and RBC counts (Solecki et al., 1991). The anemia observed in this study may have been secondary to blood loss associated with the ulcerative lesions in the large intestine. However, methylmercuric chloride at a low dose (0.1 mg Hg/kg/day for 2 years) given in the diet for 2 years caused no changes in hematological parameters (Verschuuren et al., 1976).

Other Effects

Mercury has been found to have the potential for inducing genotoxicity (Ghosh et al., 1991), carcinogenicity (Solecki et al., 1991; NTP, 1993), immunotoxicity (Thuvander et al., 1996), and endocrine, reproductive and developmental toxicity (Fuyuta et al., 1979; Castoldi et al., 2008; Liang et al., 2009; Tan et al., 2009; Vitalone et al., 2010; Lisón et al., 2016; Ni et al., 2017).

DIAGNOSIS

Presently there are reliable and accurate ways to measure mercury levels in the body, using an atomic absorption spectrometer and inductively coupled plasma (ICP) or ICP-mass spectrometer (ICP-MS). Mercury analysis is usually performed on blood, urine, milk, hair, nail, liver, and kidney. Mercury in urine is determined to test for exposure to metallic or inorganic mercury, while whole blood or hair values are used to determine exposure to methylmercury. Mercury levels in the blood provide more useful information after recent exposures than after long-term exposures. Levels found in blood, urine and hair may be used together to predict possible health effects that may be caused by the different forms of mercury. The kidney is an ideal specimen for mercury analysis from dead animals.

TREATMENT

Activated charcoal (1−3 g/kg body weight, po) is very effective in reducing further absorption of mercury from the GI tract. Specific treatment of mercury poisoning rests with the use of chelators, along with protein solutions to bind and neutralize mercury compounds. The use of a particular chelator is dependent upon the type of mercury exposure. Among several chelators, dimercaprol (BAL, 3 mg/kg, im) has been found to be the most effective against mercury poisoning. However, chelation releases mercury from soft tissues which can be redistributed to the brain. Oral administration of sodium thiosulfate (1 g/kg) can assist in eliminating mercury. Recently, Takemoto et al. (2015) mentioned that living animals are equipped with a set of endogenous defense mechanisms against Hg, such as vitamin E, vitamin K, selenium, metallothioneine, 17B-estradiol, and brain derived neurotrophic factor. Animal studies suggest that antioxidants (particularly vitamin E) may be useful for decreasing the toxicity of mercury. Improved chelation and drug therapies for treating acute and chronic mercury poisonings are greatly needed.

CONCLUDING REMARKS AND FUTURE DIRECTIONS

Toxicity by mercury depends upon the form of mercury, dose, duration and route of exposure. Organic mercury tends to bioaccumulate in the higher food chain, and as a result the maximum concentrations are found in the meat of fish, marine mammals and fish-eating birds and wildlife. Methylmercury is the most toxic among the mercury species because of its volatility and its ability to pass through biological membranes such as the BBB and the placental barrier. The nervous system and kidneys are the two major target organs. Not all forms of mercury cross the BBB (e.g., inorganic mercury), but in all forms it accumulates in the kidney and thereby causes damage to this organ. Chelation therapy appears to be the best treatment. Oral administration of activated charcoal is very effective in reducing the further absorption of mercury from the GI tract.

REFERENCES

Al-Saleem, T., 1976. Levels of mercury and pathologic changes in patients with organomercury poisoning. Bull. World Health Org. 53 (Suppl.), 99−104.

Arito, H., Takahashi, M., 1991. Effect of methylmercury on sleep patterns in the rat. In: Suzuki, T., Imura, N., Clarkson, T.W. (Eds.), Advances in Mercury Toxicology. Plenum Press, New York, NY, pp. 381−394.

Ashe, W., Largent, E., Dutra, F., et al., 1953. Behaviour of mercury in the animal organism following inhalation. Arch. Ind. Hyg. Occup. Med. 17, 19−43.

ATSDR, Agency for Toxic Substances and Disease Registry, 1999. Toxicological Profile for Mercury. U.S. Department of Health and Human Services, Atlanta, GA.

ATSDR, Agency for Toxic Substances and Disease Registry, 2011. Priority list of hazardous substances. Available online at: www.atsdr.cdc.gov/spl.

Bernhoft, R.A., 2012. Mercury toxicity and treatment: a review of the literature. J. Environ. Publ. Health. 2012, Article ID 460508, 10 pages.

Berthoud, H.R., Garman, R.H., Weiss, B., 1976. Food intake, body weight, and brain histopathology in mice following chronic methylmercury treatment. Toxicol. Appl. Pharmacol. 36, 19–30.

Bressa, G., Cima, L., Costa, P., 1988. Bioaccumulation of Hg in the mushroom Pleurotus ostreatus. Ecotoxicol. Environ. Saf. 16, 85–89.

Carmignani, M., Boscolo, P., Artese, L., et al., 1992. Renal mechanism in the cardiovascular effects of chronic exposure to inorganic mercury in rats. Br. J. Ind. Med. 49 (4), 226–232.

Castoldi, A.F., Johansson, C., Onishchenko, C., et al., 2008. Human developmental neurotoxicity of methylmercury: impact of variables and risk modifiers. Regul. Toxicol. Pharmacol. 51, 201–214.

Ceccatelli, S., Dare, E., Moors, M., 2010. Methylmercury-induced neurotoxicity and apoptosis. Chem. Biol. Interact. 188, 301–308.

Chang, L., Hartman, H.A., 1972. Ultrastructural studies of the nervous system after mercury intoxication. Acta Neuropathol. (Berlin). 20, 122–138.

Chang, L.W., Yamaguchi, S., Dudley, J.A.W., 1974. Neurological changes in cats following long-term diet of mercury contaminated tuna. Acta Neuropathl. (Berlin). 27, 171–176.

Cheung, M.K., Verity, M.A., 1985. Experimental methylmercury neurotoxicity: locus of mercurial inhibition of brain protein synthesis in vivo and in vitro. J. Neurochem. 44, 1799–1808.

Choi, C.M., Lapham, L.W., Amin-Zaki, L., et al., 1978. Abnormal neuronal migration, deranged cerebral cortical organization and diffuse white matter astrocytosis of human fetal brain: a major effect of methylmercury poisoning in utero. J. Neuropathol. Exp. Neurol. 37, 719–732.

Clarkson, T.W., 1987. Metal toxicity in the central nervous system. Environ. Health Perspect. 75, 59–64.

Deiter, M.P., Boorman, G.A., Jameson, C.W., et al., 1992. Development of renal toxicity in F344 rats gavaged with mercuric chloride for 2 weeks, or 2, 4, 6, 15, 24 months. J. Toxicol. Environ. Health. 24, 319–340.

Eriksson, P., Fischer, C., Stenerlöw, B., et al., 2010. Interaction of gamma-radiation and methyl mercury during a critical phase of neonatal brain development in mice exacerbates developmental neurobehavioral effects. NeuroToxicology. 31, 223–229.

Farina, M., Aschner, M., Rocha, J.B.T., 2011a. Oxidative stress in meHg-induced neurotoxicity. Toxicol. Appl. Pharmacol. 256, 405–417.

Farina, M., Campos, F., Vendrell, I., et al., 2009. Probucol increases glutathione peroxidase-1 activity and displays long-lasting protection against methylmercury toxicity in cerebellar granule cells. Toxicol. Sci. 112, 416–426.

Farina, M., Rocha, J.B.T., Aschner, M., 2011b. Mechanisms of methylmercury-induced neurotoxicity: evidence from experimental studies. Life Sci. 89, 555–563.

Fehling, C., Abdulla, M., Brun, A., et al., 1975. Methylmercury poisoning in the rat: a combined neurological, chemical, and histopathological study. Toxicol. Appl. Pharmacol. 33, 27–37.

Franco, J.L., Posser, T., Dunkley, P.R., et al., 2009. Methylmercury neurotoxicity is associated with inhibition of the antioxidant enzyme glutathione peroxidase. Free Radic. Biol. Med. 47, 449–457.

Fuyuta, M., Fujimoto, T., Hirata, S., 1978. Embryotoxic effects of methylmercuric chloride administered to mice and rats during organogenesis. Teratology. 18, 353–366.

Fuyuta, M., Fujimoto, T., Kiyofuji, E., 1979. Teratogenic effects of a single oral administration of methylmercuric chloride in mice. Acta Anat. 104, 356–362.

Ghosh, A.K., Sen, S., Sharma, A., et al., 1991. Effect of chlorophyllin on mercuric chloride-induced clastogenicity in mice. Food Chem. Toxicol. 29, 777–779.

Hansen, J.C., Danscher, G., 1995. Quantitative and qualitative distribution of mercury in organs from arctic sledge dogs: an atomic absorption spectrophotometric and histochemical study of tissue samples from natural long-termed high dietary organic mercury-exposed dogs for Thule, Greenland. Toxicol. Appl. Pharmacol. 77, 189–195.

Hultman, P., Enestrom, S., 1992. Dose–response studies in murine mercury-induced autoimmunity and immune-complex disease. Toxicol. Appl. Pharmacol. 113, 199–208.

Hwang, G.-W., 2012. Role of intracellular defense factors against methylmercury toxicity. Biol. Pharm. Bull. 35, 1881–1884.

Inouye, M., Murakami, U., 1975. Teratogenic effects of orally administered methylmercuric chloride in rats and mice. Cong. Abnormal. 15, 1–9.

Jacobs, J.M., Carmichael, N., Cavanagh, J.B., 1977. Ultrastructural changes in the nervous system of rabbits poisoned with methylmercury. Toxicol. Appl. Pharmacol. 39, 249–261.

Kaur, P., Schulz, K., Aschner, M., Syversen, T., 2007. Role of docosahexaenoic acid in modulating methylmercury-induced neurotoxicity. Toxicol. Sci. 100, 423–432.

Kirkpatrick, M., Benoit, J., Everett, W., et al., 2015. The effects methylmercury exposure on behaviour and biomarkers of oxidative stress in adult mice. NeuoToxicology. 50, 170–178.

Kishi, R., Hashimoto, K., Shimizu, S., et al., 1978. Behavioral changes and mercury concentrations in tissues of rats exposed to mercury vapor. Toxicol. Appl. Pharmacol. 46, 555–566.

Lecavalier, P.R., Chu, I., Villeneuve, D., et al., 1994. Combined effects of mercury and hexachlorobenzene in rat. J. Environ. Sci. Health. 29, 951–961.

Liang, J., Inskip, M., Newhook, D., Messier, C., 2009. Neurobehavioral effect of chronic and bolus doses of methylmercury following prenatal exposure in C57BL/6 weanling mice. Neurotoxicol. Teratol. 31, 372–381.

Lisón, F., Espin, S., Aroca, B., et al., 2016. Assessment of mercury exposure and maternal-fetal transfer in *Miniopterus schreibersii* (Chiroptera: Miniopteridae) from southeastern Iberian Peninsula. Environ. Sci. Pollut. Res. Available from: http://dx.doi.org/10.1007/s11356-016-8271-z.

MacDonald, J.S., Harbison, R.D., 1977. Methylmercury-induced encephalopathy in mice. Toxicol. Appl. Pharmacol. 39, 195–205.

Magos, L., Brown, A.W., Sparrow, S., et al., 1985. The comparative toxicology of ethyl and methylmercury. Arch. Toxicol. 57, 260–267.

Magos, L., Peristianis, G.C., Clarkson, T.W., et al., 1980. The effect of lactation on methylmercury intoxication. Arch. Toxicol. 45, 143–148.

Matsumoto, H., Koya, G., Takeuchi, T., 1965. Fetal Minamata disease – a neuropathological study of two cases of intrauterine intoxication by a methylmercury compound. J. Neuropathol. Exp. Neurol. 24, 563–574.

Mitsumori, K., Hirano, M., Ueda, H., et al., 1990. Chronic toxicity and carcinogenicity of methylmercury chloride in B6C3F1 mice. Fund. Appl. Toxicol. 14, 179–190.

Mitsumori, K., Maita, K., Saito, T., et al., 1981. Carcinogenicity of methylmercury chloride in ICR mice: preliminary note on renal carcinogenesis. Cancer Lett. 12, 305–310.

Miyakawa, T., Murayama, E., Sumiyoshi, S., et al., 1976. Late changes in human sural nerves in Minamata disease and in nerves of rats with experimental organic mercury poisoning. Acta Neuropathol. Berlin. 35, 131–138.

Ni, M., Li, X., dos Santos, A.P.M., et al., 2017. Mercury. In: Gupta, R. C. (Ed.), Reproductive and Developmental Toxicology. Academic Press/Elsevier, Amsterdam, pp. 583–594.

NTP, 1993. Toxicology and Carcinogenesis Studies of Mercuric Chloride (CAS No. 7487-94-7) in F344/N Rats and B6C3F1 Mice (Gavage Studies). National Toxicology Program, U.S. Department of Health and Human Service, National Institutes of Health, Research Triangle Park, NC. NTP TR 408. NIH Publication No. 91-3139.

Pletz, J., Sánchez-Bayo, F., Tennekes, H.A., 2016. Dose-response analysis indicating time-dependent neurotoxicity caused by organic and inorganic mercury- Implications for toxic effects in the developing brain. Toxicology. 347, 1–5.

Puls, R., 1994. Mineral Levels in Animal Health: Diagnostic Data. second ed. Sherpa International, Clearbrook, BC, pp. 184–191.

Ray, P.D., Yoshim, A., Fry, R.C., 2014. Incorporating epigenetic data into the risk assessment process for the toxic metals arsenic, cadmium, chromium, lead, and mercury: strategies and challenges. Front. Genet. 5, 201.

Sager, P.R., Doherty, R.A., Olmsted, J.B., 1983. Interaction of methylmercury with microtubules in cultured cells and in vitro. Exp. Cell Res. 146, 127–137.

Schuh, J.C.L., Ross, C., Meschter, C., 1988. Concurrent mercuric blister and dimethyl sulfoxide (DMSO) application as a cause of mercury toxicity in two horses. Equine Vet. J. 20, 68–71.

Sharma, B., Singh, S., Siddiqi, N.J., 2014. Biomedical implications of heavy metals induced imbalances in redox systems. Biomed. Res. Int. 640754.

Sokolowski, K., Falluel-Morel, A., Zhou, X., et al., 2011. Methylmercury (MeHg) elicits mitochondrial-dependent apoptosis in developing hippocampus and acts at low exposures. NeuroToxicology. 32, 535–544.

Solecki, R., Hothorn, L., Holzweissig, M., et al., 1991. Computerized analysis of pathological findings in long-term trials with phenylmercuric acetate in rats. Arch. Toxicol. 14 (Suppl.), 100–103.

Taber, K.H., Hurley, R.A., 2008. Mercury exposure: effects across the lifespan. J. Neuropsychiatr. Clin. Neurosci. 20, 384–389.

Takemoto, T., Ishihara, Y., Ishida, A., et al., 2015. Neuroprotection elicited by nerve growth factor and brain-derived neurotrophic factor released from astrocytes in response to methylmercury. Environ. Toxicol. Pharmacol. 40, 199–205.

Tan, S.W., Meiller, J.C., Mahaffey, K.R., 2009. The endocrine effects of mercury in humans and wildlife. Crit. Rev. Toxicol. 39, 228–269.

Thuvander, A., Sundberg, J., Oskarsson, A., 1996. Immunomodulating effects after perinatal exposure to methylmercury in mice. Toxicology. 114, 163–175.

Tsubaki, T., Krukuyama, K., 1977. Minamata Disease. Elsevier Scientific Publ. Co, Amsterdam.

Tsubaki, T., Takahashi, H., 1986. Recent Advances in Minamata Disease Studies. Kodansha, Tokyo.

Vahter, M., Mottet, N.K., Friberg, L., et al., 1994. Speciation of mercury in the primate blood and brain following long-term exposure to methylmercury. Toxicol. Appl. Pharmacol. 124, 221–229.

Verschuuren, H.G., Kroes, R., Den Tonkelaar, E.M., et al., 1976. Toxicity of methylmercury chloride in rats. III. Long-term toxicity study. Toxicology. 6, 107–123.

Vitalone, A., Catalani, A., Cinque, C., et al., 2010. Long-term effects of developmental exposure to low doses of PCB 126 and methylmercury. Toxicol. Lett. 197, 38–45.

Wakita, Y., 1987. Hypertension induced by methylmercury in rats. Toxicol. Appl. Pharmacol. 89, 144–147.

Willes, R.F., Truelove, J.F., Nera, E.A., 1978. Neurotoxic response of infant monkeys to methylmercury. Toxicology. 9, 125–135.

Yilmaz, F.M., Yilmaz, H., Tutkun, E., et al., 2014. Serum biochemical markers of central nervous system damage in children with acute elemental mercury intoxication. Clin. Toxicol. 52, 32–38.

Chapter 32

Molybdenum

Jeffery O. Hall

INTRODUCTION

Molybdenum (Mo) is an essential nutrient in plants and animals. Thorough reviews on Mo have been published (Dick, 1956; Underwood, 1977; Ward, 1978; Friberg and Lener, 1986; Mills and Davis, 1987; Rajagopalan, 1988; Nielsen, 1996; Johnson, 1997; NRC, 2006; Gould and Kendall, 2011). In plants and microbes, reduction of nitrate to nitrite and nitrogen fixation requires Mo (Williams and daSilva, 2002). Higher animals require Mo for oxygen transfer reactions of aldehyde oxidase, sulfite oxidase, and xanthine oxidase, where Mo is bound to a pterin nucleus (Johnson et al., 1980). Although dietary clinical deficiencies have not been reported under natural conditions (Mills and Davis, 1987), deficiency has been produced in animals fed purified Mo deficient diets (Mills and Bremner, 1980; Anke et al., 1985). Functional Mo deficiency has been caused by genetic disorders in humans (Reiss, 2000) and competitive replacement of tungsten for Mo in enzymes (Nell et al., 1980). Iatrogenic Mo deficiency, resulting in aberrant sulfur-containing amino acid metabolism, has been reported following prolonged total parenteral nutrition (Abumrad et al., 1981).

Mo toxicity is intricately tied to interactions with copper and sulfur. Predominant manifestations of Mo poisoning are associated with secondary copper deficiency, but not all clinical signs are alleviated by copper supplementation, as some of the effects can be related to direct thiomolybdate binding to the copper dependent enzyme systems (Gould and Kendall, 2011). The copper–sulfur–molybdenum interactions are complex and vary greatly in degree of severity among species.

BACKGROUND

Mo is a transition metal within group VI of the periodic table. It has an atomic number of 42, an atomic weight of 95.95, and has seven different naturally occurring atomic masses from 92 to 100 (Rosman and Taylor, 1998). Mo can occur in a variety of oxidation states that range from (-II) to (VI) (IMOA, 2006), but valence states IV, V, and VI are the most common in biological systems (Johnson, 1997). Mo is utilized in the production of oxidation catalysts, pigments, corrosion-resistant steel, smoke suppressants, lubricants, fertilizers, and metal alloys. Although uniformly found in nature, the United States has the greatest producible Mo reserves.

Mo is commonly found in low concentrations in most dietary constituents (Rajagopalan, 1988), but excess intake can occur from plants grown on soils naturally high in Mo or from areas contaminated by mining or smelting operations. Naturally high soil and forage molybdenum concentrations have been reported in localized areas of several states in the western United States, as well as Canada, England, Australia, and New Zealand but likely occurs in other countries as well. In addition, high molybdenum forages have been identified from contaminated areas associated with mining and industrial operations (King et al., 1984). Daily dietary requirements for all species are such that requirements are met, even with low intake.

PHARMACOKINETICS/TOXICOKINETICS

Absorption

Mo absorption differs between monogastrics and ruminants. In monogastrics, Mo absorption occurs from the stomach throughout the intestinal tract (Bell et al., 1964; Miller et al., 1972; Nielsen, 1996). In contrast, ruminant absorption likely depends on the chemical form of the molybdenum. Historically, Mo absorption in ruminants was thought to occur in the intestinal tract, as an extensive delay in peak blood concentration would indicate that rumen absorption did not occur. However, some delay in overall total Mo absorption could be due to the time necessary for the conversion of the molybdates to thiomolybdates in the rumen, as preformed thiomolybdates

Veterinary Toxicology. DOI: http://dx.doi.org/10.1016/B978-0-12-811410-0.00032-5

administered into the rumen of sheep appeared in the plasma within minutes (Kelleher et al., 1983). The mucosal absorption of molybdate is via an active carrier-mediated process that is also utilized by sulfate (Mason and Cardin, 1977). Absorption is quite efficient, ranging from 40% to 90% (Friberg and Lener, 1986; Turnlund et al., 1995). However, Mo absorption does not appear to be regulated at the point of mucosal absorption, as increasing Mo concentrations presented to the mucosa result in concomitant increased absorption (Miller et al., 1972; Turnlund et al., 1995).

Dietary constituents can limit Mo absorption. Dietary sulfate present at the point of absorption can competitively inhibit molybdate uptake (Mason and Cardin, 1977). Furthermore, in the presence of sulfur/sulfates, the reductive rumen metabolism results in di-, tri-, and tetra-thiomolybdates, which can then bind copper and form a nonabsorbable cupric thiomolybdate complex (Dick, 1956; Price et al., 1987; Gooneratne et al., 1989).

Distribution

Mo is widely distributed in tissues but has highest concentrations in the liver, kidney, and bone (Schroeder et al., 1970; Friberg and Lener, 1986). In light of the essential nature of Mo, it is somewhat unusual that very little tissue retention/reserve is maintained. Postabsorptive circulation occurs by transport bound to the red blood cell proteins or as free ionic molybdate (Allway et al., 1968; Versieck et al., 1981). However, absorbed or systemically produced thiomolybdates can bind copper and result in circulating copper–thiomolybdate complexes which are not biologically available for tissue utilization. Some of the circulating or tissue thiomolybdates may also be bound to copper dependent enzyme systems, resulting in functional inhibition (Gould and Kendall, 2011).

Elimination

Mo is eliminated from the body fairly rapidly, with little, and only short-term, tissue retention. Although urinary is the primary route of elimination, biliary elimination also occurs (Friberg and Lener, 1986; Vyskocil and Viau, 1999; NRC, 2006) and likely is the primary route of elimination in ruminants (Grace and Suttle, 1979; Pott et al., 1999). Urinary elimination is concentration dependent, resulting in relatively rapid elimination even with very large exposures. In lactating animals, Mo is excreted in the milk with content being dependent on the concentration being ingested (Archibald, 1951; Anke et al., 1985). Thus, exposure can be approximated by analysis of urine or milk for Mo content across time and extrapolating back to the time of exposure (Lesperance et al., 1985). Just as sulfate can inhibit gastrointestinal absorption of Mo, it can also compete for reabsorption sites in the renal tubules and enhance the rate of elimination (Friberg and Lener, 1986).

MECHANISM OF ACTION

The mechanism by which Mo is active in biological systems is through its redox activity in functional molybdoenzymes (Mills and Davis, 1987). The readily changeable oxidation states of Mo lend it to functional utilization in these types of reactions.

The primary mechanisms by which Mo is toxic are directly tied to its interactions with sulfur and copper. These interactions result in overt or functional copper deficiency, including inhibition of copper dependent enzyme systems. However, these interactions differ significantly among species, with ruminants being much more susceptible than monogastrics, due to the ruminal production of thiomolybdates. The reducing environment of the rumen converts sulfate or sulfur from sulfur-containing amino acids to sulfide, which then forms mono-, di-, tri-, and tetra-thiomolybdates (Price et al., 1987; Spears, 2003). Thiomolybdates' binding of copper in the digestive tract prevents absorption of ingested copper, while systemic binding renders it nonbioavailable for tissue utilization (Gooneratne et al., 1989; Suttle, 1991). These cupric thiomolybdate complexes also result in enhanced copper excretion (Howell and Gooneratne, 1987). Price et al. (1987) found that the ruminal binding was predominantly via tri- and tetra-thiomolybdates, while systemic effects were predominantly via di- and tri-thiomolybdates. In practical terms, the thiomolybdates serve as effective chelators of copper, preventing copper absorption and depleting functional body stores. As the rumenal microbial populations can differ significantly among ruminant species, the relative sensitivity among species could be related to the overall conversion to thiomolybdates or the relative abundances of the mono-, di-, tri-, and tetra-thiomolybdates produced.

Most of the clinical syndromes of Mo poisoning can be tied to deficiencies in copper-containing enzyme system functions via overt deficiencies (NRC, 2006) or inhibition of enzyme systems (Gould and Kendall, 2011). Although most clinical effects of Mo poisoning are reversed by supplementation of copper, Mo as thiomolybdates can have some direct toxic effects on copper dependent enzymes. It is also possible that permanent tissue damage, caused by severe copper depletion, may result in a nonresponse to copper supplementation in some clinically affected animals. The exact mechanisms of some noncopper responsive toxic effects of Mo are poorly defined or investigated, but it has been observed that high Mo concentrations can inhibit the in vivo activity of biological enzymes, such as succinic acid oxidase, sulfide oxidase, glutaminase, cholinesterase, cytochrome oxidase (Venugopal and Luckey, 1978), ceruloplasmin, superoxide dismutase, ascorbate oxidase, catechol activity, and other copper dependent enzyme systems (Gould and Kendall, 2011).

TOXICITY

Both acute and chronic toxicity of Mo varies greatly among species. Ruminant animals are much more sensitive than monogastric animals, due to the rumen metabolism of sulfur to sulfides and formation of thiomolybdates. The relative tolerance to Mo has been ranked: horses > pigs > rats > rabbits > guinea pigs > sheep > cattle (Venugopal and Luckey, 1978), but more recent literature suggests horses may be more sensitive (Ladefoged and Sturup, 1995). In total, the toxicity of Mo needs to be evaluated with consideration of dietary sulfur/sulfates and copper. This is with the knowledge that sulfates competitively inhibit molybdate uptake from the intestinal tract, but metabolism in the rumen results in the formation of thiomolybdates, which enhances the toxic effects on copper status.

Natural toxic effects of Mo are primarily via ingestion, but toxicity has been demonstrated by both inhalation and injection in laboratory rodents. The intraperitoneal LD_{50} of Mo in rats ranges from 22.8 to 99 mg/kg body weight (Venugopal and Luckey, 1978), with similar lethal doses in mice and guinea pigs. Chronic inflammatory lesions and hyaline degeneration within the respiratory tree was induced by Mo trioxide exposure of 10–100 mg/m^3 6 h per day, 5 days a week (Chan et al., 1998). Increased incidence of respiratory adenomas was also seen in the rats and mice.

Concentrations of Mo required to produce acute poisoning orally differ significantly among species. For cats, rabbits and guinea pigs, the oral LD_{100} for Mo is 1310, 1020, and 1200 mg/kg body weight, respectively, while the oral LD_{50} for rats is 125–370 mg/kg body weight (Venugopal and Luckey, 1978). Little acute toxicity data are available for domestic animals, but cattle have been acutely poisoned with feed containing 7400 mg Mo/kg diet (group average intake of 31 mg Mo/kg body weight/day) and Mo was acutely lethal in sheep at 132–137 mg Mo/kg body weight/day for 2–3 days (Swan et al., 1998).

Clinical signs and pathologic lesions in acutely poisoned animals differ from those seen with more chronic poisonings. Acutely poisoned cattle and sheep developed feed withdrawal, lethargy, weakness, hind limb ataxia that progressed to the front limbs and recumbency (Swan et al., 1998). The cattle also had profuse salivation, ocular discharge and mucoid feces. Hydropic hepatocellular degeneration/necrosis and hydropic degeneration/necrosis of the proximal and distal renal tubules was observed in both cattle and sheep.

Subacute to chronic toxicity of Mo is just as species dependent as acute poisoning. Oral lethal doses of Mo administered chronically to laboratory animals (rats, mice, guinea pigs and rabbits) range from 60 to 333 mg Mo/kg body weight/day, while cattle are poisoned with as little as 3 mg Mo/kg body weight/day (NRC, 2006). Literature reports of toxic dietary Mo content range from 10 to 1200 ppm for rats, 300–8000 ppm for poultry, 200–4000 ppm for rabbits, 1000–8000 ppm for guinea pigs, 2.5–20 ppm for sheep, and 2–400 ppm for cattle (Pitt, 1976). Ruminants commonly succumb to molybdenosis when Mo intake is greater than 20 ppm in the diet. However, due to the intrinsic nature of the molybdenum–copper–sulfur interactions, chronic Mo poisoning in ruminants can be divided into three classes: dietary Mo greater than 20 ppm, low Cu:Mo ratio (<2:1) and high dietary sulfur with normal copper and Mo (Ward, 1978). The desired Cu:Mo ratio in ruminants is between 6:1 and 10:1 (Thompson et al., 1991). Thus, Mo toxicosis can occur at much low concentrations in association with copper deficient forages than those with diets adequate in copper.

Most clinical signs of chronic Mo poisoning are associated with induction of overt or functional copper deficiency. Commonly, the first recognized clinical sign of chronic Mo poisoning is severe diarrhea (Dick, 1956; Pitt, 1976; Pitt et al., 1980; Underwood, 1977; Ward, 1978; Friberg and Lener, 1986; Mills and Davis, 1987; Rajagopalan, 1988; Nielsen, 1996; Johnson, 1997; Coppock and Dziwenka, 2004; NRC, 2006). "Teart" is used to refer to soil or plants that contain unusually high amounts of Mo, thus the term teart scours is commonly used to describe the diarrhea associated with excessive Mo intake. Although the exact mechanism is not well defined, copper supplementation alleviates this clinical sign. Other common clinical signs of chronic Mo poisoning include poor body weight gain, weight loss, anemia, poor immune function, decreased milk production, achromotrichia, alopecia, limb deformities, bone fractures, periostosis, lameness, poor reproductive performance, lack of libido, and ataxia. Abortions have been reported in horses.

Pathologic alterations of chronic Mo poisoning are not specifically diagnostic. These lesions are secondary to induced copper deficiency and include emaciation, periostosis and epiphyseal plate growth abnormalities. Because of the nature of chronic Mo poisoning, primary copper deficiency must always be ruled out when these lesions are identified.

TREATMENT

The two primary mechanisms for treating Mo toxicosis involve removal from the source of high Mo and copper supplementation, but administration of sulfate to monogastrics will enhance elimination rates. Administration of sulfates to ruminants would not be recommended, as ruminal reduction to sulfide could potentially result in greater thiomolybdate concentrations and worsen the clinical disease. With rapid clearance from the body, removal from the high Mo source will quickly remove excess Mo from the body. However, permanent damage may be present that results in sustained animal deaths for weeks to several months' postexposure (Swan et al., 1998). Supplementation of copper in Mo-poisoned animals must be done with care, especially in sheep, to prevent excessive copper accumulation and subsequent copper toxicosis.

CONCLUDING REMARKS AND FUTURE DIRECTIONS

The known mechanisms of Mo poisoning are a complex interaction with sulfur and copper that differ significantly across animal species. However, some clinical effects of Mo poisoning have not been related to absolute or functional copper deficits, as replenishment of copper does not result in cessation of clinical effects. Some of the copper-refractory clinical effects could be simply a direct inhibition of functional enzymes by thiomolybdates. These refractory clinical effects of Mo poisoning need further investigation to delineate the exact mechanism by which Mo produces adverse animal health.

REFERENCES

Abumrad, N.N., Schneider, A.J., Steel, D., et al., 1981. Amino acid intolerance during prolonged total parenteral nutrition reversed by molybdate therapy. Am. J. Clin. Nutr. 34, 2551–2559.

Allway, W.H., Kubota, J., Losee, F., et al., 1968. Selenium, molybdenum, and vanadium in human blood. Arch. Environ. Health. 16, 342–349.

Anke, M., Groppel, B., Grun, M., 1985. Essentiality, toxicity, requirement and supply of molybdenum in human and animals. In International Symposium on Trace Elements in Man and Animals, Mills CT, Brenner I, ChestersVol. 5. Commonwealth Agriculture Bureaux, Farnham Royal, UK.

Archibald, J.G., 1951. Molybdenum in cow's milk. J. Dairy Sci. 34, 1026–1029.

Bell, M.D., Diggs, G.B., et al., 1964. Comparison of Mo^{99} metabolism in swine and cattle as affected by stable molybdate. J. Nutr. 84, 367–372.

Chan, P.C., Herbert, R.A., Roycroft, J.H., et al., 1998. Lung tumor induction by inhalation exposure to molybdenum trioxide in rats and mice. Toxicol. Sci. 45, 58–65.

Coppock, R., Dziwenka, M.M., 2004. Molybdenum. In: Plumlee, K.H. (Ed.), Clinical Veterinary Toxicology. Mosby, St. Louis, MO, pp. 211–214.

Dick, A.T., 1956. Molybdenum in animal nutrition. Soil. Sci. 81, 229–258.

Friberg, L., Lener, J., 1986. Molybdenum. In: Friberg, L., Nordberg, G.F., Vouk, V. (Eds.), Handbook on the Toxicology of Metals, second ed. Elsevier Science, New York, p. 446.

Gooneratne, S.R., Buckley, W.T., Christensen, D.A., 1989. Review of copper deficiency and metabolism in ruminants. Can. J. Anim. Sci. 69, 819–845.

Gould, L., Kendall, N.R., 2011. Role of the rumen in copper and thiomolybdate absorption. Nutr. Res. Rev. 24, 176–182.

Grace, N.D., Suttle, N.F., 1979. Some effects of sulfur intake on molybdenum metabolism in sheep. Br. J. Nutr. 41, 125–136.

Howell, J.M., Gooneratne, S.R., 1987. The pathology of copper toxicity in animals. In: Howell, J.M., Gawthorne, J.M. (Eds.), Copper in Animals and Man. CRC Press, Boca Raton, FL, pp. 53–78.

IMOA (International Molybdenum Association), 2006. Available at <http://www.imoa.info>.

Johnson, J.L., 1997. Molybdenum. In: O'Dell, B.L., Sunde, R.A. (Eds.), Handbook of Nutritionally Essential Mineral Elements. Marcel Dekker, New York, pp. 413–438.

Johnson, J.L., Hainline, B.E., Rajagopalan, K.V., 1980. Characterization of the molybdenum cofactor of sulfite oxidase, xanthine oxidase, and nitrate reductase. J. Biol. Chem. 255, 1783–1786.

Kelleher, C.A., Ivan, M., Lamand, M., et al., 1983. The absorption of labeled molybdenum compounds in sheep fitted with re-entrant cannulae in the ascending duodenum. J. Comp. Pathol. 93, 83–92.

King, K.A., Leleux, J., Mulhern, B.M., 1984. Molybdenum and copper levels in white-tailed deer near uranium mines in Texas. J. Wildlife Manag. 48 (1), 267–270.

Ladefoged, O., Sturup, S., 1995. Copper deficiency in cattle, sheep, and horses caused by excess molybdenum. Vet. Hum. Tocicol. 37, 63.

Lesperance, A.L., Bohman, V.R., Oldfield, J.E., 1985. Interactions of molybdenum, sulfate, and alfalfa in the bovine. J. Anim. Sci. 60, 791–802.

Mason, J., Cardin, C.J., 1977. The competition of molybdate and sulfate ions for a transport system in the ovine small intestine. Res. Vet. Sci. 22, 313–315.

Miller, J.K., Moss, B.R., Bell, M.C., et al., 1972. Comparison of Mo^{99} metabolism in young cattle and swine. J. Anim. Sci. 34, 846–850.

Mills, C.F., Bremner, I., 1980. Nutritional aspects of molybdenum in animals and man. In: Coughlan, M.P. (Ed.), Molybdenum and Molybdenum Containing Enzymes. Pergamon, Oxford, pp. 517–542.

Mills, C.F., Davis, G.K., 1987. Molybdenum. In: Mertz, W. (Ed.), Trace Elements in Human and Animal Nutrition, fifth ed. Academic Press, New York, pp. 429–465.

National Research Council (NRC), 2006. Molybdenum, Mineral Tolerance of Animals. second ed. National Academies Press, Washington, DC, pp. 262–275.

Nell, J.A., Annison, E.F., Balnave, D., 1980. The influence of tungsten on the molybdenum status of poultry. Br. Poult. Sci. 21, 193–202.

Nielsen, F.H., 1996. Other trace elements. In: Ziegler, E.E., Filer, L.J. (Eds.), Present Knowledge in Nutrition, seventh ed. International Life Science Institute Press, Washington, DC, pp. 353–377.

Pitt, M., Fraser, J., Thurley, D.C., 1980. Molybdenum toxicosis in sheep: epiphysiolysis, exostoses and biochemical changes. J. Comp. Path. 90, 567–576.

Pitt, M.A., 1976. Molybdenum toxicity: interactions between copper, molybdenum, and sulfate. Agent Action. 6, 758–769.

Pott, E.B., Henry, P.R., Zanetti, M.A., et al., 1999. Effects of high dietary molybdenum concentration and duration of feeding time on molybdenum and copper metabolism in sheep. Anim. Feed Sci. Technol. 79, 93.

Price, J., Will, A.M., Paschaleris, G., et al., 1987. Identification of thiomolybdates in digesta and plasma from sheep after administration of Mo99-labeled compounds into the rumen. Br. J. Nutr. 58, 127–138.

Rajagopalan, K.V., 1988. Molybdenum: an essential trace element in human nutrition. Ann. Rev. Nutr. 8, 401–427.

Reiss, J., 2000. Genetics of molybdenum cofactor deficiency. Hum. Genet. 106, 157–163.

Rosman, K.J.R., Taylor, P.D.P., 1998. Isotopic composition of the elements 1997. Pure Appl. Chem. 70, 217–235.

Schroeder, H.A., Balassa, J.J., Tipton, I.H., 1970. Essential trace metals in man: molybdenum. J. Chron. Dis. 23, 481–499.

Spears, J.W., 2003. Trace mineral bioavailability in ruminants. J. Nutr. 133, 1506S–1509S.

Suttle, N.F., 1991. The interactions between copper, molybdenum, and sulfur in ruminant nutrition. Annu. Rev. Nutr. 11, 121–140.

Swan, D.A., Creeper, J.H., White, C.L., et al., 1998. Molybdenum poisoning in feedlot cattle. Aust. Vet. J. 76, 345–349.

Thompson, L.J., Hall, J.O., Meerdink, G.L., 1991. Toxic effects of trace element excess. Vet. Clin. N. Am. Food Anim. Pract. 7, 277–306.

Turnlund, J.R., Keyes, W.R., Peiffer, G.L., et al., 1995. Molybdenum absorption, excretion, and retention studied with stable isotopes in young men during depletion and repletion. Am. J. Clin. Nutr. 61, 1102–1109.

Underwood, E.J., 1977. Molybdenum. In: Underwood, E.J. (Ed.), Trace Elements in Human and Animal Nutrition, fourth ed. Academic Press, New York, pp. 429–465.

Venugopal, B., Luckey, T.D., 1978. Molybdenum. Metal Toxicity in Mammals 2: Chemical Toxicity of Metals and Metalloids. Plenum Press, New York, pp. 253–257.

Versieck, J., Hoste, J., Vanballengerghe, L., et al., 1981. Serum molybdenum in diseases of the liver and biliary system. J. Lab. Clin. Med. 97, 535–544.

Vyskocil, A., Viau, C., 1999. Assessment of molybdenum toxicity in humans. J. Appl. Toxicol. 19, 185–192.

Ward, G.M., 1978. Molybdenum toxicity and hypocuprosis in ruminants: a review. J. Anim. Sci. 46, 1078–1085.

Williams, R.J.P., daSilva, J.J.R.F., 2002. The involvement of molybdenum in life. Biochem. Biophys. Res. Comm. 292, 293–299.

Chapter 33

Selenium

Jeffery O. Hall

INTRODUCTION

Selenium is an essential nutrient that has a relatively narrow window between ingested amounts that result in deficiencies and those that cause toxicoses. Historically, occurrences of livestock disease that mimic clinical presentation of chronic selenium poisoning were recorded in the 13th century (Martin, 1973). Marco Polo wrote of such cases in western China in 1295. In 1560, Father Simon Pedro described human cases of presumably chronic selenosis in Columbia (Benavides and Mojica, 1965). The first documented record of selenium poisoning in livestock was reported in 1860 by a US Army surgeon (Martin, 1973). T.W. Madison described a fatal disease of horses that grazed near Fort Randall, South Dakota. It also has been speculated that the horse illness that slowed General Custer's Cavalry relief may have been due to selenium, but chronic selenosis generally takes weeks to develop.

Selenium deficiency had been historically linked to a variety of clinical effects. Since 1949, vitamin E, cysteine and a "factor 3" were known to protect rats from fatal liver necrosis (Schwarz and Foltz, 1957). When rats were fed torula, a brewer's yeast, they developed liver necrosis that could be avoided by use of baker's yeast (*Saccharomyces* sp.). It was postulated that "factor 3," an essential nutrient, was deficient in torula. After much research, the active, preventive element present in "factor 3" was identified as selenium. Several metabolic diseases of previously unknown origin were later found to relate to selenium deficiency, including "white muscle disease" in calves and lambs (Muth et al., 1958; Godwin and Fraser, 1966), hepatosis dietetica in pigs (Eggert et al., 1957), exudative diathesis in poultry (Patterson et al., 1957), and pancreatic degeneration in poultry (Thompson and Scott, 1969).

Since its first discovery as an essential nutrient, selenium has been found to act in numerous body systems. In 1973, Se was identified as an essential component of glutathione peroxidase (GSH) enzyme (Flohe et al., 1973; Rotruck et al., 1973). Selenium was shown to be essential in humans when added dietary selenium prevented a cardiomyopathy known as "Keshan disease" (Chen, 1986). Selenium supplementation may also be protective against certain types of cancer (Combs, 1997), cardiovascular disease (Duthie et al., 1989) and viral infections (Schrauzer, 1994; Levander, 2000). Because of the essential nature of selenium, poisoning cases from both natural plant accumulations of selenium and nutritional overdoses are encountered.

The identified essential functions of selenium are still increasing. The most notable is GSH, where selenocysteine is a required component of the enzyme system (Brown and Arthur, 2001). Reduced GSH is the primary physiologic first defense against free radical damage to tissues, helping to maintain functional membrane integrity. Several subclasses of GSH are now recognized (Cohen and Avissar, 1994; Sunde, 1994). To date, more than 30 selenoproteins have been identified, many of which have vital enzymatic functions (Tiwary, 2004). Thioredoxin reductase I, II, and III (Brown and Arthur, 2001), 5′ triiodothyronine deiodinase (Arthur and Beckett, 1994) and "selenoprotein" are also selenium dependent. In addition, selenium plays several roles in normal immune function, reproductive function, hepatic biotransformation reactions, neurotransmitter turnover, and anticarcinogenic functions.

BACKGROUND

Selenium is a member of the nonmetallic elements within group VIa of the periodic table. It has an atomic number of 34, an atomic weight of 78.96, and has six different naturally occurring stable isotopic masses from 74 to 82 (Rosman and Taylor, 1997). Selenium has four natural oxidation states: −2 (selenides), 0 (elemental), +4 (selenites), and +6 (selenates) (Barceloux, 1999). Selenium was first identified in 1817 by Jons Jakob Berzelius, a Swedish chemist, who investigated worker illnesses in a sulfuric acid plant at Gripsholm, Sweden (Fredga, 1972).

Veterinary Toxicology. DOI: http://dx.doi.org/10.1016/B978-0-12-811410-0.00033-7

He named this element after "Selene," the green moon goddess.

Many areas within the northern Great Plains of the United States, such as the Dakotas, eastern Wyoming, eastern Montana, eastern Colorado, western Nebraska, and western Kansas, have high soil selenium content (4–5 ppm selenium or more), resulting in high plant uptake and subsequent Se toxicosis in herbivores (Rosenfeld and Beath, 1964). High soil selenium also occurs in alkaline soils of some localities in Algeria, Argentina, Australia, Bulgaria, Canada, China, Columbia, Ireland, Israel, Mexico, Morocco, New Zealand, South Africa, the former Soviet Union, Spain, and Venezuela (NRC, 1983). However, total soil selenium is not the best indicator of potential selenium poisonings, as Hawaii and Puerto Rico have areas of high soil selenium that is not available to the plants due to the acidic soil types, which result in lowered water solubility and bioavailable selenium for plant uptake (Lakin, 1961).

Inorganic forms of selenium are the primary form in soil. Only the water soluble forms are readily available for plant uptake, with the greatest absorption being in the form of selenate via the sulfate transporter. Elemental selenium and precipitated metal-selenides are not bioavailable for plant uptake. Some "indicator plants" or "obligatory selenium accumulator plants" can accumulate several thousand ppm selenium and are often found in selenium-rich areas, since they require high selenium for growth (Rosenfeld and Beath, 1964). These plants include genera such as *Astragalus* (milk vetch), *Xylorhiza*, *Machaeranthera* (woody aster), *Haplopappus* (golden weed)—formerly known as *Oonopsis*, and *Stanleya* (prince's plume). Selenium content as high as 14,990 ppm have been reported for a sample of *Astragalus racemosus* (Beath, 1937). Although these indicator plants have poor palatability, during times of limited forage, they are eaten. Secondary or facultative accumulating plants can survive with high selenium content, but do not require it for growth. These plants are often more palatable than the indicator plants and include *Aster*, *Atriplex* (salt bush), *Castilleja* (paintbrush), *Gutierrezia* (snakeweed), *Grindelia* (gumweeds), *Sideranthus* (ironweed), *Eurotia* (winter fat), *Mentzelia*, *Machaeranthera*, and *Gyria* sp. as well as some crop plants such as western wheat grass, barley, wheat, alfalfa, onions, and Swiss chard (Beath et al., 1935; Williams and Byers, 1936). It should be noted that studies on ingestion of high selenium forages has found that as concentrations increase there appears to be an aversion to consumption in cattle and sheep, but that initial consumption may not be affected (Pfister et al., 2014).

Most of the selenium in nonindicator plants and other biological matrices is in an organic form, but small amounts of inorganic selenate and selenite can also be present. The vast majority of plant selenium, especially in nonindicator plants, is in the form of selenomethionine, but selenocysteine and a variety of other seleno-amino acid derivatives can also be found (Peterson and Butler, 1962; Olson et al., 1970; Whanger, 2002). In contrast, the majority of selenium in indicator plants, such as *Astragalus*, is a water soluble Se-methyl-selenocysteine (Shrift, 1973), but can also have selenocystathionine (Lewis, 1976). Garlic was found to contain significant selenomethionine as well as glutamyl-Se-methyl-selenocysteine and possibly gamma-glutamyl-selenomethionine (Kotrebai et al., 1999). The nonprotein associated selenium compounds may be a protective mechanism of the plants to prevent excessive replacement of methionine or other sulfur-containing amino acids with seleno-amino acids in plant proteins resulting in loss of disulfide bonds, misfolding and altered protein properties (Peterson and Butler, 1962). Some microbial populations, as well as plants, can reduce selenium to volatile chemical forms (Shrift, 1973).

PHARMACOKINETICS/TOXICOKINETICS

Absorption

The majority of ingested selenium compounds are absorbed from the duodenum, with lesser amounts in the jejunum and ileum (Wright and Bell, 1966; Whanger et al., 1976). Little to no absorption reportedly occurs from the stomach and rumen. However, one report suggests that minimal absorption of selenomethionine occurs through the rumen wall and into the blood (Hidiroglou and Jenkins, 1973).

The chemical form of selenium greatly impacts the overall absorption. Selenite absorption is via passive diffusion through the brush-border membranes (Vendeland et al., 1992, 1994). In contrast, selenate has little affinity for the brush-border membranes. Selenate is absorbed via a sodium cotransport system that is also utilized by sulfate (Wolffram et al., 1988). Selenium in the form of seleno-amino acids, selenomethionine and selenocysteine, are absorbed through active amino acid transport mechanisms and are more bioavailable than selenite or selenate (McConnell and Cho, 1967; Ammerman and Miller, 1974; Vendeland et al., 1994). The selenium status did not affect overall absorption, indicating that absorption was not under homeostatic regulation.

In monogastrics, the relative selenium absorption is greater than in ruminants, ranging from 45% to 95% (Thomson and Stewart, 1974; Furchner et al., 1975; Bopp et al., 1982). And organic forms of selenium are better absorbed (Robinson et al., 1978). In ruminants, the relative absorption ranges from 29% to 50% (Wright and Bell, 1966; Suttle and Jones, 1989). The decreased absorption in ruminants is due to microbial reduction of selenium forms in the rumen to selenides and elemental selenium, which are not bioavailable (Cousins and Cairney, 1961; Whanger et al., 1968; Peter et al., 1982). This reduction in bioavailability is generally exacerbated by high carbohydrate diets but can be altered by differing rumen microbial populations (Hudman and Glenn, 1984; Koenig et al., 1997). Some rumen microbes more efficiently reduce selenium, while others effectively incorporate it into selenium-containing amino acids. The incorporation of selenium into microbial proteins as well as systemic absorption, can be competitively inhibited by natural methionine and cysteine (Serra et al., 1996).

Distribution

Tissue distribution is dependent on the chemical form of selenium absorbed. Selenium is generally utilized for synthesis of selenoproteins, incorporated into tissue proteins or eliminated. Selenomethionine can be nonspecifically incorporated into tissue proteins in place of methionine (Awadeh et al., 1998), but selenocysteine cannot (Burk et al., 2001), with highest incorporation occurring in tissues with high rates of protein synthesis (Hansson and Jacobsson, 1966). The nonspecific incorporation of selenomethionine effectively serves as a pool of selenium reserve with a long biological half-life (Schroeder and Mitchener, 1972a). Highest total selenium content is typically found in the kidney and liver, with lesser amounts in all other tissues (Muth et al., 1967; Levander, 1987; Echevarria et al., 1988; Davidson and Kennedy, 1993). Both specific and nonspecific selenium incorporation into proteins was greater in selenium-deficient animals.

Time to peak tissue concentrations is tissue dependent. Peak selenium content of blood, liver, muscle, kidney, spleen, and lung was reached within 24 h after an injection of ^{75}Se as selenite (Muth et al., 1967). Peak serum and blood concentrations in sheep were achieved in 12 h or fewer for selenate, selenium from western aster, selenomethionine, and methylselenocysteine (Davis et al., 2011). In contrast, brain, thymus, and reproductive organs do not reach maximal content until much later (Brown and Burk, 1973; McConnell et al., 1979; Smith et al., 1979; Behne et al., 1988). Peak hair accumulation of selenium in poisoned steers was reached at 22 days pot-exposure (Davis et al., 2012).

Selenium is efficiently transferred across the placenta into feti during gestation. The overall maternal selenium content is positively correlated with fetal and newborn selenium status (McConnell and Roth, 1964). Although they get the vast majority of selenium in utero, newborns do get minimal amounts of selenium from milk, with much higher content in colostrums than in milk later in lactation.

Metabolism

Selenite is metabolized in red blood cells to hydrogen selenide (Gasiewicz and Smith, 1978). Sequential methylation reactions result in the formation of monomethylselenide, dimethylselenide and trimethylselenide (Kajander et al., 1991; Itoh and Suzuki, 1997). These reactions utilize *S*-adenosylmethionine for methyl groups that are transferred by methyltransferases (Kajander et al., 1991). These sequential reactions can deplete available *S*-adenosylmethionine, which would limit the degree of methylation. In rats given selenomethionine, trimethylselenide occurred in the urine more rapidly than in rats given sodium selenite or selenocysteine, indicating that selenomethionine may be converted to methylselenol, which is easily further methylated.

Selenomethionine is metabolized by demethylation to selenocysteine. This set of pathways is similar to the metabolism of methionine. The selenocysteine is then metabolized by selenocysteine-beta-lyase in the liver and kidney to alanine and selenide (Soda et al., 1987).

Elimination

Selenium is primarily excreted in the urine and feces, but the form and extent of elimination by different routes are dose and species dependent. In monogastric animals, urinary elimination predominates, irrespective of the route of exposure (Leng et al., 2000), with less than 10% recovered in feces (Burk et al., 1972). Some literature suggests that urinary eliminated selenium is predominantly metabolites of selenium, with trimethylselenide predominating at higher doses (McConnell and Roth, 1966; Palmer et al., 1969; Zeisel et al., 1987; Itoh and Suzuki, 1997), but monomethylselenide is more abundant at lower doses. Human elimination is tri-exponential for selenite and selenomethionine (Alexander et al., 1987). The terminal elimination phase was 8–20 and 230 days for selenite and selenomethionine, respectively. Overall selenium retention and maintenance of adequate seleno-enzymes are for much longer time periods in animals supplemented with selenomethionine than selenite. Elimination rate is dose dependent, with half-lives of 19.5 and 1.2 days with selenite of 0.1 and 1.0 ppm in the diet, respectively (Burk et al., 1972). Elimination rates in sheep also differ significantly depending on the chemical form of selenium ingested (Davis et al., 2011). Individual tissue elimination rates were found to be different in steers that ingested selenium accumulator plants at a mine contamination site, with serum and liver having terminal elimination half-lives of 40.5 and 38.2 days while whole blood and skeletal muscle had half-lives of 115.6 and 98.5 days (Davis et al., 2012). The longer elimination half-lives for whole blood and skeletal muscle likely represent red blood cell turnover rates and protein turnover rates for muscle tissue.

Due to nonspecific protein incorporation of selenomethionine, urinary and fecal recovery after dosing was less than 30% of that for equal selenium doses from selenite or selenate (Thomson, 1998).

The literature suggests that the predominant selenium elimination in ruminants is fecal when ingested, but urinary with parenteral administration or in nonruminating young animals. This is actually an error in terminology, as the fecal loss of selenium is primarily in the form of elemental selenium and precipitated selenides from ruminal reduction (Langlands et al., 1986). Thus, this selenium is nonabsorbed material and is not truly being eliminated from the central compartment. However, a small amount of metabolized selenium excesses is excreted in the bile (Cousins and Cairney, 1961). The selenium metabolites eliminated in the urine follow a similar pattern to that seen with monogastrics. Urinary elimination is predominant with parenteral administrations and in nonruminating young animals (NRC, 1983).

Renal selenium elimination is dependent of glomerular filtration and degree of reabsorption. Increasing renal fluid absorption did not increase the selenium content in urine, indicating a tubular reabsorptive process (Oster and Prellwitz, 1990). Thus, dehydration or renal insufficiency would decrease rates of elimination. Excretion and renal clearance rates correlate with creatinine, indicating glomerular filtration is the mechanism of elimination.

Some selenium is eliminated via respired air, but the relative importance of this route is dose dependent. At normal intake, only about 10% or less is eliminated from the respiratory tract (Burk et al., 1972), but as dose increases the percent eliminated in respired air increases (Jacobsson, 1966; McConnell and Roth, 1966). Dimethylselenide and dimethyldiselenide are the predominant forms eliminated in respired air at toxic doses. Dimethylselenide predominates when mice were dosed with selenite or selenocysteine, while dimethyldiselenide is most abundant when rats were dosed with selenomethionine. Respiratory elimination is primary when renal elimination thresholds are maximized, which results in most respiratory elimination occurring in a short-time period soon after exposure to toxic doses (McConnell and Roth, 1966; Tiwary et al., 2005).

MECHANISM OF ACTION

Although much research has been conducted with regard to selenium poisoning, the exact mechanism of the toxic effects in the body are still not clear. With acute poisoning, one theory is the depletion of intermediate substrates, such as glutathione and *S*-adenosylmethionine, which disturbs their respective enzyme activities (Vernie et al., 1978). Another potentially interactive theory is the production of free radicals by the reaction of selenium with thiols, causing subsequent oxidative tissue damage (Hoffman, 2002; Kaur et al., 2003; Balogh et al., 2004). A third theory is the incorporation of selenium compounds in place of sulfur, such as in proteins, in which it disrupts normal cellular functions (Raisbeck, 2000). This is an especially likely mechanism for the hair and hoof lesions of chronic selenium poisoning, with the loss of disulfide bridges that provide structural integrity to these tissues. This would also apply to inhibition of DNA methylation by *S*-adenosylmethionine or indirect inhibition by increased *S*-adenosyl homocysteine content (Hoffman, 1977). And, it is possible that each of these proposed mechanisms is valid with respect to specific chemical forms of selenium. It has been observed that tissues requiring selenium to prevent deficiency-associated disease (immune system, reproductive organs and muscular tissues) also tend to accumulate more selenium with excess exposure and are the primary tissues of toxic effects.

TOXICITY

Selenium poisoning cases generally fall into three types of exposure history. The first is from ingestion of selenium in plants that have accumulated it from naturally seleniferous soils. The second is from accidental overdoses by injection or errors in feed mixing. And the third is from environmental contamination, which often results in exposure from plant accumulation and/or contaminated waters. With each of these types of poisonings, one may see acute, subacute or chronic selenium poisoning, depending upon the daily exposure rate. However, one must understand that an animal's age plays a role in susceptibility to selenium poisoning, as young animals are less tolerant than adults (Raisbeck, 2000).

Doses for acute selenium toxicosis vary significantly across species, but also by route of exposure, with injectable routes of exposure being more toxic than oral. Acute oral selenium poisoning occurs with sudden exposure ranging from 2.2 mg/kg (Rosenfeld and Beath, 1964) to greater than 20 mg/kg body weight (Miller and Williams, 1940; Mahan and Moxon, 1984) across species. The relative oral acute toxicity of selenium-containing compounds is dependent on their solubility, with poorly soluble selenides and elemental selenium being much less toxic than soluble selenates, selenites and organic selenium (NRC, 2005). Minimum lethal dose for rabbits, rats, dogs and cats is 1.5–3 mg/kg body weight (NRC, 1983). The LD_{50} for oral selenite has been estimated to be 1.9–8.3 mg/kg body weight in ruminants (Grace, 1994), but other references suggest it to be 9–20 mg/kg body weight (Puls, 1994). In poultry, the acute oral LD_{50} of selenium is 33 mg/kg body weight. Injectable selenium is more acutely toxic than oral, with intramuscular LD_{50} of 0.5 mg/kg in lambs (Caravaggi et al., 1970).

Subcutaneous LD_{50} of selenium is 1 mg/kg in lambs and 1.9 mg/kg in adult cattle (Grace, 1994). In 2009, 21 horses from Venezuela that were in Florida for an international polo match died from selenium overdose (Florida Department of Agriculture and Consumer Services, 2009; Desta et al., 2011). The selenium was misformulated in a compounded intravenous vitamin-mineral product, resulting in a 100 fold overdose and an IV selenium exposure of 4–5 mg/kg BW. The horses developed clinical signs within hours of the administration and died within 3–18 h.

Clinical manifestation of acute selenium poisoning begins as early as 8–10 h, but can be delayed for up to 36 h (Franke and Moxon, 1936; NRC, 1983; Raisbeck, 2000; Tiwary et al., 2006; Davis et al., 2012). Onset as early as 1.5 h occurred with IV exposure (Desta et al., 2011). Early in the clinical syndrome, one can detect the garlicky smell of dimethylselenide on the breath. Clinical signs that follow include respiratory distress, restlessness or lethargy, head down, droopy ears, anorexia, gaunt appearance, salivation, watery diarrhea, fever, sweating, tachycardia, teeth grinding, stilted gait, tetanic spasms, and/or death. Clinical signs tend to progress quickly after they are first observed. Gross and histologic lesions include systemic congestion, pulmonary edema, skeletal muscle necrosis, myocardial necrosis, and petechial hemorrhages in and on the myocardium.

"Blind staggers" has historically been associated with subacute to chronic selenium poisoning. However, this association was due to its occurrence in known seleniferous areas. The areas with seleniferous soils also tend to have highly alkaline soils with high potential for excessive sulfur exposure. It has been stated that blind staggers cannot be reproduced with pure selenium compounds alone and likely involves other factors, such as alkaloid poisoning, starvation or polioencephalomalasia (O'Toole and Raisbeck, 1995). However, one can still find references that tie it to selenium (Underwood and Suttle, 1999; NRC, 2005).

Chronic selenosis, often referred to as "alkali disease," is the result of long-term ingestion of seleniferous forages (NRC, 1983, 2005; Raisbeck, 2000). High selenium intake is generally for greater than 30 days and, due to plant selenium content, is usually associated with facultative accumulators, not indicator plants, although chronic selenosis can also be reproduced by long-term feeding of high inorganic selenium (Kaur et al., 2003). Calves were chronically poisoned with selenite at 0.25 mg/kg body weight daily for 16 weeks. In a similar study in yearlings, selenium as selenite at 0.8 mg/kg/day and as selenomethionine at 0.28 mg/kg/day resulted in alkali disease (O'Toole and Raisbeck, 1995). However, other studies did not produce alkali disease with selenium doses as high as 11.9 mg/kg of diet in feeders or 118 mg/kg body weight daily for 128 days in dairy cows (Ellis et al., 1997; Lawler et al., 2004). Differences in susceptibility to chronic selenium poisoning may be a product of historical exposure, variability in rumen microbial population and/or age-associated susceptibility. As stated previously, certain microbes can reduce selenium to nonbioavailable forms, resulting in decreased systemic absorption. Pigs develop chronic selenosis with exposure to selenium as low as 8 mg/kg of diet (Goehring et al., 1984; Mahan and Magee, 1991; Stowe and Herdt, 1992). And horses exposed to 20 mg Se/kg DM for 3 weeks developed lesions (Stowe and Herdt, 1992).

Clinical signs of chronic selenosis include depression, weakness, emaciation, anemia, hair loss, hoof abnormalities, anorexia, diarrhea, weight loss, lameness, reproductive failure, and death (Rosenfeld and Beath, 1964; O'Toole and Raisbeck, 1995; Underwood and Suttle, 1999; Raisbeck, 2000; Davis et al., 2014; Davis, 2016). Hoof wall abnormalities are frequently identified in cattle, horses and pigs, and include swelling of the coronary band, hoof deformities and/or separation and sloughing of the hoof wall. Hair loss from the base of the tail and switch in cattle, horses and mules is sometimes referred to as "bobtail disease." Interestingly, sheep do not develop the alopecia or hoof lesions that are seen in cattle, but they have decreased wool growth rates. In pigs, goats and horses, there may be a general alopecia (Franke, 1934). Pigs also develop neurologic signs of paralysis (Goehring et al., 1984).

Pathologic lesions of chronic selenium poisoning are generally related to hoof lesions and to the effects of starvation (Raisbeck, 2000). Lesions of nephritis, hepatic cirrhosis, and myocardial necrosis can be expected. In pigs, bilateral malacia of the gray matter in the spinal cord can be seen.

Reproductive abnormalities are seen (Davis and Hall, 2017; Davis, 2016) in several species when excessive selenium is ingested. Field reports indicate that reproductive performance can be reduced without the other typical signs of alkali disease at 5–10 ppm Se in diet (Olson et al., 1970), but direct experimental evidence in large animals has been lacking (Raisbeck, 2000). A recent set of studies found failure of conception occurred in ewes fed 10 and 30 ppm plant origin selenium, while abnormal sperm and sperm motility occurred in rams fed 25 ppm plant origin selenium (Davis, 2016). Decreased conception rate and an increased fetal resorption rate in cattle, sheep and horses were observed when they were fed natural diets containing 20–50 mg Se/kg diet (Harr and Muth, 1972). Both rats exposed to 3 ppm Se as seleniferous wheat (Musnell et al., 1936) and mice exposed to 3 ppm selenate in their drinking water (Schroeder and Mitchener, 1972b) had abnormally low rates of conception. Both deficiencies and excesses of selenium have been shown to adversely affect spermatogenesis, motility and viability in rodent models (Kaur and Bansal, 2005; Shalini and Bansal, 2007, 2005; Boitani and Puglisi, 2008). If other species have similar effects, this could negatively affect herd reproductive performance. In addition, it must be noted that Se accumulates in the fetus at the expense of the dam (Puls, 1994). Thus, higher accumulation of selenium in the fetus may result in abortions, stillbirths or weak/lethargic calves. Yeager et al. (1998) reported a 7% abortion rate in a beef herd where cows had selenium concentrations suggestive of chronic selenosis and fetal hepatic selenium concentrations suggestive of toxicosis, but in a dosing study they only had one weak calf born that died shortly after birth. Although teratogenic effects of selenium poisoning are well documented in avian species, historical reports are all that are available for horses and sheep (Smith et al., 1936; Beath et al., 1939). However, toxic plants in the environment may have also played roles. At least some of the adverse effects on reproduction caused by excess selenium in ruminants are caused by interference with absorption and retention of copper that results in copper deficiency.

Selenosis in poultry and other avian species has major effects in reproduction. Poor hatchability, embryonic deformities and embryonic death are common sequelae to selenium poisoning (Hoffman, 2002; Latshaw et al., 2004; Hamilton, 2004).

TREATMENT

The most effective treatment is to prevent excessive exposure. Although the maximal tolerable level for selenium was once set at 2 mg/kg of diet per day for all species, this has now been changed to 5 mg/kg of diet per day for ruminants (NRC, 2005). It is stated that this new tolerance for ruminants is appropriate for horses as well. Swine have a maximum tolerance level of 4 mg/kg of diet, for poultry it is set at 3 mg/kg of diet, and for fish it is set at 2 mg/kg of diet.

As there is no specific mechanism of chelation and removal of selenium in animals, the primary treatment protocol is of supportive care with both acute and chronic selenium poisoning. With chronic poisoning, it is important to understand the long-term commitment necessary to allow an animal with hoof lesions time to regrow the hoof wall once exposure has been stopped. Especially with organic selenium's incorporation into body proteins, the time necessary to just decrease the body load of selenium, once excessive exposure has stopped, is quite long.

CONCLUDING REMARKS AND FUTURE DIRECTIONS

Selenium deficiency and toxicity are problems that veterinarians, nutritionists, and animal owners need to understand. The small difference between deficiency and toxicity in terms of dietary intake makes the risk of accidental selenium poisoning high. Many areas of the world have seleniferous soils that can cause poisoning via ingestion of natural forages grown on them. As there is no specific treatment for selenium toxicosis, it is critical that appropriate education be utilized in order to minimize the risks to the livestock industry.

Future research needs to address the mechanisms of physiologic damage caused by both acute and chronic selenium poisoning with differing chemical forms of selenium. With an understanding of the cellular mechanisms of selenium poisoning, more specific means of treatment might be developed. In addition, a clearer understanding of thresholds for chronic selenium poisoning is needed. With the knowledge that certain ruminal microbes can reduce various forms of selenium to nonabsorbable forms, preventive use of these microbes in seleniferous areas to prevent systemic accumulation and poisonings should be investigated.

REFERENCES

Alexander, J., Hogberg, J., Thomassen, Y., et al., 1987. Selenium. In: Seiler, H.G. (Ed.), Handbook on Toxicity of Inorganic Compounds. Marcel Dekker, New York, p. 585.

Ammerman, C.B., Miller, S.M., 1974. Selenium in ruminant nutrition: a review. J. Dairy Sci. 58, 1561–1576.

Arthur, J.R., Beckett, G.J., 1994. New metabolic roles for selenium. Proc. Nutr. Soc. 53, 615–624.

Awadeh, F.T., Rahman, A., Kincaid, R.L., et al., 1998. Effect of selenium supplements on the distribution of selenium among serum proteins in cattle. J. Dairy Sci. 81, 1089–1094.

Balogh, K., Weber, M., Erdelyi, M., et al., 2004. Effects of excess selenium supplementation on the glutathione redox system in broiler chickens. Acta Vet. Hung. 52, 403–411.

Barceloux, D.G., 1999. Selenium. Clin. Toxicol. 37, 145–172.

Beath, O.A., 1937. The occurrence of selenium and seleniferous vegetation in Wyoming. II. Seleniferous vegetation. Wyo. Agric. Exp. Sta Bull. Laramie, WY. 221, 29–64.

Beath, O.A., Eppson, H.F., Gilbert, C.S., 1935. Selenium and other toxic minerals in soils and vegetation. Wyo. Agric. Exp. Sta Bull. Laramie, WY. 206, 1–55.

Beath, O.A., Eppson, H.F., Gilbert, C.S., et al., 1939. Poisonous plants and livestock poisoning. Wyo. Agric. Exp. Sta Bull. 231, 1–104.

Behne, D., Hillmert, H., Scheid, S., et al., 1988. Evidence for specific target tissues and new biologically important SelP. Biochim. Biophys. Acta. 966, 12–21.

Benavides, S.T., Mojica, F.S., 1965. Selenosis, 2nd edn. Instituto Geografico Augustin Codazzi, Bogota, Columbia.

Boitani, C., Puglisi, R., 2008. Selenium, a key element in spermatogenesis and male fertility. In: Cheng, C.Y. (Ed.), Molecular Mechanisms in Spermatogenesis. Landes Bioscience and Springer Science Business, Austin, Texas, pp. 65–73.

Bopp, B.A., Sonders, R.C., Kesterson, J.W., 1982. Metabolic fate of selected selenium compounds in laboratory animals and man. Drug Metab. Rev. 13, 271–318.

Brown, D.G., Burk, R.F., 1973. Selenium retention in tissues and sperm of rats fed a torula yeast diet. J. Nutr. 103, 102–108.

Brown, K.M., Arthur, J.R., 2001. Selenium, selenoproteins and human health: a review. Public Health Nutr. 4, 593–599.

Burk, R.F., Brown, D.G., Seely, R.J., et al., 1972. Influence of dietary and injected selenium on whole-body retention, route of excretion, and tissue retention of 75SeO322 in the rat. J. Nutr. 102, 1049–1055.

Burk, R.F., Hill, K.E., Motley, A.K., 2001. Plasma selenium in specific and non-specific forms. Biofactor 14, 107–114.

Caravaggi, C., Clark, F.L., Jackson, A.R.B., 1970. Acute selenium toxicity in lambs following intramuscular injection of sodium selenite. Res. Vet. Sci. 11, 146–149.

Chen, X., 1986. Selenium and cardiomyopathy (Keshan disease). Acta Pharmacol. Toxicol. 59, 325–330.

Cohen, H.J., Avissar, N., 1994. Extracellular glutathione peroxidase: a distinct selenoprotein. In: Burk, R.F. (Ed.), Selenium in Biology and Human Health. Springer-Verlag, New York, pp. 79–92.

Combs, G.F., 1997. Selenium and cancer prevention. In: Garewal, H.A. (Ed.), Antioxidants and Disease Prevention. CRC Press, New York, pp. 97–113.

Cousins, F.B., Cairney, I.M., 1961. Some aspects of selenium metabolism in sheep. Aust. J. Agric. Res. 12, 927–933.

Davidson, W.B., Kennedy, D.G., 1993. Synthesis of [75Se] selenoproteins is greater in selenium-deficient sheep. J. Nutr. 123, 689–694.

Davis, Z., 2016. Effects of high selenium forage on reproduction in sheep. Abstract 1771. Joint Annual Meeting American Society of Animal Science. Salt Lake City, UT.

Davis, T.Z., Hall, J.O., 2017. Selenium. In: Gupta, R.C. (Ed.), Reproductive and Development Toxicology, second ed. Academic Press/Elsevier, New York, pp. 595–605.

Davis, T.Z., Stegelmeier, B.L., Green, B.T., et al., 2011. Acute toxicity of selenium compounds commonly found in selenium accumulator plants. In: Riet-Correa, F., Pfister, J., Schild, A.L., Wierenga, T. (Eds.), Poisonings by Plants, Mycotoxins, and Related Toxins. CAB International, Cambridge, MA, pp. 525–531.

Davis, T.Z., Stegelmeier, B.L., Panter, K.E., et al., 2012. Toxicokinetics and pathology of plant-associated selenium toxicosis in steers. J. Vet. Diag. Inv. 24 (2), 319–327.

Davis, T.Z., Stegelmeier, B.L., Hall, J.O., 2014. Analysis of horse hair as a means of evaluating selenium toxicosis and long term exposure. J. Agri. Food Chem. 62, 7393–7397.

Desta, B., Maldonado, G., Reid, H., et al., 2011. Acute selenium toxicosis in polo ponies. J. Vet. Diagn. Invest. 23 (3), 623–628.

Duthie, G.G., Wahle, K.W.J., James, W.P.J., 1989. Oxidants, antioxidants and cardiovascular disease. Nutr. Res. Rev. 2, 51–62.

Echevarria, M., Henry, P.R., Ammerman, C.B., et al., 1988. Effects of time and dietary selenium concentration as sodium selenite on tissue selenium uptake by sheep. J. Anim. Sci. 66, 2299–2305.

Eggert, R.O., Patterson, E., Akers, W.J., et al., 1957. The role of vitamin E and selenium in the nutrition of the pig. J. Anim. Sci. 16, 1037–1045.

Ellis, R.G., Herdt, T.H., Stowe, H.D., 1997. Physical, hematologic, biochemical, and immunological effects of supranutritional supplementation with dietary selenium in Holstein cows. Am. J. Vet. Res. 58, 760–764.

Flohe, L., Gunzler, W.A., Shock, H.H., 1973. Glutathione peroxidase: a selenoenzyme. FEBS Lett. 32, 132–134.

Florida Department of Agriculture and Consumer Services. Polo horses likely died from selenium overdose. http://www.doacs.state.fl.us/press/2009/04282009.html. April 2009.

Franke, K.W., 1934. A new toxicant occurring naturally in certain samples of plant foodstuffs. I. Results obtained in preliminary feeding trials. J. Nutr. 8, 597–608.

Franke, K.W., Moxon, A.L., 1936. A comparison of the minimum fatal doses of selenium, tellurium, arsenic, and vanadium. J. Pharm. Exptl. Therap. 58, 454–459.

Fredga, A., 1972. Organic selenium chemistry. Ann. NY Acad. Sci. 192, 1–9.

Furchner, J.E., London, J.E., Wilson, J.S., 1975. Comparative metabolism of radionuclides in mammals – IX. Retention of 75Se in the mouse, rat, monkey and dog. Health Phys. 29, 641–648.

Gasiewicz, T.A., Smith, J.C., 1978. The metabolism of selenite by intact rat erythrocytes in vitro. Chem. Biol. Interact. 21, 299–313.

Godwin, K.O., Fraser, F.J., 1966. Abnormal electrocardiograms, blood pressure changes, and some aspects of the histopathology of selenium deficiency in lambs. Quart. J. Exp. Physiol. 51, 94–102.

Goehring, T.B., Palmer, I.S., Olson, O.E., et al., 1984. Effects of seleniferous grains and inorganic selenium on tissue and blood composition of and growth performance of rats and swine. J. Anim. Sci. 59, 725–732.

Grace, N.D., 1994. Selenium. In: Grace, N.D. (Ed.), Managing Trace Element Deficiencies. New Zealand Pastoral Agricultural Research Institute, Simon Print, Palmerston North, New Zealand.

Hamilton, S.J., 2004. Review of selenium toxicity in the aquatic food chain. Sci. Total Environ. 326, 1–31.

Hansson, E., Jacobsson, S.O., 1966. Uptake of [75Se] selenomethionine in the tissues of the mouse studied by whole-body autoradiography. Biochim. Biophys. Acta. 115, 285–293.

Harr, J.R., Muth, O.H., 1972. Selenium poisoning in domestic animals and its relationship to man. Clin. Toxicol. 5, 175–186.

Hidiroglou, M., Jenkins, K.J., 1973. Absorption of 75Se-selenomethionine from the rumen of sheep. Can. J. Anim. Sci. 53, 345–347.

Hoffman, D.J., 2002. Role of selenium toxicity and oxidative stress in aquatic birds. Aquat. Toxicol. 57, 11–26.

Hoffman, J.L., 1977. Selenite toxicity, depletion of liver S-adenosylmethionine, and inactivation of methionine adenosyltransferase. Arch. Biochem. Biophys. 179, 136–140.

Hudman, J.F., Glenn, A.R., 1984. Selenite uptake and incorporation by selenomonas ruminantium. Arch. Microbiol. 140, 252–256.

Itoh, M., Suzuki, K.T., 1997. Effects of dose on the methylation of selenium to monomethylselenol and trimethyl selenonium ion in rats. Arch. Toxicol. 71, 461–466.

Jacobsson, S.O., 1966. Excretion of a single dose of selenium in sheep. Acta Vet. Scand. 7, 226–239.

Kajander, E.O., Harvima, R.J., Elonranta, T.O., et al., 1991. Metabolism, cellular actions, and cytotoxicity of selenomethionine in cultured cells. Biol. Trace Elem. Res. 28, 57–68.

Kaur, P., Bansal, M.P., 2005. Effect of selenium-induces oxidative stress on the cell kinetics in testis and reproductive ability of male mice. Nutrition 21, 351–357.

Kaur, R., Sharma, S., Rampal, S., 2003. Effects of subchronic selenium toxicosis on lipid peroxidation, glutathione redox cycle, and antioxidant enzymes in calves. Vet. Hum. Toxicol. 45, 190–192.

Koenig, K.M., Rode, L.M., Cohen, R.D.H., et al., 1997. Effect of diet and chemical form of selenium in sheep. J. Anim. Sci. 75, 817–827.

Kotrebai, M., BirringerTyson, J.F., Block, E., et al., 1999. Identification of the principal selenium compounds in selenium-enriched natural sample extracts by ion-pair liquid chromatography with inductively coupled plasma and electrospray ionization-mass spectrometric detection. Anal. Commun. 36, 249–252.

Lakin, H.W., 1961. Geochemistry of selenium in relation to agriculture. Selenium in Agriculture. US Department of Agriculture, Agric Handb 2001. U.S. Government Printing Office, Washington, DC.

Langlands, J.P., Bowles, J.E., Donald, G.E., et al., 1986. Selenium excretion in sheep. Aust. J. Agric. Res. 37, 201–209.

Latshaw, D.J., Morishita, T.Y., Sarver, C.F., et al., 2004. Selenium toxicity in breeding ring-necked pheasants (*Phasianus colchicus*). Avian. Dis. 48, 935–939.

Lawler, T.L., Taylor, J.B., Finley, J.W., et al., 2004. Effects of supranutritional and organically bound selenium on performance, carcass characteristics, and selenium distribution in finishing beef steers. J. Anim. Sci. 82, 1488–1493.

Leng, L., Boldizarova, K., Faix, S., et al., 2000. The urinary excretion of selenium in sheep treated with a vasopressin analogue. Vet. Res. 31, 499–505.

Levander, O.A., 1987. Selenium. In: fifth edn Mertz, W. (Ed.), Trace Elements in Human and Animal Nutrition, vol. 2. Academic Press, New York, pp. 209–279.

Levander, O.A., 2000. The selenium-coxsackievirus connection: chronicle of collaboration. J. Nutr. 130, 485S–488S.

Lewis, B.G., 1976. Selenium in biological systems, and pathways for its volatilization in higher plants. In: Nriagu, J.O. (Ed.), Environmental Biogeochemistry. Ann Arbor Science, Ann Arbor, MI, pp. 389–409.

Mahan, D.C., Magee, P.L., 1991. Efficacy of dietary sodium selenite and calcium selenite provided in the diet at approved, marginally toxic, and toxic levels to growing swine. J. Anim. Sci. 69, 722–725.

Mahan, D.C., Moxon, A.L., 1984. Effect of inorganic selenium supplementation on selenosis in post-weaning swine. J. Anim. Sci. 58, 216–221.

Martin, J.L., 1973. Selenium compounds in nature and medicine. In: Klayman, D.L., Gunther, W.H.H. (Eds.), Organic Selenium Compounds: Their Chemistry and Biology. John Wiley & Sons, New York, pp. 663–691.

McConnell, K.P., Burton, R.M., Kute, T., et al., 1979. Selenoproteins from rat testis cytosol. Biochim. Biophys. Acta 588, 13–19.

McConnell, K.P., Cho, G.J., 1967. Active transport of L-selenomethionine in the intestine. Am. J. Physiol. 213, 50–56.

McConnell, K.P., Roth, D.M., 1964. Passage of selenium across the placenta and also into the milk of the dog. J. Nutr. 84, 40–44.

McConnell, K.P., Roth, D.M., 1966. Respiratory excretion of selenium. Proc. Soc. Exp. Biol. Med. 123, 19–21.

Miller, W.T., Williams, K.T., 1940. Minimum lethal dose of selenium as sodium selenite for horses, mules, cattle and swine. J. Agric. Res. 60, 53–73.

Musnell, H.E., Devaney, G.M., Kennedy, M.H., 1936. Toxicity of food containing selenium as shown by its effect on the rat, USDA Tech Bull No 534, USDA Washington, DC, 25 pp.

Muth, O.H., Oldfield, J.E., Remmert, L.F., et al., 1958. Effects of selenium and vit. E on white muscle disease. Science 128, 1090–1097.

Muth, O.H., Pendell, H.W., Watson, C.R., et al., 1967. Uptake and retention of parenterally administered 75Se in ewes on different selenium regimens. Am. J. Vet. Res. 28, 397–406.

National Research Council (NRC), 1983. Selenium in Nutrition, revised edn. Subcommittee on Selenium, Committee on Animal Nutrition, Washington, DC.

National Research Council (NRC), 2005. Selenium. In Mineral Tolerance of Animals. second ed. National Academies Press, Washington, DC, pp. 321–347.

O'Toole, D., Raisbeck, M.F., 1995. Pathology of experimentally induced chronic selenosis ("alkali disease") in yearling cattle. J. Vet. Diagn. Invest. 7, 64–73.

Olson, O.E., Novacek, E.J., Whitehead, E.I., et al., 1970. Investigations on selenium in wheat. Phytochem 9, 181–190.

Oster, O., Prellwitz, W., 1990. The renal excretion of selenium. Biol. Trace Elem. Res. 24, 19–46.

Palmer, I.S., Fischer, D.D., Halverson, A.W., et al., 1969. Identification of a major selenium excretory product in rat urine. Biochim. Biophys. Acta 177, 336–342.

Patterson, E.L., Milstrey, R., Stokstad, E.L.R., 1957. Effect of selenium in preventing exudative diathesis in chicks. Proc. Soc. Exp. Biol. Med. 95, 17–20.

Peter, D.W., Whanger, P.D., Lindsay, J.P., et al., 1982. Excretion of selenium, zinc and copper by sheep receiving continuous intraruminal infusions of selenite or selenomethionine. Proc. Nutr. Soc. 7, 78.

Peterson, P.J., Butler, G.W., 1962. The uptake and assimilation of selenite by higher plants. Aust. J. Biol. Sci. 15, 26–46.

Pfister, J.A., Davis, T.Z., Hall, J.O., 2014. Effects of selenium concentrations on feed preference by cattle and sheep. J. Anim. Sci. 91 (12), 5970–5980.

Puls, R., 1994. Mineral Levels in Animal Health, second ed. Diagnostic data Sherpa International, British Columbia, Canada.

Raisbeck, M.F., 2000. Selenosis. Vet. Clin. North Am. Food Anim. Prac. 16 (3), 465–480.

Robinson, M.F., Rea, R.M., Friend, G.M., et al., 1978. On supplementing the selenium intake of New Zealanders. 2. Prolonged metabolic experiments with daily supplements of selenomethionine, selenite and fish. Br. J. Nutr. 39, 89–95.

Rosenfeld, I., Beath, O.A., 1964. Selenium: Geobotany, Biochemistry, Toxicity, and Nutrition. Academic Press, New York.

Rosman, K.J.R., Taylor, P.D.P., 1997. Isotopic composition of the elements. Pure Appl. Chem. 70, 217–235.

Rotruck, J.T., Pope, A.L., Ganther, H.E., et al., 1973. Selenium: biochemical role as a component of glutathione peroxidase. Science 179, 588–590.

Schrauzer, G.N., 1994. Selenium in the maintenance and therapy of HIV-infected patients. Chem Biol Interact. 91, 199–205.

Schroeder, H.A., Mitchener, M., 1972a. Selenium and tellurium in mice. Effects on growth, survival and tumors. Arch. Environ. Health 24, 66.

Schroeder, H.A., Mitchener, M., 1972b. Selenium and tellurium in rats: effect on growth, survival, and tumors. J. Nutr. 101, 1531–1540.

Schwarz, K., Foltz, C.M., 1957. Selenium as an integral part of Factor 3 against dietary necrotic liver degeneration. J. Am. Chem. Soc. 78, 3292.

Serra, A.B., Serra, S.D., Fujihara, T., 1996. Influence of dietary protein on the fractionation of selenium in the rumen of sheep. Biol. Trace Elem. Res. 9, 557–562.

Shalini, S., Bansal, M.P., 2005. Role of selenium in regulation of spermatogenesis: involvement of activator protein 1. Biofactors 23, 151–162.

Shalini, S., Bansal, M.P., 2007. Dietary selenium deficiency as well as excess supplementation induces multiple defects in mouse epididymal spermatozoa: understanding the role of selenium in male fertility. Int. J. Androl. 31, 438–449.

Shrift, A., 1973. Selenium compounds in nature and medicine. In: Klayman, D.L., Gunther, W.H. (Eds.), Organic Selenium Compounds: Their Chemistry and Biology. Wiley-Interscience, New York, pp. 763–814.

Smith, D.G., Senger, P.L., McCutchan, J.F., et al., 1979. Selenium and glutathione peroxidase distribution in bovine semen and selenium-75 retention by the tissues of the reproductive tract in the bull. Biol. Reprod. 20, 377.

Smith, M.I., Franke, K.W., Westfall, B.B., 1936. The selenium problem in relation to public health. A preliminary survey to determine the possibility of selenium intoxication in the rural population living on seleniferous soil. U.S. Public Health Rept. 51, 1496–1505.

Soda, K., Esaki, N., Nakamura, T., et al., 1987. Selenocysteine-lyase: an enzymological aspect of mammalian selenocysteine metabolism. In Selenium in Biology and Medicine. Part A. Proceedings of the Third International Symposium on Selenium in Biology and Medicine. May 27–June 1, 1984 at Beijing, China. AVI Book Pub by Van Nostrand Reinhold Co., New York, pp. 160–171.

Stowe, H.D., Herdt, T.H., 1992. Clinical assessment of selenium status of livestock. J. Anim. Sci. 70, 3928–3933.

Sunde, R.A., 1994. Intracellular glutathione peroxidases—structure regulation and function. In: Burk (Ed.), Selenium in Biology and Human Health. Springer-Verlag, New York, pp. 45–77.

Suttle, N.F., Jones, D.G., 1989. Recent developments in trace element metabolism and function: trace elements, disease resistance and immune responsiveness in ruminants. J. Nutr. 119, 1055–1061.

Thompson, J.M., Scott, M.L., 1969. Role of selenium in the nutrition of the chick. J. Nutr. 97, 335–342.

Thomson, C.D., 1998. Selenium speciation in human body fluids. Analyst 123, 827–831.

Thomson, C.D., Stewart, R.D.H., 1974. The metabolism of [75Se] in young women. Br. J. Nutr. 32, 47–57.

Tiwary, A.K., 2004. Differences Between Inorganic and Organic Selenium Toxicosis in Sheep. Masters Thesis, Utah State University, Logan, UT.

Tiwary, A.K., Panter, K.E., Stegelmeier, B.L., et al., 2005. Evaluation of respiratory elimination kinetics of selenium after oral administration in sheep. Am. J. Vet. Res. 66, 1–7.

Tiwary, A.K., Stegelmei, B.L., Panter, K.E., et al., 2006. Comparative toxicosis of sodium selenite and selenomethionine in lambs. J. Vet. Diag. Invest. 18, 60–69.

Underwood, E.J., Suttle, N.F., 1999. The Mineral Nutrition of Livestock, third ed. Wallingford, Oxon, UK.

Vendeland, S.C., Butler, J.A., Whanger, P.D., 1992. Intestinal absorption of selenite, selenate and selenomethionine in the rat. J. Nutr. Biochem. 3, 359–365.

Vendeland, S.C., Deagen, J.T., Butler, J.A., et al., 1994. Uptake of selenite, selenomethionine and selenate by brush border membrane vesicles isolated from rat small intestine. Biometals 7, 305–312.

Vernie, L.N., Ginjarr, H.B., Wilders, I.T., et al., 1978. Amino acid incorporation in a cell-free system derived from rat liver studied with the aid of selenodiglutathione. Biochem. Biophys. Acta 518, 507–517.

Whanger, P.D., 2002. Selenocompounds in plants and animals and their biological significance. J. Am. Coll. Nutr. 21, 223–232.

Whanger, P.D., Pedersen, N.D., Hatfield Weswig, P.H., 1976. Absorption of selenite and selenomethionine from ligated digestive tract segments in rats. Proc. Soc. Exp. Biol. Med. 153, 295.

Whanger, P.D., Weswig, P.H., Muth, O.H., 1968. Metabolism of 75Se-selenite and 75Se-selenomethionine by rumen microorganisms. Fed. Proc. 27, 418.

Williams, K.T., Byers, H.G., 1936. Se compounds in soils. Ind. Eng. Chem. 28, 912.

Wolffram, S., Grenacher, B., Scharrer, E., 1988. Transport of selenate and sulphate across the intestinal brush-border membrane of pig jejunum by two common mechanisms. Q. J. Exp. Physiol. 73, 103–111.

Wright, P.L., Bell, M.C., 1966. Comparative metabolism of selenium and tellurium in sheep and swine. Am. J. Physiol. 211, 6–10.

Yaeger, M.J., Neiger, R.D., Holler, L., et al., 1998. The effect of subclinical selenium toxicosis on pregnant beef cattle. J. Vet. Diagn. Invest. 10, 268–273.

Zeisel, S.H., Ellis, A.L., Sun, X.F., et al., 1987. Dose–response relations in urinary excretion of trimethylselenonium ion in the rat. J. Nutr. 117, 1609–1614.

Chapter 34

Sodium Chloride (Salt)

Larry J. Thompson

INTRODUCTION

Sodium chloride is often referred to as table salt, common salt, or just simply salt. Salt is an essential nutrient and can give an attractive taste to foods and feeds. It has been stated that salt is the only mineral compound for which animals can truly develop a craving.

Salt is a necessary nutrient for the health of animals and many nutrition texts divide it into separate requirements for sodium (Na) and chloride (Cl). Daily requirements for salt will increase due to lactation, exertion and increases in ambient temperatures. These same conditions will also require an increase in water intake, which must always be considered in any discussion concerning salt intake.

An excess of salt intake can lead to the condition known by various names including salt poisoning, hypernatremia, sodium ion toxicosis, and water deprivation–sodium ion intoxication. The last name in this list is the most descriptive, giving both the result (sodium ion intoxication) and the most common predisposing condition (water deprivation).

BACKGROUND

Sodium is the main cation and chloride is the main anion in the regulation of osmotic balance in the extracellular fluid (ECF) of the body. Serum sodium concentration and serum osmolarity are normally maintained under precise control by homeostatic mechanisms involving thirst, antidiuretic hormone and renal reabsorption of filtered sodium. Normal reference ranges for serum sodium in adult animals (given in mmol/L) include porcine 135–150, bovine 132–152, canine 141–152, feline 147–156, and equine 132–146 (Kaneko et al., 1997). For sodium concentration measurement, mmol/L = mEq/L and can be used interchangeably. Hyponatremia is the result of the loss of excess sodium compared to loss of water and can be the result of a large number of disease processes and conditions. For a more complete explanation on the recognition and correction of hyponatremia the reader is directed to other references (Angelos and Van Metre, 1999).

Salt is normally present in animal diets at 0.5%–1%. Production animals are often given free access to salt blocks or mineral mixes as supplements to the diet. Additional sources of salt may include high-saline ground water, brine or seawater. The use of whey as a feed or to produce wet mash can add dramatically to sodium intake. High concentrations of salt in the diet (up to 13%) have been used to limit feed intake of cattle. In general, animals can tolerate high concentrations of salt in the feed if they have free access to fresh water. Salt-deprived animals or animals not acclimated to high-salt feeds can overconsume these feeds making the animal prone to hypernatremia. Improperly formulated or improperly mixed feed can be an additional source of excess salt. Companion animal exposures to excess salt have included the use of salt as an emetic (this practice is no longer recommended) and the consumption of various salt-containing objects including rock salt and dough-salt mixtures. Dogs can develop hypernatremia during prolonged exercise and play in the ocean surf, especially if insufficient fresh water is available. Hypernatremia has also been reported in animals treated with improperly mixed oral electrolyte solutions and remedies for diarrhea. Other causes of hypernatremia in dogs can be found in Goldkamp and Schaer (2007).

Excess ingested salt can be irritating to mucosal surfaces and can result in anorexia, vomiting or diarrhea. Ingested dietary salt is approximately 90% absorbed across the gastrointestinal tract. Ingestion of excess sodium on an acute basis can result in hypernatremia with this condition being variously termed direct sodium ion toxicosis, acute sodium ion toxicosis or acute hypernatremia. Clinical signs develop within 1–2 days. The more common form of hypernatremia develops due to restricted water intake and is termed indirect sodium ion toxicosis, chronic sodium ion toxicosis or chronic hypernatremia. Clinical signs will develop over a period of 4–7 days but the early changes may be missed or ignored. There are several common reasons for restricted water intake

Veterinary Toxicology. DOI: http://dx.doi.org/10.1016/B978-0-12-811410-0.00034-9

including frozen water sources, unpalatable water sources, mechanical failure, overcrowding or naive animals, and owner neglect.

PHARMACOKINETICS AND MECHANISM OF ACTION

An increase in sodium intake leads to a rise in sodium concentration in the serum and a rapid distribution throughout the body. Osmolarity of the ECF is monitored by osmoreceptors in the hypothalamus and the body reacts to increases by stimulating thirst for increased water intake. Additionally, the release of antidiuretic hormone from the posterior pituitary will cause increased water retention by the kidneys. These responses should function to quickly restore normal osmolarity but may only be effective if the osmolar changes are gradual and sufficient water is available to the animal. As the sodium ion concentration of the serum increases, water will move out of the interstitium and intracellular fluid into the ECF along the osmotic gradient. Sodium will passively diffuse across the blood–brain barrier increasing the sodium concentration of the cerebral spinal fluid above the normal range (135–150 mmol/L). During this developing hypernatremia, the cells of the brain will also increase their intracellular osmolarity to prevent excess water loss to the ECF, which would cause cell shrinkage. If the hypernatremia develops too quickly and this protective mechanism fails, significant cell shrinkage occurs and the entire brain shrinks and pulls away from the calvarium resulting in the disruption of the blood supply to the brain. This can result in subarachnoid, subdural or intravascular hemorrhages (Hardy, 1989). In severe cellular dehydration, the result can be seizure-like activity and death. If the increase in sodium concentration of the brain cells continues, there will be an inhibition of glycolysis and a decrease in the energy available in the cell. While sodium will passively diffuse into the brain, it is an energy-requiring active process that transports sodium out. Thus the brain response to a rapid decrease in serum sodium is delayed and the developing osmotic gradient will cause water to move into the brain causing swelling, cerebral edema, and the development of clinical signs.

Changes in cellular osmolarity will occur in both acute and chronic hypernatremia situations, but changes to osmolarity on a chronic basis will involve the accumulation of more osmotically active organic compounds, termed idiogenic osmoles. These include taurine, myoinositol, glycerophosphoryl-choline, glutamate, glutamine, betaine, and phosphocreatine. Maximum concentrations of idiogenic osmoles occur within 48–72 h and can account for 60% of the change in cellular osmolarity. Once the hypernatremia situation is corrected, the idiogenic osmoles will take 48–72 h to decrease back to normal levels. As in the acute situation, a rapid decrease in serum sodium will develop an osmotic gradient causing water to move into the brain with resulting cerebral edema and the development of clinical signs.

TOXICITY

In all situations involving salt intake, the intake of water will have great impact and must also be considered. The acute toxic dose of sodium chloride is approximately 2.2 g/kg in swine, equine and bovine species with the ovine toxic dose approximately 6 g/kg (Osweiler et al., 1985). Swine appear to be the most sensitive domestic animal and involve the greatest number of clinical reports. Both swine and poultry can be severely affected when water intake is greatly restricted or with high-salt diets and only moderate water restriction. Increased water requirements will increase the susceptibility of lactating cows and sows to salt poisoning, making them more sensitive to sudden restrictions in water. The acute toxic dose of sodium chloride in dogs is given as 4 g/kg, but clinical signs have been reported for lesser ingestions (Barr et al., 2004) and an ingestion greater than this was reported with only mild clinical signs. Cats and dogs can safely tolerate 3.7% salt in the diet if fresh water is continuously available (NRC, 2005). Horses appear to be rarely affected with classic salt poisoning but can develop it with conditions of increased salt intake and sudden water restriction. Horses are, however, subject to dehydration and electrolyte abnormalities especially under conditions of exercise and high ambient temperatures (Cohen et al., 1993).

Clinical signs have best been described in swine and include loss of appetite, thirst, restlessness, pruritus and constipation. These early clinical signs can progress over several days to aimless wandering, head pressing, circling or pivoting around a limb. The animal may display seizure-like activity and assume a dog-sitting position, draw its head back in a jerking motion and fall over on its side (Osweiler et al., 1985; Niles, 2004). Terminally, the animal will be in lateral recumbency with paddling and opisthotonus. Cattle with acute excess salt intake may develop gastroenteritis, weakness, dehydration, tremors, and ataxia. The cattle may appear to be blind and develop seizure-like activity or partial paralysis including knuckling over at the fetlocks. Terminally, cattle can also be in lateral recumbency with paddling and opisthotonus. Cattle can die within 24 h following the appearance of severe clinical signs. Recovered animals may drag the rear feet or knuckle over at the rear fetlock without exhibiting pain (Osweiler et al., 1985). Poultry and other birds may exhibit clinical signs of depression, weakness, dyspnea and sudden death. Excess salt intake in the dog will result in vomiting within several hours of ingestion. The clinical signs can progress to diarrhea, muscle tremors and seizure-like activity. Increased severity of clinical signs in the dog have been seen when serum sodium levels have been above 180 mEq/l (Barr et al., 2004).

Postmortem examination of salt-poisoned animals may include some degree of gastric irritation, including ulceration and hemorrhages. The content of the gastrointestinal tract may be abnormally dry. Histopathologic lesions may be limited to the brain and include cerebral edema and inflammation of the meninges. In swine, the appearance of eosinophilic perivascular cuffing is seen if the animal dies early in the syndrome with the lesion not found after 48 h. Brain sodium concentrations above 2000 ppm are considered diagnostic in cattle and swine. Upper normal brain sodium concentrations are 1600 ppm for cattle and 1800 ppm for swine, both on a wet weight basis. There is a paucity of data on normal brain sodium concentrations in other common domestic species but normal ranges should be similar. Serum sodium concentrations taken from the live animal will be significantly above the normal ranges listed previously. Postmortem analysis of aqueous humor, vitreous humor or cerebral spinal fluid will show a significant increase over values from normal animals (Osweiler et al., 1995). Optimally, the values obtained should be compared to normal values for that species generated by the same laboratory.

TREATMENT

Prior to the onset of clinical signs, the acute ingestion of salt can best be treated by allowing the animal full access to water and closely observing the animal for several hours. Emetics may be used in the dog if known ingestions occur and the animal is not yet showing clinical signs. However, most cases are discovered long after the excess salt ingestion or the water deprivation has occurred and the affected animals are showing obvious clinical signs. The overriding concept of treatment is to slowly return the animal to normal water and electrolyte balance over a period of 2–3 days. Quickly lowering the serum sodium concentration will increase the osmotic gradient between the serum and the brain with water following the gradient into the brain increasing the likelihood of severe cerebral edema. The prognosis for an animal hypernatremic from salt ingestion/water deprivation with significant clinical signs on either an acute or chronic basis should be guarded at best.

On a herd basis with large animals, water intake should be limited to 0.5% of body weight at hourly intervals until normal hydration is accomplished. Monitoring serum sodium concentration is the first step in treatment on an individual animal basis. This information can be used to correct the free water deficit (*FWD*) in the animal, based on the following formula:

$$FWD\,(1) = 0.6 \times \text{body weight (kg)} \times [(\text{measured serum Na}/\text{normal serum Na}) - 1]$$

Not more than 50% of the *FWD* should be replaced in the first 24 h with the remaining deficit replaced in the following 24–48 h. Serum sodium levels should be lowered at a rate of 0.5–1.0 mEq/L/h, with the slower rate recommended for cases of chronic hypernatremia (Schaer, 2000). In dogs with acute hypernatremia, the use of warm water enemas (6.6–11 mL/kg) repeated every 1–2 h has been suggested (Donaldson, 2003; Howard, 2007). In acute hypernatremia without clinical dehydration, the use of 5% dextrose solution in combination with a loop diuretic has been suggested at 3.7 mL/kg/h to decrease serum sodium at 1 mEq/L/h (Barr et al., 2004). Diuretics such as furosemide can be used to prevent the development of pulmonary edema during fluid therapy. The use of slightly hypertonic intravenous fluids has been recommended to reduce the likelihood of cerebral edema developing. Intravenous fluids should be made to approximate the serum sodium concentration of the animal, or the clinician may start with a solution containing 170 mEq/L of sodium and decrease this concentration as clinical signs improve (Angelos and Van Metre, 1999; Niles, 2004). If brain edema is suspected, the use of mannitol, dexamethasone, or dimethyl sulfoxide may aid in control.

CONCLUDING REMARKS AND FUTURE DIRECTIONS

While the term "salt poisoning" may not be the most accurate way to describe the above syndrome, it is certainly in common usage. A similar and confusing term, "water intoxication," has been used to describe the situation of excess water intake or infusion over a short period of time, which can dramatically decrease the serum sodium concentration and make the serum hypoosmolar. Water intoxication has been used to describe the exacerbation of cerebral edema when the correction of hypernatremia occurs too quickly. Water intoxication has also been used to describe the brain swelling and seizure-like activity which occurs when a normal animal drinks excessive amounts of water over a short period of time. In addition to the possible neurological effects, hemolysis has also been described (Middleton et al., 1997). In the above situations, acute and dramatic osmotic changes are the cause.

REFERENCES

Angelos, S.M., Van Metre, D.C., 1999. Treatment of sodium balance disorders. In: Roussel Jr, A., Constable, P.D. (Eds.), Veterinary Clinics of North America: Food Animal Practice, vol. 15. W.B. Saunders Co, Philadelphia, PA, pp. 587–607.

Barr, J.M., Khan, S.A., McCullough, S.M., et al., 2004. Hypernatremia secondary to homemade play dough ingestion in dogs: a review of 14 cases from 1998 to 2001. J. Vet. Emerg. Crit. Care 14, 196–202.

Cohen, N.D., Roussel, A.J., Lumsden, J.H., et al., 1993. Alterations of fluid and electrolyte balance in thoroughbred racehorses following strenuous exercise during training. Can. J. Vet. Res. 57, 9–13.

Donaldson, C.W., 2003. Paintball toxicosis in dogs. Vet. Med. 98, 995–998.

Goldkamp, C., Schaer, M., 2007. Hypernatremia in dogs. Compend. Contin. Educ. Vet. 29, 148–161.

Hardy, R.M., 1989. Hypernatremia. In: Schaer, M. (Ed.), Veterinary Clinics of North America: Small Animal Practice, Vol. 19. W.B. Saunder Co., Philadelphia, PA, pp. 231–240.

Howard, J., 2007. Paintball toxicosis. Vet. Technician 28, 336–338.

Kaneko, J., Harvey, J., Bruss, M., 1997. Appendices VII and VIII. In: Kaneko, J., Harvey, J., Bruss, M. (Eds.), Clinical Biochemistry of Domestic Animals, fifth ed. Academic Press, San Diego, CA, p. 894.

Middleton, J.R., Katz, L., Angelos, J.A., et al., 1997. Hemolysis associated with water administration using nipple bottle for human infants in juvenile pygmy goats. J. Vet. Intern. Med. 11, 382–384.

Niles, G., 2004. Sodium. In: Plumlee, K.H. (Ed.), Clinical Veterinary Toxicology. Mosby, St. Louis, MO, pp. 218–221.

NRC, 2005. Sodium Chloride. In Mineral Tolerance of Animals: Second Revised Edition. National Research Council. Washington, DC: The National Academies Press, pp. 357–371.

Osweiler, G.D., Carson, T.L., Buck, W.B., Van Gelder, G.A., 1985. Water deprivation-sodium salt, Clinical and Diagnostic Veterinary Toxicology, third edn. Kendall/Hunt Publishing Co., Dubuque, IA, pp. 167–170.

Osweiler, G.D., Carr, T.F., Sanderson, T.P., et al., 1995. Water deprivation-sodium ion intoxication in cattle. J. Vet. Diagn. Invest. 7, 583–585.

Schaer, M., 2000. Hyperkalemia and hypernatremia. In: Ettinger, S.J., Feldman, B.F. (Eds.), Textbook of Veterinary Internal Medicine, fifth ed. W.B. Saunders Co, Philadelphia, PA, pp. 227–232.

Chapter 35

Sulfur

Jeffery O. Hall

INTRODUCTION

Sulfur is a necessary dietary component that can be toxic at excessive concentrations. Animal bodies are about 0.15% sulfur by weight (NRC, 1989, 2006). Sulfur is incorporated into many essential molecules, including biotin, chondroitin sulfate, cartilage mucopolysaccharides, coenzyme A, fibrinogen, glutathione, heparin, lipoic acid, mucins, and thiamine (NRC, 1989, 1998, 2006). In addition to these biologically active compounds, sulfur is an intricate component of sulfur-containing amino acids, such as methionine, cysteine, cystine, homocysteine, and taurine. With the exception of thiamine and biotin, all sulfur-containing compounds in the body can be synthesized from methionine (NRC, 1996). Thus, thiamine, biotin, and methionine are essential nutrients in the diet of monogastric animals, but ruminant microbes can synthesize these compounds from inorganic sulfate in the diet (Block et al., 1951). Species differences are such that cats cannot synthesize taurine from methionine, making it an essential nutrient in their diets. Recommended daily dietary intakes of sulfur are 0.15%, 0.14%–0.26%, 0.15%–0.2%, and 0.2%–0.25% of the diet for horses, sheep, beef cattle, and dairy cattle, respectively (NRC, 1985, 1988, 1989, 1996).

Ruminants tend to be more sensitive to the toxic effects of dietary sulfur/sulfate due to efficient microbial conversion to bioactive sulfur species in the rumen. But both dietary and water sources of sulfur/sulfate have similar toxic potential and must be factored into the total daily intake in order to establish potential risk. Dietary feed sources that can contain high sulfur concentrations, which are frequently overlooked, include distiller's byproducts, wet and dry distiller's grains and gluten feeds. These products can also have significant batch-to-batch variability in sulfur content, even from the same production plant. Due to their relative inexpensive nature, compared to grains, these potentially high sulfur materials are more and more frequently being added to ruminant diets.

In addition to dietary sulfur, other sulfur-containing compounds can be toxic. Sulfur dioxide gas from industrial waste gas, as well as hydrogen sulfide gas from manure pits, natural gas production and crude oil production, can be toxic to livestock. The toxic effects of these gaseous forms of sulfur are better summarized separately from the dietary toxicoses.

Plants can accumulate high sulfur concentrations. High sulfate water can cause a dual increase in total daily sulfur intake by way of the water and ingested proximal vegetation. Plant sulfur concentrations have been shown to increase with increasing sulfate in the soil (Reddy et al., 1981; Hardt et al., 1991; Leustek and Saito, 1999). In soil matrices, sulfate can be actively reduced and precipitated; however, this only sequesters the sulfur until environmental change allows the reoxidation of sulfur back to sulfate. During drought conditions, precipitated sulfur in the subsurface soil is exposed to greater oxygen and potentially reoxidized. The resultant sulfate is then bioavailable for plant uptake during subsequent periods of normal or high precipitation.

BACKGROUND

Sulfur is a nonmetal within group VIA of the periodic table. This group is sometimes referred to as the chalcogenides or ore-formers, since many metal ores are sulfide or sulfate salts. Sulfur has an atomic number of 16, an atomic weight of 32.07, and has four different naturally occurring atomic masses from 32 to 36 (Rosman and Taylor, 1998). It can occur in four different oxidation states: −2 (sulfide), 0 (elemental sulfur), +4 (sulfite), and +6 (sulfate). All valence states, except elemental sulfur, are found in biologic molecules. Sulfur is utilized in the production of sulfuric acid, fertilizers, pigments, dyes, drugs, explosives, rubber, insecticides and detergents, as well as many inorganic salts and esters. Although uniformly found in nature, industrialized countries are the largest users of sulfur materials.

Veterinary Toxicology. DOI: http://dx.doi.org/10.1016/B978-0-12-811410-0.00035-0

PHARMACOKINETICS/TOXICOKINETICS

When evaluating the absorption of sulfur, the chemical form must be considered. The intestinal mucosal absorption of sulfate is via an active carrier-mediated process that is also utilized by molybdate (Mason and Cardin, 1977). Active intestinal absorption of sulfate has been shown in sheep, rats, dogs, rabbits, and hamsters (Bird and Moir, 1971). Similarly, the sulfur-containing amino acids and other sulfur-containing compounds are absorbed via specific transporter mechanisms across the intestinal mucosa (NRC, 2006). These specific transport processes are specific for the individual compounds. Rumen microbes convert a percentage of dietary sulfur-containing compounds to sulfide, which can then be incorporated into microbial sulfur-containing amino acids, thiamine, biotin, other microbial sulfur metabolites, or absorbed as sulfide. In addition to gastrointestinal absorption of sulfides, hydrogen sulfide can be absorbed across respiratory epithelium. Large amounts of sulfide, as hydrogen sulfide, produced in the rumen can be eructated, inhaled and absorbed (Dougherty et al., 1965). Inhaled sulfide is important in sulfur toxicosis, as sheep that had their trachea blocked to prevent eructation and inhalation of sulfide did not succumb while those without tracheal block were poisoned (NRC, 2006).

Sulfur is widely distributed in the body. All tissues in the body have significant sulfur components, with the body being made up of approximately 0.15% sulfur (NRC, 2006). Absorbed sulfides and thiomolybdates, the primary toxic sulfur metabolites, are well distributed in the body. This is evidenced by the fact that thiomolybdate can deplete tissue stores of copper, and sulfides can cross the blood–brain barrier causing neurological effects.

Sulfur-containing amino acids and sulfate are extensively metabolized in order to produce biologically utilized sulfur compounds. In comparison, absorbed sulfide is efficiently metabolized in the liver to sulfate, with a high first pass clearance (NRC, 2006). Inhaled sulfide would not be subject to the rapid hepatic removal that occurs for that absorbed from the gastrointestinal tract. This results in increased circulating concentrations that can expose neuronal tissues and result in toxic neurologic effects.

Sulfur-containing compounds are eliminated by both renal and biliary routes. Just as molybdate can compete for the intestinal absorption sites for sulfate, it can also compete for reabsorption sites in the renal tubules (Friberg and Lener, 1986). The relative quantities of sulfur elimination from renal and biliary routes can differ depending on the form ingested. In sheep, Bird (1972) found the greatest percent elimination of sulfate was via urine, while that from taurine was predominantly eliminated in the bile. Intestinally absorbed sulfide efficiently undergoes hepatic metabolism to sulfate, which is eliminated in the urine (NRC, 2006).

MECHANISM OF ACTION

Acute oral poisoning with elemental sulfur results in the formation of hydrogen sulfide, as well as many other potential metabolites. The gastric and respiratory effects are postulated to be due to the coagulative effects of rumen-produced sulfurous acids and the irritating effects of hydrogen sulfide, respectively (Julian and Harrison, 1975; Kandylis, 1984; Gunn et al., 1987). However, the exact mechanisms are not well delineated. Inhaled ruminal sulfide at high concentrations may act in a similar mechanism to high concentrations of exogenous hydrogen sulfide gas, causing acute respiratory paralysis.

The mechanism of subacute sulfur poisoning has been more extensively researched. This condition is correlated with the reduction of the sulfate or other forms of sulfur to sulfide in the rumen (Gould et al., 1991, 1997; Loneragan et al., 1998). The current literature suggests that inhibition of cytochrome C oxidase, which is essential for cellular respiration, is the primary mechanism of poisoning (Smith et al., 1977; Beauchamp et al., 1984). However, cerebral vasospasms and regional ischemia could also account for the localization of the lesions (Siesjo, 1984; McAllister, 1991). Although once thought to be associated with a true thiamine deficiency from either inhibition of rumen microbial production or cleavage of thiamine (Edwin and Jackman, 1982), it has been shown that systemic thiamine concentrations are within the normal range for most animals (Olkowski et al., 1992; Gould, 2000). However, more recent research has implicated low brain concentrations of thiamine pyrophosphate, one of the biologically active forms of the vitamin that is important in several metabolic pathways (Amat et al., 2013). A slight decline in the blood thiamine concentration can also be seen in some animals (Olkowski et al., 1991). However, thiamine supplementation in the presence of high sulfate/sulfur-associated PEM suppresses the clinical disease (Olkowski et al., 1992). This would indicate that the sulfide or some other sulfur metabolite is either competitively inhibiting the cellular uptake/utilization of thiamine, or therapeutic doses of thiamine diminish the effects of sulfide on the cytochrome C oxidase enzyme.

The subacute to chronic, indirect effects of excessive sulfur are seen in ruminants, due to the efficient conversion of sulfur compounds to sulfide. The sulfide can form insoluble salts with copper and zinc (Suttle, 1974), but it can also react with molybdenum and form thiomolybdate complexes, which efficiently bind copper making it nonbioavailable (Suttle, 1991). Systemic copper decreases, associated with increased sulfur/sulfate, have been reported in sheep (Moshtaghi-Nia et al., 1989; Van Niekerk and Van Niekerk, 1989a,b) and cattle (Wittenberg and Boila, 1988). High forage and water sulfur have also been associated with selenium deficiency (Ivancic and Weiss, 2001). Decreased serum and wool selenium have been reported with increasing dietary sulfate (White and Somers, 1977; White, 1980). In addition, increased soil sulfate inhibits plant uptake of selenium, thereby increasing the potential for inducing a selenium deficiency in ingesting herbivores (Newman and Schreiber, 1985), which may be an important mechanism in grazing animals.

TOXICITY

Toxicity of sulfur can be divided into three main categories that are likely to be encountered. The first is acute oral poisoning. The second is subacute to chronic direct toxicosis. And the third is subacute to chronic indirect toxicosis, as a secondary interference with other essential minerals that result in deficiencies.

Reports of acute oral sulfur poisoning are scarce in the literature. In a group of Holstein heifers, sulfur ingested at 0.85–3.8 g/kg body weight resulted in high morbidity and moderate mortality (Gunn et al., 1987), while 20 heifers given 250 g sulfur in grain had high mortality (Julian and Harrison, 1975). Ewes fed a barley-sulfur mix that provided approximately 40–45 g sulfur/ewe were poisoned (White, 1964). Five horses administered 300 g sulfur succumbed to sulfur poisoning (Ales, 1907).

Clinical and pathological manifestations of acute oral sulfur poisoning are similar across species (White, 1964; Julian and Harrison, 1975; Gunn et al., 1987). Abdominal pain, colic, rumen stasis, fetid diarrhea, dehydration, metabolic acidosis, tachypnea, recumbency, and hydrogen sulfide smell are expected clinical signs. Irritation, edema, and hemorrhage of the gastrointestinal tract and respiratory tract also should be expected. In addition, renal tubular necrosis can be seen.

Monogastric animals are much less susceptible to the subacute direct and indirect toxic effects of excessive sulfur intake than ruminants. Pigs can tolerate 1000 mg/L sulfur in the drinking water with only a mild cathartic effect (Paterson et al., 1979), and 0.42% in the diet for several months without adverse effects (Dale et al., 1973). Similarly, chicks had decreased growth rates at 1.2% dietary sulfur (Leach et al., 1960), and chickens had decreased egg production, decreased feed intake and deaths at 4000 mg/L sulfate in their drinking water (Adams et al., 1975). Since the indirect toxic effects of excessive sulfur, related to the interferences with other essential minerals, are related to rumen conversion to sulfides, these effects are not observed in monogastric animals.

In contrast, for sheep, beef cattle and dairy cattle the maximum tolerable content of sulfur in the total diet is 0.4% (NRC, 1985, 1988, 1996, 2001), while concentrations slightly below this tolerable content (0.36%) have resulted in toxic effects (Gould et al., 1991). When 0.36% sulfur was fed in a high concentrate ration that slightly decreased rumen pH, which can enhance the formation of hydrogen sulfide. In a review of the toxicology of sulfur in ruminants, it was stated that concentrations of sulfur greater than 0.3%–0.4% may cause toxic effects (Kandylis, 1984). Since dietary toxicity of sulfur is not mutually exclusive to the various sulfur-containing compounds, as different chemicals containing sulfur can have the same clinical effects, total doses of sulfur/sulfate from both water and dietary material must be taken into account when evaluating potential toxicity (Suttle, 1974). For example, water sulfate content of 500 mg/L would provide approximately half of the recommended maximal daily intake for ruminants. In ruminants, the typical clinical presentation of subacute sulfur poisoning is one of ataxia, weakness, blindness, recumbency, seizures, and death.

Subacute ingestion of toxic doses of sulfate/sulfur has been associated with Polioencephalomalacia (PEM), a necrotizing lesion of the brain (Beke and Hironaka, 1991; Gould et al., 1991; Olkowski et al., 1992; Hamlen et al., 1993; McAllister et al., 1997). Gross and histologic lesions are primarily in the brain, but ruminal changes can be observed. Gross pathologic lesions include a darkening of the rumen contents from precipitated sulfide salts, swelling of the cerebral hemispheres, softening of the cerebral hemispheres, and yellow discoloration of the cortical gray matter. Histological lesions include necrosis of the cortical gray matter and occasional areas of necrosis in the thalamus or midbrain. The clinical condition can be an additive effect of the total sulfur in the diet and sulfate in the drinking water (Beke and Hironaka, 1991). PEM has been reported to be associated with high sulfur/sulfate ingestion in cattle (Beke and Hironaka, 1991; Gould et al., 1991; Hamlen et al., 1993), pigs (Dow et al., 1963), and sheep (Olkowski et al., 1992). However, sodium ion poisoning in the pigs was likely the primary causative factor, as the exposure was to sodium sulfate.

The peak rumen production of hydrogen sulfide can be somewhat delayed from the time of initiating high sulfur intake. Peak rumen gas cap sulfide occurred at 1–3 weeks after placing cattle on a high sulfur diet (Gould et al., 1997). But, continuing exposure resulted in a gradual decline in the gas cap sulfide content. This would indicate an adaptation of the rumen microbes to favor direct utilization of the sulfide or diminished rates of production.

Subacute to chronic sulfur-induced mineral deficiencies can result in severe health problems. Copper deficiency can cause poor growth, weakness, poor immune function, poor reproductive function, and death. In addition, sulfur-induced copper deficiency may play a role in PEM (Gooneratne et al., 1989). Severe copper deficiency also causes myelin degeneration (enzootic ataxia) in lambs, deer, and other ruminants (Cordy, 1971; Faye et al., 1991; Audige et al., 1995). Sulfate-induced selenium deficiency can cause poor growth, weakness, poor immune function, poor reproductive function, damage to the cardiac or skeletal muscles and death.

TREATMENT

Treatment for acute sulfur poisoning is predominantly supportive in nature, with removal of the causative material, as well as administration of fluids and electrolytes. However, the human literature points to successful treatment of acute hydrogen sulfide poisoning by induction of methemoglobinemia with nitrite to allow for the formation of sulfmethemoglobin, similar to therapeutic protocols for treatment of cyanide poisoning (Stine et al., 1976; Peters, 1981). This type of therapy may also be beneficial in the treatment of subacute direct sulfur poisoning. Since sulfides act on and split disulfide bridges, the use of oxidized glutathione or other simple disulfide compounds could be protective or antidotal (Smith and Abbanat, 1966). The use of thiamine in the treatment of PEM is beneficial, even though there is no overt thiamine deficiency. The primary treatment of indirect mineral deficiencies resultant from high sulfur intake would also include enhanced supplementation of copper and potentially selenium. In some cases in which limitation of water or forage sulfur intake is not possible, use of chelated copper and selenium becomes important in order to bypass the sulfide binding/precipitation of essential minerals in the rumen and competitive inhibition of selenate from the intestinal tract.

In addition to direct treatment, management can play a role in the prevention of sulfur poisoning. Testing of water and dietary materials will identify high sulfur prior to utilization. With this information, management strategies can be utilized that would incorporate the sulfur at a gradually increasing content in an attempt to allow for microbial adaptation.

CONCLUDING REMARKS AND FUTURE DIRECTIONS

Although much is known about the different clinical disease conditions that excessive sulfur can cause, treatment remains only somewhat effective. Thus, it is important to evaluate the use of nitrite- or disulfide-containing compounds in the treatment of domestic animals.

REFERENCES

Adams, A.W., Cunningham, F.E., Munger, L.L., 1975. Some effects on layers of sodium sulfate and magnesium sulfate in their drinking water. Poult. Sci. 54, 707–714.

Ales, 1907. Case of poisoning by sulfur in the horse. Vet. J. 63, 524.

Amat, S., McKinnon, J.J., Olkowski, A.A., et al., 2013. Understanding the role of sulfur-thiamine interaction in the pathogenesis of sulfur-induced polioencephalomalacia in beef cattle. Res. Vet. Sci. 95, 1081–1087.

Audige, L., Wilson, P.R., Morris, R.S., et al., 1995. Osteochondrosis, skeletal abnormalities and enzootic ataxia associated with copper deficiency in a farmed red deer (*Cervus elaphus*) herd. N. Zeal. Vet. J. 43 (2), 70–76.

Beauchamp Jr, R.O., Bus, J.S., Popp, J.A., et al., 1984. A critical review of the literature on hydrogen sulfide toxicity. Crit. Rev. Toxicol. 13, 25–97.

Beke, G.J., Hironaka, R., 1991. Toxicity to beef cattle of sulfur in saline well water: a case study. Sci. Total Environ. 101 (3), 281–290.

Bird, P.R., 1972. Sulfur metabolism and excretion studies in ruminants: VII. Secretion of sulfur and nitrogen in sheep pancreatic and bile fluids. Aust. J. Biol. Sci. 25, 817–834.

Bird, P.R., Moir, R.J., 1971. Sulfur metabolism and excretion studies in ruminants. I. The absorption of sulfate in sheep after intraruminal or intraduodenal infusions of sodium sulfate. Aust. J. Biol. Sci. 24, 1319–1328.

Block, R.J., Stekol, J.A., Loosli, J.K., 1951. Synthesis of sulfur amino acids from inorganic sulfate by ruminants. II. Synthesis of cystine and methionine from sodium sulfate by the goat and by the microorganisms of the rumen of the ewe. Arch. Biochem. 33, 353–363.

Cordy, D.R., 1971. Enzootic ataxia in California lambs. J. Am. Vet. Med. Assoc. 158 (11), 1940–1942.

Dale, S.E., Ewan, R.C., Speer, V.C., et al., 1973. Copper, molybdenum, and sulfate interaction in young swine. J. Anim. Sci. 37, 913–917.

Dougherty, R.W., Mullenax, C.H., Allison, M.J., 1965. Physiological phenomena associated with eructation in ruminants. In: Dougherty, R.W. (Ed.), Physiology of Digestion in the Ruminant. Buttersworth, Washington, DC, p. 159.

Dow, C., Lawson, G.H.K., Todd, J.R., 1963. Sodium sulfate toxicity in pigs. Vet. Rec. 75, 1052–1055.

Edwin, E.E., Jackman, R., 1982. Ruminant thiamine requirement in retrospect. Vet. Res. Commun. 5, 237–250.

Faye, B., Grillet, C., Tessema, A., et al., 1991. Copper deficiency in ruminants in the Rift Valley of East Africa. Trop. Anim. Health Prod. 23 (3), 172–180.

Friberg, L., Lener, J., 1986. Molybdenum. In: Friberg, L., Nordberg, G.F., Vouk, V.B. (Eds.), Handbook on the Toxicology of Metals, second ed. Elsevier/North-Holland Biomedical Press, New York, pp. 446–461.

Gooneratne, S.R., Olkowski, A.A., Klemmer, R.G., et al., 1989. High sulfur related thiamine deficiency in cattle: a field study. Can. Vet. J. 30, 139–146.

Gould, D.H., 2000. Update on sulfur-related polioencephalomalacia. Vet. Clin. North Am. Food Anim. Pract. 16, 481–496.

Gould, D.H., McAllister, M.M., Savage, J.C., et al., 1991. High sulfide concentrations in rumen fluid associated with nutritionally induced polioencephalomalasia. Am. J. Vet. Res. 52, 1164–1169.

Gould, D.H., Cummings, B.A., Hamar, D.W., 1997. In vivo indicators of pathologic ruminal sulfide production in steers with diet-induced polioencephalomalacia. J. Vet. Diagn. Invest. 9, 72–76.

Gunn, M.F., Baird, J.D., Wilke, J.S.N., 1987. Accidental sulfur poisoning in a group if Holstein heifers. Can. Vet. J. 28, 188–192.

Hamlen, H., Clark, E., Janzen, E., 1993. Polioencephalomalasia in cattle consuming water with elevated sodium sulfate levels: a herd investigation. Can. Vet. J. 34, 153–158.

Hardt, P.F., Ocumpaugh, W.R., Greene, L.W., 1991. Forage mineral concentration, animal performance, and mineral status of heifers grazing cereal pastures fertilized with sulfur. J. Anim. Sci. 69, 2310–2320.

Ivancic Jr, J., Weiss, W.P., 2001. Effects of dietary sulfur and selenium concentrations on selenium balance of lactating Holstein cows. J. Dairy Sci. 84, 225–232.

Julian, R.J., Harrison, K.B., 1975. Sulfur poisoning in cattle. Can. Vet. J. 16, 28–29.

Kandylis, K., 1984. Toxicology of sulfur in ruminants: review. J. Dairy Sci. 67, 2179–2187.

Leach, R.M., Ziegler, T.R., Norris, L.C., 1960. The effects of dietary sulfate in the growth rate of chicks fed purified a diet. Poult. Sci. 39, 1577–1582.

Leustek, T., Saito, K., 1999. Sulfate transport and assimilation in plants. Plant. Physiol. 120, 637–644.

Loneragan, G.H., Gould, D.H., Callan, R.J., et al., 1998. Association of excess sulfur intake and an increase in hydrogen sulfide concentrations in the ruminal gas cap of recently weaned beef calves with polioencephalomalacia. J. Am. Vet. Med. Assoc. 213, 1599–1604.

Mason, J., Cardin, C.J., 1977. The competition of molybdate and sulphate ions for a transport system in the ovine small intestine. Res. Vet. Sci. 22 (3), 313–315.

McAllister, M.M., 1991. Sulfur Toxicosis and Polioencephalomalasia in Ruminants. PhD Dissertation, Colorado State University, Fort Collins, CO.

McAllister, M.M., Gould, D.H., Raisbeck, M.F., et al., 1997. Evaluation of ruminal sulfide concentrations and seasonal outbreaks of polioencephalomalacia in beef cattle in 1992a feedlot. J. Am. Vet. Med. Assoc. 211 (10), 1275–1279.

Moshtaghi-Nia, S.A., Devlin, T.J., Phillips, G.D., 1989. Influence of dietary copper, molybdenum, and sulfur on copper metabolism of sheep. Can. J. Anim. Sci. 69, 187–194.

Newman, J.R., Schreiber, R.K., 1985. Effects of acidic deposition and other energy emissions on wildlife: a compendium. Vet. Hum. Toxicol. 27, 394–401.

NRC, 1985. Nutrient Requirements of Sheep. sixth revised ed. National Academic Press, Washington, DC, p. 15.

NRC, 1988. Nutrient Requirements of Dairy Cattle. sixth revised ed. National Academic Press, Washington, DC, pp. 28–29.

NRC, 1989. Nutrient Requirements of Horses. sixth revised ed. National Academic Press, Washington, DC, pp. 28–29.

NRC, 1996. 1Nutrient Requirements of Beef Cattle. seventh revised ed. National Academic Press, Washington, DC, pp. 60–61.

NRC, 1998. Nutrient Requirements of Swine. tenth revised ed. Natinal Academic Press, Washington, DC, pp. 60–61.

NRC, 2001. Nutrient Requirements of Dairy Cattle. seventh revised ed. National Academic Press, Washington, DC, pp. 131–132.

NRC, 2006. Molybdenum. In Mineral Tolerance of Animals. second ed. National Academies Press, Washington, DC, pp. 262–275.

Olkowski, A.A., Rousseaux, C.G., Christensen, D.A., 1991. Association of sulfate-water and blood thiamine concentration in beef cattle: field studies. Can. J. Anim. Sci. 71, 825–832.

Olkowski, A.A., Gooneratne, S.R., Rousseaux, C.G., et al., 1992. Role of thiamine in sulfur induced polioencephalomalacia in sheep. Res. Vet. Sci. 52, 78–85.

Paterson, D.W., Wahlstrom, R.C., Libal, G.W., et al., 1979. Effects of sulfate water on swine reproduction and young pig performance. J. Anim. Sci. 49, 664–667.

Peters, J.W., 1981. Hydrogen sulfide poisoning in a hospital setting. J. Am. Med. Assoc. 246, 1588–1589.

Reddy, G.D., Alston, A.M., Tiller, K.G., 1981. Effects of fertilizer on concentrations of copper, molybdenum, and sulfur in subterranean clover (Trifilium subterraneum). Aust. J. Exp. Anim. Husb. 21, 491–497.

Rosman, K.J.R., Taylor, P.D.P., 1998. Isotopic composition of the elements 1997. Pure Appl. Chem. 70, 217–235.

Siesjo, B.K., 1984. Cerebral circulation and metabolism. J. Neurosurg. 60, 883–908.

Smith, L., Kruszyana, H., Smith, R.P., 1977. The effects of methemoglobin on the inhibition of cytochrome c oxidase by cyanide, sulfide, and azide. Biochem. Pharmacol. 26, 2247–2250.

Smith, R.P., Abbanat, R.A., 1966. Protective effects of oxidized glutathione in acute sulfide poisoning. Toxicol. Appl. Pharmacol. 9, 209–217.

Stine, R.J., Slosberg, B., Beacham, B.E., 1976. Hydrogen sulfide intoxication: a case report and discussion of treatment. Ann. Intern. Med. 85, 756–758.

Suttle, N.F., 1974. Effects of organic and inorganic sulfur on the availability of dietary copper to sheep. Br. J. Nutr. 32, 559–568.

Suttle, N.F., 1991. The interactions between copper, molybdenum, and sulfur in ruminant nutrition. Annu. Rev. Nutr. 11, 121–140.

Van Niekerk, F.E., Van Niekerk, C.H., 1989a. Effects of high levels of dietary molybdenum and sulfate on SA Mutton Merino sheep. I. Mineral status and haematologic parameters. S. Afr. Tydskr Veek. 19, 107–113.

Van Niekerk, F.E., Van Niekerk, C.H., 1989b. Effects of high levels of dietary molybdenum and sulfate on SA Mutton Merino sheep. II. Certain aspects of the oestrous cycle and pregnancy. S. Afr. Tydskr Veek. 19, 114–120.

White, C.L., 1980. Sulfur–selenium studies in sheep. Effect of dietary sulfur deficiency on selenium and sulfur metabolism in sheep fed varying levels of selenomethionine. Aust. J. Biol. Sci. 33, 699–707.

White, C.L., Somers, M., 1977. Sulfur–selenium studies in sheep. The effect of varying dietary sulfate and selenomethionine on sulfur, nitrogen, and selenium metabolism in sheep. Aust. J. Biol. Sci. 30, 47–56.

White, J.B., 1964. Sulfur poisoning in ewes. Vet. Rec. 76, 278–279.

Wittenberg, K.M., Boila, R.J., 1988. Supplementary copper for growing cattle consuming diets high in molybdenum or molybdenum plus sulfur. Can. J. Anim. Sci. 68, 1143–1154.

Chapter 36

Zinc

Tam Garland

INTRODUCTION

Zinc (Zn) is a transitional metal in group XII on the periodic chart and is the fourth most commonly used metal today. It is a moderately reactive metal with a common valence state of +2. It is also an essential element in mammals and birds and is a component of approximately 200 metalloenzymes. Although zinc has an essential role in nutrition and consequences of nutritional deficiency (Chasapis et al., 2012; Oteiza, 2012; Marchan et al., 2012; Marger et al., 2014; Mayward and Rink, 2015), this chapter will focus on its toxicity.

BACKGROUND

As the fourth most commonly used metal it is expected to be found in a variety of places with a multitude of uses. Zinc is an economical metal to use and is relatively nontoxic. Table 36.1 details some of those uses. Since zinc has nutritional qualities, it is not uncommon to find it added as a supplement to feed. Problems with toxicity generally occur when the levels are 1000 parts per million (ppm) or greater.

PHARMACOKINETICS/TOXICOKINETICS

Ingested zinc is primarily absorbed from the duodenum and the intestine by a carrier-mediated mechanism. Approximately 25%–50% of ingested zinc is absorbed. However, absorption of zinc in influenced by many factors, including whether or not food is in the stomach. Plant phytates can bind zinc and in an alkaline pH environment can form insoluble complexes. Similarly, zinc absorption is decreased in the presence of phosphates and calcium in the diet. However, the presence of some peptides, amino acids, and ethylenediamine tetra acetic acid disodium (EDTA) may cause an increase in absorption. Generally, the stomach acid provides for rapid release of zinc from ingested metallic objects.

Once zinc has been absorbed it is bound to plasma albumin and to macroglobulins, and transported to the liver. Zinc is extracted by the liver and returned to the bloodstream for distribution to the liver, pancreas, kidney, and spleen, all of which rapidly accumulate the zinc. These tissues, as well as muscle and prostate, are induced to synthesize metallothionein in the cells.

Under normal dietary conditions, excess zinc is excreted through the feces. Nevertheless, excretion of zinc, especially in toxic situations, is limited. Excretion occurs through the bile and feces but may also occur through urine (Abdel-Mageed and Oehme, 1990) and saliva.

MECHANISM OF ACTION

The mechanism of action producing clinical signs is not well defined or understood. The characteristic clinical signs are more easily recognized. The most recognized abnormality observed is severe intravascular hemolysis and gastroenteritis. This may be a result of excess zinc interfering with copper and iron storage and utilization, resulting in a suppression of hematopoiesis.

Diets high in zinc interfere with hepatic copper storage and may compete with calcium for intestinal absorption.

TOXICITY

The different forms of zinc have different toxicities. The zinc salts have a median lethal dose (LD_{50}) of approximately 100 mg/kg body weight. Zinc oxides are less toxic. Zinc oxides are frequently found in ointments, such as for preventing sunburn or treating diaper rash. Dogs often ingest it when it is applied topically to them or to someone they can lick it off. Dogs also ingest the ointment by chewing on the tube container. It has been estimated that the toxic dose is approximately 108 g of zinc for dogs (Breitschwerdt et al., 1986).

Veterinary Toxicology. DOI: http://dx.doi.org/10.1016/B978-0-12-811410-0.00036-2

TABLE 36.1 Uses and Purposes of Zinc

Zinc is used in:	Its purpose is:
Galvanized steel	Prevents corrosion
Parkerized steel	Prevents rust and corrosion
Used in numerous metal alloys	Brass, nickeled silver, typewriter metal, various soldering formulas, German silver
Primary metal	American pennies, nuts, and bolts
Die casting	Automotive industry
Zinc oxide	Paints, sun protectants, rubber activator, diaper rash ointments
Wall tiles	Germicidal properties
Zinc chloride	Wood preservative and deodorant
Zinc methyl ($Zn(CH_3)_2$)	Number of organic syntheses
Zinc stearate	A lubricative plastic additive

The ingestion of pennies, which are 96% zinc (Latimer et al., 1989) and may be as high as 97.5% zinc (https://www.usmint.gov/coins/coin-medal-programs/circulating-coins/penny), by dogs has resulted in the development of a subacute zinc toxicosis. The pennies remain in the acidic environment of the stomach and slowly release metallic zinc. It is unclear how many pennies are required to produce a toxicosis. The size of the animal, lack of food in the stomach, and the number of pennies will all be factors in how quickly zinc toxicities develop. The pennies can be vomited or passed in the feces prior to presentation at the veterinary clinic.

Other forms of zinc-containing hardware such as transport kennel bolts or machine nuts and bolts have caused problems in animals. Analysis of these objects has shown them to be about 97% zinc (Breitschwerdt et al., 1986; Torrance and Fulton, 1987). They remain in the stomach, producing a subclinical toxicosis or are vomited or passed out prior to the animal's presentation.

Other sources of toxicity have been galvanized wire used in cages in aviaries (Reece et al., 1986) and for housing ferrets (Straube et al., 1980). The toys an animal selects may be made almost entirely of zinc (Bexfield et al., 2007), and may not necessarily be a toy designed for animals. In addition to galvanized wire, avian food dishes and toys such as bells and other shiny toys may contain zinc. Birds, such as parrots may be able to chip the exterior of the feeding container or bend the toy bells and be exposed to zinc (Center for Avian & Exotic Medicine).

An additional component of zinc toxicosis is acute renal failure observed in some dogs (Breitschwerdt et al., 1986). The clinical findings include hypercreatinemia, azotemia, hyperphosphatemia, and granular casts in the urine (Breitschwerdt et al., 1986; Torrance and Fulton, 1987; Latimer et al., 1989). Other signs of acute intoxication are pancreatitis and acute arthritis. Also, non-viable newborns may be observed with zinc intoxication.

Foals are susceptible to zinc intoxication. It appears to be a chronic zinc toxicosis. Initially, the foals have non-painful joint enlargement lasting 7–21 days. They are reluctant to rise and have stiff gait and increased joint fluid (Gunson et al., 1982).

Other livestock have early signs of lethargy and anorexia followed by diarrhea. Later, they display a decreased rate of gain or decreased milk production. As the toxic condition progresses, the animals have anemia and icterus. Other signs include exophthalmia, polydipsia, polyphagia, and seizures.

Generally most species display some degree of hemolytic anemia, often with an erythrocytic regenerative response. Additionally, there is renal damage with hematuria, urinary casts, and proteinuria. Diagnostically, there may be a radiodense area in the gastrointestinal tract indicating the presence of zinc or some other metal such as lead. Postmortem lesions include renal tubular necrosis, hepatocyte necrosis, and gastroenteritis.

TREATMENT

As with many metal intoxications, removal of the source of the toxin from the animal, followed by supportive therapy, are critical to the patient's recovery. This procedure with zinc will result in dramatic drops in serum and tissue levels within a relatively short time. Removal of the source will allow the normal excretory pathways to work appropriately.

Particularly when treating foals it is important to evaluate the copper status of the animal. Copper and zinc seem to work in tandem and adding copper to copper-deficient animals may help decrease the overriding effects of zinc.

Supportive care is critically important as the gastroenteritis and anemia must be addressed. Activated charcoal is not recommended as it is ineffective at absorbing elemental zinc. The vomiting, in species capable of vomiting, has usually resulted in severe gastroenteritis. Vomiting may be controlled with metoclopramide (0.2–0.4 mg/kg) administered every 6 h intramuscularly (IM), subcutaneously (SQ) or per os. Decreasing zinc absorption may be accomplished by decreasing gastric acidity (Meurs, 1995). Use of H2-receptor blockers, such as famotidine (0.5 mg/kg orally, SQ, intramuscularly, or intravenously (IV)) should be administered once or twice daily (Plumb, 1999) until the serum zinc has decreased.

Blood transfusions may be necessary to address the anemia. Fluid therapy with a balanced solution such as lactated Ringer's solution is appropriate. Good supportive care includes continuous monitoring of various blood parameters such as red blood cells, platelets, packed cell volume and serum chemistries including liver enzymes, serum urea nitrogen, and electrolytes. Treatment efforts must be directed at correcting pancreatic, renal, and/or liver dysfunctions, which are closely associated with zinc intoxication.

A radiograph of the animal should help locate the offending object. Removing the offending object or objects is important in decreasing the serum zinc concentrations. If the patient is asymptomatic, inducing emesis may remove the object. The offending agent should be removed, either by surgery or retrieval by endoscopy. Serum zinc levels should decrease when the offending object is removed from the patient. However, dogs may die as a result of complications from anemia or kidney failure even after a penny or other zinc object is removed (Latimer et al., 1989).

Evaluate the serum zinc levels after removal of what is believed to be the offending object. If the zinc levels have not dropped, then all of the offending objects have not been removed from the gastrointestinal tract or the renal insufficiency has prevented zinc excretion. If either of these situations is present, then chelation therapy (see below paragraph) is inappropriate and contraindicated as it may increase gastrointestinal or intestinal absorption of any remaining zinc, and the chelated metal is potentially nephrotoxic.

Chelation therapy is an option in the patient's care. Chelation therapy is effective but not without risk and some controversy (see above paragraph) so must be evaluated with regard to the patient's overall condition. Patient conditions requiring evaluation include the hydration status, the degree of dysfunction of the excretory organs, especially the kidneys, and the severity of the serum zinc concentration. While chelation therapy can increase zinc elimination and speed recovery, chelation treatment may increase absorption of zinc from the intestines (Cahill-Morasco, 2016). Hence, removal of the offending item prior to chelation therapy is critical. The most commonly suggested chelator is calcium disodium EDTA. Calcium disodium EDTA is most commonly used to treat lead intoxication and the dose for zinc intoxication has thus been extrapolated (100 mg/kg and may be given IV or SQ, divided into four doses per day for 3 days. It may be diluted in 5% dextrose or in sterile water to decrease local irritation) but may exacerbate zinc-induced nephrotoxicity. Especially with chelation therapy, daily monitoring of the patient is essential to determine the length of therapy.

CONCLUDING REMARKS AND FUTURE DIRECTIONS

Evidence of pancreatitis, liver, and kidney dysfunction must be considered along with gastroenteritis and a hemolytic event when considering the differentials. The clinical sign of acute gastroenteritis is common to viral and bacterial diseases, parasitic diseases, and various neoplasms. Gastroenteritis and a hemolytic event must be differentiated from other metal intoxications such as copper poisoning. Additional considerations include acetaminophen or onion intoxication, mustard poisoning, immune-mediated diseases and certain snake bites.

As zinc is a very economically useful metal it is likely to be found in more products that animals are exposed to in various fashions. It would be beneficial to have a larger array of safe chelation products. Unfortunately, the importance of chelation therapy outweighs the available markets for the product. Therefore it is unlikely research dollars will be directed at finding new chelation therapies.

Online Contents

Center for Avian &Exotic Medicine <https://avianandexoticvets.com/top-toxins-to-pet-birds/>.

US Mint <https://www.usmint.gov/coins/coin-medal-programs/circulating-coins/penny>.

REFERENCES

Abdel-Mageed, A.B., Oehme, F.W., 1990. A review of the biochemical roles, toxicity and interactions of zinc, copper and iron: 1. Zinc. Vet. Hum. Toxicol. 32 (1), 34–39.

Bexfield, N., Archer, J., Herrtage, M., 2007. Heinz body haemolytic anaemia in a dog secondary to ingestion of a zinc toy: a case report. Vet. J. 174 (2), 414–417.

Breitschwerdt, E.B., Armstrong, P.J., Robinette, C.L., et al., 1986. Three cases of acute zinc toxicosis in dogs. Vet. Hum. Toxicol. 28, 109.

Cahill-Morasco, R., 2016. Zinc toxicosis. In: Aiello, S., Moses, M.A. (Eds.), The Merck Veterinary Manual, eleventh ed. Merck & Co, Inc, New Jersey, pp. 3088–3089.

Chasapis, C.T., Loutsidou, A.C., Spiliopoulou, C.A., et al., 2012. Zinc and human health: an update. Arch. Toxicol. 86, 521–534.

Gunson, D.E., Kowalczyk, D.F., Shoop, C.R., et al., 1982. Environmental zinc and cadmium pollution associated with generalized osteochondrosis, osteoporosis, and nephrocalcinosis in horses. J. Am. Vet. Med. Assoc. 180 (3), 295–299.

Latimer, K.S., Jain, A.V., Inglesby, H.B., et al., 1989. Zinc-induced hemolytic anemia caused by ingestion of pennies by a pup. J. Am. Vet. Med. Assoc. 195 (1), 77–80.

Marchan, R., Cadenas, C., Bolt, H.M., 2012. Zinc as a multipurpose trace element. Arch. Toxicol. 86, 519–520.

Marger, L., Schubert, C.R., Bertrand, D., 2014. Zinc: an underappreciated modulatory factor of brain function. Biochem. Pharmacol. 91, 426–435.

Mayward, M., Rink, L., 2015. Zinc homeostasis and immunosenescence. J. Trace Elment. Med. Biol. 29, 24–30.

Meurs, K.M., 1995. CVT Update: zinc toxicity. In: Bonagura, J.D. (Ed.), Kirk's Current Veterinary Therapy XII Small Animal Practice. W.B Saunders, Pennsylvania, pp. 238–239.

Oteiza, P.I., 2012. Zinc and the modulation of redox homeostasis. Free Rad Biol. Med. 53, 1748–1759.

Plumb, D.C., 1999. Veterinary Drug Handbook. third ed. Iowa State University Press, Iowa (pp 134, 218–219, 221–223, 264).

Reece, R.L., Dickson, D.B., Burrowes, P.J., 1986. Zinc toxicity (new wire disease) in aviary birds. Aust. Vet. J. 63, 199.

Straube, E.F., Schuster, N.H., Sinclair, A.J., 1980. Zinc toxicity in the ferret. J. Comp. Pathol. 90, 355.

Torrance, A.G., Fulton, R.B., 1987. Zinc-induced hemolytic anemia in a dog. J. Am. Vet. Med. Assoc. 191, 443.

Section VI

Insecticides

Chapter 37

Organophosphates and Carbamates

Ramesh C. Gupta, Magdalini Sachana, Ida M. Mukherjee, Robin B. Doss, Jitendra K. Malik and Dejan Milatovic

INTRODUCTION

Organophosphates (OPs) and carbamates (CMs) are commonly used in agriculture, industry and around homes/gardens throughout the world. In addition, these chemicals are used in veterinary and human medicine. Both types of chemicals produce their toxicity by virtue of inhibition of the acetylcholinesterase (AChE) enzyme, which terminates the action of the neurotransmitter acetylcholine (ACh) at the synapses in nervous tissue and at the neuromuscular junctions (NMJs). These chemicals are referred to as "anticholinesterase agents". OPs, with strong AChE inhibiting potential, are also used as nerve agents or nerve gases in chemical warfare.

Many compounds of both classes are extremely toxic and lack species selectivity. Their inadvertent/accidental use continues to pose a threat to human and animal health, wildlife and aquatic systems, and the environment. Small animals often encounter poisoning with these insecticides via malicious activity or accidental exposure, while livestock may ingest freshly sprayed crop or contaminated feed. Although these compounds are neurotoxicants, they produce a variety of cholinergic and noncholinergic effects. The latest evidence suggests that while cholinergic mechanisms play a critical role in the initial stage of toxicity, neuronal damage/death appears to occur through noncholinergic mechanisms. OPs and CMs are discussed together here because they produce similar toxic effects in poisoned animals. This chapter describes various aspects of toxicity of OP and CM compounds and therapeutic interventions in animals. For more details, readers are referred to publications elsewhere (Gupta, 2006; Satoh and Gupta, 2010; Gupta and Milatovic, 2012; Gupta et al., 2017).

BACKGROUND

Tetraethyl pyrophosphate was the first OP compound synthesized in 1854 by Philipe de Clermont. In 1932, Lange and Kruger described the synthesis of dimethyl and diethyl phosphorofluoridate. Based on the chemistry of these compounds, Gerhard Schrader (a chemist at the I.G. Farbenindustrie) led the exploration of the OP class of compounds that could be used as insecticides. One of the earliest OP insecticides synthesized by Schrader was parathion, which is still used worldwide. Prior to World War II, the German Ministry of Defense developed highly toxic OPs of the G series (tabun, sarin and soman) and diisopropyl phosphorofluoridate. In the 1950s, OP compounds with super toxicity of the V series, such as VX and VR, were synthesized in the United Kingdom and the Soviet Union. Since World War II, thousands of OPs have been synthesized in the search for compounds with species selectivity, i.e., more toxicity to insects and less toxicity to mammals. Malathion is an example, as it has been used for more than half a century as the most popular insecticide. Today, more than 200 OPs are in use for a variety of purposes, such as protection of crops, grains, gardens, homes and public health.

The first carbamate compound, physostigmine (eserine alkaloid), was isolated from calabar beans (ordeal poison) of a perennial plant *Physostigma venenosum* in the mid-1860s. The compound was used to treat glaucoma. About 50 years later, an aromatic ester of carbamic acid, neostigmine, was synthesized and used in the treatment of myasthenia gravis. Most of the carbamates (esters of carbamic acid) that are used as pesticides were synthesized in the 1960s and 1970s. Carbaryl was the first CM compound used as an insecticide. The most toxic compound of this class, aldicarb, was synthesized by mimicking the structure of ACh. Like OPs, thousands of CMs have been synthesized, but fewer than two dozen compounds have been used practically. Today, CMs are preferred for pesticide use over OPs because some OPs have been found to be extremely neurotoxic, while others cause delayed neuropathy in animals as well as in humans. In essence, both OPs and CMs have broad applications in agriculture and veterinary medicine and as a result of their indiscriminate use acute poisonings often result in animals, birds, fish, and wildlife.

Veterinary Toxicology. DOI: http://dx.doi.org/10.1016/B978-0-12-811410-0.00037-4

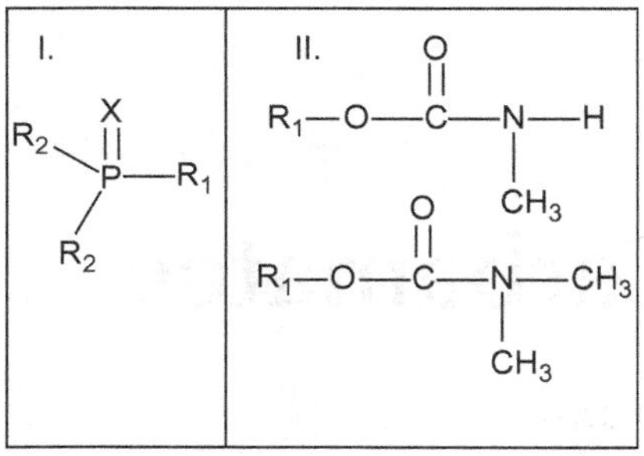

FIGURE 37.1 General structure for organophosphorus (I) and carbamate (II) insecticides. *Adapted from Timchalk, C., 2006. Physiologically based pharmacokinetic modeling of organophosphorus and carbamate pesticides. In R.C. Gupta (Ed.), Toxicology of Organophosphate and Carbamate Compounds. Academic Press/Elsevier, Amsterdam, pp. 103–125*

Basic structures of OPs and CMs are shown in Fig. 37.1. There are at least 13 types of OPs (Table 37.1). Despite differences in chemical structures, all OPs share one thing in common: they all have a pentavalent phosphorus atom and a characteristic phosphoryl bond (PO) or thiophosphoryl bond (PS). Essentially, OPs are esters of phosphoric acid with varying combinations of oxygen, carbon, sulfur and/or nitrogen attached. Of course, the chemistry of these compounds is much more complex. The OPs that are derivatives of phosphoric or phosphonic acid possess anticholinesterase activity, unlike those that are derivatives of phosphinic acid. Usually, OP compounds have two alkyl substituents and an additional substituents group (the leaving group, which is more labile to hydrolysis than the alkyl group). Some OPs, such as dichlorvos, monocrotophos and trichlorfon, are direct AChE inhibitors, while those of the phosphorothioates type, such as bromophos, diazinon, fenthion and parathion, possess minimal anticholinesterase (anti-AChE) activity and require desulfuration to analogous oxon before acquiring anti-AChE activity and hypercholinergic effects. Also, OPs that are used as defoliants (*S,S,S*-tributyl phosphorotrithioate and *S,S,S*-tributyl phosphorotrithioite), herbicides (glyphosate and gluphosinate), flame retardants, and plasticizers are of very low mammalian toxicity.

OP PESTICIDES

The majority of OP compounds are used as pesticides. Chemical descriptions for commonly used compounds and their toxicity are given in Table 37.2. Chemical structures of some of the commonly used OP pesticides are shown in Fig. 37.2.

OP NERVE AGENTS/GASES

OP nerve agents include tabun (GA), sarin (GB), soman (GD), cyclosarin (GF), venom toxin (VX), and Russian VX (VR). These compounds are highly toxic and pose continuous threats to the lives of humans as well as animals since they can be used as chemical weapons of mass destruction (CWMD). Unlike so many incidents in humans, animals have also been victims in some incidents of military operations. These compounds produce toxicity by directly inhibiting AChE, and are much more potent than OP pesticides. Their chemical structures are shown in Fig. 37.3. For details of toxicity of these compounds, refer to Watson et al. (2006, 2015) and Rembovskiy et al. (2015).

CARBAMATES

The carbamate (CM) compounds are esters of carbamic acid. Unlike OPs, CM compounds are not structurally complex. Chemical structures of some commonly used CM insecticides are shown in Fig. 37.4, and brief toxicological data of CMs is provided in Table 37.3. For the details of CMs, readers are referred to Gupta (2006) and Gupta and Milatovic (2012). Currently, the volume of CMs used exceeds OPs because of their relative safety.

PHARMACOKINETICS OF OPs AND CMs

Pharmacokinetics deals with the rate limiting processes of absorption, distribution, metabolism and excretion (ADME). The ADME of some OP and CM insecticides in animals have been described (Tomokuni et al., 1985; Gupta, 1994; Wu et al., 1996; Timchalk, 2006, 2010; Gupta and Milatovic, 2012; Gupta et al., 2017). These insecticides gain entry into the body mainly through oral, dermal, or inhalation exposure. Ingestion of food contaminated with pesticides residue is common, while dermal exposure is more relevant when these insecticides are used as ectoparasiticides in the form of dust, dip, or oily solution. Inhalation of airborne insecticides occurs during or soon after aerial spray, particularly due to chemical drift. Once the insecticide reaches a portal of entry, it is available for absorption. It is established that following absorption, these insecticides are well distributed in tissues throughout the body. Being lipophilic, maximum levels of these compounds are usually found in the adipose tissue and brain.

In terms of metabolism, OP insecticides may follow either activation and/or detoxification. Activation implies that the metabolite is more toxic than the parent compound, e.g., the conversion of malathion to malaoxon. This process is often called "lethal synthesis." On the other hand, detoxification implies that the metabolite is less toxic than the parent compound, e.g., the conversion of malathion to malathion monoacid and malathion diacid. Unlike OPs, CMs are metabolized to less toxic or

TABLE 37.1 Types of Organophosphates

Type of OP	Chemical Structure	Example
Phosphates	O ‖ RO—P—OR | OR	Chlorfenvinphos, Dichlorvos, Monocrotophos
Phosphonates	O ‖ RO—P—R | OR	Trichlorfon
Phosphinates	O ‖ R—P—R | OR	Gluphosinate
Phosphorothioates (S)	S ‖ RO—P—OR | OR	Bromophos, Diazinon, Fenthion, Parathion, Pirimiphos-methyl
Phosphonothioates (S)	S ‖ RO—P—R | OR	EPN, Leptophos
Phosphorothioates (S-substituted)	O ‖ RS—P—OR | OR	Demeton-S-methyl, Echothiophate
Phosphonothioates (*S*-substituted)	O ‖ RS—P—R | OR	VX
Phosphorodithioates	O ‖ RS—P—SR | OR or S ‖ RS—P—OR | OR	Azinphos-ethyl, Azinphos-methyl, Dimethoate, Disulfoton, Malathion, Methidathion
Phosphorotrithioates	O ‖ RS—P—SR | SR	DEF (tribufos)
Phosphoramidates	O ‖ RO—P—N(R)(R) | OR	Fenamiphos
Phosphoramidothioates	S ‖ RO—P—N(R)(R) | OR or O ‖ RS—P—N(R)(R) | OR	Methamidophos, Isofenphos

(*Continued*)

TABLE 37.1 (Continued)

Type of OP	Chemical Structure	Example
Phosphorofluoridates	$RO{-}P(=O)(OR){-}F$	Diisopropyl phosphorofluoridate (DFP)
Phosphonofluoridates	$RO{-}P(=O)(R){-}F$	Cyclosarin, Sarin, Soman

Source: Adapted from Marrs, T.C., 1993. Organophosphate poisoning. Pharmacol. Ther. 58: 51–66.

TABLE 37.2 A Brief Chemical Description of Commonly Used OP Pesticides and Their Toxicity

Chemical	Chemical Name	Mol. wt.	Oral LD_{50} in Rat (mg/kg)	Dermal LD_{50} in rabbit (mg/kg)
Acephate	*O,S*-dimethyl acetylamidothiophosphate	183.17	866	>2000
Azinphos-ethyl	*O,O*-diethyl *S*-[(4-oxo-1,2,3-benzotriazin-3(4*H*)-yl) methyl] dithiophosphate	345.38	13	250
Azinphos-methyl	*O,O*-dimethyl *S*-[(4-oxo-1,2,3-benzotriazin-3(4*H*)-yl) methyl] dithiophosphate	317.32	5	220
Bromophos	*O*-(4-bromo-2,5-dichlorophenyl) *O,O*-dimethyl thiophosphate	366.00	1600	2188
Cadusaphos	*S,S*-di-*sec*-butyl *O*-ethyl dithiophosphate	270.40	391	143
Carbophenothion	*S*-{[(4-chlorophenyl)thio] methyl} *O,O*-diethyl dithiophosphate	342.87	6	22
Chlorethoxyphos	*O,O*-diethyl *O*-(1,2,2,2-tetrachloroethyl) thiophosphate	336.00	1.8	12.5
Chlorfenvinphos	2-chloro-1-(2,4-dichloro-phenyl)vinyl diethyl phosphate	359.57	12	3200
Chlorpyrifos	*O,O*-diethyl *O*-(3,5,6-trichloropyridin-2-yl) thiophosphate	350.59	135	2000
Chlorpyrifos-methyl	*O,O*-dimethyl *O*-(3,5,6-trichloropyridin-2-yl) thiophosphate	322.53	941	2000
Coumaphos	*O*-(3-chloro-4-methyl-2-oxo-2*H*-chromen-7-yl) *O,O*-diethyl thiophosphate	362.77	13	–
Crotoxyphos	1-phenylethyl (2*E*)-3-[(dimethoxyphosphoryl)oxy]but-2-enoate	314.27	125	385
Cyanophos	*O*-(4-cyanophenyl) *O,O*-dimethyl thiophosphate	243.22	610	800
Demeton-O	*O,O*-diethyl *O*-[2-(ethylthio)ethyl] thiophosphate	258.34	2.5	8
Diazinon	*O,O*-diethyl *O*-(2-isopropyl-6-methylpyrimidin-4-yl) thiophosphate	304.35	300	379
Dichlorvos	2,2-dichlorovinyl dimethyl phosphate	220.98	25	59

(*Continued*)

TABLE 37.2 (Continued)

Chemical	Chemical Name	Mol. wt.	Oral LD_{50} in Rat (mg/kg)	Dermal LD_{50} in rabbit (mg/kg)
Dicrotophos	(1*E*)-3-(dimethylamino)-1-methyl-3-oxoprop-1-en-1-yl dimethyl phosphate	237.19	22	223
Dimethoate	*O,O*-dimethyl *S*-[2-(methylamino)-2-oxoethyl] dithiophosphate	229.26	250	400
Disulfoton	*O,O*-diethyl *S*-[2-(ethylthio)ethyl] dithiophosphate	274.40	2	6
Ethion	*O,O,O′,O′*-tetraethyl *S,S′*-methylene bis (dithiophosphate)	384.48	27	915
Famphur	*O*-{4-[(dimethylamino)sulfonyl]phenyl} *O,O*-dimethyl thiophosphate	325.34	35	2730
Fenamiphos	ethyl 3-methyl-4-(methylthio)phenyl isopropylamidophosphate	303.36	15.3	–
Fenitrothion	*O,O*-dimethyl *O*-(3-methyl-4-nitrophenyl) thiophosphate	277.23	250	1300
Fenthion	*O,O*-dimethyl *O*-[3-methyl-4-(methylthio)phenyl] thiophosphate	278.33	255	330
Fonofos	*O*-ethyl *S*-phenyl ethylphosphonodithioate	246.33	8	25
Glyphosate	*N*-(phosphonomethyl)-glycine	169.07	4300	>5000
Gluphosinate ammonium	2-amino-4-[hydroxy(methyl)phosphoryl]butanoic acid ammoniate	198.16	2000	>4000
Glyphosine	*N,N*-bis(phosphonomethyl)glycine	263.08	3925	>5010
Isazophos	*O*-(5-chloro-1-isopropyl-1*H*-1,2,4-triazol-3-yl) *O,O*-diethyl thiophosphate	313.75	40	>3100
Isofenphos	isopropyl 2-{[ethoxy(isopropylamino) phosphorothioyl]oxy}benzoate	345.40	32	162
Malathion	diethyl 2-[(dimethoxyphosphorothioyl)thio] succinate	330.36	885	4000
Methamidophos	*O,S*-dimethyl amidothiophosphate	141.13	13	110
Methidathion	*S*-[(5-methoxy-2-oxo-1,3,4-thiadiazol-3(2*H*)-yl) methyl] *O,O*-dimethyl dithiophosphate	302.33	25	200
Methyl parathion	*O,O*-dimethyl *O*-(4-nitrophenyl) thiophosphate	263.21	9	63
Mevinphos	methyl (2*E*)-3-[(dimethoxyphosphoryl)oxy]but-2-enoate	224.15	3	16
Monocrotophos	dimethyl (1*E*)-1-methyl-3-(methylamino)-3-oxoprop-1-en-1-yl phosphate	223.16	8	354
Omethoate	*O,O*-dimethyl *S*-[2-(methylamino)-2-oxoethyl] thiophosphate	213.19	50	1400
Paraoxon	diethyl 4-nitrophenyl phosphate	275.19	1.8	–
Parathion	*O,O*-diethyl *O*-(4-nitrophenyl) thiophosphate	291.26	3	6.8
Phenthoate	ethyl [(dimethoxyphosphorothioyl)thio] (phenyl) acetate	320.36	200	4000
Phorate	*O,O*-diethyl *S*-[(ethylthio)methyl] dithiophosphate	260.38	1.6	2.5
Phosmet	*S*-[(1,3-dioxo-1,3-dihydro-2*H*-iso-indol-2-yl)methyl] *O,O*-dimethyl dithiophosphate	317.32	147	3160
Phosphamidon	(1*Z*)-2-chloro-3-(diethylamino)-1-methyl-3-oxoprop-1-en-1-yl dimethyl phosphate	299.69	15	125

(*Continued*)

TABLE 37.2 (Continued)

Chemical	Chemical Name	Mol. wt.	Oral LD_{50} in Rat (mg/kg)	Dermal LD_{50} in rabbit (mg/kg)
Phoxim	phenylglyoxylonitrile oxime, *O,O*-diethyl phosphorothioate	289.30	1845	1126
Profenofos	*O*-(4-bromo-2-chlorophenyl) *O*-ethyl *S*-propyl thiophosphate	373.63	400	472
Propetamphos	isopropyl (2*E*)-3-{[(ethylamino)(methoxy) phosphorothioyl]oxy}but-2-enoate	281.31	82	2300
Quinalphos	*O,O*-diethyl *O*-quinoxalin-2-yl thiophosphate	298.30	65	340
Ronnel	*O,O*-dimethyl *O*-(2,4,5-trichlorophenyl) thiophosphate	321.55	1250	2000
Sulfotepp	*O,O,O,O*-tetraethyl dithiodiphosphate	322.32	5	–
Sulprofos	*O*-ethyl *O*-[4-(methylthio)phenyl] *S*-propyl dithiophosphate	322.45	107	820
Terbufos	*S*-[(*tert*-butylthio)methyl] *O,O*-diethyl dithiophosphate	288.43	1.6	1
Triazophos	*O,O*-diethyl *O*-(1-phenyl-1*H*-1,2,4-triazol-3-yl) thiophosphate	313.32	83	280
Trichlorfon	dimethyl (2,2,2-trichloro-1-hydroxyethyl)phosphonate	257.44	630	>2100

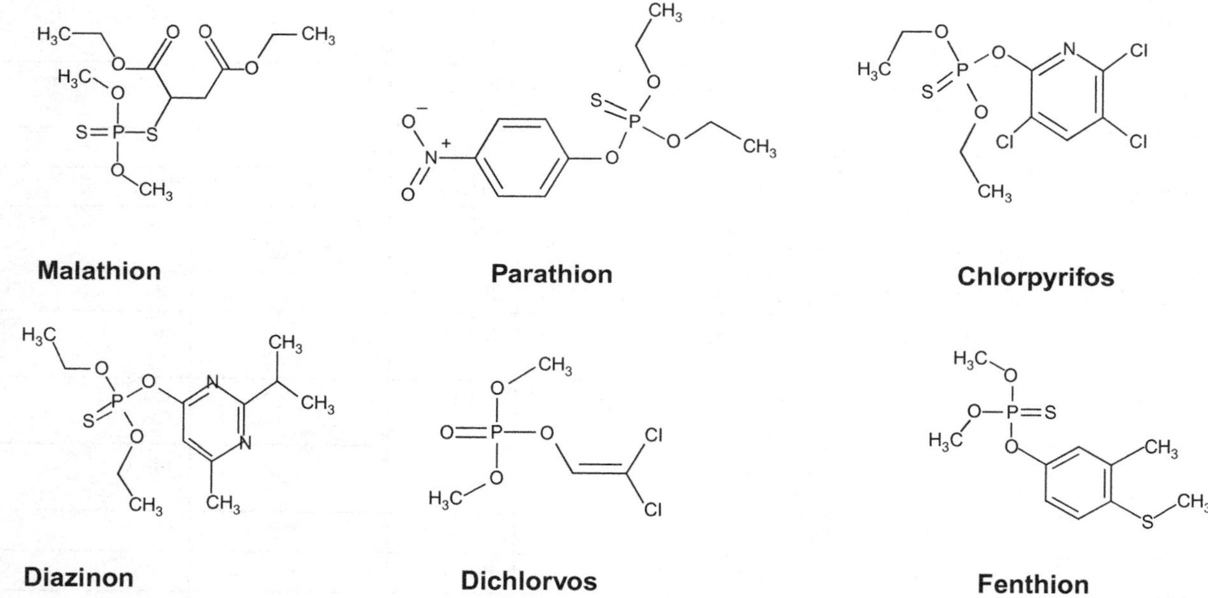

FIGURE 37.2 Chemical structures of commonly used OP pesticides.

nontoxic metabolites. There are some metabolites of CMs that are quite toxic. For example, the two major metabolites (3-hydroxycarbofuran and 3-ketocarbofuran) of carbofuran have a significant impact on overall toxicity of carbofuran (Gupta, 1994).

A bulk of the metabolic activation and detoxification of OPs and CMs occurs within the liver (Tang et al., 2006; Sogorb and Vilanova, 2010; Vacondio et al., 2010; Gupta and Milatovic, 2012). Due to extensive metabolism of these insecticides in the body, only a few

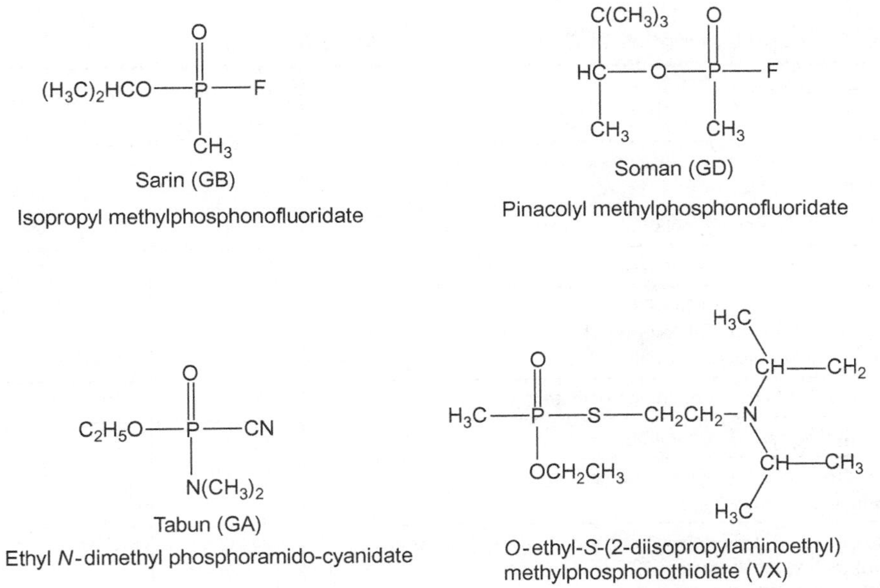

Sarin (GB)
Isopropyl methylphosphonofluoridate
Soman (GD)
Pinacolyl methylphosphonofluoridate
Tabun (GA)
Ethyl *N*-dimethyl phosphoramido-cyanidate
O-ethyl-*S*-(2-diisopropylaminoethyl) methylphosphonothiolate (VX)

FIGURE 37.3 Chemical structures of OP nerve agents.

Carbaryl
Carbofuran
Aldicarb
Oxamyl
Methomyl
Propoxur

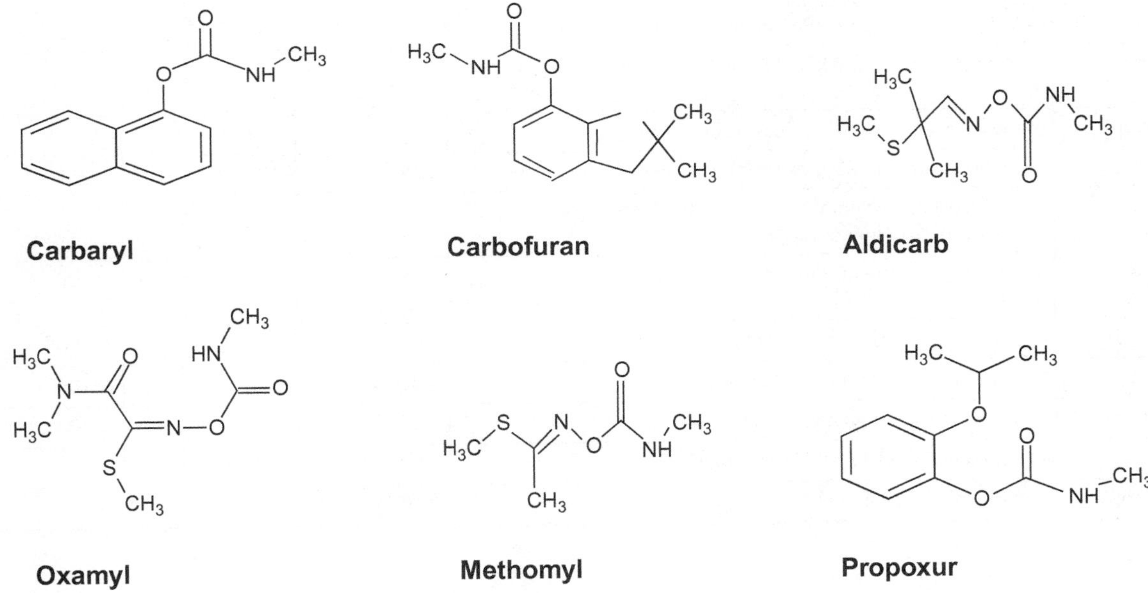

FIGURE 37.4 Chemical structures of commonly used CM pesticides.

metabolites are excreted in the urine that can be used as biomarkers of insecticides exposure (Gupta and Milatovic, 2014; Mangas et al., 2017). Residues of some OPs and CMs can also be detected in the feces, saliva and milk. In dead animals, residues of OPs and CMs are likely to be detected in the GI content (following ingestion), adipose tissue and brain.

MECHANISM OF ACTION

OP and CM insecticides share a common mode of toxicological action associated with their ability to inhibit the AChE enzyme within the nervous tissue and at the NMJs. Both types of insecticides have a high affinity for binding to and inhibiting AChE, an enzyme specifically responsible for the hydrolysis of the neurotransmitter ACh. Since

TABLE 37.3 A Brief Chemical Description of Commonly Used CM Pesticides and Their Toxicity

Chemical	Chemical Name	Molecular Weight	Oral LD_{50} in Rat (mg/kg)	Dermal LD_{50} in Rabbit (mg/kg)
Aldicarb	(1*E*)-2-methyl-2-(methylthio)propanal *O*-[(methylamino) carbonyl] oxime	190.26	0.9	5
Aminocarb	4-(dimethylamino)-3-methylphenyl methylcarbamate	208.26	30	275
Bendiocarb	2,2-dimethyl-1,3-benzodioxol-4-yl methylcarbamate	223.23	34	566
Benfuracarb	2,3-dihydro-2,2-dimethyl-7-benzofuranyl N-[n[2-(ethylcarbonyl) ethyl]-*N*-isopropyl sulfenamoyl]-*N*-methylcarbamate	410.53	138	>2000
BPMC	2-*sec*-butylphenyl *N*-methylcarbamate	422.87	340	4200
Carbaryl	1-naphthyl methylcarbamate	201.22	307	2000
Carbofuran	2,2-dimethyl-2,3-dihydro-1-benzofuran-7-yl methylcarbamate	221.25	8	2550
Carbosulfan	2,3-dihydro-2,2-dimethyl-7-benzofuranyl-[(di-butylamino) thio] methyl carbamate	380.55	209	>2000
Croneton	2-[(ethylthio)methyl]phenyl methyl carbamate	225.31	200	1000
Fenoxycarb	ethyl [2-(4-phenoxyphenoxy)ethyl] carbamate	301.34	10,000	2000
Isoprocarb	2-isopropylphenyl methyl carbamate	193.24	450	–
Methiocarb	3,5-dimethyl-4-(methylthio)phenyl methyl carbamate	225.31	15	2000
Methomyl	methyl (1*E*)-*N*-{[(methylamino) carbonyl]oxy} ethanimidothioate	162.21	17	5000
Metolcarb	3-methylphenyl methyl carbamate	165	268	–
Mexacarbate	4-(dimethylamino)-3,5-dimethylphenyl methyl carbamate	222.28	15	5000
Oxamyl	methyl 2-(dimethylamino)-*N*-{[(methyl-amino)carbonyl] oxy}-2-oxoethan-imidothioate	219.26	5	710
Pirimicarb	2-(dimethylamino)-5,6-dimethyyrimidin-4-yl dimethylcarbamate	238.29	147	>500
Promecarb	3-isopropyl-5-methylphenyl methyl carbamate	207.27	61	>1000
Propoxur	2-isopropoxyphenyl methyl carbamate	209.24	95	>1000
Trimethacarb	3,4,5-trimethylphenyl methyl carbamate	193.24	125	>2000
XMC	3,5-dimethylphenyl methyl carbamate	179.22	542	–
Xylylcarb	3,4-dimethylphenyl methyl carbamate	179.22	384	–

the cholinergic system is widely distributed within both the central and peripheral nervous systems, chemicals that inhibit AChE are known to produce a broad range of well-characterized symptoms of anticholinesterases. A graphic representation for the comparison of the AChE inhibition dynamics for the interaction of ACh, carbaryl (CM) or chlorpyrifos-oxon (OP) with AChE is shown in Fig. 37.5 (Timchalk, 2006). The cholinesterases (ChEs) are serine hydrolases that catalyze the breakdown of ACh through an acyl-transfer, where water is the acceptor molecule to which the substrate acyl moiety is transferred. A serine oxygen of the active site gorge in ChEs carries out a nucleophilic attack on the electrophilic carbon of the carbonyl group of ACh, resulting in an acetylated enzyme intermediate and the release of choline. Deacetylation occurs when an attacking water molecule (hydroxyl ion) acts as a more effective nucleophile, thereby releasing acetate. The molecular interactions between OPs and AChE (Fig. 37.6) have been studied in much more detail than those between CMs and AChE. The rates of hydrolysis and reactivation of AChE following carbamylation and phosphorylation of the active site appears to be markedly slower than for the hydrolysis of the acetylated enzyme. The turnover time for ACh is of the order of ~150 μs,

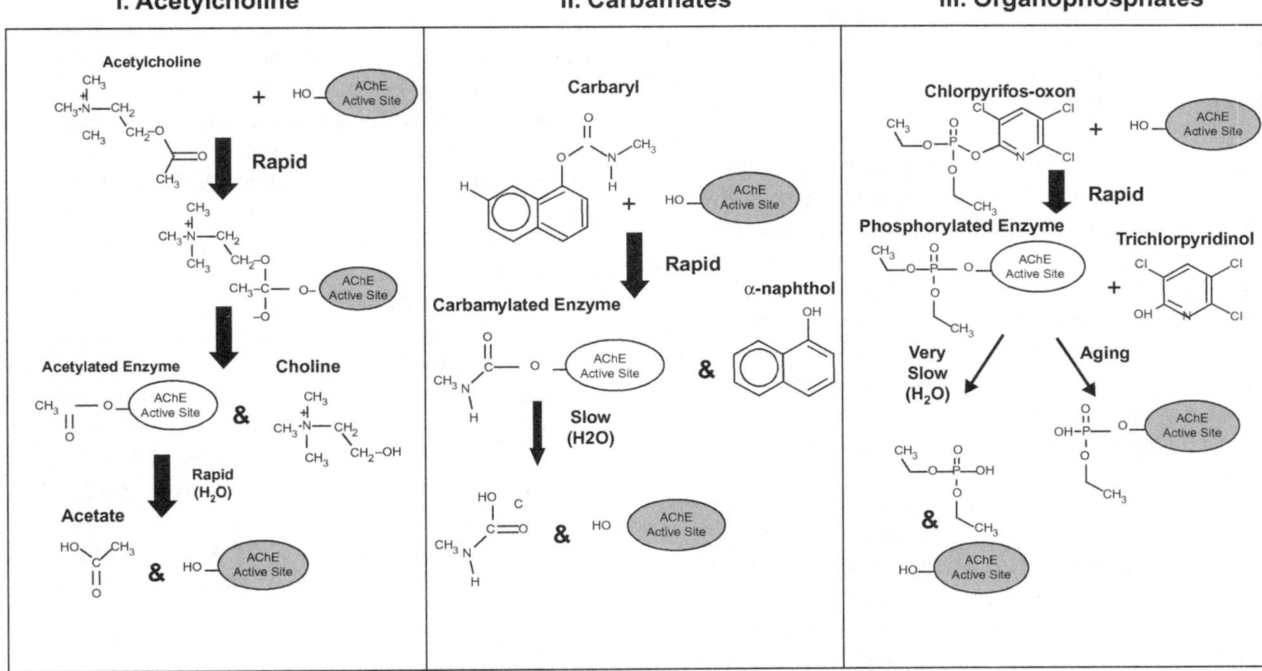

FIGURE 37.5 Interaction of acetylcholine (I), the carbamate carbaryl (II), and the organophosphate chlorpyrifos-oxon (III) with the active site of acetylcholinesterase (AChE). The general rate of bound AChE hydrolysis is ACh > carbaryl > chlorpyrifos-oxon (Timchalk, 2006).

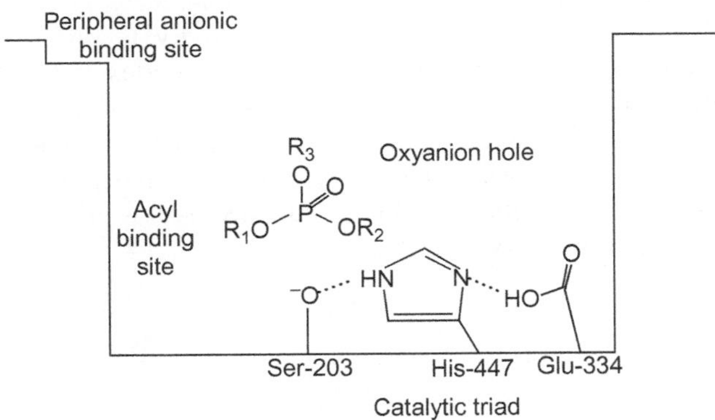

FIGURE 37.6 Schematic drawing of the active site gorge of AChE, with the entry of an OP molecule. R_1 and R_2 on the OP are usually identical alkyl chains, whereas R_3 is the leaving group. The catalytic triad consists of Ser203, His447 and Glu334. The acyl binding site is likely important in positioning the inhibitor for the nucleophilic attack from Ser203 (Ordentlich et al., 1996), whereas the oxyanion hole may polarize the PO bond, thereby facilitating the nucleophilic attack (Ordentlich et al., 1998). Binding of ligand to the peripheral anionic site can lead to inhibition or activation. Additionally, the peripheral anionic site plays an important role in the stereoselectivity of AChE toward methylphosphonates (Ordentlich et al., 2004). *Adapted from Sultatos, L.G., 2006. Interactions of organophosphorus and carbamate compounds with cholinesterases. In Gupta, R.C. (Ed.), Toxicology of Organophosphate and Carbamate Compounds. Academic Press/Elsevier, Amsterdam, pp. 209–218.*

whereas the carbamylated enzyme $t_{½}$ for hydrolysis is substantially slower (~15–30 min). The phosphorylated enzyme is highly stable ($t_{½}$ ~days), and further dealkylation of the phosphorylation group produces an "aged" AChE that is irreversibly inhibited (Taylor, 2006; Timchalk, 2006). In general, OPs and CMs are considered as irreversible and reversible AChE inhibitors, respectively. Details of ChEs, interaction of OPs and CMs with ChEs, and reactivation/regeneration of ChEs, are described elsewhere (Radic and Taylor, 2006; Sultatos, 2006; Timchalk, 2006; Jokanovic, 2010; Gupta and Milatovic, 2012; Mangas et al., 2017).

By now, it is established that OP/CM-induced seizures and lethality are also associated with noncholinergic mechanisms, such as *N*-methyl-D-aspartate (NMDA) receptors, and adenosinergic, gamma-aminobutyric (GABAergic), monoaminergic systems, and others (Gupta, 2004; Gupta et al., 2007; Dekundy and Kaminski, 2010; Myhrer, 2010; Gupta and Milatovic, 2012; Marrs and Maynard, 2013; Kaur et al., 2014). Furthermore, the persistence of excitotoxicity for more than an hour can lead to oxidative and nitrosative stress, neuroinflammation and neurodegeneration in cortex, amygdala and hippocampus, which are the areas of brain primarily involved in initiation and propagation of convulsions and seizures (Gupta, 2004; Gupta et al., 2007; Gupta and Milatovic, 2012).

TOXICITY

Most animal poisoning cases in the field are acute in nature. Onset of clinical signs usually occurs within 15 min to 1 h, followed by signs of maximal severity. However, timings of maximal severity signs tend to vary depending upon the OP/CM compound and its dose, and species. For example, onset of clinical signs is delayed with chlorpyrifos (Dursban) and dimethoate (Rogor). Clinical signs observed in poisoned animals can be divided into local and systemic effects. The local effects involve the eyes and the lungs, owing to their exposure to vapors or droplets of the insecticides. These effects, however, are of significance in the case of animals only when exposure is via spraying. The systemic effects are primarily on the brain, skeletal muscles, lungs, heart and other organs.

The clinical signs can also be classified as muscarinic, nicotinic and central. Fig. 37.7 describes the sequence of events involved in OP/CM toxicity. Muscarinic ACh receptor (mAChR)-associated effects are manifested by vomiting, abdominal pain, salivation, lacrimation, urination, diarrhea (SLUD), miosis (pinpoint pupils), tracheobronchial secretion, lung edema, and cyanosis. The nicotinic ACh receptor (nAChR)-associated effects are produced on autonomic ganglia and skeletal muscles, and the affected animals show twitching of muscles, tremors, followed by convulsions and seizures. This condition may lead to paralysis. The central effects include apprehension and stimulation, followed by depression. The affected animals may also show restlessness, ataxia, stiffness of the neck, and coma. Death occurs due to respiratory failure and cardiac arrest. It is important to mention that not all poisoned animals show all the clinical signs (as described above) with every OP or CM compound. Furthermore, at nonlethal doses, the signs of toxicity caused by each OP or CM can vary widely. This can be due to the fact that each OP or CM reacts not only with AChE but also with other targets, such as butyrylcholinesterase, carboxylesterases, neuropathy target esterase (NTE), acylpeptide hydrolase, arylformamidase, proteases, trypsin, chymotrypsin, cannabinoid CB1 receptor, albumin, and many other enzymes, receptors, and proteins (Gupta, 2004; Lockridge and Schopfer, 2006; Gupta and Milatovic, 2012; Mangas et al., 2017). While surviving animals usually recover within 3–6 h with CMs and within 24 h with OPs; animals exposed to OP nerve agents may show signs of toxicity for several days.

Poisoning cases of OP or CM are usually diagnosed based on clinical signs and quantified levels of AChE inhibition in blood from a live animal and brain from a dead animal. Inhibition of AChE activity >70% is considered a positive case of poisoning. It should be noted that great species variability exists in normal values of AChE activity (Table 37.4). In addition, there is more than a sixfold variability in AChE activity in different brain areas with preference given to the cortex and not the striatum for AChE analysis (Gupta, 2004). Therefore, interpretation should be made with great caution. Residue analysis of an insecticide and/or its metabolite(s), and by confirmation with GC/MS or LC/MS, seems an ideal approach for diagnosis.

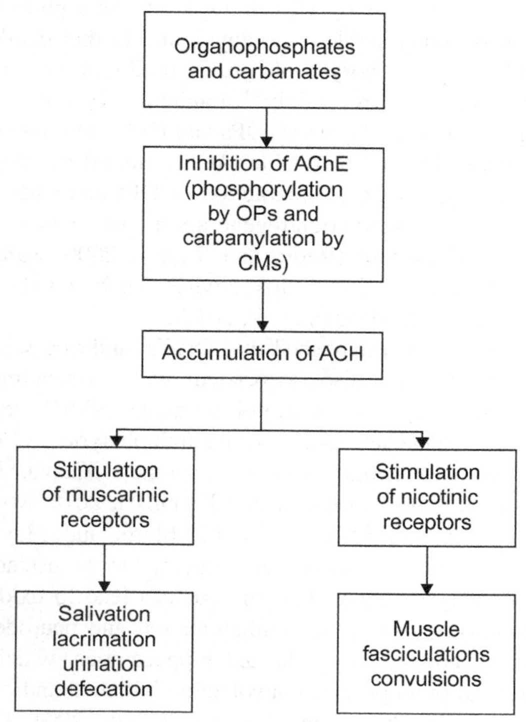

FIGURE 37.7 Important steps involved in mechanism of toxicity of OPs and CMs.

TABLE 37.4 Normal Acetylcholinesterase (AChE) Activity in Brain Cortex of Different Species

Species	AChE (μmol/g/h)
Cattle	160
Swine	163
Sheep	170
Horse	124
Chicken	1098
Dog	200
Rat	255

TREATMENT OF ACUTE POISONING

Before instituting antidotal therapy, monogastric animals, such as the dog, should be given gastric lavage. Animals of any species can be given activated charcoal to stop further absorption of OP/CM insecticides. Animals should be washed thoroughly with water if they are exposed to insecticides dermally. Intravenous fluid therapy is always beneficial.

In the case of OP poisoning, antidotal treatment requires the combined use of atropine sulfate and pyridine-2-aldoxime methochloride (2-PAM). Atropine sulfate acts by blocking the mAChRs from ACh. In ruminants, one-fourth of the total recommended dose (0.5 mg/kg) can be given as a slow IV injection, and the remainder through IM or SC injection (Gupta, 1984). The total dose of atropine sulfate for an average size horse is about 65 mg, and for a dog is about 2 mg. Atropine sulfate treatment can be repeated at an interval of every hour until all hypersecretory signs have subsided. 2-PAM reactivates the AChE inhibited by OPs. The recommended therapeutic dose of 2-PAM is 20 mg/kg, IV. The injection of 2-PAM can be repeated once after 1 h at half of its initial dose. Care should be taken that only a freshly prepared solution of 2-PAM be used. It needs to be emphasized that the combined therapy of atropine sulfate and 2-PAM is superior to any other treatment to date in the case of OP poisoning. Although many other oximes have been tested against many OPs, none has been proven to be better than 2-PAM. Furthermore, the depressant drugs, such as morphine and barbiturates, are contraindicated, since they aggravate the condition. Diazepam without atropine sulfate also accentuates the toxicity of OPs.

Unlike OP poisoning, 2-PAM and other oximes are ineffective in CM poisoning cases. In fact, in the case of some carbamates, such as carbaryl and carbofuran, 2-PAM therapy accentuates toxicity. Some anticonvulsant drugs, such as barbiturates and diazepam, also aggravate the toxicity of CMs. Therefore, atropine sulfate, with doses as described for OPs, is the only preferred antidote. However, when the animals are exposed to very high doses of carbamates, atropine sulfate does not appear to be a life-saving antidote.

OP-INDUCED INTERMEDIATE SYNDROME

OP insecticide-induced intermediate syndrome (IMS) was reported for the first time in human patients in Sri Lanka in 1987 (Senanayake and Karalliedde, 1987). The observations were made in 10 patients who presented 24–96 h after acute cholinergic crisis from exposure to methamidophos, fenthion, dimethoate, and monocrotophos. This syndrome has also been diagnosed in OP-poisoned patients in South Africa (1989), Turkey (1990), Belgium (1992), the United States (1992), Venezuela (1998), France (2000), and in many other countries. To date, OPs that are known to cause IMS include bromophos, chlorpyrifos, diazinon, dicrotophos, dimethoate, disulfoton, fenthion, malathion, methamidophos, methyl parathion, monocrotophos, omethoate, parathion, phosmet, and trichlorfon. IMS is usually observed in individuals who have ingested a massive dose of an OP insecticide either accidentally or in a suicide attempt. A small number of human case studies have also suggested that some CMs (carbaryl and carbofuran) can cause IMS (Paul and Mannathukkaran, 2005; Indira et al., 2013).

IMS is clearly a separate clinical entity from acute toxicity and delayed polyneuropathy. Clinically, IMS is characterized by acute paralysis and weakness in the areas of several cranial motor nerves, neck flexors and facial, extraocular, palatal, nuchal, proximal limb and respiratory muscles 24–96 h after poisoning. Generalized weakness, depressed deep tendon reflexes, ptosis, and diplopia are also evident. These symptoms may last for several days or weeks depending on the OP involved. A similar syndrome has also been observed in dogs and cats poisoned maliciously or accidentally with massive doses of certain OPs and CMs (Myberg and Gupta, 2007; Tinson et al., 2017). It should be noted that despite severe AChE inhibition, muscle fasciculations and muscarinic receptor-associated hypersecretory activities are absent.

Although the exact mechanism involved in the pathogenesis of IMS is unclear, studies suggest that decrease of AChE and nAChR mRNA expression occur after oral poisoning with disulfoton in rats. Involvement of oxidative stress is also suggested (Dandapani et al., 2003). Based on electromyographic (EMG) findings from OP-poisoned patients and experimental studies on laboratory animals, it has been found that the defect in IMS is at the neuromuscular endplate and postsynaptic level, but the effects of neural and central components in producing muscular weakness have not been ruled out. It seems clear that some OPs are greatly distributed to muscles and have a higher affinity for nAChRs. Currently, very little is known about the type of damage at the motor endplate or about risk factors contributing to its development. There is no specific treatment, and therapy relies upon atropine sulfate and 2-PAM. The administration of atropine sulfate and 2-PAM should be continued for a long period, even if efficacy of these drugs on the development of IMS appears to be limited. For further details about IMS, readers are referred to Gupta (2005), De Bleecker (2006) and Gupta and Milatovic (2012).

CHRONIC TOXICITY

Chronic toxicity is a major concern with OP pesticides. OP compounds that produce delayed neurotoxic effects are esters of phosphorus-containing acids. Almost half a century ago, tri-*o*-cresyl phosphate (TOCP) was known to produce delayed neurotoxic effects in man and chickens, characterized by ataxia and weakness of the limbs, developing 10–14 days after exposure (Johnson, 1969). This syndrome was called OP-induced delayed neuropathy (OPIDN). In recent literature, the syndrome has been renamed OP-induced delayed polyneuropathy (OPIDP). OPIDP is characterized by distal degeneration of long and large-diameter motor and sensory axons of both peripheral nerves and spinal cord. Among all animal species the hen appears to be the most sensitive and is therefore used as an animal model. TOCP and certain other compounds have minimal or no anti-AChE property; however, they cause phosphorylation and aging (dealkylation) of a protein in neurons called neuropathy target esterase (NTE), and subsequently lead to OPIDP (Gupta and Milatovic, 2012). Studies on the sensitivity of the target enzymes of a variety of OPs showed that the comparative inhibitory power of OPs against hen AChE and NTE in vitro correlates with their comparative effects in vivo (i.e., delayed neuropathy or death). The relationship between the degree of NTE inhibition and the severity of OPIDP changes according to the compound involved and the source of NTE. For example, certain compounds cause OPIDP with a minimum of 70% NTE inhibition, while others require almost complete inhibition to cause OPIDP. Inhibition of peripheral nerve NTE is required to develop OPIDP and no clinical deficits appear if only brain NTE is inhibited. For neuropathy to occur, a second reaction called "aging" of NTE must take place and this involves cleavage of the lateral side chain from the phosphorylated NTE. This reaction is called aging because it is a slow progressive process and the product is no longer responsive to nucleophilic reactivating agents, such as oximes. The cascade of events from NTE inhibition/aging to impairment of retrograde axonal transport and axonal degeneration is yet to be explained (Moretto and Lotti, 2006; Gupta and Milatovic, 2012; Mangas et al., 2017). Today, many compounds, such as DFP, *N,N′*-diisopropyl phosphorodiamidic fluoride (mipafox), tetraethyl pyrophosphate (TEPP), parathion, *o*-cresyl saligenin phosphate, and haloxon, are known to produce this syndrome. Some OPs as well as non OP inhibitors (such as carbamates and sulfonyl fluorides) also covalently react with NTE but cannot undergo the aging reaction. As a result, these inhibitors do not cause OPIDP, and when given to experimental animals prior to neuropathic OP, may protect from OPIDP when they occupy at least 30% of the NTE active site. For the details of OPIDP syndrome, readers are referred to Morreto and Lotti (2006) and Wu and Chang (2010). Treatment of this syndrome is symptomatic.

TOLERANCE DEVELOPMENT

Tolerance development to the toxicity of OPs was noted more than half a century ago. Following prolonged exposure to an OP, the physiological effects often diminish more than expected from the degree of AChE inhibition or repeated additions of OP give lower responses with time. Tolerance to AChE inhibiting OPs (such as DFP, disulfoton, methyl parathion, and others) has been observed using different forms of administration and in different species, such as mice, rats, guinea pig, and man (Fonnum and Sterri, 1981, 2006; Gupta and Dettbarn, 1986; Gupta et al., 1986; Gupta, 2004).

Tolerance to OP toxicity can develop in several ways. Most often, it occurs due to receptor changes either in the number of receptors or by decreased affinity of the receptor molecule. However, it can also occur due to the presence of other proteins that can bind or inactivate the inhibitor and thereby make it less readily available. Some of the examples for binding to the OPs are carboxylesterases, butyrylcholinesterases, lysophospholipase, acetylhydrolase, or other binding proteins such as albumin (Sogorb and Vilanova, 2010; Mangas et al., 2017). In addition, tolerance can be achieved through more rapid metabolism of the OP compounds by OP-hydrolyzing enzymes such as paraoxonases (PONs), DFPase, and somanases (Costa et al., 2006; Fonnum and Sterri, 2006).

ACh receptors (both mAChRs and nAChRs) are involved in the development of tolerance to OP toxicity. Treatment with a cholinergic agonist for a prolonged time leads to a decrease in the mAChRs. This is common for G protein-linked receptors. In some studies, OPs have been found to cause a decrease in the numbers of mAChRs in the brain, while in others both the number of mAChRs and the affinity to the ligand in ileum and striatum.

Significant reductions in nAChRs numbers (B_{max}), without change in affinity (K_D), have been found in brain of tolerant rats treated with disulfoton (Costa and Murphy, 1983) and in skeletal muscle of rats treated with DFP (Gupta et al., 1986; Gupta and Dettbarn, 1986). In tolerant rats, significant recovery of CarbEs and BuChEs has also been found. In essence, tolerance development following subchronic or chronic treatment with AChE inhibiting OPs occurs through multiple mechanisms.

CONCLUDING REMARKS AND FUTURE DIRECTIONS

OPs and CMs constitute a large number of chemicals that are used in agriculture primarily as insecticides and in veterinary medicine as parasiticides. These chemicals exert a broad range of toxic effects, varying from mild effects such as salivation and tremors to serious effects such as convulsions, seizures, paralysis, and death. Basically, OPs and CMs are neurotoxicants, but directly or indirectly several vital organs are affected. These chemicals produce a variety of toxicological effects on the central nervous system, peripheral nervous system and cardiovascular, pulmonary, ocular, neurobehavioral, immunological, reproductive, placental, cutaneous, and other body systems. In addition, these insecticides cause neurodegeneration, oxidative stress, neuroinflammation, endocrine disruption, and many other complications. In general, OPs produce more serious and lingering health effects than CMs. These devastating effects, including a complex syndrome like OPIDP, are yet to be mechanistically characterized and fully defined. It is expected that newer compounds of both OP and CM classes with greater selective toxicity as well as improved antidotes effective in patients with OPIDP or against CMs will be developed.

REFERENCES

Costa, L.G., Murphy, S.D., 1983. [3H]-nicotine binding in rat brain: Alteration after chronic acetylcholinesterase inhibition. J. Pharmacol. Exp. Ther. 226, 392–397.

Costa, L.G., Cole, T.B., Vitalone, A., Furlong, C.E., 2006. Paraoxonase polymorphisms and toxicity of organophosphates. In: Gupta, R.C. (Ed.), Toxicology of Organophosphate and Carbamate Compounds. Academic Press/Elsevier, Amsterdam, pp. 247–255.

Dandapani, M., Zachariah, A., Kavitha, M.R., et al., 2003. Oxidative damage in intermediate syndrome of acute organophosphorus poisoning. Indian J. Med. Res. 117, 253–259.

De Bleecker, J., 2006. Intermediate syndrome in organophosphate poisoning. In: Gupta, R.C. (Ed.), Toxicology of Organophosphate and Carbamate Compounds. Academic Press/Elsevier, Amsterdam, pp. 371–380.

Dekundy, A., Kaminski, R.M., 2010. Central mechanisms of seizures and lethality following anticholinesterase pesticide exposure. In: Satoh, T., Gupta, R.C. (Eds.), Anticholinesterase Pesticides: Metabolism, Neurotoxicity, and Epidemiology. John Wiley & Sons, Hoboken, pp. 149–164.

Fonnum, F., Sterri, S.H., 1981. Factors modifying the toxicity of organophosphorus compounds including soman and sarin. Fund. Appl. Toxicol. 1, 143–147.

Fonnum, F., Sterri, S.H., 2006. Tolerance development to toxicity of cholinesterase inhibitors. In: Gupta, R.C. (Ed.), Toxicology of Organophosphate and Carbamate Compounds. Academic Press/ Elsevier, Amsterdam, pp. 257–267.

Gupta, R.C., 1984. Acute malathion toxicosis and related enzymatic alterations in Bubalus bubalis: antidotal treatment with atropine, 2-PAM, and diazepam. J. Toxicol. Environ. Health. 14, 291–303.

Gupta, R.C., 1994. Carbofuran toxicity. J. Toxicol. Environ. Health. 42, 383–418.

Gupta, R.C., 2004. Brain regional heterogeneity and toxicological mechanisms of organophosphates and carbamates. Toxicol. Mechan. Meth. 14, 103–143.

Gupta, R.C., 2005. Organophosphate poisoning, intermediate syndrome. In: Wexler, P. (Ed.), Encyclopedia of Toxicology, 2nd edn. Academic Press, San Diego, CA, pp. 306–308.

Gupta, R.C., 2006. Classification and uses of organophosphates and carbamates. In: Gupta, R.C. (Ed.), Toxicology of Organophosphate and Carbamate Compounds. Academic Press/Elsevier, Amsterdam, pp. 5–24.

Gupta, R.C., Dettbarn, W.-D., 1986. Role of uptake of [14C]valine into protein in the development of tolerance to diisopropyl phosphorofluoridate (DFP) toxicity. Toxicol. Appl. Pharmacol. 84, 551–560.

Gupta, R.C., Milatovic, D., 2012. Toxicity of organophosphates and carbamates. In: Marrs, T.C. (Ed.), Mammalian Toxicology of Insecticides. Royal Society of Chemistry Publ, Cambridge, pp. 104–136.

Gupta, R.C., Milatovic, D., 2014. Insecticides. In: Gupta, R.C. (Ed.), Biomarkers in Toxicology. Academic Press/Elsevier, Amsterdam, pp. 389–407.

Gupta, R.C., Patterson, G.T., Dettbarn, W.-D., 1986. Mechanisms of toxicity and tolerance to diisopropyl phosphorofluoridate at the neuromuscular junction of the rat. Toxicol. Appl. Pharmacol. 84, 541–550.

Gupta, R.C., Milatovic, S., Dettbarn, W.-D., et al., 2007. Neuronal oxidative injury and dendritic damage induced by carbofuran: protection by memantine. Toxicol. Appl. Pharmacol. 219, 97–105.

Gupta, R.C., Miller Muhkerjee, I., Doss, R.B., et al., 2017. Organophosphate and carbamate pesticides. In: Gupta, R.C. (Ed.), Reproductive and Developmental Toxicology, 2nd edn. Academic Press/Elsevier, Amsterdam, pp. 609–631.

Indira, M., Andrews, M.A., Rakesh, T.P., 2013. Incidence, predictors, and outcome of intermediate syndrome in cholinergic insecticide poisoning: A prospective observational cohort study. Clin. Toxicol. 51, 838–845.

Johnson, M.K., 1969. Delayed neurotoxic action of some organophosphorus compounds. Br. Med. Bull. 25, 231–235.

Jokanovic, M., 2010. Medical treatment of poisoning by organophosphates and carbamates. In: Satoh, T., Gupta, R.C. (Eds.), Anticholinesterase Pesticides: Metabolism, Neurotoxicity, and Epidemiology. John Wiley & Sons, Hoboken, pp. 583–597.

Kaur, S., Singh, S., Chahal, K.S., Prakash, A., 2014. Potential pharmacological strategies for the improved treatment of organophosphate-induced neurotoxicity. Can. J. Physiol. Pharmacol. 92, 893–911.

Lockridge, O., Schopfer, L.M., 2006. Biomarkers of organophosphorus pesticide poisoning. In: Gupta, R.C. (Ed.), Toxicology of Organophosphate and Carbamate Compounds. Academic Press/ Elsevier, Amsterdam, pp. 703–711.

Mangas, I., Estevez, J., Vilanova, E., et al., 2017. New insights on molecular interactions of organophosphorus pesticides with esterases. Toxicology. 376, 30–43.

Marrs, T.C., 1993. Organophosphate poisoning. Pharmacol. Ther. 58, 51–66.

Marrs, T.C., Maynard, R.L., 2013. Neurotransmission systems as targets for toxicants: a review. Cell Biol. Toxicol. 29, 381–396.

Moretto, A., Lotti, M., 2006. Peripheral nervous system effects and delayed neuropathy. In: Gupta, R.C. (Ed.), Toxicology of Organophosphate and Carbamate Compounds. Academic Press/ Elsevier, Amsterdam, pp. 361–370.

Myberg J, Gupta RC. 2007. Intermediate syndrome: muscle weakness after organophosphate poisoning in dogs and cats. Vet News South Africa.

Myhrer, T., 2010. Identification of neuronal target areas for nerve agents and speciation of receptors for pharmacological treatment. Neurotoxicology. 31, 629–638.

Ordentlich, A., Barak, D., Kronman, C., et al., 1996. The architecture of human acetylcholinesterase active center probed by interactions with selected organophosphate inhibitors. J. Biol. Chem. 271, 11953–11962.

Ordentlich, A., Barak, D., Kronman, C., et al., 1998. Functional characteristics of the oxyanion hole in human acetylcholinesterase. J. Biol. Chem. 273, 19509–19517.

Ordentlich, A., Barak, D., Sod-Moriah, G., et al., 2004. Stereoselectivity toward VX is determined by interactions with residues of the acyl pocket as well as of the peripheral anionic site of AChE. Biochemistry. 43, 11255–11265.

Paul, N., Mannathukkaran, T.J., 2005. Intermediate syndrome following carbamate poisoning. Clin. Toxicol. 43, 867–868.

Radic, Z., Taylor, P., 2006. Structure and function of cholinesterases. In: Gupta (Ed.), Toxicology of Organophosphate and Carbamate Compounds. Academic Press/Elsevier, Amsterdam, pp. 161–186.

Rembovskiy, V., Radilov, A., Savelieva, E., et al., 2015. Russian VX. In: Gupta, R.C. (Ed.), Handbook of Toxicology of Chemical Warfare Agents, 2nd edn. Academic Press/Elsevier, Amsterdam, pp. 111–130.

Satoh, T., Gupta, R.C., 2010. Anticholinesterase Pesticides: Metabolism. Neurotoxicity, and Epidemiology. John Wiley & Sons, Hoboken, pp. 1–597.

Senanayake, N., Karalliedde, L., 1987. Neurotoxic effects of organophosphorus insecticides. An intermediate syndrome. N. Engl. J. Med. 316, 761–763.

Sogorb, M.A., Vilanova, E., 2010. Detoxication of anticholinesterase pesticides. In: Satoh, T., Gupta, R.C. (Eds.), Anticholinesterase Pesticides: Metabolism, Neurotoxicity, and Epidemiology. John Wiley & Sons, Hoboken, pp. 121–132.

Sultatos, L.G., 2006. Interactions of organophosphorus and carbamate compounds with cholinesterases. In: Gupta, R.C. (Ed.), Toxicology of Organophosphate and Carbamate Compounds. Academic Press/ Elsevier, Amsterdam, pp. 209–218.

Tang, J., Rose, R.L., Chambers, J.E., 2006. Metabolism of organophosphorus and carbamate pesticides. In: Gupta, R.C. (Ed.), Toxicology of Organophosphate and Carbamate Compounds. Academic Press/ Elsevier, Amsterdam, pp. 127–143.

Taylor, P., 2006. Anticholinesterase agents. In: Brunton, L.L., Lazo, J.S., Parker, K.L. (Eds.), Goodman and Gilmam's The Pharmacological Basis of Therapeutics. McGraw-Hill, New York, NY, pp. 201–216.

Timchalk, C., 2006. Physiologically based pharmacokinetic modeling of organophosphorus and carbamate pesticides. In: Gupta, R.C. (Ed.), Toxicology of Organophosphate and Carbamate Compounds. Academic Press/Elsevier, Amsterdam, pp. 103–125.

Timchalk, C., 2010. Biomonitoring of pesticides: pharmacokinetics of organophosphorus and carbamate insecticides. In: Satoh, T., Gupta, R. C. (Eds.), Anticholinesterase Pesticides: Metabolism, Neurotoxicity, and Epidemiology. John Wiley & Sons, Hoboken, pp. 267–287.

Tinson, E., Boller, E., Davis, M., 2017. A suspected case of intermediate syndrome in a dog with carbamate toxicosis. Aust. Vet. J. 95 (6), 201–206.

Tomokuni, K., Gasegawa, T., Hirai, Y., et al., 1985. The tissue distribution of diazinon and the inhibition of blood cholinesterase activities in rats and mice receiving a single intraperitoneal dose of diazinon. Toxicology. 37, 91–98.

Vacondio, F., Silva, C., Mor, M., et al., 2010. Qualitative structure–metabolism relationship in the hydrolysis of carbamates. Drug. Metab. Rev. 42, 551–589.

Watson, A., Bakshi, K., Opresko, D., et al., 2006. Cholinesterase inhibitors as chemical warfare agents: community preparedness guidelines. In: Gupta, R.C. (Ed.), Toxicology of Organophosphate and Carbamate Compounds. Academic Press/Elsevier, Amsterdam, pp. 47–68.

Watson, A., Opresko, D., Young, R., et al., 2015. Organophosphate nerve agents. In: Gupta, R.C. (Ed.), Handbook of Toxicology of Chemical Warfare Agents, 2nd edn. Academic Press/Elsevier, Amsterdam, pp. 87–109.

Wu, H.X., Evereux-Gros, C., Descotes, J., 1996. Diazinon toxicokinetics, tissue distribution and anticholinesterase activity in the rat. Biomed. Environ. Sci. 9, 359–369.

Wu, Y.-J., Chang, P.-A., 2010. Molecular toxicology of neuropathy target esterase. In: Satoh, T., Gupta, R.C. (Eds.), Anticholinesterase Pesticides: Metabolism, Neurotoxicity, and Epidemiology. John Wiley & Sons, Hoboken, pp. 109–120.

FURTHER READING

Gupta, R.C., 2015. Introduction. In: Gupta, R.C. (Ed.), Handbook of Toxicology of Chemical Warfare Agents, 2nd edn. Academic Press/ Elsevier, Amsterdam, pp. 3–5.

Chapter 38

Organochlorines

Steve M. Ensley

INTRODUCTION

The organochlorines (OCs) are still causing adverse health effects in humans and animals in 2017. Most OCs were banned in the United States in the 1980s. Despite the ban these chemicals are still causing adverse health in animals in the United States and worldwide.

Historically many methods have been used and developed to control or eliminate insects and other plant and animal pests that have threatened man and his food supply. Chemicals used in the past to control insects include sulfur (used before 1000 BC and is still used today), vinegar, whale oil and arsenic (used in the 1500s), nicotine (used in the 1600s), rotenone from the plant *Derris eliptica*, pyrethrum from *Chrysanthemum cinerariaefolium*, copper arsenate (used in the 1800s) and calcium and lead arsenate (used in the early 1900s). There were major changes in the development of insecticides in the 1930s when the synthetic organic chemical industry began developing compounds to control insects. Chlorinated compounds such as aldrin and dieldrin, used as insecticides, became available for use in the 1940s. Dichlorodiphenyltrichloroethane (DDT) became available during World War II and was used extensively as an insecticide worldwide. OCs were effective because they persist in the environment (Leonard et al., 1999; Hites et al., 2004; Hoekstra et al., 2005). Because of that persistence, most have been eliminated from use today. Lindane (gamma-hexachlorocyclohexane) and endosulfan are the most biodegradable OCs and are still used today.

The diphenyl aliphatic OCs, such as DDT, affect the peripheral nerves and brain by slowing sodium (Na^+) influx and inhibiting potassium (K^+) outflow. This results in excess intracellular K^+ in the neuron, which partially depolarizes the cell.

In the 1980s, the mechanism of toxicity for the cyclodiene OC insecticides was determined. These compounds were found to be noncompetitive antagonists acting on the chloride ion channel of the gamma-aminobutyric acid A (GABA) receptor.

BACKGROUND

Even though DDT was first synthesized by Othmar Zeidler in 1874, it was another 40 years before this compound was used as an insecticide. Paul Mueller, a Swiss chemist, rediscovered DDT in 1939 while investigating insecticides for use against clothes moths and carpet beetles. Mueller won the Nobel Prize in 1948 for this work. "This pleasant smelling, greasy white powder (DDT) has had an influence on human ecology perhaps unmatched by any other chemical discovery including gunpowder, sulfanilamide, penicillin, and plutonium" (Metcalf, 1973).

The insecticidal properties of technical HCH (*t*-hexachlorocyclohexane; commonly known as benzene hexachloride) and the first cyclodiene insecticides (e.g., aldrin, dieldrin, chlordane) were discovered as a result of the commercial interest in new uses for chlorine and hydrocarbons such as cyclopentadiene and benzene. The first use of the chlorinated hydrocarbons was for dielectrics and as fire retardants. The use of these compounds as insecticides occurred when benzene was added to liquid chlorine in the field and it was noted that the product killed insects.

As with many insecticides there are many unintended secondary targets for every insecticide (Uzoukwu and Sleight, 1972; Furie and Trubowitz, 1976; Hathway, 1977). Hexachlorocyclopentadiene, a raw material used in manufacturing chemicals, was known to be stable and was found to react easily with cyclopentadiene in a Diels-Alder reaction, which leads to the production of chlordane. It was discovered later to react with norbornadiene (a bicyclic hydrocarbon) to produce aldrin. Allylic chlorination of chlordane produces heptachlor. The intermediate hexachloronorbornadiene reacts with cyclopentadiene to produce isodrin and after epoxidation, dieldrin, and endrin are produced. Technical hexachlorocyclohexane (*t*-HCH) can be used to produce the gamma isomer lindane. One of the problems with the production of lindane is the inefficiency of the process; for every ton of lindane produced,

Veterinary Toxicology. DOI: http://dx.doi.org/10.1016/B978-0-12-811410-0.00038-6

8–10 tons of the inactive alpha and beta isomers are formed. Because of the widespread use of *t*-HCH, the environment has become contaminated with the inactive alpha and beta-HCH isomers.

Overcoming the problem of insect resistance to the OCs has also been associated with toxicity. A major mechanism of insect resistance to DDT was found to be enzymatic dechlorination of DDT to dichlorodiphenyldichloroethylene (Bonner and Yarbrough, 1988). While working to overcome resistance to DDT, it was discovered that certain nontoxic DDT analogs and other compounds suppressed resistance when coapplied with DDT. Toxicity to parent compounds as well as congeners has been associated with use of the OCs.

The beginning of the science of toxicology can be traced to the problems associated with use of DDT and the subsequent impact on man and the environment. Rachel Carson's book *Silent Spring* brought the problems associated with the use of DDT to national attention in 1962. OCs continue to be an environmental contaminant as evident in this 2010 study (Ding et al., 2010).

The structures of various OC insecticides are shown in Fig. 38.1.

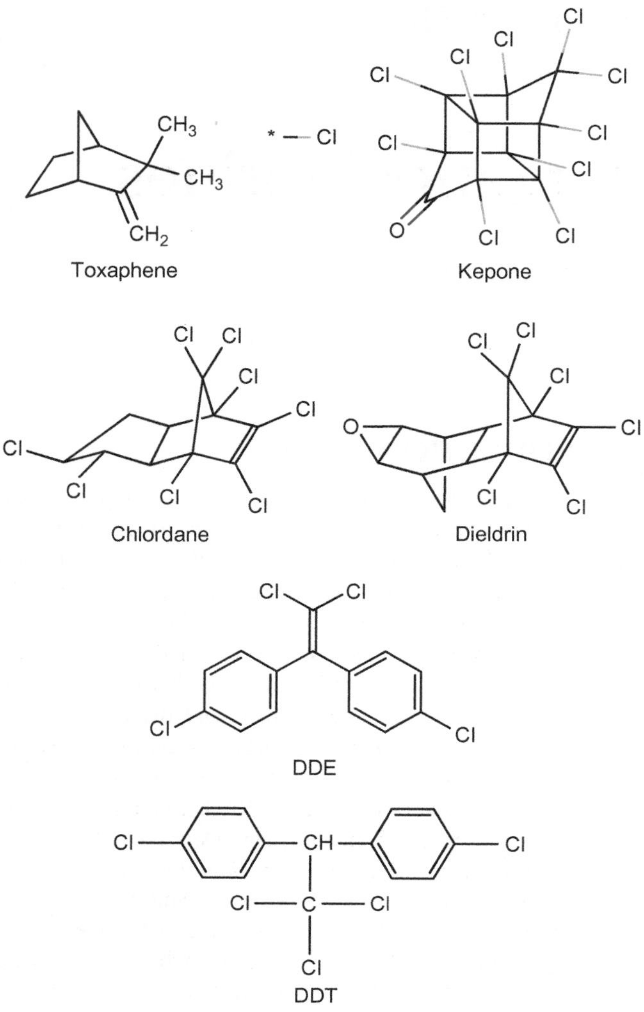

PHARMACOKINETICS/TOXICOKINETICS

OC insecticides can be absorbed orally and topically, with absorption being rapid due to the lipid solubility of these compounds (Buck et al., 1976; Marth et al., 1989). In the presence of animal or vegetable fat the gastrointestinal absorption is increased. OC insecticides are not highly volatile, so inhalation is not a normal route of exposure (Jaeger et al., 1973). Absorption of the OCs after inhalation exposure occurs primarily by mucocillary trapping followed by gastrointestinal absorption. Distribution is to the liver, kidney, brain, and adipose tissue (Buck and Van Note, 1968; Buck, 1970; Booth and McDowell, 1975; Mrema et al., 2013). The acute toxicity caused is of concern, but bioaccumulation from chronic exposures is equally important (Starr and Clifford, 1972). Chlorinated hydrocarbons are highly lipid soluble and persist in the environment; as a result, bioaccumulation occurs in the food chain from the environment to animals and humans (Mount et al., 1980; Oehme, 1991; Safe and Krishnan, 1995; Watanabe et al., 1999; Backer et al., 2001; Smith and Gangolli, 2002; Harris et al., 2005).

As with all xenobiotics, the toxicity of the OCs is related to absorption, distribution, metabolism and elimination (Jaeger et al., 1975; Beasley et al., 1994).

Tissue distribution of endosulfan in a human consuming 100 mL of endosulfan is presented in Table 38.1 (Quick, 1992).

The diphenyl aliphatics, such as DDT, are dechlorinated by mixed function oxidases (MFOs). Aryl hydrocarbons, like paradichlorobenzene, undergo glucuronidation and sulfation. The cyclodiene insecticides, such as endrin, are rapidly converted to epoxides by MFOs. Methoxychlor is rapidly eliminated compared to DDT by

Toxaphene

Kepone

Chlordane

Dieldrin

DDE

DDT

FIGURE 38.1 Structures of common organochlorines.

TABLE 38.1 Tissue Distribution of Endosulfan

Tissue	Endosulfan (ppb)
Adipose tissue	4105
Liver	<50
Brain	80
Kidney	59
Stomach content	3541

dechlorination and oxidation. The intermediates of OC insecticide production may be more toxic than the parent compound.

The major excretory route of OCs is from bile into the digestive tract, and as a result enterohepatic recycling can occur. Metabolites are also lipophilic, will move into adipose tissue and are released slowly from lipid depot storage (Sell et al., 1977). The half-life of some diphenyl aliphatics, such as DDT and the cyclodienes, may range from days to years (Council for Agricultural Science and Technology, 1974). Elimination can sometimes be explained by a two-compartment model, where the first phase is rapid elimination and the second is prolonged.

Excretion of OCs does not follow first order kinetics. As the body stores get lower, the half-life of the remaining OC increases dramatically. This is due to lipoprotein binding, where different forms of the OC exhibit different dissociation kinetics. Aldrin is biotransformed in cattle to dieldrin, this is stored in adipose tissue. Dieldrin in fat is slowly biotransformed to hydroxydieldrin that can be conjugated and excreted in urine (Casteel et al., 1993).

MECHANISM OF ACTION

There are at least two different mechanisms of action for OC insecticides (Shankland, 1982; Narahashi, 1987; Osweiler, 1996; Smith, 2012). DDT-type OC (dichlorodiphenylethanes) insecticides affect the peripheral nerves and brain by slowing sodium (Na^+) influx and inhibiting potassium (K^+) efflux. This results in excess intracellular K^+ in the neuron, which partially depolarizes the cell. The threshold for another action potential is decreased, resulting in premature depolarization of the neuron.

The aryl hydrocarbons and cyclodienes, in addition to decreasing action potentials, may inhibit the postsynaptic binding of GABA (Bloomquist and Soderlund, 1985; Lummis et al., 1990; French-Constant, 1993; Hahn, 1998; Carr, et al., 1999; Mrema et al., 2013). The cyclodiene OC insecticides act by competitive inhibition of the binding of GABA at its receptor, causing stimulation of the neuron, as described below (Joy, 1976, 1982; Gandolfi et al., 1984).

GABA is a neurotransmitter in the mammalian and insect central nervous system and the inhibitory neurotransmitter for insects at the neuromuscular junction. $GABA_A$ receptors, present in mammalian and insect synapse, are ligand gated chloride ion channels. In mammals, $GABA_B$ receptors are coupled to calcium and potassium channels and the action of GABA is mediated by G-proteins. $GABA_B$ receptors are not important in insect physiology. When GABA is released in the synapse it diffuses to the presynaptic terminal of another nerve, where it binds to a $GABA_A$ receptor. This causes chloride ions to enter the synapse resulting in hyperpolarization of the terminal and inhibition of release of other neurotransmitters. Because of this inhibition, postsynaptic stimulation of other nerves by other transmitters (e.g., acetylcholine) is reduced. When GABA is inhibited, there is no synaptic downregulation, and other neurotransmitters can be released in excess. The inhibitory mechanism of GABA explains the cholinergic effects (over stimulation by acetylcholine) of dieldrin and lindane on some species.

A description of the $GABA_A$ receptor in the human brain is presented in Figs. 38.2 and 38.3 to clearly describe the chloride ion channel. The $GABA_A$ receptor of the human brain consists of four or five 50–60 kDa glycoprotein subunits, each of which contains four (M_1–M_4) hydrophobic domains. The five M_2 domains are arranged to form a 5.6 Å diameter ion channel.

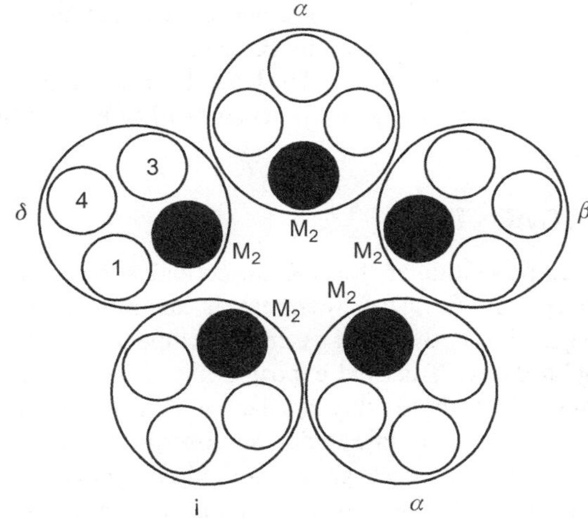

FIGURE 38.2 Illustration of the $GABA_A$ receptor of the mammalian brain. The M_2 segments form the chloride ion channel (McDonald and Olsen, 1994).

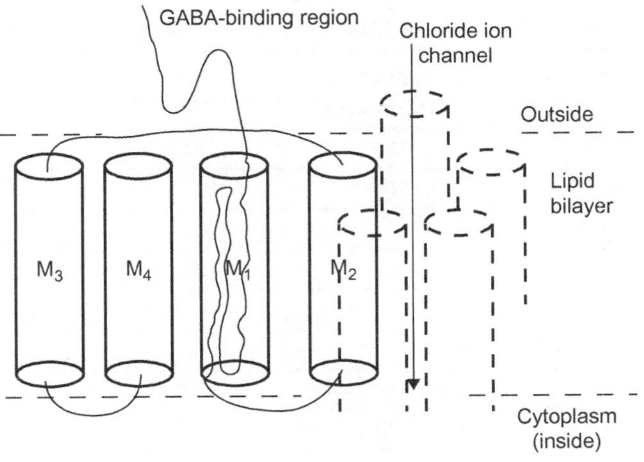

FIGURE 38.3 Illustration of the $GABA_A$ receptor of the mammalian brain (McDonald and Olsen, 1994).

TOXICITY

Cats are the most sensitive species to OC insecticides, with the LD_{50} for endrin in cats of 3–6 mg/kg. The cyclodiene OC insecticides cause more seizure activity and have a lower LD_{50} than the DDT-type insecticides in most species.

The oral LD_{50} for DDT in rats is 113–2500 mg/kg and the IV LD_{50} is 47 mg/kg. In humans, toxic signs from oral exposure to OCs can be observed at 10 mg/kg.

The acute toxicity to rats and rabbits of other chlorinated insecticides is shown in Table 38.2.

In addition to the effects on the nervous system, DDT metabolites can inhibit the output of the adrenal gland by selective necrosis of the zona fasciculata and the zona reticularis.

Following an acute or chronic exposure, OCs can produce a variety of reproductive and developmental effects in animals as well as humans (Gupta, 2009; Malik et al., 2017). Chronic exposure to DDT has been documented to cause eggshell thinning and reduced fertility in wild birds.

TREATMENT

No specific antidotes for OC insecticides are available (Osweiler, 1996). The treatment is mainly supportive. Detoxification is the most essential component of therapy for OC toxicity. If dermal exposure has occurred, the animal should be thoroughly washed with a detergent and water to remove the insecticide so absorption ceases. The hair of heavily contaminated long-haired animals should be clipped. Personnel treating animals should exercise caution and prevent themselves from becoming contaminated with the insecticide by wearing gloves, aprons, or raincoats.

TABLE 38.2 Toxicity Data for Some Organochlorines

Compound	Rat Acute Oral LD_{50} (mg/kg)	Rabbit Dermal LD_{50} (mg/kg)
Lindane	76–190	500
Aldrin	39–60	65
Dieldrin	40	65
Endrin	3	12
Chlordane	283–1100	580
Endosulfan	18–76	74
Mirex	235– > 3000	800
Kepone	95–125	345
Toxaphene	40–127	600

For oral exposure to OCs, activated charcoal (1–2 g/kg) should be administered orally. An alternative but less effective treatment is mineral oil. The insecticide can dissolve in mineral oil, which decreases its absorption systemically. The approximate oral dose of mineral oil is 2–6 mL in cats, 5–15 mL in dogs, and 1–3 L in large animals. Charcoal or nonabsorbable oils are most effective when given within 4 h of ingestion of the pesticide (Aslani, 1996).

General supportive care includes the use of antiseizure medications such as diazepam, phenobarbital or pentobarbital. Animals should be placed in a warm and comfortable area to minimize trauma when they are seizuring. Animals recovering from OC insecticide exposure may have to be monitored long-term because OCs can persist in the body for months or years. The source of the exposure must be identified and removed to stop exposure. One decontamination strategy is to reduce feed intake so that the animal loses body fat, thereby reducing OC residues in adipose tissue. Lactating animals rapidly eliminate OC residues because the residues are excreted in milk. An additional treatment option in large animals is to feed activated charcoal (500–1000 g/day) to reduce enterohepatic recycling.

CONCLUDING REMARKS AND FUTURE DIRECTIONS

The use of OC insecticides is decreasing in the United States but they are still used worldwide. In the United States, with the ability of these compounds to persist in the environment and bioaccumulate, the OC insecticides will continue to be an important toxicant for many years (Custer et al., 2005).

REFERENCES

Aslani, M.R., 1996. Endosulfan toxicosis in calves. Vet. Hum. Toxicol. 38, 364.

Backer, L.C., Grindem, C.B., et al., 2001. Pet dogs as sentinels for environmental contamination. Sci. Total Environ. 274, 161–169.

Beasley, V.R., Dorman, D.C., Fikes, F.D., et al., 1994. A Systems Approach to Veterinary Toxicology. University of Illinois, Champagne, IL.

Bloomquist, J.R., Soderlund, D.M., 1985. Neurotoxic insecticides inhibit GABA-dependent chloride uptake by mouse brain vesicles. Biochem. Biophys. Res. Commun. 133, 37–43.

Bonner, J.C., Yarbrough, J.D., 1988. Vertebrate cyclodiene insecticide resistance: role of gamma-aminobutyric acid and diazepam binding sites. Arch. Toxicol. 62, 311–315.

Booth, N.H., McDowell, J.R., 1975. Toxicity of hexachlorobenzene and associated residues in edible animal tissues. J. Am. Vet. Med. Assoc. 166, 591–595.

Buck, W.B., 1970. Lead and organic pesticide poisonings in cattle. J. Am. Vet. Med. Assoc. 156, 1468–1472.

Buck, W.B., Van Note, W., 1968. Aldrin poisoning resulting in dieldrin residues in meat and milk. J. Am. Vet. Med. Assoc. 153, 1472–1475.

Buck, W.B., Osweiler, G.D., VanGelder, G.A., 1976. Clinical and Diagnostic Veterinary Toxicology. second ed. Kendall/Hunt Publishing, Dubuque, IA.

Carr, R.L., Couch, T.A., et al., 1999. The interaction of chlorinated alicyclic insecticides with brain GABA(A) receptors in channel catfish (*Ictalurus punctatus*). J. Toxicol. Environ. Health A. 56, 543–553.

Casteel, S.W., Stalowich, F.T., Kendall, J.D., 1993. Aldrin intoxication and clearance of associated dieldrin residues in a group of feedlot cattle. JAVMA. 202, 83–85.

Council for Agricultural Science and Technology, 1974. Aldrin and dieldrin in agriculture. Report No. 34.

Custer, C.M., Custer, T.W., et al., 2005. Exposure and effects of 2,3,7,8-tetrachlorodibenzo-p-dioxin in tree swallows (*Tachycineta bicolor*) nesting along the Woonasquatucket River, Rhode Island, USA. Environ. Toxicol. Chem. 24, 93–109.

Ding, Y.P., Harwood, A.D., Foslund, H.M., et al., 2010. Distribution and toxicity of sediment-associated pesticides in urban and agricultural waterways from Illinois, USA. Environ. Toxicol. Chem. 29, 149–157.

French-Constant, R.H., 1993. Cloning of a putative GABAA receptor from cyclodiene-resistant Drosophila: a case study in the use of insecticide-resistant mutants to isolate neuroreceptors. Comp. Mol. Neurobiol. Exs. 63, 210–223.

Furie, B., Trubowitz, S., 1976. Insecticides and blood dyscrasias. J. Am. Med. Assoc. 235, 1720–1722.

Gandolfi, O., Cheney, D.L., et al., 1984. On the neurotoxicity of chlordecone: a role for gamma-aminobutyric acid and serotonin. Brain Res. 303, 117–123.

Gupta, R.C., 2009. Toxicology of the placenta. In: Ballantyne, B., Marrs, T.C., Syversen, T. (Eds.), General and Applied Toxicology, third ed. John Wiley & Sons, Chichester, pp. 2003–2039.

Hahn, M.E., 1998. The aryl hydrocarbon receptor: a comparative perspective. Comp. Biochem. Physiol. C Pharmacol. Toxicol. Endocrinol. 121, 23–53.

Harris, M.L., Wilson, L.K., et al., 2005. An assessment of PCBs and OC pesticides in eggs of double-crested (*Phalacrocorax auritus*) and Pelagic (*P. pelagicus*) cormorants from the west coast of Canada, 1970 to 2002. Ecotoxicology. 14, 607–625.

Hathway, D.E., 1977. Comparative mammalian metabolism of vinyl chloride and vinylidene chloride in relation to oncogenic potential. Environ. Health Perspect. 21, 55–59.

Hites, R.A., Foran, J.A., et al., 2004. Global assessment of organic contaminants in farmed salmon. Science. 303, 226–229.

Hoekstra, P.F., O'Hara, T.M., et al., 2005. Concentrations of persistent organochlorine contaminants in bowhead whale tissues and other biota from northern Alaska: implications for human exposure from a subsistence diet. Environ. Res. 98, 329–340.

Jaeger, R.J., Conolly, R.B., et al., 1973. Diurnal variation of hepatic glutathione concentration and its correlation with 1,1-dichloroethylene inhalation toxicity in rats. Res. Commun. Chem. Pathol. Pharmacol. 6, 465–471.

Jaeger, R.J., Conolly, R.B., et al., 1975. Biochemical toxicology of unsaturated halogenated monomers. Environ. Health Perspect. 11, 121–128.

Joy, R., 1976. The alteration by dieldrin of corticol excitability conditioned by sensory stimuli. Toxicol. Appl. Pharm. 38, 357–368.

Joy, R.M., 1982. Mode of action of lindane, dieldrin and related insecticides in the central nervous system. Neurobehav. Toxicol. Teratol. 4, 813–823.

Leonard, A.W., Hyne, R.V., et al., 1999. Effect of endosulfan runoff from cotton fields on macroinvertebrates in the Namoi river. Ecotoxicol. Environ. Saf. 42, 125–134.

Lummis, S.C., Buckingham, S.D., et al., 1990. Blocking actions of heptachlor at an insect central nervous system GABA receptor. Proc. R Soc. Lond. B Biol. Sci. 240, 97–106.

Malik, J.K., Aggarwal, M., Kalpana, S., Gupta, R.C., 2017. Chlorinated hydrocarbons and pyrethrins/pyrethroids. In: Gupta, R.C. (Ed.), Reproductive and Developmental Toxicology, second ed. Academic Press/Elsevier, Amsterdam, pp. 633–655.

Marth, E., Stunzner, D., et al., 1989. Toxicokinetics of chlorinated hydrocarbons. J. Hyg. Epidemiol. Microbiol. Immunol. 33 (Suppl. 4), 514–520.

McDonald, R.L., Olsen, R.W., 1994. GABAa-receptor channels. Ann. Rev. Neurosci. 17, 569–602.

Metcalf, R.L., 1973. A century of DDT. J. Agr. Food Chem. 21, 511–519.

Mount, M.E., Traffas, V., Milleret, R.J., Oehme, F.W., 1980. An unusual occurrence of toxaphene poisoning in swine. J. Am. Vet. Med. Assoc. 177, 445–447.

Mrema, E.J., Rubino, F.M., Brambilla, G., et al., 2013. Persistent organochlorinated pesticides and mechanisms of their toxicity. Toxicology. 307, 74–88.

Narahashi, T., 1987. Nerve membrane ion channels as the target site of environmental toxicants. Environ. Health Perspect. 71, 25–29.

Oehme, M., 1991. Dispersion and transport paths of toxic persistent organochlorines to the Arctic – levels and consequences. Sci. Total Environ. 106 (1–2), 43–53.

Osweiler, G.D., 1996. Toxicology. Williams and Wilkins, Philadelphia, PA.

Quick, M.P., 1992. Suspected cases of bromocyclen poisoning. Vet. Hum. Toxicol. 34, 455–457.

Safe, S., Krishnan, V., 1995. Chlorinated hydrocarbons: estrogens and antiestrogens. Toxicol. Lett. 82–83, 731–736.

Sell, J.L., Davison, K.L., Bristol, D.W., 1977. Depletion of dieldrin from turkeys. Poult. Sci. 56, 2045–2051.

Shankland, D.L., 1982. Neurotoxic action of chlorinated hydrocarbon insecticides. Neurobehav. Toxicol. Teratol. 4, 805–811.

Smith, A.G., 2012. DDT and other chlorinated insecticides. In: Marrs, T.C. (Ed.), Mammalian Toxicology of Insecticides. RSC Publ, Cambridge, pp. 37–103.

Smith, A.G., Gangolli, S.D., 2002. Organochlorine chemicals in seafood: occurrence and health concerns. Food Chem. Toxicol. 40, 767–779.

Starr, H.G., Clifford, N.J., 1972. Acute lindane intoxication. Arch. Environ. Health. 25, 374–375.

Uzoukwu, M., Sleight, S.D., 1972. Effects of dieldrin in pregnant sows. J. Am. Vet. Med. Assoc. 160, 1641–1643.

Watanabe, M., Tanabe, S., et al., 1999. Contamination levels and specific accumulation of persistent organochlorines in Caspian seal (*Phoca caspica*) from the Caspian sea, Russia. Arch. Environ. Contam. Toxicol. 37, 396–407.

Chapter 39

Pyrethrins and Pyrethroids

Steve M. Ensley

INTRODUCTION

Pyrethrins are the insecticidal compounds obtained from the flowers of the plant *Tanacetum cinerariaefolium*, also called *Chrysanthemum cinerariaefolium* or *Pyrethrum cinerariaefolium*. Pyrethrum comes from extracts from the flowers that contain the active pyrethrin compounds (Proudfoot, 2005). The use of pyrethrum in insecticide preparations dates back to Persia, about 400 BC. Pyrethroids are synthetic analogs of pyrethrins. Because of stability problems with the natural pyrethrins, these insecticides were replaced by the more stable organophosphate and organochlorine insecticides developed after World War II (Valentine, 1990). As a result of the toxicity and environmental contamination associated with the organophosphate and organochlorine insecticides, interest in the use of pyrethrins and pyrethroids reemerged in the 1970s. Pyrethrin and pyrethroid insecticides are effective against a variety of insect pests on companion animals and livestock, and are used on farms, in the home and garden and have many public health applications because of the safety associated with these compounds. The pyrethroids are considerably safer than the organochlorines. The neonicotinoids were developed to replace the pyrethrins.

BACKGROUND

There are six compounds that comprise the natural pyrethrins: pyrethrin I and II, jasmolin I and II, and cinerin I and II. Synthetic pyrethroids have been developed because the natural pyrethrins tend to break down quickly when exposed to air, light and heat. The synthetic pyrethroids can be classified as first and second generation. First-generation pyrethroids are esters of chrysanthemic acid and an alcohol, having a furan ring and terminal side chain moieties. Second-generation pyrethrins have 3-phenoxybenzyl alcohols derivatives in the alcohol moiety and have had some of the terminal side chain moieties replaced with a dichlorovinyl or dibromovinyl substitute and aromatic rings. The addition of the alpha-cyano group to the 3-phenoxybenzyl alcohol group in the second-generation pyrethroids has increased the insecticidal potency and stability of these compounds.

Pyrethrins cause hyperexcitability with very little cytotoxicity. The molecular targets of the pyrethrins and pyrethroids are similar in mammals and insects and include voltage-gated sodium, chloride and calcium channels, GABA-gated chloride channels, nicotinic receptors, membrane depolarization and intercellular gap junctions (Forshaw and Ray, 1990; Song and Narahashi, 1996a). Mammals are less susceptible to pyrethrin and pyrethroid toxicoses than insects primarily because they have a faster metabolic clearance, higher body temperatures and a lower affinity for the pyrethrins/pyrethroids (Song and Narahashi, 1996b; Gammon et al., 2012).

PHARMACOKINETICS/TOXICOKINETICS

Determination of the toxicity of pyrethroids in vivo is difficult because they have low water solubility, easily partition into lipids and will bind to plastics and glass. The reported toxicity of this class of insecticides has high variability.

Most pyrethrin and pyrethroid products are applied dermally in animals, but because of grooming, there can be oral and inhalation exposures, too (Anadón et al., 2013). Less than 2% of topically applied pyrethrin and pyrethroid insecticides are absorbed dermally (Wollen et al., 1992). One study confirmed that absorption of cypermethrin across human skin is minimal and peak excretion rates after dermal application were not observed until 12–36 h after dosing. Pyrethrins may be sequestered in the skin and slowly released into the systemic circulation (He et al., 1989). Oral or inhalation exposure results in faster systemic exposure (Anadon et al., 1996, 2013).

Approximately 40%–60% of an orally ingested dose is absorbed. When cypermethrin was administered orally to six adult male volunteers, oral absorption ranged from

Veterinary Toxicology. DOI: http://dx.doi.org/10.1016/B978-0-12-811410-0.00039-8

27% to 57% of the administered dose and peak excretion rates were measured in the urine between 8 and 24 h after dosing. When adult males were exposed to cyfluthrin at 160 μg/m^3, 93% of the metabolites were excreted within the first 24 h with peak excretion rates ranging from 0.5 to 3 h.

Pyrethroids are lipophilic and will distribute to tissues with high lipid content such as fat and nervous tissue in addition to liver, kidney and milk. Kim et al. (2008) described the pharmacokinetics and tissue distribution of deltamethrin in adult rats following oral or intravenous administration. Utilizing a physiologically based toxicokinetic model, GI absorption of deltamethrin was rapid, but bioavailability was low. Deltamethrin in blood was largely present in plasma. A very small proportion of the absorbed doses reached or remained in the brain. Fat, skin and muscle ultimately accumulated large amounts of this highly lipophilic insecticide.

Pyrethroids and pyrethrins are rapidly hydrolyzed in the gastrointestinal tract. Once absorbed these compounds are metabolized by mixed function oxidases and esterases. Metabolism of the pyrethroids results in water-soluble metabolites. Metabolism includes hydrolysis of the central ester bond, oxidation at several sites and conjugation with glycine, sulfate, glucuronide, or glucosides. Cleavage of the ester bond results in substantial reduction in toxicity. The presence of the alpha-cyano group, as in type II pyrethroids, will decrease the rate of hydrolysis of the ester bond. Cleavage of the alpha-cyano group results in rapid conversion of the cyano group to thiocyanate. For the detailed metabolism of different pyrethroids, readers are referred to Gammon et al. (2012).

Pyrethroids are eliminated by first order kinetics and most of the dose is eliminated in the first 12–24 h after absorption. The pyrethroids are rapidly metabolized to inactive metabolites, which are primarily excreted in the urine (Fig. 39.1).

MECHANISM OF ACTION

Pyrethroids primarily affect the sodium channel of cells, but chloride and calcium channels are also affected (Gammon et al., 2012; Soderlund, 2012; Meijer et al., 2014). Pyrethrins and pyrethroids slow the opening and closing of the sodium channels, resulting in excitation of the cell (Marban et al., 1989; Conley and Brammar, 1999). The increase of sodium in the sodium channels results in a cell that is in a stable, hyperexcitable state. The duration of the sodium action potential is much longer for type II pyrethroids than for type I. Type I pyrethroids result in primarily repetitive charges with membrane depolarization predominating in type II pyrethroids. Paresthesia results from the direct action of pyrethroids on sensory nerve endings, causing repetitive firing of these fibers. Less than 1% of sodium channels must be modified by pyrethroids to produce neurological signs. High concentrations of type II pyrethroids may also act on GABA-gated chloride channels (Bloomquist et al., 1986).

Pyrethrins also affect the voltage-dependent chloride channels. These channels are found in the brain, nerve, muscle, and salivary gland, and control cell excitability. There are many different functional types of chloride channels in contrast to sodium channels. Most pyrethroid-sensitive channels belong to the Maxi chloride channel class. Maxi channels are activated by depolarization, have high conductance, are calcium independent and are activated by protein kinase C phosphorylation. Pyrethroids cause a decrease in the Maxi chloride channel current, which increases excitability of the cell just as the action of pyrethroids on the sodium channel.

The decreased sensitivity of mammals to this class of compounds compared to insects is due to several factors. Pyrethroids bind more strongly with the sodium channel at low temperatures than at high temperatures. Insects' ambient temperature is approximately 25°C compared to mammals at 37°C. Mammalian sodium channels are at least 1000 times less sensitive to pyrethroids than insect sodium channels. Mammalian sodium channels recover much more quickly from depolarization than do insect sodium channels and are much more likely to detoxify pyrethroids before they reach their target site than are insects.

Pyrethroids cause a phenomenon in insects called "knockdown" (Narahashi, 1985). Knockdown is caused by inhibiting the cell but does not cause a lethal effect. This is caused from the ability of the sodium channels to retain many of the normal functions, such as selectivity for sodium ions and conductance after exposure to pyrethroids. After exposure to moderate doses of pyrethroids, cells function in a new state of hyperexcitability. If the level of sodium in the ion channel does not exceed the ability of the sodium pump to remove it, the cell continues to function normally. High concentrations of pyrethroids or hyperactivity beyond what the cell can sustain will cause depolarization and conduction block. The pyrethroids that hold the sodium channel open the longest will cause the greatest amount of depolarization.

There is marked stereospecificity of the action of pyrethroids on the sodium channel; some isomers are more toxic than others (Soderlund, 1985, 2012; Meacham et al., 2008). The *cis* isomers are usually more toxic than the *trans* isomers. As an example, the 1*R* and 1*S cis* isomers bind competitively to one site, and the 1*R* and 1*S trans* isomers bind noncompetitively to another (Narahashi, 1986). In mammals the 1*R* isomers are active and the 1*S* isomers inactive, making the 1*S* isomers nontoxic. Deltamethrin has been produced using stereospecificity to

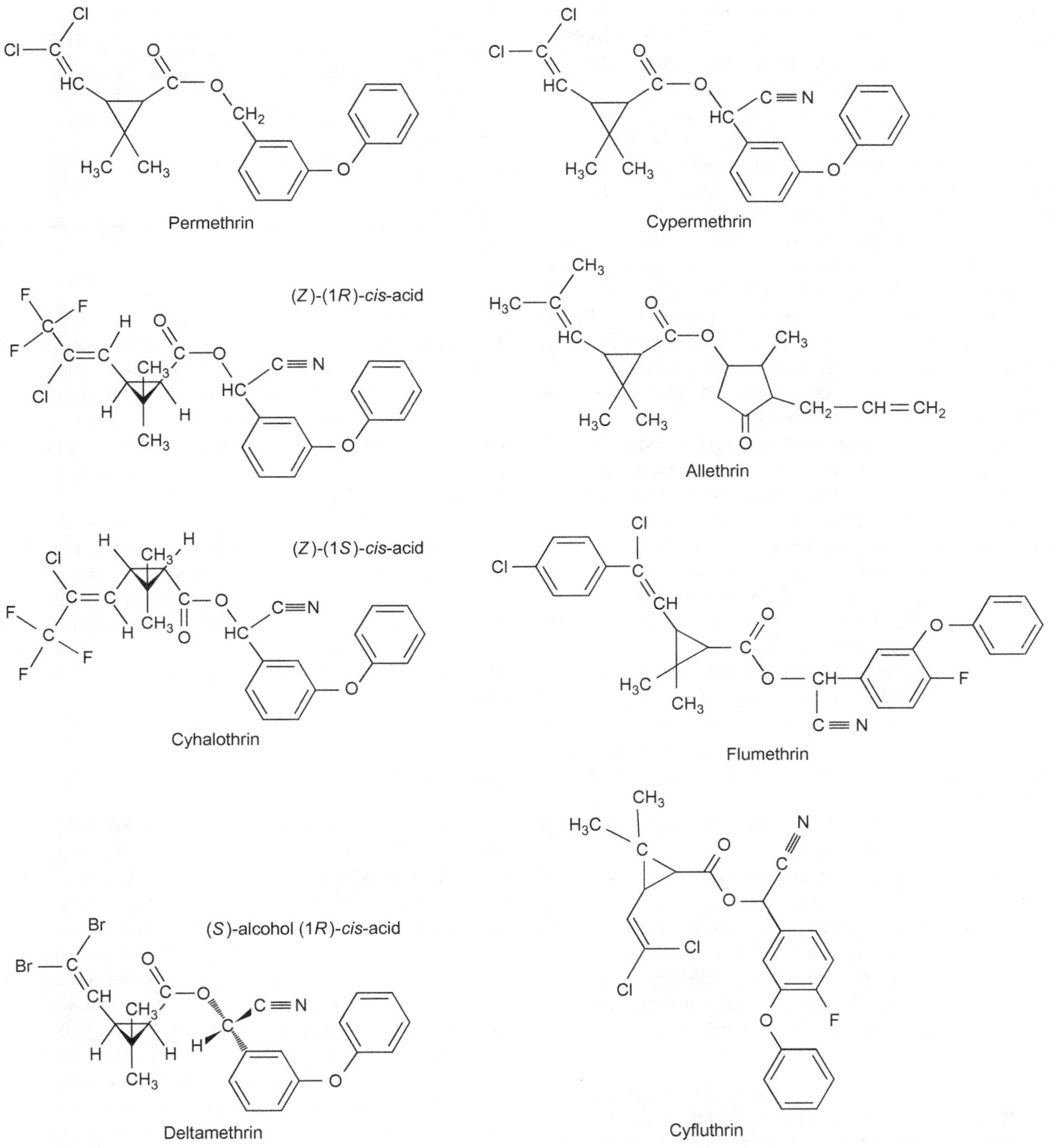

FIGURE 39.1 Structures of selected pyrethrins and pyrethroids.

produce a high degree of selective toxicity. This is the reason that the toxicity of different batches of pyrethroids can vary from batch to batch. The rat oral LD_{50} of commercial permethrin can vary from 430 to 8900 mg/kg, with toxicity depending on the amount of *cis* isomer present in the batch.

TOXICITY

Dermal exposure to pyrethroids is most common (Osweiler, 1996; Gammon et al., 2012; Anadon et al., 2013). In humans, the bioavailability of pyrethroids applied dermally is approximately 1%. Absorption after oral exposure in humans is 36%, mostly from the stomach. Once absorbed, the pyrethroids are rapidly distributed due to their lipophilicity. Systemic distribution produces effects that can be difficult to control and may be confused with poisoning by other pesticides, such as organophosphates, which also cause increased salivation and hyperexcitability. Many pyrethroid formulations also contain solvents, which can also cause toxicity. Cats are very sensitive to pyrethroid exposure (Meyer, 1999; Malik et al., 2010).

The half-life of pyrethroids in general in plasma is in hours, while oral exposure can be equally short. Cyfluthrin has a plasma half-life of 19–86 min. Intravenous LD_{50}s for pyrethroids range from 0.5 to 250 mg/kg. The major neurotoxicity observed in adults with pyrethroid toxicity is acute toxicity with no chronic or cumulative toxicity being caused. The excitatory motor signs are generated at the spinal level.

Fish are highly sensitive to pyrethrin and pyrethroid products, and contamination of lakes, streams, ponds or any aquatic habitat should be avoided (Bradbury and Coats, 1986, 1989; Ansari and Kumar, 1988). Household exposure of fish can occur when the premise is sprayed or fogged with insecticides and the aquarium aerator is left on. The tank and aerator should be covered during use of insecticides and the home should be well ventilated before uncovering and starting the pump.

Most avian species are thought to be tolerant of pyrethrin and pyrethroid products but carriers or propellants in spray formulations may be hazardous (Bradbury and Coats, 1982). There is very little literature about pyrethrin or pyrethroid toxicity of exotic avian species, reptiles or lagomorphs.

Tables 39.1 and 39.2 reference the oral toxicity of some type I and II pyrethroids.

In dogs, cats and large animals the clinical signs are similar for both type I and II compounds. Clinical signs include salivation, vomiting, hyperexcitability, tremors, seizures, dyspnea, weakness, prostration and death (Murphy, 1996). In rats with type I toxicity there is an increased response to stimulation, muscle tremors, excitement and paralysis (Beasley et al., 1994). These clinical signs can also be compatible with strychnine toxicities. Type II overexposure will cause increased salivation, weakness, and choreoathetosis. The concomitant use of pyrethrins and pyrethroids with synergists such as piperonyl butoxide, organophosphorus compounds or carbamates may increase toxicity by mechanisms involving inhibition of microsomal oxidation (Anadon et al., 2009, 2013).

These insecticides, in addition to neurotoxicity, can also produce hepatic, renal, dermal, cardiac, neurobehavioral, endocrine disruption, reproductive, and developmental effects in animals and humans (Vijverberg and van den Bercken, 1990; Wolansky and Harrill, 2007; Gupta, 2009; Drago et al., 2014; Atmaca and Aksoy, 2015; Hossain et al., 2015; Botnariu et al., 2016; Slima et al., 2016; Malik et al., 2017).

TABLE 39.1 Toxicity of Selected type I Pyrethroids

Type I Compounds	Oral LD_{50} (mg/kg body wt.) in Rat
Pyrethrin I	900
Allethrin	680
Tetramethrin	4640
Resmethrin	100
Permethrin	2000

TABLE 39.2 Toxicity of Selected type II Pyrethroids

Type II Compounds	Oral LD_{50} (mg/kg body wt.) in Rat
Cypermethrin	500
Deltamethrin	31
Fenvalerate	450
Fluvalinate	1000

TREATMENT

There is no specific antidote for pyrethroid toxicity; animals should be treated symptomatically. The main treatment for dermal exposure is to wash the animal with a mild detergent and water. Do not use any shampoos that contain additional insecticides as this could increase exposure to insecticides. Large and small animals should be treated the same. The pyrethroids bound to the skin cannot be removed by washing with soap and water, but dermal paresthesia can be reduced by applying corn oil to the site(s) of application. For oral exposure, emetics or gastric lavage can be used to empty the stomach, if done within 1–2 h of ingestion. Activated charcoal and a saline or sorbitol cathartic will reduce oral absorption and increase elimination.

Supportive therapy using diazepam or barbiturates to control hyperexcitability or seizures can be used. Phenothiazine tranquilizers should not be used because they can lower the threshold for seizures. Atropine can be used to control excess salivation or gastrointestinal hypermotility.

The prognosis for pyrethroid toxicity is usually good because of the low toxicity.

CONCLUDING REMARKS AND FUTURE DIRECTIONS

Pyrethroid insecticides, being of plant origin, are attractive to people that prefer to use organic insecticides on their companion animals or livestock, or who are engaged in organic food production. Pyrethrin insecticides, while toxic to selected species, have a wider margin of safety than organophosphate or organochlorine insecticides. Biomarkers of exposure to pyrethroids are being investigated (Gupta and Milatovic, 2014). Urine is the matrix that is being most heavily investigated to determine which metabolites can be used to identify exposure to the parent compound. Advances in analytical methods to detect low concentrations of the pyrethroid metabolites will allow improved assessment of exposure in the future.

REFERENCES

Anadon, A., Martinez Larranage, M.R., Fernandez Cruz, M.L., et al., 1996. Toxicokinetics of deltamethrin and its 4′-HO-metabolite in the rat. Toxicol. Appl. Pharmacol. 141, 8–16.

Anadon, A., Martinez-Larranaga, M.R., Martinez, M.A., 2009. Use and abuse of pyrethrins and synthetic pyrethroids in veterinary medicine. Vet. J. 182, 7–20.

Anadon, A., Arés, I., Martíinez, M.A., et al., 2013. Pyrethrins and synthetic pyrethroids:use in veterinary medicine. In: Ramawat, K.G., Mérillon, J.M. (Eds.), Natural Products. Springer-Verlag, Berlin, pp. 4061–4086.

Ansari, B.A., Kumar, K., 1988. Cypermethrin toxicity: effect on the carbohydrate metabolism of the Indian catfish, Heteropneustes fossilis. Sci. Total Environ. 72, 161–166.

Atmaca, E., Aksoy, A., 2015. D-phenothrin-induced oxidative DNA damage in rat liver and kidney determined by HPLC-ECD/DAD. Environ. Toxicol. 30, 607–613.

Beasley, V.R., Dorman, D.C., Fikes, F.D., et al., 1994. A Systems Approach to Veterinary Toxicology. University of Illinois, Champagne, IL.

Bloomquist, J.R., Adams, P.M., Soderlund, D.M., 1986. Inhibition of gamma-aminobutyric acid-stimulated chloride flux in mouse brain vesicles by polychloroalkane and pyrethroid insecticides. Neurotoxicology. 7, 11–20.

Botnariu, G., Birsan, C., Podoleanu, C., et al., 2016. Skin necrosis caused by prallethrin, a worldwide used insecticide. Environ. Toxicol. Pharmacol. 43, 103–104.

Bradbury, S.P., Coats, J.R., 1982. Toxicity of fenvalerate to bobwhite quail (Colinus virginianus) including brain and liver residues associated with mortality. J. Toxicol. Environ. Health. 10, 307–319.

Bradbury, S.P., Coats, J.R., 1986. Toxicokinetics of fenvalerate in rainbow trout (Salmo gairdneri). Environ. Toxicol. Chem. 5, 567–576.

Bradbury, S.P., Coats, J.R., 1989. Comparative toxicology of the pyrethroid insecticides. Reviews of Environmental Contamination and Toxicology, US Environmental Res. LabVol. 108. Springer-Verlag, New York, pp. 133–177.

Conley, E.C., Brammar, W.J., 1999. The Ion Channel Facts Book. Academic Press, San Diego, CA.

Drago, B., Shah, N.S., Shah, S.H., 2014. Acute permethrin neurotoxicity: variable presentations, high index of suspicion. Toxicol. Rep. 1, 1026–1028.

Forshaw, P.J., Ray, D.E., 1990. A novel action of deltamethrin on membrane resistance in mammalian skeletal-muscle and non-myelinated nerve-fibers. Neuropharmacology. 29, 75–81.

Gammon, D.W., Chandrasekaran, A., AlNaggar, S.F., 2012. Comparative metabolism and toxicology of pyrethroids in mammals. In: Marrs, T.C. (Ed.), Mammalian Toxicology of Insecticides. RSC Publ, Cambridge, pp. 137–183.

Gupta, R.C., 2009. Toxicology of the placenta. In: Ballantyne, B., Marrs, T.C., Syversen, T. (Eds.), General and Applied Toxicology, third ended. John Wiley and Sons, Chichester, pp. 2003–2039.

Gupta, R.C., Milatovic, D., 2014. Insecticides. In: Gupta, R.C. (Ed.), Biomarkers in Toxicology. Academic Press/Elsevier, Amsterdam, pp. 389–407.

He, F.S., Wang, S.G., Liu, L.H., et al., 1989. Clinical manifestations and diagnosis of acute pyrethroid poisoning. Arch. Toxicol. 63, 54–58.

Hossain, M.M., DiGicco-Bloom, E., Richardson, J.R., 2015. Hippocampal ER stress and learning deficits following repeated pyrethroid exposure. Toxicol. Sci. 143 (1), 220–228.

Kim, K.-B., Anand, S.S., Kim, H.J., et al., 2008. Toxicokinetics and tissue distribution of deltamethrin in adult Sprague-Dawley rats. Toxicol. Sci. 101, 197–205.

Malik, R., Ward, M.P., Seavers, A., et al., 2010. Permethrin spot-on intoxication of cats literature review and survey of veterinary practitioners in Australia. J. Feline Med. Surg. 12, 5–14.

Malik, J.K., Aggarwal, M., Kalpana, S., Gupta, R.C., 2017. Chlorinated hydrocarbons and pyrethrins/pyrethroids. In: Gupta, R.C. (Ed.), Reproductive and Developmental Toxicology, second ed. Academic Press/Elsevier, Amsterdam, pp. 633–655.

Marban, E., Yamagishi, T., Tomaselli, G.F., 1989. Structure and function of voltage-gated sodium channels. J. Physiol. 508, 647–657.

Meacham, C.A., Brodfuehrer, P.D., Watkins, J.A., Shafer, T.J., 2008. Developmentally-regulated sodium channel subunits are differentially sensitive to -cyano containing pyrethroids. Toxicol. Appl. Pharmacol. 231, 273–281.

Meijer, M., Dingemans, M.M.L., van den Berg, M., et al., 2014. Inhibition of voltage-gated calcium channels as common mode of action for (mixture of) distinct classes of insecticides. Toxicol. Sci. 141 (1), 103–111.

Meyer, K.E., 1999. Toxicosis in cats erroneously treated with 45 to 65% permethrin products. J. Am. Vet. Med. Assoc. 215, 198–203.

Murphy, M., 1996. A Field Guide to Common Animal Poisons. State University Press, Ames, IA.

Narahashi, T., 1985. Nerve membrane ionic channels as the primary target of pyrethroids. Neurotoxicology. 6, 3–22.

Narahashi, T., 1986. Mechanisms of action of pyrethroids on sodium and calcium channel gating. In: Ford, G.G., Lunt, G.G., Reay, R.C., Usherwood, P.N.R. (Eds.), Neuropharmacology of Pesticide Action. Ellis Horwood, Chichester, pp. 36–40.

Osweiler, G.D., 1996. Toxicology. Williams and Wilkins, Philadelphia, PA.

Proudfoot, A.T., 2005. Poisoning due to pyrethrins. Toxicol. Rev. 24, 107–113.

Slima, A.B., Chtourou, Y., Barkallah, M., et al., 2016. Endocrine disrupting potential and reproductive dysfunction in male mice exposed to deltamethrin. Hum. Exp. Toxicol. 2016, 1–9.

Soderlund, D.M., 1985. Pyrethroid-receptor interactions: stereospecific binding and effects on sodium channels in mouse brain preparations. Neurotoxicology. 6, 35–46.

Soderlund, D.M., 2012. Molecular mechanisms of pyrethroid insecticide neurotoxicity: recent advances. Arch. Toxicol.165–181.

Song, J.H., Narahashi, T., 1996a. Differential effects of the pyrethroid Tetramethrin on tetrodotoxin-sensitive and tetrodotoxin-resistant single sodium channels. Brain Res. 712, 258–264.

Song, J.H., Narahashi, T., 1996b. Modulation of sodium channels of rat cerebellar Purkinji neurons by the pyrethroid Tetramethrin. J. Pharmacol. Exp. Ther. 277, 445–453.

Valentine, W.M., 1990. Pyrethrin and pyrethroid insecticides. Vet. Clin. N Am. Sm. An. Pract. 20, 375–382.

Vijverberg, H.P.M., van den Bercken, J., 1990. Neurotoxicological effects and the mode of action of pyrethroid insecticides. Crit. Rev. Toxicol. 21, 105–126.

Wolansky, M.J., Harrill, J.A., 2007. Neurobehavioral toxicology of pyrethroid insecticides in adult animals: a critical review. Neurotoxicol. Teratol. 30, 55–78.

Wollen, B.H., Marsh, J.R., Laird, W.J.D., Lesser, J.E., 1992. The metabolism of cypermethrin in man – differences in urinary metobolite profiles following oral and dermal administration. Xenobiatica. 22, 983–991.

Chapter 40

Neonicotinoids

Steve M. Ensley

INTRODUCTION

Neonicotinoids are a relatively new class of insecticides with widespread use in veterinary medicine and crop production. The neonicotinoid insecticides include imidacloprid, acetamiprid, dinotefuran, thiamethoxam, and clothianidin. In the last decade neonicotinoid insecticides have been the fastest growing class of insecticides in modern crop protection because of the widespread use against a broad spectrum of sucking and certain chewing pests (Jeschke et al., 2010). Neonicotinoids have a relatively low risk for nontarget organisms and the environment, a high-target specificity to insecticide, and versatility in application methods (Cresswell, 2011). The neonicotinoids have been implicated in the Colony Collapse disorder in bees but this has not been proven definitively (Lundin et al., 2015). Neonicotinoids have been shown to affect the immunocompetence of honey bees (Brandt et al., 2016). Recently, some concerns have also been raised about adverse effects of imidacloprid in birds and aquatic life (Zeng et al., 2013; Sánchez-Bayo, 2014).

Imidacloprid is a neonicotinoid compound that is used as an insecticide for dermal application on animals, for termite and grub control and as an insecticide for crop protection. The neonicotinoids act on nicotinic receptors in insects and vertebrates. To reduce toxicity to mammals and increase toxicity to insects, neonicotinic compounds have been selected that are highly specific for subtypes of nicotinic receptors that occur in insects (Kagabu, 2011; Tomizawa et al., 2011). The neonicotinoids do not readily pass the blood–brain barrier (BBB), further reducing the potential for mammalian toxicity (Yamamoto et al., 1995).

Imidacloprid does not accumulate in the body, and it is not carcinogenic, mutagenic, teratogenic nor a reproductive toxicant. Imidacloprid has a high margin of safety due to the high insecticidal specificity and low mammalian toxicity (Nagata et al., 1999). This chapter describes toxicity of neonicotinoids in animals.

BACKGROUND

The neonicotinoids were developed in the late 1970s by chemists at Shell Chemical Company doing research with the heterocyclic nitromethylenes for use as insecticides (Soloway et al., 1978; Schroeder and Flattum, 1984). The neonicotinoids and chloronicotinyls are a separate class of compounds from the nicotinoids (Tomizawa and Yamamoto, 1993). Chemists at Nihon Bayer Agrochem discovered imidacloprid in 1984 when the 3-pyridylmethyl group was added to the nitromethylene heterocyclic parent molecule. This addition to nitromethylene greatly increased the insecticidal activity and reduced mammalian toxicity. After imidacloprid was discovered several other analogs with the 6-chloro-3-pyridylmethyl moiety have been developed, such as acetamiprid, nitenpyram and thiacloprid (Takahashi et al., 1992; Minamida et al., 1993; Yamada et al., 1999). Fig. 40.1 shows the structure of imidacloprid.

PHARMACOKINETICS/TOXICOKINETICS

When administered orally, imidacloprid is rapidly absorbed, metabolized primarily in the liver and excreted primarily in urine. Absorption and distribution of imidacloprid in rats occurs within 1 h following oral administration. Imidacloprid is not distributed to the central nervous system (CNS), fatty tissues or bone. This indicates that the BBB allows little distribution to the CNS for imidacloprid in particular and the neonicotinoids in general. There are two routes of imidacloprid metabolism in mammals. The first route of metabolism involves oxidative cleavage of imidacloprid to imidazolidine and 6-chloronicotinic acid. The imidazolidine moiety is excreted in the urine. The 6-chloronicotinic acid is further degraded by glutathione conjugation to a derivative of mercapturic acid, then to methyl mercaptonicotinic acid. The mercaptonicotinic acid is then conjugated with glycine to form a hippuric acid conjugate that is excreted.

Veterinary Toxicology. DOI: http://dx.doi.org/10.1016/B978-0-12-811410-0.00040-4

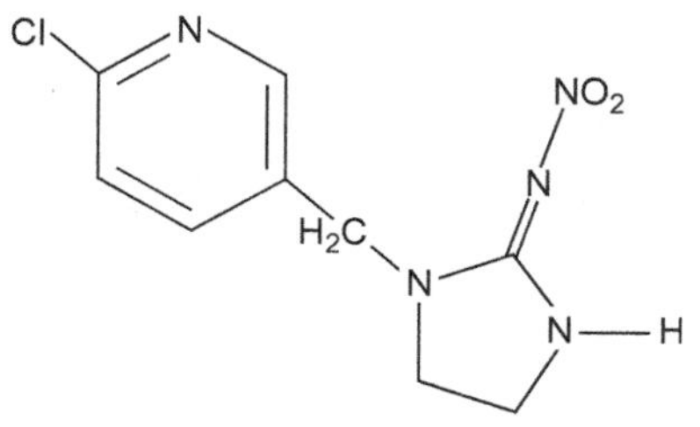

FIGURE 40.1 Structure of imidacloprid.

A second route of metabolism involves hydroxylation of the imidazolidine ring followed by elimination of water and formation of an unsaturated metabolite. In rats, more than 90% of a dose of imidacloprid is eliminated within 24 h. Approximately 80% of the dose is excreted by the urine with the remainder eliminated in the feces. Specific information on the toxicokinetics of the rat and other species can be found in Thyssen and Machemer (1999) and Rose (2012).

MECHANISM OF ACTION

The neonicotinoids act on postsynaptic nicotinic receptors (Buckingham et al., 1997). These receptors are located entirely in the CNS of insects. Imidacloprid acts on at least three different subtypes of nicotinic receptors in the cockroach. Neonicotinoids cause a bi-phasic response: an initial increase in the frequency of spontaneous discharge followed by a complete block to nerve propagation. Insecticidal activity is increased by adding synergists that inhibit oxidative degradation (Liu and Casida, 1993).

Mammalian tissue also contains multiple subtypes of nicotinic receptors. The various subtypes are formed from different combinations of nine α, four β, γ, δ, and ε subunits (Tomizawa et al., 1999). Nicotinic receptors in mammals are located in the autonomic ganglia, skeletal muscle, spinal cord, and in different regions of the brain. Neonicotinoids have much lower activity in vertebrates compared to insects due to the different binding properties of the various receptor subtypes (Yamamoto et al., 1998; Tomizawa and Casida, 2011). Acute toxicity of the neonicotinoids in mammals is related to the potency at the α_7 nicotinic receptor subtype with the activity at the α_4, β_2, α_3, and α_1 receptors having a decreasing effect on toxicity. Toxicity in mammals involves complex interactions at multiple receptor sites with some of the receptor types even having a combination of agonist and antagonist effects on the synapse.

TOXICITY

The following studies were conducted by Bayer CropScience (Sheets, 2001). Acute oral toxicity of imidacloprid in rats has been demonstrated at doses above 300 mg/kg with 100% mortality at 500 mg/kg. At doses in rats above 300 mg/kg, clinical signs were observed within 15 min of dosing and recovery was observed within 8–24 h. A subchronic 13-week oral dosing study of imidacloprid in rats also demonstrated toxicity at a dose of 300 mg/kg in male rats. At a dose of 300 mg/kg in male rats, hypertrophy of hepatocytes and sporadic cell necrosis was observed in the liver. This mild liver damage was not observed after a 4-week recovery period. Serum alkaline phosphatase and alanine aminotransferase were elevated in male and female rats treated at 300 mg/kg and above. In dogs, a 13-week oral dose of imidacloprid at 15 mg/kg and above produced a tremor that increased with dose. A 52-week study in dogs at oral doses up to 72 mg/kg/day of imidacloprid did not produce tremors. The no observed effective level for this chronic oral exposure dog study was 15 mg/kg. Carcinogenicity was not observed in rats dosed orally at doses up to 103 mg/kg for 2 years. Studies confirm that imidacloprid is nonmutagenic, nonembryotoxic, and nonteratogenic.

In a developmental and neurobehavioral toxicity study, Abou-Donia et al. (2008) treated timed pregnant Sprague-Dawley rats on day nine of gestation with a single large ip dose of imidacloprid (337 mg/kg), and on postnatal day 30 evaluated male and female offspring for histopathological, neurochemical and behavioral alterations. The offspring exhibited significant sensorimotor impairments during behavioral assessment. These changes were associated with increased acetylcholinesterase activity in the midbrain, cortex, and brainstem. Ligand binding densities for [^{3}H]cytosine for $\alpha4\beta2$ type nicotinic acetylcholine receptors did not show any significant change, whereas [^{3}H] AFDX 384, a ligand for m2 muscarinic acetylcholine receptors, was significantly increased in the cortex. Histopathological evaluation of brain regions did not show any alteration in surviving neurons. On the other hand, there was a rise in glial fibrillary acidic protein immunostaining in motor cortex layer III, CA1, CA3, and the dentate gyrus subfield of the hippocampus. Recently, Sheets et al. (2016) reviewed the neonicotinoids for developmental neurotoxicity and found the decreased body weight of F1 animals during development (e.g., delayed sexual maturation, decreased brain weight, and morphometric measurements) and acute toxicity (decreased motor activity associated with peak exposure via the diet and milk).

In a recent experimental study, male rats exposed to an LD_{50} dose of imidacloprid (170 mg/kg, ip) showed susceptibility to the genotoxic effects of imidacloprid (Arslan et al., 2016). In another study, Pandit et al. (2016) exposed mice to imidacloprid orally at 1/20th of LD_{50} dose for 30 days. Semiquantitative histopathology revealed lung injury without any change in the expression of TLR-4 and TNF-α both at mRNA and protein levels.

The most common adverse effects observed with dosing of neonicotinoids at low levels is decreased activity and tremors, impaired pupillary function (dilated or pinpoint pupils), and uncoordinated gait; hypothermia is observed at higher doses. At lethal doses, deaths are observed within 4 h of dosing. If death did not occur, recovery was observed within 8–24 h of dosing.

TREATMENT

There is no specific antidote to treatment of overdoses of imidacloprid. Treatment is symptomatic. If the exposure is dermal, washing the affected animal with soap and water is indicated. If the exposure is oral, emetics, adsorbents, or cathartics could be used depending on whether vomiting is occurring spontaneously or not. Absorption and elimination of imidacloprid is rapid, so immediate supportive care should allow for rapid recovery.

CONCLUDING REMARKS AND FUTURE DIRECTIONS

The neonicotinoids have a wide safety margin in mammals, and the insecticidal activity can be targeted so this class of compounds can have wide future use as an insecticide. The neonicotinoids have been restricted in many parts of Europe since 2013 because of the association with the colony collapse syndrome in bees. The European Union is reviewing the restrictions on the neonicotinoids and the review will conclude in 2017.

REFERENCES

Abou-Donia, M.B., Goldstein, L.B., Bullman, S., et al., 2008. Imidacloprid induces neurobehavioral deficits and increases expression of glial fibrillary acidic protein in the motor cortex and hippocampus in offspring rats following *in utero* exposure. J. Toxicol. Environ. Health Part A. 71, 119–130.

Arslan, M., Sevgiler, Y., Buyukleyla, M., et al., 2016. Sex-related effects of imidacloprid modulated by piperonyl butoxide and menadione in rats. Part II: genotoxic and cytotoxic potential. Drug Chem. Toxicol. 39 (1), 81–86.

Brandt, A., Gorenflo, A., Siede, R., et al., 2016. The neonictotinoids thiacloprid, imidacloprid, and clothianidin affect the immunocompetence of honey bees (*Apis mellifera* L.). J. Insect. Physiol. 86, 40–47.

Buckingham, S.D., Lapied, B., LeCorronc, H., et al., 1997. Imidacloprid actions on insect neuronal acetylcholine receptors. J. Exp. Biol. 200, 2685–2692.

Cresswell, J.E., 2011. A meta-analysis of experiments testing the effects of a neonicotinoid insecticide (imidacloprid) on honey bees. Ecotoxicology. 20, 149–157.

Jeschke, P., Nauen, R., Schindler, M., et al., 2010. Overview of the status and global strategy for neonicotinoids. Symposium on the Strategic Molecular Design of Neonicotinoid Insecticides at the 239th Meeting of the American Chemical Society, San Francisco, California, USA, 21–25: 2897–2908.

Kagabu, S., 2011. Discovery of imidacloprid and further developments from strategic molecular designs. J. Agr. Food Chem. 59, 2887–2896.

Liu, M.-Y., Casida, J.E., 1993. High affinity binding of [3H] Imidacloprid in the insect acetylcholine receptor. Pestic. Biochem. Physiol. 46, 40–46.

Lundin, O., Rundlöf, M., Smith, H.G., et al., 2015. Neonicotinoid insecticides and heir impacts on bees: a systematic review of research approaches and identification of knowledge gap. PLoS One. Available from: http://dx.doi.org/10.1371/journal.pone.0136928.

Minamida, I., Iwanaga, K., Tabuchi, T., et al., 1993. Synthesis and insecticidal activity of acyclic nitroethene compounds containing a heteroarylmethylamino group. J. Pestic. Sci. 18, 41.

Nagata, K., Aoyama, E., Ikeda, T., et al., 1999. Effects of nitenpyram on the neuronal nicotinic acetylcholine receptor-channel in rat phaeochromocytoma PC12 cells. J. Pestic. Sci. 24, 143–148.

Pandit, A.H., Choudhary, S., et al., 2016. Imidacloprid induced hitomorphological changes and expression of TLR-4 and TNFα in lung. Pestic. Biochem. Physiol. 131, 9–17.

Rose, P.H., 2012. Nicotine and the nicotinoids. In: Marrs, T.C. (Ed.), Mammalian Toxicology of Insecticides. RSC Publ, Cambridge, pp. 184–220.

Sánchez-Bayo, F., 2014. The trouble with neonicotinoids. Science. 346, 806–807.

Schroeder, M.E., Flattum, R.F., 1984. The mode of action and neurotoxic properties of the nitromethylene heterocycle insecticides. Pest Biochem. Physiol. 22, 148–160.

Sheets, L.P., 2001. The neonicotinoid insecticides. In: Massaro, E. (Ed.), Handbook of Neurotoxicology, vol. 1. Humana Press, pp. 79–87.

Sheets, L.P., Li, A.A., Minnema, D.J., 2016. A critical review of neonicotinoid insecticides for developmental neurotoxicity. Crit. Rev. Toxicol. 46, 153–190.

Soloway, S.B., Henry, A.C., Kollmeyer, W.D., et al., 1978. Nitromethylene insecticides. Adv. Pestic. Sci. 4, 206–217.

Takahashi, H., Mitsui, J., Takakusa, N., et al., 1992. Ni-25, a new type of systemic and broad spectrum insecticide. In Brighton Crop Protection Conferences B Pest and Diseases, vol. 1: 89–96.

Thyssen, J., Machemer, L., 1999. Imidacloprid: toxicology and metabolism. In: Yamamoto, I., Casida, J.E. (Eds.), Nicotinoid Insecticides and the Nicotinic Acetylcholine Receptor. Springer-Verlag, Tokyo, pp. 213–222.

Tomizawa, M., Casida, J.E., 2011. Unique neonicotinoid binding conformations conferring selectin inceptor interactions. J. Agri. Food Chem. 59, 2825–2828.

Tomizawa, M., Yamamoto, I., 1993. Structure–activity relationships of nicotinoids and imidacloprid analogs. J. Pestic. Sci. 18, 91–98.

Tomizawa, M., Latli, B., Casida, J.E., 1999. Structure and function of insect nicotinic acetylcholine receptors studied with nicotinoids insecticide affinity probes. In: Yamamoto, I., Casida, J.E. (Eds.), Nicotinoid Insecticides and the Nicotinic Acetylcholine Receptor. Springer-Verlag, Tokyo, pp. 271–292.

Tomizawa, M., Kagabu, S., Casida, J.E., 2011. Receptor structure-guided neonicotinoid design. J. Agr. Food Chem. 59, 2918–2922.

Yamada, T., Takashi, H., Hatano, R., 1999. A novel insecticide, acetamiprid. In: Yamamoto, I., Casida, J.E. (Eds.), Nicotinoid Insecticides and the Nicotinic Acetylcholine Receptor. Springer-Verlag, Tokyo, pp. 149–176.

Yamamoto, I., Yabuta, G., Tomizawa, M., et al., 1995. Molecular mechanism for selective toxicity of nicotinoids and neonicotinoids. J. Pestic. Sci. 20, 33–40.

Yamamoto, I., Tomizawa, M., Saito, T., et al., 1998. Structural factors contributing to insecticidal and selective actions of neonicotinoids. Arch. Insect. Biochem. Physiol. 37, 24–32.

Zeng, G., Chen, M., Zeng, Z., 2013. Risks of neonicotinoid pesticides. Science. 340, 1403.

FURTHER READING

Tomizawa, M., Casida, J.E., 1999. Minor structural changes in nicotinoids insecticides confer differential subtype selectivity for mammalian nicotinic acetylcholine receptors. Br. J. Pharmacol. 127, 115–122.

Chapter 41

Amitraz

Ayhan Filazi and Begum Yurdakok-Dikmen

INTRODUCTION

Amitraz (*N*,*N*′-[(Methylimino)dimethylidyne]di-2,4-xylidine) (Fig. 41.1), is a formamidine derivative pesticide (USEPA, 1996). Although it is particularly significant with its acaricide effects, today, amitraz is widely used as a pesticide for various purposes. Many formulations such as wettable powder (WP), emulsified concentrate (EC), soluble concentrate/liquid or impregnated collar (for dogs) are available for insecticide purposes (USEPA, 1996). It is used widely to control all stages of plant parasites and as an ectoparasiticide in cattle, sheep, pigs, and dogs exclusively topically (Peter et al., 2006). It has been reported that other animal species such as horses, cats, and dog breeds like Chihuahua and Pomeranian should not be treated with amitraz because of its adverse effects (Tarallo et al., 2009). Despite this, due to its effectiveness, low price and malpractice of the veterinary surgeon, it might still be used in these species and cause poisonings. As a result of this, many cases of poisoning have been reported for horses, cats, dogs, and humans (Grossman, 1993; Gunaratnam et al., 1993; Yilmaz and Yildiztas, 2003). In this chapter, amitraz poisonings that occur in animals will be discussed.

BACKGROUND

Amitraz is a broad-spectrum insecticide and acaricide that is used globally in agriculture and veterinary medicine. It has a rapid effect on the control of animal ectoparasites such as scabies, ticks, and lice. Tick collars that contain 9% of amitraz are rather widely used in veterinary medicine (Hugnet et al., 1996). All dip solutions containing amitraz that are used for tick infestations in cattle and sheep contain xylene and 12.5%–20% amitraz as an active substance. While amitraz is also used to control ectoparasites in cattle, sheep, goat, and pigs, it is not recommended for use in horses, cats, and small breed dogs such as Chihuahua and Pomeranian (Peter et al., 2006; Tarallo et al., 2009). Also, amitraz should not be used in diabetic animals because it adversely affects glucose and insulin levels even if it used topically (Hsu and Schaffer, 1988). Mainly, the stimulation of α-adrenergic receptors is held responsible for its adverse effects in mammals. Low blood pressure, hypothermia, lethargy, anorexia, vomiting, high blood glucose levels, and digestive tract disorders may develop in exposed animals. Dogs may also develop cutaneous or mucosal irritations resulting itching, eczema, alopecia, or conjunctivitis due to the collars containing this substance (Grossman, 1993; Peter et al., 2006; Tarallo et al., 2009).

PHARMACOKINETICS/TOXICOKINETICS

Amitraz is absorbed rapid and easily by dermal or oral administration due to its highly lipophilic property; which makes it potentially hazardous for animals and humans.

Studies on the pharmacokinetics of amitraz in different species have shown that 53%–80% is excreted in urine when it is delivered orally in mice, rats, dogs, baboons, and humans within the first 24 h. Two hours after oral application in mice and rats, the highest residual concentrations were detected in the liver, kidney, and muscle tissues, and its levels rapidly decreased afterward. Gender did not affect the excretion route or speed. It was shown that 92% of the amitraz applied to rats topically could be cleansed by washing the skin even after 10 h postapplication, that only 3% remains on the skin for 24 h and that this ratio drops to 1.4% after 5 days. A small portion of amitraz was absorbed during these 5 days (approximately 3%–8% of the amitraz applied) which is excreted in urine and feces (USEPA, 1996).

The metabolism of amitraz is quite similar in rats, mice, cats, dogs, baboons, cows, and humans. It is initially hydrolyzed into *N*-(2,4-dimethylphenyl)-*N*′-methyl formamidine (BTS-27271) and 2,4-dimethyl formanilide (BTS-27919). The compounds contain a 2,4-dimethylaniline (2,4-DMA) ring. The end product of its metabolism is 4-amino-3-methylbenzoic acid (BTS-28369) that is rapidly conjugated and excreted. Besides these, it also

Veterinary Toxicology. DOI: http://dx.doi.org/10.1016/B978-0-12-811410-0.00041-6

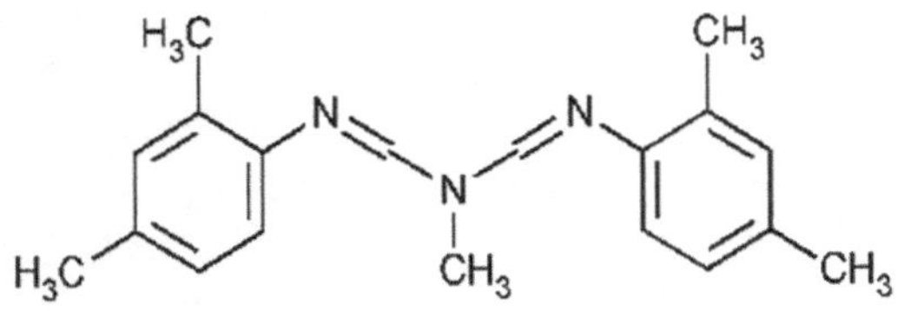

FIGURE 41.1 The chemical structure of amitraz.

transforms into 4-formamido-3-methylbenzoic acid (BTS-39098), BTS-28369 and some unknown metabolites that contain DMA rings, where all of these metabolites can be found in urine (Knowles and Benezet, 1981). BTS-27271 and BTS-27919 are the primary metabolites of amitraz, and they are a cause of concern because they may have developmental or genotoxic effects and because they contain a 2,4-dimethylaniline ring (USEPA, 1996).

When amitraz is administered orally, it is absorbed in significant levels, and it has a long excretion half-life in dogs (Hugnet et al., 1996). It has been shown that the concentration of amitraz and clinical signs are strongly associated in both cats (Marafon et al., 2010) and dogs (Hugnet et al., 1996). In dogs, the clinical signs of amitraz poisoning usually start 1 h after oral intake and/or when it reaches a plasma concentration of 5 mg/L which lasts until the concentration of amitraz drops below this level (Hugnet et al., 1996).

In an experimental study (Pass and Mogg, 1995), it was shown that the metabolism rate of amitraz to BTS-27271 and/or the excretion rate of unmetabolized amitraz is higher in sheep than it is in ponies and that amitraz can remain in the plasma of ponies for longer. This study is an important indicator of the sensitivity of horses to amitraz.

MECHANISM OF ACTION

Amitraz shows its effects in mammals mainly by activating α_2-adrenergic receptors (Costa et al., 1988). Both amitraz and BTS-27271 change the secretion of insulin and glucagon by stimulating the pancreatic α_2-adrenergic receptors of rats in vitro (Abu-Basha et al., 1999). With the stimulation of α_2-adrenergic receptors, the intracellular adenylate cyclase enzyme is also inhibited, and the cAMP levels were found to decrease (Chen and Hsu, 1994).

Amitraz was also found to activate α_1-adrenergic receptors in vitro in the forebrain of mice (Costa et al., 1988), and in vivo in dogs (Cullen and Reynoldson, 1990) slightly through partial agonist effects. Therefore, vascular α_1 and α_2-adrenergic receptors contribute to the vasopressor effect of amitraz causing hypotension and central nervous system (CNS) depression through the stimulation of the central α_2-adrenergic receptors (Cullen and Reynoldson, 1990). All of this data indicate that the effects of amitraz are sometimes mediated solely through α_2 receptors and sometimes through both receptor types. It is also predicted that the signs related to α_1 adrenergic receptors expected to appear during poisoning could be masked by α_2-agonist effects (Del Pino et al., 2015).

Amitraz blocks H1 receptors in the ileum of guinea pig strongly in vitro (Pass and Mogg, 1991), but in rat brains weakly in vivo (Costa et al., 1988). A strong histaminergic effect was achieved with BTS-27271 in the ileum of guinea pigs (Pass and Mogg, 1991). Besides this, the fact that the intestinal stagnation obtained by intravenous delivery of amitraz and BTS-27271 to separate sheep was partially reversed by an H1 agonist, and it was completely reversed by an α_2-adrenergic receptor antagonist suggests that amitraz is a weak inhibitor of H1 receptors and that this effect is a seconder result of amitraz's stimulation of α_2-adrenergic receptors (Pass and Mogg, 1991).

The behavioral disorders (Godar et al., 2014), infertility (Mihalik et al., 2010), and neurotoxic signs (Del Pino et al., 2011) that develop in amitraz poisoning are explained by its effect on the monoamine oxidase (MAO) enzyme. Studies indicate that amitraz mainly inhibits MAO-A and BTS-27271 inhibit MAO-B (Moser and MacPhail, 1989).

TOXICITY

Acute Toxicity

The acute lethal dose-50 (LD_{50}) or lethal concentration-50 (LC_{50}) values of amitraz and some of its metabolites delivered by inhalation, orally, or dermal routes are described in Table 41.1 (Krieger, 2010; Del Pino et al., 2015; CALEPA, 1995). USEPA has classified amitraz as class III mildly toxic by the oral or inhalation route, as class II, moderately toxic by dermal route, and as class IV, nonirritating to the skin and only mildly irritating if it contacts the eyes, and as "nonsensitizing to skin" (USEPA, 1996). However, because amitraz poisoning mostly occurs due to contact with products that contain, it would be more appropriate to provide the toxicity data of these products. In a risk assessment performed by California EPA, amitraz formulated with 50% of a soil-derived carrier (Mitac 50% WP), a surfactant and a dispersive agent and a 12.5% amitraz product prepared using a petrol distillate (Taktic 12.5% EC) were found to be less poisonous in rats. Twenty percent amitraz product prepared with a petrol distillate (Mitac 20% EC) caused more toxicity (Table 41.1) (CALEPA, 1995). The acute oral LD_{50} of an amitraz formulation that contains xylene prepared in the laboratory (12.5% EC) was found to be higher than the LD_{50} of technical amitraz. In this case, it was concluded that xylene increased the toxicity of

TABLE 41.1 Acute Toxicity of Amitraz

Species	Route	LC50 or LC50	Mitac EC	Taktic	Mitac 50 WP
		Amitraz (Technical)	Amitraz (20% Emulsifiable Concentrate)	Amitraz (12.5% Emulsifiable Concentrate)	Amitraz (50% Wettable Powder)
Mouse	Oral	>1600 mg/kg	–	–	–
	Intraperitoneal	>100 mg/kg	–	–	–
Rat	Oral	400–938 mg/kg	200–400 mg/kg	2000 mg/kg	1427 mg/kg
	Dermal	>1600	–	2043 mg/kg	–
	Inhalation (6 h)	65 mg/L	2.3 mg/L		>1.6 mg/L (4 h)
	Intraperitoneal	800 mg/kg	–	–	–
Guinea pig	Oral	400–800 mg/kg	–	–	–
	Dermal sensitizasyon	Negative	Negative	–	–
Dog	Oral	100 mg/kg	–	–	–
Rabbit	Oral	>100 mg/kg	–	–	–
	Dermal	>200 mg/kg	>1000 mg/kg	–	>2000 mg/kg
	Dermal irritation	Negative	Moderate	Moderate	Mild
	Eye irritation	Negative	Moderate-severe	Mild	Moderate
Baboon	Oral	100–250 mg/kg	–	–	–
Mallard ducks	Diet (8 day)	7000 mg/kg/day	–	–	–
Japanese quail	Diet (8 day)	1800 mg/kg/day	–	–	–
Bobwhite quail	Oral	788 mg/kg	–	–	–
Rainbow trout	96-h exposure	2.7-4 mg/L	–	–	–
Bluegill sunfish	96-h exposure	1.3 mg/L	–	–	–
Harlequin fish	96-h exposure	3.2–4.2 mg/L	–	–	–
Daphnia	96-h exposure	35 μg/L	–	–	–
Bee	Oral	12 μg/bee	–	–	–
	Direct spraying	3.6 mg/L	–	–	–

amitraz. Another important aspect is the gender difference where the sensitivity to the formulation was found to be higher in females (by nearly 30%). The fact that no such difference occurred when technical amitraz was used alone indicates that the difference between sensitivity was caused by the solvent and the excipients (Filazi et al., 1998a). One other assessment that supports this hypothesis suggested that xylene is more toxic to kidneys in females than it is in males (Jones, 1990).

Acute amitraz poisonings are encountered most in cats and dogs. Although poisonings mostly occur by oral intake, dermal or inhalation exposure may also be the cause. After the oral intake, clinical signs are expected to appear within 30 min to 2 h. Gastrointestinal disorders, nausea, vomiting, hypersalivation, ataxia, lethargy, sedation, CNS and respiratory depression, bradycardia, mydriasis, hypotension, and hypothermia are the most common signs of acute poisoning. It has been reported that geriatric animals and those younger than 3 months are more susceptible. Besides this, it is not recommended to apply amitraz to toy breeds such as Chihuahua and Pomeranian, and to horses and cats because of species specific susceptibility (Andrade et al., 2006; Bonsall and Turnbull, 1983; Cullen and Reynoldson, 1990; Grossman, 1993).

In biochemical analyses, hyperglycemia and increased liver enzyme (transaminase) activity were detected. Amitraz was found to cause damage in the liver by oxidative stress due to cellular membrane damage (Filazi et al., 1998b). Amitraz and its BTS-27271 were found to inhibit the secretion of insulin from beta cells of the pancreas and increase the secretion of glucagon from the alpha cells in the Langerhans islets (Abu-Basha et al., 1999) in vitro. Therefore, clinical signs may worsen in diabetic animals. It has been reported that amitraz delivered once orally to mice leads to a dose-related decrease in hematocrit and hemoglobin values and leukocyte count, a decrease of erythrocyte numbers, and an increase in neutrophil and basophil ratios (Filazi et al., 2003).

Different clinical and necropsy signs are observed by amitraz poisoning in dogs. QT interval on the electrocardiographic examination of English Bulldogs were found to be prolonged in amitraz poisoning (Malmasi and Ghaffari, 2010). Cortical necrosis and hemorrhages were observed in the kidney of a Scottish Terrier breed dog that died from acute kidney failure after drinking a bathing liquid that contained amitraz (Oglesby et al., 2006).

In an experimental poisoning induced by intravascular administration of 1 mg/kg of amitraz in cats, showed that the blood profile, urea, creatinine, alanine aminotransferase, and aspartate aminotransferase were unaffected, but sedation, loss of reflexes, hypothermia, bradycardia, bradyarrhythmia, hypotension, bradypnea, mydriasis, hyperglycemia, hypoinsulinemia, and reduced cortisol levels occurred (Andrade et al., 2007). In an experimental study, cats poisoned by external administration of a bathing solution containing 0.4% amitraz caused reduced heart and respiratory rates. Although the signs of poisoning in cats started 30 min after the administration of the bathing solution that contains amitraz, it was reported that the most critical signs developed within approximately 2–4 h and that it could become difficult to treat cats not intervened within this period (Marafon et al., 2010).

Clinical signs such as depression, ataxia, stupor, and coma that occur in amitraz formulations are mainly related to its xylene or propylene oxide content (Jones, 1990). Hydropic degeneration and fatty changes in the liver are more significant and no kidney lesions appear in mice poisoned by technical amitraz, but that degeneration and necrosis develop in the tubular epithelial cells in the kidneys of the mice poisoned by amitraz-containing xylene indicates that xylene increases the toxicity of amitraz (Filazi et al., 2004).

In horses, it was reported that a 3-year-old mare was brought to the clinic 2 days after the topical administration of a nondiluted veterinary preparation that contains 12.5% of amitraz with the complaints of anorexia, anxiety, perspiration, nondefecation and anuria, the clinical examination performed revealed depression, pawing, chewing, ataxia, and moderate abdominal distension (Phetudomsinsuk et al., 2014).

In cattle, it was reported that anorexia, depression, scleral congestion, abdominal distension and the loss of pupillary reflexes developed right after the accidental intramuscular administration of a 12.5% amitraz formulation to a 7-year-old cow and a 1-year-old heifer (19 and 10 mL, respectively) (Kizil et al., 2008).

Animals that are not treated may enter a coma or die due to respiratory failure. Animals that survive recover from nearly all symptoms within 7–10 days even if they are exposed to high doses (Bonsall and Turnbull, 1983).

Chronic Toxicity

Amitraz was found to have endocrine disrupting effects and that cause reproductive and developmental toxicity. As a α_2-adrenergic agonist, amitraz attaches to presynaptic α_2-adrenergic receptors in the hypothalamus and adversely impacts the reproductive system of mammals and inhibits the secretion of noradrenaline and reduces the secretion of gonadotropin releasing hormone (Altobelli et al., 2001). Some in vivo and in vitro studies have confirmed that amitraz is a fertility poison (Young et al., 2005).

According to the studies in mice (Al-Thani et al., 2003) and rats (Omoja et al., 2016), mice were more susceptible to the reproductive toxicity of amitraz than rats. Whereas, in general rats are more sensitive to amitraz toxicity according to the LD_{50} values (Table 41.1). Since the LD_{50} of BTS-27271 is lower in mice than it is in rats, it is predicted that BTS-27271 is more involved in the reproductive toxicity of amitraz that amitraz itself.

European Medicines Agency (EMEA) defined NOAEL dose for developmental toxicity of amitraz as 1.5 mg/kg/day in general (EMEA, 2004). It has also been shown that amitraz and its metabolite 2,4-dimethylaniline are teratogenic for frog embryos (*Xenopus laevis*) (Osano et al., 2002). Since the developmental toxicity studies of amitraz have many deficiencies according to the Federal

Insecticide, Fungicide, and Rodenticide Act (FIFRA) guideline such as an insufficient number of animals, lack of clinical observations, the dose levels not being verified along with inadequate tissue examinations, they are not accepted by the USEPA yet (USEPA, 1996, 2013; CALEPA, 1995).

Although studies about the genotoxic (mutagenic) effects of amitraz have contradicting results, in general, it is accepted that the compound does not have any genotoxic potential nor it causes DNA damage. Meanwhile, the metabolite 2,4-dimethylaniline is genotoxic (Osano et al., 2002).

DIAGNOSIS

In general, amitraz poisonings in animals are acute cases. Diagnosis is generally based on anamnesis, the visualization of collar pieces on stomach examination by abdominal radiography, the development of clinical signs related to the stimulation of α_2-adrenergic receptors, and the analyses of residues. Since it has a long half-life, the residues of amitraz and its main metabolites can be detected in the body fluids (such as plasma, stomach contents, urine) and hair by chromatographic methods (Hugnet et al., 1996).

TREATMENT

In most cases, symptomatic and supportive treatment are sufficient. Firstly, the source of amitraz that caused the poisoning must be moved away from animal. If mild or temporary sedation occurs after contact with amitraz treatment is not needed. If mild signs are observed after topical administration of amitraz, washing the skin with plenty of warm water is sufficient.

In case of mild clinical symptoms are seen in dogs and cats after eating the collar or pieces of the collar, vomiting should be induced immediately. If inducing vomiting fails or if small pieces of the collar remain in the small intestines, they can be removed by endoscopic interventions. In such cases, in asymptomatic and mildly symptomatic patients, oral active charcoal can be delivered if the collar cannot be removed completely. In addition, to accelerate the excretion of the source of amitraz salty laxatives such as sodium or magnesium sulfate may also be delivered. In patients that manifest moderate or significant clinical findings, specific α_2-adrenergic receptor antagonists (atipamezole or yohimbine) should be immediately delivered (Hugnet et al., 1996; Andrade et al., 2006).

For dehydration, supportive fluids are also necessary. By these means, with good care and aggressive treatment, severe cases of poisoning can be even treated. In cases of severe poisoning, the heart rate, blood pressure, body temperature, urine production, and serum glucose levels should be monitored for at least 24–72 h as a precaution for potential disease relapse. When treatment is initiated immediately, the prognosis is good. It has been reported that fewer dogs die of amitraz poisoning ($<5\%$), and that prognosis is less favorable in cats.

Warnings

In case of atropine treatment for bradycardia of amitraz poisoning, practitioners should remember that atropine will increase the heart rate and induce hypertension. Increased myocardial oxygen consumption following atropine would predispose the patients for cardiac arrhythmias, so extra care should be considered. It also decreases the GI motility. If the patient is sedated, vomiting should not be induced. It is also not recommended to perform gastrostomy to remove the collar in cases where the collar swallowed is the source of the amitraz poisoning. In such conditions, there is a risk for the development of gastric dilatation.

CONCLUDING REMARKS AND FUTURE DIRECTIONS

Amitraz is a widely used pesticide in agricultural products as well as in veterinary medicine. Due to its widespread use, poisonings in human and animals (especially in cats and dogs) are very common. It exerts its toxic effects, through the stimulation of α_2-adrenergic receptors, and inhibition of MAO enzyme and prostaglandins. Acute poisonings include clinical signs such as lethargy, sedation, ataxia, bradycardia, hypothermia, tachypnea/dyspnea, mydriasis, vomiting, hypersalivation, dehydration, hypoperfusion, seizures, gastrointestinal stasis, hypertension, or hypotension. In chronic cases, endocrine disrupting effects leading reproductive and developmental toxicity are seen. The diagnosis is based on clinical signs and the detection of amitraz along with its metabolites in biological fluids. For treatment, α_2-adrenergic receptor antagonists (yohimbine or atipamezole) should be used, and symptomatic and supportive substances should be applied.

REFERENCES

Abu-Basha, E.A., Yibchok-Anun, S., Hopper, D.L., et al., 1999. Effects of the pesticide amitraz and its metabolite BTS 27271 on insulin and glucagon secretion from the perfused rat pancreas: involvement of alpha2D-adrenergic receptors. Metabolism 48, 1461–1469.

Al-Thani, R.K., Al-Thani, A.S., Elbetieha, A., et al., 2003. Assessment of reproductive and fertility effects of amitraz pesticide in male mice. Toxicol. Lett. 138, 253–260.

Altobelli, D., Martire, M., Maurizi, S., et al., 2001. Interaction of formamidine pesticides with the presynaptic alpha(2)- adrenoceptor regulating. Toxicol. Appl. Pharmacol. 172, 179–185.

Andrade, S.F., Sakate, M., Laposy, C.B., et al., 2006. Yohimbine and atipamezole on the treatment of experimentally induced amitraz intoxication in cats. Int. J. Appl. Res. Vet. Med. 4, 200–208.

Andrade, S.F., Sakate, M., Laposy, C.B., et al., 2007. Effects of experimental amitraz intoxication in cats. Arq. Brasil de Med. Vet. Zoot. 59, 1236–1244.

Bonsall, J.L., Turnbull, G.J., 1983. Extrapolation from safety data to management of poisoning with reference to amitraz and xylene. Hum. Toxicol. 2, 587–592.

CALEPA (California Environmental Protection Agency), 1995. Amitraz Risk Characterization Document, vol. 1. Health Assessment Section, Medical Toxicology Branch, Department Pesticide Regulation, California Environmental Protection Agency, Sacramento, CA.

Chen, T.H., Hsu, W.H., 1994. Inhibition of insulin release by a formamidine pesticide amitraz and its metabolites in a rat beta-cell line: an action mediated by alpha-2 adrenoceptors, a GTP-binding protein and a decrease in cyclic AMP. J. Pharmacol. Exp. Ther. 271, 1240–1245.

Costa, L.G., Olibet, G., Murphy, S.D., 1988. Alpha-2 adrenoceptors as a target for formamidine pesticides. In vitro and in vivo studies in mice. Toxicol. Appl. Pharmacol. 93, 319–328.

Cullen, L.K., Reynoldson, J.A., 1990. Central and peripheral alpha-adrenoceptor actions of amitraz in the dog. J. Vet. Pharmacol. Ther. 13, 86–92.

Del Pino, J., Martinez, M.A., Castellano, V.J., et al., 2011. Effects of prenatal and postnatal exposure to amitraz on norepinephrine, serotonin and dopamine levels in brain regions of male and female rats. Toxicology 287, 145–152.

Del Pino, J., Moyano-Cires, P.V., Anadon, M.J., et al., 2015. Molecular mechanisms of amitraz mammalian toxicity: a comprehensive review of existing data. Chem. Res. Toxicol. 28, 1073–1094.

EMEA (European Medicines Agency), 2004. Amitraz (Extrapolation to goats). Summary Report. Committee for Medicinal Products for Veterinary Use. EMEA/MRL/872/03-Final.

Filazi, A., Kaya, S., Kum, C., et al., 1998a. Investigation of amitraz toxicosis in mice: 1. Assessment of the oral acute lethal dose-50 levels and therapeutic alternatives in toxicosis. Ankara Univ. Vet Fakul Dergisi. 45, 259–265.

Filazi, A., Yarsan, E., Kaya, S., et al., 1998b. Investigation of amitraz toxicosis in mice: 2. Liver malondialdehyde levels in acute poisoning. Ankara Univ. Vet Fakul Dergisi. 45, 267–271.

Filazi, A., Sireli, M., Kalkan, F., 2003. The influence of amitraz on biochemical parameters in mice. Hum. Exp. Toxicol. 22, 99–101.

Filazi, A., Güvenç, T., Kum, C., et al., 2004. Pathological findings in acute amitraz intoxication in mice. Turkish J. Vet. Anim. Sci. 28, 873–878.

Godar, S., Bortolato, M., Castelli, M.P., et al., 2014. The aggression and behavioral abnormalities associated with monoamine oxidase A deficiency are rescued by acute inhibition of serotonin reuptake. J. Psychiatr. Res. 56, 1–9.

Grossman, M.R., 1993. Amitraz toxicosis associated with ingestion of an acaricide collar in a dog. J. Am. Vet. Med. Assoc. 203, 55–57.

Gunaratnam, P., Wilkinson, G.T., Seawright, A.A., 1993. A study of amitraz toxicity in cats. Austr. Vet. J. 60, 278–289.

Hsu, W.H., Schaffer, D.D., 1988. Effects of topical application of amitraz on plasma glucose and insulin concentrations in dogs. Am. J. Vet. Res. 49, 130–131.

Hugnet, C., Buronrosse, F., Pineau, X., et al., 1996. Toxicity and kinetics of amitraz in dogs. Am. J. Vet. Res. 57, 1506–1510.

Jones, R.D., 1990. Xylene/amitraz: a pharmacologic review and profile. Vet. Hum. Toxicol. 32, 446–448.

Kizil, O., Balikçi, E., Dabak, M., et al., 2008. Amitraz intoxication in two cattle. Rev. Méd. Vét. 159 (3), 166–168.

Knowles, C.O., Benezet, H.J., 1981. Excretion balance, metabolic fate and tissue residues following treatment of rats with amitraz and N′-(2,4-dimethylphenyl)-N-methylformamidine. J. Environ. Sci. Health, Part B. 16, 547–555.

Krieger, R., 2010. Hayes' Handbook of Pesticide Toxicology, third ed. vol. 1. Academic Press, Inc, New York, NY.

Malmasi, A., Ghaffari, M.S., 2010. Electrocardiographic abnormalities in an English bulldog with amitraz toxicity. Comp. Clin. Pathol. 19, 103–105.

Marafon, C.M., Delfim, C.I., Valadao, C.A., et al., 2010. Analysis of amitraz in cats by gas chromatography. J. Vet. Pharmacol. Ther. 33, 411–414.

Mihalik, J., Maslankova, J., Spakovska, T., et al., 2010. Impact of 2 doses of clorgyline on the rat preimplantation embryo development and the monoamine levels in urine. Repr. Sci. 17, 734–741.

Moser, V.C., MacPhail, R.C., 1989. Investigations of amitraz neurotoxicity in rats. III. Effects on motor activity and inhibition of monoamine oxidase. Fund. Appl. Toxicol. 12, 12–22.

Oglesby, P.A., Joubert, K.E., Meiring, T., 2006. Canine renal cortical necrosis and hemorrhage following ingestion of an amitraz-formulated insecticide dip. J. South Afr. Vet. Assoc. 77, 160–163.

Omoja, V.U., Anika, S.M., Asuzu, I.U., 2016. The effects of sub-chronic administration of sub-lethal doses of amitraz/xylene on selected reproductive parameters of male Wistar rats. Iran J. Vet. Res. 17, 277–280.

Osano, O., Oladimeji, A.A., Kraak, M.H.S., et al., 2002. Teratogenic effects of amitraz, 2,4-dimethylaniline, and paraquat on developing frog (Xenopus) embryos. Arch. Environ. Cont. Toxicol. 43, 42–49.

Pass, M.A., Mogg, T.D., 1991. Effect of amitraz and its metabolites on intestinal motility. Comp. Biochem. Physiol. Part C: Comp. Pharmacol. 99, 169–172.

Pass, M.A., Mogg, T.D., 1995. Pharmacokinetics and metabolism of amitraz in ponies and sheep. J. Vet. Pharmacol. Ther. 18, 210–215.

Peter, R., de Bruin, C., Odendaal, D., et al., 2006. The use of a pour-on and spray dip containing Amitraz to control ticks (Acari: Ixodidae) on cattle. J. South Afr. Vet. Assoc. 77, 66–69.

Phetudomsinsuk, K., Soontornsook, N., Phanusaweekul, N., et al., 2014. Amitraz toxicity in a horse. Chiang. Mai. Vet. J. 12, 231–236.

Tarallo, V.D., Lia, R.P., Sasanelli, M., et al., 2009. Efficacy of amitraz plus metaflumizone for the treatment of canine demodicosis associated with Malassezia pachydermatis. Paras. Vect. 2, 13.

USEPA (United States Environmental Protection Agency), 1996. Amitraz Reregistration Eligibility Decision (RED), Case 0234 (EPA-738-F-96-031). US Environmental Protection Agency, Office of Prevention, Pesticide and Toxic Substances, Washington, DC.

USEPA (United States Environmental Protection Agency), 2013. Amitraz Proposed Tolerance Actions, Federal Register, Vol. 78, Number 54. US Environmental Protection Agency, Office of Prevention, Pesticide and Toxic Substances, Washington, DC.

Yilmaz, H.L., Yildizdas, D.R., 2003. Amitraz poisoning, an emerging problem: epidemiology, clinical features, management, and preventive strategies. Arch. Dis. Childhood. 88, 130–134.

Young, F.M., Menadue, M.F., Lavranos, T.C., 2005. Effects of the insecticide amitraz, an α2-adrenergic receptor agonist, on human luteinized granulosa cells. Hum. Reprod. 20, 3018–3025.

FURTHER READING

Hsu, W.H., Lu, Z.X., Hembrough, F.B., 1986. Effects of amitraz on heart rate and aortic blood pressure in conscious dogs: influence of atropine, prazosin, talazoline, and yohimbine. Toxicol. Appl. Pharmacol. 84, 418–422.

Kim, J.C., Shin, J.Y., Yang, Y.S., et al., 2007. Evaluation of developmental toxicity of amitraz in Sprague-Dawley rats. Arch. Environ. Cont. Toxicol. 52, 137–144.

FURTHER READING

Chapter 42

Fipronil

Ramesh C. Gupta and Arturo Anadón

INTRODUCTION

Fipronil is a member of a new class of insecticides called phenylpyrazoles. Chemically, it is a (5-amino-1-[2,6-dichloro-4-(trifluoromethyl)phenyl]-4-[(trifluoromethyl)sulfinyl]-1*H*-pyrazole). The chemical structure of fipronil is shown in Fig. 42.1. Fipronil is an active ingredient of one of the popular ectoparasiticide products, Frontline. Fipronil is also present in other ectoparasiticide products, such as Certifect and Parastar Plus. There are currently two forms of Frontline preparation commercially available (a spray and a spot-on topical application) for dogs and cats. The product is meant to kill fleas and all stages of brown dog ticks, American dog ticks, lone star ticks, which may carry Lyme disease, and mites (Cutler, 1998; Hutchinson et al., 1998; Anonymous, 2000). Fipronil is used in combination with methoprene (9.8% fipronil/11.8% methoprene for cats; 9.8% fipronil/8.8% methoprene for dogs) for additional control of immature flea stages. Fipronil is also formulated as insect bait for roaches, ants and termites; as sprays for pets; and as a granular turf product to control mole crickets. Presently, fipronil is widely used in agriculture for soil treatment and seed coating.

Currently, fipronil-based products with various trade names (Chipco, Choice, ICON 6.2FS, and Over n' Out, TeckPac, Frontline) have gained popularity worldwide for pest management, including residential insect control, rice and cotton production, and turf-grass management. The EPA has determined fipronil to be safe for use on dogs and cats, with no harm to humans who handle these animals. Poisoning cases from accidental use or misuse of fipronil may occur in animals. This chapter describes the toxicity of fipronil in various species of animals, birds and fish.

BACKGROUND

Fipronil was first discovered by Rhone-Poulenc Agro in 1987 and is used worldwide in agriculture. It represents the second generation of insecticides that acts through a different mechanism compared to other conventional insecticides (Narahashi, 2000; Narahashi et al., 2007, 2010). It is poorly soluble in water, delivered in very small amounts and does not leach into groundwater. In 1996, it was registered as a pesticide in the United States (Bobe et al., 1998). It can be formulated as roach or ant baits, flea and tick sprays for pets, and in granular turf products to control mole crickets (Kidd and James, 1991; EPA, 1996). In addition, fipronil is used for soil treatment and to protect crops from insects. Unlike many modern pesticides, fipronil and its derivatives are moderately persistent in the environment (EPA, 1996; Gunasekara et al., 2007). It is currently used worldwide and has good adulticide activity against fleas and ticks. It has significant residual activity and for small animal use is available as a spray or spot-on product. Sunlight, immersion in water and bathing do not significantly impact the performance of this compound and it kills adult fleas within 24 h (Kunkle, 1997). Fipronil has also been used to treat some mite infections.

Most fipronil poisoning cases occur in dogs and cats due to accidental ingestion or licking the product Frontline, Certifect, or Parastar Plus. Frontline preparation for dogs contains 132 mg fipronil in a 1.34 mL tube that is meant for topical application. In humans, poisoning is mainly due to accident or suicidal attempt. In a published report, the Paris Poison Center, France, recorded 81 human cases of fipronil exposure from 1994 to 1999. Out of these 81 cases, 57 involved veterinary ectoparasiticides and seven used domestic insecticide preparations (Gasmi et al., 2001).

PHARMACOKINETICS/TOXICOKINETICS

Fipronil in Frontline (132 mg in 1.34 mL liquid), Certifect (9.8% of 4.28 mL), or Parastar Plus (9.8% of 2.68 mL) is placed between the dog's shoulder blades at the nape of the neck. After application, fipronil spreads and sequesters in the lipids of the skin and hair follicles, and continues to be released onto the skin and coat, resulting

Veterinary Toxicology. DOI: http://dx.doi.org/10.1016/B978-0-12-811410-0.00042-8

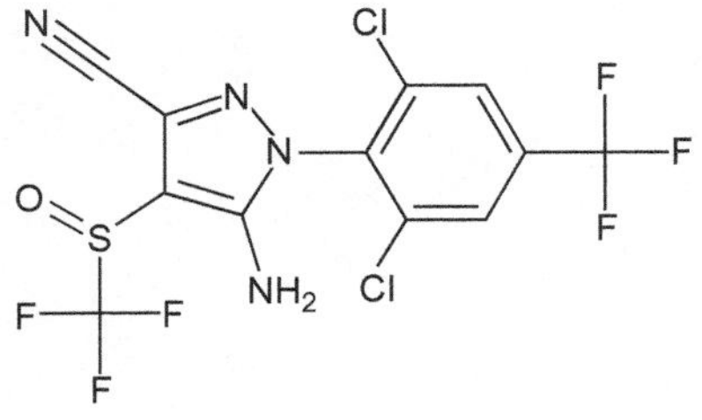

FIGURE 42.1 Chemical structure of fipronil.

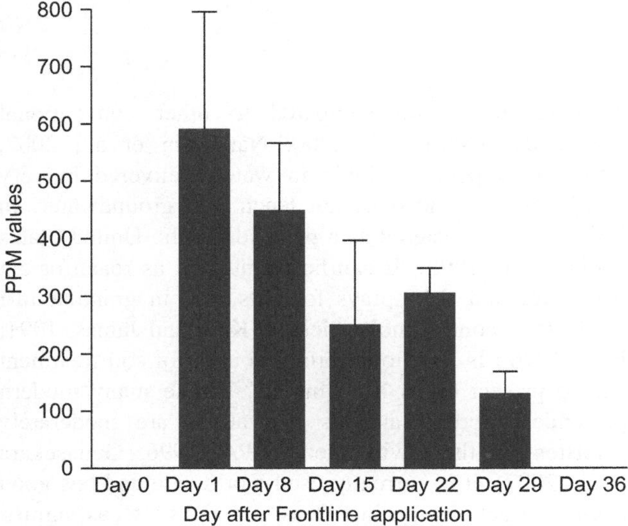

FIGURE 42.2 Transferable residue of fipronil from the dog coat after a single application of Frontline Spot-On.

in long-lasting residual activity against fleas and ticks. Residue of fipronil lasts on a dog's hair coat for about 1 month. The maximum concentration of fipronil on the canine hair coat is found 24 h after a single application of Frontline Top Spot (Jennings et al., 2002) or Parastar Plus (Case et al., 2016), and 72 h after Certifect (Nichols et al., 2014). With a descending concentration trend, fipronil residue can be detected on a dog's hair coat for a period of up to 29 days (Fig. 42.2). Although fipronil binds to the lipids of the skin cells and hair follicles, the transferable residue can be detected up to a month after application. Studies have revealed that in rats, fipronil is excreted mainly in the feces (45%–75%) and small amounts in the urine (5%–25%).

In rats, after oral administration of fipronil, maximum blood concentrations are achieved after approximately 6 h. Once absorbed, fipronil is rapidly metabolized, and then the biotransformation products are widely distributed in tissues. Significant amounts of metabolites can persist in the tissues, particularly in fat and fatty tissues, for 1 week after treatment. The metabolite concentrations in fat and other tissues are greater with repeated low doses or a single high dose than with a single low dose. The long half-life (183 h in male and 245 h in female) of fipronil in blood may reflect slow release of metabolites from fat (Woodward, 2012). The compounds identified in feces and urine are the parent compound and sulfone, the amide derived from the nitrile group and a cleavage product of sulfone and its derivatives formed by further metabolism. Sulfone is the major metabolite in fat and tissues. In essence, fipronil can be metabolized through three major pathways. Fipronil can be metabolized to fipronil sulfone by oxidation at the sulfinyl moiety, to fipronil sulfide by reduction at the sulfinyl moiety, and to fipronil amide by hydrolysis of the cyano moiety (Wang et al., 2016).

In another pharmacokinetics study, rats received either a single oral dose of a labeled compound (^{14}C-fipronil-desulfinyl) at 1 or 10 mg/kg body wt or daily oral doses of unlabeled compound at 1 mg/kg body wt/day for 14 days, followed by a single oral labeled dose. In animals of both sexes, elimination of the radiolabeled fipronil was much greater in the feces (46%–70% of the dose) than in the urine with all dosing regimens. Appreciable metabolic products were found in the tissues 1 week after treatment with the highest concentrations being present in the fat and fatty tissues. The long half-life in blood was 183–195 h and fat: plasma ratio of the radiolabel compound was increased. Numerous metabolites or conjugates of fipronil desulfinyl were present in the urine and feces. Only unchanged fipronil desulfinyl was identified in the liver, fat, skin and body. There was no appreciable difference between male and female rats in the absorption, distribution, metabolism or excretion of fipronil after oral administration. Fipronil is degraded by sunlight to produce a variety of metabolites, one of which is fipronil desulfinyl. This metabolite is extremely stable, bioaccumulates in the fatty tissues and is more toxic than the parent compound in insects (EPA, 1998). Information on other metabolites of fipronil in living and nonliving systems can be found elsewhere (Feung and Yenne, 1997; Aajoud et al., 2003; Wang et al., 2016). This photoproduct exerts high neurotoxicity by blocking the $GABA_A$-regulated chloride channels. Fipronil has a greater specificity for the $GABA_A$ receptor (β3 subunit) found in insects than mammalian $GABA_A$ receptors. Fortunately, this metabolite is not formed in mammals. However, it does have a high affinity towards the insect's GABA system, thereby contributing to fipronil's selective toxicity toward insects (Narahashi et al., 2007, 2010).

It is known that fipronil is an effective inducer of CYP450 isoforms (Roques et al., 2012; Wang et al., 2016). Fipronil can inhibit testosterone metabolism by CYP3A4. Since fipronil is a hepatotoxicant at doses somewhat above those required for induction, the decrease may represent one of the initial toxic effects, with CYP3A4 induction being more sensitive than

CYP1A1 induction. Fipronil has the potential to interact with a wide range of xenobiotics or endogenous chemicals that are CYP3A4 substrates. In the case of possible metabolic interactions based on the induction or inhibition of xenobiotic metabolizing enzymes, concentrations of fipronil at the active site(s) become crucial (Wang et al., 2016).

MECHANISM OF ACTION

In mammalian systems, the mechanism of fipronil is quite different from other classes of insecticides, and it is better understood in insects than in mammals. Fipronil sulfone is a major metabolite of fipronil in mammals and insects. In invertebrates (insects), fipronil or its metabolite noncompetitively inhibits γ-aminobutyric acid ($GABA_A$)-induced ion influx by targeting the $GABA_A$-regulated chloride channels (Cole et al., 1993; Narahashi et al., 2007, 2010; Wang et al., 2016). Consequently, fipronil binding blocks the inhibitory action of $GABA_A$, leading to neural hyperexcitation, and at sufficient concentrations, paralysis and death (Bobe et al., 1998; Wang et al., 2016). Fipronil exhibits >500-fold selective toxicity to insects over mammals, primarily because of affinity differences in receptor binding between insect and mammalian receptors (Cole et al., 1993; Grant et al., 1998; Hainzl et al., 1998; Kamijima and Casida, 2000; Ratra et al., 2001; Zhao et al., 2005; Narahashi et al., 2007, 2010). In essence, fipronil binds more tightly to $GABA_A$ receptors (β3 subunit) in insects than in mammals. It is important to note this, since the fipronil sulfone metabolite forms rapidly. Both in vivo and in vitro studies suggest that the majority of toxicological effects are more likely due to fipronil sulfone than fipronil itself (Zhao et al., 2005; Romero et al., 2016; Wang et al., 2016). Recent reports indicate that fipronil and its metabolite(s) can cause toxicity in liver, kidney and other vital organs by dysregulating mitochondrial bioenergetics (by inhibiting mitochondrial respiratory chain) and calcium homeostasis, oxidative and nitrosative stress, as well as damage to DNA and proteins (Badgujar et al., 2015; de Medeiros et al., 2015; Khan et al., 2015; Tavares et al., 2015; Wang et al., 2016). Cell death can occur due to apoptosis or autophagy (Zhang et al., 2015; Wang et al., 2016).

The toxicity of fipronil desulfinyl is qualitatively similar to that of fipronil, but the dose–effect curve for neurotoxic effects appears to be steeper for fipronil desulfinyl. Also, fipronil desulfinyl appears to have a much greater tendency than fipronil to bind to sites in the chloride ion channel of the rat brain $GABA_A$ receptor. This finding appears to be consistent with the greater toxicity of fipronil desulfinyl, relative to fipronil, in the central nervous system (CNS) of mammals.

Different studies have shown that fipronil reveals thyroid disrupting properties in rats (Leghait et al., 2009; Roques et al., 2012), but not in sheep (Leghait et al., 2010). The differences between rat and sheep for thyroid disruption might be related to the difference in exposure to the toxicant, the actual exposure to the sulfone metabolite of fipronil being lower in sheep than in rats. Mechanistic investigations conducted with fipronil in rats suggest that it does not interfere with the incorporation of iodine into thyroxine (T4), but it does interfere with the biliary clearance of this hormone. This may trigger an increase in the concentration of thyroid-stimulating hormone by interference with the feedback mechanism and decreased T4 concentrations. Roques et al. (2012) stated that the potential of fipronil sulfone to act as a thyroid disruptor is more critical because it persists much longer in the organism than fipronil itself.

TOXICITY

Fipronil produces toxicity in insects and mammals by the same mechanism; however, due to selective action, toxicity is much more severe in insects than in mammals. Fipronil and other phenylpyrazole compounds exert neurotoxicity by blocking transmission of signals by inhibitory neurotransmitter $GABA_A$. These compounds bind within the chloride channels and consequently inhibit the flux of chloride ions into the nerve cell, resulting in hyperexcitation.

There are numerous reports regarding the effects of fipronil in small animals, birds and fish (http://www.cdpr.ca.gov/docs/empm/pubs/fatememo/fipronil.pdf).

Laboratory Animals

Adequate acute toxicity data are available for laboratory animals. Fipronil is moderately hazardous to rats (LD_{50} = 97 mg/kg body wt) and mice (LD_{50} = 95 mg/kg body wt). In rats, signs of toxicity and death were delayed for up to 4 days after a single dose or repeated oral doses of 75 mg/kg body wt/day for up to 5 days. Fipronil has moderate inhalation toxicity with an acute LC_{50} of 0.682 mg/L in rats (EPA, 1996).

It is nontoxic to slightly toxic via the dermal route, with a reported dermal LD_{50} of greater than 2000 mg/kg in rats (EPA, 1996). In rabbits, fipronil was found to be moderately hazardous after dermal application (LD_{50} = 354 mg/kg body wt; WHO, 1998–99). In general, dermal absorption of fipronil is less than 1% after 24 h and therefore dermal toxicity is considered very low. In a dermal toxicity study, fipronil was applied (0.5% in carboxymethylcellulose) to the intact skin of rabbits for 6 h/day, 5 days a week, for 3 weeks at doses of 0, 0.5, 1, 5 or 10 mg/kg body wt/day. No dermal irritation was observed. At 10 mg/kg body wt/day, body weight gains and food consumption were reduced in animals of either sex. Some animals showed hyperactivity. The NOAEL was calculated to be 5 mg/kg body wt/day. Primary dermal irritation in rabbits was examined in two studies. Fipronil was slightly irritating when moistened with corn oil before application, but was not irritating when moistened with water. Fipronil was slightly irritating in two studies of primary ocular irritation in rabbits. It did not sensitize the skin of guinea pigs when tested by the Buehler method, but was a weak sensitizer in guinea pigs when tested by the Magnusson-Kligman method (WHO, 1998–99). This product was reported to be contraindicated in rabbits because deaths occurred when a spray formulation of fipronil was used. Extra-label use in rabbits could produce anorexia, lethargy, convulsions and death. In rabbits, fipronil produces serious adverse reactions, suggesting that this species is unusually sensitive to fipronil. Young rabbits are particularly more sensitive than adults. Frontline has been considered to be improper for rabbits.

One reproductive toxicity study was performed in rabbits (WHO, 1998–99). Rabbits treated with fipronil by gavage at doses of 0, 0.1, 0.2, 0.5 or 1 mg/kg body wt/day during gestation days 6–19 showed no developmental toxicity, but there were some signs of maternal toxicity (decreased body weight gain, decreased food consumption and reduced efficiency of food use at all doses). The NOAEL for developmental toxicity was identified to be 1 mg/kg body wt/day. In a number of experimental studies, fipronil has been found to be a reproductive and developmental neurotoxicant, and effects appeared to be due to alterations in either the GABAergic system or via endocrine disruption (Ohi et al., 2004; Stehr et al., 2006; Lassiter et al., 2009; Sidiropoulou et al., 2011; Roques et al., 2012; Udo et al., 2014; Khan et al., 2015).

Dogs and Cats

Several subacute and chronic toxicity studies of fipronil have been performed in dogs (WHO, 1998–99). In a subacute toxicity study, fipronil was administered in gelatin capsules to dogs for 13 weeks at doses of 0, 0.5, 2 or 10 mg/kg body wt/day. Inappetence and decreased body weight gain and food consumption were noted in females at 2 and 10 mg/kg body wt/day. The NOAEL was reported to be 0.5 mg/kg body wt/day.

In a chronic study, fipronil was administered to dogs in gelatin capsules for 1 year at doses of 0, 0.2, 2 or 5 mg/kg body wt/day. At 2 mg/kg body wt/day and higher, there were clinical signs of neurotoxicity (convulsions, twitching, tremors, ataxia, unsteady gait, rigidity of limbs, nervous behavior, hyper- or hypoactivity, vocalization, nodding, aggression, resistance to dosing, inappetence and abnormal neurological responses) in animals of both sexes. One animal at 2 mg/kg body wt/day was humanely euthanized because of poor condition related to treatment. The NOAEL was identified to be 0.2 mg/kg body wt/day. In another study, fipronil was administered in the diet at doses of 0, 0.075, 0.3, 1 or 3 mg/kg body wt/day for 1 year. At 1 mg/kg body wt/day, clinical signs of neurotoxicity (whole body twitching and extensor rigidity of limbs) were noted in females. There were no effects on T3 or T4 levels. The NOAEL was identified to be 0.3 mg/kg body wt/day.

A neurotoxicity study was performed in female dogs (WHO, 1998–99). In this study, dogs received fipronil in capsules at doses of 0 (one animal) or 20 mg/kg body wt/day (four animals) until the appearance of neurotoxic signs in each animal, after which they were allowed to recover for 28 days. Severe neurotoxic signs were observed at a dose of 20 mg/kg body wt/day during the treatment phase. Most animals appeared to recover, although one had exaggerated reflex responses and was excitable at the end of the recovery period.

Poisoning cases of fipronil occur in dogs and cats due to accidental ingestion/licking of Frontline product. There is some indication that dogs are more severely affected than cats. Application of Frontline Spot-On, Certifect or Parastar Plus to dogs and cats can cause skin irritation and/or hair loss at the site of application. Dermal hypersensitivity reactions may also occur. In a series of clinical studies, dogs topically treated with fipronil-containing ectoparasiticide products (Frontline Spot-On, Certifect or Parastar Plus) did not show any skin reactions (Jennings et al., 2002; Nichols et al., 2014; Case et al., 2016). Common clinical signs of fipronil toxicosis are of CNS hyperexcitability, including tremors, convulsions, seizures and death (Grant et al., 1998; Hainzl et al., 1998; Kamijima and Casida, 2000).

Domestic Animals

In a subacute study, buffalo calves orally exposed with fipronil (0.5 mg/kg body wt/day) produced toxic signs including salivation, lacrimation, dullness, depression, decreased body weight gain, muscle weakness, alopecia and sunken eyes. Fipronil-exposed animals recovered within 2 weeks after discontinuation of treatment (Gill and Dumka, 2013).

Birds and Fish

On an acute and subchronic level, fipronil is practically nontoxic to slightly toxic in waterfowl with an acute oral LC_{50} of >2000 mg/kg and a 5-day dietary LC_{50} of >5000 mg/kg in mallard ducks. The oral LC_{50} for bobwhite quail is 11.3 mg/kg, and the LC_{50} for 5-day dietary is 49 mg/kg (EPA, 1996). The sulfone metabolite is more toxic than the parent compound to certain bird species. This metabolite has shown a very high toxicity in game birds and a moderate toxicity in waterfowl (EPA, 1996; Bobe et al., 1997). Fipronil is highly toxic to rainbow trout and very highly toxic to bluegill sunfish with an LC_{50} of 0.246 mg/L and 0.083 mg/L, respectively. Fipronil is moderately toxic to freshwater daphnids ($LC_{50} = 190\ \mu g/L$) and crayfish ($LC_{50} = 14-20\ \mu g/L$), and is extremely toxic to estuarine mysids ($LC_{50} = 0.14\ \mu g/L$). Fipronil was reported to adversely affect development, fertility, and reproduction of copepods (*Amphiascus tenuiremis*) (Chandler et al., 2004). WHO classifies fipronil as a Class II moderately hazardous pesticide.

DIAGNOSIS

Diagnosis of a fipronil poisoning can be based on circumstantial evidence, clinical manifestations and chemical confirmation. Residue of fipronil or its metabolites (predominantly fipronil sulfone) can be detected in the blood, tissue, fat, or hair using GC/MS, and can be used as a biomarker of fipronil exposure (Gupta and Milatovic, 2014). The long half-life (183–245 h) of fipronil in blood may reflect its slow release from fat. Transferable residue of fipronil can be detected on a dog's hair coat up to 4 weeks after a single spot-on application (Fig. 42.2). In a recent study, Huang et al. (2014) reported microRNA–155 (*miR–155*) in Zebrafish as a potential novel toxicological biomarker for fipronil exposure. Clinical signs and symptoms and pathological changes in liver are not specific, and are of little value in terms of toxicological biomarkers and diagnosis.

TREATMENT

There is no specific treatment for the toxicity of fipronil, and therefore treatment relies upon symptomatic and supportive measures. If a dog or cat shows an adverse reaction to topical application of fipronil-containing ectoparasiticide (Frontline, Certifect or Parastar Plus), decontamination by washing at the site of application is advisable. The ingestion of any fipronil topical veterinary product should be treated by the ingestion of water or milk. The most recommended methods of internal decontamination include gastric lavage, and administration of activated charcoal (1–4 g/kg) and a cathartic agent within 3–4 h.

If hypersensitivity skin reactions occur after application of any topical product, the animals should be submitted for a bath with a noninsecticidal shampoo and symptomatic treatment (e.g., antihistamines, hydrocortisone or antibiotics).

CONCLUDING REMARKS AND FUTURE DIRECTIONS

Fipronil elicits neurotoxicity in mammals by inhibition of $GABA_A$-gated chloride channels, producing hyperexcitability of the CNS. Overdosage due to accidental ingestion often leads to serious toxicosis in dogs and cats. There is no specific antidote for the toxicity of fipronil. The manufacturer warns that the product may be harmful to debilitated, aged, pregnant or nursing animals and also states that fipronil must not be used on kittens less than 12 weeks of age and on puppies less than 10 weeks of age.

ACKNOWLEDGMENTS

Authors would like to thank Ms. Robin B. Doss for her assistance in preparation of this chapter.

REFERENCES

Aajoud, A., Ravanel, P., Tissut, M., 2003. Fipronil metabolism and dissipation in a simplified aquatic ecosystem. J. Agric. Food Chem. 51, 1347–1352.

Anonymous, 2000. Fipronil. Pesticide News. 48, 20.

Badgujar, P.C., Pawar, N.N., Chandratre, G.A., et al., 2015. Fipronil induced oxidative stress in kidney and brain of mice: protective effect of vitamin E and vitamin C. Pest Biochem. Physiol. 118, 10–18.

Bobe, A., Coste, C.M., Cooper, J., 1997. Factors influencing the adsorption of fipronil on soils. J. Agric. Food Chem. 45, 4861–4965.

Bobe, A., Meallier, P., Copper, J., et al., 1998. Kinetics and mechanisms of abiotic degradation of fipronil. J. Agric. Food Chem. 46, 2834–2839.

Case, K.M., Vega, N.M., Gupta, R.C., et al., 2016. Safety evaluation of Parastar® Plus in dogs and assessment of transferable residue of fipronil and cyphenothrin from dogs to humans. Front Vet. Med. 3, 1–8.

Chandler, G.T., Cary, T.L., Volz, D.C., et al., 2004. Fipronil affects on estuarine copepod (*Amphiascus tenuiremis*) development, fertility, and reproduction: a rapid life-cycle assay in 96-well microplate format. Environ. Toxicol. Chem. 23 (1), 117–124.

Cole, L.M., Nicholson, R., Casida, J.E., 1993. Action of phenylpyrazole insecticides at the GABA-gated chloride channel. Pestic. Biochem. Physiol. 46, 47–54.

Cutler, S.L., 1998. Ectopic psoroptes cuniculi infestation in a pet rabbit. J. Small Anim. Pract. 39, 86–87.

de Medeiros, H.C., Constantin, J., Ashii-Iwamoto, E.L., et al., 2015. Effect of fipronil on energy metabolism in the perfused rat liver. Toxicol. Lett. 236, 34–42.

Environmental Protection Agency, 1996. New Pesticide Fact Sheet. PB96-181516. epa 737-F-96-005. U.S. EPA Office of Prevention, Pesticides and Toxic Substances. May 1996.

Environmental Protection Agency, 1998. Office of Prevention, Pesticides and Toxic Substances. Washington, DC. 90.

Feung, C.S., Yenne, S.P., 1997. Fipronil: aerobic aquatic metabolism. Rhone-Poulenc Agricultural Limited. Data Package ID No. 169043. DPR Document No. 52062-180.

Gasmi, A., Chataigner, D., Garnier, R., et al., 2001. Toxicity of fipronil-containing insecticides. Report of 81 cases from the Paris Poison Center. Vet. Hum. Toxicol. 43, 247.

Gill, K.K., Dumka, V.K., 2013. Biochemical alterations induced by oral subchronic exposure to fipronil, fluoride and their combination in buffalo calves. Environ. Toxicol. Pharmacol. 36, 1113–1119.

Grant, D.B., Chalmers, A., Wolff, M., et al., 1998. Fipronil: action at the GABA receptor. Rev. Toxicol. 2, 147–156.

Gunasekara, A.S., Trong, T., Goh, K.S., et al., 2007. Environmental fate and toxicology of fipronil. J. Pestic. Sci. 32 (3), 189–199.

Gupta, R.C., Milatovic, D., 2014. Insecticides. In: Gupta, R.C. (Ed.), Biomarkers in Toxicology. Academic Press/Elsevier, Amsterdam, pp. 389–407.

Hainzl, D., Cole, L.M., Casida, J.E., 1998. Mechanism for selective toxicity of fipronil insecticide and its sulfone metabolite and desulfinyl photoproduct. Chem. Res. Toxicol. 11, 1529–1535.

Huang, H., Zhang, K., Zhou, Y., et al., 2014. MicroRNA-155 targets *cyb561d2* in zebrafish in response to fipronil exposure. Environ. Toxicol. 31, 877–886.

Hutchinson, M.J., Jacobs, D.E., Fox, M.T., et al., 1998. Evaluation of flea control strategies using fipronil on cats in a controlled simulates home environment. Vet. Rec. 142, 356–357.

Jennings, K.A., Canerdy, T.D., Keller, R.J., et al., 2002. Human exposure to fipronil from dogs treated with Frontline. Vet. Human. Toxicol. 44, 301–303.

Kamijima, M., Casida, J.E., 2000. Regional modification of [3H]ethynylbicyclo-orthobenzoate binding in mouse brain GABAA receptor by endosufan, fipronil, and avermectin B1a. Toxicol. Appl. Pharmacol. 160, 188–194.

Khan, S., Jan, M.H., Kumar, D., et al., 2015. Fipronil induced spermotoxicity is associated with oxidative stress, DNA damage and apoptosis in male rats. Pest Biochem. Physiol. 124, 8–14.

Kidd, H., James, D., 1991. The Agrochemicals Handbook, third ed. Royal Society of Chemistry Information Services, Cambridge, UK.

Kunkle, G., 1997. An updated review of actoparasiticide treatments in dogs and cats. J. Vet. Pharmacol. Ther. 20 (Suppl. 1), 110–120.

Lassiter, T.L., MacKillop, E.A., Ryde, I.T., et al., 2009. Is fipronil safer than chlorpyrifos? Comparative developmental neurotoxicity modeled in PC12 cells. Brain Res. Bull. 78, 313–322.

Leghait, J., Gayrard, V., Toutain, P.L., et al., 2009. Fipronil-induced disruption of thyroid function in rats is mediated by increased total and free thyroxine clearances concomitantly to increased activity of hepatic enzymes. Toxicology 255, 38–44.

Leghait, J., Gayrard, V., Toutain, P.L., et al., 2010. Is the mechanisms of fipronil-induced thyroid disruption specific of the rat: re-evaluation of fipronil thyroid toxicity in sheep? Toxicol. Lett. 194, 51–57.

Narahashi, T., 2000. Neuroreceptors and ion channels as the basis for drug action: past, present, and future. J. Pharmacol. Exp. Ther. 294, 1–26.

Narahashi, T., Zhao, X., Ikeda, T., et al., 2007. Differential actions of insecticides on target sites: basis for selective toxicity. Hum. Exp. Toxicol. 26, 361–366.

Narahashi, T., Zhao, X., Ikeda, T., et al., 2010. Glutamate-activated chloride channels: unique fipronil targets present in insects but not in mammals. Pest Biochem. Physiol. 97, 149–152.

Nichols, H., Gupta, R.C., Doss, R.B., et al., 2014. Residue of fipronil, s-methoprene, and amitraz in dog blood and in gloves from topical Certifect® application: toxicity and safety considerations. J. J. Vet. Sci. Res. 2014 (1), 9.

Ohi, M., Dalsenter, P.R., Andrade, A.J.M., et al., 2004. Reproductive adverse effects of fipronil in Wistar rats. Toxicol. Lett. 146, 121–127.

Ratra, G., Kamita, S.G., Casida, J.E., 2001. Role of human GABAA receptor β3 subunit in insecticide toxicity. Toxicol. Appl. Pharmacol. 172, 233–240.

Romero, A., Ramos, E., Ares, I., et al., 2016. Fipronil sulfone induced higher cytotoxicity than fipronil in SH-SY5Y cells: protection by antioxidants. Toxicol. Lett. 252, 42–49.

Roques, B.B., Lacroix, M.Z., Puel, S., et al., 2012. CYP450-dependent biotransformation of the insecticide fipronil into fipronil sulfone can mediate fipronil-induced thyroid disruption in rats. Toxicol. Sci. 127 (1), 29–41.

Sidiropoulou, E., Sachana, M., Flasko, J., et al., 2011. Fipronil interferes with the differentiation of mouse N2a neuroblastoma cells. Toxicol. Lett. 201, 86–91.

Stehr, C.M., Linbo, T.L., Incardona, J.P., et al., 2006. The developmental neurotoxicity of fipronil: notochord degeneration and locomotor defects in zebrafish embryos and larvae. Toxicol. Sci. 92, 270–278.

Tavares, M.A., Palma, I.D.F., Medeiros, H.C.D., et al., 2015. Comparative effects of fipronil and its metabolites sulfone and desulfinyl on the isolated rat liver mitochondria. Environ. Toxicol. Pharmacol. 40, 206–214.

Udo, M.S.B., Sandini, T.M., Reis, T.M., et al., 2014. Prenatal exposure to a low fipronil dose disturbs maternal behavior and reflex development in rats. Neurotoxicol. Teratol. 45, 27–33.

Wang, X., Martínez, M.A., Wu, Q., et al., 2016. Fipronil insecticide toxicology: oxidative stress and metabolism. Crit. Rev. Toxicol. 46, 1–24.

WHO, 1998–99. Classification of pesticides by hazard. International Program on Chemical Safety. WHO/IPCS/98.21.

Woodward, K.N., 2012. Veterinary pesticides. In: Marrs, T.C. (Ed.), Mammalian Toxicology of Insecticides. RSC Publ, Cambridge, pp. 348–426.

Zhang, B., Xu, Z., Zhang, Y., et al., 2015. Fipronil induces apoptosis through caspase-dependent mitochondrial pathways in Drosophila S2 cells. Pest Biochem. Physiol. 119, 81–89.

Zhao, X., Yeh, J.Z., Salgado, V.L., et al., 2005. Sulfone metabolite of fipronil blocks GABA- and glutamate-activated chloride channels in mammalian and insect neurons. Toxicol. Sci. 84, 401–402.

Chapter 43

Macrocyclic Lactone Endectocides

Sharon M. Gwaltney-Brant, Camille DeClementi and Ramesh C. Gupta

INTRODUCTION

Macrocyclic lactones (MLs) consist of several compounds (doramectin, eprinomectin, ivermectin, milbemycin, moxidectin, and selamectin) that are commonly used as insecticides, acaricides, and nematicides in various animal species. Chemical structures of these MLs are shown in Figs. 43.1–43.6. Ivermectin, a semisynthetic ML, was the first to be obtained from *Streptomyces avermitilis*. Ivermectin/abamectin is a mixture of two homologs, ivermectin B_{1a} and ivermectin B_{1b} (Fig. 43.1). It was introduced to the market in 1981 as a potent antiparasitic animal health drug. It has been found to be effective against virtually all external and internal parasites thus far tested, except for trematodes and cestodes. Ivermectin is approved at a very low dosage for the control of parasites in many animal species (cattle, sheep, swine, horse, cat, and dog), but in many countries it is not approved for use in lactating cows, sheep, and goats. In agriculture, ivermectin is used for its miticidal, insecticidal, and acaricidal activities.

Although ML poisoning has been reported in many animal species due to inadvertent overdose or misuse (Godber et al., 1995; Haldrick et al., 1995), a major concern of ML toxicosis is in individuals of certain dog breeds, such as collies (Paul et al., 1987), which are very sensitive to this class of drug due to genetic defects in the blood–brain barrier (BBB). To date, over 11 dog breeds (Houston et al., 1987; Geyer et al., 2007; Mosher and Court, 2010), Murray Grey cattle (Seaman et al., 1987), and young animals have also been reported to be more sensitive to ML toxicosis. This chapter describes the toxicity of ML endectocides in animals.

BACKGROUND

Currently, there are many MLs available on the market for their wide applications as insecticides, nematicides, and acaricides. Ivermectin and its derivatives are most popular because of their efficacy and wide margin of safety. Ivermectin/abamectin is a mixture of two homologs, i.e., not less than 80% of 22,23-dihydroavermectin B_{1a} and not more than 20% of 22,23-dihydroavermectin B_{1b}. The B_{1a} and B_{1b} components differ from each other by a single methylene group, have very similar biological and toxicological properties, and can, for all practical purposes, be considered equipotent (Campbell, 1989). The mixture is sold commercially as abamectin. It is a drug of choice because of its broad spectrum nematicidal, insecticidal, and acaricidal properties, and it has been approved for prophylactic use against heartworm (*D. immitis*) infection in dogs.

Ivermectin is utilized at relatively low dosages. It is effective against a wide range of helminths in sheep and cattle in a single oral or parenteral dose of 0.1 mg/kg body weight (Egerton et al., 1979). Ivermectin is approved for use in sheep, goats, swine, beef cattle, horses, and reindeer at dosages ranging from 0.2 to 0.5 mg/kg orally, topically, or subcutaneously (Bimectin, Duocare, Ecomectin, Equell, Eqvalan, Iver-On, Iversol, Ivomec, Noromectin, Primectin, Privermectin, Phoenectin, SparMectin-E, Ziimecterin). The tolerances for American bison, beef cattle, reindeer, swine, and sheep are 15, 15, 15, 20 and 30 ppb of dihydroavermecin B_{1a}, respectively, for liver, and 20 ppb (swine) and 650 ppb (cattle) for muscle (CFR, 1998). Ivermectin is not approved for lactating animals whose milk will enter the food chain. Ivermectin is approved for use in ranch-raised foxes at a dosage of 0.2 mg/kg subcutaneously for control of ear mites (Ivomec). Ivermectin is approved in cats as a heartworm preventative, and for control of internal helminths at a monthly dosage of 24 μg/kg (Heartgard), and as an otic preparation to control ear mites (Acarexx). In dogs, ivermectin is approved for prevention of heartworms, and control of internal helminths at an oral dosage of 6 μg/kg (Heartgard, Advantage, Iverhart, Tri-Heart).

Selamectin, a novel semisynthetic avermectin, is marketed as Revolution (Pfizer). Revolution is a topical antiparasitic preparation recommended for use in dogs and

Veterinary Toxicology. DOI: http://dx.doi.org/10.1016/B978-0-12-811410-0.00043-X

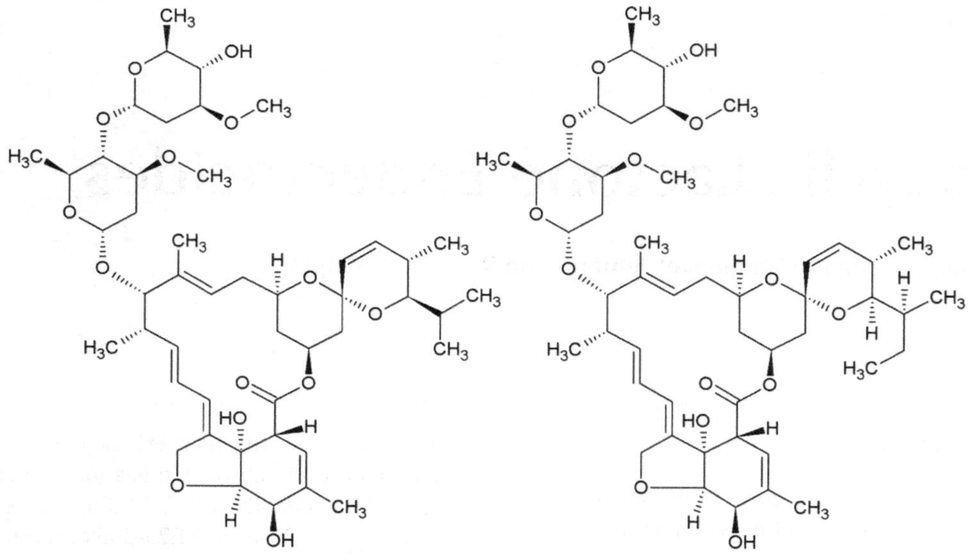

FIGURE 43.1 Chemical structure of abamectin (right, ivermectin B_{1a}; and left, ivermectin B_{1b}).

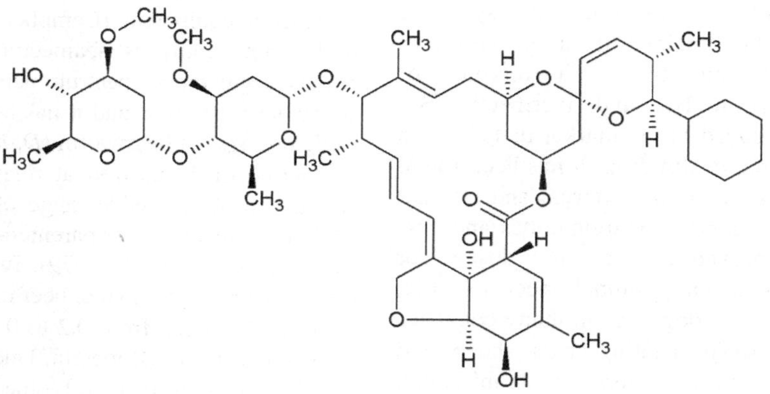

FIGURE 43.2 Chemical structure of doramectin.

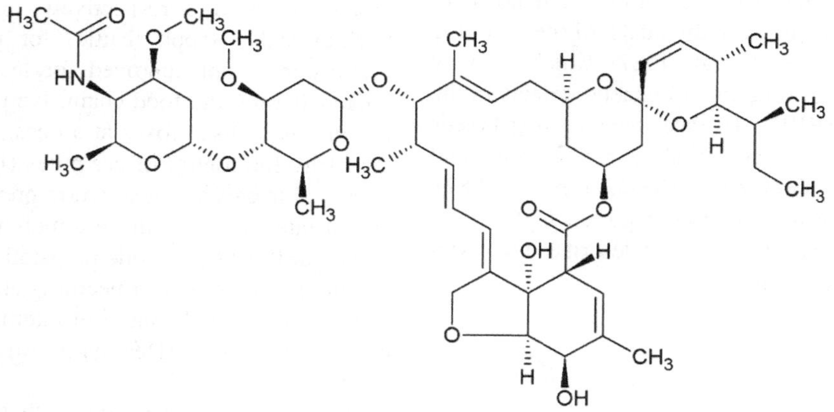

FIGURE 43.3 Chemical structure of eprinomectin.

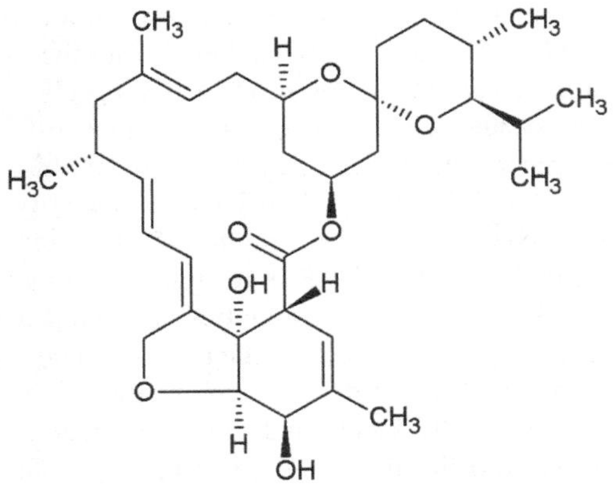

FIGURE 43.4 Chemical structure of milbemycin.

cats 6 weeks of age and older. Selamectin is used to kill fleas (Ctenocephalides felis) and ear mites (Otodectis cynotis) in dogs and cats. It is also indicated for the treatment and control of sarcoptic mange (Sarcoptes scabiei) and for the control of tick (Dermacentor variabilis) infestations in puppies, as well as for the treatment of hookworm (Ancylostoma tubaeforme) and roundworm (Toxocara cati) infections in kittens. Selamectin is also used to prevent heartworm disease caused by Dirofilaria immitis. Most recently, Jacsó et al. (2010) reported the efficacy of selamectin in the treatment of subcutaneous dirofilariosis in dogs caused by Dirofilaria repens. Topical application of selamectin (Revolution) at 6 mg/kg body weight has a broad range of efficacy against many external and internal parasites of dogs and cats (Jacobs, 2000; Dryden et al., 2001). Following topical administration to a single site on the skin, selamectin is absorbed, enters the bloodstream and the gastrointestinal tract (GI) tract, and it is ingested by the external and internal parasites as they feed on the treated host. Selamectin has a direct parasiticidal effect following ingestion (Bishop et al., 2000; Pfizer, 2001).

Other MLs are variously used as injectable, oral, and topical products in livestock, including abamectin (Duotin, injectable) and doramectin (Dectomax, injectable and pour-on). Doramectin tolerances for cattle are 100 ppb in liver and 30 ppb in muscle, and 160 ppb for liver of swine (CFR, 1998). Eprinomectin is approved for use in beef and dairy cattle as a pour-on (Eprinex) and injectable solution (Longrange); tolerances for marker residue eprinomectin B_{1a} are 1.5 ppb in liver, 100 ppb in muscle, and 12 ppb in milk (CFR, 1998). Milbemycin (Interceptor, Sentinel, Trifexis) is used as an oral heartworm preventative in dogs at dosages of 500 μg/kg and cats at dosages of 2000 μg/kg; it is also used as an otic solution for control of ear mites in cats (Milbemite). Moxidectin is utilized as heartworm preventative for cats at 2 mg/kg topically (Advantage-Multi) and as heartworm and internal parasiticide/preventative for dogs at dosages of 3 μg/kg orally (Interceptor), 17 μg/kg subcutaneously (sustained-release injection, ProHeart6), and 2.5 mg/kg topically (Advantage-Multi). In livestock, moxidectin is used as an oral, injectable and pour-on parasiticide in dosages ranging from 200 to 1000 μg/kg (Cydectin, Quest). Moxidectin tolerances for cattle are 900 ppb in fat, 200 ppb in liver, 50 ppb in muscle and 40 ppb in milk; tolerances for sheep are 900 ppb in fat, 200 ppb in liver, and 50 ppb in muscle (CFR, 1998).

As a class, MLs have a wide margin of safety when used in the appropriate species and at appropriate dosages. Toxicoses generally occur due to accidental or intentional overdoses or when products are misused, such as using a livestock formulation in a small companion animal (Merola and Eubig, 2012).

PHARMACOKINETICS/TOXICOKINETICS

The extended antiparasitic activity of MLs in mammals is due to the unique pharmacokinetic profile of this class of compounds. MLs tend to have prolonged tissue and plasma residence times due to their relatively slow absorption, wide tissue distribution, low rate of metabolism, and slow rate of elimination (Lanusse et al., 2009). Characteristics of MLs that influence these kinetic properties include strong adsorption to gastrointestinal particulate digesta, extensive and reversible plasma-tissue exchanges, relatively high degree of lipophilicity, extensive biliary and *p*-glycoprotein mediated intestinal secretion, and extensive enterohepatic recycling. With most MLs, the pharmacokinetic properties are dose-dependent and highly dependent upon the formulation of the individual compounds. For instance, when injected subcutaneously, ivermectin formulations that are oil-based have a slower absorption than those based in glycerol or propylene glycol (Gonzalez et al., 2007).

In general, MLs are well absorbed following injection, oral or topical administration, although species differences in absorption and bioavailability have been noted for some MLs. For instance, the bioavailability of selamectin following topical administration was 4.4% in dogs and 74% in cats, while the oral bioavailability in dogs and cats was 62% and 109%, respectively (Sarasola et al., 2002). Moxidectin absorption is enhanced by coadministration of lipid in most species, but not in dogs (Lallemand et al., 2007). Additionally, within species, sex-related differences in absorption or bioavailability have been reported, including increased absorption of ivermectin and doramectin in female bovines (Toutain et al., 1997).

MLs distribute widely throughout the body and tend to have long tissue residence times, resulting in prolonged antiparasitic activity. The degree of body fat can play a major role in the distribution of MLs, which in turn controls the terminal half-life of the individual animal; for

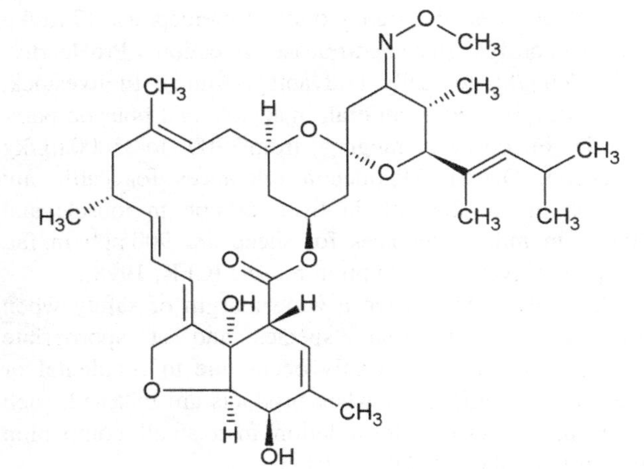

FIGURE 43.5 Chemical structure of moxidectin.

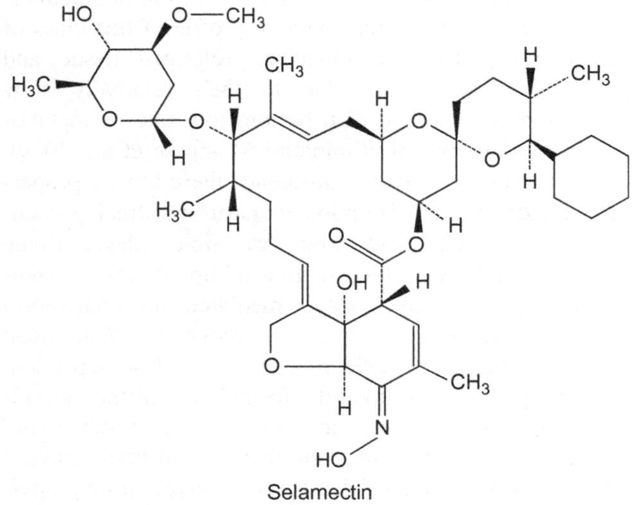

FIGURE 43.6 Chemical structure of selamectin.

instance, the elimination half-life of moxidectin in dogs with a high body fat content is longer than the half-life in leaner dogs (Lallemand et al., 2007). ML levels in tissues such as the gastrointestinal mucosa, lungs, and skin may exceed that of plasma for days to weeks following administration (Lanusse et al., 2009). Doramectin achieves high concentrations in pulmonary tissue of cattle, making it highly effective against the lungworm *Dictyocaulus viviparus.* Following topical administration, selamectin is absorbed into the bloodstream and excreted via the bile into the intestinal tract, where it is reabsorbed and selectively distributed to the sebaceous glands in the skin (Gupta et al., 2005; Gupta, 2007). This unique multiphasic distribution accounts for the ability of selamectin to control hematogenous, gastrointestinal, and integumentary parasites following topical administration.

Although they have widespread distribution to most body tissues, MLs are largely excluded from the mammalian brain through the action of the BBB's *p*-glycoprotein transport system (P-GP) (Fig. 43.7). The P-GP is a 170 kDa transmembrane protein coded for by the ABCB1 (formerly MDR1) gene and is located primarily in the intestine, liver, kidney, and brain (Mosher and Court, 2010). The function of P-GP is to limit the systemic and brain uptake of certain xenobiotics and enhance their elimination from the body (Shen and Zhang, 2010). Alterations in P-GP function can result in increased systemic xenobiotic levels and enhanced penetration of xenobiotics into the brain. MLs comprise one family of drugs that serve as substrates for P-GP; therefore, animals with defects within the P-GP system may have increased absorption and decreased elimination of MLs, as well as an influx of MLs into the central nervous system (CNS), where ML-sensitive gamma-aminobutyric acid (GABA)-gated chloride channels reside. Such animals will be hypersensitive to the neurologic effects of MLs at levels well below those tolerated by animals with intact P-GP, and will show signs of toxicosis at relatively low levels.

Alteration of P-GP function may occur via genetically mediated abnormalities or drug–drug interactions. In addition to its role in the BBB, P-GP within cells of the intestine, liver, and biliary canaliculi can influence the absorption and elimination of substrate xenobiotics (Martinez et al., 2008). The administration of drugs that alter P-GP function can also increase the sensitivity of an individual to the neurologic effects of MLs. P-GP inhibiting drugs such as ketoconazole can increase absorption and decrease elimination of MLs, increasing the likelihood of neurotoxicosis (Hugnet et al., 2007). Spinosad, a ML antiparasitic agent unrelated to the avermectin family, is a potent inhibitor of P-GP that can increase the level of circulating ivermectin by increasing absorption and/or decreasing clearance (Dunn et al., 2011); this alteration of ivermectin pharmacokinetics increases the risk of ivermectin toxicosis when the two drugs are administered concomitantly. Interestingly, similar adverse interaction between spinosad and milbemycin was not detected when the compounds were coadministered (Merola and Eubig, 2012).

In dogs, a 4 base-pair deletion resulting in a frame-shift mutation in the ABCB1 gene has been identified within several breeds (Mosher and Court, 2010). Affected dogs possess truncated, nonfunctional P-GP and are extremely sensitive to the effects of xenobiotics that serve as substrates for P-GP (Mealey, 2004). First identified in collies, the ABCB1 defect has also been identified in over 11 breeds of dogs, as well as mixes of these breeds (Geyer et al., 2007; Mosher and Court, 2010). Table 43.1 lists the breeds in which ABCB1 defects have been identified. Interestingly, although increased brain penetration of

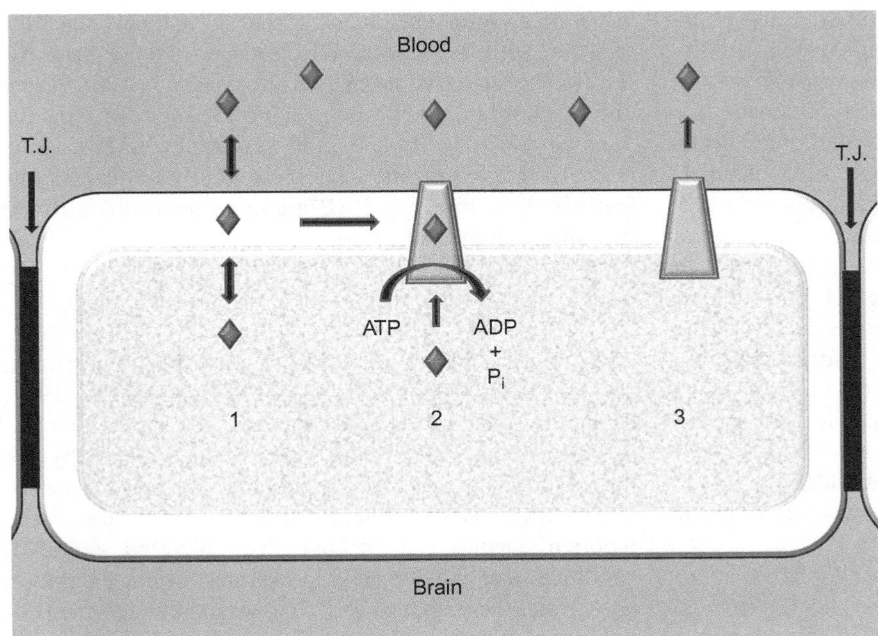

FIGURE 43.7 Cartoon of normal *p*-glycoprotein function within the blood–brain barrier (BBB). P-glycoprotein is a transmembrane pump (gray trapezoids) located on the apical (blood-facing) side of endothelial cells that form the BBB. These endothelial cells are joined through tight junctions (T.J.) that prevent diffusion of substances between the cells. (1) P-glycoprotein substrates (diamonds) diffuse into and out of the endothelial cells through the lipid bilayer of the cell membrane. (2) Substrates within the cell or cell membrane are taken up by the *p*-glycoprotein molecule, an active process requiring ATP for energy. (3) Once taken up by the *p*-glycoprotein, substrates are ejected back into the bloodstream. Defects in *p*-glycoprotein structure and/or function can result in increased concentrations of substrates within the endothelial cell, and egress of substrates out the basal side of the cell into the brain. Please see color plate section.

TABLE 43.1 Dog Breeds in Which ABCB1 Mutations Have Been Identified

Australian shepherd
Border collie
Collie
English shepherd
German shepherd
Longhaired whippet
McNab
Old English sheepdog
Shetland sheepdog
Silken windhound
Wäller
White Swiss shepherd

Reported by Geyer, J., Klintsch, S., Meerkamp, K., et al., 2007. Detection of the nt230 (del4) MDR1 mutation in white Swiss shepherd dogs: case reports of doramectin toxicosis, breed predisposition, and microsatellite analysis. J. Vet. Pharmacol. Therap. 30:482–485; Mosher, C.M., Court, M.H., 2010. Comparative and veterinary pharmacogenomics. In Comparative and Veterinary Pharmacology, Handbook of Experimental Pharmacology, Cunningham F, Elliott J, Lees P (eds). Springer-Verlag, Berlin, pp. 50–78.

xenobiotics has been demonstrated in dogs with the ABCB1 mutation, pharmacokinetic studies have shown no significant differences in oral bioavailability or elimination between dogs with mutant ABCB1 and wild-type dogs (Mealey et al., 2010). Affected dogs develop clinical effects of ML toxicosis at levels that do not cause clinical signs in dogs with normal P-GP. Recently, a novel insertion mutation in the ABCB1 gene was found to be associated with ivermectin sensitivity in a border collie that lacked the previously described deletion mutation (Han et al., 2010), suggesting that more than one genotypic abnormality may result in a similar phenotypic expression.

Although MLs undergo some metabolism, the majority are excreted unchanged in the feces via the bile. This excretion into the intestine results in reabsorption and enterohepatic recycling of up to 20% of the total dose of ML administered (Lanusse et al., 2009). The fact that parenterally administered ML ultimately ends up being secreted into the bile and thereby enters the intestinal tract to undergo some degree of enterohepatic recycling largely explains the efficacy of injected MLs against intestinal parasites. Up to 95% of an ML dose is excreted unchanged in the feces and the half-lives for the various MLs are in the range of days to weeks rather than hours. Half-lives for the various MLs vary widely depending on formulation, dose administered and species, as well as the relative amount of body fat (Lo et al., 1985; Fink and Porras, 1989; Lallemand et al., 2007).

There have been many ML pharmacokinetic/toxicokinetic studies conducted in dogs, cats, sheep, goats, cattle, horses, and pigs (Tway et al., 1981; Lo et al., 1985; Prichard et al., 1985; Alvinerie et al., 1987, 1993; Marriner et al., 1987; Bogan and McKeller, 1988; Toutain et al., 1988, 1997; Fink and Porras, 1989; Scott and McKeller, 1991; Godber et al., 1995; Sarasola et al., 2002; Gupta et al., 2005). It is evident from many of these studies that ivermectin and its derivatives are excreted in the milk.

MECHANISM OF ACTION

The MLs exert their toxic actions through their high affinity for ligand-gated chloride channels, particularly those mediated through the neurotransmitters GABA and glutamate, with higher concentrations required for GABA-mediated effects than for glutamate-mediated actions (Lanusse et al., 2009). Glutamate-gated channels are unique to invertebrates (Trailovic and Nedelijovic, 2011). Binding of MLs to glutamate-gated chloride channels causes increased conductance of chloride through the cell membrane, resulting in hyperpolarization and flaccid paralysis of invertebrate musculature, particularly in nematodes and arthropods (Lanusse et al., 2009). Paralysis of pharyngeal pump musculature decreases the ingestion of nutrients while paralysis of somatic musculatures impedes the ability of the parasite to remain at its site of predilection in the host, resulting in death of the parasites. Additionally, effects on the GABA and glutamate-mediated activity of the musculature of the female reproductive system result in decreases in oviposition (Fellowes et al., 2000).

Glutamate-mediated chloride channels sensitive to MLs are found uniquely in nematodes and arthropods. Cestodes and trematodes lack ML binding sites, and are therefore unaffected by MLs. In mammals, ML-sensitive GABA-mediated chloride channels are restricted to the CNS, from which the MLs are largely excluded through the action of a *p*-glycoprotein efflux pump (see MLs and *p*-glycoprotein defective animals in previous section). When the *p*-glycoprotein transporter is overwhelmed (e.g., in overdose situations), defective (e.g., ABCB1 defect), or compromised (e.g., pharmacologically inhibited), entry of MLs into the mammalian CNS may lead to signs of toxicosis.

TOXICITY

Toxicity Data

At the doses used as parasiticides in veterinary medicine, MLs have low levels of toxicity to most animal species with at least a 10-fold margin of safety for ruminants, horses, swine, and dogs with normal P-GP (Campbell et al., 1983; Bennett, 1986; Lanusse et al., 2009). For example, the dosage of ivermectin used to prevent heartworms and intestinal nematodes in dogs is 6 μg/kg body weight, which is over 30 times less than the dosage of 200–600 μg/kg that is often used in dogs to manage ectoparasites such as *Demodex* mites. Dogs with ABCB1 defects would not be expected to show clinical signs until levels of 80–100 μg/kg of ivermectin were administered, while most dogs with normal P-GP can generally tolerate dosages of 200 μg/kg/day, although some dogs may show mild signs at that dosage (Merola et al., 2009; Merola and Eubig, 2012). In beagle dogs, the oral LD_{50} of ivermectin is 80,000 μg/kg body weight (Pullium et al., 1985). Toxic and therapeutic dosages for some MLs are listed in Table 43.2. Some chelonians appear to be highly sensitive to MLs, with the leopard tortoise (*Geochelone pardalis*) developing signs at dosages as low as 25 μg/kg (Teare and Bush, 1983). White lions appear to be more sensitive than tawny lions (Lobetti and Caldwell, 2012). Young animals in general may be more sensitive than adults because their immature BBB are more permeable to ivermectin (Sanford et al., 1988).

Clinical Effects

The clinical signs of ML toxicosis have been reported in several studies (Pullium et al., 1985; Paul et al., 1987; Tranquilli et al., 1987) as well as case reports of toxicosis in various species. In most species, signs generally are those of CNS depression, although in some species, GABA-mediated cholinergic effects have also been reported. Ocular effects have been reported with ML overdoses and include mydriasis, miosis (less common), absent menace response and blindness. Although multifocal retinal edema and separation were described in two dogs (Kenny et al., 2008), other cases in cats, dogs, and horses did not show abnormalities on fundic examinations (Meekins et al., 2015; Pollio et al., 2016). In all reported cases, vision returned upon recovery from toxicosis.

After ingesting ivermectin at about 200 μg/kg of an ivermectin anthelmintic paste, a dog with the ABCB1 mutation exhibited dehydration, bradycardia, respiratory depression, cyanosis, mydriasis, and a diminished gag reflex (Heit et al., 1989). Signs of ML toxicosis in dogs may also include hypersalivation, vomiting, lethargy, ataxia, tremors, hyperthermia or hypothermia, disorientation, lack of menace response, blindness, head-pressing, seizures, coma, and death (Merola and Eubig, 2012). Signs reported with ML toxicosis in cats include mild diarrhea, posterior ataxia, miosis or mydriasis, vocalization, ataxia, tremors, sternal recumbency, coma, and death. (Song, 1991; Merola and Eubig, 2012). ML toxicosis in calves can cause depression, ataxia, diarrhea, dyspnea, tachycardia, recumbency, increased respiratory rates, muscular fasciculations, mydriasis, extensor rigidity of the limbs, and miosis or mydriasis (Gupta, 2007). In sheep, ML toxicosis is characterized by depression and incoordination. In horses, ataxia, depression, mydriasis, depressed respiratory rate and drooping lower lip visual impairment have been reported (Leaning, 1983).

Ten lions that were administered 0.2–0.5 mg/kg of doramectin subcutaneously and then subsequently fed the carcass of a horse that had recently received doramectin via injection developed ataxia, hallucinations, and mydriasis 3–5 days following doramectin administration; two affected lions died (Lobetti and Caldwell, 2012). Post mortem lesions consisted of cyanosis, pulmonary edema, pleural effusion and pericardial effusion, and brain and

TABLE 43.2 Toxicity of Various Macrocyclic Lactone Endectocides

Agent	Species	Therapeutic Dose (Route)	NOAEL	Toxic Dose (LOEL or MTD Unless Otherwise Stated)	Comments/References
Abamectin	Cattle	0.2 mg/kg, SC		2–8 mg/kg, SC	Not recommended for calves <4 mo; Lanusse et al. (2009)
	Dog (beagle)	N/A	0.25 mg/kg/d × 12 mo, PO		Stevens and Breckenridge (2001)
	Mouse			14–80 mg/kg (PO, LD_{50})	Extoxnet (1994)[a]
	Mouse (CF-1, pregnant)		0.05 mg/kg/day, PO	0.075 mg/kg/day, PO	Stevens and Breckenridge (2001)
	Mouse (CD-I)		4–8 mg/kg/day × 18 mo, PO		Stevens and Breckenridge (2001)
	Rabbit (pregnant)		1 mg/kg/day, PO	2 mg/kg/day, PO	Stevens and Breckenridge (2001)
	Rat	N/A		11 mg/kg (PO, LD_{50})	Extoxnet (1994)[a]
	Rat (SD)	N/A	1.5–2 mg/kg/d × 53 weeks, PO		Stevens and Breckenridge (2001)
	Rat (SD, pregnant)	N/A	1.6 mg/kg/day, PO	2.0 mg/kg/day PO	Stevens and Breckenridge (2001)
Doramectin	Camelids	0.2 mg/kg IM, SC			Fowler (2010)[b]
	Cattle	0.2 mg/kg IM, SC	2.5 mg/kg, SC × 3 d		Lanusse et al. (2009)
		0.5 mg/kg, Topical			FDA (1997)[c]
	Cattle (breeding)	0.2 mg/kg, SC	0.6 mg/kg, SC		Lanusse et al. (2009)
	Dogs (beagle)	N/A	2 mg/kg/day × 14 d		INCHEM (2010)[d]
	Dogs (collie)	N/A	0.25 mg/kg, PO	0.5 mg/kg, PO	INCHEM (2010)[d]
	Goats	0.2 mg/kg IM, SC			Pfizer (2006)[e]
	Lions	0.2–0.5 mg/kg IM, SC		0.2 mg/kg SC, IM	Lobetti and Caldwell (2012)
	Pigs	0.3 mg/kg IM	3 mg/kg, IM	7.5 mg/kg, IM	Lanusse et al. (2009); EMEA (1997)[f]
	Rats	0.2 mg/kg q 24 h × 4 d, PO			Oege et al. (2000)[g]
	Sheep	0.2 mg/kg IM, SC	0.6 mg/kg, SC		Lanusse et al. (2009); EMEA (1997)[f]
Eprinomectin	Camelids	0.5 mg/kg, topical			Plant et al. (2007)[h]
	Cattle	0.5 mg/kg, topical	2.5 mg/kg, topical		Lanusse et al. (2009)
	Dogs	N/A	1 mg/kg/d × 14 d, PO	1.6 mg/kg/d × 14 d, PO	EMEA (1996)[i]
	Horses	0.5 mg/kg, topical			Ural et al. (2008)[j]
	Goats	1 mg/kg, topical			Scheuerle et al. (2009)[k]
	Mice	N/A		75 mg/kg, PO (LD_{50}), 35 mg/kg, IP (LD_{50})	EMEA (1996)[i]
	Rats	N/A	5 mg/kg/d × 14 d, PO	55 mg/kg, PO (LD_{50}), 35 mg/kg, IP (LD_{50})	EMEA (1996)[i]
	Sheep	0.5 mg/kg, topical			Kircali Sevimli et al. (2007)[l]

(*Continued*)

TABLE 43.2 (Continued)

Agent	Species	Therapeutic Dose (Route)	NOAEL	Toxic Dose (LOEL or MTD Unless Otherwise Stated)	Comments/References
Ivermectin	Camelids	0.2–0.6 mg/kg, SC			Fowler (2010)[b]
	Cats	0.024–0.4 mg/kg, PO	0.75 mg/kg, PO	1.0 mg/kg, PO	FDA (1996)[m]; Lanusse et al. (2009)
	Cattle	0.5 mg/kg, topical, 0.2 mg/kg, SC	5 mg/kg, topical	0.6 mg/kg, SC	Lanusse et al. (2009); Gupta (2007)
	Dogs	0.006–0.6 mg/kg, PO		80 mcg/kg (ABCB1 defective);0.2–1 mg/kg (ABCB1 normal)	Plumb (2009)[o]; Merola et al. (2009)
	Frogs (*Dendrobates* spp.)	0.2–0.4 mg/kg PO		0.2 mg/kg PO	Clayton et al. (2012)
	Goats	0.4 mg/kg, PO			Lanusse et al. (2009)
	Horses	0.2 mg/kg, PO		1.2–2 mg/kg, PO	Lanusse et al. (2009); Gupta (2007)
	Pigs	0.1 mg/kg/d′7 d, PO			Lanusse et al. (2009)
	Sheep	0.2 mg/kg, PO			Lanusse et al. (2009)
Milbemycin	Cats	2 mg/kg, PO			Lanusse et al. (2009)
	Dogs	0.5 mg/kg, PO	0.6 mg/kg (ABCB1 defective)	5 mg/kg (ABCB1 defective)	Lanusse et al. (2009); Barbet et al. (2009)[n]; Tranquilli et al. (1991)[o]
Moxidectin	Cattle	0.2–1 mg/kg SC, Topical	2 mg/kg		Lanusse et al. (2009)
	Dogs	0.003–0.17 mg/kg, PO			Lanusse et al. (2009)
	Horses	0.4 mg/kg, PO		1 mg/kg	Lanusse et al. (2009); Khan et al. (2002)[p]
	Pigs	0.3 mg/kg, SC			Lanusse et al. (2009)
	Sheep	0.2–1 mg/kg PO, SC			Lanusse et al. (2009)
Selamectin	Cats	6 mg/kg, topical	60 mg/kg, topical		Lanusse et al. (2009)
	Dogs	6 mg/kg, topical	60 mg/kg, topical		Lanusse et al. (2009)

[a] *ExToxNet, 1994. Abamectin. Pesticide Information Profile. Cornell University. Accessed via web 2/2011. http://pmep.cce.cornell.edu/profiles/extoxnet/24d-captan/abamectin-ext.html.*
[b] *Fowler, M.E., 2010. Parasites.* In Medicine and Surgery of Camelids, *Fowler ME (ed.). Wiley Blackwell, p. 259.*
[c] *FDA (1997) Dectomax® Approval Letter, FOIA.*
[d] *INCHEM, 2010. International Programme on Chemical Safety. Accessed via web 2/2011. http://www.inchem.org/documents/jecfa/jecmono/v36je02.htm*
[e] *Pfizer, 2006. Dectomax® Label Information. Pfizer Animal Health, New York.*
[f] *EMEA, 1997. Doramectin (pigs and sheep). European Agency for the Evaluation of Medicinal Products, Veterinary Medicines Evaluation Unit. EMEA/MRL/186/97-FINAL. Accessed via web 3/2011: http://www.ema.europa.eu/docs/en_GB/document_library/Maximum_Residue_Limits_-_Report/2009/11/WC500013916.pdf.*
[g] *Oege, H., Ayaz, E., Dalgic, S., 2000. The effect of doramectin, moxidectin and netobimin against natural infections of* Syphacia muris *in rats. Vet. Parasitol. 88, 299–303.*
[h] *Plant, J.D., Kutzler, M.A., Cebra, C.K., 2007. Efficacy of topical eprinomectin in the treatment of* Chorioptes sp. *infestation in alpacas and llamas. Vet. Dermatol. 18, 59–62.*
[i] *EMEA, 1996. Eprinomectin. European Agency for the Evaluation of Medicinal Products, Veterinary Medicines Evaluation Unit. EMEA/MRL/114/96-FINAL. Accessed via web 3/2011: http://www.ema.europa.eu/docs/en_GB/document_library/Maximum_Residue_Limits_-_Report/2009/11/WC500014177.pdf.*
[j] *Ural, K., Ulutas, B., Kar, S., 2008. Eprinomectin treatment of psoroptic mange in hunter/jumper and dressage horses: a prospective, randomized, double-blinded, placebo-controlled clinical trial. Vet. Parasitol. 156, 353–357.*
[k] *Scheuerle, M.C., Mahling, M., Pfister, K., 2009. Anthelminthic resistance of* Haemonchus contortus *in small ruminants in Switzerland and Southern Germany. Wien Klin Wochenschr 121, 46–49.*
[l] *Kırcalı Sevimli, F., Kozan, E., Dolan, N., 2011. Efficacy of eprinomectin pour-on treatment in sheep naturally infected with* Dictyocaulus filaria *and* Cystocaulus ocreatus. *J. Helminthol. 7, 1–4.*
[m] *FDA, 1996. Heartgard® for Cats Original Approval. Accessed via web: http://www.fda.gov/AnimalVeterinary/Products/ApprovedAnimalDrugProducts/FOIADrugSummaries/ucm116793.htm.*
[n] *Barbet, J.L., Snook, T., Gay, J.M., Mealey, K.L., 2009. ABCB1-1 Delta (MDR1-1Delta) genotype is associated with adverse reactions in dogs treated with milbemycin oxime for generalized demodicosis. Vet. Dermatol. 20, 111–114.*
[o] *Tranquilli, W.J., Paul, A.J., Todd, K.S., 1991. Assessment of toxicosis induced by high-dose administration of milbemycin oxime in collies. Am. J. Vet. Res. 52, 1170–1172.*
[p] *Khan, S.A., Kuster, D.A., Hansen, S.R., 2002. A review of moxidectin overdose cases in equines from 1998–2000. Vet. Hum. Toxicol. 44, 232–235.*

liver tissues had elevated levels of doramectin. The remaining lions made full recoveries. Dendrobatid frogs administered ivermectin orally via micropipette (attempted dosage 0.2 mg/kg) developed clinical signs of toxicosis 24–48 h following administration (Clayton et al., 2012). Signs included ataxia, reduced/absent reflexes, lack of righting reflex, reduced/absent buccal pumping, hydrocoelom, and unresponsiveness; overall mortality was 68% and surviving frogs remained symptomatic for up to 3 weeks.

In a reproduction study, Wise et al. (1997) demonstrated that at a high dose, emamectin benzoate (derivative of avermectin B_1) exposure during gestation and lactation in rats produced evidence of neurotoxicity in the F_1 offspring. A no observed adverse effect level for developmental neurotoxicity of emamectin was determined to be 0.6 mg/kg/day.

Diagnosis

Diagnosis of ivermectin, selamectin, and other MLs can be based on history of exposure to a product, clinical signs, and residue analysis in the body tissue or fluids. These compounds are analyzed using high-performance liquid chromatograph coupled with a UV, fluorescence, or photodiode array detector (Reising et al., 1988; Maynard and Maynard, 1989; Rabel et al., 1993; Payne et al., 1995; Anastaseo et al., 2002; Gupta et al., 2005). GI content, liver, fat, and feces are usually the specimens analyzed for MLs residue, while brain tissue would be utilized for confirming toxicosis.

Fatal doramectin toxicosis in two lions (*Panthera leo*) was associated with brain doramectin concentrations of 0.082 and 0.183 ppm (Lobetti and Caldwell, 2012). Brain ivermectin concentrations reported in clinically normal cattle are low (e.g., ~0.004 ppm), while concentrations of 0.056 ppm have been associated with clinical toxicosis (Seaman et al., 1987). In dogs, 0.134 ppm of ivermectin in brain tissue was associated with fatal toxicosis (Pullium et al., 1985), while in horses 0.131 ppm was associated with ivermectin-induced fatality (Swor et al., 2009).

TREATMENT

Treatment for intoxication with MLs should include limiting systemic absorption of the xenobiotic, monitoring for possible clinical effects, and managing any signs that develop. Symptomatic patients should be stabilized prior to performing decontamination procedures. For oral exposures, emesis, lavage and/or administration of activated charcoal should be considered. If the exposure was by a recent subcutaneous injection and life-threatening toxicosis is possible, surgical excision of the injection site can be considered if the bleb can still be palpated (Beasley et al., 1999).

For patients that can safely vomit, emesis may be effective if performed within 2 h of ingestion (Mealey, 2006). If the patient is unable to safely vomit (e.g., is a species that cannot vomit or is symptomatic), gastric lavage can be considered. Activated charcoal should be considered in addition to, or instead of, emesis or lavage. It is important to mention that with xenobiotics like the MLs, which are excreted in the bile, activated charcoal can be of benefit regardless of the route of the exposure. Thus if a patient received an overdose of injectable ML subcutaneously, activated charcoal will still be a very valuable decontamination option. The ML molecules will be carried to the GI by the bile.

MLs undergo enterohepatic recycling; therefore, multiple doses of activated charcoal will likely be beneficial. In addition, the MLs are substrates for the *p*-glycoprotein transport system (P-GP) that transports some drugs across cell membranes. In the intestine, the MLs enter the enterocyte by absorption from the GI. However, once in the cell, the P-GP acts to move the ML across the membrane and back into the gastrointestinal lumen. This cycling allows the ML molecules to have multiple opportunities to bind with the repeated doses of activated charcoal (Mealey, 2006). When repeated doses are indicated, half the original dose should be given at 4–8 h intervals, often for 2–3 days (Peterson, 2006).

The patient should be monitored for the development of CNS effects including ataxia, lethargy, recumbency, tremors and seizing. Also monitor for bradycardia, gastrointestinal upset, and respiratory depression. No specific chemistry panel changes are expected. If activated charcoal is given, serial serum sodium tests should be run to check for elevations, as hypernatremia has been associated with repeated doses of activated charcoal (Ball, 2014).

There is no specific antidote for ML toxicosis, so treatment is symptomatic and supportive. Patients who are recumbent or comatose will require good nursing care including thermoregulation, soft bedding, and frequent turning to prevent decubital ulcers and urine scalding since the patient may be immobile for multiple days (Mealey, 2006). Patients that are experiencing tremors or seizures can be treated with methocarbamol. Minimize sensory stimuli since these patients can be hyperesthetic. Nutritional support through tube feeding may also be necessary (Mealey, 2006). Intravenous fluids should be given as needed for cardiovascular support and atropine can be used for bradycardia. A respirator may be necessary if significant respiratory depression develops. Picrotoxin and pysostigmine have both been used to treat ivermectin toxicosis, but have been associated with significant adverse effects including seizures (Crandell and Weinberg, 2009).

A promising new therapy, intravenous infusion of a lipid emulsion (ILE), has been used to treat ML toxicosis in dogs, cats, and horses (Crandell and Weinberg, 2009; Jourdan et al., 2015; Pollio et al., 2016). Lipid emulsions are made from purified soybean oil in water, are commonly used in medicine to provide intravenous (parenteral) nutrition, and are the delivery mechanism for certain hydrophobic drugs like propofol.

The mechanism by which ILE is effective at treating toxicoses is not yet fully understood. However, the fact that ILE seems to be most effective in treating overdosage of lipid soluble medications suggests that the infusion expands the amount of plasma lipid, which acts as a sink in which the offending xenobiotic can gather, thus reducing free drug concentrations. In theory the xenobiotic is trapped in the plasma lipid so it is not available to act on other tissues (Crandell and Weinberg, 2009; O'Brien et al., 2010; Clarke et al., 2011).

The ASPCA Animal Poison Control Center uses the following dosing protocol for ILE. Using a 20% product, give an initial bolus of 1.5 mL/kg slowly then start a continuous rate infusion (CRI) of 0.25 mL/kg/min for 30–60 min (Merola and Eubig, 2012). Four hours after the CRI is finished, check the serum for hyperlipemia and to see if the serum is orange or yellow. If the serum looks normal, repeat the initial bolus and CRI again. If hyperlipemia or a color change is present, check the serum for resolution every 2 h. Repeat the initial bolus and CRI once the hyperlipemia or color change resolves. If a third dose is needed, follow the above directions beginning 4 h after the second CRI finishes. Do not give more than three doses if there has been no significant response.

Possible side effects of administering ILE include induction of pancreatitis, creation of a fat embolism, immunosuppression, phlebitis, thrombosis, hypertriglyceridemia, and hepatic lipidosis (Crandell and Weinberg, 2009; O'Brien et al., 2010).

CONCLUDING REMARKS AND FUTURE DIRECTIONS

MLs are commonly used as insecticides, nematicides, and acaricides in animals. Among all MLs, acute toxicosis is more often encountered with ivermectin. Poisoning occurs in dogs (especially collies) and cats due to inadvertent or misuse of the product meant for another species. In general, young animals are affected with a greater frequency than adults. Clinical signs are those of CNS toxicity. Treatment relies upon symptomatic and supportive therapies.

ACKNOWLEDGMENTS

One of the authors (RCG) would like to thank Mrs. Robin B. Doss for her assistance in the preparation of this chapter.

REFERENCES

Alvinerie, M., Sutra, J.F., Galtier, P., Toutain, P.L., 1987. Determination of invermectin in milk by high performance liquid chromatography. Ann. Rech. Vet. 18, 269–274.

Alvinerie, M., Sutra, J.F., Galtier, P., 1993. Ivermectin in goat plasma and milk after subcutaneous injection. Ann. Rech. Vet. 24, 417–421.

Anastaseo, A., Esposito, M., Amorena, M., et al., 2002. Residue study of ivermectin in plasma, milk, and mozzarella cheese following subcutaneous administration to buffalo (*Bubalus bubalis*). J. Agric. Food Chem. 50, 5244–5245.

Ball, A., 2014. Managing hypernatremia after activated charcoal administration. Vet. Med. 109, 128–130.

Beasley, V.R., Dorman, D.C., Fikes, J.D., Diana, S.G., 1999. A Systems Affected Approach to Toxicology. University of Illinois College of Veterinary Medicine, Urbana, pp. 249–252.

Bennett, D.G., 1986. Clinical pharmacology of ivermectin. J. Am. Vet. Med. Assoc. 189, 100–104.

Bishop, B.F., Bruce, C.I., Evans, N.A., et al., 2000. Selamectin: a novel broad spectrum endoctocide for dogs and cats. Vet. Parasitol. 91, 163–176.

Bogan, J.A., McKellar, Q.A., 1988. The pharmacokinetics of ivermectin in sheep and cattle. J. Vet. Pharmacol. Ther. 11, 260–268.

Campbell, W.C., 1989. Ivermectin and Abamectin. Springer Verlag, New York, NY.

Campbell, W.C., Fisher, M.H., Stapley, E.O., et al., 1983. Avermectin: a potent new antiparasitic agent. Science 222, 823.

Clarke, D.L., Lee, J.A., Murphy, L.A., Reineke, E.L., 2011. Use of intravenous lipid emulsion to treat ivermectin toxicosis in a Border Collie. JAVMA 239, 1328–1333.

Clayton, L.A., Nelson, J., Payton, M.E., et al., 2012. Presumptive ivermectin overdose in a group of dendrobatid frogs. J. Herpet. Med. Surg. 22, 5–11.

Code of Federal Regulations, 1998. Title 21, Sec. 556.344. U.S. Government Printing Office, Washington, DC. Available at: http://www.ecfr.gov/cgi-bin/text-idx?c=ecfrandtpl=/ecfrbrowse/Title21/21cfr556_main_02.tpl (accessed 27.02.17.).

Crandell, D.E., Weinberg, M.D., 2009. Moxidectin toxicosis in a puppy successfully treated with intravenous lipids. J. Vet. Emerg. Crit. Care. 19, 181–186.

Dryden, M.W., Atkins, C.E., Evans, N.A., et al., 2001. Insight: new perceptions for veterinary innovators. (Sym.). Pfizer, pp. 7–55.

Dunn, S.T., Hedges, L., Sampson, K.E., et al., 2011. Pharmacokinetic interaction of the antiparasitic agents ivermecin and spinosad. Drug Metab. Dispos. 39, 789–795.

Egerton, J.R., Ostlind, D.A., Blair, L.S., et al., 1979. Avermectins, new family of potent anthelmintic agents: efficacy of the B_{1a} component. Antimicrob. Agents Chemother. 15, 372–378.

Fellowes, R.A., Maule, A.G., Martin, R.J., et al., 2000. Classical neurotransmitters in the ovijector of Ascaris suum: localization and modulation of muscle activity. Parasitology 1221, 325–336.

Fink, D.W., Porras, A.G., 1989. Pharmacokinetics of ivermectin in animals and humans. In: Campbell, W.C. (Ed.), Ivermectin and Abamectin. Springer-Verlag, New York, NY, pp. 113–130.

Geyer, J., Klintsch, S., Meerkamp, K., et al., 2007. Detection of the nt230 (del4) MDR1 mutation in white Swiss shepherd dogs: case reports of doramectin toxicosis, breed predisposition, and microsatellite analysis. J. Vet. Pharmacol. Therap. 30, 482–485.

Godber, L.M., Derksen, F.J., Williams, J.F., Mahmoud, B., 1995. Ivermectin toxicosis in a neonatal foal. Aust. Vet. J. 72, 191–192.

Gonzalez, A., Sahagun, A., Diez, M.J., et al., 2007. Bioavailability of a commercial formulation of ivermectin after subcutaneous administration to sheep. Am. J. Vet. Res. 68, 101–105.

Gupta, R.C., 2007. Ivermectin and selamectin. In: Gupta, R.C. (Ed.), Veterinary Toxicology: Basic and Clinical Principles. Academic Press, San Diego, CA, pp. 508–513.

Gupta, R.C., Masthay, M.B., Canerdy, T.D., et al., 2005. Human exposure to selamectin from dogs treated with Revolution™: methodological consideration for selamectin isolation. Toxicol. Mechan. Methods 15, 317–321.

Haldrick, M.K., Bunch, S.C., Kornegay, J.N., 1995. Ivermectin toxicosis in two Australian shepherds. Am. J. Vet. Med. Assoc. 206, 1147–1150.

Han, J.I., Son, H.W., Park, S.C., Na, K.J., 2010. Novel insertion mutation of ABCB1 gene in an ivermectin sensitive border collie. J. Vet. Sci. 11, 341–344.

Heit, J.E., Tranquili, W.J., Paul, A.J., et al., 1989. Clinical management of ivermectin toxicosis in a collie dog. Compan. Anim. Pract. 19, 3–7.

Houston, D.M., Parent, J., Matushek, K.J., 1987. Ivermectin toxicosis in a dog. J. Am. Vet. Med. Assoc. 191, 78–80.

Hugnet, C., Lespine, A., Alvinerie, M., 2007. Multiple oral dosing of ketoconazole increases dog exposure to ivermectin. J. Pharm. Pharmaceut. Sci. 10, 311–318.

Jacobs, D.E., 2000. Selamectin – a novel endoctocide for dogs and cats. Vet. Parasitol. 91, 161–162.

Jacsó, O., Fok, E., Kiss, G., et al., 2010. Preliminary findings on the efficacy of selamectin in the treatment of dogs naturally infected with *Dirofilaria repens*. Acta Vet. Hung. 58, 405–412.

Jourdan, G., Boyer, G., Raymond-Letron, I., et al., 2015. Intravenous lipid emulsion therapy in 20 cats accidentally overdosed with ivermectin. J. Vet. Emerg. Crit. Care. 25, 667–671.

Kenny, P.J., Vernau, K.M., Puschner, B., 2008. Retinopathy associated with ivermectin toxicosis in two dogs. J. Am. Vet. Med. Assoc. 233, 279–284.

Lallemand, E., Lespine, A., Alvinerie, M., et al., 2007. Estimation of absolute oral bioavailability of moxidectin in dogs using a semi-simultaneous method: influence of lipid co-administration. J. Vet. Pharmacol. Ther. 30, 375–380.

Lanusse, C.E., Lifschitz, A.L., Imperiale, F.A., 2009. Macrocyclic lactones: endectocide compounds. In: Reviere, J.E., Papich, M.G. (Eds.), Veterinary Pharmacology and Therapeutics. Wiley-Blackwell, Ames, IA, pp. 1119–1144.

Leaning, W.H.D., 1983. The efficacy and safety evaluation of ivermectin as a parenteral and oral antiparasitic agent in horses. Proc. Am. Assoc. Equine Pract. 29, 319–1780.

Lo, P.K.A., Fink, D.W., Williams, J.B., Blodinger, J., 1985. Pharmacokinetic studies of ivermectin: effects of formulation. Vet. Res. Commun. 9, 251–268.

Lobetti, R.G., Caldwell, P., 2012. Doramectin toxicity in a group of lions (*Panthera leo*). J. South Afr. Vet. Assoc. 83, Art #509; http://dx.doi.org/10.4102/jsava.v83i1.509.

Marriner, S.C., McKinnon, I., Bogan, J.A., 1987. The pharmacokinetics of ivermectin after oral and subcutaneous administration to sheep and horses. J. Vet. Pharmacol. Ther. 10, 175–179.

Martinez, M., Modric, S., Sharkey, M., et al., 2008. The pharmacogenomics of P-glycoprotein and its role in veterinary medicine. J. Vet. Pharmacol. Therap. 31, 285–300.

Maynard, M.S., Maynard, H.D., 1989. HPLC assay for avermectin B1a and its two photoisomers using a photo diode array detector. Bull. Environ. Contam. Toxicol. 43, 499–504.

Mealey, K.L., 2004. Therapeutic implications of the MDR-1 gene. J. Vet. Pharmacol. Therap. 27, 257–264.

Mealey, K.L., 2006. Toxicological decontamination. In: Peterson, M.E., Talcott, P.A. (Eds.), Small Animal Toxicology, second ed. Elsevier Inc, St. Louis, pp. 785–793.

Mealey, K.L., Waiting, D., Raunig, D.L., et al., 2010. Oral bioavailability of P-glycoprotein substrate drugs do not differ between ABCB1-1⊗ and ABCB1 wild type dogs. J. Vet. Pharmacol. Therap. 33, 453–460.

Meekins, J.M., Guess, S.C., Rankin, A.J., 2015. Retinopathy associated with ivermectin toxicosis in five cats. J. Am. Vet. Med. Assoc. 246, 1238–1241.

Merola, V.M., Eubig, P.A., 2012. Toxicology of avermectins and milbemycins (macrocyclic lactones) and the role of P-glycoprotein in dogs and cats. Vet. Clin. Small Anim. 42, 313–333.

Merola, V.M., Khan, S.A., Gwaltney-Brant, S.M., 2009. Ivermectin toxicosis in dogs: a retrospective study. J. Am. Anim. Hosp. Assoc. 45, 106–111.

Mosher, C.M., Court, M.H., 2010. Comparative and veterinary pharmacogenomics. In: Cunningham, F., Elliott, J., Lees, P. (Eds.), Comparative and Veterinary Pharmacology, Handbook of Experimental Pharmacology. Springer-Verlag, Berlin, pp. 50–78.

O'Brien, T.Q., Clark-Price, S.C., Evans, E.E., et al., 2010. Infusion of a lipid emulsion to treat lidocaine intoxication in a cat. J. Am. Vet. Med. Assoc. 237, 1455–1458.

Paul, A.J., Tranquilli, W.J., Seward, R.L., et al., 1987. Clinical observations in collies given ivermectin orally. Am. J. Vet. Res. 48, 684–685.

Payne, L.D., Hicks, M.B., Wehner, T.A., 1995. Determination of abamectin and/or ivermectin in cattle feces at low parts per billion levels using HPLC with fluorescence detection. J. Agric. Food Chem. 43, 1233–1235.

Peterson, M.E., 2006. Toxicological decontamination. In: Peterson, M. E., Talcott, P.A. (Eds.), Small Animal Toxicology, second ed. Elsevier Inc, St. Louis, pp. 127–141.

Pfizer, 2001. Revolution: mechanism of action. http://www.revolution-vet.com/action3.htm (accessed 28.10.02.).

Pollio, D., Michau, T.M., Weaver, E., Kuebelbeck, K.L., 2016. Electroretinographic changes after intravenous lipid emulsion therapy in a dog and a foal with ivermectin toxicosis. Vet. Ophthalmol. 1–6, http://dx.doi.org/10.1111/vop.12410.

Prichard, R.K., Steel, J.W., Lacey, E., Hennessy, D.R., 1985. Pharmacokinetics of ivermectin in sheep following intravenous, intra-abomasal or intra-ruminal administration. J. Vet. Pharmacol. Ther. 8, 88–94.

Pullium, J.D., Seward, R.L., Henry, R.T., Steinberg, S.A., 1985. Investigating ivermectin toxicity in collies. Vet. Med. 80, 33–40.

Rabel, S.R., Stobaugh, J.F., Heining, R., Bostick, J.M., 1993. Improvements in detection sensitivity for the determination of ivermectin in plasma using chromatographic techniques and laser-induced fluorescence detection with automated derivatization. J. Chromatogr. 617, 79–86.

Reising, K.P., Migdal, N., Benedetto, D., 1988. Solid-phase extraction cleanup for ivermectin in liver tissue. AOAC Intl. 81, 484–487.

Sanford, S.E., Rehmtulla, A.J., Josephson, G.K.A., 1988. Ivermectin overdose and toxicosis in neonatal pigs. Can. Vet. J. 29, 735–736.

Sarasola, P., Jernigan, A.D., Walker, D.K., et al., 2002. Pharmacokinetics of selamectin following intravenous oral and topical administration in cats and dogs. J. Vet. Pharmacol. Ther. 25, 265–272.

Scott, E.W., McKellar, O.A., 1991. Pharmacokinetics and pharmacodynamics of ivermectin administered subcutaneously to pigs. Proc. 5th Cong. Eur. Assoc. Vet. Pharm. Tox.383–384.

Seaman, T.J., Eagleson, J.S., Carrigan, M.J., Web, R.F., 1987. Avermectin B, toxicity in a herd of Murray Grey cattle. Aust. Vet. J. 64, 284.

Shen, S., Zhang, W., 2010. ABC transporters and drug efflux at the blood–brain barrier. Rev. Neurosci. 21, 29–53.

Song, M.D., 1991. Using ivermectin to treat feline dermatoses caused by external parasites. Vet. Med. 86, 498–502.

Stevens, J., Breckenridge, C.B., 2001. The avermectins: insecticidal and antiparasitic agents. In: Krieger, R. (Ed.), Handbook of Pesticide Toxicology, second ed. Academic Press, San Diego, CA, pp. 1157–1168.

Swor, T.M., Whittenburg, J.L., Chaffin, M.K., 2009. Ivermectin toxicosis in three adult horses. J. Am. Vet. Med. Assoc. 235, 558–562.

Teare, J.A., Bush, M., 1983. Toxicity and efficacy of ivermectin in chelonians. J. Am. Vet. Med. Assoc. 183, 1195–1197.

Toutain, P.L., Chapman, M., Galtier, P., Alvinerie, M., 1988. Kinetic and insecticidal properties of ivermectin residues in the milk of dairy cows. J. Vet. Pharmacol. Ther. 11, 288–291.

Toutain, P.L., Upson, D.W., Terhune, T.N., McKenzie, M.E., 1997. Comparative pharmacokinetics of doramectin and ivermectin in cattle. Vet. Parasitol. 72, 3–8.

Trailovic, S.M., Nedelijovic, J.T., 2011. Central and peripheral neurotoxic effects of ivermectin in rats. J. Vet. Med. Sci. 73 (2), 591–599.

Tranquilli, W.J., Paul, A.J., Seward, R.L., et al., 1987. Response to phystostigmore administration on collie dogs exhibiting ivermectin toxicosis. J. Vet. Pharmacol. Ther. 10, 96–100.

Tway, P.C., Woods, J.S., Downing, G.V., 1981. Determination of ivermectin in cattle and sheep tissue using high performance liquid chromatography with fluorescence detection. J. Agric. Food Chem. 29, 1059–1063.

Wise, L.D., Allen, H.L., Hoe, C.M.L., et al., 1997. Developmental neurotoxicity evaluation of the avermectin pesticide, emamectin benzoate, in Sprague-Dawley rats. Neurotoxicol. Teratol. 19, 315–326.

FURTHER READING

Easby, S.M., 1984. Ivermectin in the dog. Vet. Rec. 115, 45.

Section VII

Herbicides and Fungicides

Chapter 44

Toxicity of Herbicides

Pawan K. Gupta

INTRODUCTION

Herbicides, also commonly known as weed killers, are chemical substances used to control unwanted plants. They are phytotoxic chemicals used for destroying various weeds or inhibiting their growth. They have variable degrees of specificity. The worldwide consumption of herbicides is almost 48% of the total pesticides usage. The consumption of herbicides in developing countries is low because weed control is mainly done by hand weeding (Gupta, 2004). Early chemicals used as herbicides include sulfuric acid, sodium chlorate, arsenic trioxide, sodium arsenate, and petroleum oils. Iron and copper sulfate or sodium borate were generally difficult to handle and/or toxic, relatively nonspecific, or phytotoxic to the crop as well as the unwanted plant life if not applied at exactly the proper time (Gupta, 2016a,b). During the last few decades, the herbicides have represented the most rapidly growing section of the pesticide industry due in part to (1) movement into monoculture practices and (2) mechanization of agricultural practices because of increased labor costs. The result has been a plethora of chemically diverse structures rivaling the innovative chemistry so as to develop synthetic organic herbicides and biopesticides that are quite selective for specific plants and have low mammalian toxicity. The aim is to protect desirable crops and obtain high yields by selectively eliminating unwanted plant species, thereby reducing the competition for nutrients (Gupta, 2006).

Most of the animal/human health problems that result from exposure to herbicides are due to their improper use or careless disposal of containers (Gupta, 2010a). Very few problems occur when these chemicals are used properly. However, there is increased concern about the effects of herbicides on animal health because of runoff from agricultural applications and entrance into drinking water supply (Gupta, 1986, 1988).

BACKGROUND

The first discovery in the field of selective weed control was the introduction of 2,4-dinitro-*o*-cresol (DNOC) in France in 1933. This is very toxic to mammals and can cause bilateral cataract in humans. In 1934, phenoxy herbicides were developed and 2,4-dichlorophenoxyacetic acid (2,4-D) was introduced (Gupta, 2010b). During World War II, considerable effort was directed toward the development of effective, broad-spectrum herbicides with a view to both increasing food production and finding potential chemical warfare agents (Gupta, 1989). One chemical class of phenoxy derivatives including the acids, salts, amines, and esters represents the first commercially available products evolving from this research in 1946. Some other herbicides used from this class include 4-(2,4-dichlorophenoxy) butyric acid (2,4-DB), 2-(2,4-dichlorophenoxy propionic acid) (dichlorprop), 2-(2-methyl-4-chlorophenoxy) propionic acid (MCPP or mecoprop), and 2-methyl-4-chlorophenoxyacetic acid (MCPA) (Kennepohl et al., 2010). This class of herbicides has been in continuous, extensive, and uninterrupted use since 1947 and is the most widely used family of herbicides. Another chemical class of herbicides deserving particular attention is the bipyridyl group, especially paraquat and diquat. Weidel and Russo first described the structure of paraquat in 1882. In 1933, Michaelis and Hill discovered its redox properties and called the compound methyl viologen. Its herbicidal properties were discovered by ICI in 1955, and it became commercially available in 1962 (Smith, 1997; Lock and Wilks, 2010).

The first urea herbicide, *N*,*N*-dimethyl-*N*′-(4-chlorophenyl)-urea, was introduced in 1952 by DuPont under the common name of monuron. In subsequent years, many more derivatives of this class of compounds have been marketed (Liu, 2010).

Protopyrinogen oxidase (Protox)-inhibiting herbicides have been used since the 1960s and currently represent a relatively large and growing segment of the herbicide

Veterinary Toxicology. DOI: http://dx.doi.org/10.1016/B978-0-12-811410-0.00044-1

market. Nitrofen was the first Protox-inhibiting herbicide to be introduced for commercial use in 1964. This diphenyl ether (DPE) herbicide was eventually recognized as a relatively weak inhibitor of Protox, but it was a lead compound of an entire class of structurally related herbicides that were much more active. Subsequently, several DPE herbicides have been successfully commercialized (Nandihalli et al., 1992; Anderson et al., 1994).

Substituted aniline, an alachlor herbicide, was registered and introduced in 1967 for the preplant or preemergent control of a broad spectrum of grass, sedge and broadleaf weeds (Heydens et al., 2010). Subsequently, inhibitors of aromatic acid biosynthesis herbicides (organic phosphorus) such as glyphosate, broad-spectrum, nonselective, postemergent, systemic herbicide with activity on essentially all annual and perennial plants have been developed. Monsanto discovered the herbicidal properties of glyphosate in 1970, and the first commercial formulation was introduced in 1974 under the Roundup brand name. Other triazine and triazole herbicides have been extensively used in agriculture in the United States and other areas of the world for more than 50 years. The triazines inhibit photosynthesis by blocking photosynthetic electron transport (Gysin and Knuesli, 1960; Steven and Summer, 1991; Breckenridge et al., 2010). Dicamba, which was first registered in the United States in 1967, is another organic (benzoic) acid herbicide that acts by mimicking the effects of auxins (i.e., natural plant growth hormones), causing enhanced but uncontrolled growth rates, alterations in plant function homeostasis and death (Harp, 2010). Another class of synthetic chemical compounds called the imidazolinone herbicides was discovered in the 1970s, with the first US patent awarded in 1980 for imazamethabenzmethyl. New families of herbicides introduced since the 1970s account for increasing shares of use and include bipyridyl (paraquat), bentazon, fenaxalactogen, oxyfluorfen, clomazone, clorpyralid, fluazifop, and norfluorazon. Today, the use of newer compounds that have low toxicity is quite common (Osteen and Padgitt, 2002).

TOXICOKINETICS

Toxicokinetics studies provide important data on the amount of toxicant delivered to a target as well as species-, age- and gender-specific metabolism. Animals are exposed to herbicides of different chemical classes. In general, liver is the primary site for biotransformation and may include activation as well as detoxification reactions through the cytochrome P450-dependent monooxygenase system, the flavin-containing monooxygenase, esterases and a variety of transferases, most notably the glutathione (GSH) *S*-transferases (Hodgson and Meyer, 1997).

2,4-D is the most extensively studied phenoxy acid derivative herbicide. Absorption of 2,4-D occurs rapidly from the gastrointestinal (GI) tract, and peak levels are reached in 10 min to 24 h depending on species, dose and chemical form. Following oral exposure to 2,4-D, plasma half-life ranges from 3.5 to 18 h. Dermal absorption was reported to occur rapidly but was usually less than 6%. The compound is protein bound in vivo and is rapidly distributed to the liver, kidneys, lung and brain. 2,4-D has also been reported to cross the placental barrier in laboratory animals and pigs. 2,4-D is not metabolized to reactive intermediates, does not accumulate in tissues and is excreted predominantly as the parent compound in urine. However, the rate of excretion via urine is inversely proportional to dose. 2,4-D has been detected in the milk of lactating rats dosed with 2,4-D. The salts and esters of 2,4-D undergo acid and/or enzymatic hydrolysis to form 2,4-D acid, and small amounts may be conjugated with glycine or taurine. Excretion can be markedly enhanced by ion trapping using alkaline agents because most of these herbicides are organic acids (Erne, 1966a,b; Pelletier et al., 1989; Kennepohl et al., 2010).

Another organic acid herbicide, dicamba, is rapidly and nonselectively distributed to most of the organs; however, dermal absorption is minimal. Ninety percent of excretion is through urine, and a small amount is excreted in feces. Dicamba is mostly unmetabolized but may be conjugated with glucuronic acid or glycine. Elimination occurs rapidly, and there is no evidence of bioaccumulation in the mammalian system (Harp, 2010).

Bipyridyl derivative paraquat is rapidly but incompletely absorbed from the GI tract of laboratory animals and humans, with plasma concentration of 30–90 min, and it is poorly absorbed through contact with skin. It has been reported that dogs absorb more paraquat than do rats, resulting in greater susceptibility of dogs toward paraquat toxicity (Lock and Wilks, 2010). Paraquat is very poorly metabolized, and bulk is excreted unchanged in the urine and feces. The transport mechanism for organic cations in renal proximal tubular cells is not fully understood; however, two membrane proteins, organic cation transporter 1 (OCT1) and organic cation transporter 2 (OCT2), have been isolated from rat kidney. OCT1, located at the basolateral membrane, transports tetraethylammonium, and this can be inhibited by other organic cations such as quinine. OCT2 stimulates the uptake of tetraethylammonium, and this can be markedly inhibited by cimetidine. The transport of paraquat can be blocked by the addition of the divalent cation quinine, cimetidine and, to a lesser extent, tetraethylammonium, suggesting that paraquat may be transported by both transport systems, an electro neutral organic cation/H^+ exchange and P-glycoprotein (Chan et al., 1998). It was found that the hMATE1-mediated transport of agmatine was inhibited by paraquat, which indicates the involvement of MATE-1 (multidrug and toxin extrusion) in paraquat renal transport (Winter et al., 2011). It is clear that paraquat can enter a renal cell via OCT2 and, to a lesser extent, OCT1 and then be transported out of the cell by MATE-1. However, whether MATE-2k can transport paraquat is not known (Chan et al., 1998; Lock and Wilks, 2010; Winter et al., 2011). A schematic representation of the proposed transport systems for paraquat across renal tubular cells is shown in Figs. 44.1 and 44.2.

Unlike paraquat, diquat does not accumulate in the lungs; however, it is observed in liver, kidney, plasma and adrenal gland. Diquat does not enter the brain (Rose et al., 1976). Following oral administration, 90%–98% of the dose is eliminated via the urine (Daniel and Gage, 1966). Metabolism studies indicate some unidentified metabolites of diquat in the urine of rabbits and guinea pigs. In rats, diquat monopyridone has been identified in the feces, at approximately 5% of an oral dose, whereas diquat–dipyridone has been detected in urine. These results indicate that diquat is probably metabolized by GI bacteria (JMPR, 1993).

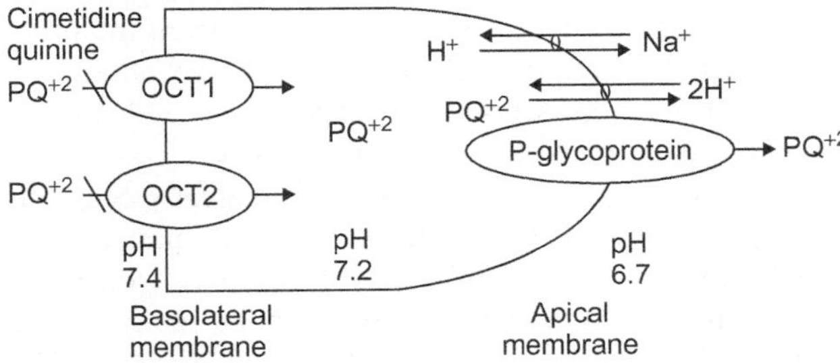

FIGURE 44.1 Schematic representation of the proposed transport systems for paraquat across renal tubular cells. The transporters are OCT1 and OCT2 at the basolateral membrane and P-glycoprotein and the cation/H^+ exchange system at the brush border membrane. *Reproduced with permission from Chan, B.S.H., Lazzaro, V.A., Seale, J.P., Duggin, G.G., 1998. The renal excretory mechanisms and the role of organic cations in modulating the renal handling of paraquat. Pharmacol. Ther. 79, 193–203.*

Ureas and thioureas such as diuron are readily absorbed through the GI tract in rats and dogs and are mainly metabolized by dealkalization of the urea methyl groups. The predominant metabolite of diuron in urine is *N*-(3,4-dichlorophenyl)-urea. Diuron is partially excreted unchanged in feces and urine. The storage of diuron does not occur in tissues (Boehme and Ernst, 1965; Hodge et al., 1967; Liu, 2010).

Organophosphorus herbicides such as glyphosate and glufosinate are poorly absorbed both orally and via the dermal route. There is rapid elimination, and these are not biotransformed and do not accumulate in tissues. More than 70% of an orally administered dose of glyphosate is rapidly eliminated through feces and 20% through urine. The main metabolite of glyphosate is aminomethylphosphonic acid (AMPA); AMPA is of no greater toxicological concern than its parent compound (JMPR, 2004).

The proton class of oxidase inhibitor herbicides is either not readily absorbed or is rapidly degraded by metabolism and/or excreted. In mammals, there are remarkable species differences in the levels of porphyrin accumulation resulting from exposure to Protox inhibitors. There is no bioaccumulation risk to animals. The carboxyester group of the triazolinone herbicide carfentrazone ethyl is initially metabolized to a carboxylic acid group. Other metabolites identified in rats and lactating goats include hydroxymethylpropionic acid and cinnamic acid derivatives, which are further metabolized to yield a benzoic acid derivative (Aizawa and Brown, 1999).

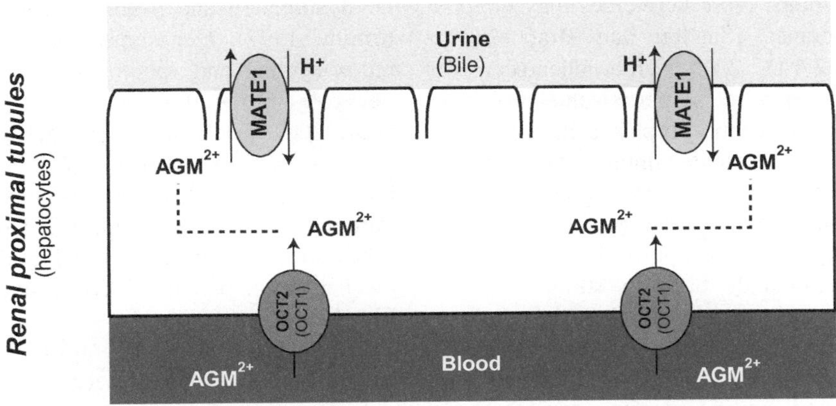

FIGURE 44.2 Proposed mechanism of agmatine transport in tissues (i.e., kidney and liver) widely recognized to express OCT1, OCT2 and MATE-1. Organic cation transporter (OCT) 1 and 2 mediate the facilitated influx transport of organic cations at the basolateral membrane of hepatocytes and renal proximal tubule cells, respectively. The multidrug and toxic compound extrusion (MATE) transporter 1, an H^+/cation antiporter, is critical in the efflux elimination of various organic cations from the brush border and canalicular membrane of the kidney and liver, respectively. (Descriptions in parentheses refer to equivalent structures in the liver.) *Reproduced with permission from Winter, T.N., Elmquist, W.F., Fairbanks, C.A., 2011. OCT2 and MATE1 provide bidirectional agmatine transport. Mol. Pharm. 8, 133–142.*

Substituted anilines are well absorbed in rats orally. The dermal penetration in monkeys is relatively slow. The metabolism of alachlor in rats is complex due to extensive biliary excretion, intestinal microbial metabolism and enterohepatic circulation of metabolites. The main routes of excretion are urine and feces, and nearly 90% of the dose is eliminated in 10 days. Dimethenamid, an amide derivative, is slowly but well absorbed after oral administration (90% in rats) and is extensively metabolized in rats. The maximum concentration in blood is not achieved until approximately 72 h. Excretion is primarily via bile. By 168 h after treatment, an average of 90% of the administered dose is eliminated. In rats, the triazolopyrimidine compounds are rapidly absorbed and urinary elimination is rapid, with half-lives ranging from 6 to 12 h. Excretion is mainly through urine, and small amounts are excreted in feces.

MECHANISM OF ACTION

There are a number of biochemical changes or free radical-mediated processes; some may also be produced by other mechanisms that have been used to assess tissue injury. For example, the loss of tissue GSH may reflect alkylation reactions, not oxidation. Furthermore, some free radical-mediated changes that may cause injury are also the result of injury. In most situations, it is difficult to pinpoint the exact mechanism of action. The mechanism of action of phenoxy derivatives, triazines, triazolopyrimidines, imidazolinones, dinitroaniline, and many other classes of herbicides is not precisely known. However, phenoxy compounds are known to depress ribonuclease synthesis, uncouple oxidative phosphorylation and increase the number of hepatic peroxisomes. The relationship of these biochemical changes to clinical effect is not clear. In dogs, these herbicides may directly affect muscle membranes (Sandhu and Brar, 2000). Herbicides such as 2,4-D, 2,4,5-trichlorophenoxyacetic acid (2,4,5-T) and dicamba act as peroxisome proliferators. Oxadiazinon causes hepatic porphyria in both mice and rats. The phenyl urea herbicides linuron and monuron are rodent liver carcinogens. Chloroacetanilide and metolachlor have shown weak hepatocarcinogenicity in female rats and are nongenotoxic, suggesting a tumor-promoting action. The dinitro compounds markedly stimulate respiration while simultaneously impairing adenosine triphosphate synthesis. The main toxic action is uncoupling of oxidative phosphorylation, converting all cellular energy in the form of heat and causing extreme hyperthermia. In addition, the gut flora in ruminants is able to further reduce the dinitro compounds to diamine metabolites, which are capable of inducing methemoglobinemia.

The available information on substituted anilines indicates that there is a nongenotoxic mechanism of action and lack of relevance to humans for the nasal turbinate, stomach and/or thyroid oncogenic effects produced in rats. The data support grouping of alachlor, acetochlor, and butachlor with respect to a common mechanism of toxicity for nasal turbinate and thyroid tumors, and grouping of alachlor and butachlor for stomach tumors (Heydens et al., 2010).

The mechanism of action of paraquat and diquat is very similar at the molecular level and involves cyclic reduction–oxidation reactions, which produce reactive oxygen species and depletion of nicotinamide adenine dinucleotide phosphate hydrogen (NADPH). However, the critical target organ differs for the two compounds, so the mammalian toxicity is quite different. Although both herbicides affect kidneys, paraquat is selectively taken up in the lungs. Paraquat causes pulmonary lesions as a result of type I and type II pneumocytosis. The primary event in the mechanism of toxicity within cells is paraquat's ability to undergo a single electron reduction from the cation to form a free radical that is stable in the absence of oxygen. If oxygen is present, a concomitant reduction of oxygen takes place to form superoxide anion (O_2^-). Superoxide radical, in turn, is nonenzymatically converted to singlet oxygen, which attacks polyunsaturated lipids associated with cell membranes to form lipid hydroperoxides. Lipid hydroperoxides are normally converted to nontoxic lipid alcohols by the selenium-containing GSH-dependent enzyme, GSH peroxidase. Selenium deficiency, deficiency of GSH, or excess lipid hydroperoxides allows the lipid hydroperoxides to form lipid-free radicals. Lipid hydroperoxides are unstable in the presence of trace amounts of transition metal ions and decompose to free radicals, which in turn cause further peroxidation of polyunsaturated lipid in a process that is slowed by vitamin E. Peroxidation of the membranes could in turn cause cellular dysfunction and hence lead to cell damage or death (Smith, 1997). Genes associated with oxidative stress, redox cycling and apoptosis have been shown to play a key role in the development of lung fibrosis (Tomita et al., 2007; Lock and Wilks, 2010). The neurotoxicity of paraquat is under debate (Lock and Wilks, 2010), but its involvement in neurodegenerative diseases like Parkinson's is well established (Jones et al., 2014). A schematic diagram incorporating these elements of the mechanism of paraquat-induced lung toxicity is shown in Fig. 44.3.

The mechanism of action of diquat differs somewhat from that of paraquat because it undergoes alternate reduction followed by reoxidation—a process known as redox recycling. Like paraquat, diquat can redox cycle, with the major difference being that diquat can more readily accept an electron than can paraquat (Gage, 1968). The major target organs are the GI tract, the liver and the kidneys. Unlike paraquat, diquat shows no special

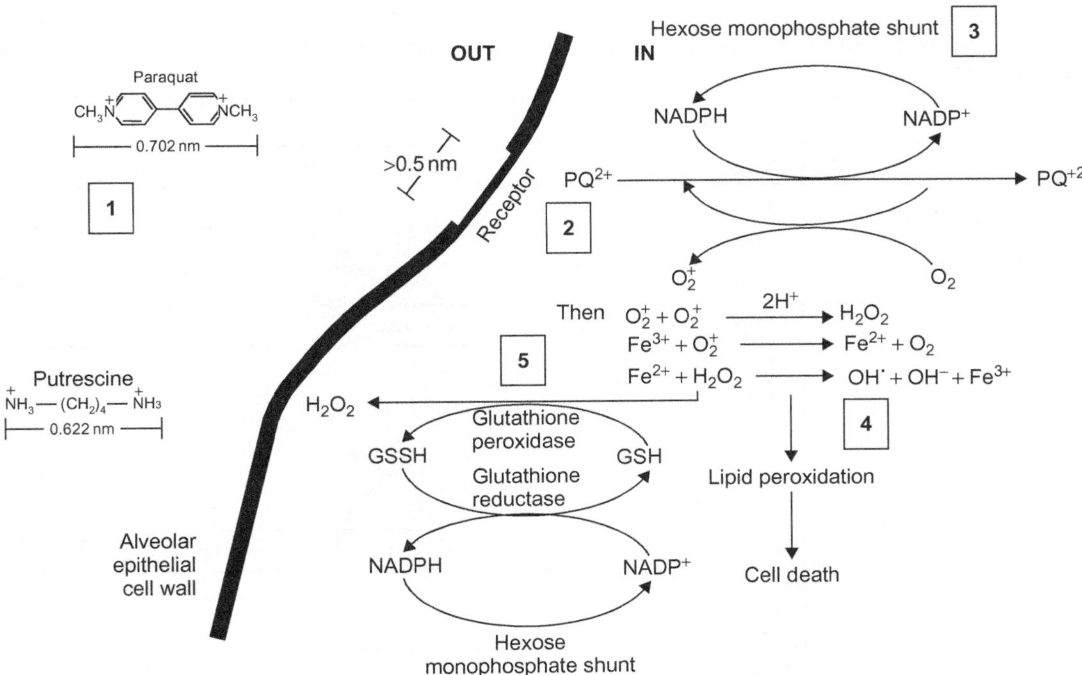

FIGURE 44.3 Schematic representation of mechanism of toxicity of paraquat. (1) Structure of paraquat and putrescine; (2) putative accumulation receptor; (3) redox cycling of paraquat utilizing NADPH; (4) formation of hydroxyl radical (OH•) leading to lipid peroxidation; and (5) detoxication of H_2O_2 via GSH reductase peroxidase couple, utilizing NADPH. *Reproduced with permission from Smith, L.L., 1997. Paraquat. In: Sipes, I.G., McQueen, C.A., Gandolfi, A.J. (Eds.), Comprehensive Toxicology: Toxicology of the Respiratory System, vol. 8. Pergamon, New York, NY, pp. 581–589.*

affinity for the lung and does not appear to involve the same mechanism that selectively concentrates paraquat in the lung (Rose and Smith, 1977).

Glyphosate, a member of the phosphonomethyl amino acid group, selectively inhibits the enzyme 5-enolpyruvoylshikimate 3-phosphate synthetase. The enzyme plays a key role in the biosynthesis of the intermediate, chorismate, which is necessary for the synthesis of the essential amino acids phenylalanine, tyrosine and tryptophan. This aromatic amino acid biosynthesis pathway is found in plants as well as in fungi and bacteria but not in insects, birds, fish, mammals and humans, thus providing a specific selective toxicity to plant species (Franz et al., 1997).

TOXICITY

More than 200 active ingredients are used as herbicides; however, some are believed to be obsolete or have been discontinued. Of these, several have been evaluated for their toxic potential, and acceptable daily intake has been recommended by the Joint Meeting on Pesticide Residues (IPCS, 2002). In general, with a few exceptions, most of the newly developed chemicals have a low order of toxicity to mammals. However, there is increasing experimental and anecdotal evidence that exposure to herbicides also affects at least some form of development and/or reproduction in one or more species of animals. Some herbicides have been associated with birth defects in humans. For example, 2,4-D in combination with 2,4,5-T or dioxin, oryzalin, butiphos, picloram, Silvex (2-(2,4,5-trichlorophenoxy) propionic acid) and TCDD (2,3,7,8-tetrachlorodibenzo-*p*-dioxin) are known to cause reproductive problems/malformations in humans. A non-exhaustive list of herbicides that cause developmental toxicity in experimental animals is presented in Table 44.1.

Inorganic Herbicides and Organic Arsenicals

Substances such as sodium arsenite, arsenic trioxide, sodium chlorate, ammonium sulfamate and borax were formerly used on a large scale. The disadvantage of such herbicides from an agricultural standpoint is that they are nonselective; thus, their use has declined due to the availability of better and selective organic preparations (Marrs, 2004; Gupta, 2016a,b).

Phenoxy Acid Derivatives

This class of herbicides includes 2,4-D, 2,4,5-T, 2,4-DB, dalapon, dichlorprop or 2,4-DP, mecoprop or MCPP, MCPA and Silvex. Some of the phenoxy derivatives are

TABLE 44.1 Nonexhaustive List of Herbicides That Are Known to Cause Developmental Toxicity in Experimental Animals (Gupta, 2017)

Chemical	Malformations
Atrazine	Disruption of ovarian cycle and induced repetitive pseudopregnancy (rats, at high doses)
Buturon	Cleft palate, increased fetal mortality (mice)
Butiphos	Teratogenic (rabbit)
Chloridazon	Malformations
Chlorpropham	Malformations or other developmental toxicity (mice)
Cynazine	Malformations such as cyclopia and diaphragmatic hernia (rabbits). Skeletal variations in rats
2,4-D[a], 2,4,5-T[a] alone or in combination	Malformations such as cleft palate, hydronephrosis, teratogenic (mice, rats)
Dichlorprop	Teratogenic (mice), affects postnatal behavior (rats)
Dinoseb[b]	Multiple defects (mice, rabbits)
Dinoterb	Skeletal malformations (rats), skeletal, jaw, head and visceral (rabbits)
Linuron	Malformations (rats)
Mecoprop	Malformations (mice)
Monolinuron	Cleft palate (mice)
MCPA	Teratogenic and embryotoxic (rats), teratogenic (mice)
Prometryn	Head, limbs and tail defects (rat)
Propachlor	Slightly teratogenic (rats)
Nitrofen[b]	Malformations (mice, rats, hamsters)
Silvex	Teratogenic (mice)
TCDD[a]	Malformations/teratogenic (fetotoxicity in chicken, rats, mice, rabbits, guinea pigs, hamsters and monkeys)
Tridiphane	Malformations such as cleft palate (mice), skeletal variations (rats)

[a]*TCDD is a common contaminant of 2,4-D and 2,4,5-T.*
[b]*Obsolete.*

no longer agents of choice because of the formation of chlorinated dibenzofurans and dibenzodioxins, particularly TCDD, as a consequence of poorly monitored manufacturing practices. Some formulations of 2,4,5-T contain dioxin contaminants that increase the toxicity of technical-grade herbicides and therefore the safe use of phenoxy herbicides has been questioned. Reports indicate the occurrence of three rare forms of cancer (Hodgkin's disease, soft tissue carcinoma, and non-Hodgkin's lymphoma) in workers exposed to these herbicides contaminated with dioxins (Kennepohl et al., 2010). However, 2,4-D contains less than the quantitation limits of dioxins set by regulatory agencies (e.g., USEPA). 2,4-D is permitted for use in many countries throughout the world, including the United States and Canada.

As a group, these are essentially nontoxic, and acute oral/dermal exposure to phenoxy herbicides is slightly to moderately hazardous in normal use. Dermal irritation in rabbits is considered slight for the acid form of 2,4-D and minimal for the salt and ester forms. Eye irritation in rabbits, on the other hand, is severe for the acid and salt forms, but it is minimal for the ester. The oral LD_{50} for phenoxy acid derivatives in dogs is 100–800 mg/kg body weight (BW). The dog is more sensitive and may develop myotonia, ataxia, posterior weakness, vomiting, bloody diarrhea and metabolic acidosis because of difficulty in the renal elimination of such organic acids (Gehring et al., 1976). Kidney effects consisting of reduced cytoplasmic eosinophilia of the epithelial cells lining and some convoluted tubules have been reported in dog. 2,4-D does not produce any testicular/ovarian damage or induce any abnormal reproductive disorders. However, some of the molecules of this class have been reported to cause teratogenic effects in animals at maternally toxic doses (Table 44.1) and reproductive problems in humans (Gupta, 2017). The group of compounds neither induces adverse effects in the nervous and immune systems nor has any potential to induce cancer or mutagenicity in laboratory animals. 2,4-D was found to be noncarcinogenic to rats, mice and dogs. Dogs are the most sensitive animals, whereas sheep, cattle and poultry are less sensitive (Yano et al., 1991a,b; Munro et al., 1992; Kennepohl et al., 2010).

In dogs and pigs, GI signs of toxicity include anorexia, rumen atony, diarrhea, ulceration of oral mucosa, bloat and rumen stasis in cattle and vomiting, diarrhea, salivation, etc. Neuromuscular signs include depression and muscular weakness in cattle and ataxia, posterior weakness (particularly the pelvic limbs) and periodic clonic spasms (at high doses) in dogs. Silvex is unusual for this group because it is very toxic and small doses (2–6 mg/kg BW) may cause ill effects in dogs (Sandhu and Brar, 2000).

Bipyridyl Derivatives

This chemical class of herbicides includes paraquat (1,1′-dimethyl-4,4′-bipyridylium dichloride) and diquat (1,1′-ethylene-2,2′-bipyridylium dibromide). Paraquat is usually formulated as dichloride salt (also known as methyl viologen). The bis(methyl sulfate) salt is no longer commercialized. Paraquat is nonselective and is a fast-acting contact herbicide. This compound is one of the most toxic of the commonly used herbicides, and the toxicity varies in different animals depending on the formulation and species used. The toxic doses (oral LD_{50}) of paraquat and diquat in rats are 150 and 231 mg/kg BW, respectively, and this class of herbicides is classified as moderately hazardous. Paraquat is a skin and eye irritant but not a skin sensitizer in animals. Mice are less sensitive than rats to orally administered paraquat, whereas guinea pigs, cats, monkeys and rabbits are more sensitive (Murray and Gibson, 1972; Bus et al., 1976a,b; Nagata et al., 1992; Lorgue et al., 1996; JMPR, 2003; Lock and Wilks, 2010). Cattle and sheep are more sensitive than other species.

As indicated previously, paraquat and diquat have somewhat different mechanisms of action. Diquat exerts most of its harmful effects in the GI tract. The major cause of death after exposure to paraquat is lung damage. However, rabbits do not show signs of respiratory distress. Immediate toxic effects include convulsions or depression and incoordination, gastroenteritis and, finally, difficult respiration due to pulmonary edema and alveolar fibrosis (2–7 days). Animals that survive the first few days develop dehydration, pallor or cyanosis, tachycardia, tachypnea, harsh respiratory sounds and emphysema or pneumomediastinum.

Upon long-term exposure, there is progressive pulmonary fibrosis and increased respiratory distress. The morphological changes seen in animals include degeneration and vacuolization of pneumocytes, damage to type I and type II alveolar epithelial cells, destruction of the epithelial membranes and proliferation of fibrotic cells. The animals die as a consequence of reduced gas exchange and the development of severe hypoxia.

Gross lesions include pulmonary congestion, edema and hemorrhages. Lingual ulcers may be seen. Other findings include failure of lungs to collapse when chest is opened and areas of hemorrhages, fibrosis and atelectasis. Microscopic lesions include necrosis of type I alveolar epithelial cells followed by progressive alveolar and intestinal fibrosis and alveolar emphysema. Renal proximal tubular degeneration and moderate centrilobular hepatic degeneration may also be seen (Smith, 1997). In mice, paraquat did not readily cross the placenta, whereas in rats it readily crossed the placenta, being detected in fetuses within 30 min of an intravenous injection to pregnant rats (Lock and Wilks, 2010). It has neither carcinogenic nor mutagenic potential; however, high doses injected into pregnant rats and mice on various days of gestation may cause significant maternal toxicity but do not produce teratogenic effects (Bus and Gibson, 1975).

Diquat is formulated as dibromide salt and is slightly less toxic to dogs than is paraquat. After chronic exposure, the major target organs are the GI tract, the liver and the kidneys; however, lungs are not affected (Hayes, 1982). The presence of cataracts in both dogs and rats has been observed. Similar signs of toxicity have been seen in mice, guinea pigs, rabbits, dogs, and monkeys. Diquat has no effect on fertility, is not teratogenic and produces fetotoxicity only at doses that are maternally toxic. In a multigeneration study, at high doses, cataracts were observed in rats (FAO/WHO, 1993).

Ureas and Thioureas

The ureas and thioureas (polyureas) are available under different names, such as diuron, fluometuron, isoproturon, linuron, buturon, chlorbromuron, chlortoluron, chloroxuron, difenoxuron, fenuron, methiuron, metobromuron, metoxuron, monuron, neburon, parafluron, siduron, tebuthiuron, tetrafluron and thidiazuron.

In general, polyureas have low acute toxicity and are unlikely to present any hazard in normal use, with the exception of tebuthiuron, which may be slightly hazardous.

Diuron and monuron are potent inducers of hepatic metabolizing enzymes compared to those polyurea herbicides with one or no halogen substitutions (chlortoluron and isoproturon). Male rats are more sensitive than females to the enzyme-inducing activity of diuron, and this can lead to detoxication of EPN and O-demethylation of *p*-nitro anisole. N-demethylation of aminopyrine increases for 1–3 weeks and then returns to normal (Hodgson and Meyer, 1997). Recovery from diuron intoxication is quick (within 72 h), and no signs of skin irritation or dermal sensitization have been reported in guinea pigs. Linuron in sheep causes erythrocytosis and leukocytosis with hypohemoglobinemia and hypoproteinemia, hematuria and ataxia, enteritis, degeneration of the liver and muscular dystrophy (Liu, 2010). In chickens, it leads to loss of weight, dyspnea, cyanosis and diarrhea. It is nontoxic to fish (Lorgue et al., 1996). Fluometuron is less toxic than diuron. In sheep, depression, salivation, grinding of teeth, chewing movements of the jaws, mydriasis, dyspnea, incoordination of movements and drowsiness are commonly seen. On histopathology, severe congestion of red pulp with corresponding atrophy of the white pulp of the spleen and depletion of the lymphocyte elements have been reported (Mehmood et al., 1995). The acute LD_{50} of isoproturon in rats is similar to that of diuron and does not produce any overt signs of toxicity, except at very high doses. A single oral dose of isoproturon in mice may produce some neurotoxic effects at very high doses and may reduce spontaneous and forced locomotor activity (Sarkar and Gupta, 1993a,b).

Polyurea herbicides have been suspected to have some mutagenic effects but do not have carcinogenic potential (Liu, 2010). In general, the compounds do not cause developmental toxicity; however, buturon, linuron and monolinuron are known to cause some teratogenic abnormalities in experimental animals (Table 44.1). Isoproturon has been reported to cause maturational malformation of sperm and decreased spermatogenesis in rats (Liu, 2010).

Phosphonomethyl Amino Acids or Inhibitors of Aromatic Acid Biosynthesis

Two organophosphorus compounds, glyphosate (Roundup and Vision; *N*-(phosphonomethyl) glycine) and glufosinate (Basta; *N*-(phosphonomethyl)homoalanine), are broad-spectrum, nonselective systemic herbicides. Although they exist as free acids, due to their low solubility, they are marketed as the isopropyl amine or trimethylsulfonium salts of glyphosate and the ammonium salt of glufosinate.

Glyphosate has low acute oral toxicity in mice and rats and is unlikely to pose acute hazard in normal use. The LD_{50} of trimethylsulfonium salt is 750 mg/kg BW. The animals most affected are cattle, sheep and dogs. Dogs and cats show eye, skin and upper respiratory tract signs when exposed during or subsequent to an application to weeds or grass. Nausea, vomiting, staggering and hind leg weakness have been reported in dogs and cats that were exposed to fresh chemical on treated foliage (Susan, 2003). Glyphosate is not a dermal irritant and does not induce photosensitization; and formulations can cause severe occupational contact dermatitis. Glyphosate is an ocular irritant in the rabbit and human, with minor to moderate conjunctival irritation and slight iritis that usually disappears within 48 h after exposure (Acquavella et al., 1999; JMPR, 2004). Formulations of glyphosate can cause intoxication in humans, which may be due to the presence of surfactants such as polyoxyethyleneamine. This class of surfactants has been associated with hemolysis and with GI tract and central nervous system (CNS) effects (Talbot et al., 1991). There is no evidence of mutagenic or carcinogenic potential of glyphosate. Several investigations do indicate the teratogenicity and reproductive toxicity of glyphosate. However, there is further need to conduct such studies and other parameters involving risk assessment of these compounds (Antoniou et al., 2012). It does not have adverse effects on reproductive performance in animals, except at very high doses maternal toxicity has been reported (JMPR, 2004). The testicular seminiferous tubules of rats treated with glyphosate indicated decreased epithelium lengths. The commercial formulation of glyphosate (Roundup, Monsanto Co.) is a potent endocrine disruptor in vivo and causes disturbances in the reproductive development of rats (Romano et al., 2010) and may lead to human breast cancer cells growth via estrogen receptors (Thongprakaisang et al., 2013).

The acute oral toxicity of glufosinate is low, and glufosinate is slightly more hazardous than glyphosate. Common signs of toxicity include CNS excitation and hypothermia in animals (Ebert et al., 1990; Hack et al., 1994). Glufosinate ammonium formulation has been involved in a number of poisoning cases (cardiovascular and CNS adverse effects) possibly due to surfactant-induced penetration into the CNS (Watanabe and Sano, 1998). The compound is not considered to be mutagenic, teratogenic, or carcinogenic, except in whole-embryo culture. Teratogenic effects in mice have been observed, resulting in apoptosis in the neuroepithelium of the developing embryo (Watanabe, 1997).

Protoporphyrinogen Oxidase Inhibitors

In the past, the Protox-inhibiting herbicides were often termed "DPE-type herbicides," and almost all of the Protox inhibitors were DPEs. This nomenclature led to confusion concerning the classification of these herbicides because other DPE herbicides have an entirely different molecular site of action (i.e., inhibition of acetyl-CoA carboxylase). Since then, many other structurally related Protox inhibitors have been commercialized. In general, the newer products are more potent Protox inhibitors, resulting in lower application rates than those of the older herbicides of this class. Some of them appear to be analogs of the substrate or a substrate/product transition state of the enzyme (Reddy et al., 1998; Dayan and Duke, 2010).

After the first generation of Protox inhibitors (with the exception of oxadiazon), which were based on the DPE, numerous other nonoxygen-bridged compounds (non-DPE Protox inhibitors) with the same site of action (carfentrazone, JV 485 and oxadiargyl) were commercialized (Dayan and Duke, 2010). Protox inhibitors have little acute toxicity and are unlikely to pose any acute hazard in normal use. These compounds increase the porphyrin levels in animals when administered orally, and the porphyrin levels return to normal within a few days. Rats and mice are sensitive and variegate porphyria-like symptoms can be generated in mice with high doses of Protox inhibitors. The majority of these compounds are neither mutagenic nor carcinogenic in nature, and the developmental toxicity correlates with Protox accumulation. Most Protox inhibitors, except bifenox and oxyfluorfen, are non- to moderately toxic to aquatic wildlife (Dayan and Duke, 2010). It has been reported in rats that prenatal exposure to sulfentrazone leads to neurodevelopmental effects (de Castro et al., 2007).

Triazines and Triazoles

These herbicides are inhibitors of photosynthesis and include both the asymmetrical and the symmetrical triazines. Examples of symmetrical triazines are chloro-*S*-triazines (atrazine, simazine, propazine, terbuthylazine and cyanazine); the thiomethyl-*S*-triazines (ametryn, prometryn and terbutryn), and the methoxy-*S*-triazine (prometon) (Breckenridge et al., 2010). The commonly used asymmetrical triazine is metribuzin.

These herbicides have low oral toxicity and are unlikely to pose acute hazards in normal use, except for ametryn and metribuzin, which may be slightly to moderately hazardous. They are generally neither irritants to the skin or eye nor skin sensitizers. The exceptions are atrazine, which is a skin sensitizer in guinea pigs, and cyanazine, which is toxic by the oral route. However, sensitivity of sheep and cattle to these herbicides is appreciably high. The main symptoms are anorexia, hemotoxia, hypothermia, locomotor disturbances, irritability, tachypnea and hypersensitivity (Sandhu and Brar, 2000). Doses of 500 mg/kg of simazine or 30 mg/kg atrazine for 30–60 days are lethal to sheep. Deaths have been reported in sheep and horses grazing triazine-treated pasture 1–7 days after spraying. Cumulative effects are not seen. Metribuzin is slightly more toxic than simazine, but it does not produce any harmful effects in dogs fed at 100 ppm in the diet. Simazine is excreted in milk, so it is a public health concern (Susan, 2003). Atrazine is more toxic to rats but comparatively less toxic to sheep and cattle than is simazine. These herbicides are classified as liver microsomal enzyme inducers and are converted to *N*-dealkylated derivatives. In contrast to simazine, it is not excreted in milk. Triazines seem to have no potential to be mutagenic or to produce carcinogenicity in animals. However, feeding of very high levels of some triazines resulted in mammary tumors in rats. Terbutryn also caused thyroid and liver tumors in female rats (Breckenridge et al., 2010). The exception is cyanazine, which is more acutely toxic, weak mutagenic, and results in developmental toxicity, presumably because of the presence of cyano moiety (Hodgson and Meyer, 1997).

Substituted Anilines

Substituted anilines are used as systemic herbicides. The commonly used herbicides are alachlor, acetochlor, butachlor, metolachlor and propachlor.

This class of herbicides is slightly hazardous, except butachlor, which is not likely to pose any hazard. The compounds are nonirritant to eyes, slight to moderate skin irritant, and produce skin sensitization in guinea pigs. Lower doses in rats and dogs do not produce any adverse effects; however, long-term exposure in dogs causes hepatotoxicity and splenic effects. The ocular lesions (progressive uveal degenerative syndrome) produced by alachlor are considered to be unique to the Long–Evans rat because the response has not been observed in other strains of rats, mice, or dogs. At high oral doses, it may lead to maternal and fetal toxicity but may not cause any adverse effect on reproduction. It is neither teratogenic nor produces any microbial genotoxicity. Alachlor has the potential to produce thyroid tumors and adenocarcinomas of the stomach and nasal turbinates of Long–Evans rats and in the lungs (bronchoalveolar) of CD-1 mice at high doses. It is considered to be a human carcinogen (Ahrens, 1994; Monsanto, 1997a,b; Heydens et al., 2010).

Long-term exposure of acetochlor to rats has no adverse effects on reproductive performance. Acetochlor is converted into a rat-specific metabolite that may be related to the nasal and thyroid tumors, thus posing no genetic or carcinogenic hazard to humans (Ashby et al., 1996). Butachlor does not adversely affect reproductive performance or pup survival. It is nongenotoxic. Butachlor induced multiple tumors in SD rats but not in F344 rats or CD-1 mice (Heydens et al., 2010). Metolachlor can increase the incidence of liver tumors in rats and has been classified as a possible human carcinogen (Monsanto, 1991; Wilson and Takei, 1999; Heydens et al., 2010).

Compared to other substituted anilines, propachlor is severely irritating to the eye and slightly irritating to the skin. Propachlor produces skin sensitization in guinea pigs. In rats, high doses of propachlor produce erosion, ulceration, and hyperplasia of the gastric mucosa; herniated mucosal glands in the pyloric region of the stomach; hypertrophy; and necrosis of the liver. In dogs, there is poor diet palatability, which results in weight loss and poor consumption of food. Propachlor may produce slight developmental or adverse reproductive effects (Table 44.1). It is not genotoxic or clastogenic in mammals. However, there is evidence that it produces benign hepatic tumors in male mice (Heydens et al., 2010). The previously discussed data support grouping alachlor, acetochlor and butachlor based on a common mechanism of toxicity for evaluation of risk assessment to humans and animals (Heydens et al., 2010).

Amides and Acetamides

The commonly used amides and acetamides include bensulide, dimethenamid-P and propanil and are slightly to moderately hazardous in normal use. Dimethenamid is a racemic mixture of the M and P stereoisomers, whereas P isomer has useful herbicidal activity. Both substances produce only mild reversible skin and eye irritation and skin sensitization in guinea pigs. Comparison of racemic dimethenamid with dimethenamid-P indicates that there is little difference in their toxicological profiles. The signs of toxicity in mice, rats and dogs are similar, with reduced BW gain and liver enlargement with induction of liver xenobiotics metabolizing enzyme. There is strong binding to hemoglobin in rats, but this has no relevance to humans. Dimethenamid can reduce fetal BW but is not teratogenic. There is no compound-related mutagenic or carcinogenic potential (JMPR, 2005).

Dinitrophenol Compounds

Several substituted dinitrophenols alone or as salts, such as DNP (2,4-dinitrophenol), DNOC (dinitro-*o*-cresol) and dinoseb (2-(1-methylpropyl)-4,6-dinitro), are used as herbicides. The main source of poisoning in animals is human negligence in removing the preparation if it spills, in disposing of the containers and in preventing animals access to treated fields.

In general, the dinitro compounds are not very water-soluble and are highly hazardous to animals. The oral acute LD_{50} of DNOC in mice, guinea pigs, rabbits, hens, dogs, pigs and goats ranges from 25 to 100 mg/kg BW. In sheep, a dosage of 25 mg/kg/day causes toxicosis in 2−5 days. Clinical signs include fever, dyspnea, acidosis, oliguria, muscular weakness, tachycardia and convulsions followed by coma and death with a rapid onset of rigor mortis. Abortions have been reported in sows. In cattle and ruminants, methemoglobinemia, intravascular hemolysis and hemoproteinemia have been observed. Cataract can occur with chronic dinitrophenol intoxication. Exposure to these compounds may cause yellow staining of skin, conjunctiva, or hair (Lorgue et al., 1996).

Triazolopyrimidine Herbicides

Triazolopyrimidine herbicides include cloransulam-methyl, diclosulam, florasulam, penoxsulam, flumetsulam, metosulam, and pyroxsulam. The generic structure of the triazolopyrimidine herbicides connected to a substituted phenyl ring through a sulfonamide bridge is shown in the second edition of this book.

The acute oral toxicity of triazolopyrimidine herbicides is very low. On repeated exposure, the primary organs are the kidney (rat and mouse), liver (rat, mouse, and dog) and thyroid (rat) (Billington et al., 2010). In dogs, the target organ is eye as compared to other species (Timchalk et al., 1996). No adverse effects on neurotoxicity, reproductive performance and mutagenic abnormalities have been observed. The compound has no carcinogenic potential in humans (EPA, 1997a,b).

Imidazolinones

Imidazolinone herbicides include imazapyr, imazamethabenzmethyl, imazapic, imazethapyr, imazamox, and imazaquin. These are selective broad-spectrum herbicides discovered in the 1970s.

These herbicides are relatively nontoxic. Results from primary eye irritation studies range from no irritation (imazaquin) to slightly irritating (imazamethabenzmethyl) and moderately irritating (imazapic and imazethapyr), showing complete recovery within 7 days postdosing. The rabbit primary irritation study with imazapyr showed irreversible irritation. Toxicological effects of imidazolinone herbicides are slight to moderate skeletal myopathy and/or slight anemia in dogs occurring in the 1-year dietary toxicity studies with three structurally similar imidazolinones (imazapic, imazaquin and imazethapyr). There is no evidence of any adverse effect on reproductive performance and on fetal abnormalities in the rat and the rabbit. Neither mutagenicity nor any carcinogenicity has been reported in either of these species (Hess et al., 2010).

Benzoic Acids

The herbicides in this group include chloramben, dicamba, and naptalam. These have a low order of toxicity.

In practice, dicamba is often combined with other herbicides and is used to control a wide spectrum of weeds. The signs and lesions are similar to those described for the chlorophenoxy acids. Poisoning after normal use has not been reported in domestic animals. Dicamba either alone or combined with another herbicide induced significant levels of apoptosis in mouse preimplantation embryo assay (Greenlee et al., 2004). It is a skin and eye irritant, and high doses may cause neurobehavioral symptoms in rats and rabbits. The compound did not show any adverse effects in a three-generation study in rats (Harp, 2010).

Dicamba induces peroxisomal enzymes in rat liver and causes transcription up-regulation of the peroxisome proliferator-activated receptor. Long-term exposure to dicamba may induce tumors in rats due to its action as a peroxisome proliferator; however, the implications of these findings are not clear and may require further study (Espandiari et al., 1998). Dicamba-induced oxidative stress-mediated cytogenotoxicity has been demonstrated in an in vitro cell model (Gonzalez et al., 2009; Harp, 2010).

Carbamates, Thiocarbamates and Dithiocarbamate Compounds

The compounds in this category include derivatives of carbamic acid (asulam, barban, chlorpropham, chlorbufam, karbutilate and phenmedipham), derivatives of thiocarbamic acid (butylate, cycloate, diallate, EPTC, molinate and triallate) and derivatives of dithiocarbamic acid (metham sodium). These herbicides have low to moderate toxicity in rats and do not pose acute hazards. They are used at low concentrations, and poisoning problems have not been reported. In general, these herbicides do not produce skin or eye irritation. With repeated exposure, there is a possibility of alopecia for some time after ingestion (Lorgue et al., 1996; Hurt et al., 2010).

In ruminants, diallate results in anorexia, ataxia, muscular contractions, exhaustion, prostration, and alopecia in sheep, which is an indication of chronic poisoning. Thiobencarb has induced toxic neuropathies in neonatal and adult laboratory rats. It appears to increase permeability of the blood–brain barrier. The nonspecific lesions include hepatic, renal and pulmonary congestion, enteritis, ascites, and hydrothorax (Susan, 2003).

Others

Bromacil and terbacil are commonly used methyluracil compounds. These compounds can cause mild toxic signs at levels of 50 mg/kg BW in sheep, 250 mg/kg BW in cattle and 500 mg/kg BW in poultry when given daily for 8–10 days. Signs of toxicity include bloat, incoordination, depression and anorexia. Toxic doses of bromacil can be hazardous, especially for sheep, but no field cases of toxicity have been reported.

The nitrile herbicides, ioxynil and bromoxynil, may uncouple and/or inhibit oxidative phosphorylation. Ioxynil, presumably due to its iodine content, causes enlargement of the thyroid gland in the rat (Marrs, 2004). Members of polycyclic alkanoic acids (diclofop, fenoxaprop, fenthiaprop, fluazifop and haloxyfop) have moderately low toxicity, whereas haloxyfop-methyl is an exception, and has high toxicity. They tend to be more toxic if exposure is dermal. The dermal LD_{50} of diclofop in rabbits is only 180 mg/kg (Susan, 2003). Some members of the amide group, such as bensulide and propanil, are used as plant growth regulators, and some of them are more toxic than others. A lethal dose of bensulide for dogs is 200 mg/kg.

The prominent clinical sign is anorexia; other signs and lesions are not definitive and are similar to those of chlorophenoxy acid poisoning. Hemolysis, methemoglobinemia and immunotoxicity have occurred after experimental exposure to propanil (Lorgue et al., 1996). The toxicity of sulfonylureas (chlorsulfuron, sulfometuron, metsulfuron, chloremuron, and kensulfuron) appears to be quite low (Susan, 2003).

A number of substances are used as defoliants in agriculture, including sulfuric acid to destroy potato haulms and two closely related trialkylphosphorothioates (DEF and merphos) to defoliate cotton. A notable feature of the latter is that they produce organophosphate-induced delayed neuropathy in hens (Baron and Johnson, 1964). Chlomequat is used as a growth regulator on fruit trees. The signs of toxicity in experimental animals indicate that it is a partial cholinergic agonist (JMPR, 2000).

ENDOCRINE DISRUPTION

In both males and females, some herbicides affect reproduction through different mechanisms of action of endocrine disruption; exogenous agents interfere with reproduction and the development process. In males, normal reproductive function involves interaction of the hypothalamic-pituitary-testis axis and the thyroid gland. In females, increased concentrations of xenoestrogens may affect ovarian function through the disruption of feedback mechanisms in the hypothalamus-pituitary-gonadal axis (Flaws and Hirshfield, 1997; Bretveld et al., 2006). Herbicides, like other chemicals, may disrupt all stages of hormonal function of the reproductive system. In females, during pregnancy and, to a greater extent, during lactation, a portion of the maternal body burden of these chemicals is transferred to the offspring. For example, herbicides such as linuron produce hypothyroidism (Gupta, in press). The herbicide glyphosate in low nontoxic concentrations caused disruption of the aromatase enzyme in human placental cells in vitro. It reduced the aromatase enzyme activity responsible for the synthesis of estrogens (Richard et al., 2005). A study indicated that male reproductive toxicity of glyphosate is due to the inhibition of a StAR protein and an aromatase enzyme, which caused an in vitro reduction in testosterone and estradiol synthesis. The study further suggested that commercial formulation of glyphosate (glyphosate–Roundup Transorb, Monsanto) is a potent endocrine disruptor in vivo because it caused disturbances in the reproductive development of rats when the exposure was performed during the puberty period (Romano et al., 2010). From various experimental studies, it has been concluded that herbicides can disturb reproduction and developmental processes of both males and females through endocrine signals in organisms indirectly exposed during prenatal or early postnatal life. Such effects during fetal development may be permanent and irreversible.

According to one estimate, eight herbicides (2,4-D, 2,4,5-T, alachlor, amitrole, atrazine, metribuzin, trifluralin and nitrofen) were identified as endocrine disruptors. Most of these were identified accidentally rather than as a result of an exhaustive screening process (Pocar et al., 2003).

TREATMENT

The successful management of herbicide poisoning depends on (1) the clinicians' understanding of the mechanism of herbicide toxicity and applying that understanding to the treatment options, (2) accurate diagnosis and assessment of the severity of intoxication, (3) maintenance of vital body functions and adequate clinical monitoring, (4) minimization of further absorption of the compound, and (5) appropriate use of specific treatment. Treatment is usually symptomatic and supportive. Intravenous fluid should be given to promote diuresis. Toxicity of paraquat is enhanced by selenium/vitamin E deficiency, oxygen, and low tissue GSH peroxidase activity. Therefore, vitamin E and selenium with supportive therapy may be useful in the early stages of paraquat intoxication. Excretion of bipyridyl compounds may be accelerated by forced diuresis induced by mannitol infusion and furosemide administration. Oxygen therapy and fluid therapy are contraindicated (Clark, 1971; Smith et al., 1974). Dinis-Oliveira et al. (2006, 2007, 2008, 2009) experimentally found dexamethasone, sodium salicylate and lysine acetylsalicylate to be an effective treatment for paraquat-induced toxicity. These authors concluded that the antioxidant properties of these agents might be responsible for their effectiveness.

An effective antidote for dinitrophenol compounds is not known. Affected animals should be cooled and sedated to help control hyperthermia. Phenothiazine tranquilizers are contraindicated; however, diazepam can be used to calm the animal. Atropine sulfate, aspirin, and antipyretics should not be used; rather, physical cooling measures such as cool baths or sponging and keeping the animal in a shaded area are advocated. Intravenous administration of large doses of sodium bicarbonate (in carnivores) solutions, parenteral vitamin A, and intense oxygen therapy, where possible, may be useful. If the herbicide is ingested and the animal is alert, an emetic should be administered; if the animal is depressed, gastric lavage should be performed. Treatment with activated charcoal should follow. Dextrose–saline infusions in combination with diuretics and tranquilizers (not barbiturates) are very useful. In ruminants, for methemoglobinemia, methylene blue solution and administration of ascorbic acid are useful (Lorgue et al., 1996).

CONCLUDING REMARKS AND FUTURE DIRECTIONS

Herbicides are routinely used to control noxious plants. Most of these chemicals, particularly the synthetic organic herbicides, are quite selective for specific plants and have low toxicity for mammals; other less selective compounds (e.g., arsenicals, chlorates and dinitrophenols) are more toxic to animals. Most animal health problems including reproduction, which is affected by endocrine disruption, result from exposure to excessive amounts of herbicides because of improper or careless use or disposal of containers. The residue potential for most of these chemicals is low.

REFERENCES

Acquavella, J.F., Weber, J.A., Cullen, M.R., et al., 1999. Human ocular effects from self-reported exposure to roundup herbicides. Hum. Exp. Toxicol. 18, 479–486.

Ahrens, W.H., 1994. Herbicide Handbook of the Weed Society of America. seventh ed. Weed Science Society America, Champaign, IL.

Aizawa, K., Brown, H.M., 1999. Mechanism and degradation of porphyrin biosynthesis inhibitor herbicide. In: Boger, P., Wakbayashi, K. (Eds.), Peroxidizing Herbicides. Spring-Verlag, Berlin, pp. 371–383.

Anderson, R.J., Norris, A.E., Hess, F.D., 1994. Synthetic organic chemicals that act through the porphyrin pathway. Am. Chem. Soc. Symp. Ser. 559, 18–33.

Antoniou, M., Habib, M.E.M., Howard, C.V., et al., 2012. Teratogenic effects of glyphosate-based herbicides: divergence of regulatory decisions from scientific evidence. J. Environ. Anal. Toxicol. S4, 006.

Ashby, J., Kier, L., Wilson, A.G.E., et al., 1996. Evaluation of the potential carcinogenicity and gene toxicity to humans of the herbicide acetochlor. Hum. Exp. Toxicol. 15, 702–735.

Baron, R.L., Johnson, C.H., 1964. Neurological disruption produced in hens by two organophosphate esters. Br. J. Pharmacol. 23, 295–304.

Billington, R., Gehen, S.C., Hanley Jr, T.R., 2010. Toxicology of triazolopyrimidine herbicides. In: Krieger, R. (Ed.), Hayes' Handbook of

Pesticide Toxicology, third ed., vol. 2. Elsevier, San Diego, CA, pp. 1865–1885.

Boehme, C., Ernst, W., 1965. The mechanism of urea–herbicides in the rat: diuron and linuron. Food Cosmet. Toxicol. 3, 797–802 (in German).

Breckenridge, C.B., Eldridge, J.C., Stevens, J.T., Simpkins, J.W., 2010. Symmetric triazine herbicides: a review of regulatory toxicity endpoints. In: Krieger, R. (Ed.), Hayes' Handbook of Pesticide Toxicology, third ed., vol. 2. Elsevier, San Diego, CA, pp. 1711–1723.

Bretveld, R.W., Thomas, C., Scheepers, M.G., et al., 2006. Pesticide exposure: the hormonal function of the female reproductive system disrupted? Reprod. Biol. Endocrinol. 4, 30–43.

Bus, J.S., Gibson, J.E., 1975. Postnatal toxicity of chronically administered paraquat in mice and interactions with oxygen and bromobenzene. Toxicol. Appl. Pharmacol. 33, 461–470.

Bus, J.S., Aust, S.D., Gibson, J.E., 1976a. Paraquat toxicity: proposed mechanism of action involving lipid peroxidation. Environ. Health Perspect. 16, 139–146.

Bus, J.S., Cagen, S.Z., Olgard, M., Gibson, J.E., 1976b. Paraquat toxicity: a mechanism of paraquat toxicity in mice and rats. Toxicol. Appl. Pharmacol. 35, 501–513.

Chan, B.S.H., Lazzaro, V.A., Seale, J.P., Duggin, G.G., 1998. The renal excretory mechanisms and the role of organic cations in modulating the renal handling of paraquat. Pharmacol. Ther. 79, 193–203.

Clark, D.G., 1971. Inhibition of the absorption of paraquat from the gastrointestinal tract by absorbents. Br. J. Ind. Med. 28, 186–188.

Daniel, J.W., Gage, J.C., 1966. Absorption and excretion of diquat and paraquat in rats. Br. J. Ind. Med. 23, 133–136.

Dayan, F.E., Duke, S.O., 2010. Protophyrinogen oxidase-inhibiting herbicides. In: Krieger, R. (Ed.), Hayes' Handbook of Pesticide Toxicology, third ed. Elsevier, San Diego, CA, pp. 1733–1751.

de Castro, V.L.S.S., Destefani, C.R., Diniz, C., Poli, C., 2007. Evaluation of neurodevelopmental effects on rats exposed prenatally to sulfentrazone. Neurotoxicology 28, 1249–1259.

Dinis-Oliveira, R.J., Duarte, J.A., Remião, F., et al., 2006. Single high dose dexamethasone treatment decreases the pathological score and increases the survival rate of paraquat-intoxicated rats. Toxicology 227, 73–85.

Dinis-Oliveira, R.J., Sousa, C., Remião, F., et al., 2007. Full survival of paraquat exposed rats after treatment with sodium salicylate. Free Radic. Biol. Med. 42, 1017–1028.

Dinis-Oliveira, R.J., Duarte, J.A., Sánchez-Navarro, A., et al., 2008. Paraquat poisonings: mechanisms of lung toxicity, clinical features, and treatment. Crit. Rev. Toxicol. 38, 13–71.

Dinis-Oliveira, R.J., Pontes, H., Bastos, M.L., et al., 2009. An effective antidote for paraquat poisonings: the treatment with lysine acetylsalicylate. Toxicology 255, 187–193.

Ebert, E., Leist, K.H., Mayer, D., 1990. Summary of safety evaluation of toxicity study of glufosinate ammonium. Food Chem. Toxicol. 28, 339–349.

EPA, U.S. Environmental Protection Agency, 1997a. Cloransulam-Methyl: Pesticide Fact Sheet. OPPTS 7501C.

EPA, U.S. Environmental Protection Agency, 1997b. Cloransulam-methyl: pesticide tolerances. 40 CR 180. Fed. Reg. 62 (182).

Erne, K., 1966a. Distribution and elimination of chlorinated phenoxyacetic herbicides in animals. Acta Vet. Scand. 7, 240–256.

Erne, K., 1966b. Studies on animal metabolism of phenoxyacetic herbicides. Acta Vet. Scand. 7, 264–271.

Espandiari, P., Ludewig, G., Glauert, H.P., et al., 1998. Activation of hepatic NF-κB by the herbicide dicamba (2-methoxy-3,6-dichlorobenzoic acid) in female and male rats. J. Biochem. Mol. Toxicol. 12, 339–344.

FAO/WHO, Food and Agriculture Organization/World Health Organization, 1993. Diquat. Evaluation 1993. Part II – Toxicology, Pesticide Residues in Food. Food and Agricultural Organization of the United Nations, Rome.

Flaws, J.A., Hirshfield, A.N., 1997. Reproductive, development, and endocrinology toxicology. In: Boekelheide, K., Chapin, R., Hoyer, P., Harris, C. (Eds.), Reproductive and Endocrine Toxicology, vol. 10. Pergamon/Elsevier, New York, NY, pp. 283–291.

Franz, J.E., Mato, M.K., Sikorski, J.A., 1997. Glyphosate: A Unique Global Herbicide. ACS Monograph No. 189. American Chemical Society, Washington, DC.

Gage, J.C., 1968. The action of paraquat and diquat on the respiration of liver cell fractions. Biochem. J. 109, 757–761.

Gehring, P.J., Watanabe, P.G., Blau, G.E., 1976. Pharmacokinetic studies in evaluation of the toxicological and environmental hazard of chemicals. In: Mehlman, M.A., Shapiro, R.E., Blumenthal, L.L. (Eds.), New Concepts in Safety Evaluation. Wiley, New York, NY, pp. 195–270.

Gonzalez, N.V., Soloneski, S., Larramendy, M.L., 2009. Dicamba-induced genotoxicity in Chinese hamster ovary (CHO) cells is prevented by vitamin E. J. Hazard. Mater. 163, 337–343.

Greenlee, A.R., Ellis, T.M., Berg, R.L., 2004. Low-dose agrochemicals and lawn-care pesticides induce developmental toxicity in murine preimplantation embryos. Environ. Health Perspect. 112, 703–709.

Gupta, P.K., 1986. Pesticides in the Indian Environment. Interprint, New Delhi.

Gupta, P.K., 1988. Veterinary Toxicology. Cosmo, New Delhi.

Gupta, P.K., 1989. Pesticide production in India: an overview. In: Mishra, P.C. (Ed.), Soil Pollution and Soil Organisms. Ashish, New Delhi, pp. 1–16.

Gupta, P.K., 2004. Pesticide exposure – Indian scene. Toxicology 198, 83–90.

Gupta, P.K., 2006. WHO/FAO guidelines for cholinesterase-inhibiting pesticide residues in food. In: Gupta, R.C. (Ed.), Toxicology of Organophosphate and Carbamate Compounds. Academic Press/Elsevier, Amsterdam, pp. 643–654.

Gupta, P.K., 2010a. Epidemiological studies of anticholinesterase pesticides poisoning in India. In: Satoh, T., Gupta, R.C. (Eds.), Anticholinesterase Pesticides: Metabolism, Neurotoxicity, and Epidemiology. Wiley, New York, NY, pp. 417–431.

Gupta, P.K., 2010b. Pesticides. In: Gupta, P.K. (Ed.), Modern Toxicology: Adverse Effects of Xenobiotics, vol. 2. Pharma Med Press/BSP, Hyderabad, India, pp. 1–60.

Gupta, P.K., 2016a. Fundamental of Toxicology: Essential Concepts Sand Applications. Elsevier-BSP, Elsevier/Academic Press, USA, p. 398.

Gupta, P.K., 2016b. Herbicide poisoning. In: Aiello, S.E. (Ed.), The Merck Veterinary Manual, 11th ed. Merck & Co Inc, USA, pp. 2969–2999.

Gupta, P.K., 2017. Herbicides and fungicides. In: Gupta, R.C. (Ed.), Reproductive and Developmental Toxicology, 2nd ed., Academic Press/Elsevier, San Diego, USA, 657–679.

Gysin, H., Knuesli, E., 1960. Chemistry and herbicidal properties of triazine derivatives. In: Metcalf, R. (Ed.), Advances in Pest Control Research, vol. 3. Wiley Interscience, New York, NY, pp. 289–358.

Hack, R., Ebert, E., Ehling, G., 1994. Glufosinate ammonium – some aspects of its mode of action in mammals. Food Chem. Toxicol. 32, 461–470.

Harp, P.R., 2010. Dicamba. In: Krieger, R. (Ed.), Hayes' Handbook of Pesticide Toxicology, third ed., vol. 2. Elsevier, San Diego, CA, pp. 1849–1852.

Hayes Jr, W.J., 1982. Pesticide Studies in Man. Williams & Wilkins, Baltimore, MD.

Hess, F.G., Harris, J.E., Pendino, K., Ponnock, K., 2010. Imidazolinones. In: Krieger, R. (Ed.), Hayes' Handbook of Pesticide Toxicology, third ed., vol. 2. Elsevier, San Diego, CA, pp. 1853–1863.

Heydens, W.F., Lamb, I.C., Wilson, A.G.E., 2010. Chloracetanilides. In: Krieger, R. (Ed.), Hayes' Handbook of Pesticide Toxicology, third ed., vol. 2. Elsevier, San Diego, CA, pp. 1753–1769.

Hodge, H.C., Downs, W.L., Panner, B.S., et al., 1967. Oral toxicity and metabolism of diuron (N-3,4-dichlorophenyl-N9,N9-dimethylurea) in rats and dogs. Food Cosmet. Toxicol. 5, 513–531.

Hodgson, E., Meyer, S.A., 1997. Pesticides. In: Sipes, I.G., McQueen, C. A., Gandolfi, A.J. (Eds.), Comprehensive Toxicology: Hepatic and Gastrointestinal Toxicology, vol. 9. Pergamon, New York, NY, pp. 369–387.

Hurt, S., Ollinger, J., Arce, G., et al., 2010. Dialkylthiocarbamates (EBDCs). In: Krieger, R. (Ed.), Hayes' Handbook of Pesticide Toxicology, third ed., vol. 2. Elsevier, San Diego, CA, pp. 1689–1710.

IPCS, International Programme on Chemical Safety, 2002. The WHO Recommended Classification of Pesticides by Hazard and Guidelines to Classification 2002–2003. World Health Organization, Geneva.

JMPR, Joint FAO/WHO Meeting on Pesticide Residues, 1993. Pesticide residues in food. Evaluation: Part II. Toxicological. Joint Meeting of the FAO Panel of Experts on Pesticide Residues in Food and the Environment and a WHO Expert Group on Pesticide Residues. WHO/PCS/94.4. World Health Organization, Geneva.

JMPR, Joint FAO/WHO Meeting on Pesticide Residues, 2000. Pesticide residues in food. Evaluation: Part II. Toxicological. Joint Meeting of the FAO Panel of Experts on Pesticide Residues in Food and the Environment and a WHO Expert Group on Pesticide Residues, WHO/PCS/01.3. World Health Organization, Geneva.

JMPR, Joint FAO/WHO Meeting on Pesticide Residues, 2003. Paraquat. Joint Meeting of the FAO Panel of Experts on Pesticide Residues in Food and the Environment and the WHO Core Assessment Group. World Health Organization, Geneva, pp. 203–266.

JMPR, Joint FAO/WHO Meeting on Pesticide Residues, 2004. Pesticide residues in food. Report of the Joint Meeting of the FAO Panel of Experts on Pesticide Residues in Food and the Environment and a WHO Expert Group on Pesticide Residues, FAO Plant Production and Protection Paper, 178. Food and Agriculture Organization, Rome.

JMPR, Joint FAO/WHO Meeting on Pesticide Residues, 2005. Pesticide residues in food. Report of the Joint Meeting of the FAO Panel of Experts on Pesticide Residues in Food and the Environment and a WHO Expert Group on Pesticide Residues, FAO Plant Production and Protection Paper, 179. Food and Agriculture Organization, Rome.

Jones, B.C., Huang, X., Mailman, R.B., et al., 2014. The perplexing paradox of paraquat: the case for host-based susceptibility and postulated neurodegenerative effects. J. Biochem. Mol. Toxicol. 28, 191–197.

Kennepohl, E., Munro, I.C., Bus, J.S., 2010. Phenoxy herbicides (2,4-D). In: Krieger, R. (Ed.), Hayes' Handbook of Pesticide Toxicology, third ed., vol. 2. Elsevier, San Diego, CA, pp. 1829–1847.

Liu, J., 2010. Phenylurea herbicides. In: Krieger, R. (Ed.), Hayes' Handbook of Pesticide Toxicology, third ed., vol. 2. Elsevier, San Diego, CA, pp. 1725–1731.

Lock, E.A., Wilks, M.F., 2010. Paraquat. In: Krieger, R. (Ed.), Hayes' Handbook of Pesticide Toxicology, third ed., vol. 2. Elsevier, San Diego, CA, pp. 1771–1827.

Lorgue, G., Lechenet, J., Riviere, A., 1996. Clinical Veterinary Toxicology (English version by MJ Chapman). Blackwell, Oxford.

Marrs, T.C., 2004. Toxicology of herbicides. In: Marrs, T.C., Ballantyne, B. (Eds.), Pesticide Toxicology and International Regulation. Wiley, Chichester, pp. 305–345.

Mehmood, O.S.A., Ahmed, K.E., Adam, S.E.I., Idris, O.F., 1995. Toxicity of cotoran (fluometuron) in desert sheep. Vet. Hum. Toxicol. 37, 214–216.

Monsanto, 1991. Material Data Sheet: Butachlor Technical. Monsanto, St. Louis, MO.

Monsanto, 1997a. Material Data Sheet: Alachlor Technical. Monsanto, St. Louis, MO.

Monsanto, 1997b. Material Data Sheet: Acetochlor Technical. Monsanto, St. Louis, MO.

Munro, I.C., Carlo, G.L., Orr, J.C., et al., 1992. A comprehensive, integrated review and evaluation of the scientific evidence relating to the safety of the herbicide 2,4-D. J. Am. Coll. Toxicol. 11, 559–664.

Murray, R.E., Gibson, J.E., 1972. A comparative study of paraquat intoxication in rats, guinea pigs and monkeys. Exp. Med. Pathol. 17, 317–325.

Nagata, T., Kono, I., Masaoka, T., Akahori, F., 1992. Acute toxicological studies on paraquat pathological findings in beagle dogs following single subcutaneous injections. Vet. Hum. Toxicol. 34, 105–112.

Nandihalli, U.B., Duke, M.V., Duke, S.O., 1992. Quantitative structure–activity relationships of protoporphyrinogen oxidase inhibiting diphenyl ether herbicides. Pestic. Biochem. Physiol. 43, 193–211.

Osteen, C.D., Padgitt, M., 2002. Economic issues of agricultural pesticide use and policy in the United States. In: Wheeler, W.B. (Ed.), Pesticides in Agriculture and the Environment. Dekker, New York, NY, pp. 59–95.

Pelletier, O., Ritter, L., Caron, J., Somers, D., 1989. Disposition of 2,4-dichlorophenoxyacetic and dimethylamine salt by Fischer 344 rats dosed orally and dermally. J. Toxicol. Environ. Health. 28, 221–234.

Pocar, P., Brevini, T.A.L., Fischer, B., Gandolfi, F., 2003. The impact of endocrine disruptors on oocyte competence. Reproduction 125, 313–325.

Reddy, K.N., Dayan, F.E., Duke, S.O., 1998. QSAR analysis of protoporphyrinogen oxidase inhibitors. In: Devillers, J. (Ed.), Comparative QSAR. Taylor & Francis, London, pp. 197–234.

Richard, S., Moslemi, S., Sipahutar, H., et al., 2005. Differential effects of glyphosate and Roundup on human placental cells. Environ. Health Perspect. 113, 716–720.

Romano, R.M., Romano, M.A., Bernardi, M.M., et al., 2010. Prepubertal exposure to commercial formulation of the herbicide glyphosate alters testosterone levels and testicular morphology. Arch. Toxicol. 84, 309–317.

Rose, M.S., Smith, L.L., 1977. The relevance of paraquat accumulation by tissues. In: Autor, A.P. (Ed.), Biochemical Mechanism of Paraquat Toxicity. Academic Press, San Diego, CA, pp. 71–91.

Rose, M.S., Lock, E.A., Smith, L.L., Wyatt, I., 1976. Paraquat accumulation. Tissue and species specificity. Biochem. Pharmacol. 25, 419–423.

Sandhu, H.S., Brar, R.S., 2000. Textbook of Veterinary Toxicology. Kalyani, Ludhiana.

Sarkar, S.N., Gupta, P.K., 1993a. Feto-toxic and teratogenic potential of substituted phenylurea herbicide, isoproturon in rats. Ind. J. Exp. Biol. 31, 280–282.

Sarkar, S.N., Gupta, P.K., 1993b. Neurotoxicity of isoproturon, a substituted phenylurea herbicide in mice. Ind. J. Exp. Biol. 31, 977–981.

Smith, L.L., 1997. Paraquat. In: Sipes, I.G., McQueen, C.A., Gandolfi, A.J. (Eds.), Comprehensive Toxicology: Toxicology of the Respiratory System, vol. 8. Pergamon, New York, NY, pp. 581–589.

Smith, L.L., Wright, A., Rose, M.S., 1974. Effective treatment of paraquat poisoning in rats and its relevance to the treatment of paraquat poisoning in man. Br. Med. J. 4, 569–571.

Steven, J.T., Summer, D.D., 1991. Herbicides. In: Hayes, W.J., Laws, E.R. (Eds.), Handbook of Pesticide Toxicology, vol. 3. Academic Press, San Diego, CA, pp. 1317–1408.

Susan, E.A., 2003. The Merck Veterinary Manual. eighth ed. Merck, Whitehouse Station, NJ.

Talbot, A.R., Shiaw, M.H., Haung, J.S., 1991. Acute poisoning with a glyphosate-surfactant herbicide (Roundup): a review of 93 cases. Hum. Exp. Toxicol. 10, 1–8.

Thongprakaisang, S., Thiantanawat, A., Rangkadilok, N., et al., 2013. Glyphosate induces human breast cancer cells growth via estrogen receptors. Food Chem. Toxicol. 59, 129–136.

Timchalk, C., Dryzga, M.D., Johnson, K.A., et al., 1996. Comparative pharmacokinetics of 14C metosulam (N[2,6-dichloro-3-methylphenyl]-5,7-dimethoxy-1,2,4-triazolo-[1,5a]-pyrimidine-2-sulfonamide) in rats, mice and dogs. J. Appl. Toxicol. 17, 9–21.

Tomita, M., Okuyam, T., Katsuyama, H., et al., 2007. Mouse model of paraquat-poisoned lungs and its gene expression profile. Toxicology 231, 200–209.

Watanabe, T., 1997. Apoptosis induced by glufosinate ammonium in the neuro-epithelium of developing mouse in culture. Neurosci. Lett. 222, 17–20.

Watanabe, T., Sano, T., 1998. Neurological effects of glufosinate poisoning with a brief review. Hum. Exp. Toxicol. 17, 35–39.

Wilson, A.G.E., Takei, A.S., 1999. Summary of toxicology studies with butachlor. J. Pestic. Sci. 25, 75–83.

Winter, T.N., Elmquist, W.F., Fairbanks, C.A., 2011. OCT2 and MATE1 provide bidirectional agmatine transport. Mol. Pharm. 8, 133–142.

Yano, B.L., Cosse, P.F., Atkin, L., Corley, R.A., 1991a. 2,4-D Isopropylamine Salt (2,4-D IPA): A 13-Week Dietary Toxicity Study in Fischer 344 Rats, HET m-004725-006. Dow Elanco, Indianapolis, IN.

Yano, B.L., Cosse, P.F., Markham, D.A., Atkin, L., 1991b. 2,4-D Tri-Isopropylamine Salt (2,4-D IPA): A 13-Week Dietary Toxicity Study in Fischer 344 Rats, K-008866-006. Dow Elanco, Indianapolis, IN.

Chapter 45

Toxicity of Fungicides

Pawan K. Gupta

INTRODUCTION

Fungicides are agents that are used to prevent or eradicate fungal infections from plants or seeds. Numerous substances having widely varying chemical constituents are used as fungicides (Gupta, 1988, 2016). Fungicides have been classified according to chemical structures or have been categorized agriculturally and horticulturally according to their mode of action (Ballantyne, 2003). According to the mode of application, fungicides are grouped as foliar, soil, and dressing fungicides. Foliar fungicides are applied as liquids or powders to the aerial green parts of plants, producing a protective barrier on the cuticular surface and systemic toxicity in the developing fungus. Soil fungicides are applied as liquids, dry powders, or granules, acting either through the vapor phase or by systemic properties. Dressing fungicides are applied to the post-harvest crop as liquids or dry powders to prevent fungal infestation of the crop, particularly if stored under less than optimum conditions of temperature and humidity. Thus, effective fungicides must be protective, curative, or eradicative and should possess the following properties: (1) low toxicity to the plant/animal but high toxicity to the particular fungus; (2) activity per se or the ability to convert themselves (by plant or fungal enzymes) into toxic intermediates; (3) the ability to penetrate fungal spores or the developing mycelium to reach the site of action; (4) low ecotoxicity; and (5) the ability to form a protective, tenacious deposit on the plant surface that will be resistant to weathering from sunlight, rain, and wind (Phillips, 2001). With a few exceptions, most of the newly developed chemicals have a low order of toxicity to mammals. Public concern has focused on the positive mutagenicity tests obtained with many fungicides and the predictive possibility of both teratogenic and carcinogenic potential. The quantity of fungicides used on major crops is estimated to have increased 2.3-fold between 1964 and 1997. Use of inorganics (primarily copper compounds) and dithiocarbamates has declined since the 1960s, but captan, chlorothalonils, and other organic materials now account for 90% of fungicide use. Newer groups, such as benzimidazoles, conazoles, dicarboximides, and metal organic compounds, account for approximately 10% of fungicide use (Osteen and Padgitt, 2002). In this chapter, fungicides are discussed using a chemical classification system.

BACKGROUND

The earliest fungicides were inorganic materials such as sulfur, lime, copper and mercury compounds. The use of elemental sulfur as a fungicide was recommended as early as 1803. It has become an important component of integrated pest management systems because it can be used in "organic farming." There are an increasing number of instances of dermatitis in human farmworkers and diseases in ruminants caused by exposure to high levels of sulfur (Gammon et al., 2010). The mercury-containing fungicides have been responsible for many deaths or permanent neurological disability. Some of the earlier inorganic metallic fungicides have been withdrawn in many countries because of their toxicity and adverse environmental effects (Ballantyne, 2003). Another compound, hexachlorobenzene (HCB), was extensively used from the 1940s through the 1950s as a fungicidal dressing applied to seed grains as a dry powder. Between 1955 and 1959, an epidemic of poisoning occurred in Turkey and resulted in a syndrome called black sore and caused more than 4000 deaths. Although use of this agent has greatly diminished, it is still being used in developing countries. It is a highly toxic compound and can lead to severe skin manifestations including hypersensitivity (Hayes, 1982; Gupta, 2010a). Carbamic acid derivatives, including ethylenebisdithiocarbamates (EBDCs), are a group of fungicides that have been used widely throughout the world since the 1940s. The important members of this class include mancozeb, maneb, metiram, zineb and nabam. All the members have an EBDC backbone, with different metals associated with

Veterinary Toxicology. DOI: http://dx.doi.org/10.1016/B978-0-12-811410-0.00045-3

the individual compounds. Captan, folpet and captafol have been in use for more than 55 years. These compounds belong to the chloroalkylthiodicarboximide class of fungicides due to the presence of chlorine, carbon, and sulfur in the side chain. Related compounds associated with this fungicide class are dichlofluanid and tolylfluanid. These two compounds have a fluorine atom substituted for one of the terminal chlorine atoms. Another compound, chlorothalonil, which is a halogenated benzonitrile fungicide, was first registered for use as an agrochemical in the United States in 1966. Chlorothalonil also has wider biocidal applications, including use in paints and lubricant fluids. The benzimidazole fungicides, benomyl, and carbendazim, have been in use for more than 40 years, whereas anilinopyrimidines, a new class of fungicides (cyprodinil, mepanipyrim, and pyrimethanil), were introduced in 1993 for application on cereal grains (Ollinger et al., 2010).

TOXICOKINETICS

Toxicokinetic studies provide important data on the amount of toxicant delivered to a target as well as species-specific metabolism. Animals are exposed to fungicides through ingestion or they are absorbed through the skin or the respiratory system. Different factors regulate their absorption, distribution, metabolism, and excretion. In general, the liver is the primary site for biotransformation and may include detoxification as well as activation reactions (Gupta, 1986). Some fungicides do not undergo any metabolism and bind with other active binding sites. The aryl organomercurials methyl- and ethylmercury chloride are poorly excreted and tend to accumulate in muscle, brain and other tissues, whereas the aryl organomercurial phenylmercury is more readily excreted via the kidney and less likely to accumulate in brain and muscles. Similarly, HCB possesses all the properties of chemical stability, slow degradation and biotransformation, environmental persistence and bioaccumulation in adipose tissue and organs containing a high content of lipid membranes (Costa, 2008). The newly introduced class of fungicides are rapidly absorbed, metabolized and excreted and do not accumulate in tissues, but some of them are partially absorbed from the gastrointestinal (GI) tract. For example, absorption of chlorothalonil from the GI tract is on the order of 30%–32% of the administered dose. At least 80% of the administered dose is excreted in feces within 96 h. The highest concentrations are observed in the kidneys—approximately 0.1% of the dose. Gut microflora plays a role in the disposition and metabolism in rats. Glutathione conjugation plays a central role in the metabolism and subsequent complex metabolic processing of these conjugates, resulting in selective renal uptake and urinary excretion of thiol-derived metabolites. Hepatic glutathione levels are decreased, and renal glutathione levels are elevated. The depletion of hepatic glutathione is considered a direct consequence of glutathione conjugation within the liver utilizing tissue resources. The increase in renal glutathione content is more difficult to explain, but it may be a consequence of urinary excretion of glutathione conjugates (Parsons, 2010).

Captan is rapidly degraded to 1,2,3,6-tetrahydrophthalimide (THPI) and thiophosgene (via thiocarbonyl chloride) in the stomach before reaching the duodenum. THPI has a half-life of 1–4 s, and thiophosgene is detoxified via reaction with cysteine or glutathione and is rapidly excreted. No captan is detected in blood or urine. It is therefore unlikely that these compounds or even thiophosgene would survive long enough to reach systemic targets such as the liver, uterus, or testes. Due to rapid elimination, meat, milk, or eggs from livestock/poultry would be devoid of the parent materials. Humans appear to metabolize captan in a similar manner to other mammals (Krieger and Thongsinthusak, 1993; JMPR, 2004; Gordon, 2010).

Cyprodinil, an anilinopyrimidine class fungicide, is rapidly absorbed from the GI tract into systemic circulation in rats. Approximately 48%–68% of the administered dose is excreted in the urine, whereas 29%–47% is found in the feces. Total excretions reach 92%–97% of the administered dose within 48 h. Cyprodinil is almost completely metabolized. No unchanged parent molecule is found in urine, whereas minor amounts of unchanged cyprodinil are found in feces. Most of the administered cyprodinil is metabolized by sequential oxidation of the phenyl and pyrimidine ring (Fig. 45.1). In urine and feces, there is no difference in the metabolite patterns of the phenyl or pyrimidyl labeled cyprodinil. Seven urinary, two biliary, and two fecal metabolites have been identified, which in total account for 65%–80% of the administered dose. Cyprodinil is absorbed in goats to a lesser extent and more slowly than in rats. The major route of excretion is in urine and feces, whereas excretion via milk is minimal. In laying hens, cyprodinil is rapidly and completely eliminated. Residues in eggs and edible tissues are very low. The metabolic pathways of cyprodinil in lactating goats and laying hens are similar to those observed in rats (Waechter et al., 2010).

Carbamic acid derivative fungicides, such as EBDCs, are only partially absorbed, and then are rapidly metabolized and excreted with no evidence of long-term bioaccumulation. Absorption of oral doses is rapid, and doses are excreted within 24 h with approximately half eliminated in the urine and half in the feces. Their common metabolite is ethylenethiourea (ETU). Only low-level residues are found in tissues, particularly the thyroid. Another compound in this class, propamocarb, is rapidly and nearly completely absorbed and distributed with a concentration reaching peak levels within 1 h. Elimination from tissues is rapid; with a

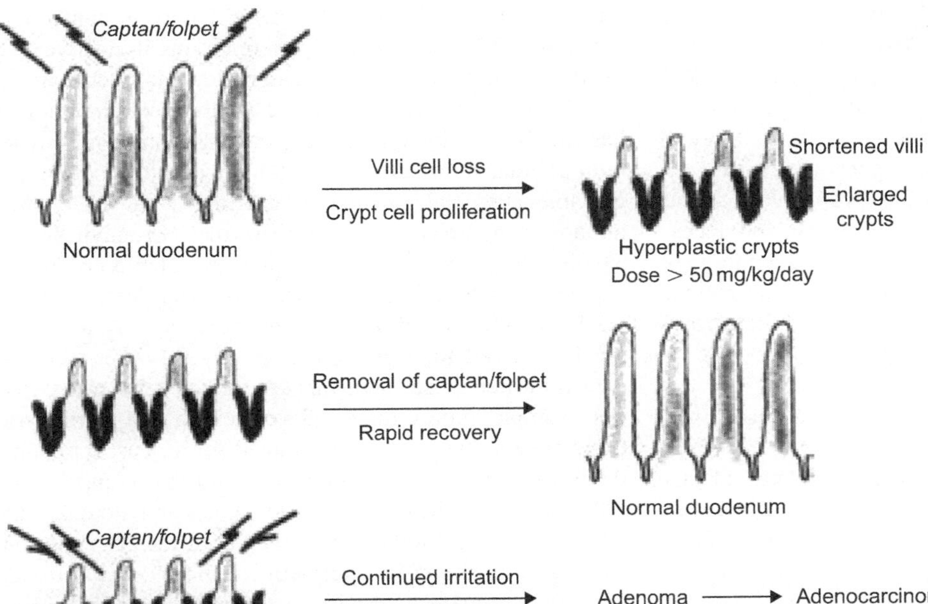

FIGURE 45.1 Mode of action for captan and folpet in the mouse duodenum. *Reproduced with permission from Gordon, E.B., 2010. Captan and folpet. In: Krieger, R. (Ed.), Hayes' Handbook of Pesticide Toxicology, third ed., vol. 2. Elsevier, New York, NY, pp. 1915–1949.*

half-life ranging from 11 to 26 h, urine is the main route of excretion (~75%–91% within 24 h). Up to 6% of the administered dose is excreted in feces. Propamocarb is extensively metabolized, and only small quantities are unchanged in urine. Metabolism involves aliphatic oxidation of the propyl chain (to form hydroxyl propamocarb) and N-oxidation and N-demethylation of the tertiary amine resulting in propamocarb *N*-oxide and mono demethyl propamocarb, respectively. Both benomyl and carbendazim are well absorbed after oral exposure (80%–85%) but poorly absorbed after dermal exposure (1% or 2%) in rats, mice, dogs, and hamsters. The major pathway of clearance is urinary elimination in rats and mice, but in dogs the majority of the dose (83.4%) is eliminated via feces, with only 16.2% of the dose eliminated in the urine after 72 h of dosing. In animals, benomyl is converted into carbendazim through the loss of the *n*-butylcarbamyl side chain prior to further metabolism. In dogs and rats, carbendazim undergoes aryl hydroxylation–oxidation at the fifth and sixth positions of the benzimidazole ring, followed by sulfate or glucuronide conjugation before elimination. The urinary excretion half-life of carbendazim in both male and female rats is approximately 12 h. Benomyl, carbendazim and their metabolites are cleared rapidly from blood and exhibit minimal potential for bioaccumulation in rats exposed orally or intravenously (Gardiner et al., 1974; JMPR, 2005).

Similarly, amide fungicides are rapidly absorbed and eliminated. Metalaxyl-M and metalaxyl can lead to stimulation of hepatic and renal cytochrome P450 and some other drug metabolizing enzymes. Tolylfluanid is rapidly and extensively absorbed, followed by rapid metabolism and almost complete excretion, mainly in the urine and to a lesser extent in the bile, within 48 h. High tissue concentrations have been seen soon after dosing in the kidney and liver, with lower concentrations in the perirenal fat, brain, gonads, and thyroid. In most species, the concentration of fluoride in the bone and teeth increases in a dose-related manner (JMPR, 2002, 2005).

Following an oral dose, conazole fungicides such as triadimenol and triadimefon are rapidly absorbed and widely distributed in the liver and kidney. Excretion and metabolism are rapid and extensive, predominantly through oxidation of the *t*-butyl methyl group. Propiconazole indicates rapid and extensive absorption (80% of the administered dose) and is widely distributed, having the highest concentration in liver and kidney. Excretion is more than 95% in the urine and feces within 48 h. There is extensive enterohepatic recirculation. The compound is extensively metabolized with oxidation of the propyl side chain, hydroxylation of phenyl and triazole rings, and conjugation. The cleavage of dioxolane is significantly different according to species and sex (JMPR, 2004). The other compound, fludioxonil, is rapidly and extensively (80%) absorbed, widely distributed, extensively metabolized and rapidly excreted, primarily in feces (80%), with a small amount being excreted in the urine (20%). The maximum blood concentration is reached within 1 h of administration. Elimination is biphasic, with half-lives of between 2 and 5 h for the first phase and between 30 and 60 h for the second phase. The compound is extensively metabolized primarily involving oxidation of the pyrrole ring (57% of the administered dose) and a minor oxo-pyrrole metabolite (4% of the administered dose), followed by glucuronyl and sulfate conjugation. There is no potential of accumulation in the tissues. Trifloxystrobin is rapidly absorbed (66%) in 48 h and is widely distributed, with highest concentrations in blood, liver and kidney. Within 72 h, 72%–96% of the administered dose is eliminated in the urine and feces. Metabolism is extensive, and the compound undergoes hydroxylation, O-demethylation, oxidation, conjugation, chain shortening and cleavage between glyoxylphenyl and trifluoromethyl moieties (JMPR, 2004).

MECHANISM OF ACTION

There are a series of biochemical changes or free radical-mediated processes; some may also be produced by other mechanisms that have been used to assess tissue injury. This is exemplified by the phenomenon of lipid peroxidation, which has been invoked as a toxic mechanism in many situations and also occurs subsequent to cell death and membrane lysis. However, in most situations, it is difficult to identify the exact mechanism of action. For example, in fungicides containing mercury, the mercury ions inhibit the sulfhydryl group of enzymes involved in the transfer of amino acids across the blood–brain barrier (BBB) and then interfere with protein synthesis. Organomercurials can also release some mercury ions in the body, but their toxicity is not believed to be a primary action of mercury ions (Sandhu and Brar, 2009). There are several theories regarding the mechanism by which sulfur produces its toxic action. The oxidized sulfur theory attributes toxicity to its oxidation products, such as sulfur dioxide, sulfur trioxide, thiosulfuric acid, or pentathionic acid. The reduced sulfur theory ascribes toxicity to hydrogen sulfide. A direct action theory suggests toxicity due to crosslinking of proteins, formation of other cellular components by free radicals of sulfur or polysulfides, or extensive oxidation of thiol groups leading to loss of function or structural integrity of proteins. Pentachlorophenol (PCP), a halogenated substituted monocyclic aromatic, acts cellularly to uncouple oxidative phosphorylation, with the target enzyme being Na^+/K^+-ATPase. Oxygen consumption is increased, whereas adenosine triphosphate (ATP) formation is decreased. The energy is lost as heat instead of being stored as high-energy phosphate bonds. The electron transport chain responds by using increasingly more available oxygen (increased oxygen demand) in an effort to produce ATP, but much of the free energy is lost as body heat. This leads to depletion of energy reserves (Eaton and Gallagher, 1997). Similarly, organotin compounds, particularly triethyltin, uncouple oxidative phosphorylation, whereas other agents (e.g., sulfur) in the presence of sulfiting agents such as sulfur dioxide uncouple oxidative phosphorylation. Thiamine is cleaved into its constituent pyrimidine and thiazole moieties, rendering it inactive.

Although the biochemical and molecular mechanism(s) by which captan and its analogs exert their cellular toxicity has not been fully established, captan is known to react with cellular thiols to produce thiophosgene, a potent and unstable chemical capable of reacting with sulfhydryl-, amino-, or hydroxyl-containing enzymes (Cremlyn, 1978). Thiols reduce the potency of captan. A volatile product of captan is responsible for mutagenic activity, the intermediate being short-lived and formed more quickly at higher levels at an alkaline pH. There are several other mechanisms by which these chemicals can induce cellular toxicity. For example, mouse tumors develop with oral administration above a threshold if maintained for at least 6 months. As shown in Fig. 45.1, epithelial cells that comprise the villi are damaged by exposure to captan and sloughed off into the intestinal lumen at an increased rate. Second, the basal cells in the crypt compartment that normally divide at a rate commensurate with the normal loss of villi cells from the tips of the villi increase, resulting in high cell proliferation, which is not carcinogenic per se but does play a role in tumor development. However, there appears to be no treatment-related duodenal tumor incidence of captan in rats or dogs. Some of the data have been compiled in reviews, and a task force and framework have been evolving for evaluation of the mode of toxicity and tumorogenicity findings in mice bioassay and human relevance for risk assessment purposes (Arce et al., 2010; Cohen et al., 2010; Gordon, 2010).

Chlorothalonil fungicide is a reactive molecule toward thio (–SH) groups. It is a soft electrophile with a preference for sulfur nucleophiles rather than nitrogen/oxygen nucleophiles. Such chemicals tend to show reactivity toward proteins containing critical S electrophiles rather than toward DNA (containing critical O and N nucleophiles). A mechanistic interpretation for the carcinogenicity of chlorothalonil has been published by Wilkinson and Killeen (1996). Repeated administration of chlorothalonil causes hyperplasia in the forestomach of rats and mice. The data are consistent with a temporal sequence of events starting with increased cell proliferation, multifocal ulceration and erosion of the forestomach mucosa, regenerative hyperplasia and hyperkeratosis, and ultimately progressing to the formation of gastric tumors within the forestomach. In dogs, there is no evidence of either neoplastic development or the occurrence of preneoplastic lesions in the kidney or stomach. The absence of stomach lesions in dogs is attributable to the anatomical differences between rodents and dogs: dogs do not possess a forestomach. Continued administration of chlorothalonil leads to the development of a regenerative hyperplasia within the renal proximal tubular epithelium. Continued regenerative hyperplasia ultimately results in progression of the kidney lesion to tubular adenoma and carcinoma. Initial cytotoxicity and regenerative hyperplasia within the proximal tubular epithelium are essential prerequisites for subsequent tumor development. The proposed mode of action for the induction of renal toxicity in rodents is outlined in Fig. 45.2.

The toxicology database supporting mechanism of action of carbamic acid derivatives such as EBDCs and their common metabolite ETU has been explained using modern studies with mancozeb, maneb and metiram because the principal target organ is the thyroid. These compounds inhibit the synthesis of thyroid hormone, thyroxine (T4), and triiodothyronine (T3), leading to elevated levels of thyroid-stimulating hormone (TSH) via feedback stimulation of the hypothalamus and pituitary (Atterwill and Aylard, 1995). Prolonged and continuous elevation of TSH levels results in hypertrophy and hyperplasia of the thyroid follicular cells in rats, mice, hamsters, monkeys, and dogs, leading to development of follicular nodular hyperplasia, adenoma and/or carcinoma in rats and mice (Ollinger et al., 2010). Conazoles such as propiconazole have a phenobarbital-type mode of action, leading to cell proliferation, increased liver weight, and microsomal enzyme induction (JMPR, 2004).

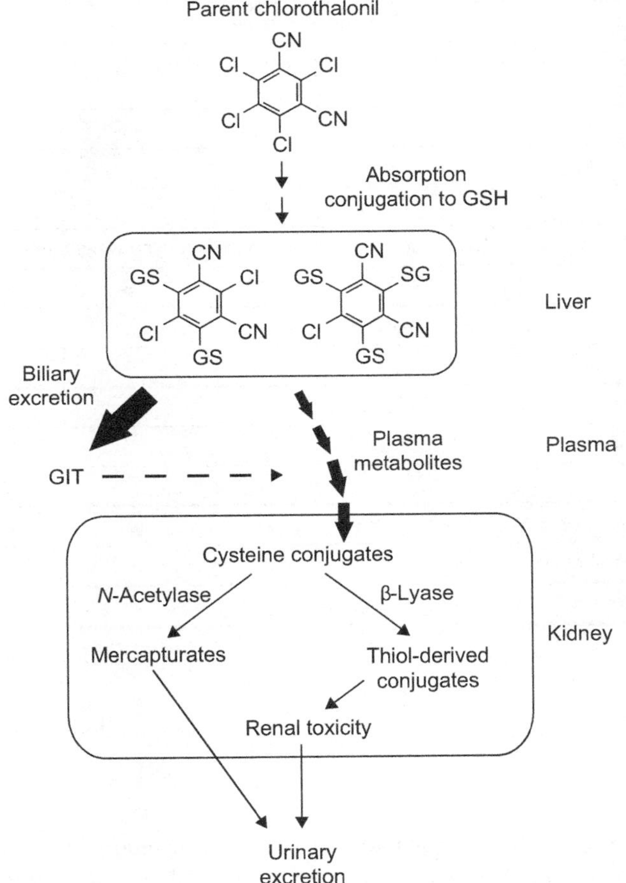

FIGURE 45.2 Schematic outlining potential pathways of chlorothalonil metabolism in the rat that leads to formation of toxic metabolites within the kidney. Following absorption from the GI tract, chlorothalonil is conjugated to glutathione in the liver. Further metabolic processing results in the formation of cysteine conjugates that may be detoxified via *N*-acetylase or activated to toxic thiol-derived species. *GIT*, gastrointestinal tract; *GSH*, glutathione. *Reproduced with permission from Parsons, P.P., 2010. Mammalian toxicokinetics and toxicity of chlorothalonil. In: Krieger, R. (Ed.), Hayes' Handbook of Pesticide Toxicology, third ed., vol. 2. Elsevier, New York, NY, pp. 1951–1966.*

TOXICITY

There is a wide and diverse spectrum of chemical structures of fungicides, covering both inorganic and organic substances, thus leading in toxicity to livestock. Some of these fungicides are believed to be obsolete or discontinued. To date, several fungicides have been evaluated by WHO for their toxic potential and acceptable daily intake has been recommended by the Joint Meeting on Pesticide Residues (JMPR). A number of livestock poisoning cases from fungicides result from treated grains or potatoes, etc. Most of the available toxicity data are from laboratory animals; little information is available for farm animals and pets. In general, newer classes of fungicides have low to moderate toxicity. However, the toxicity of fungicides may vary due to the presence of other ingredients (e.g., surfactants and emulsifiers) present in the formulation. The details of guidelines for their hazard evaluation and their classification have previously been summarized (IPCS, 2002; Gupta, 2006). There is increasing experimental and anecdotal evidence that exposure to fungicides also affects at least some form of development and/or reproduction in one or more species of animals. A nonexhaustive list of fungicides that cause developmental toxicity in experimental animals is presented in Table 45.1. More than 80% of all oncogenic risk from the use of pesticides derives from a few fungicides; however, only a small proportion of pesticide-related deaths from fungicides have been reported (NAS, 1987; Costa, 1997).

Inorganic Fungicides

This class of fungicides includes potassium azide, potassium thiocyanate, and titrated or sublimed sulfur. Sulfur had been in use throughout the 19th and early 20th centuries. Elemental sulfur and crude lime sulfur (calcium polysulfide and barium polysulfide) are commonly used as fungicides. The most notable chemical property of sulfur is its tendency to spontaneously oxidize. This property is responsible for sulfur's effects on the eyes, skin, and respiratory tract. Safety concerns presented by combustion of sulfur can be mitigated by avoiding its use during

TABLE 45.1 Select Fungicides That Cause Developmental Toxicity in Experimental Animals

Chemicals	Malformations
Ammonium salts, manganese and zinc	Multiple defects (rats)
Benomyl	Skeletal malformations, increased mortality (rats), multiple anomalies (mice), small renal papillae but no malformations (rabbits)
Bis(tri-*n*-butyltin)oxide	Cleft palate and developmental toxicity (rats, mice)
Bitertanol	Tail, palate, jaw, eye defects (rat)
Captafol, folpet	CNS, rib, tail and limb defects (hamsters); no teratogenic effects in other four species
Captan	Multiple defects, CNS and rib (rabbits, hamsters)
Carbendazim	Limb malformations, postnatal behavior alterations, postural reflex, open field behavior (rat)
Conazoles	Variable multiple defects[c]
Cycloheximide[a]	Skeletal defects, dactyly, hydrocephaly or other developmental defects
Dinocap[b]	Multiple malformations, hyprocephaly (rabbit)/experimental teratogen
EBDCs (maneb and zineb metabolites, monosulfide and ETU)	Multiple malformations and embryo–fetotoxic effects
Fenpropimorph	Developmental toxicity and malformations
Ferbam	Soft tissue and skeletal (rats)
Flusilazole	Multiple malformations
Hexachlorobenzene	Variety of defects, renal and palate (hamsters, mice), rib variation and reduced weight (rats)
Mancozeb	Variety of defects
Methylmercury	Multiple malformations and embryotoxic
Polycarbacin	Embryotoxic, malformations
Probineb	Multiple malformations
Propioconazole	Developmental toxicant
Thiram	Multiple malformations
Triadimenol	Developmental toxicity
Triadimefon	Scapula malformations (rabbits)
Tridemorph	Cleft palate, other malformations and developmental toxicity (rats, mice)

EBDCs, ethylenebisdithiocarbamates; *ETU*, ethylenethiourea.
[a]*Obsolete.*
[b]*Withdrawn by manufacturer.*
[c]*Variable: results need further study; from Gupta (2011).*

periods of high ambient temperature. In general, the use of sulfur does not present a toxicological problem. Only micronized sulfur is responsible for sulfur poisoning. Lethal doses are as follows: cattle, 100–1000 mg/kg body weight (BW); sheep, 1000–1500 mg/kg BW; and horses, 1000–1500 mg/kg BW. The most affected animals are cattle, sheep, goats, and dogs. In ruminants, excessive sulfur ingestion may lead to polioencephalomalacia, which is also called cerebrocortical necrosis. It involves softening of gray matter of the brain. Sulfur poisoning may lead to GI tract, neurological and pulmonary effects. On postmortem, congestion of the stomach and intestine, hemorrhagic effusions and petechiae along the GI tract and occasionally on the surface of the bladder have been observed (Jensen et al., 1956; Low et al., 1996; Gammon et al., 2010). Negative effects in humans, especially on the skin, eyes and respiratory tract, have been reported (Gammon et al., 2010). Currently, its use has declined due to the availability of organic fungicides. Another fungicide, barium polysulfide, after reaction with gastric acid yields barium chloride, which is a super purgative (Lorgue et al., 1996; Ballantyne, 2003; Sandhu and Brar, 2009).

Metallic Fungicides

Inorganic metallic fungicides were first used in agriculture. They are protective and preventive. Mercuric and mercurous compounds have been withdrawn because of their toxicity. Ethylmercury phosphate, 2-methoxyethylmercury chloride, phenylmercury chloride and phenylmercury acetate are used as seed treatments for cereals and fodder beet (Lorgue et al., 1996). Cattle, sheep, and pigs are the most affected species. Oral LD_{50} ranges from 10 to 500 mg/kg BW, depending on the species and the particular compound involved. The organic metallic fungicides are both aliphatic and aromatic. Many are of moderate to high mammalian toxicity, with several being immunotoxic and neurotoxic. Livestock exposed to mercurials may develop central nervous system (CNS) and skin changes. The CNS signs include incoordination and ataxia, body swaying followed by prostration, convulsions and death. CNS stimulation is seen in calves, dogs, cats, rats, and humans. However, other species (adult cattle, swine, and fowl) manifest CNS depression. Other signs associated with organomercurials are bronchopneumonia, hyperpyrexia, epistasis, mucous membrane hemorrhages, hematuria and bloody feces. Skin lesions include eczema, pustules, ulceration, keratinization, dehydration, weakness, and death (Sandhu and Brar, 2009). Typical organotins are di- and trialkyl and triphenyltins. In general, they are severely irritating to the skin, eyes and mucosa, and several are hepatorenotoxic and immunotoxic. They have been shown to increase susceptibility to infection, decrease lymphopoiesis and decrease T lymphocyte production. Trialkyl tins cross the BBB and are centrally neurotoxic (WHO, 1990).

Halogenated Substituted Monocyclic Aromatics

This class of chemicals includes chlorothalonil, dicloran, HCB, quintozene, PCP, dichlorophen, dinocap, tecnazene and chloroneb. Chlorothalonil is a nontoxic halogenated benzonitrile fungicide. Dermal irritation has been observed following repeated exposure in the rat and rabbit. Chlorothalonil causes irreversible and severe ocular lesions in rabbits. Signs of toxicity include decreased BW and decreased hematological parameters, increased absolute kidney weight, vacuolar degeneration in the proximal tubular epithelium, and hyperplasia of the forestomach. Chlorothalonil is not genotoxic in vivo. Treatment-related increase in renal tubular adenoma and carcinoma, squamous cell adenoma, and carcinomas of the forestomach of both species have been reported. Chlorothalonil is not a developmental or reproductive toxicant when tested up to doses that cause significant maternal toxicity and maternal death; however, a significant increase in the incidence of postimplantation loss due to early embryonic death has been observed (Parsons, 2010). Tecnazene has an oral LD_{50} of 2047 mg/kg BW in the rat and is a mild irritant in the rabbit eye. The compound has the potential to produce pulmonary adenoma, but it is neither embryotoxic nor teratogenic in mice (Ballantyne, 2003). Chloroneb, quintozene, and dicloran have low toxicity, and dinocap is a moderate eye irritant and has a human skin sensitizing potential. HCB, like other organochlorine compounds, possesses all the properties of chemical stability, slow degradation, and biotransformation with potential to accumulate in adipose tissues and organs containing a high content of lipid membranes, and it has the ability to induce a range of tissue cytochrome P450 as well as conjugate enzymes. Repeated exposure in animals results in hepatomegaly and porphyria as well as focal alopecia with itching and eruptions, followed by pigmented scars, anorexia and neurotoxicity expressed as irritability, ataxia and tremors. The compound can increase hepatic and thyroid tumors in hamsters and is teratogenic in mice (renal and palate malformations) and in rats (increased incidence of 14th rib). HCB is also toxic to developing perinatal animals (Table 45.1) and causes adverse effects on the immune system (Costa, 2008). PCP has oral LD_{50} of 150–210 mg/kg BW in the rat. Common signs of toxicity are increased respiration, increased body temperature, tremors, convulsions, loss in righting reflex, and asphyxial spasms. Corneal injury may result from splashes or vapor overexposure. Toxicity is more often due to contamination of commercial-grade PCP. Technical-grade PCP causes hepatic porphyria, increased microsomal monooxygenase activity and increased liver weight. Lethal dose in cattle and sheep is in the range of 120–140 mg/kg BW. Chronic toxicity leads to emaciation, weight loss, reduced productivity (milk, eggs, meat, etc.), and increased mortality in poultry (ATSDR, 1994; Lorgue et al., 1996).

Chloroalkylthiodicarboximides (Phthalimides)

This class of chemicals contains broad-spectrum fungicides (captan, folpet, captafol, etc.) used as surface protectants on many crops. They are usually nontoxic to mammals. The oral LD_{50} in rats is as follows: captan, >9000 mg/kg BW; folpet, $>10,000$ mg/kg BW; and captafol, >5000 mg/kg BW. However, a low-protein diet makes the animal more sensitive. Of this class of chemicals, folpet and captafol, which are true phthalimides, have been deregistered; only captan, being structurally different with a cyclohexene ring, is being used. The compound is a severe eye irritant because of its high reactivity. Folpet induces incidences of diarrhea, vomiting, salivation, reduced food intake, and reduced BW gain. Testes weights are reduced in dogs. A single dose applied to the skin results in mild to low irritation. Long-term exposure to rats causes hyperkeratosis and acanthosis of the esophagus and stomach, particularly after folpet exposure. Among ruminants, cattle are the most affected, and captan produces toxicity (oral TD, 250–500 mg/kg BW) with labored respiration, anorexia, depression, hydrothorax, ascites and gastroenteritis (Sandhu and Brar, 2009). Mutagenicity may be associated with these agents in vitro at exceptionally high doses required to elicit biological effects. These compounds degrade extremely rapidly in the presence of thiols, with a plasma half-life of only a few seconds. However, duodenal tumors in mice have been reported, which were considered to be due to the irritation potential of compounds to the GI tract of rats (Gordon, 2010). Some compounds of this class cause developmental effects (Table 45.1), whereas others are not proven because of, and/or masked by, maternal toxicity and possible nutritional deficits (Costa, 2008). Captan induces hyperplasia of the crypt cells. Following treatment with folpet, immune function is reduced, villi length is reduced and crypt compartments are expanded, thereby reducing the villi-to-crypt ratio in mice (JMPR, 1990; Tinston, 1995; Waterson, 1995; Gordon, 2010). The most characteristic pathologic finding consists of necrotizing and proliferative changes in the nonglandular portion of the stomach, dilation of the small intestine and focal epithelial hyperplasia in the proximal part of the small intestine in mice following treatment with captan (Gordon, 2010). Captafol differs from captan and folpet in a number of ways, including structure and chemical activity. Both of them have low acute toxicity. They are not carcinogenic, mutagenic, or teratogenic. They are neither selective developmental toxins nor reproductive toxins. They are an irritant of mucus membranes, especially after repeated exposures (Gordon, 2010).

Anilinopyrimidines

The anilinopyrimidine class of fungicides includes cyprodinil, mepanipyrim and pyrimethanil. The compounds have low toxicity and are unlikely to present acute hazards in normal use. Cyprodinil produces hepatomegaly with hepatocellular hypertrophy and increased thyroid weights associated with follicular cell hypertrophy and hypochromasia in rats. Subchronic exposure results in kidney lesions in rats. The compound also causes single cell necrosis in male mice and depletion of glycogen in female mice, whereas in dogs, increased blood platelets have been observed at high doses. Mepanipyrim causes hepatocellular fatty vacuolation and lipofuscin deposition in Kupffer cells and hepatocytes of dogs, whereas such changes are not observed in cyprodinil-treated rats (Terada et al., 1998). Pyrimethanil produces thyroid follicular cell tumors in rats and enhancement of hepatic thyroid hormone metabolism, which may be responsible for thyroid tumorigenesis (Hurlety, 1998). The findings in the thyroid were considered to be secondary to liver changes. Enhancement of hepatic thyroid hormone metabolism and excretion are considered to be the mode of action of thyroid tumorigenesis (Hurlety, 1998; Waechter et al., 2010). Cyprodinil induced microsomal protein and cytochrome P450 contents along with ethoxyresorufin *O*-deethylase, pentoxyresorufin *O*-depentylase and lauric acid 11- and 12-hydroxylase, as well as cytosolic glutathione *S*-transferase activities in rats (Waechter et al., 2010). Cyrodinil and mepanipyrim induce the opposite effects on liver and blood lipid parameters in rats. In general, anilinopyrimidines do not have adverse effects on developmental toxicity, they are neither genotoxic nor have any carcinogenic potential (Waechter et al., 2010).

Carbamic Acid Derivatives

The carbamic acid class of fungicides includes dithiocarbamates (ferbam, thiram, ziram, propamocarb, etc.) and EDBCs (maneb, mancozeb, zineb, nabam, metiram, etc.). In general, carbamic acid derivatives, except nabam, have low or moderate acute toxicity via the oral, dermal and respiratory routes. The main features of toxicity include anorexia, diarrhea, and flatulence followed by neurological effects, ataxia, muscular contractions and prostration. With repeated ingestion, there is a possibility of cutaneous effects, alopecia and a risk of antithyroid effects, especially with maneb. Certain compounds inhibit ovulation and egg laying (thiram and ziram). On histopathology, hepatic, renal and pulmonary congestion is common. Occasionally, hepatic degeneration, ascites, enteritis, and hydrothorax have been observed (Lorgue et al., 1996). Propamocarb is nonirritating to the eyes or skin. It induces sensitization in a Magnusson–Kligman maximization test. The signs of toxicity include hypokinesia, lethargy, hunched posture, body tremors, clonic convulsions, nasal hemorrhages, piloerection, staggering gait, and ataxia. Vacuolar changes in various tissues including choroid plexus in the brain and reduction in organ weights have been observed in rats and dogs. Common development and reproductive abnormalities include reduction in copulation index (female rats) and BW, retardation in ossification (rat), and increased postimplantation loss (rabbit) (JMPR, 2005). The principal target organ upon repeated exposure to EBDCs is the thyroid. These fungicides alter thyroid hormone levels and/or weights. The developmental toxicity includes malformations and embryo–fetotoxic effects at maternally toxic dose levels with EBDCs in rats (Table 45.1) (Ollinger et al., 2010).

Benzimidazoles

The major benzimidazole fungicides include benomyl, carbendazim, and fuberidazole. Benomyl and carbendazim have low toxicity, whereas fuberidazole has moderate toxicity. Both benomyl and carbendazim produce reproductive and developmental toxic effects in laboratory animals at high oral doses (Table 45.1). Reproductive toxic effects include decreased sperm count, decreased testicular weights and histopathological changes, whereas developmental toxicity effects include reduced fetal weight and anomalies of the eyes (microphthalmia or anophthalmia), skull, and head (hydrocephaly). The effects observed on the oocytes and uterine weight in female rats is direct and is not mediated by endocrine changes (Jeffay et al., 1996; Spencer et al., 1996). A high dose of carbendazim causes an increased incidence of diffuse proliferation of parafollicular cells of the thyroid in female rats. Both of these compounds are not carcinogenic in rats; however, lifetime exposure in mice shows benign (not malignant), hepatocellular neoplasms and adenomas. Carbendazim is a developmental toxicant and teratogen (JMPR, 2005).

Conazoles

The conazole class of fungicides includes cyproconazole, diniconazole, triadimefon, triadimenol, propiconazole, and imazalil and has low to moderate acute toxicity. Triadimenol is triazole, and triadimefon is closely related chemically to triadimenol, with increasing toxicity for increasing isomer A ratios (isomer B is less toxic). Triadimenol is nonirritating, whereas technical-grade triadimefon is sensitizing. The other symptoms of toxicity include liver toxicity and CNS effects (general restlessness, alternating phases of increased and reduced motility, and aggressive behavior). Liver adenomas have been observed in female mice. Developmental toxicity indicates increased ovary and testes weights, increased supernumerary lumbar ribs with triadimenol, and increased scapula malformations at maternal toxic doses in rabbits after triadimefon exposure (JMPR, 2004). Propiconazole is not an eye irritant in rabbits, but it is irritating to rabbit skin and a skin sensitizer in guinea pigs. The compound causes reduction in BW, liver toxicity, and adverse changes in erythrocytes (rat) and the stomach (dog). Following long-term exposure, liver hypertrophy and tumors (mice), uterine lumen dilation (rats), and developmental toxicity indicative of reduced pup weight at parenterally toxic dose and skeletal variations in laboratory animals have been observed (JMPR, 2004).

Morpholines

The class of morpholine fungicides includes dodemorph, fenpropimorph, and tridemorph. Dodemorph and fenpropimorph are unlikely to cause acute hazards, whereas tridemorph is moderately hazardous. Dodemorph acetate is moderately irritating to rabbit skin and a severe irritant to rabbit eye. Fenpropimorph is a mild irritant to rabbit skin, whereas tridemorph is a nonirritant. Tridemorph and fenpropimorph lead to developmental toxicity (Table 45.1), with an increase in the total number of malformations (JMPR, 2004).

Amides

Commonly used amide fungicides are fenhexamid, benalaxyl, metalaxyl, flutolanil, tolylfluanid, and dichlofluanid. These compounds are of low toxicity, except for metalaxyl, which is slightly hazardous. With long-term exposure, benalaxyl causes liver steatosis and hematological changes in rats and atrophy of seminiferous tubules in dogs. In mice, increased mortality associated with amyloidosis has been observed. Reproductive abnormalities in rats include decreased BW gain, increased liver weight of pups and delayed ossification of cranial bones. Minor skeletal deviations at maternally toxic levels have been reported in rabbits (JMPR, 2005). Metalaxyl is a 1:1 mixture of the R-enantiomer and S-enantiomer. Technical-grade metalaxyl-M consists of a minimum of 97% of the R-enantiomer and 3% of the S-enantiomer. The two compounds are used as fungicides and are severe irritants to rabbits. The dog is the most sensitive species, with the liver as the target organ. Both substances cause hepatocellular enlargement in rats, whereas dogs show changes in blood biochemical parameters indicative of hepatocellular damage (JMPR, 2002). Dichlofluanid and tolylfluanid have a fluorine atom substituted for one of the three chlorine atoms on the trichloromethylthio moiety of captan and folpet. These two compounds do not share a common mechanism of action with captan and folpet with regard to mouse duodenal tumors, principally because they do not induce these tumors. Flutolanil is slightly irritating to the eye. Following long-term exposure, it leads to enlargement of the liver, decreased BW and mild hematological disturbances, with evidence of increased thyroid weight in rats and dogs. On long-term exposure to fenhexamid, the major target organ is the kidney in rats and mice and the hematopoietic system (increase in Heinz bodies) and adrenal gland in dogs. At higher doses, delayed ossification has been observed in rabbits but is not teratogenic (JMPR, 2005). Tolylfluanid is a skin sensitizer and can lead to sedation, decreased motility, disturbed behavior and dyspnea. After intraperitoneal injection, signs consistent with local irritation, altered liver enzyme activity, increased liver weight, and histopathological changes that are indicative of liver toxicity in mice, rats and dogs have been reported. At higher doses, signs of renal toxicity and discoloration of bones and teeth, particularly the skull cap and incisors, have been observed. Alterations in thyroid hormone levels have also been observed in a number of studies in rats. The compound causes decreased pup viability at maternally toxic doses but is not teratogenic. These amides are neither genotoxic nor do they have any carcinogenic potential in animals (JMPR, 2002).

Others

Several other antibiotic substances, thiocarbonates, and cinnamic acid derivatives are used as fungicides. Sodium tetrathiocarbonate, a thiocarbonate fungicide, is moderately toxic. The rat oral LD_{50} is 631 mg/kg BW. It is a severe irritant to rabbit skin and a marked irritant to rabbit eyes. Another compound, cycloheximide, is extremely toxic, including development toxicity (Table 45.1), with mutagenic potential. Dimethomorph has low oral toxicity in rats, is not an irritant to rabbit skin and is a minimal irritant to rabbit eyes. The acute oral LD_{50} of fenpyroximate is 245 and 480 mg/kg BW in male and female rats, respectively. The compound may cause developmental toxicity in rats. Fludioxonil, a phenylpyrrole fungicide, and trifloxystrobin have low acute toxicity in rats. Fludioxonil is a slight eye irritant in rabbits, but it is neither a skin irritant in rabbits nor a skin sensitizer in guinea pigs. On long-term exposure, it causes liver necrosis, kidney nephropathy and mild anemia, and blue coloration of the urine and perineal fur. Reproductive toxicity indicates decreased pup weight gains in rats at parenterally toxic doses. Trifloxystrobin is nonirritating but may be a skin sensitizer. Toxic symptoms are associated with liver toxicity, changes in kidney weight, atrophy of the pancreas, and spleen abnormalities. Developmental toxicity indicates decreased BW gain of pups accompanied by delayed eye opening at parenterally toxic doses (JMPR, 2004).

ENDOCRINE DISRUPTION

In both males and females, some fungicides affect reproduction through different mechanisms of action by endocrine disruption: exogenous agents interfere with normal reproduction and development processes. In males, normal reproductive function involves interaction of the hypothalamic-pituitary-testis axis and the thyroid gland. In females, increased concentrations of xenoestrogens may affect ovarian function through the disruption of feedback mechanisms in the hypothalamus-pituitary-gonadal axis (Flaws and Hirshfield, 1997; Bretveld et al., 2006). Fungicides, like other chemicals, may disrupt all stages of hormonal function of the reproductive system. In females, during pregnancy, and to a greater extent during lactation, a portion of the maternal body burden of these chemicals is transferred to the offspring. Fungicides that are toxic to endocrine cells and that delete germ cells are beyond the scope of this chapter. However, it is well established that some fungicides affect male and female reproduction through different mechanisms of action by endocrine disruption. For example, fenarimol, prochloraz and chlorothalonil cause infertility in male and female rats through inhibition of CYP450 enzymes involved in steroid metabolism and alter sexual differentiation through antagonism of the androgen receptor(s) (Ankley et al., 2005; Noriega et al., 2005). The fungicide vinclozolin was shown to have endocrine-modulating effects in male offspring when rat dams were treated during the last one-third of gestation through postnatal day 3. The anogenital distance was reduced, and there were cleft phallus, hypospadias and other malformations in the offspring (Gray et al., 1994). Procymidone has antiandrogenic properties. Long-term exposure of rats to procymidone had different effects on the pituitary–gonadal axis in vivo and on Leydig cell steroidogenesis ex vivo. The disruption of hormonal feedback could be due to its antiandrogenic action through activation of the endocrine axis, thereby causing hypergonadotropic activation of testicular steroidogenesis (Svechnikov et al., 2005). From experimental studies, it has been concluded that fungicides can disturb the reproduction and development processes of both males and females through endocrine signals in organisms indirectly exposed during prenatal or early postnatal life. Such effects during fetal development may be permanent and irreversible. They may act through hormone receptors and enhance or diminish the activity normally controlled by endogenous hormones. According to one estimate in 2003, eight fungicides (benomyl, hexachlorobenzene, mancozeb, maneb, metriam complex, tributyltin, zineb, and ziram) were identified as potentially causing endocrine disruption in animals. Most of these were identified accidentally rather than as a result of an exhaustive screening process (Pocar et al., 2003). Recently, in an in vitro study endocrine activity of five conazole compounds solely based on potency or interference with steroidogenesis (assay based on H295R cells) indicated their ranking as follows:

Decreased estradiol production:
prochloraz > epoxiconazole > ketoconazole ≈ propiconazole ≈ tebuconazole

Decreased testosterone production:
prochloraz > ketoconazole > tebuconazole > epoxiconazole > propiconazole

Increased progesterone production:
prochloraz > epoxiconazole = propiconazole > ketoconazole > tebuconazole

Aromatase inhibition:
prochloraz > ketoconazole ≈ propiconazole ≈ epoxiconazole > tebuconazole.

It is therefore concluded that conazole compounds may alter the synthesis of sex hormones (Dreisig et al., 2013).

TREATMENT

In some cases, there is no treatment, whereas in others supportive therapy as required by condition is indicated:

(1) in the initial stages, the use of emetics, gastric lavage, or activated charcoal may be helpful for removal of residual material from the GI tract; (2) oxygen should be provided immediately to meet oxygen demand; (3) body temperature should be lowered (use of cool baths, cool sponging, or placing the animal in the shade or in a cool, quiet room); (4) phenothiazine tranquilizers IM are advised to decrease exertion and stress and to facilitate handling of the animal; however, these should not be used to sedate or comatose the animal; (5) balanced electrolyte solution should be administered to prevent dehydration; and (6) the animal should be removed immediately from the exposure site. In the case of metallic poisoning, there is no satisfactory treatment of organomercurial toxicosis in farm or pet animals. Once developed, brain lesions are irreversible, and treatment in such cases is meaningless. Traditional chelators such as dimercaprol (BAL) or sodium thiosulfate have been recommended for many years but have little or no value due to their poor affinity for organomercury compounds (Gupta, 2010b).

CONCLUDING REMARKS AND FUTURE DIRECTIONS

Fungicides have a low to moderate toxicity. However, several fungicides, such as alkyldithiocarbamic acid (manganese, zinc and ammonium salts), halogenated substituted monocyclic aromatics (dinocap), carbamic acid derivatives (maneb and zineb metabolites and ethylenethiuram monosulfide), ferbam, mancozeb and maneb metabolites, HCB, benzimidazoles (benomyl and carbendazim), bis(tri-*n*-butyltin)oxide, chloroalkylthiodicarboximides (captafol and folpet), and tridemorph are known to cause developmental toxicity and oncogenesis. More than 80% of all oncogenic risk from the use of pesticides derives from a few fungicides; only a small number of pesticide-related deaths from fungicides have been reported. Some fungicides are known to disrupt the endocrine system and may lead to reproductive and developmental abnormalities. Based on teratogenicity, several fungicides including cycloheximide have been deregistered or banned in many countries but are still used in other, less regulated areas of the world. Other fungicides are undergoing reevaluation because of changing regulatory policies; suspected toxicity, particularly as carcinogenic, mutagenic, or toxic to reproduction; and incomplete or outdated toxicity database.

REFERENCES

Ankley, G.T., Kathleen, M., Jensen, K.M., et al., 2005. Effects of two fungicides with multiple modes of action on reproductive endocrine function in the fathead minnow (*Pimephales promelas*). Toxicol. Sci. 86, 300–308.

Arce, G.T., Gordon, E.B., Cohen, S.M., Singh, P., 2010. Genetic toxicology of folpet and captan. Crit. Rev. Toxicol. 40 (6), 546–574.

ATSDR, Agency for Toxic Substances and Disease Registry, 1994. Toxicological Profile for Pentachlorophenol. U.S. Department of Health and Human Services, Agency for Toxic Substances and Disease Registry, Atlanta, GA.

Atterwill, C.P., Aylard, S.P., 1995. Endocrine toxicology of the thyroid for industrial compounds. In: Thomas, H., Hess, R., Waechter, F. (Eds.), Toxicology of Industrial Compounds. Taylor & Francis, London, pp. 257–280.

Ballantyne, B., 2003. Toxicology of fungicides. In: Marrs, T.C., Ballantyne, B. (Eds.), Pesticide Toxicology and International Regulation. John Wiley & Sons, Ltd, Chichester, UK. Available from: http://dx.doi.org/10.1002/0470091673.ch6

Bretveld, R.W., Thomas, C., Scheepers, M.G., et al., 2006. Pesticide exposure: the hormonal function of the female reproductive system disrupted? Reprod. Biol. Endocrinol. 4, 30–43.

Cohen, S.M., Gordon, E.B., Singh, P., et al., 2010. Carcinogenic mode of action of folpet in mice and evaluation of its relevance to humans. Crit. Rev. Toxicol. 40 (6), 531–545.

Costa, L.G., 1997. Basic toxicology of pesticides. Occup. Med. State Art Rev. 12, 251–268.

Costa, L.G., 2008. Toxic effects of pesticides. In: Klaassen, C.D. (Ed.), Casarett and Doull's Toxicology: The Basic Science of Poisons, 76th ed. McGraw-Hill, New York, NY, pp. 883–933.

Cremlyn, R., 1978. Pesticides: Preparation and Mode of Action. Wiley, Hoboken.

Dreisig, S., Taxvig, K.C., Birkhøj, K.M., et al., 2013. Predictive value of cell assays for developmental toxicity and embryotoxicity of conazole fungicides. ALTEX 30, 319–330.

Eaton, D.L., Gallagher, E.P., 1997. Introduction to the principles of toxicology. In: Glenn, S., Charlene, I., McQueen, A., Gandolfi, J. (Eds.), Comprehensive Toxicology: General Principles. Pergamon, New York, NY, pp. 1–38.

Flaws, J.A., Hirshfield, A.N., 1997. Reproductive, development, and endocrinology toxicology. In: Boekelheide, K., Chapin, R., Hoyer, P.B., Harris, C., McQueen, C.A., Gandolfi, A.J., Sipes, I.G. (Eds.), Reproductive and Endocrine Toxicology. Pergamon, New York, NY.

Gammon, D.W., Moore, T.B., O'Malley, M.A., 2010. A toxicological assessment of sulfur as a pesticide. In: Krieger, R. (Ed.), Hayes' Handbook of Pesticide Toxicology, third ed., vol. 2. Elsevier, New York, NY, pp. 1889–1901.

Gardiner, J.A., Kirkland, J.J., Klopping, H.L., Sherman, H., 1974. Fate of benomyl in animals. J. Agric. Food Chem. 22 (3), 419–427.

Gordon, E.B., 2010. Captan and folpet. In: Krieger, R. (Ed.), Hayes' Handbook of Pesticide Toxicology, third ed., vol. 2. Elsevier, New York, NY, pp. 1915–1949.

Gray, L.E., Ostby, J.S., Kelce, W.R., 1994. Developmental effects of an environmental antiandrogen: the fungicide vinclozin alters sex differentiation of the male rat. Toxicol. Appl. Pharmacol. 125, 46–52.

Gupta, P.K., 1986. Pesticides in the Indian Environment. Interprint, New Delhi.

Gupta, P.K., 1988. Veterinary Toxicology. Cosmo, New Delhi.

Gupta, P.K., 2006. WHO/FAO guidelines for cholinesterase-inhibiting pesticide residues in food. In: Gupta, R.C. (Ed.), Toxicology of Organophosphate and Carbamate Compounds. Academic Press/Elsevier, Amsterdam, pp. 643–654.

Gupta, P.K., 2010a. Principles of nonspecific therapy. In: Gupta, P.K. (Ed.), Modern Toxicology: Immuno and Clinical Toxicology, vol. 3. Pharma Med Press/BSP, Hyderabad, pp. 210–243.

Gupta, P.K., 2010b. Pesticides. In: Gupta, P.K. (Ed.), Modern Toxicology: Adverse Effects of Xenobiotics, vol. 2. Pharma Med Press/BSP, Hyderabad, India, pp. 1–60.

Gupta, P.K., 2016. Fundamental of Toxicology: Essential Concepts Sand Applications. Elsevier-BSP, Elsevier/Academic Press, USA, p. 398.

Gupta, P.K., Herbicides and fungicides. In: Gupta, R.C., (Ed.), Reproductive and Developmental Toxicology, second ed. Academic Press/Elsevier, Amsterdam, The Netherlands, 2011, p. 503–521.

Hayes Jr, W.J., 1982. Pesticide Studies in Man. Williams & Wilkins, Baltimore, MD.

Hurlety, P.M., 1998. Mode of carcinogenic action of pesticides inducing thyroid follicular cell tumors in rodents. Environ. Health Perspect. 106, 437–445.

IPCS, International Programme on Chemical Safety, 2002. The WHO Recommended Classification of Pesticides by Hazard and Guidelines to Classification 2000–2002. World Health Organization, Geneva.

Jeffay, S., Libbus, B., Barbee, R., Perreault, S., 1996. Acute exposure of female hamsters to carbendazim (MBC) during meiosis results in aneuploid oocytes with subsequent arrest of embryonic cleavage and implantations. Reprod. Toxicol. 10 (3), 183–189.

Jensen, R., Griner, L.A., Adams, O.R., 1956. Polioencephalomalacia of cattle and sheep. J. Am. Vet. Med. Assoc. 129, 311–321.

JMPR, Joint FAO/WHO Meeting on Pesticide Residues, 1990. Pesticide Residues in Food. Report of the Joint Meeting of the FAO Panel of Experts on Pesticide Residues in Food and the Environment and a WHO Expert Group on Pesticide Residues. FAO Plant Production and Protection Paper 102. Food and Agriculture Organization, Rome.

JMPR, Joint FAO/WHO Meeting on Pesticide Residues, 2002. Pesticide Residues in Food. Report of the Joint Meeting of the FAO Panel of Experts on Pesticide Residues in Food and the Environment and a WHO Expert Group on Pesticide Residues. FAO Plant Production and Protection Paper 176. Food and Agriculture Organization, Rome.

JMPR, Joint FAO/WHO Meeting on Pesticide Residues, 2004. Pesticide Residues in Food. Report of the Joint Meeting of the FAO Panel of Experts on Pesticide Residues in Food and the Environment and a WHO Expert Group on Pesticide Residues. FAO Plant Production and Protection Paper 178. Food and Agriculture Organization, Rome.

JMPR, Joint FAO/WHO Meeting on Pesticide Residues, 2005. Pesticide Residues in Food. Report of the Joint Meeting of the FAO Panel of Experts on Pesticide Residues in Food and the Environment and a WHO Expert Group on Pesticide Residues. FAO Plant Production and Protection Paper 179. Food and Agriculture Organization, Rome.

Krieger, R.I., Thongsinthusak, T., 1993. Captan metabolism in humans yields two biomarkers, tetrahydrophthalimide (THPI) and thiazolidine-2-thione-4-carboxylic acid (TTCA), in urine. Drug Chem. Toxicol. 16 (2), 207–225.

Lorgue, G., Lechenet, J., Rivière, A., Chapman, M.J., Whitehead, A., 1996. Clinical veterinary toxicology. In: Lorgue, G., Lechenet, J., Rivière, A. (Eds.), Précis de toxicologie clinique vétérinaire, science, vol. VI. Blackwell, Oxford, 210 pp. ISBN: 0632032693 (English translation by M.J. Chapman).

Low, J.C., Scott, P.R., Howie, F., et al., 1996. Sulfur-induced polioencephalomalacia in lambs. Vet. Rec. 138, 327–329.

NAS, National Academy of Sciences, 1987. Regulating Pesticides in Food. The Delaney Paradox. Report of the Committee on Scientific and Regulatory Issues. Unlikely Pesticide Use Patterns. National Academic Press, Washington, DC.

Noriega, N.C., Ostby, J., Lambright, C., et al., 2005. Late gestational exposure to the fungicide prochloraz delays the onset of parturition and causes reproductive malformations in male but not female rat offspring. Biol. Reprod. 72, 1324–1335.

Ollinger, S.J., Arce, G., Bui, Q., Tobia, A.J., Ravenswaay, B.V., 2010. Dialkyldithiocarbamates (EBDCs). In: Krieger, R. (Ed.), Hayes' Handbook of Pesticide Toxicology, third ed., vol. 2. Elsevier, New York, NY, pp. 1689–1710.

Osteen, C.D., Padgitt, M., 2002. Economic issues of agricultural pesticide use and policy in the United States. In: Wheeler, W.B. (Ed.), Pesticides in Agriculture and the Environment. Dekker, New York, NY, pp. 59–95.

Parsons, P.P., 2010. Mammalian toxicokinetics and toxicity of chlorothalonil. In: Krieger, R. (Ed.), Hayes' Handbook of Pesticide Toxicology, third ed., vol. 2. Elsevier, New York, NY, pp. 1951–1966.

Phillips, S.D., 2001. Fungicides and biocides. In: Sullivan, J.B., Krieger, G.R. (Eds.), Clinical Environmental Health and Toxic Exposures, second ed., vol. 2. Lippincott Williams & Wilkins, Philadelphia, PA, pp. 1109–1125.

Pocar, P., Brevini, T.A.L., Fischer, B., Gandolfi, F., 2003. The impact of endocrine disruptors on oocyte competence. Reproduction. 125, 313–325.

Sandhu, H.S., Brar, R.S., 2009. Textbook of Veterinary Toxicology, second ed. Kalyani, Ludhiana.

Spencer, F., Chi, L., Zhu, M., 1996. Effect of benomyl and carbendazim on steroid and molecular mechanisms in uterine decidual growth in rats. J. Appl. Toxicol. 16, 211–214.

Svechnikov, K., Supornsilchai, V., Strand, M.L., et al., 2005. Influence of long-term dietary administration of procymidone, a fungicide with anti-androgenic effects, or the phytoestrogen genistein to rats on the pituitary–gonadal axis and Leydig cell steroidogenesis. J. Endocrinol. 187, 117–124.

Terada, M., Mizuhashi, F., Tomita, T., et al., 1998. Mepanipyrim induced fatty liver in rats but not in mice and dogs. J. Toxicol. Sci. 23, 223–234.

Tinston, D.J., 1995. Captan: Investigation of Duodenal Hyperplastic in Mice, Report CTL/4532. Central Toxicology Laboratory, Alderley Park.

Waechter, F., Weber, E., Herner, T., May-Hertl, U., 2010. Cyprodinil: a fungicide of the anilinopyrimidine class. In: Krieger, R. (Ed.), Hayes' Handbook of Pesticide Toxicology, third ed., vol. 2. Elsevier, New York, NY, pp. 1903–1913.

Waterson, L., 1995. Folpet: Investigation of the Effects on the Duodenum of Male Mice after Dietary Administration for 28 Days with Recovery, Report MBS 45/943003. Huntingdon Research Centre, Huntingdon.

WHO, World Health Organization, 1990. Methylmercury. Environmental Health Criteria No. 101, International Program on Chemical Safety. World Health Organization, Geneva.

Wilkinson, C.F., Killeen, J.C., 1996. A mechanistic interpretation of the oncogenicity of chlorothalonil in rodents and an assessment of human relevance. Regul. Toxicol. Pharmacol. 24, 69–84.

Section VIII

Rodenticides

Chapter 46

Anticoagulant Rodenticides

Michael J. Murphy

INTRODUCTION

The origin of oral anticoagulant therapy and anticoagulant rodenticides traces back to investigations of moldy sweet clover poisoning in the 1920s. This cattle disease was characterized by high mortality and internal bleeding; investigations revealed that the cattle had been fed moldy sweet clover hay.

An association between vitamin K and coagulopathies was made in the mid 1930s (Dam, 1935; Fieser et al., 1939). Soon thereafter, Professor Link reported the discovery of dicoumarol in moldy hay (Last, 2002). Naturally occurring coumarin in the sweet clover hay is reportedly converted by fungi to dicoumarol. Dicoumarol was found to be the causative agent of moldy sweet clover toxicosis. The elements of the toxicosis were coumarin-containing plant material plus conversion of coumarin to dicoumarol by mold; subsequently, a range of molecules were synthesized, one of which, named warfarin, became popular as both an oral anticoagulant and a rodenticide. (Duxbury and Poller, 2001) Warfarin takes its name, in part, from the Wisconsin Alumni Research Foundation.

Sweet clover requires the action of molds to cause a toxicosis giant fennel does not.

Giant fennel, *Ferula communis*, grows in Mediterranean countries. It has a naturally occurring anticoagulant effect. An association between the plant and anticoagulation was first reported in the 1950s (Costa, 1950a,b; Carta, 1951), then further investigated in Italy (Cannava, 1958; Mazzetti and Cappelletti, 1957; Corticelli and Deiana, 1957; Corticelli et al., 1957) and Israel (Shlosberg and Egyed, 1983). The anticoagulant activity of the plant in Morocco has recently been reviewed (Lamnaouer, 1999).

Five coumarins and 11 daucane derivatives have been isolated from *F. communis*. (Arnoldi et al., 2004). Previously identified chemicals included allohedycaryol, fercoperol (Miski et al., 1986), and ferulenol.

The toxicity of ferulenol in rats, mice, and sheep has been reported. It is a 4-hydroxycoumarin, with the expected anticoagulation effects (Fraigui et al., 2002). The single oral LD_{50} of ferulenol in albino mice is 2100 mg/kg (Fraigui et al., 2002). This value is similar to oral LD_{50} values of 1650 and 2000 for rats and mice, respectively, using fessoukh, the resinous gum of *Ferula* (Fraigui et al., 2001). These reports supported prior studies in rats (Tagliapietra et al., 1989; Aragno et al., 1988).

Anticoagulation activity of the plant in sheep was reported in 1985 (Shlosberg and Egyed, 1985). Subsequently, ferulenol has been measured in the serum of sheep experimentally dosed with 600 g of powdered plant material (Tligui et al., 1994). Ferulenol was detected at 6 h after dosing and for about 12 h after cessation of dosing. The prothrombin time (PT) was elevated to 6 times normal about 70 h after the last dose, then returned to normal by day 5 postdosing (Tligui and Ruth, 1994; Tligui et al., 1994).

Ferula has also been examined for chemotherapy (Poli et al., 2005), antimycobacterial (Appendino et al., 2004; Mossa et al., 2004), microtubule effects (Bocca et al., 2002) and testicular and epididymal changes in rams (Gil et al., 2002), much like the warfarin and other oral anticoagulants now have. It is found in Morocco (Fraigui et al., 2001), Israel (Shlosberg and Egyed, 1983), and Italy (Tagliapietra et al., 1989).

The phrase oral anticoagulants normally refer to these chemicals when used therapeutically. The oral anticoagulants are briefly discussed before the detailed discussion of the application of the progeny of dicoumarol as anticoagulant rodenticides.

Warfarin, and its congeners, are still used as therapeutic agents. Oral anticoagulants available therapeutically in Europe include warfarin, phenprocoumaron, and nicoumalone—also called acenocoumarol (Shetty et al., 1993). Oral anticoagulants are used therapeutically to reduce thromboembolic events. Warfarin examples include a reduction in catheter-related thrombosis (Magagnoli et al., 2006; Guidry et al., 1991), early venous thrombosis after operations (Pan et al., 2005; Calnan and

Veterinary Toxicology. DOI: http://dx.doi.org/10.1016/B978-0-12-811410-0.00046-5

Allenby, 1975), including hip surgery, atrial fibrillation (Reiffel, 2000; Middlekauff et al., 1995), and myocardial infarction (Asperger and Jursic, 1970). Dicoumarol is also used in the therapy of thrombotic occlusion of intracoronary stents (Alonso Martin et al., 1997), prosthetic valves (Dalla, 1994), and other types of venous thromboses (Ferlito, 1996; Piovella et al., 1995) or thrombophlebitis (Creutzig, 1993; Byrne, 1970).

Warfarin has been reported to be associated with a reduction of the recurrence of malignant melanoma (Thornes et al., 1994) or small cell lung cancer (Aisner et al., 1992). This antimetastatic activity may be associated with distribution of metastatic cells on thrombi (Smith et al., 1988; McNiel and Morgan, 1984).

Low-dose warfarin therapy has been adopted by the United States, Europe, and the World Health Organization (Duxbury and Poller, 2001). International normalized ratio (INR) is now used to measure therapeutic anticoagulation (Duxbury and Poller, 2001).

Oral anticoagulants have been used for decades, and a number of adverse events have been recognized, most of which are related to drug interactions (Dayton and Perel, 1971). A controversy exists as to whether acetaminophen induces an adverse effect on warfarinized patients in therapeutic doses (Toes et al., 2005). The acetaminophen metabolite NAPQI (*N*-acetyl-para-benzoquinoneimine) seems to interfere with vitamin K-dependent gamma carboxylase. Such interference may lead to potentiation of the anticoagulant effect of warfarin (Thijssen et al., 2004). COX-2 inhibitors may also interfere with control of warfarin anticoagulation in elderly patients (Savage, 2005), and rifampin may interfere with P-450 associated warfarin metabolism (Finch et al., 2002; Strayhorn et al., 1997). Inconsistent anticoagulation has been recognized in generic versus prescription warfarin (Burns, 1999), and a single case of hemothorax with eosinophilia has been reported in a warfarin overdose (Nasilowski and Krenke, 2002).

Complementary or alternative medical therapies may also interfere with warfarin metabolism (Wood et al., 2003; Tumova, 2000). For example, passionflower, hydroalcoholic extracts, juniper, and verbena contain vitamin K_1, so they can lessen the anticoagulation effect of warfarin therapy (Argento et al., 2000). On the other hand, genoderma, japonicum, papaw, *Salvia miltiorrhiza*, ginseng, devil's claw, garlic, quinine, ginkgo, ginger, red clover, and horse chestnut may reinforce the anticoagulant effect of warfarin by various mechanisms (Argento et al., 2000).

A "coumarin-induced hepatitis" has been reported a number of times in warfarinized patients (Ehrenforth et al., 1999; Hohler et al., 1994; Matsukawa et al., 1994; Bamanikar and Hiremath, 2002; Biagini et al., 2006; Bint and Burtt, 1980; Rehnqvist, 1978; Tanaka et al., 1985). Liver damage has also been reported in a brushtail possum (*Trichosurus vulpecula*) dosed with the anticoagulant rodenticide pindone (Jolly et al., 1994). Pindone has also been associated with an increased frequency of sex chromosome loss in *Drosophila melanogaster* (Santoro et al., 1993). The remainder of the chapter is devoted to the application of the chemical progeny of dicoumarol as anticoagulant rodenticides.

HISTORY AND CHEMICAL CLASSES

In the 1940s, a small British pharmaceutical company suggested that dicoumarol might have rodenticide properties. Trials carried out by Armour and Barnett (1950) supported that idea, starting the era of anticoagulant rodenticides. Warfarin was the first anticoagulant rodenticide introduced into the market shortly after World War II, and became widely used in many countries. Other anticoagulant compounds with potency similar to that of warfarin were also synthesized. These early anticoagulant rodenticides have often been called "first-generation anticoagulant rodenticides." These first-generation compounds generally have moderate toxicity, with acute LD_{50} values ranging from 10 to 50 mg/kg body wt. They often needed continuous bait exposure for effective rodent control.

Many rodent species developed a resistance to warfarin (Jackson et al., 1975), presumably associated with continuous bait exposure and widespread use. Consequently, new chemical structures were synthesized and used as anticoagulant rodenticides. These newer compounds are generally more toxic than warfarin, with acute LD_{50}s of 0.2–3.9 mg/kg body wt. For example, a bait concentration of only 50 ppm of brodifacoum is adequate to give control in a single feeding for most rodents and noncommensal species (Matolesy et al., 1988). These newer compounds were often referred to as "second-generation anticoagulant rodenticides," and are often now referred to as "superwarfarins" in the contemporary medical literature (Chong et al., 1986; Chua and Friedenberg, 1998; Dolin et al., 2006; Exner et al., 1992; Gallo, 1998; Greeff et al., 1987; Hui et al., 1996; Pavlu et al., 2005; Rauch et al., 1994; Routh et al., 1991; Sharma and Bentley, 2005; Swigar et al., 1990; Tecimer and Yam, 1997; Wallace et al., 1990; Wilton, 1991).

Anticoagulant rodenticides are also categorized by chemical structure. The chemical structure of currently marketed products fits in one of two chemical classes: (1) hydroxycoumarins and (2) indanediones.

1. Hydroxycoumarins. This group of compounds have a 4-hydroxycoumarin ring, with different side-chain substituents at the 3-position. Commonly used anticoagulant rodenticides in this group are bromadiolone, brodifacoum, coumafuryl, coumatetralyl, difenacoum, and warfarin.

2. Indanediones. This group of compounds has a 1,3-indanedione structure, with different side-chain substituents at the 2-position. The most common anticoagulant rodenticides in this group are chlorophacinone and diphacinone. Examples of each of these compounds are briefly summarized.

A few representative chemicals are described below. A number of other chemicals have now been developed.

Hydroxycoumarins

Bromadiolone

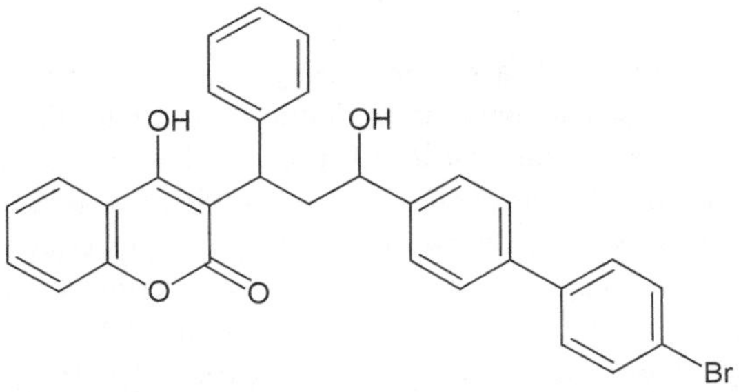

Bromadiolone {3-(3-(4′ bromobiphenyl-4-yl)-3-hydroxy-1-phenyl propyl)-4-hydroxycoumarin} was synthesized and marketed by the French company Lipha S.A. during the mid-1970s. It is used widely for control of commensal and field rodents in many countries. Technical grade bromadiolone is a 97% pure yellowish powder and stable up to 2000°C. It is very soluble in dimethylformamide (730 g/L), less soluble in ethyl acetate (25 g/L) and ethanol (8.2 g/L), and sparingly soluble in water (0.019 g/L). Bromadiolone is considered more palatable to rodents than most other anticoagulants; its concentration in baits is usually 50 ppm. Although bromadiolone is considered a "second-generation" anticoagulant rodenticide, resistance in *Rattus norvegicus* and *Mus musculus* has been reported in the United Kingdom and Denmark (Rowe et al., 1981).

Brodifacoum

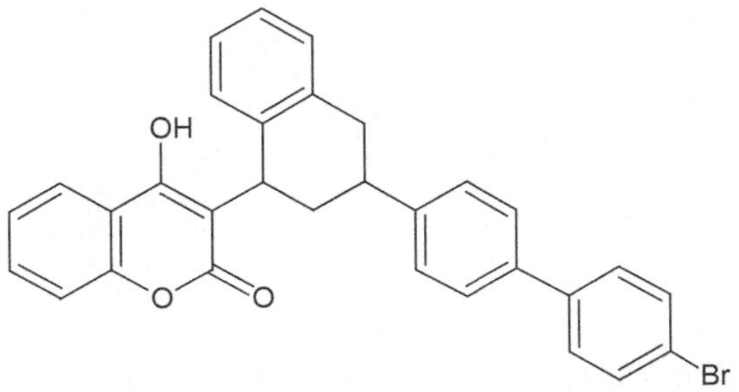

Brodifacoum {3-(3-(4′ bromobiphenyl-4-yl)-1,2,3,4-tetrahydro naphth-1-yl)-4-hydroxycoumarin} is one of the newer and more potent second-generation anticoagulant rodenticides. It was introduced in 1977 by Sorex Ltd. of London, then developed by the Imperial Chemicals Incorporated (ICI) Plant Protection Division (Chalermchaikit et al., 1993).

Pure brodifacoum is off-white to fawn-colored powder, with a solubility of 6–20 g/L in acetone, 3 g/L in chloroform, 0.6–6 g/L in benzene, and less than 10 mg/L in water. It is very stable in the environment, with no loss after 30 days of exposure to direct sunlight (Chalermchaikit et al., 1993).

Brodifacoum has been marketed in several countries for the control of a wide range of rodent pest species. It is available as a 0.005% pellet for rat and house mouse controls, a smaller 0.001% pellet for field rodent control, and as 29 g wax blocks for sewer rat control. It was the only anticoagulant rodenticide reported to produce 100% mortality in most rodent species after a 24 h dose. Although brodifacoum was effective against warfarin-resistant rats and mice in 1984, the possibility of resistance has been raised (Lund, 1984).

Variation occurs in the susceptibility of species to brodifacoum. The average pig, sheep, or chicken must consume considerable quantities of prepared bait to be endangered; however, dogs are susceptible, and are commonly exposed to potentially toxic quantities. According to the recent report by Feinstein et al. (2017), brodifacoum presents a danger to public health in the United States.

Coumatetralyl

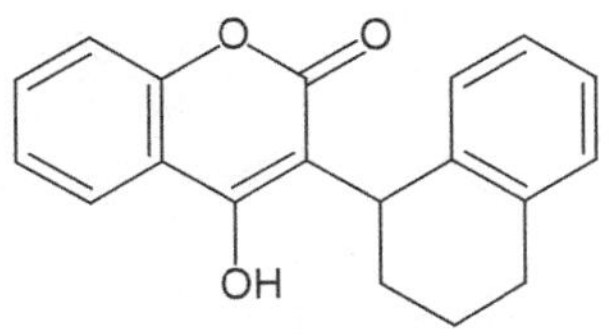

Coumatetralyl {3-(alpha-tetralyl-4-hydroxycoumarin} was introduced by Bayer AG with the trademark name of Racumin. It has been used for commensal control in many countries. It is formulated as a dry bait (0.0375%), a liquid bait of its sodium-salt, and a 0.75% tracking dust (Chalermchaikit et al., 1993).

Pure coumatetralyl is a colorless powder, which is stable at temperatures below 150°C. Its solubility is 20–50 g/L in propan-2-ol, 50–100 g/L in methylene dichloride, and 4 mg/L in water. The acute and chronic LD_{50}s to *R. norvegicus* are 16.5 and 0.3 mg/kg for five consecutive doses, respectively. Chickens are quite resistant to coumatetralyl, with a chronic LD_{50} of 50 mg/kg for eight consecutive doses. Signs did not appear in fish until the concentration of coumatetralyl reached 1000 mg/L in water.

In spite of its low toxicity, coumatetralyl is reported to be a little more effective than warfarin against *R. norvegicus*, apparently due to a higher palatability. Coumatetralyl was introduced after the detection of warfarin-resistant rat populations, and showed considerable success for a number of years, but resistant pests have been reported in the United Kingdom and Denmark (Rowe and Redfern,1968).

Coumafuryl

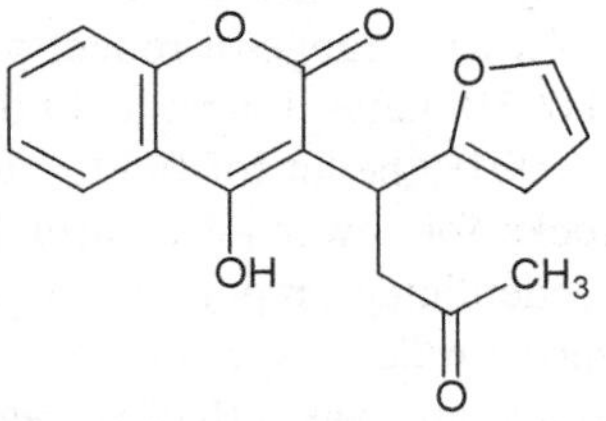

Coumafuryl {3-(alpha-acetonylfurfuryl)-4-hydroxycoumarin} is an anticoagulant rodenticide that was introduced in Germany in 1952, and is used at 0.025%–0.05% in baits. Its toxicity is considered equal to warfarin for *R. norvegicus*, but slightly less efficient against *M. musculus*. The chronic LD_{50} in *R. norvegicus* is 1.4 mg/kg for five repeated doses. Cats and dogs seem to be almost as susceptible as rats, with dogs experiencing toxicosis after 2 mg/kg for five repeated doses and cats after 10 mg/kg for four repeated doses (Chalermchaikit et al., 1993).

Difenacoum

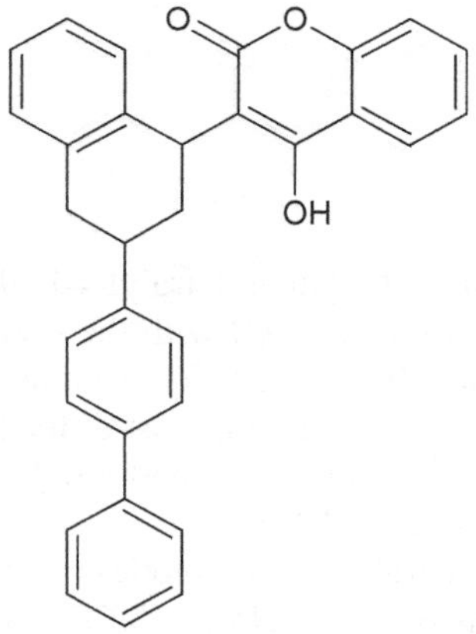

Difenacoum {3-(3-*p*-diphenyl-1,2,3,4-hydronaphth-1-yl)-4-hydroxycoumarin} was synthesized in the United Kingdom and marketed in 1975 by Sorex Ltd. under the trademark "Neosorexa." It was marketed under the trademark "Ratak" by the ICI Plant Protection Division as a 0.005% pelleted bait and as a wax block. Pure difenacoum is an off-white powder with a solubility of greater than 50 g/L in acetone, 600 mg/L in benzene, and less than 10 mg/L in water. It is more toxic than warfarin, but less palatable. Difenacoum is still effective against many populations of warfarin-resistant rats (Desideri et al., 1979), but resistance may be developing in the United Kingdom (Greaves et al., 1982).

Warfarin

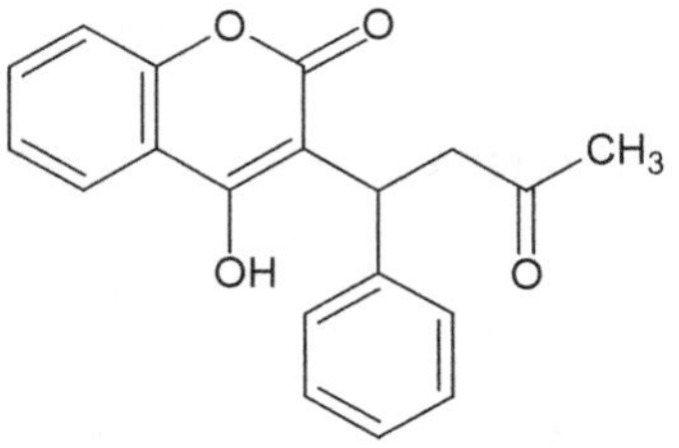

Warfarin {3-(a-acetonylbenzyl)-4-hydroxycoumarin} was the first anticoagulant rodenticide introduced, as discussed above. Warfarin is still used widely, especially for the control of *R. norvegicus*, in areas where resistance has not developed. In its racemic form, warfarin is colorless and crystalline, insoluble in water, but readily soluble in acetone, dioxane, and moderately soluble in alcohols. Warfarin is formulated as dry bait (0.005%–0.05%) as well as a liquid bait, based on the sodium salt, and a tracking dust (0.5%–1.0%). It is generally applied as the S-isomer, which is 10 times more toxic than the R-isomer. The acute and chronic LD_{50}s for *R. norvegicus* are around 10–12 mg/kg and 0.75 mg/kg for five repeated doses, respectively (Colvin and Wang, 1974).

Warfarin is sometimes combined with an antibacterial agent, sulfaquinoxaline, intended to reduce the bacterial production of vitamin K in the rat intestine, but effectiveness of this combination has not been reported. Warfarin is considered one of the safest anticoagulants to domestic and other nontarget animals; however, serious resistance has been reported in Europe. It has recently been evaluated against sewer rats in London (Channon et al., 2000) (Table 46.1).

Indanedione Group

Chlorophacinone

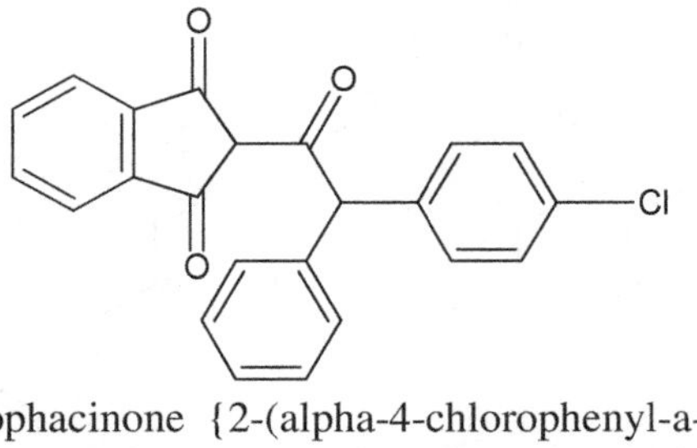

Chlorophacinone {2-(alpha-4-chlorophenyl-a-phenylacetyl)-1,3-indandione} was first introduced during the mid-1960s by S.A. Lipha of France, at concentrations of

TABLE 46.1 The Oral LD_{50} Values (mg/kg body weight) of Some Anticoagulant Rodenticides

Animals	Bromadiolone	Brodifacoum	Difenacoum
Rat (acute)	0.65	0.27	1.8
Rat (chronic)	(0.06–0.14) × 5	(0.05–0.08) × 5	0.15 × 5
Mouse	0.99	0.4	0.8
Rabbit	1.0	0.2	2.0
Pig	3.0	10.0	80.0
Dog	10.0	3.5	50.0
Cat	25.0	25.0	100.0
Chicken	5.0	10.0–20.0	50.0
Guinea pig	2.8	–	–
Opossum	–	0.17	–
Sheep	–	10.0	100.0

0.05% in baits and 0.2% in tracking dust. Pure chlorophacinone is a yellow crystalline solid, which is very soluble in acetone, ethanol, ethyl acetate, but sparingly soluble in water. It is quite stable, and resistant to weathering. Chlorophacinone does not induce "bait-shyness," and is compatible with cereals, fruits, roots, and other potential bait substances. Its acute LD_{50} in *R. norvegicus* is about 20.5 mg/kg, which is less toxic than warfarin, but it has a stronger initial effect on rats and mice. For control of house mice populations, a prolonged feeding period is needed. Chlorophacinone may not be effective against warfarin-resistant rodents (Chalermchaikit et al., 1993).

Diphacinone

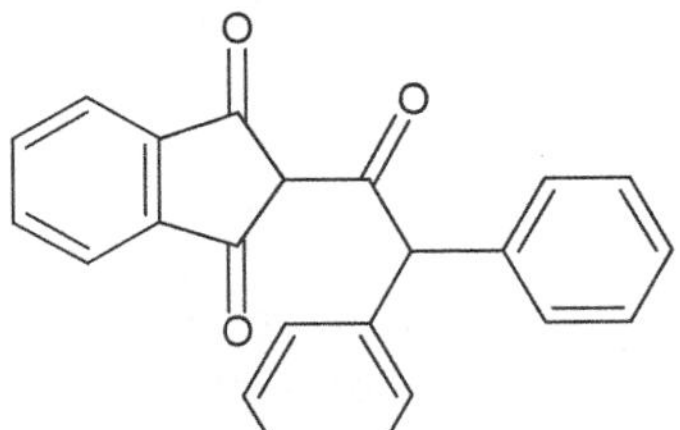

Diphacinone (2-diphenylacetyl-1,3-indandione) is an anticoagulant rodenticide introduced by Vesicol Chemical Corp. and the Upjohn Co. It has been produced and used primarily in the United States as 0.005% dry or liquid bait. Pure diphacinone is a yellow powder that is very soluble in chloroform (204 g/kg), toluene (73 g/kg), xylene (50 g/ kg), and acetone (29 g/kg), but sparingly soluble in water (0.30 g/L). It will decompose in water due to sunlight. The acute LD_{50}s in *R. norvegicus* are 22.7 mg/kg in females and 43.3 mg/kg in males. It is more toxic than warfarin to rats, mice, and dogs, but its palatability is somewhat lower. Diphacinone may not be effective against warfarin-resistant rodents (Chalermchaikit et al., 1993).

The anticoagulant rodenticides are marketed to have efficacy against a number of target pest species. These species are listed in Table 46.1 by chemical compound.

PRIMARY MECHANISM OF ACTION AND METABOLISM

Primary Mechanism of Action

The biochemical mechanism, metabolism, and kinetics of the anticoagulant rodenticides are summarized. The mechanism of action of all anticoagulant rodenticides is similar to that of warfarin (i.e., inhibition of vitamin K_1 epoxide reductase) (Park et al.,1979; Leck and Park, 1981; Breckenridge et al., 1985). In the coagulation cascade, the clotting factors II, VII, IX, and X bind calcium ions to be most active in clot formation. Ca^{2+} binding ability requires posttranslational modification of glutamyl residues on precursors of these clotting factors to gamma-carboxyl glutamyl residues by carboxylation. This carboxylation uses vitamin K_1 hydroquinone as a cofactor. This vitamin K-dependent carboxylase reaction converts vitamin K_1 hydroquinone to its epoxide form, vitamin K_1 2,3-epoxide. In the normal cycle, vitamin K_1 2,3-epoxide is reduced to vitamin K_1 (phylloquinone) by enzyme epoxide reductase, and is thus, recycled.

Anticoagulant rodenticides produce some biochemical effect by interfering with the enzyme vitamin K_1 epoxide reductase, resulting in the depletion of vitamin K_1 and, subsequently, impairing the synthesis of gamma-carboxylated clotting factors II, VII, IX, and X (Craciun et al., 1997, 1998). Clinical coagulopathy soon follows the depletion of vitamin K_1. Since these clotting factors have finite plasma half-lives of, e.g., 41, 6.2, 13.9, and 16.5 h in the dog, respectively, a lag time of 3–5 days is commonly observed between ingestion of bait and the onset of clinical signs (Jackson and Suttie, 1977; Suttie, 1986; Murphy and Gerken, 1989). The interrelationship of vitamin K, prothrombin, and gamma-carboxyglutamic acid are reviewed in Stenflo (1978). The interaction of warfarin and vitamin K reviewed in Suttie (1990).

Microsomal vitamin K dependent carboxylase, vitamin K epoxidase, vitamin K_1 epoxide reductase, and cytosolic vitamin K reductase (DT-diaphorase) are involved in vitamin K reduction (Hildebrandt and Suttie, 1982). The physiologically important site of action of the anticoagulant rodenticides has been reported to be vitamin K_1 epoxide reductase (Hildebrandt and Suttie, 1982). Anticoagulant rodenticides act by inhibiting vitamin K_1-2,3 epoxide reductase and, consequently, the synthesis of clotting factors II, VII, IX and X. S-warfarin and difenacoum are more potent in complete inhibition of clotting factor synthesis than racemic warfarin, R-warfarin, or brodifacoum (Breckenridge et al., 1985).

The greater potency and duration of action of the long-acting or "superwarfarins" has been attributed to (1) a greater affinity for vitamin K_1-2,3-epoxide reductase, (2) ability to inhibit the vitamin K_1 epoxide cycle at more than one point, (3) hepatic accumulation, and (4) unusually long half-lives due to lipid solubility, enterohepatic circulation, or both (Watt et al., 2005). The two diastereomers of brodifacoum may have different conformational alignment with vitamin K epoxide reductase (Cort and Cho, 2009).

As it turns out, rat liver has two pathways for vitamin K reduction. One is responsible for the therapeutic effect of vitamin K_1 therapy. This pathway is DT-diaphorase (EC.1.6.99.2) and a microsomal dehydrogenase that has 3.6 fold higher activity with NADH than with NADPH. It is not a cytochrome P-450 or cytochrome-b5 reductase (Wallin, 1986). Although dicoumarol, warfarin, and diphenadione inhibit NADPH in rat liver in vitro, only dicoumarol inhibited the enzyme in rats dosed in vivo (Schor et al., 1983).

Pathway I is inactive in warfarin- and difenacoum-intoxicated rats. Vitamin K_1 epoxide reductase was also inactive, so this may be part of Pathway I in vivo. Pathway II mediates the therapeutic effect of vitamin K_1 and resulting carboxylation in vitro (Wallin, 1986).

Vitamin K and vitamin K_1 epoxide can be measured in serum (Bjornsson et al., 1979; Donnahey et al., 1979) and tissue. A number of vitamin K detection methods have been reported (Haroon et al., 1987; Haroon and Hauschka, 1983; Haroon et al., 1980; Haroon et al., 1986, Hart et al., 1984; Williams et al., 1972), including detection in human plasma (Langenberg and Tjaden, 1984) and serum (Lefevere et al., 1979) using HPLC with electrochemical detection (Takani and Suttie, 1983), or fluorimetric detection in liver (Usui et al., 1989). The mode of action of vitamin K has been reviewed (Olson, 1966).

Because anticoagulant rodenticides inhibit the vitamin K_1 reductase reaction (Pelz et al., 2005) vitamin K_1 epoxide is elevated and vitamin K_1 is reduced. For example, diphenadione- (Mount and Kass, 1989) and warfarin-exposed dogs (Carlisle and Blaschke, 1981) have elevated vitamin K_1 epoxide after SC vitamin K_1 administration.

Also, vitamin K_1 concentrations are low-to-nondetectable in rats 24 h after exposure to difenacoum (Winn et al., 1987). Measurement of the epoxide in serum has been proposed as a method to detect surreptitious exposure (Bechtold et al., 1983; Bechtold and Jahnchen, 1979). The disposition of vitamin K in anticoagulant rodenticide poisoning was examined some years ago (Park et al., 1984).

Other mechanism of action: The anticoagulant rodenticides and oral anticoagulants are also of interest in cancer research. In part, because catalyzing obligatory two-electron reductions of quinones to hydroquinones, NAD (P)H: quinone reductase (QR1) protects cells against the deleterious effects of redox cycling of quinones and their ability to deplete glutathione and produce neoplasia (Dinkova and Talalay, 2000). DT-diaphorase and coenzyme Q appear to have both antioxidant and prooxidant functions in quinone metabolism (Cadenas, 1995; Beyer, 1994), and have recently been investigated as modulators of inflammation.

Metabolism

Warfarin is metabolized by CYP 2C9 and 2C19 in humans (Brandon et al., 2005; Goldstein, 2001). The CYP 2C9 enzyme has several inherited polymorphisms (Kirchheiner and Brockmoller, 2005). Chlorophacinone elimination may be enhanced by phenobarbital administration (Burocoa et al., 1989; Lagrange et al., 1999), perhaps due to CYP induction. The effect of phenobarbitone on vitamin K_1 metabolism (Wilson and Park, 1984) can be compared to that of the rabbit (Winn et al., 1988) (Fig. 46.1).

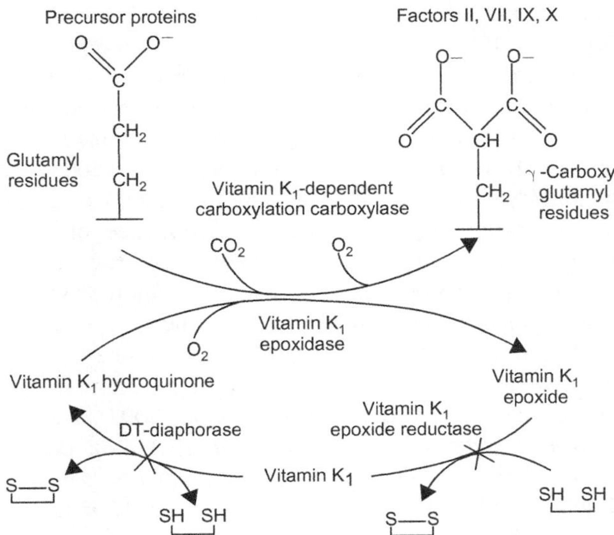

FIGURE 46.1 Liver metabolism of vitamin K. The dithiol-dependent vitamin K_1 epoxide reduction and vitamin K_1 (Phylloquinone) reduction are the metabolic steps inhibited by anticoagulant rodenticides.

TOXICITY

TOXICOKINETICS

Bioavailability

Most anticoagulant rodenticide toxicoses occur after oral exposure. However, a diphacinone-induced coagulopathy has been reported after dermal exposure to a liquid preparation (Spiller et al., 2003), and an unusual case is reported after exposure to brodifacoum after transplantation of multiple organs (Ornstein et al., 1999).

The oral bioavailability of warfarin, chlorophacinone, and bromadiolone were estimated at 79%, 92%, and 88%, respectively, in sheep. These anticoagulants degraded by about 15% over 24 h in rumen extracts. The bioavailability of warfarin is influenced by dietary protein (Barber and Colvin, 1980).

Distribution

Sixty percent of ^{14}C-labeled diphacinone is eliminated in feces and 10% in urine over 4 days in mice and 8 days in rats (Yu et al., 1982). Tissue distribution indicated that liver had the most ^{14}C activity, with the lowest amounts in brain, muscle, blood, and fat (Yu et al., 1982). The disposition and pharmacodynamic properties of brodifacoum have also been characterized in rats (Bachmann, Sullivan, 1983). Similarly, 30% of ^{14}C-labeled fluocoumafen is eliminated in feces and less than 3% in urine within 3 days in rats (Huckle et al., 1988). About 60% of ^{14}C fluocoumafen is liable to beta-glucuronidase, and most radioactivity is found unchanged in the liver. Elimination is biphasic, with a rapid phase of 5 days, then a prolonged phase of 100 days in Japanese quail (Huckle et al., 1989a,b).

Alteration of parental behavior was speculated to be a cause of 54% lethality in offspring in the face of 40% lethality of lactating female albino rats dosed with coumatetralyl (Marchini and Turillazzi, 1978). However, passage into milk is an alternative theory.

Elimination

The different chemical structures give different elimination kinetics for the various anticoagulant rodenticides. Elimination kinetics is estimated from human or animal clinical cases in many instances. Such cases are presented for the 4-hydroxycoumarins warfarin, brodifacoum, difenacoum, bromadiolone, difethialone, and chlorophacinone.

Warfarin has a terminal half-life of 5.6 + 0.7 h, with a mono-exponential decay (Breckenridge et al., 1985). Brodifacoum and difenacoum have a bi-exponential decay of 60 ± 1.9 and 83 ± 10 h, respectively, in rabbits (Breckenridge et al., 1985). An estimated median half-life of brodifacoum elimination in dogs has been estimated to be 2.4 days (Robben et al., 1998), although the data may reflect only the first elimination phase. Plasma half-life for brodifacoum was reported to initially be 0.75 days, with a terminal half-life of 24.3 days in a patient with hematuria requiring 4 months of phytonadione treatment.

A 41-year-old man had a terminal half-life of 11.7 days for difenacoum after covert administration of an unknown amount of the drug (McCarthy et al., 1997). A second individual had a peak serum concentration of 600 ng/mL (Butcher et al., 1992).

A peak serum concentration of 440 ug/L, then an elimination half-life of 140 h, was reported in a 55-year-old man who ate an unknown amount of bromadiolone (Grobosch et al., 2006). Elimination half-lives of 2.2 and 3.2 days have been reported in 2 dogs with difethialone exposure, respectively (Robben et al., 1998). A half-life of 5 days is reported in sheep dosed with pindone (Robinson et al., 2005).

Duration

Despite reported elimination half-lives, the duration of the anticoagulant effect provides an indication of the clinically relevant treatment times. Brodifacoum and difenacoum cases seem to have the longest duration of anticoagulant effect in animals and humans.

Rabbits are anticoagulated 6 weeks after oral exposure to 1 mg/kg body wt. brodifacoum (Park and Leck, 1982). Although clotting times were prolonged for 7 months after a person's exposure to an unknown amount of difenacoum (McCarthy et al., 1997), elevated concentrations of vitamin K_1 2,3-epoxide were detected for 18 months after exposure of two factory workers to brodifacoum and difenacoum despite normal PTs (Park et al., 1986).

Duration of treatment has also been reported for bromadiolone and chlorophacinone cases, as well as pindone-dosed sheep. A patient exposed to bromadiolone had to be treated for 6 months (Haug et al., 1992). An 18-year-old woman's PT normalized 7 weeks after deliberate ingestion of 100 mg chlorophacinone (Vogel et al., 1988). Pindone has been detected for up to 14 days in blood, 17 days in fat, and 39 days in liver of sheep dosed with it (Robinson et al., 2005).

TOXICITY

Target Species

By Chemical

Brodifacoum: One day of feeding on a 0.005% brodifacoum or difenacoum bait is reportedly successful in controlling the lesser bandicoot rat (*Bandicota bengalensis*) in Burma (Brooks et al., 1980). Within 3 days, a 0.005% brodifacoum bait gave complete control of golden hamsters (*Mesocricetus auratus*) resistant to 0.005% warfarin and difenacoum (Bradfield and Gill, 1984). A 20 ppm brodifacoum bait gave virtually complete control of Norway rats (*R. norvegicus*) in 21–73 days after other treatments had failed (Greaves et al., 1982). Among 35 analyzed target and nontarget small mammals, Norway rats (*R. norvegicus*) from both baited and nonbaited farms had residues of brodifacoum or bromadiolone, and a single vole had hepatic residues (18.6 μ/g). Brodifacoum has recently been used to control brown-necked ravens (*Corvus ruficollis*) in the Suez Canal region (El-Bahrawy et al., 2007). At a 0.005% bait concentration brodifacoum was more effective at 8 days in controlling *Meriones shawi* than warfarin at 0.025%, coumatetralyl at 0.0375%, difenacoum at 0.005%, and bromadiolone at 0.005% (Gill and Redfern, 1983). Brodifacoum's efficacy has also been shown for *Tatera indica* (Rehman and Ahmad, 1983), *T. indica*, *Nesokia indica*, *B. bengalensis* (Greaves and Rehman, 1977), field mice (*Mus Booduga* Gray) (Balasubramanyam et al., 1984), *Rattus rattus* and *B. bengalensis* (Deobhankar, 1985), eight rodent species (Lund, 1981, 1988), the Egyptian spiny mouse (*Acomys cahirinus*) (Mahmoud and Redfern, 1981), nonresistant (Mosterd and Thijssen, 1991), and warfarin-resistant rats (Rennison and Dubock, 1978). A number of early studies were conducted under the designation WBA 8119 (Rowe and Bradfield, 1976; Rowe et al., 1978). A number of different rodenticides have been tested for efficacy against rodents in cucumber (*Cucumis sativus*) plantings (Sabhlok et al., 1997).

Bromadiolone: Bromadiolone has been effective against warfarin-resistant rats and mice (Redfern and Gill, 1980). It is effective against the Norway rat (*R. norvegicus*) (Richards, 1981; Kamil, 1987). It was recently reported as being effective in a standard 4-day no-choice study of the Norway rat, *Rattus norvegicus,* and the roof rat, *R. rattus* Egypt. Bromadiolone residues have been examined in tissues of *Arvicola terreteris* (Giraudoux et al., 2006) and coypu (*Myocastor coypus*) (Jeantet et al., 1991) after field use. Its effects on the breeding performance of house mice have also been investigated (Twigg and Kay, 1995).

Chlorophacinone: The efficacy of chlorophacinone against mice, voles, and squirrels has been reported. At a 25 ppm bait concentration, chlorophacinone is more effective than coumachlor in controlling common mice (*M. musculus*) in Egypt (Mesban et al., 2003), and can control common voles (*Microtus arvalis*) (Nikodemusz et al., 1981), palm squirrels (*Funambulus pennanti*) (Mathur and Prakash, 1980), and house mice (*M. musculus*) (Lund, 1971).

Coumafuryl: Coumafuryl is more effective on *R. rattus*, *R. norvegicus*, and *B. bengalensis* than fumarin and warfarin when used in liquid form (Renapurkar, 1982). It was effective in controlling the cotton rat (*Sigmodon hispidus*) at concentrations used to control *R. rattus* and *R. norvegicus* (Gill and Redfern, 1980) and *M. natalensis* (Gill and Redfern, 1979).

Coumatetralyl: Median survival time was 4.7 and 11.2 days in *B. bengalensis* and *R. rattus* exposed to 0.0375% coumatetralyl bait, respectively (Chopra and Parshad, 1985).

Diphacinone: Diphacinone has been shown to control rats (Elias and Johns, 1981), vampire bats (Thornton, 1980; Burns and Bullard, 1979, 1980), *B. bengalensis* (Brooks et al., 1980), and coyotes (Sterner, 1979; Szuber and Diechtiar, 1968).

Difenacoum: Fifty percent of male mice exposed to 0.5 mg difenacoum/kg body wt. died within 9 days, whereas no female mice died (Winn et al., 1989). Norway rats (*R. norvegicus*) fed 25 ppm difenacoum bait for 5, 10, or 20 days had whole carcass residues of 0.52–0.74 mg/kg body wt., with the higher amount being present after the longer feeding period (Atterby et al., 2005; Redfern and Gill, 1980; Rennison and Hadler, 1975). A symptom-dependent taste aversion of the brown rat (*R. norvegicus*) has been reported because the taste aversion is only present when signs are present in the animal (Smith et al., 1994).

Flocoumafen: Flocoumafen has been demonstrated to control *R. rattus*, *B. bengalensis* (Parshad and Chopra, 1986), *R. norvegicus* (Buckle, 1986), and the house mouse (*M. musculus*) (Rowe et al., 1985a, b). Flocoumafen gave a quicker and equally effective kill of 68 mice (*M. musculus*) exposed to a 0.005% oatmeal bait when compared to difenacoum, bromadiolone, and brodifacoum at the same bait concentrations (Rowe et al., 1985a,b). A nonbiliary intestinal elimination of flocoumafen has been reported in rats (Huckle et al., 1989a,b), and metabolic and toxicological studies have been reported (Veenstra et al., 1991). Accumulation of flocoumafen in rats after repeated exposure has been examined (Huckle et al., 1988).

Flupropadine: Flupropadine is nearly as effective as calciferol/warfarin in control of the house mouse (*M. musculus*) (Rowe et al., 1985a,b).

Warfarin: The efficacy of warfarin has been evaluated against squirrels (Chambers and Chambers, 1983) and a host of other species.

Fenacoum has recently been reported to be effectively reduced in rats that serve as a reservoir of Leishmania in Saudi Arabia.

Resistance

Resistance to anticoagulant rodenticides has been recognized for decades. Initial investigators postulated that a genetic mutation in the resistant rodents produced an epoxide reductase with reduced binding affinity for warfarin and similar anticoagulants, resulting in resistance to warfarin (Bell and Caldwell, 1973; Zimmerman and Matschiner, 1974; Hadler and Shadbolt, 1975; Misenheimer et al., 1994); a number of such mutations have been reported.

Eight different mutations in the vitamin K reductase reaction have been identified in laboratory strains of brown rats and house mice, and in wild-caught brown rats. Mutations at Leu128Gln, Tyr139Ser, Tyr139Cys, Tyr139Phe, and Leu120Gln have been reported to impact the efficacy of anticoagulant rodenticides in the United Kingdom (Pelz et al., 2005; Buckle, 2013), and substitutions at Leu128Ser, Tyr139Cys, and a linked sequence change Arg12Trp/Ala26Ser/Ala48Thr/Arg61Leu are reported in Germany (Pelz et al., 2012). The genomic assignment of the warfarin-resistant locus (Kohn and Pelz, 1999) and a gene-anchored map of the rat warfarin-resistant locus (Kohn and Pelz, 2000) have been reported. These followed on reports of the biochemical basis of warfarin and bromadiolone resistance in house mice (Misenheimer et al., 1994).

Literature often refers to these mutations generally as VKOR activity or coding (Endepols et al., 2013; Endepols et al., 2012; Jacob et al., 2012; Pelz et al., 2012). Rodents with these mutations are reported as being resistant to effective control with warfarin, bromadiolone (Endepols et al., 2012), difethialone (Lefevre et al., 2016) and, perhaps, difenacoum (Buckle et al., 2013); however, control with brodifacoum may be achieved (Buckle et al., 2012).

Control problems not associated with Vkore1 coding have been recently encountered (Endepols et al., 2013) and previously postulated (Bell et al., 1976), so other resistance mechanisms continue to be considered. An absolute requirement for vitamin K_1 in Danish Norway rats (*Rattus norvegicus*) (Markussen et al., 2003), increased expression of P450 (CYP) (Ishizuha et al., 2008), and the potential for differential absorption or accumulation of chlorophacinone (Vein et al., 2013) have recently been reported.

Pest Management Approaches

Newly integrated pest management approaches are being proposed for the use of anticoagulant rodenticides, in part because those that retain utility for Norway rat control at an operational level may be impossible to actually use because of restrictions (Buckle, 2013). One proposal for water vole (*Arvicola terrestris*) control includes use of trapping or limited chemical treatment when pests are at low densities, with consideration of mechanical destruction of vole tunnels, mole control, landscape management, and predator fostering (Coeurdassier et al., 2014).

An innovative use of PVC hoops ("Hula Hoops") was used to examine bait densities in aerially applied brodifacoum in a biodiversity center's efforts to eradicate invasive black rats (Engeman et al., 2013). Successful eradication of alien-invasive rabbits and mice occurred in 1 and 6 months, respectively, in the Natural Park of Madeira, using about 17,000 individual brodifacoum baiting points. Mitigated adverse impacts of the eradication program on nontarget species was balanced with adverse effects of these invasive species on the island's ecosystem.

NONTARGET EXPOSURES

Recently, the United States Environmental Protection Agency provided notice of intent to cancel registration of, and notice of denial of, applications for certain rodenticide products. The affected products are anticoagulant rodenticide pesticides containing warfarin, brodifacoum, or difethialone (Federal Register Volume 78, No 24, Tuesday, February 5, 2013).

Unfortunately, nontarget species may also be exposed to anticoagulant rodenticides because they are a potential hazard to all species of mammals and birds. The prevalence of exposure to nontarget species in the environment, insects, birds, and mammals are briefly summarized.

Prevalence: In the United States, anticoagulant rodenticides are the most common rodenticide exposure of dogs (Murphy and Hornfeldt), and the most common toxin seen in many US veterinary practices (Murphy et al., 2006; Beasley and Trammel, 1989). A recent retrospective study of 123 dogs tested for anticoagulant rodenticides reported that 75 (60.9%) dogs tested positive and 48 did not. Brodifacoum, diphacinone, and chlorophacinone were detected at concentrations ranging from trace amounts to 1120 parts per billion, but were not correlated with any recorded parameter. Dogs with toxicosis had a survival rate of 98.7%. The most common diagnoses in 48 dogs without detectable anticoagulant rodenticides were neoplasia (15), immune-mediated disease (7), and gastrointestinal bleeding (5) (Waddell et al., 2013).

Prevalence of nontarget animal exposures has also been reported in the Netherlands, Spain, France, and Mongolia. Dogs suspected of anticoagulant rodenticide poisoning in the Netherlands had brodifacoum (19), bromadiolone (14), difenacoum (8), difethialone (6), and chlorophacinone (1) (Robben et al., 1997). Assessment of potential toxicity of pindone for domestic animals has also been made (Martin et al., 1991). Anticoagulant rodenticides were detected in the liver of 401 wild and domestic animals found dead in Spain, including two species of reptiles ($n = 2$), 42 species of birds ($n = 271$), and 18 species of mammals ($n = 128$) (Sánchez-Barbudo et al., 2012). Hernandez-Moreno et al. (2013) reported the deaths of three birds in an ornithological zoo in Galicia (NW Spain) by difenacoum and brodifacoum. A retrospective analysis of French human and animal poison control center data from 2004 to 2007 reported no mortality in humans, and less than 1% mortality in domestic animals. Dogs represented 60% of domestic species, while hares and rabbits represented 50% of wildlife cases, followed by predators and scavengers. In wildlife, bromadiolone and chlorophacinone were most frequently observed (Berny et al., 2010 a,b). In 2002, hundreds of nontarget wildlife deaths reportedly occurred in Mongolia following aerial applications of bromadiolone to control eruptive Brandt's vole (*Microtus brandti*) populations.

Environmental Approximately 700 kg of cereal bait containing 20 ppm of the anticoagulant rodenticide brodifacoum was spilled into a southern New Zealand lake in 2010 from a helicopter being used to transport containers of brodifacoum bait for an aerial baiting operation. In the month after the spill, no residual brodifacoum was detected in samples of lake water, sediment, benthic invertebrates, eels, and two birds (Fisher et al., 2012).

Anticoagulant rodenticides may be detected in water, soil, and invertebrates. A method of detecting warfarin in water has recently been reported (Badia and Diaz-Garcia, 1999), perhaps since anticoagulant rodenticides are used in rice paddies (Baskaran et al., 1995), and accidental discharges of brodifacoum bait may occur in fresh water or marine environments (Primus et al., 2005). The toxicity of anticoagulant rodenticides in soil may be related to the portion not bound to humic acid. Testing for the halogenated biphenyl side chain has been suggested as a way to determine soil exposure to rodenticides (Townsend et al., 1995).

Insects: Diphacinone ranging from 0.8 to 2.5 and from 1.3 to 4.0 ppm has been detected in snails and slugs, respectively, in Hawaii (Primus et al., 2006). The mean brodifacoum concentration in cockroaches immediately after bait exposure of 262 ± 131 μg/kg wet weight decreased quickly in the following 2 weeks, and then continued at a slower rate over the following 4 weeks. Woodlice recorded a similar brodifacoum concentration and a similar time course for the postexposure decline. Diphacinone has been detected in snails after broadcast, (Johnston et al., 2005) and a concentration of 0.39 μg/g has been reported from a pool of carrion beetles (*Dermestes* spp.) in a nonbaited farm area.

Birds: A number of experimental and field studies of bird exposures to anticoagulant rodenticides have been reported.

Experimental: Owls, kestrels, and stone martens have been experimentally exposed.

Eastern screech-owls (*Megascops asio*) fed 10 μg diphacinone/g wet weight food for 7 days were monitored for 21-day postexposure. Liver and kidney diphacinone elimination was initially rapid, then followed by slower loss rate, with overall half-lives of 11.7 and 2.1 days, respectively (Rattner et al., 2014; Rattner et al., 2012). The acute oral toxicity of diphacinone was found to be more than 20 times greater in American kestrels (*Falco sparverius*) with a median lethal dose of 96.8 mg/kg body weight compared to Northern bobwhite (*Colinus virginianus*) and mallards (*Anas platyrhynchos*). Chlorophacinone has also been studied in captive kestrels (Radvanyi et al., 1988), and bromadiolone-poisoned mice in stone martens (*Martes foina*) (Lund and Rasmussen, 1986). Diphacinone, dicoumarol, and pival have all been shown to increase the PT in chicks (Charles et al., 1966), and a 100% mortality occurred in 1-week-old chicks fed coumestral in wood-straw mats (Munger et al., 1993). A "no observed effect" concentration of chlorophacinone of 1 mg chlorophacinone/kg feed is reported for Japanese quail (*Coturnix japonica*) (Riedel et al., 1990).

Six owls fed difenacoum-intoxicated mice survived and coagulation times returned to normal in 5–23 days; however, four of six owls fed brodifacoum-intoxicated mice died 6–17 days after feeding. Dead owls had 630–1250 ng/g brodifacoum in their livers (Newton et al., 1990).

Field: Numerous studies of birds exposed to anticoagulant rodenticides in the field have been reported. These studies are summarized here, transitioning from those birds that primarily ingest grain to birds of prey to present the author's inferences of the potential routes of exposure to the anticoagulant rodenticide bait.

Exposure of quail, sparrows, duck, turkeys, and Poouli have been reported. Emaciated California quail (*Callopepla californica*) were found to have impacted crops due to parafinized chlorophacinone pellets attributed to the paraffin, since PT times were normal (Blus et al., 1985). A study of two adjacent working farms reports that house sparrows (*Passer domesticus*) readily entered brodifacoum or bromadiolone bait stations and fed on unloaded bait. Cases of brodifacoum toxicity in white winged wood duck (James et al., 1998) and mortality of wild turkeys (*Meleagris gallopavo*) associated with use of chlorophacinone for prairie dog (*Cynomys* spp.) control have been reported (Ruder et al., 2011). In Hawaii, broadcast diphacinone has been implicated in toxicoses of the endangered bird Poouli. A 3% and 8% probability of mortality was reported for adult and juvenile Poouli 5 days post broadcast, respectively; residues in snails apparently increased exposure in juvenile birds (Johnston et al., 2005).

Ten of 71 Great Bustard (*Otis tarda*) carcasses collected from 1991 to 2010 are reported to contain residues of chlorophacinone or flocoumafen associated with vole control.

Studies reporting exposure and toxicosis of birds of prey following exposure to anticoagulant rodenticides have been reported for the United States, England, Canada, Norway, Denmark, France, and Australia.

United States: In the New York area, brodifacoum, diphacinone, bromadiolone, chlorophacinone, and coumatetralyl are reportedly implicated in poisoning of nontarget wildlife in 80% of 55 animals investigated; exposure of great horned owls (*Bubo virginianus*) and red-tailed hawks (*Buteo jamaicensis*) constituted half the cases (Stone et al., 1999). In Massachusets, exposure and toxicosis of red-tailed hawks (*B. jamaicensis*), barred owls (*Strix varia*), eastern screech owls (*M. asio*), and great horned owls (*B. virginianus*) presented to a wildlife clinic were reported. Of 161 birds tested, 86% had liver residues, 99% of which were brodifacoum; toxicosis was diagnosed in 6% of these birds. No indications of sublethal effects of exposure were found, and no association between liver brodifacoum concentration and toxicosis were reported. In New Jersey, residues of one or more anticoagulant rodenticides were detected in 81% of red-tailed hawks (*B. jamaicensis*) and 82% of great horned owls (*B. virginianus*) sampled. Brodifacoum and bromadiolone were detected in 76% and 20% of red-tailed hawks and 73% and 27% of great horned owls, respectively. The only other anticoagulant rodenticide reported was difenacoum in one great horned owl (Stansley et al., 2014).

England: Ten percent of barn owls collected in England had detectable residues of difenacoum or brodifacoum in their livers. Liver concentrations of difenacoum and brodifacoum ranged from 5 to 106 ng/g and 19 to 515 ng/g, respectively (Newton et al., 1990). Of 114 red kites (*Milvus milvus*) sampled, 70% contained residues and 10% reportedly died as a result of rodenticide exposure (Hughes et al., 2013).

Canada: A compilation of 164 stringiformes collected in Western Canada between 1988 and 2003 showed that 70% had residues of at least one rodenticide, and of these, 41% had more than one. Barred owls (*S. varia*) were most frequently exposed (92%), with liver concentration of brodifacoum ranging from 0.001 to 0.927 mg/kg and bromadiolone ranging from 0.002 to 1.012 mg/kg (Albert et al., 2010). A logistic regression analysis of published data on hepatic rodenticide residues and associated symptoms of anticoagulant poisoning from 270 birds of prey reports an estimated probability of toxicosis associated with different liver residue concentrations. Exposure was also evaluated by analyzing 196 livers from great horned owls (*B. virginianus*) and red-tailed hawks (*B. jamaicensis*) found dead at locations across Canada.

Norway: Flocoumafen, difethialone, difenacoum, bromadiolone, and brodifacoum were reported in the livers of five species of raptors found dead between 2009 and 2011. Brodifacoum, bromadiolone, difenacoum, and flocoumafen were detected in about 70% of golden eagle (*Aquila chrysaetos*) and about 50% of eagle owl (*Bubo bubo*) livers at concentrations between 11 and 255 ng/g (Langford et al., 2013).

Denmark: Exposure rates and concentrations of five anticoagulant rodenticides in liver samples from five raptors and six owls are reported. Of a total of 430 birds, at least one rodenticide was detected in 84%–100% of individual birds within each species, and multiple rodenticides were detected in 73% of all birds. The average number of rodenticides detected in individual birds was 2.2, with no differences between owls and raptors. Difenacoum, bromadiolone, and brodifacoum were the most prevalent substances, and occurred in the highest concentrations. Concentrations were lower in rough-legged buzzard (*Buteo lagopus*) and long-eared owl (*Asio otus*) than in barn owl (*Tyto alba*), buzzard (*B. buteo*), kestrel (*Falco tinnunculus*), or tawny owl (*Strix aluco*) (Christensen et al., 2012).

France and Australia: Bromadiolone has been detected in buzzards (*Buteo buteo*) in France (Berny et al., 1997), and anticoagulant rodenticide toxicosis of birds has been reported in Australia (Reece et al., 1985).

Sparrowhawks: Interestingly, sparrowhawks (*Accipiter nisus*), which prey almost exclusively on birds, have recently been reported to have similar exposure rates to species which prey on rodents (Hughes et al., 2013).

Mammals

Exposure to nontarget mammals is summarized as nontarget wildlife and humans; domestic animals were discussed above.

Nontarget wildlife: Questions of the risks of anticoagulant rodenticide toxicosis in nontarget animals have been raised for some time (Eason et al., 2002). Recent studies report detection of anticoagulant rodenticides in polecats, mink, and fox in the wild.

Polecats: Recently, difenacoum and bromadiolone were detected in 35% of male (13 of 37) and 38% of female (5 of 13) polecats (*Mustela putorius*) collected in England and Wales in areas where the baits had been used (Shore et al., 2003). Spatial and temporal residues in polecats in Britain have been reported (Shore et al., 2003), consistent with a previous study reporting difenacoum in 7 of 24 livers analyzed (Shore et al., 1996).

Mink: In France, populations of the free-ranging European mink (*Mustela lutreola*) have declined. Investigators found bromadiolone and chlorophacinone residues in the livers of four species of free-ranging mink, and raised the question of the risk to these mink (Fournier-Chambrillon et al., 2004).

Fox: Secondary poisoning of fox after broadcast of anticoagulant rodenticides for voles has been proposed (Raoul et al., 2003). Recently, a comparison of liver residues in fox (*Vulpes vulpes*) in Northern Ireland (NI) was made with those in Great Britain. Residues were detected in 84% of fox livers, more than in comparable samples from Scotland and similar to England and Wales. Bromadiolone toxicosis of coypu has also been reported (Morin et al., 1990). Bromadiolone has also been detected in fox (*Vulpes vulpes*) in France (Berny et al., 1997). Experimentally dosed fox had bromadiolone residues in feces beginning at 15 h after exposure that remained detectable at 26 days; residues in plasma showed a similar pattern but were not detectable as long.

Stoats and weasels: Examination of five anticoagulant rodenticides in livers from 61 stoats (*Mustela erminea*) and 69 weasels (*Mustela nivalis*) revealed exposure in 97% of stoats and 95% of weasels, with 79% of the animals having more than one substance. Difenacoum had the highest prevalence (82% in stoats and 88% in weasels), but bromadiolone was detected in the highest concentrations in stoats (1.290 μg/g ww) and weasels (1.610 μg/g ww).

Hedgehogs: Exposure of 120 European hedgehogs (*Erinaceus europaeus*) throughout Britain is reported to be 3%–13% per compound and 23% overall.

Badger and Prairie dogs: Badger tissues collected in California contained brodifacoum and bromadiolone (Quinn et al., 2012). Black-tailed prairie dogs (*Cynomys ludovicianus*) exposed to 0.005% chlorophacinone had hepatic concentrations of 0.44–7.56 μg/g (Vyas et al., 2012).

Anticoagulant rodenticides have also been reported in other nontarget wildlife in both urban and rural settings. Brodifacoum, diphacinone, bromadiolone, chlorophacinone, and coumatetralyl have been implicated in exposures of nontarget wildlife in the New York area, including grey squirrels (*Scirurus carolinensis*), raccoons (*Procyon lotor*), and white-tailed deer (*Odocoileus virginianus*) (Stone et al., 1999).

Humans

Most cases of human anticoagulant rodenticide toxicosis follow either accidental or intentional oral exposure to the bait, although cases of potential occupational (Voĭtsekhovskiĭ et al., 2012), transdermal (Binks and Davies, 2007), and food exposure have been reported.

The potential for exposure to anticoagulant rodenticides through food has been examined for chickens, pigs, and sheep.

Chickens: A toxicosis in 6000 laying hens caused by the malicious addition of coumatetralyl bait, as well as the insecticides aldicarb, methomyl, and imidacloprid in the drinking water, was investigated. Coumatetralyl in the yolk was detected at levels of 0.0057 mg/kg and 0.0052 mg/kg on the second and fourth day of exposure, respectively (Shimshoni et al., 2013). Experimentally, laying hens were divided into four groups of 12 animals. Groups I and II received orally a single dose of bromadiolone 10 mg/kg, group III received a single dose of bromadiolone 60 mg/kg, and group IV was the control. Following 10 and 60 mg/kg treatment, bromadiolone was not detected in albumen but was present in yolk from day 4 to 5 and from day 2 to 9, respectively.

Pigs: Cooking feral pig tissues containing diphacinone had little effect on residual diphacinone. Coumatetralyl poisoning has been reported in pigs (Dobson, 1973) and pest species (Greaves and Ayres, 1969; Rowe and Redfern, 1968).

Sheep: Sheep dosed orally with 10, 3, or 2 mg/kg body wt. pindone developed coagulopathies (Robinson et al., 2005).

Pediatric Versus Adult Exposures

Pediatric: Most anticoagulant rodenticide toxicoses are accidental; however, some are intentional (Mack, 1994) in both humans and animals (Misra et al., 2010). In the United States in 2004, 16,054 cases of exposure were reported as accidental ingestions by children; of these, 4576 patients were hospitalized, 23 had major adverse outcomes, and one died (Binks and Davies, 2007). Pediatric exposures are common, but are usually asymptomatic without significant coagulopathy. Spontaneous hemorrhage after accidental brodifacoum exposure in a child is rarely known to occur (Travis et al., 1993; Watts et al., 1990; Beriain Rodríguez et al., 2008); however, it may occur after intentional dosing (Babcock et al., 1993).

Adult: Iatrogenic toxicosis cases in adults occur with more frequency (Walker and Beach, 2002; Waien et al., 2001; Weitzel et al., 1990; Hong et al., 2010; Moery and Pontious, 2009), and combinations of anticoagulant rodenticides and glass (Tsutaoka et al., 2003), ethylene glycol (Seidelmann et al., 1995), and drugs of abuse (Spahr et al., 2007) have been reported. As many as three different compounds have been detected in one woman (Zolcinski et al., 2008). Human bromadiolone toxicosis has recently been reported in China (Shi et al., 2005), and is known elsewhere (Shanberge, 1988). Cases of intentional exposures in adults with major depressive disorders (Yu et al., 2013), attempts at potentiating self-mutilation (Centorino et al., 2012), and suicide have recently been reported (Altay et al., 2012).

Toxicosis should be considered in any adult who presents with an unexplained coagulopathy with extreme elevation of PT and partial thromboplastin time with associated depletion of vitamin K dependent factors. If toxicosis is confirmed, intentional ingestion should be considered (Watson et al., 2012).

DIAGNOSIS

History

A clinical diagnosis of anticoagulant rodenticide poisoning is most often dependent on a history of exposure, clinical signs, evidence of a coagulopathy, and response to vitamin K_1 therapy. The most pragmatic approach for determining the specific anticoagulant rodenticide involved is to read the product package. This approach alone is not definitive, because as much as 25% of anticoagulant rodenticide-intoxicated dogs do not have the anticoagulant in serum the owners suspect.

A 25-year-old man attempted suicide by eating four 42-g boxes of 0.005% brodifacoum bait, and succeeded in developing a coagulopathy (Kruse and Carlson, 1992). A 33-year-old man ate 1875 mg of chlorophacinone (Lagrange et al., 1999) and an 18-year-old female deliberately ingested 100 mg chlorophacinone (Vogel et al., 1988), and both became anticoagulated.

Rodenticides may be more toxic when repeatedly ingested over several days than when an equal amount is consumed in a single feeding (Dorman, 1990). Susceptibility may be greater in hypoprothrombinemic juveniles or animals with malabsorption syndromes. Also, the concurrent administration of highly protein-bound drugs (e.g., phenylbutazone, aspirin, or disease states, such as chronic renal disease, may increase the susceptibility of individuals to anticoagulant rodenticide poisoning) (Beasley and Buck, 1983; Mount et al., 1985).

A point-of-care test kit was evaluated and found to be able to detect warfarin at concentrations below the manufacturer's recommended limit of detection, but was unable to detect pindone, chlorphacinone, brodifacoum, bromethalin, or its metabolite desmethylbromethalin (Istvan et al., 2014).

Identification of dye in fecal material may be used to raise a question about potential ingestion of a pesticide. For example, a 57-year-old woman ingested red-dyed pellets of anticoagulant rodenticide containing difethialone and warfarin, as well as tablets of nitrazepam. Although she presented to the hospital in a comatose state, notable pink-colored excreta hinted at the consumption of anticoagulant rodenticide.

Clinical Signs

A history of exposure to anticoagulant rodenticides is not always available, or reliable, so toxicosis is occasionally inferred from symptoms in humans and clinical signs in animals. Clinical symptoms and signs have been reported in a number of human and animal cases.

Most clinical observations are interpreted as an acquired coagulopathy (Huic et al., 2002; Humphry, 1989). The onset of the coagulopathy is, however, delayed. Dogs exposed to toxic doses of anticoagulant rodenticides remain asymptomatic until depletion of the active clotting factors occurs, so clinical signs are not generally observed until 1–2 days (Dorman, 1990) or 3–5 days (Murphy and Gerken, 1989) postexposure.

Symptoms in humans: Epistaxis, gingival bleeding, widespread bruising, hematomas, hematuria, menorrhea, GI bleeding, rectal bleeding, hemorrhage into any body organ, and anemia have been reported (Watt et al., 2005). Cases of abdominal pain, hematuria, red blood in feces, diffuse cutaneous hematomas, hemoperitoneum, urethral hematoma on tomography (Terneu et al., 2003; Barlow et al., 1982; Berry et al., 2000), and diffuse alveolar hemorrhage (Barnett et al., 1992) may be observed. Hemoperitoneum after fluconazole administration (Kim et al., 2010), hematuria in 8 of 9 patients (Wu et al., 2009; Nelson et al., 2006), hemarthrosis (Kotsaftis et al., 2007), and red sputum (Grobosch et al., 2006) have been reported.

Symptoms do not normally help identify the anticoagulant rodenticide involved. For example, hemoperitoneum and intramural hematoma of the small intestine (Soubiron et al., 2000), epistaxis, hematoma, purpuria, and bruising (McCarthy et al., 1997; Laposata et al., 2007), hematuria (Butcher et al., 1992; Fang et al., 2012), neck pain, and cervical hematoma have also been observed in humans with diphenacoum exposure (Nighoghossian et al., 1990).

Pleural, pericardial, mediastinal, and subarachnoid hemorrhages (Kruse and Carlson, 1992), gastric and pulmonary hemorrhage (Olmos and López, 2007), hematemesis (Dolin et al., 2006), and hemoperitoneum (Morgan et al., 1996; Kim et al., 2010) have been reported in brodifacoum toxicosis cases.

Gastrointestinal hemorrhage after endoscopic cold mucosal biopsy (Zhao et al., 2010) and intestinal obstruction (Nie et al., 2010) have been reported. A number of other cases of brodifacoum (Braithwaite, 1982; Bruno et al., 2000; Casner, 1998; Corke, 1997; Stanziale et al., 1997), bromadiolone (Chow et al., 1992), chlorophacinone (Dusein et al., 1984; Murdoch, 1983) and other anticoagulant rodenticide exposure are present in the human literature (Ross et al., 1992).

Misdiagnosis of rodenticide poisoning as ectopic pregnancy (Wu et al., 2012), and successful treatment of pregnant women with anticoagulant rodenticide toxicosis, have been reported (Yan et al., 2013, Franco et al., 2013), although in one case, the neonate that showed evidence of fetal coagulopathy died at 4 days of age (Mehlhaff et al., 2013).

Bilateral ureteral and renal pelvis thrombus leading to acute obstructive nephropathy (Reese et al., 2012), renal pelvic thrombus, (Pais, 2012), bruising, hematuria, and abdominal pain secondary to a perinephric hematoma have been reported (Kapadia and Bona, 2008).

Clinical signs in animals: Clinical signs in animals are largely from canine cases (Woody et al., 1992). Sometimes, the only clinical signs in anticoagulant-poisoned animals are dyspnea, lethargy, or anorexia, but, more often, depression, weakness, pallor, and ventral hematomas are present (DuVall et al., 1989). In addition, pulmonary edema, pleural effusion, pericardial effusion (Schulman et al., 1986), intratracheal hemorrhage (McGuire et al., 1999), thymic hemorrhage (Elsinghorst, 2003), laryngeal obstruction (Peterson and Streeter, 1996), pericardial effusion and cardiac tamponade (Petrus and Henik, 1999), renal subcapsular hemorrhage (Radi and Thompson, 2004), and hematometra (Padgett et al., 1998) have been reported.

Additional cases of diphacinone (Troy, 1988; Schulman et al., 1986) and brodifacoum toxicosis (Baker et al., 2002; Booth, 1989; Grayson, 1982; McSporran and Phillips, 1983) in dogs have been reported. Horses have been exposed experimentally (Boermans et al., 1991) and in the field (Ayala et al., 2007) to these rodenticides. Brodifacoum may have been observed in neonatal puppies (Munday and Thompson, 2003), and has been successfully treated in a pregnant bitch (Hornfeldt and Phearman, 1996).

In clinical settings, prolonged bleeding from injection sites is usually noticed. A few clinical signs are reported that are not directly attributable to the coagulopathy. A paradoxical venous thrombosis was reported in a person with chlorophacinone exposure (Papin et al., 2007). Death, reduced breeding performance, stillborn, and nonviable lambs, as well as reduced sperm motility of rams is reported in sheep dosed with pindone (Robinson et al., 2005).

Coagulopathy

Evidence of a coagulopathy is the second element of the diagnosis. Coagulation tests are normally run on live animals, and a necropsy on dead animals, to support the presence of a coagulopathy. The basic mechanisms of clotting have been reviewed (Seegers, 1969).

Hematology: As discussed above, the anticoagulant rodenticides reduce activity of factors II, VII, IX, and X in circulation. For example, activities of 5% for factor II, 8% for factor VII, 4% for factor IX, and 6% for factor X have been reported in a brodifacoum case (Kim et al., 2010; Wu et al., 2009) The one-stage prothrombin time (OSPT) for evaluating factor VII is normally the most sensitive tool for early diagnosis because factor VII has the shortest half-life of the vitamin K_1-dependent clotting factors, e.g., about 6.2 h in dogs. Activated partial thromboplastin time (APTT) tests for all coagulation factors, except factor VII, are usually used in conjunction with OSPT. Activated coagulation time (ACT) is used in the same way as the APTT. ACT is easiest to use in a veterinary clinic setting since it only requires diatomaceous earth tubes and a heater block or water bath (Byrne, 1970).

Laboratory test results of abnormally prolonged OSPT, APTT, and ACT in the presence of normal thrombin time (TT), fibrinogen, circulating fibrin degradation products (FDPs), and platelet counts is consistent with anticoagulant rodenticide poisoning. Occasionally, however, animals with severe anemia may have elevated FDPs and reduced platelet counts. An INR is frequently measured in human coagulopathy cases (Boettcher et al., 2011; Schmeits et al., 2009); rarely, thrombosis is reported (De Paula et al., 2009; Papin et al., 2007).

The diagnostic protocol based on these coagulation factor evaluation tests (OSPT, APTT, ACT) cannot differentiate between short- and long-acting anticoagulant rodenticide poisoning. The ability to recognize long-acting anticoagulants is critical, since therapeutic success may be based, at least in part, on the duration of vitamin K_1 treatment. The ability to identify the specific anticoagulant rodenticide involved using analytical chemistry is discussed below.

Coagulation testing is not always indicated after minor exposure. Of 110 children ingesting anticoagulant rodenticides, eight had prolonged PTs. Seventeen percent (6 of 34) were prolonged 48 h after exposure, while only 1.9%

(2 of 104) at 24 h after exposure. The recommended times to check for prothrombin in children is 24 and 48 h after exposure (Smolinske et al., 1989). Routine measurement of the INR is unnecessary in young children because the amount of rodenticide ingested is invariably small (Watt et al., 2005).

Although some bias in pediatric brodifacoum exposure data (Osterhoudt and Henretig, 2003) is suspected, prospective studies of acute, unintentional, pediatric superwarfarin ingestions managed without (Ingels et al., 2002) or with (Smolinske et al., 1989) decontamination have been conducted. Some argue against the need for a PT in unintentional pediatric superwarfarin exposures (Mullins et al., 2000). See also cases of acute pediatric brodifacoum ingestions (Shepherd et al., 2002). Although less treatment is often better (Kanabar and Volans, 2002) for accidental pediatric brodifacoum exposures, rare pediatric cases have coagulopathies despite early treatment (Montanio et al., 1993).

In all other cases, the INR should be measured 36–48 h postexposure. If the INR is normal at this time, even in the case of long-acting formulations, no further action is required (Watt et al., 2005).

The most significant elevation of PT, PTT and PIVKA was observed 72 hours after a single dose of diphacinone of 2 mg/kg in ground squirrels (*Spermophilus beecheyi*), although elevations were seen at 24 h (Whisson and Salmon, 2002). The increase in ACT, APTT, and OSPT are often used to support a clinical diagnosis of anticoagulant rodenticide poisoning in dogs (Dorman, 1990). Coagulation factor synthesis may be inhibited for up to 30 days in diphacinone-exposed dogs (Mount and Feldman, 1983).

PT should be checked 48 h after stopping vitamin K_1 therapy to detect any recurrence of coagulopathy (Chataigner et al., 1989). PT times in sheep were stable in samples stored at 0, 20, and 30 degrees for 24 h.

Vitamin K-dependent factor activity has been suggested for rapid identification of surreptitious brodifacoum poisoning (Miller et al., 2006).

Necropsy/Autopsy

Pleural, pericardial, mediastinal, and subarachnoid hemorrhages have been reported in humans with brodifacoum exposure (Kruse and Carlson, 1992; Tahir et al., 2008).

Hemoperitoneum, hemothorax, and pulmonary hemorrhage are the most common necropsy findings in dogs and cats with anticoagulant rodenticide residues in liver (DuVall et al., 1989; Rickman and Gurfield, 2009). Pulmonary edema, pleural effusion, pericardial effusion (Schulman et al., 1986), and intratracheal hemorrhage are reported as well (McGuire et al., 1999).

Many cases of anticoagulant poisoning are subacute in nature, but sudden death may occur as the result of acute internal hemorrhage. Evidence of external hemorrhage, such as melena, epistaxis, hematemesis, hematuria, gingival bleeding, or excessive bleeding from an open wound, may or may not be seen. However, internal hemorrhage involving the lungs, pleural and/or peritoneal cavities, and facial planes are commonly reported (Murphy and Gerken, 1989; DuVall et al., 1989). Massive tracheal and esophageal hemorrhage 2 days after bait ingestion was reported in a dog (Stowe et al., 1983). In New Zealand, where brodifacoum was used in control of wild rabbits, 43 rabbit carcasses were found with massive hemorrhage in the abdominal cavity (52%) and thoracic cavity (17%), and the remaining 31% of cases were found with hemorrhage of muscles, cecum, stomach, kidney, mesentery, and placenta of pregnant does (Rammell et al., 1984). Postmortem findings in warfarin poisoning have been described similarly by Dakin (1968).

Response to Vitamin K_1 Treatment

Remission of the coagulopathy 24 h after vitamin K_1 treatment supports a clinical diagnosis of a vitamin K_1 responsive coagulopathy (Tvedten, 1989). A clinical diagnosis is not sufficient in all cases. Some cases require that an etiological diagnosis be made. Analytical chemistry testing is required in such cases.

Treatment

General, supportive, and specific treatments are available for anticoagulant rodenticide toxicosis. Prospective study of the outcome of patients with excessive warfarin exposure is described by Hylek et al. (2000).

General

Emetic, adsorbent, and cathartic therapies are indicated if the ingestion of the anticoagulant rodenticide has occurred within the last few hours (e.g., peak serum brodifacoum concentrations occur 2 h after oral dosing of dogs).

Clinical coagulopathy normally occurs 2–5 days after oral exposure, so emetics and cathartic at the time of presentation is not normally indicated if clinical signs are present. Oral-activated charcoal therapy, however, may be useful for those chemicals that undergo enterohepatic circulation.

Supportive

Recommendations for humans with anticoagulant rodenticide toxicosis have recently been reported by Watt et al. (2005). If active bleeding occurs, prothrombin complex concentrate (which contains factors II, VII, IX and X) 50 units/kg, recombinant activated factor VII 1.2-4.8 mg or fresh frozen plasma 15 mL/kg if no concentrate is available, and phytomenadione 10 mg IV (100 μg/kg body wt. in a child) is recommended to be given. If there is no active bleeding and the INR is $<$ or $=$ 4.0, no treatment is recommended; if INR is $\geq$4.0 phytomenadione 10 mg should be administered intravenously (Watt et al., 2005).

Animals with severe clinical bleeding, or markedly reduced PCVs, should receive fresh plasma or blood transfusions because of the 4–8 h often required to increase clotting factor activity following vitamin K_1 therapy (Chalermchaikit et al., 1993; Terneu et al., 2003; Soubiron et al., 2000; McCarthy et al., 1997).

Specific

Vitamin K_1 therapy is recommended in humans (Terneu et al., 2003; Soubiron et al., 2000; McCarthy et al., 1997; Boettcher et al., 2011) and animals with elevated coagulation times after exposure to anticoagulant rodenticides (Robben et al., 1998; Murphy et al., 1989; Mount et al., 1982). Vitamin K_1 (phylloquinone) is the most effective form for the treatment of anticoagulant rodenticide intoxication because of its immediate availability for the synthesis of new clotting factors (Chalermchaikit et al., 1993).

The pharmacological half-life of vitamin K_1 is $1.7 + 0.1$ h in rabbits dosed with brodifacoum (Park and Leck, 1982). Prothrombin activity reaches peak improvement 4 h after administration of vitamin K_1 to rabbits anticoagulated with brodifacoum or difenacoum (Park and Leck, 1982).

The duration of vitamin K_1 treatment is prolonged (Butcher et al., 1992) for the longer-acting chemicals. It may be required for up to 2 weeks in diphacinone-exposed dogs (Mount and Feldman, 1983). Daily doses of vitamin K_1 in the range of 0.25–2.5 mg/kg for 1 week are recommended for exposure to short-acting rodenticides, and 2.5–5.0 mg/kg for 3–4 weeks is recommended for exposure to long-acting rodenticides (Mount et al., 1985). Prolonged anticoagulation in rat poisoning has been reported by Jones et al. (1984) and Lipton and Klass (1984). Treatment for 48 days has been reported in a human case of flocoumafen exposure in which a half-life of 6.7 days was estimated (Boettcher et al., 2011). In intentional poisoning cases in humans, vitamin K_1 treatment may be required for 2 (Dolin et al., 2006) or 3 months (Wu et al., 2009), or. A brodifacoum case had a 56 day half-life (Olmos and López, 2007). Another report is of two concurrent cases at a clinical toxicology service that required prolonged treatment with oral vitamin K to achieve normalization of coagulation studies. Case 1 had a brodifacoum elimination half-life of 33 days, and was treated with vitamin K (100 mg) for 6 months. Case 2 was treated with vitamin K_1 (100 mg) for 3 months, with a half-life of 15 days.

The two most commonly recommended routes of vitamin K_1 administration are oral and subcutaneous. Intramuscular injections in a hypoprothrombinemic animal can produce hematoma, and intravenous administration of vitamin K_1 has been associated with anaphylaxis; therefore, these routes are discouraged in the therapeutic regimen (Clark and Halliwell, 1963).

Vitamin K_1 therapy may be reduced in a step-wise manner as long as the PT remains normal (Robben et al., 1998). The length of treatment is presently decided by evaluation of OSPT values for 2 days after the cessation of vitamin K_1 administration. If prolonged OPST is found, treatment is commonly continued for another week, but if it remains normal for 5–6 days, the vitamin K_1 treatment is usually terminated (Murphy et al., 1989).

DIAGNOSIS

Diagnostic approach to the bleeding patient has been described by Johnstone (1989). A diagnostic protocol should utilize more than one coagulation test, since it is necessary to differentiate rodenticide poisoning from other coagulopathies, such as disseminated intravascular coagulopathy, congenital factor deficiencies, hyperviscosity syndromes, platelet deficiencies or functional defects, von Willebrand's disease, and canine ehrlichiosis. Hypovitaminosis K-associated bleeding has been reported in cats with malabsorption syndrome (Edwards and Russell, 1987).

Analytical Chemistry

A number of analytical methods have been reported for detecting anticoagulant rodenticides in various matrices. Warfarin-specific analytical methods were generally not adequate for the subsequently developed rodenticides, so a number of other methods were developed. These methods include thin layer chromatography (TLC), high pressure liquid chromatography (HPLC), mass spectroscopy (MS), and antibody-mediated tests. Coumarin anticoagulant rodenticides were initially detected using TLC (Lau-Cam and Chu-Fong, 1972; Mallet et al., 1973); then, an immunoassay was developed to detect diphacinone and chlorophacinone (Mount et al., 1988). Enantiomers of warfarin, coumachlor, and coumafuryl were separated chromatographically (Armstrong et al., 1993) to assist identification.

Extraction and cleanup procedures often vary on the matrix. For example, a dispersive solid-phase extraction (dSPE) technique for multiple anticoagulant rodenticides was recently reported for blood or tissue matrices. Methods for bait and technical material, environmental samples, liquid, and solid biological samples are briefly summarized.

Bait formulation and technical material: HPLC methods to detect chlorophacinone (Vigh et al., 1981; Grant and Pike, 1979), difenacoum (Hadler and Shadbolt, 1975), and Rozol (Kawano and Chang, 1980) in bait formulation have been reported. Recently, NMR has been used to detect source-to-source and batch-to-batch variations in distereomer ratios of brodifacoum (Cort et al., 2012).

Air, soil, or water environmental samples: A recent method quantifies brodifacoum in workplace air 0.2 ~ 10.0 μg/mL, with a detection limit of 0.08 μg/mL and minimum detectable concentration of 0.00067 mg/m^3 (Fu et al., 2013). An LC-ESI-MS analytical method is reported to determine chlorophacinone, bromadiolone, pindone, diphacinone, warfarin, coumatetralyl, brodifacoum, fluocoumafen, and difenacoum residues with limits of detection and quantitation of 0.09 and 2.2 μg/kg in soil and 0.08 and 1.7 μg/L in water (Hernández et al., 2013a).

Food: An interesting new method uses HPLC to detect anticoagulant rodenticides in soft drinks (Dimuccio et al., 1991), an ion pair LC method to detect chlorophacionone and diphacinone in oats (Primus et al., 1998), and a cell culture/ELISA assay to detect anticoagulant rodenticides in treated grain (Lawley et al., 2006) have all been reported.

Exposed Animals: Liquid (Serum, Blood, Urine)

Methods to detect anticoagulant rodenticides in exposed animals were initially focused on individual compounds, then expanded to detection of groups of compounds in the same method. Matrices from exposed animals are commonly either liquids, such as urine, blood or serum, or solids, such as tissues. Methods are presented similarly.

Warfarin: Early fluorimetric and GC methods were for serum (Corn and Berberich, 1967; Fasco et al., 1977; Hanna et al., 1978; Lee et al., 1981; Lewis et al., 1970; O'Reilly et al., 1962; Vesell and Shivley, 1974; Welling et al., 1970; Mildha et al., 1974).

Brodifacoum: Numerous HPLC methods for detection of brodifacoum (Murphy and Gerken, 1989; Koubek et al., 1979; Hoogenboom and Rammell, 1983; Keiboom and Rammel, 1981; Ray et al., 1989; Hong et al., 2010; Kim et al., 2010; Fu et al., 2012) or bromadiolone (Subbiah et al., 2005; Hunter and Sharp, 1988) in serum or plasma have been reported. One method reports the use of difenacoum as the internal standard (O'Bryan and Constable, 1991).

Difenacoum: An HPLC method distinguishes cis and trans isomers with detection limits of 5 ng/mL (Kelly et al., 1993).

Various detection methods have also been used historically, including a postcolumn pH shift to enhance fluorescence detection (Hunter, 1985; Hunter and Sharp, 1988), as well as other fluorescent methods (Mundy and Machin, 1982; AOAC, 1976a,b) for diphacinone (Bullard et al., 1975, 1976), bromadiolone (Deepa and Mishra, 2005), and brodifacoum (Fu et al., 2006). Diode array (Yang et al., 2001) and rapid fluorimetric methods for detection of chlorophacinone or diphacinone (Cai et al., 2011) in human serum based on formation of histidine complexes have also been reported.

Increasingly, methods are developed to look for many, if not all, anticoagulant rodenticides in a single method. An early example extracted and detected eight anticoagulant rodenticides in serum or liver using fluorescence and UV detection with detection of 4-hydroxycoumains to about 1 ng/mL of serum and 1 ng/g of liver; and indanediones down to 10 ng/mL of serum and 10 ng/g of liver (Chalermchaikit et al., 1993; Felice et al., 1991; Felice and Murphy, 1989). A number of methods for simultaneous detection of multiple rodenticides in serum (Kuijpers et al., 1995), with detection limits of 3–12 ng/mL for fluorescence and 20–75 ng/mL for UV detection (Kuijpers et al., 1995; McCarthy et al., 1997; Mura et al., 1992; Feng et al., 1999; Jin et al., 2007) or less than 10–851 ng/L for brodifacoum, difethialone, and difenacoum (Robben et al., 1998), were reported.

Solid: (Hair, Feces, Tissues and Food)

A high performance TLC method with an estimated detection limit of 200 ppb and 87% recovery from liver has been reported (Berny et al., 1995). HPLC methods for chlorophacinone (Hunter, 1984), difethiolone (Goldade et al., 1998), difenacoum (Mundy and Machin, 1977), brodifacoum (Hagenboom and Rammell, 1983), and bromadiolone (Nahas, 1986) in tissue have been reported.

Methods for detection of multiple molecules from tissue samples, such as a solid phase cartridge extraction from liver, with recoveries ranging from 52% for difenacoum to 78% for warfarin, with limits of detection of about 10 ppb for warfarin and difenacoum and 110 ppb for chlorophacinone (Fauconnet et al., 1997; Jones, 1996; Addison, 1982), were reported. HPLC: method reports simultaneous determination of bromadiolone, brodifacoum, coumachlor, coumafuryl, coumatetralyl, difenacoum, flocoumafen, and warfarin in liver (Armentano et al., 2012).

Many recent methods use mass spectroscopy. For example, for indandiones diphacinone and chlorophacinone in whole blood or urine, and the 4-hydroxy coumarins, bromadiolone, brodifacoum, coumachlor, coumatetralyl, difenacoum, and warfarin, in whole blood specimens (Schaff and Montgomery, 2013), or LC-IT/MS method with limits of detection of 5–25 ng/mL in plasma.

Various internal standards have been reported, including a LC-EI-MS/MS method using warfarin-D5 (Yan et al., 2012) and another using Chloro-warfarin.

Contemporary mass spectroscopy methods have been reported for use on solid samples such as hair or tissues. The limits of detection (LODs) for bromadiolone and brodifacoum in human hair were recently reported as 0.010 and 0.025 ng/mg, respectively (Zhu et al., 2013).

Recent LC-ESI-MS methods have been reported for the analysis of up to 10 anticoagulant rodenticides, with a limit of quantitation of about 5 μg/L (Grobosch et al., 2006; Jin et al., 2007, Jin and Chen, 2006). Other LC MS-MS methods include warfarin (Marquet et al., 2003) and flocoumafen (Boettcher et al., 2011), with an LC-ESI-MS and HPLC-UV method to detect anticoagulant rodenticides as low as 20 ng on column (Mesmer and Flurer, 2000).

One of the earlier MS methods used a direct probe technique to detect indandione residues in food animals (Braselton et al., 1992). Methods applicable to edible tissues include an HPLC-Ion Trap/MS for indandiones (Chen et al., 2010) and LC-MS/MS. Edible tissues, including bovine muscle, bovine liver, bovine fat, swine muscle, salmon, eel, freshwater clam, egg, milk, and honey, spiked at 0.0005–0.001, with limits of quantitations of 0.0005 mg/kg for brodifacoum, 0.001 mg/kg for warfarin, coumatetralyl, and bromadiolone. Finally, an LC-DAD-FLD-MS method is reported to detect the indandione chlorophacinone, and 4-hydroxy coumarins, bromadiolone, brodifacoum and difenacoum in liver, intestine, and muscle using FLD-DAD-ESI-MS, with limits of detection and quantification ranging from 9 to 89 μg/kg (FLD-DAD) and 0.6 to 4.6 μg/kg (ESI-MS) (Hernández et al., 2013b).

CONCLUDING REMARKS AND FUTURE DIRECTIONS

Warfarin was the first anticoagulant rodenticide introduced into the market soon after World War II, and was widely used in many countries. Many other anticoagulant rodenticides with similar potency to that of warfarin were also synthesized (LD_{50}s ranging from 10 to 50 mg/kg BW). These compounds were recognized as the first-generation anticoagulant rodenticides. Due to the problem of tolerance development in rodents, newer compounds with a greater toxicity (acute LD_{50}s of 0.2–3.9 mg/kg) were developed. These compounds are called second-generation anticoagulant rodenticides, or superwarfarins. Based on chemical structures, anticoagulant rodenticides are classified into two categories: hydroxycoumarins and indanediones. Common examples of the former group are brodifacoum, bromadiolone, coumatetralyl, difenacoum, and warfarin; examples of the latter group are chlorophacinone and diphacinone. Whereas intentional poisoning is common in dogs, secondary poisoning is common in avian and wildlife species. The mechanism of action of all anticoagulant rodenticides is similar to that of warfarin—i.e., inhibition of vitamin K_1 epoxide reductase, resulting in the depletion of vitamin K_1. Subsequently, this impairs the synthesis of normal clotting factors II, VII, IX, and X, and, ultimately, coagulopathy ensues due to depletion of vitamin K_1 in the liver. Diagnosis is based on history of rodenticide exposure, clinical signs of hemorrhage and coagulopathy, and chemical confirmation in body tissues or fluids. Treatment includes vitamin K_1 and blood transfusion.

REFERENCES

Addison, J.B., 1982. Improved method for HPLC determination of chlorophacinone in mouse tissue. J. Assoc. Off. Anal. Chem. 65, 1299–1301.

Aisner, J., Goutsou, M., Maurer, L.H., Cooper, R., Chahinian, P., Carey, R., et al., 1992. Intensive combination chemotherapy, concurrent chest irradiation, and warfarin for the treatment of limited-disease small-cell lung cancer: a Cancer and Leukemia Group B pilot study. J. Clin. Oncol. 10 (8), 1230–1236.

Albert, C.A., Wilson, L.K., Mineau, P., Trudeau, S., Elliott, J.E., 2010. Anticoagulant rodenticides in three owl species from western Canada, 1988–2003. Arch. Environ. Contam. Toxicol. 58 (2), 451–459.

Alonso Martin, J.J., Duran Hernandez, J.M., Gimeno de Carlos, F., de la Fuente Galan, L., Munoz San Jose, J.C., Fernandez-Aviles, F., 1997. Post-implant antithrombotic treatment after intracoronary stents. Thrombotic occlusion. Rev. Esp. Cardiol. 50 (Suppl 2), 31–43.

Altay, S., Velibey, Y., Cakmak, H.A., et al., 2012. Prolonged coagulopathy related to coumarin rodenticide in a young patient: superwarfarin poisoning. Cardiovasc. J. Afr. 23 (9), e9–e11.

AOAC, 1976a. Determination of chlorophacinone by ultraviolet spectroscopy, Chlorophacinone EPA-1, May 1977. Supplement to EPA Manual of Chemical Methods for Pesticides and Devices. AOAC, Arlington, VA.

AOAC, 1976b. Determination of diphacinone by high pressure liquid chromatography using paired-ion chromatography, Diphacinone EPA-2, May 1978. Supplement to E PA Manual of Chemical Methods for Pesticides and Devices. AOAC, Arlington, VA.

Appendino, G., Mercalli, E., Fuzzati, N., Arnoldi, L., Stavri, M., Gibbons, S., et al., 2004. Antimycobacterial cou-marins from the Sardinian giant fennel (*Ferula communis*). J. Nat. Prod. 67 (12), 2108–2110.

Aragno, M., Tagliapietra, S., Nano, G.M., Ugazio, G., 1988. Experimental studies on the toxicity of *Ferula communis* in the rat. Res. Commun. Chem. Pathol. Pharmacol. 59 (3), 399–402.

Argento, A., Tiraferri, E., Marzaloni, M., 2000. Oral anticoagulants and medicinal plants: an emerging interaction [in Italian]. Ann. Ital. Med. Int. 15 (2), 139–143.

Armentano, A., Iammarino, M., Lo Magro, S., et al., 2012. Validation and application of multi-residue analysis of eight anticoagulant rodenticides by high-performance liquid chromatography with fluorimetric detection. J. Vet. Diagn. Invest. 24 (2), 307–311.

Armour, C.J., Barnett, S.A., 1950. The action of dicoumarol on laboratory and wild rats and its effect on feeding behavior. J. Hyg. Cambridge. 48, 158–171.

Armstrong, D.W., Reid 3rd, G.L., Hilton, M.L., Chang, C.D., 1993. Relevance of enantiomeric separations in environmental science. Environ. Pollut. 79 (1), 51–58.

Arnoldi, L., Ballero, M., Fuzzati, N., Maxia, A., Mercalli, E., Pagni, L., 2004. HPLC-DAD-MS identification of bioactive secondary metabolites from *Ferula communis* roots. Fitoterapia. 75 (3–4), 342–354.

Asperger, Z., Jursic, M., 1970. Prolonged administration of anticoagulants after myocardial infarct [in Croatian]. Lijec. Vjesn. 92 (3), 369–374.

Atterby, H., Kerins, G.M., MacNicoll, A.D., 2005. Whole-carcass residues of the rodenticide difenacoum in anticoagulant-resistant and -susceptible rat strains (*Rattus norvegicus*). Environ. Toxicol. Chem. 24 (2), 318–323.

Ayala, I., Rodríguez, M.J., Martos, N., Zilberschtein, J., Ruíz, I., Motas, M., 2007. Fatal brodifacoum poisoning in a pony. Can. Vet. J. 48 (6), 627–629.

Babcock, J., Hartman, K., Pedersen, A., Murphy, M., Alving, B., 1993. Rodenticide-induced coagulopathy in a young child. A case of Munchausen syndrome by proxy. Am. J. Pediatr. Hematol. Oncol. 15 (1), 126–130.

Bachmann, K.A., Sullivan, T.J., 1983. Disposition and pharmacodynamic characteristics of brodifacoum in warfarin-sensitive rats. Pharmacology. 27, 281–288.

Badia, R., Diaz-Garcia, M.E., 1999. Cyclodextrin-based optosensor for the determination of warfarin in waters. J. Agric. Food. Chem. 47 (10), 4256–4260.

Baker, J.T., Graversen, C.H., Files, J.E., 2002. Brodifacoum toxicity. J. Miss. State. Med. Assoc. 43 (4), 106–107.

Balasubramanyam, M., Christopher, M.J., Purushotham, K.R., 1984. Laboratory trials of three anticoagulant rodenticides for use against the Indian field mouse, Mus booduga Gray. J. Hyg. London. 93 (3), 575–578.

Bamanikar, A., Hiremath, S., 2002. Hepatotoxic reaction to warfarin in a recovering hepatitis patient with hypoalbuminenia. J. Assoc. Physicians. India. 50, 1456.

Barber, D.L., Colvin Jr, H.W., 1980. Influence of dietary protein on the response of rats receiving toxic levels of warfarin. Toxicol. Appl. Pharmacol. 56 (1), 8–15.

Barlow, A.M., Gay, A.L., Park, B.K., 1982. Difenacoum (Neosorexa) poisoning. Br. Med. J. 285 (6341), 541.

Barnett, V.T., Bergmann, F., Humphrey, H., Chediak, J., 1992. Diffuse alveolar hemorrhage secondary to superwarfarin ingestion. Chest. 102 (4), 1301–1302.

Baskaran, J., Kanakasabai, R., Neelanarayanan, P., 1995. Evaluation of two rodenticides in the paddy fields during Samba and Thaladi seasons. Indian J. Exp. Biol. 33 (2), 113–121.

Beasley, V.R., Buck, W.B., 1983. Warfarin and other anticoagulant poisoning. In: Kirk, R.W. (Ed.), Current Veterinary Therapy VIII. Saunders, Philadelphia, pp. 101–106.

Beasley, V.R., Trammel, H.L., 1989. Incidence of poisoning in small animals. In: Kirk, R.W. (Ed.), Current Veterinary Therapy X. Saunders, Philadelphia, pp. 97–113.

Bechtold, H., Jahnchen, E., 1979. Quantitative analysis of vitamin K_1 and vitamin K_1-2,3-epoxide in plasma by electron capture gas–liquid chromatography. J. Chromatogr. 164, 85–90.

Bechtold, H., Trenk, D., Jahnchen, E., Meinertz, T., 1983. Plasma vitamin K_1-2,3-epoxide as diagnostic aid to detect surreptitious ingestion of oral anticoagulant drugs. Lancet. 1, 596–597.

Bell, R.G., Caldwell, P.T., 1973. Mechanism of warfarin resistance: warfarin and the metabolism of vitamin K_1. Biochemistry. 12, 1759–1762.

Bell, R.G., Caldwell, P.T., Holm, E.E., 1976. Coumarins and the vitamin K-K epoxide cycle: lack of resistance to coumatetralyl in warfarin-resistant rats. Biochem. Pharmacol. 25 (9), 1067–1070.

Beriain Rodríguez, M., Gómez Cortés, B., Benito Fernández, J., Mintegi Raso, S., 2008. Accidental ingestion of superwarfarins [in Spanish]. An. Pediatr. Barcelona. 68 (5), 503–506.

Berny, P.J., Buronfosse, T., Lorgue, G., 1995. Anticoagulant poisoning in animals: a simple new high-performance thin-layer chromatographic (HPTLC) method for the simultaneous determination of eight anticoagulant rodenticides in liver samples. J. Anal. Toxicol. 19 (7), 576–580.

Berny, P.J., Buronfosse, T., Buronfosse, F., Lamarque, F., Lorgue, G., 1997. Field evidence of secondary poisoning of foxes (*Vulpes vulpes*) and buzzards (*Buteo buteo*) by bromadiolone: a 4-year survey. Chemosphere. 35 (8), 1817–1829.

Berry, R.G., Morrison, J.A., Watts, J.W., Anagnost, J.W., Gonzalez, J.J., 2000. Surreptitious superwarfarin ingestion with brodifacoum. South. Med. J. 93 (1), 74–75.

Beyer, R.E., 1994. The relative essentiality of the antioxidative function of coenzyme Q: the interactive role of DT-diaphorase. Mol. Aspects. Med. 15 (Suppl.), s117–s129.

Berny, P., Caloni, F., Croubels, S., Sachana, M., Vandenbroucke, V., Davanzo, F., et al., 2010a. Animal poisoning in Europe. Part 2: Companion animals . Vet. J. 183, 255–259.

Berny, P., Velardo, J., Pulce, C., D'Amico, A., Kammerer, M., Lasseur, R., 2010b. Prevalence of anticoagulant rodenticide poisoning in humans and animals in France and substances involved. Clin. Toxicol. 48, 935–941.

Biagini, C.P., Boissel, E., Borde, F., Bender, V.E., Bouskila, M., Blazy, F., et al., 2006. Investigation of the hepatotoxicity profile of chemical entities using Liverbeads and WIF-B9 *in vitro* models. Toxicol. In. Vitro. 20 (6), 1051–1059.

Binks, S., Davies, P., 2007. Case of the month: "Oh! Drat! A case of transcutaneous superwarfarin poisoning and its recurrent presentation". Emerg. Med. J. 24 (4), 307–308.

Bint, A.J., Burtt, I., 1980. Adverse antibiotic drug interactions. Drugs. 20 (1), 57–68.

Bjornsson, T.D., Meffin, R.J., Swezey, S.E., Blascke, T.F., 1979. Effects of clofibrate and warfarin alone and in combination on the disposition of vitamin K_1. J. Pharmacol. Exp. Ther. 210, 322–326.

Blus, L.J., Henny, C.J., Grove, R.A., 1985. Effects of pelletized anticoagulant rodenticides on California quail. J. Wildl. Dis. 21 (4), 391–395.

Bocca, C., Gabriel, L., Bozzo, F., Miglietta, A., 2002. Microtubule-interacting activity and cytotoxicity of the prenylated coumarin ferulenol. Planta. Med. 68 (12), 1135–1137.

Boermans, H.J., Johnstone, I., Black, W.D., Murphy, M., 1991. Clinical signs, laboratory changes and toxicokinetics of brodifacoum in the horse. Can. J. Vet. Res. 55 (1), 21–27.

Boettcher, S., Wacker, A., Moerike, K., Kopp, H.G., Jaschonek, K., Grobosch, T., et al., 2011. Acquired coagulopathy caused by intoxication with the superwarfarin-type anticoagulant rodenticide flocoumafen. Eur. J. Haematol. 86 (2), 173–175.

Booth, K., 1989. Brodifacoum poisoning in a dog. N. Z. Vet. J. 37 (2), 74–75.

Bradfield, A.A., Gill, J.E., 1984. Laboratory trials of five rodenticides for the control of *Mesocricetus auratus* Waterhouse. J. Hyg. London. 93 (2), 389–394.

Braithwaite, G.B., 1982. Vitamin K and brodifacoum. J. Am. Vet. Med. Assoc. 181 (6), 531–534.

Brandon, E.F., Meijerman, I., Klijn, J.S., den Arend, D., Sparidans, R. W., Lazaro, L.L., et al., 2005. *In-vitro* cytotoxicity of ET-743 (Trabectedin, Yondelis), a marine anti-cancer drug, in the Hep G2 cell line: influence of cytochrome P450 and phase II inhibition, and cytochrome P450 induction. Anticancer Drugs. 16 (9), 935–943.

Braselton Jr, W.E., Neiger, R.D., Poppenga, R.H., 1992. Confirmation of indandione rodenticide toxicoses by mass spectrometry/mass spectrometry. J. Vet. Diagn. Invest. 4 (4), 441–446.

Breckenridge, A.M., Cholerton, S., Hart, J.A., Park, B.K., Scott, A.K., 1985. A study of the relationship between the pharmacokinetics and the pharmacodynamics of the 4-hydroxycoumarin anticoagulants warfarin, difenacoum and brodifacoum in the rabbit. Br. J. Pharmacol. 84 (1), 81–91.

Brooks, J.E., Htun, P.T., Naing, H., 1980. The susceptibility of *Bandicota bengalensis* from Rangoon, Burma to several anticoagulant rodenticides. J. Hyg. London. 84 (1), 127–135.

Bruno, G.R., Howland, M.A., McMeeking, A., Hoffman, R.S., 2000. Long-acting anticoagulant overdose: brodifacoum kinetics and optimal vitamin K dosing. Ann. Emerg. Med. 36 (3), 262–267.

Buckle, A., 2013. Anticoagulant resistance in the United Kingdom and a new guideline for the management of resistant infestations of Norway rats (*Rattus norvegicus* Berk.). Pest. Manag. Sci. 69 (3), 334–341.

Buckle, A.P., 1986. Field trials of flocoumafen against warfarin-resistant infestations of the Norway rat (*Rattus norvegicus* Berk.). J. Hyg. London. 96 (3), 467–473.

Buckle, A.P., Klemann, N., Prescott, C.V., et al., 2012. Brodifacoum is effective against Norway rats (*Rattus norvegicus*) in a tyrosine139-cysteine focus of anticoagulant resistance in Westphalia, Germany. Pest. Manag. Sci. 68 (12), 1579–1585.

Buckle, A.P., Endepols, S., Klemann, N., et al., 2013. Resistance testing and the effectiveness of difenacoum against Norway rats (*Rattus norvegicus*) in a tyrosine139cysteine focus of anticoagulant resistance, Westphalia, Germany. Pest. Manag. Sci. 69 (2), 233–239.

Bullard, R.W., Holguin, G., Peterson, J.E., 1975. Determination of chlo-rophacinone and diphenadione residues in biological materials. J. Agric. Food. Chem. 23 (1), 72–74.

Bullard, R.W., Thompson, R.D., Holguin, G., 1976. Diphacinone residues in tissues of cattle. J. Agric. Food. Chem. 24, 261–263.

Burns, M., 1999. Management of narrow therapeutic index drugs. J. Thromb. Thrombolysis. 7 (2), 137–143.

Burns, R.J., Bullard, R.W., 1979. Diphacinone residue from whole bodies of vampire bats: a laboratory study. Bull. Pan. Am. Health. Organ. 13 (4), 365–369.

Burns, R.J., Bullard, R.W., 1980. Residues of diphacinone in cadavers of vampire bats: a laboratory study [in Spanish]. Bol. Oficina. Sanit. Panam. 88 (5), 396–401.

Burocoa, Ch, Mura, P., Robert, R., Boinot, C., Bouset, S., Piriou, A., 1989. Chlorophacinone intoxication, a biological and toxicological study. Clin. Toxicol. 27, 78–89.

Butcher, G.P., Shearer, M.J., MacNicoll, A.D., Kelly, M.J., Ind, P.W., 1992. Difenacoum poisoning as a cause of haematuria. Hum. Exp. Toxicol. 11 (6), 553–554.

Byrne, J.J., 1970. Thrombophlebitis in pregnancy. Clin. Obstet. Gynecol. 13 (2), 305–320.

Cadenas, E., 1995. Antioxidant and prooxidant functions of DT-diaphorase in quinone metabolism. Biochem. Pharmacol. 49 (2), 127–140.

Calnan, J.S., Allenby, F., 1975. The prevention of deep vein thrombosis after surgery. Br. J. Anaesth. 47 (2), 151–160.

Cannava, A., 1958. Is 3-methyl-4-hydroxycoumarin the active principal to which we attribute the hypoprothrombinizing action of Ferula communis? Boll. Chim. Farm. 97 (4), 207–212.

Carlisle, D.M., Blaschke, T.F., 1981. Vitamin K1 epoxide and warfarin interrelationships in dog. Biochem. Pharmacol. 30, 2931–2936.

Carta, A., 1951. Ferulosis; isolation of the substance with hypoprothrombinemizing action from the galbanum of *Ferula communis*. Boll. Soc. Ital. Biol. Sper. 27 (5), 690–693.

Casner, P.R., 1998. Superwarfarin toxicity. Am. J. Ther. 2, 117–120.

Centorino, M.B., Sanchez, D.L., Catalano, G., et al., 2012. The use of bromadiolone to potentiate self-mutilatory bleeding: a case report. Psychosomatics. 53 (5), 489–493.

Chalermchaikit, T., Felice, L.J., Murphy, M.J., 1993. Simultaneous determination of eight anticoagulant rodenticides in blood serum and liver. J. Anal. Toxicol. 17 (1), 56–61.

Chambers, C.M., Chambers, P.L., 1983. Warfarin and the grey squirrel. Arch. Toxicol. Suppl. 6, 214–221.

Channon, D., Cole, M., Cole, L., 2000. A long-term study of *Rattus nor-vegicus* in the London borough of Enfield using baiting returns as an indicator of sewer population levels. Epidemiol. Infect. 125 (2), 441–445.

Charles, O.W., Dilworth, B.C., Bushong Jr, R.D., Day, E.J., 1966. The effect of dicumarol, diphacinone and pivalyl upon blood prothrombin time of chicks. Poul. Sci. 45 (2), 387–393.

Chataigner, D., Garnier, R., Elmalem, J., Efthymiou, M.L., 1989. Prolonged hypocoagulability following the ingestion of anticoagulant raticides [in French]. Ann. Med. Int. Paris. 139 (8), 537–541.

Chen, Y., Wenjun, Y., Wang, Z., Peng, Y., Li, B., Ahang, L., et al., 2010. Deposition of melamine in eggs from laying hens exposed to melamine contaminated feed. J. Agric. Food. Chem. 58, 3512–3516.

Chong, L.L., Chau, W.K., Ho, C.H., 1986. A case of "superwarfarin" poisoning. Scand. J. Haematol. 36 (3), 314–315.

Chopra, G., Parshad, V.R., 1985. Evaluation of coumatetralyl against two predominant murid species. J. Hyg. London. 94 (3), 327–330.

Chow, E.Y., Haley, L.P., Vickars, L.M., Murphy, M.J., 1992. A case of bro-madiolone (superwarfarin) ingestion. CMAJ. 147 (1), 60–62.

Christensen, T.K., Lassen, P., Elmeros, M., 2012. High exposure rates of anticoagulant rodenticides in predatory bird species in intensively managed landscapes in Denmark. Arch. Environ. Contam. Toxicol. 63 (3), 437–444.

Chua, J.D., Friedenberg, W.R., 1998. Superwarfarin poisoning. Arch. Intern. Med. 158 (17), 1929–1932.

Clark, W.T., Halliwell, R.E.W., 1963. The treatment with vitamin K preparation of warfarin poisoning in dogs. Vet. Rec. 75, 1210–1213.

Coeurdassier, M., Riols, R., Decors, A., et al., 2014. Unintentional Wildlife Poisoning and Proposals for Sustainable Management of Rodents. Conserv. Biol. Jan 9, 2014. 28, 315–321.

Colvin Jr, H.W., Wang, W.L., 1974. Toxic effects of warfarin in rats fed different diets. Toxicol. Appl. Pharmacol. 28 (3), 337–348.

Corke, P.J., 1997. Superwarfarin (brodifacoum) poisoning. Anaesth. Intensive Care. 25 (6), 707–709.

Corn, M., Berberich, R., 1967. Rapid fluorometric assay for plasma warfarin. Clin. Chem. 13, 126–131.

Cort, J.R., Cho, H., 2009. (1)H and (13)C NMR chemical shift assignments and conformational analysis for the two diastereomers of the vitamin K epoxide reductase inhibitor brodifacoum. Magn. Reson. Chem. 47 (10), 897–901.

Cort, J.R., Alperin, P.J., Cho, H., 2012. Measurement and analysis of diastereomer ratios for forensic characterization of brodifacoum. Forensic. Sci. Int. 214 (1-3), 178–181.

Corticelli, B., Deiana, S., 1957. Electrophoretic behavior of serous and plasmatic proteins of the rabbit poisoned by *Ferula communis*. Boll. Soc. Ital. Biol. Sper. 33 (5), 625–628.

Corticelli, B., Deiana, S., Palmas, G., 1957. Protective and antihemorrhagic effects of vitamin K-1 in poisoning by *Ferula communis*. Boll. Soc. Ital. Biol. Sper. 33 (5), 629–631.

Costa, A., 1950a. Hemorrhagic diathesis from juice of the roots of *Ferula communis*; behavior of the V factor of Owren. Boll. Soc. Ital. Biol. Sper. 26 (7), 1043–1044.

Costa, A., 1950b. Hemorrhagic diathesis from the juice of the roots of *Ferula communis*; behavior of the fibrinogen. Boll. Soc. Ital. Biol. Sper. 26 (7), 1041–1042.

Craciun, A.M., Groenen-van Dooren, M.M., Vermeer, C., 1997. Nutritional vitamin K-intake and urinary gamma-carboxyglutamate excretion in the rat. Biochim. Biophys. Acta. 1334 (1), 44–50.

Craciun, A.M., Groenen-van Dooren, M.M., Thijssen, H.H., Vermeer, C., 1998. Induction of prothrombin synthesis by K-vitamins compared in vitamin K-deficient and in brodifacoum-treated rats. Biochim. Biophys. Acta. 1380 (1), 75–81.

Creutzig, A., 1993. Thrombophlebitis: basic principles of treatment [in German]. Z. Kardiol. 82 (Suppl. 2), 41–47.

Dakin, G., 1968. Post-mortem toxicological findings in a case of warfarin poisoning. Vet. Rec. 83 (25), 664.

Dalla, V.S., 1994. Valvular prosthesis: indications and updated protocols for thrombosis prophylaxis [in Italian]. Cardiologia. 39 (12 Suppl. 1), 331–340.

Dam, H., 1935. The antihemorrhagic vitamin of the chick. Biochem. J. 29, 1273–1285.

Dayton, P.G., Perel, J.M., 1971. Physiological and physicochemi-cal bases of drug interactions in man. Ann. N. Y. Acad. Sci. 179, 67–87.

De Paula, E.V., Montalvao, S.A., Madureira, P.R., Jose Vieira, R., Annichino-Bizzacchi, J.M., Ozelo, M.C., 2009. Simultaneous bleeding and thrombosis in superwarfarin poisoning. Thromb. Res. 123 (4), 637–639.

Deepa, S., Mishra, A.K., 2005. Fluorescence spectroscopic study of serum albumin–bromadiolone interaction: fluorimetric determination of bromadiolone. J. Pharm. Biomed. Anal. 38 (3), 556–563.

Deobhankar, P.B., 1985. Field evaluation of brodifacoum against *Rattus rattus* and *Bandicota bengalensis* in Bombay. J. Commun. Dis. 17 (2), 151–161.

Desideri, D., Aldighieri, R., Le Louet, M., Tardieu, A., 1979. Murine resistance to anticoagulants in the port of Marseille: response to difenacoum [in French]. Bull. Soc. Pathol. Exot. Filiales. 72 (3), 278–283.

Dimuccio, A., Camoni, I., Vergori, L., Dommarco, R., Attard Barbini, D., Vergori, F., et al., 1991. Screening for coumatetralyl in soft drinks by solid-matrix extraction and high-performance liquid chromatography with diode-array detection. J. Chromatogr. 553 (1–2), 305–309.

Dinkova, K.A.T., Talalay, P., 2000. Persuasive evidence that quinone reductase type 1 (DT diaphorase) protects cells against the toxi-city of electrophiles and reactive forms of oxygen. Free. Radic. Biol. Med. 29 (3–4), 231–240.

Dobson, K.J., 1973. Coumatetralyl poisoning in pigs and effectiveness of vitamin K_1. Aust. Vet. J. 49 (2), 98–100.

Dolin, E.K., Baker, D.L., Buck, S.C., 2006. A 44-year-old woman with hematemesis and cutaneous hemorrhages as a result of superwarfarin poisoning. J. Am. Osteopath. Assoc. 106 (5), 280–284.

Donnahey, P.L., Burt, V.T., Rees, H.H., Pennock, J.F., 1979. High performance liquid chromatography of menaquinone-4,2,3-epoxyme-naquinone-4, demethyl/menaquinone 4 and related compounds. J. Chromatogr. 170, 272–277.

Dorman, D.C., 1990. Anticoagulant, cholecalciferol, and brometha-lin-based rodenticides. Vet. Clin. North. Am. Small. Anim. Pract. 20, 339–352.

DuVall, M.D., Murphy, M.J., Ray, A.C., Reagor, J.C., 1989. Case studies on second-generation anticoagulant rodenticide toxicities in non-target species. J. Vet. Diagn. Invest. 1 (1), 66–68.

Dusein, P., Manigand, G., Taillandier, J., 1984. Severe, prolonged hypoprothrombinemia following poisoning by chlorophacinone [in French]. Presse. Med. 13 (30), 1845.

Duxbury, B.M., Poller, L., 2001. The oral anticoagulant saga: past, present, and future. Clin. Appl. Thromb. Hemost. 7 (4), 269–275.

Eason, C.T., Murphy, E.C., Wright, G.R., Spurr, E.B., 2002. Assessment of risks of brodifacoum to non-target birds and mammals in New Zealand. Ecotoxicology. 11 (1), 35–48.

Edwards, D.F., Russell, R.G., 1987. Probable vitamin K-deficient bleeding in two cats with malabsorption syndrome secondary to lymphocytic–plasmacytic enteritis. J. Vet. Int. Med. 1, 97–101.

Ehrenforth, S., Schenk, J.F., Scharrer, I., 1999. Liver damage induced by coumarin anticoagulants. Semin. Thromb. Hemost. 25 (1), 79–83.

El-Bahrawy, A.A., Vijver, M.G., De Snoo, G.R., 2007. Threats and control of the brown necked ravens (*Corvus ruficollis*) in Egypt. Commun. Agric. Appl. Biol. Sci. 72 (2), 221–232.

Elias, D.J., Johns, B.E., 1981. Response of rats to chronic ingestion of diphacinone. Bull. Environ. Contam. Toxicol. 27 (4), 559–567.

Elsinghorst, T.A., 2003. First cases of animal diseases published since 2000: 1. Dogs. Vet. Q. 25 (3), 112–123.

Endepols, S., Klemann, N., Buckle, A.P., 2012. Resistance tests and field trials with bromadiolone for the control of Norway rats (*Rattus norvegicus*) on farms in Westphalia, Germany. Pest. Manag. Sci. 68 (3), 348–354.

Endepols, S., Klemann, N., Song, Y., et al., 2013. Vkorc1 variation in house mice during warfarin and difenacoum field trials. Pest. Manag. Sci. 69 (3), 409–413.

Engeman, R.M., Pitt, W.C., Berentsen, A.R., et al., 2013. Assessing spatial variation and overall density of aerially broadcast toxic bait during a rat eradication on Palmyra Atoll. Environ. Sci. Pollut. Res. Int. 20 (1), 480–487.

Exner, D.V., Brien, W.F., Murphy, M.J., 1992. Superwarfarin ingestion. CMAJ. 146 (1), 34–35.

Fang, Y., Ye, D., Zhang, J., et al., 2012. Superwarfarin rodent poisons and hemorrhagic disease. Epidemiology. 23 (6), 932–934.

Fasco, M.J., Piper, L.J., Kaminsky, L.S., 1977. Biochemical applications of a quantitative HPLC assay of warfarin and its metabolites. J. Chromatogr. 131, 365–373.

Fauconnet, V., Pouliquen, H., Pinault, L., 1997. Reversed-phase HPLC determination of eight anticoagulant rodenticides in animal liver. J. Anal. Toxicol. 21 (7), 548–553.

Feinstein, D.L., Brodsky, S., Weinberg, G., et al., 2017. Brodifacoum poisoning: a clear and present danger to public health in the USA. Toxicol. Lett. 268, 71–72.

Felice, L.J., Murphy, M.J., 1989. The determination of the anticoagulant rodenticide brodifacoum in blood serum by liquid chromatogra-phy with fluorescence detection. J. Anal. Toxicol. 13, 229–231.

Felice, L.J., Chalermchaikit, T., Murphy, M.J., 1991. Multicomponent determination of 4 hydroxycoumarin anticoagulant rodenticides in blood serum by liquid chromatography with fluorescence detection. J. Anal. Toxicol. 15, 126–129.

Feng, S.Z., Zhou, H.Z., Li, Y.L., Wang, F.L., Sun, J., Liu, Y., 1999. SPE analysis of 4 rodenticides in whole blood and liver by HPLC [in Chinese]. Fa. Yi. Xue. Za. Zhi. 15 (1), 21–22.

Ferlito, S., 1996. Main antithrombotic drugs in the therapy and prevention of arterial and venous thrombosis [in Italian]. Minerva. Cardioangiol. 44 (6), 299–312.

Fieser, L.F., Campbell, W.P., Fry, E.M., Gates Jr, M.D., 1939. Naphthoquinones of vitamin K_1 type of structure. J. Am. Chem. Soc. 61, 3216–3223.

Finch, C.K., Chrisman, C.R., Baciewicz, A.M., Self, T.H., 2002. Rifampin and rifabutin drug interactions: an update. Arch. Intern. Med. 162 (9), 985–992.

Fisher, P., Funnell, E., Fairweather, A., et al., 2012. Accidental discharge of brodifacoum baits into a freshwater lake: a case study. Bull. Environ. Contam. Toxicol. 88 (2), 226–228.

Fournier-Chambrillon, C., Berny, P.J., Coiffier, O., Barbedienne, P., Dasse, B., Delas, G., et al., 2004. Evidence of secondary poisoning of free-ranging riparian mustelids by anticoagulant rodenticides in France: implications for conservation of European mink (*Mustela lutreola*). J. Wildl. Dis. 40 (4), 688–695.

Fraigui, O., Lamnaouer, D., Faouzi, M.Y., Cherrah, Y., Tijjane, M., 2001. Acute and chronic toxicity of fessoukh, the resinous gum of *Ferula communis* L, compared to warfarin. Vet. Hum. Toxicol. 43 (6), 327–330.

Fraigui, O., Lamnaouer, D., Faouzi, M.Y., 2002. Acute toxicity of ferule-nol, a 4-hydroxycoumarin isolated from *Ferula communis* L. Vet. Hum. Toxicol. 44 (1), 5–7.

Fu, Z.H., Huang, X.X., Xiao, H.R., 2006. Determination of serum brodifacoum with high performance liquid chromatography [in Chinese]. Zhonghua. Lao. Dong. Wei. Sheng. Zhi. Ye. Bing. Za. Zhi. 24 (5), 295.

Fu, Z.H., et al., 2012. Determination of brodifacoum in rat plasma by HPLC. Zhonghua. Lao. Dong. Wei. Sheng. Zhi. Ye. Bing. Za. Zhi. 30 (2), 135–136.

Fu, Z.H., Xu, J.-N., Yu, W.-L., et al., 2013. Method for determining brodifacoum in workplace air by high-performance liquid chromatography. Chin. J. Ind. Hyg. Occup. Dis. 31 (8), 625–626.

Gallo, J., 1998. Brodifacoum. Anaesth. Intensive Care. 26 (6), 708–709.

Gil, M.C., Gomez, L., Roy, T.J., Prieto, L., Pena, F.J., Garcia, L., 2002. Testicular and epididymal changes in rams following intoxication by Ferula communis. Vet. Rec. 150 (1), 24–25.

Gill, J.E., Redfern, R., 1979. Laboratory test of seven rodenticides for the control of *Mastomys natalensis*. J. Hyg. London. 83 (2), 345–352.

Gill, J.E., Redfern, R., 1980. Laboratory trials of seven rodenticides for use against the cotton rat (*Sigmodon hispidus*). J. Hyg. London. 85 (3), 443–450.

Gill, J.E., Redfern, R., 1983. Laboratory tests of seven rodenticides for the control of *Meriones shawi*. J. Hyg. London. 91 (2), 351–357.

Giraudoux, P., Tremollieres, C., Barbier, B., Defaut, R., Rieffel, D., Bernard, N., et al., 2006. Persistence of bromadiolone anticoagulant rodenticide in *Arvicola terrestris* populations after field control. Environ. Res. 55, 439–448.

Goldade, D.A., Primus, T.M., Johnston, J.J., Zapien, D.C., 1998. Reversed-phase ion-pair high-performance liquid chromatographic quantitation of difethialone residues in whole-body rodents with solid-phase extraction cleanup. J. Agric. Food. Chem. 46 (2), 504–508.

Goldstein, J.A., 2001. Clinical relevance of genetic polymorphisms in the human CYP2C subfamily. Br. J. Clin. Pharmacol. 52 (4), 349–355.

Grant, R.G., Pike, R.K., 1979. High pressure liquid chromatographic determination of chlorophacinone in formulations. J. Assoc. Off. Anal. Chem. 62, 1001–1003.

Grayson, J.L., 1982. Brodifacoum poisoning in a dog. N. Z. Vet. J. 37 (4), 173.

Greaves, J.H., Ayres, P., 1969. Some rodenticidal properties of coumatetralyl. J. Hyg. London. 67 (2), 311–315.

Greaves, J.H., Rehman, A.B., 1977. The susceptibility of *Tatera indica, Nesokia indica* and *Bandicota bengalensis* to three anticoagulant rodenticides. J. Hyg. London. 78 (1), 75–84.

Greaves, J.H., Shepherd, D.S., Quy, R., 1982. Field trials of second-generation anticoagulants against difenacoum-resistant Norway rat populations. J. Hyg. London. 89 (2), 295–301.

Greeff, M.C., Mashile, O., MacDougall, L.G., 1987. Superwarfarin (bro-modialone) poisoning in two children resulting in prolonged anticoagulation. Lancet. 2 (8570), 1269.

Grobosch, T., Angelow, B., Schonberg, L., Lampe, D., 2006. Acute bromadiolone intoxication. J. Anal. Toxicol. 30 (4), 281–286.

Guidry, J.R., Raschke, R.A., Morkunas, A.R., 1991. Toxic effects of drugs used in the ICU. Anticoagulants and thrombolytics: risks and benefits. Crit. Care Clin. 7 (3), 533–554.

Hadler, M., Shadbolt, R.S., 1975. Novel 4-hydroxycoumarin anticoagulants active against resistant rats. Nature. 253, 275–277.

Hagenboom, J.J.L., Rammell, C.G., 1983. Improved HPLC method for determining brodifacoum in animal tissues. Bull. Environ. Contam. Toxicol. 31, 239–244.

Hanna, S., Rosen, M., Eisenberger, P., Rasero, L., Lachman, L., 1978. GLC determination of warfarin in human plasma. J. Pharm. Sci. 67, 84–86.

Haroon, Y., Hauschka, P.V., 1983. Application of high-performance liquid-chromatography to assay phylloquinone (vitamin K_1) in rat liver. J. Lipid. Res. 24, 481–484.

Haroon, Y., Shearer, M.J., Barkhan, P., 1980. Resolution of phylloquinone (vitamin K_1), phylloquinone 2,3-epoxide, 2-chloro-phylloquinone and their geometric isomers by high-performance liquid chromatography. J. Chromatogr. 200, 293–299.

Haroon, Y., Bacon, D.S., Sadowski, J.A., 1986. Liquid-chromatography determination of vitamin K_1 in plasma, with fluorometric detection. Clin. Chem. 32, 1925–1929.

Haroon, Y., David, S.B., Sadowski, J.A., 1987. Chemical reduction system for the detection of phylloquinone (vitamin K_1) and menaquinones (vitamin K_2). J. Chromatogr. 384, 383–389.

Hart, J.A.D., Haynes, B.P., Park, B.K., 1984. A study of factors which determine the pharmacological response to vitamin K in coumarin anticoagulated rabbit. Biochem. Pharmacol. 33, 3013–3029.

Haug, B., Schjodt-Iversen, L., Rygh, J., 1992. Poisoning with long-acting anticoagulants [in Norwegian]. Tidsskr. Nor. Laegeforen. 112 (15), 1958–1960.

Hernández, A.M., Bernal, J., Martin, M.T., et al., 2013a. Simultaneous determination of nine anticoagulant rodenticides in soil and water by LC-ESI-MS. J. Sep. Sci. 36 (16), 2593–2601.

Hernández, A.M., Bernal, J., Bernal, J.L., et al., 2013b. Analysis of anticoagulant rodenticide residues in *Microtus arvalis* tissues by liquid chromatography with diode array, fluorescence and mass spectrometry detection. J. Chromatogr. B. Analyt. Technol. Biomed. Life. Sci. 925, 76–85.

Hernandez-Moreno, D., De La Casa-Resino, I., Lopez-Beceiro, A., et al., 2013. Secondary poisoning of non-target animals in an ornithological zoo in Galicia (NW Spain) with anticoagulant rodenticides: a case report. Vet. Med. 58, 553–559.

Hildebrandt, E.F., Suttie, J.W., 1982. Mechanism of coumarin action: sensitivity of vitamin K metabolizing enzymes of normal and warfarin-resistant rat liver. Biochemistry. 21 (10), 2406–2411.

Hohler, T., Schnutgen, M., Helmreich-Becker, I., Mayet, W.J., Mayer Zum Buschenfelde, K.H., 1994. Drug-induced hepatitis: a rare complication of oral anticoagulants. J. Hepatol. 21 (3), 447–449.

Hong, J., Yhim, H.Y., Bang, S.M., Bae, S.H., Yuh, Y.J., Yoon, S.S., et al., 2010. Korean patients with superwarfa-rin intoxication and their outcome. J. Korean. Med. Sci. 25 (12), 1754–1758.

Hoogenboom, J.J., Rammell, C.G., 1983. Improved HPLC method for determining brodifacoum in animal tissues. Bull. Environ. Contam. Toxicol. 31 (2), 239–243.

Hornfeldt, C.S., Phearman, S., 1996. Successful treatment of brodifacoum poisoning in a pregnant bitch. J. Am. Vet. Med. Assoc. 209, 1690–1691.

Huckle, K.R., Hutson, D.H., Warburton, P.A., 1988. Elimination and accumulation of the rodenticide flocoumafen in rats following repeated oral administration. Xenobiotica. 18 (12), 1465–1479.

Huckle, K.R., Morrison, B.J., Warburton, P.A., 1989a. The percutaneous fate of the rodenticide flocoumafen in the rat: role of non-biliary intestinal excretion. Xenobiotica. 19 (1), 63–74.

Huckle, K.R., Warburton, P.A., Forbes, S., Logan, C.J., 1989b. Studies on the fate of flocoumafen in the Japanese quail (*Coturnix coturnix japonica*). Xenobiotica. 19 (1), 51–62.

Hughes, J., Sharp, E., Taylor, M.J., et al., 2013. Monitoring agricultural rodenticide use and secondary exposure of raptors in Scotland. Ecotoxicology. 22 (6), 974–984.

Hui, C.H., Lie, A., Lam, C.K., Bourke, C., 1996. "Superwarfarin" poisoning leading to prolonged coagulopathy. Forensic. Sci. Int. 78 (1), 13–18.

Huic, M., Francetic, I., Bakran, I., Macolic-Sarinic, V., Bilusic, M., 2002. Acquired coagulopathy due to anticoagulant rodenticide poisoning. Croat. Med. J. 43 (5), 615–617.

Humphry, N.F., 1989. Anticoagulant rodenticides. Med. J. Aust. 150 (12), 727–728.

Hunter, K., 1984. Reversed-phase ion-pair liquid chromatographic determination of chlorophacinone residues in animal tissues. J. Chromatogr. 299, 405–414.

Hunter, K., 1985. High-performance liquid chromatographic strategies for the determination and confirmation of anticoagulant rodenticide residues in animal tissues. J. Chromatogr. 321 (2), 255–272.

Hunter, K., Sharp, E.A., 1988. Modification to procedures for the determination of chlorophacinone for multi-residue analysis of rodenticides in animal tissues. J. Chromatogr. 437, 301–305.

Hylek, E.M., Chang, Y.C., Skates, S.J., Hughes, R.A., Singer, D.E., 2000. Prospective study of the outcomes of ambulatory patients with excessive warfarin anticoagulation. Arch. Intern. Med. 160 (11), 1612–1617.

Ingels, M., Lai, C., Tai, W., Manning, B.H., Rangan, C., Williams, S.R., et al., 2002. A prospective study of acute, unintentional, pediatric superwarfarin inges-tions managed without decontamination. Ann. Emerg. Med. 40 (1), 73–78.

Ishizuka, M., Tanikawa, T., Tanaka, K.D., Heewon, M., Okajima, F., Sakamoto, K.Q., et al., 2008. Pesticide resistance in wild mammals: mechanisms of anticoagulant resistance in wild rodents. J. Toxicol. Sci. 33 (3), 283–291.

Istvan, S.A., Marks, S.L., Murphy, L.A., et al., 2014. Evaluation of a point-of-care anticoagulant rodenticide test for dogs. J. Vet. Emerg. Crit. Care. 24, 168–173.

Jackson, C.M., Suttie, J.W., 1977. Recent developments in understanding the mechanism of vitamin K and vitamin K–antagonist drug action and the consequences of vitamin K action in blood coagulation. Prog. Haematol. 10, 333–359.

Jackson, W.B., Brooks, J.E., Bowerman, A.M., 1975. Anticoagulant resistance in Norway rats. Pest. Control. 43, 14–23.

Jacob, J., Endepols, S., Pelz, H.-J., et al., 2012. Vitamin K requirement and reproduction in bromadiolone-resistant Norway rats. Pest. Manag. Sci. 68 (3), 378–385.

James, S.B., Raphael, B.L., Cook, R.A., 1998. Brodifacoum toxicity and treatment in a white-winged wood duck (*Cairina scutulata*). J. Zoo. Wildl. Med. 29 (3), 324–327.

Jeantet, A.Y., Truchet, M., Naulleau, G., Martoja, R., 1991. Effects of bro-madiolone on some organs and tissues (liver, kidney, spleen, blood) of coypu (*Myocastor coypus*) [in French]. C. R. Acad. Sci. III. 312 (4), 149–156.

Jin, M., Chen, X., Li, X., 2007. Determination of five 4-hydroxycoumarin rodenticides in whole blood by high performance liquid chromatography with fluorescence detection [in Chinese]. Se. Pu. 25 (2), 214–216.

Jin, M.C., Chen, X.H., 2006. Rapid determination of three anticoagulant rodenticides in whole blood by liquid chromatography coupled with electrospray ionization mass spectrometry. Rapid. Commun. Mass. Spectrom. 20 (18), 2741–2746.

Jin, M.C., OuYang, X.K., Chen, X.H., 2007. High-performance liquid chromatography coupled with electrospray ionization tandem mass spectrometry for the determination of flocou-mafen and brodifacoum in whole blood. J. Appl. Toxicol. 27 (1), 18–24.

Johnston, J.J., Pitt, W.C., Sugihara, R.T., Eisemann, J.D., Primus, T.M., Holmes, M.J., et al., 2005. Probabilistic risk assessment for snails, slugs, and endangered honeycreepers in dipha-cinone rodenticide baited areas on Hawaii, USA. Environ. Toxicol. Chem. 24 (6), 1557–1567.

Johnstone, T.B., 1989. Diagnostic approach to the bleeding patient. In: Kirk, R.W. (Ed.), Current Veterinary Therapy X. Saunders, Philadelphia, pp. 436–442.

Jolly, S.E., Eason, C.T., Frampton, C., Gumbrell, R.C., 1994. The anticoagulant pindone causes liver damage in the brushtail possum (*Trichosurus vulpecula*). Aust. Vet. J. 71 (7), 220.

Jones, A., 1996. HPLC determination of anticoagulant rodenticide residues in animal livers. Bull. Environ. Contam. Toxicol. 56 (1), 8–15.

Jones, E.C., Growe, G.H., Naiman, S.C., 1984. Prolonged anticoagulation in rat poisoning. J. Am. Med. Assoc. 252, 3005–3007.

Kamil, N., 1987. Kinetics of bromadiolone, anticoagulant roden-ticide, in the Norway rat (*Rattus norvegicus*). Pharmacol. Res. Commun. 19 (11), 767–775.

Kanabar, D., Volans, G., 2002. Accidental superwarfarin poisoning in children: less treatment is better. Lancet. 360 (9338), 963.

Kapadia, P., Bona, R., 2008. Acquired deficiency of vitamin K-dependent clotting factors due to brodifacoum ingestion. Conn. Med. 72 (4), 207–209.

Kawano, Y., Chang, W., 1980. Spectrophotometric determination of Rozol in paraffinized formulations. J. Assoc. Off. Anal. Chem. 63, 996–998.

Keiboom, P.J., Rammel, C.G., 1981. Detection of brodifacoum in animal tissues by high performance liquid chromatography. Bull. Environ. Toxicol. 26, 674–678.

Kelly, M.J., Chambers, J., MacNicoll, A.D., 1993. Simple and rapid method for the determination of the diastereomers of difenacoum in blood and liver using high-performance liquid chromatogra-phy with fluorescence detection. J. Chromatogr. 620 (1), 105–112.

Kim, S.Y., Cho, S.Y., Lee, H.J., Suh, J.T., Oh, S.H., Lee, W.I., et al., 2010. Superwarfarin intoxication of unknown etiology accompanying hemoperitoneum in a patient on fluconazole therapy. Ann. Clin. Lab. Sci. 40 (3), 300–303.

Kirchheiner, J., Brockmoller, J., 2005. Clinical consequences of cytochrome P450 2C9 polymorphisms. Clin. Pharmacol. Ther. 77 (1), 1–16.

Kohn, M.H., Pelz, H.J., 1999. Genomic assignment of the warfarin resistance locus, Rw, in the rat. Mamm. Genome. 10 (7), 696–698.

Kohn, M.H., Pelz, H.J., 2000. A gene-anchored map position of the rat warfarin-resistance locus, Rw, and its orthologs in mice and humans. Blood. 96 (5), 1996–1998.

Kotsaftis, P., Girtovitis, F., Boutou, A., Ntaios, G., Makris, P.E., 2007. Haemarthrosis after superwarfarin poisoning. Eur. J. Haematol. 79 (3), 255–257.

Koubek, K.G., Ussary, J.P., Saulsee, R.E., 1979. High performance liquid chromatographic determination of the rodenticide brodifacoum in rat tissue. J. Assoc. Off. Anal. Chem. 62, 1297–1301.

Kruse, J.A., Carlson, R.W., 1992. Fatal rodenticide poisoning with brodifacoum. Ann. Emerg. Med. 21 (3), 331–336.

Kuijpers, E.A., den Hartigh, J., Savelkoul, T.J., de Wolff, F.A., 1995. A method for the simultaneous identification and quantitation of five superwarfarin rodenticides in human serum. J. Anal. Toxicol. 19 (7), 557–562.

Lagrange, F., Corniot, A.G., Titier, K., Bedry, R., Pehourcq, F., 1999. Toxicological management of chlorophacinone poisoning. Acta. Clin. Belg. Suppl. 1, 13–16.

Lamnaouer, D., 1999. Anticoagulant activity of coumarins from *Ferula communis* L [in French]. Therapie. 54 (6), 747–751.

Langenberg, J.P., Tjaden, U.R., 1984. Determination of (endogenous) vitamin K_1 in human plasma by reversed-phase HPLC using fluorometric detection after post-column electro-chemical reduction. J. Chromatogr. 305, 61–72.

Langford, K.H., Reid, M., Thomas, K.V., 2013. The occurrence of second generation anticoagulant rodenticides in non-target raptor species in Norway. Sci. Total Environ. 450-451, 205–208.

Laposata, M., Van Cott, E.M., Lev, M.H., 2007. Case records of the Massachusetts General Hospital. Case 1-2007. A 40-year-old woman with epistaxis, hematemesis, and altered mental status. N. Engl. J. Med. 356 (2), 174–182.

Last, J.A., 2002. The missing link: the story of Karl Paul Link. Toxicol. Sci. 66 (1), 4–6.

Lau-Cam, C.A., Chu-Fong, I., 1972. Thin-layer chromatography of coumarin anticoagulant rodenticides. J. Pharm. Sci. 61, 1303–1306.

Lawley, W.J., Charlton, A.J., Hughson, E.J., Grundy, H.H., Brown, P.M., Jones, A., 2006. Development of a cell culture/ELISA assay to detect anticoagulant rodenticides and its application to analysis of rodenticide treated grain. J. Agric. Food Chem. 54 (5), 1588–1593.

Leck, J.B., Park, B.K., 1981. A comparative study of the effects of warfarin and brodifacoum on the relationship between vitamin K_1 metabolism and clotting factor activity in warfarin-susceptible and warfarin-resistant rats. Biochem. Pharmacol. 30, 123–128.

Lee, S.H., Field, L.R., Howard, W.N., Trager, W.F., 1981. High performance liquid chromatographic separation and fluorescence detection of warfarin and its metabolites by postcolumn acid base manipulation. Anal. Chem. 53, 467–471.

Lefevere, M.F., Leenheer de, A.P., Claeys, A.E., 1979. High performance liquid chromatographic assay of vitamin K in human serum. J. Chromatogr. 186, 749–762.

Lefevre, S., Rannou, B., Besse, S., et al., 2016. Origin of the gender differences of the natural resistance to antivitamin K anticoagulants in rats. Toxicology. 344–346, 34–41.

Lewis, R.J., Ilnicki, L.P., Carlstrom, M., 1970. The assay of warfarin in plasma or stool. Biochem. Med. 4, 376–382.

Lipton, R.A., Klass, E.M., 1984. Human ingestion of a superwarfarin rodenticide resulting in prolonged anticoagulant effect. J. Am. Med. Assoc. 252, 3004–3005.

Lund, M., 1971. The toxicity of chlorophacinone and warfarin to house mice (*Mus musculus*). J. Hyg. London. 69 (1), 69–72.

Lund, M., 1981. Comparative effect of the three rodenticides warfarin, difenacoum and brodifacoum on eight rodent species in short feeding periods. J. Hyg. London. 87 (1), 101–107.

Lund, M., 1984. Resistance to the second-generation anticoagulant rodenticides. Proceedings of the 11th Vertebrate Pest Conference, Sacramento, CA, p. 89.

Lund, M., 1988. Anticoagulant rodenticides. In: Prakash, I. (Ed.), Rodent Pest Management. CRC Press, Boca Raton, FL, pp. 342–351.

Lund, M., Rasmussen, A.M., 1986. Secondary poisoning hazards in stone martens (*Martes foina*) fed bromadiolone-poisoned mice. Nord. Vet. Med. 38 (4), 241–243.

Mack, R.B., 1994. Not all rats have four legs: superwarfarin poisoning. N. C. Med. J. 55 (11), 554–556.

Magagnoli, M., Masci, G., Castagna, L., Pedicini, V., Poretti, D., Morenghi, E., et al., 2006. Prophylaxis of central venous catheter-related thrombosis with minidose warfarin in patients treated with high-dose chemotherapy and peripheral-blood stem-cell transplantation: retrospective analysis of 228 cancer patients. Am. J. Hematol. 81 (1), 1–4.

Mahmoud, W., Redfern, R., 1981. The response of the Egyptian spiny mouse (*Acomys cahirinus*) and two other species of commensal rodents to anticoagulant rodenticides. J. Hyg. London. 86 (3), 329–334.

Mallet, V., Surette, D., Brun, G.L., 1973. Detection of naturally fluorescent pesticides on silica gel layers. J. Chromatogr. 79, 217–222.

Marchini, S., Turillazzi, P.G., 1978. Effect of an anticoagulant rodenticide on the female albino rat with offspring [in Italian]. Parassitologia. 20 (1–3), 59–70.

Markussen, M.D., Heiberg, A.C., Nielsen, R., Leirs, H., 2003. Vitamin K requirement in Danish anticoagulant-resistant Norway rats (*Rattus norvegicus*). Pest. Manag. Sci. 59 (8), 913–920.

Marquet, P., Saint-Marcoux, F., Gamble, T.N., Leblanc, J.C., 2003. Comparison of a preliminary procedure for the general unknown screening of drugs and toxic compounds using a quadrupole-linear ion-trap mass spectrometer with a liquid chromatography-mass spectrometry reference technique. J. Chromatogr. B. Analyt. Technol. Biomed. Life. Sci. 789 (1), 9–18.

Martin, G.R., Sutherland, R.J., Robertson, I.D., Kirkpatrick, W.E., King, D.R., Hood, P.J., 1991. Assessment of the potential toxicity of a poison for rabbits, pindone (2-pivalyl 1,3 indandione), to domestic animals. Aust. Vet. J. 68 (7), 241–243.

Mathur, R.P., Prakash, I., 1980. Laboratory evaluation of anticoagulant-treated baits for control of the northern palm squirrel, *Funambulus pennanti* Wroughton. J. Hyg. London. 85 (3), 421–426.

Matolesy, Gy, Nadasy, M., Andriaska, V., 1988. Rodenticides. Pesticide Chemistry. Elsevier, Amsterdam, pp. 261–271.

Matsukawa, R., Uemura, S., Fukuchi, S., Tsuruta, Y., Murakami, S., 1994. Thrombosed St. Jude Medical prosthesis with drug induced hepatitis due to warfarin potassium: a case report [in Japanese]. Nippon. Kyobu. Geka. Gakkai. Zasshi. 42 (3), 413–415.

Mazzetti, G., Cappelletti, G.A., 1957. Effect of the active principle of *Ferula communis* on blood coagulation; thromboelastographic study. Arch. Sci. Med. Torino. 104 (3), 236–245.

McCarthy, P.T., Cox, A.D., Harrington, D.J., Evely, R.S., Hampton, E., al-Sabah, A.I., et al., 1997. Covert poisoning with difenacoum: clinical and toxicological observations. Hum. Exp. Toxicol. 16 (3), 166–170.

McGuire, N.C., Williams, J., Marks, S.L., 1999. What is your diagnosis? Rodenticide poisoning in a dog. J. Am. Vet. Med. Assoc. 214 (8), 1157–1158.

McNiel, N.O., Morgan Jr, L.R., 1984. Effects of sodium warfarin and sodium heparin plus anticancer agents on growth of rat C6 gli-oma cells. J. Natl. Cancer. Inst. 73 (1), 169–176.

McSporran, K.D., Phillips, C.A., 1983. Brodifacoum poisoning in a dog. N. Z. Vet. J. 31 (10), 185–186.

Mehlhaff, K.M., Baxter, C.C., Rudinsky, K., et al., 2013. Lethal neonatal coagulopathy after maternal ingestion of a superwarfarin. Obstet. Gynecol. 122 (2 Pt 2), 500–502.

Mesban, H.A., Tayeb, E.H., Mourad, A.K., Younis, L.K., el Zaher, M.A., Aly, M.T., 2003. Toxicology and histopathology of some rodenticides and palatable food items combinations on the common mice *Mus musculus* var. *albus* in Egypt. Commun. Agric. Appl. Biol. Sci. 68 (4 Pt B), 771–787.

Mesmer, M.Z., Flurer, R.A., 2000. Determination of chlorophacinone and diphacinone in commercial rodenticides by liquid chromatography-UV detection and liquid chromatography-elec-trospray ionization mass spectrometry. J. Chromatogr. A. 891 (2), 249–255.

Middlekauff, H.R., Stevenson, W.G., Gornbein, J.A., 1995. Antiarrhythmic prophylaxis vs warfarin anticoagulation to prevent thromboembolic events among patients with atrial fibrillation: a decision analysis. Arch. Intern. Med. 155 (9), 913–920.

Mildha, K.K., McGitveray, I.J., Cooper, J.K., 1974. GLC determination of plasma levels of warfarin. J. Pharm. Sci. 63, 1725–1729.

Miller, M.A., Levy, P.D., Hile, D., 2006. Rapid identification of surreptitious brodifacoum poisoning by analysis of vitamin K-dependent factor activity. Am. J. Emerg. Med. 24 (3), 383.

Misenheimer, T.M., Lund, M., Baker, E.M., Suttie, J.W., 1994. Biochemical basis of warfarin and bromadiolone resistance in the house mouse. Mus musculus domesticus Biochem. Pharmacol. 47 (4), 673–678.

Miski, M., Mabry, T.J., Bohlmann, F., 1986. Fercoperol, an unusual cyclic-endoperoxynerolidol derivative from *Ferula communis* subsp. *communis*. J. Nat. Prod. 49 (5), 916–918.

Misra, D., Bednar, M., Cromwell, C., Marcus, S., Aledort, L., 2010. Manifestations of superwarfarin ingestion: a plea to increase awareness. Am. J. Hematol. 85 (5), 391–392.

Moery, S., Pontious, J.M., 2009. Coagulopathy associated with superwarfarin exposure. J. Okla. State. Med. Assoc. 102 (10), 323–325.

Montanio, C.D., Wruk, K.M., Kulig, K.W., Riggs, B.S., Rumack, B.H., 1993. Acute pediatric warfarin (Coumadin) ingestion: toxic effects despite early treatment. Am. J. Dis. Child. 147 (6), 609–610.

Morgan, B.W., Tomaszewski, C., Rotker, I., 1996. Spontaneous hemoperitoneum from brodifacoum overdose. Am. J. Emerg. Med. 14 (7), 656–659.

Morin, M.F., Merlet, N., Naulleau, G., Dore, M., 1990. Primary toxicity of bromadiolone on the coypu. Bull. Environ. Contam. Toxicol. 44 (4), 595–601.

Mossa, J.S., El-Feraly, F.S., Muhammad, I., 2004. Antimycobacterial constituents from *Juniperus procera*, *Ferula communis* and *Plumbago zeylanica* and their *in vitro* synergistic activity with isonicotinic acid hydrazide. Phytother. Res. 18 (11), 934–937.

Mosterd, J.J., Thijssen, H.H., 1991. The long-term effects of the rodenticide, brodifacoum, on blood coagulation and vitamin K metabolism in rats. Br. J. Pharmacol. 104 (2), 531–535.

Mount, M.E., Feldman, B.F., 1983. Mechanisms of diphacinone rodenticide toxicosis in dog and its therapeutic implications. Am. J. Vet. Res. 44, 2009–2017.

Mount, M.E., Kass, P.H., 1989. Diagnostic importance of vitamin K_1 and its epoxide measured in serum of dogs exposed to an anticoagulant rodenticide. Am. J. Vet. Res. 50, 1704–1709.

Mount, M.E., Feldman, B.F., Buffington, T., 1982. Vitamin K and its therapeutic importance. J. Am. Vet. Med. Assoc. 180 (11), 1354–1356.

Mount, M.E., Woody, M.J., Murphy, M.J., 1985. The anticoagulant rodenticides. In: Kirk, R.W. (Ed.), Current Veterinary Therapy I.X. Saunders, Philadelphia, pp. 156–165.

Mount, M.E., Kurth, M.J., Jackson, D.Y., 1988. Production of antibodies and development of an immunoassay for the anticoagulant, diphacinone. J. Immunoassay. 9 (1), 69–81.

Mullins, M.E., Brands, C.L., Daya, M.R., 2000. Unintentional pediat-ric superwarfarin exposures: do we really need a prothrombin time? Pediatrics. 105 (2), 402–404.

Munday, J.S., Thompson, L.J., 2003. Brodifacoum toxicosis in two neonatal puppies. Vet. Pathol. 40 (2), 216–219.

Mundy, D.E., Machin, A.F., 1977. Determination of the rodenticide difenacoum in biological materials by high-pressure chro-matography with confirmation of identity by mass spectrome-try. J. Chromatogr. 139 (2), 321–329.

Mundy, D.E., Machin, A.F., 1982. The multi-residue determination of coumarin-based anticoagulant rodenticides in animal materials by HPLC. J. Chromatogr. 234, 427–435.

Munger, L.L., Su, J.J., Barnes, H.J., 1993. Coumafuryl (Fumarin) toxicity in chicks. Avian. Dis. 37 (2), 622–624.

Mura, P., Piriou, A., Papet, Y., Lochon, D., Reiss, D., 1992. Rapid high-performance liquid chromatographic assay of chlorophacinone in human serum. J. Anal. Toxicol. 16 (3), 179–181.

Murdoch, D.A., 1983. Prolonged anticoagulation in chlorphacinone poisoning. Lancet. 1 (8320), 355–356.

Murphy, M.J., Gerken, D.F., 1989. The anticoagulant rodenticides. In: Kirk, R.W. (Ed.), Current Veterinary Therapy X. Saunders, Philadelphia, pp. 143–146.

Murphy, P.A., Hendrich, S., Landgren, C., et al., 2006. Food mycotoxins: an update. J. Food Sci. 71 (5), 51–65.

Murphy, M.J., Ray, A.C., Bailey, E.M., 1989. A high-performance liquid chromatographic method for the detection of brodifacoum in serum. Vet. Hum. Toxicol. 31, 228–231.

Nahas, K., 1986. Analysis of bromadiolone (an anticoagulant rodenticide) in plasma, liver and kidney of the rat. J. Chromatogr. 369 (2), 445–448.

Nasilowski, J., Krenke, R., 2002. Hemothorax with high number of eosinophils following warfarin overdose. Pneumonol. Alergol. Pol. 70 (9–10), 496–503.

Nelson, A.T., Hartzell, J.D., More, K., Durning, S.J., 2006. Ingestion of superwarfarin leading to coagulopathy: a case report and review of the literature. Med. Gen. Med. 8 (4), 41.

Newton, I., Wyllie, I., Freestone, P., 1990. Rodenticides in British barn owls. Environ. Pollut. 68 (1–2), 101–117.

Nie, H., Wei, W., Cao, Y., Du, X.D., 2010. Superwarfarin poisoning as a cause of intestinal obstruction. Clin. Toxicol. Philadelphia. 48 (3), 238–239.

Nighoghossian, N., Ruel, J.H., French, P., Froment, J.C., Trouillas, P., 1990. Cervicodorsal subdural hematoma caused by coumarinic roden-ticide poisoning. Rev. Neurol. Paris. 146 (3), 221–223.

Nikodemusz, E., Nechay, G., Imre, R., 1981. Histopathological changes resulting by some pesticides in the common vole (*Microtus arvalis pallas*). Acta. Vet. Acad. Sci. Hung. 29 (3), 317–326.

Olmos, V., López, C.M., 2007. Brodifacoum poisoning with toxicokinetic data. Clin. Toxicol. Philadelphia. 45 (5), 487–489.

Olson, R.E., 1966. Studies on the mode of action of vitamin K. Adv. Enzyme. Regul. 4, 181–196.

Ornstein, D.L., Lord, K.E., Yanofsky, N.N., Cornell, C.J., Zacharski, L. R., 1999. Successful donation and transplantation of multiple organs after fatal poisoning with brodifacoum, a long-acting anticoagulant rodenticide: case report. Transplantation. 67 (3), 475–478.

Osterhoudt, K.C., Henretig, F.M., 2003. Bias in pediatric brodifacoum exposure data. Pediatr. Emerg. Care. 19 (1), 62.

O'Bryan, S.M., Constable, D.J., 1991. Quantification of brodifacoum in plasma and liver tissue by HPLC. J. Anal. Toxicol. 15, 144–147.

O'Reilly, R.A., Aggeler, P.M., Hoag, M.S., Leong, L., 1962. Studies on the coumarin anticoagulant drugs: the assay of warfarin and its biological application. Thromb. Diath. Haemorrh. 8, 82–86.

Padgett, S.L., Stokes, J.E., Tucker, R.L., Wheaton, L.G., 1998. Hematometra secondary to anticoagulant rodenticide toxicity. J. Am. Anim. Hosp. Assoc. 34 (5), 437–439.

Pais Jr, V.M., 2012. In a well presented report of bilateral renal pelvic thrombus formation with subsequent bilateral ureteral obstruction. Clin. Nephrol. 78 (4), 253.

Pan, K., Xia, L.G., Chen, X.C., Zhong, K.L., Jiang, H.X., 2005. Diagnosis and treatment of mesenteric venous thrombosis early after operation. Zhonghua. Wei. Chang. Wai. Ke. Za. Zhi. 8 (1), 50–52.

Papin, F., Clarot, F., Vicomte, C., Gaulier, J.M., Daubin, C., Chapon, F., et al., 2007. Lethal paradoxical cerebral vein thrombosis due to suspicious anticoagulant rodenticide intoxication with chlorophacinone. Forensic. Sci. Int. 166 (2–3), 85–90.

Park, B.K., Leck, J.B., 1982. A comparison of vitamin K antagonism by warfarin, difenacoum and brodifacoum in rabbit. Biochem. Pharmacol. 31, 3635–3639.

Park, B.K., Leck, J.B., Wilson, A., Breckenridge, A.M., 1979. Investigation of anticoagulants and vitamin K1 in the rabbit. In *Vitamin K Metabolism and Vitamin K Dependent Protein*, Suttie JW (ed.), Proceedings of the 8th Steenbock Symposium. University of Wisconsin, Madison, pp. 348–353.

Park, B.K., Scott, A.K., Wilson, A.C., Haynes, B.P., Breckenridge, A. M., 1984. Plasma disposition of vitamin K1 in relation to anticoagulant poisoning. Br. J. Clin. Pharmacol. 18 (5), 655–662.

Park, B.K., Choonara, I.A., Haynes, B.P., Breckenridge, A.M., Malia, R.G., Preston, F.E., 1986. Abnormal vitamin K metabolism in the presence of normal clotting factor activity in factory workers exposed to 4-hydroxycoumarins. Br. J. Clin. Pharmacol. 21 (3), 289–293.

Parshad, V.R., Chopra, G., 1986. The susceptibility of Rattus rattus and Bandicota bengalensis to a new anticoagulant rodenticide, flocoumafen. J. Hyg. London. 96 (3), 475–478.

Pavlu, J., Harrington, D.J., Voong, K., Savidge, G.F., Jan-Mohamed, R., Kaczmarski, R., 2005. Superwarfarin poisoning. Lancet. 365 (9459), 628.

Pelz, H.J., Rost, S., Hunerberg, M., Fregin, A., Heiberg, A.C., Baert, K., et al., 2005. The genetic basis of resistance to anticoagulants in rodents. Genetics. 170 (4), 1839–1847.

Pelz, H.J., Rost, S., Müller, E., et al., 2012. Distribution and frequency of VKORC1 sequence variants conferring resistance to anticoagulants in *Mus musculus*. Pest. Manag. Sci. 68 (2), 254–259.

Peterson, J., Streeter, V., 1996. Laryngeal obstruction secondary to brodifacoum toxicosis in a dog. J. Am. Vet. Diag. Invest. 208, 352–353.

Petrus, D.J., Henik, R.A., 1999. Pericardial effusion and cardiac tamponade secondary to brodifacoum toxicosis in a dog. J. Am. Vet. Med. Assoc. 215 (5), 647–648.

Piovella, F., Siragusa, S., Barone, M., Beltrametti, C., Carbone, S., Vicentini, L., et al., 1995. Secondary prophylaxis of venous thromboem-bolism: rational use of oral anticoagulants. Haematologica. 80 (Suppl. 2), 87–91.

Poli, F., Appendino, G., Sacchetti, G., Ballero, M., Maggiano, N., Ranelletti, F.O., 2005. Antiproliferative effects of daucane esters from *Ferula communis* and *F. arrigonii* on human colon cancer cell lines. Phytother. Res. 19 (2), 152–157.

Primus, T., Wright, G., Fisher, P., 2005. Accidental discharge of brodifacoum baits in a tidal marine environment: a case study. Bull. Environ. Contam. Toxicol. 74 (5), 913–919.

Primus, T.M., Griffin, D.L., Volz, S.A., Johnston, J.J., 1998. Reversed-phase ion-pair liquid chromatographic determination of chlorophacinone and diphacinone in steam-rolled oat baits and steam-rolled oat/wax baits. J. AOAC. Int. 81 (2), 349–357.

Primus, T.M., Kohler, D.J., Johnston, J.J., 2006. Determination of dipha-cinone residues in Hawaiian invertebrates. J. Chromatogr. Sci. 44 (1), 1–5.

Quinn, J.H., Girard, Y.A., Gilardi, K., et al., 2012. Pathogen and rodenticide exposure in American badgers (*Taxidea taxus*) in California. J. Wildl. Dis. 48 (2), 467–472.

Radi, Z.A., Thompson, L.J., 2004. Renal subcapsular hematoma associated with brodifacoum toxicosis in a dog. Vet. Hum. Toxicol. 46 (2), 83–84.

Radvanyi, A., Weaver, P., Massari, C., Bird, D., Broughton, E., 1988. Effects of chlorophacinone on captive kestrels. Bull. Environ. Contam. Toxicol. 41 (3), 441–448.

Rammell, C.G., Cotter, M., Williams, J.M., Bell, J., 1984. Brodifacoum residues in target and non-target animals following rabbit poisoning trials. N. Z. J. Exp. Agric. 12, 107–111.

Raoul, F., Michelat, D., Ordinaire, M., Decote, Y., Aubert, M., Delattre, P., et al., 2003. *Echinococcus multilocularis*: secondary poisoning of fox population during a vole outbreak reduces environmental contamination in a high endemicity area. Int. J. Parasitol. 33 (9), 945–954.

Rattner, B.A., Horak, K.E., Lazarus, R.S., et al., 2012. Assessment of toxicity and potential risk of the anticoagulant rodenticide diphacinone using Eastern screech-owls (*Megascops asio*). Ecotoxicology. 21 (3), 832–846.

Rattner, B.A., Horak, K.E., Lazarus, R.S., et al., 2014. Toxicokinetics and coagulopathy threshold of the rodenticide diphacinone in eastern screech-owls (*Megascops asio*). Environ. Toxicol. Chem. 33 (1), 74–81.

Rauch, A.E., Weininger, R., Pasquale, D., Burkart, P.T., Dunn, H.G., Weissman, C., et al., 1994. Superwarfarin poisoning: a significant public health problem. J. Community Health. 19 (1), 55–65.

Ray, A.C., Murphy, M.J., DuVall, M.D., Reagor, M.D., 1989. Determination of brodifacoum and bromadiolone residues in rodent and canine liver. Am. J. Vet. Res. 50, 546–550.

Redfern, R., Gill, J.E., 1980. Laboratory evaluation of bromadiolone as a rodenticide for use against warfarin-resistant and non-resistant rats and mice. J. Hyg. London. 84 (2), 263–268.

Reece, R.L., Scott, P.C., Forsyth, W.M., Gould, J.A., Barr, D.A., 1985. Toxicity episodes involving agricultural chemicals and other substances in birds in Victoria, Australia. Vet. Rec. 117 (20), 525–527.

Reese, J., Tausch, T., Barnwell, M., et al., 2012. Spontaneous bilateral renal pelvis thrombus formation presenting as anuric acute renal failure. Clin. Nephrol. 78 (4), 312–315.

Rehman, A.B., Ahmad, S.I., 1983. Comparative haematological studies on *Tatera indica* with three anticoagulant compounds. J. Pak. Med. Assoc. 33 (8), 203–207.

Rehnqvist, N., 1978. Intrahepatic jaundice due to warfarin therapy. Acta Med. Scand. 204 (4), 335–336.

Reiffel, J.A., 2000. Drug choices in the treatment of atrial fibrillation. Am. J. Cardiol. 85 (10A), 12D–19D.

Renapurkar, D.M., 1982. A comparative assessment of efficacy of three anticoagulant rodenticides. J. Hyg. Epidemiol. Microbiol. Immunol. 26 (2), 125–130.

Rennison, B.D., Dubock, A.C., 1978. Field trials of WBA 8119 (PP 581, brodifacoum) against warfarin-resistant infestations of *Rattus norvegicus*. J. Hyg. London. 80 (1), 77–82.

Rennison, B.D., Hadler, M.R., 1975. Field trials of difenacoum against warfarin-resistant infestations of *Rattus norvegicus*. J. Hyg. London. 74 (3), 449–455.

Richards, C.G., 1981. Field trials of bromadiolone against infestations of warfarin-resistant *Rattus norvegicus*. J. Hyg. London. 86 (3), 363–367.

Rickman, B.H., Gurfield, N., 2009. Thymic cystic degeneration, pseudoepitheliomatous hyperplasia, and hemorrhage in a dog with brodifacoum toxicosis. Vet. Pathol. 46 (3), 449–452.

Riedel, B., Grun, G., Clausing, P., 1990. The subacute and subchronic toxicity of chlorophacinone in Japanese quail (*Coturnix c. japonica*) [in German]. Arch. Exp. Veterinarmed. 44 (3), 341–346.

Robben, J.H., Mout, H.C., Kuijpers, E.A., 1997. Anticoagulant rodenticide poisoning in dogs in The Netherlands [in Dutch]. Tijdschr. Diergeneeskd. 122 (17), 466–471.

Robben, J.H., Kuijpers, E.A., Mout, H.C., 1998. Plasma superwarfarin levels and vitamin K_1 treatment in dogs with anticoagulant rodenticide poisoning. Vet. Q. 20 (1), 24–27.

Robinson, M.H., Twigg, L.E., Wheeler, S.H., Martin, G.R., 2005. Effect of the anticoagulant, pindone, on the breeding performance and survival of merino sheep. Ovis aries Comp. Biochem. Physiol. B Biochem. Mol. Biol. 140 (3), 465–473.

Ross, G.S., Zacharski, L.R., Robert, D., Rabin, D.L., 1992. An acquired hemorrhagic disorder from long-acting rodenticide ingestion. Arch. Intern. Med. 152 (2), 410–412.

Routh, C.R., Triplett, D.A., Murphy, M.J., Felice, L.J., Sadowski, J.A., Bovill, E.G., 1991. Superwarfarin ingestion. Am. J. Hematol. 36, 50–54.

Rowe, F.P., Bradfield, A., 1976. Trials of the anticoagulants rodenticide WBA 8119 against confined colonies of warfarin-resistant house mice (*Mus musculus* L.). J. Hyg. London. 77 (3), 427–431.

Rowe, F.P., Redfern, R., 1968. Comparative toxicity of the two anticoagulants, coumatetralyl and warfarin, to wild house mice (*Mus musculus* L). Ann. Appl. Biol. 62, 355–361.

Rowe, F.P., Swinney, T., Plant, C., 1978. Field trials of brodifacoum (WBA 8119) against the house mouse (*Mus musculus* L.). J. Hyg. London. 81 (2), 197–201.

Rowe, F.P., Plant, C.J., Bradfield, A., 1981. Trials of the anticoagulant rodenticides bromadiolone and difenacoum against the house mouse (*Mus musculus* L.). J. Hyg. London. 87 (2), 171–177.

Rowe, F.P., Bradfield, A., Swinney, T., 1985a. Pen and field trials of a new anticoagulant rodenticide flocoumafen against the house mouse (*Mus musculus* L.). J. Hyg. London. 95 (3), 623–627.

Rowe, F.P., Bradfield, A., Swinney, T., 1985b. Pen and field trials of flupropadine against the house mouse (*Mus musculus* L.). J. Hyg. London. 95 (2), 513–518.

Sabhlok, V.P., Pasahan, S.C., Kumar, P., Singal, R.K., 1997. Evaluation of different rodenticidal baits against rodent population in cucumber (*Cucumis sativus*) crop fields. Indian J. Exp. Biol. 35 (6), 670–672.

Sánchez-Barbudo, I.S., Camarero, P.R., Mateo, R., 2012. Primary and secondary poisoning by anticoagulant rodenticides of non-target animals in Spain. Sci. Total Environ. 420, 280–288.

Santoro, P., Parisi, G., Copetti, S., 1993. Mutagenic effect of pindone on *D. melanogaster* [in Italian]. Boll. Soc. Ital. Biol. Sper. 69 (4), 237–241.

Savage, R., 2005. Cyclo-oxygenase-2 inhibitors: when should they be used in the elderly? Drugs Aging. 22 (3), 185–200.

Schaff, J.E., Montgomery, M.A., 2013. An HPLC-HR-MS-MS method for identification of anticoagulant rodenticides in blood. J. Anal. Toxicol. 37 (6), 321–325.

Schmeits, P.C., Péquériaux, N.C., van Geest-Daalderop, J.H., Ouwehand, M.E., Coremans, A.M., Hermans, M.H., et al., 2009. Investigating unexpected INRs: in search of the culprit – adherence, interactions, genetics, and superwarfarin. Neth. J. Med. 67 (2), 76–78.

Schor, N.A., Huddleson, R.L., Kane, G.M., Lee, G., 1983. Effects of the administration of anticoagulants on the activity of the enzyme-reduced NAD(P)H dehydrogenase in rat livers, hepatomas and precarcinomatous rat liver lesions. Enzyme. 30 (4), 244–251.

Schulman, A., Lusk, R., Lippincott, C.L., Ettinger, S.J., 1986. Diphacinone-induced coagulopathy in the dog. J. Am. Vet. Med. Assoc. 188 (4), 402–405.

Seegers, W.H., 1969. Blood clotting mechanisms: three basic reactions. Annu. Rev. Physiol. 31, 269–294.

Seidelmann, S., Kubic, V., Burton, E., Schmitz, L., 1995. Combined superwarfarin and ethylene glycol ingestion: a unique case report with misleading clinical history. Am. J. Clin. Pathol. 104 (6), 663–666.

Shanberge, J.N., 1988. Bromodialone poisoning. Lancet. 1 (8581), 363–364.

Sharma, P., Bentley, P., 2005. Of rats and men: superwarfarin toxicity. Lancet. 365 (9459), 552–553.

Shepherd, G., Klein-Schwartz, W., Anderson, B.D., 2002. Acute, unintentional pediatric brodifacoum ingestions. Pediatr. Emerg. Care. 18 (3), 174–178.

Shetty, H.G., Woods, F., Routledge, P.A., 1993. The pharmacology of oral anticoagulants: implications for therapy. J. Heart Valve Dis. 2 (1), 53–62.

Shi, H.P., Liu, Y., Ma, D.Y., 2005. One case of acute severe bromadiolone poisoning. Zhonghua Lao Dong Wei. 23, 469–470.

Shimshoni, J.A., Soback, S., Cuneah, O., et al., 2013. New validated multiresidue analysis of six 4-hydroxy-coumarin anticoagulant rodenticides in hen eggs. J. Vet. Diagn. Invest. 25 (6), 736–743.

Shlosberg, A., Egyed, M.N., 1983. Examples of poisonous plants in Israel of importance to animals and man. Arch. Toxicol. Suppl. 6, 194–196.

Shlosberg, A., Egyed, M.N., 1985. Experimental *Ferula communis* (giant fennel) toxicosis in sheep. Zentralbl. Veterinarmed. A. 32 (10), 778–784.

Shore, R.F., Birks, J.D., Freestone, P., Kitchener, A.C., 1996. Second-generation rodenticides and polecats (*Mustela putorius*) in Britain. Environ. Pollut. 91 (3), 279–282.

Shore, R.F., Birks, J.D., Afsar, A., Wienburg, C.L., Kitchener, A.C., 2003. Spatial and temporal analysis of second-generation anticoagulant rodenticide residues in polecats (*Mustela putorius*) from throughout their range in Britain, 1992–1999. Environ. Pollut. 122 (2), 183–193.

Smith, G.F., Neubauer, B.L., Sundboom, J.L., Best, K.L., Goode, R.L., Tanzer, L.R., et al., 1988. Correlation of the in vivo anticoagulant, antithrombotic, and antimetastatic efficacy of warfarin in the rat. Thromb. Res. 50 (1), 163–174.

Smith, P., Inglis, I.R., Cowan, D.P., Kerins, G.M., Bull, D.S., 1994. Symptom-dependent taste aversion induced by an anticoagulant rodenti-cide in the brown rat (*Rattus norvegicus*). J. Comp. Psychol. 108 (3), 282–290.

Smolinske, S.C., Scherger, D.L., Kearns, P.S., Wruk, K.M., Kulig, K.W., Rumack, B.H., 1989. Superwarfarin poisoning in children: a prospective study. Pediatrics. 84 (3), 490–494.

Soubiron, L., Hantson, P., Michaux, I., Lambert, M., Mahieu, P., Pringot, J., 2000. Spontaneous haemoperitoneum from surreptitious inges-tion of a rodenticide. Eur. J. Emerg. Med. 7 (4), 305–307.

Spahr, J.E., Maul, J.S., Rodgers, G.M., 2007. Superwarfarin poisoning: a report of two cases and review of the literature. Am. J. Hematol. 82 (7), 656–660.

Spiller, H.A., Gallenstein, G.L., Murphy, M.J., 2003. Dermal absorption of a liquid diphacinone rodenticide causing coagulaopathy. Vet. Hum. Toxicol. 45 (6), 313–314.

Stansley, W., Cummings, M., Vudathala, D., et al., 2014. Anticoagulant rodenticides in Red-Tailed hawks, *Buteo jamaicensis*, and great horned owls, *Bubo virginianus*, from New Jersey, USA, 2008-2010. Bull. Environ. Contam. Toxicol. 92 (1), 6–9.

Stanziale, S.F., Christopher, J.C., Fisher, R.B., 1997. Brodifacoum roden-ticide ingestion in a patient with shigellosis. South. Med. J. 90 (8), 833–835.

Stenflo, J., 1978. Vitamin K, prothrombin, and gamma-carboxy-glutamic acid. Adv. Enzymol. Relat. Areas. Mol. Biol. 46, 1–31.

Sterner, R.T., 1979. Effects of sodium cyanide and diphacinone in coyotes (*Canis latrans*): applications as predacides in livestock toxic collars. Bull. Environ. Contam. Toxicol. 23 (1–2), 211–217.

Stone, W.B., Okoniewski, J.C., Stedelin, J.R., 1999. Poisoning of wildlife with anticoagulant rodenticides in New York. J. Wildl. Dis. 35 (2), 187–193.

Stowe, C.M., Metz, A.L., Arendt, T.D., Schulman, J., 1983. Apparent brod-ifacoum poisoning in a dog. J. Am. Vet. Med. Assoc. 182 (8), 817–818.

Strayhorn, V.A., Baciewicz, A.M., Self, T.H., 1997. Update on rifampin drug interactions, III. Arch. Intern. Med. 157 (21), 2453–2458.

Subbiah, D., Kala, S., Mishra, A.K., 2005. Study on the fluorescence characteristics of bromadiolone in aqueous and organized media and application in analysis. Chemosphere. 61 (11), 1580–1586.

Suttie, J.W., 1986. Vitamin K-dependent carboxylase and coumarin anticoagulant action. In: Seegers, W.H., Walz, D.A. (Eds.), Prothrombin and Other Vitamin K Proteins. CRC Press, Boca Raton, FL, pp. 17–47.

Suttie, J.W., 1990. Warfarin and vitamin K. Clin. Cardiol. 13, 16–18.

Swigar, M.E., Clemow, L.P., Saidi, P., Kim, H.C., 1990. "Superwarfarin" ingestion: a new problem in covert anticoagulant overdose. Gen. Hosp. Psychiatr. 12 (5), 309–312.

Szuber, T., Diechtiar, M., 1968. Studies of the effectiveness of the anticoagulant rodenticide diphacinone (2-diphenylacetyl-1,3-indiandone) using the conditioning method [in Polish]. Rocz. Panstw. Zakl. Hig. 19 (3), 343–353.

Tagliapietra, S., Aragno, M., Ugazio, G., Nano, G.M., 1989. Experimental studies on the toxicity of some compounds isolated from *Ferula communis* in the rat. Res. Commun. Chem. Pathol. Pharmacol. 66 (2), 333–336.

Tahir, M., Khan, M.F., Tourbaf, K., 2008. Impending compartment syndrome and hemothorax after brodifacoum ingestion. South. Med. J. 101 (12), 1277.

Takani, U., Suttie, J.W., 1983. High performance liquid chromatography-reductive electrochemical detection analysis of serum trans-phylloquinone. Anal. Biochem. 133, 63–67.

Tanaka, N., Matsushita, E., Morimoto, H., Kobayashi, K., Hattori, N., 1985. Toxic hepatitis induced by cardiovascular agents [in Japanese]. Nippon. Rinsho. 43 (6), 1172–1175.

Tecimer, C., Yam, L.T., 1997. Surreptitious superwarfarin poisoning with brodifacoum. South. Med. J. 90 (10), 1053–1055.

Terneu, S., Verhelst, D., Thys, F., Ketelslegers, E., Hantson, P., Wittebole, X., 2003. An unusual cause of abdominal pain. Acta Clin. Belg. 58 (4), 241–244.

Thijssen, H.H., Soute, B.A., Vervoort, L.M., Claessens, J.G., 2004. Paracetamol (acetaminophen) warfarin interaction: NAPQI, the toxic metabolite of paracetamol, is an inhibitor of enzymes in the vitamin K cycle. Thromb. Haemost. 92 (4), 797–802.

Thornes, R.D., Daly, L., Lynch, G., Breslin, B., Browne, H., Browne, H. Y., et al., 1994. Treatment with coumarin to prevent or delay recurrence of malignant melanoma. J. Cancer. Res. Clin. Oncol. 120 (Suppl), S32–S34.

Thornton, H., 1980. An ingenious method of destroying the vampire bats which transmit rabies to cattle. Cent. Afr. J. Med. 26 (9), 207–209.

Tligui, N., Ruth, G.R., 1994. *Ferula communis* variety *brevifolia* intoxication of sheep. Am. J. Vet. Res. 55 (11), 1558–1563.

Tligui, N., Ruth, G.R., Felice, L.J., 1994. Plasma ferulenol concentration and activity of clotting factors in sheep with *Ferula communis* variety *brevifolia* intoxication. Am. J. Vet. Res. 55 (11), 1564–1569.

Toes, M.J., Jones, A.L., Prescott, L., 2005. Drug interactions with paracetamol. Am. J. Ther. 12 (1), 56–66.

Townsend, M.G., Entwisle, P., Hart, A.D., 1995. Use of two halogenated biphenyls as indicators of non-target exposure during rodenti-cide treatments. Bull. Environ. Contam. Toxicol. 54 (4), 526–533.

Travis, S.F., Warfield, W., Greenbaum, B.H., Molokisher, M., Siegel, J.E., 1993. Spontaneous hemorrhage associated with accidental brodifacoum poisoning in a child. J. Pediatr. 122 (6), 982–984.

Troy, G.C., 1988. Diphacinone toxicity, von Willebrand's disease, and *Ehrlichia canis* in a dog. Vet. Clin. North. Am. Small. Anim. Pract. 18 (1), 255–257.

Tsutaoka, B.T., Miller, M., Fung, S.M., Patel, M.M., Olson, K.R., 2003. Superwarfarin and glass ingestion with prolonged coagulo-pathy requiring high-dose vitamin K1 therapy. Pharmacotherapy. 23 (9), 1186–1189.

Tumova, L., 2000. Interactions between herbal medicines and drugs. Ceska. Slov. Farm. 49 (4), 162–167.

Tvedten, H., 1989. Hemostatic abnormalities. In: Willard, M.D., Tvedten, H., Turnwald, G.A. (Eds.), Small Animal Clinical Diagnosis by Laboratory Methods. Saunders, Philadelphia, pp. 86–102.

Twigg, L.E., Kay, B.J., 1995. The effect of sub-lethal doses of bromadiolone on the breeding performance of house mice (*Mus domesticus*). Comp. Biochem. Physiol. C. Pharmacol. Toxicol. Endocrinol. 110 (1), 77–82.

Usui, U., Nishjmura, N., Kobayashi, N., Okanoue, T., Kimoto, M., Ozawa, K., 1989. Measurement of vitamin K in human liver by gradient elution high performance liquid chromatography using platinum-black catalyst reduction and fluorometric detection. J. Chromatogr. 489, 291–301.

Veenstra, G.E., Owen, D.E., Huckle, K.R., 1991. Metabolic and toxicolog-ical studies on the anticoagulant rodenticide, flocoumafen. Arch. Toxicol. Suppl. 14, 160–165.

Vein, J., Vey, D., Fourel, I., et al., 2013. Bioaccumulation of chlorophacinone in strains of rats resistant to anticoagulants. Pest. Manag. Sci. 69 (3), 397–402.

Vesell, E.S., Shivley, C.A., 1974. Liquid chromatographic assay of warfarin: similarity of warfarin half-lives in human subjects. Science. 184, 466–468.

Vigh, Gy, Varga-Puchony, l, Papp-Hites, E., Hlavay, J., 1981. Determination of chlorophacinone in formulations by reversed-phased ion-pair chromatography. J. Chromatogr. 214, 335–341.

Vogel, J.J., de Moerloose, P., Bouvier, C.A., Gaspoz, J., Riant, P., 1988. Prolonged anticoagulation following chlorophacinone poisoning [in French]. Schweiz. Med. Wochenschr. 118 (50), 1915–1917.

Voĭtsekhovskiĭ, V.V., Pivnik, A.V., Bitiutskaia, L.G., et al., 2012. Acquired hemorrhagic coagulopathy due to contact with the rodenticide brodifacoum in the Nutcracker bait. Ter. Arkh. 84 (7), 66–71.

Vyas, N.B., Hulse, C.S., Rice, C.P., 2012. Chlorophacinone residues in mammalian prey at a black-tailed prairie dog colony. Environ. Toxicol. Chem. 31 (11), 2513–2516.

Waddell, L.S., Poppenga, R.H., Drobatz, K.J., et al., 2013. Anticoagulant rodenticide screening in dogs: 123 cases (1996-2003). J. Am. Vet. Med. Assoc. 242 (4), 516–521.

Waien, S.A., Hayes Jr, D., Leonardo, J.M., 2001. Severe coagulopathy as a consequence of smoking crack cocaine laced with rodenticide. N. Engl. J. Med. 345 (9), 700–701, Erratum in *N Engl J Med* 2001 Dec 20; 345(25): 1860.

Walker, J., Beach, F.X., 2002. Deliberate self-poisoning with rodenticide: a diagnostic dilemma. Int. J. Clin. Pract. 56, 223–224.

Wallace, S., Worsnop, C., Paull, P., Mashford, M.L., 1990. Covert self poisoning with brodifacoum, a "superwarfarin". Aust. N. Z. J. Med. 20 (5), 713–715.

Wallin, R., 1986. Vitamin K antagonism of coumarin anticoagula-tion: a dehydrogenase pathway in rat liver is responsible for the antagonistic effect. Biochem. J. 236 (3), 685–693.

Watson, K.S., Mills, G.M., Burton, G.V., 2012. Superwarfarin intoxication: two case reports and review of pathophysiology and patient management. J. La. State. Med. Soc. 164 (2), 70–72.

Watt, B.E., Proudfoot, A.T., Bradberry, S.M., Vale, J.A., 2005. Anticoagulant rodenticides. Toxicol. Rev. 24 (4), 259–269.

Watts, R.G., Castleberry, R.P., Sadowski, J.A., 1990. Accidental poisoning with a superwarfarin compound (brodifacoum) in a child. Pediatrics. 86 (6), 883–887.

Weitzel, I.N., Sadowski, J.A., Furie, B.C., Morosee, R., Kim, H., Mount, M.E., et al., 1990. Hemorrhagic disorder caused by surreptitious ingestion of long acting vitamin K antagonist/ rodenticide, brodifacoum. Blood. 76, 2555–2559.

Welling, P.G., Lee, K.P., Khanna, U., Wagner, J.G., 1970. Comparison of plasma concentrations of warfarin measured by both simple extraction and thin-layer liquid chromatographic methods. J. Pharm. Sci. 59, 1621–1625.

Whisson, D.A., Salmon, T.P., 2002. Effect of diphacinone on blood coagulation in *Spermophilus beecheyi* as a basis for determining optimal timing of field bait applications. Pest. Manag. Sci. 58 (7), 736–738.

Williams, R.C., Schmit, J.A., Henry, R.A., 1972. Quantitative analysis of the fat-soluble vitamins by high-speed liquid chromatography. J. Chromatogr. Sci. 10, 494–501.

Wilson, A.C., Park, B.K., 1984. The effect of phenobarbitone pre-treatment on vitamin K_1 disposition in the rat and rabbit. Biochem. Pharmacol. 33 (1), 141–146.

Wilton, N.M., 1991. "Superwarfarins" as agents of accidental or deliberate intoxication. Aust. N. Z. J. Med. 21 (4), 491.

Winn, M.J., Clegg, J.A., Park, B.K., 1987. An investigation of sex-linked differences to the toxic and to the pharmacological actions of difenacoum: studies in mice and rats. J. Pharm. Pharmacol. 39 (3), 219–222.

Winn, M.J., Cholerton, S., Park, B.K., 1988. An investigation of the pharmacological response to vitamin K_1 in the rabbit. Br. J. Pharmacol. 94 (4), 1077–1084.

Winn, M.J., White, P.M., Scott, A.K., Pratt, S.K., Park, B.K., 1989. The bio-availability of a mixed micellar preparation of vitamin K1, and its procoagulant effect in anticoagulated rabbits. J. Pharm. Pharmacol. 41 (4), 257–260.

Wood, M.J., Stewart, R.L., Merry, H., Johnstone, D.E., Cox, J.L., 2003. Use of complementary and alternative medical therapies in patients with cardiovascular disease. Am. Heart. J. 145 (5), 806–812.

Woody, B.J., Murphy, M.J., Ray, A.C., Green, R.A., 1992. Coagulopathic effects and therapy of brodifacoum toxicosis in dogs. J. Vet. Intern. Med. 6 (1), 23–28.

Wu, L., Lu, K., Yin, R., et al., 2012. Misdiagnosis of rodenticide poisoning as ectopic pregnancy: a case report. Eur. J. Obstet. Gynecol. Reprod. Biol. 163 (1), 120–121.

Wu, Y.F., Chang, C.S., Chung, C.Y., Lin, H.Y., Wang, C.C., Shen, M.C., 2009. Superwarfarin intoxication: hematuria is a major clinical manifestation. Int. J. Hematol. 90 (2), 170–173.

Yan, H., Xiang, P., Zhu, L., et al., 2012. Determination of bromadiolone and brodifacoum in human blood using LC-ESI/MS/MS and its application in four superwarfarin poisoning cases. Forensic. Sci. Int. 222 (1-3), 313–317.

Yan, J., Shi, Y., Sun, C., et al., 2013. Vitamin K treatment of brodifacoum poisoning in a pregnant woman. Int. J. Gynaecol. Obstet. 122 (2), 162–163.

Yang, S.Y., Pan, G.M., Meng, G.F., Zhang, D.M., 2001. Study of diphaci-none in biological samples by high performance liquid chroma-tography/diode array detector. Se. Pu. 19 (3), 245–247.

Yu, C.C., Atallah, Y.H., Whitacre, D.M., 1982. Metabolism and disposition of diphacinone in rats and mice. Drug. Metab. Dispos. 10 (6), 645–648.

Yu, H.Y., Lin, J.-L., Fu, J.-F., et al., 2013. Outcomes of patients with rodenticide poisoning at a far east poison center. Springerplus. 3. 2, 505.

Zhao, S.L., Li, P., Ji, M., Zong, Y., Zhang, S.T., 2010. Upper gastrointestinal hemorrhage caused by superwarfarin poisoning. World. J. Gastroenterol. 16 (13), 1680–1682.

Zhu, L., Yan, H., Shen, B., et al., 2013. Determination of bromadiolone and brodifacoum in human hair by liquid chromatography/tandem mass spectrometry and its application to poisoning cases. Rapid. Commun. Mass. Spectrom. 27 (4), 513–520.

Zimmerman, A., Matschiner, J.T., 1974. Biochemical basis of hereditary resistance to warfarin in the rat. Biochem. Pharmacol. 23, 1033–1040.

Zolcinski, M., Padjas, A., Musial, J., 2008. Intoxication with three different superwarfarin compounds in an adult woman. Thromb. Haemost. 100 (1), 156–157.

Chapter 47

Non-Anticoagulant Rodenticides

Ramesh C. Gupta

STRYCHNINE

Introduction

Strychnine is an alkaloid derived from the seeds and bark of a tree, *Strychnos nux-vomica* is native to Southeast Asia (India, West Indies, Sri Lanka, and Indonesia) and Australia. Strychnine is also found in *Strychnos ignatii*. It's a white, odorless, crystalline powder that has the chemical formula $C_{21}H_{22}N_2O_2$ and a molecular weight of 334.41. Its structural formula is shown in Fig. 47.1.

Nux-vomica/strychnine has been used for at least five centuries for both pests and people. Its major use is as a pesticide (rodenticide, avicide, and insecticide), but it is also used as a therapeutic agent in human ailments (laxative, appetizer, and central nervous system (CNS) stimulant). In addition, strychnine in small amounts is known to be added to lysergic acid diethylamide (LSD), heroin, cocaine, and other "street drugs," and has been known to cause poisoning (O'Callaghan et al., 1982). Strychnine has many names, and is sold under various trade names, including Boomer-Rid, Certox, Dog-button, Dolco mouse Ceral, Gopher Bait, Gopher Gitter, Kwik-kill, Stricnina, Mole death, Mouse-nots, Mouse-rid, Mouse-tox, Ro-dex, Strychnos, and Sanaseed. Strychnine poisoning in animals occurs from ingestion of baits designed for use against rodents. The most common domestic animal to be affected is the dog, either through accidental ingestion or through intentional poisoning.

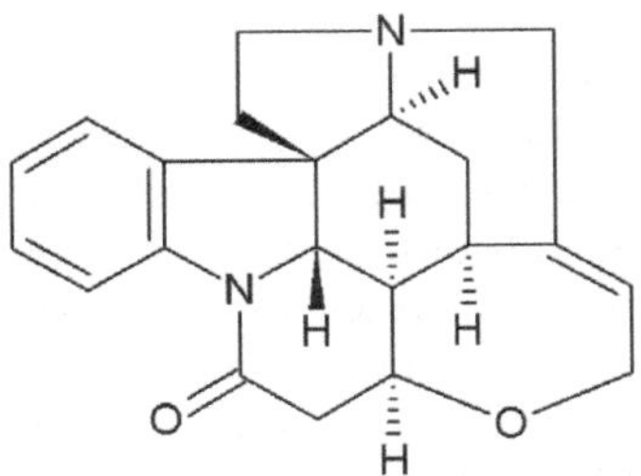

FIGURE 47.1 Structural formula of strychnine.

Background

Strychnine was first discovered in Saint-ignatii (*S. ignatii*) beans in 1818 by two French scientists (Joseph-Bienaime Caventou and Pierre-Joseph Pelletier). *S. ignatii* is a woody climbing shrub found in the Philippines. In general, the beans have the same properties as the species *S. nux-vomica*. Strychnine is also found in other species of *Strychnos* (i.e., *S. colubrine* and *S. tieute*), and is accompanied by another alkaloid brucine. The ripe seeds of *Strychnos* look like flattened discs, which are very hard and covered with satiny hairs. The properties of strychnine are substantially those of the nux-vomica. Strychnine is an extremely toxic alkaloid primarily used to kill rodents, moles, predatory animals, and birds, or used to trap fur-bearing animals. Pharmaceutically, strychnine is an unjustifiable component of traditional tonics, cathartic pills, and CNS stimulants.

Toxicokinetics

Following ingestion, strychnine is readily absorbed in the gastrointestinal (GI) tract, but mainly in the small intestine. Soon after absorption, it readily distributes to various tissues within 5 min (Reynolds, 1982). Strychnine is readily metabolized in the liver. In fact, the metabolism is rapid enough that approximately two lethal doses can be given over 24 h without cumulative effects. Its half-life has been reported to be approximately 10 h in humans. Elimination of strychnine is also rapid, as its unchanged residue can be detected in the urine within a few minutes of exposure. The elimination constant ($K_{el} = 0.07\ h^{-1}$) indicates that 7% of the strychnine in the serum at any one moment would be eliminated in 1 h (Edmunds et al., 1986). Following exposure to a sublethal dose of strychnine, approximately 50% of the dose is eliminated within 6 h (Boyd et al., 1983), 10%–20% within 24 h, and almost completely in 48–72 h (Cooper, 1974).

Veterinary Toxicology. DOI: http://dx.doi.org/10.1016/B978-0-12-811410-0.00047-7

Mechanism of Action

Pharmacologically, because of its bitter taste, strychnine strongly stimulates salivary and gastric secretions. This increases appetite, and as a result, strychnine has been used for a long time to counteract the loss of appetite associated with illnesses.

Strychnine is a potent convulsant. The convulsant action of strychnine is due to interference with the post-synaptic inhibition that is mediated by the amino acid glycine. Glycine is an inhibitory transmitter to motor neurons and interneurons in the spinal cord. Strychnine acts as a selective competitive antagonist to block the inhibitory effects of glycine at the glycine receptors. Studies indicate that strychnine and glycine interact with the same receptor, but at different sites. It increases reflex excitability in the spinal cord, which results in a loss of the normal inhibition of spread of motor cell stimulation, so that all muscles contract simultaneously. There is also evidence of an increase in brain levels of glutamic acid, an amino acid that acts as a transmitter for excitatory nerve impulses that excite muscle contraction. The result of these effects is that skeletal muscles become hyperexcitable. With a little sound or touch, uncontrollable convulsions and seizures become eminent, followed by suffocation and death. Death occurs due to respiratory failure.

TABLE 47.1 Acute Toxicity Data for Strychnine

Species	Route of Administration	LD_{50} (mg/kg)
Rat	Oral	2.30
Rat	i.p.	2.50
Rat	s.c.	1.20
Rat	i.v.	0.96
Mice	Oral	2.00
Mice	i.p.	0.98
Mice	s.c.	0.474
Mice	i.v.	0.41
Duck	Oral	3.00
Pigeon	Oral	21.00

i.p., intraperitoneal; i.v., intravenous; s.c., subcutaneous.
Source: From NIOSH (1983–1984).

Toxicity

Strychnine has been studied for acute toxicity in many species, and all species that have been tested have been found to be sensitive. Strychnine is an extremely toxic substance, with an LD_{50} of 2.3 mg/kg in rats, 2 mg/kg in mice, 0.6 mg/kg in rabbits, and 0.5 mg/kg in cats and dogs. An approximate lethal dose for a dog is 0.75 mg/kg body weight. Thus, 5-g bait having 0.3% strychnine could be enough to kill a 20-kg dog. Toxicity data of strychnine for various animal species are given in Table 47.1.

Among animals, poisoning occurs with greatest frequency in dogs due to accidental ingestion or malicious intent. The onset of signs can occur within 15–30 min or, occasionally, 60 min after oral exposure, depending on whether the stomach is empty or full. The clinical signs are associated with CNS effects. Onset of signs includes restlessness, anxiety, muscle twitching, and stiffness of the neck. The poisoned dogs usually show the signs of mydriasis, tonic convulsions, contractions of striated muscles, seizures, opisthotonus, and death. The animal becomes sensitive to touch, sound, noise, or any other sudden change in the environment. A minor stimulation can trigger violent convulsions. Muscular contractions are easily triggered by external stimuli, accompanied by hypothermia, lactic acidosis, rhabdomyolysis and, consequently, nephrosis, which may result in renal failure (Gupta and Crissman, 2012).

Although strychnine has no direct effects on skeletal muscles, all voluntary muscles contract simultaneously (as discussed earlier). The increase in muscle tone is caused by the central action of strychnine. The most powerful effects are seen on the muscles of joints. Respiratory muscles (diaphragm, thoracic, and abdominal) contract, respiration ceases and, eventually, death ensues due to respiratory failure.

Birds poisoned by strychnine exhibit the signs of ataxia, ruffled feathers, wing droop, salivation, tremors, and convulsions. Death occurs due to respiratory failure. On postmortem, lesions are only observed in the lungs—i.e., pinpoint hemorrhages resulting from death due to asphyxia. Rigor mortis occurs soon after death and persists for days. Occasionally, wildlife species are also inadvertently poisoned by strychnine.

There is no evidence of cumulative toxicity from strychnine (Gosselin et al., 1984). From animal studies, there is no evidence that strychnine has potential for reproductive and developmental toxicity or mutagenic and carcinogenic activity.

Diagnosis

Diagnosis of strychnine poisoning is based on (1) history of exposure to a strychnine bait or the presence of cracked corn in the digestive tract; (2) clinical signs of tetanic convulsions, seizures, hypersensitivity to external stimuli, and muscle stiffness; and (3) chemical identification of strychnine in the stomach content, blood, urine, or visceral organs (liver and kidney). Strychnine residue can be detected and quantified using gas chromatography (GC)–flame ionization detector or

GC–mass spectrometry (GC-MS). It is important to note that strychnine causes elevation of serum enzymes, including glutamic oxaloacetic transaminase, creatine phosphokinase, and lactate dehydrogenase. In addition, lactic acidosis, hyperkalemia, and leukocytosis are the characteristic laboratory findings. In differential diagnosis, tetanus must be ruled out.

Treatment

There is no specific antidote for strychnine poisoning, so treatment rests with symptomatic and supportive therapies. Seizures need to be controlled as soon as possible with diazepam or phenobarbital. Artificial respiration can be used for apnea. Once the seizures are controlled, detoxification can be performed using gastric lavage with potassium permanganate. Give activated charcoal with a saline cathartic to stop further absorption in the GI tract. Animals should be kept in a quiet environment and protected from any secondary sensory input.

Conclusion

Strychnine is an extremely toxic plant alkaloid that is primarily used as rodenticide. Due to inadvertent use or malicious intent, the poisoning is frequently encountered in dogs. Onset of clinical signs occurs very quickly, and the poisoning is characterized by convulsions, seizures, and hypersensitivity to any external stimulus. Treatment is symptomatic, and warranted immediately.

BROMETHALIN

Introduction

Chemically, bromethalin is a diphenylamine compound with an appearance of a pale, odorless, and solid crystalline powder. It has a chemical formula of $C_{14}H_{17}Br_3F_3N_3O_4$, with a molecular weight of 577.93. Its chemical structure is shown in Fig. 47.2. It is commonly used as rodenticide for the control of rats and mice. Bromethalin has many other names, and is sold under brand names such as Assault, Trounce, Vengeance, and Wipe Out.

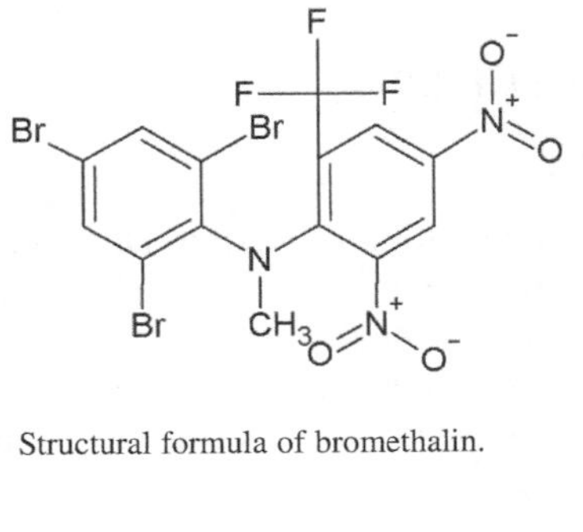

FIGURE 47.2 Structural formula of bromethalin.

Background

Bromethalin was developed for use against warfarin-resistant rodents. It is a restricted-use rodenticide used in and around buildings and sewers and inside transportation and cargo vehicles. It is extremely toxic, and only a single dose of bromethalin is needed to cause death in rats and mice. Bromethalin is marketed in a 0.01% formulation (2.84 mg of bromethalin per ounce of bait), and comes in bait pellets, bars, and packs. It is important to note that bromethalin cannot be distinguished from other rodent baits by color or appearance alone. Secondary poisoning usually occurs in dogs and cats that eat a mouse killed by bromethalin. There are few cases of bromethalin poisoning in humans following accidental exposure or suicidal intent (Pasquale-Styles et al., 2006; Huntington et al., 2016).

Toxicokinetics

Toxicokinetic information on bromethalin is available from laboratory animals such as rats. Bromethalin is rapidly absorbed following oral ingestion. Plasma concentration peaks in approximately 4 h. Metabolism takes place in the liver, where bromethalin undergoes N-demethylation, forming desmethyl bromethalin. This metabolite is toxic, as its LD_{50} is 7.5 mg/kg body weight. The plasma half-life of bromethalin is approximately 6 days (Dorman et al., 1990c), suggesting slow elimination. Excretion occurs mainly in bile, as it enters into enterohepatic circulation.

Mechanism of Action

Bromethalin is a neurotoxicant, and affects the CNS. It uncouples oxidative phosphorylation in the mitochondria, thereby decreasing ATP synthesis. With a marked depletion of ATP, very little energy is available to maintain Na^+/K^+-ATPase pump. As a result, cells lose their ability to maintain osmotic control, Na^+ is retained intracellularly, and the cells swell with water. This leads to fluid accumulation within myelin sheaths and vacuolation of the nervous system, resulting in nerve conduction impairment. Damage to neuronal axons and increased intracranial pressure occur, followed by convulsions, paralysis, and death (Van Lier and Cherry, 1988; Dorman et al., 1992).

Toxicity

Bromethalin is a single-dose rodenticide. It is classified as highly toxic if swallowed, inhaled, or absorbed through skin. The acute oral LD_{50} of bromethalin is 2.38–5.6 mg/kg in bait for dogs and 0.4–0.71 mg/kg in bait for cats (Dorman et al., 1990c). Its LD_{50} is 2 mg/kg in mice, 5 mg/kg in rats, 13 mg/kg in rabbits, and 0.25 mg/kg in pigs.

In field cases, most often, poisoning occurs in pets, including dogs and cats. Signs of bromethalin appear within 10 h to several days after exposure, and may last up to 12 days. In most cases, the poisoning is acute in nature, characterized by cerebral edema and paralysis of the hind limbs. In general, clinical signs in pets include severe muscle tremors, hyperexcitability, hyperesthesia (hypersensitivity to touch), and seizures. Symptoms with mild exposure to bromethalin occur with slow progress in several days, and they include loss of ability to bark, loss of appetite, vomiting, depression, lethargy, tremors, paralysis, lateral recumbency, coma, and death. Following exposure to a large dose of bromethalin, animals can show signs of muscle tremors and seizures, hyperexcitability, ataxia and paddling, hyperthermia, potential loss of vocalization, loss of tactile sensation, forelimb extensor rigidity (Schiff–Sherrington posture), and death occurs within 2–4 days. Death can occur with a low or high dose, and is usually caused by respiratory paralysis. Poisoned dogs show the signs of tremors, ataxia, depression, tachypnea, hyperreflexia of the hind limbs, loss of vocalization, recumbency, anorexia, vomiting, and death (Dorman et al., 1990a). Poisoned cats exhibit the signs of ataxia, seizures, vocalization, rigidity, decreased proprioception, abdominal distension, recumbency, depression, and death (Dorman et al., 1990b, 1992). Other signs of poisoning include generalized seizures, head pressing, hyperesthesia, coma, hyperexcitability, ataxia, extensor rigidity, nystagmus, hyperthermia, cyanosis, miosis, and drooling (Moorman, 2003). Overall, cats are much more sensitive than dogs to bromethalin.

Histopathological changes have been described in dogs receiving a single oral dose of bromethalin (6.25 mg/kg). Histologic lesions included diffuse white matter spongiosis, mild microgliosis, optic nerve vacuolization, mild thickening of Bowman's capsule, and occasional splenic megakaryocytes. Ultramicroscopic examination of the mid brain stem revealed occasional swollen axons, intramyelinic vacuolization, and myelin splitting at the intraperiod line (Dorman et al., 1990c). Dorman et al. (1992) also reported histopathological changes in cats induced by bromethalin. In brief, ultrastructural changes include separation of myelin lamellae at the interperiod lines, with the formation of intramyelinic vacuoles (intramyelinic edema), rupture and coalescence of intramyelinic vacuoles into larger extracellular spaces (spongy change), and pronounced cytosolic edema of astrocytes and oligodendroglial cells. Histopathology of the brain and spinal cord of rodents receiving multiple low or sublethal doses of bromethalin revealed a spongy degeneration of the white matter that was shown upon ultramicroscopic examination to be intramyelinic edema (Van Lier and Cherry, 1988).

According to the World Health Organization and the US Environmental Protection Agency, bromethalin is considered carcinogenic.

Diagnosis

Diagnosis of bromethalin poisoning is based on history of exposure to bromethalin bait, clinical signs, and identification of bromethalin in bait, GI content, brain, and visceral organs. Residue of bromethalin, or its major metabolite (desmethyl bromethalin), can be quantified using GC coupled with electron capture detector (Dorman et al., 1990c) or high-performance liquid chromatography (HPLC), coupled with ultraviolet detector or with negative-ion atmospheric pressure chemical ionization–mass spectrometric detector (Mesmer and Flurer, 2001). The highest concentrations of bromethalin are found in the fat, liver, kidney, and brain. Differential diagnosis should rule out lead, ethylene glycol, organophosphates, strychnine, metaldehyde, zinc phosphide, and tremorgenic mycotoxins.

Treatment

There is no specific antidote for bromethalin poisoning (Coppock, 2013). Symptoms can be treated with corticosteroids, but clinical studies indicate that symptoms return as soon as the corticosteroids are discontinued. Emesis should be induced using apomorphine or 3% hydrogen peroxide if the animal is not exhibiting signs of convulsions and seizures. Alternatively, perform gastric lavage and give activated charcoal with saline cathartic. Activated charcoal needs to be repeated if the dog or cat is exposed to a large dose of bromethalin. The animal needs to be monitored and treated for cerebral edema. Intravenous fluids can be administered with great caution so as not to worsen cerebral edema. The seizures in dogs can be somewhat refractory to diazepam; thus, a barbiturate can be given to control seizures.

Conclusion

Bromethalin is a commonly used rodenticide that is encountered in poisoning in dogs and cats. Bromethalin exerts toxicity by uncoupling oxidative phosphorylation in mitochondria, thereby decreasing ATP synthesis. The CNS is the target organ, and toxicity is characterized by cerebral edema, convulsions, and paralysis. There is no specific antidote, so treatment is symptomatic and supportive.

CHOLECALCIFEROL

Introduction

Cholecalciferol is a form of vitamin D, also called vitamin D_3, that is commonly used as rodenticide. Vitamin D_3 is a secosteroid, and structurally similar to other steroids, such as cholesterol, testosterone, and cortisol. It has chemical formula $C_{27}H_{44}O$, with a molecular weight of 384.64. Its

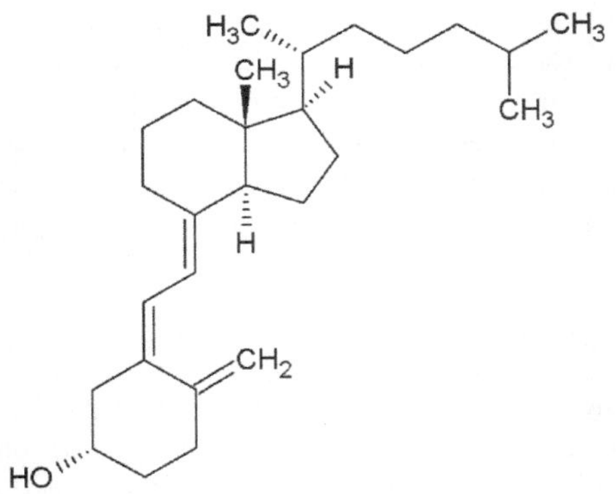

FIGURE 47.3 Structural formula of cholecalciferol.

structural formula is shown in Fig. 47.3. Cholecalciferol has other names, and is marketed as a rodenticide under the brand names Quintox, True Grit Rampage, and Ortho Rat-B-Gone; it is also marketed as a feed additive under the name Viactive.

Background

Cholecalciferol is a rodenticide that is used in and around buildings and inside transport vehicles. Vitamin D_3, as such, does not have significant biological activity but, in two steps, is metabolized in the body to make an active form. In the liver, cholecalciferol is hydroxylated to 25-hydroxycholecalciferol (calcifedion) by the enzyme 25-hydroxylase. In the kidney, 25-hydroxycholecalciferol serves as a substrate for 1-α-hydroxylase, forming 1,25-dihydroxycholecalciferol (calcitriol), which is the biologically active form. Cholecalciferol is formulated in the granular form (0.075% bait), and is very effective against Norway rats, roof rats, and house mice.

Toxicokinetics

Very little information is available on the toxicokinetics of cholecalciferol. Cholecalciferol is transported in blood bound to carrier proteins. The major carrier protein is a vitamin D-binding protein. The half-life of 25-hydroxycholecalciferol is several weeks, whereas that of 1,25-dihydroxycholecalciferol is just a few hours.

Mechanism of Action

Ingestion of cholecalciferol-containing bait is known to cause a marked increase in calcium level in blood and tissues. Cholecalciferol not only increases the absorption of calcium, but also mobilizes calcium and phosphorus from bones to the circulation. High calcium causes heart problems and bleeding secondary to mineralization of the vessels, kidneys, stomach wall, and lungs. Mineralization of the kidney leads to renal failure and death. Cholecalciferol and its metabolites exert their effects by binding to vitamin D receptors in tissues. 1,25-Dihydrocholecalciferol is the most metabolically active form, with 500 times greater binding to the vitamin D receptors than that of 25-hydroxycholecalciferol and 1000 times greater binding than that of cholecalciferol.

Toxicity

Cholecalciferol is of low toxicity to mammalian species, as it is classified as a class III toxic chemical. The oral LD_{50} of cholecalciferol in rats is 43.6 mg/kg and 42.5 mg/kg in mice. The dermal LD_{50} in rabbits is 2000 mg/kg. Studies suggest that cholecalciferol is of low toxicity to birds (oral LD_{50} is $>$2000 mg/kg in mallard ducks and dietary LC_{50} is 4,000 ppm in mallard ducks and 2000 ppm in bobwhite quail).

Pets such as dogs are poisoned by ingesting rodenticide bait, whereas farm animals are affected by overdose of additive vitamin D_3 in the feed. Signs and symptoms of poisoning are similar to those of hypercalcemia, such as anorexia, fatigue, headache, itching, weakness, nausea, vomiting, and diarrhea. In acute cases, cholecalciferol causes severe polyneuropathy. Dogs poisoned with cholecalciferol-containing rodenticide bait usually show signs of depression, anorexia, vomiting, bloody diarrhea, cardiac irregularities, hypertension, seizures, and death. In dogs, signs of poisoning may occur with as little as a 2 mg/kg dose, and death may occur with a 10 mg/kg dose of cholecalciferol.

Treatment

Decontamination, including induction of emesis, gastric lavage, and administration of activated charcoal, is beneficial. Administration of intravenous fluids helps reduce serum calcium levels by increasing urine production and calcium excretion. Biphosphonate pamidronate disodium is used to decrease serum calcium levels. Seizures can be controlled by diazepam or barbiturates. Treatment needs to be continued for 2 or 3 weeks because the elimination half-life of cholecalciferol is more than 2 weeks. Poisoned animals should receive feed devoid of vitamin D_3.

Conclusion

Cholecalciferol is a single- or multiple-dose rodenticide that has low toxicity to mammalian and avian species. It produces toxicity by marked increases in calcium and mineralization of tissues. Once animals develop severe signs, they usually die.

RED SQUILL

Introduction

Red squill, which is also known as sea onion, is obtained in the powder form from the plant *Urginea maritima*. The plant is native to the Mediterranean region. It resembles an onion, and its bulb extracts and dried powders have been used for the control of rodents since the 13th century. Although red squill has many alkaloids, scilliroside is the most toxic, and provides rodenticidal activity. It has the chemical formula $C_{32}H_{44}O_{12}$ and a molecular weight of 620.7. Its structural formula is shown in Fig. 47.4. The compound is sparingly soluble in water and thermostable. Scilliroside is formulated in the powder form (Dethdiet) and liquid extract (Rodine), and it has many other names, including Sea squill, Scilla maritima, Silmurin, Silmine, Sea onion, and Squill. It was demonstrated long ago by Winton (1927b) that only red squill, not white squill, has rodenticide activity. The red squill is mixed in baits and applied at a 10% concentration and mixed with meat, fish, and cereals (Thomson, 1991–1992).

Background

Red squill bulbs were an ancient source of rodenticide products replaced later by warfarin and other modern anticoagulant rodenticides. Because rats have developed resistance to such products, there is renewed interest in the red squill. Studies suggest that the white squill drug is used as a diuretic, stimulant, and expectorant, whereas the red squill is used mostly as a rat poison. Many glycosides and aglycones have been isolated from the red squill bulb. Krenn et al. (1994) and Pascual-Villalobos (2002) isolated five different bufadienolides as pure substances (proscillaridin A, scillaren A, scilliroside, gammabufotalin, and scillirosidin). Scilliroside is the most toxic bufadienolide glycoside (Verbiscar et al., 1986a,b).

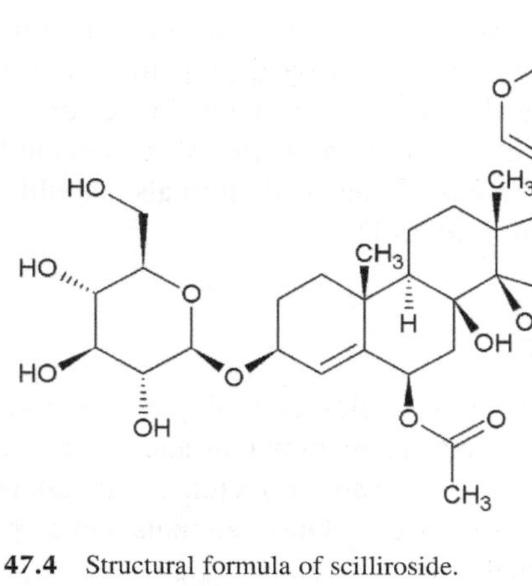

FIGURE 47.4 Structural formula of scilliroside.

Scilliroside has an emetic property; thus, if rodents ingest a product containing scilliroside, because they are incapable of vomiting, they develop glycoside intoxication and pulmonary edema. However, it has rarely been associated with toxicity in humans because humans are capable of vomiting and exhibit poor GI absorption.

Toxicokinetics

Scilliroside is inefficiently absorbed from the GI tract. Its metabolism is not well-studied, although the unmetabolized scilliroside is rapidly excreted in the urine.

Mechanism of Action

Red squill bulbs contain many glycosides, but scilliroside is the major component that has a rodenticidal property. The compound is cardiotoxic, similar to digitalis; i.e., injection of scilliroside induces cardiac impulse condition and arrhythmias. In very early experiments, red squill preparations administered to rats induced convulsions and paralysis (Winton, 1927a). Female rats succumb to red squill at half the dose that is required to kill males.

Toxicity

The red squill plant (mainly the bulb) contains scilliroside, a highly toxic bufadienolide glycoside. It adversely affects cardiovascular and CNSs, causing convulsions and death. The oral LD_{50} of scilliroside is 0.7 mg/kg in male rats, 0.43 mg/kg in female rats, and 0.35 mg/kg in mice. Studies found that pigs and cats survived doses of 16 mg/kg and fowls survived 400 mg/kg (Worthing, 1983). It is classified as class I—i.e., a highly toxic chemical.

Red squill contains several compounds that have emetic properties. Due to poor GI absorption and decreased potency, red squill has seldom been associated with toxicity in humans, dogs, cats, and pigeons. However, rats and mice are unable to vomit, and they die within a few hours after ingesting a lethal dose of scilliroside.

In toxic doses, red squill produces inflammation of the GI and genitourinary tracts, manifested by nausea, vomiting, abdominal pain, and purging. Other signs of poisoning include convulsions, hypothermia, enfeebled circulation, blurred vision and, sometimes, death. Convulsions are seen in humans, and they have also been observed in rats. Higher doses of red squill can cause serious heart rhythm alterations, resulting in death. Farm animals require large quantities for intoxication. There are field cases in which dogs, cats, and pigs have been poisoned. Signs of poisoning include vomiting, ataxia, and hyperesthesia, followed by paralysis, depression, or convulsions. Cardiac arrest occurs due to bradycardia and cardiac arrhythmias.

Generally, animals exposed to a sublethal dose can recover in less than 48 h.

Treatment

Treatment is based on symptomatic and supportive therapies. In case a significant amount of red squill is retained in the stomach, decontamination (gastric lavage with saline cathartic) is rewarding. The patient must be monitored for cardiac arrhythmias and conduction disturbances. Atropine sulfate given subcutaneously at 6- to 8-h intervals may prevent cardiac arrest. Phenytoin at 35 mg/kg, TID, should be given to dogs to suppress arrhythmias.

Conclusions

Red squill is a botanical rodenticide, and exerts toxicity due to cardiac effects. Treatment is symptomatic and supportive.

FLUOROACETATE

Introduction

Sodium fluoroacetate (compound 1080) is an extremely toxic white powder that has been used as a rodenticide throughout the world. The compound has the chemical formula $C_2H_2FO_2.Na$, with a molecular weight of 100.02. Its structural formula is shown in Fig. 47.5. It is used to control rats, mice, squirrels, prairie dogs, foxes, wolves, coyotes, and rabbits. The compound is also used to control brush-tail possums, deer, wild pigs, wallabies, and rooks. It is very toxic to birds, domestic animals, and carnivores. Secondary poisoning is very common in birds and carnivores from eating poisoned carcasses.

Sodium fluoroacetate has many other names, and is sold under trade names such as Nissol, 1080 gel, 1080 paste, 1080 solution, Tenate, and Tenate 1080. The commercial products are provided with a black dye called nigrosine (0.5%).

Background

Sodium fluoroacetate was discovered by German military chemists during World War II. However, it was not until later that American chemists discovered its use as a rodenticide. The name "1080" refers to the catalog number of the poison, which became its brand name. The compound is an extremely toxic substance, which is commonly used as a rodenticide. Inhalation of dust or swallowing can also be fatal. The compound can also be absorbed through cuts or abrasions in the skin and lead to poisoning.

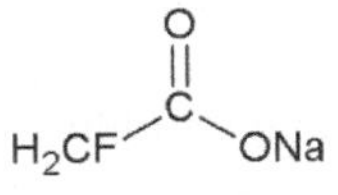

It is important to note that sodium fluoroacetate is also formed naturally in approximately 40 plants that are native to Australia, Brazil, and Africa after fluoride uptake from soil, water, or air. Examples of plants that contain sodium fluoroacetate are *Dichapetalum cymosum*, *Dichapetalum toxicarum*, *Chailletia toxicaria*, *Gastrolobium grandiflorum* ("poison peas"), *Oxylobium parviflorum*, and *Acacia georginae*. Consumption of these plants has resulted in many serious cases of livestock poisoning and high stock losses (Oelrichs and McEwan, 1962). Poisoning has also been documented in field workers exposed to fluoroacetate (Suh et al., 1970).

$$H_2CF{-}C({=}O){-}ONa$$

FIGURE 47.5 Structural formula of sodium fluoroacetate.

Toxicokinetics

Sodium fluoroacetate (1080) is rapidly absorbed from the GI tract. Dust formulations are easily absorbed by inhalation, which is not usually the route for poisoning cases. Compound 1080 is not readily absorbed through intact skin, but it can be absorbed in the case of cuts, abrasions, or dermatitis (Brockman et al., 1955). It is reported that sublethal doses of compound 1080 are completely metabolized and excreted in 4 days.

The bioavailability of sodium fluoroacetate appears to be similar for oral, injected, and inhaled doses. Dermal absorption is lower because a subcutaneous LD_{50} is 10- to 15-fold higher than the oral dose. Distribution studies suggest that the plasma levels of sodium fluoroacetate are twice those of tissues. Sheep receiving sodium fluoroacetate (0.1 mg/kg) contained the residue in plasma, kidney, heart, muscle, spleen, and liver as 0.098, 0.057, 0.052, 0.042, 0.026, and 0.021, respectively (Eason et al., 1993). The plasma $t_{½}$ is 3.6–6.9 h in goats, 6.6–13.3 h in sheep, 1.1 h in rabbits, and 1.6–1.7 h in mice (Eason et al., 1993; Gooneratne et al., 1995). Metabolism of fluoroacetate (i.e., defluorination) takes place in the liver. Fluoroacetate and fluorocitrate salts are excreted mainly in the urine.

Mechanism of Action

In the body, fluoroacetate (1080) is converted to fluorocitrate, which is a potent inhibitor of the enzyme aconitase in the tricarboxylic acid cycle (Krebs cycle) (Elliot and Kalnitsky, 1996). As a result, the elevated levels of citrate in the blood become observable 30 min after administration and maximum levels at 4 h after administration. It has been shown that citrate levels are directly influenced by the thyroid hormone (i.e., free T_3; Maruo et al., 1992). Accumulation of citrate causes toxicity due to reduction of ATP levels by inhibiting energy production in most cells of the body, leading to a slow and painful death as the body "suffocates from within." Compound 1080 causes damage to tissue of high energy needs, such as brain, heart, lungs, and fetus. Accumulated levels of citrate cause chelation of divalent metal ions, especially Ca^{2+}. Depletion of these ions in the CNS may be responsible for seizures in certain species (Hornfeldt and Larson, 1990).

Fluoroacetate/fluorocitrate also affects activities of other enzymes, including mitochondrial citrate carriers, pyruvate dehydrogenase kinase (Taylor et al., 1977), succinate dehydrogenase (Mehlman, 1967), glutamine synthetase, phosphofructokinase (Godoy and del Carmen Villarruel, 1974), and ATP-citrate lyase (Rokita and Walsh, 1983).

Toxicity

Severity of signs is dose-related, and the oral route is the most important in cases of compound 1080 poisoning. Most species are sensitive to fluoroacetate (1080); however, rodents and dogs are the most sensitive species. The oral LD_{50} of 1080 is 0.1–0.22 mg/kg in rats, 0.1 mg/kg in mice, 0.34 mg/kg in rabbits, and 0.3 mg/kg in guinea pigs. The oral LD_{50}s of this compound in the house sparrow, red-winged blackbird, starling, and golden eagle are 3.0, 4.22, 2.37, and 1.25–5 mg/kg, respectively. Measured LD_{50} of this rodenticide in mammalian wildlife is 0.22–0.44 mg/kg in mule deer, 1.41 mg/kg in male ferrets, and 0.5–1.0 mg/kg in bears.

In general, fluoroacetate is very toxic to mammalian, bird, and wildlife species, whereas it is of low toxicity to fish. Toxicity of 1080 is different according to route of exposure (i.e., ingestion or inhalation), and symptoms vary widely among species. Species have been categorized into four groups according to symptomatology:

1. Rabbit, goat, horse, sheep, and spider monkey: CNS effects are not observed, and death is due to cardiac effects with ventricular fibrillation.
2. Cat, pig, rhesus monkey, and human: Heart and CNS are affected, and death usually results from respiratory failure during convulsions, but is occasionally due to ventricular fibrillation.
3. Dog and guinea pig: Epileptiform convulsions predominate, with death being due to cessation of respiratory activity following running movements such as those of strychnine poisoning.
4. Rat and hamster: Respiratory depression and delayed bradycardia are the main features.

In general, 1080 produces convulsions, involuntary urination, vomiting, and ventricular fibrillation. The onset of symptoms of poisoning is usually between 30 min and 4 h after exposure. The common symptoms are vomiting, involuntary hyperextension of the limbs, convulsions and, finally, cardiac and respiratory failure. Dogs usually show CNS signs such as convulsions and uncontrollable running, whereas sheep and cattle show predominantly cardiac signs. Dogs appear to be highly sensitive to fluoroacetate, and mass poisonings of dogs eating contaminated poultry have been documented (Egyed, 1979).

The main target organs affected are the central nervous, cardiovascular, and respiratory systems. This causes metabolic derangement that includes alteration in transaminase, calcium, and glucose levels apart from acidosis and renal failure. Clinical effects are associated with neurological and cardiac systems. CNS effects include tremulousness, hallucinations, convulsions, and respiratory depression. Cardiac effects include arrhythmias, ventricular fibrillation, and cardiac arrest. If the patient survives the first 24 h after ingestion of sodium fluoroacetate, recovery is favorable. Acute exposure often results in complete recovery or death. Of course, in some cases, exposure results in cardiac damage.

The fluorocitric acid is, itself, highly toxic, and therefore, sodium fluoroacetate can cause secondary poisoning—i.e., poisoning in an organism that has consumed a part of an organism already poisoned.

The development of tolerance to increasing doses of fluoroacetate has been reported in rats and mice, whereby a dose of 0.5 mg/kg protects rats against a dose of 5 mg/kg for a period of 48 h (Chenoweth, 1949). The mechanism of fluoroacetate resistance in certain species is not well-understood, but the rate of defluorination does not appear to play a significant role (Mead et al., 1985).

Studies suggest that sodium fluoroacetate has no carcinogenic, mutagenic, or teratogenic potential.

Diagnosis

Diagnosis is based on evidence of exposure, clinical signs, necropsy findings, and chemical confirmation. Samples for chemical confirmation should include suspected bait, vomitus, stomach content, liver, and kidney. Testing for compound 1080 should be performed on the vomited stomach content. In the case of ruminants, rumen content needs to be analyzed for fluoroacetate. Significant elevation of citric acid levels in blood and kidney is a reliable biochemical marker of fluoroacetate or fluorocitrate poisoning (Bosakowski and Levin, 1986). Hyperglycemia, hypocalcemia, and hypokalemia are characteristic laboratory findings. Other metabolic/biochemical changes include metabolic acidosis resulting from a buildup of citric acid, lactic acid, and ammonium in blood and organs. Metabolic acidosis is also associated with elevated serum creatinine and transaminase levels.

Differential diagnosis should include lead, strychnine, chlorinated hydrocarbons, and plant alkaloids.

Treatment

There is no specific antidote for compound 1080 poisoning. Use of glyceryl monoacetate has shown some positive results because it provides acetate ions to allow continuation of the cellular respiration process, which is interrupted by compound 1080. Other symptomatic and supportive measures following decontamination procedures (to prevent further absorption by activated charcoal) include use of anticonvulsants, muscle relaxants, and mechanical ventilation. Induction of emesis is contraindicated because of potential arrhythmias and convulsions. Special attention should be paid to stabilize cardiac and CNS functions.

Acetate and ethanol have been found to be potentially effective in mice, guinea pigs, and rabbits, but not in dogs. A combination of calcium gluconate and sodium succinate has proven effective in mice (Omara and Sisodia, 1990). Calcium chloride has antidotal effects in cats (Roy et al., 1980).

Conclusion

Fluoroacetate converts to fluorocitrate, which is an extremely toxic metabolite. Symptoms vary markedly between species. For example, carnivores exhibit more signs related to the CNS, herbívores exhibit signs related to cardiac effects, and omnivores show signs of both CNS and cardiac effects. Treatment relies on symptomatic and supportive measures.

ALPHA-NAPHTHYL THIOUREA

Introduction

Alpha-naphthyl thiourea (ANTU) is a colorless, odorless, crystalline powder that is exclusively used as rodenticide. The technical product is gray powder. Its chemical formula is $C_{11}H_{10}N_2S$, and it has a molecular weight of 220.28. Its structural formula is shown in Fig. 47.6. ANTU has several other names, including alpha-naphthyl thiocarbamide, 1-naphthyl-thiourea, *N*(1-naphthyl)-2 thiourea, Alrato, Anturat, Bantu, Dirax, Krysid, Rat-tu, and Rattrack.

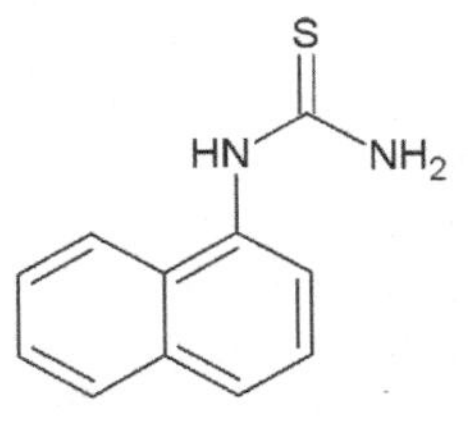

S
HN NH2

FIGURE 47.6 Structural formula of alpha-naphthyl thiourea.

Toxicokinetics and Mechanism of Action

Following ingestion, ANTU is rapidly absorbed from the GI tract. The exact mechanism of action of ANTU is not known. ANTU stimulates the sympathetic nervous system, and causes a major increase in the permeability of the lung capillaries; consequently, extensive pleural effusion and pulmonary edema develop. This results in respiratory failure.

Toxicity

All animal species are susceptible to ANTU, but lethal doses differ widely. Lethal doses of ANTU (in mg/kg) in various species are as follows: rats (3), dogs (10), pigs (25), horses (30), cows (50), cats (75), and fowl (2500).

Clinical signs of poisoning due to ANTU include vomiting, abdominal pain, dyspnea, shortness of breath, seizures, bluish discoloration, coarse pulmonary rales, pulmonary edema, and liver damage. In a time-course study, ANTU at a dose rate of 5 mg/kg induced lung edema in adult albino rats (Vivet et al., 1983). After 6 h, pulmonary extravascular water increased by 50% in ANTU-treated rats, and the volume of the pulmonary effusion reached 3.4 ± 0.1 mL. The most characteristic feature is the absence of hypoxemia in ANTU-intoxicated rats. The absence of hypoxemia is common with normobaric oxygen. ANTU can produce hyperglycemia of three times normal in 3 h.

Chronic sublethal exposure to ANTU may cause enlarged thyroid gland (goiter) and interfere with normal thyroid function. Repeated sublethal doses in rats lead to the development of tolerance so that resistance to several lethal doses develops (Peoples, 1970).

Diagnosis

Diagnosis of ANTU poisoning is based on evidence of rodenticide exposure, clinical signs, lung and liver damage, and chemical confirmation. ANTU can be quantified using HPLC.

Treatment

There is no specific antidote; therefore, treatment relies on symptomatic and supportive measures. Induce vomition if the patient is not showing convulsions and seizures. The decontamination procedure includes administration of activated charcoal.

ZINC PHOSPHIDE

Introduction

Zinc phosphide is an inorganic compound with the appearance of gray crystalline powder and a decaying fish or garlic odor. It has the chemical formula Zn_3P_2, with a molecular weight of 258.1. Its structural formula is shown in Fig. 47.7. Zinc phosphide was first synthesized in 1740, and was first used as a rodenticide in 1911–12 in Italy. It was not used in the United States until 1939. In the 1970s, there was a renewed interest in zinc phosphide for rodent control in agriculture. Currently, zinc phosphide is used worldwide for the control of a range of animals, including mice, rats, voles, ground squirrels, prairie dogs, moles, muskrats, rabbits, and gophers. Pelleted zinc phosphide is sold extensively under brand names such as Arrex, Blue-ox, Gopha-rid, Kil-rat, Mous-con, Phosvin, Pollux, Ratol, Ridall, Rodenticide AG, Zinc-tox, and ZP. It is also used on crop/noncrop areas, including lawns, golf courses, and around wetlands.

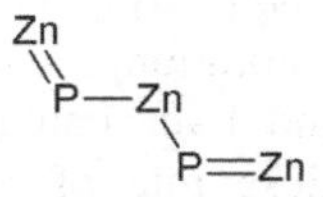

Zn
P—Zn
P=Zn

FIGURE 47.7 Structural formula of zinc phosphide.

Background

The history of the use of zinc phosphide as a rodenticide dates back approximately a century. In the early years, technical zinc phosphide and highly concentrated paste were sold in shops and used by consumers to make their own baits for rodents. This led to use of the technical material for suicide and to accidental deaths in small children and pets.

Zinc phosphide is recognized as the slowest acting of the commonly used rodenticides. It can cause toxicity and death in rodents after one feeding if adequate dose is consumed. However, bait must be continuously available to be effective. In fact, zinc phosphide is recommended as the rodenticide of choice because it is fairly specific for rodents and secondary poisoning is rare, except in dogs and cats.

Rodenticide-grade zinc phosphide usually comes as a black powder containing 75% zinc phosphide and 25% antimony potassium tartrate, an emetic to cause vomiting if the material is accidentally ingested by humans or domestic animals.

Toxicokinetics

Zinc phosphide can be absorbed into the body by oral ingestion, inhalation, and through damaged skin. Following oral ingestion, zinc phosphide reacts in the stomach and intestine with water and hydrochloric acid to liberate phosphine gas. Metabolism of zinc phosphide can occur via oxidation of the phosphorus to various phosphorus oxyacids or via reduction of the phosphorus to phosphine gas. Zinc phosphide excretes in the urine either as a hypophosphite or as dissolved phosphine. The presence of strong reducing substance in the urine is a common feature of poisoning with zinc phosphide. Other metabolites include phosphoric acid and phosphate. Phosphine gas is also exhaled from the lungs.

Mechanism of Action

The overall toxicity of zinc phosphide is due to both zinc and phosphine gas, but it is primarily from phosphine. It needs to be pointed out that animals can have access to phosphine gas from the feed/forage fumigated with phosphine or aluminum phosphide (Easterwood et al., 2010; Nath et al., 2011). Phosphine can cause irritation of the alimentary tract. It can enter the bloodstream and exert toxicity through multiple mechanisms, including acetylcholinesterase inactivation, mitochondrial disruption, and oxidative stress (Nath et al., 2011). Phosphine adversely affects the lungs, liver, kidneys, heart, and CNS. It causes CNS depression, irritation of the lungs, damage to the blood vessels and erythrocyte membranes and, eventually, cardiovascular collapse.

Toxicity

Zinc phosphide is an extremely toxic compound. The oral LD_{50} in rats is 41 mg/kg body weight. In sheep, the LD_{50} ranges from 60 to 70 mg/kg. It is also very toxic to cows, sheep, goats, pigs, rabbits, and other species. Following oral ingestion, both zinc phosphide and phosphine are absorbed from the GI tract, although the majority of acute effects are caused by phosphine. Zinc phosphide causes damage to the liver and kidney. Phosphine causes CNS depression, irritation of the lungs, and damage to the liver, kidney, heart, and CNS. Death occurs as a result of cardiac arrest or, more commonly, pulmonary edema. In addition, there are reports of cardiac arrest accompanied by kidney damage. Following a large dose, death usually occurs within 1 h, whereas with smaller doses, death can occur between 4 and 72 h. Symptoms usually appear 20–25 min after exposure. Animals are prostrated with deep, slow respiration, finally terminating in convulsions. Following repeated exposure, cumulative effects occur in the liver, kidney, and lungs.

Zinc phosphide is highly toxic to wild animals, birds, and to freshwater fish. The most sensitive bird species that has been evaluated is geese (LD_{50} of 7.5 mg/kg). Pheasants, mourning doves, quails, mallard ducks, and horned larks are also very sensitive to this rodenticide. The fish species that have been found sensitive to zinc phosphide include bluegill sunfish, rainbow trout, and carp.

Diagnosis

Diagnosis of zinc phosphide in animals is based on detection of zinc phosphide, phosphine, and zinc in body tissues and fluids. At necropsy, stomach content smells like acetylene. A zinc phosphide level of 50 ppm or higher in stomach content is considered significant, and is indicative of zinc phosphide poisoning.

Treatment

There is no specific antidote, and treatment is mainly symptomatic. Vomiting should be induced as soon as possible after ingestion, followed by gastric lavage or administration of activated charcoal. Sodium bicarbonate can be given orally to stop liberation of phosphine gas. Calcium gluconate and sodium lactate can be given intravenously to combat acidosis.

Conclusion

Zinc phosphide is a slow-acting but highly toxic rodenticide. At acidic pH in stomach, zinc phosphide generates phosphine gas, which is responsible for the majority of toxic effects. There is no specific antidote, and treatment is symptomatic (emesis, gastric lavage or administration of activated charcoal).

THALLIUM

Introduction

Thallium (Tl) is a bluish-white heavy metal that occurs naturally in the earth's crust. The word thallium derives from the Greek word *thallos*, which means a young twig or shoot. Tl enters the environment from natural and anthropogenic sources. Natural sources of Tl are less bioavailable, and therefore, of less toxicological concern than anthropogenic sources. The largest anthropogenic sources of Tl are related to coal combustion and heavy metal (primarily zinc and cadmium) smelting and refining. Tl salts were introduced as pesticides in Germany in 1920. The sulfate salt is most common, and has been widely used as a rodenticide and ant killer. In the past, TI was also used for medicinal purpose against dysentery with violent or persistent diarrhea, syphilis, gonorrhea, gout, mycosis of the scalp, and as an inhibitor of sweat secretion in tuberculosis patients. Approximately 50 years ago, Tl was frequently referred to as the poison of choice because Tl is as toxic as arsenic or lead. Tl is banned in many countries, but it is still widely available in developing countries as a rodenticide. The possibility also exists for Tl to be used as a chemical warfare agent (Thompson, 2015). In general, Tl poisoning cases are on the decline, but diagnostic labs still receive suspected baits and tissues from poisoned animals, especially dogs, on a regular basis.

Background

Thallium is a toxic heavy metal that was discovered by Sir William Crookes in 1961 by burning the dust from a sulfuric acid industrial plant. It forms two kinds of compounds: monovalent thallo- and trivalent thalli-compounds. The monovalent Tl resembles potassium, and trivalent Tl resembles aluminum. Tl tends to form stable complexes with soft ligand donors, such as sulfur-containing compounds. Inorganic TI (I) compounds are more stable than Tl (III) analogs in aqueous solution at neutral pH. In contrast, organothallium compounds are stable only in the trivalent form. Tl is particularly toxic in its Tl (I) compounds, such as sulfate (Tl_2SO_4), acetate (CH_3COOTl), and carbonate (Tl_2CO_3). The sulfide (Tl_2S) and iodide (Tl I) are both poorly soluble and, therefore, much less toxic. Today, Tl is recognized as one of the most toxic heavy metals, with an LD_{50} of 30 mg/kg in rats and 8–12 mg/kg in humans.

Toxicokinetics

The water-soluble Tl compounds are rapidly absorbed following oral, inhalation, and dermal exposure. After absorption, Tl compounds are widely distributed to the body tissues, including brain, heart, kidney, skeletal muscle, and testes. Both monovalent and divalent Tl appear to distribute in tissues in a similar manner. In blood, Tl is found slightly more within erythrocytes than in plasma. Following an acute exposure, the maximal concentration of Tl is found in the kidneys, preferentially in the medulla. Studies conducted in rats show lower concentrations of Tl in renal tissue of young compared to adult. Tl^+ and K^+ are monovalent cations with similar ionic radii, but Tl^+ accumulates intracellularly more than K^+ because of its greater affinity for certain enzymes and protein. Because of its large volume of distribution and low free plasma concentration, renal excretion of Tl is slow, and its residue can be detected in the tissues for months. Organic Tl compounds, such as thallous malonate, show a higher elimination rate constant, but are similar in toxicity and distribution pattern compared to the inorganic Tl compounds, such as thallous sulfate (Aoyama, 1989). The elimination half-life is between 8 and 30 days. Tl is excreted in urine, bile, feces, saliva, tears, and milk. In mammals, Tl excretion via the GI tract is twice that of the kidneys because of its involvement in enterohepatic circulation. Tl is known to pass in the milk of poisoned female rats, mice, guinea pigs, and humans. A significant fraction of free plasma Tl also crosses the placental barrier. A small amount of Tl can also be found in hair. Following chronic exposure, Tl can be deposited in the bones, which may account for its cumulative toxicity.

Mechanism of Action

Tl produces toxicity in mammals through multiple mechanisms. Tl^+ and K^+ have common cellular targets and receptor sites associated with biological activity and toxicity. Tl^+ replaces K^+ in the intracellular environment, and shows a 10-fold greater affinity over K^+ for Na^+/K^+-ATPase. Tl at higher concentrations competitively inhibits Na^+/K^+-ATPase activity. Mitochondria have an abundance of Na^+/K^+-ATPase, and are particularly susceptible to the effects of Tl. Tl inhibits the influx and efflux of K^+ in mitochondria without causing any alterations in movement of Na^+. In addition, Tl inactivates sulfhydryl groups, including those affecting the permeability of the outer mitochondrial membrane. As a result of mitochondrial dysfunction, a variety of morphological changes, including mitochondrial swelling and vacuolization, occur in mitochondria in kidney, liver, brain, pancreas, and other tissues of mammals. Tl compromises mitochondrial energy production by inhibiting pyruvate dehydrogenase complex and succinate dehydrogenase by uncoupling oxidative phosphorylation. Tl is also known to disrupt normal cell metabolism by stimulating several K^+-dependent enzymes such as phosphatase, homoserine dehydrogenase, vitamin B_{12}-dependent diol dehydrogenase, L-threonine dehydratase, and AMP deaminase.

Tl has been demonstrated to increase the levels of hydrogen peroxide and decrease the levels of glutathione, which leads to enhanced lipid peroxidation, oxidative stress, and energy depletion primarily in the brain (Hasan and Ali, 1981; Hanzel and Verstraeten, 2005). Tl-induced changes, such as cellular energy loss, depletion of flavoproteins, and binding of Tl to active sulfhydryl sites of enzymes, are the proposed mechanisms for Tl neuropathy. The complexing of Tl to cysteine appears to inhibit cross-linking of proteins, and thereby, causes inhibition of keratinization of hair. Tl blocks formation of the disulfide bonds in keratin and, thus, leads to hair loss (Mulkey and Oehme, 1993). Most evidence supports direct involvement of Tl with the hair follicles as the mechanism of hair loss.

Toxicity

Tl toxicity has been studied extensively in rats, mice, guinea pigs, rabbits, dogs, and humans. In general, Tl compounds are extremely toxic to humans and animals. Tl has been classified as the most toxic cumulative metal cation. A single dose of 15 mg Tl/kg body weight has been found to be lethal in guinea pigs, dogs, and humans. The LD_{50} is 15 mg/kg in rats and 16–27 mg/kg in mice. Of course, these values vary depending on the form of Tl (Mulkey and Oehme, 1993).

Onset of signs and symptoms of Tl poisoning is slow (i.e., within 48 h). The signs and symptoms of Tl toxicity (thallotoxicosis) can vary depending on the species, age, form of Tl, dose, and acute versus chronic exposure. Gastroenteritis, polyneuropathy, and hair loss are the dominant features of Tl poisoning (Mulkey and Oehme, 1993). Acutely poisoned animals show abdominal pain, vomiting, and constipation or diarrhea. At a high-dose exposure, neurologic signs dominate with peripheral neuropathy. Sensory disturbances include pain, ataxia, and paresthesia, which progress to muscle atrophy. Muscle fibers can show myopathic changes with abnormal central nucleoli, striated transverse fibers disappearance, necrosis, and fibrosis. Cats dosed with Tl at 4 mg/kg body weight developed hypotonia and ataxia mainly due to pathological changes in sensory neurons (Sager, 1994). Dogs and cats exposed to Tl also showed hemorrhagic gastroenteritis and hepatic and renal damage.

Surviving animals usually show signs of alopecia, bloody lesions of the skin, tremors, neuropathy (involving both central and peripheral nervous systems), and paralysis of muscles. In addition, Tl causes structural and functional changes in the heart and kidneys. Evidence from experimental animal studies suggests that the reproductive system is highly susceptible to Tl. Humans and animals accumulate Tl in testes, where morphological and biochemical changes occur. Tl is embryotoxic and teratogenic in chick embryo, causing achondroplasia, leg bone curvature, beak deformity, microcephaly, and decreased fetal size. However, teratological investigations in mammals have produced conflicting results (Gregotti and Faustman, 1998). For further details on Tl toxicity, refer to Mulkey and Oehme (1993) and Galvan-Arzate and Santamaria (1998).

Diagnosis

Diagnosis of Tl poisoning is based on evidence of Tl exposure, clinical signs, and chemical confirmation in body tissue/fluid. Quantitative analysis for Tl in urine, serum, feces, saliva, or hair is performed to assess the extent of Tl exposure and to monitor treatment. Tl residue analysis at diagnostic labs is commonly carried out using atomic absorption spectrometer, inductively coupled plasma (ICP), or ICP–mass spectrometer-based methods. Tl-induced hematological changes may include anemia, leukocytosis, eosinophilia, and lymphocytopenia. Decreased creatinine clearance, elevated BUN, and proteinuria indicate renal function impairment. Alopecia is usually observed 3 or 4 weeks postexposure, thus diminishing the timely treatment.

Treatment

Therapy for Tl poisoning should be instituted as early as possible. In the case of acute oral ingestion, supportive care should include induction of vomiting, followed by gastric lavage and use of laxatives to remove Tl as much as possible from the GI tract. Prussian blue (potassium ferric hexacyanoferrate (II)) is the treatment of choice for Tl exposure. Prussian blue acts by binding to Tl in the GI tract, making it unavailable for absorption or reabsorption. Hemodialysis and hemoperfusion can be used to remove Tl from the circulation. At later stages of the treatment, potassium can be used to mobilize Tl from the tissues. Maintenance of vital organ functions should be a priority, especially in acute cases. If Tl poisoning is diagnosed and treated early, the chance for full recovery is good.

Conclusion

Tl is one of the most toxic heavy metals used as a rodenticide. It produces a wide range of toxic effects involving multiple organs and mechanisms. Neurological, renal, and GI effects are of primary concern. Exposure with a high dose is often fatal. Surviving animals often show complex signs of Tl poisoning, especially polyneuropathy, renal impairment, and hair loss. The diagnosis of Tl poisoning is based on clinical signs and Tl detection in urine, serum, or other biological tissue/fluids. Timely therapy with Prussian blue, as well as supportive measures can lead to full recovery.

REFERENCES

Aoyama, H., 1989. Distribution and excretion of thallium after oral and intraperitoneal administration of thallous malonate and thallous sulfate in hamsters. Bull. Environ. Contam. Toxicol. 42, 456–463.

Bosakowski, T., Levin, A.A., 1986. Serum citrate as a peripheral indication of fluoroacetate and fluorocitrate toxicity in rats and dogs. Toxicol. Appl. Pharmacol. 85, 428–436.

Boyd, R.E., Brennan, P.T., Deng, J.F., et al., 1983. Strychnine poisoning. Am. J. Med. 74, 507–512.

Brockman, J.L., McDowell, A.W., Leeds, W.G., 1955. Fatal poisoning with sodium fluoroacetate. J. Am. Med. Assoc. 159, 1529–1532.

Chenoweth, M.B., 1949. Monofluoroacetic acid and related compounds. J. Pharmacol. Exp. Ther. 102, 21–49.

Cooper, P., 1974. Poisoning by Drugs and Chemicals. Alchemist, London, pp. 193–194.

Coppock, R., 2013. Advisory: bromethalin rodenticide- no known antidote. Can. Vet. J. 54, 557–558.

Dorman, D.C., Parker, A.J., Buck, W.B., 1990a. Bromethalin toxicosis in the dog: Part I. Clinical effects. JAAHA. 26, 589–594.

Dorman, D.C., Parker, A.J., Dye, J.A., et al., 1990b. Bromethalin toxicosis in the cat. Prog. Vet. Neurol. 1, 189–196.

Dorman, D.C., Simon, J., Harlin, K.A., et al., 1990c. Diagnosis of bromethalin toxicosis in the dog. J. Vet. Diagn. Invest. 2, 123–128.

Dorman, D.C., Zachary, J.F., Buck, W.B., 1992. Neuropathologic findings of bromethalin toxicosis in cat. Vet. Pathol. 29, 139–144.

Eason, C.T., Gooneratne, R., Fitzgerald, H., et al., 1993. Persistence of sodium monofluoroacetate in livestock animals and risk to humans. Hum. Exp. Toxicol. 13 (2), 119–122.

Easterwood, L., Chaffin, M.K., Marsh, P.S., et al., 2010. Phosphine intoxication following oral exposure of horses to aluminium phosphide-treated feed. J. Am. Vet. Med. Assoc. 236 (4), 446–450.

Edmunds, M., Sheehan, T.M., Van't Hoff, W., 1986. Strychnine poisoning: clinical and toxicological observations. J. Toxicol. Clin. Toxicol. 24, 245–255.

Egyed, M.N., 1979. Mass poisoning in dogs due to meat contaminated by sodium fluoroacetate or fluoroacetamide: special reference to the differential diagnosis. Fluoride 12 (2), 76–84.

Elliot, W.B., Kalnitsky, G., 1996. Mechanism for Fluoroacetate Inhibition. Govt. Reports Announcements & Index (GRA&I), Issue 02.

Galvan-Arzate, S., Santamaria, A., 1998. Thallium toxicity. Toxicol. Lett. 99, 1–13.

Godoy, H.M., del Carmen Villarruel, M., 1974. Myocardial adenine nucleotides, hexose phosphates and inorganic phosphate, and the regulation of phosphofructokinase activity during fluoroacetate poisoning in the rat. Biochem. Pharmacol. 23, 3179–3189.

Gooneratne, S.R., Eason, C.T., Dickson, C.J., et al., 1995. Persistence of sodium monofluoroacetate in rabbits and risk to non-target species. Hum. Exp. Toxicol. 14, 212–216.

Gosselin, R.E., Smith, R.P., Hodge, H.C., 1984. Clinical Toxicology of Commercial Products. fifth ed. Williams & Wilkins, Baltimore, MD, pp. 375–379.

Gregotti, C., Faustman, E.M., 1998. Reproductive and developmental toxicity of thallium. In: Nriagu, J.O. (Ed.), Thallium in the Environment. Wiley, New York, NY, pp. 201–214.

Gupta, R.C., Crissman, J.W., 2012. Agricultural chemicals. In: Haschek-Hock, W.M., Rousseaux, C.G., Wallig, M.A. (Eds.), Handbook of Toxicologic Pathology, third ed. Elsevier, Amsterdam, pp. 1349–1372.

Hanzel, C.E., Verstraeten, S.V., 2005. Thallium induces hydrogen peroxide generation by impairing mitochondrial function. Toxicol. Appl. Pharmacol. 216, 485–492.

Hasan, M., Ali, F.S., 1981. Effects of thallium, nickel and cobalt administration on the lipid peroxidation in different brain regions of the rat brain. Toxicol. Appl. Pharmacol. 57, 8–13.

Hornfeldt, C.S., Larson, A.A., 1990. Seizures induced by fluoroacetic acid and fluorocitric acid may involve chelation of divalent cations in the spinal cord. Eur. J. Pharmacol. 179, 307–313.

Huntington, S., Fenik, Y., Vohra, R., et al., 2016. Human bromethalin exposures reported to a U.S. statewide poison control system. Clin. Toxicol. 54 (3), 277–281.

Krenn, L., Kopp, B., Deim, A., et al., 1994. About the bufadienolide complex of red squill. Planta Med. 60, 63–69.

Maruo, T., Katayama, K., Barnea, E.R., et al., 1992. A role for thyroid hormone in the induction of ovulation and corpus luteum function. Horm. Res. 37 (Suppl. 1), 12–18.

Mead, R.J., Moulden, D.L., Twigg, L.E., 1985. Significance of sulfhydryl compounds in the manifestation of fluoroacetate toxicity to the rat, brush-tailed possum, woylie and western grey kangaroo. Aust. J. Biol. Sci. 38, 139–149.

Mehlman, M.A., 1967. Inhibition of pyruvate carboxylation by fluorocitrate in rat kidney mitochondria. J. Biol. Chem. 243, 1919–1925.

Mesmer, M.Z., Flurer, R.A., 2001. Determination of bromethalin in commercial rodenticides found in consumer product samples by HPLC-UV-Vis spetrophotometry and HPLC-negative-ion APCI-MS. J. Chromatogr. Sci. 39, 49–53.

Moorman, M., 2003. Bromethalin: it's not what you think. Vet. Techn. 24, 484–487.

Mulkey, J.P., Oehme, F.W., 1993. A review of thallium toxicity. Vet. Hum. Toxicol. 35, 445–453.

Nath, N.S., Bhattacharya, I., Tuck, A.G., 2011. Mechanisms of phosphine toxicity. A review. J. Toxicol. 2011, 1–9.

NIOSH, National Institute for Occupational Safety and Health, 1983–1984. Registry of Toxic Effects of Chemical Substances. Cumulative Supplement to the 1981–1982 edition. Advanced Engineering and Planning Corp., Rockville, MD, pp. 1738–1739.

O'Callaghan, W.G., Joyce, N., Counihan, H.E., et al., 1982. Unusual strychnine poisoning and its treatment: report of eight cases. Br. Med. J. 185, 478.

Oelrichs, P.B., McEwan, T., 1962. The toxic principle of *Acacia georginae*. Queensland. J. Agric. Sci. 19, 1–16.

Omara, F., Sisodia, C.S., 1990. Evaluation of potential antidotes for sodium fluoroacetate in mice. Vet. Hum. Toxicol. 32 (5), 427–431.

Pascual-Villalobos, M.J., 2002. Anti-insect activity of bufadienolides from *Urginea maritima*. In: Janick, J., Whipkey, A. (Eds.), Trends in New Crops and New Uses. ASHS Press, Alexandria, VA, pp. 564–566.

Pasquale-Styles, M.A., Sochaski, M.A., et al., 2006. Fatal bromethalin poisoning. J. Forens. Sci. 51, 1154–1157.

Peoples, S.A., 1970. The pharmacology of rodenticides. Proceedings of the 4th Vertebrate Pest Conference. University of Nebraska, Lincoln, NE, pp. 1–18.

Reynolds, J.E.F., 1982. Martindale: The Extra Pharmacopoeia. Pharmaceutical Press, London, pp. 319–320, 995–1000.

Rokita, S.E., Walsh, C., 1983. Turnover and inactivation of bacterial citrate lyase with 2-fluorocitrate and 2-hydroxycitrate stereoisomers. Biochemistry 22, 2821–2828.

Roy, A., Taitelman, U., Bursztein, S., 1980. Evaluation of the role of ionized calcium in sodium fluoroacetate ("1080") poisoning. Toxicol. Appl. Pharmacol. 56, 216–220.

Sager, M., 1994. Thallium. Toxicol. Environ. Chem. 45, 11–32.

Suh, D., Kim, K., Hong, D., Hong, S., 1970. Acute intoxication due to agricultural chemicals. Taeham Naekwa Hakkoe Chapci. 13 (3), 197–206.

Taylor, W.M., D'Costa, M., Angel, A., et al., 1977. Insulin-like effects of fluoroacetate on lipolysis and lipogenesis in adipose tissue. Can. J. Biochem. 55, 982–987.

Thompson, L.J., 2015. Thallium. In: Gupta, R.C. (Ed.), Handbook of Toxicology of Chemical Warfare Agents, second ed. Elsevier, Amsterdam, pp. 167–170.

Thomson, W.T., 1991–1992. Agricultural Chemicals Book 3: Fumigants, Growth Regulators, Seed Safeners, Repellents, Fish Toxicants, Bird Toxicants, Pheromones, Rodenticides, and Others. Thomson, Fresno, CA, pp. 157–158.

Van Lier, R.B., Cherry, L.D., 1988. The toxicity and mechanism of action of bromethalin: a new single-feeding rodenticide. Fundam. Appl. Toxicol. 11, 664–672.

Verbiscar, A.J., Patel, J., Banigan, T.F., et al., 1986a. Scilliroside and other scilla compounds in red squill. J. Agric. Food Chem. 34, 973–979.

Verbiscar, A.J., Banigan, T.F., Gentry, H.S., 1986b. Recent research on red squill as a rodenticide. In: Salmon, T.P. (Ed.), Proceedings of the 25th Vertebrate Pest Conference. University of California, Davis, CA, pp. 51–56.

Vivet, P., Brun-Pascaud, M., Mansour, H., et al., 1983. Non-hypoxaemic pulmonary edema induced by alpha-naphthyl thiourea in the rat. Br. J. Exp. Pathol. 64, 361–366.

Winton, F.R., 1927a. The rat-poisoning substance in red squill. J. Pharmacol. Exp. Ther. 31, 123–136.

Winton, F.R., 1927b. A contrast between the actions of red and white squills. J. Pharmacol. Exp. Ther. 31, 137–144.

Worthing, C.R., 1983. The Pesticide Manual. A World Compendium, seventh ed. British Crop Protection Council, Croydon.

FURTHER READING

Gray, S.L., Lee, J.A., Hovda, L.R., et al., 2011. Potential zinc phosphide rodenticide toxicosis in dogs: 362 cases (2004–2009). J. Am. Vet. Med. Assoc. 239 (5), 646–651.

Section IX

Gases, Solvents and Other Industrial Toxicants

Chapter 48

Toxic Gases and Vapors

Rhian Cope

INTRODUCTION

For the purposes of this chapter, a gas is defined as a state of matter consisting of molecules that have neither a defined volume nor shape at standard temperatures and pressures. A vapor is the gaseous phase of substances that are either solid or liquid at standard temperatures and pressures. As a general rule, the toxicology of gases is also broadly applicable to the toxicology of vapors.

This chapter is divided into two sections: general principles and specific toxic gases. The general principles section covers gas toxicokinetics and basic dosimetric adjustments for human risk assessment. The specific toxic gases section covers specific toxic gases that are of veterinary clinical and veterinary occupational relevance (carbon monoxide (CO), hydrogen sulfide, oxides of nitrogen (silo filler's disease), gaseous ammonia (including anhydrous ammonia), and smoke inhalation).

GENERAL PRINCIPLES

Toxicokinetics

Absorption and Distribution

Depending on their physicochemical properties, gases can produce site-of-first-contact effects or systemic toxicity following absorption or a combination of both. The usual driving force for the systemic absorption (i.e., entry into the central circulation) and tissue distribution of inhaled gases is diffusion down concentration gradients (although cellular uptake and protein binding can alter this dynamic; Rozman and Klaassen, 2001; Witschi and Last, 2001; Renwick, 2008; Valentine and Kennedy, 2008). These relationships can be described at a high level by a series of simplified toxicokinetic equilibria and related equilibrium constants (K):

$$\text{Air} \overset{K}{\leftrightarrow} \text{Systemic Circulation} \overset{K}{\leftrightarrow} \text{Tissues}$$

The absorption of a gas will continue until equilibria are established in the various compartments. In a closed system, once the equilibria are established, no net absorption will occur unless there is loss from the system (i.e., metabolism), reaction with tissue molecules, or excretion through nonrespiratory pathways (e.g., renal excretion). It is critical to note that just because the equilibria have been established does not mean that the concentrations in the different compartments are equal. Rather, once the equilibria are established, the concentration ratios between the various compartments will remain constant provided that saturation of the system and/or other system perturbations do not occur, i.e., the air:blood:tissue(s) concentration ratios remain constant.

Absorption of the gas will continue if "losses" from the system occur. If the substance is lost through metabolism, the rate of continued absorption once the equilibria have been established is effectively the rate of metabolism of the substance. This mass–balance relationship is the basis of closed respirometry measures of oxygen consumption and metabolic rate (pioneered by Laplace and Lavoisier in the 1770s). If the substance is lost from the system solely through nonrespiratory excretion once the equilibria have been established, the rate of continued absorption is equivalent to the rate of nonrespiratory excretion.

If the concentration of the gas in the tissue(s) is higher than that in the respiratory airspaces (e.g., if the inhalation exposure is stopped or the concentration in the inhaled air is reduced), the net diffusive force will drive the movement of the gas from the tissue(s) into the air. An example is the excretion of carbon dioxide produced by aerobic metabolism in the tissues that is largely driven by simple diffusion. This is also the basis for the net excretion of a nonmetabolized gas once exposure has ceased, e.g., the recovery from gaseous anesthesia.

In normal circumstances, gas diffusion is not rate limiting for the systemic absorption because: (1) generally ionized, hydrophilic molecules that are apt to be diffusion-limited across biological membranes have low volatility, i.e., their concentration in normal air is usually very low; (2) alveolar type I pneumocytes are very thin and are in intimate contact with the pulmonary capillaries,

Veterinary Toxicology. DOI: http://dx.doi.org/10.1016/B978-0-12-811410-0.00048-9

effectively resulting in extremely short diffusion distances; and (3) gases absorbed through the alveoli are rapidly removed by the blood, thus maintaining the diffusion concentration gradient (Rozman and Klaassen, 2001; Witschi and Last, 2001; Renwick, 2008; Valentine and Kennedy, 2008). There are two exceptions: (1) CO absorption is diffusion limited (the basis for its use in the lung diffusion capacity test or determination of the DLCO; referred to as the TLCO or transfer capacity in Europe), and (2) the presence of interstitial lung disease that increases the pulmonary diffusion distance, resulting in diffusion-limited absorption for gases (notably oxygen).

In a broad sense, the rate of establishment of the equilibrium between the respiratory airspaces and the bloodstream depends on: (1) whether or not uptake of the gas is perfusion limited; and (2) whether or not the uptake of the gas is ventilation limited (Rozman and Klaassen, 2001; Witschi and Last, 2001; Renwick, 2008; Valentine and Kennedy, 2008). These innately characteristic properties of a substance are directly related to the blood:gas partition coefficient, an innate physicochemical property of the substance. The blood:gas partition coefficient is the ratio of the substance's concentration in the gaseous phase and the blood phase at equilibrium. For substances with low blood:gas partition coefficients (i.e., substances that have a low affinity for dissolving in blood), the ability of blood in blood:gas exchange regions of the lungs to absorb the substance is rapidly saturated, and thus only a small amount of the substance in the respiratory tract is removed by blood during passage through the pulmonary circulation. In such circumstances, changes in the respiratory minute volume have relatively little effect on the rate of transfer of the gas from the alveolar spaces to the bloodstream. However, small changes in the rate of flow of blood through the respiratory tract (i.e., pulmonary perfusion) have proportionally large effects on the rate of transfer of the gas from the respiratory system to the blood; i.e., increasing pulmonary perfusion results in more rapid removal of the gas from the site of equilibration (the alveolar membranes) and thus a proportionally more rapid rate of transfer of the gas from the respiratory system to the bloodstream occurs and vice versa. Thus, for gases with a low blood:gas partition coefficient, blood gas equilibration occurs relatively quickly (~8–21 min for relatively blood-insoluble gases), and the absorption of such gases is described as being perfusion limited. As a general rule, perfusion-limited gases tend to be sparingly soluble in water, are relatively lipophilic and hydrophobic, and have high octanol:water partition coefficients (Fiserova-Bergerova and Diaz, 1986). However, other factors, such as the affinity of the particular gas to protein and other elements in blood, may also significantly impact the blood:gas partition coefficient (Veltman et al., 2009). Notably, alteration in the level of lipid components in the blood (particularly blood triglycerides) can significantly increase the blood:gas partition coefficient of lipophilic xenobiotics and thus affect their inhalation absorption kinetics (Lin et al., 2002). Ingestion of a high-fat meal during or before inhalation may result in an increased absorbed dose of an inhaled lipophilic gas and affect the rate of excretion by exhalation of such substances.

The alternate extremes are gases that are ventilation limited (Rozman and Klaassen, 2001; Witschi and Last, 2001; Renwick, 2008; Valentine and Kennedy, 2008). Ventilation-limited gases are highly soluble in blood (tend to be hydrophilic or, in rare cases, zwitterion-like) and often have low octanol:water partition coefficients (Fiserova-Bergerova and Diaz, 1986). Again, other factors, such as the affinity of the particular gas to protein and other elements in blood, may also significantly impact the blood:gas partition coefficient, e.g., a high affinity for erythrocytes or blood proteins may result in a high blood:gas partition coefficient irrespective of other physicochemical properties (Veltman et al., 2009). The majority of a ventilation-limited gas present in alveoli is removed during each respiratory cycle because of its high affinity for blood, i.e., replenishment of the gas in the gas-exchange regions is dependent on the subsequent inhalation of fresh gas. In this situation, relatively small changes in respiratory minute volume can produce relatively large effects on the rate of transfer of the gas from the respiratory system to the blood and tissues. The rate of pulmonary blood perfusion has little effect on the rate of transfer of the gas from the respiratory system to the blood because virtually all of the gas is removed from the gas-exchange site during each pulmonary circulation, i.e., increasing the rate of blood flow through the lung during each circulation would result in little additional gas absorption and decreasing the rate of blood flow through the lung would result in little reduction of absorption. The time to blood:gas equilibration for gases that are ventilation limited is at least 1 h and often much longer (days or, in some cases, never).

Gases may also be absorbed in the upper respiratory tract, particularly the nasal cavity (Rozman and Klaassen, 2001; Witschi and Last, 2001; Renwick, 2008; Valentine and Kennedy, 2008; Morris and Buckpitt, 2009). In this case, gases may be systemically reversibly absorbed via diffusion processes in which the mucus:blood:tissue:air partition equilibria (and associated coefficients) are important; alternatively, the gas may react with tissue macromolecules in the upper respiratory tract (including enzymes with subsequent metabolism). In general, gases that are absorbed in the upper respiratory tract tend to be highly soluble in aqueous solutions (particularly in the mucous lining of the upper respiratory tract), or highly reactive (i.e., site-of-first-contact toxicants), or both (Renwick, 2008). In such cases, the nasal cavity can be regarded as being analogous to a "gas scrubber" that prevents or limits the exposure of the deeper respiratory tract tissues (i.e., a protective mechanism). As with any "gas scrubber," the capacity to remove a gas from the inhaled air can be "overcome" if the scrubbing capacity becomes saturated due to high concentrations and/or long durations of exposure. As a general rule, gases that are poorly water soluble and are not highly reactive are generally poorly absorbed/scrubbed out in the upper respiratory tract. A further general rule is that relatively little gas exchange occurs in the conducting airways (anatomic dead space) areas of the respiratory tract. However, adverse site-of-contact effects can certainly still occur in these anatomic dead spaces of the respiratory system.

Metabolism

Metabolism of gases can occur locally in the respiratory tract or at other distant sites (discussed elsewhere in this book). As a generalization, biotransformation of gases within the respiratory tract primarily occurs at two main locations: within the epithelia of the nasal cavity and within the club cells of the lung (Bogdanffy et al., 1986, 1987; Castranova et al., 1988; Baron and Voigt, 1990; Bogdanffy, 1990; Keller et al., 1990; Hukkanen et al., 2002; Castell et al., 2005). Phase I biotransformation also occurs to a lesser degree in type II pneumocytes and in pulmonary macrophages (although there are important examples of metabolic toxication by type II pneumocytes and/or alveolar macrophages). The immunohistochemical distribution and biochemical activity of biotransformation enzymes in the rat nasal cavity are shown in Table 48.1. As can be seen from the table, biotransformation potential is predominantly located in the olfactory and respiratory epithelia of the nasal cavity. Whether or not metabolism in the olfactory or respiratory epithelium predominates depends on which enzymes are involved and the particular substrate. Although it is notable that both phase I and phase II biotransformation reactions occur in the nasal cavity, the biotransformation capacity of the nasal cavity is a prime source of local toxication of many inhaled (and noninhaled) xenobiotics (Bogdanffy, 1997).

Numerous studies have demonstrated that club cells are a rich source of cytochrome P450-dependent mixed-function oxidases and a prime site for P450-mediated phase I metabolism and toxication in the lung (Devereux, 1984; Devereux et al., 1985; Baron and Voigt, 1990; Hukkanen et al., 2002; Castell et al., 2005).

Excretion via the Respiratory Tract

Simple single-phase excretion (single compartment kinetics) of inhaled gases through the respiratory tract is in many ways dependent on the same factors as gas

TABLE 48.1 Distribution of Biotransformation Enzymes in the Rat Nasal Cavity

Tissue Type	AldH	CarbE	FdH	NBE	P450 red	P450	EH	GSHt	BαPOH
Squamous epithelium	Low	No data	No data	Low	No data	No data	No data	No data	No data
Respiratory epithelium	High	High	Present	Moderate	Present	Present	Present	Present	Present
Seromucous glands	No data	No data	No data	Low	Present	Present	Present	Present	Present
Olfactory sustentacular cells	Absent	Present in olfactory mucosa	Present	Moderate	Present	Present	Present	Present	Present
Olfactory nerves	Absent		Present	Absent	Absent	Absent	Absent	Absent	Absent
Bowman's glands	Low		Present	High	Present	Present	Present	Present	Present

AldH, acetaldehyde dehydrogenase; *CarbE*, carboxylesterase; *FdH*, formaldehyde dehydrogenase; *NBE*, alpha-naphthyl butyrate esterase; *P450 red*, NADPH–cytochrome P450 reductase; *P450*, cytochrome P450s; *EH*, epoxide hydrolase; *GSHt*, glutathione-*S*-transferases; *BαPOH*, benzo(a)pyrene hydroxylase.
Source: Data from Bogdanffy, M.S., Randall, H.W., Morgan, K.T., 1986. Histochemical localization of aldehyde dehydrogenase in the respiratory tract of the Fischer-344 rat. Toxicol. Appl. Pharmacol. 82:560–567; Bogdanffy, M.S., Kee, C.R., Hinchman, C.A., Trela, B.A., 1991. Metabolism of dibasic esters by rat nasal mucosal carboxylesterase. Drug Metab. Dispos. 19:124–129; Bogdanffy, M.S., 1990. Biotransformation enzymes in the rodent nasal mucosa: the value of a histochemical approach. Environ. Health Perspect. 85:177–186 (Bogdanffy et al., 1991); Keller, D.A., Heck, H.D., Randall, H.W., Morgan, K.T., 1990. Histochemical localization of formaldehyde dehydrogenase in the rat. Toxicol. Appl. Pharmacol. 106:311–326; Trela, B.A., Bogdanffy, M.S., 1991a Carboxylesterase-dependent cytotoxicity of dibasic esters (DBE) in rat nasal explants. Toxicol. Appl. Pharmacol. 107:285–301; Trela, B.A., Bogdanffy, M.S., 1991b. Cytotoxicity of dibasic esters (DBE) metabolites in rat nasal explants. Toxicol. Appl. Pharmacol. 110:259–267 (Trela and Bogdanffy et al., 1991a,b); and Bogdanffy, M.S., Taylor, M.L., 1993. Kinetics of nasal carboxylesterase-mediated metabolism of vinyl acetate. Drug Metab. Dispos. 21:1107–1111 (Bogdanffy and Taylor, 1993).

absorption by inhalation. Gases with a high blood:gas partition coefficient tend to be slowly excreted by exhalation due to the relatively large amount of the substance dissolved in the blood volume and the high affinity of the gas for blood relative to its affinity for air. Gases with a low blood:gas partition coefficient tend to be excreted by exhalation relatively rapidly because of the relatively small amount present in the blood volume and the greater affinity of the gas for air than for blood. However, respiratory excretion of gases that have a high affinity for lipophilic tissue compartments (including the adipose tissues), may be biphasic (have two compartment excretion kinetics or even more complex patterns of excretion). This is most commonly observed with lipophilic gases that have a low blood:gas partition coefficient and a tendency for tissue sequestration (i.e., large volumes of distribution exceeding 1 L/kg). The initial phase of excretion is relatively rapid due to the fast removal of the gas from the blood tissue compartment during exhalation. This is followed by an often much slower phase as the gas slowly redistributes from lipophilic tissue compartments and/or sites of sequestration into the bloodstream, with subsequent excretion by exhalation.

Regional Gas Dose Ratios for Human Risk Assessment Based on Animal Data

Human health risk assessment for gases commonly involves extrapolation from animal data to humans, i.e., the calculation of a human equivalent concentration (HEC). The general formula for this calculation is:

$$\text{HEC (mg/m}^3) = \text{NOAEL (mg/m}^3) \times \text{RGDR}$$

RGDR, regional gas dose ratio.

For the purposes of derivation of RGDR values, gases, and vapors can be categorized into three general classes (US EPA, 2009):

- *Category 1 gases*: These gases are highly water soluble and/or irreversibly reactive in the surface liquid/tissues of the extrathoracic and tracheobronchial regions of the respiratory tract. Most of the toxicological effects of these substances will occur at sites of first contact within the respiratory system. Relevant examples include hydrogen fluoride, chlorine, and acrolein.
- *Category 2 gases*: These gases are moderately water soluble, rapidly and reversibly reactive, and/or moderately to slowly irreversibly metabolized within respiratory tissues. These intermediate gases have the potential for both sites of contact and systemic toxic effects, i.e., effects will likely occur both within the respiratory tract and at remote sites following systemic absorption. Examples include the vapors of acetonitrile, xylene, propanol, and isoamyl alcohol.
- *Category 3 gases*: These gases are relatively insoluble in water and are not reactive in the extrathoracic and tracheobronchial regions of the respiratory tract. These gases are not "scrubbed out" in the upper respiratory tract and conducting airways and thus penetrate into the deep pulmonary areas, where they are available for absorption into the systemic circulation. Examples include benzene and most of the common anesthetic gases and vapors.

Based on the above categorization, the following equations can be used to derive RGDRs:

$$\text{RGDR}_{\textit{Extra}\text{ Thoracic}} = \frac{\left(\frac{V_e}{\text{SA}_{\text{ETh}}}\right)\text{animal}}{\left(\frac{V_e}{\text{SA}_{\text{ETh}}}\right)\text{human}}$$

$$\text{RGDR}_{\text{Tracheobronchial}} = \frac{\left(\frac{V_e}{\text{SA}_{\text{TB}}}\right)\text{animal}}{\left(\frac{V_e}{\text{SA}_{\text{TB}}}\right)\text{human}}$$

$$\text{RGDR}_{\text{Pulmonary}} = \frac{\left(\frac{Q_{\text{alv}}}{\text{SA}_{\text{PU}}}\right)\text{animal}}{\left(\frac{Q_{\text{alv}}}{\text{SA}_{\text{PU}}}\right)\text{human}}$$

$$\text{RGDR}_{\text{Systemic}} = \frac{H_{\text{B/G}}\text{ animal}}{H_{\text{B/G}}\text{ human}}$$

- *Abbreviations:*
  - Extrathoracic region: upper respiratory tract comprising the nose, mouth, oropharynx, laryngopharynx and larynx.
  - Tracheobronchial region: conducting areas of the respiratory tract distal to the larynx including the trachea, bronchi and bronchioles (to the terminal bronchioles).
  - Pulmonary region: gas exchange areas of the lung including the respiratory bronchioles, alveolar ducts, alveolar sacs and alveoli.
  - V_e, respiratory minute volume.
  - SA_{ET}, extrathoracic surface area.
  - SA_{TB}, tracheobronchial surface area.
  - SA_{PU}, pulmonary surface area.
  - Q_{alv}, alveolar ventilation rate ($\approx 0.7 \times V_e$ for rats).
  - $H_{B/G}$, blood gas partition coefficient.

Extrapolating Duration of Exposure for Human Risk Assessment

The duration of exposure in animal studies rarely correlates with the exact duration of interest in terms of human risk assessment. Haber's Law is commonly used to compensate for these differences in human health risk assessment. Ernest Warren and Fritz Haber noted during their studies of the acute (exposure durations between 1 and 120 min) lethality effects of poison gases (specifically gas weapons in the case of Fritz Haber, notably phosgene, methylchloroformate, cyanide gas, chloracetone, xylybromide, and chlorine) that exposure to a low concentration of a poisonous gas for a long time often had the same effect (death) as exposure to a high concentration for a short time. They discovered that, in general, a simple mathematical relationship applied: $C \times t = k$, where C is the concentration of the poisonous gas, t is the time of exposure, and k (the "toxic load" required to produce the effect) is a constant (Haber, 1924; Lohs, 1990; Witschi, 1999, 2000). If different concentrations and times of exposure are used, this implies that $C_1 \times t_1 = C_2 \times t_2$. This relationship, in theory, can also be used to extrapolate concentration values between short-term and long-term exposures, i.e.,

$$C_2 = \frac{C_1 \times t_1}{t_2}$$

In modern risk assessment, the ten Berge modification of Haber's law is commonly used: $C^n \times t = k$ (ten Berge et al., 1986). The exponential n is a regression coefficient for the exposure concentration–exposure duration relationships for the relevant effect. In general, the value of n lies between 1 and 3. If suitable data are not available to derive n, a default value of $n = 1$ is used for extrapolating from shorter to longer exposure durations and a default value of $n = 3$ is used for extrapolating from longer to shorter exposure durations. Using the ten Berg modification, the Haber's law equation becomes:

$$C_2 = \frac{C_1^n \times t_1}{t_2}$$

However, note that there are many cases in which Haber's law and the ten Berge-modified Haber's law do not accurately describe the dose–time relationships for the toxicological effects of gases. The use of these simple relationships may seriously over- or under-estimate the degree of toxicological effects, particularly when there are large extrapolations in terms of the time of exposure (Weller et al., 1999; Miller et al., 2000; Hoyle et al., 2010). High-quality data for the specific duration of exposure of interest are often preferable to the use of Haber's law or the ten Berge modification.

SPECIFIC TOXIC GASES

Carbon Monoxide

Overview, Uses, and Sources of Exposure

CO is colorless, odorless and virtually undetectable without the use of gas detection technologies, hence its reputation as a "silent killer" (Weaver, 2004). CO is ubiquitous and most commonly produced by incomplete hydrocarbon combustion. A component of CO poisoning is almost always present in cases of smoke inhalation injury (Alarie, 2002; Jones, 2003; Fitzgerald et al., 2006). CO is also produced by the mixed function oxidase-mediated biotransformation of methylene chloride (dichloromethane), a common solvent component present in paint strippers and degreasers (Weaver, 2004). The combustion of methylene chloride produces phosgene. CO is also produced endogenously as a byproduct of erythropoiesis.

CO commonly causes poisoning and high-mortality in humans in the United States (Sadovnikoff et al., 1992; Meredith, 1993; McGuigan, 1999; Hampson and Stock, 2006; Harduar-Morano and Watkins, 2011). Epidemics of CO poisoning in humans and animals are notoriously associated with the occurrence of storms, cold snaps or other severe weather, particularly when such events are accompanied by a loss of electrical power and/or the failure of heating systems. Veterinarians, farm workers, and animals are at risk of exposure to CO in intensive animal production units that are heated by hydrocarbon combustion. Both acute lethal and sublethal CO poisonings are well-known problems in intensive pig operations, particularly those relying on gas heating systems (Boller, 1976; Keller, 1976; Wood, 1979; Stuart and Oehme, 1982; Dominick and Carson, 1983; Morris et al., 1985a,b; Pejsak et al., 2008). CO in engine fumes may also reduce egg hatchability (Swarbrick, 1989).

CO has also been investigated as a veterinary euthanasia agent, and has some utility when mass euthanasia of poultry is necessary (Moreland, 1974; Simonsen et al., 1981; Chalifoux and Dallaire, 1983; Lambooy et al., 1985; Enggaard Hansen et al., 1991; Kingston et al., 2005; Gerritzen et al., 2006). However, there are substantial operator safety concerns with the use of CO for this purpose. CO treatment has also been used for improving the color of muscle foods (Hamling et al., 2008; Mantilla et al., 2008; Jeong and Claus, 2010, 2011). Again, strict safety standards are necessary to protect human workers in such circumstances.

Toxic Dose

At physiological equilibrium, an atmospheric CO level of 50 ppm produces a carboxyhemoglobin (COHb) level of 8% in humans, which is the basis for the US Occupational Safety and Health Administration PEL 8-h time-weighted average level of 50 ppm (Weaver, 2004). Reduction in cognitive performance occurs in humans exposed to levels as low as 17 ppm for 1.5–2.5 h (COHb level of 2%). Situations that result in lower alveolar oxygen partial pressure (e.g., high altitudes), increased alveolar ventilation (e.g., higher metabolic rates and increased activity), preexisting cardiovascular or cerebrovascular disease, cardiac insufficiency, increased affinity of hemoglobin (Hb) for CO (e.g., fetal Hb), and decrease blood oxygen carrying capacity will reduce the tolerance to CO (Weaver, 2004). CO exposure is a noted cause of angina in humans with preexisting cardiovascular disease.

Exposure of pregnant sows to CO levels of 150–400 ppm for 48–96 h results in stillbirth rates of 6.7%–80.0% (Dominick and Carson, 1983). The risk of stillbirth increases significantly when COHb concentration is greater than 23%. Notably, piglets that are born live in such circumstances usually have hypoxic/ischemic leukoencephalopathy. There is evidence that preweaning pigs have some capacity to adapt to high air CO levels given that exposure to 200 ppm of CO for the first 21 days of life has no adverse effect on any performance or behavioral characteristics in weanling pigs; however, exposure to 300 ppm in such circumstances results in reduced growth and production performance (Morris et al., 1985a, b). Perinatal exposure to 250 ppm of CO resulting in a COHb level of approximately 20% produced detrimental effects in neonatal pigs.

Toxicokinetics and Toxicodynamics

CO is one of the few diffusion-limited gases during respiratory absorption. Despite this, CO is rapidly absorbed through the respiratory tract (Weaver, 2004). Approximately 85% of absorbed CO binds to Hb with an affinity approximately 200–300 times higher than that of oxygen, i.e., it has a high blood:gas partition coefficient and a high degree of sequestration. The remainder binds to myoglobin in muscle and to blood proteins. Very small amounts are metabolized to carbon dioxide, and subsequently exhaled. Free (unbound) CO is excreted primarily through the respiratory tract with a whole body half-life ($t_{½}$) of 3 or 4 h in adult humans.

Treatment with 100% oxygen shortens the adult human CO $t_{½}$ to approximately 30–126 min, and treatment with hyperbaric oxygen further shortens this to about 23 min (Weaver, 2004). The human COHb $t_{½}$ is much longer at 7 h.

Pathophysiology

The principal mode of action of CO is tissue hypoxia secondary to reduced blood oxygen carrying capacity, i.e., it acts as a chemical asphyxiant (Weaver, 2004). Reduced blood oxygen carrying capacity occurs because of the preferential binding of CO rather than oxygen to Hb. The presence of COHb also results in a left shift of the oxygen:Hb dissociation curve, further exacerbating tissue hypoxia. Organs and tissues with poorly developed anastomotic networks and high metabolic rates (e.g., the heart and brain) are especially susceptible to CO-induced hypoxia. Venous blood has a high level of COHb and is classically described as being "cherry red" in color.

Myoglobin also has a higher affinity for CO compared with oxygen (Weaver, 2004). Cardiac myoglobin is particularly vulnerable to this effect, and the result is direct myocardial depression. CO–myoglobin is described as having a bright pink to red coloration. CO also binds to cytochrome oxidases in vitro although at lower affinity than oxygen. Thus, the in vivo relevance of this effect is uncertain. However, such metabolic effects may have some relevance under conditions of tissue hypoxia.

CO exposure produces substantial endovascular oxidative stress (Weaver, 2004). CO triggers the release of oxygen radicals from neutrophils and triggers nitric oxide (NO) release from platelets with the subsequent formation of peroxynitrate. CO also triggers brain neuronal apoptosis, particularly in the hippocampus, which contributes to the common amnesic effects of the gas.

Vulnerable Populations

Vulnerable populations include any life stage in which fetal Hb is present, pregnant individuals, and individuals with preexisting cardiovascular disease, anemia or any other factor resulting in reduced blood oxygen carrying capacity (Weaver, 2004).

Clinical Presentation

The most common clinical presentation is that the animal is found either unconscious or dead following acute high-level CO exposure. Nonpigmented mucous membranes, nails, and skin may have "cherry red" color. Humans with CO poisoning have been described as looking "pink-cheeked and healthy" (Weaver, 2004). Unfortunately, cherry red coloration of the mucous membranes, skin, and nails is not a reliable diagnostic sign, and very often "cherry red means dead." When CO is used as a euthanasia agent in dogs, short periods of vocalization and agitation can occur, even when the animal is apparently unconscious (Chalifoux and Dallaire, 1983).

With nonlethal exposures, any body system, organ, or tissue can be affected (Weaver, 2004). Most commonly, clinical signs pertain to hypoxic central nervous system (CNS) damage and may include apparent weakness, fatigue, depression, transient loss of consciousness, and seizure disorders. Cardiovascular signs and effects usually pertain to the effects of reduced blood oxygen carrying capacity, tissue hypoxia, and direct effects on the myocardium and may include exercise intolerance, dyspnea, syncope, and cardiac arrhythmias. Other noted effects include retinal hemorrhage, hearing loss, rhabdomyolysis, peripheral neuropathies, vomiting, and nausea. Permanent CNS injury, particularly to the hippocampus, caudate nucleus, globus pallidus, and the substantia nigra (bilaterally), as well as the cerebellum, cerebral cortex, and dorsal thalamus, can be expected in animals that survive significant CO poisoning (Kent et al., 2010).

In pigs, the most common clinically observable effects are abortion storms, stillbirth, increases in perinatal mortality, and reduced neonatal growth rates (Wood, 1979; Dominick and Carson, 1983; Morris et al., 1985a,b). Reduced hatching rates may be observed in poultry (Swarbrick, 1989). Critically, human workers in these facilities may also experience symptoms of CO poisoning, the most common of which are headache, nausea, dizziness, vomiting, and weakness.

Diagnostic Testing

Elevated blood COHb is the most definitive form of testing (Weaver, 2004). The presence of COHb cannot be determined by normal pulse oximetry because these instruments cannot discriminate between COHb and oxyhemoglobin. Specific CO pulse oximeters are necessary. The presence of fetal Hb may give falsely elevated COHb levels during the use of CO pulse oximeters. Electrocardiography is recommended because of the likely presence of cardiac arrhythmias and myocardial damage. Computerized tomography (CT) and magnetic resonance imaging of the brain may reveal brain neurological injury (particularly in the globus pallidus and other basal ganglia and the hippocampus); however, CT images may be normal in the early stages of poisoning.

Postmortem Findings

Common gross lesions include cherry red discoloration of the subcutaneous tissues, muscle, blood, and viscera. Unlike cases of cyanide poisoning, the cherry red discoloration does not fade relatively quickly over time. Histopathology findings include focal leukoencephalomalacia and other lesions that resemble brain ischemic hypoxia, particularly in the basal ganglia (especially the globus pallidus), cerebral cortex, and cerebral white matter.

Treatment

The immediate treatment priority is the prompt removal of the patient from the source of exposure. Rescuers need to take great care not to become casualties in such circumstances. The administration of 100% oxygen may be helpful because this reduces the CO $t_{½}$. Hyperbaric oxygen therapy may offer some additional benefits, but it is rarely available in veterinary practice (Stoller, 2007).

Prognosis

In cases of significant poisoning, the prognosis is typically poor. Although few data are available from the veterinary literature, human data indicate that a high proportion of survivors of significant CO poisoning develop long-term or permanent neurological, neurocognitive, and neuropsychiatric sequelae (Hampson et al., 2001; Weaver, 2004; Hopkins and Woon, 2006; Tapeantong and Poungvarin, 2009).

Prevention

The best form of prevention is the effective use of CO monitors and alarms in addition to well-adjusted heating equipment and good ventilation.

Hydrogen Sulfide

Overview, Uses, and Sources of Exposure

Note that polioencephalomalacia in ruminants due to excessive intakes of sulfur (which is converted to hydrogen sulfide by rumen microflora-mediated metabolism) is discussed in other chapters of this textbook. Within the veterinary context, hydrogen sulfide (H_2S; "sewer gas," "swamp gas," "sour gas," and "stink damp") is most commonly encountered as a byproduct of the decomposition of sulfur-containing organic material, particularly with manure tanks, septic tanks, sludge pits, cesspools or settling ponds, or enclosed spaces containing decomposing feed (Caravati, 2004; Chou et al., 2006). H_2S may also be produced when hydrochloric acid and/or sulfuric acid are used to clean drains or when wool, hair, and hides are burned. H_2S is also a byproduct of petroleum refining, tanning, rubber vulcanizing, coal and gas production, and a number of other industrial processes. H_2S is colorless, heavier than air (concentrates in low-lying areas), flammable, and explosive.

H_2S is a common and important cause of sudden death in humans, and carries with it the (somewhat exaggerated) mantra "one breath means death" (Caravati, 2004). Within the farm context, agitation of solutions containing dissolved H_2S may greatly increase the level in air (Hooser et al., 2000). This is of great importance in the case of manure tanks, septic tanks, sludge pits, and settling ponds. Exposure of confined cattle to H_2S liberated by agitation of a manure pit has resulted in significant mortality. A common cause of human casualties due to H_2S poisoning involves misguided rescue attempts (referred to as the "H_2S lemmings over the cliff phenomenon").

Toxic Dose

Relevant dose thresholds for H_2S are summarized in Table 48.2. A critical point in the dose response is the onset of odor fatigue and paralysis of the olfactory nerves (Caravati, 2004). At this point, individuals can no longer readily detect that they are being exposed to H_2S. Furthermore, the capacity of humans to detect the odor of H_2S is genetically determined, i.e., a proportion of the human population is unable to detect the odor at all. Odor detection is not an adequate method of determining exposure.

TABLE 48.2 Dose Thresholds for Hydrogen Sulfide (H_2S)

Concentration (ppm)	Effect
0.02	Human odor threshold
10	Obvious unpleasant odor + mild eye irritation
20	US OSHA PEL 15-min ceiling limit
50	Definite conjuctival irritation
50–100	Mild respiratory irritation
100	Olfactory fatigue
150–200	Olfactory nerve paralysis
250	Prolonged exposure results in pulmonary edema
300–500	Imminent threat to life plus pulmonary edema plus potentially apnea
500	30- to 60-min exposure results in excitement, staggering, unconsciousness, apnea, and respiratory failure
500–1000	Acts primarily as a systemic poison producing unconsciousness and death due to respiratory paralysis
700	Rapid unconsciousness and death if not rescued immediately
5000	Sudden death

Source: Data from Beauchamp, R.O. Jr., Bus, J.S., Popp, J.A., et al., 1984. A critical review of the literature on hydrogen sulfide toxicity. Crit. Rev. Toxicol. 13:25–97.

Toxicokinetics and Toxicodynamics

H_2S is rapidly absorbed through the lungs, although respiratory excretion is minimal (Caravati, 2004; Chou et al., 2006). Metabolic detoxification to sulfate within erythrocytes and hepatocyte mitochondria occurs relatively rapidly. Sulfate is primarily eliminated in urine. Approximately 85% of an acutely lethal dose is eliminated per hour.

Pathophysiology

The classical pathophysiology is essentially the same as that for cyanide poisoning, i.e., it produces histotoxic anoxia (Reiffenstein et al., 1992; Smith, 1997; Milby and Baselt, 1999; Albin, 2000; Caravati, 2004; Woodall et al., 2005; Chou et al., 2006; Khoshniat, 2008; Oesterhelweg and Puschel, 2008; Ballerino-Regan and Longmire, 2010). H_2S binds to the ferric moiety of cytochrome *c* oxidase, thus disrupting the mitochondrial electron transport chain and blocking of cellular aerobic energy generation. Anaerobic metabolism then predominates, resulting in lactate accumulation and metabolic acidosis. At lower concentrations, H_2S is an eye, mucous membrane, and respiratory irritant (Caravati, 2004). The respiratory effects of H_2S (initial respiratory stimulation followed by apnea) are produced by direct central respiratory effects and/or by sulfide stimulation of the chemoreceptors of the carotid body, which results in initial respiratory hypocapnia followed by reflex apnea that may be sustained and/or lethal if significant hypocapnia is present (Beauchamp et al., 1984). This results in the classical H_2S knockdown effects in humans. Death from H_2S poisoning is usually due to respiratory arrest and hypoxia (Caravati, 2004). Individuals who survive the initial exposure may subsequently die from the effects of pulmonary edema/acute respiratory distress syndromes.

Vulnerable Populations

Fetuses and neonates are assumed to be more vulnerable than adults (Caravati, 2004).

Clinical Presentation

The H_2S knockdown or "one breath means death" phenomenon occurs with exposures greater than 750 ppm and is characterized by apnea, sudden collapse, loss of consciousness and death (Reiffenstein et al., 1992; Smith, 1997; Milby and Baselt, 1999; Albin, 2000; Caravati, 2004; Woodall et al., 2005; Chou et al., 2006; Khoshniat, 2008; Oesterhelweg and Puschel, 2008; Ballerino-Regan and Longmire, 2010). Individuals may occasionally recover from H_2S knockdown if exposure ceases, although permanent neurological damage is the usual sequel. Acute respiratory distress due to pulmonary edema occurs following prolonged exposures to greater than 250 ppm (Caravati, 2004). At lower levels of exposure, upper respiratory and ocular irritation ("gas eye") effects may dominate the clinical picture. Sulfur deposits may be detectable on the eye lashes. Reactive airway disease, bronchiolitis obliterans, and pulmonary interstitial fibrosis have been reported in humans with chronic irritant exposures. Cardiac arrhythmias, nausea, vomiting, diarrhea, and abdominal pain are also common.

Diagnostic Testing

Measurements of H_2S metabolites, such as sulfide and thiosulfate in whole blood and/or urine as well as breathing zone air sampling/monitoring, are useful (Caravati, 2004).

Postmortem Findings

Greenish discoloration of gray matter, viscera, and bronchial secretions is a classical indicator in fresh tissues, but the coloration is lost with formalin fixation (Park et al., 2009). Fresh tissues may also have a distinctive sulfide smell and may undergo accelerated decomposition.

Treatment

The immediate treatment priority is the prompt removal of the patient from the source of exposure (Reiffenstein et al., 1992; Smith, 1997; Milby and Baselt, 1999; Albin, 2000; Caravati, 2004; Woodall et al., 2005; Chou et al., 2006; Khoshniat, 2008; Oesterhelweg and Puschel, 2008; Ballerino-Regan and Longmire, 2010). Rescuers need to take great care not to become casualties in such circumstances. The next treatment priority is resuscitation and provision of 100% oxygen (Caravati, 2004). Induction of methemoglobinemia by administration of nitrites, based on the predilection of sulfide to bind to ferric ions forming sulfmethemoglobin and thus potentially removing the sulfide from cytochrome oxidase and reactivating aerobic metabolism, has been suggested as an antidotal therapy. In clinical reality, induction of methemoglobinemia is only of benefit if performed within seconds to minutes of exposure. Hydroxycobalamin has been proposed as an antidote for H_2S poisoning on the basis that the pathophysiology resembles that of acute cyanide poisoning (Truong et al., 2007; Fujita et al., 2011). This antidote seems to have some effect under laboratory conditions. However, its effectiveness under field conditions has not been adequately investigated. Hyperbaric oxygen has also been proposed as being beneficial; however, it is rarely available in veterinary practice (Smilkstein et al., 1985; Whitcraft et al., 1985; Lindenmann et al., 2010).

Prognosis

The prognosis is variable depending on the duration of apnea and the degree of CNS hypoxia (Caravati, 2004). A few individuals appear to recover without any subsequent problems; however, a significant proportion of survivors will develop subsequent neurological problems associated with brain hypoxia.

Prevention

Losses of detection ability (odor fatigue and/or olfactory nerve paralysis), ill-advised entries into closed spaces, and misguided attempts to rescue casualties have all been associated with many deaths. The use of electronic exposure monitors (both personal and in spaces) and the immediate availability of personal protective equipment have saved many lives. Great care should be taken not to stir or agitate manure tanks, septic tanks, sludge pits, cesspools, or settling ponds. The use of hydrochloric acid and/or sulfuric acid-based drain cleaners should be avoided.

Oxides of Nitrogen (Silo Filler's Disease)

Overview, Uses, and Sources of Exposure

The main gas involved is nitrogen dioxide (NO_2), although other reactive oxides of nitrogen may also be present (Lowry and Schuman, 1956; Jonas, 1984; Pladson, 1984; Douglas et al., 1989; Epler, 1989; Gurney et al., 1991; Zwemer et al., 1992; Leavey et al., 2004). NO_2 has a bleach-like odor, a reddish-brown to yellow color, and leaves a yellow stain on silage, wood, or other contact materials. It is heavier than air. The most commonly encountered source in veterinary medicine is from silos that have been recently filled with fresh organic material (notably corn or other grains) or from silage pits. NO_2 is formed when NO in fresh silage or silo contents comes in contact with oxygen in the air. Silage gas also typically contains carbon dioxide. Silo gas has been a cause of mortality in dairy cattle (Haynes, 1963; Verhoeff et al., 2007).

Toxic (and potentially lethal) levels of NO_2 can develop within hours on top of the material in the silo or silage pit (Groves and Ellwood, 1989). Within silos, the gas tends to seep down through the silo chute. The risk is highest when feedstuffs that are high in nitrates are ensiled or used for silage. Gas production typically peaks at approximately 24 h, but it may last for several days. Other veterinary-relevant sources of NO_2 include kerosene heaters, unvented gas stoves, gas heaters, and tobacco smoke.

Toxic Dose

The US EPA National Ambient Air Quality Standards lists 0.053 ppm as the 24-h time-weighted average upper limit for NO_2 in air. Levels of 25.9 ppb (SD, 18.1 ppb) are known to increase the risk of pediatric asthma in humans (Belanger et al., 2006). Brief exposures to 200 ppm can be fatal, and exposure to 50 ppm can result in significant pulmonary edema. A 1-h exposure to 1 ppm is associated with deleterious effects in the lung. The human odor threshold is approximately 0.1–0.2 ppm.

Toxicokinetics and Toxicodynamics

NO_2 is relatively water insoluble, and accumulation in the upper respiratory tract is limited (Jonas, 1984; Douglas et al., 1989; Epler, 1989; Gurney et al., 1991; Leavey et al., 2004). The high levels of carbon dioxide present in silage gas may stimulate deeper inspiration of the gas, resulting in a higher delivered dose in the deep lung, i.e., it behaves as a typical EPA Category 1 gas that produces site-of-contact effects in the deep lung/gas exchange areas. Prolonged and/or high level exposure can also result in systemic effects (notably the formation of nitrosyl hemoglobin and methemoglobinemia).

Pathophysiology

NO_2 dissolves in water to produce nitrous and nitric acids, which are irritant and corrosive (Jonas, 1984; Douglas et al., 1989; Epler, 1989; Gurney et al., 1991; Leavey et al., 2004). Free radical generation and associated damage are also important parts of the pathophysiology. The acids are also immunosuppressive and result in a reduced resistance to infection. With prolonged or high levels of exposure, NO_2 is absorbed. Absorbed NO_2 binds with high affinity to hemoglobin, forming nitrosyl hemoglobin, which is further oxidized to methemoglobin. This results in chemical asphyxia. Methemoglobinemia produces a left shift of the hemoglobin:oxygen disassociation curve, further impairing tissue oxygen delivery.

Vulnerable Populations

Individuals with preexisting reactive airway disorders, asthma, and lung disease are likely to be at greater risk.

Clinical Presentation

Clinical disease is usually with harvest season and the presentation depends on the concentration and duration of exposure (Jonas, 1984; Pladson, 1984; Douglas et al., 1989; Epler, 1989; Gurney et al., 1991; do Pico, 1992; Zwemer et al., 1992; Stepanek et al., 1998; Leavey et al., 2004). High level exposures can produce sudden death due to bronchiolar spasm, laryngeal spasm, reflex respiratory arrest, and/or asphyxia. Lower exposures may be asymptomatic, or produce mild, self-limiting effects, or result in eye irritation, pulmonary edema, and/or acute respiratory distress syndromes. Mucous membrane irritation is uncommon because NO_2 does not tend to dissolve onto wet mucous membrane surfaces.

Failure to adequately treat significant NO_2 exposure with corticosteroids results in bronchiolitis obliterans, particularly in the small airways and alveolar ducts, and permanent restrictive lung disease. Bronchiolitis obliterans can develop weeks or months following the initial exposure.

Diagnostic Testing

Apart from air sampling/monitoring, there are no specific diagnostic tests. Occasionally, red gaseous material can be observed being released from freshly filled silos and red staining of surfaces near silo chutes can be observed.

Postmortem Findings

Chemical pneumonitis and pulmonary edema primarily located in the deep lung are the predominant findings. Emphysema may be present, depending on the duration of the toxidrome. Typically, type I pneumocytes, pulmonary mast cells, and ciliated airway cells are the most affected cell types. Delayed effects include bronchiolitis obliterans.

Treatment

The immediate treatment priority is the prompt removal of the patient from the source of exposure. Rescuers need to take great care not to become casualties in such circumstances. The next treatment priority is the administration of 100% oxygen and resuscitation. Pulmonary edema may develop up to 48 h following exposure, so volume expanders and fluid therapy must be used with great caution during this period. Corticosteroids are important for reducing the risk of bronchiolitis obliterans. The use of broad-spectrum antibiotics with the objective of preventing bronchopneumonia may be justified. Subsequent follow-up management of reactive airway syndromes and asthma may be required.

Prognosis

The prognosis depends entirely on the degree of lung damage and whether or not bronchiolitis obliterans and restrictive lung disease develop (Jonas, 1984; Douglas et al., 1989; Epler, 1989; Gurney et al., 1991; Zwemer et al., 1992; Leavey et al., 2004). In many cases, the toxidrome is mild and self-limiting; however, it may take months for pulmonary function to return to normal. Permanent mild loss of pulmonary function is relatively common.

Prevention

The following methods can prevent exposure: stay out of silos during the 2-week danger period after the initial filling; close all silo doors before filling; use outside ladders rather than internal ladders in silos; if the silo is not completely full, remove the doors that lead down to the silage; enter the silo only with a complete oxygen support system; ventilate the silo by opening the cover flaps and running the silo blower for 24–48 h before entering; never enter the silo alone or without a lifeline for rescue during the danger period; use a personal air monitor; and install air monitors in areas where NO_2 is likely to concentrate.

Gaseous Ammonia

Overview, Uses, and Sources of Exposure

Within the veterinary context, ammonia (NH_3) is most commonly encountered anywhere decaying organic matter is present, particularly urine and feces (Roney et al., 2004). In this context, it is ubiquitous within intensive animal production facilities. Swine and poultry production facilities are notorious for containing toxic levels of ammonia that are often higher than acceptable human threshold limit values (Sigurdarson et al., 2004; Davis and Morishita, 2005; McDonnell et al., 2008). Ammonia is lighter than air and will thus tend to rise from manure pits (Roney et al., 2004). Ammonia is still used as a refrigerant, and leaks in such systems remain a common cause of serious incidents. The burning of nylon, silk, wood, and melamine also results in considerable production of NH_3. NH_3 is a major component of many common household cleaning and bleaching products, and the mixing of these products with those that contain chlorine results in the liberation of chloramines, which are highly irritant and potentially dangerous (Pascuzzi and Storrow, 1998).

High-pressure anhydrous ammonia gas is a commonly used fertilizer in some locations because it is often the cheapest source of nitrogen. Errors in handling (often associated with its illicit use for the production of methamphetamine) and leakage represent a substantial risk (George et al., 2000; Fitzgerald and Flood, 2006; Welch, 2006).

Anhydrous ammonia is an important component in the manufacture of methamphetamines (Bloom et al., 2008). Theft of anhydrous ammonia from farms is common and has resulted in numerous serious incidents (Amshel et al., 2000; Latenser and Lucktong, 2000; Lessenger, 2004; Welch, 2006). Due to the unique chemical properties of anhydrous ammonia, it can exert extremely high pressures even at relatively low temperatures; thus, specialized containers and equipment are required for safe handling of the gas. Attempts at anhydrous ammonia theft often involve the use of propane tanks that are not designed to handle the physicochemical properties of anhydrous ammonia, and the risk of explosion of these types of containers is high. Veterinarians and farmers should be extremely cautious around apparently empty propane tanks that have blue- or green-discolored valves or if the tanks have frost on them. Anhydrous ammonia may have been inappropriately stored in such containers, and the container's brass, copper, or galvanized valve fittings may be compromised.

Liquid anhydrous ammonia expands to many times its original volume when released into air and forms large, highly dangerous vapor clouds. Aerosolized liquid anhydrous ammonia may behave as a dense gas and accumulate in low-lying spaces, even though it is normally lighter than air.

Toxic Dose

The concentration of NH_3 in well-ventilated animal production facilities should remain below 30 ppm. The human odor threshold is approximately 10 ppm. The human dose response to NH_3 is shown in Table 48.3. Adverse effects occur at concentrations greater than approximately 75 ppm.

TABLE 48.3 Dose Thresholds for Gaseous Ammonia

Concentration (ppm)	Effect
Source: ≤25	Eight-hour time weighted average human exposure limit
25–50	Detectable odor; unlikely to experience adverse effects
50–100	Mild eye and upper respiratory tract irritation; may develop tolerance in 1 or 2 weeks with no adverse effects thereafter
140	Moderate eye irritation; no long-term sequelae in exposures of less than 2 h
400	Moderate throat irritation
500	Immediately dangerous to life and health (human)
700	Immediate eye injury
1000	Severe airway injury
1700	Immediate laryngospasm
2500–6500	Sloughing and necrosis of airway mucosa, chest pain, acute lung injury, and bronchospasm
5000	Rapidly fatal

Source: Data from Roney, N., Llados, F., Little, S.S., Knaebel, D.B., 2004. ATSDR Toxicological Profile for Ammonia. ATSDR, Atlanta.

Anhydrous ammonia has an 8-h time-weighted average maximum acceptable exposure of 25 ppm, a short-term exposure limit of 35 ppm, and an immediately dangerous to life and health level of 500 ppm.

Toxicokinetics and Toxicodynamics

NH_3 is highly water soluble and thus tends to primarily affect the upper respiratory tract, mucous membranes, and the eye (Close et al., 1980; O'Kane, 1983; Robinson et al., 1990; Chao and Lo, 1996; Brautbar et al., 2003; Makarovsky et al., 2008). However, deeper structures may be affected if the upper respiratory tract scrubbing is overwhelmed.

Pathophysiology

NH_3 is irritant and/or corrosive depending on the concentration. NH_3 reacts with tissue water to produce ammonium hydroxide, a strong alkali (Close et al., 1980; Robinson et al., 1990; Chao and Lo, 1996; Brautbar et al., 2003; Makarovsky et al., 2008). The reaction is exothermic and capable of producing significant tissue burns. Ammonium hydroxide produces typical alkaline liquefaction necrosis. Alkali liquefaction necrosis results in deeper tissue damage than that caused by an acid of similar pH reserve. In addition, ammonium hydroxide tissue breakdown liberates water, aiding the further conversion of NH_3 to ammonium hydroxide. Mild exposure primarily affects the upper respiratory tract and eyes, whereas more severe exposure may affect the entire respiratory tract. The degree of damage to the respiratory tract is dependent on the depth of inhalation, duration of exposure, concentration, and the pH change of the tissue fluids. Even mild levels of exposure can reduce pulmonary clearance and potentially increase the risk of infections of the respiratory tract. Within animal facilities, ammonia is generally adsorbed by dust particles, which enable deeper penetration of the lung compared with gaseous NH_3 (Kim et al., 2008). In such circumstances, the toxicological thresholds for adverse effects may be lower than for gaseous NH_3.

Liquid anhydrous ammonia (−33°C) freezes tissue on contact and can produce deep, irreversible skin damage (Amshel et al., 2000; Latenser and Lucktong, 2000; Lessenger, 2004; Welch, 2006).

Vulnerable Populations

Individuals with preexisting lung disease, reactive airway syndromes, and/or asthma are at significantly greater risk.

Clinical Presentation

Clinical signs associated with relatively low-level exposures pertain to eye and upper respiratory tract irritation: shallow breathing, excessive lacrimation, nasal discharge, keratoconjunctivitis, corneal opacity, atrophic rhinitis, dyspnea, hemoptysis, hoarse voice, dysphagia, reduced production values, and possibly increased rates of respiratory infections. Higher exposures can result in severe pulmonary disease and possibly acute respiratory distress.

Diagnostic Testing

Air monitoring is the most effective form of diagnostic testing.

Postmortem Findings

Irritation and possibly corrosion of the respiratory tract, particularly the upper tract, and exposed surfaces of the eye dominate the gross findings. Histological findings may include hyperplasia of the bronchiolar and alveolar epithelium.

Treatment

The immediate treatment priority is the prompt removal of the patient from the source of exposure. Rescuers need to take great care not to become casualties in such circumstances. Copious skin and eye irrigation should be performed for at least 20 min (taking care to avoid hypothermia). Patients should then be treated for acute respiratory distress and/or burns. In animal production facilities, the best treatment is to improve ventilation and to reduce the accumulation of animal wastes within the facilities.

Prognosis

The prognosis depends on the severity, depth, and chronicity of respiratory tract injury. Reactive airway diseases and asthma are common following NH_3 exposures. Chronic respiratory sequelae may occur with severe exposures.

Prevention

Improved ventilation and removal of wastes is the most effective form of prevention within intensive animal facilities. The use of air monitors (personal and space) and personal protective equipment has reduced human casualties. Veterinarians and farmers should have a very high degree of suspicion regarding areas where high levels of NH_3 might be present, particularly enclosed spaces. Improved security of liquid anhydrous ammonia storage facilities has been recommended.

Smoke Inhalation

Overview, Uses, and Sources of Exposure

Smoke inhalation injury results from a combination of exposure to gaseous combustion products, particulate matter (which may be superheated), and superheated air (Lee-Chiong, 1999; Alarie, 2002; Enkhbaatar and Traber, 2004; Fitzgerald et al., 2006; Lee and Mellins, 2006; Schnepp, 2006; Sicoutris and Holmes, 2006; Stefanidou et al., 2008). Thus, the syndrome results from a combination of thermal, gas, and particle effects. Smoke inhalation always involves some degree of CO and cyanide poisoning. Combustion of plastics, polyurethane, wool, silk, nylon, nitriles, rubber, and paper leads to the production of cyanide gas. Other combustion products may include acrolein and other reactive aldehydes (organic combustion) and also chlorine, ammonia, ketones, hydrocarbons, and various acids (combustion of rubber and plastics).

Toxic Dose

The toxic dose depends on the source.

Pathophysiology

Thermal damage primarily occurs in the upper respiratory tract, particularly in the oropharyngeal area, due to the poor heat conductivity of air and high dissipation of heat in the upper airways (Clark et al., 1989, 1990; Clark, 1992; Lee-Chiong, 1999; Alarie, 2002; Enkhbaatar and Traber, 2004; Fitzgerald et al., 2006; Lee and Mellins, 2006; Schnepp, 2006; Sicoutris and Holmes, 2006; Stefanidou et al., 2008). Both pulmonary irritation and systemic effects occur. Systemic effects occur primarily due to direct and chemical asphyxiation. Chemical asphyxiation most commonly occurs as a result of a combination of CO and cyanide (CN) poisoning. Methemoglobinemia occurs due to direct heat denaturation of hemoglobin, as well as the inhalation of nitrites.

Vulnerable Populations

Individuals with preexisting lung disease, reactive airway syndromes, and/or asthma are at significantly greater risk.

Clinical Presentation

Any individual with facial burns is likely also to have concurrent smoke inhalation injury. Individuals who no longer have eyelashes are very likely to have concurrent ocular injury. Common early clinical signs of respiratory tract injury include hoarseness and a change in voice, carbonaceous nasal discharge or sputum, coughing, tachypnea, and use of accessory respiratory muscles (Clark et al., 1989, 1990; Clark, 1992; Lee-Chiong, 1999; Alarie, 2002; Enkhbaatar and Traber, 2004; Fitzgerald and Flood, 2006; Lee and Millens, 2006; Schnepp, 2006; Sicoutris and Holmes, 2006; Stefanidou et al., 2008). Later clinical signs are related to progressive pulmonary decline and acute respiratory distress.

Diagnostic Testing

Bronchoscopy is the definitive diagnostic procedure. Clinical chemistry may indicate metabolic acidosis resulting from a combination of hypoxia, CO poisoning, CN poisoning, and methemoglobinemia. Elevated serum lactate is a relatively sensitive indication of cyanide poisoning. Patients may have lowered blood cholinesterases because the pyrolysis products of many phosphorus-based fire retardants are anticholinesterases. Pulse oximetry may provide misleading information due to the presence of COHb and methemoglobinemia. If available, pulse cooximetry is preferable.

Chest radiographs are common normal after smoke inhalation, and the diagnostic accuracy of the technique is low. Chest computerized tomography (CCT) is a preferable imaging technique. CCT abnormalities include ground-glass opacities in a peribronchial distribution and/or patchy peribronchial consolidations. Such abnormal CCT findings may be present within a few hours following smoke inhalation. Pulmonary function tests are sensitive indicators of smoke inhalation injury, but they are rarely readily available in veterinary practice.

Treatment

The immediate treatment priority is the prompt removal of the patient from the source of exposure. Rescuers need to take great care not to become casualties in such circumstances. The next treatment priority is the administration of 100% oxygen, resuscitation, and maintenance of airway patency (Clark et al., 1989, 1990; Clark, 1992).

Unfortunately, there is no specific treatment for the tissue damage and increased risk of infection associated with smoke inhalation. Studies in humans have indicated that positive pressure ventilation with low tidal volumes (3–5 mL/kg) and positive end-expiratory pressure may increase short-term survival (Cancio, 2009). High-frequency percussive ventilation, whole-body hypothermia, and hyperbaric oxygen may also decrease mortality (Reper et al., 1998; Thom et al., 2001). Unfortunately, none of these techniques are readily available in veterinary medicine. Induction of methemoglobinemia for the treatment of CN poisoning may be dangerous if significant CO poisoning is also present. However, the use of hydroxocobalamin (Cyanokit) in combination with low-dose sodium thiosulfate as a CN antidote may be considered (Borron et al., 2007a,b). Bronchodilator therapy is almost always indicated in cases of smoke inhalation.

Patients with significant smoke inhalation commonly require concurrent treatment for burns, a subject that is beyond the scope of this chapter.

Prognosis

The prognosis is entirely dependent on the degree of smoke injury and associated injury. Significant smoke inhalation always has a guarded prognosis.

CONCLUDING REMARKS AND FUTURE DIRECTIONS

The toxic gases of veterinary importance are likely to continue as ongoing human health and veterinary production problems. Further research is required to determine the levels of chronic exposure to these gases that do not result in production losses. High morbidity/mortality epizootics in intensive animal production facilities will inevitably continue to occur following breakdowns in the management of such facilities. Ongoing areas of research include the development of a better understanding of xenobiotic metabolism in the lung and improved methods of experimentally replicating/modeling real world exposures. Both of these areas are necessary for the future high-quality risk assessments of gases of toxicological importance.

REFERENCES

Alarie, Y., 2002. Toxicity of fire smoke. Crit. Rev. Toxicol. 32, 259–289.

Albin, R.L., 2000. Basal ganglia neurotoxins. Neurol. Clin. 18, 665–680.

Amshel, C.E., Fealk, M.H., Phillips, B.J., Caruso, D.M., 2000. Anhydrous ammonia burns case report and review of the literature. Burns. 26, 493–497.

Ballerino-Regan, D., Longmire, A.W., 2010. Hydrogen sulfide exposure as a cause of sudden occupational death. Arch. Pathol. Lab. Med. 134, 1105.

Baron, J., Voigt, J.M., 1990. Localization, distribution, and induction of xenobiotic-metabolizing enzymes and aryl hydrocarbon hydroxylase activity within lung. Pharmacol. Ther. 47, 419–445.

Beauchamp Jr, R.O., Bus, J.S., Popp, J.A., et al., 1984. A critical review of the literature on hydrogen sulfide toxicity. Crit. Rev. Toxicol. 13, 25–97.

Belanger, K., Gent, J.F., Triche, E.W., et al., 2006. Association of indoor nitrogen dioxide exposure with respiratory symptoms in children with asthma. Am. J. Respir. Crit. Care Med. 173, 297–303.

Bloom, G.R., Suhail, F., Hopkins-Price, P., Sood, A., 2008. Acute anhydrous ammonia injury from accidents during illicit methamphetamine production. Burns. 34, 713–718.

Bogdanffy, M.S., 1990. Biotransformation enzymes in the rodent nasal mucosa: the value of a histochemical approach. Environ. Health Perspect. 85, 177–186.

Bogdanffy, M.S., 1997. Mechanisms of chemical toxicity to the nasal cavity. Mutat. Res. 380, 1–2.

Bogdanffy, M.S., Taylor, M.L., 1993. Kinetics of nasal carboxylesterase-mediated metabolism of vinyl acetate. Drug Metab. Dispos. 21, 1107–1111.

Bogdanffy, M.S., Randall, H.W., Morgan, K.T., 1986. Histochemical localization of aldehyde dehydrogenase in the respiratory tract of the Fischer-344 rat. Toxicol. Appl. Pharmacol. 82, 560–567.

Bogdanffy, M.S., Randall, H.W., Morgan, K.T., 1987. Biochemical quantitation and histochemical localization of carboxylesterase in the nasal passages of the Fischer-344 rat and B6C3F1 mouse. Toxicol. Appl. Pharmacol. 88, 183–194.

Bogdanffy, M.S., Kee, C.R., Hinchman, C.A., Trela, B.A., 1991. Metabolism of dibasic esters by rat nasal mucosal carboxylesterase. Drug Metab. Dispos. 19, 124–129.

Boller, E., 1976. Carbon monoxide poisoning in a pig-breeding unit due to wrongly adjusted propane gas infrared radiation. Schweiz Arch. Tierheilkd. 118, 127–129.

Borron, S.W., Baud, F.J., Barriot, P., et al., 2007a. Prospective study of hydroxocobalamin for acute cyanide poisoning in smoke inhalation. Ann. Emerg. Med. 49, 794–801.

Borron, S.W., Baud, F.J., Megarbane, B., Bismuth, C., 2007b. Hydroxocobalamin for severe acute cyanide poisoning by ingestion or inhalation. Am. J. Emerg. Med. 25, 551–558.

Brautbar, N., Wu, M.P., Richter, E.D., 2003. Chronic ammonia inhalation and interstitial pulmonary fibrosis: a case report and review of the literature. Arch. Environ. Health. 58, 592–596.

Cancio, L.C., 2009. Airway management and smoke inhalation injury in the burn patient. Clin. Plast. Surg. 36, 555–567.

Caravati, E.M., 2004. Hydrogen sulfide. In: Dart, R.C., Caravati, E.M., McGuigan, M.A., Whyte, I.M., Dawson, A.H., Seifert, S.A., et al., Medical Toxicology. Lippincott Williams & Wilkins, Philadelphia, pp. 1169–1173.

Castell, J.V., Donato, M.T., Gomez-Lechon, M.J., 2005. Metabolism and bioactivation of toxicants in the lung. The in vitro cellular approach. Exp. Toxicol. Pathol. 57 (Suppl 1), 189–204.

Castranova, V., Rabovsky, J., Tucker, J.H., Miles, P.R., 1988. The alveolar type II epithelial cell: a multifunctional pneumocyte. Toxicol. Appl. Pharmacol. 93, 472–483.

Chalifoux, A., Dallaire, A., 1983. Physiologic and behavioral evaluation of CO euthanasia of adult dogs. Am. J. Vet. Res. 44, 2412–2417.

Chao, T.C., Lo, D.S., 1996. Ammonia gassing deaths: a report on two cases. Singapore Med. J. 37, 147–149.

Chou, S., Fay, M., Keith, S., Ingerman, L., Chappell, L., 2006. ATSDR Toxicological Profile for Hydrogen Sulfide. ATSDR, Atlanta.

Clark Jr, W.R., 1992. Smoke inhalation: diagnosis and treatment. World J. Surg. 16, 24–29.

Clark, W.R., Bonaventura, M., Myers, W., 1989. Smoke inhalation and airway management at a regional burn unit: 1974 to 1983. I: diagnosis and consequences of smoke inhalation. J. Burn. Care Rehabil. 10, 52–62.

Clark, W.R., Bonaventura, M., Myers, W., Kellman, R., 1990. Smoke inhalation and airway management at a regional burn unit: 1974 to 1983. II. Airway management. J. Burn. Care Rehabil. 11, 121–134.

Close, L.G., Catlin, F.I., Cohn, A.M., 1980. Acute and chronic effects of ammonia burns on the respiratory tract. Arch. Otolaryngol. 106, 151–158.

Davis, M., Morishita, T.Y., 2005. Relative ammonia concentrations, dust concentrations, and presence of Salmoneua species and *Escherichia coli* inside and outside commercial layer facilities. Avian Dis. 49, 30–35.

Devereux, T.R., 1984. Alveolar type II and Clara cells: isolation and xenobiotic metabolism. Environ. Health Perspect. 56, 95–101.

Devereux, T.R., Diliberto, J.J., Fouts, J.R., 1985. Cytochrome P-450 monooxygenase, epoxide hydrolase and flavin monooxygenase activities in Clara cells and alveolar type II cells isolated from rabbit. Cell Biol. Toxicol. 1, 57–65.

do Pico, G.A., 1992. Hazardous exposure and lung disease among farm workers. Clin. Chest. Med. 13, 311–328.

Dominick, M.A., Carson, T.L., 1983. Effects of carbon monoxide exposure on pregnant sows and their fetuses. Am. J. Vet. Res. 44, 35–40.

Douglas, W.W., Hepper, N.G., Colby, T.V., 1989. Silo-filler's disease. Mayo Clin. Proc. 64, 291–304.

Enggaard Hansen, N., Creutzberg, A., Simonsen, H.B., 1991. Euthanasia of mink (Mustela vison) by means of carbon dioxide (CO_2), carbon monoxide (CO) and nitrogen (N_2). Br. Vet. J. 147, 140–146.

Enkhbaatar, P., Traber, D.L., 2004. Pathophysiology of acute lung injury in combined burn and smoke inhalation injury. Clin. Sci. London. 107, 137–143.

Epler, G.R., 1989. Silo-filler's disease: a new perspective. Mayo Clin. Proc. 64, 368–370.

Fiserova-Bergerova, V., Diaz, M.L., 1986. Determination and prediction of tissue-gas partition coefficients. Int. Arch. Occup. Environ. Health. 58, 75–87.

Fitzgerald, K.T., Flood, A.A., 2006. Smoke inhalation. Clin. Tech. Small Anim. Pract. 21, 205–214.

Fitzgerald, S.D., Grooms, D.L., Scott, M.A., et al., 2006. Acute anhydrous ammonia intoxication in cattle. J. Vet. Diagn. Invest. 18, 485–489.

Fujita, Y., Fujino, Y., Onodera, M., et al., 2011. A fatal case of acute hydrogen sulfide poisoning caused by hydrogen sulfide: hydroxocobalamin therapy for acute hydrogen sulfide poisoning. J. Anal. Toxicol. 35, 119–123.

George, A., Bang, R.L., Lari, A.R., et al., 2000. Liquid ammonia injury. Burns. 26, 409–413.

Gerritzen, M.A., Lambooij, E., Stegeman, J.A., Spruijt, B.M., 2006. Slaughter of poultry during the epidemic of avian influenza in The Netherlands in 2003. Vet. Rec. 159, 39–42.

Groves, J.A., Ellwood, P.A., 1989. Gases in forage tower silos. Ann. Occup. Hyg. 33, 519–535.

Gurney, J.W., Unger, J.M., Dorby, C.A., et al., 1991. Agricultural disorders of the lung. Radiographics. 11, 625–634.

Haber, F., 1924. Zur Geschichte de Gas Kriegs. Fuenf Vortraege Aus Den Jahren. Julius Springer, Berlin.

Hamling, A.E., Jenschke, B.E., Calkins, C.R., 2008. Effects of dark storage and retail display on beef chuck and round muscles enhanced with ammonium hydroxide, salt, and carbon monoxide. J. Anim. Sci. 86, 972–981.

Hampson, N.B., Stock, A.L., 2006. Storm-related carbon monoxide poisoning: lessons learned from recent epidemics. Undersea Hyperb. Med. 33, 257–263.

Hampson, N.B., Mathieu, D., Piantadosi, C.A., et al., 2001. Carbon monoxide poisoning: interpretation of randomized clinical trials and unresolved treatment issues. Undersea Hyperb. Med. 28, 157–164.

Harduar-Morano, L., Watkins, S., 2011. Review of unintentional non-fire-related carbon monoxide poisoning morbidity and mortality in Florida, 1999–2007. Public Health Rep. 126, 240–250.

Haynes, N.B., 1963. "Silo filler's disease" in dairy cattle. J. Am. Vet. Med. Assoc. 143, 593–594.

Hooser, S.B., Van Alstine, W., Kiupel, M., Sojka, J., 2000. Acute pit gas (hydrogen sulfide) poisoning in confinement cattle. J. Vet. Diagn. Invest. 12, 272–275.

Hopkins, R.O., Woon, F.L., 2006. Neuroimaging, cognitive, and neurobehavioral outcomes following carbon monoxide poisoning. Behav. Cogn. Neurosci. Rev. 5, 141–155.

Hoyle, G.W., Chang, W., Chen, J., et al., 2010. Deviations from Haber's law for multiple measures of acute lung injury in chlorine-exposed mice. Toxicol. Sci. 118, 696–703.

Hukkanen, J., Pelkonen, O., Hakkola, J., Raunio, H., 2002. Expression and regulation of xenobiotic-metabolizing cytochrome P450 (CYP) enzymes in human lung. Crit. Rev. Toxicol. 32, 391–411.

Jeong, J.Y., Claus, J.R., 2010. Color stability and reversion in carbon monoxide packaged ground beef. Meat Sci. 85, 525–530.

Jeong, J.Y., Claus, J.R., 2011. Color stability of ground beef packaged in a low carbon monoxide atmosphere or vacuum. Meat Sci. 87, 1–6.

Jonas, D.O., 1984. Silo filler's disease. Mil. Med. 149, 481–485.

Jones, R., 2003. Smoke inhalation: assessing and managing patients. Emerg. Nurse. 11, 18–23.

Keller, D.A., Heck, H.D., Randall, H.W., Morgan, K.T., 1990. Histochemical localization of formaldehyde dehydrogenase in the rat. Toxicol. Appl. Pharmacol. 106, 311–326.

Keller, H., 1976. Stillbirths in a pig breeding unit due to high carbon monoxide content of the air. Schweiz Arch. Tierheilkd. 118, 425–428.

Kent, M., Creevy, K.E., Delahunta, A., 2010. Clinical and neuropathological findings of acute carbon monoxide toxicity in Chihuahuas following smoke inhalation. J. Am. Anim. Hosp. Assoc. 46, 259–264.

Khoshniat, H., 2008. H2S: the silent killer. Occup. Health Saf. 77, 55.

Kim, K.Y., Ko, H.J., Kim, H.T., et al., 2008. Effect of manual feeding on the level of farmer's exposure to airborne contaminants in the confinement nursery pig house. Ind. Health. 46, 138–143.

Kingston, S.K., Dussault, C.A., Zaidlicz, R.S., et al., 2005. Evaluation of two methods for mass euthanasia of poultry in disease outbreaks. J. Am. Vet. Med. Assoc. 227, 730–738.

Lambooy, E., Roelofs, J.A., van Voorst, N., 1985. Euthanasia of mink with carbon monoxide. Vet. Rec. 116, 416.

Latenser, B.A., Lucktong, T.A., 2000. Anhydrous ammonia burns: case presentation and literature review. J. Burn Care Rehabil. 21, 40–42.

Leavey, J.F., Dubin, R.L., Singh, N., Kaminsky, D.A., 2004. Silo-filler's disease, the acute respiratory distress syndrome, and oxides of nitrogen. Ann. Intern. Med. 141, 410–411.

Lee, A.S., Mellins, R.B., 2006. Lung injury from smoke inhalation. Paediatr. Respir. Rev. 7, 123–128.

Lee-Chiong Jr, T.L., 1999. Smoke inhalation injury. Postgrad. Med. 105, 55–62.

Lessenger, J.E., 2004. Anhydrous ammonia injuries. J. Agromed. 9, 191–203.

Lin, Y.S., Smith, T.J., Wypij, D., et al., 2002. Association of the blood/air partition coefficient of 1,3-butadiene with blood lipids and albumin. Environ. Health Perspect. 110, 165–168.

Lindenmann, J., Matzi, V., Anegg, U., et al., 2010. Hyperbaric oxygen in the treatment of hydrogen sulphide intoxication. Acta Anaesthesiol. Scand. 54, 784–785.

Lohs, K., 1990. The history of toxicology of the "Haber's constant.". Z. Gesamte. Hyg. 36, 130–131.

Lowry, T., Schuman, L.M., 1956. Silo-filler's disease; a syndrome caused by nitrogen dioxide. J. Am. Med. Assoc. 162, 153–160.

Makarovsky, I., Markel, G., Dushnitsky, T., Eisenkraft, A., 2008. Ammonia: when something smells wrong. Isr. Med.Assoc. J. 10, 537–543.

Mantilla, D., Kristinsson, H.G., Balaban, M.O., et al., 2008. Carbon monoxide treatments to impart and retain muscle color in tilapia fillets. J. Food Sci. 73, C390–C399.

McDonnell, P.E., Coggins, M.A., Hogan, V.J., Fleming, G.T., 2008. Exposure assessment of airborne contaminants in the indoor environment of Irish swine farms. Ann. Agric. Environ. Med. 15, 323–326.

McGuigan, M.A., 1999. Common culprits in childhood poisoning: epidemiology, treatment and parental advice for prevention. Paediatr. Drugs. 1, 313–324.

Meredith, T.J., 1993. Epidemiology of poisoning. Pharmacol. Ther. 59, 251–256.

Milby, T.H., Baselt, R.C., 1999. Hydrogen sulfide poisoning: clarification of some controversial issues. Am. J. Ind. Med. 35, 192–195.

Miller, F.J., Schlosser, P.M., Janszen, D.B., 2000. Haber's rule: a special case in a family of curves relating concentration and duration of exposure to a fixed level of response for a given endpoint. Toxicology. 149, 21–34.

Moreland, A.F., 1974. Carbon monoxide euthanasia of dogs: chamber concentrations and comparative effects of automobile engine exhaust and carbon monoxide from a cylinder. J. Am. Vet. Med. Assoc. 165, 853–855.

Morris, G.L., Curtis, S.E., Simon, J., 1985a. Perinatal piglets under sublethal concentrations of atmospheric carbon monoxide. J. Anim. Sci. 61, 1070–1079.

Morris, G.L., Curtis, S.E., Widowski, T.M., 1985b. Weanling pigs under sublethal concentrations of atmospheric carbon monoxide. J. Anim. Sci. 61, 1080–1087.

Morris, J.B., Buckpitt, A.R., 2009. Upper respiratory tract uptake of naphthalene. Toxicol. Sci. 111, 383–391.

Oesterhelweg, L., Puschel, K., 2008. "Death may come on like a stroke of lightening:" phenomenological and morphological aspects of fatalities caused by manure gas. Int. J. Legal. Med. 122, 101–107.

O'Kane, G.J., 1983. Inhalation of ammonia vapour: a report on the management of eight patients during the acute stages. Anaesthesia. 38, 1208–1213.

Park, S.H., Zhang, Y., Hwang, J.J., 2009. Discolouration of the brain as the only remarkable autopsy finding in hydrogen sulphide poisoning. Forensic. Sci. Int. 187, e19–e21.

Pascuzzi, T.A., Storrow, A.B., 1998. Mass casualties from acute inhalation of chloramine gas. Mil. Med. 163, 102–104.

Pejsak, Z., Zmudzki, J., Wojnicki, P., 2008. Abortion in sows associated with carbon monoxide intoxication. Vet. Rec. 162, 417.

Pladson, T.R., 1984. Silo emptiers' diseases. Minn. Med. 67, 265–269.

Reiffenstein, R.J., Hulbert, W.C., Roth, S.H., 1992. Toxicology of hydrogen sulfide. Ann. Rev. Pharmacol. Toxicol. 132, 109–134.

Renwick, A.G., 2008. Principles of toxicology. Toxicokinetics. In: Hayes, A.W. (Ed.), Principles and Methods of Toxicology. CRC Press, New York, pp. 179–230. Part 1.

Reper, P., Dankaert, R., van Hille, F., et al., 1998. The usefulness of combined high-frequency percussive ventilation during acute respiratory failure after smoke inhalation. Burns. 24, 34–38.

Robinson, F.R., Runnels, L.J., Conrad, D.A., Teclaw, R.F., Thacker, H. L., 1990. Pathologic response of the lung to irritant gases. Vet. Hum. Toxicol. 32, 569–572.

Roney, N., Llados, F., Little, S.S., Knaebel, D.B., 2004. ATSDR Toxicological Profile for Ammonia. ATSDR, Atlanta.

Rozman, K.K., Klaassen, C.D., 2001. Unit 2: disposition of toxicants. Absorption, distribution and excretion of toxicants. In: Klaassen, C.D. (Ed.), Casarett & Doull's Toxicology: The Basic Science of Poisons. McGraw-Hill, New York, pp. 107–132.

Sadovnikoff, N., Varon, J., Sternbach, G.L., 1992. Carbon monoxide poisoning: an occult epidemic. Postgrad. Med. 92 (86–88), 92–96.

Schnepp, R., 2006. Cyanide: sources, perceptions, and risks. J. Emerg. Nurs. 32, S3–S7.

Sicoutris, C.P., Holmes, J.H.T., 2006. Fire and smoke injuries. Crit. Care Nurs. Clin. North Am. 18, 403–417.

Sigurdarson, S.T., O'Shaughnessy, P.T., Watt, J.A., Kline, J.N., 2004. Experimental human exposure to inhaled grain dust and ammonia: towards a model of concentrated animal feeding operations. Am. J. Ind. Med. 46, 345–348.

Simonsen, H.B., Thordal-Christensen, A., Ockens, N., 1981. Carbon monoxide and carbon dioxide euthanasia of cats: duration and animal behaviour. Br. Vet. J. 137, 274–278.

Smilkstein, M.J., Bronstein, A.C., Pickett, H.M., Rumack, B.H., 1985. Hyperbaric oxygen therapy for severe hydrogen sulfide poisoning. J. Emerg. Med. 3, 27–30.

Smith, R.P., 1997. Sulfide poisoning. J. Toxicol. Clin. Toxicol. 35, 305–306.

Stefanidou, M., Athanaselis, S., Spiliopoulou, C., 2008. Health impacts of fire smoke inhalation. Inhal. Toxicol. 20, 761–766.

Stepanek, J., Capizzi, S., Edell, E., 1998. Case in point: silo fillers lung. Hosp. Pract. Minneapolis. 33, 70.

Stoller, K.P., 2007. Hyperbaric oxygen and carbon monoxide poisoning: a critical review. Neurol. Res. 29, 146–155.

Stuart, L.D., Oehme, F.W., 1982. Environmental factors in bovine and porcine abortion. Vet. Hum. Toxicol. 24, 435–441.

Swarbrick, O., 1989. Reduced hatchability associated with engine fumes. Vet. Rec. 125, 444–445.

Tapeantong, T., Poungvarin, N., 2009. Delayed encephalopathy and cognitive sequelae after acute carbon monoxide poisoning: report of a case and review of the literature. J. Med. Assoc. Thai. 92, 1374–1379.

Ten Berge, W.F., Zwart, A., Appelman, L.M., 1986. Concentration-time mortality response relationship of irritant and systematically acting vapours and gases. J. Haz. Mat. 13, 301–309.

Thom, S.R., Mendiguren, I., Fisher, D., 2001. Smoke inhalation-induced alveolar lung injury is inhibited by hyperbaric oxygen. Undersea. Hyperb. Med. 28, 175–179.

Trela, B.A., Bogdanffy, M.S., 1991a. Carboxylesterase-dependent cytotoxicity of dibasic esters (DBE) in rat nasal explants. Toxicol. Appl. Pharmacol. 107, 285–301.

Trela, B.A., Bogdanffy, M.S., 1991b. Cytotoxicity of dibasic esters (DBE) metabolites in rat nasal explants. Toxicol. Appl. Pharmacol. 110, 259–267.

Truong, D.H., Mihajlovic, A., Gunness, P., et al., 2007. Prevention of hydrogen sulfide (H_2S)-induced mouse lethality and cytotoxicity by hydroxocobalamin (vitamin B(12a)). Toxicology. 242, 16–22.

US EPA, US Environmental Protection Agency, 2009. Risk Assessment Guidance for Superfund Volume I: Human Health Evaluation Manual. US EPA, Washington, DC (Part F, Supplemental Guidance for Inhalation Risk Assessment).

Valentine, R., Kennedy, G.L., 2008. Methods. Inhalation toxicology. In: Hayes, A.W. (Ed.), Principles and Methods of Toxicology. CRC Press, New York, pp. 1407–1464. Part 3.

Veltman, K., McKone, T.E., Huijbregts, M.A., Hendriks, A.J., 2009. Bioaccumulation potential of air contaminants: combining biological allometry, chemical equilibrium and mass-balances to predict accumulation of air pollutants in various mammals. Toxicol. Appl. Pharmacol. 238, 47–55.

Verhoeff, J., Counotte, G., Hamhuis, D., 2007. Nitrogen dioxide (silo gas) poisoning in dairy cattle. Tijdschr Diergeneeskd. 132, 780–782.

Weaver, L.K., 2004. Carbon monoxide. In: Dart, R.C., Caravati, E.M., McGuigan, M.A., Whyte, I.M., Dawson, A.H., Seifert, S.A., et al., Medical Toxicology. Lippincott Williams & Wilkins, Philadelphia, pp. 1146–1154.

Welch, A., 2006. Exposing the dangers of anhydrous ammonia. Nurse Pract. 31, 40–45.

Weller, E., Long, N., Smith, A., et al., 1999. Dose-rate effects of ethylene oxide exposure on developmental toxicity. Toxicol. Sci. 50, 259–270.

Whitcraft 3rd, D.D., Bailey, T.D., Hart, G.B., 1985. Hydrogen sulfide poisoning treated with hyperbaric oxygen. J. Emerg. Med. 3, 23–25.

Witschi, H., 1999. Some notes on the history of Haber's law. Toxicol. Sci. 50, 164–168.

Witschi, H., 2000. Fritz Haber: December 9, 1868–January 29, 1934. Toxicology. 149, 3–15.

Witschi, H.R., Last, J.A., 2001. Unit 4 Target organ toxicity. Toxic responses of the respiratory system. In: Klaassen, C.D. (Ed.), Casarett & Doull's Toxicology: The Basic Science of Poisons. McGraw-Hill, New York, pp. 515–534.

Wood, E.N., 1979. Increased incidence of stillbirth in piglets associated with levels of atmospheric carbon monoxide. Vet. Rec. 104, 283–284.

Woodall, G.M., Smith, R.L., Granville, G.C., 2005. Proceedings of the Hydrogen Sulfide Health Research and Risk Assessment Symposium October 31–November 2, 2000. Inhal. Toxicol. 17, 593–639.

Zwemer Jr, F.L., Pratt, D.S., May, J.J., 1992. Silo filler's disease in New York State. Am. Rev. Respir. Dis. 146, 650–653.

FURTHER READING

Derelanko, M.J., Hollinger, M.A., 2001. Handbook of Toxicology. second ed. CRC Press, Boca Raton, FL.

Chapter 49

Alcohols and Glycols

Szabina Stice, Mary A. Thrall and Dwayne W. Hamar

INTRODUCTION

Alcohols are organic compounds containing hydroxyl (−OH) group(s). Alcohols that have one hydroxyl group are called monohydric. These include the three alcohols most commonly responsible for alcohol toxicosis: methanol, ethanol, and isopropanol. Alcohols are also classified as primary, secondary, or tertiary, according to the number of carbon atoms bonded to the carbinol carbon atom (the carbon atom to which the hydroxyl group is bonded). As such, ethanol is classified as a primary alcohol and isopropanol a secondary alcohol. Methanol, in which the carbinol carbon is bonded to no other carbon, is not a primary alcohol per se, but shares many of the reactivity patterns of primary alcohols. Alcohols with two hydroxy groups are called diols or glycols. Ethylene glycol (EG) is the most common glycol responsible for poisonings; EG poisoning is significantly more common in domestic animals than is alcohol toxicosis. Propylene glycol and butylene glycol poisonings are rarer and they are much less toxic than EG.

Alcohols and glycols are initially metabolized by hepatic alcohol dehydrogenase (ADH). Toxicosis from alcohols and glycols results in central nervous system (CNS) depression, ranging from decreased motor function to decreased consciousness, hypothermia, hypotension, coma, and death from respiratory depression, and cardiovascular collapse. However, metabolites of the alcohols and glycols vary greatly in their toxicity. Metabolites of EG are nephrotoxic and they may result in acute renal failure. In primates, metabolites of methanol may cause blindness and permanent neurologic abnormalities. This chapter describes toxicity and treatment of alcohols and glycols in animals.

BACKGROUND

Reports of alcohol toxicosis are relatively rare in domestic animals compared to the reported incidence in humans. Ethanol, methanol, and isopropanol poisoning are all quite common in humans. Methanol and isopropanol are usually ingested by adults as a substitute for ethanol or in an attempt to commit suicide. In children ingestion is usually accidental. Propylene glycol toxicosis is relatively rare in both humans and domestic animals. Butylene glycol toxicosis is also rare and was only reported in humans after use as a "recreational" drug. EG toxicosis is relatively common, both in humans and in domestic animals (Barton and Oehme, 1981; Mueller, 1982; Rowland, 1987; Hornfeldt and Murphy, 1998). In humans, it is ingested either accidentally, as a substitute for ethanol, or to commit suicide; approximately 5000 episodes are reported in the United States each year (Mowry et al., 2015). The vast majority of these poisonings are unintentional, and approximately one-third of the cases occur in children.

Most incidents of EG toxicosis in domestic animals are also accidental, although malicious poisonings also occur. The mortality rate in dogs is reported to range from 50% to 70% (Barton and Oehme, 1981; Rowland, 1987; Connally et al., 1996), and it is likely even higher in cats. EG intoxication is the second most common cause of fatal poisoning in animals, according to the American Association of Poison Control Centers (Hornfeldt and Murphy, 1998).

The first reported case of EG intoxication in a human occurred in 1930 (Anonymous, 1930), but the toxicity of EG was not fully realized until more than 100 people died after consuming an elixir of sulfanilamide containing 96% diethylene glycol (Ballentine, 1981). This incident hastened final enactment in 1938 of the Federal Food, Drug, and Cosmetic Act, the statute that today remains the basis for FDA regulation of these products. Since then, many reports of EG poisoning in humans and animals have been published.

ALCOHOL TOXICOSES

Ethanol Toxicosis

Ethanol (ethyl alcohol or grain alcohol, CH_3CH_2OH) is the alcohol used in mouth washes, perfumes, and alcoholic

Veterinary Toxicology. DOI: http://dx.doi.org/10.1016/B978-0-12-811410-0.00049-0

beverages. Ethanol toxicosis in dogs has been associated with ingestion of bread dough (Thrall et al., 1984a; Suter, 1992; Means, 2003). Uncooked bread dough contains *Saccharomyces cerevisiae* (common brewer's and baker's yeast) that metabolizes carbohydrate substrates to ethanol and carbon dioxide. Ethanol poisoning in dogs has also been associated with rotten apples (Kammerer et al., 2001) and alcoholic beverages (van Wuijckhuise and Cremers, 2003). Ethanol is also an ingredient in many liquid formulations of various medications; some products contain as much as 25% ethanol (Papich, 1990). Although it is unlikely that a pet would ingest enough ethanol from these preparations to produce ethanol toxicosis, the alcohol may augment the depressive effects of other ingredients. Ethanol toxicosis can also occur in dogs and cats when ethanol is given intravenously (i.v.) as a competitive substrate to treat EG toxicosis (Thrall et al., 1998). Ethanol intoxication was also reported in a litter of 6-week-old puppies shampooed with an alcohol-based detergent (Del Mar, 1984). The median lethal dose (LD_{50}) of 100% ethanol in dogs is 4.1–4.9 g/kg after ingestion (Du Jardin-Beaumet, 1875).

Toxicokinetics

Ethanol is rapidly absorbed from the gastrointestinal (GI) tract; the rate of absorption can be slowed by the presence of food in the stomach or small intestine. Most of the ethanol is metabolized in the liver to acetaldehyde (a toxic metabolite) by ADH and then to acetate by aldehyde dehydrogenase (Fig. 49.1). The end products of ethanol metabolism are carbon dioxide and water.

Clinical findings in dogs and cats with ethanol intoxication can be correlated with blood ethanol concentration (BEC). Clinical signs include ataxia, lethargy, sedation, hypothermia, metabolic acidosis, vomiting, diarrhea, and poor breathing (Kovalkovicova et al., 2009). Levels of 2–4 mg/mL in adult dogs have produced clinical signs ranging from ataxia and coma (Valentine, 1990). The time of onset of clinical signs is dependent on the dose ingested and the amount of food present in the GI tract, but it usually occurs within an hour of ingestion.

Mechanism of Action

The mechanism of action of alcohol on the CNS is related in part to its interactions with biomembranes and its probable inhibition of gamma-aminobutyric acid receptors (Valentine, 1990).

Diagnosis and Treatment

A diagnosis can be made based on history, clinical signs, increased plasma osmolality and osmole gap, metabolic acidosis, and BEC. If rapid BEC cannot be obtained, the animal has to be treated based on clinical signs. It is important to differentiate EG toxicosis from alcohol toxicosis as the clinical signs and early laboratory findings can be similar. However, patients with EG toxicosis must be given ADH inhibitors such as 4-methylpyrazole to prevent the formation of toxic metabolites, whereas patients with ethanol toxicosis can be treated supportively. Heart and respiratory rate should be monitored. Respiratory depression may require the administration of Doxapram (a respiratory stimulant) or in severe cases mechanical ventilation. Emesis should not be induced in dogs or cats with severe ataxia or CNS depression as the animal could become recumbent or comatose quickly and aspiration

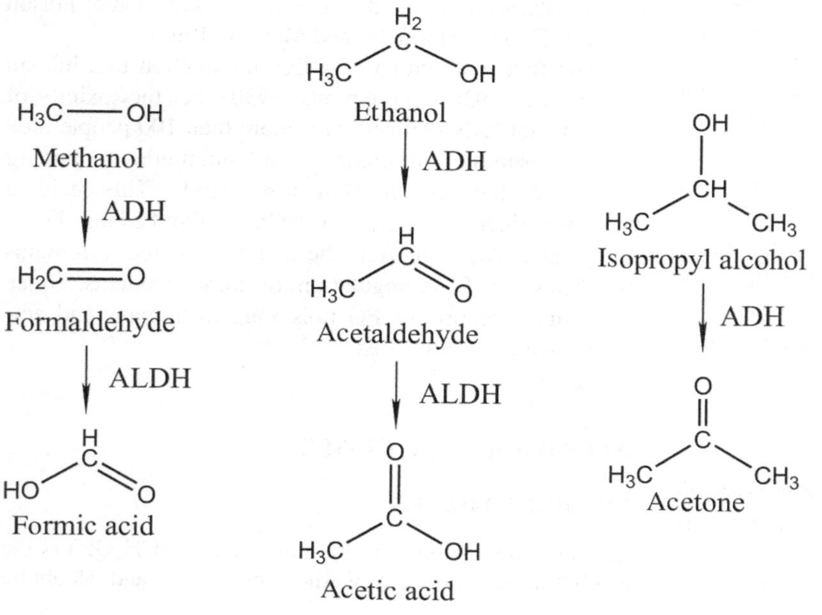

FIGURE 49.1 Pathways of formation of toxic metabolites for methanol, ethanol, and isopropyl alcohol.

could occur (Means, 2003). Hypothermia may develop, and alterations in hydration, electrolyte, and acid–base status should be corrected (Richardson, 2006).

Methanol Toxicosis

Methanol (methyl alcohol or wood alcohol, CH_3OH) is widely used as a solvent, fuel (Sterno), gasoline additive, antifreeze, and windshield washer fluid (30–40% methanol). The minimum lethal dose (MLD) in dogs is between 3.9 and 8.9 g/kg, and in rats, rabbits, rhesus monkeys, and human beings it is 9.5, 7, 3, and 0.99 g/kg, respectively, indicating a variation in species susceptibility to methanol toxicosis (Valentine, 1990; Gilger and Potts, 1955). Methanol toxicosis is rare in dogs, but it has been reported in a dog that chewed open a bottle of 98% methanol antifreeze (Hurd-Kuenzi, 1983).

Toxicokinetics

Ingested methanol is absorbed quickly from the GI tract, and peak methanol concentrations occur within 30–60 min following ingestion (Barceloux et al., 2002). Toxicosis has also been reported following inhalation or dermal absorption. The rate of elimination of methanol from the blood is slower than that of ethanol. Methanol is metabolized by ADH to formaldehyde, which is oxidized to formic acid by formaldehyde dehydrogenase (Fig. 49.1). In mammals other than primates, formic acid is detoxified relatively rapidly to yield carbon dioxide and water. Formic acid is metabolized less efficiently in primates. This may lead to the accumulation of formic acid, which plays a major part in the development of acidosis observed in primates. Consequently, methanol is more toxic to humans and nonhuman primates that it is to other mammals.

Mechanism of Action

Formic acid is responsible for ocular and CNS lesions in primates as a result of the inhibition of cytochrome oxidase (Roe, 1982). Blindness and permanent neurological abnormalities are common sequelae in primates.

Diagnosis and Treatment

Clinical signs in animals other than primates are similar to those seen with ethanol toxicosis and are primarily related to CNS depression. Vomiting and abdominal pain may be seen. In primates, following the initial nausea and CNS depression, a latent period of approximately 12–24 h is followed by metabolic acidosis and impaired visual function. Coma, other CNS signs, and death (20–30 h) may follow after significant exposures. Laboratory findings in primates include hyperosmolality, increased anion gap, and severe metabolic acidosis (Bischoff, 2006a). Diagnosis can be made by history and measurement of blood methanol concentrations (or formic acid in primates).

Treatment in nonprimates is symptomatic and similar to treatment for ethanol toxicosis. Primates are treated with 4-methylpyrazole to compete with ADH to inhibit the bioactivation of methanol (Barceloux et al., 2002) or, alternatively, with ethanol. It is probably inappropriate to treat methanol toxicosis in nonprimates with ethanol because ethanol contributes to the sedation, and the metabolites of methanol do not cause blindness in nonprimates, as they do in primates. Hemodialysis is also used to remove formic acid. Folic acid is given i.v. to enhance formic acid metabolism.

Isopropanol Toxicosis

Isopropanol (isopropyl alcohol or IPA, $CH_3CH(OH)CH_3$) is found in rubbing alcohol (70%), antifreeze, detergents, window cleaning products, and disinfectants. Ingestion is the usual cause of poisoning in humans, although toxicity from inhalation and topical absorption has been reported. Isopropanol toxicosis is rare in domestic animals, possibly due to its bitter taste. It has been reported in a horse that was mistakenly administered isopropanol via nasogastric intubation for colic; the isopropanol was mistaken for mineral oil (Somerville and Plumlee, 1996).

Toxicokinetics

Isopropanol is approximately twofold more toxic than ethanol in dogs, rabbits, and rats (Lehman and Chase, 1944) and about as toxic as methanol when taken orally. On the other hand, it is safer after dermal exposure as it does not pass through the skin as easily as methanol. It is rapidly absorbed from the GI tract, and approximately 80% is metabolized to acetone, which is also a CNS depressant, but acetone has a much longer half-life (16–20 h) than does alcohol (Fig. 49.1). Acetone is further metabolized to CO_2. The metabolism of IPA appears equivalent across species.

Diagnosis and Treatment

Clinical signs associated with isopropanol toxicosis are similar to those for ethanol toxicosis and include CNS depression, hypotension, vomiting, and abdominal pain due to severe gastritis, which is secondary to direct irritation. The breath of patients who have ingested isopropanol has a characteristic acetone-like odor (Somerville and Plumlee, 1996). Treatment is supportive and includes fluids, correction of acid-base abnormalities, and assisted respiration, if necessary (Oehme and Kore, 2006). Hemodialysis is effective in removing isopropanol and acetone, and 4-methylpyrazole will prevent the metabolism of isopropanol to acetone.

GLYCOL TOXICOSES

Propylene Glycol Toxicosis

Propylene glycol (1,2-propanediol, $CH_3CH(OH)CH_2OH$) is one of the least toxic of the glycols. It is used as automotive antifreeze, an industrial and pharmaceutical solvent, in cosmetics, and as an additive in processed food for human and animal consumption. Although it is considered nontoxic compared to EG, it causes CNS depression and lactic acidosis when ingested in large quantities. When used as an additive in semimoist cat food, it caused Heinz body formation in erythrocytes (inclusions within red blood cells composed of denatured hemoglobin) but did not cause anemia when ingested in small quantities (Christopher et al., 1989a,b; Weiss et al., 1990; Bauer et al., 1992a,b). However, cats eating such diets were more susceptible to other additional causes of oxidative injury, and although overt anemia may not occur, red cells with Heinz bodies have a reduced life span. Consequently, the use of propylene glycol in cat foods is prohibited in the United States.

The oral median lethal dose for propylene glycol in dogs has been reported to be as low as 9 mL/kg ($\approx$8.7 g/kg) (Bischoff, 2006b). Fatal cases of malicious propylene glycol toxicosis have been reported in dogs (Bischoff, 2006b). It is considered relatively unpalatable to dogs (Marshall and Doty, 1990). Fatal propylene glycol toxicosis was reported in a horse that was inadvertently given 7.6 mL/kg ($\approx$7.3 g/kg) propylene glycol orally instead of mineral oil for potential grain overload (Dorman and Hascheck, 1991). Cause of death was presumed to be from respiratory arrest. Propylene glycol toxicosis has been reported in at least two other horses with colic in which propylene glycol was mistakenly administered instead of mineral oil (Myers and Usenik, 1969; McClanahan et al., 1998); both horses survived: they were both given approximately 6 mL/kg ($\approx$5.8 g/kg) body weight via nasogastric tube. Heinz body formation also occurs in horses ingesting propylene glycol (McClanahan et al., 1998). Propylene glycol may be used to treat and prevent bovine ketosis, which may partially explain the availability and apparent ease with which it is confused with mineral oil.

Toxicokinetics

In mammals, part of the propylene glycol dose is eliminated unchanged by the kidney and part is metabolized by the liver to lactic acid (responsible for metabolic acidosis) by ADH and further metabolized to pyruvic acid; in mammals, with the exception of cats, the remainder is conjugated with glucuronic acid and eliminated in the urine (Fig. 49.2). The CNS depression resulting from large, single doses of propylene glycol is probably due to the excessive presence of propylene glycol and not to its metabolic products (Cavender and Sowinski, 1994).

Diagnosis and Treatment

Clinical signs depend on the quantity ingested and may include depression, ataxia, muscle fasciculations, hypotension, osmotic diuresis, respiratory arrest, and circulatory collapse. Clinical signs in ruminants are similar to those seen in other species and include ataxia, depression, and recumbency (Pintchuck et al., 1993). Laboratory findings include metabolic acidosis, increased anion gap, hyper osmolality of the plasma, and the presence of Heinz bodies in cats and horses. Diagnosis is usually based on history of exposure and can be confirmed by measuring propylene glycol concentrations in urine and serum by gas chromatography. Treatment for all species is supportive and includes correction of hydration and acid-base abnormalities. Most animals recover within 24–27 h with supportive care. To slow the production of toxic metabolites 4-methylpyrazole may be given. Dialysis may be used after significant exposure in dogs.

Butylene Glycol Toxicosis

Butylene glycol (1,2-, 1,3-, and 1,4-butanediol,$C_4H_{10}O_2$) is used as antifreeze, as an industrial cleaner, and in cosmetics. Although no published reports of butylene glycol toxicosis in domestic animals were found in the literature, there are numerous reports of human intoxications from butylene glycol or the metabolite gamma-hydroxybutyrate (Dyer, 1991; Mack, 1993). Butylene glycol and the metabolite gamma-hydroxybutyrate are used as "recreational" drugs and were once marketed by health food stores as a food additive for bodybuilders and to treat depression and insomnia.

1,3-Butanediol has been used as an antidote for experimental EG toxicosis in dogs because it is a competitive substrate for ADH (Thrall et al., 1982; Murphy et al., 1984; Cox et al., 1992). Although it was found to be a more effective antidote than ethanol, in that more unmetabolized EG was excreted in the urine in patients treated with 1,3-butanediol, CNS depression was as severe or more severe than that induced by ethanol therapy, and plasma hyperosmolality and metabolic acidosis were more severe than with ethanol therapy (Thrall et al., 1982).

Toxicokinetics

Butylene glycol is metabolized by ADH to acetoacetate and gamma-hydroxybutyrate, the so-called "date rape" drug.

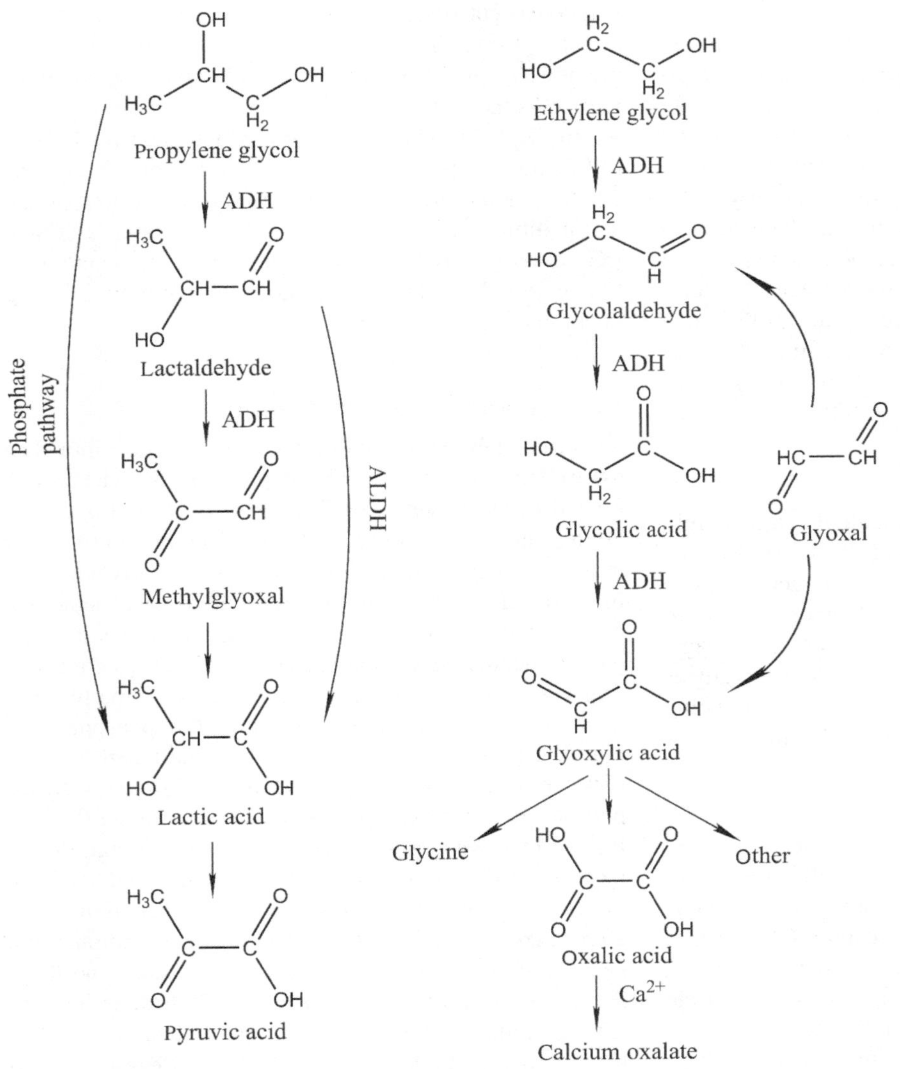

FIGURE 49.2 Pathways of formation of toxic metabolites for propylene glycol and ethylene glycol.

Mechanism of Action

Butylene glycol is a CNS depressant much like ethanol, due to the effect of the metabolite gamma-hydroxybutyrate on the CNS. In large quantities butylene glycol can result in seizures and respiratory arrest.

Treatment

Therapy for butylene glycol toxicosis in humans is supportive, similar to therapy for ethanol toxicosis.

Ethylene Glycol Toxicosis

EG (1,2-ethanediol, $HOCH_2CH_2OH$) is used primarily as an antifreeze and a windshield deicing agent. It is also used as a cryoprotectant for embryo preservation, in the manufacture of polyester compounds, as a solvent in the paint and plastic industries, and as an ingredient in photographic developing solutions, hydraulic brake fluid and motor oil, and inks and wood stains (Davis et al., 1997). The most readily available source of EG in the home is antifreeze solutions, which consist of approximately 95% EG. Because of its sweet taste, EG is often consumed unintentionally by children and animals. Aversive bittering agents may be added to EG containing antifreeze to try to prevent ingestions by making the antifreeze unpalatable.

The MLDs reported in the literature for humans, rats, dogs, and cats are 1.57, 3.8–11, 6.7–7.3, and 1 g/kg, respectively (LaKind et al., 1999). Based on the MLDs, on a body weight basis, EG appears to be more acutely toxic to humans and cats than to other experimental animals.

Toxicokinetics

Before it is metabolized, EG is no more toxic than ethanol, although EG is a more potent CNS depressant than ethanol (Berger and Ayyar, 1981). However, EG is biotransformed to highly toxic metabolites that results in severe metabolic acidosis and acute renal failure, hallmarks of EG poisoning (Thrall et al., 1984b; Dial et al., 1994a,b; Davis et al., 1997). EG is initially oxidized to glycoaldehyde by ADH, and glycoaldehyde is then oxidized to glycolic acid, and then to glyoxylic acid (Fig. 49.2). Glyoxylic acid is primarily converted to oxalic acid but may follow other metabolic pathways; end products may also include glycine, formic acid, hippuric acid, oxalomalic acid, and benzoic acid. Oxalic acid forms calcium oxalate crystals with calcium. Cats are unusually sensitive to EG due to their high baseline production of oxalic acid (LaKind et al., 1999).

Mechanism of Action

EG and its first metabolite, glycoaldehyde, are mainly responsible for CNS toxicity (LaKind et al., 1999). The accumulation of glycolic acid and glyoxylic acid leads to metabolic acidosis. Acidosis is also thought to lead to altered levels of consciousness and cerebral damage. Calcium oxalate crystal deposition in various organs is widespread but is most severe in the kidney producing renal damage. Renal toxicity may also be due to the cytotoxicity of other EG metabolites.

Clinical Signs

Initial symptoms (Stage I, 30 min to 12 h after ingestion) may be similar to drunkenness, but without the characteristic breath odor of alcohol. EG also causes GI irritation and high EG blood concentrations. Symptoms in Stage I include nausea, vomiting, ataxia and knuckling, muscle fasciculations, decreased withdrawal reflexes and righting ability, hypothermia, and osmotic diuresis with resultant polyuria and polydipsia (Grauer et al., 1984; Thrall et al., 1984b; Connally et al., 1996). As CNS depression increases in severity, dogs drink less but osmotic diuresis persists, resulting in dehydration. In dogs, CNS signs abate after approximately 12 h, and patients may briefly appear to have recovered. Cats usually remain markedly depressed and do not exhibit polydipsia. Animals may be severely hypothermic. Stage II is characterized by pulmonary toxicity. Symptoms may include tachycardia, tachypnea, pulmonary edema, hyperventilation, and shallow and rapid breathing. Over time, as a result of glycolic and glyoxylic acid accumulation during metabolism, profound acidosis will present. Glycolic acid accumulates because the lactic dehydrogenase enzyme that metabolizes glycolic to glyoxylic acid becomes saturated. As glycolic acid is further metabolized to oxalic acid, which then crystalizes with calcium, hypocalcemia may occur along with the precipitation of calcium oxalate crystals in the kidney, which will produce renal toxicity in Stage III. Crystalluria is a consistent finding in animals producing urine (Grauer et al., 1984; Thrall et al., 1984b). As mentioned previously, renal toxicity may also be due to the cytotoxicity of other EG metabolites. Renal failure is evident by 36–72 h following ingestion in dogs and by 12–24 h following ingestion in cats. Anuria often develops 72–96 h after ingestion. The kidneys are often swollen and painful, particularly in cats. The three stages of acute EG toxicity may overlap depending on the amount of EG ingested. Delayed neurological symptoms, though uncommon, may present.

Early Laboratory Abnormalities

Abnormal laboratory findings can be divided into those associated with early EG intoxication, which may be related to the presence of EG per se or to its toxic metabolites, and those associated with late EG intoxication, most of which are related to renal failure. Early abnormalities are primarily due to the presence of acid metabolites of EG in the serum that result in metabolic acidosis and include decreased plasma bicarbonate (HCO_3^-) concentration and increased anion gap. In addition, hyperphosphatemia may occur due to ingestion of a phosphate rust inhibitor present in some commercial antifreeze products (Grauer et al., 1984; Connally et al., 1996). The decreased plasma HCO_3^- concentration can be seen as early as 1 h following EG ingestion. Metabolites of EG significantly increase the pool of unmeasured anions and cause an increased anion gap. The anion gap is increased by 3 h after ingestion, peaks at 6 h after EG concentration, which peaks 1–6 h following ingestion. EG is usually no longer detectable in the serum or urine 48–72 h after ingestion (Thrall et al., 1982; Grauer et al., 1984; Dial et al., 1994a, b). Kits (e.g., Ethylene Glycol Test Kit, PRN Pharmacol, Pensacola, Florida) are available that accurately estimate blood EG concentrations with a minimum detection limit of 50 mg/dL, and the results correlate well with other established methods of measuring EG concentrations such as gas chromatography (Dasgupta et al., 1995), although the presence of propylene glycol or glycerol in the blood may cause a false-positive test result. Ethanol and methanol do not result in a false-positive test result. Cats may be intoxicated with a lethal dose of EG that is below the 50 mg/dL detectable level of the EG test kit. Therefore, if the test kit is negative and historical findings as well as clinical signs are compatible with EG ingestion, the recommendation is to initiate appropriate therapy for EG intoxication as well as submit a serum sample to a reference laboratory capable of determining a quantitative concentration.

Determination of serum osmolality is also useful for diagnosing early EG toxicosis, although other osmotically active, low-molecular-weight alcohols and glycols could also increase serum osmolality. Serum osmolality is increased within an hour of EG ingestion, increasing in parallel with serum EG concentrations (Dial et al., 1994a,b). When measured serum osmolality (by osmometry) is compared to calculated serum osmolality, the difference is referred to as the osmole or osmolal gap. Normal serum osmolality is 280–310 mOsm/kg, and the normal osmole gap is less than 10 mOsm/kg. Serum osmolality as high as 450 mOsm/kg and an osmole gap as high as 150 mOsm/kg may be seen 3 h after ingestion, depending on the quantity of antifreeze ingested (Jacobsen et al., 1982b; Grauer et al., 1984). Both the gap and the measured osmolality may remain significantly high for approximately 18 h after ingestion. Multiplication of the osmole gap by five yields an approximate serum EG concentration in mg/dL (Burkhart and Kulig, 1990). Each 100 mg/dL increment increase in EG concentration contributes approximately 16 mOsm/kg H_2O to the serum osmolality (Eder et al., 1998). Simultaneous or sequential increases in osmole and anion gaps are very suggestive of EG intoxication. As EG is metabolized, its contribution to the osmole gap diminishes because the accumulating negatively charged metabolites do not contribute to the osmole gap (Eder et al., 1998). Two types of instruments are used to measure osmolality: freezing point osmometers and vapor pressure osmometers. Because EG is nonvolatile (boiling point, 197°C), it is detected by either the freezing point or vapor pressure methods. However, methanol, ethanol, and other volatile compounds, although contributing to serum osmolality, may go undetected if assayed by the vapor pressure method. Most clinical laboratories use the freezing point method (Kruse and Cadnapaphornchai, 1994). Osmolality can be measured using serum or plasma; if the latter is used, heparin is the preferred anticoagulant. Other anticoagulants, such as EDTA, can markedly increase osmolality and can result in spurious increases in the osmole gap (Kruse and Cadnapaphornchai, 1994).

Dogs are isosthenuric (urine specific gravity of 1.008–1.012) by 3 h following ingestion of EG due to osmotic diuresis and serum hyperosmolality-induced polydipsia (Grauer et al., 1984; Dial et al., 1994a). The urine specific gravity in cats is also decreased by 3 h after ingestion but may be above the isosthenuric range (Dial et al., 1994b; Fogazzi, 1996). Calcium oxalate crystalluria is a common finding and may be observed as early as 3 and 6 h after ingestion in the cat and dog, respectively, as a result of oxalic acid combining with calcium (Dial et al., 1994a,b). Calcium oxalate monohydrate crystals are variably sized, clear, six-sided prisms (Fig. 49.3) (Scully et al., 1979; Terlinsky et al., 1981; Jacobsen et al., 1982a; Kramer et al., 1984; Thrall et al., 1985). In animals and people poisoned with EG, the monohydrate form is observed more frequently than the dihydrate form, which appears as an envelope or Maltese cross (Connally et al., 1996; Eder et al., 1998). Dumbbell or sheaf-shaped crystals are observed infrequently. The detection of calcium oxalate crystalluria, particularly the monohydrate form, provides strong supporting evidence for the diagnosis of EG poisoning (Fogazzi, 1996). Urinary pH consistently decreases following EG ingestion.

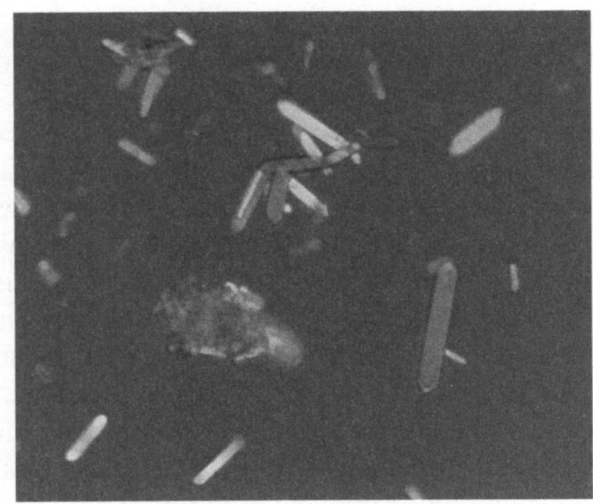

FIGURE 49.3 Calcium oxalate monohydrate crystals (polarized light) from a dog with EG toxicosis.

Another diagnostic procedure that may be helpful in detecting early EG intoxication is examination of the oral cavity, face, paws, vomitus, and urine with a Wood's lamp to determine whether they appear fluorescent. Many antifreeze solutions manufactured today contain sodium fluorescein, a fluorescent dye that aids in the detection of leaks in vehicle coolant systems. The dye is excreted in the urine for up to 6 h following ingestion of the antifreeze (Winter et al., 1990). A negative test does not eliminate the possibility of EG ingestion because not all antifreeze solutions contain the dye.

Late Laboratory Abnormalities

With the onset of renal damage and subsequent decreased glomerular filtration, serum creatinine and blood urea nitrogen (BUN) concentrations increase. In the dog, these increases begin to occur between 24 and 48 h following EG ingestion. In the cat, BUN and creatinine begin to increase approximately 12 h after ingestion; however, because cats do not develop polydipsia, this may be in part due to dehydration. Serum phosphorus concentrations increase at this time due to decreased glomerular filtration. Hyperkalemia develops with the onset of oliguria and anuria. Serum calcium concentration is decreased in approximately half of patients (Thrall et al., 1984b; Connally et al., 1996) and is due to the formation of insoluble calcium oxalate. Clinical signs of hypocalcemia are infrequently observed because acidosis results in a shift to the ionized, physiologically active form of calcium. Serum glucose concentration is increased in approximately 50%

of dogs and cats (Thrall et al., 1984b; Connally et al., 1996) and is attributed to inhibition of glucose metabolism by aldehydes, increased epinephrine and endogenous corticosteroids, and uremia. Animals presenting with late EG poisoning are likely to have little or no osmole gap increase but will have an increased osmolality (whether calculated or measured) because of the azotemia and hyperglycemia. Animals remain isosthenuric in the later stages of toxicosis due to renal dysfunction and impaired ability to concentrate urine. Calcium oxalate crystalluria persists for as long as animals are producing urine. Urine abnormalities associated with renal damage may include hematuria, proteinuria, and glucosuria. Granular and cellular casts, white blood cells, red blood cells, and renal epithelial cells may be observed in the urine sediment of some patients (Thrall et al., 1984b; Connally et al., 1996).

Treatment

Therapy for EG poisoning is aimed at preventing absorption, increasing excretion, and preventing metabolism of EG. Supportive care to correct fluid, acid–base, and electrolyte imbalances is also helpful. Although therapeutic recommendations have traditionally included induction of vomiting, gastric lavage, and administration of activated charcoal (Thrall et al., 1995, 1998), it is likely that these procedures are not beneficial because of the rapidity with which EG is absorbed (Davis et al., 1997). The most critical aspect of therapy is based on prevention of EG oxidation by ADH, the enzyme responsible for the initial reaction in the EG metabolic pathway (Parry and Wallach, 1974). Typically, dogs must be treated within 8 h following ingestion and cats must be treated within 3 h for treatment to be successful (Dial et al., 1994a,b). However, this is somewhat dependent on the amount of EG ingested. Historically, treating EG toxicosis has been directed toward inhibiting EG metabolism with ethanol, a competitive substrate that has a higher affinity for ADH than EG (Penumarthy and Oehme, 1975; Bostrom and Li, 1980). Ethanol has numerous disadvantages because it enhances many of the metabolic effects of EG. Both ethanol and EG are CNS depressants, and it is the compounded CNS depression that most limits the usefulness of ethanol as an antidote. Additional disadvantages of ethanol treatment include its metabolism to acetaldehyde, which impairs glucose metabolism and is a cerebral irritant. Ethanol also contributes to metabolic acidosis by enhancing the formation of lactic acid from pyruvate and may potentiate hypocalcemia (Money et al., 1989). Moreover, ethanol compounds the effects of EG-induced osmotic diuresis and serum hyperosmolality (Kruse and Cadnapaphornchai, 1994).

4-Methylpyrazole (fomepizole) has become the preferred antidote in dogs (Grauer et al., 1987; Dial et al., 1989; Connally et al., 1996) and cats (Thrall et al., 2006; Connally et al., 2010). Fomepizole is an ADH inhibitor, not a competitive substrate, and it does not induce CNS depression (in dogs), diuresis, or hyperosmolality at the recommended dosage. The recommended dose of fomepizole for dogs is 20 mg/kg body weight i.v. initially, followed by 15 mg/kg i.v. at 12 and 24 h and 5 mg/kg i.v. at 36 h (Grauer et al., 1987; Connally et al., 1996; Thrall et al., 2006). Cats must be given a much higher dose of fomepizole than dogs because feline ADH is less effectively inhibited by fomepizole than is canine ADH (Connally et al., 2000, 2010). Cats are initially treated with 125 mg/kg fomepizole i.v. followed by 31.25 mg/kg i.v. fomepizole at 12, 24, and 36 h. The only adverse clinical sign that the authors have observed is CNS depression that appears to be fomepizole related (Connally et al., 2010). If ingestion of a large dose of EG is suspected, repeating serum quantification tests can be performed to determine whether continuation of therapy beyond 36 h is necessary. Alternatively, additional doses of fomepizole can be administered empirically. Appropriate therapy also consists of i.v. fluids to correct dehydration, increase tissue perfusion, and promote diuresis. The fluid volume administered should be based on the maintenance, deficit, and continuing loss needs of the patient. Frequent measurement of urine production, serum urea nitrogen and creatinine, and blood pH, bicarbonate, ionized calcium, and electrolytes daily or twice daily will help guide fluid and electrolyte therapy (Grauer, 1998). Bicarbonate should be given slowly i.v. to correct the metabolic acidosis. Hypothermia can be controlled with blankets or the use of a pad with circulating warm water.

In animals that are azotemic and in oliguric renal failure on presentation, almost all of the EG has been metabolized, and treatment to inhibit ADH is likely to be of little benefit. However, ADH inhibitors should be given up to 36 h following ingestion to prevent the metabolism of any residual EG. Fluid, electrolyte, and acid–base disorders should be corrected and diuresis established, if possible. Diuretics, particularly mannitol, may be helpful. The tubular damage caused by EG may be reversible, but tubular repair can take weeks to months. Animals may take up to 1 year following EG toxicosis to regain concentrating ability, and some remain isosthenuric. Supportive care to maintain the patient during the period of renal tubular regeneration is necessary, and peritoneal dialysis may be useful (Shahar and Holmberg, 1985; Fox et al., 1987; Crisp et al., 1989). Hemodialysis has been attempted in dogs with EG-induced renal failure (DiBartola et al., 1985) and has been shown to have a relatively good success rate in cats with acute renal failure (Langston et al., 1997). Renal transplantation has also been used with variable success in cats with renal failure (Mathews and Gregory, 1997) and has been described in dogs (Nemeth et al., 1997).

Prognosis

EG has a very high potential for a lethal outcome, but with early recognition of the syndrome and timely institution of therapy, animals can be saved. The quantity of EG ingested, rate of absorption, and time interval prior to institution of therapy are variables that affect the prognosis. The prognosis is excellent in dogs treated with fomepizole within 5 h of ingesting EG. In a retrospective study of dogs with confirmed EG poisoning, all of the dogs that were azotemic when initially treated died. Of the dogs that did not have azotemia when initially treated, approximately 90% survived (Connally et al., 1996). The prognosis for cats is reasonably good if treatment is instituted within 3 h following ingestion (Dial et al., 1994b). In contrast, the prognosis in humans who survive the initial syndrome of severe acidosis is very good. Terminal renal failure in humans is rare, and most human patients regain renal function by 2 months following EG poisoning (Davis et al., 1997) likely due to the effectiveness of hemodialysis therapy in humans (Christiansson et al., 1995).

CONCLUDING REMARKS AND FUTURE DIRECTIONS

Ethanol, methanol, isopropanol, propylene glycol, and butylene glycol toxicosis can produce ataxia and other CNS signs similar to those seen in acute EG poisoning but are much less common than EG toxicosis. These disorders can be differentiated by the diagnostic laboratory tests discussed previously. Other causes of an increased anion gap include diabetic ketoacidosis and lactic acidosis; these disorders can also be differentiated by appropriate laboratory tests. Other causes of increased osmolality include ethanol, isopropanol, methanol, and propylene glycol toxicosis. Ethanol, like EG, can also produce hypocalcemia (Money et al., 1989). Other differentials for acute renal failure include leptospirosis, ibuprofen, and other nonsteroidal antiinflammatory drug toxicosis, aminoglycoside antibiotics, hemolyticuremic syndrome, cholecalciferol toxicosis, grape and raisin toxicosis in dogs, and ingestion of oxalate-containing plants such as philodendron and lily toxicosis in cats (Brown et al., 1985; Gunther et al., 1988; Peterson et al., 1991; Holloway et al., 1993; Vaden et al., 1997a,b; Poortinga and Hungerford, 1998; Forrester and Troy, 1999; Adin and Cowgill, 2000; Hovda, 2000; Rumbeiha et al., 2000; Langston, 2002; Tefft, 2004). The majority of dogs with grape and raisin toxicosis are hypercalcemic, as are animals with cholecalciferol toxicosis (Fooshee and Forrester, 1990; Gwaltney-Brant et al., 2001); hypercalcemia is not associated with EG toxicosis (Thrall et al., 1984b; Connally et al., 1996). Acute renal failure must be differentiated from acutely decompensated chronic renal failure. Carbamylated hemoglobin concentration has been shown to be useful in making this differentiation (Vaden et al., 1997b; Heiene et al., 2001). In addition, animals with chronic renal failure may be anemic and in poor body condition. A history of the duration of clinical signs is also helpful. Continuing to increase the awareness of the toxicity of EG, as well as other alcohols and glycols, will aid in preventing exposure and result in earlier treatment of animals.

REFERENCES

Adin, C.A., Cowgill, L.D., 2000. Treatment and outcome of dogs with leptospirosis: 36 cases (1990–1998). J. Am. Vet. Med. Assoc. 216, 371–375.

Anonymous, 1930. Possible death from drinking ethylene glycol ("Prestone"): queries and minor notes. J. Am. Med. Assoc. 94, 1940.

Ballentine, C., 1981. Sulfanilamide disaster. FDA Consumer magazine.

Barceloux, D.G., Bond, G.R., Krenzelok, E.P., et al., 2002. American Academy of Clinical Toxicology practice guidelines on the treatment of methanol poisoning. Clin. Toxicol. 40, 415–446.

Barton, J., Oehme, F.J., 1981. The incidence and characteristics of animal poisonings seen at Kansas State University from 1975 to 1980. Vet. Hum. Toxicol. 23, 101–102.

Bauer, M.C., Weiss, D.J., Perman, V., 1992a. Hematologic alterations in adult cats fed 6 or 12% propylene glycol. Am. J. Vet. Res. 53, 69–72.

Bauer, M.C., Weiss, D.J., Perman, V., 1992b. Hematological alterations in kittens induced by 6 and 12% dietary propylene glycol. Vet. Hum. Toxicol. 34, 127–131.

Berger, J.R., Ayyar, D.R., 1981. Neurological complications of ethylene glycol intoxication: report of a case. Arch. Neurol. 38, 724–726.

Bischoff, K., 2006a. Methanol. In: Peterson, M., Talcott, P. (Eds.), Small Animal Toxicology. Saunders, St. Louis, MO, pp. 840–844.

Bischoff, K., 2006b. Propylene glycol. In: Peterson, M., Talcott, P. (Eds.), Small Animal Toxicology. Saunders, St. Louis, MO, pp. 996–1001.

Bostrom, W.F., Li, T., 1980. Alcohol dehydrogenase enzyme. In: Jakoby, W.B. (Ed.), Enzyme Basis of Detoxification. Academic Press, New York, pp. 231–248.

Brown, S.A., Barsanti, J.A., Crowell, W.A., 1985. Gentamicin-associated acute renal failure in the dog. J. Am. Vet. Med. Assoc. 186, 686–690.

Burkhart, K.K., Kulig, K.W., 1990. The other alcohols. Emerg. Med. Clin. North Am. 8, 913–928.

Cavender, F.L., Sowinski, E.J., 1994. Glycols. In: Calayton, G.D., Clayton, F.E. (Eds.), Patty's Industrial Hygiene and Toxicology. Vol. 2F: Toxicology, fourth rev. ed. Wiley, New York, pp. 4645–4719.

Christiansson, L.K., Kaspersson, K.E., Kulling, P.E., et al., 1995. Treatment of severe ethylene glycol intoxication with continuous arteriovenous hemofiltration dialysis. J. Toxicol. Clin. Toxicol. 33, 267–270.

Christopher, M.M., Perman, V., Eaton, J.W., 1989a. Contribution of propylene glycol-induced Heinz body formation to anemia in cats. J. Am. Vet. Med. Assoc. 194, 1045–1056.

Christopher, M.M., Perman, V., White, J.G., 1989b. Propylene glycol-induced Heinz body formation and d-lactic acidosis in cats. Prog. Clin. Biol. Res. 319, 69–87.

Connally, H.E., Thrall, M.A., Forzney, S.D., et al., 1996. Safety and efficacy of 4-methylpyrazole as treatment for suspected or confirmed ethylene glycol intoxication in dogs: 107 cases (1983–1995). J. Am. Vet. Med. Assoc. 209, 1880–1883.

Connally, H.E., Hamar, D.W., Thrall, M.A., 2000. Inhibition of canine and feline alcohol dehydrogenase activity by fomepizole. Am. J. Vet. Res. 61, 450–455.

Connally, H.E., Thrall, M.A., Hamar, D.W., 2010. Safety and efficacy of high dose fomepizole compared to ethanol as therapy for ethylene glycol intoxication in cats. J. Vet. Emerg. Crit. Care. 20 (2), 191–206.

Cox, S.K., Ferslew, K.E., Boelen, L.J., 1992. The toxicokinetics of 1,3 butylene glycol versus ethanol in the treatment of ethylene glycol poisoning. Vet. Hum. Toxicol. 34, 36–42.

Crisp, M.S., Chew, D.J., DiBartola, S.P., et al., 1989. Peritoneal dialysis in dogs and cats: 27 cases (1976–1987). J. Am. Vet. Med. Assoc. 195, 1262–1266.

Dasgupta, A., Blackwell, W., Griego, J., et al., 1995. Gas chromatographic–mass spectrometric identification and quantitation of ethylene glycol in serum after derivatization with perfluorooctanoyl chloride: a novel derivative. J. Chromatogr. B Biomed. Appl. 666, 63–70.

Davis, D.P., Bramwell, K.J., Hamilton, R.S., et al., 1997. Ethylene glycol poisoning: case report of a record-high level and a review. J. Emerg. Med. 15, 653–657.

Del Mar, E., 1984. Apparent ethanol poisoning in puppies shampooed in dishwashing detergent. Vet. Med. Small Anim. Clin. 79 (3), 318–320.

Dial, S.M., Thrall, M.A., Hamar, D.W., 1989. 4-Methylpyrazole as treatment for naturally acquired ethylene glycol intoxication in dogs. J. Am. Vet. Med. Assoc. 195, 73–76.

Dial, S.M., Thrall, M.A., Hamar, D.W., 1994a. Efficacy of 4-methylpyrazole for treatment of ethylene glycol intoxication in dogs. Am. J. Vet. Res. 55, 1762–1770.

Dial, S.M., Thrall, M.A., Hamar, D.W., 1994b. Comparison of ethanol and 4-methylpyrazole as therapies for ethylene glycol intoxication in the cat. Am. J. Vet. Res. 55, 1771–1782.

DiBartola, S.P., Chew, D.J., Tarr, M.J., et al., 1985. Hemodialysis of a dog with acute renal failure. J. Am. Vet. Med. Assoc. 186, 1323–1326.

Dorman, D.C., Hascheck, W.M., 1991. Fatal propylene glycol toxicosis in a horse. J. Am. Vet. Med. Assoc. 198, 1643–1644.

Dujardin-Beaumetz, M.M., 1875. Acad. Sci. 81, 192, Cited by Ratcliff, R.C., Zuber, R.M. Acute ethyl alcohol poisoning in dogs. Aust. Vet. J. 1977; 53:48–49.

Dyer, J.E., 1991. Gamma-hydroxybutyrate: a health-food product producing coma and seizure-like activity. Am. J. Emerg. Med. 9, 321–324.

Eder, A.F., McGrath, C.M., Dowdy, Y.G., et al., 1998. Ethylene glycol poisoning: toxicokinetic and analytical factors affecting laboratory diagnosis. Clin. Chem. 44, 168–177.

Fogazzi, G.B., 1996. Crystalluria: a neglected aspect of urinary sediment analysis. Nephrol. Dial. Transplant. 11, 379–387.

Fooshee, S.K., Forrester, S.D., 1990. Hypercalcemia secondary to cholecalciferol rodenticide toxicosis in two dogs. J. Am. Vet. Med. Assoc. 196, 1265–1268.

Forrester, S.D., Troy, G.C., 1999. Renal effects of nonsteroidal antiinflammatory drugs. Compend. Contin. Educ. Pract. Vet. 21, 910–919.

Fox, L.E., Grauer, G.F., Dubielzig, R.R., et al., 1987. Reversal of ethylene glycol-induced nephrotoxicosis in a dog. J. Am. Vet. Med. Assoc. 191, 1433–1435.

Gilger, A.P., Potts, A.M., 1955. Studies on the Visual Toxicity of Methanol*: V. The Role of Acidosis in Experimental Methanol Poisoning. Am. J. Ophthalmol. 39 (2), 63–86.

Grauer, G.F., 1998. Fluid therapy in acute and chronic renal failure. Vet. Clin. North Am. Small Anim. Pract. 28, 609–622.

Grauer, G.F., Thrall, M.A., Henre, B.A., et al., 1984. Early clinicopathologic findings in dogs ingesting ethylene glycol. Am. J. Vet. Res. 45, 2299–2309.

Grauer, G.F., Thrall, M.A., Henre, B.A., et al., 1987. Comparison of the effects of ethanol and 4-methylpyrazole on the pharmacokinetics and toxicity of ethylene glycol in the dog. Toxicol. Lett. 35, 307–314.

Gunther, R., Felice, L.J., Nelson, R.K., et al., 1988. Toxicity of a vitamin D3 rodenticide to dogs. J. Am. Vet. Med. Assoc. 193, 211–214.

Gwaltney-Brant, S., Holding, J.K., Donaldson, C.W., et al., 2001. Renal failure associated with ingestion of grapes or raisins in dogs. J. Am. Vet. Med. Assoc. 218, 1555–1556.

Heiene, R., Vulliet, P.R., Williams, R.L., et al., 2001. Use of capillary electrophoresis to quantitate carbamylated hemoglobin concentrations in dogs with renal failure. J. Am. Vet. Res. 62, 1302–1306.

Holloway, S., Senior, D., Roth, L., et al., 1993. Hemolytic uremic syndrome in dogs. J. Vet. Intern. Med. 7, 220–227.

Hornfeldt, C.A., Murphy, M.J., 1998. American Association of Poison Control Centers report on poisonings of animals, 1993–1994. J. Am. Vet. Med. Assoc. 212, 358–361.

Hovda, L., 2000. Common plant toxicities. In: Ettinger, S.J., Feldman, E.C. (Eds.), Textbook of Veterinary Internal Medicine, fifth ended. Saunders, Philadelphia.

Hurd-Kuenzi, L.A., 1983. Methanol intoxication in a dog. J. Am. Vet. Med. Assoc. 183, 882–883.

Jacobsen, D., Akesson, I., Shefter, E., 1982a. Urinary calcium oxalate monohydrate crystals in ethylene glycol poisoning. Scand. J. Clin. Lab. Invest. 42, 213–234.

Jacobsen, D., Bredesen, J.E., Eide, I., 1982b. Anion and osmolal gaps in the diagnosis of methanol and ethylene glycol poisoning. Acta Med. Scand. 212, 17–20.

Kammerer, M., Sachot, E., Blanchot, D., 2001. Ethanol toxicosis from the ingestion of rotten apples by a dog. Vet. Hum. Toxicol. 43, 349–350.

Kovalkovičová, N., Šutiaková, I., Pistl, J., et al., 2009. Some food toxic for pets. Interdiscipl. Toxicol. 2 (3), 169–176.

Kramer, J.W., Bistline, D., Sheridan, P., et al., 1984. Identification of hippuric acid crystals in the urine of ethylene glycol-intoxicated dogs and cats. J. Am. Vet. Med. Assoc. 184, 584.

Kruse, J.A., Cadnapaphornchai, P., 1994. The serum osmole gap. J. Crit. Care. 9, 185–197.

LaKind, J.S., McKenna, E.A., Hubner, R.P., et al., 1999. A review of the comparative mammalian toxicity of ethylene glycol and propylene glycol. Crit. Rev. Toxicol. 29 (4), 331–365.

Langston, C.E., 2002. Acute renal failure caused by lily ingestion in six cats. J. Am. Vet. Med. Assoc. 220, 49–52.

Langston, C.E., Cowgill, L.D., Spano, J.A., 1997. Applications and outcome of hemodialysis in cats: a review of 29 cases. J. Vet. Intern. Med. 11, 348–355.

Lehman, A.J., Chase, H.F., 1944. The acute and chronic toxicity of isopropyl alcohol. J. Lab. Clin. Med. 29 (6), 561–567.

Mack, R.B., 1993. Love potion number 8½: gamma-hydroxybutyrate poisoning. North Carol. Med. J. 54, 232–233.

Marshall, D.A., Doty, R.L., 1990. Taste responses of dogs to ethylene glycol, propylene glycol, and ethylene glycol-based antifreeze. J. Am. Vet. Med. Assoc. 197, 1599–1602.

Mathews, K.G., Gregory, C.R., 1997. Renal transplants in cats: 66 cases (1987–1996). J. Am. Vet. Med. Assoc. 211, 1432–1436.

McClanahan, S., Hunter, J., Murphy, M., et al., 1998. Propylene glycol toxicosis in a mare. Vet. Hum. Toxicol. 40, 294–296.

Means, C., 2003. Bread dough toxicosis in dogs. J. Vet. Emerg. Crit. Care. 3, 39–41.

Money, S.R., Petroianu, A., Kimura, K., et al., 1989. Acute hypocalcemic effect of ethanol in dogs:alcoholism. Clin. Exp. Res. 13, 453–456.

Mowry, J.B., Spyker, D.A., Brooks, D.E., et al., 2015. 2014 Annual Report of the American Association of Poison Control Centers' National Poison Data System (NPDS): 32nd Annual Report. Clin. Toxicol. 53 (10), 962–1147.

Mueller, D.H., 1982. Epidemiologic considerations of ethylene glycol intoxication in small animals. Vet. Hum. Toxicol. 24, 21–24.

Murphy, M.J., Ray, A.C., Jones, L.P., et al., 1984. Butanedial treatment of ethylene glycol toxicosis in dogs. Am. J. Vet. Res. 45, 2293–2295.

Myers, V.S., Usenik, E.A., 1969. Propylene glycol intoxication of horses. J. Am. Vet. Med. Assoc. 155, 1841.

Nemeth, T., Toth, J., Balogh, L., et al., 1997. Principles of renal transplantation in the dog: a review. Acta Vet. Hung. 45, 213–226.

Oehme, F.W., Kore, A.M., 2006. Miscellaneous indoor toxicants. In: Peterson, M., Talcott, P. (Eds.), Small Animal Toxicology. Saunders, St. Louis, MO, pp. 223–243.

Papich, M.G., 1990. Toxicoses from over-the-counter human drugs. Vet. Clin. North Am. Small Anim. Pract. 20 (2), 431–451.

Parry, M.F., Wallach, R., 1974. Ethylene glycol poisoning. Am. J. Med. 57 (1), 143–150.

Penumarthy, R., Oehme, F.W., 1975. Treatment of ethylene glycol toxicosis in cats. Am. J. Vet. Res. 36, 209–212.

Peterson, E.N., Kirby, R., Sommer, M., 1991. Cholecalciferol rodenticide intoxication in a cat. J. Am. Vet. Med. Assoc. 199, 904–906.

Pintchuck, P.A., Galey, F.D., George, L.W., 1993. Propylene toxicity in adult dairy cows. J. Vet. Intern. Med. 7, 150.

Poortinga, E.W., Hungerford, L.L., 1998. A case–control study of acute ibuprofen toxicity in dogs. Prevent Vet. Med. 35, 115–124.

Richardson, J.A., 2006. Ethanol. In: Peterson, M., Talcott, P. (Eds.), Small Animal Toxicology. Saunders, St. Louis, MO, pp. 698–701.

Roe, O., 1982. Species differences in methanol poisoning. Crit. Rev. Toxicol. 10, 275–286.

Rowland, J., 1987. Incidence of ethylene glycol intoxication in dogs and cats seen at Colorado State University Veterinary Teaching Hospital. Vet. Hum. Toxicol. 29, 41–44.

Rumbeiha, W.K., Braselton, W.E., Nachreiner, R.F., et al., 2000. The postmortem diagnosis of cholecalciferol toxicosis: a novel approach and differentiation from ethylene glycol toxicosis. J. Vet. Diagn. Invest. 12, 426–432.

Scully, R.E., Galbadine, J.J., McNeely, B.V., 1979. Case records of the Massachusetts General Hospital, Case 38-1979. N. Engl. J. Med. 30, 650–657.

Shahar, R., Holmberg, D.L., 1985. Pleural dialysis in the management of acute renal failure in two dogs. J. Am. Vet. Med. Assoc. 187 (9), 952–954.

Somerville, B.A., Plumlee, K.H., 1996. Acute isopropyl alcohol intoxication in a horse. Can. Vet. J. 37, 359–360.

Suter, R.J., 1992. Presumed ethanol intoxication in sheep dogs fed uncooked pizza dough. Aust. Vet. J. 69, 20.

Tefft, K.M., 2004. Lily nephrotoxicity in cats. Compend. Contin. Educ. Pract. Vet. 26, 149–156.

Terlinsky, A.S., Grochowski, J., Geoly, K.L., et al., 1981. Identification of atypical calcium oxalate crystalluria following ethylene glycol ingestion. Am. J. Clin. Pathol. 76, 223–226.

Thrall, M.A., Grauer, G.F., Mero, K.N., 1982. Ethanol, 1,3-butanediol, pyrazole, and 4-methylpyrazole therapy in dogs with experimental ethylene glycol intoxication [Abstract]. Proc. Am. Soc. Vet. Clin. Pathol.

Thrall, M.A., Freemyer, F.G., Hamar, D.W., et al., 1984a. Ethanol toxicosis secondary to sourdough ingestion in a dog. J. Am. Vet. Med. Assoc. 184, 1513–1514.

Thrall, M.A., Grauer, G.F., Mero, K.N., 1984b. Clinicopathologic findings in dogs and cats with ethylene glycol intoxication. J. Am. Vet. Med. Assoc. 184, 37–41.

Thrall, M.A., Dial, S.M., Winder, D.R., 1985. Identification of calcium oxalate monohydrate crystals by X-ray diffraction in urine of ethylene glycol-intoxicated dogs. Vet. Pathol. 22, 625–628.

Thrall, M.A., Grauer, G.F., Dial, S.M., 1995. Antifreeze poisoning. In: Bonagura, J.D. (Ed.), Kirk's Current Veterinary Therapy XII, Small Animal Practice. Saunders, Philadelphia, pp. 232–237.

Thrall, M.A., Connally, H.E., Grauer, G.F., 1998. Don't freeze up! Quick response is key in ethylene glycol poisoning. Vet. Tech. 19, 557–567.

Thrall, M.A., Connally, H.E., Grauer, G.F., et al., 2006. Ethylene glycol. In: Peterson, M., Talcott, P. (Eds.), Small Animal Toxicology. Saunders, St. Louis, MO, pp. 702–726.

Vaden, S.L., Gookin, J., Trogdon, M., et al., 1997a. Use of carbamylated hemoglobin concentration to differentiate acute from chronic renal failure in dogs. Am. J. Vet. Res. 58, 1193–1196.

Vaden, S.L., Levine, J., Breitschwerdt, E.B., 1997b. A retrospective case–control of acute renal failure in 99 dogs. J. Vet. Intern. Med. 11, 58–64.

Valentine, W.M., 1990. Toxicology of selected pesticides, drugs, and chemicals: short chain alcohols. Vet. Clin. North Am. 20, 515–523.

van Wuijckhuise, L., Cremers, G.G., 2003. Alcohol poisoning in dogs. Tijdschr Diergeneeskd. 128, 284–285.

Weiss, D.J., McClay, C.B., Christopher, M.M., 1990. Effects of propylene glycol-containing diets on acetaminophen-induced methemoglobinemia in cats. J. Am. Vet. Med. Assoc. 196, 1816–1819.

Winter, M.L., Ellis, M.D., Snodgrass, W.R., 1990. Urine fluorescence using a Wood's lamp to detect the antifreeze additive sodium fluorescein: a qualitative adjunctive test in suspected ethylene glycol ingestions. Ann. Emerg. Med. 19, 663–667.

Chapter 50

Petroleum

Robert W. Coppock and Ralph G. Christian

INTRODUCTION

Intoxication of birds and animals with petroleum and chemicals used by the petroleum industry does occur. This chapter essentially focuses on terrestrial animals and especially livestock. Land used for agriculture and lands used by wildlife are used for oil and gas production. Land used by the upstream oil and gas industry include well sites, tank battery sites, sweet and sour gas plants, compressor stations, and pipelines. Crude petroleum and chemicals used in the oilfields can be spilled, and livestock and other animals can be poisoned by dermal, inhalation, and oral routes of exposure. Air emissions from oil and gas facilities also occur. The production of sour gas, natural gas containing hydrogen sulfide (H_2S), and the removal of sulfur (sour gas processing plants) present toxicology issues when substances are released.

OIL AND GAS WELL DRILLING AND COMPLETING

Drilling

Oil and gas wells are vertically and horizontally drilled into oil, gas and bitumen producing formations. During drilling operations, drilling fluids are used to cool and lubricate the drill bit, support the walls of the bore hole, control subsurface pressure in the drill stem, move the cuttings to surface and expose the borehole to various chemicals that assist in the drilling operation. Drilling fluids generally are complex mixtures and the composition varies with the different geologic zones and target formation. Water-based drilling fluid and the nonaqueous drilling fluids are the two basic types of drilling fluids used (Coppock and Christian, 2012). Water-based drilling fluids generally consist of bentonite clay and barium sulfate for increasing density and other chemicals are added to give desired properties such as lubrication, reduce foaming. and bore wall stabilization. Brine or fresh water can be used in water-based drilling fluids. The nonaqueous drilling fluids (invert drilling fluids) have fresh or brine water emulsified in a hydrocarbon phase. Hydrocarbons used include diesel oil, distillates. and hydrotreated mineral oil (low in polycyclics). Drilling mud can also contain metals and metalloids and have a high alkaline pH. Biocides that can be added to drilling muds include glutaraldehyde and quaternary ammonium salts. If naturally occurring radioactive materials (NORMs) are encountered in the formations, radioactive metals and gas can contaminate drilling fluids and drill cuttings.

Fracking

Oil and gas bearing formations are porous with oil, gas and water filling the pores. Flow to the borehole is stimulated by fracking. Hydraulic fracturing is performed by pumping water containing chemicals and proppants down the bore hole under high pressure and the formation is fractured. Propping agents are used to reduce the closure of the fractures. The United States Environmental Protection Agency (USEPA, 2016) estimates that fracking, a typical horizontal well for shale gas uses 15 million liters of water. Three are over 1000 different chemicals used in fracking operations that have been listed by the USEPA. Toxicology issues associated with fracking chemicals are known (Carpenter, 2016). Earthquakes are associated with fracking and deep well disposal of unwanted oilfield liquids.

SOURCES OF TOXIC SUBSTANCES

Toxicological issues are associated with chemicals used in drilling, fracking and the crude petroleum. Crude natural gas as it comes from the wellhead may have volatile liquids (condensate), produced water, NORMs, and may contain H_2S and other forms of sulfur. Sour petroleum can have the H_2S removed and disposed of by burning in a flare stack.

Veterinary Toxicology. DOI: http://dx.doi.org/10.1016/B978-0-12-811410-0.00050-7

Air Emissions

Air emissions from the upstream oil and gas industry are from burning unwanted products, production testing of gas wells, controlled and uncontrolled releases of volatile substances, and emissions from internal combustion engines and emissions from tank heaters. After gaswell completion, production testing is done to estimate productivity and remove corrosive fracking chemicals from the formation. During production testing the total production from the well is generally burned in a flare or incinerator. Burned emissions contain various levels of products of combustion, products of incomplete combustion (PICs) and may be a source of halogenated dibenzodioxins (Martinez-Guijarro et al., 2017). Polyaromatic hydrocarbons (PAHs) and particulates can also be formed. Sulfur dioxide, reduced sulfur compounds (including carbon disulfide and carbonyl sulfide) PAHs and other compounds are produced by burning sour well emissions by flaring (Strosher, 1996). Tank heaters are used in the production of heavy oil and bitumen. If the tanks are vented to atmosphere, heating the petroleum in the tank can drive off a variety of hydrocarbons and water into the atmosphere.

Flowback and Produced Water

Flowback fluid is the liquid that flows back during staged drilling, fracking and completion operations. During the flowback period, the fluids coming from the well are drilling and fracking liquids. Water from the formation brought to the surface during production of crude oil and natural gas is called produced water. It is estimated that unconventional wells produce 1.7–14.3 million liters of brine water/well over the first 5–10 years of production. Produced water is the largest waste stream generated in the oil and gas industry and contains inorganic and organic compounds (Ahmaduna et al., 2009). Produced water is separated from crude petroleum and natural gas and becomes a waste product and can be high in total dissolved solids. Ingestion of production water can induce poisoning. Produced water can contain heavy metals and metalloids. Both flowback water and produced water can contain NORMs, predominantly radium ($^{228\ \&\ 236}Ra$) and with barium can form radioactive pipe scale. Production water generally has a unique ratio of ions and this ratio is generally distinctly different from the ratio of ions found in ground water. Leaks of produced water can contaminate ground and surface water and soil (Carpenter, 2016). Depending on the redox potential, produced water can be very corrosive and corrosion of oilfield equipment can be a cause of leaks. Produced water disposal is variable depending on its chemical and NORMs composition. Produced water that is an environmental hazard is often disposed by returning it to the formation or injection underground using disposal wells. Tremors are being associated with disposal wells. Produced water can damage soil. Coalbed methane can be a large source of produced water (Moore, 2012).

Well Rework

Reworking a well can include dewaxing, descaling, replacement of downhole equipment, replacing location of downhole equipment and several other procedures. Reworking can include stimulation of the formation and fracking to increase flow to the well bore. Surfactants, acids, dewaxing solvents, biofilm inhibitors and numerous other chemicals can be used during rework operations. Some of these compounds are intrinsically toxic, and can enhance the toxicity of other substances in a mixture. Chelating and descaling agents may increase the bioavailability of chemicals that otherwise would be considered to have a low order of toxicity. Spillage of rework chemicals can occur and livestock poisonings have been reported (Monlux et al., 1971). Down-hole equipment can be laid out at unsecured sites and cattle will investigate and lick the petroleum and other substances from the equipment.

Sumps

Earthen pits have been used for the disposal of upstream oilfield waste by burning (flare pits). Many jurisdictions have limited the use of sumps and do not allow sump contents to be buried. Old buried sumps can be a hidden source of surface and subsurface chemical contamination. Sumps also may be remote to oil and gas well sites (Heitman, 1986). Although environmental practices have changed, old sumps can be a cause of surface and subsurface issues because they may contain a variety of contaminants inclusive of salts, acids, and heavy metals and metalloids (Heitman, 1986; Gleason and Tangen, 2014). Extrusions from a drilling sump containing petroleum hydrocarbons have been linked with maladies in cattle and sheep (Mostrom et al., 1993; Adler et al., 1992). Extrusions from an invert sump contaminated a pasture. Cows grazing this pasture had calves that were stunted. Necropsy findings were: abnormal epiphyseal plates in the long bones and myeloid-like bodies in the proximal tubular cells of the kidney. The activities of hepatic polysubstrate mixed function oxidase enzymes were also elevated. Sheep have been poisoned following extensive rains that caused extrusion of natural gas condensate from the soil. Sumps and old oilfield equipment can contain nonpesticide organophosphorus esters used to prevent foaming of lubricating oils. Reviews of the neurotoxicity and pathology of the tri-alkyl/aryl phosphate esters have been published (Coppock et al., 1995a; Maxie and Youssef, 2007; Coppock and Christian, 2012).

SELECTED TOXIC SUBSTANCES

Antihydrates and Antifreezes

Chemicals are used in the upstream oil and gas industry to prevent the formation of hydrates and freezing of water. Surfactants, polymers (e.g., polyvinylcaprolactam) and antifreezes are used as antihydrate and antifreezing agents. Methanol can be used to prevent freezing of water in pipes, and to prevent hydrate formation in gas wells and pipelines. Intoxication of cattle by methanol has been reported (Rousseaux et al., 1982). A herd of 600 cows had access to methanol barrels stored on a lease and two cows were found dead. Rumen contents from the two dead cows contained 370 mg of methanol/100 mL of rumen fluid. Clinical signs of experimentally induced methanol poisoning in cattle were like those reported for field exposures (Fritz and Coppock, 1992). Diethylene glycol is used in oil and gas operations. Research has shown that cattle are a species sensitive to diethylene glycol (Fritz and Coppock, 1992; Khan et al., 1992). A dose of 1.5 mL/kg of body weight is fatal to a cow. Diethylene glycol is toxic to the eye, liver, kidney, and nervous system. Diethylene glycol induced ocular changes that are similar in appearance to those of pinkeye. Diethylene glycol causes a unique lace-like hypertrophy of the perineuronal amphicytes in the Gasserian ganglion in cattle. This lesion has not been reported in laboratory animals. Other glycols such as monoethylene glycols and ethylene glycol are used in oil and gas production (see Chapter 49 entitled Alcohols and Glycol).

Grease and Motor Oil

Lithium (Li) grease intoxication has occurred in cattle. Wallace and Blodgett (1996) reported Li poisoning in one cow after the animal consumed Li-grease, and Johnson et al. (1980) reported on Li poisoning in 19 out of 90 animals. In both incidents, the source of Li-grease was in discarded drums that had been used previously for transporting and storing grease. In the incident reported by Wallace and Blodgett (1996), the cow was euthanized and in the incident reported by Johnson et al. (1980), all 19 animals died. In the animals that consumed Li-grease, clinical signs included muscular tremors, ataxia, stiffness, apparent disorientation, ptyalism, diarrhea, rapid respiration, and periodic seizure-like activity. The concentrations of Li in grease for the incidents reported were 2050 μg of Li/g of grease and 1250 μg of Li/g of grease, respectively (Wallace and Blodgett, 1996; Johnson et al., 1980). Lithium can also be present in produced water. Grease can contain other metallic substances. Lead grease has excellent water repellence properties. Lead grease is also a hazard to livestock. Motor oils generally contain additives to prevent foaming, to keep carbon deposits in suspension and to reduce friction and wear of parts at high temperatures, viscosity improvers, pour-point improvers and antioxidants. Synthetic oils can contain molybdenum and surfactants. Antiwear additives such as zinc diakyldithiophosphate compounds are added to lubricants to reduce friction. Micronized metals can be added to lubricating oils. Many additives are mixtures of substances and most companies closely guard their intellectual property.

VETERINARY MEDICAL USE OF PETROLEUM

Uses of mineral oils in the food industry include lubricants in manufacturing of human foodstuffs, direct addition to foodstuffs and as a pharmaceutic. Mineral oils are highly refined naphthenic or paraffinic distillates free from unsaturated and aromatic compounds, and other substances that influence color, taste and render unacceptable properties. As a prophylactic for bloat in ruminants, purified mineral oils are mixed with surfactants (pasture spray oil) and sprayed on alfalfa (lucerne) forage before grazing. Spray oil formulations have been used for over 100 years as pesticides. Prolonged oral exposure to mineral oil can deplete fat soluble vitamins. There is historical record of various crude, refined petroleum fractions and waste petroleum being used as veterinary medicaments. Lamp paraffin (kerosene) and other kerosene-like products were used as a veterinary medicament for treating animals with intestinal helminths, frothy bloat and diarrhea, and crude oil was used as an aperient. Used motor oil has been used for tick control. The unpredictable adverse reactions of orally administered kerosene are anorexia, ptyalism, indigestion, irritation of the digestive tract, respiratory difficulties, and death.

TOXICOLOGY OF PETROLEUM

Ingestion of Petroleum by Livestock

Numerous reports that exist in the scientific literature show that cattle ingest crude petroleum and other oilfield substances (Coppock et al., 1995b). Cattle are attracted to and will ingest several gallons of petroleum (Monlux et al., 1971; Oehme, 1977). Deaths have occurred after cattle drank tractor paraffin and vaporizing oil (Eaton, 1943). Heifers drank gasoline (Albert and Ramey, 1964), and Messerli (1969) reported that cattle greedily ingested diesel oil flowing from a storage tank. Cattle have drunk from petroleum puddles near a tank battery, from slush pits, from puddles of volatile petroleum and petroleum distillate (Edwards et al., 1979). Crude oil spilled by a pipeline break has been consumed by cattle, and cattle have drunk from puddles of road-oil after it was applied for dust suppression (Bumstead, 1949; Coale, 1947). Cattle have drunk used motor oil (Gardner, 1977), and have also ingested petroleum-contaminated forage (Beck et al., 1977; Stober, 1962). An entire herd of heifers was irreversibly poisoned by ingesting water from a stream that was contaminated with aviation turbine fuel (Barber et al., 1987). Monlux et al. (1971) reported that most animals avoid oil, but in some instances, the entire herd, especially feeder calves, can be attracted to oil. Cattle have ingested sump oil with adverse effects on health (Ballantyne, 1950, 1955). Cattle were attracted to soil saturated with crude condensate and sore feet were observed in many of the animals. Other species also ingest petroleum. Sheep have ingested Bunker "C" fuel oil (No. 6 Heavy Fuel Oil) following the sinking of a tanker ship in Chedabucto Bay (MacIntyre, 1970). Ingestion of surface water contaminated with extrusions by rain water of natural gas condensate has caused fatalities in sheep (Adler et al., 1992). Voluntary ingestion of kerosene by two goats was reported by Pathan (1961). In Iran, goats ingested diesel fuel leaking from an overturned truck tanker (Toofanian et al., 1979). Sheep and goats were reported to drink liquids accumulating around petroleum well heads (Batista et al., 2013). Dogs have been reported to have liver pathology secondary to the ingestion of motor oil (Chalifoux et al., 1973). An experimental study demonstrated that cows on a balanced diet with water ad libitum are attracted to crude petroleum, and will ingest it (Coppock et al., 1992). The most frequent method of ingesting oil was by licking; the cyclic pattern suggested that cattle will go on oil-licking "binges." Rowe et al. (1973) found that calves will drink sweet and sour crude oils. After water was withheld for 48 h, calves drank 4 L of either a sweet or sour crude oil, but would not repeat the ingestion of crude oil after water had been withheld for a total of 96 h. Two of the calves that drank oil had previously been administered per gavage kerosene in a previous study. Calves that were not water deprived did not drink oil. These findings suggest that cattle may acquire some aversion to drinking crude petroleum.

TABLE 50.1 Clinical Signs of Petroleum Poisoning in Cattle

Acute Signs (Within 24 h)	Subacute Signs (After 24 h)	Chronic Signs
Ruminal tympanites[a]	Depression	Lethargy
Emesis	Pneumonia	Anorexia
Postural weakness	Anorexia	Loss of condition
Ataxia and incoordination	Constipation	Impaired reproductive performance
Seizures	Coughing	Chronic cough
Hyperthermia	Ileus	Abortion
Dyspnea	Recumbency	Laminitis (walking in petroleum puddles)
Bloody diarrhea	Ruminal atony	Loss of body weight
Strong petroleum-like odor to breath/feces	Abortion	Chest/abdominal pain
Ruminal atony	Loss of weight	Cachexia
Depression	Sweet petroleum-like odor to breath and feces	
Death	Lethargy	

[a]*Ruminal tympanites is not a consistent finding.*

Clinical Signs and Pathology Observed in Field Incidents

Varied clinical signs have been observed in field incidents of petroleum poisoning (Table 50.1). A herd of 58 yearling steers had access to crude petroleum distillate (condensate) on an oil-lease property (Edwards and Zinn, 1979). Following oral exposure, 17 animals became sick and nine died. The sick cattle had petroleum distillate dripping from the nostrils and oil in their feces. Surviving animals had varied signs including anorexia and weight loss, and some of these animals died. Edwards and Zinn (1979) also described clinical signs in 18 out of 135 animals that had access to a slush pit. The surviving animals lost weight and were unthrifty. These authors also reported that, of 200 steers with access to petroleum in puddles, 12 were found dead, and 13 died 24 h later. Oehme (1977) attributed abortions to ingestion of petroleum products. Loss of body condition can also result from petroleum ingestion-linked chronic pneumonia and pleural adhesions. Cattle attracted to an area saturated with petroleum condensate can have sore feet mimicking signs of laminitis. Ballantyne (1950) reported that a 545 kg cow, representative of a malady observed in 20 other cows from a large herd, was necropsied. After ingestion of oil this cow had a reduction in body weight. Necropsy findings were: visible oil in the rumen, the mucous membranes of the abomasum were stained black, and areas of inflammation were observed in the gut. There was 213 mL of oil/L of rumen contents. In another report (Bumstead, 1949), cattle drank from a pool of oil. Two animals died, and all animals that had wandered into the pool of oil showed clinical signs of intoxication. One heifer had severe enteritis, was dehydrated and had cachexia. All animals receiving veterinary medical intervention consisting of rapidly removed oil from the digestive tract, and prophylactic treatment with an antimicrobial chemotherapeutic recovered. In another report (Coale, 1947), five dairy cows drank crude oil that had escaped from a broken pipeline and were sold 90 days later because of lost productivity. Gibson and Linzell (1948) reported that dairy cows drank petroleum after 5 gal (23 L) were mistakenly dumped in a water trough. Clinical signs in six out of eight cows were central nervous system (CNS) depression including coma, coughing, salivating, head shaking, hypothermia, and petroleum odor on respired air and from the milk. The diesel-like odor on the breath and from the milk persisted for 5 days. Three animals died at 12, 24, and 48 h, respectively, after exposure. During the interval between exposure and death, all the animals would eat and ruminate and were dull in temperament and were constipated. Forty-eight hours after ingestion, two cows had abnormal respiratory sounds, which persisted for 14 days in one cow. The pathological findings were chemical pneumonia, and evidence of inflammation in the mammary gland. Eaton (1943) reported clinical signs of vomiting and death after a lactating Shorthorn animal ingested approximately 1 gal (4.55 L) of tractor paraffin. Clinical signs of anorexia and constipation were reported after cattle ingested tractor vaporizing oil (tractor distillate) (Parker and Williamson, 1951). Pathological findings were fatty changes in the liver, degeneration of the kidney, and multiple small hemorrhages in the lungs. Barber et al. (1987) reported an environmental incident with aviation turbine fuel. Fifty-one heifers 12–18 months old were exposed to water in a stream that had been contaminated with aviation turbine fuel. The duration of exposure was not determined and, when discovered, the contaminated waterway was immediately fenced, and the heifers were provided an alternative source of drinking water. At the initial examination, two heifers were dead, ataxia was observed in five animals. Over 3 weeks, eight heifers died or were euthanized in extremis. Animals that survived were dull, did not show interest in strangers walking about the field, and had marked weight loss, and increased respiratory rate was observed in some animals. Six weeks after the initial examination, 41 of the surviving animals appeared unhealthy. At 121 days after the initial examination, the heifers were compared to siblings, and were found to have lost 50–100 kg. Because of apparent chronic, poor health, 41 of the heifers were slaughtered approximately 124 days after the initial exposure and tissues submitted for histopathology. One heifer died during transport to slaughter.

Experimental Studies

Bystrom (1989) studied the acute toxicity of crude oil in cattle. The treatment groups (four animals in each group) received 20, 40, 60 or 80 mL of sweet crude oil/kg of body weight, or 80 mL of potable water/kg of body weight, respectively, administered per gavage. The analytical data for the crude oil has previously been described (Coppock and Christian, 2012). Following exposure, daily mean rectal body temperatures were normal. Ruminal motility was decreased after animals were dosed with oil and slowly increased to pretreatment values by day 8. Vomiting occurred in 10 out of 12 of the animals dosed with oil and, in some animals, vomiting was characterized by a projectile expulsion of oil. Emesis recurred after forage or water was ingested. Ruminal tympanites was observed in most the animals, but did not require medical intervention. Neurological abnormalities were not observed in control animals. Central nervous signs expressed by nystagmus, muscular tremors, and "petit mal-like" seizures were observed in treated animals. Depression was the most common clinical sign observed. These effects were attributed to the anesthetic-like effects of the volatile hydrocarbons. The neurological effects contributed to aspiration pneumonia. Oil was identified in feces at 23 h after dosing for the 20 and 40 mL /kg groups, at 7–31 h for the 60 mL /kg group, and at 5–19 h for the 80 mL /kg group. Feces from the control animals did not contain oil. Head-space analysis on filled blood tubes showed that volatile hydrocarbon constituents from the oil were present in blood. *N*-heptane was used as a representative hydrocarbon. Semiquantitative values for total light naphtha were estimated as high as 10 mg/L of blood. Aspiration of oil into the lungs, based on pathology findings, increased the levels of *N*-heptane in the blood. Rowe et al. (1973) found that sweet crude oil was more toxic in cattle than was sour crude oil. Administration of 8 mL of sweet crude oil/kg body weight/day caused death within 7–14 days in four out of five calves. For the same dose of sour crude oil, five of five calves died between days 16 and 24; for kerosene, five of five calves died between days 9 and 23. Administration of 37 mL of sweet crude oil/kg was fatal within a few minutes. Most of the surviving animals developed pneumonia. Considerable variations have been reported for the dose-response of cattle to petroleum substances. These effects can be due to presence of surfactants or emulsifiers, and additives in refined petroleum. A 200 mL single oral dose of odorless kerosene administered to a mature dairy cow caused a 90.3% reduction in dry matter intake, and the same dose of Stanvac odorless solvent caused a 42.5% reduction in dry matter intake for a 3-day period (Reid, 1957). Emulsification of kerosene with a nonionic surfactant decreased the interval between exposure and the onset of effects. Similar findings were observed when kerosene was placed directly into the omasum. Fistulation of the rumen did not alter the response to kerosene or solvent. Studies in cattle on a heavy liquid paraffin (mineral oil) to control bloat showed that the oil can reduce blood and milk butter fat levels of fat soluble vitamins (McGillivray et al., 1959).

TOXICOPATHOLOGY OF PETROLEUM AND OILFIELD CHEMICALS

Clinical Pathology

Barber (1987) reported on the toxicology of aviation turbine fuel in heifers. Ten animals were considered to have elevated serum activity of aspartate aminotransferase, interpreted as a reflection of acute hepatic dysfunction, activates of γ-glutamyl transpeptidase (GGT) were within the normal range. Elevated concentrations of nonesterified fatty acids were observed in 11 of the animals, two had elevated concentrations of blood urea nitrogen and five had a leukocytosis. Six weeks after the initial farm visit, 41 of 41 animals had elevated serum activity of GGT. Bystrom (1989) found that acute sweet crude oil intoxication did not alter hematological parameters. There was a correlation between the severity of clinical signs and increased concentrations of plasma fibrinogen. The activity of hepatocellular enzymes in serum and serum glucose were not consistently increased after acute exposure to sweet crude oil, but serum calcium and potassium values consistently decreased and bilirubin values consistently increased. Rowe et al. (1973) found that hematological parameters, especially leukocyte numbers, were increased as clinical signs of chemical pneumonia increased. A single dose of sour crude oil caused a constant decline in plasma glucose. A transient decline in plasma glucose was also observed in calves given sweet crude oil or kerosene. Exposure to nitrates from drilling fluids can cause methemoglobinemia. The concentration of nitrates can be determined in rumen fluid, aqueous humor (anterior chamber of the eye), urine, and plasma. Uterine and fetal fluids can also be used.

Pulmonary Pathology of Petroleum

The lung is a target especially for unweathered petroleum. Hydrocarbon-induced chemical (inhalation) pneumonia can occur after petroleum is inhaled. Aspiration of oil during emesis is the most common mechanism of inhalation exposure to liquid petroleum (Coppock et al., 1996; Coppock and Christian, 2012). Necropsy findings of oil-induced chemical pneumonia have been described (Dungworth, 1993). Generally, the cranioventral lobes of the lungs are affected first. During necropsy, oil may be identified in the lungs by oil discoloration and a petroleum odor, visible oil in the lung, oil floating to the surface when a piece of lung is immersed in water or formalin, or oil layering on the surface of the supernatant when a piece of lung is homogenized. The pulmonary histopathology for unweathered petroleum is similar for the various forms of petroleum. Histopathological changes are proliferative, and macrophages, with a foamy-appearing cytoplasm, are found in and tend to fill the alveoli (Dungworth, 1993). In the pathogenesis, oil-containing macrophages are found in the lymphatics, especially those adjacent to blood vessels around bronchi. Fibrosis and proliferation of type II macrophages are prominent features. Foamy macrophages may be incorporated into the alveolar septa by fibroblastic proliferation. As determined by histochemistry and special stains, lipids are found in both intracellular and extracellular sites, and oil can be identified in the alveolar spaces. In the early stages, the lesion may be an acute necrotizing fibrinous bronchopneumonia. Generally, neutrophils, lymphocytes, and plasma cells surround the necrotic areas. Fibrinous exudate, inflammatory cells, and amorphous eosinophilic and oily material can fill the alveolar spaces. Empty spaces in the tissues suggest that liquid foreign material may have been absorbed and subsequently washed out by tissue processing. Plant material from aspirated ingesta may also be seen in alveoli. Fibrin hemorrhages and a mixed population of mononuclear cells may be observed on the pleural surface. Extensive coagulative necrosis and suppuration may be observed in the consolidated areas. Bacteria may be present in the necrotic areas and alveoli. Hematogenous exposure of the lungs to petroleum hydrocarbons also occurs. Volatile components of petroleum are absorbed by the gastrointestinal tract and are volatilized from the blood in the lungs. An oil embolism can occur in the lungs through absorption of oil from the gastrointestinal tract. These oil embolisms can block the small blood vessels in the lungs and brain. Oil embolisms in blood vessels of the lungs and brain have not been reported in cattle intoxicated with crude petroleum. The pathogenesis and observed lesions may be altered by concurrent bacterial infection and cytotoxicity of the oil.

There are reports of field and experimental-induced petroleum intoxication. Ulceration of the ventral aspect of the trachea can occur in kerosene poisoning and the ulcers may be covered with a pseudomembrane (Rowe et al., 1973). Areas of the lung can be consolidated and have a dark purple, reddened or tan-gray, mottled discoloration. The areas of consolidation often have a nodular appearance. Fibrinous pleural adhesions and serofibrinous pleural exudate can occur. Pulmonary abscesses can also be observed (Rowe et al., 1973). Pulmonary pathology was observed after cattle were administrated a sweet crude oil per gavage (Bystrom, 1989). Many of the animals, especially those in the high dose groups had black discoloration of the lungs. Visible oil was present in the cranioventral lobes. In one animal, it was estimated that 80% of the lungs were affected by black discoloration, and visible oil was observed. Pathological diagnoses included pulmonary consolidation, fiibronecrotizing pneumonia, pleuritis, emphysema, atelectasis, multifocal interstitial pneumonia, proliferative alveolitis, bronchopneumonia, and alveolitis. In animals that survived 8 days, hyperplasia of type II epithelial cells was observed, and the alveoli were filled with foamy, alveolar macrophages. Multiple small hemorrhages were observed in the lungs of cattle poisoned with tractor vaporizing oil (Parker and Williamson, 1951). Chemical pneumonia was reported in cattle dying from diesel fuel poisoning (Gibson and Linzell, 1948). Pneumonia and pulmonary abscesses containing Gram-negative organisms were found in cattle that died acutely from drinking water contaminated with aviation turbine engine fuel (Barber et al., 1987). The rumen contents smelled of oil. Microscopic examination of tissues from the animals that died in the first 3 weeks showed fatty degeneration of hepatocytes and focal areas of hepatitis, and one out of four had tubulointerstitial nephrosis and renal vascular thrombi. A diagnosis of pneumonia, and abscesses containing gram-negative organisms was made in two out of four of the animals. Approximately 124 days after the ingestion of aviation turbine fuel-contaminated water, the remaining cattle were necropsied. At slaughter, the lungs of the cattle were considered abnormal, and were characterized by enlargement and gray-blue areas of varying and abnormal firmness. Histopathological abnormalities in tissues taken at slaughter were not observed in lung, liver, and kidneys. Infection in the lungs can occur rapidly following chemical injury. Cattle that survive for 6 weeks or longer usually have marked loss of weight and have chronic ill health (Rowe et al., 1973). Pulmonary lesions have been observed in sheep following a 1-day exposure to natural gas condensate-contaminated water (Adler et al., 1992). Gross pathological observations included severe bilateral consolidations and tan to gray mottling of the ventral lobes. Histological diagnosis of the lesions was a necrotizing bronchopneumonia. There were extensive areas of coagulation necrosis bordered by a dense zone of neutrophils and lesser numbers of lymphocytes, plasmacytes and macrophages. The alveoli were filled with fibrinous exudate and amorphous eosinophilic material. Plant material was also observed in the pulmonary parenchyma. The pleural surface was coated with fibrin, hemorrhages and mononuclear cells. Pathogenic and potentially pathogenic bacteria (*Pasteurella haemolytica, Klebsiella pneumoniae, Fusobacterium necrophorum, Actinomyces pyogenes, Escherichia coli*, and *Pseudomonas* spp.) were isolated from the lungs of some of the sheep. Lung lesions can also occur after animals are exposed to gaseous petroleum and sour gas. Mostrom and Campbell (1996) reported lesions of hyperplasia of the submucosal glands in the trachea of cattle exposed to emissions from a multiphase sour gas leak. Other lesions observed included hyperplasia of tracheal, bronchial and bronchiolar glands, metaplasia of the tracheal mucosa, and loss of cilia from the respiratory epithelium.

Hepatic Pathology of Petroleum

Hepatic pathology has been observed following exposure to oil. Bystrom (1989) observed swelling and increased weight of the liver, increased friability and centrilobular congestion in cattle that were administered a sweet crude oil per gavage. Histopathology showed vacuolization of numerous hepatocytes and these vacuoles were thought to have previously contained oil. Parker and Williamson (1951) reported fatty changes in the liver from a cow that had ingested tractor vaporizing oil. Fatty degenerative changes and focal areas of hepatitis were observed in cattle following ingestion of water contaminated with aviation turbine engine fuel (Barber et al., 1987). An abnormal-appearing liver in a heifer was attributed to the ingestion of gasoline 15 months previously (Albert and Ramey, 1964). Hepatic pathology observed in sheep poisoned by natural gas condensate was fatty degeneration, biliary hyperplasia, periportal fibrosis, and periportal infiltration of lymphocytes and plasma cells (Adler et al., 1992). Wallace and Blodgett (1996) reported the histopathological changes in the liver of a cow that consumed lithium grease containing 2050 μg lithium/g of grease were vacuolated and atrophied hepatocytes. Experimental oral exposure of cattle to lithium has been reported to cause periportal fibrosis (Johnson et al, 1980).

Gastrointestinal Pathology of Petroleum

Petroleum, in acute exposures, can be observed in the gastrointestinal tract and petroleum odor can be detected. Kerosene-induced ulcers of the esophagus have been reported (Rowe et al., 1973). Bystrom (1989) reported pyloric ulcers of the abomasum of cattle exposed to unweathered sweet crude oil. Bumstead (1949) reported oil to be very irritating to the intestinal tract of cattle. Sheep, after ingestion of natural gas condensate, were observed to have reddening of the serosal surface of the gastrointestinal tract and intraluminal hemorrhage (Adler et al., 1992). Histopathology was submucosal and mucosal congestion, and mucosal and serosal hemorrhage and inflammation in all areas of the gastrointestinal tract. Isolated necrosis of enterocytes, superficial erosions, mild acute cryptitis and neutrophilic and lymphocytic exudates were also observed.

Renal Pathology of Petroleum

Renal lesions have been observed in cattle dosed with a light crude oil (Bystrom, 1989). These lesions were shrunken or collapsed glomeruli (2–5 in a 4× field), mild focal necrosis of epithelial cells in the collecting ducts, and inflammatory cells that were observed in the renal cortex. Parker and Williamson (1951) reported degeneration of the kidney in cattle after they consumed tractor vaporizing oil. Tubulointerstitial nephrosis with renal vascular thrombi observed in 1 out of 51 cattle following environmental exposure to aviation turbine engine fuel (Barber et al., 1987). Renal lesions were not observed in surviving animals slaughtered 124 days later. Renal histopathology was observed in sheep poisoned by ingestion of natural gas condensate (Adler et al., 1992). The lesions were tubular epithelial necrosis, granular eosinophilic casts (negative for hemoglobin), protein droplet filled Bowman's space, and in many renal tubules, inflammatory cells were observed around tubular casts.

Nervous System Pathology of Petroleum

Histopathology of the CNS was observed in sheep poisoned by ingestion of natural gas condensate (Adler et al., 1992). Mild perivascular hemorrhage was seen in the pia matter and white matter of the cerebellum and cerebrum. Increased separation between the pia and arachnoid membranes was prominent, and edema was observed in the stroma of the choroid plexus.

Cardiac Pathology of Petroleum

Adler et al. (1992). observed cardiac pathology in sheep that ingested natural gas condensate. Gross pathological changes included epicardial hemorrhages, serosanguineous pericardial fluid, pale-appearing myocardium, and reddened endocardium. Histopathology was segmental myocardial necrosis and calcification. The myofibrils had loss of cross striations and a beaded appearance. There were multifocal areas infiltrated with lymphocytes, macrophages, and occasional neutrophils. The cardiac blood vessels were congested.

Pathological Effects of Petroleum in Embryos

Studies on the embryotoxicity of Prudhoe Bay Crude Oil (PBCO) have been reported. Couillard and Leighton (1989, 1990a,b) showed that PBCO was embryotoxic and that the toxicity was different from hypoxia induced by sealing the eggs with wax. Mineral oil (USP) was not toxic to chicken embryos. On day 9 of incubation, PBCO was applied below the airspace to the surface of the egg shell. Dosages ranged from 2 to 30 μL PBCO/egg. Hepatic lesions were observed 2 days after treatment, and renal and splenic lesions observed on the third day. The livers were observed to have superficial yellowish zones that were multifocal to diffuse. These yellowish zones and mineralization corresponded to areas of hepatocellular necrosis. Hepatic histopathology was hepatocellular vacuolization, hepatocellular necrosis with mineralization, and perivascular and multifocal accumulations of heterophils. Hepatocellular necrosis was dose-dependent. The number of mitotic figures in the liver increased with the dose of PBCO.

Renal lesions were primarily limited to the mesonephros. The capillaries of the glomeruli were distended and cellular casts and mineralization were observed in the renal tubules. Splenic lesions were limited to increased granulopoietic cells arranged in distinct cords. Other pathological findings were ascites and subcutaneous edema. Edema fluid was more pronounced after the third day of incubation. In another study, the toxicity of PBCO was evaluated in chicken embryos (Lusimbo and Leighton, 1996). The chicken embryos were exposed to oil on day 9 of incubation. The oil was placed on the eggshell over a prominent blood vessel of the chorioallantoic membrane. Dosages ranged from 0 to 16 μL PBCO/egg, and embryonal mortality was dose-dependent. Lesions were observed in the liver, subcutaneous tissues, bursa of Fabricius and pipping muscle (musculus complexus). Hepatic lesions were multifocal to locally extensive areas of hepatic necrosis and mineralization. Large fluid-filled vesicles were observed on the dorsocaudal aspect of 5% and 16% of embryos dosed with 1 and 2 μL of PBCO, respectively. The bursa of Fabricius had depleted lymphoid tissue and the interstitium was infiltrated with heterophils. Lesions in the pipping muscle were edema and hemorrhage, sparse multifocal fragmentation, and occasional vacuolation of the myofibers. Exposure to PBCO at 4 μL decreased weight gains during a 3-week posthatching observation period.

TOXICOLOGY OF SOUR PETROLEUM

Sour petroleum can be defined as petroleum that contains more than 0.5% sulfur (mass/mass). Sweet crude oil generally has a sulfur content of <0.5%. A common constituent in sour petroleum is H_2S, which has the odor of rotten eggs. Sour gas at the wellhead can have greater than 20% hydrogen sulfide. Sour petroleum can be burned for a variety of reasons including production testing of wells, pipeline breaks and to prevent exposure to H_2S during uncontrolled releases (blowouts). The toxicology of sour petroleum is often indexed on the toxicology of H_2S for well emissions and on sulfur dioxide (SO_2) for products of combustion from burning sour petroleum. These assumptions ignore the toxicology of a complex chemical mixture.

Sour gas is crude natural gas that contains H_2S and other sulfur compounds (Coppock and Christian, 2012). Uncontrolled releases of sour gas constitute a unique hazard to humans and other animals. Uncontrolled release of sour gas into the environment can be 4.2×10^6 m^3/day and the release of sulfur compounds equivalent to 900–1400 metric tons of elemental sulfur/day. The gas well emissions from uncontrolled releases are a complex mixture of chemicals generally containing condensate, produced water and other substances. The wells may be set on fire and the emissions are a complex mixture of products of combustion and PIC. In the blowout incidents, which have been reported in the literature, cattle were confined by fences, corrals, etc., and generally could not escape the air-borne emissions. Ranchers and their families generally have been forced to evacuate the danger area leaving cattle and other livestock unattended or were not allowed to attend to livestock confined in the cordoned off area. These events can cause major disruptions in basic animal husbandry. Sour gas is heavier than air and settles into low areas especially during cool temperatures. Low areas tend to be sheltered from the wind and less dilution of the sour gas occurs. The toxic effects of sour gas have been summarized in Table 50.2. Livestock exposed to sour gas do not have clinical signs that are uniquely different from infectious diseases.

TABLE 50.2 Summary of Observed Effects of Gaseous Petroleum Emissions in Cattle

Incident	Observation	References
Canada	Watery discharge from eyes and nostrils. Post exposure pneumonia was observed	EPS (1973)
Canada, Lodgepole Blowout	Ocular and respiratory irritation, abortions, other reproductive problems	Round (1992)
	Number of aborted fetuses and diagnostic trends did not change for the Provincial Laboratory (Edmonton) during and after the blowout	Klavano and Christian (1992)
	Maladies in cattle increased with decreasing distance from the well and were increased in geographically low areas. Maladies associated with trace mineral deficiency were observed. Other maladies observed were changes in hair color, *inertia uteri*, calves born with deformed feet, failure to thrive following birth, decreased growth of replacement heifers, and 20% reduction in milk production by dairy cows, increased calving interval. Herds returned to pre- exposure level of health problems	Harris (1992)
	Significant reduction in weaning weights of calves that were exposed as cow-calf pairs	Whitelock (1992)
	The conclusions from this study were: physical examinations were within the expected normal variation, pathological findings were of varied diagnosis, and were not considered to be unique, three calves from these cows raised at the laboratory grew at average to above-average rates, parameters used may not have been sensitive enough to detect irreversible toxicological effects, and the owner may have been biased in his evaluation of long-term effects	Church (1992)
Mississippi (USA)	Post exposure observations were irritation of the eyes and respiratory tract, respiratory distress, and intolerance to exercise	Edwards (1992)
Canada	Clinical signs mimicked shipping fever, but infective agents or clinical evidence of infection were not detected, exposed feedlot cattle had extended feeding time to finish, loss of stamina in cattle, exercise intolerance in horses, exposure to sour gas may have contributed to shipping fever in recently weaned calves, and claims of reproductive failures were not established	Anon (1986)
Canada, multiphase pipeline leak	Observed effects were ocular and nasal irritation, evidence of immune and nervous system dysfunction, abnormal aggressive behavior in cows, *in estrus* behavior of pregnant cows, above average mortalities in cows and calves, calves lacked sucking instinct, cows failed to nurture new born calves, and lesions in lymph nodes and trachea	Mostrom and Campbell (1996)

Experimental Studies on Hydrogen Sulfide

Hydrogen sulfide is a toxic gas. It also has been shown to be produced endogenously at micromolar levels in all organ systems and performs regulatory functions in cell cycles, apoptosis, is important in reducing oxidative stress and functions as a gasotransmitter (Olas, 2015). Toxicity studies on H_2S have shown that it has a steep dose response curve, is an irritating gas and uncouples mitochondrial electron transport at the cytochrome c oxidase target (Khan et al., 1990; Haouzi et al., 2016). There is evidence to suggest that H_2S interactions with cysteine can be an important factor in acute H_2S poisoning. Exposure to high level of H_2S causes abolishment of cardiac contractions while rhythmic contractions persist. Hydrogen sulfide poisoning inhibits L-type calcium channels and the effects on the heart mimic poisoning by calcium channel blockers.

Goats were essentially continuously exposed to H_2S during a 96-h interval in an exposure-hood delivery system (Hayes, 1972). The exposure hood sealed around the head and neck and the animals could eat and drink. Exposure concentrations of H_2S were 0.0 ppm, four goats; 10 ppm, four goats; 50 ppm, four goats; and 100 ppm, five goats. Goats exposed to 50 or 100 ppm H_2S trembled during physical activity. At 50 ppm of exposure, epiphora occurred 24 h after exposure, and persisted for the remainder of the exposure interval. Epiphora also occurred with exposure to 100 ppm H_2S, and ocular injury was visible following 24–48 h of exposure. Corneal opacities, considered to be reversible, caused partial loss of vision. There was an inverse relationship between exposure levels and the decrease intake of feed and water. Plasma concentrations of cortisol were increased 48% and 55% in the 50 and 100 ppm groups, respectively. Respiratory and heart rates, and blood pressure were recorded each day at 08:00, 10:00, 13:00 and 16:00 h. These data suggest that initial exposure to H_2S at the 10 and 20 ppm levels caused a decrease in respiratory rate on day 1 of exposure. The 0.0 and 10 ppm treatment groups were not different for respiratory rate; exposure to 50 ppm significantly decreased respiration from 19.8 respirations/min on exposure day 2–16.5 respirations/min on day 3; goats exposed to 100 ppm had a significant decrease in respiratory rate on the last 2 days of exposure. Exposure to H_2S did not significantly alter heart rate, blood pressure, or rectal temperature; however, there was a trend for rectal temperature to increase during the exposure period.

Pathology of Hydrogen Sulfide

Detailed reports on the pathology of H_2S and sour gas in livestock do not appear to exist in the scientific literature. There are reports on the toxicopathology of H_2S in other species. Lopez et al. (1988a) exposed rats to 0, 83, and 439 ppm H_2S for 4 h. Rats exposed to 439 ppm H_2S showed perivascular and pulmonary edema 1 h postexposure. The edema cleared postexposure at hour 18. The olfactory epithelium is considered a sensitive target for H_2S (Lopez et al., 1988b; Dorman et al., 2004). Ciliated cells in the nasal passages, trachea, and bronchi are also sensitive targets for airborne irritants including H_2S and SO_2. Ciliated cells transport mucus or foreign particulate matter from the lower respiratory tract toward the pharynx where it is swallowed, and from the nasal passages to exit at the nares.

Exposure to Environmental Sulfur

Sulfur removed from sour petroleum can be stored in large stockpiles. The impact of elemental sulfur on cattle, especially to producers near sulfur stockpiles, is a concern to cattle producers. A study was done on the impact in cattle of fugitive sulfur and other pollution from sulfur mines in Poland (Janowski and Chmielowiec, 1981). The principal pollutants were sulfur dust, sulfur gases, SO_2, and sulfur hydride. Fifty-five cattle within 1 km of the mine were evaluated during the summer months on pasture, and during the winter months when the cattle were predominantly stabled. The control group of 27 cattle was kept in an area that was free of sulfur pollution, 20 km from the mine. Clinical findings in the polluted area were: decreased occurrences of infestation with external parasites and mycotic skin infections (ringworm), increased body temperature, heart and respiratory rates, and decreased excitement response to pain. Other findings were abnormal eyes (90.4%), respiratory disease (94.2%), and digestive disorders (21.1%). Clinical findings in the eye were epiphora, erythema of the conjunctiva, and edema of the eyelids. Abnormal findings of the respiratory system included dyspnea, coughing, mucopurulent nasal discharge, and abnormal pulmonary sounds. Digestive disorders included abnormal ruminal motility and diarrhea. Cattle were healthier when kept indoors. Cattle in areas polluted with sulfur, as compared to controls, had a decreased burden of parasites in the digestive tract. Pathological findings in the sulfur-exposed cattle were: the respiratory tract contained gray-yellow tinged mucus, inflammation of the trachea, thinning of cellular layers in the bronchi, almost to the point of squamous metaplasia, and interstitial inflammation. The authors concluded that sulfur pollution produces intoxication in the form of a chronic disease.

Toxicology of Sulfur Dioxide in Cattle

Inhalation studies (head-only exposure) on SO_2 in cattle showed that SO_2 adversely affects the immune system and metabolism, and cold ambient temperature modulates

SO_2 toxicity (Komarnisky, 2003). A summary of this study is given. Eight steers were progressively exposed to room air containing 1 ppm SO_2 for 10 days, 5 ppm SO_2 for 7 days, and 20 ppm for 7 days. Four steers were exposed to SO_2 at room temperature (approximently18°C), and four steers were exposed to SO_2 at −16°C. In the cold environment, the metabolic rate was increased by 33%, 39%, and 44% at 1, 5, and 20 ppm of SO_2, respectively. Exposure to SO_2 in the warm environment did not significantly alter metabolic rate. For a 500-kg steer intermittently exposed to 1 ppm of SO_2, the extra feed required for maintenance and growth would be equivalent to 1.5 kg/day of additional grain or 2.1 kg/day of additional hay. Sulfur dioxide was shown to have adverse immunotoxic effects in cattle. Exposure of steers to 5 and 20 ppm in the cold environment decreased the respiratory bursts in neutrophils. Exposure to SO_2 in the cold environment decreased the threshold dose for shedding of respiratory epithelial cells into bronchoalveolar lavage (BAL) fluid. Neutrophil numbers in BAL were increased by exposure to SO_2, and exposure to cold temperature further increased neutrophil numbers. Exposure to SO_2 decreased the number of pulmonary macrophages in BAL fluid. At the 20-ppm level, lactate dehydrogenase was increased in the BAL fluid.

ANALYTICAL TOXICOLOGY

The matrix containing petroleum and the chemicals associated with petroleum and oil—gas field operations can be assayed. The most common approach used is to match chromatographic finger prints. The organic substances assayed generally are extracts from specimens and samples submitted to the laboratory. Chemicals in petroleum that are resistant to biodegradation can be used as biomarkers (e.g., phytane and pristine). Many of the biomarkers in crude petroleum are sensitive to petroleum refining and up-grading processes and may not be found in refined products. Gas found in ground water contaminated by petroleum wells may be different from the endogenous gas or the ratio of gases found in ground water. Ions and heavy metal pollutants can be assayed in produced water and ground and surface water suspected of being contaminated with water chemicals from oilfield operations. The ratio of substances in ground water can be compared to the ratio found in produced water or other contaminating substances. During necropsy, samples and specimens need to be taken for analytical toxicology. The best procedure is to phone the laboratory in advance and request instructions for sampling containers and methods of preservation. The specimens that should be collected at necropsy are rumen and stomach contents, contents from various areas of the gastrointestinal tract, liver, kidney, lung (including description of the lobe), perirenal or bone marrow fat, brain, soiled hair or feathers. Environmental samples include suspect liquid petroleum, contaminated soil, and water.

DIFFERENTIAL DIAGNOSIS

The diagnosis of petroleum toxicity can be straight forward or very difficult depending on the circumstances. If the exposure is current or recent and there is direct evidence of toxic substances in or on the animals and obvious detrimental effects, the diagnosis may still require careful assessment and testing, but should be accomplished relatively easily. However, if the exposure has not been recent and clinical signs are not specific or are ones that may have several possible causes, the diagnosis can be very difficult. Pneumonic lesions associated with crude oil toxicity are easier to interpret if oil is still present in the gastrointestinal tract or identified in the lungs. The presence of vacuolated macrophages is helpful in differentiation from infectious causes of pneumonia. Pneumonia initiated by toxic gases is difficult to diagnose because the initial site of injury is at the broncho-alveolar junction, the same location as the initial site of infection for several viral and bacterial pathogens. The bronchial and alveolar reactions of necrosis, edema and cellular infiltration can be indistinguishable between toxic gas responses and infectious agent responses. In addition, toxic gases can interfere with the normal functions of cells lining the trachea and bronchi leading to reduced resistance to infection (Dungworth, 1993). Multiple toxic agents may also be present at the same time, making the determination of the initial cause impossible. Acute neurological signs may result from sodium ion toxicity or the acute effects of volatile hydrocarbons. The differential includes thiamine responsive polioencephalomalacia, which results in brain lesions that are indistinguishable, and lead poisoning. The analysis for sodium levels in rumen content is essential and serum osmolarity may be helpful. Exposure to high sulfates in water is linked to thiamine responsive polioencephalomalacia. The occurrence of delayed neurotoxicity signs requires an in-depth investigation of potential causes, including the tri-alkyl/aryl phosphate esters and pesticides, to determine possible exposure. The occurrence of ocular and respiratory irritation in the presence of toxic gases is a typical sign. However, similar irritation may result from dry, dusty and windy conditions and from irritating particles in feed. The measurement of toxic gas levels near the livestock is seldom possible and assumptions of exposure based on data from the emission source and nearby monitoring sites may be the only data available. Differentiation from infectious pinkeye may be made by isolating the infectious agent and ruling out toxic gas exposure.

Poor growth and weight loss may have many possible causes including nutritional deficiency, parasitism, chronic pneumonia, chronic intestinal disease, mycotoxicosis and others. Temporal connection to petroleum sources such as crude oil and previous acute cases is important in the differentiation. The possible role of adverse effects of petroleum compounds on the immune system increasing susceptibility to infectious disease further complicates the situation. Decreased reproductive performance may have multiple causes. The time delay often present between exposure and clinical signs makes diagnosis very difficult, if not impossible. Abortions that result during an acute toxic episode are the easiest to associate with the exposure incident. The potential hormonal disruption from chemicals that disturb the endocrine hormone system relating to conception and pregnancy may not be possible to determine days or weeks after the exposure.

EPIDEMIOLOGICAL STUDIES: CATTLE

Scott and colleagues used licensed SO_2 emissions from sour gas plants to estimate the exposure of cattle to air emissions from oil and gas fields (Scott et al., 2003a–d). Using Alberta Agriculture extension survey data for beef cattle, these authors found that there was no association for annual risk of culling, calf crop delivered, stillbirth, twinning, mortality, and calf crop weaned and estimated exposures to SO_2. For dairy herds using Dairy Herd Improvement data, there was no association with time to culling and no association for annual culling risks and mortality. There was a small risk for increased calving interval with high estimated exposure levels. Geographic area was interactive, suggesting the effect of emissions is subject to modification by soil type, vegetation, and climate. A study was done in the high density petroleum production and cow-calf area of Alberta (Waldner et al., 2001a,b). Seven beef herds were nonrandomly selected for study, and herds with health problems previously identified with oil and gas field pollution were not included in the study. Associations were identified for exposure to unaudited industry reported oil and gas field pollution and increased calving interval, increased calf mortality, decreased cow productivity, and increased risk of stillbirth. Lead dioxide-impregnated gauze in Petri plates and filter paper impregnated with zinc acetate were used as static monitors to measure SO_2 and H_2S, respectively. These static monitors were assayed every 30 days for sulfate and sulfide. Total sulfation increased the risk of odds of nonpregnancy and increased the risk of twinning. Increased H_2S increased the calving-to-calving interval and increased the risk of nonpregnancy and abortion. The relationship between nonaudited industrial reported emissions and total sulfation was not reported.

A large epidemiologic study was done on the effects of oil and gas pollution in beef cattle (Waldner, 2008a–d; WISSA, 2006). Static monitors were used to determine predominantly monthly averages of selected emissions from oil and gas field operations, including sour gas plants, gas gathering plants, and batteries (Burstyn et al., 2007). Assessing exposure parameters for pollutants that are complex chemical mixtures over a wide area is difficult. A substantial portion of the variability in analytical values occurred in sampling and analytical techniques. Distance from the wells rapidly decreases the concentrations of H_2S, and the number of sour gas wells increases the expected concentration of H_2S. Including flaring and sourness (sulfur content) of the wells improved the model fit. The primary predictor of SO_2 was the distance of the sampler to gas processing plants. The results suggest that SO_2 levels peaked during December to March. There was poor correlation between the logarithms of H_2S and SO_2, suggesting that SO_2 levels are not a good predictor for H_2S levels. Sampling equipment was operating close to the lower range of sensitivity.

The positive associations with exposure to oil and gas field pollutants that have been reported are given (Waldner, 2008a–d; Waldner and Clark, 2009; Waldner and Stryhn, 2008; Waldner et al., 2010). Calving interval in mature cows exposed to greater than 0.236 μg benzene/m^3 was estimated to increase by 3 days compared to that of mature cows exposed to less than 0.236 μg benzene/m^3. Exposure to SO_2 at the time of calving also increased the risk of calf mortality. Exposure to SO_2, H_2S, and volatile organic compounds measured as benzene or toluene was associated with a minor increased likelihood of calf treatment after the first month of life. There was a linear relationship between H_2S exposure and the risk of treatment. The proximity to sour gas flares was not examined. In calves that died, increasing postnatal exposures to benzene and toluene were associated with increased odds of respiratory lesions in calves older than 3 weeks. Increasing prenatal exposure to SO_2 increased the odds of lesions in skeletal muscle or myocardium. The odds were higher in calves exposed to levels greater than 9 ppb SO_2. Thyroid lesions of several types, including hypoplasia and lack of colloid, necrosis and degeneration, and hyperplasia, were recorded in calves aborted, stillborn and calves dying postnatally. Changes were most common in stillborn calves and least in calves born alive. Calves with thyroid lesions often had other pathology as well.

Immune parameters in yearling cattle from 22 herds were examined for effects of ambient $PM_{1.0}$ and selected PAHs. Immune parameters were peripherally circulating B lymphocytes and CD4, CD8, γδ, and WC1 T-lymphocyte subtypes (Bechtel et al., 2009a). The antibody response to rabies vaccine was also evaluated. No associations between $PM_{1.0}$ and selected PAHs were demonstrated in the epidemiologic models employed. In another model, in which exposures to SO_2, H_2S, benzene, and toluene were examined, exposure to toluene was associated with significant CD4 T lymphocytopenia (Bechtel et al., 2009b). The number of CD4 T lymphocytes was 30% lower in cattle exposed to 0.823 $\mu g/m^3$ toluene than in cattle exposed to less than 0.406 $\mu g/m^3$ toluene. In a similar model, 360 newborn calves (24 h to 7 days of age) were studied (Bechtel et al., 2009c). The exposure period examined was from breeding date to birth. The circulating CD4 and CD8 T lymphocyte numbers were 42% and 43% lower, respectively, in calves exposed to 0.378 $\mu g/m^3$ or greater of benzene compared with calves exposed to less than 0.276 $\mu g/m^3$ benzene. Also, CD4 T lymphocytes were 40% lower in calves exposed to 0.713 $\mu g/m^3$ or greater of toluene compared to calves exposed to less than 0.348 $\mu g/m^3$ toluene.

CONCLUDING REMARKS AND FUTURE DIRECTIONS

The petroleum industry uses and produces many mixtures of chemicals in the upstream extraction of petroleum resources. Lands used by the petroleum industry are also used by wildlife and agriculture. Domestic and wild animals inhale and ingest petroleum and chemicals used in the exploration and production of oil and gas. Contamination of surface and ground water can occur. Great care by the petroleum industry and other users of the landscape is required to prevent domestic and wild animals from being exposed to toxic substances. The emissions and effluents from petroleum extraction are complex mixtures. Most of these complex mixtures are unique to each exposure incident. Toxicity is not limited to the substances used to assess exposure. The petroleum industry is often positioned in areas of food production. Contamination of feed and food and water must be avoided. The medical community must be more aware of the possibility of toxicities and continue to develop better diagnostic capacity. In the one-medicine approach, animals are sentinels for environmental toxicology and impacts on human health.

REFERENCES

Adler, R., Boermans, H.J., Moulton, J.E., et al., 1992. Toxicosis in sheep following ingestion of natural gas condensate. Vet. Pathol. 29, 11–20.

Ahmaduna, F.-R., Pendashteh, A., Chuah Abdullah, L., et al., 2009. Review of technologies for oil and gas produced water treatment. J. Hazard Mater. 170, 530–551.

Albert, T.F., Ramey, D.B., 1964. Abomasal displacement associated with ingestion of gasoline. J. Am. Vet. Med. Assoc. 145, 460–461.

Anon, 1986. A Report on The Field Investigation into Livestock Health Complaints Subsequent to The Drummond 6-30 Sour Gaswell Blowout: September 24-28, 1984. Publication AECV86-R3. Alberta Environmental Centre, Vegreville, AB.

Batista, J.S., Carmara, A.C.L., Almeida, R.D., et al., 2013. Poisoning by crude oil in sheep and goats. Rev. Méd. Vét. 164, 517–520.

Ballantyne, E.E., 1950. Crude Petroleum Oil Poisoning. Annual Report: Veterinary Services Branch. Alberta Agriculture, Edmonton, AB.

Ballantyne, E.E., 1955. Oilwell Poisoning. Annual Report: Veterinary Services Branch. Alberta Agriculture, Edmonton, AB.

Barber, D.L.M., Cousin, D.A.H., Seawright, D., 1987. An episode of kerosene poisoning in dairy heifers. Vet. Rec. 120, 462–463.

Beck, B.E., Wood, C.D., Whenham, G.R., 1977. Triaryl phosphate poisoning in cattle. Vet. Pathol. 14, 128–137.

Bechtel, D.G., Waldner, C.L., Wickstrom, M., 2009a. Associations between immune function in yearling beef cattle and airborne polycyclic aromatic hydrocarbons and $PM_{1.0}$ near oil and natural gas field facilities. Arch. Environ. Occup. Health. 64, 47–58.

Bechtel, D.G., Waldner, C.L., Wickstrom, M., 2009b. Associations between immune function in yearling beef cattle and airborne emissions of sulfur dioxide, hydrogen sulfide, and VOCs from oil and natural gas facilities. Arch. Environ. Occup. Health. 64, 73–86.

Bechtel, D.G., Waldner, C.L., Wickstrom, M., 2009c. Associations between *in utero* exposure to airborne emissions from oil and gas production and processing facilities and immune system outcomes in neonatal beef calves. Arch. Environ. Occup. Health. 64, 59–71.

Bumstead, W.A., 1949. Unusual case of crude oil poisoning of cattle. North Am. Vet. 30, 712.

Burstyn, I., Senthilselvan, A., Kim, H.M., et al., 2007. Industrial sources influence air concentrations of hydrogen sulfide and sulfur dioxide in rural areas of western Canada. J. Air. Waste Manag. Assoc. 57, 1241–1250.

Bystrom, J.M., 1989. Study of The Acute Toxicity of Ingested Crude Petroleum Oil to Cattle (M.Sc. Thesis). University of Saskatchewan, Faculty of Graduate Studies, Saskatoon, SK.

Carpenter, D.O., 2016. Hydraulic fracturing for natural gas: impact on health and environment. Rev. Environ. Health. 31, 47–51.

Chalifoux, A., Bonneau, N., Major, P., et al., 1973. Poisoning by ingestion of motor oil in a dog. dystrophy of hepatocytes and secondary cholestasis. Can. Vet. J. 14, 68–70.

Church, T.L., 1992. Field investigation findings of the long-term effects in Alberta livestock exposed to acid forming emissions: a case study report. In: Coppock, R.W., Lillie, L.E. (Eds.), Proceedings, International Workshop on Effects of Acid Forming Emissions in Livestock (Publication AECV92-P2). Alberta Environmental Centre, Vegreville, AB.

Coale, A.J., 1947. Drinking of crude oil by cattle. North Am. Vet. 28, 221.

Coppock, R.W., Christian, R.G., 2012. Petroleum. In: Gupta, R.C. (Ed.), Veterinary Toxicology Basic and Clinical Principles, second ed. Elsevier, Toronto.

Coppock, R.W., Florence, L.Z., Miller, C.G., et al., 1992. Study on the ethology of crude oil ingestion by cattle. Toxicologist. 12, 336.

Coppock, R.W., Mostrom, M.S., Khan, A.A., et al., 1995a. A review of nonpesticide phosphate ester-induced neurotoxicity in cattle. Vet. Hum. Toxicol. 37, 576–579.

Coppock, R.W., Mostrom, M.S., Khan, A.A., et al., 1995b. Toxicology of oilfield pollutants in cattle: a review. Vet. Hum. Toxicol. 37, 569–576.

Coppock, R.W., Mostrom, M.S., Stair, E.L., et al., 1996. Toxicopathology of oilfield poisoning in cattle: a review. Vet. Hum. Toxicol. 38, 36–42.

Couillard, C.M., Leighton, F.A., 1989. Comparative pathology of Prudhoe Bay crude oil and inert shell sealants in chicken embryos. Fundam. Appl. Toxicol. 13, 165–173.

Couillard, C.M., Leighton, F.A., 1990a. The toxicopathology of Prudhoe Bay crude oil in chicken embryos. Fundam. Appl. Toxicol. 14, 30–39.

Couillard, C.M., Leighton, F.A., 1990b. Sequential study of the pathology of Prudhoe Bay crude oil in chicken embryos. Ecotoxicol. Environ. Safety. 19, 17–23.

Dorman, D.C., Struve, M.F., Gross, E.A., et al., 2004. Respiratory tract toxicity of inhaled hydrogen sulfide in Fischer-344 rats, Sprague-Dawley rats, and B6C3F1 mice following subchronic (90-day) exposure. Toxicol. Appl. Pharmacol. 198, 29–39.

Dungworth, D.L., 1993. The respiratory system. In: fourth ed. Jubb, K.V.F., Kennedy, P.C., Palmer, N. (Eds.), Pathology of Domestic Animals, vol. 2. Academic Press, Toronto, pp. 507–509.

Eaton, G., 1943. Paraffin poisoning in cattle. Vet. Rec. 55, 19.

Edwards, W.C., 1992. Investigation of animal health effects of sour gas acid forming emissions. In: Coppock, R.W., Lillie, L.E. (Eds.), Proceedings, International Workshop on Effects of Acid Forming Emissions in Livestock (Publication AECV92-P2). Alberta Environmental Centre, Vegreville, AB.

Edwards, W.C., Zinn, L.L., 1979. Petroleum hydrocarbon poisoning. Vet. Med. Small Anim. Clin. 74, 1516–1518.

Edwards, W.C., Coppock, R.W., Zinn, L.L., 1979. Toxicosis related to the petroleum industry. Vet. Hum. Toxicol. 21, 328–337.

Environmental Protection Services (EPS), 1973. Report of New Norway Scientific Committee Regarding A Gaswell Blowout October 2, 1973 Near Camrose. Alberta Environmental Protection Services, Edmonton, AB.

Fritz, D.L., Coppock, R.W., 1992. Toxicopathy of diethylene glycol in cattle. Toxicologist. 12, 119.

Gardner, D.L., 1977. Toxicology of waste petroleum products in cattle. Vet. Med. Small Anim. Clin. 72, 1874–1875.

Gibson, E.A., Linzell, J.L., 1948. Diesel oil poisoning in cattle. Vet. Rec. 60, 60–61.

Gleason, R.A., Tangen, B.A. (Eds.), 2014. Brine Contamination to Aquatic Resources from Oil and Gas Development in the Williston Basin, United States (U.S. Geological Survey Scientific Investigations Report 2014–5017). U.S. Geological Survey, Reston, VA.

Haouzi, P., Sonobe, T., Judenherc-Haouzi, A., 2016. Developing effective countermeasures against acute hydrogen sulfide intoxication: challenges and limitations. Ann. NY Acad. Sci. 1374, 29–40.

Harris, B., 1992. Field investigation findings of the long-term effects in Alberta livestock exposed to acid forming emissions: survey following the Lodgepole blowout. In: Coppock, R.W., Lillie, L.E. (Eds.), Proceedings, International Workshop on Effects of Acid Forming Emissions in Livestock (Publication AECV92-P2). Alberta Environmental Centre, Vegreville, AB.

Hayes, F.L., 1972. Studies on the Effects of Atmospheric Hydrogen Sulfide in Animals (Ph.D. Thesis). University of Missouri Graduate School, Columbia, MO.

Heitman, J.F., 1986. Chemical stratification and environmental concerns of Oklahoma off-site disposal pits. In: Kamat, R.E. (Ed.), Proceedings of A National Conference on Drilling Muds. Environmental Groundwater Institute, Norman, OK.

Janowski, T.M., Chmielowiec, J., 1981. Sulfuroza bydla. Med. Weter. 37, 265–268.

Johnson, J.H., Crookshank, H.R., Smalley, H.E., 1980. Lithium toxicity in cattle. Vet. Hum. Toxicol. 22, 248–251.

Klavano, G.G., Christian, R.G., 1992. Findings of a retrospective survey conducted after the Lodgepole sour gaswell blowout to determine if the natural occurrence of bovine abortions and fetal abnormalities increased. In: Coppock, R.W., Lillie, L.E. (Eds.), Proceedings, International Workshop on Effects of Acid Forming Emissions in Livestock (Publication AECV92-P2). Alberta Environmental Centre, Vegreville, AB.

Khan, A.A., Schuler, M.M., Prior, M.G., et al., 1990. Effects of hydrogen sulfide exposure on lung mitochondrial respiratory chain enzymes in rats. Toxicol. Appl. Pharmacol. 103, 482–490.

Khan, A.A., Coppock, R.W., Schuler, M.M., 1992. Hepatic biochemical effects in cattle exposed to methanol and diethylene glycol. Toxicologist. 12, 338.

Komarnisky, L., 2003. The Effect of Sulfur Dioxide and Cold Stress on Cattle (Ph.D. Thesis). University of Alberta, Edmonton, AB.

Lopez, A., Prior, M., Lillie, L.E., et al., 1988a. Histologic and ultrastructural alterations in lungs of rats exposed to sub-lethal concentrations of hydrogen sulfide. Vet. Pathol. 25, 376–384.

Lopez, A., Prior, M., Yong, S., et al., 1988b. Nasal lesions in rats exposed to hydrogen sulfide for four hours. Am. J. Vet. Res. 49, 1107–1111.

Lusimbo, W.S., Leighton, F.A., 1996. Effects of Prudhoe Bay crude oil on hatching success and associated changes in pipping muscles in embryos of domestic chicken (*Gallus gallus*). J. Wildl. Dis. 32, 209–215.

MacIntyre, T.M., 1970. Effect of Bunker "C" oil on sheep. Can. J. Anim. Sci. 50, 748–749.

Martinez-Guijarro, K., Ramadan, A., Gevao, B., 2017. Atmospheric concentration of polychlorinated dibenzo-p-dioxins, polychlorinated dibenzofurans (PCDD/Fs) and dioxin-like polychlorinated biphenyls (Dl-PCBs) at Umm-Al-Aish Oil Field-Kuwait. Chemosphere. 168, 147–154.

Maxie, M.G., Youssef, S., 2007. Nervous system. In: fourth ed. Maxie, M.G. (Ed.), Jubb, Kennedy and Palmer's Pathology of Domestic Animals, vol. 1. Elsevier, Toronto, pp. 281–457.

McGillivray, W.A., McDowall, F.H., Reid, C.S.W., 1959. Effects of ingestion of paraffins by ruminants. VI. Ingestion of heavy liquid paraffin by cows near parturition in relation to milk yield and composition and to fat-soluble vitamin content of the butterfat during the lactation. NZ J. Agric. Res. 2, 35–46.

Messerli, V.W., 1969. Vergiftungen in einer rinderherde durch dieselol. Schweizer Arch. Fur. Tierheilkunde. 111, 642–644.

Monlux, A.W., Schoeppel, R.J., Pearson, C.C., et al., 1971. The effect of oilfield pollutants on vegetation and farm animals. Am. J. Vet. Res. 158, 1379–1390.

Moore, T.A., 2012. Coalbed Methane: a review. Int. J. Coal. Geol. 101, 36–81.

Mostrom, M.S., Campbell, C.A.J., 1996. 1994 Livestock Field Investigation of Two Ranches Associated with A Pipeline Break (Publications Office, Communications Division). Agriculture Food and Rural Development, Edmonton, AB.

Mostrom, M.S., Khan, A.A., Fritz, D.L., et al., 1993. Alterations in xenobiotic metabolizing enzymes and tissue ultrastructure in a calf with exposure to oil field chemicals. Toxicologist. 13, 267.

Oehme, F.W., 1977. Veterinary toxicology: the epidemiology of poisonings in domestic animals. Clin. Toxicol. 10, 1–21.

Olas, B., 2015. Hydrogen sulfide in signaling pathways. Clin. Chim. Acta. 439, 212–218.

Parker, W.H., Williamson, T.F., 1951. Paraffin poisoning in cattle. Vet. Rec. 63, 430–432.

Pathan, M.H., 1961. A case record of kerosene poisoning in two goats. Ind. Vet. J. 38, 559–561.

Reid, C.S.W., 1957. Effects of ingestion of paraffins by ruminants. 1. The effect of different liquid paraffins on the feed intake of nonlactating monozygotic twin cows. NZ J. Sci. Technol. 38, 825–838.

Rousseaux, C.R., Audette, R.J., Ellefson, G., 1982. Methyl alcohol toxicity in cattle. Can. Vet. J. 23, 252.

Round, J., 1992. Clinical syndromes in livestock associated with acid forming emissions. In: Coppock, R.W., Lillie, L.E. (Eds.), Proceedings, International Workshop on Effects of Acid Forming Emissions in Livestock (Publication AECV92-P2). Alberta Environmental Centre, Vegreville, AB.

Rowe, L.D., Dollahite, J.W., Camp, B.J., 1973. Toxicity of two crude oils and of kerosene to cattle. J. Am. Vet. Med. Assoc. 162, 61–66.

Scott, H.M., Soskolne, C.L., Lissemore, K.D., et al., 2003a. Associations between air emissions from sour gas processing plants and indices of cow retainment and survival in dairy herds in Alberta. Can. J. Vet. Res. 67, 1–11.

Scott, H.M., Soskolne, C.L., Martin, S.W., et al., 2003b. Lack of associations between air emissions from sour-gas processing plants and beef cow–calf herd health and productivity in Alberta, Canada. Prev. Vet. Med. 57, 35–68.

Scott, H.M., Soskolne, C.L., Martin, S.W., et al., 2003c. Comparison of two atmospheric-dispersion models to assess farm-site exposure to sour-gas processing-plant emissions. Prev. Vet. Med. 57, 15–34.

Scott, H.M., Soskolne, C.L., Martin, S.W., et al., 2003d. Air emissions from sour-gas processing plants and dairy-cattle reproduction in Alberta, Canada. Prev. Vet. Med. 57, 69–95.

Stober, V.M., 1962. Vetraglichkeitsprufungen mit roh- und Heizol an Rindern. Deutsche Tierarztliche Wochenschrift. 69, 386–390.

Strosher, M., 1996. Investigations of Flare Gas Emissions in Alberta. Alberta Research Council, Edmonton, AB.

Toofanian, F., Aliakbari, S., Ivoghli, B., 1979. Acute diesel fuel poisoning in goats. Trop. Anim. Health Prod. 11, 98–101.

USEPA (U.S. Environmental Protection Agency), 2016. Hydraulic Fracturing for Oil and Gas: Impacts from the Hydraulic Fracturing Water Cycle on Drinking Water Resources in the United States (US EPA Report No. EPA-600-R-16-236Fa). US EPA, Washington, DC.

Waldner, C.L., 2008a. Western Canada study of animal health effects associated with exposure to emissions from oil and natural gas field facilities. Study design and data collection I. Herd performance records and management. Arch. Environ. Occup. Health. 63, 167–184.

Waldner, C.L., 2008b. Western Canada study of animal health effects associated with exposure to emissions from oil and natural gas field facilities. Study design and data collection II. Location of study herds relative to the oil and gas industry in western Canada. Arch. Environ. Occup. Health. 63, 187–199.

Waldner, C.L., 2008c. Western Canada study of animal health effects associated with exposure to emissions from oil and natural gas field facilities. Study design and data collection III. Methods of assessing animal exposure to contaminants from the oil and gas industry. Arch. Environ. Occup. Health. 63, 201–219.

Waldner, C.L., 2008d. The association between exposure to the oil and gas industry and beef calf mortality in western Canada. Arch. Environ. Occup. Health. 63, 220–240.

Waldner, C.L., Clark, E.G., 2009. Association between exposure to emissions from the oil and gas industry and pathology of the immune, nervous, and respiratory systems, and skeletal and cardiac muscle in beef calves. Arch. Environ. Occup. Health. 64, 6–27.

Waldner, C.L., Stryhn, H., 2008. Risk of nonpregnancy, risk of disposal for pregnant cows, and duration of the calving interval in cow–calf herds exposed to the oil and gas industry in western Canada. Arch. Environ. Occup. Health. 63, 241–261.

Waldner, C.L., Ribble, C.S., Janzen, E.D., et al., 2001a. Associations between total sulfation, hydrogen sulfide deposition, and beef-cattle breeding outcomes in western Canada. Prev. Vet. Med. 50, 19–33.

Waldner, C.L., Ribble, C.S., Janzen, E.D., et al., 2001b. Associations between oil- and gas-well sites, processing facilities, flaring, and beef cattle reproduction and calf mortality in western Canada. Prev. Vet. Med. 50, 1–17.

Waldner, C.L., Kennedy, R.I., Rosengren, L.B., et al., 2010. Gross postmortem and histologic examination findings from abortion losses and calf mortalities in western Canadian beef herds. Can. Vet. J. 51, 1227–1238.

Wallace, M.A., Blodgett, D.J., 1996. Lithium toxicosis in a cow. Vet. Hum. Toxicol. 138, 99–100.

Whitelock, C., 1992. Producer's observations of the short-term effects of acid forming emissions in cattle. In: Coppock, R.W., Lillie, L.E. (Eds.), Proceedings, International Workshop on Effects of Acid Forming Emissions in Livestock (Publication AECV92-P2). Alberta Environmental Centre, Vegreville, AB.

WISSA (Western Interprovincial Scientific Studies Association), 2006. Western Canada Study of Animal Health Effects Associated with Exposure to Emissions from Oil and Natural Gas Field Facilities, Technical Summary. Western Interprovincial Scientific Studies Association, Calgary, Calgary, AB.

Chapter 51

Polychlorinated Biphenyls, Polybrominated Biphenyls, Polychlorinated Dibenzo-*p*-Dioxins, and Polychlorinated Dibenzofurans

Prasada Rao S. Kodavanti, Matthew C. Valdez, Jae-Ho Yang and Margarita Curras-Collazo

INTRODUCTION

Polychlorinated biphenyls (PCBs), polybrominated biphenyls (PBBs), polychlorinated dibenzo-*p*-dioxins (PCDDs), and polychlorinated dibenzofurans (PCDFs) belong to a group of organic compounds that are well-known for their contamination in the global environment, bioaccumulating and biomagnifying in the food chain, and exerting toxic effects in wildlife, veterinary animals, and humans (Huwe, 2002; Schecter et al., 2006; Kodavanti et al., 2014a,b; Kodavanti and Loganathan, 2017). PCBs and PBBs were produced commercially for a variety of applications, while the PCDDs and PCDFs occur as byproducts of industrial and natural processes. PCBs and PBBs are structurally similar, and are formed by substituting chlorine or bromine, respectively, for hydrogen on the biphenyl molecule (Fig. 51.1). Theoretically, there are 209 possible PCB and PBB congeners considering the five chlorine- or bromine- binding sites on each ring. Each congener has been assigned a unique number from 1 to 209 in accordance with the rules of the International Union of Pure and Applied Chemistry. Commercial PCB and PBB products were mixtures of congeners that differed with respect to the number and positions of chlorination or bromination. PCDDs are composed of two benzene rings connected by two oxygen atoms and contain four to eight chlorines, for a total of 75 congeners (Fig. 51.1). PCDFs are also composed of two connected benzene rings. The rings have one oxygen molecule between them and have four chlorine binding sites available on each ring (Fig. 51.1). There are 135 different PCDF congeners (Huwe, 2002; Kodavanti et al., 2014a,b; Loganathan and Masunaga, 2015).

Certain approximate stereoisomers in this group, often collectively referred to as dioxins and dioxin-like compounds, induce a common suite of effects and have a common mechanism of action mediated by binding of the polyhalogenated aromatic hydrocarbons (PHAHs) ligand to a specific high-affinity cellular protein. This group of chemicals includes seven PCDD congeners, 10 PCDF congeners, and 12 PCB congeners. While the PBB congeners analogous to the 12 PCB congeners could also be considered dioxin-like chemicals, the relatively short commercial lifespan and restricted environmental distribution of PBBs generally precludes them from consideration. The prototype for the dioxins is 2,3,7,8-tetrachlorodibenzo-*p*-dioxin (TCDD). Toxicity and persistence of the PHAHs are determined by structure, with lateral substitutions on the ring, resulting in the highest degree of toxicity. For the PCDDs and PCDFs, congeners with chlorines in the 2, 3, 7, and 8 positions fall into this category. The TCDD-like PCB congeners are the non-*ortho*- and mono-*ortho*-substituted compounds with no chlorines or no more than one chlorine on the 2, 2′, 6, or 6′ position (Schecter et al., 2006; Kodavanti et al., 2014a,b).

The PCDDs, PCDFs, and PCBs are widely distributed into the global environment due to long-range transport and are very resistant to environmental degradation (Kodavanti et al., 2014a,b). As a result, they readily accumulate in the food chain with the greatest tissue concentrations in species at the higher trophic levels. Residues have been detected in a variety of animal species, including humans (Safe, 1998; Loganathan and Lam, 2012). In some situations, the concentrations of these chemicals in the environment are high enough to

Veterinary Toxicology. DOI: http://dx.doi.org/10.1016/B978-0-12-811410-0.00051-9

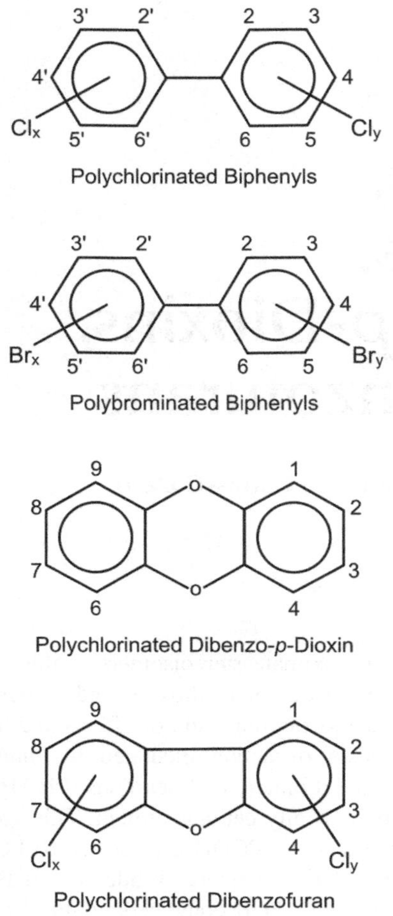

Polychlorinated Biphenyls

Polybrominated Biphenyls

Polychlorinated Dibenzo-*p*-Dioxin

Polychlorinated Dibenzofuran

FIGURE 51.1 Core structures of polychlorinated biphenyls (PCBs), polybrominated biphenyls (PBBs), polychlorinated dibenzo-*p*-dioxins (PCDDs) and polychlorinated dibenzofurans (PCDFs). The letters (o), (m), and (p) indicate *ortho-*, *meta-*, and *para-* substitutions for halogen side groups. The numbers indicate position of halogens.

pose a health risk. Because of this risk, efforts should be made to minimize exposure to these environmental contaminants.

HISTORICAL BACKGROUND

Sources

Commercial production of PCBs for a variety of uses began in the United States in 1929 and continued until 1977 (Kimbrough, 1995; Headrick et al., 1999). PCBs were used in closed systems such as electrical transformers, capacitors, and heat transfer and hydraulic systems. For a period of time, PCBs also had a large number of open-ended applications, including paints, polymers, and adhesives, as lubricants, plasticizers, fire retardants. and immersion oils, vehicles for pesticide application, and as agents for the suspension of pigments in carbonless copy paper (Headrick et al., 1999; Loganathan and Lam, 2012). The PCB products in the United States had the trade name Aroclor followed by four digits that identified the particular mixture. The first two digits referred to the 12 carbon atoms of the biphenyl molecule, and the last two digits referred to the percent of chlorine in the mixture, by weight (i.e., Aroclor 1254 has 54% chlorine by weight). Similar commercial PCB mixtures were produced by other manufacturers worldwide, including the Clophens (Germany), Phenoclors and Pyralenes (France), Fenclors (Italy), and Kanechlors (Japan) (Kimbrough, 1995; Safe, 1994; Kodavanti et al., 2014a,b).

The physical and chemical properties of PCBs, such as high stability, inertness, and dielectric properties, which were advantageous for many industrial purposes, led to the indiscriminate use of PCBs in large quantities (Loganathan and Lam, 2012; Kodavanti et al., 2014a,b). For example, the estimated cumulative production of PCBs in the United States between 1930 and 1975 was 700,000 tons. About 1.2 million tons were estimated to have been produced worldwide (Kimbrough, 1995; Tanabe, 1988). As a result of widespread use, PCBs were identified in environmental media and biota. Due to their widespread environmental contamination in the 1970s, PCB production decreased, and eventually, ceased (Loganathan and Kannan, 1994). Nevertheless, PCBs are still found in the environment, as well as in biological tissues due to their persistence. About 31% (370,000 tons) of all the PCBs produced is present in the global environment. Also, it is estimated that 780,000 tons are still available in older electric equipment and other products deposited in landfills or in storage (Tanabe, 1988).

PBBs were manufactured for use as flame retardants in industrial and consumer products (Damstra et al., 1982; Kodavanti et al., 2014a,b). It is estimated that approximately 13 million pounds were produced in the United States from 1970 to 1976, and used for incorporation into plastic products that included business machine housings, radios, televisions, thermostats, electric shavers, hand tools, and various automotive parts (DiCarlo et al., 1978; Headrick et al., 1999). Three commercial PBB products were manufactured in the United States: hexabromobiphenyl, octabromobiphenyl, and decabromobiphenyl (DiCarlo et al., 1978; Hardy, 2000). Hexabromobiphenyl was the predominant product, with approximately 11.8 million pounds being produced. More than 98% of the hexabromobiphenyl was produced as FireMaster BP-6, with the remainder being produced as FireMaster FF-1 (Hesse and Powers, 1978) after addition of an anticaking agent to FireMaster BP-6; production of PBBs ceased in 1974 (DiCarlo et al., 1978).

PCDDs and PCDFs are byproducts that are formed during the synthesis of certain industrial halogenated aromatic chemicals, byproducts from other commercial processes, and byproducts of combustion (Safe, 1990; Kodavanti et al., 2001). Some of the important industrial sources of PCDDs and PCDFs have included their formation as byproducts in the production of PCBs, chlorinated phenols and chlorinated phenol-derived chemicals, hexachlorobenzene, technical hexachlorocyclohexanes, and chlorides of iron, aluminum, and copper. PCDDs and PCDFs have also been identified in wastes and finished paper products from the pulp and paper industry. Emissions from municipal and hazardous waste incinerators, as well as home heating systems that use wood and coal, diesel engines, forest and grass fires, and agricultural and backyard burning contain PCDDs and PCDFs (Safe, 1990; Huwe, 2002; Loganathan and Masunaga, 2015). In addition, these compounds might come from naturally formed PCDD/Fs, which have been detected in deep soils and clays (Safe, 1990; Huwe, 2002).

Environmental Fate

The release of PCBs into the environment primarily has been the result of leaks, spills, and improper disposal. As stated earlier, it is estimated that approximately 370,000 tons of PCBs are present in the global environment (Tanabe, 1988). The volatility of PCBs allows their evaporation from source containers and movement through the atmosphere, resulting in widespread environmental dispersal (Headrick et al., 1999). PCDDs and PCDFs are released into the atmosphere primarily by combustion sources and by evaporation from PCDD/PCDF-containing soils and water. Similar to PCBs, the PCDDs and PCDFs can be transported long distances by winds, contributing both to general background concentrations and contamination of remote areas far from the original source. PCBs, PCDDs, and PCDFs are removed from the atmosphere by physical processes such as wet and dry deposition and vapor uptake, and are deposited on soils, surface waters, and plant surfaces. Once bound to soil and sediment, these chemicals generally remain fixed, except for bulk transport due to soil erosion, flooding, and dredging (Dickson and Buzik, 1993). Ingestion of these compounds by animals results in their preferential bioaccumulation and biomagnification in the food chain (Safe, 1994). Due to their restricted manufacturing and use, PBBs are not considered to be a significant environmental contaminant, with the exception of specific locations in Michigan. Like PCBs, PCDDs, and PCDFs, PBBs are very stable and lipophilic compounds and, therefore, persist in the environment and bioaccumulate in the food chain (Damstra et al., 1982). Also, PBBs have a high affinity for soil, and can translocate into vegetation (Fries, 1985). PCBs, PBBs, PCDDs, and PCDFs in environmental extracts are complex mixtures of congeners that can vary by lot due to various physical and biological processes. Thus, the impacts of these chemicals on the environment and biota are due to the individual components of these mixtures, their additive, and/or nonadditive (synergistic/antagonistic) interactions with themselves and other classes of pollutants (Safe, 1994; Loganathan and Masunaga, 2015).

Exposure

There are a number of ways by which animals can be, and have been, exposed to PCBs, PCDDs/PCDFs, and PBBs. Some of the scenarios involve ingestion of low concentrations of these chemicals through consumption of environmentally or accidentally contaminated feed or feed components. During the 1940s and 1950s, silos constructed with concrete were sealed with a PCB-containing paint, which eventually peeled off from the walls, resulting in contaminated silage. Dairy and beef cattle were exposed to the paint in the feed, resulting in accumulation of PCBs in adipose tissue. As a result, food products such as milk and meat contained detectable concentrations of PCBs. Examples of other exposure incidents resulting in PCB residues in food animals include consumption of tar paper by veal calves, consumption of fish viscera by swine, pullet consumption of feed containing PCB-contaminated fat added during processing, exposure of chickens to contaminated ceiling and fiberglass insulation, and treatment of boars with a topical pesticide containing PCB-contaminated oil (Headrick et al., 1999).

Several dioxin contamination incidents have occurred in Europe. In 1998, during routine monitoring, dairy products were identified that had dioxin concentrations that were 2–4 times higher than background concentrations. The source of the contamination was traced to contaminated citrus pulp used in cattle feed, which was immediately removed from the market. In another incident, PCB/PCDD/PCDF-contaminated oil was added to recycled fat used as an additive in animal feeds. The affected feeds contaminated Belgian poultry, dairy, and meat, and were discovered only after toxic effects characteristic of "chick edema disease" were seen in chickens (Bernard et al., 2002; Huwe, 2002).

PBB Incident in Michigan

FireMaster BP-6 was a mixture of PBB congeners containing 2–8 bromines with major constituents of 2,2′,4,4′,5,5′-hexabromobiphenyl (56%) and 2,2′,3,4,4′,5,5′-heptabromobiphenyl (27%) (Damstra et al., 1982). In 1972, the formulation was changed by grinding BP-6 and adding 2% calcium silicate as an anticaking agent. This new formulation, now called FireMaster FF-1, was a white powder as opposed to brown flakes, which was the appearance of BP-6 (Fries, 1985). In May 1973, 650 pounds of FF-1 were mistakenly included in a shipment of feed-grade magnesium oxide (NutriMaster), which had an appearance identical to FireMaster FF-1, to a feed mill in Climax, MI. Most of the high-level exposures occurred during the fall of 1973 before sale of the initial batch of feed was stopped in December 1973 because of dairy producer complaints of animal health problems. Shortly after PBBs were identified as the feed contaminant, the US Food and Drug Administration (FDA) set a temporary guideline of 1 ppm PBBs in milk fat, meat, and poultry, 0.1 ppm in whole eggs, and 0.3 ppm in animal feeds. In response to increasing concerns about the effects of PBBs on human and animal health, the Michigan legislature lowered the PBB tolerance to 0.02 ppm in body fat of all dairy cattle offered for slaughter in 1977. A small number of dairy producers who had repopulated after the initial quarantine in 1974 continued to have violative cattle because of residual contamination on their facilities, although this number was less than 2% of all culled cows.

TOXICOKINETICS

PCBs and PBBs

Because commercial PCB and PBB products are mixtures of individual congeners that differ in the number and position of chlorine or bromine atoms and, thus, differ in terms of their biological activities, it is difficult to accurately assess their absorption, distribution, metabolism, and elimination. A number of experiments have been conducted with a variety of species, including cows, pigs, rats, and birds on the absorption, distribution, metabolism, and elimination of the commercial PBB mixture, FireMaster BP-6, which have been summarized in an extensive review by Fries (1985). Because of the similarities between PCBs and PBBs, information pertaining to one can generally be applied to the other.

In general, PBBs are rapidly and extensively absorbed, with absorption being inversely dependent on the number of bromine atoms (Damstra et al., 1982; Fries, 1985). PBBs are widely distributed throughout the body of all species studied. Initial concentrations are generally greatest in the liver, and especially, adipose tissue (Damstra et al., 1982; Fries, 1985). Concentrations of PBBs in muscle and other tissues are usually an order of magnitude lower (Fries, 1985) compared to adipose tissue. Generally, differences in concentration between tissues can be attributed, at least in part, to variations in their fat content. Individual PBB congeners in FireMaster BP-6 and related PCBs undergo hydroxylation by metabolic routes in a manner that is dependent on the position of bromine atoms on the ring and secondarily by the bromine content of the molecule (Damstra et al., 1982). In vivo studies suggest that, like PCBs, metabolism can occur if there are two adjacent unbrominated positions (Fries, 1985).

Accumulation of individual PBB congeners into animal tissues is inversely dependent on their rate of elimination. PBBs are eliminated primarily by biliary excretion into the feces, but fecal concentrations are low compared to whole-body concentrations (Damstra et al., 1982; Fries, 1985). For example, less than 7% of an intravenous dose of 2,2′,4,4′,5,5′-hexabromobiphenyl was eliminated by rats over a 42-day period (Matthews et al., 1977; Fries, 1985), and rhesus monkeys excreted on a daily basis approximately 0.5% of a single oral dose of the same congener from 10 to 42 days postdosing (Rozman et al., 1982; Fries, 1985).

Placental transfer of PBBs occurs to some extent, but the levels in fetal or offspring tissues are relatively lower compared to levels in maternal tissues. In contrast, transfer of PBBs to the offspring during nursing results in much greater whole-body. For example, pigs that were fed PBBs during gestation and lactation had a fivefold increase in body burden during the 4-week lactation period, with residues accumulated during lactation, accounting for 95% of the total body burden (Werner and Sleight, 1981; Fries, 1985). Concentrations of PBBs in milk fat generally exceed dietary levels, with concentrations in bovine milk fat exceeding dietary levels by three- to fourfold (Damstra et al., 1982; Fries, 1985). Thus, milk seems to be the major route of elimination of PBBs for lactating mammals, inadvertently transferring PBBs from one animal to another.

PBBs can have a relatively long biological half-life in animals. Data suggested that only 10% of the total dose of 2,2′,4,4′,5,5′-hexabromobiphenyl would be eliminated during the lifetime of a rat (Matthews et al., 1977; DiCarlo et al., 1978). Rats receiving a single dose of ^{14}C-octabromobiphenyl had biphasic fecal excretion, with the initial half-life being less than 24 h and second-phase half-life being greater than 16 days (Norris et al., 1975; DiCarlo et al., 1978). Studies with cows suggested biphasic elimination of PBBs via the milk, with an initial half-life of 11 days and a second half-life of 58 days (Gutenmann and Lisk, 1975; DiCarlo et al., 1978). In cases where observation periods were long, a biological half-life of 180 days was estimated for lactating cows (Fries, 1985). It was estimated that the concentration of FireMaster BP-6 in bovine milk fat would decrease from approximately 300 to 0.3 ppm in 120 weeks (DiCarlo et al., 1978). The half-life of hexabromobiphenyl was 28 days, and that of heptabromobiphenyl was 20 days in chicken eggs (DiCarlo et al., 1978). Using the eggs of chickens fed a diet containing FireMaster FF-1 half-lives of 17 days and 31 days were calculated for chick muscle and liver, respectively, and the concentration of PBBs in adipose tissue was essentially unchanged after 56 days (Ringer and Polin, 1977; Polin and Ringer, 1978a, b).

PCDDs and PCDFs

The absorption, distribution, metabolism, and elimination of PCDDs and PCDFs have been extensively reviewed by Van den Berg et al. (1994). Absorption from the gastrointestinal tract of mammals is effective, and can exceed 75% of the dose for the lower chlorinated congeners. With increasing molecular size, absorption from the intestines is greatly reduced, which is most apparent for the hepta- and octa-chlorinated congeners. The liver and adipose tissue are the major storage sites of PCDDs and PCDFs for most mammalian and avian species. Whole-body half-lives of 2,3,7,8-substituted congeners in rodents range from a few to more than 100 days. The extent of absorption of TCDD or related compounds is variable, depending on the vehicle and the substitution pattern of the congener. There appear to be no differences between species in terms of absorption of these compounds through the gastrointestinal tract. Studies with rats, mice, hamsters, guinea pigs, cows, and chickens, in general, indicate that tetra- and penta-chlorinated congeners are well absorbed from the gastrointestinal tract (50%–90%), but octa is absorbed only to a limited extent (2%–15%) (Van den Berg et al., 1994).

As in mammals, the liver and adipose tissue of avian species are the major sites for storage and accumulation of 2,3,7,8-substitiuted PCDDs and PCDFs. Hepatic deposition of 2,3,7,8-substituted PCDDs and PCDFs appeared to increase with increasing chlorination, resulting in a limited transfer of the more highly chlorinated congeners to the egg (Van den Berg et al., 1994). In mammals, the liver and adipose tissue are the major compartments for the deposition of PCDDs and PCDFs. The elimination of polar metabolites of 2,3,7,8-substituted PCDDs and PCDFs occurs predominantly via the bile and feces, with urinary excretion playing a minor role. As chlorine content increases, the rate of elimination of PCDDs and PCDFs decreases (Pohjanvirta and Tuomisto, 1994; Van den Berg et al., 1994).

Interspecies differences in toxicity can only be partly explained by differences in toxicokinetics. The guinea pig is most sensitive to the acute effects of TCDD and has the slowest metabolism and elimination of TCDD, suggesting that toxicokinetics, in part, explains the unique sensitivity of the guinea pig to the acute toxicity of TCDD and 2,3,7,8-TCDF (Van den Berg et al., 1994). The hamster is the species most resistant to the acute toxicity of TCDD. Although the elimination rate of TCDD is two- to three-fold greater in the hamster than the rat and mouse, this does not explain entirely the 10- to 100-fold difference in acute toxicity between the hamster and other rodent species.

TOXICITY

Exposure to PBBs, PCBs, PCDDs, and PCDFs has been linked with a broad spectrum of effects, both in vivo and in vitro, which vary depending on method/age of exposure, sex of the individual, and dose/duration of exposure (Steinberg et al., 2008). Fetal and early developmental exposures to these chemicals are particularly devastating, and can have different outcomes from adult exposure (Crews et al., 2000).

Male Reproductive Effects

TCDD and related compounds decrease testis and accessory sex organ weight, cause abnormal testicular morphology, decrease spermatogenesis, and reduce fertility when given to adult animals in doses sufficient to reduce food intake and/or body weight. Some of these effects have been reported in chickens, rhesus monkeys, rats, guinea pigs, and mice treated with toxic doses of these chemicals. Effects on reproductive hormones in human males have also been characterized (Makey et al., 2016a). TCDD effects on spermatogenesis are characterized by loss of germ cells, the appearance of degenerating spermatocytes and mature spermatozoa within the lumens of seminiferous tubules, and a reduction in the number of tubules. Effects of TCDD on the male reproductive system are thought to be due, in part, to an androgen deficiency, caused by decreased plasma testosterone and dihydrotestosterone levels concomitant with unchanged plasma clearance of androgens and luteinizing hormone (LH) (Peterson et al., 1993; Safe, 1994). Pflieger-Bruss et al. (2004) provide a review of the effects of various endocrine-disrupting chemicals, including PCBs/PCDDs/PCDFs, on the male reproductive system.

Foster et al. (2010) state that decreased sperm counts are considered to be the most sensitive outcome of the reproductive/developmental effects of TCDD. A single exposure of pregnant rats to 0.064 μg TCDD/kg body weight on gestational day (GD) 15 resulted in a significant decrease (36%) in epididymal sperm counts (Mably et al., 1992). The World Health Organization (WHO) used this endpoint to establish a tolerable daily intake for TCDD of approximately 2 pg/kg body weight/day (Foster et al., 2010). Further reports show that developmental exposure to PCBs and the plasticizer di(2-ethylhexyl) phthalate (DEHP) alters adult F1 males' reproductive health. Both dioxin-like and nondioxin-like PCB can alter the timing of puberty in males (Burns et al., 2016). High exposure of PCBs in humans during their lifetime have been associated with significantly increased rates of disomy in male sperm (Perry et al., 2016). The DEHP/PCB mixture reduced testis weight more than DEHP or PCB alone, while all treatments significantly lowered intratesticular testosterone levels similarly. DEHP or PCB exposure reduced the number of Leydig cells and reduced the ratio of Group 1–2 seminiferous tubules. DEHP or PCB reduced sperm viability, epididymal sperm count, or daily sperm production. When testing sperm cells from treated and control mice offspring, the predominant effect reported was an 80%–90 % reduction by DEHP in the ability of embryos to reach the blastocyst stage, indicating predominant effects on development capacity of semen (Fiandanese et al., 2016).

Female Reproductive Effects

TCDD and approximate stereoisomers have been shown to affect female reproductive endpoints in a variety of animal studies. Among the effects reported are a decrease in the number of females mated in rats, mink, and monkeys, fewer completed pregnancies in rats, mink, and monkeys, lower maternal weight gain during pregnancy in rats, rabbits, and monkeys, decreased litter size in rats, rabbits, mink, and swine, effects on female gonads in guinea pigs and mice, and altered estrous and menstrual cycles in mice, rats, and monkeys.

Consumption of PCB-contaminated fish from Lake Ontario by women of reproductive age has been associated with reduced fecundity and menstrual cycle length (Mendola et al., 1997; Buck et al., 2000). Irregular menstrual cycle length and abnormal menstrual bleeding has been associated with consumption of rice oil contaminated with PCBs and PCDFs in Yucheng, Taiwan, between 1978 and 1979 (Yu et al., 2000) and with greater placental toxic-equivalency PCDD/PCDF concentrations in Taiwanese women (Chao et al., 2007). In utero exposure to PCBs and PCDFs during the Yucheng incident and serum dioxin levels in women from Seveso, Italy, are associated with a dose-related reduced fertility and/or prolonged time to pregnancy (Yang et al., 2008; Eskenazi et al., 2010). A recent study using the human choriocarcinoma cell line JAR and the human endometrial cell line Ishikawa in vitro model for human embryo implantation, has shown that PCBs impair the endometrial receptivity. Environmental-relevant concentrations of the PCB mixture Aroclor 1254 (2.5, 12.5, and 62.5 mM) dose-dependently reduced the adhesion of JAR spheroid attachment and increased the spheroid outgrowth (Cai et al., 2016).

Rier et al. (1993) were the first to report an association between chronic exposure to TCDD-like chemicals and endometriosis in rhesus monkeys. Findings from subsequent human epidemiological studies are inconclusive about the association between body burden of TCDD and PCBs and the incidence of endometriosis (Bruner-Tran and Osteen, 2010). TCDD-induced ovarian toxicity appears to be strain-dependent and can lead to infertility. Long-Evans rats exposed to 1 μg TCDD/kg body weight on GD 8 had reduced ovarian weight, a decline in fertility and persistent vaginal estrous. Recently, Baldridge et al. (2015) reported that TCDD at femtomolar levels significantly decreases E2 (estradiol-17β) production by human luteinizing granulose cells obtained from women stimulated for in vitro fertilization. It has been suggested that in utero exposure to TCDD results in placental hypoxia. Li et al. (2015) reported that TCDD suppresses proliferation and migration of human umbilical cord vein and artery endothelial cells and inhibits fetoplacental angiogenesis, leading to negative pregnancy outcomes.

Fenton et al. (2002) reported that in utero and lactational exposure of Long-Evans rats to TCDD (1 μg/kg body weight) on GD 15 (but not GD 20) delayed maturation of the mammary gland and could increase the incidence of breast cancer due to increased susceptibility of the gland to carcinogens. Brown et al., (1998) treated Sprague-Dawley rats prenatally with 1 μg TCDD/kg body weight, which resulted in more of the less-mature terminal end buds and less lobules II in mammary gland at postnatal day (PND) 50 compared to controls. This may explain the increased propensity for developing mammary adenocarcinomas after prenatal TCDD exposure is followed by exposure to chemical carcinogens like dimethylbenzanthracene (Brown et al., 1998). Prenatal exposure to non-*ortho* PCB congeners also results in similar effects (Muto et al., 2002).

The mammary gland is also susceptible to exposure to TCDD-like chemicals during pregnancy as the gland prepares for lactation (Fenton, 2006). Vorderstrasse et al. (2004) reported that pregnant C57B1/6 mice exposed to 5 μg TCDD/kg body weight had stunted gland growth, decreased branching, and poor formation of lobular alveolar structures. In addition, expression of a specific milk protein in the gland was suppressed, and all pups born to TCDD-treated dams died within 24 h of birth. TCDD has been implicated in impaired mammary differentiation and lactation since TCDD directly blocks lactogenesis in isolated mammary epithelial cells of mouse. The study suggested a model in which aryl hydrocarbon receptor repressor (AhRR) induction by TCDD promotes formation of AhRR/AhR nuclear translocator (ARNT) heterodimers, which transcriptionally inhibits β-casein production (Basham et al., 2015).

Developmental and Teratogenic Effects

Exposure to TCDD during pregnancy causes prenatal mortality in the mouse, rat, guinea pig, hamster, rabbit, mink, and monkey. The time period during which exposure of the embryo/fetus to TCDD occurs is just as important as the dose of TCDD administered in terms of prenatal mortality. In most laboratory mammals, gestational exposure to TCDD produces a characteristic pattern of fetotoxic responses that consist of thymic hypoplasia, subcutaneous edema, decreased fetal growth, and prenatal mortality, as well as other effects of TCDD that are highly species-specific. In the mouse, hydronephrosis is the sensitive sign of prenatal toxicity, followed by cleft palate formation and atrophy of the thymus at higher doses, and by subcutaneous edema and mortality at maternally toxic doses. In the rat, TCDD prenatal toxicity is characterized by intestinal hemorrhage, subcutaneous edema, decreased fetal growth, and mortality. Structural abnormalities occur in the rat only at relatively large doses. In the hamster fetus, hydronephrosis and renal congestion are the most sensitive effects, followed by subcutaneous edema and mortality. In the rabbit, an increased incidence of extra ribs and prenatal mortality is found, whereas in the guinea pig and rhesus monkey, prenatal mortality is seen (Dickson and Buzik, 1993; Peterson et al., 1993).

Studies characterizing the developmental cardiovascular toxicity of TCDD in mammalian species have focused on mice. Since fetal exposure to TCDD in mice does not cause overt toxicity and mortality when exposure occurs after the fusion of the palate, studies assessing the developmental effects of TCDD on the heart have conducted exposures on GD 14.5, a developmental window of cardiomyocyte proliferation (Kopf and Walker, 2009). Fetal heart-to-body weight ratio is decreased on GD 17.5, with a reduction in myocyte proliferation. This decreased heart-to-body weight ratio persisted, with a trend in PND 7 pups. However, PND 21 pups from TCDD-treated litters exhibited a significant increase in heart-to-body weight ratios, decreased basal heart rate, and a concomitant increase in mRNA expression of atrial natriuretic factor, an indicator of cardiac stress and hypertrophy (Thackaberry et al., 2005; Kopf and Walker, 2009). Expression of extracellular matrix remodeling and cardiac hypertrophy genes were dysregulated in both fetal (GD 17.5) and adult (3 months) hearts, suggestive of cardiac remodeling that persists into adulthood. Additionally, adult mice exposed to TCDD in utero had increased left ventricle weight, mild hydronephrosis, and decreased plasma volume (Aragon et al., 2008).

The teratogenic responses induced by TCDD-like chemicals are species- and strain-specific. The induction of terata is one of the most sensitive indicators of TCDD toxicity in mice, as hydronephrosis and cleft palate are induced at doses below those resulting in either maternal or embryo/fetal toxicity (Couture et al., 1990). Hydronephrosis is induced in the absence of palatal clefting; thus, the urinary tract is more sensitive to TCDD than is the secondary palate (Birnbaum et al., 1989; Couture et al., 1990). In addition, while palatal sensitivity to TCDD increases with gestational age at days 6–12 in the C57BL/6N mouse, the urinary tract appears to be equally sensitive throughout the major period of organogenesis (Couture et al., 1990).

Cleft palate in mice has been studied extensively (Abbott and Birnbaum, 1991; Abbott et al., 1992; Moriguchi et al., 2003). TCDD-exposed murine palatal shelves grow and make contact, but the subsequent process of epithelial-to-mesenchyme transformation does not occur. Therefore, a cleft is formed as the palatal shelves continue to grow without fusing (Bock and Köhle, 2006). Human embryonic palatal shelves are similarly affected, but at a much higher TCDD concentration (Abbott and Birnbaum, 1991). The observation that humans are less sensitive than mice is supported by studies with AhR-transgenic "humanized" mice (Moriguchi et al., 2003).

Neuroendocrine Effects

PCBs are the most studied class of endocrine-disrupting chemicals, yet the neuroendocrine effects of PCBs have not enjoyed the same attention. The reproductive and thyroid axes are organized with hierarchical control at hypothalamic, pituitary, and organ levels. Neuroendocrine systems within the hypothalamus depend on a relatively more porous blood–brain barrier at the hypothalamic-pituitary interface, and are subject to negative feedback from peripheral hormones. Therefore, it is likely that PCBs produce part of their actions via neuroendocrine disruption. Early-life PCB exposure results in long-term changes in reproductive capacity. There is mounting evidence that PCBs impact reproductive function via neurotoxic actions on multiple aspects of hypothalamic neuroendocrine circuitry. In combination, the evidence suggests that neurotransmitters, neurotrophic factors, steroid hormone receptors, and metabolic factors involved in the control of gonadotropin-releasing hormone (GnRH) activity are altered by PCB exposure (Bell, 2014).

PCBs can increase the responsiveness of the pituitary gland to GnRH in female sheep. In utero and lactational exposure to PCB 153 can significantly enhance LH secretion induced by GnRH in PND60 offspring (Kraugerud et al., 2012). These effects may result from interactions with developmental processes, with adult functions, or a combination of both. Estrogenic PCBs can also suppress LH levels on proestrus, the day of the preovulatory GnRH/gonadotropin surge in F2 female Sprague-Dawley rats. These profound transgenerational effects of PCBs on the reproductive axis of female rats may represent epigenetic reprogramming actions of their estrogenic activity (Steinberg et al., 2008).

Hypothyroid and hyperthyroid actions of PCBs have been reported, suggesting complex interaction between PCBs and the thyroid axis. For example, low-chlorinated PCB exposure during late gestation and lactation may significantly decrease total triiodothyronine (T3) levels in 3-week-old children (Darnerud et al., 2010). In contrast, exaggerated circulating T3 has been shown in adolescent children belonging to baby-mother pairs to be associated with high body burdens of dioxin like-PCBs in the Netherlands from 1987 to 1991 (Leijs et al., 2012). The latter finding suggests that developmental effects of PCBs on thyroid function may continue to impact physiology in adolescence. Studies on experimental animals suggest that inhibitory and stimulatory actions of PCBs arise due to reduction in circulating thyroid hormone (TH) levels, reducing pituitary sensitivity to thyrotropin-releasing hormone (TRH) and/or TH receptor agonism, respectively (Bansal and Zoeller, 2008).

PCBs share a striking structural similarity with THs, making it likely that PCBs interfere with biosynthesis and metabolism, transport of THs, and/or action at TH receptors. Chlorinated hydrocarbons, such as PCBs, result in T3 reduction and a compensatory increase in thyroid-stimulating hormone (TSH) secretion, as well as thyroid hypertrophy and increased incidence of tumors (Capen, 1994). In contrast, acute oral exposure of adult male Sprague-Dawley rats to PCB 126 (75 and 275 μg/kg body weight) increased serum TSH and reduced serum thyroxine (T4) and T3 (Fisher et al., 2006). Administration of 2,3,6,2′,5′-pentachlorinated biphenyl (PCB 95; 32 mg/kg/day, i.p) to early-weaned male rats on PND 15 and 16 reduced serum concentrations of T4, T3 and increased serum concentration of TSH at PND 17 and 18 compared to controls. This negative correlation between organohalogens and serum T4 has also been demonstrated in a North American human cohort (Makey et al., 2016b). This hypothyroid state was correlated with higher serum concentrations of leptin, adiponectin, and lower serum concentrations of insulin compared with the control group, pointing to a possible link between PCB-induced hypothyroidism and metabolic disease (Ahmed, 2013).

Fetal and neonatal neurons express TH receptors before the fetal thyroid is functional, suggesting a role for maternal THs. An important question is whether developmental exposure to PCBs interferes with TH signaling indirectly by producing maternal hypothyroidism or directly by disrupting the hypothalamic-pituitary-thyroid axis (HPT) of the offspring. Nevertheless, maternal exposure to PCBs is associated with lower TSH during pregnancy, warning of adverse consequences for maternal health and fetal development (Lv et al., 2015). In the case of hydroxylated PCB isomers, neonatal TSH has been positively associated with maternal exposure during the first trimester of pregnancy (Hisada et al., 2014). Several other studies showed no changes in TSH even though free and total T4 and T3 concentrations were suppressed (Morse et al., 1996; Khan et al., 2002). The varied outcomes of these studies is likely due to differences in the PCB mixtures and doses used, length and time of exposure, and gender differences. It is unclear if altered TSH levels resulting after PCB exposure is due, in part, to a reduction of neuroendocrine stimulation by TRH, or from an increase in the peripheral metabolism of THs through induction of hepatic microsomal enzymes or by other mechanisms.

PCBs appear to have direct agonist action on TH receptors. Gestational exposure to Aroclor 1254 (1 and 4 mg/kg/day) produced stimulatory actions on TH-responsive genes (RC3/neurogranin, Oct-1) in the fetal cortex of GD 16 rat embryos (Gauger et al., 2004). These effects are contradictory to those seen in exposed pregnant dams (reduced T3 and T4), suggesting that PCBs can have direct stimulatory actions on the fetus aside from inhibitory actions produced via maternal hypothyroidism.

Exposure to PCBs and related compounds causes a reduction in THs in developing and adult animals (Kodavanti et al., 1998; Kodavanti and Curras-Collazo, 2010). Several mechanisms have been summarized (Kashiwagi et al., 2009; Kodavanti and Loganathan, 2014) to explain how PCBs and related chemicals alter thyroid function. Since these chemicals are structurally similar to THs, PCBs, especially those that are nondioxin-like bind to transthyretin (TTR) and displace T4 (Chauhan et al., 2000). This free T4 in serum is subjected to hepatic metabolism and elimination. PCBs that are bound to TTR will be transported to the target sites, where it can bind to TH receptors to elicit a physiological response. Dioxin-like PCBs act through the AhR. These PCBs can bind to the AhR in the liver and induce hepatic uridine diphosphate glucuronyl transferases, leading to biliary excretion and elimination of T4. Consistent with these multiple modes of action of PCBs on the thyroid axis and the importance of thyroid status during neural development, functional studies have also demonstrated delayed hippocampal and cerebellar development and altered dendritogenesis after neonatal exposure to Aroclor 1254 (Lein et al., 2007; Royland et al., 2008; Yang et al., 2008). Disruption of dendritic growth by PCBs could explain, in part, the impairment in learning and memory after perinatal exposure (Yang et al., 2008; Parent et al., 2011).

Neurobehavioral Effects

In humans as well as wildlife, laboratory along with epidemiological studies have shown that exposure to TCDD-like compounds can impair cognitive functions, motor development, as well as gender-related behavior (Schantz et al., 2003). Furthermore, these studies have indicated that the behavioral effects associated with PCB exposure appear to be species-independent, and that the most susceptible period of exposure is during development and nursing. In several studies conducted in Michigan and North Carolina, there were correlations between the PCB exposure levels in mothers who consumed fish contaminated with PCBs and impairment of their children in terms of behavioral test performance and display of fine motor skills (Jacobson and Jacobson, 1996; Stewart et al., 2000, 2008). However, unlike their children, the mothers exhibited no effects of the exposure. Similar signs have been observed in children exposed to PCBs in the Faroe Islands, Germany, and the Netherlands, where in nearly all cases there was a negative correlation between PCB exposure and cognition in children (Schantz et al., 2003).

Several epidemiological studies have indicated that exposure to PCBs can contribute to hyperactivity, and may contribute to the prevalence of attention deficit hyperactivity disorder (ADHD) in humans (Bowman et al., 1981; Rice, 2000; Hardell et al., 2002). Exposure to PCBs during brain development has been shown to increase activity levels in rats and mice, indicating that PCB exposure could potentially lead to ADHD-like symptoms (Eriksson and Fredriksson, 1998; Berger et al., 2001; Branchi et al., 2005).

Mechanism of Action

Dioxin-like Chemicals

The AhR is a ligand-activated transcription factor that is involved in the regulation of a number of genes, including those for enzymes that play a role in the metabolism of xenobiotics as well as genes involved in cell growth regulation and differentiation (Safe, 1994; Denison and Nagy, 2003; Mandal, 2005; Kodavanti and Loganathan, 2014). The AhR plays an important role in the altered gene expression and species- and tissue-specific toxicity resulting from exposure to specific PCB congeners and PCDD and PCDF isomers. The toxicity of individual isomers and congeners is closely related to the affinity with which these compounds bind to the AhR, with the most toxic compounds being those that bind with the greatest affinity (Okey et al., 1994). There are large species and strain differences in sensitivity to TCDD and related chemicals. Mouse and rat strain differences in sensitivity to TCDD can be partially explained by differences in the ligand-binding affinity of their polymorphic AhR variants.

The AhR is a basic helix-loop-helix (bHLH) and Per-Arnt-Sim (PAS)-containing transcription factor (Denison and Nagy, 2003). In the absence of a ligand, AhR occurs as a soluble multiprotein complex in the cytosol of the cell. The chaperone proteins are two molecules of hsp90 (a heat shock protein of 90 kDa): the X-associated protein 2 (XAP2) and p23 (a co-chaperone protein of 23 kDa). When TCDD or another ligand diffuses across the plasma membrane and binds to the AhR, the ligand AhR complex undergoes a conformational change that exposes a nuclear localization sequence (Fig. 51.2). The complex translocates into the nucleus of the cell and the chaperone proteins dissociate from the complex. The AhR–ligand then binds to the bHLH-PAS nuclear protein, AhR nuclear translocator or ARNT. The formation of this heterodimer initiates conversion of the complex into a form that binds to DNA with high affinity on a specific recognition site called the dioxin responsive element (DRE). Binding of the ligand–AhR–ARNT complex to the DRE stimulates transcription of genes encoding cytochrome P450 enzymes in the CYP1A1 (Cytochrome P450, family 1, member A1) subfamily and other AhR-responsive genes that are located upstream of the DRE (Denison and Nagy, 2003). Continuous and inappropriate modulation of gene expression is thought to be responsible for a series of biochemical and cellular changes that result in toxicity characteristic of TCDD and related chemicals (Mandal, 2005).

Nondioxin-like Chemicals

The disruption of Ca^{2+}-homeostasis may have a significant effect on other signal transduction pathways (e.g., inositol phosphate (IP) and arachidonic acid (AA) second messengers) regulated or modulated by Ca^{2+}. The *ortho*-substituted PCB, 2,2′-dichlorobiphenyl (DCBP), but not the non-*ortho*-substituted PCB, 3,3′,4,4′,5-pentachlorobiphenyl (PCBP), affected basal and carbachol (CB)-stimulated IP accumulation in cerebellar granule cells (Kodavanti et al., 1994). AA is released intracellularly following activation of membrane phospholipases, and AA is an important second messenger in releasing Ca^{2+} from endoplasmic reticulum (Striggow and Ehrlich, 1997). Aroclor 1254 and noncoplanar PCB congener increased [^{3}H]-AA release in cerebellar granule cells while coplanar PCB did not (Kodavanti and Derr-Yellin, 1999); this is in agreement with previous structure-activity relationship (SAR) studies on Ca^{2+} buffering and protein kinase C (PKC) translocation (Kodavanti and Tilson, 1997). A similar increase in [^{3}H]-AA was observed with structurally similar chemicals such as PBDE mixtures (Kodavanti and Derr-Yellin, 2002).

One of the downstream effects of perturbed Ca^{2+}-homeostasis is translocation of PKC from the cytosol to the membrane, where it is activated (Trilivas and Brown, 1989). [3H]-Phorbol ester ([^{3}H]-PDBu) binding has been used as an indicator of PKC translocation. The noncoplanar PCB congener increased [^{3}H]-PDBu binding in a concentration-dependent manner in cerebellar granule

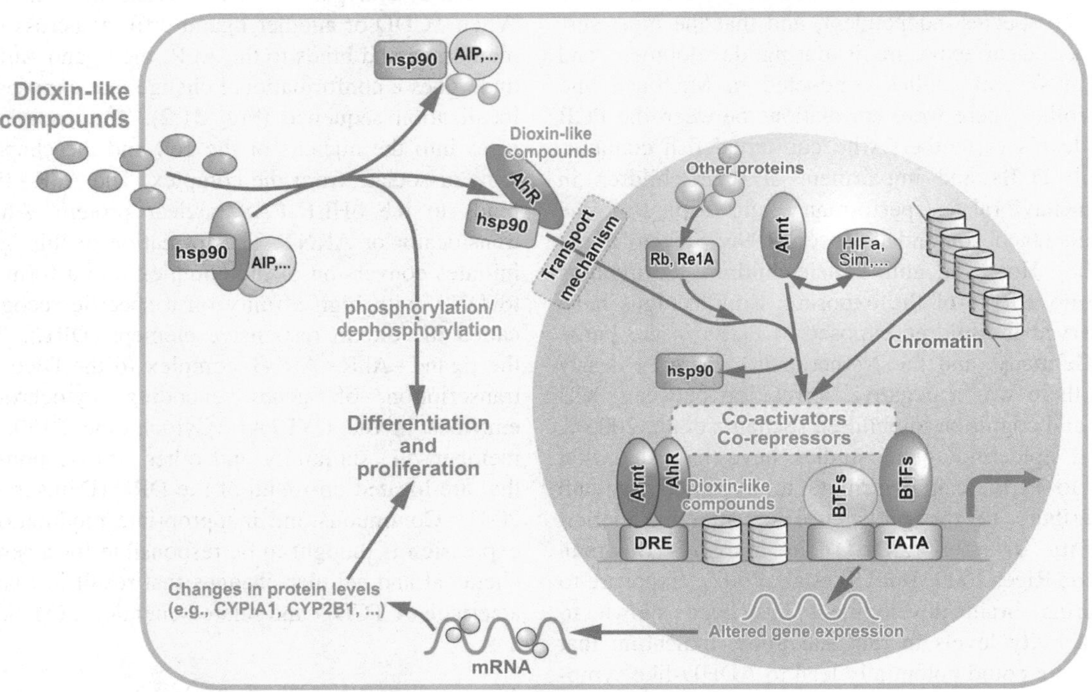

FIGURE 51.2 The proposed molecular mechanism of action of 2,3,7,8-tetrachorinated dibenzo-*p*-dioxin (TCDD) and TCDD-like chemicals. Schematic representation of functioning of the AhR (aryl hydrocarbon receptor) pathway. After entering the cell, the TCDD-like compounds bind to a protein complex in the cytoplasm consisting of AhR, Hsp90, AIP. Upon ligand binding AIP is released, exposing nuclear localization signal on AhR and leading to translocation of AhR from the cytoplasm to the nucleus. Within the nucleus, Hsp90 are released and AhR heterodimerizes with the Aryl Receptor Nuclear Translocator (ARNT). The AhR-ARNT complex then binds to multiple enhancer elements in the promotor region of the responsive genes in the AhR battery such as CYP1A. Source: *Adapted from Denison, M.S., Nagy, S.R., 2003. Activation of the aryl hydrocarbon receptor by structurally diverse exogenous and endogenous chemicals. Ann. Rev. Pharmacol. Toxicol. 43, 309–334.*

cells, while coplanar PCB had no effect even at 100 μM (Kodavanti and Tilson, 2000). Experiments with several pharmacological agents revealed that the effects of PCBs are additive with glutamate, and none of the channel (glutamate, calcium, and sodium) antagonists blocked the response of 2,2′-DCB (Kodavanti et al., 1994). Immunoblots of PKC-alpha and epsilon indicated that noncoplanar *ortho*-PCB decreased the cytosolic form and increased the membrane form significantly at 25 μM (Yang and Kodavanti, 2001). Subsequent SAR studies indicated that congeners that are noncoplanar increased PKC translocation, while coplanar congeners did not (for review, see Kodavanti and Tilson, 1997, 2000). This was further strengthened by observations with structurally similar chemicals such as polychlorinated diphenyl ethers (Kodavanti et al., 1996). Nitric oxide (NO), which is produced by nitric oxide synthase (NOS), is a gaseous neurotransmitter. NO has an important role as a retrograde messenger in long-term potentiation (LTP), learning and memory processes, and endocrine function (Schuman and Madison, 1994). The congener 2,2′-DCB, but not 4,4′-DCB, inhibited both cytosolic (nNOS) and membrane (eNOS) forms of NOS (Sharma and Kodavanti, 2002).

These in vitro studies clearly demonstrated that second messenger systems involved in the development of the nervous system, LTP, and learning and memory are sensitive targets for the *ortho*-substituted PCBs and related chemicals. Fig. 51.3 illustrates the intracellular signaling events affected by these chemicals (*ortho*-PCBs and commercial PCB mixtures) at low micromolar concentrations and shorter exposure periods, where cytotoxicity is not evident. These signaling pathways include calcium homeostasis and PKC translocation. The rise of intracellular free Ca^{2+} is slow, but steady following exposure. This free Ca^{2+} rise could be due to increased calcium influx, inhibited Ca^{2+} buffering mechanisms, and/or calcium release from intracellular stores by the products of membrane phospholipases. This increase in free Ca^{2+} could cause translocation of PKC. The coplanar non-*ortho*-PCBs have marginal effects on calcium homeostasis and

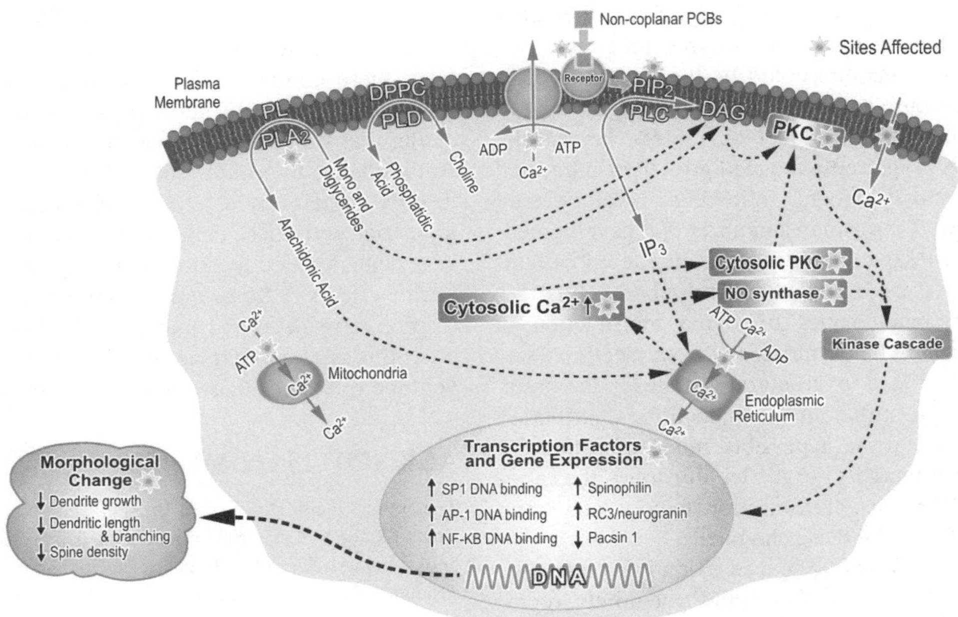

FIGURE 51.3 Schematic showing calcium and kinase signaling as a mode of action for noncoplanar PCBs. The processes by which these compounds disrupt calcium homeostasis and kinase signaling are as follows. First, chemicals bind to the cell surface receptors and activate membrane phospholipases such as phospholipase C (PLC), phospholipase A2 (PLA2), phospholipase D (PLD). This will result in several second messengers such as arachidonic acid, inositol triphosphate (IP3) which will release calcium from intracellular stores such as endoplasmic reticulum. Following blockage of calcium sequestration mechanisms in mitochondria and endoplasmic reticulum, cytosolic free calcium levels rise. Increased cytosolic calcium levels translocate protein kinases from cytosol to the membrane where they are activated. This will result in the activation of kinase cascade triggering transcription of genes which will result in a morphological change. Source: *Adapted from Kodavanti, 2004. Intracellular signaling and developmental neurotoxicity. In: N.H. Zawia (Ed.), Molecular Neurotoxicology: Environmental agents and transcription-transduction coupling. (pp 151–182). CRC Press.*

no effects on PKC translocation. Literature reports indicate that at slightly higher concentrations, commercial PCB mixtures (Aroclors 1221 and 1254) have been able to alter neurite outgrowth in PC12 cells (Angus and Contreras, 1995) and in hypothalamic cells (Gore et al., 2002). The possible mode of action for this structural change could be due to changes in intracellular signaling by these chemicals.

In vivo effects of PCBs have been studied with a commercial PCB mixture, Aroclor 1254, given orally from GD 6 through PND 21. Both calcium homeostasis and PKC activities were significantly affected following developmental exposure to Aroclor 1254 (Kodavanti et al., 2000). Developmental exposure to PCBs also caused significant hypothyroxinemia and age-dependent alterations in the translocation of PKC isozymes; the effects were significant at PND 14 (Yang et al., 2003). The changes in PKC and other second messengers were associated with changes in transcription factors such as Sp1 (specificity protein 1) and NF-kB (nuclear factor kappa-light-chain-enhancer of activated B cells), indicating changes in gene expression following developmental exposure to PCBs (Riyaz Basha et al., 2006). Considering the significant role of PKC signaling in motor behavior, learning, and memory, altered subcellular distribution of PKC isoforms at critical periods of brain development may be associated with activation of transcription factors and subsequent gene expression, and may be a possible mechanism of PCB-induced neurotoxic effects. Proteomic studies indicated that Aroclor 1254-like chemicals may alter protein networks related to energy metabolism and intracellular signaling (Kodavanti et al., 2011).

Further studies focused on the structural outcome for changes in the intracellular signaling pathway following developmental PCB exposure. Detailed brain morphometric evaluation was performed by measuring neuronal branching and spine density. Developmental exposure to PCBs affected normal dendritic development of Purkinje cells and CA1 pyramids (Lein et al., 2007). The branching area was significantly smaller in the PCB-exposed rats. When the rats become adults, there is continued neurostructural disruption of the CA1 dendritic arbor following PCB exposure; however, the branching area of the Purkinje cells returned to normal level. Developmental exposure to PCBs also resulted in a significantly smaller spine density in hippocampus, but not in cerebellum. This dysmorphic cytoarchitecture could be the structural basis for long-lasting neurocognitive deficits in PCB-exposed rats (Lein et al., 2007; Yang et al., 2009). Previously, Pruitt et al. (1999) reported a reduced growth of intra- and infrapyramidal mossy fibers following developmental exposure to PCBs. These studies indicate that developmental exposure to a PCB mixture resulted in altered cellular distribution of PKC isoforms, which can subsequently disrupt the normal maintenance of signal transduction in developing neurons. The perturbations in intracellular signaling events could lead to structural changes in the brain. These findings suggest that altered subcellular distribution of PKC isoforms may be a possible mode of action for PCB-induced neurotoxicity. Fig. 51.1 illustrates the intracellular signaling events, transcription factors, and brain morphometry affected by these chemicals.

PCBs have been shown to induce oxidative stress (Lee and Opanashuk, 2004), and this could potentially represent one mechanism of the deleterious effects of PCBs. Recently it has been shown that exposure to PCB 126, PCB 153, or binary mixtures can increase the occurrence of DNA oxidative adducts in Sprague Dawley rat hepatocytes which, in turn, can influence the prevalence of liver cancer (Mutlu et al., 2016)

CONCLUDING REMARKS AND FUTURE DIRECTIONS

PCBs, PBBs, PCDDs, and PCDFs belong to a group of compounds that are structurally related and environmentally and biologically persistent. These chemicals have a tendency to bioaccumulate and biomagnify in the food chain. Residues of these chemicals have been detected in remote areas of the world and in a variety of animal species, including humans. Exposure to these chemicals has been linked to a broad spectrum of effects. Fetal and early developmental exposures are particularly sensitive, and can have different outcomes from adult exposure. Latent effects of early exposures include, but are not limited to, depressed circulating TH levels and abnormal thyroid cytology; developmental effects on the heart, palate and kidney; delayed cognitive development; altered sensory and motor abilities; and reproductive impairment and compromised neural function. Although AhR activation has been attributed to several dioxin-like coplanar compounds, some PCBs that are noncoplanar in nature seem to exert their toxic effects through different mechanisms, including calcium signaling, oxidative stress, TH perturbations, and neurotransmitter imbalance. While certain congeners and isomers can pose a very serious threat to the health of animals and humans, environmental exposure situations are generally such that risks of health effects are generally low. The most significant problem from these compounds involve accidental poisoning via food supply and consumption of contaminated food indicating that oral ingestion was a major route of exposure. Additionally, there are areas of the environment that are heavily contaminated by these chemicals because of past industrial activities. Animals and humans residing in or near contaminated locations certainly are at risk of serious health effects. Efforts must continue to reduce exposure to protect wildlife and humans. The best way to accomplish this is to modernize technological processes to prevent the release of these chemicals into the environment.

ACKNOWLEDGMENTS

The authors thank Drs. Steven Bursian, John Newsted, and Matthew Zwiernik for the material provided in the previous edition of this book chapter. Also, Dr. Michael F. Hughes of USEPA, Research Triangle Park, NC and Dr. Ramesh Gupta of Murray State University, Hopkinsville, KY are acknowledged for the constructive review of this book chapter. The contents of this chapter have been reviewed by the National Health and Environmental Effects Research Laboratory of the US Environmental Protection Agency, and approved for publication. Approval does not signify that the contents necessarily reflect the views and policies of the Institute or Agency, nor does mention of trade names or commercial products constitute endorsement or recommendation for use.

REFERENCES

Abbott, B.D., Birnbaum, L.S., 1991. TCDD exposure of human embryonic palatal shelves in organ culture alters the differentiation of medial epithelial cells. Teratology. 43 (2), 119–132.

Abbott, B.D., Harris, M.W., Birnbaum, L.S., 1992. Comparisons of the effects of TCDD and hydrocortisone on growth factor expression provide insight into their interaction in the embryonic mouse palate. Teratology. 45 (1), 35–53.

Ahmed, R.G., 2013. Early weaning PCB 95 exposure alters the neonatal endocrine system: thyroid adipokine dysfunction. J. Endocrinol. 219 (3), 205–215.

Angus, W.G., Contreras, M.L., 1995. Aroclor 1254 alters the binding of 125 I-labeled nerve growth factor in PC12 cells. NeurosciLetter. 191 (1), 23–26.

Aragon, A.C., Kopf, P.G., Campen, M.J., et al., 2008. In utero and lactational 2, 3, 7, 8-tetrachlorodibenzo-p-dioxin exposure: effects on fetal and adult cardiac gene expression and adult cardiac and renal morphology. Toxicol. Sci. 101 (2), 321–330.

Baldridge, M.G., Marks, G.T., Rawlins, R.G., et al., 2015. Very low-dose (femtomolar) 2, 3, 7, 8-tetrachlorodibenzo-p-dioxin (TCDD) disrupts steroidogenic enzyme mRNAs and steroid secretion by human luteinizing granulosa cells. Reprod. Toxicol. 52, 57–61.

Bansal, R., Zoeller, R.T., 2008. Polychlorinated biphenyls (Aroclor 1254) do not uniformly produce agonist actions on thyroid hormone responses in the developing rat brain. Endocrinology. 149 (8), 4001–4008.

Basha, M.R., Braddy, N.S., et al., 2006. Ontogenetic alterations in prototypical transcription factors in the rat cerebellum and hippocampus following perinatal exposure to a commercial PCB mixture. Neurotoxicology. 27, 118–124.

Basham, K.J., Leonard, C.J., Kieffer, C., et al., 2015. Dioxin exposure blocks lactation through a direct effect on mammary epithelial cells mediated by the aryl hydrocarbon receptor repressor. Toxicol. Sci. 143 (1), 36–45.

Bell, M.R., 2014. Endocrine-disrupting actions of PCBs on brain development and social and reproductive behaviors. Curr. Opin. Pharmacol. 19, 134–144.

Berger, D.F., Lombardo, J.P., Jeffers, P.M., et al., 2001. Hyperactivity and impulsiveness in rats fed diets supplemented with either Aroclor 1248 or PCB-contaminated St. Lawrence river fish. Behav. Brain Res. 126 (1), 1–11.

Bernard, A., Broeckaert, F., De Poorter, G., et al., 2002. The Belgian PCB/dioxin incident: analysis of the food chain contamination and health risk evaluation. Environ. Res. 88 (1), 1–18.

Birnbaum, L.S., Harris, M.W., Stocking, L.M., et al., 1989. Retinoic acid and 2, 3, 7, 8-tetrachlorodibenzo-p-dioxin selectively enhance teratogenesis in C57BL/6N mice. Toxicol. Appl. Pharmacol. 98 (3), 487–500.

Bock, K.W., Köhle, C., 2006. Ah receptor: dioxin-mediated toxic responses as hints to deregulated physiologic functions. Biochem. Pharmacol. 72 (4), 393–404.

Bowman, R.E., Heironimus, M.P., Barsotti, D.A., 1981. Locomotor hyperactivity in PCB-exposed rhesus monkeys. Neurotoxicology. 2 (2), 251–268.

Branchi, I., Capone, F., Vitalone, A., et al., 2005. Early developmental exposure to BDE 99 or Aroclor 1254 affects neurobehavioural profile: interference from the administration route. Neurotoxicology. 26 (2), 183–192.

Brown, N.M., Manzolillo, P.A., Zhang, J.X., et al., 1998. Prenatal TCDD and predisposition to mammary cancer in the rat. Carcinogenesis. 19 (9), 1623–1629.

Bruner-Tran, K.L., Osteen, K.G., 2010. Dioxin-like PCBs and endometriosis. Syst. Biol. Reprod. Med. 56 (2), 132–146.

Buck, G.M., Vena, J.E., Schisterman, E.F., et al., 2000. Parental consumption of contaminated sport fish from Lake Ontario and predicted fecundability. Epidemiology. 11 (4), 388–393.

Burns, J.S., Lee, M.M., Williams, P.L., et al., 2016. Associations of peripubertal serum dioxin and polychlorinated biphenyl concentrations with pubertal timing among Russian boys. Environ. Health Perspect. 124 (11), 1801.

Cai, J.L., Liu, L.L., Hu, Y., et al., 2016. Polychlorinated biphenyls impair endometrial receptivity in vitro via regulating mir-30d expression and epithelial mesenchymal transition. Toxicology. 365, 25–34.

Capen, C.C., 1994. Mechanisms of chemical injury of thyroid gland. Progr. Clin. Biol. Res. 387, 173–191.

Chao, H.R., Wang, S.L., Lin, L.Y., et al., 2007. Placental transfer of polychlorinated dibenzo-p-dioxins, dibenzofurans, and biphenyls in Taiwanese mothers in relation to menstrual cycle characteristics. Food Chem. Toxicol. 45 (2), 259–265.

Chauhan, K.R., Kodavanti, P.R.S., McKinney, J.D., 2000. Assessing the role of ortho-substitution on polychlorinated biphenyl binding to transthyretin, a thyroxine transport protein. Toxicol. Appl. Pharmacol. 162 (1), 10–21.

Couture, L.A., Abbott, B.D., Birnbaum, L.S., 1990. A critical review of the developmental toxicity and teratogenicity of 2,3,7,8-tetrachlorodibenzo-p-dioxin: recent advances toward understanding the mechanism. Teratology. 42, 619–627.

Crews, D., Willingham, E., Skipper, J.K., 2000. Endocrine disruptors: present issues, future directions. Q. Rev. Biol. 75, 243–260.

Damstra, T., Jurgelski Jr., W., Posner, H.S., et al., 1982. Toxicity of polybrominated biphenyls in domestic and laboratory animals. Environ. Health Perspect. 44, 1765–1788.

Darnerud, P.O., Lignell, S., Glynn, A., et al., 2010. POP levels in breast milk and maternal serum and thyroid hormone levels in mother-child pairs from Uppsala, Sweden. Environ. Int. 36, 180–187.

Denison, M.S., Nagy, S.R., 2003. Activation of the aryl hydrocarbon receptor by structurally diverse exogenous and endogenous chemicals. Ann. Rev. Pharmacol. Toxicol. 43, 309–334.

DiCarlo, F.J., Seifter, J., DeCarlo, V.J., 1978. Assessment of the hazards of polybrominated biphenyls. Environ. Health Perspect. 23, 351–365.

Dickson, L.C., Buzik, S.C., 1993. Health risks of "dioxins": a review of environmental and toxicological considerations. Vet. Human Toxicol. 35, 68–77.

Eriksson, P., Fredriksson, A., 1998. Neurotoxic effects in adult mice neonatally exposed to 3,3′,4,4′,5-pentachlorobiphenyl or 2,3,3′,4,4′-pentachlorobiphenyl. Changes in brain nicotinic receptors and behaviour. Environ. Toxicol. Pharmacol. 5, 17–27.

Eskenazi, B., Warner, M., Marks, A.R., et al., 2010. Serum dioxin concentrations and time to pregnancy. Epidemiology. 21 (2), 224–231.

Fenton, S.E., 2006. Endocrine-disrupting compounds and mammary gland development: early exposure and later life consequences. Endocrinology. 147, S18–S24.

Fenton, S.E., Hamm, J.T., Birnbaum, L.S., et al., 2002. Persistent abnormalities in the rat mammary gland following gestational and lactational exposure to 2,3,7,8-tetrachlorodibenzo- p-dioxin (TCDD). Toxicol. Sci. 67, 63–74.

Fiandanese, N., Borromeo, V., Berrini, A., et al., 2016. Maternal exposure to a mixture of di (2-ethylhexyl) phthalate (DEHP) and polychlorinated biphenyls (PCBs) causes reproductive dysfunction in adult male mouse offspring. Reprod. Toxicol. 65, 123–132.

Fisher, J.W., Campbell, J., Muralidhara, S., et al., 2006. Effect of PCB 126 on hepatic metabolism of thyroxine and perturbations in the hypothalamic-pituitary-thyroid axis in the rat. Toxicol. Sci. 90, 87–95.

Foster, W.G., Maharaj-Briceno, S., Cyr, D.G., 2010. Dioxin-induced changes in epididymal sperm count and spermatogenesis. Environ. Hhealth Perspect. 118, 458–464.

Fries, G.F., 1985. The PBB episode in Michigan: an overall appraisal. Crit. Rev. Toxicol. 16, 105–156.

Gauger, K.J., Kato, Y., Haraguchi, K., et al., 2004. Polychlorinated biphenyls (PCBs) exert thyroid hormone-like effects in the fetal rat brain but do not bind to thyroid hormone receptors. Environ. Health Perspect. 112, 516–523.

Gore, A.C., Wu, T.J., Oung, T., et al., 2002. A novel mechanism for endocrine-disrupting effects of polychlorinated biphenyls: direct effects on gonadotropin-releasing hormone neurones. J. Neuroendocrinol. 14, 814–823.

Gutenmann, W.H., Lisk, D.J., 1975. Tissue storage and excretion in milk of polybrominated biphenyls in ruminants. J. Agri. Food Chem. 23, 1005–1007.

Hardell, L., Lindstrom, G., Van Bavel, B., 2002. Is DDT exposure during fetal period and breast-feeding associated with neurological impairment? Environ. Res. 88, 141–144.

Hardy, M.L., 2000. The toxicity of the commercial polybrominated diphenyl oxide flame retardants: DBDPO, OBDPO, PeBDPO. Organohal. Comp. 47, 41–44.

Headrick, M.L., Hollinger, K., Lovell, R.A., et al., 1999. PBBs, PCBs, and dioxins in food animals, their public health implications. Vet. Clin. North Am. Food Anim. Pract. 15, 109–131.

Hesse, J.L., Powers, R.A., 1978. Polybrominated biphenyl (PBB) contamination of the Pine River, Gratiot and Midland Counties, Michigan. Environ. Health Perspect. 23, 19–25.

Hisada, A., Shimodaira, K., Okai, T., et al., 2014. Associations between levels of hydroxylated PCBs and PCBs in serum of pregnant women and blood thyroid hormone levels and body size of neonates. Int. J. Hyg. Environ. Health. 217, 546–553.

Huwe, J.K., 2002. Dioxins in food: a modern agricultural perspective. J. Agri. Food Chem. 50, 1739–1750.

Jacobson, J.L., Jacobson, S.W., 1996. Dose–response in perinatal exposure to polychlorinated biphenyls (PCBs): the Michigan and North Carolina cohort studies. Toxicol. Industr. Health. 12, 435–445.

Kashiwagi, K., Furuno, N., Kitamura, S., et al., 2009. Disruption of thyroid hormone function by environmental pollutants. J. Health Sci. 55, 147–160.

Khan, M.A., Lichtensteiger, C.A., Faroon, O., et al., 2002. The hypothalamo-pituitary-thyroid (HPT) axis: a target of nonpersistent *ortho*-substituted PCB congeners. Toxicol. Sci. 65, 52–61.

Kimbrough, R.D., 1995. Polychlorinated biphenyls (PCBs) and human health: an update. Crit. Rev. Toxicol. 25, 133–163.

Kodavanti, P.R., Tilson, H.A., 1997. Structure-activity relationships of potentially neurotoxic PCB congeners in the rat. NeuroToxicology. 18, 425–442.

Kodavanti, P.R.S., 2004. Intracellular signaling and developmental neurotoxicity. In: Zawia, N.H. (Ed.), Molecular Neurotoxicology: Environmental agents and transcription-transduction coupling. CRC Press, Boca Raton, FL, pp. 151–182.

Kodavanti, P.R.S., Curras-Collazo, M.C., 2010. Neuroendocrine actions of organohalogens: thyroid hormones, arginine vasopressin, and neuroplasticity. Front. Neuroendocrinol. 31, 479–496.

Kodavanti, P.R.S., Derr-Yellin, E.C., 1999. Activation of calcium-dependent and –independent phospholipase A2 by non-coplanar polychlorinated biphenyls in rat cerebellar granule neurons. Organohal. Comp. 42, 449–453.

Kodavanti, P.R.S., Derr-Yellin, E.C., 2002. Differential effects of polybrominated diphenyl ethers and polychlorinated biphenyls on [^{3}H] arachidonic acid release in rat cerebellar granule neurons. Toxicol. Sci. 68, 451–457.

Kodavanti, P.R.S., Loganathan, B.G., 2014. PCBs, PBBs and brominated flame retardants. In: Gupta, R.C. (Ed.), Biomarkers in Toxicology. Academic Press/Elsevier, Amsterdam, pp. 433–450.

Kodavanti, P.R.S., Loganathan, B.G., 2017. Organohalogen pollutants and Huma Health. In: second ed. Quah, S.R., Cockerham, W.C. (Eds.), The International Encyclopedia of Public Health, vol 5. Academic Press, Oxford, pp. 359–366.

Kodavanti, P.R.S., Tilson, H.A., 2000. Neurochemical effects of environmental chemicals: in vitro and in vivo correlations on second messenger pathways. Ann. NY Acad. Sci. 919, 97–105.

Kodavanti, P.R.S., Shafer, T.J., Ward, T.R., et al., 1994. Differential effects of polychlorinated biphenyl congeners on phosphoinositide hydrolysis and protein kinase C translocation in rat cerebellar granule cells. Brain Res. 662, 75–82.

Kodavanti, P.R.S., Ward, T.R., McKinney, J.D., et al., 1996. Increased [3H]phorbol ester binding in rat cerebellar granule cells and inhibition of 45Ca2 + sequestration by polychlorinated diphenyl ether congeners and analogs: structure-activity relationships. Toxicol. Appl. Pharmacol. 138, 251–261.

Kodavanti, P.R.S., Derr-Yellin, E.C., Mundy, W.R., et al., 1998. Repeated exposure of adult rats to Aroclor 1254 causes brain region-specific changes in intracellular Ca2 + buffering and protein kinase C activity in the absence of changes in tyrosine hydroxylase. Toxicol. Appl. Pharmacol. 153, 186–198.

Kodavanti, P.R.S., Mundy, W.R., Derr-Yellin, E.C., et al., 2000. Developmental exposure to Aroclor 1254 alters calcium buffering and protein kinase C activity in the brain. Toxicol. Sci. 54, 76–77.

Kodavanti, P.R.S., Kannan, N., Yamashita, N., et al., 2001. Differential effects of two lots of Aroclor 1254: congener-specific analysis and neurochemical endpoints. Environ. Health Perspect. 109, 1153–1161.

Kodavanti, P.R.S., Osorio, C., Royland, J.E., et al., 2011. Aroclor 1254, a developmental neurotoxicant, alters energy metabolism- and intracellular signaling-associated protein networks in rat cerebellum. Toxicol. Appl. Pharmacol. 256, 290–299.

Kodavanti, P.R.S., Loganathan, B., Kurunthachalam, S.K., et al., 2014a. Organohalogen Pollutants and Human Health. Reference Module in Biomedical Sciences. Elsevier.

Kodavanti, P.R.S., Royland, J.E., Sambasiva Rao, K.R.S., 2014b. Article 403: toxicology of Persistent Organic Pollutants (POPs). Reference Module in Biomedical Research. Elsevier.

Kopf, P.G., Walker, M.K., 2009. Overview of developmental heart defects by dioxins, PCBs, and pesticides. J. Enviro. Sci. Health Part C. 27, 276–285.

Kraugerud, M., Aleksandersen, M., Nyengaard, J.R., et al., 2012. In utero and lactational exposure to PCB 118 and PCB 153 alter ovarian follicular dynamics and GnRH-induced luteinizing hormone secretion in female lambs. Environ. Toxicol. 27, 623–634.

Lee, D.W., Opanashuk, L.A., 2004. Polychlorinated biphenyl mixture Aroclor 1254-induced oxidative stress plays a role in dopaminergic cell injury. Neurotoxicology. 25, 925–939.

Leijs, M.M., Ten Tusscher, G.W., Olie, K., et al., 2012. Thyroid hormone metabolism and environmental chemical exposure. Environ. Health. 11 (Suppl. 1), S10.

Lein, P.J., Yang, D., Bachstetter, A.D., et al., 2007. Ontogenetic alterations in molecular and structural correlates of dendritic growth after developmental exposure to polychlorinated biphenyls. Environ. Health Perspect. 115, 556–563.

Li, Y., Wang, K., Zou, Q.Y., et al., 2015. 2,3,7,8-Tetrachlorodibenzo-p-dioxin differentially suppresses angiogenic responses in human placental vein and artery endothelial cells. Toxicology. 336, 70–78.

Loganathan, B.G., Kannan, K., 1994. Global organochlorine contamination trends: an Overview. AMBIO, J. Human Environ. 23, 187–191.

Loganathan, B.G., Lam, P.K.S., 2012. Global contamination trends of persistent organic chemicals: an overview. In: Loganathan, B.G., Lam, P.K.S. (Eds.), Global Contamination Trends of Persistent Organic Chemicals. CRC Press, Boca Raton, FL, pp. 3–31. (Chapter 1).

Loganathan, B.G., Masunaga, S., 2015. PCBs, dioxins, and furans: human exposure and health effects. In: Gupta, R.C. (Ed.), Handbook of Toxicology of Chemical Warfare Agents, second ed. Academic Press/Elsevier, Amsterdam, pp. 239–247.

Lv, Q.X., Wang, W., Li, X.H., et al., 2015. Polychlorinated biphenyls and polybrominated biphenyl ethers in adipose tissue and matched serum from an E-waste recycling area (Wenling, China). Environ. Poll. 199, 219–226.

Mably, T.A., Bjerke, D.L., Moore, R.W., et al., 1992. In utero and lactational exposure of male rats to 2,3,7,8-tetrachlorodibenzo- p-dioxin. 3. Effects on spermatogenesis and reproductive capability. Toxicol. Appl. Pharmacol. 114, 118–126.

Makey, C.M., McClean, M.D., Braverman, L.E., et al., 2016a. Polybrominated diphenyl ether exposure and reproductive hormones in North American men. Repr. Toxicol. 62, 46–52.

Makey, C.M., McClean, M.D., Braverman, L.E., et al., 2016b. Polybrominated diphenyl ether exposure and thyroid function tests in North American Adults. Environ. Health Perspect. 124 (4), 420.

Mandal, P.K., 2005. Dioxin: a review of its environmental effects and its aryl hydrocarbon receptor biology. J. Comp. Physiol. B. 175, 221–230.

Matthews, H.B., Kato, S., Morales, N.M., et al., 1977. Distribution and excretion of 2,4,5,2′,4′,5′-hexabromobiphenyl, the major component of Firemaster BP-6®. J. Toxicol. Environ. Health. 3, 599–605.

Mendola, P., Buck, G.M., Seve, L.E., et al., 1997. Consumption of PCB-contaminated freshwater fish and shortened menstrual cycle length. Am. J. Epidemiol. 146, 955–960.

Moriguchi, T., Motohashi, H., Hosaya, T., et al., 2003. Distinct responses to dioxin in an aryl hydrocarbon receptor (AhR)-humanized mouse. Proc. Nat. Acad. Sci. USA. 100, 5652–5657.

Morse, D.C., Seegal, R.F., Borsch, K.O., et al., 1996. Long-term alterations in regional brain serotonin metabolism following maternal polychlorinated biphenyl exposure in the rat. NeuroToxicology. 17, 631–638.

Mutlu, E., Gao, L., Collins, L.B., et al., 2016. Polychlorinated biphenyls induce oxidative DNA adducts in female Sprague–Dawley rats. Chem. Res. Toxicol. 29 (8), 1335–1344.

Muto, T., Wakui, S., Imano, N., et al., 2002. Mammary gland differentiation in female rats after prenatal exposure to 3,3′,4,4′,5-pentachlorobiphenyl. Toxicology. 177, 197–205.

Norris, J.M., Kociba, R.J., Schwetz, B.A., et al., 1975. Toxicology of octabromobiphenyl and decabromobiphenyl oxide. Environ. Health Perspect. 11, 153–161.

Okey, A.B., Riddick, D.S., Harper, P.A., 1994. The Ah receptor: mediator of the toxicity of 2,3,7,8-tetrachlorodibenzo- p-dioxin (TCDD) and related compounds. Toxicol. Lett. 70, 1–22.

Parent, A.S., Naveau, E., Gerard, A., et al., 2011. Early developmental actions of endocrine disruptors on the hypothalamus, hippocampus, and cerebral cortex. J. Toxicol. Environ. Health Part B Crit. Rev. 14, 328–345.

Perry, M.J., Young, H.A., Grandjean, P., et al., 2016. Sperm aneuploidy in Faroese men with lifetime exposure to dichlorodiphenyldichloroethylene (p, p-DDE) and polychlorinated biphenyl (PCB) pollutants. Environ. Health Prspect. 124 (7), 951.

Peterson, R.E., Theobald, H.M., Kimmel, G.L., 1993. Developmental and reproductive toxicity of dioxins and related compounds: cross-species comparisons. Crit. Rev. Toxicol. 23, 283–335.

Pflieger-Bruss, S., Schuppe, H.C., et al., 2004. The male reproductive system and its susceptibility to endocrine disrupting chemicals. Andrologia. 36, 337–345.

Pohjanvirta, R., Tuomisto, J., 1994. Short-term toxicity of 2,3,7,8-tetrachlorodibenzo- p-dioxin in laboratory animals: effects, mechanisms, and animal models. Pharmacol. Rev. 46, 483–549.

Polin, D., Ringer, R.K., 1978a. PBB fed to adult female chickens: its effect on egg production, viability of offspring, and residues in tissues and eggs. Environ. Health Perspect. 23, 283–290.

Polin, D., Ringer, R.K., 1978b. Polybrominated biphenyls in chicken eggs vs. hatchability. Proc. Soc. Exp. Biol. Med. 159, 131–135.

Pruitt, D.L., Meserve, L.A., Bingman, V.P., 1999. Reduced growth of intra- and infra-pyramidal mossy fibers is produced by continuous exposure to polychlorinated biphenyl. Toxicology. 138, 11–17.

Rice, D.C., 2000. Parallels between attention deficit hyperactivity disorder and behavioral deficits produced by neurotoxic exposure in monkeys. Environ. Health Perspect. 108, 405–408.

Rier, S.E., Martin, D.C., Bowman, R.E., et al., 1993. Endometriosis in rhesus monkeys (*Macaca mulatta*) following chronic exposure to 2,3,7,8-tetrachlorodibenzo- p-dioxin. Fund. Appl. Toxicol. 21, 433–441.

Ringer, R.K., Polin, D., 1977. The biological effects of polybrominated biphenyls in avian species. Fed. Proc. 36, 1894–1898.

Royland, J.E., Parker, J.S., Gilbert, M.E., 2008. A genomic analysis of subclinical hypothyroidism in hippocampus and neocortex of the developing rat brain. J. Neuroendocrinol. 20, 1319–1338.

Rozman, K.K., Rozman, T.A., Williams, J., et al., 1982. Effects of mineral oil and/or cholestryamine in the diet on biliary and intestinal elimination of 2,2′,4,4′,5,5′-hexachlorobiphenyl in the rhesus monkey. J. Toxicol. Environ. Health. 9, 611–618.

Safe, S., 1990. Polychlorinated biphenyls (PCBs), dibenzo-p-dioxins (PCDDs), dibenzofurans (PCDFs), and related compounds: environmental and mechanistic considerations which support the development of toxic equivalency factors (TEFs). Crit. Rev. Toxicol. 21, 51–88.

Safe, S., 1994. Polychlorinated biphenyls (PCBs): environmental impact, biochemical and toxic responses, and implications for risk assessment. Crit. Rev. Toxicol. 24, 87–149.

Safe, S., 1998. Development validation and problems with the toxic equivalency factor approach for risk assessment of dioxins and related compounds. J. Anim. Sci. 76, 134–141.

Schantz, S.L., Widholm, J.J., Rice, D.C., 2003. Effects of PCB exposure on neuropsychological function in children. Environ. Health Perspect. 111, 357–376.

Schecter, A., Birnbaum, L., Ryan, J.J., et al., 2006. Dioxins: an overview. Env. Res. 101, 419–428.

Schuman, E.M., Madison, D.V., 1994. Nitric oxide and synaptic function. Ann. Rev. Neurosci. 17, 153–183.

Sharma, R., Kodavanti, P.R.S., 2002. *In vitro* effects of polychlorinated biphenyls and hydroxy metabolites on nitric oxide synthases in rat brain. Toxicol. Appl. Pharmacol. 178, 127–136.

Steinberg, R.M., Walker, D.M., Juenger, T.E., et al., 2008. Effects of perinatal polychlorinated biphenyls on adult female rat reproduction: development, reproductive physiology, and second generational effects. Biol. Reprod. 78, 1091–1101.

Stewart, P., Pagano, J., Sargent, D., et al., 2000. Effects of Great Lakes fish consumption on brain PCB pattern, concentration, and progressive-ratio performance. Environ. Res. 82, 18–32.

Stewart, P.W., Lonky, E., Reiman, J., et al., 2008. The relationship between prenatal PCB exposure and intelligence (IQ) in 9 year old children. Environ. Health Perspect. 116, 1416–1422.

Striggow, F., Ehrlich, B.E., 1997. Regulation of intracellular calcium release channel function by arachidonic acid and leukotriene B4. Biochem. Biophys. Res. Commun. 237, 413–418.

Tanabe, S., 1988. PCB problems in the future: foresight from current knowledge. Environ. Poll. 50, 5–28.

Thackaberry, E.A., Nunez, B.A., Ivnitski-Steele, I.D., et al., 2005. Effect of 2,3,7,8-tetrachlorodibenzo-p-dioxin on murine heart development: alteration in fetal and postnatal cardiac growth, and postnatal cardiac chronotropy. Toxicol. Sci. 88, 242–249.

Trilivas, I., Brown, J.,H., 1989. Increases in intracellular Ca2 + regulate the binding of [3H]phorbol 12,13-dibutyrate to intact 1321N1 astrocytoma cells. J. Biol. Chem. 264, 3102–3107.

Van den Berg, M., De Jongh, J., Poiger, H., et al., 1994. The toxicokinetics and metabolism of polychlorinated dibenzo- p-dioxins (PCDDs) and dibenzofuran (PCDFs) and their relevance for toxicity. Crit. Rev. Toxicol. 24, 1–74.

Vorderstrasse, B.A., Fenton, S.E., Bohn, A.A., et al., 2004. A novel effect of dioxin: exposure during pregnancy severely impairs mammary gland differentiation. Toxicol. Sci. 78, 248–257.

Werner, P.R., Sleight, S.D., 1981. Toxicosis in sows and their pigs caused by feeding rations containing polybromonated biphenyls to sows during pregnancy and lactation. Am. J. Vet. Res. 42, 183–189.

Yang, C.H., Wang, Y.J., Chen, P.C., et al., 2008. Exposure to a mixture of polychlorinated biphenyls and polychlorinated dibenzofurans resulted in a prolonged time to pregnancy in women. Environ. Health Perspect. 116, 599–604.

Yang, D., Kim, K.H., Phimister, A., et al., 2009. Developmental exposure to polychlorinated biphenyls interferes with experience-dependent dendritic plasticity and ryanodine receptor expression in weanling rats. Environ. Health Perspect. 117, 426–435.

Yang, J.H., Kodavanti, P.R.S., 2001. Possible molecular targets of halogenated aromatic hydrocarbons in neuronal cells. Biochem. Biophys. Res. Commun. 280, 1372–1377.

Yang, J.H., Derr-Yellin, E.C., Kodavanti, P.R.S., 2003. Alterations in brain protein kinase C isoforms following developmental exposure to polychlorinated biphenyl mixture. Mol. Brain Res. 111, 123–135.

Yu, M.L., Guo, Y.L.L., Hsu, C.C., et al., 2000. Menstruation and reproduction in women with polychlorinated biphenyl (PCB) poisoning: long-term follow-up interviews of the women from the Taiwan Yucheng cohort. Int. J. Epidemiol. 29, 672–677.

Chapter 52

Brominated Flame Retardants and Perfluorinated Chemicals

Prasada Rao S. Kodavanti, Matthew C. Valdez and Nobuyoshi Yamashita

INTRODUCTION

During the past several decades, concern has been raised regarding exposure and harmful health effects of synthetic organohalogen compounds, especially chlorine-containing compounds such as chlorinated pesticides and polychlorinated biphenyls (PCBs) in domestic animals, wildlife, and humans (Kodavanti et al., 2008, 2014; Loganathan and Masunaga, 2015). There is mounting evidence that bromine- and fluorine-containing organohalogens are emerging as new pollutants that pose a threat on the global scale for present and future adverse health effects in animals and humans (Roth and Wilks, 2014; Shaw and Kannan, 2009; Shaw et al., 2010; Tanabe and Minh, 2010). Polybrominated diphenyl ethers (PBDEs) along with brominated bisphenols and cyclododecanes are three major groups of chemicals of brominated flame retardants (BFRs) predominantly used in numerous industrial and consumer products to make these materials more fire resistant (Alaee et al., 2003; Blum, 2010). The general chemical formula for PBDEs is $C_{12}H_{10-x}Br_xO$, and molecular weight ranges from 233 to 943.

Perfluorinated compounds (PFCs) such as perfluorooctane sulfonate/sulfonic acid (PFOS) and related compounds are used as surfactants and have a wide range of industrial and commercial applications. The chemical formula for PFOS is $C_8HF_{17}O_3S$, and its molecular weight is 500. The structures of selected PBDEs and PFCs are shown in Figs. 52.1–52.3. Unlike chlorinated compounds such as DDT (1,1,1-trichloro-2,2-bis[*p*-chlorophenyl]-ethane) and other pesticides (hexachlorobenzene, hexachlorocyclohexanes, etc.) that are used as agricultural/public health insecticides, use of BFRs and/or PFCs has never resulted in direct exposure to farm, domestic and/or pet animals. However, due to their unique physicochemical and biochemical properties, both BFRs and PFCs persist and pervade every component of the global ecosystem, leading to exposure of animals and humans and contributing to negative health effects (Linares et al., 2015; Blum, 2010; Loganathan, 2012). The Stockholm Convention on persistent organic pollutants (POPs) included some of the PBDEs and PFCs in the POPs list (Stockholm Convention Secretariat, 2010). Although the production and use of PBDEs and PFCs are restricted, environmental contamination and harmful effects to animals and humans continue. In this chapter, the historical background of BFRs and PFCs, physicochemical properties, exposure, pharmacokinetics, mechanism of action, and effects are discussed with emphasis on domestic and pet animals.

BACKGROUND

Of the brominated compounds still on the market, brominated bisphenols, diphenyl ethers, and cyclododecanes are three major classes that are still produced in large volumes (Fig. 52.1; Shaw and Kannan, 2009). It is estimated that more than one million metric tons of PBDEs have been produced. Although the manufacture of penta- and octa-bromo mixtures has ceased, the production of decabromodiphenyl ether (decaBDE) continues in some countries (Guo et al., 2011). DecaBDE was banned in Sweden and followed by partial bans in four US states (Washington, Maine, Oregon, and Vermont) in 2007, the European Union in 2008, and Canada in 2009. The REACH (Registration, Evaluation, Authorization, and Restriction of Chemical Substances) program in the European Union announced in February 2011 the ban of hexabromocyclododecane (HBCD) used with all polystyrene in building insulation (REACH, 2011). In general, PBDEs and other brominated and chlorinated flame retardants in use are HBCD, decabromodiphenyl ether, tetrabromobisphenol-A (TBBPA), tris(1-chloro-2-propyl)-phosphate, tris(2-chloroethyl)-phosphate, and Dechlorane

Veterinary Toxicology. DOI: http://dx.doi.org/10.1016/B978-0-12-811410-0.00052-0

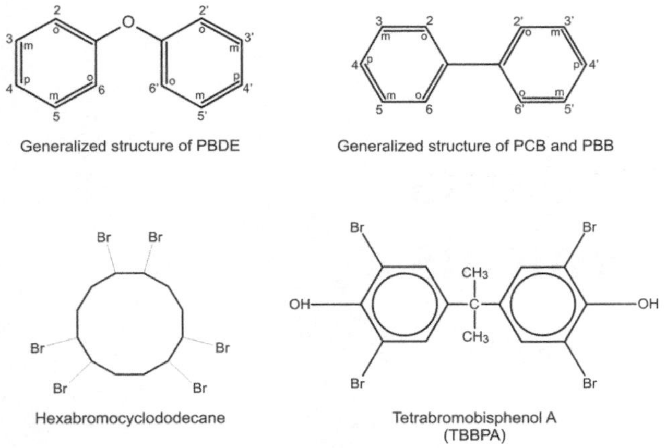

FIGURE 52.1 Chemical structures of brominated flame retardants. Structural similarities between polybrominated diphenyl ethers (PBDEs), polychlorinated biphenyls (PCBs), and polybrominated biphenyls (PBBs) are shown that are relevant to their mode of action. The letters "o," "m," and "p" respectively indicate *ortho*, *meta*, and *para* substitutions for chlorines or bromines. The numbers indicate the positions of halogens.

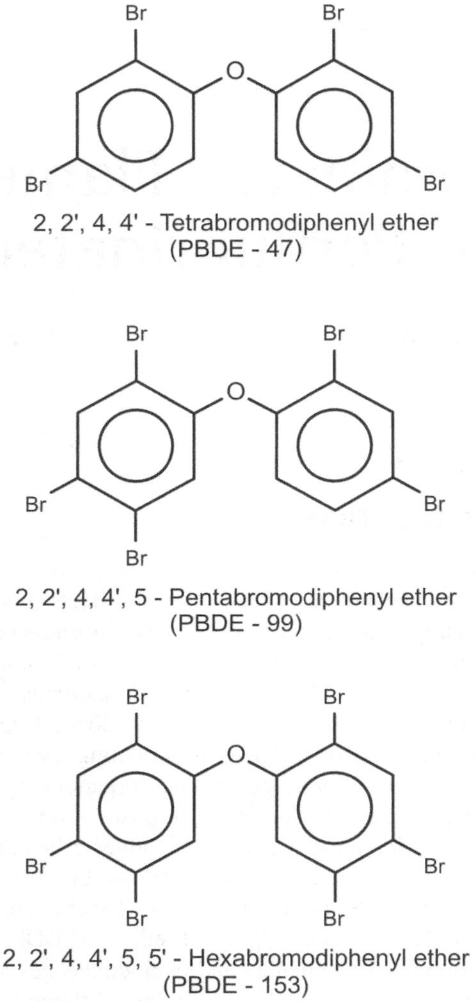

FIGURE 52.2 Chemical structures of predominant PBDEs found in commercial mixtures as well as biological and environmental samples.

Plus. These compounds are used in furniture, textiles, polyurethane foam, plastics used in electric and electronic equipment, printed circuit boards, curtains, carpets, etc. to meet fire safety standards (Alaee et al., 2003; Stapleton et al., 2009; De Wit et al., 2010; Guo et al., 2011). The high production volume and the structural similarities of these brominated chemicals to other well-known toxic environmental contaminants such as DDTs and PCBs are the main concerns for environmental and human/animal health. Furthermore, polybrominated dioxins (PBDDs)/dibenzofurans (PBDFs), formed during heating or incineration of BFRs, have toxicological profiles similar to those of their chlorinated homologs (Birnbaum et al., 2003; DiGangi et al., 2010), but they are more toxic than PBDEs. Like other organohalogens, BFRs are ubiquitous in the environment, bioaccumulate, and are toxic to animals and humans (Dye et al., 2007; Kodavanti et al., 2008; Kierkegaard et al., 2009; Ounnas et al., 2010; Shaw et al., 2010; Guo et al., 2011). A recent study pointed out that the contribution of diet to total intake is high in Germany and the United Kingdom, while in the United States, the high concentrations of PBDEs in dust resulted in a notably smaller proportion of the intake being attributed to diet as far as toddlers and adult exposures are concerned (Fromme et al., 2016).

PFCs are another class of persistent organohalogens. PFCs differ from brominated and chlorinated organohalogens by virtue of all hydrogen atoms, except those in the functional groups being substituted by fluorine atoms (Fig. 52.3). PFCs have been used in a variety of specialized consumer and industrial products for more than 60 years (Lau, 2015). The applications of PFCs include heat-, chemical-, and abrasion-resistive coatings on utensils; they are also used as dispersion, wetting, or water protection for paper and surface treatments. In particular, PFCs are used in metal-plating baths, surfactants, cleaning products, rust inhibitors, fire-fighting applications, starting materials for polymers, herbicide and insecticide formulations, cosmetics, shampoos, pharmaceuticals, lubricants, paints, polishes, upholstery, textiles, carpets, soil/stain resistance coatings, mining and oil well surfactants, acid mist suppressants, electronic etching baths, alkaline cleaners, floor polishes, photographic film, and denture cleaners and adhesives (Senthilkumar, 2005; Kodavanti et al., 2008; Yamashita et al., 2011). PFCs are also used in paper protection, including food contact applications (plates, food containers, bags, and wraps) and nonfood contact applications (folding cartons, carbonless forms, and masking papers) (Kannan et al., 2002).

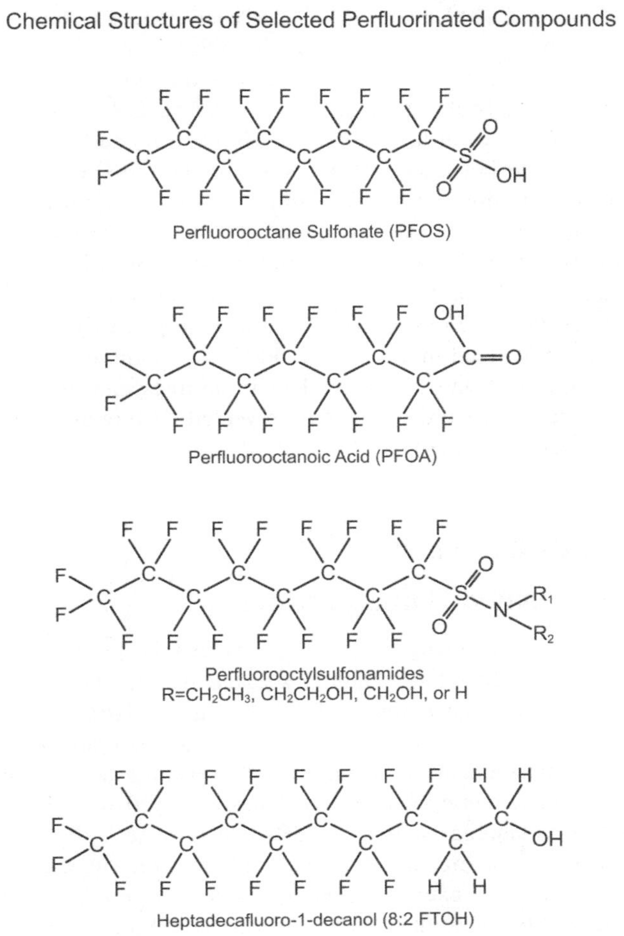

Chemical Structures of Selected Perfluorinated Compounds

Perfluorooctane Sulfonate (PFOS)

Perfluorooctanoic Acid (PFOA)

Perfluorooctylsulfonamides
R=CH_2CH_3, CH_2CH_2OH, CH_2OH, or H

Heptadecafluoro-1-decanol (8:2 FTOH)

FIGURE 52.3 Chemical structures of predominant perfluorinated chemicals, PFOS (perfluorooctane sulfonic acid) and PFOA (perfluorooctanoic acid). The metabolites perfluorooctylsulfonamide and heptadecafluoro-1-decanol are shown for structural comparison.

As a result of widespread use of these compounds, concern regarding PFC contamination has increased. PFOS and perfluorooctanoic acid (PFOA) have been consistently detected in environmental matrices, animals, and human tissues (Kannan et al., 2004, 2005a,b). Although PFOCs have been produced since the late 1950s, these compounds were first reported to occur on a global scale in 2001 (Giesy and Kannan, 2001). Perfluorinated contaminants, such as perfluorobutanesulfonate, perfluorohexanesulfonate (PFHxS), perfluorononanoic acid (PFNA), perfluorodecanoic acid (PFDA), perfluoroundecanoic acid (PFUnDA), perfluorododecanoic acid (PFDOA), and perfluorooctanesulfonamide (PFOSA), are less frequently detected in biota than are PFOS and PFOA. Studies suggest that PFCs accumulate in farm and pet animals such as chicken, cattle, goats, horses, pigs, and other vertebrates (Kennedy et al., 2004; Guruge et al., 2008).

PHYSICOCHEMICAL PROPERTIES

Brominated Flame Retardants

TBBPA (Fig. 52.1), the highest volume flame retardant worldwide, is primarily a reactive BFR (90%) covalently bound to the polymer structure and less likely to be released into the environment than are additive flame retardants (Birnbaum and Bergman, 2010). TBBPA is used in several types of circuit board polymers. TBBPA is highly lipophilic (log $K_{ow} = 4.5$) and has low water solubility (0.72 mg/mL). TBBPA has been measured in the air (Zweidinger et al., 1979), soil, and sediment (Watanabe et al., 1983), but it is generally not found in water samples. TBBPA is found in eggs of birds, human milk, and umbilical cord serum. TBBPA derivatives such as ethers are reported to be biologically active, which may lead to health effects (Legler, 2008; Birnbaum and Bergman, 2010). HBCD (Fig. 52.1) is a nonaromatic brominated cyclic alkane with a molecular weight of 641.7, and it is mainly used as an additive flame retardant in thermoplastic polymers with final applications in styrene resins (National Research Council, 2000). Like other BFRs, HBCD is highly lipophilic, with a log K_{ow} of 5.6, and it has low water solubility (0.0034 mg/L) (MacGregor and Nixon, 1997). The melting point is 185–195°C, and vapor pressure is 4.7×10^{-7} mmHg. Studies have shown that HBCD is highly persistent, with a half-life of 3 days in air and 2025 days in water (Lyman, 1990), and it is bioaccumulative, with a bioconcentration factor of approximately 18,100 in fathead minnows (Veith and Defoe, 1979).

PBDEs are composed of two phenyl rings linked by an oxygen (thus the designation as "ether"; Figs. 52.1 and 52.2). The phenyl rings may have 1–10 bromine atoms, leading to the formation of 209 possible congeners. The exact identity and pattern of various congeners in various commercial mixtures depend on the manufacturer and the specific product. Among these, the commercial "penta" mixture generally consists of PBDE congeners 99 (pentaBDE) and 47 (tetraBDE) as the major constituents (Fig. 52.2), which comprise approximately 70% of the mixture (Huber and Ballschmiter, 2001). PBDE congener 100 (pentaBDE) is present at less than 10%, with PBDE congeners 153 and 154 (hexaBDEs) at less than 5% each. The commercial "octa" mixture is 10%–12% hexaBDE, 43%–44% heptaBDE, 31%–35% octaBDE, 9%–11% nonaBDE, and 0%–1% decaBDE. The "deca" commercial mixture consists of 98% decaBDE, with a small percentage of nonaBDEs (World Health Organization, 1994; LaGuardia et al., 2006).

PBDEs are structurally similar to PCBs (Fig. 52.1) and elicit adverse effects similar to those of PCBs on nervous, immune, and endocrine systems. They also influence metabolism of chemicals endogenous to the body as well as that of foreign chemicals. Compared to chlorine atoms, bromine atoms are in general lost more easily from the molecule (more "reactive"), rendering PBDEs more susceptible to various types of degradation and metabolism than PCBs (Table 52.1). Trace analysis of these commercial mixtures for other brominated contaminants revealed the presence of PBBs and PBDFs, but not PBDDs, at levels above the limit of detection (Hanari et al., 2006). It is known that PBDEs, upon pyrolysis at 900°C, release PBDFs and PBDDs, and the amount of these contaminants depends on the conditions of pyrolysis (Buser, 1986; Thoma et al., 1986; Shaw et al., 2010).

Perfluorinated Compounds

Perfluorinated compounds have ionic and neutral characters. Because of their thermodynamically strong covalent carbon–fluorine bonds, these compounds were initially considered as nontoxic and nonmetabolizable. It is apparent that the carbon–fluorine bond has maximum energy compared to other bonds. Most of them were also considered to have little volatility. PFCs with considerable volatility are fluorotelomer alcohols (FTOHs or hydroxylated PFCs), which together with some sulfonamide-based PFCs may undergo transformation in the environment to form more persistent PFOA or similar perfluoroalkyl carboxylic or sulfonic acids (Buck, 2015). PFCs are water soluble in the several parts per million range (Table 52.2). PFCs with unique surface modification properties readily bind to surfaces including blood globulins (Kodavanti et al., 2008).

The stability of the carbon–fluorine bond contributes to the persistence of PFCs in the environment and their ability to bioaccumulate and biomagnify in higher trophic levels of a food chain. PFOS has been shown to bioconcentrate from water into benthic invertebrates by three orders of magnitude and to bioaccumulate in top predators by 5- to 20-fold (Kannan et al., 2005a). PFCs are also detected in wildlife and human tissues. Bald eagles, river otters, and bottlenose dolphins accumulate PFOS in their livers at microgram per gram tissue concentrations (Senthilkumar, 2005; Houde et al., 2006). Furthermore, fluorinated acids are even found in ocean waters, Arctic ice, and Antarctic environment and biota (Yamashita et al., 2011). Physical and chemical properties of PFCs are summarized in Table 52.2. PFCs are ubiquitous in the environment and bioaccumulate in animals and humans; their toxic properties are being revealed (Gill et al., 2004; Stein et al., 2014).

TOXICOKINETICS

Brominated Flame Retardants

The major pathway of TBBPA exposure is through diet, despite its low levels in the average diet in the United States. The bioavailability of TBBPA in circulation is very low even after administration of a high dose to rats due to rapid metabolism, indicating its low potential to bioaccumulate and cause toxic effects (Shaw et al., 2010). TBBPA or its metabolites such as TBBPA-glucuronide, a diglucuronide, and a mixed glucuronide-sulfate were detected in bile and were excreted predominantly in feces; however, metabolites were also found in urine (Hakk et al., 2000). After intravenous injection into rats, TBBPA was also rapidly cleared, and the majority of the intravenous dose was also recovered in the feces (Kuester et al., 2007). Kinetic studies in rodents and humans suggest low absorption of TBBPA from the gastrointestinal tract and rapid

TABLE 52.1 Physical and Chemical Properties of Polybrominated Diphenyl Ethers

Property	PBDEs (penta-, octa-, and deca-PBDE)
Physical state at room temperature	Pale yellow liquid to white powder
Molecular weight	564–959.2
Water solubility (μg/L at 25°C)	1
Boiling point (°C)	<300 to >400
Melting point (°C)	85–306
Vapor pressure at 25°C (mmHg)	2.2×10^{-7} to 9×10^{-10}
Log K_{ow}	5.7–8.27
Henry's law constant (atm m³/mol)	7.5×10^{-8} to 1.2×10^{-5}

Source: Data from ATSDR (Agency for Toxic Substances and Disease Registry), 2004. Toxicological Profile for Polybrominated Diphenyl Ethers and Polybrominated Biphenyls (ATSDR, 2004) and De Wit, C.A., 2002. An overview of brominated flame retardants in the environment. Chemosphere, 46, 583–624 (De Wit, 2002).

TABLE 52.2 Physical and Chemical Properties of Perfluorinated Compounds

Compound	Boiling Point (°C)	Melting Point (°C)	Vapor Pressure at 20°C (Pa)	Water Solubility (mg/L)	pK_a	Henry's Law Constant (atm m^3 mol^{-1})
Perfluorooctane sulfonyl fluoride (POSF)	154–155		221			
Perfluorooctane sulfonic acid (PFOS)	149	70–100				
Perfluorooctane sulfonate potassium salt (PFOS K)		<400	3.31×10^{-4}	570		7.2×10^{-9}
N-ethyl-perfluorooctanesulfonamide (*N*-EtFOSA)	~110	~90	0.16			
Perfluorobutanoic acid (PFBA)	120	−19.5	1333			
Perfluoropentanoic acid (PFPeA)	127					
Perfluorohexanoic acid (PFHxA)	157	12–14				
Perfluoroheptanoic acid (PFHpA)	175–177					
Perfluorooctanoic acid (PFOA)	189–192	55	100	3400	2.5	4.6×10^{-6}
Perfluorononanoic acid (PFNA)		71–77				
Perfluorodecanoic acid (PFDA)	218	83–85				
Perfluoroundecanoic acid (PFUnDA)	160	96–101				
Perfluorododecanoic acid (PFDoDA)	245	107–109				
8:2 fluorotelomer alcohol (8:2 FTOH)	95–105	42–44	356 at 25°C	0.14		9.6×10^{-2}

Source: Data from U.S. EPA, U.S. Environmental Protection Agency, 2000. Perfluorooctayl Sulfonates; Proposed Significant New Use Rule. Fed. Reg., 65 62319–62333 (U.S. EPA, 2000), Giesy, J.P., Kannan, K., 2001. Global distribution of perfluorooctane sulfonate in wildlife. Environ. Sci. Tech. 35, 1339–1342, and Yamashita, N., Young, L.Y.W., Taniyasu, S., et al., 2011. Global distribution of PFOS and related chemicals. In B. Loganathan, P.K.S. Lam (Eds.), Global Contamination Trends of Persistent Organic Chemicals. Boca Raton, Florida: CRC Press.

metabolism of the absorbed TBBPA by conjugation (Schauer et al., 2006; Kuester et al., 2007). Studies also indicated that primary route of elimination 72 h following ^{14}C-labeled TBBPA administration was in feces (94%–99%) with low levels in urine (0.2%–2%) and tissues (<0.1%) (Knudsen et al., 2014). A recent study that is based on the parallelogram calculation indicated that up to 6% of the dermally applied TBBPA may be bioavailable to humans exposed to TBBPA (Knudsen et al., 2015). Information on the toxicokinetics of HBCD is limited. A recent review article discussed the toxicokinetics and toxicodynamics of three diastereomers (α, β, and γ) of HBCD and discussed the toxicity outcomes (Koch et al., 2015). HBCD is absorbed from the gastrointestinal tract, and major sources of human exposure are food and dust intake. There are three main diastereoisomers in the commercial HBCD mixture, denoted as α, β, and γ, with the γ-diastereoisomer predominating (>70%) (Heeb et al., 2005). High levels of HBCD in some top predators indicate the persistence and biomagnification of HBCD. However, most early studies did not examine individual HBCD diastereoisomers but only the commercial HBCD mixture. Further studies have shown that there is a predominance of the most persistent stereoisomer, α-HBCD, in biota

(Covaci et al., 2006; Law et al., 2006) and that individual diastereomers have different physical and chemical properties. There is a growing need to understand the individual diastereomers that make up the commercial mixture.

There are significant differences in the pharmacokinetic behavior of individual PBDE congeners and mixtures. These differences in absorption, distribution, metabolism, and excretion depend on the test animal species and the degree of bromination. As the number of bromine atoms increases from 4 to 10 bromines (tetraBDE to decaBDE), there are decreases in oral absorption, which leads to shortened half-lives and increased elimination in both urine and feces. DecaBDE is poorly absorbed, with greater than 90% of the dose excreted in feces within 48 h (Morck et al., 2003). Workers occupationally exposed to decaBDEs have shown decaBDE half-lives of approximately 15 days (Thuresson et al., 2006), which is considerably shorter than those of other lower brominated congeners. DecaBDE has been found in the blood and breast milk of humans in the general population, but at lower levels than other PBDE congeners (Hendriks and Westerink, 2015; Lorber, 2008).

Lower brominated PBDEs, in contrast to decaBDE, are more readily absorbed and persist in the body for many years because they are mainly stored in body fat. PBDE-47 and PBDE-99 are well absorbed and highly distributed to lipophilic tissues, such as adipose, skin, and liver tissue (Hakk et al., 2002; Staskal et al., 2005). In rats, tetra- and pentaBDEs are metabolized and eliminated slowly (Hakk et al., 2002), whereas in mice, PBDE-47 is well absorbed and distributed, but its elimination is also rapid (Staskal et al., 2005). Uptake efficiencies of PBDE-47, PBDE-99, and PBDE-153 by pike fed trout injected with the congeners were 90%, 62%, and 40%, respectively (Burreau et al., 1997).

Perfluorinated Compounds

Very limited information is available on the pharmacokinetics and toxicokinetics of perfluorochemicals in farm or domestic animals. Laboratory animal studies have shown that PFOS and PFOA are well absorbed orally, not metabolized, and poorly eliminated (Ophaug and Singer, 1980; DuPont Company, 1982; Johnson et al., 1984; Vanden Heuvel et al., 1991; Guruge et al., 2006; Chang et al., 2012; Butenhoff and Rodricks, 2015). Upon ingestion, these compounds are distributed primarily to the liver, kidney, and serum, with liver concentrations being the highest (Seacat et al., 2002, 2003; Hundley et al., 2006). PFOS and PFOA tend to bind to β-lipoproteins (Jones et al., 2003), albumin, and liver fatty acid binding protein (Luebker et al., 2002). Perfluoroalkyl sulfonates (PFSAs) such as PFHxS and PFOS are transported into hepatocytes in both sodium-dependent and sodium-independent manners (Zhao et al., 2015,2017). Elimination rates and half-lives of PFCs vary with carbon chain length and animal species and gender tested. Hanhijarvi et al. (1988) reported that male hamsters excrete PFOA more rapidly than do females. In dogs, the half-life of PFOA is 20–30 days in males and 8–13 days in females. However, gender differences are not discernible in mice or rabbits (Hundley et al., 2006; Lau et al., 2006). The cause for gender and species differences in elimination of PFCs is not elucidated. Buist and Klaassen (2004) attributed these differences to the functions of organic anion transporters in the kidney because several transporter proteins are expressed differentially in male and female adult rats. Due to gender and species differences in elimination of PFCs, careful consideration must be given to compare toxicological effects. Further studies with emphasis on body burden rather than administered dose are warranted.

MECHANISM OF ACTION AND TOXICITY

Brominated Flame Retardants

TBBPA is of high ecotoxicologic concern due to its acute and chronic toxicity in several biota (U.S. EPA, 2008; Lyche et al., 2015). TBBPA has been shown to be rapidly metabolized by mammalian livers and eliminated in bile, urine, and feces (Schauer et al., 2006). TBBPA has been detected in various environmental media and biota, including air, soil, water, sediment, and bird muscle from electronic waste processing regions of China (Shi et al., 2009; Liu et al., 2016), and also in bottlenose dolphins and bull sharks from the Florida coast (Johnson-Restripo et al., 2008). Currently, no restrictions are placed on the production and use of TBBPA. TBBPA is a cytotoxicant, immunotoxicant, and thyroid hormone (TH) agonist, and it has the potential to disrupt estrogen signaling (Birnbaum and Staskal, 2004). TBBPA is also toxic in rat brain cells in vitro, where it causes oxidative stress, calcium influx, and inhibits dopamine uptake (Reistad et al., 2007). In vivo studies indicate that neonatal TBBPA exposure causes hearing deficits in rat offspring, similar to those observed following developmental exposure to PCBs (Lilienthal et al., 2008). Nakajima et al. (2009) reported the presence of TBBPA in brain along with behavioral alterations following acute treatment of TBBPA. Disruption of TH homeostasis is proposed to be the primary toxic effect of TBBPA and other BFRs. TBBPA has a closer structural relation to thyroxine (T_4) than to PCBs and binds to transthyretin (TTR) with greater affinity than it does to T_4 (Meerts et al., 2000). A study utilizing F344 rats and B6C3F1/N mice conducted by the U.S. National Toxicology Program (NTP), showed a significant fall in serum total T_4 levels at the 500 and 1000 mg/kg doses in both males and females (NTP,

2014). This decrease T_4 was not concomitant with any detectable thyroid lesions. The detailed mechanism by which BFRs can disrupt TH homeostasis is discussed later (Fig. 52.4).

Experimental studies showed that HBCD, the second most used flame retardant, has negative effects on endocrine and reproductive processes (Birnbaum and Staskal, 2004). Many effects of HBCDs seem to occur during development. During developmental exposure, HBCDs have been shown to decrease bone density and retinoids and to enhance immune response to sheep red blood cells (van der Ven et al., 2009). HBCD isomers are endocrine disruptors with antiandrogenic properties that inhibit aromatase and interact with steroid hormone receptors (Hamers et al., 2006). Like other BFRs, HBCDs may disrupt TH homeostasis, resulting in decreased T_4 levels and increased thyroid-stimulating hormone (TSH) (Ema et al., 2007). Studies indicate that a low dose of HBCD can potentially disrupt TH hormone receptor-mediated transactivation and impairs cerebellar Purkinje cell dendritogenesis (Ibhazehiebo et al., 2011).

PBDE residues have been detected in indoor air, house dust, and foods (Schecter et al., 2006; Sjodin et al., 2008). Sewage treatment plant effluents and biosolids are considered a major source of PBDEs (Rieck, 2004). More than half of the sewage sludge produced annually in the United States is applied to land as fertilizer (U.S. EPA, 1999). Agricultural land that has been treated with sewage sludge can be highly contaminated with PBDEs. Thus, application of sewage sludge may represent a source of exposure by direct contact or uptake through plants. In grazing animals including cattle, soil ingestion leads to contamination of meat and dairy products. In dairy cattle, the major intake of organohalogens occurs via spontaneous soil ingestion during grazing (Fries, 1995). Cows ingest up to 1000 g of soil per day (i.e., several micrograms of halogenated compounds daily) depending on several factors, including season, climate, and density of grass (Laurent et al., 2005).

There are a few reports indicating high levels of serum PBDEs in household cats because of their high exposure to house dust (Dye et al., 2007). In captive giant and red pandas, the tissue levels of PBDEs ranged from 38 to 2158 ng/g lipid weight (lw) (Hu et al., 2008). Kierkegaard et al. (2009) reported PBDE levels in cow milk (1100–2600 pg/g lw) and fat (1300–2600 pg/g lw). In Arctic fox, the levels of PBDEs are very low, ranging from 26 to 31 ng/g lw (De Wit et al., 2010). Whereas the levels of PBDEs in the liver of California sea otter are 2423 ng/g lw (Kannan et al., 2008), the levels are much higher in blubber of California sea lions, ranging from 569 to 24343 ng/g lw (Stapleton et al., 2006). In adipose tissue of polar bears in Canada, Muir et al. (2006) reported levels of PBDEs ranging from 4.6 to 11 ng/g lw, and these levels were lower than those reported from polar bear fat samples from Svalbard and East Greenland. PBDE levels in domestic, pet, and wild animals are presented in Table 52.3.

Exposure to PBDEs in domestic/pet animals and humans may occur via multiple sources (air, water, dust, and food). Levels of PBDEs in animal and human tissues have increased exponentially since the 1970s in several countries, including the United States, Canada, and Sweden (Schecter et al., 2005; Guo et al., 2011). Elevated levels of PBDEs in North America have been attributed to the greater use of the pentaBDE mixture compared to its use throughout the rest of the world. Like other lipophilic compounds, PBDEs readily cross the placenta into the fetus, providing an opportunity for PBDEs to interfere with human and animal developmental processes (Frederiksen et al., 2010).

Because PBDEs are predominantly used indoors, data on their effects on wildlife and farm animals are limited and exposure seems to be more through nondietary sources (Caspersen et al., 2016). A few studies indicate that PBDE exposure at environmentally relevant concentrations increases nestling growth (Fernie et al., 2006) and causes changes in reproductive courtship behaviors in adult American kestrels (Fernie et al., 2008). However, a number of studies on laboratory animals have indicated that commercial PBDE mixtures as well as the individual PBDE congeners that compose them affect the nervous, endocrine, reproductive, and immune systems (Lyche et al., 2015). Tseng et al. (2006) did not find effects on sperm count or function at high concentrations of PBDE-209 (500–1500 mg/kg/day from postnatal day (PND) 21 to 70) in mice, but they did find indications of oxidative stress in sperm. In a subsequent study, Tseng et al. (2013) found significant changes in the male offspring in anogenital distance, sperm heads, and testicular histopathology following exposure to PBDE-209. Few studies have indicated association of PBDEs with pregnancy- related outcomes such as longer time to pregnancy in women (Harley et al., 2010) and enhanced risk of developing gestational diabetes mellitus (Smarr et al., 2016). With regard to neurotoxic effects, several studies have indicated that HBCD and PBDEs cause permanent aberrations in spontaneous behavior and habituation capability in mice after a single exposure at PND 10 (a period of rapid brain growth development). It is interesting to note that the effects seen on this behavioral paradigm with PBDEs are identical to those produced by PCBs (Eriksson and Fredriksson, 1996). Mice exposed to a single dose of PBDE 47 on PND 10 demonstrated delayed ontogeny of neuromotor function and hyperactivity when they attained adult age without any alterations in circulating TH levels (Gee and Moser, 2008; Gee et al., 2008). Other studies showed developmental delays in the acquisition of the palpebral reflex following neonatal exposure to PBDE 209 along with changes in circulating T_4 levels (Rice et al.,

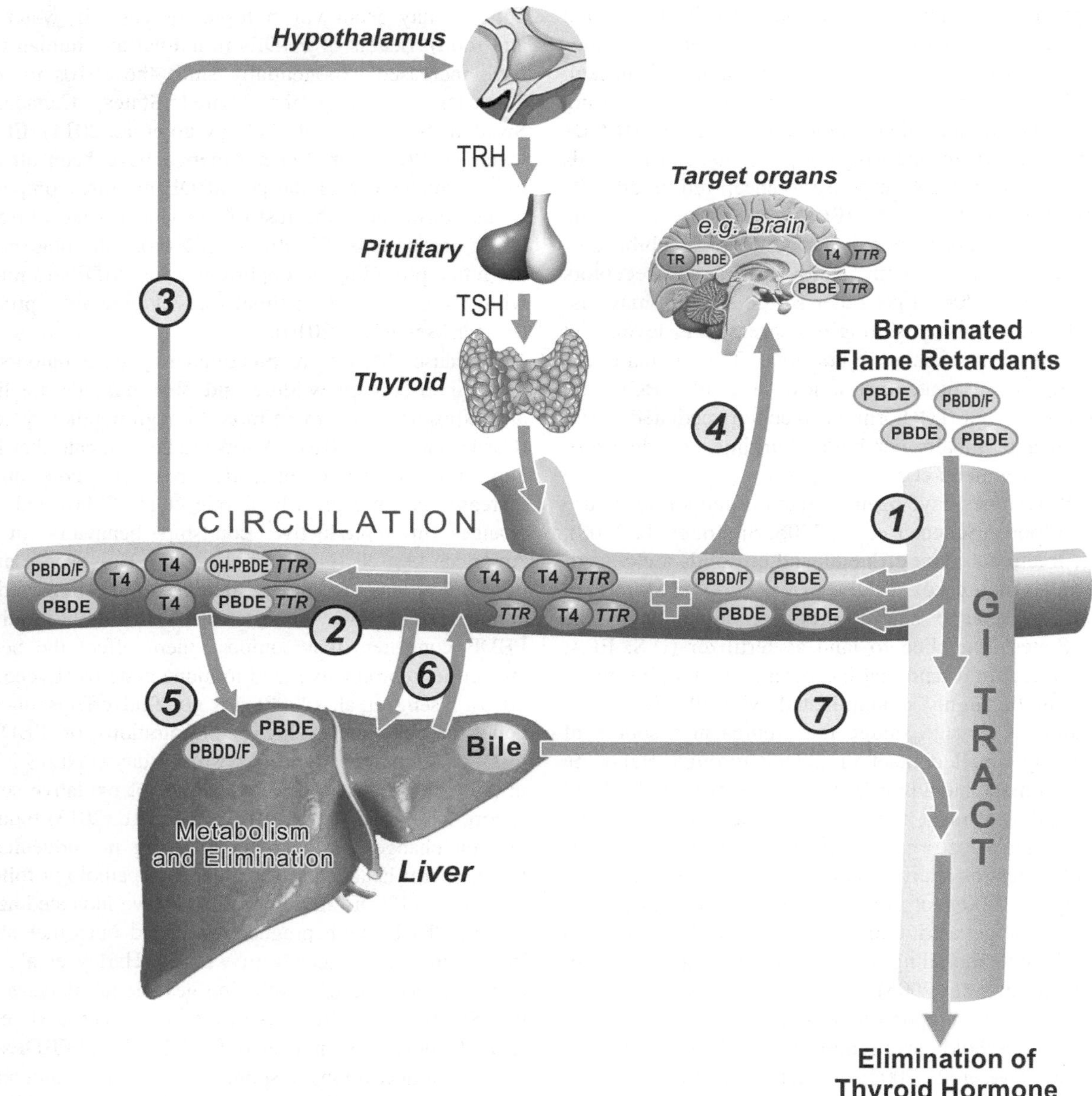

FIGURE 52.4 Possible mechanisms by which BFRs can disrupt thyroid hormone (TH) homeostasis. PBDE is shown as an example of all BFRs. (1) BFRs as well as their contaminants enter the circulation from the gastrointestinal (GI) tract. (2) BFRs (parent compound as well as metabolites) can displace thyroxine (T4) from serum binding proteins such as transthyretin (TTR). The resulting free T4 will be subjected to hepatic metabolism and elimination. (3) Reduced circulating T4 levels trigger the hypothalamic–pituitary axis to synthesize and secrete more T4 by thyroid. (4) BFRs bound to TTR along with T4 will reach target organs including brain, where they can bind to TH receptor to elicit a biological/toxicological response. (5) After entering liver activate nuclear receptors, BFRs initiate transcription of xenobiotic-metabolizing enzymes for T4 metabolism and elimination. (6) Influx transporters further increase the T4 uptake and metabolism. (7) Efflux transporters eliminate T4 or its conjugates from liver into either serum or the bile. Figure is not to scale. *Adapted from Kodavanti, P.R.S., Curras-Collazo, M.C., 2010. Neuroendocrine actions of organohalogens: thyroid hormones, arginine vasopressin, and neuroplasticity. Front. Neuroendo. 31, 479–496 (Kodavanti and Curras-Collazo, 2010).*

TABLE 52.3 Polybrominated Diphenyl Ether Levels in Domestic, Pet, and Wild Animals

Animal	Sample	Total PBDE Concentration	Unit	Age (years)	References
Household cat[a]	Serum	4.3 ± 1.5 (3.5)	ng/mL	1.25–5	Dye et al. (2007)
	Serum	10.5 ± 3.5 (5.9)	ng/mL	8–15	Dye et al. (2007)
	Serum	12.7 ± 3.9 (6.2)	ng/mL	10–18	Dye et al. (2007)
Captive giant and red panda	Liver, Kidney, brain, gonad, muscle, adipose tissues	38.4–2158	ng/g lw	NA	Hu et al. (2008)
Cow	Fat tissue	1300–2700	pg/g lw	NA	Kierkegaard et al. (2009)
Cow	Milk	1100–2600	pg/g lw	NA	Kierkegaard et al. (2009)
Moose	Liver	0.24–26 (PBDE-47) 0.26–34 (PBDE-99)	ng/g lw		De Wit et al. (2010)
Arctic fox	Subcutaneous adipose tissue	26.3	ng/g lw	NA	De Wit et al. (2010)
Arctic fox	Abdominal adipose tissue	31.6	ng/g lw	NA	De Wit et al. (2010)
California sea lion	Blubber	569–24,343	ng/g lw	NA	Stapleton et al. (2006)
Polar bear	Adipose tissue	4.6–11	ng/g lw		Muir et al. (2006)
California sea otter	Liver	2,423 ($n = 6$)	ng/g lw		Kannan et al. (2008)
Silver perch	Whole fish	337 ($n = 2$)	ng/g lw		Sajwan et al. (2008)

NA, not available.
[a]*Total PBDE concentrations in parentheses indicate median;* lw, *lipid weight.*

2007). Because of these differential reports, the role of hypothyroxinemia with regard to the behavioral effects of PBDEs is unclear. However, the mechanisms by which PBDEs or other BFRs disrupt TH homeostasis are shown in Fig. 52.4. BFRs as well as their contaminants enter the circulatory system from the gastrointestinal tract. T_4 is synthesized and released into circulation by the thyroid gland. In circulation, BFRs (parent compound as well as metabolites) can displace T_4 from serum binding proteins such as TTR. The resulting free T_4 will be subjected to hepatic metabolism and elimination. The reductions in circulating T_4 levels increase TSH production via reduced negative feedback on the hypothalamic–pituitary axis, which induces increased synthesis and secretion of T_4 by the thyroid gland. BFRs bound to TTR along with T_4 will reach target organs including the brain, in which they can bind to the TH receptor to elicit a biological/toxicological response. In the liver, BFRs activate nuclear receptors, initiating transcription of xenobiotic metabolizing enzymes for T_4 metabolism and elimination. Influx transporters further increase the T_4 uptake and metabolism, whereas efflux transporters eliminate T_4 or its conjugates from the liver into either serum or the bile (Fig. 52.4). Recent studies indicate that PBDE 47 (2,2′,4,4′-tetrabromodiphenyl ether) inhibited iodine uptake suggesting its effects on TH synthesis (Wu et al., 2016). Given the key role of TH in development, BFR-induced perturbations in TH homeostasis might play a role in the outcome of adverse effects associated with BFR exposure.

Studies indicate that a commercial pentabrominated mixture (DE-71), when administered during development, did not alter maternal or male offspring body weights. However, female offspring were smaller compared to controls from PND 35 to 60. Exposure to DE-71 also resulted in accumulation of PBDE congeners in various tissues including brain, suggesting that PBDEs cross the blood–placenta and blood–brain barriers, causing subtle changes in some parameters of neurobehavior and dramatic changes in circulating TH levels, as well as changes in both male and female reproductive end points (Kodavanti et al., 2010). Further studies using the same cohort of animals focused on proteomic analysis indicated that energy metabolism and processes related to neuroplasticity and growth may be involved in the developmental neurotoxicity of PBDEs (Kodavanti et al., 2015).

In addition to the effects on TH, there is evidence that PBDEs affect the cholinergic neurotransmitter system (Viberg et al., 2003a,b), which is involved in memory and motor function, among others. Several PBDE congeners have been compared to PCBs with regard to their ability to affect intracellular signaling in a cerebellar (brain) culture system (Kodavanti and Ward, 2005; Kodavanti et al., 2005; Fan et al., 2010). The Ca/protein kinase C signaling pathways are also proposed as mechanisms of neurotoxicity for a number of chemicals, including PCBs and PBDEs. The order of potency for their effects on intracellular signaling was DE-71 (a commercial mixture of tetra-, penta-, and hexaBDEs) >PBDE-47 > PBDE-100 > PBDE-99. On a molar basis, DE-71 was equipotent with Aroclor 1254; the most widely used commercial PCB mixture. A Swedish study found that PBDE-99 and PCB-52 produced effects on behavior when given together but not at the same dose given alone (Eriksson et al., 2006). These results suggest that there may be little difference in neurotoxic potency between PBDEs and PCBs, and that effects of PCBs and PBDEs are additive. This implies that body burdens of PCBs and PBDEs in humans may need to be added when assessing risk.

The NTP published results of the 2-year bioassay on the reportedly nonpersistent BFR, TBBPA, and found a significant treatment-related increase in uterine carcinoma incidence in Wistar Han rats (NTP, 2014). In fact, using longitudinal and transverse sections of the female reproductive tract, Malignant Mixed Müllerian Tumors were diagnosed and were found to have a 76% metastatic rate (MR) compared to those rats diagnosed with endometrial adenocarcinoma alone (MR = 24%) (Dunnick et al., 2015). There was an overall dose related increase in endometrial adenocarcinoma in the study ($n = 50$/grp); 0 (12%), 250 (22%), 500 (32%), and 1000 (38%) mg/kg TBBPA. Other sites demonstrating TBBPA-enhanced tumor risk in the rat were the testis, and in the B6C3F1 mice, large intestine (males), liver, and vascular system. Although the mechanism for these tumors is not well understood, there was a significant correlation of increased Her2 expression and Tp53 mutation in the tumors; markers of aggressive endometrial cancer in women (Harvey et al., 2015). Other studies have assessed the effects of TBBPA on estrogenic outcomes and have found no effect on ERα or ERβ activity (Molina-Molina et al., 2013; Dorosh et al., 2011), but report interactions with the thyroid receptor and PPARγ (Kitamura et al., 2002; Riu et al., 2011; Molina-Molina et al., 2013). Recent work found 5 days of 250 mg/kg TBBPA in Wistar Han adult rats induced significant decreases in serum T4, altered nuclear receptor gene expression in liver and uterine samples, and caused a striking increase in uterine CYP1B1, UGT1A1, and IGF-1, with corresponding decreases in liver SULT 2A1 and 1E1, solidifying its role as an endocrine disruptor (Sanders et al., 2016). In prior studies, neither persistence nor accumulation of ^{14}C-labeled TBBPA was observed in uterine tissue following repeated oral administration to adult female Wistar Han rats (Knudsen et al., 2014), suggesting metabolic/endocrine disrupting effects as primary modes of action.

Perfluorinated Compounds

Table 52.4 summarizes PFC concentrations in farm and pet/captive animals. Detectable levels of PFCs were found in serum samples from chicken, pigs, cattle (Jack Black), horses, dogs, and goats from Japan (Guruge et al., 2008). Among several PFCs measured, PFOS and PFOA concentrations were consistently higher in almost all samples. The serum PFOS and PFOA concentrations ranged from 0.57 to 4.9 ng/g wet weight and from less than 0.05 to 2.5 ng/g wet weight, respectively (Table 52.4). Serum samples of Amur tigers, giant pandas, and red pandas from China also contained detectable concentrations of PFCs (Dai et al., 2006; Li et al., 2008). As observed in farm animals, Amur tiger and panda serum samples had comparatively higher concentrations of PFOS than other PFCs, including PFOA. Animal tissue samples from remote locations, such as polar bear liver samples from Svalbard and serum samples from bottlenose dolphin from Bermuda, also showed relatively high concentrations of PFOS compared to other PFCs (Table 52.4). Polar bear liver contained 1290 ng/g wet weight of PFOS and 2940 ng/g wet weight of PFHxS (Kannan et al., 2005b).

Perfluorinated chemicals (PFCs), especially PFOS and PFOA, were associated with liver enlargement and hepatocellular adenomas in rats (Lau et al., 2007). Lau and coworkers suggested that agonism of the peroxisome proliferator-activated receptor-α (PPAR-α) may be involved in tumor (primarily liver) induction by a number of nongenotoxic carcinogens in the rodents. Following this, a number of studies were conducted to determine whether the PPAR-α agonistic mode of action is involved in the liver toxicity and hepatocellular adenomas observed in rats treated with PFOS and PFOA. Several short-term studies in rats and mice have revealed that PFOS and PFOA are capable of inducing peroxisome proliferation, and the first key event in this mode of action is activation of PPAR-α (Ikeda et al., 1987; Berthiaume and Wallace, 2002; 3M Company, 2004; Vanden Huevel et al., 2006). Because several PFCs can activate PPAR-α, these

TABLE 52.4 Perfluorinated Compound Concentrations in Farm and Pet/Captive Animals in Different Countries

			PFC conc., (ng/mL wet wt.)					
Species/Tissue	*N*	Location	PFOS	PFHxS	PFDA	PFNA	PFOA	References
Chicken/serum	7	Japan	4.9	0.07	0.06	0.22	0.44	Guruge et al. (2008)
Pig/serum	6	Japan	0.57	0.04	0.07	0.12	0.23	Guruge et al. (2008)
Cattle, Jack Black/serum	5	Japan	1.5	0.01	0.48	0.04	0.01	Guruge et al. (2008)
Horse/serum	2	Japan	0.82	<0.01	0.5	0.04	<0.05	Guruge et al. (2008)
Dog/serum	10	Japan	25	10	0.28	1.5	2.5	Guruge et al. (2008)
Goat/plasma	5	Japan	2.4	0.05	1.0	1.2	0.13	Guruge et al. (2008)
Amur tiger/serum	100	China	1.41	0.11	0.07	0.32	0.11	Li et al. (2008)
Polar bear/liver[a]	NR	Svalbard	1290	2940	43	102	21	Kannan et al. (2005b)
Giant panda/serum	9	China	11.10	NA	NA	NA	0.80	Dai et al. (2006)
Red panda/serum	12	China	15.65	NA	NA	NA	2.29	Dai et al. (2006)
Bottlenose dolphin/serum	2	Bermuda	49	5.9	9.6	17	0.8	Giesy and Kannan (2001)

NA, not available.
[a]*Indicates levels found in liver compared to others reported in serum.*

compounds may also induce peroxisome proliferation by perturbing lipid metabolism and transport. Maloney and Waxman (1999) reported that PPAR-α was activated by endogenous cellular fatty acids. Based on these observations, Lau et al. (2007) suggested that displacement of endogenous ligands from L-FABP may be one of the mechanisms by which PFOS induces peroxisome proliferation. In addition, Yang et al. (2002a,b) showed that the activation of PPAR-α by PFOA was consistent with a significant increase in liver weight in wild-type mice exposed to dietary PFOA or WY-14,643, a classical peroxisome proliferator, at 0.02% and 0.125% (wt/wt), respectively, for 7 days.

Because PPAR-α controls lipid metabolism and transport, the hepatomegaly observed in PPAR-α in null mice was attributed to accumulation of lipid droplets or accumulation of PFOA in the liver (Yang et al., 2006). Guruge et al. (2006) studied gene expression profiles in rat liver with PFOA and showed that the largest categories of induced genes are those participating in metabolism and transport of lipids (fatty acids). PFOA not only exhibits properties of a peroxisome proliferator but also possesses the properties of a mixed-type enzyme-inducing agent, as demonstrated by marked induction of CYP2B2, CYP3A4, and CYP4A1 in liver microsomes (Elcombe et al., 2007). Kudo et al. (2000) studied the induction of peroxisomal β-oxidation by perfluorochemicals in rat livers by administration of PFCs at doses ranging from 2.5 to 20 mg/kg/day for 5 days and found that in male rats, all compounds except PFHA induced the activity of peroxisomal β-oxidation. However, in female rats, PFNA and PFDA induced the activity. Differences in accumulation of these compounds in the rat livers may be responsible for the different hepatic responses observed between various PFCs with different carbon chain length and between sexes. PFOA is currently being replaced by 2,3,3,3-tetrafluoro-2-(heptafluoropropoxy)-propanoate, which emerging evidence suggests that this compound also produces detectable changes in parameters affected by PFOAs including increased liver weights (Rushing et al., 2017).

In multicellular organisms, cells communicate (exchange ions, send messages, and exchange small molecules) by a process known as gap junctional intercellular communication (GJIC). GJIC maintains tissue homeostasis and is involved in growth, development, and differentiation (Lau et al., 2007). Trosko and Rush (1998) suggested that loss of GJIC plays a role in carcinogenesis. Hu et al. (2002) showed that rats exposed orally (5 mg/kg) for 3 days or 3 weeks inhibit GJIC, and GJIC is also inhibited in a dose-dependent manner in rat liver and dolphin kidney cell lines. However, the pathophysiological significance of GJIC inhibition with regard to the carcinogenic mode of action for PFOS and PFOA is unclear.

It is important to mention that PBDEs, PFOS, and PFOA have strong potential for reproductive and developmental toxicity (Johansson et al., 2009; Abdelouahab et al., 2011; Costa et al., 2014; Berghuis et al., 2015; Kodavanti et al., 2017).

CONCLUDING REMARKS AND FUTURE DIRECTIONS

BFRs and perfluorinated compounds are considered emerging environmental pollutants. During the past few decades, there has been a great deal of progress in understanding the distribution of these pollutants in the global environment, wildlife, and humans (Kodavanti and Loganathan, 2016). Although monitoring studies have clearly shown the presence of BFRs and PFCs worldwide, environmental/biological transformation and toxicology, pathways, and mode of action are not fully understood or described. Furthermore, contamination levels and potential negative effects of these toxic pollutants on domestic and pet animals have been largely ignored. Laboratory animal studies and accidental poisoning case studies have shown that exposure to BRRs and/or PFCs may result in serious health effects, including endocrine disruption leading to reproductive and immune dysfunction, birth defects, neurotoxicity, and certain types of cancers. Based on laboratory and field study results, environmental exposure of farm animals to BFRs and PFCs is of great concern because these compounds can affect animal health as well as serve as a source for human exposure via consumption of contaminated meat and/or dairy products. Although some BFRs have been banned or voluntarily withdrawn by manufacturers, human/animal exposure to these chemicals will continue for a long time, as is the case with chlorinated organic chemicals that exist in large quantities in consumer products (Shaw et al., 2010). Therefore, research is needed to address the long-term consequences of exposure to these chemicals even as new brominated replacement chemicals enter into the market.

ACKNOWLEDGMENTS

We thank Dr. Suryanarayana Vulimiri of National Center for Environmental Assessment of USEPA, Research Triangle Park, NC and Dr. Ramesh Gupta of Murray State University, Hopkinsville, KY for their excellent comments on an earlier version of this chapter. The contents of this article have been reviewed by the National Health and Environmental Effects Research Laboratory of the U.S. Environmental Protection Agency and approved for publication. Approval does not signify that the contents necessarily reflect the views and policies of the Agency, nor does mention of trade names or commercial products constitute endorsement or recommendation for use.

REFERENCES

3M Company, 2004. Comparative molecular biology of perfluorooctanesulfonate (PFOS, T-6295), N-ethyl perfluorooctane-sulfanamido ethanol (N-EtFOSE, T-6316), N-ethyl perfluorooctanesulfonamide (FOSAA, T-6868), perfluorooctanesulfonamido acetate (FOSAA T-7071), and/or perfluorooctanesulfonamide (FOSA, T-7132) in rats and guinea pigs following oral dosing. Final Report, July 16, 2004. *U.S. EPA Administrative Record*, AR-226-1813.

Abdelouahab, N., AinMelk, Y., Takser, L., 2011. Polybrominated diphenyl ethers and sperm quality. Reprod. Toxicol. 31, 546–550.

Alaee, M., Arias, P., Sjodin, A., et al., 2003. An overview of commercially used brominated flame retardants, their applications, their use patterns in different countries/regions and possible modes of release. Environ. Int. 29, 683–689.

ATSDR, Agency for Toxic Substances and Disease Registry, 2004. Toxicological Profile for Polybrominated Diphenyl Ethers and Polybrominated Biphenyls.

Berghuis, S.A., Bos, A.F., Sauer, P.J., et al., 2015. Developmental neurotoxicity of persistent organic pollutants: an update on childhood outcome. Arch. Toxicol. 89 (5), 687–709.

Berthiaume, J., Wallace, K.B., 2002. Perfluorooctanoate, perfluorooctanesulfonate and N-ethyl perfluorooctanesulfonamido ethanol: peroxisome proliferation and mitochondrial biogenesis. Toxicol. Lett. 129, 23–32.

Birnbaum, L.S., Bergman, A., 2010. Brominated and chlorinated flame retardants: the San Antonio Statement. Environ. Health Perspect. 118, A514–A515.

Birnbaum, L.S., Staskal, D.F., 2004. Brominated flame retardants: cause for concern? Environ. Health Perspect. 112, 9–17.

Birnbaum, L.S., Staskal, D.F., Diliberto, J.J., 2003. Health effects of polybrominated dibenzo-p-dioxins (PBDDs) and dibenzofurans (PBDFs). Environ. Int. 29, 855–860.

Blum, A., 2010. Toxicity of flame retardants in buildings: what can be done about it? Lecture at Green Building. McCormick Place West, Chicago, November 18, 2010.

Buck, R.C., 2015. Toxicology Data for Alternative "Short-Chain" Fluorinated Substances. Toxicological Effects of Perfluoroalkyl and Polyfluoroalkyl Substances. Springer Int. Publishing, pp. 451–477.

Buist, S.C.N., Klaassen, C.D., 2004. Rat and mouse differences in gender-predominant expression of organic anion transporter (OATI-3; SLC22A6-8) mRNA levels. Drug. Metab. Disp. 32, 620–625.

Burreau, S., Axelman, J., Broman, D., et al., 1997. Dietary uptake in pike (*Esox lucius*) of some polychlorinated biphenyls, polychlorinated naphthalenes and polybrominated diphenyl ethers administered in natural diet. Environ. Tox. Chem. 16, 2508–2513.

Buser, H.R., 1986. Polybrominated dibenzofurans and dibenzo-p-dioxins: thermal reaction products of polybrominated diphenyl ether flame retardants. Environ. Sci. Tech. 20, 404–408.

Butenhoff, J.L., Rodricks, J.V., 2015. Human health risk assessment of perfluoroalkyl acids. Toxicological Effects of Perfluoroalkyl and Polyfluoroalkyl Substances. Springer Int. Publishing, pp. 363–418.

Caspersen, I.H., Kvalem, H.E., Haugen, M., et al., 2016. Determinants of plasma PCB, brominated flame retardants, and organochlorine pesticides in pregnant women and 3 year old children in The Norwegian Mother and Child Cohort Study. Environ. Res. 146, 136–144.

Chang, S.C., Noker, P.E., Gorman, G.S., et al., 2012. Comparative pharmacokinetics of perfluorooctanesulfonate (PFOS) in rats, mice, and monkeys. Reprod. Toxicol. 33 (4), 428–440.

Costa, L.G., de Laat, R., Tagliaferri, S., et al., 2014. A mechanistic view of polybrominated diphenyl ether (PBDE) developmental neurotoxicity. Toxicol. Lett. 230 (2), 282–294.

Covaci, A., Gerecke, A.C., Law, R.J., et al., 2006. Hexabromocyclododecanes (HBCDs) in the environment and humans: a review. Environ. Sci. Tech. 40 (12), 3679–3688.

Dai, J., Li, M., Jin, Y., et al., 2006. Perfluorooctane sulfonate and perfluorooctanoate in red panda and giant panda from China. Environ. Sci. Tech. 40, 5647–5652.

De Wit, C.A., 2002. An overview of brominated flame retardants in the environment. Chemosphere. 46, 583–624.

De Wit, C.A., Herzke, D., Vorkamp, K., 2010. Brominated flame retardants in the Arctic environment: trends and new candidates. Sci. Total Environ. 408, 2885–2918.

DiGangi, J., Blum, A., Bergman, A., et al., 2010. San Antonio statement on brominated and chlorinated flame retardants. Environ. Health Perspect. 118, A516–A518.

Dorosh, A., Děd, L., Elzeinová, F., et al., 2011. Assessing oestrogenic effects of brominated flame retardants hexabromocyclododecane and tetrabromobisphenol A on MCF-7 cells. Folia Biol. 57, 35–39.

Dunnick, J.K., Sanders, J.M., Kissling, G.E., et al., 2015. Environmental chemical exposure may contribute to uterine cancer development: studies with tetrabromobisphenol A. Toxicol. Pathol. 43 (4), 464–473.

DuPont Company, 1982. Excretion and Disposition of 14C-Ammonium Perfluorooctanoate in Male and Female Rats, Mice, Hamsters and Rabbits. Haskell Laboratory, DuPont, Newark, DE, unpublished report.

Dye, J.A., Venier, M., Zhu, L., et al., 2007. Elevated PBDE levels in pet cats: sentinels for humans? Environ. Sci. Tech. 41 (18), 6350–6356.

Elcombe, C.R., Elcombe, B.M., Foster, J.R., et al., 2007. Characterization of the heptomegaly induced by ammonium perfluorooctanoic acid (APFO) in rats. Toxicologist. 96, 179.

Ema, M., Fujii, S., Hirata-Koizumi, M., et al., 2007. Two-generation reproductive toxicity study of the flame retardant hexabromocyclododecane in rats. Reprod. Toxicol. 25, 335–351.

Eriksson, P., Fredriksson, A., 1996. Developmental neurotoxicity of four ortho-substituted polychlorinated biphenyls in the neonatal mouse. Environ. Toxicol. Pharm. 1, 155–165.

Eriksson, P., Fischer, C., Fredriksson, A., 2006. Polybrominated diphenyl ethers, a group of brominated flame retardants, can interact with polychlorinated biphenyls in enhancing developmental neurobehavioral defects. Toxicol. Sci. 94, 302–309.

Fan, C.-Y., Besas, J., Kodavanti, P.R.S., 2010. Changes in mitogen-activated protein kinase in cerebellar granule neurons by polybrominated diphenyl ethers and polychlorinated biphenyls. Toxicol. Appl. Pharmacol. 245, 1–8.

Fernie, K.J., Shutt, J.L., Ritchie, I.J., et al., 2006. Changes in the growth, but not the survival, of American kestrels (*Falco sparverius*) exposed to environmentally relevant polybrominated diphenyl ethers. J. Toxicol. Environ. Health. Part A. 69, 1541–1554.

Fernie, K.J., Shutt, J.L., Letcher, R.J., et al., 2008. Changes in reproductive courtship behaviors of adult American kestrels (*Falco sparverius*) exposed to environmentally relevant levels of the polybrominated diphenyl ether mixture, DE-71. Toxicol. Sci. 102, 171–178.

Fries, G.F., 1995. A review of the significance of animal food products as potential pathways of human exposure to dioxins. J. Anim. Sci. 73, 1639–1650.

Frederiksen, M., Vorkamp, K., Mathiesen, L., et al., 2010. Placental transfer of the polybrominated diphenyl ethers BDE-47, BDE-99 and BDE-209 in a human placenta perfusion system: an experimental study. Environ. Health. 9 (1), 32.

Fromme, H., Becher, G., Hilger, B., et al., 2016. Brominated flame retardants – exposure and risk assessment for the general population. Int. J. Hyg. Environ. Health. 219, 1–23.

Gee, J.R., Moser, V.C., 2008. Acute exposure to brominated diphenyl ether 47 delays neuromotor ontogeny and alters motor activity in mice. Neurotoxicol. Teratol. 30, 79–87.

Gee, J.R., Hedge, J.M., Moser, V.C., 2008. Lack of alterations in thyroid hormones following exposure to polybrominated diphenyl ether 47 during a period of rapid brain development in mice. Drug Chem. Toxicol. 31, 245–254.

Giesy, J.P., Kannan, K., 2001. Global distribution of perfluorooctane sulfonate in wildlife. Environ. Sci. Tech. 35, 1339–1342.

Gill, U., Chu, I., Ryan, J., et al., 2004. Polybrominated diphenyl ethers: human tissue levels and toxicology. Rev. Environ. Contam. Toxicol. 183, 55–97.

Guo, Y., Shaw, S., Kannan, K., 2011. Spatial and temporal trends of polybrominated diphenyl ethers. In: Loganathan, B., Lam, P.K.S. (Eds.), Global Contamination Trends of Persistent Organic Chemicals. CRC Press, Boca Raton, FL.

Guruge, K.S., Yeung, L.W.Y., Yamanaka, N., et al., 2006. Gene expression profiles in rat liver treated with perfluorooocatanoic acid (PFOA). Toxicol. Sci. 89, 93–107.

Guruge, K.S., Manage, P.M., Yamanaka, N., et al., 2008. Species-specific concentrations of perfluoroalkyl contaminants in farm and pet animals in Japan. Chemosphere. 73 (1), S210–S215.

Hakk, H., Larsen, G., Bergman, A., et al., 2000. Metabolism, excretion and distribution of the flame retardant tetrabromobisphenol-A in conventional and bile-duct cannulated rats. Xenobiotica. 30, 881–890.

Hakk, H., Larsen, G., Klasson-Wehler, E., 2002. Tissue disposition, excretion and metabolism of 2,2′,4,4′,5-pentabromodiphenyl ether (BDE-99) in the male Sprague–Dawley rat. Xenobiotica. 32, 369–382.

Hamers, T., Kamstra, J.H., Sonneveld, E., et al., 2006. In vitro profiling of the endocrine-disrupting potency of brominated flame retardants. Toxicol. Sci. 92 (1), 157–173.

Hanari, N., Kannan, K., Miyake, Y., et al., 2006. Occurrence of polybrominated biphenyls, polybrominated dibenzo-dioxins, and polybrominated dibenzofurans as impurities in commercial polybrominated diphenyl ether mixtures. Environ. Sci. Tech. 40, 4400–4405.

Hanhijarvi, H., Ylinen, M., Haarenen, T., et al., 1988. A proposed species difference in the renal excretion of perfluorooctanoic acid in the beagle dog and rat. In: Baynen, A.C., Solleveid, H.A. (Eds.), New Development in Biosciences: Their Implications for Laboratory Animal Sciences. Martinus Nijhoff, Dodrecht, Netherlands, pp. 409–412.

Harley, K.G., Marks, A.R., Chevrier, J., et al., 2010. PBDE concentrations in women's serum and fecundability. Environ. Health Perspect. 118 (5), 699.

Harvey, J.B., Osborne, T.S., Hong, H.H.L., et al., 2015. Uterine carcinomas in tetrabromobisphenol A–exposed Wistar Han Rats Harbor Increased Tp53 Mutations and Mimic High-grade Type I Endometrial Carcinomas in Women. Toxicol. Pathol. 43 (8), 1103–1113.

Heeb, N.V., Schweizer, W.B., Kohler, M., et al., 2005. Structure elucidation of hexabromocyclododecanes: a class of compounds with a complex stereochemistry. Chemosphere. 61, 65–73.

Hendriks, H.S., Westerink, R.H., 2015. Neurotoxicity and risk assessment of brominated and alternative flame retardants. Neurotoicol. Teratol. 52, 248–269.

Houde, M., Bujas, T.A., Small, J., et al., 2006. Biomagnification of perfluoroalkyl compounds in the bottlenose dolphin (*Tursiops truncatus*) food web. Environ. Sci. Tech. 40 (13), 4138–4144.

Hu, G.C., Luo, X.J., Dai, J.Y., et al., 2008. Brominated flame retardants, polychlorinated biphenyls, and organochlorine pesticides in captive giant panda (*Ailuropoda melanoleuca*) and red panda (*Ailurus fulgens*) from China. Environ. Sci. Tech. 42 (13), 4704–4709.

Hu, W., Jones, P.D., Upham, B.L., et al., 2002. Inhibition of gap junctional intercellular communication by perfluorinated compounds in rat liver and dolphin kidney epithelial cell lines in vitro and Sprague–Dawley rats in vivo. Toxicol. Sci. 68, 429–436.

Huber, S., Ballschmiter, K., 2001. Characterization of five technical mixtures of brominated flame retardants. Fresenius' J. Analyt Chem. 371, 882–890.

Hundley, S.G., Sarrif, A.M., Kennedy, G.L., 2006. Absorption, distribution, and excretion of ammonium perfluorooctanoate (APFO) after oral administration to various species. Drug Chem. Toxicol. 29, 137–145.

Ibhazehiebo, K., Iwasaki, T., Shimokawa, N., et al., 2011. 1,2,5,6,9,10-α-Hexabromocyclododecane (HBCD) impairs thyroid hormone-induced dendrite arborization of Purkinje cells and suppresses thyroid hormone receptor-mediated transcription. Cerebellum. 10, 22–31.

Ikeda, T., Fukuda, K., Mori, I., et al., 1987. Induction of cytochrome P-450 and peroxisome proliferation in rat liver by perfluorinated octanesulfonic acid. In: Fahimi, H.D., Sies, H. (Eds.), Peroxisomes in Biology and Medicine. Springer-Verlag, New York, pp. 304–308.

Johansson, N., Eriksson, P., Viberg, H., 2009. Neonatal exposure to PFOS and PFOA in mice results in changes in proteins which are important for neuronal growth and synaptogenesis in the developing brain. Toxicol. Sci. 108, 412–418.

Johnson, J.D., Gibson, S.J., Ober, R.E., 1984. Cholestyramine-enhanced fecal elimination of carbon-14 in rats after administration of ammonium [14C]perfluorooctanoate or potassium [14C]perfluorooctanesulfonate. Fund. App. Tox. 4, 972–976.

Johnson-Restripo, B., Adams, D.H., Kannan, K., 2008. Tetrabromobisphenol A (TBBPA) and hexabromocyclododecanes (HBCDs) in tissues of humans, dolphins, and sharks from the United States. Chemosphere. 70, 1935–1944.

Jones, P.D., Hu, W., De Coen, W., et al., 2003. Binding of perfluorinated fatty acids to serum proteins. Environ. Toxicol. Chem. 22, 2639–2649.

Kannan, K., Newsted, J., Halbrook, R.S., et al., 2002. Perfluorooctanesulfonate and related fluorinated hydrocarbons in mink and river otters from the United States. Environ. Sci. Tech. 36, 2566–2571.

Kannan, K., Corsolini, S., Falandysz, J., et al., 2004. Perfluorooctanesulfonate and related fluorochemicals in human blood from several countries. Environ. Sci. Tech. 38, 4489–4495.

Kannan, K., Tao, L., Sinclair, E., et al., 2005a. Perfluorinated compounds in aquatic organisms at various trophic levels in a Great Lakes food chain. Arch. Env. Contam. Toxicol. 48, 559–566.

Kannan, K., Yun, S.H., Evans, T.I., 2005b. Chlorinated, brominated and perfluorinated contaminants in livers of polar bears from Alaska. Environ. Sci. Tech. 39, 9057–9063.

Kannan, K., Moon, H.-B., Yun, S.H., et al., 2008. Chlorinated, brominated and perfluorinated compounds, polycyclic aromatic hydrocarbons and trace elements in livers of sea otters from California, Washington, Alaska (USA) and Kamchatka (Russia). J. Environ. Monitor. 10, 552–558.

Kennedy, G.L., Butenhoff, J.L., Olsen, G.W., et al., 2004. The toxicology of perfluorooctanoate. Crit. Rev. Toxicol. 34 (4), 351–384.

Kierkegaard, A., De Wit, C., Asplund, L., et al., 2009. A mass balance of tri-hexabromodiphenyl ethers in lactating cows. Environ. Sci. Tech. 43, 2602–2607.

Kitamura, S., Jinno, N., Ohta, S., et al., 2002. Thyroid hormonal activity of the flame retardants tetrabromobisphenol A and tetrachlorobisphenol A. Biochem. Biophys. Res. Comm. 293 (1), 554–559.

Knudsen, G.A., Sanders, J.M., Sadik, A.M., et al., 2014. Disposition and kinetics of tetrabromobisphenol A in female Wistar Han rats. Toxicol. Rep. 1, 214–223.

Knudsen, G.A., Hughes, M.F., McIntosh, K.L., et al., 2015. Estimation of tetrabromobisphenol A (TBBPA) percutaneous uptake in humans using the parallelogram method. Toxicol. Appl. Pharmacol. 289 (2), 323–329.

Koch, C., Schmidt-Kotters, T., Rupp, R., et al., 2015. Review of hexabromocyclododecane (HBCD) with a focus on legislation and recent publications concerning toxicokinetics and –dynamics. Environ. Poll. 199, 26–34.

Kodavanti, P.R.S., Curras-Collazo, M.C., 2010. Neuroendocrine actions of organohalogens: thyroid hormones, arginine vasopressin, and neuroplasticity. Front. Neuroendo. 31, 479–496.

Kodavanti, P.R.S., Ward, T.R., 2005. Differential effects of commercial polybrominated diphenyl ether and polychlorinated biphenyl mixture on intracellular signaling in rat brain in vitro. Toxicol. Sci. 85, 952.

Kodavanti, P.R.S., Loganathan, B.G., 2016. Brominated flame retardants: spatial and temporal trends in the environment and biota from the pacific basin countries. In: Loganathan, B., et al., (Eds.), Persistent Organic Chemicals in the Environment: Status and Trends in the Pacific Basin Countries II. Temporal Trends. ACS Symposium Series, American Chemical Society, Washington, DC, pp. 21–48.

Kodavanti, P.R.S., Ward, T.R., Ludewig, G., et al., 2005. Polybrominated diphenyl ether (PBDE) effects in rat neuron cultures: 14C-PBDE accumulation, biological effects, and structure – activity relationships. Toxicol. Sci. 88, 181–192.

Kodavanti, P.R.S., Senthilkumar, K., Loganathan, B.G., 2008. Organohalogen pollutants and human health. In: Heggenhougen, K., Quah, S. (Eds.), International Encyclopedia of Public Health, Vol. 4. Academic Press, San Diego, pp. 686–693.

Kodavanti, P.R.S., Coburn, C.G., Moser, V.C., et al., 2010. Developmental exposure to a commercial PBDE mixture, DE-71: neurobehavioral, hormonal, and reproductive effects. Toxicol. Sci. 116, 297–312.

Kodavanti, P.R.S., Sambasiva Rao, K.R.S., Royland, J.E., 2014. Article 403: toxicology of Persistent Organic Pollutants (POPs), Reference Module in Biomedical Research. third ed. Elsevier, pp. 1–9.

Kodavanti, P.R.S., Royland, J.E., Osorio, C., et al., 2015. Developmental exposure to a commercial PBDE mixture: effects on protein networks in the cerebellum and hippocampus of rats. Environ. Health Perspect. 123, 428–436.

Kodavanti, P.R.S., Szabo, Stoker, T.E., Fenton, S.E., 2017. Brominated flame retardants. In: Gupta, R.C. (Ed.), Reproductive and Developmental Toxicology, second ed. Academic Press/Elsevier, Amsterdam, pp. 681–710.

Kudo, N., Bandi, N., Suzuki, E., et al., 2000. Induction by perfluorinated fatty acids with different carbon chain length of peroxisomal beta-oxidation in the liver of rats. Chemico. Biol. Interact. 124, 119–132.

Kuester, R.K., Solyom, A.M., Rodriguez, V.P., et al., 2007. The effects of dose, route, and repeated dosing on the disposition and kinetics of tetrabromobisphenol A in male F-344 rats. Toxicol. Sci. 96, 237–245.

LaGuardia, M., Hale, R., Harvey, E., 2006. Detailed polybrominated diphenyl ether (PBDE) congener composition of the widely used *penta-*, *octa-*, and *deca-*PBDE technical flame-retardant mixtures. Environ. Sci. Tech. 40, 6247–6254.

Lau, C., 2015. Perfluorinated compounds: an overview. Toxicological Effects of Perfluoroalkyl and Polyfluoroalkyl Substances. Springer International Publishing, Cham, pp. 1–21.

Lau, C., Thibodeaux, J.R., Hanson, R.G., et al., 2006. Effects of perfluorooctanoic acid exposure during pregnancy in the mouse. Toxicol. Sci. 90, 510–518.

Lau, C., Anitole, K., Hodes, C., et al., 2007. Perfluoroalkylacids: a review of monitoring and toxicological findings. Toxicol. Sci. 99, 366–394.

Laurent, C., Feidt, C., Laurent, F., 2005. Contamination des Soils. EDP Sciences/ADEME, Les Ulis Cedex A, France.

Law, K., Palace, V.P., Halldorson, T., et al., 2006. Dietary accumulation of hexabromocyclododecane diastereoisomers in juvenile rainbow trout (*Oncorhynchus mykiss*): I. Bioaccumulation parameters and evidence of bioisomerization. Environ. Toxicol. Chem. 25, 1757–1761.

Legler, J., 2008. New insights into the endocrine disrupting effects of brominated flame retardants. Chemosphere. 73, 216–222.

Li, X., Yeung, L.W.Y., Taniyasu, S., et al., 2008. Perfluorooctane sulfonate and related fluorochemicals in the Amur tiger (*Panthera tigris altaica*) from China. Environ. Sci. Tech. 42, 7078–7083.

Lilienthal, H., Verwer, C.M., van der Ven, L.T., et al., 2008. Exposure to tetra-bromobisphenol A (TBBPA) in Wistar rats: neurobehavioral effects in offspring from a one-generation reproduction study. Toxicology. 246, 45–54.

Linares, V., Bellés, M., Domingo, J.L., 2015. Human exposure to PBDE and critical evaluation of health hazards. Arch Tox. 89 (3), 335–356.

Liu, K., Li, J., Yan, S., et al., 2016. A review of status of tetrabromobisphenol A (TBBPA) in China. Chemosphere. 148, 8–20.

Loganathan, B.G., 2012. Global contamination trends of persistent organic chemicals: an overview. In: Loganathan, B., Lam, P.K.S. (Eds.), Global Contamination Trends of Persistent Organic Chemicals. CRC Press, Boca Raton, FL, pp. 3–32.

Loganathan, B.G., Masunaga, S., 2015. PCBs, dioxins and furans: human exposure and health effects. In: Gupta, R.C. (Ed.), Handbook of Toxicology of Chemical Warfare Agents, second ed. Academic Press/Elsevier, Amsterdam, pp. 239–247.

Lorber, M., 2008. Exposure of Americans to polybrominated diphenyl ethers. J. Expos. Sci. Environ. Epidemiol. 18, 2–19.

Luebker, D.J., Hansen, K.J., Bass, N.M., et al., 2002. Interactions of fluorochemicals with rat liver fatty acid-binding protein. Toxicology. 176, 175–185.

Lyche, J.L., Rosseland, C., Berge, G., et al., 2015. Human health risk associated with brominated flame-retardants (BFRs). Environ. Int. 74, 170–180.

Lyman, W.J., 1990. Handbook of Chemical Property Estimation Methods. American Chemical Society, Washington, DC.

MacGregor, J.A., Nixon, W.B., 1997. Hexabromocyclododecane (HBCD): Determination of n-Octanol/Water Partition Coefficient. Brominated Flame Retardant Industry Panel, Chemical Manufacturers Association. Wildlife International 439C-104, Arlington, VA.

Maloney, E.K., Waxman, D.J., 1999. Trans-activation of PPARalpha and PPARgamma by structurally diverse environmental chemicals. Toxicol. Appl. Pharmacol. 161, 209–218.

Meerts, I.A., van Zanden, J.J., Luijks, E.A.C., et al., 2000. Potent competitive interactions of some brominated flame retardants and related compounds with human transthyretin *in vitro*. Toxicol. Sci. 56, 95–104.

Molina-Molina, J.M., Amaya, E., Grimaldi, M., et al., 2013. In vitro study on the agonistic and antagonistic activities of bisphenol-S and other bisphenol-A congeners and derivatives via nuclear receptors. Toxicol. Appl. Pharmacol. 272 (1), 127–136.

Morck, A., Hakk, H., Orn, U., et al., 2003. Decabromodiphenyl ether in the rat: absorption, distribution, metabolism and excretion. Drug Metab. Disp. 31, 900–907.

Muir, D.C., Backus, S., Derocher, A.E., et al., 2006. Brominated flame retardants in polar bears (*Ursus maritimus*) from Alaska, the Canadian Arctic, East Greenland, and Svalbard. Environ. Sci. Tech. 40, 449–455.

Nakajima, A., Saigusa, D., Tetsu, N., et al., 2009. Neurobehavioral effects of tetrabromobisphenol A, a brominated flame retardant, in mice. Toxicol. Lett. 189, 78–83.

National Research Council, 2000. Toxicological Risks of Selected Flame-Retardant Chemicals. National Academies Press, Washington, DC.

National Toxicology Program, 2014. Technical Report on the toxicology studies of tetrabromobisphenol A (CAS NO. 79–94–7) in F344/NTac rats and B6C3F1/N mice and toxicology and carcinogenesis study of tetrabromobisphenol A in Wistar Han [Crl: WI (Han)] rats and B6C3F1/N mice (gavage studies). National Institutes of Health, Research Triangle Park, NC.

Ophaug, R.H., Singer, L., 1980. Metabolic handling of perfluorooctanoic acid in rats. Proc. Soc. Exp. Biol. Med. 163, 19–23.

Ounnas, F., Feidt, C., Toussaint, H., 2010. Polychlorinated biphenyl and low polybrominated diphenyl ether transfer to milk in lactating goats chronically exposed to contamination soil. Environ. Sci. Tech. 44, 2682–2688.

Reach, 2011. Commission Regulation (EU) No 143/2011 of 17 February 2011 amending Annex XIV to Regulation (EC) No 1907/2006, O.J. L 44, 18.2.2011, p. 2–6, Special edition in Croatian: Chapter 13 Volume 054 P. 238–242. Retrieved from http://data.europa.eu/eli/reg/2011/143/oj.

Reistad, T., Mariussen, E., Fonnum, F., 2007. In vitro toxicity of tetrabromobisphenol A on cerebellar granule cells: cell death, free radical formation, and calcium influx and extracellular glutamate. Toxicol. Sci. 96, 268–278.

Rice, D.C., Reeve, E.A., Herlihy, A., et al., 2007. Developmental delays and locomotor activity in the C57BL6/J mouse following neonatal exposure to the fully brominated PBDE, decabromodiphenyl ether. Neurotoxicol. Teratol. 29, 511–520.

Rieck, R.H., 2004. Polybrominated diphenyl ether analysis in fish tissue and other matrices by GC-ECD. LCGC North Am. 22, 914–925.

Riu, A., le Maire, A., Grimaldi, M., et al., 2011. Characterization of novel ligands of ERα, ERβ, and PPARγ: the case of halogenated bisphenol A and their conjugated metabolites. Toxicol. Sci. 122, 372–382.

Roth, N., Wilks, M.F., 2014. Neurodevelopmental and neurobehavioural effects of polybrominated and perfluorinated chemicals: a systematic review of the epidemiological literature using a quality assessment scheme. Toxicol. Lett. 230 (2), 271–281.

Rushing, B.R., Hu, Q., Franklin, J.N., et al., 2017. Evaluation of the Immunomodulatory Effects of 2, 3, 3, 3-Tetrafluoro-2-(Heptafluoropropoxy)-Propanoate in C57BL/6 Mice. Toxicol. Sci. 156 (1), 179–189.

Sajwan, K.S., Kumar, K.S., Nune, A., et al., 2008. Persistent organochlorine pesticides, polychlorinated biphenyls, polybrominated diphenyl ethers in fish from coastal waters off Savannah, GA, USA. Toxicol. Environ. Chem. 90, 81–96.

Sanders, J.M., Coulter, S.J., Knudsen, G.A., et al., 2016. Disruption of estrogen homeostasis as a mechanism for uterine toxicity in Wistar Han rats treated with tetrabromobisphenol A. Toxicol. Appl. Pharmacol. 298, 31–39.

Schauer, U.M., Volkel, W., Dekant, W., 2006. Toxicokinetics of tetrabromobisphenol A in humans and rats after oral administration. Toxicol. Sci. 91, 49–58.

Schecter, A., Papke, O., Tung, K., et al., 2005. Polybrominated diphenyl ether flame retardants in the U.S. population: current levels, temporal trends, and comparison with dioxins, dibenzofurans, and polychlorinated biphenyls. J. Occup. Env. Med. 47, 199–211.

Schecter, A., Papke, O., Harris, T.R., et al., 2006. Polybrominated diphenyl ether (PBDE) levels in an expanded market basket survey of U. S. food and estimated PBDE dietary intake by age and sex. Environ. Health Perspect. 114, 1515–1520.

Seacat, A.M., Thomford, P.J., Hansen, K.J., et al., 2002. Sub-chronic toxicity studies on perfluorooctanesulfonate potassium salt in cynomolgus monkeys. Toxicol. Sci. 68, 249–264.

Seacat, A.M., Thomford, P.J., Hansen, K.J., et al., 2003. Subchronic dietary toxicity of potassium perfluorooctanesulfonate in rats. Toxicology. 183, 117–131.

Senthilkumar, K., 2005. Fluorinated organic chemicals: a review. Res. Chem. Environ. 8, 50–79.

Shaw, S.D., Kannan, K., 2009. Polybrominated diphenyl ethers in marine ecosystems of the American continents: foresight from current knowledge. Rev. Environ. Health. 24, 157–229.

Shaw, S.D., Blum, A., Weber, R., et al., 2010. Halogenated flame retardants: do the fire safety benefits justify the health and environmental risks? Rev. Environ. Health. 25 (4), 261–305.

Shi, T., Chen, S.J., Luo, X.J., et al., 2009. Occurrence of brominated flame retardants other than polybrominated diphenyl ethers in environmental and biota samples from southern China. Chemosphere. 74 (7), 910–916.

Sjodin, A., Papke, O., McGahe, E., et al., 2008. Concentrations of polybrominated diphenyl ethers (PBDEs) in household dust from various countries. Chemosphere. 73 (Suppl. 1), S131–S136.

Smarr, M.M., Grantz, K.L., Zhang, C., et al., 2016. Persistent organic pollutants and pregnancy complications. Sci. Total Environ. 551, 285–291.

Stapleton, H.M., Dodder, N.G., Kucklick, J.R., et al., 2006. Determination of HBCD, PBDEs, and MeO-BDEs in California sea lion (*Zalophus califronianus*) stranded between 1993 and 2003. Marine Poll. Bul. 52, 522–531.

Stapleton, H.M., Klosterhaus, S., Eagle, S., et al., 2009. Detection of organophosphate flame retardants in furniture foam and U.S. house dust. Environ. Sci. Tech. 43, 7490–7495.

Staskal, D.F., Diliberto, J.J., DeVito, M.J., et al., 2005. Toxicokinetics of BDE 47 in female mice: effect of dose, route of exposure, and time. Toxicol. Sci. 83, 215–223.

Stein, C.R., Savitz, D.A., Elston, B., et al., 2014. Perfluorooctanoate exposure and major birth defects. Reprod. Toxicol. 47, 15–20.

Stockholm Convention Secretariat, 2010. What Are POPs? Retrieved from http://chm.pops.int/Convention/The%20POPs/tabid/673/language/en-US/Default.aspx.

Tanabe, S., Minh, T.-B., 2010. Dioxins and organohalogen contaminants in the Asia-Pacific region. Ecotoxicology. 19, 463–478.

Thoma, H., Rist, S., Hauschulz, G., et al., 1986. Polybrominated dibenzodioxins and -furans from the pyrolysis of some flame retardants. Chemosphere. 15, 649–652.

Thuresson, K., Höglund, P., Hagmar, L., et al., 2006. Apparent half-lives of hepta- to decabrominated diphenyl ethers in human serum as determined in occupationally exposed workers. Environ. Health Perspect. 114, 176–181.

Trosko, J.E., Rush, R.J., 1998. Cell–cell communication in carcinogenesis. Front. Biosci. 3, D208–D236.

Tseng, L.H., Lee, C.W., Pan, M.H., et al., 2006. Postnatal exposure of the male mouse to 2, 2′, 3, 3′, 4, 4′, 5, 5′, 6, 6′-decabrominated diphenyl ether: decreased epididymal sperm functions without alterations in DNA content and histology in testis. Toxicology. 224 (1), 33–43.

Tseng, L.H., Hsu, P.C., Lee, et al., 2013. Developmental exposure to decabrominated diphenyl ether (BDE-209): effects on sperm oxidative stress and chromatin DNA damage in mouse offspring. Environ. Toxicol. 28 (7), 380–389.

U.S. EPA, U.S. Environmental Protection Agency, 1999. Biosolids Generation, Use and Disposal in the United States, EPA530-R-99-009. U.S. Environmental Protection Agency, Washington, DC.

U.S. EPA, U.S. Environmental Protection Agency, 2000. Perfluorooctayl Sulfonates; Proposed Significant New Use Rule. Fed. Reg. 65, 62319–62333.

U.S. EPA, U.S. Environmental Protection Agency, 2008. Flame Retardants in Printed Circuit Boards. Available at http://www.epa.gov/dfe/pubs/projects/pcb/index.htm.

Vanden Heuvel, J.P., Kuslikis, B.I., Van Ragelghem, M.L., et al., 1991. Tissue distribution, metabolism, and elimination of perfluorooctanoic acid in male and female rats. J. Biochem. Mol. Toxicol. 6, 83–92.

Vanden Huevel, J.P., Thompson, J.T., Frame, S.R., et al., 2006. Differential activation of nuclear receptors by perfluorinated fatty acid analogs and natural fatty acid: a comparison of human, mouse and rat peroxisome proliferator-activated receptor-alpha, beta, and gamma liver X receptor-beta, and retinoid X receptor-alpha. Toxicol. Sci. 92, 476–489.

van der Ven, L.T., van de Kuil, T., Leonards, P.E., et al., 2009. Endocrine effects of hexabromocyclododecane (HBCD) in a one-generation reproduction study in Wistar rats. Toxicol. Lett. 185 (1), 51–62.

Veith, G.D., Defoe, D.L., 1979. Measuring and estimating the bioconcentration factor of chemicals in fish. J. Fish Res. B. Canada. 36, 1040–1048.

Viberg, H., Fredriksson, A., Eriksson, P., 2003a. Neonatal exposure to polybrominated diphenyl ether (PBDE 153) disrupts spontaneous behaviour, impairs learning and memory, and decreases hippocampal cholinergic receptors in adult mice. Toxicol. Appl. Pharmacol. 192, 95–106.

Viberg, H., Fredriksson, A., Jakobsson, E., et al., 2003b. Neurobehavioral derangements in adult mice receiving decabrominated diphenyl ether (PBDE 209) during a defined period of neonatal brain development. Toxicol. Sci. 76, 112–120.

Watanabe, I., Kashimoto, T., Tatsukawa, R., 1983. The flame retardant tetrabromobisphenol A and its metabolite found in river and marine sediments in Japan. Chemosphere. 12, 1533–1539.

World Health Organization, 1994. Environmental Health Criteria: Brominated Diphenyl Ethers, vol. 162. World Health Organization, Geneva.

Wu, Y., Beland, F.A., Fang, J.L., 2016. Effect of triclosan, triclocarban, 2,2′,4,4′-tetrabromodiphenyl ether, and bisphenol A on the iodide uptake, thyroid peroxidase activity, and expression of genes involved in thyroid hormone synthesis. Toxicol. In Vitro. 32, 310–319.

Yamashita, N., Young, L.Y.W., Taniyasu, S., et al., 2011. Global distribution of PFOS and related chemicals. In: Loganathan, B., Lam, P. K.S. (Eds.), Global Contamination Trends of Persistent Organic Chemicals. CRC Press, Boca Raton, FL.

Yang, Q., Xie, Y., Alexson, S.H.E., et al., 2002a. Involvement of the peroxisome proliferator-activated receptor alpha in the immunomodulation caused by peroxisome proliferators in mice. Biochem. Pharm. 63, 1893–1900.

Yang, Q., Abedi-Valugerdi, M., Xie, Y., et al., 2002b. Potent suppression of the adaptive immune response in mice upon dietary exposure to the potent peroxisome proliferator, perfluorooctanoic acid. Int. Immunopharm. 2, 289–397.

Yang, Q., Karotani, R., Yamada, A., et al., 2006. PPARα activation during pregnancy severely impairs mammary lobulalveolar development in mice. Endocrinology. 147, 4772–4780.

Zhao, W., Zitzow, J.D., Ehresman, D.J., et al., 2015. Na + /taurocholate cotransporting polypeptide and apical sodium-dependent bile acid transporter are involved in the disposition of perfluoroalkyl sulfonates in humans and rats. Toxicol. Sci. 146 (2), 363–373.

Zhao, W., Zitzow, J.D., Weaver, Y., et al., 2017. Organic Anion Transporting Polypeptides Contribute to the Disposition of Perfluoroalkyl Acids in Humans and Rats. Toxicol. Sci. 156 (1), 84–95.

Zweidinger, R.A., Cooper, S.D., Erickson, M.D., et al., 1979. Sampling and analysis for semi volatile brominated organics in ambient air. In: Schuetzle, D. (Ed.), Monitoring Toxic Substances ACS Symposium Series, vol. 94. American Chemical Society, Washington, DC, pp. 217–231.

Section X

Avian and Aquatic Toxicology

Chapter 53

Avian Toxicology

Arya Sobhakumari, Robert H. Poppenga and Snehal Tawde

INTRODUCTION

There are approximately 30 orders of birds in the Aves class, with approximately 2000 genera and 10,000 species. Obviously, such a large class of animals possesses a bewildering array of unique physiologic adaptations, behaviors, and ecologic niches. Thus, a discussion of a broad topic such as avian toxicology presents a daunting task. This chapter provides an overview of toxicologic hazards to three subsets of birds: pet and aviary birds, poultry and other farm-raised birds, and wild birds. Given the breadth of the topic, this chapter is not an exhaustive treatise but, it is hoped, provides an overview of major avian toxicologic hazards.

Environment as a Toxicological Risk Factors in Birds

The increase in popularity of pet birds and their confinement in a home environment exposes them to toxicants that poultry and wild birds are unlikely to come into contact with, such as the pyrolysis products from Teflon-coated cookware. Alternatively, pet birds can be exposed to toxicants to which poultry and wild birds are also exposed but that are in different forms or from different sources. For example, pet birds can be intoxicated by lead, most often in the form of lead-based paint or lead objects such as drapery weights or toys, whereas wild birds are frequently intoxicated following ingestion of lead ammunition or lead-containing fishing gear.

Wild birds exist in a much less well-controlled environment than do pet birds or poultry and are therefore exposed to a greater variety of potential toxicants. One unique aspect of wild bird toxicology is the potential exposure of wild birds to toxicants via their prey. Raptors and scavengers such as turkey vultures or condors are often poisoned as a result of feeding on animal carcasses contaminated with pesticides or lead. Thus, secondary or relay toxicosis is a more common occurrence in wild birds than in pet birds or poultry.

Most commercial poultry are raised in well-controlled environments and are provided quality feed and water. Thus, their potential for exposure to toxicants is more limited. However, poultry can become intoxicated following exposure to common feed additives such as ionophores, if feed misformulations occur. Obviously, free-ranging poultry are potentially exposed to a greater variety of hazardous chemicals.

Physiologic Differences of Birds Relevant to Toxicology

Respiratory System

The unique physiology of a bird's respiration makes them more susceptible to some inhaled toxicants, such as carbon monoxide (CO) and pyrolysis products from overheated Teflon. The sensitivity of birds to inhaled toxicants brings to mind the image of the canary in the coal mine. Several physiologic differences of birds increase their sensitivity to inhaled toxicants, such as a higher mass–specific minute ventilation, a higher mass–specific ventilation of gas-exchange tissues, cross-current and countercurrent gas-exchange mechanisms, and a gas-diffusion barrier one-half the thickness of that of mammals (Brown and Wang, 1997). These physiologic adaptations are a result of high metabolic rates of birds and the concomitant need for a high ventilatory capacity.

Metabolic System

A number of studies have examined the metabolism of xenobiotics in a variety of avian species and compared metabolic capabilities of birds and mammals (Pan and Fouts, 1978; Dalvi et al., 1987). Organophosphate (OP) insecticides are more toxic to birds than mammals, and the basis for this difference is primarily due to differences in OP metabolism. For example, dimethoate is 20 times

Veterinary Toxicology. DOI: http://dx.doi.org/10.1016/B978-0-12-811410-0.00053-2

more toxic to pheasants than rats. Dimethoate is metabolized by pheasants to a toxic metabolite, whereas the toxic metabolite is detoxified by rats (Pan and Fouts, 1978). In addition, there are differences between bird species and between sexes and ages. Geese, chickens, and turkeys had similar liver aniline hydroxylase activity compared with that of rats, whereas quail and ducks had lower activities (Dalvi et al., 1987).

Excretion

Birds have several unique excretory pathways for xenobiotics. Many metals are incorporated into feathers, which are subsequently molted. In addition, incorporation of toxicants into eggs provides a significant excretory pathway for female birds.

GENERAL COMMENTS ABOUT DIAGNOSING AVIAN INTOXICATIONS

Although most diagnostic approaches for documenting intoxication in mammals are applicable to birds, there are several unique aspects that bear mentioning. Given the small size of many birds, obtaining a sufficient amount of sample for testing can sometimes present a challenge. For example, it is not unusual to be able to obtain only 100 μL (sometimes less) of whole blood or serum antemortem for lead and zinc testing, respectively. Quantities of gastrointestinal contents or tissues such as liver are sometimes limiting, especially if multiple tests are desired. The availability of less than optimal sample sizes often decreases the sensitivity of toxicologic testing, so it is possible that low toxicant concentrations are not detected. In the case of wild bird die-offs, pooling of samples from several dead birds is often required.

Antemortem, whole blood is most often requested from mammals for cholinesterase activity determinations. However, in birds, there is little cholinesterase activity that is associated with the red blood cell. Therefore, for avian species, plasma is preferred. Feathers and egg samples are sometimes useful for diagnosing either exposure to or intoxication from toxicants.

Investigation of wild bird die-offs is often a challenge from the standpoint that frequently birds are not discovered until significant postmortem autolysis and/or predation has occurred. Postmortem autolysis often precludes thorough pathologic and microbiologic testing. However, for the vast majority of toxicologic tests, the condition of the tissue or fluid sample is of less concern, and severely autolyzed samples may be perfectly suitable for toxicologic testing.

As is the case for any suspected intoxication related to feed, it is critical to obtain a representative feed sample. For example, feed-related mycotoxicoses are common concerns in poultry. However, the distribution and concentration of a mycotoxin in a feed can be quite variable. Therefore, it is important to obtain a number of samples that can then be pooled and subsampled. Other toxicants for which obtaining representative feed samples are critical include drugs; growth promotants such as ionophores; sodium chloride; and nutritionally important minerals such as copper, zinc, and selenium.

Because malicious poisonings of wild birds are common, and state or federal laws protect some poisoned birds, the potential for litigation should always be of concern. Therefore, it may be critical to obtain and submit samples following chain-of-custody procedures.

NATURAL TOXICANTS

Algal Toxins

Cyanobacterial blooms and cyanotoxins have been linked to the death of animals throughout the world. The more popular cyanotoxins are anatoxin-a and microcystins, produced by cyanobacteria belonging to various genera such as Anabaena, Microcystis, Coelosphaerium, and Plankothrix. There are few documented instances of intoxication of birds, mostly in wild birds because they are more likely to be exposed to cyanobacterial toxins than pet birds or poultry given their water sources such as lakes, reservoirs, and rivers. However, it is possible that zoo birds or production birds such as poultry, game birds, or waterfowl can be exposed via their water depending on its source and if conditions conducive to algal blooms are present. Anatoxin-a(s) was believed to have been the cause of bird mortality in several Danish lakes where *Anabaena lemmermannii* dominated the blooms, and anatoxin-a(s) was detected (Henriksen et al., 1997). Similarly a bloom of *Microcystis aeurginosa* in a pond in Japan was believed to have played a role in the death of approximately 20 spot-billed ducks (Matsunaga et al., 1999).

Clinical signs may vary depending on the cyanotoxin though birds are often found dead in mass mortality events occurring along water sources. Anatoxin-a is a potent agonist at nicotinic acetylcholine receptors (nAChRs) and poisoning may result in clinical signs of muscle fasciculations or seizures. Microcystins are hepatotoxic, which on ingestion of an acutely toxic dose can result in fulminant liver failure. Brevetoxins produced by the dinoflagellate *Karenia brevis* has been attributed to clinical signs such as disorientation, inability to stand, ataxia, seizures (Fauquier et al., 2013) and the death of sea birds along the west Florida coast in 2005 and 2006. Necropsy findings are typically absent in anatoxin intoxications whereas microcystins exposed birds may present a hemorrhagic, necrotic, severely jaundiced, and dark-green colored liver (Matsunaga et al., 1999).

A diagnosis of cyanobacterial intoxications is often by detection of the toxin in the gastrointestinal contents and confirmation of its presence in the algal blooms.

In addition to anatoxins and microcystins produced by cyanobacteria, the death of lesser flamingos in East African Rift Valley revealed another class of potent cyanobacterial toxins the β-*N*-methylamino-L-alanine and 2,4-diaminobutyric acid. These are neurotoxic amino acids produced by the cyanobacteria belonging to the family Arthrospira (Metcalf et al., 2013).

Avian Vacuolar Myelinopathy

Avian vacuolar myelinopathy (AVM) is a disease of birds that has sporadically caused mortality of bald eagles (*Haliaeetus leucocephalus*), American coots (*Fulica americana*), and other waterbirds in several reservoirs in the southeastern Unites States. Studies have demonstrated an association between bird mortality and the presence of the invasive plant hydrilla (*Hydrilla verticillata*) (Wilde et al., 2005). Earlier, the cyanobacteria belonging to Stigonematales was suspected to be the causative agent. However, recent studies have shown that cyanobacterial species belonging to *Aetokthonus hydrillicola* gen. et sp. nov., described recently, has been found to be associated with the hydrilla plant (Dodd, 2016). AVM was reproduced using mallard ducks and chickens exposed to *Stigonematales* blooms previously. It is believed that a currently uncharacterized algal neurotoxin is the etiology. AVM is characterized by widespread, bilaterally symmetrical vacuolation of the white matter of the brain and spinal cord.

Plants

A number of plants are recognized for their toxicity in birds (Table 53.1). Plants contain a large variety of biologically active constituents, including volatile oils, resins, alkaloids, polysaccharides, phenols, glycosides, and fixed oils.

The susceptibility of different bird species to specific toxic plants is variable. In addition, birds may be unaffected by plants that are toxic to other animals such as mammals. For example, cedar waxwings and house finches can consume fruit from the pepper tree (*Capsicum annuum*) that is toxic to mammals (Navarro, 1992). Feeding behaviors also influence the susceptibility to intoxication. For example, it has been suggested that parrots can consume otherwise toxic plants because they remove the outer covering of fruits and seeds, which can contain high concentrations of toxins, before consumption.

Mycotoxins

Independent chapters pertaining to mycotoxins are presented elsewhere in this book; therefore, select information pertaining to avian mycotoxicoses is presented in this section.

Aflatoxins

Aflatoxins are secondary fungal metabolites produced by *Aspergillus flavus*, *Aspergillus parasiticus*, and *Aspergillus nomius*. There are different toxin types designated by letters: B1, B2, G1, and G2. Of these aflatoxin B1 is the most frequently occurring and toxic member of the group. Although peanuts and corn are commonly known substrates for the growth of aflatoxin-producing fungi, other grains and nuts have been implicated as well. Economic losses attributed to aflatoxin exposure in poultry often stem from reductions in growth rate, hatchability, feed efficiency, and immunocompetence.

Poultry, especially turkeys, are extremely sensitive to the toxic effects of AFB_1, with quail being intermediate and chickens being comparatively resistant (Lozano and Diaz, 2006). Mortality events have been reported in migrating wild birds such as cranes, ducks, Canada geese, teals and other free ranging birds following consumption of grains in damaged, fungus infested standing crops (Friend and Franson, 1999).

Clinical signs in birds include lethargy, depression, blindness, inability to fly, tremors, and wing flapping, although birds can also simply be found dead. Lethal aflatoxicoses in ducklings occurred as inappetence, reduced growth, abnormal vocalization, feather picking, purple discoloration of leg and feet, and lameness. Ataxia, convulsions, and opisthotonus preceded death (Carnaghan, 1961). Turkeys develop inappetence, reduced spontaneous activity, unsteady gait, recumbency, anemia, and death. Aflatoxicosis in chickens closely resembles the clinical signs in ducks and turkeys. Chronic effects, which include appetite loss, weight loss/reduced weight gain, and general ill health due to immunosuppression, can be more insidious and difficult to definitively relate to aflatoxin exposure.

Acute exposures over a relatively short period lead to pale, swollen, and enlarged livers (and kidneys), occasional gallbladder distension, thickening of crop and proventricular mucosa, and hemorrhages in internal organs especially GI tract (blackish red). Chronic exposure produces a shrunken, fibrous liver with regenerative nodules or tumors. Microscopically, the hepatocytes show fatty changes, proliferation of bile ductules, and extensive fibrosis, accompanied by vascular and degenerative lesions in pancreas and kidney.

Measurement of aflatoxin concentrations in suspected feed, ingesta, or the liver is crucial for confirming diagnosis. Representative sampling and adequate precautions (e.g., freezing samples) to avoid fungal growth and toxin

TABLE 53.1 Plants Reported to be Toxic to Birds

Common Name	Scientific Name	Toxin	Plant Part Demonstrated to be Toxic	Mechanism of Toxic Action	Primary Organ System Affected	Species/Bird Type Reported to be Affected	References
Avocado	*Persea americana*	Persin	Fruit, leaves	Unknown	Cardiovascular system	Budgerigars (*Melopsittacus undulates*), canaries (*Serinus canaria*), cockatiels, ostriches (*Struthio camelus*)	Burrows and Tyrl (2013); Shropshire et al. (1992)
Black locust	*Robinia pseudoacacia*	Unknown; possibly glycoprotein lectins, proteins	Leaves, bark	Unknown	Cardiovascular system, gastrointestinal tract	Budgerigars (*Melopsittacus undulates*)	Burrows and Tyrl (2013); Shropshire et al. (1992)
Bladder pod, rattlebox, coffeeweed, daubentonia, others	*Sesbania* spp.	Saponins, others	Seeds	Smooth muscle inhibition, vasodilation	Nervous system, gastrointestinal tract, kidneys	Chickens	Flory and Hebert (1984)
Cacao	*Theobroma cacao*	Theobromine, caffeine	Seeds	Adenosine receptor antagonism, increased intracellular Ca^{2+} concentrations	Nervous system, cardiovascular system	Chickens	Day and Dilworth (1984)
Canola (also referred to as rapeseed), mustards	*Brassica* spp.	Glucosinolates, others	Seeds	Accumulation of trimethylamine affects eggs (odor and taste); liver and muscle damage due to unknown mechanism	Eggs, liver, muscle, cardiovascular system	Chickens, turkeys, ducks	Burrows and Tyrl (2013)
Cassava	*Manihot* spp.	Cyanide	Root	See section on cyanide			
Castor bean	*Ricinus communis*	Ricin	Seeds	Protein synthesis inhibition	Gastrointestinal tract, liver	Ducks	Jensen and Allen (1981)
Coffee senna, sickle pod, coffeeweed, others	*Senna* spp. (previously *Cassia* spp.)	Anthraquinones	Fruit, seeds	Irritation, mitochondrial myopathy	Gastrointestinal tract, skeletal muscle	Chickens	Burrows and Tyrl (2013)
Corn cockle	*Agrostemma githago*	Saponins	Seeds	Irritation	Gastrointestinal tract	Chickens	Burrows and Tyrl (2013)

Cottonseed	*Gossypium* spp.	Gossypol	Seeds	Unknown	Gastrointestinal tract, kidneys, liver, egg production	Poultry	Brown and Julian (2003)
Coyotillo	*Karwinskia humboldtiana*	Anthracenones	Seeds	Uncoupling of oxidative phosphorylation, inhibition of axoplasmal transport	Nervous system	Poultry	Burrows and Tyrl (2013)
Day jessamine, day cestrum, wild jasmine, Chinese inkberry	*Cestrum diurnum*	Analog of 1,25-dihydroxycholecalciferol	Leaves	Hypercalcemia, dystrophic tissue calcification	Cardiovascular system, kidneys	Chickens	Sarkar et al. (1981)
Death camas, others	*Zygadenus* spp.	Alkaloids	Seeds, stems, roots	Increase reflex activity, stimulate afferent pathway receptors, increase and extend negative after potentials	Nervous system	Poultry	Burrows and Tyrl (2013)
Dieffenbachia	*Dieffenbachia* spp.	Insoluble oxalates	Leaves	Physical irritation	Gastrointestinal tract	Canaries (*Serinus canaria*)	Arai et al. (1992)
Digitalis	*Digitalis purpurea*	Cardiac glycosides	Leaves	Inhibit $Na^+ - K^+$ ATPase	Cardiovascular system	Canaries (*Serinus canaria*)	Arai et al. (1992)
Eucalyptus	*Eucalyptus cladocalyx*	Cyanide	Leaves	Inhibit cytochrome oxidase *c*	Multiorgan	Poultry	Brown and Julian (2003)
Jimsonweed, thorn apple	*Datura* spp.	Tropane alkaloids	Seeds	Cholinergic (muscarinic) receptor antagonism	Nervous system	Chickens	Day and Dilworth (1984)
Jojoba	*Simmondsia chinensis*	Simmondsin	Seeds	Inhibition of appetite via unknown mechanism	Overall growth rate	Chickens	Arnouts *et al.*, (1993)
White popinac, lead tree, guacis, jumby bean	*Leucaena leucocephala*	Mimosine	Seeds	Inhibit reactions requiring pyridoxine, inhibit DNA and RNA synthesis	Bone, depressed growth	Poultry	Burrows and Tyrl (2013)
Lily of the valley	*Convallaria majalis*	Cardenolides	Leaves, rhizomes, roots	Inhibit $Na^+ - K^+$ ATPase	Cardiovascular system	Poultry	Burrows and Tyrl (2013)

(*Continued*)

TABLE 53.1 (Continued)

Common Name	Scientific Name	Toxin	Plant Part Demonstrated to be Toxic	Mechanism of Toxic Action	Primary Organ System Affected	Species/Bird Type Reported to be Affected	References
Lupine	*Lupinus* spp.	Quinolizidine alkaloids	Leaves	Cholinergic receptor agonists	Nervous system	Canaries (*Serinus canaria*)	Arai et al. (1992); Burrows and Tyrl (2013)
Milkweed	*Asclepias* spp.	Cardenolides, uncharacterized neurotoxin	Entire plant, latex sap	Inhibit $Na^+ - K^+$ ATPase, uncertain for neurotoxic effect	Cardiovascular system, nervous system		Burrows and Tyrl (2013)
Nightshades, potato	*Solanum* spp.	Steroidal glycosides (chaconine, solanine, others)	Immature seeds, foliage	Saponin-induced irritation, AChE inhibition	Gastrointestinal tract, nervous system	Chickens	Burrows and Tyrl (2013)
Oak	*Quercus* spp.	Tannins	Leaves, early buds	Astringent effect (protein precipitation), direct cell damage	Gastrointestinal tract, kidneys (*Casuarius casuarius*)	Double-wattled cassowary	Burrows and Tyrl (2013)
Oleander	*Nerium oleander*	Oleandrin	Leaves	Inhibit $Na^+ - K^+$ ATPase	Cardiovascular system	Budgerigars (*Melopsittacus undulates*), canaries (*Serinus canaria*), geese (species not identified)	Arai et al. (1992); Shropshire et al. (1992)
Oxalates, soluble	Many plants (*Halogeton* spp., *Sarcobatus* spp., others)	Calcium or potassium oxalates	Leaves, stems	Hypocalcemia, calcium oxalate precipitation in renal tubules	Cardiovascular system, kidneys	Poultry	Burrows and Tyrl (2013)
Parsley	*Ammi majus*	Furanocoumarins	Seeds, leaves	Primary photosensitization, other (calcium channel inhibition)	Skin, liver, kidneys	Ducks, geese; chickens and turkeys are less sensitive	Burrows and Tyrl (2013)
Poison hemlock	*Conium maculatum*	Pyridine alkaloids including coniine, *N*-methylconiine, γ-coniceine	Seeds	Nicotinic receptor agonist	Nervous system	Range turkeys (species not identified)	Burrows and Tyrl (2013)
Pokeberry	*Phytolacca americana*	Saponins, oxalates	Berries	Irritation	Gastrointestinal tract	Turkeys	Burrows and Tyrl (2013)

Rattlebox, others	*Crotalaria* spp.	Pyrrolizidine alkaloids	Seeds, leaves, stems	Inhibition of protein and RNA synthesis, alkylate DNA, inhibit mitosis	Liver	Chickens, geese	Burrows and Tyrl (2013)
Ragwort, groundsel	*Senecio* spp.						
Sweet pea	*Lathyrus* spp.	Amino acids, nitriles, β-aminoproprionitrile	Seeds	Glutamate receptor agonism, inhibition of lysyl oxidase	Nervous system, reproduction (decrease ovarian activity), eggs	Chickens, turkeys	Burrows and Tyrl (2013)
Tobacco	*Nicotiana* spp.	Nicotine, nornicotine, anabasine	Leaves and stems	Nicotinic receptor stimulation, teratogen	Nervous system, embryo development	Poultry	Burrows and Tyrl (2013)
Velvetweed	Abutilon theophrasti			Affects egg yolks due to unknown mechanism	Eggs	Poultry	Brown et al. (1997)
Vetch	*Vicia* spp.	Cyanogenic glycosides (probably not toxic), β-cyano-L-alanine	Seeds	Cyanide inhibits cytochrome oxidase *c*; signs similar to pyridoxine deficiency	Nervous system	Chickens	Burrows and Tyrl (2013)
Virginia creeper	*Parthenocissus quinquefolia*		Leaves	Unknown	Gastrointestinal system	Budgerigars (*Melopsittacus undulates*)	Burrows and Tyrl (2013); Shropshire et al. (1992)
Yew	*Taxus* spp.	Taxine	Leaves, seeds	Alter atrioventricular conduction via inhibition of $Na^+ - Ca^{2+}$ fluxes and possible K^+ channel effects	Cardiovascular system	Budgerigars (*Melopsittacus undulates*), canaries (*Serinus canaria*), emus (*Dromaius novaehollandiae*)	Burrows and Tyrl (2013); Shropshire et al. (1992)

production secondary to improper postcollection storage and shipping are necessary.

Steps to minimize crop damage and mold growth are crucial. Suspected feed sources should be removed from the diet. Since aflatoxin contamination of feedstuff is nearly universal, various chemopreventive and enterosorptive approaches such as addition of synthetic zeolites and sodium calcium aluminosilicate in the feed, and administration of the hepatoprotective agent silymarin have been shown to be protective (Kubena et al., 1998; Tedesco et al., 2004).

The Food and Drug Administration (FDA) has set a current guidance level for AFB_1 concentrations in corn and peanut products intended for immature and mature poultry at 20 and 100 parts per billion (ppb), respectively.

Fusariotoxins

Fungi belonging to *Fusarium* spp. and several other genera produce chemically distinct mycotoxins in feed grains and nuts. Type A and type B trichothecenes, zearalenone (ZEN), and fumonisins are fusariotoxins of relatively greater importance from a poultry-production and health perspective (Girgis and Smith, 2010). Type A trichothecenes include T-2 toxin, HT-2 toxin and diacetoxyscirpenol; type B trichothecenes include deoxynivalenol (DON, vomitoxin), 3- and 15-acetyl-DON, nivalenol, and fusarenon-X. Of these, DON is the most commonly encountered fusariotoxin.

Fusariotoxins differ from other mycotoxins in that they tend to be produced during the colder seasons of the year. Common substrates involved in fusariotoxin production include corn, wheat, barley, oats, and peanuts. ZEN often occurs with DON in naturally contaminated cereals, and it is responsible for reproductive disorders due to its estrogenic effect at suitable concentrations in susceptible livestock and avian populations. However, in general, ZEN has limited toxicity to birds.

T-2 toxin: T-2 toxin is a type A trichothecene mycotoxin produced by *Fusarium sporotrichioides*, *Fusarium poae*, and *Fusarium acuinatum* and detected less frequently in grain and other agricultural products (Li et al., 2011; Murphy et al., 2006). However, T-2 is one of the most acutely toxic mycotoxins of the trichothecene family. In 7-day-old broilers, the LD_{50} of T-2 toxin is 4.97 mg/kg, and it is more toxic than aflatoxin ($LD_{50} = 6.8$ mg/kg), HT-2 toxin ($LD_{50} = 7.22$ mg/kg), and DON ($LD_{50} = 140$ mg/kg) (Summers, 1995).

In poultry, toxicological effects of T-2 are observed on the liver and digestive system, nervous system, and skin due to its cytotoxic and genotoxic potential, leading to impairment of performance. Incoordination, seizures, eggshell thinning, reduced egg production, decreased feed intake and weight gain, comb cyanosis, depigmentation of the skin on legs, and necrohemorrhagic dermatitis are common clinical signs (Wyatt et al., 1973). T-2 toxin can induce necrosis and depletion of lymphoid cells in the thymus, spleen, and lymph nodes of chickens and pullets. A major postmortem finding is necrotic damage characterized by white-yellowish bulges containing caseous–necrotic material in various areas of the mouth, gizzard, intestinal mucosa, and liver (Wyatt et al., 1973).

Diagnosis is based on history, postmortem findings including necrotic lesions in the digestive system, and detection of T-2 at significant concentrations in the suspected feed. Total amount of all trichothecenes including T-2 toxin in poultry feed should preferably not exceed 0.5 mg/kg, based on a compilation of data including occurrence, toxicity, and clinical signs in poultry (Eriksen and Pettersson, 2004).

Deoxynivalenol (vomitoxin): DON is the least acutely toxic tricothecene mycotoxin to poultry but a more commonly occurring grain contaminant (Rotter et al., 1996). Diversion of DON-infected cereals to poultry feed is commonly believed to be a significant route of exposure.

The effects of DON on performance are highly variable but reduced weight gain and feed refusal are established findings. DON can cause significant lipid peroxidation, oxidative stress and DNA damage indicating the genotoxic potential and possibly explaining its effects on various body systems. The immune and intestinal epithelial cells are particularly sensitive to the toxic effects of DON. Erosions in the mucosa of the gizzard, corrugations in the gastric mucosa, duodenitis, jejunitis, intestinal bleeding, and necrosis are significant postmortem findings associated with DON exposure. Reduced immune responses to Newcastle disease vaccine infectious bronchitis virus have been observed in laying hens and broilers due to feeding DON-contaminated grains (Harvey et al., 1991).

The FDA has established a 10 mg/kg advisory concentration for DON in grain or grain byproducts destined for chickens, with the added recommendation that such feed may not exceed 50% of the total diet.

Fumonisins: Fumonisins are produced by *Fusarium verticillioides* and occur as a contaminant of corn and other agricultural products. Fumonisins exert their toxic effects by disruption of sphingolipid metabolism. Ducks are very sensitive to toxicity, whereas turkeys are more resistant.

Fumonisins in excess of 100 mg/kg in the diet have been shown to reduce weight gain, cause diarrhea and hepatotoxicity. In day-old broiler chicks fed 0–400 mg/kg FB_1 for 21 days and 30 mg/kg for 14 days hepatic necrosis, biliary hyperplasia, and thymic cortical atrophy were noted postmortem (Brown et al., 1992).

The FDA guidance concentration for fumonisins in poultry feed is set at 50 ppm in the total ration. Feed containing elevated fumonisin concentrations may be disposed or diluted with suitable feed sources.

Ochratoxin and Citrinin

These nephro- and hepatotoxic mycotoxins are produced by multiple species of *Aspergillus* and *Penicillium*, and occur in feedstuffs worldwide. Ochratoxin A (OTA) is comparatively ten times more toxic than citrinin and has been studied extensively, although both may co-occur. Avian species vary in their sensitivity to OTA; the LD_{50} in chickens is reported to be 2–4 mg/kg, whereas ducks and Japanese quail are susceptible to 0.5–16.5 mg/kg body weight (BW) (Peckham et al., 1971).

OTA inhibits protein biosynthesis, causes oxidative stress, accelerates lipid peroxidation, and reacts with enzymes-utilizing phenylalanine as a substrate, thereby exerting its toxic effects. The nephrotoxic effect of OTA is due to its action on the organic anion transport system, located in basolateral and brush border membranes of the proximal tubule cells of the nephron and also involved in the absorption/reabsorption and excretion of OTA in the kidney.

Field outbreaks of ochratoxicosis typically result in decreased feed consumption, efficiency, growth rate, and increased mortality. Hepatotoxicity is characterized by a significant increase in γ-glutamyl transferase activity, decrease in serum total protein, albumin, globulin, cholesterol, triglyceride, and increase in the weight of liver. An elevation in serum uric acid, creatinine, postmortem degenerative changes, and an increase in the weight of kidney were considered to be indicative of nephrotoxicity (Huff et al., 1988). For details on mechanism and toxicity of OTA and citrinin refer to Chapter 74, Tremorgenic Mycotoxins.

To detoxify and reduce the concentration of OTAs, various probiotic bacteria, yeast or gamma-irradiation have been used (Biernasiak et al., 2006).

Zootoxins

There are few reports of bird intoxication resulting from exposure to zootoxins. Snakebite was believed to have been responsible for the deaths of two red-tailed hawks (*Buteo jamaicensis*) and a Cooper's hawk (*Accipiter cooperii*) based on the carcasses being found in the vicinity of venomous snakes and gross findings of hemorrhages, muscle degeneration, and gangrenous necrosis of a limb (Heckel et al., 1994). Chickens, turkeys, and ducks have also reportedly been killed by snakes based on bite sites that were identified on postmortem examination and compatible gross organ lesions (Lawal et al., 1992). For further details on zootoxins, see Chapter 59, Chemical-Induced Estrogenicity.

Bacterial Toxins

Botulinum Toxin

Avian botulism results from the ingestion of botulinum toxin produced by the anaerobic bacterium *Clostridium botulinum*. There are eight antigenically distinct toxin types designated as A, B, C (alpha and beta), D, E, F, and G; with Type C alpha cultures producing three toxins designated C1–C3. A number of factors play a role in the occurrence of an outbreak of botulism, including optimal environmental conditions for spore germination and bacterial growth, availability of suitable material to support bacterial replication such as decomposing carcasses, and a means for toxin transfer to birds. Type C toxin–producing bacterial spores are ubiquitous in wetland environments inhabited by bird populations.

Botulinum toxin is one of the most toxic biotoxins known, although for any given species, toxicity varies by toxin type and age. For example, chickens, turkeys, pheasants, and peafowl are susceptible to types A, B, C, and E but not to types D or F (Gross and Smith, 1971). As broiler chickens age, they become less susceptible to type C toxin. Most outbreaks of botulism in birds are due to exposure to type C1 toxin. Avian botulism is one of the most important diseases of migratory birds. Exposure occurs when waterfowl feed on contaminated zooplankton, and carcass-feeding maggots or raptors feed on carcasses. Poultry and production birds are also exposed through wound contamination by spores. Vultures and other carrion eaters are resistant to botulinum toxin, perhaps, in part, due to the production of antibodies to botulinum toxin, which does not occur in sensitive species such as chickens and ducks (Ohishi et al., 1979).

Clinical signs are consistent with neuromuscular paralysis. Affected waterfowl are unable to sustain flight, hold their head erect (limberneck) and present with paralysis of nictitating membrane. Waterfowl often drown; affected terrestrial birds die from respiratory and cardiac failure. In chickens, an ascending flaccid paralysis is noted with symptoms similar to waterfowl. Postmortem lesions are generally not observed; in affected waterfowl, lesions may be consistent with drowning.

A presumptive diagnosis is based on characteristic clinical signs, environmental conditions conducive to bacterial growth and toxin production, and detection of toxin in serum and tissues. Treatment of affected birds with antitoxin is helpful in waterfowl but not in other species such as coots, shorebirds, gulls, and grebes (Friend and Franson, 1999). Prevention and control of outbreaks are critical to minimize losses. Removing organic and decaying material in wetlands, and proper disposal of animal carcasses can interrupt bacterial growth and toxin production.

Feed Additives

Sodium

Sodium ion intoxication is a significant problem in poultry production. Intoxication can result from excessive sodium in the feed and/or water deprivation as in commercial poultry, or ingestion of saline waters or precipitation of salt on feathers in waterfowls (Gordus et al., 2002). The most common form of sodium associated with intoxication is sodium chloride. High dietary sodium can be well tolerated if access to water is not restricted.

A number of factors influence the toxicity of the sodium ion, including bird age, bird species, dietary factors, water quality, and accessibility. Young birds are more sensitive to sodium ion toxicity, most likely due to a less-developed renal function. Turkeys are more susceptible to intoxication than are chickens (Berger, 1993). In addition, birds have less ability to excrete salts in excess of water, so their ability to reduce high-plasma osmolality is limited. In general, the addition of 1% salt (as sodium chloride) to poultry rations is safe, even for very young birds. A level of 0.25% salt in drinking water is considered to be safe (Berger, 1993).

At high sodium intakes, birds develop acute, severe diarrhea and dehydration, dyspnea, weight loss, and die. Ascites, edema, fluid in the lungs, hydropericardium, cardiac hypertrophy (right-sided in chickens and bilateral in poults), and dilatory cardiomyopathy (poults) are found on postmortem examination. Most microscopic lesions are secondary to cardiac failure, although bilaterally symmetrical areas of cerebral necrosis, vascular congestion, and edema were noted in intoxicated tom turkeys (Wages et al., 1995). Significant gross and microscopic lesions in ruddy ducks intoxicated by sodium include conjunctivitis, lens opacity, cataract formation, vascular congestion in multiple organs, especially in the meninges; and myocardial and skeletal muscle degeneration (Gordus et al., 2002).

Sodium concentrations in both the feed and the water need to be considered in assessing sodium exposure. A diagnosis of sodium ion intoxication relies on detection of high dietary and/or water, serum, and/or brain sodium concentrations in conjunction with other historical, clinical, and postmortem findings. Serum sodium concentrations greater than 150 mEq/L are elevated, and brain sodium concentrations greater than 2000 ppm wet weight are highly suggestive of intoxication (Puls, 1994).

Ionophores

Monensin, lasalocid, salinomycin, narasin, maduramicin, and semduramicin are some of the ionophore antibiotics used in poultry. Accidental or intentional off-label use has resulted in adverse reactions in adult poultry (laying hens), ostriches, and ornamental or game birds. In addition, interactions with other drugs used in target and nontarget species can occur. Various antibiotics have been reported to potentiate ionophore toxicity. The most frequently reported drug interaction is with the pleuromotilin derivative and tiamulin. This antibiotic interferes with the metabolic degradation of monensin in the liver, causing accumulation at toxic concentrations.

Excessive monensin exposure was reported in a 42-week broiler flock due to feed mixing error. There was high mortality and affected birds exhibited feed refusal, decreased water consumption, diarrhea and severe paralysis that ranged from abnormal gait to complete inability to move (Zavala et al., 2011). Another case report of monensin intoxication on a commercial ostrich farm in northern Greece described similar clinical signs along with elevated concentrations of serum aspartate aminotransferase, creatine kinase, and lactate dehydrogenase (Dedoussi et al., 2007). In layers, there will be a loss of egg production, hatchability, infertile eggs, early embryonic death, and weak ataxic chicks (Perelman and Smith, 1993). Reported cases of salinomycin intoxication in birds were associated with high mortality, signs of dyspnea, drowsiness, sternal recumbency with legs extended posteriorly, inability to stand, stiffness, and weakness (Andreasen and Schleifer, 1995). Gross postmortem findings may be absent or limited to hydropericardium, pale myocardium, hepatic congestion and enteritis. However, significant findings occur histologically and, include extensive fragmentation and necrosis of skeletal and myocardial muscle fibers (Dedoussi et al., 2007; Zavala et al., 2011).

Though avoidance of feed mixing errors and off-label use is the mainstay of prevention, results from few in vitro studies have been promising and show the protective effect of the herbal flavonolignan compound silybin from *Silybum marinum* against the toxicity of salinomycin, lasalocid, monensin and narasin in chicken hepatoma cell lines (Cybulski et al., 2015; Radko et al., 2013).

Pesticides

A tabulation of the toxicity of a number of pesticides for birds is provided in Table 53.2.

Insecticides

Organochlorine Insecticides

Historically, OCs were widely used from the 1940s to the 1970s in agriculture and forestry and for mosquito control. The most widely used organochlorines included the dichlorodiphenylethanes (DDT, methoxychlor, and dicofol), cyclodienes (aldrin, dieldrin, heptachlor, chlordane, and endosulfan), and hexachlorocyclohexanes (lindane and benzene hexachloride). Although some of these insecticides are no longer used in the United States, Canada, and Europe, they continue to be used in developing countries. These compounds are highly lipophilic and, in

TABLE 53.2 Rodenticides, Avicides, and Molluscicides Toxic for Avian Species

Rodenticides/ Avicides/ Molluscicides	Uses	Formulations	Avian Toxicity	Mechanism of Toxic Action	Clinical Signs	Species Affected	References
4-Aminopyridine (Avitrol)	Control red-winged blackbirds, blackbirds, grackles, pigeons, sparrows	Powder concentrate; 0.5%–3.0% grain baits; 3% cracked corn bait for agricultural use diluted to 0.03% with untreated grain; 1% whole corn diluted to 0.1% for crows; 0.5% bait for pigeons	Highly toxic for most species, including birds; LD_{50}s for birds range from 1.4 to 8.1 mg/kg	Blocks potassium ion channels and increases release of ACh	Distress cries, aerial distress displays, seizures, coma	Potentially all birds	Bischoff et al. (2001); Schell (2004b)
Bromethalin	Rodenticide	0.01% tan or green grain-based pellets in 16- to 42.5 g place packs	Not determined	Uncouples oxidative phosphorylation	Not described in birds; clinical signs in mammals dependent on ingested dose, with CNS excitation noted with high doses and paralysis noted with lower doses	Potentially all birds	Dorman (2004)
3-Chloro-*p*-toluidine hydrochloride (Starlicide)	Control ravens, starlings, crows, pigeons, cowbirds, grackles, magpies, certain gull species	98% powder used to prepare baits; 0.1% ready-to-use product	Highly toxic for most species including birds; LD_{50}s for birds of 1.8–3.8 mg/kg BW	Unknown	Decreased activity, tachypnea, dyspnea, renal failure	Potentially all birds	Schell (2004a)
Fluoroacetate (1080)	Rodenticide, coyote control	Use restricted to livestock protection collars (LPCs); LPCs for sheep and goats contain 30 mL at 1%	Oral LD_{50}s for magpies are 1.78–2.3 mg/kg BW	Blocks tricarboxylic acid cycle resulting in cell energy depletion	Vary depending on species; not well described in birds; CNS, gastrointestinal, and cardiovascular signs likely; skeletal muscle necrosis reported in mallard ducks	Potentially all birds; proper use of LPCs appears to present little or no intoxication risk to avian scavengers	Burns and Connolly (1995); Parton (2004)

(*Continued*)

TABLE 53.2 (Continued)

Rodenticides/ Avicides/ Molluscicides	Uses	Formulations	Avian Toxicity	Mechanism of Toxic Action	Clinical Signs	Species Affected	References
Metaldehyde	Control slugs and snails	Pelleted baits, granules, liquids, or wettable powders containing 5% metaldehyde	Minimum lethal doses for chickens and ducks are 500 and 300 mg/kg BW, respectively	Decreases GABA in the brain; alterations of other brain neuro-transmitters	Restlessness, anxiety, tachypnea, seizures, hyperthermia	Potentially all birds; secondary poisoning not reported	Talcott (2004a)
Strychnine	Controlling ground squirrels, meadow and deer mice, prairie dogs, porcupines, chipmunks, rabbits, pigeons	Colored grain-based baits with 0.5%–1.0% strychnine sulfate	Reported oral LD_{50}s for golden eagles, sage grouse, and pheasants are 5–10, 42.5, and 8.5–24.7 mg/kg, respectively	Blocks inhibitory actions of glycine of spinal cord anterior horn cells and inhibits neurotransmitter release from Renshaw cells	Nervousness, apprehension, anxiety, tachypnea, muscle spasms, stiffness, tonic extensor muscle contractions, death due to respiratory impairment	Potentially all birds	Talcott (2004b)
					Secondary toxicity reported		
Zinc phosphide	Used to control rats, mice, voles, ground squirrels, prairie dogs, nutrias, muskrats, rabbits, opossums, gophers	Grain-based bait, scrap bait, paste, or tracking powder; baits generally contain 0.5%–2.0% zinc phosphide; paste up to 10%	Oral LD_{50}s for wild birds and ducks reported to be 23.7–37.5 mg/kg; oral LD_{50} in chickens reported to be 25 mg/kg	Phosphene released from zinc or aluminum phosphide blocks cytochrome oxidase	Often found dead; dullness, tachypnea, dyspnea, tremors, paralysis, seizures, death	Potentially all birds	Poppenga et al. (2005); Tiwary et al. (2005)
	Aluminum phosphide used as a fumigant				Secondary toxicity unlikely		

general, have long environmental and body half-lives. Because of their lipophilic and persistent nature, they biomagnify within food webs. They were banned due to their environmental persistence, concern about their impact on human health and wildlife health, and widespread insect resistance.

Cholinesterase Inhibitors (Organophosphorus and Carbamate Insecticides)

Due to their more rapid breakdown in the environment, OP and carbamate insecticides replaced the OC pesticides as the latter were banned for use in North America and Europe in the 1960s and 1970s. A number of different formulations are available for use either in the environment (e.g., agricultural or residential use) or on animals (e.g., livestock dips or sprays). The more toxic insecticides of each group are generally restricted to agricultural uses, whereas less-toxic members are approved for use on animals or in residential environments.

Birds are exposed to cholinesterase inhibitors in different ways. Pet and production birds can be exposed via their diets, via home or premise use, or via direct application. Inhalation exposure is also possible from the use of dichlorvos-impregnated pest strips or premise spraying or fogging. Acute OP and carbamate intoxications are common in wild birds, and exposures can occur via ingestion of treated seeds or vegetation (accidental, intentional, or misuse of a product), poisoned insects or animals (impaired live animals or carcasses), product (especially granular formulations), or contaminated water (Friend and Franson, 1999). Inhalation or dermal exposure is also possible from spraying or spills. With avian wildlife, there can be some degree of seasonality to OP or carbamate intoxications as a result of seasonal patterns of insecticide use.

The acute oral toxicity of individual OPs and carbamates vary considerably within classes and between species. A number of other factors can influence toxicity, including age, sex, diet, body condition, and product formulation.

Although chemically distinct, the OPs and carbamates have a common mechanism of toxic action, namely the inhibition of cholinesterase enzymes. Inhibition of acetylcholinesterase (AChE) is primarily responsible for the clinical signs associated with intoxication. The onset of clinical signs and death can be rapid; birds are often found dead. Death is most often due to respiratory failure and hypoxia. OP inhibition of AChE activity can be irreversible, thus necessitating synthesis of new enzyme before recovery can occur. Carbamates do not irreversibly inhibit AChE, and spontaneous regeneration of enzyme activity is rapid. Clinical signs can persist for days in OP intoxicated animals, whereas recovery from carbamate intoxication is generally completed within 2 or 3 days. Gross and histopathologic lesions in dead birds are usually minimal and nonspecific.

Some OPs, including insecticides such as leptophos, mipafox, and cyanofenphos and industrial chemicals such as tri-*ortho*-cresyl-phosphate, cause a delayed neurotoxic effect referred to as OP-induced delayed neuropathy (OPIDN) or OP-induced delayed polyneuropathy (OPIDPN). OPIDN occurs as a result of inhibition of neurotoxic esterase (NTE), an enzyme found in peripheral nerves. OP insecticides are tested for their ability to cause OPIDN in adult hens as a result of their unique sensitivity to this effect. Also, pheasants and mallard ducklings are highly susceptible to delayed neurotoxicity (Brown and Julian, 2003). Most OPIDN-inducing insecticides are no longer on the market.

A diagnosis of intoxication is dependent on measuring reduced activity of cholinesterase along with identification of a specific insecticide in suitable antemortem or postmortem samples. In birds, plasma is suitable for cholinesterase activity determinations. Brain cholinesterase activity can be measured in dead birds. It is important to note that because carbamate-induced inhibition of cholinesterase activity is readily reversible, even after death, care must be taken when interpreting laboratory results. In general, cholinesterase activity less than 70% of normal suggests significant exposure to an OP or carbamate (activity is often $<20\%$ of normal following lethal exposures) (Hill, 1988). Normal plasma/whole blood and brain cholinesterase activities are quite variable among bird species, and interpretation of cholinesterase activity should be based on species-specific and, when possible, laboratory-specific reference ranges. Gastrointestinal contents should be examined carefully because the presence of granules or dye may suggest pesticide exposure. Often, given the rapidity of death, there is freshly ingested food in the upper GI tract.

Fortunately, the overall adverse impact of agricultural pesticide use in general, and OPs and carbamate use more specifically, on avian wildlife has lessened during approximately the past decade due primarily to the replacement of older, more toxic insecticides with newer, less-toxic ones such as pyrethrins/pyrethroids and neonicotinoids.

Pyrethrins/Pyrethroids

Naturally occurring pyrethrins (derived from chrysanthemum flowers) and synthetic pyrethroid insecticides are currently estimated to make up more than 25% of insecticide use worldwide. Their popularity is due to their lack of environmental persistence and relatively low toxicity for birds and mammals (they are highly toxic for fish). They are used to control a variety of agricultural, home, and animal pests and are available in a large number of formulations, including sprays, dusts, dips, shampoos, spot-ons, foggers, ear tags, wettable powders, granules, soluble powders, and emulsifiable concentrates. They are often combined with synergists such as piperonyl butoxide to enhance their insecticidal activity.

Pyrethrins and pyrethroids are neurotoxic as a result of their ability to alter sodium, chloride, and calcium channels and cause repetitive nervous discharges or membrane depolarization. At relatively high concentrations, they also have effect on GABA-gated chloride channels (Anadón et al., 2009). Clinical signs associated with acute intoxication are related to nervous system stimulation such as restlessness, pecking feathers, and abrupt movements (Zwart, 1988). There does not appear to be any reports on adverse behavioral effects on avian wildlife following sublethal exposures to pyrethrins/pyrethroids, similar to those reported for OPs or carbamates, which would cause mortality due to increased predation or inability to obtain food. Gross and histopathological findings are usually absent.

The diagnosis of pyrethrin and pyrethroid toxicosis is dependent on exposure history and development of compatible clinical signs. Serum samples antemortem and gastrointestinal contents, brain or liver postmortem can confirm exposure but not necessarily intoxication.

Neonicotinoids

Neonicotinoids, a new class of insecticide, are nicotinic receptor agonists. They initially stimulate the receptor and cause a depolarizing blockade later leading to death as a result of paralysis. This class includes acetamiprid, clothianidin, dinotefuran, imidacloprid, nitenpyram, thiacloprid, and thiamethoxam. They are considered to have low toxicity for vertebrates because of relatively low affinity for vertebrate nicotinic receptors compared to insect nicotinic receptors (Tomizawa and Casida, 2011). However recent studies have shown decline in insectivorous bird populations in association with widespread usage of the neonicotinoid drug imidacloprid possibly due to depletion of insect food resource though a less possible-direct consumption toxicity has also been proposed (Hallmann et al., 2014).

Rodenticides

Anticoagulants

Anticoagulant rodenticides are widely used to control rodent pests in urban and agricultural settings. Avian species that feed primarily on small rodents are at greatest risk of poisoning. Wild birds and raptors have likelihood of exposure following ingestion of baits and exposed and/or intoxicated prey. Commercial poultry have a less chance of exposure due to their controlled environments whereas free-roaming poultry are more likely to be exposed. The second-generation anticoagulant rodenticides (brodifacoum, bromodiolone, difenacoum, and difethialone) are acutely toxic and have longer tissue half-lives resulting in bioaccumulation and risk of secondary poisoning. Soon after the introduction of second-generation anticoagulants, the potential for secondary intoxication of raptor species such as owls and hawks was investigated and residues have been measured in a number of bird species (Thomas et al., 2011). Although anticoagulant intoxication has been documented in a number of individual birds, population impacts are less clear.

Anticoagulant rodenticides bind and inhibit vitamin K epoxide reductase and halt the recycling of vitamin K thereby affecting both intrinsic and extrinsic pathways of the coagulation system. Initial clinical signs are nonspecific, and coagulopathies develop as vitamin K–dependent clotting factors deplete. Observable clinical signs of poisoning are depression, mucous membrane pallor, increased capillary refill time and bleeding from superficial wounds. On postmortem, extensive subcutaneous, intramuscular, pulmonary, pericardial and intracoelomic hemorrhages, and pallor of internal organs are noted (Murray, 2011).

Diagnosis of intoxication is dependent on antemortem and/or postmortem evidence of a coagulopathy and the detection of an anticoagulant in blood, serum, or liver samples. Merely finding a residue of an anticoagulant in an animal is not sufficient for a diagnosis of intoxication because residues are often found in the absence of a coagulopathy.

Vitamin K_1 is antidotal treatment, although there is some delay before coagulopathy resolves. Dosing regimens have not been well defined in avian species, but vitamin K_1 at 2.5 mg/kg given subcutaneously every 12 h along with oxygen therapy has been found to be curative in a red-tailed hawk (Murray and Tseng, 2008). Once stabilized, vitamin K_1 given at similar doses once daily for 2 weeks or longer is indicated.

Avicides

A number of chemicals have been investigated for their ability to repel birds (Clark, 1998). Avicides are marketed primarily to control pest bird species such as blackbirds, pigeons, and grackles. Two commonly used avicides are 4-aminopyridine (4-AP, Avitrol) and 3-chloro-4-methylbenzenamine hydrochloride (Starlicide). 4-AP is designed to be placed on grain for baiting in such a way as to only affect a few individuals in a flock. The clinical signs exhibited by affected birds (distress cries and aerial distress displays) are such that unaffected birds are scared away. Repellants such as methyl anthranilate are generally not associated with lethal intoxication.

4-AP is rapidly absorbed from gastrointestinal tract and clinical signs develop within a short duration of

15–30 min. Frequent vocalization, incoordination, tremors and seizures are the common clinical signs reported in birds (Bischoff et al., 2001). There are no specific postmortem lesions associated with 4-AP poisoning.

Diagnosis is usually confirmed by the detection of 4-AP in the grain/bait, gastrointestinal contents, or liver.

METALS

Lead

Occurrences of lead exposure and intoxication in birds continue to be detected worldwide along with increasing awareness and regulation. Though wild raptors, waterfowl, and upland game birds are groups that have been subjected to lead intoxication, there are few reports of lead exposure in backyard chickens (Bautista et al., 2014; Trampel et al., 2003). Various species-specific and habitat-linked factors of lead exposure are unique to birds. Often, birds consume lead shot or other lead objects mistaken as seed or grit. The curious nature of pet birds leads them to ingest shiny objects easily. Temporal and spatial patterns of lead intoxication in California condors coinciding with anthropogenic activities such as big game hunting have been recorded (Cade, 2007).

Inorganic lead salts and organic forms are more bioavailable than elemental lead; however, the acidic environment in the proventriculus and ventriculus increases the solubility of elemental lead. Lead is actively transported across the GI tract through the same transport mechanism used for calcium absorption. Irrespective of its form, ingested lead is mostly excreted in the feces without being absorbed. Red blood cells contain a majority of the absorbed lead, with smaller amounts being bound to albumin or existing as free lead in plasma. Bone is a long-term storage depot for lead and bone remodeling can result in release of stored lead. In chickens, a significant amount of lead can result in eggs especially shells since divalent lead (Pb^{2+}) can alternate for calcium (Ca^{2+}) during shell formation.

Clinical signs consistent with lead intoxication are related to nervous, GI, hematopoietic, and renal systems. Signs of intoxication can also be nonspecific and limited to regurgitation, anorexia, weakness, and weight loss (Puschner and Poppenga, 2009). Lethargy, wing droop, leg paresis, changes in phonation, head tilt, ataxia, blindness, circling, head tremors, and seizures are notable signs related to nervous system dysfunction. GI signs include regurgitation and decreased motility of the upper GI tract (esophagus, proventriculus, and ventriculus) resulting in impaction and greenish diarrhea that stains feathers around the vent. Anemia as a result of increased erythrocyte fragility and decreased erythrocyte replacement is observed in affected birds. Whole blood lead concentration does not always correlate with the severity of clinical signs.

Emaciation, atrophy of breast muscles, hydropericardium, pale musculature or viscera consistent with anemia, renal or visceral gout, air sacculitis, and fat atrophy have been reported in various avian species. Bile stasis leading to an engorged gallbladder, dark-green viscous bile, bile-stained gastric and intestinal mucosa, and a greenish appearance to the liver have been reported in raptors (Locke and Thomas, 1996). Histologically, myelin degeneration of peripheral nerves, renal necrosis with or without intranuclear inclusion bodies, hemosiderosis in liver, lung, and kidneys, and patchy necrosis of gizzard muscles may be observed (Dvm et al., 2016; Locke and Thomas, 1996).

Measurement of whole blood lead concentration in live birds or in the liver and kidney of dead birds is employed for diagnosis and is widely available. A whole blood lead concentration of 0.20 ppm (20 μg/dL) or greater is considered to be consistent with lead exposure. Because lead associates with red blood cells, serum and plasma are not appropriate for testing. Generally, 4 ppm wet weight or greater lead concentration in the avian liver and kidney is likely to be significant.

Various chelation therapies are employed for the treatment of lead intoxication. Several chelators can effectively bind lead, including $CaNa_2EDTA$, succimer, D-penicillamine, and British anti-Lewisite (BAL). $CaNa_2EDTA$ and succimer are currently the chelators of choice, although no veterinary-approved forms are available. Symptomatic and supportive care including seizure control, fluid and electrolyte therapy for birds experiencing diarrhea, and vitamin supplementation may further aid in patient stabilization and therapy.

Zinc

Galvanized cage wires and accessories, pennies minted after 1982, and contaminated soil, water, and feed are some of the documented sources of zinc associated with avian toxicosis (Puschner and Poppenga, 2009). Zinc is absorbed in the proventriculus and small intestine. Postabsorption, zinc is distributed to pancreas, liver, kidneys, intestinal mucosa, and brain where it binds to metallothionein.

The toxic effects of zinc are observed on the GI tract, liver, kidneys, pancreas, red blood cells, and brain. High intracellular zinc concentrations lead to increased cellular reactive oxygen species production, reduced cellular ATP concentrations, and loss of mitochondrial membrane potential (Dineley et al., 2003).

Clinically affected birds may exhibit neurological signs such as intermittent head bobbing and ataxia. Other signs are lethargy, anorexia, polyuria, polydipsia, hematuria, regurgitation, pallor, dark or bright green diarrhea, paresis, seizures, and sudden death. In acute cases, corrosive lesions in the GI tract leading to associated disturbances, and injury to the liver, kidneys, and pancreas may be observed. In chronic cases, erythrocyte abnormalities and anemia may be commonly observed due to oxidative damage to the erythrocyte hemoglobin and cell membrane proteins (Luttgen et al., 1990). Common findings on gross examination of birds that have died from zinc toxicosis include greenish, mucoid feces in the ileum, colon, or cloaca and wasting of pectoral muscles. Microscopically, pancreas may reveal severe apoptosis, loss of acinar structure, necrosis of individual acinar cells, and interstitial fibrosis (Wight et al., 1986). Hemosiderosis in the liver, accompanied by hepatic biliary retention and multifocal, necrotizing hepatitis, may be observed. In GI, hemorrhagic enteritis, hemorrhagic ventriculitis, and ventricular koilin degeneration are noted (Puschner et al., 1999).

Diagnosis of zinc intoxication can be challenging. History of exposure (e.g., exposure to a new cage, feeding and/or watering utensils, or metallic toys), radiographic imaging, measurement of zinc in plasma/serum (live birds) and liver / kidney (dead birds) and histopathology can aid diagnosis. For most psittacines, a physiologic, nontoxic zinc concentration in serum or plasma is 2 ppm (0.2 mg/dL) or less. However physiologic concentrations are slightly higher of up to 3.5 ppm (0.35 mg/dL) for cockatoos and up to 2.5 ppm (0.25 mg/dL) for eclectus parrots (Puschner et al., 1999). Postmortem, liver zinc concentrations exceeding 100 ppm are toxic.

If a radio-dense zinc object is identified by radiography, removal of the zinc source results in the rapid decline of body concentrations. If immediate removal is not possible or delays are expected, reducing the further absorption of zinc in the GI tract may be achieved by administering antacids such as calcium carbonate (Van der Merwe and Tawde, 2009). Chelation of zinc is possible with $CaNa_2EDTA$, although its efficacy and safety in the treatment of zinc intoxication in birds have not been evaluated.

Mercury

Mercury exists in nature in different forms ranging from inorganic elemental forms to complex organic forms. One of the most toxic forms is methylercury (MeHg) which is the major source of intoxication in fish-eating birds such as loons, mergansers, and bald eagles. Consumption of MeHg-containing diets at environmentally realistic concentrations has been demonstrated to cause behavioral, neurological, hormonal, and reproductive changes in birds, fish, and mammals (Scheuhammer et al., 2007). MeHg is metabolized and excreted more slowly than other organomercurials. The lipophilic nature of MeHg allows it to penetrate the blood–brain barrier, where the majority of toxic effects are expressed. Selenium can modify the toxicity of MeHg by forming nontoxic mercury–selenium complexes, preventing the attachment of mercury with sulfhydryl groups of enzymes and other bioligands (Sugiura et al., 1976), when the average molar ratio Hg:Se is approximately 1.0–1.5 and total mercury concentrations exceeded about 50 μg/g as reported in eagles, loons and marine or freshwater fishes (Luten et al., 1980; Scheuhammer et al., 2008).

Clinical signs due to mercury intoxication are similar in multiple species of birds and are characterized by reduced food intake, emaciation, weakness in wings and legs, with difficulty flying, walking, and standing. Reproductively, MeHg exposure leads to shell-less eggs, decrease in mean egg weight, early embryonic mortality and an increase in unfertilized eggs. Most important pathological findings in birds are atrophy of fat deposits, muscles, demyelination and necrosis of nerves in the peripheral and central nervous system, and necrosis of renal tubular epithelium.

The diagnosis of mercury intoxication should not be based on tissue concentrations of mercury alone but necessarily address corresponding selenium concentrations, the presence or absence of compatible clinical signs and necropsy findings. There are no successful treatment approaches reported in birds to reverse damage due to mercury intoxication. Feeding uncontaminated food and water is the most practical approach. Selenium and vitamin E supplementation can additionally be utilized to reduce the toxic potential of mercury before the appearance of expected signs.

Iron

Increased hepatic iron storage or iron storage disease (ISD) is a serious condition noted in captive birds especially in some species belonging to families Paradiseadae (birds-of-paradise), Ramphastidae (toucans), and Sturnidae (starlings) (Pavone et al., 2014). Avian species that have been evolved to tolerate relatively low iron content in their diet have very efficient iron absorption and do not downregulate their iron absorption when body stores are saturated or on feeding of high-iron containing diets (Klasing et al., 2012). Many commercial diets intended for captive birds have been formulated using the nutritional requirements of poultry and are not optimal for the low-iron tolerating species. In addition, the use of animal byproducts significantly affects the nutritional interactions and bioavailability of iron. Absorption of iron from animal byproducts (heme-based iron sources) may be three times higher than that from nonheme products containing equivalent iron concentrations. Thus excessive dietary iron, nutritional interactions increasing the bioavailability and genetically or physiologically regulated increased iron uptake in sensitive species are all contributing factors to this condition (Cork, 2000; Sheppard, 2002). A diet containing 50–100 mg/kg iron on a dry matter basis has been recommended for sensitive avian species.

Increasing cellular iron concentrations leads to lysosomal injury and release of ionic iron, causing oxidative damage to membranes and proteins. Liver, heart, and spleen are most commonly affected. Clinically, dyspnea, abdominal distension, weight loss, and depression are major signs. Fibrotic changes in the liver affect its function, commonly leading to ascites, hypoalbuminemia, and icteric symptoms. The accumulation of hemosiderin in the lysosome of ISD-susceptible species is a common finding in birds (Cork, 2000; Klasing et al., 2012).

Diagnosis is by radiography (enlargement of liver, heart, and spleen), elevation in liver enzymes and transferrin concentrations. A liver biopsy might help in antemortem diagnosis. To treat the condition, chelation with deferiprone (75 mg/kg, PO, once daily for 90 days) (Sandmeier et al., 2012), CaEDTA and BAL have been utilized. Prophylactically, testing the iron content of the ingredients, choosing ingredients with low bioavailability of iron and feeding a low-iron diet with natural chelators such as tannins, phytates and fiber might be useful.

ENVIRONMENTAL TOXICANTS

Petroleum

Exposure of avian wildlife to crude oil is a significant cause of morbidity and mortality. Although oil spills involving large tanker accidents such as the grounding of the Exxon Valdez in Alaska or Deepwater Horizon received public attention, other scenarios related to oil drilling and production, off-loading of oil from tankers, production, processing, and refining of oil, road transport, and improper disposal of waste oil and petroleum products result in considerable wildlife exposure (Jessup and Leighton, 1996). Because oil floats on the surface of water, birds that live on water or dive through water for food are more likely to be exposed during spills. Marine birds and bird species that utilize environments near to shore are also likely to be exposed to oil if spills reach shorelines. Raptors such as peregrine falcons that feed on other birds can be exposed to oil from contaminated prey (Zuberogoitia et al., 2006).

Crude oil and petroleum products are complex mixtures of chemicals, including a variety of aromatic and aliphatic compounds. The toxicity of crude oils and petroleum products varies depending on their chemical compositions. Another complicating factor in assessing the toxicity of crude oil is the fact that soon after environmental release, the process of "weathering" occurs, which changes its chemical and physical properties.

Crude oil and other petroleum products affect birds in several ways. First, loss of insulating properties of the feathers results in rapid hypothermia. Oiled birds lose their ability to fly, and they frequently die from starvation, exhaustion, or drowning (Friend and Franson, 1999). Second, crude oil and other petroleum products are irritating to skin, mucous membranes, and the respiratory tract. Aspiration of oil into the respiratory tract and lungs can cause aspiration pneumonia. Third, systemic absorption of chemicals found in crude oil or petroleum products causes adverse effects on several organ systems, including reproductive, hematopoietic, nervous, immune, and hepatobiliary systems. Lastly, petroleum is extremely toxic to bird embryos. Exposed birds are often emaciated. On postmortem, presence of oil in the respiratory or GI tracts, intestinal congestion, and swelling of salt glands are noted sometimes (Friend and Franson, 1999).

Diagnosing petroleum intoxication as a cause of death can be challenging. There are no characteristic gross or histopathologic lesions specific to petroleum intoxication. A diagnosis is based on a history or evidence of exposure and compatible clinical and postmortem findings. Exposed birds, especially those with white or light-colored feathers, are easily identified because of the persistence of oil on feathers and skin. Feathers, skin, or organs of birds that do not have external evidence of exposure can be analyzed for the presence of chemicals typically found in crude oil or petroleum products (Jessup and Leighton, 1996).

Cyanide

Cyanide (hydrocyanic acid) poisoning often occurs following ingestion of a cyanide salt or inhalation of hydrogen cyanide gas. Avian wildlife intoxications have occurred following exposure to cyanide from gold or silver mining processes (Friend and Leighton, 1999). Birds are most often intoxicated by ingesting cyanide-contaminated water from tailings ponds. Most mortality events occur in the spring and fall as migratory birds pass through mining areas. Large-scale cyanide spills have caused widespread contamination of rivers in Europe and South America.

Cyanide is a rapidly acting cellular poison and it binds to ferric (Fe^{+3}) iron of mitochondrial cytochrome oxidase. This enzyme mediates the transfer of electrons to molecular oxygen, which is the last step in oxidative phosphorylation (Delaney, 2001). Cells are unable to use oxygen, resulting in tissue anoxia, increased anaerobic metabolism, and rapid development of lactic acidosis. The acute oral toxicity of sodium cyanide has been studied in several bird species. LD_{50}s ranged from 4.0 to 21 mg/kg BW (Wiemeyer et al., 1986).

Cyanide is a rapidly acting toxicant; most intoxicated birds are found dead. Grossly, dead animals often have bright red blood and multiorgan congestion (Woldemeskel and Styer, 2010).

A diagnosis is based on the history of exposure and measurement of cyanide in blood, heart, liver, or brain. Samples should be stored and shipped frozen to avoid the loss of cyanide before analysis. Denying birds access to cyanide-contaminated water is the best preventive approach.

TOXIC GASES

Ammonia

Exposure to toxic concentrations of ammonia mostly occur in chickens as a result of decomposition of poultry waste and poor ventilation in confined poultry houses (Brown et al., 1997). Ammonia readily dissolves in water to form ammonium hydroxide, which is an alkaline irritant. Thus, contact with the moist mucous membranes of the eyes and respiratory tract results in corneal and epithelial cell damage. High ambient air concentrations of ammonia (50–75 ppm) reduce feed consumption, growth rate, and egg production in poultry. Toxic air concentrations cause keratoconjunctivitis, corneal ulceration, blindness, photophobia, tracheitis, tachypnea, and dyspnea. Prolonged exposure can result in increased mucous secretion and hyperplasia of the bronchiolar and alveolar epithelium.

Maintenance of adequate ventilation and prompt removal of poultry waste alleviate problems associated with excessive ammonia. Ambient ammonia air concentrations should not be greater than 25 ppm for poultry (Brown and Julian, 2003).

Carbon Monoxide

Toxic exposure to carbon monoxide, CO (a product of incomplete combustion of hydrocarbon-based fuels) often results from use of defective gas catalytic or open-flame brooders, furnaces or internal combustion engines in poorly ventilated spaces, or confinement in an operating vehicle with poor ventilation. Of all the species, canaries are known to be susceptible to the toxic effects of CO. Harris hawks (*Buteo unicinctus*) are also very sensitive and many deaths have been reported following transport in enclosed pick-up trucks (Redig and Arent, 2008).

CO competes with oxygen to form carboxyhemoglobin which reduces the oxygen carrying ability of red blood cells, and the oxygen dissociation curve shifts to the left, resulting in tissue hypoxia. Affected birds exhibit drowsiness, labored breathing, weakness, and ataxia, with seizures occurring before death (Brown and Julian, 2003). Birds may be found dead when blood carboxyhemoglobin concentrations approach 60%–70% (Osweiler et al., 1985). Ambient CO concentrations of 600 ppm for 30 min cause clinical signs in chickens; concentrations of 2000 ppm or greater are lethal within 1.5–2 h (Brown and Julian, 2003).

Diagnosis of CO intoxication is based on a history compatible with CO production, compatible clinical signs, and measurement of ambient air CO and blood carboxyhemoglobin concentrations. Treatment is generally limited to provision of fresh air or oxygen; pet birds can be placed in oxygen cages.

Polytetrafluoroethylene: Teflon

Polytetrafluoroethylene (PTFE) is a synthetic polymer that is widely used as a nonstick surface in cookware and as a coating on heat lamp bulbs. Heated to high temperatures ($\geq$280°C), PTFE releases toxic pyrolysis products that can cause rapid death of birds. Although all birds are likely to be susceptible to intoxication, most spontaneous cases involve pet birds such as cockatiels, parrots, finches, and budgerigars. PTFE pyrolysis products contain toxic particulates of respirable size ($<$1 μm diameter) that can penetrate the alveoli. Lung damage is believed to be due to direct irritation and oxidative damage (Johnston et al., 1996; Wells et al., 1982). Although there is little comparative toxicity information among avian species, budgerigars were more sensitive than quail in one experimental study.

After exposure, the onset of clinical signs is rapid. Eyelid blinking is an early sign and may be related to a direct irritant effect on the conjunctiva and cornea. Eyelid movements could also be secondary to hypoxia-induced somnolence. Tachypnea, dyspnea, anxiety, cage wire biting, incoordination, and inability to perch or stand may be due to hypoxia secondary to lung damage. In many cases, the bird may be found dead with no other clinical signs noted. Grossly, the lungs are severely edematous, congested and hemorrhagic. Histologically, there is extensive, severe, necrotizing, and hemorrhagic pneumonitis. Amorphous, elongate particles may also be noted (Wells and Slocombe, 1982).

A diagnosis is generally based on a history of exposure and characteristic postmortem lesions. Currently, there is no analytical test available to confirm exposure to the pyrolysis products. The rapidity of onset of severe signs and subsequent death most often precludes treatment. Awareness of the hazard and avoiding housing birds near PTFE coatings is the best prevention.

CONCLUDING REMARKS AND FUTURE DIRECTIONS

Given the number and diversity of avian species and their environments and the diversity of chemicals to which they are exposed, assessing the impact of toxicants on individuals and populations is a daunting task. Toxicants can have direct toxic effects or, more subtly, indirect effects on the availability of important prey items. In addition, birds are commonly exposed to toxicants that accumulate in their prey (e.g., mercury and anticoagulant rodenticides). Although the diagnosis of acute intoxication is frequently straightforward, the challenge in avian toxicology is twofold. First, it is sometimes difficult to determine the sublethal impact of more chronic exposure to toxicants on bird health. For example, does exposure to methylmercury predispose susceptible birds to sublethal effects on reproduction or altered fledgling success? Second, although the impact of toxicant exposure on individuals might be easily determined, it is more difficult to assess whether individual effects translate into adverse effects on populations. There is no doubt that many raptor species are exposed to anticoagulant rodenticides. However, the population impacts of such exposures are largely unknown. Better defining the effects of chronic, low-level toxicant exposures and toxicant effects on the long-term stability of avian populations are future challenges.

REFERENCES

Anadón, A., Martinez-Larrañaga, M.R., Martínez, M.A., 2009. Use and abuse of pyrethrins and synthetic pyrethroids in veterinary medicine. Vet. J. 182 (1), 7–20.

Andreasen Jr., J.R., Schleifer, J.H., 1995. Salinomycin toxicosis in male breeder turkeys. Avian. Dis. 39 (3), 638–642.

Arai, M., Stauber, E., Shropshire, C.M., 1992. Evaluation of selected plants for their toxic effects in canaries. J. Am. Vet. Med. Assoc. 200 (9), 1329–1331.

Arnouts, S., Buyse, J., Cokelaere, M.M., et al., 1993. Jojoba meal (*Simmondsia chinensis*) in the diet of broiler breeder pullets: physiological and endocrinological effects. Poult. Sci. 72 (9), 1714–1721.

Bautista, A.C., Puschner, B.P., Poppenga, R.H., 2014. Lead exposure from backyard chicken eggs: a public health risk? J. Med. Toxicol. 10 (3), 311–315.

Berger, L.L., 1993. Salt and Trace Minerals for Livestock, Poultry and Other Animals. Salt Institute, Alexandria, VA, pp. 1–52.

Biernasiak, J., Piotrowska, M., Libudzisz, Z., 2006. Detoxification of mycotoxins by probiotic preparation for broiler chickens. Mycotoxin. Res. 22 (4), 230–235. Available from: http://dx.doi.org/10.1007/BF02946747.

Bischoff, K., Morgan, S., Chelsvig, J., et al., 2001. 4-aminopyridine poisoning of crows in the Chicago area. Vet. Hum. Toxicol. 43 (6), 350–352.

Brown, R.E., Brain, J.D., Wang, N., 1997. The avian respiratory system: a unique model for studies of respiratory toxicosis and for monitoring air quality. Environ. Health Perspect. 105 (2), 188–200.

Brown, T., Julian, R., 2003. Other toxins and poisons. In: Barnes, H.J., Saif, Y.M., Glisson, J.R. (Eds.), Diseases of Poultry, eleventh ed. Iowa State University Press, Ames, IA, pp. 1133–1159.

Brown, T.P., Rottinghaus, G.E., Williams, M.E., 1992. Fumonisin mycotoxicosis in broilers: performance and pathology. Avian Dis. 36 (2), 450–454.

Burns, R.J., Connolly, G.E., 1995. Assessment of potential toxicity of compound 1080 from livestock protection collars to canines and scavenging birds. Int. Biodeterior. Biodegrad. 36, 161–167.

Burrows, G.E., Tyrl, R.J., 2013. Toxic Plants of North America. second ed. Wiley-Blackwell, Singapore.

Cade, T., 2007. Exposure of California condors to lead from spent ammunition. J. Wildl. Manage. 71 (7), 2125–2133.

Carnaghan, A., 1961. The toxicity of certain groundnut meals for poultry with special reference to their effect on ducklings and chickens. Vet. Rec. 73, 1215–1219.

Clark, L., 1998. Review of bird repellants. Paper presented at the Proceedings of the 18th Vertebral Pesticides Conference, University of California, Davis, CA.

Cork, S.C., 2000. Iron storage diseases in birds. Avian Pathol. 29 (1), 7–12.

Cybulski, W., Radko, L., Rzeski, W., 2015. Cytotoxicity of monensin, narasin and salinomycin and their interaction with silybin in HepG2, LMH and L6 cell cultures. Toxicol. In Vitro. 29 (2), 337–344.

Dalvi, R.R., Nunn, V.A., Juskevich, J., 1987. Studies on comparative drug metabolism by hepatic cytochrome P-450-containing microsomal enzymes in quail, ducks, geese, chickens, turkeys and rats. Comp. Biochem. Physiol. C. 87 (2), 421–424.

Day, E.J., Dilworth, B.C., 1984. Toxicity of jimson weed seed and cocoa shell meal to broilers. Poult. Sci. 63 (3), 466–468.

Dedoussi, A., Roubies, N., Tserveni-Goussi, A., 2007. Monensin toxicity in ostriches on a farm in northern Greece. Vet. Rec. 161 (18), 628–629.

Delaney, K.A., 2001. Cyanide. In: Ford, M., Delaney, K.A., Ling, L.J. (Eds.), Clinical Toxicology. Saunders, Philadelphia, pp. 705–711.

Dineley, K.E., Votyakova, T.V., Reynolds, I.J., 2003. Zinc inhibition of cellular energy production: implications for mitochondria and neurodegeneration. J. Neurochem. 85 (3), 563–570.

Dodd, S.R., Haynie, R.S., Williams, S.M., et al., 2016. Alternate food-chain transfer of the toxin linked to avian vacuolar myelinopathy and implications for the endangered Florida snail kite (Rostrhamus Sociabilis). J. Wildl. Dis. 52 (2), 335–344.

Dorman, D., 2004. Bromethalin. In: Plumlee, K. (Ed.), Clinical Veterinary Toxicology. Mosby, St. Louis, MO, pp. 446–448.

Dvm, M.A., Oliveira, P.A., Brandao, R., et al., 2016. Lead Poisoning due to lead-pellet ingestion in griffon vultures (*Gyps fulvus*) from the Iberian peninsula. J. Avian Med. Surg. 30 (3), 274–279.

Eriksen, G.S., Pettersson, H., 2004. Toxicological evaluation of trichothecenes in animal feed. Anim. Feed Sci. Technol. 114, 205–239.

Fauquier, D.A., Flewelling, L.J., Maucher, J.M., et al., 2013. Brevetoxicosis in seabirds naturally exposed to *Karenia brevis* blooms along the central west coast of Florida. J. Wildl. Dis. 49 (2), 246–260.

Flory, W., Hebert, C.D., 1984. Determination of the oral toxicity of Sesbania drummondii seeds in chickens. Am. J. Vet. Res. 45 (5), 955–958.

Friend, M., Franson, J.C., 1999. Field Manual of Wildlife Diseases Biological Resources Division, USGS, Information and Technology Report 1999–2001. U.S. Government Printing Office, Washington, DC.

Girgis, G.N., Smith, T.K., 2010. Comparative aspects of F usarium mycotoxicoses in poultry fed diets containing naturally contaminated grains. World Poult. Sci. J. 66 (1), 665–686.

Gordus, A.G., Shivaprasad, H.L., Swift, P.K., 2002. Salt toxicosis in ruddy ducks that winter on an agricultural evaporation basin in California. J. Wildl. Dis. 38, 124–131.

Gross, W.B., Smith, L.D., 1971. Experimental botulism in gallinaceous birds. Avian Dis. 15 (4), 716–722.

Hallmann, C.A., Foppen, R.P., Van Turnhout, C.A., et al., 2014. Declines in insectivorous birds are associated with high neonicotinoid concentrations. Nature. 511 (7509), 341–343.

Harvey, R.B., Kubena, L.F., Huff, W.E., et al., 1991. Hematologic and immunologic toxicity of deoxynivalenol (DON)-contaminated diets to growing chickens. Bull. Environ. Contam. Toxicol. 46 (3), 410–416.

Heckel, J.O., Sisson, D.C., Quist, C.F., 1994. Apparent fatal snakebite in three hawks. J. Wildl. Dis. 30 (4), 616–619.

Henriksen, P., Carmichael, W.W., An, J., et al., 1997. Detection of an anatoxin-a(s)-like anticholinesterase in natural blooms and cultures of cyanobacteria/blue-green algae from Danish lakes and in the stomach contents of poisoned birds. Toxicon. 35 (6), 901–913.

Hill, E.F., 1988. Brain cholinesterase activity of apparently normal wild birds. J. Wildl. Dis. 24 (1), 51–61.

Huff, W.E., Kubena, L.F., Harvey, R.B., 1988. Progression of ochratoxicosis in broiler chickens. Poult Sci. 67 (8), 1139–1146.

Jensen, W.I., Allen, J.P., 1981. Naturally occurring and experimentally induced castor bean (*Ricinus communis*) poisoning in ducks. Avian Dis. 25 (1), 184–194.

Jessup, D.A., Leighton, F.A., 1996. Oil pollution and toxicity to wildlife. In: Fairbrother A, L.L., Hoff, G.L. (Eds.), Noninfectious Diseases of Wildlife, second ed. Iowa State University Press, Ames, IA.

Johnston, C.J., Finkelstein, J.N., Mercer, P., et al., 1996. Pulmonary effects induced by ultrafine PTFE particles. Toxicol. Appl. Pharmacol. 168, 208–215.

Klasing, K.C., Dierenfeld, E.S., Koutsos, E.A., 2012. Avian iron storage disease: variations on a common theme? J. Zoo Wildl. Med. 43 (Suppl. 3), S27–34.

Kubena, L.F., Harvey, R.B., Bailey, R.H., et al., 1998. Effects of a hydrated sodium calcium aluminosilicate (T-Bind) on mycotoxicosis in young broiler chickens. Poult Sci. 77 (10), 1502–1509.

Lawal, S., Abdu, P.A., Jonathan, G.B., et al., 1992. Snakebites in poultry. Vet. Hum. Toxicol. 34 (6), 528–530.

Li, Y., Wang, Z., Beier, R.C., et al., 2011. T-2 toxin, a trichothecene mycotoxin: review of toxicity, metabolism, and analytical methods. J. Agric. Food Chem. 59 (8), 3441–3453. Available from: http://dx.doi.org/10.1021/jf200767q.

Locke, L.N., Thomas, N.J., 1996. Lead poisoning of waterfowl and raptors. In: Fairbrother A, L.L., Hoff, G.L. (Eds.), Noninfectious Diseases of Wildlife. Iowa State University Press, Ames, IA, pp. 108–117.

Lozano, M.C., Diaz, G.J., 2006. Microsomal and cytosolic biotransformation of aflatoxin B1 in four poultry species. Br. Poult Sci. 47 (6), 734–741.

Luten, J.B., Ruiter, A., Ritskes, T.M., 1980. Mercury and selenium in marine and freshwater fish. J. Food Sci. 45 (3), 416–419.

Luttgen, P.J., Whitney, M.S., Wolf, A.M., et al., 1990. Heinz body hemolytic anemia associated with high plasma zinc concentration in a dog. J. Am. Vet. Med. Assoc. 197 (10), 1347–1350.

Matsunaga, H., Harada, K.I., Senma, M., et al., 1999. Possible cause of unnatural mass death of wild birds in a pond in Nishinomiya, Japan: sudden appearance of toxic cyanobacteria. Nat. Toxins. 7 (2), 81–84.

Metcalf, J.S., Banack, S.A., Kotut, K., et al., 2013. Amino acid neurotoxins in feathers of the Lesser Flamingo, Phoeniconaias minor. Chemosphere. 90 (2), 835–839.

Murphy, P.A., Hendrich, S., Landgren, C., et al., 2006. Food mycotoxins: an update. J. Food Sci. 71 (5), 51–65.

Murray, M., 2011. Anticoagulant rodenticide exposure and toxicosis in four species of birds of prey presented to a wildlife clinic in Massachusetts, 2006–2010. J. Zoo Wildl. Med. 42 (1), 88–97.

Murray, M., Tseng, F., 2008. Diagnosis and treatment of secondary anticoagulant rodenticide toxicosis in a red-tailed hawk (*Buteo jamaicensis*). J. Avian Med. Surg. 22 (1), 41–46.

Navarro, J.L., 1992. Capsaicin effects on consumption of food by cedar wax-wings and house finches. Wilson Bull. 104, 549–551.

Ohishi, I., Sakaguchi, G., Riemann, H., 1979. Antibodies to *Clostridium botulinum* toxins in free-living birds and mammals. J. Wildl. Dis. 15, 3–9.

Osweiler, G.D., Carson, T.L., Buck, W.B., 1985. Clinical and Diagnostic Veterinary Toxicology. third ed. Kendall-Hunt, Dubuque, IA.

Pan, H.P., Fouts, J.R., 1978. Drug metabolism in birds. Drug Metab. Rev. 7 (1), 1–253.

Parton, K.H., 2004. Sodium fluoroacetate. In: Plumlee, K. (Ed.), Clinical Veterinary Toxicology. Mosby, St. Louis, MO, pp. 451–454.

Pavone, S., Salamida, S., Pecorelli, I., et al., 2014. Deadly outbreak of iron storage disease (ISD) in Italian birds of the family Turdidae. J. Vet. Med. Sci. 76 (9), 1209–1212.

Peckham, J.C., Doupnik Jr., B., Jones Jr., O.H., 1971. Acute toxicity of ochratoxins A and B in chicks. Appl. Microbiol. 21 (3), 492–494.

Perelman, B.P.M., Smith, B., 1993. Effects of the accidental feeding of lasalocid sodium to broiler breeder chickens. Vet. Rec. 132 (11), 271–273.

Poppenga, R.H., Ziegler, A.F., Habecker, P.L., et al., 2005. Zinc phosphide intoxication of wild turkeys (*Meleagris gallopavo*). J. Wildl. Dis. 41 (1), 218–223. Available from: http://dx.doi.org/10.7589/0090-3558-41.1.218.

Puls, R., 1994. Mineral Levels in Animal Health. second ed. Sherpa International Clearbrook, BC, Canada.

Puschner, B.P., Poppenga, R.H., 2009. Lead and zinc intoxication in companion birds. Vet. Learn Compendium. Vet Learn, San Francisco, CA.

Puschner, B.P., St Leger, J., Galey, F.D., 1999. Normal and toxic zinc concentrations in serum/plasma and liver of psittacines with respect to genus differences. J. Vet. Diagn. Invest. 11 (6), 522–527.

Radko, L., Cybulski, W., Rzeski, W., 2013. The protective effect of silybin against lasalocid cytotoxic exposure on chicken and rat cell lines. Biomed. Res. Int. 2013, 783519.

Redig, P.T., Arent, L.R., 2008. Raptor toxicology. Vet. Clin. North Am. Exot. Anim. Pract. 11 (2), 261–282, vi. http://dx.doi.org/10.1016/j.cvex.2007.12.004.

Rotter, B.A., Prelusky, D.B., Pestka, J.J., 1996. Toxicology of deoxynivalenol (vomitoxin). J. Toxicol. Environ. Health. 48 (1), 1–34.

Sandmeier, P., Clauss, M., Donati, O.F., et al., 2012. Use of deferiprone for the treatment of hepatic iron storage disease in three hornbills. J. Am. Vet. Med. Assoc. 240 (1), 75–81.

Sarkar, K., Narbaitz, R., Pokrupa, R., et al., 1981. The ultrastructure of nephrocalcinosis induced in chicks by *Cestrum diurnum* leaves. Vet. Pathol. 18 (1), 62–70. Available from: http://dx.doi.org/10.1177/030098588101800107.

Schell, M.M., 2004a. 3-Chloro- p -toluidine hydrochloride. In: Plumlee, K. (Ed.), Clinical Veterinary Toxicology. Mosby, St. Louis, p. 443.

Schell, M.M., 2004b. 4-Aminopyridine. In: Plumlee, K. (Ed.), Clinical Veterinary Toxicology. Mosby, St. Louis, MO, pp. 443–444.

Scheuhammer, A.M., Meyer, M.W., Sandheinrich, M.B., et al., 2007. Effects of environmental methylmercury on the health of wild birds, mammals, and fish. Ambio. 36 (1), 12–18.

Scheuhammer, A.M., Basu, N., Burgess, N.M., et al., 2008. Relationships among mercury, selenium, and neurochemical parameters in common loons (*Gavia immer*) and bald eagles (*Haliaeetus leucocephalus*). Ecotoxicology. 17 (2), 93–101.

Sheppard, C.D.E., 2002. Iron storage disease in birds: speculation on etiology and implications for captive husbandry. J. Avian Med. Surg. 16 (3), 192–197.

Shropshire, C.M., Stauber, E., Arai, M., 1992. Evaluation of selected plants for acute toxicosis in budgerigars. J. Am. Vet. Med. Assoc. 200 (7), 936–939.

Sugiura, Y., Hojo, Y., Tamai, Y., et al., 1976. Letter: selenium protection against mercury toxicity. Binding of methylmercury by the selenohydryl-containing ligand. J. Am. Chem. Soc. 98 (8), 2339–2341.

Summers, L.D.G., 1995. Poultry Metabolic Disorders and Mycotoxins. University Books, Ontario, Canada.

Talcott, P.A., 2004a. Metaldehyde. In: Plumlee, K. (Ed.), Clinical Veterinary Toxicology. Mosby, St. Louis, MO, pp. 182–183.

Talcott, P.A., 2004b. Strychnine. In: Plumlee, K. (Ed.), Clinical Veterinary Toxicology. Mosby, Louis, MO, pp. 454–456.

Tedesco, D., Steidler, S., Galleti, S., et al., 2004. Efficacy of silymarin-phospholipid complex in reducing the toxicity of aflatoxin B1 in broiler chicks. Poult Sci. 83 (11), 1839–1843.

Thomas, P.J., Mineau, P., Shore, R.F., et al., 2011. Second generation anticoagulant rodenticides in predatory birds: Probabilistic characterisation of toxic liver concentrations and implications for predatory bird populations in Canada. Environ. Int. 37 (5), 914–920. Available from: http://dx.doi.org/10.1016/j.envint.2011.03.010.

Tiwary, A.K., Puschner, B.P., Charlton, B.R., et al., 2005. Diagnosis of zinc phosphide poisoning in chickens using a new analytical approach. Avian Dis. 49 (2), 288–291. Available from: http://dx.doi.org/10.1637/7275-090804R.

Tomizawa, M., Casida, J.E., 2011. Unique neonicotinoid binding conformations conferring selective receptor interactions. J. Agric. Food Chem. 59 (7), 2825–2828.

Trampel, D.W., Imerman, P.M., Carlson, T.L., et al., 2003. Lead contamination of chicken eggs and tissues from a small farm flock. J. Vet. Diagn. Invest. 15 (5), 418–422.

Van der Merwe, D., Tawde, S., 2009. Antacids in the initial management of metallic zinc ingestion in dogs. J. Vet. Pharmacol. Ther. 32 (2), 203–206.

Wages, D.P., Ficken, M.D., Cook, M.E., et al., 1995. Salt toxicosis in commercial turkeys. Avian Dis. 39 (1), 158–161.

Wells, R.E., Slocombe, R.F., 1982. Acute toxicosis of budgerigars (*Melopsittacus undulatus*) caused by pyrolysis products from heated polytetrafluoroethylene: microscopic study. Am. J. Vet. Res. 43 (7), 1243–1248.

Wells, R.E., Slocombe, R.F., Trapp, A.L., 1982. Acute toxicosis of budgerigars (*Melopsittacus undulatus*) caused by pyrolysis products from heated polytetrafluoroethylene: clinical study. Am. J. Vet. Res. 43 (7), 1238–1242.

Wiemeyer, S.N., Hill, E.F., Carpenter, J.W., et al., 1986. Acute oral toxicity of sodium cyanide in birds. J. Wildl. Dis. 22 (4), 538–546.

Wight, P.A., Dewar, W.A., Saunderson, C.L., 1986. Zinc toxicity in the fowl: ultrastructural pathology and relationship to selenium, lead and copper. Avian Pathol. 15 (1), 23–38.

Wilde, S.B., Murphy, T.M., Hope, C.P., et al., 2005. Avian vacuolar myelinopathy linked to exotic aquatic plants and a novel cyanobacterial species. Environ. Toxicol. 20 (3), 348–353.

Woldemeskel, M., Styer, E.L., 2010. Feeding behavior-related toxicity due to nandina domestica in cedar waxwings (*Bombycilla cedrorum*). Vet. Med. Int. 2010, 818159.

Wyatt, R.D., Hamilton, P.B., Burmeister, H.R., 1973. The effects of T-2 toxin in broiler chickens. Poult Sci. 52 (5), 1853–1859.

Zavala, G., Anderson, D.A., Davis, J.F., et al., 2011. Acute monensin toxicosis in broiler breeder chickens. Avian Dis. 55 (3), 516–521.

Zuberogoitia, I., Martinez, J.A., Iraeta, A., et al., 2006. Short-term effects of the prestige oil spill on the peregrine falcon (*Falco peregrinus*). Mar. Pollut Bull. 52 (10), 1176–1181.

Zwart, P., 1988. Poisoning caused by the pyrethroid compound deltamethrin in Gould's amadines (*Chloebia gouldiae*). Description of a case. Tijdschr. Diergeneeskd. 113 (18), 1009–1010.

Chapter 54

Aquatic Toxicology

Robert W. Coppock and P. Nick Nation

INTRODUCTION

This chapter focuses on aquatic toxicology of fish culture. Aquaculture is the production of aquatic animals in the aquatic environment for human food, replenishing fish stocks and other uses. The water may be a sheltered oceanic bay containing penned organisms, inland ponds or an indoor tank system. The more contained the aquatic rearing system, the more diligent must be monitoring and controls over the artificial ecosystem. The smaller the volume of water and the more contained the system is, the more susceptible it is to water safety issues. Issues in water safety can contribute to outbreaks of infectious diseases. The hobbyist also raises or maintains fish and other aquatic animals/plants in a variety of integrated ecosystems. Fish are also used as public displays by commercial organizations.

Chemical and physical causes of disease in aquatic organisms are generally linked to water and food because these are the primary pathways of toxic substances to animals in the aquatic environment. Noise pollution is being shown to be an important physical agent (NAS, 2016). Intoxication of fish can be acute, subacute, or chronic. Chemical-linked food safety issues can occur if chemical contamination of edible aquatic organisms occurs. The toxicity of a specific substance can vary between fish species and can change with water temperature, pH, and ion composition (Wlasow et al., 2010). In recirculation systems, waste materials and microbial degradation products can reach toxic levels. Chemical intoxication and other environmental stressors can increase the susceptibility of aquatic organisms to infectious diseases (Morley, 2010). The predisposing causes of infectious disease and larval survival can be overlooked because they may be subtle or unrecognized. The toxicology of the water column differs from that of the sediment, and these variations in the aquatic environment present different issues to various segments of the aquaculture industry (Rudolph et al., 2009).

BACKGROUND

Fish are cultured in some form of confinement such as a pen, pond, or tank. Cultured fish are usually dependent on humans for part or all of their feed and can be entirely dependent on humans for maintenance of their ecosystem. Inland aquaculture often requires at least some amount of mechanical-hydrological management to maintain the aquatic environment. Large capital investment and high operational costs are incentives to maximize stocking densities in aquaculture systems. Increased stocking densities increase sophistication and attention to details required for water management.

WATER SAFETY

Water safety is essential for maintaining healthy life. Upstream users and incidents can contaminate the water source for aquaculture. Rainstorm events creating excessive surface runoff, and fires and chemical spills can contaminate water sources. Unsafe water kills more fish in tanks and ponds than all other causes of mortality. The biology of fish can directly affect safety of the water in which they live, and their metabolic activity interacting with other aquatic biota can move water parameters from safe to unsafe. This is particularly true in recirculating systems and at high stocking densities. Sensitivity to water parameters in aquaculture varies with age of the fish and stage of development (Finn, 2007). Water parameters are interactive and dynamic, and changing one parameter always affects other factors. For example, the pH of water is important in affecting the solubility of metals (Finn, 2007). Increasing the pH generally decreases the bioavailability of metals by increasing complexes with organic matter in the water. Temperature of the water is important, and the ideal temperature can vary with life stage and genera.

Veterinary Toxicology. DOI: http://dx.doi.org/10.1016/B978-0-12-811410-0.00054-4

Nitrogen Cycle

The nitrogen cycle in aquatic systems is critically important especially in closed systems. The nitrogen cycle in an aquatic system is primarily regulated by biota. An excellent review on the geobiochemistry of the nitrogen cycle has been written (Hargreaves, 1998). The nitrogen cycle transforms organic nitrogen, ammonia, and other forms of nitrogen to nitrogen gas (N_2). The most common ionic forms of nitrogen are ammonium (NH_4^+), nitrite (NO_2^-), and nitrate (NO_3^-) (Camargo et al., 2005). Sources of these ions are atmospheric deposition, presence in surface and groundwater, nitrogen fixation, and degradation of organic matter and agricultural fertilizers. An important reactive gaseous form of nitrogen is ammonia (HN_3). Important sources of reactive nitrogen in the aquatic system are feedstuff residues, fish feces, and nitrogen compounds excreted from other aquatic animals or present in runoff and intake waters. The organisms regulating the different steps in the aquatic nitrogen cycle are remarkably independent, and products from different steps can accumulate in the system. Species of *Nitrosomonas* and *Nitrobacter* oxidize ammonia to NO_2^-. Following this, oxidation of NO_2^- to NO_3^- occurs, and species of *Nitrobacter* are the primary organisms that accomplish this. Species of *Nitrosomonas* and *Nitrobacter* are dissimilarly affected by oxygen tension, pH, temperature, etc. Species of *Nitrobacter* are the most sensitive, and when they are disadvantaged, the level of NO_2^- increases. The end step in the nitrogen cycle is reduction, with production and release of N_2 into the atmosphere. The most toxic compounds in the aquatic nitrogen cycle are NH_3 and NO_2^-. Changes in the nitrogen cycle can also be seasonal and/or related to weather conditions or changes in the indoor controlled environment. For example, NO_2^- poisoning (brown blood disease) in the southern United States is more common in the fall and spring (Durborow et al., 1997). When the concentration is less than 1 μmol NO_3^-, the water is generally considered unpolluted (Jensen, 2003).

Ammonia

Recirculation systems, for economic reasons, can have densities as high as 0.3 kg of fish/kg of water that can result in high NH_3 loads. Ammonia is very toxic to fish. Total NH_3-nitrogen requires monitoring because NH_3 is the primary and most toxic nitrogen waste excreted by freshwater fish. The best predictor of water safety is total NH_3-nitrogen (TA-N), which is the sum of $NH_3 + NH_4^+$ forms. Ammonium ion has a low order of toxicity. Estimated NH_3 production by fish is 0.02 kg of NH_3-nitrogen produced for each kilogram of feed fed and the nitrogen is excreted within 24 h (Masser et al., 1999; Ip and Chew, 2010). Ammonia gas can radially diffuse across cell membranes. The toxicity of NH_3 in water is dependent on water pH, temperature, and the species of aquatic animal. The p*K* of ammonia is approximately 9.2 and at a pH of 9.2, NH_3 is in equilibrium with $NH_4^+ + OH^-$. Lowering pH below the p*K* increases the concentration of ionized NH_4^+. Most of the NH_3 in fish blood exists as $NH_4{}^+$ ion because the pH of blood is approximately 2 pH units below the p*K* of ammonia. Most fish species excrete excess nitrogen from deaminization of amino acids as NH_3 instead of uric acid (Wilkie, 2002; Bucking, 2017). The gill excretion of NH_3 (80%–90%) occurs by simple diffusion down a concentration gradient from the fish to the ambient water. Fish have mechanisms to acidify (excretion of H^+) the boundary layer on the apical surface of the gill to favor both the formation of $NH_4{}^+$ and maintain a high diffusion gradient for NH_3 (Bucking, 2017). Increasing pH of the ambient water decreases excretion of NH_3 as does increasing the concentration of NH_3 and a reversed inward flux of NH_3 can occur. Ammonium ions can be transported in the potassium ion (K^+)/sodium ion (Na^+) by the substitution of NH_4^+ for K^+ in the Na^+/K^+ exchange mechanism to give Na^+ in/NH_4^+ out exchange occurring in the basolateral region of the brachial epithelium. The activity of Na^+/K^+-ATPase is upregulated when NH_3 is high in ambient water along with the expression for cortisol receptors (Sinha et al., 2012). Increased NH_3 in fish increases glycolysis in cytosol and decreases the TCA cycle in the mitochondria and the brain is sensitive to these effects. The NH_4^+ ion at high endogenous concentrations can substitute for K^+ in ion transporters and disrupt electrochemical physiology. Physical activity, feeding, and stress-linked increase in cortisol levels increase blood NH_3 by amino acid catabolism (Randall and Tsui, 2002). Increased blood NH_3 reduces physical activity. There appears to be metabolic dysfunction in the liver and links to disruption of neurotransmitters and electrochemistry in skeletal muscle (Randall and Tsui, 2002). Increasing water NH_3 decreases swimming ability (Wicks et al., 2002). The decrease in swimming ability is linked to depolarization of white muscles, and increasing water calcium ions (Ca^{2+}) ameliorated NH_3 toxicity. Feeding fish appears to provide some protection from toxicity by ambient NH_3 likely by decreasing gluconeogenesis (Wicks and Randall, 2002). Immune suppression can occur. Daoust and Ferguson (1984) used ambient conditions of pH 7.93 and NH_3 concentrations of 0.0, 0.215, and 0.423 ppm, respectively, for 90 days to study the toxicity of NH_3 in rainbow trout (*Oncorhynchus mykiss*) fingerlings. Signs of central nervous system disfunction were observed, no histopathology was observed in the gills and the occurrences of acidophilic droplets in epithelial cells of renal proximal convoluted tubules were increased in fish exposed to NH_3.

Benli et al. (2008) exposed Nile tilapia (*Oreochromis niloticus*) to 0.0, 1.0, 2.0, 5.0 and 10.0 mg TA-N/1 of ambient water for 6 weeks. Fish exposed to elevated TA-N had a dose response increase in severity of histopathologic lesions in the gills consisting of hyperemia, chloride cell proliferation, fusion of the secondary lamellae, and telangiectasis. Cloudy swelling and hydropic degeneration were observed in the liver, and hyperemia and glomerulonephritis were observed in the kidney. Skin lesions were not observed. Elevated TA-N reduces growth in fish. Thyroid dysfunction has been observed in fish exposed to high ambient concentrations of NH_3, and reduced expression of thyroid hormone receptor β and insulin-like growth factor 1 (Sinha et al., 2012; Nugegoda and Kibria, 2016).

Nitrite (NO_2^-)

Ammonium is oxidized to nitrate in a two-step process (from NH_4^+ to NO_2^- to NO_3^-) by aerobic bacteria. Aquatic animals, especially freshwater fish and crustacea, are more at risk for NO_2^- poisoning than are terrestrial organisms (Camargo et al., 2005). Nitrite intoxication of aquatic animals occurs when conditions exist for imbalance in the nitrogen cycle. Freshwater fish are more susceptible to NO_2^- than are saltwater fish. In freshwater fish, NO_2^- is rapidly absorbed across the gills. The generally accepted mechanism for NO_2^- absorption is by competing for chloride ion (Cl^-) uptake across the gills. Chloride ion is exchanged for bicarbonate (HCO_3^-), and this exchange occurs in the apical part of the gill epithelial cell. Nitrite has affinity for the Cl^-/HCO_3^- exchange protein and replaces Cl^- in the exchange process. Increasing the water concentration of Cl^- reduces the toxicity of NO_2^-. Fish with high Cl^- uptake, such as rainbow trout, perch (family Percidae), and northern pike (*Esox lucius*), are more susceptible to NO_2^-. Millimolar NO_2^- levels in such fish, especially if Cl^- in the water is low, can result from micromolar levels of NO_2^- exposure from water. Nitrite causes a net loss of Cl^- because there is a reduction in the influx of Cl^-, and it stimulates a net loss of K^+ from muscle, causing an extracellular hyperkalemia and increased excretion of K^+. Nitrite also enters red blood cells and oxidizes Fe^{+2} (ferrous) in hemoglobin (Hb) to Fe^{+3} (ferric), forming methemoglobin (metHb) (Grabda et al., 1974). The blood becomes discolored brown, a characteristic diagnostic feature of methemoglobinemia. The oxidation of Fe^{+2} to Fe^{+3} changes oxygen affinity of Hb and oxygen tensions in blood drop toward dissolved oxygen in ambient water. Changes in oxygen affinity and blood pH increase movement of oxygen to the swim bladder, thus affecting buoyancy. In teleost (bony) fish, there is NO_2^--mediated disruption of the Na^+/H^+ exchange mechanism in the red blood cell, which further decreases the affinity of Hb for oxygen. Decreased oxygen tensions increase anaerobic metabolism and acidosis occurs. Exposure of rainbow trout to 1 mmol NO_2^- causes vasodilation and an increased cardiac workload (Aggergaard and Jensen, 2001; Jensen and Agnisola, 2005). The fish died when the metHg was greater than 70%. Plasma NO_2^- level was 2.9 mmol at the time of death. Liver cell damage linked to mitochondrial pathology occurs, and hepatic stores of glycogen are depleted. Necrosis of the retina can occur. Under in vitro conditions, hepatocytes from rainbow trout detoxify NO_2^- by converting NO_2^- to considerably less toxic NO_3^- (Doblander and Lackner, 1996; Jensen and Hansen, 2011). Recovery from nitrite poisoning appears to take several weeks, and compensatory weight gain may or may not occur. There is a spectrum of species susceptibility to NO_2^-, which is linked to Cl^- uptake by the gills (Durborow et al., 1997; Jensen, 2003). Largemouth (*Micropterus salmoides*) and smallmouth bass (*Micropterus dolomieu*), bluegill (*Lepomis macrochirus*), and green sunfish (*Lepomis cyanellus*) are relatively resistant to high concentrations of NO_2^-. Catfish (order Siluriformes), goldfish (*Carassius auratus*), fathead minnows (*Pimephales promelas*), and tilapia (genus *Tilapia*) are sensitive to NO_2^-, and cold-water fish such as rainbow trout are highly sensitive to NO_2^-. Nitrite poisoning can be prevented by adding Cl^- to the water (Durborow et al., 1997). The most common option is to add Cl^- to the water to achieve a 10:1 ratio of Cl^- to NO_2^-. Decreased feeding rates and increased throughput of nonrecycled water are alternative methods of controlling NO_2^-. Bacterial and parasitic disease increases the sensitivity of fish to NO_2^- poisoning. The presence of concurrent infectious disease requires increasing the concentration of ambient Cl^-. Catfish producers commonly maintain 100 ppm Cl^- in the pond or tank water as insurance against an increase in NO_2^- levels or to counteract the effects of concurrent infectious disease. Dietary vitamin E may also be protective against nitrite poisoning.

Nitrate (NO_3^-)

Fish, comparing NH_3 and NO_2^-, are relatively resistant to NO_3^- intoxication. Nitrate accumulation can be >100 mg NO_3^-/L of water. Nitrate poisoning is commonly associated with accidental increases caused by nitrate rich runoff water contaminating water sources. Larval forms of fish generally are the most sensitive life stages. Chronic NO_3^- poisoning in rainbow trout was studied using 26.2 ppm NO_3^- and a static tank system (Grabda et al., 1974). Fish were observed to gather around the aeration system. Liver pathology consisting of degenerative changes and necrosis was observed, and degenerative changes were observed in the hemopoietic centers.

Chlorine

Water is not considered safe for fish if a measurable level of chlorine (Cl_2) is present, not to be confused with chloride ions (Cl^-). Morbidity can occur at 0.02 ppm Cl_2 and mortality at 0.04 ppm and tap water can contain 2 ppm Cl_2 (Hadfield et al., 2007). Chlorine, chloramines, and other chlorine compounds are used as disinfection agents in municipal water and in aquaculture to disinfect ponds and tanks. Chlorine gas added to water forms several compounds (hypochlorous acid, hydrochloric acid, and hypochlorite), with the concentration of dissociated ions depending on the pH of the water. Chloramines are also formed by the reaction of Cl_2 with NH_3 in water. Chlorine dioxide is used as a water disinfection agent and is reduced to chlorite. Chlorine dioxide is approximately 16 times more toxic to fish than is chlorite. For rainbow trout, safe levels for chlorine dioxide appear to be approximately 0.2 ppm and approximately 3 ppm for chlorite. The toxicity of Cl_2 residues is variable with temperature changes. Residual Cl_2 in the water is generally oxidative and causes irritation and damage to the gills. The acute gill lesion is necrosis of gill epithelium occurring at higher Cl_2 concentrations, whereas the subacute and chronic lesions are gill epithelial hypertrophy and hyperplasia. Gill lesions not only cause hypoxia but also affect the acid–base homeostasis of fish. In this regard, gill damage in fish is akin to a mammal suffering nephritis with concurrent pneumonia

METALS

There are numerous metals that can find their way into aquatic systems. Contaminated surface water can be a serious threat. Water conducting systems and aquaculture equipment can also be a source of metals. Some plastics also contain metals and should not use in aquatic systems.

Copper

Copper (Cu) is an essential trace nutrient for fish. There are many sources of copper ions in aquaculture systems. Runoff water from lands receiving swine and poultry manure containing Cu from dietary copper sulfate can be an important source. Copper compounds are commonly used in aquaculture as algaecides and as treatments for parasites and copper piping may be used in closed systems. In freshwater aquatic systems, Cu exists in complexes with organic matter, other chemicals and is weakly associated with water molecules (USEPA, 2007). These factors can affect the bioavailability of Cu in ambient water. USEPA uses the biotic ligand model (BLM) to assess Cu toxicity. The model assumes that free Cu and copper monohydroxide bind to a biotic ligand on the organism's surface. Death occurs when a critical amount of the total biotic ligand sites are attached to copper. Multiple studies demonstrate that gill rapidly accumulates Cu following the onset of waterborne exposure, and the accumulation of Cu results in the disturbance of multiple physiological processes. The USEPA BLM model does not consider differences in sensitivity due to size of the fish and ambient water altering the physiology of the fish (de Polo and Scrimshaw, 2012).

The uptake of copper ions across the gill of fish is dependent on many parameters, including levels of Ca^{2+} and magnesium ions (Mg^{2+}) in the water. There is generally a small margin of safety for many aquatic species for copper ions. Cupric ions (Cu^{2+}) disrupt the ATP-dependent sodium/potassium pump located in the gill chloride cells. This allows increased efflux of Na^+. Cupric ions also replace Ca^{2+} at the tight junctions, resulting in an efflux of Na^+. The net loss of Na^+ results in disruption of osmoregulation and cardiovascular collapse. Copper ions are neurotoxic in fish, disrupting the olfactory and mechanosensory-neuromast systems (Linbo et al., 2006; Sommers et al., 2016). Peripheral olfactory function is inhibited at levels as low as 5 μg copper/L ambient water, and loss of neuromast sensory cells occurs at concentrations greater than 20 μg/L. Exposure to copper ions also decreases immune function. Copper levels can be difficult to interpret because pH, carbonate ions, and dissolved organic carbon are interactive in forming unavailable forms of copper, and Mg^{2+} and Ca^{2+}compete for copper uptake by the fish. Changes in these parameters can cause a 60-fold difference in the lethal toxicity of Cu. Decreasing water pH increases the toxicity, and 100 times increase in toxicity can occur with each unit decrease in pH. Warm-water fish are more tolerant of copper than are cold-water fish.

Methylmercury

Methylmercury (meHg) is a concern with human foods from aquatic sources. The primary source of meHg in aquaculture is the use of fish byproducts in feedstuffs. Methylmercury is also formed by biota in the benthic region of the aquatic system, and it is biomagnified in the food web. In fish, meHg is bioaccumulated in skeletal muscle (80% of body burden in *Salmo salar*) (Berntssen et al., 2004). Approximately 23% of the dietary meHg and approximately 6% of dietary inorganic mercury are absorbed by fish. Fish fed diets containing 5 and 10 ppm meHg for 4 months had 1.1 and 3.1 ppm of meHg in muscle (freeze-dried), respectively. The threshold toxic level for Atlantic salmon is estimated at 0.5 ppm meHg in diet.

The threshold level of dietary meHg on spawning parameters in fathead minnows is <0.88 ppm.

MYCOTOXINS

Important genera of fungi that produce mycotoxins are *Fusarium*, *Aspergillus*, and *Penicillium* (Coppock and Jacobsen, 2009). These fungi, depending on growing conditions, can be field and/or storage fungi and produce mycotoxins. Important growing conditions for mycotoxigenic fungi are temperature and moisture. A common source of mycotoxins in fish feed is the use of grain screenings as a feed ingredient. Important mycotoxins identified in aquaculture are fumonisins (FBs), moniliformin (MON), ochratoxin A (OTA), trichothecenes, zearalenone (ZEA), and aflatoxins (AFs) (Greco et al., 2015). If one mycotoxin is identified in a feed, it is most likely that other mycotoxins are present. There are species differences between fish genera and species, and age in susceptibility to mycotoxins. To some mycotoxins, e.g., AFs, rainbow trout are uniquely sensitive.

Fumonisins and Moniliformin

Fish consuming contaminated feeds are exposed to FBs and MON (Coppock and Nation, 2012). Of the FBs, FB_1 is the most toxic. Fumonisins are structurally like sphingosine, and inhibit ceramide synthase, an enzyme in the sphingolipid synthesis pathway. The effects of FB_1 on sphinganine–sphingosine metabolism is an elevated hepatic sphinganine/ sphingosine ratio and this can occur at dietary levels of 150 mg of FB_1/kg of feed. Fish fed diets containing 20, 80, 320, or 720 mg of FB_1/kg of feed for 2 years had dose response histopathologic changes in the liver. In all fish on the FB_1 diets the lesions were swollen hepatocytes with centrally located nuclei and foci of hepatocytes containing clear cytoplasm (likely contained lipids), hepatocellular necrosis and shrunken hepatocytes, (80 mg group). The hepatocytes with clear cytoplasm were near the central vein in the 20 mg/kg group and focally dispersed in the other treatment groups.

Moniliformin inhibits pyruvate dehydrogenase in the mitochondrial respiratory chain enzymes. Nile tilapia (*O. niloticus*), using weight gains and histopathology parameters, generally are more resistant to FB_1 than catfish. Diets containing 20 mg FB_1 or MON/kg of feed fed for 2 weeks can depress growth in tilapia and catfish. MON has been reported to cause cardiac myopathy in other species studied (mammals and birds), but this does not appear to have been reported for fish species. Catfish fed 120 mg MON/kg of feed for 10 weeks had small nucula in liver cells. FB_1 is immunosuppressive in fish.

Ochratoxins

OTA is nephrotoxic and immunotoxic in mammalian and avian species. OTA decreases weight gains and feed conversion in catfish when fed at 3 ppm OTA/kg of feed for 8 weeks. A dose response was observed in histopathology in the posterior kidney and liver. The lesions were enlarged melanomacrophage centers replacing kidney and pancreatic cells. The no effect dose for OTA in diet is likely less than 1.0 mg OTA/kg of diet (See Chapter 72: Ochratoxins and Citrinin).

Trichothecenes

The trichothecene group of mycotoxins is radiomimetic in toxicity and target rapidly dividing cells and cells with high metabolic activity (Coppock and Jacobsen, 2009). The trichothecenes are also potent inhibitors of protein synthesis. All the trichothecenes studied are immunotoxic. A common observation is reduced feed intake and feed refusal. The most common trichothecene identified in fish feeds is deoxynivalenol (DON). Rainbow trout are sensitive to DON when fed at 2.0 ppm DON/kg of feed for 8 weeks. DON is immunosuppressive in fish and decreases native resistance to disease and growth. Toxicopathy of DON is subcapsular edema of the liver, fatty infiltration of hepatocytes and hyaline droplet degeneration of tubular epithelial cells of the caudal kidney. Feeding a diet containing 2 mg DON/kg of feed for 23 days induced oxidative stress in rainbow trout. T-2 toxin is a potent trichothecene mycotoxin and younger fish are at a greater risk for intoxication. Feeding diets containing 1.5–5.0 T-2 toxin/kg of feed decreases growth, feed conversion, and diets with >6.1 mg of T-2 toxin/fish (20-month-old) causes sloughing of the intestinal mucosa as casts without mortality. The hemopoietic system is a target for T-2 toxin and effects can be observed at dietary levels of 1.2 mg T-2 toxin/kg of feed. T-2 toxin, in carp, causes anemia and leukopenia, primarily a lymphopenia, at dietary levels of 5.3 mg T-2 toxin/kg of feed fed for 4 weeks. Diet containing 0.625 mg of T-2 toxin/kg of feed fed for 8 weeks cause reduction in growth. T-2 toxin-linked histopathology is stomach lesions consisting of multifocal lymphocytic infiltrates in the lamina propria and disruption of normal submucosal glandular architecture with glandular loss. In the head kidney, hemopoietic areas have decreased erythrocytic and myelocytic precursors. Macrophage aggregates are increased in head kidney.

Zearalenone

Zearalenone, a resorcylic acid lactone, is associated with DON contamination of cereal grains (Coppock and

Jacobsen, 2009). ZEA, an estrogen mimic, is also present in runoff waters from wheat and maize fields. The effect of ZEA in fish can be contradictory depending on species, life stage, dose and duration of exposure. Decreased spawning frequency and increased plasma vitellogenin is observed in zebra fish. ZEA alters iron metabolism and clotting time in rainbow trout. ZEA alters in vitro immune functions of leukocytes harvested from the head and trunk kidney of fish fed low dietary levels (332 μg/kg of feed) by upregulation and downregulates these functions at higher doses (≥0.621 μg/kg of feed). Oxygen consumption is increased in carp exposed to dietary levels (≥0.621 μg/kg of feed for 4 weeks).

Aflatoxins

Fish feeds can be contaminated with AFs. (see Chapter 69: Aflatoxins). AFB_1 is activated by the CYP enzymes in fish and important detoxification pathways in fish are the uridine diphosphate glucuronyltransferase and, to a lesser extent, glutathione S-transferase pathway. Rainbow trout are one of the most sensitive species to the carcinogenic effects of aflatoxins and carp are a relatively resistant species. Aflatoxins also cause hepatocellular necrosis and fibrosis. Differences in biotransformation of AFs likely explain the differences in species sensitivity. AFs are rapidly excreted and are not known to be biomagnified in edible fish tissues. Aflatoxicol and AFM_1 are the primary metabolites of fish that are excreted into water. Dietary ascorbic acid is protective against AFs. Aflatoxins target both the innate and adaptive immune functions. There is some evidence that immune memory is decreased by exposure to AFs. Hematocrit may be reduced in fish exposed to dietary AFs and hepatic enzymes in serum are also increased.

CONTAMINANTS IN AQUACULTURE FISH

Aquaculture animals are an important dietary source of environmentally persistent organic chemicals. These persistent chemicals are biomagnified in fish and animals consuming these products. including offal incorporated into pet foods. These compounds are also transferred to the human fetus during pregnancy and excreted in breast milk during lactation. The most sensitive life stage, including humans, for adverse effects is the prenatal and early postnatal period. Endocrine disruption and epigenetic effects have been observed depending of the specific chemical and animal species. Dietary animal protein, fat, and clays are the predominant source of POCs for cultured fish.

ACOUSTIC POLLUTION AND FISH

Sound propagation in water is strongly affected by temperature, pressure, and to a lesser extent, by salinity (NOAA, 2000). Low frequency sound can be propagated long distances in water. Fish use sound sensors for many interactions with their ambient environment and interactions with each other (NAS, 2016). Pressure sensors are also important for locomotion in the aquatic environment. Noise pollution can mask or shift hearing thresholds, damage auditory organs and cause adverse stress responses (Peng et al., 2015). Exposure of fish to noise during embryo and larval stages can cause decreased survival (Brown et al., 2016). Reduction in ability to monitor the aquatic environment is a plausible explanation.

CONCLUDING REMARKS AND FUTURE DIRECTIONS

Fish are being concentrated for aquaculture, breeding, display, and similar human-directed activities. The culture of an increasingly wide range of aquatic organisms for food is accelerating worldwide. Fish offal and oil are an important raw material for animal feeds and can be source-persistent organic chemicals that are bioconcentrated in body fat. Increasing artificiality of the aquatic environment also increases the monitoring required to maintain water safety. The safety of input water and feeds is important in maintaining the health of aquatic organisms being cultured and the safety of foods and byproducts being produced. Multiple competing uses of water resources provide an ongoing challenge to aquaculture. Securing rights for incoming water supplies is becoming increasingly competitive as are increasing requirements to return the outflow water to the environment in acceptable condition. Food and feed safety are increasing issues that requires cooperation among all the industries involved with aquaculture. An additional future research need is for rapid and accurate diagnostics in diseases caused by chemical and physical agents.

REFERENCES

Aggergaard, S., Jensen, F.B., 2001. Cardiovascular changes and physiological response during nitrite exposure in rainbow trout. J. Fish Biol. 59, 13–27.

Benli, A.C., Koksal, G., Ozkul, A., 2008. Sublethal ammonia exposure of Nile tilapia (*Oreochromis niloticus* L.): effects on gill, liver and kidney histology. Chemosphere. 72, 1355–1358.

Berntssen, M.H.G., Hylland, K., Julshamn, K., et al., 2004. Maximum limits of organic and inorganic mercury in fish feed. Aquacul. Nutr. 10, 83–97.

Brown, A.D., Sisneros, J.A., Jurasin, T., et al., 2016. Effects of hatchery rearing on the structure and function of salmonid mechanosensory systems. Adv. Exp. Med. Biol. 875, 117–124.

Bucking, C., 2017. A broader look at ammonia production, excretion, and transport in fish: a review of impacts of feeding and the environment. J. Comp. Physiol. B. 187, 1–18.

Camargo, J.A., Alonso, A., Salamanca, A., 2005. Nitrate toxicity to aquatic animals: a review with new data for freshwater invertebrates. Chemosphere. 58, 1255–1267.

Coppock, R.W., Jacobsen, B.J., 2009. Mycotoxins in animal and human patients. Toxicol. Ind. Health. 25, 637–655.

Coppock, R.W., Nation, P.N., 2012. Aquatic Toxicology. In: Gupta, R. C. (Ed.), Veterinary Toxicology Basic and Clinical Principles, second ed. Elsevier, Toronto.

Daoust, P.Y., Ferguson, H.W., 1984. The pathology of chronic ammonia toxicity in rainbow trout, *Salmo gairdneri* Richardson. J. Fish Dis. 7, 199–205.

de Polo, A., Scrimshaw, M.D., 2012. Challenges for the development of a biotic ligand model predicting copper toxicity in estuaries and seas. Environ. Toxicol. Chem. 31, 230–238.

Doblander, C., Lackner, R., 1996. Metabolism and detoxification of nitrite by trout hepatocytes. Biochim. Biophys. Acta. 1289, 270–274.

Durborow, R.M., Crosby, D.M., Burnson, M.W., 1997. Nitrate in Fish Ponds. Southern Regional Aquaculture Center, Stoneville, MS.

Finn, R.N., 2007. The physiology and toxicology of salmonid eggs and larvae in relation to water quality criteria. Aquat. Toxicol. 81, 337–354.

Grabda, E., Einszporn-Orecka, T., Felinska, C., et al., 1974. Experimental methemoglobinemia in rainbow trout. Acta Ichthyl. Piscat. 4, 43–71.

Greco, M., Pardo, A., Pose, G., 2015. Mycotoxigenic fungi and natural co-occurrence of mycotoxins in rainbow trout (*Oncorhynchus mykiss*) feeds. Toxins (Basel). 7, 4595–4609.

Hadfield, C.A., Whitaker, B.R., Clayton, L.A., 2007. Emergency and critical care of fish. Vet. Clin. North Am. Exot. Anim. Pract. 10, 647–675.

Hargreaves, J.A., 1998. Nitrogen biogeochemistry of aquaculture ponds. Aquaculture. 166, 181–212.

Ip, Y.K., Chew, S.F., 2010. Ammonia production, excretion, toxicity, and defense in fish: a review. Front. Physiol. 1, Article 134.

Jensen, F.B., 2003. Nitrite disrupts multiple physiological functions in aquatic animals. Comp. Biochem. Physiol. A Mol. Integr. Physiol. 135, 9–24.

Jensen, F.B., Agnisola, C., 2005. Perfusion of the isolated trout heart coronary circulation with red blood cells: effects of oxygen supply and nitrite on coronary flow and myocardial oxygen consumption. J. Exp. Biol. 208, 3665–3674.

Jensen, F.B., Hansen, M.N., 2011. Differential uptake and metabolism of nitrite in normoxic and hypoxic goldfish. Aquat. Toxicol. 101, 318–325.

Linbo, T.L., Stehr, C.M., Incardona, J.P., et al., 2006. Dissolved copper triggers cell death in the peripheral mechanosensory system of larval fish. Environ. Toxicol. Chem. 25, 597–603.

Masser, M.P., Rakocy, J., Losordo, T.M., 1999. Recirculating Aquaculture Tank Production Systems: Management of Recirculating Systems. Southern Regional Aquaculture Center, Stoneville, MS.

Morley, N.J., 2010. Interactive effects of infectious diseases and pollution in aquatic molluscs. Aquat. Toxicol. 96, 27–36.

National Academies of Sciences, Engineering, and Medicine, 2016. Approaches to Understanding the Cumulative Effects of Stressors on Marine Mammals. National Academies Press, Washington, DC.

NOAA, 2000. Anthropogenic Noise in the Marine Environment. Potential Impacts on The Marine Resources of Stellwagen Bank and Channel Islands National Marine Sanctuaries. National Oceanic and Atmospheric Administration, Washington, DC, http://sanctuaries.noaa.gov/management/pdfs/anthro_noise.pdf.

Nugegoda, D., Kibria, G., 2016. Effects of environmental chemicals on fish thyroid function: implications for fisheries and aquaculture in Australia. Gen. Comp. Endocrinal.. Available from: http://dx.doi.org/10.1016/j.ygcen.2016.02.021.

Peng, C., Zhao, X., Liu, G., 2015. Noise in the sea and its impacts on marine organisms. Int. J. Environ. Res. Public Health. 12, 12304–12323.

Randall, D.J., Tsui, T.K.N., 2002. Ammonia toxicity in fish. Marine Pollut. Bull. 45, 17–23.

Rudolph, A., Medina, P., Urrutia, C., et al., 2009. Ecotoxicological sediment evaluations in marine aquaculture areas of Chile. Environ. Monit. Assess. 155, 419–429.

Sinha, A.K., Diricx, M., Chan, L.P., et al., 2012. Expression pattern of potential biomarker genes related to growth, ion regulation and stress in response to ammonia exposure, food deprivation and exercise in common carp (*Cyprinus carpio*). Aquat. Toxicol. 122–123, 93–105.

Sommers, F., Mudrock, E., Labenia, J., et al., 2016. Effects of salinity on olfactory toxicity and behavioral responses of juvenile salmonids from copper. Aquat. Toxicol. 175, 260–268.

(USEPA) U.S. Environmental Protection Agency, 2007. Aquatic Life Ambient Freshwater Quality Criteria: Copper. U.S. Environmental Protection Agency, Washington, DC.

Wicks, B.J., Randall, D.J., 2002. The effect of feeding and fasting on ammonia toxicity in juvenile rainbow trout, *Oncorhynchus mykiss*. Aquat. Toxicol. 59, 71–82.

Wicks, B.J., Joensen, R., Tang, Q., et al., 2002. Swimming and ammonia toxicity in salmonids: the effect of sublethal ammonia exposure on the swimming performance of coho salmon and the acute toxicity of ammonia in swimming and resting rainbow trout. Aquat. Toxicol. 59, 55–69.

Wilkie, M.P., 2002. Ammonia excretion and urea handling by fish gills: present understanding and future research challenges. J. Exp. Zool. 293, 284–301.

Wlasow, T.K., Demska-Zakes, P., Gomulka, P., et al., 2010. Various aspects of piscine toxicology. Interdiscip. Toxicol. 3, 100–104.

Section XI

Bacterial and Cyanobacterial Toxins

Chapter 55

Botulinum Neurotoxins

Rhian B. Cope

INTRODUCTION

Botulinum toxins are exotoxins produced by *Clostridium botulinum*; a Gram-positive anaerobic rod shaped bacterium, and related *Clostridia* including *C. butyricum, C. baratii*, and *C. argentinense* (Popoff and Bouvet, 2013; Pirazzini et al., 2017). These toxins are a family of structurally similar, but antigenically and serologically distinct, neurotoxins that consist of two basic components: the neurotoxic component (light chain) and the accessory component (heavy chain). There are now eight antigenically distinct toxin serotypes (A, B, C1, C2, D, E, F, G, H; Barash and Arnon, 2014; Dover et al., 2014). Human botulism is mostly caused by serotypes A, B, E and F while serotypes C and D only cause toxicity in animals. Serotype H was recently discovered in the feces of a child suffering botulism (Barash and Arnon, 2014). Six of the serotypes have additional subtypes (Dover et al., 2014; Kalb et al., 2011).

Botulinum toxin A and B have been successfully commercialized as pharmaceuticals for the treatment of cervical dystonia, severe primary axillary hyperhidrosis, strabismus, blepharospasm, neurogenic detrusor over activity, chronic migraine, upper limb spasticity, lateral canthal lines (crow's feet) and glabellar lines. Critically, serious medication errors have occurred with different types of pharmaceutical botulinum toxins due to their different individual potencies.

Botulinum toxin A is a noted potential bioweapon. An estimated 1 g of botulinum toxin A could kill more than one million people via inhalation exposure (the preferred exposure pathway for weaponization; Arnon et al., 2001a,b). The estimated median IV lethal dose of botulinum toxin A in humans is 1 ng/kg (Gill, 1982).

SEROTYPES OF VETERINARY SIGNIFICANCE

Serotypes A, B, C1, and D have been associated with outbreaks of botulism in domestic animals, livestock, poultry, and wildlife.

BACTERIAL SYNTHESIS

Botulinum toxins are synthesized as a 150 kD progenitor toxin that is then cleaved to form an active dimer consisting of disulphide bond linked heavy and light chains (Fig. 55.1). When isolated from *Clostridia*, botulinum toxins are found in 300–500 kD complexes with hemagglutinins and other nonhemagglutinin, nontoxic proteins.

MECHANISM OF ACTION

The overall classical mode of action is to presynaptically bind to high-affinity recognition sites on the cholinergic nerve terminals, decrease the release of acetylcholine, and produce presynaptic neuromuscular blockade. Denervation muscular atrophy accompanies the neuromuscular blockade. Although effected neuromuscular junctions may eventually recover, most of the recovery from botulinum toxin neuromuscular blockade results from proximal axonal sprouting and muscle reinnervation through the synthesis of new neuromuscular junctions (de Paiva et al., 1999).

The terminal membrane acceptor-binding domain (H_c) and *N*-terminal translocation domains on the toxin heavy chain facilitate the translocation of the light chain into the neuronal cytosol via a pH dependent mechanism. Within the nerve terminal cytosol, the light chain polypeptide is separated from the heavy chain and refolded to form a Zn^{2+} metalloprotease. The light chain metalloproteases have different cellular targets in the sequence of events leading to the release of acetylcholine in to the synaptic cleft depending on the toxin serotype (Table 55.1, Fig. 55.2; Rossetto et al., 2014).

TOXICODYNAMICS

The toxicodynamics of botulinum toxins has been mostly evaluated using commercialized versions of serotype A. For this serotype, cleavage of less than 10% of SNAP-25 in the presynaptic nerve terminal results in 90% muscular paralysis (Kalandakanond and Coffield, 2001). Spontaneous cholinergic neurotransmission in cultured

Veterinary Toxicology. DOI: http://dx.doi.org/10.1016/B978-0-12-811410-0.00055-6

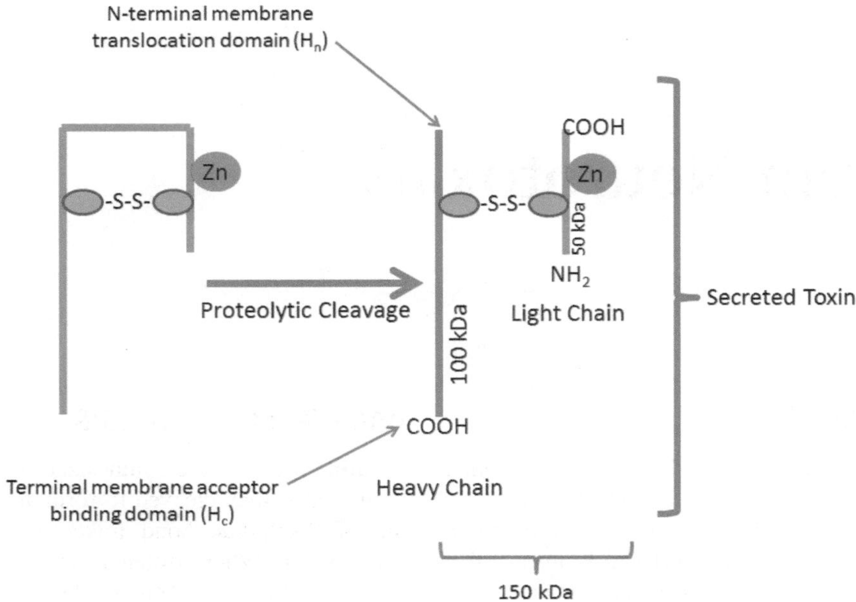

FIGURE 55.1 Botulinum toxin structure.

TABLE 55.1 Neuronal Cellular Targets of Botulinum Toxins

Botulinum Toxin Serotypes	Molecular Target of the Light Chain	Key Effect
A	Cleaves SNAP-25	SNAP-25[a] is presynaptic membrane protein required for fusion of neurotransmitter-containing vesicles
E		
B	Cleaves VAMP	VAMP (*syn:* synaptobrevin) is a small integral membrane protein found in neurotransmitter secretory vesicles. Cleavage of VAMP blocks neurotransmitter exocytosis and endocytosis
D		
F		
G		
C1	Syntaxin	The syntaxin domain contains a soluble NSF[b] attachment protein (SNARE) that acts as the docking site for SNAP-25

[a]*SNAP-25 = Synaptosomal-associated protein 25.*
[b]*NSF = N-ethylmaleimide sensitive fusion proteins.*

autonomic neurons is reduced to less than 20% (i.e., near complete synaptic paralysis) when less than 20% of presynaptic nerve terminal SNAP-25 is cleaved (Lawrence et al., 2013).

The effects of serotype A light chains on SNAP-25 lasts for about 4 days (i.e., equivalent to SNAP-25 turnover time in the synaptic terminal; Bartels et al., 1994). However, this does not correlate with the persistence of serotype A-induced paralysis which may last several months. The unusual cytosolular stability of the proteolytic form of the light chain (at least 180 days in vivo and 80 days in vitro in rodent tissues) and its resistance to proteasomal degradation are the major reasons for the long duration of botulinum toxin A-induced paralysis (Antonucci et al., 2008; Keller et al., 1999). Consistent with this conclusion is the finding that the light chains of botulinum toxin serotype E are more susceptible to proteasomal degradation, resulting in its shorter duration of action *cf* serotype A.

Overall, the major pharmacokinetic and pharmacodynamic factors that combine to cause the exquisitely high toxicity of botulinum toxins are: (1) although it is a large protein, a large fraction of ingested toxin is systemically absorbed; (2) the long elimination half-life of botulinum toxin/A in the systemic circulation acts as a allows distribution to peripheral tissues and entry into peripheral nerve terminals; (3) the relatively long persistence of

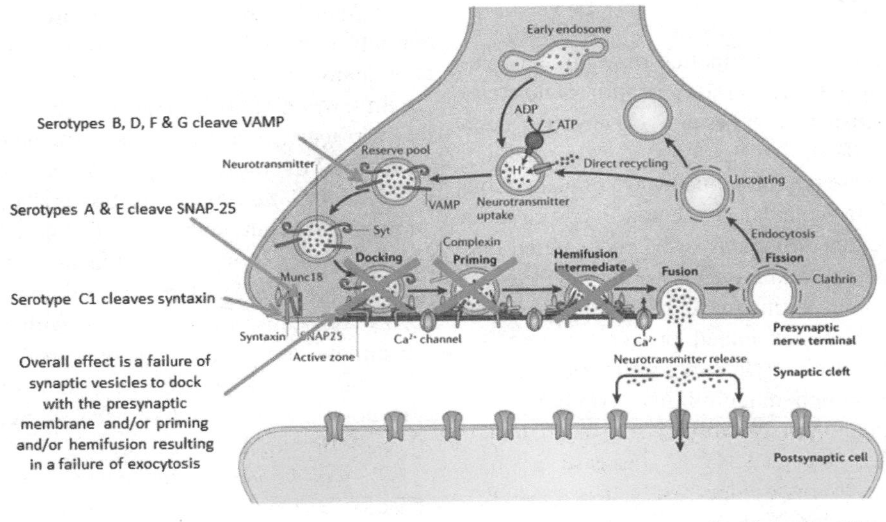

FIGURE 55.2 Botulinum toxin disruption of synaptic vesicle release. *Adapted from Rossetto, O., Pirazzini, M., Montecucco, C. Botulinum neurotoxins: genetic, structural, and mechanistic insights. Nat. Rev. Microbiol. 2014 Aug;12(8):535–549. (Cortesy of Rossetto O).*

biologically active toxin within the general circulation acts as a "holding compartment" which contributes to the severity and extent of the disease; (4) the high affinity of botulinum toxin/A heavy chain to dual ganglioside-protein acceptors at the peripheral nerve terminals; (5) the capacity of a single light chain metalloprotease to inactivate large numbers of its toxicological target proteins; (6) in the cytosol, the light chains are very stable and resistant to proteasomal degradation, resulting in long duration effects; (7) cleavage of only a small proportion of the toxicological target proteins results in a very large overall biological effect; and (8) in practical terms, recovery requires nerve sprouting and the synthesis of new neuromuscular junctions.

Botulinum toxins also affect in vitro neurotransmission associated with serotonin, dopamine, noradrenalin, glutamate, GABA, encephalin, glycine, substance P, ATP, and calcitonin gene related peptide. Botulinum toxins tend to have greater efficacy on excitatory neurotransmitters (acetylcholine, glutamate), and inhibitory transmitters (e.g., GABA), which may explain the clinical sign of "dullness" seen in some animals (notably horses; Verderio et al., 2007). Notably, the effects of botulinum toxins are not necessarily confined to neuronal synapses, e.g., botulinum toxin A inhibits the ectopic vesicular release of glutamate and ATP in olfactory receptor axons (Thyssen et al., 2010) and blocks several nonneuronal SNAP-25 dependent effects, notably insulin release from pancreatic beta cells, acetylcholine release from chromaffin cells, acetylcholine release from sciatic Schwann cells, glutamate release from astrocytes, Ca^{2+} channel and possibly other voltage gated ion channel function, receptor translocation to the plasma membrane, neurite extension and dendrite and axonal growth (which may further impair recovery from classical botulism).

Apart from its effects on motor neurons, botulinum toxins have antinociceptive effects and have been developed as potential therapies for subacute to chronic pain. These effects are, at least in part, dependent on axonal transport of the toxin into the CNS (Matak and Lacković, 2014). Botulinum toxins also undergo axonal transport in motor neurons; however the clinical significance of this is uncertain.

QUANTIFICATION OF NEUROMUSCULAR BLOCKING POTENCY

The classical, and still standard, assay of potency is the mouse bioassay. One mouse unit (MU) is the amount of botulinum toxin A required to kill 50% of a group of 20 g Swiss Webster mice within 3 days of IP injection. Approximately 1 ng of botulinum A is equivalent to 20 MU. A more pharmacologically relevant unit, the median paralysis unit (MPU) was developed in 1995 to better characterize the biological activities of the pharmaceutical versions of botulinum toxins (Pearce et al., 1995). The unit is based on a regional chemodenervation following IM injection rather than mortality. One MPU is the ED_{50} producing complete hind limb paralysis following IM injection into the mouse hind limb and is equivalent to an amount of toxin in the picogram range.

TOXICOKINETICS

While all aspects of the toxicokinetics may not be relevant to specific situations (e.g., oral absorption is not relevant to wound botulism), a general overview has been provided (Simpson, 2013).

Absorption: There are two broad pathways of absorption: oral and parenteral (via wounds). Inhalation exposure is an unusual circumstance that is unlikely to be encountered outside of bioweapon use and toxin manufacturing facilities

Release of botulinum toxins by *Clostridia* sp. is in the form of a noncovalently associated progenitor complex consisting of hemagglutinins (Has: three different classes, HA1−3), nontoxic nonhemagglutinins (NTHA: one class), and botulinum toxin. Notably, serotypes E and F do not produce HAs. HAs and NTHA increase the oral potency of botulinum toxins by decreasing their proteolysis in the gut. In particular, NTHA has been described as essentially acting as a "bioshield." There is also limited in vitro evidence that HAs may disrupt enterothelial tight junctions, thus facilitating paracellular transport. Critically, HAs are not essential for intestinal absorption.

Absorption across relevant epithelia displays the following features: (1) it is an active, receptor-dependent, endocytosis/transcytosis process that is not dependent on HAs or NTHA; (2) the critical domain for endocytosis/transcytosis across epithelia is located is associated with the carboxy terminal end of the toxin heavy chain; (3) different epithelia have different relevant receptors; and (4) the cellular handling of botulinum toxins by epithelial cells is different from what occurs in neurons.

Distribution: botulinum toxins essentially distribute to the non-CNS extracellular fluid compartment. The toxin obeys a classical 2 compartment model elimination kinetics with a distribution phase and an approximately first-order elimination phase. Botulinum toxins are highly stable within the circulation and the general circulation acts as a "holding compartment." The handling of the toxin with the neuronal compartment has been described above.

Metabolism and elimination: the metabolism and elimination of botulinum toxins remains poorly described. Critically, the persistence of biologically active toxin within the general circulation holding compartment likely contributes to the severity of the disease.

BOTULISM IN HUMANS

Food-borne botulism (Kerner's disease): the disease is due to the ingested of food containing preformed toxin. It is most common in food preserved under anaerobic conditions. While the spores of *C. botulinum* are heat-resistant, the toxin itself can be destroyed by boiling (WHO, 2013). A major objective of food preservation is the destruction of the toxin and creation of conditions unfavorable to clostridial growth.

Inhalation botulism: this form is very rare and is largely confined to the industrial toxin manufacture. It is the major route of exposure for weaponized botulinum toxin (Arnon et al., 2001a,b).

Iatrogenic botulism: this form involves the misuse or accidental overdosing of pharmaceutical botulinum toxins.

Human infant botulism: this is due to anaerobic conditions in the gut that allow for germination of ingested *C. botulinum* spores in human infants under 6 months of age (Brook, 2007). Honey containing *C. botulinum* spores is a major cause of this disease with up to 20% of honey specimens containing the spores (Nakano et al., 1990).

Adult intestinal toxemia botulism: this occurs when the normal gut flora has been altered due to antibiotic therapy or surgical procedures.

Wound botulism: this occurs with infection of deep anaerobic wounds with *C. botulinum.*

BOTULISM IN VETERINARY SPECIES

Equine Botulism

Horses are amongst the most susceptible species. Equine botulism in North America is mostly due to serotype B (>80% of equine cases) although cases involving serotypes A and C1 have been reported (Whitlock, 1996; Johnson et al., 2010). *C. botulinum* serotype B strains are ubiquitous in the soils of the northeastern and central United States (particularly a zone extending from Kentucky to the mid-Atlantic states). Serotype A strains are more prominent in the western states (California, Utah, Idaho, and Oregon) and in Ohio. Botulinum serotype C1 cases have been reported in California, Florida, the New England states, and Canada.

Horses acquire botulism in one of three ways: (1) from the ingestion of preformed toxin in contaminated foodstuffs; (2) from anaerobic wound contamination with *C. botulinum*; and (3) from the colonization of the intestinal tract with *C. botulinum* bacteria (toxicoinfection).

The ingestion of preformed toxin in spoiled or carrion-contaminated foodstuffs is the most common scenario. Contaminated feed sources such as alfalfa cubes, alfalfa hay, baled hay, wheat, oats, potatoes, bale silage, rye silage, grass clippings, oat chaff, and brewer's grains have all been purported sources (Whitlock and Buckley, 1997). Serotype B is more commonly associated with spoiled foodstuffs or moldy hay. Damp, alkaline conditions in spoiled vegetation are optimal conditions for clostridial growth, sporulation, and toxin production. For these reasons, it is recommended that silage with a pH greater than 4.5 should not be fed to horses (Whitlock and Buckley, 1997; Galey, 2001). Storage of silage and hay in large plastic bags is a risk factor.

Carrion-contaminated feed is most commonly associated with botulinum toxin C1 (Galey, 2001; Kinde et al.,

1991). Birds may act as vectors, transporting toxin or bacterial spores from a rotting carcass to nearby horse farms (Schoenbaum et al., 2000).

Wound botulism occurs from the contamination of an anaerobic wound with the *Clostridium* bacteria and is most commonly associated with botulinum toxin B. Distal limb wounds, castration sites, umbilical hernias, and injection site abscesses are the usual suspects.

Shaker foal syndrome is a form of toxicoinfectious botulism occurring in foals of around 2–5 weeks of age (Rooney and Prickett, 1967; Vaala, 1991; Whitlock, 2002). The syndrome is most common in fast-growing foals on high planes of nutrition and is most commonly associated with botulinum toxin serotype B with occasional cases involving serotype C1 (MacKay and Berkhoff, 1982). Gastrointestinal ulceration and liver abscesses have been documented postmortem in foals that succumbed to botulism (Swerczek, 1980). Exposures to stress, high nutrient diets, or corticosteriod use are reputed to play a role in susceptibility by promoting gastric ulcers that act as an anaerobic nidus for colonization. Furthermore, as in human neonatal toxicoinfection, the immature GI tract of foals may be more permissible to overgrowth by *C. botulinum*. Sand colitis or other causes of gastrointestinal irritation may be risk factors.

Equine grass sickness (EGS) is a polyneuronopathy affecting both the central and the peripheral nervous systems of grazing (mostly) horses (Pirie et al., 2014). The etiology of the disease remains uncertain although toxicoinfectious exposure to botulinum toxin C1 was proposed as a cause in the 1920s. Critically, EGS is not associated with classical botulinum toxin induced overt flaccid paresis/paralysis. There is limited evidence of: (1) a greater frequency of detection of botulinum toxin C1 in the ileal contents and/or feces of horses with EGS *cf* healthy horses; (2) low antibody status to *C. botulinum* type C as a risk factor; (3) survivors of chronic EGS have higher levels of antibodies against *C. botulinum* serotype C *cf* nonsurvivors; (4) the specific action of *C. botulinum* type C1 neurotoxin on nerve terminal syntaxin at cholinergic synapses may account for the neuroanatomical distribution of some EGS-associated neuronal dysfunctions; (5) *C. botulinum* type C can produce C2 and C3 ADP-ribosylating toxins capable of inducing ultrastructural cellular disarray; and (6) two successful vaccine trials using partly neutralized *C. botulinum* toxin, were conducted in the 1920s. However, the disease has not been experimentally reproduced with *C. botulinum* type C.

Clinical Signs, Diagnosis, and Treatment

The onset of classical equine botulism is variable with signs starting between 12 h and 10 days postexposure (i.e., gradual, acute, or peracute depending on exposure dose, duration and individual sensitivity). Adult horses that ingest low doses of toxin may show only mild dysphagia and recover with minimal treatment. Ingestion of large doses is more likely to induce peracute disease with a poor prognosis. In peracute illness, muscle paralysis progresses rapidly and the animal is recumbent within 8–12 h; ultimately, paralysis of the respiratory muscles results in death.

With the exception of EGS, the clinical presentation is not related to the botulinum toxin serotype involved (Whitlock, 1996; Whitlock and Buckley, 1997; Johnson et al., 2010). Early signs are typically progressive and include depression, exercise intolerance, difficulty with grain consumption, myasthenia, dysphagia, ataxia, gait stiffness, muscle tremors (particularly in the triceps and quadriceps muscle groups), decreased tail tone, mydriasis, ptosis, decreased pupillary light responses, and decreased palpebral reflexes. Exercise typically worsens the paresis. Dysphagia and pharyngeal weakness are often associated with secondary aspiration pneumonia. Horses often have difficulty in drinking. Stridor may develop due to pharyngeal/laryngeal paresis/paralysis. Low head carriage is noted in some cases. During the initial stages of the disease vital signs typically remain normal. However evidence of progressively worsening gut stasis (decreased borborygmi, ileus, colic, and constipation) is common with disease progression. Diarrhea is often associated with serotype C, possibly in association with C2 toxin. Urine retention with resultant bladder distention often occurs, thereby increasing the risk of urinary tract infection.

As the disease progresses, horses spend more time in sternal recumbency and ultimately become laterally recumbent. Heart and respiratory rates may increase as recumbent horses struggle to stand. In late stages, dyspnea and other signs of respiratory distress may be observed. With serotype C intoxication, an exaggerated expiration and "prolonged abdominal lift" may be noted. In the final stages of botulism, horses are laterally recumbent, demonstrate significant respiratory difficulty, and develop anoxia. As the anoxia progresses, horses may exhibit agonal paddling. At this point, the patient either dies due to respiratory failure or is euthanized.

In shaker foal syndrome, the first clinical signs are typically increased periods of recumbency and muscle tremors. Soon after the foal rises, muscle tremors are evident, and after brief periods of standing, the foal collapses from weakness. Recumbent foals appear to be bright and alert. Foals may dribble milk from their muzzles soon after nursing due to dysphagia and pharyngeal muscle paresis and aspiration pneumonia is common. Constipation and ileus are also frequently observed. Other clinical signs are similar to those observed in the adult horse.

The characteristic spectrum of EGS clinical signs are due to neuronal degeneration in the autonomic nervous system and the myenteric and submucosal plexuses of the enteric nervous system. The clinical syndromes are described as acute, subacute and chronic depending on the duration of the disease (typically the duration of survival after initial diagnosis). The syndrome almost always includes dullness, anorexia, dysphagia and tachycardia. The cranial nerves (and their CNS nuclei) involved in prehension and mastication (cranial nerves V, VII, IX, X, and XII) often become involved. Ptosis (due to denervation of sympathetic axons innervating Müller's superior tarsal muscle) and patchy sweating (due to sympathetic denervation with chemical hypersensitivity of the sweat gland and/or vasodilatation and subsequent increased sudiferous adrenaline arriving at the sweat glands and or elevated baseline plasma adrenalin) may occur. In acute cases, mild to moderate abdominal pain and large volumes of nasogastric reflux are common. Weight loss and progressive myasthenia (base-narrow stance, leaning back against walls, weight shifting of the limbs) are common findings in the chronic disease. The pathophysiological basis for the effects on muscles is uncertain. Overt botulism-like flaccid paralysis does not occur and, unlike botulism cases, affected horses to not spend progressively longer periods of time in recumbency and triceps/quadriceps fasciculations persist during periods of recumbency. Generalized small intestinal distention and colon/cecal impactions are common findings and reflect intestinal dysmotility due to enteric nervous system damage.

A tentative diagnosis of classical botulism can be made following a neurological examination and repeat neurological examinations are useful for monitoring disease progression. Routine clinical pathology examinations are usually negative but can be useful for differential diagnosis purposes. Typically normal laboratory values in the presence of neurological deficits support a diagnosis of botulism. Important differential diagnoses include: equine protozoal myeloencephalitis, equine viral encephalitis (alphaviruses: eastern and western equine encephalitis, mdariaga virus, highland virus, Venezuelan equine encephalitis, everglades virus, Ross River virus, Semliki Forrest virus, Una virus; flaviviruses: Japanese encephalitis, Murray Valley encephalitis, Kunjin virus, St. Louis encephalitis, Usutu, West Nile virus, Louping ill, Powassan, tickborn encephalitis), equine herpes virus-1, rabies, guttural pouch mycosis, and listeriosis; other toxicoses such as leukoencephalomalacia (moldy corn poisoning), ionophore poisoning (monesin, salinomycin, and narasin), yellow star thistle poisoning, yew poisoning, white snake root poisoning, and organochlorine poisoning; metabolic disorders such as equine motor neuron disease, azoturia, eclampsia, hypocalcemia, hyperkalemic periodic paralysis, and white muscle disease, and pharyngeal ulceration.

A tentative diagnosis of classical equine botulism can be confirmed by: (1) mouse bioassay detection of toxin in horse sera, gut contents, viscera, wounds, tissues or foodstuffs (the gold standard test); (2) detection of *C. botulinum* spores or toxin in suspect foodstuffs in association with clinical signs; and (3) ELISA detection of serum antitoxin antibodies in unvaccinated horses with clinical signs. However, a definitive diagnosis is usually difficult to achieve. There are no gross or pathognomonic histological lesions associated with classical botulism, and serum toxin levels in the horse are often too low to be detected by the mouse bioassay. Due to the sensitivity of horses, the mouse bioassay is most useful in early, peracute equine botulism, when higher concentrations of toxin may be present in the bloodstream. Greater diagnostic success may be achieved through detection of botulinum toxin in food using the mouse bioassay rather than detection within affected animals (Galey, 2001). Anaerobic fecal or tissue culture enrichment can be used to enhance bacterial spore numbers and toxin levels for greater detection. However, because spores may be present in the feces of healthy horses, direct detection of systemically absorbed botulinum toxin within the animal is a more reliable finding. Following a positive result from the mouse bioassay, the serotype can be identified using the mouse neutralization test.

The key diagnostic histological finding in EGS is neuronal degeneration (extensive chromatolysis, with loss of Nissl substance; eccentricity or pyknosis of the nuclei; neuronal swelling and vacuolation; accumulation of intracytoplasmic eosinophilic spheroids and axonal dystrophy; cell death followed by neuronophagia; and an apparent increase in capsule/satellite cells). The neuronal damage is most prominent in the prevertebral and paravertebral ganglia of the autonomic nervous system and in enteric neurons (myenteric and submucous plexuses). However, there is usually extensive neurological damage throughout the autonomic nervous system. The exact pathogenesis of the neuronal damage is unknown. There is evidence of elevated galanin, extensive cytoskeletal disruption with loss of the Golgi apparatus, apoptosis, accumulation of noradrenalin and/or enzymes involved in noradrenaline synthesis (tyrosine hydroxylase and dopamine-β-hydroxylase), reduction in glutamate immunostaining, and an abnormal distribution of enzymes involved in glutamate metabolism (glutamate dehydrogenase and glutamine synthase) and increased synaptophysin. Damage to the CNS nuclei associated with cranial nerves III, V, VI, VIII, XII, X as well as the accessory cuneate nucleus, the red nucleus, the reticular formation, spinal cord lower motor neurons and spinal cord intermediolateral horn neurons.

Once botulism is suspected, the patient should be confined to prevent exertion. Polyvalent antiserum (antitoxin) should be given as soon as possible; the recommended dose for an adult horse is 70,000 IU and for foals it is

30,000 IU. One dose typically provides coverage for about 60 days (Sprayberry and Carlson, 1997; Whitlock and Buckley, 1997). The use of parasympathomimetics should be avoided because these agents deplete acetylcholine stores and exacerbate paresis/paralysis. Antibiotic therapy is indicated in cases of wound botulism or secondary infections; however, aminoglycosides, tetracycline, procaine penicillin, and metronidazole are contraindicated. Aminoglycosides block neurotransmission at the neuromuscular junction and will exacerbate muscle weakness and paralysis (Barsanti, 1990). Although gram-positive anaerobes are sensitive to penicillin and metronidazole, administration of these drugs is controversial. These antimicrobials may cause more bacterial lysis, thus increasing the release of toxin (in the case of a toxicoinfection), or they may promote *C. botulinum* colonization by altering the normal intestinal flora. Drugs such as the aminopyridines and guanidines should also be avoided because they will further deplete acetylcholine stores (Critchley, 1991).

After antitoxin administration, supportive care is the mainstay of treatment. H_2 blockers and proton pump inhibitors may be indicated, especially for foals. Topical ophthalmic ointments should be used to prevent corneal abrasions and ulceration. Adult horses may require sedation with xylazine or diazepam to reduce anxiety and exertion. Patients should be muzzled between feedings to reduce the risk of aspiration pneumonia. Nutritional support should be provided to dysphagic patients. Alfalfa slurries with adequate amounts of water may be administered through a nasogastric tube to adult horses. Foals should receive milk replacer through a nasogastric tube or parenteral nutrition if ileus is present. Patients should be maintained in sternal recumbency to prevent aspiration pneumonia and checked periodically for gastric reflux because ileus may lead to the accumulation of ingesta/fluid in the stomach. If gastric reflux is not present, some authors recommend that mineral oil be administered via a nasogastric tube to alleviate ileus and constipation; however, this should be done under close supervision due to the increased risk of aspiration in these patients. Recumbent patients should be turned frequently or suspended periodically by full-body slings to prevent decubital ulcer formation, myopathies, and other complications of prolonged recumbency. Recumbent stallions and geldings should be catheterized twice daily to empty the bladder and prevent pressure necrosis or cystitis (Whitlock and Buckley, 1997).

A tracheostomy should be performed in cases of botulism in which horses show signs of upper airway obstruction as a result of paralysis of the nares or larynx. In more complicated cases, patients may require intravenous fluids to correct respiratory acidosis resulting from decreased ventilation. For foals in particular, arterial blood gases should be monitored frequently to determine the need for artificial ventilation. Intranasal oxygen insufflation and mechanical ventilation can be instituted in foals with poor arterial blood gas values and/or metabolic acidosis. Unfortunately, mechanical ventilation is not practical in the adult horse (Mitten et al., 1994).

A more optimistic prognosis is associated with low doses, slow disease progression, and mild clinical signs. A poor prognosis is associated with rapid disease onset with recumbency after 8–12 h. A positive response to antitoxin therapy is indicated by the ability to eat relatively normally within 7–10 days posttreatment and regain full strength within a month. The most common complications associated with botulism are decubital ulcers and aspiration pneumonia; these problems can be resolved with supportive care and antimicrobial therapy.

Prevention

Following recommended vaccination protocols, basic wound hygiene, and sound husbandry methods reduces the occurrence of equine botulism. Forages should be examined for carrion, and pastures should be cleared of decaying vegetation and rotting animal carcasses. To date, only serotype B toxoid vaccine is marketed for horses in the United States. In general, vaccination is only recommended for horses in endemic areas. Adult horses in endemic areas should be vaccinated annually. Mares should be boosted 4–6 weeks prior to parturition to achieve adequate antitoxin immunoglobulin (Ig) levels in colostrum. Foals born to vaccinated mares should receive a series of three vaccinations, each 1 month apart, starting at 2 or 3 months of age. Foals born to unvaccinated mares should be vaccinated at 2, 4, and 8 weeks of age (Whitlock and Buckley, 1997; Galey, 2001).

Bovine Botulism

Cattle are susceptible to botulinum toxins B, C1, and D, and the most common form of the disease is caused by ingestion of preformed toxin in spoiled silage, carrion-laden silage (typically serotype B), or silage contaminated with poultry litter (typically serotype C1 and more rarely D; Divers et al., 1986; Heider et al., 2001; Galey et al., 2000; Braun et al., 2005; Martin, 2003; McLoughin et al., 1988). Pica associated chewing on bones and carrion in area with phosphorus deficient soils and/or protein deficiencies is a noted risk factor, particularly for toxin serotype D. Carcasses of animals that have died from botulism present an ongoing risk to other animals under such circumstances. Transfer of carrion by foxes and crows has been reported overseas as an indirect method of disease spread. Outbreaks of botulism in feedlots (and other intensive animal production systems) have been associated with contamination of water supplies by rotting organic matter containing the botulism toxin or bacteria. Toxicoinfectious and wound botulism are occasional causes. As with horses wet, soil-contaminated, alkaline, anaerobic hay wrapped in plastic bags provides ideal incubation conditions for *C. botulinum* (Martin, 2003).

Clinical Signs, Diagnosis, and Treatment

Bovine botulism usually presents as a herd outbreak. The classical signs of bovine botulism resemble those in horses; however, cattle exhibit a more gradual progression of clinical signs, improving the prognosis and probability of recovery (Whitlock et al., 1989; Whitlock and Williams, 1999). The lower susceptibility of cattle to feed-associated botulism is likely due to presystemic elimination by the rumen microflora (Allison et al., 1976). The clinical course ranges from 2 to 30 days, depending on exposure dose, duration and treatment. Early botulism may be confused with milk fever because generalized muscle weakness, increased ataxia, muscle tremors and herd outbreaks may occur in both conditions. Cattle with botulism also exhibit depression, dysphagia, decreased tongue and jaw tone, hypersalivation, dehydration, decreased tail tone, decreased pupillary light responses, and mydriasis. Rumen contractions decrease and constipation may develop. Diarrhea and/or putrid-smelling faces may also be noted. Cattle with botulism tend to spend significant amounts of time in sternal recumbency. At terminal stages of botulism, cattle are laterally recumbent, exhibit abdominal breathing patterns, and finally succumb from respiratory failure. Vital signs are often normal in early stages of botulism; however, as the disease progresses, increased heart and respiratory rates may be noted, whereas body temperature may decrease.

A syndrome resembling equine dysautonomia has been described in German cattle, and a link to botulinum toxins has been proposed. These cattle may present with a subclinical to chronic "visceral" disease. Nonspecific symptoms such as weight loss, decreased milk production, depression, alternating constipation and diarrhea, edema, laminitis, ataxia, retracted abdomen, emaciation, tachypnea, and unexpected death are associated with this syndrome (Böhnel et al., 2001). In cattle exhibiting these symptoms, Böhnel and associates demonstrated the presence of both *C. botulinum* and botulinum toxin in lower GI tract contents. Furthermore, neither botulinum toxin nor *C. botulinum* was isolated from asymptomatic herds. This study hypothesized that small levels of *C. botulinum* colonized the lower intestinal tract and created a low-level, chronic exposure of botulinum toxin. This low-level of toxin may not reach the systemic circulation, and thus toxin may only disrupt nearby parasympathetic ganglionic innervation of the GI tract, altering intestinal function.

In cases of bovine botulism, clinical pathology may reveal signs of dehydration such as increases in packed cell volume and total plasma protein. Bicarbonate loss from excessive ptyalism may lead to a metabolic acidosis. Increases in muscle enzymes such as aspartate transaminase and creatinine kinase may be present due to muscle atrophy or trauma resulting from prolonged lateral recumbency. Electrolyte abnormalities and hyperglycemia may also be detected. One study documented indicators of renal failure in a herd poisoned by botulinum toxin B; increased γ-glutamyl transpeptidase, urea, creatinine, and phosphorus were also detected.

As with other species, there are no definitive gross pathological or pathognomonic histological signs of botulism. Aspiration pneumonia and pulmonary emphysema are the most frequent sequelae of botulism in cattle (Galey et al., 2000; Heider et al., 2001; Braun et al., 2005). Other lesions, such as gastric ulcerations, thickened intestinal mucosa, hepatic lipidosis, suppurative rumenitis, and renal failure, have been documented in concurrence with botulism; however, these findings are not consistent in all cases of bovine botulism.

Botulism in cattle is usually a presumptive field diagnosis made on the basis of clinical signs and the ruling out of other diseases. Differential diagnoses include hypocalcemia, hypomagnesia, hypokalemia, hypophosphatemia, listeriosis, lead poisoning, polioencephalomalacia, ionophore toxicity, nutritional or plant toxin-induced myopathies, molds, organophosphate poisoning, and tick paralysis. Clinical diagnosis is usually made through the detection of neurological deficiencies in light of relatively unremarkable laboratory diagnostic findings. The neurological examination should assess cranial nerve responses, gait, posture, and attitude. Specifically, a tongue tone test, tongue stress test, and a jaw tone test should be performed. The tongue stress test is performed by placing a hand at the base of the cow's tongue and putting pressure on the tongue followed by an assessment of muscular tone. The tongue tone test is performed as in the horse. Cattle with botulism will exhibit weak tongue strength. The jaw test is performed by grasping the mandible near the symphysis and attempting to move the mandible laterally. This test assesses the strength of the masseter muscles. A "loose" jaw is suggestive of botulism.

A definitive diagnosis is made by identifying toxin in the patient's serum, ruminal fluid, or tissues. Identification of botulinum toxin or *C. botulinum* in suspect feedstuffs previously consumed by clinically ill animals may further support a diagnosis. Isolation of botulinum toxin from the rumen may prove difficult because the toxin is often diluted by rumen contents and/or degraded by ruminal microbes. Similar to botulism in other species, the MBA is the gold standard for a definitive diagnosis in cattle; however, as in horses, the MBA is often not sensitive enough to detect the low levels of toxin in the general circulation. The MBA may also be used to detect toxin in rumen contents, the liver and other organ tissues, milk, or feedstuffs. Due to the relatively slower progression of clinical signs in cattle, diagnostic samples are often obtained long after ingestion of toxin. Thus, the level of toxin in these samples may have fallen below the level of detection. Specimens may also be cultured to isolate *C. botulinum*. An ELISA test has been developed to detect botulinum toxin C and D in cattle; however, this test is considered less sensitive than the MBA. ELISA tests for the detection of antibodies to botulinum toxins C and D in cattle have also been developed.

Supportive care is the core of therapy for bovine botulism, and treatment should only be pursued in standing cattle. Affected cattle should be kept in confinement to minimize movement and exertion. Dehydration, electrolyte deficiencies, acid–base abnormalities, and glucose deficiencies should be managed with fluid therapy. Fluids can be administered orally (via an orogastric tube) or IV. Mineral oil or sodium sulfate can be administered with care as cathartics to treat ileus; however, magnesium sulfate should be avoided because it may potentiate muscle weakness. Rumen transfaunation may also be performed. Alfalfa gruels may be administered via an orogastric tube to maintain caloric intake. Equine origin polyvalent antiserum may be administered to cattle. However, antitoxin therapy may be less efficacious in cattle because most of the toxin will have been internalized into the neuron or degraded by the time the diagnosis is made. Antibiotics may be administered for secondary complications such as aspiration pneumonia; as in horses, those that produce muscle weakness should be avoided.

Prevention

Although toxoid vaccinations for serotypes B, C, and D are the mainstay of treatment in many countries, there are no U.S. Food and Drug Administration-approved vaccinations for cattle in the United States. Animal carcasses should either be buried, or burnt and buried, or fenced off so that cattle are unable to access the burial area. This will also reduce the risk of a botulism outbreak if cattle were to chew on carrion or bones.

Other important preventative measures include: providing nutritional supplements of protein and phosphorus to reduce bone chewing among rangeland cattle, taking care with the harvesting and storage of feeds to reduce the possibility of small animals contaminating feeds, checking water sources for organic matter contamination, and high moisture feeds such as silage or brewer's grains when allowed to rot rather than ferment can provide an ideal anaerobic environment for botulism growth. High mortality incidents have been associated with the use of mixing wagons for preparing dairy rations. This allowed the toxin to be evenly distributed throughout the mix.

Since poultry litter is used as fertilizer on many farms it is important that litter stores are not accessible to cattle, that any bird carcasses are removed prior to spreading on pasture, that cattle are withheld from grazing for at least 21 days after application of poultry litter on to pastures and that poultry litters are not used as cattle feeds.

Public Health

The Food Safety Act of the United States (1990) requires that meat or milk products be withheld from market for a minimum of 14 days after the onset of the last clinical case of botulism in an affected herd (Cobb et al., 2002). However, the public health concern for transmission of toxins through milk appears to be minimal. No cases of human botulism acquired from the consumption of meat or milk from botulism-affected cattle have been reported; furthermore, it does not appear that calves acquire botulism through nursing from affected cows. Only a single study to date has been able to detect toxins in milk from a dairy cow affected with botulism (Böhnel et al., 2005). In this study, botulinum toxin serotype B was isolated in milk collected from one udder quarter that was simultaneously affected with mastitis. The toxin concentration in the milk was determined to be approximately 10^4 MU. However, the milk did not test positive for *C. botulinum* bacteria. It is likely that the concurrent mastitis infection enhanced the passage of the rather large toxin protein (150 kDa) across the normally protective blood:milk barrier by altering its permeability. This is supported by a much earlier report from Moberg and Sugiyama (1980), who isolated botulinum toxin in milk using an infected rat model. Other studies have not been able to detect the toxins in milk from affected cows using either ELISA or mouse bioassay techniques (Galey et al., 2000; Cobb et al., 2002; Moeller et al., 2003). Regardless, the pasteurization process would likely denature any toxin protein that was able to pass into milk, reducing the risk to the consumer. Note, however, that the potential for botulinum toxin contamination of milk may be more relevant in regions where unpasteurized milk is available for public consumption.

Avian Botulism

Avian botulism (limberneck, western bird disease) has been a significant problem worldwide in both domestic and wild fowl (Jensen and Price, 1987). The majority of the natural outbreaks of avian botulism have occurred in fowl (Lamana, 1987). Carnivorous, omnivorous, carrion scavengers, and insectivorous birds, as well as aquatic bottom-feeding birds, are all susceptible to botulism. At least 117 avian species, including chickens, ducks, turkeys, pheasants, and ostriches are known to be susceptible. Carrion eating birds such as vultures are reputedly less sensitive to the toxins, possibly because healthy birds often have antibodies to the toxins (Ohishi et al., 1979). Although broiler outbreaks are common, botulism is a more significant problem for waterfowl, resulting in millions of deaths worldwide. Avian species are sensitive to serotypes A, B, C1, and E, although serotype C1 is most commonly associated with outbreaks. Outbreaks of serotype C1 intoxication have been reported worldwide, whereas outbreaks of serotype A botulism have only been reported in western regions of North and South America; serotype B in the eastern United States, England, Europe, and China; and serotype E in the Great Lakes and North Sea. Interestingly, serotype A was found to be more toxic than serotype C1 when administered IV to chickens; however, when given orally, serotype C1 demonstrated greater toxicity.

The etiology of botulism among wild avian species and waterfowl differs from that observed in other animals and involves a complex cycle involving environmental contamination, toxicoinfection, bird die-offs, bacterial proliferation in bird carcasses, and invertebrate vectors. *C. botulinum* often colonizes the intestinal tract and cecum of clinically normal birds, increasing the potential for toxicoinfection in avian species (Dohms, 2003). Because these birds are already seeded with the bacteria, upon death, avian carcasses provide an excellent substrate for *C. botulinum* growth. The proliferating bacteria spread from the GI tract to other tissues, the carcass becomes flyblown, and toxin accumulates in the fly larvae. Invertebrates concentrate the bacterium or toxin after feeding on contaminated carcasses; however, due to their neurophysiological differences, botulinum toxins do not affect insects and aquatic invertebrates. Subsequently, birds ingest these animals and accumulate lethal amounts of the toxins. One gram of fly larvae may contain 1.8×10^5 MU, and ingestion of as little as eight fly larvae was sufficient to kill a pheasant. Bird and invertebrate die-offs perpetuate botulism outbreaks by increasing the levels of *C. botulinum* in soils, lakes, rivers, and estuaries. Environmental factors such as shallow alkaline waters, warm seasons/summer months, and flooding of mudflats or dried-out lakes may promote invertebrate die-offs, further enhancing environmental levels of *C. botulinum.* As *C. botulinum* levels increase in the environment, the intestinal tracts of wild birds and waterfowl become seeded with the bacteria, and any cause of bird deaths can trigger an outbreak of botulism.

Contaminated feed, water, litter, carcasses, and insects may be associated with botulism in broilers. Often, the source of the toxins cannot be identified, and toxicoinfection has been hypothesized as the perpetuating factor. *C. botulinum* has been isolated from the intestinal tract and cecum of healthy birds; furthermore, the chicken body temperature (41°C) and cecal pH (7.4) are optimum for *C. botulinum* growth (Miyazaki and Sakaguchi, 1978; Trampel et al., 2005). Most broiler outbreaks have occurred in chickens between 2 and 3 weeks of age; however, an outbreak in postcaponized chickens was documented in birds as old as 14 weeks. Coprophagy has also been implicated as a causative factor in poultry outbreaks because both botulinum toxin C1 and *C. botulinum* are secreted in cecal droppings. Broiler outbreaks are also more likely to occur in hot weather.

As in other species, morbidity and mortality of avian botulism increases with ingested dose. The onset of clinical symptoms may be from a few hours to 2 days postexposure. The mortality rate in broilers has been reported to be as high as 27%, whereas thousands to millions of birds may have been lost as a result of outbreaks in waterfowl. Botulism may be a limiting factor for waterfowl population growth in predisposed areas of the United States (Jensen and Price, 1987).

Clinical Signs, Diagnosis, and Treatment

As in other species, avian botulism is characterized by lower motor neuron deficits resulting in flaccid muscle paralysis. Paresis begins in the legs and progresses cranially to involve the wings, neck, and eyelids. Mildly affected birds may appear ataxic, reluctant to move, have a ruffled coat, and have easily epilated feathers. The wings may droop and the neck may become flaccid, hence the name "limberneck." Diarrhea is often noted in broilers. As the disease progresses, birds become recumbent. Neck muscles become paralyzed, and birds eventually lie down with necks extended out, resting on the ground. Birds may appear comatose due to eyelid paralysis. Dyspnea may develop as paralysis progresses. Birds usually die from respiratory failure and dehydration. Broilers may succumb to hyperthermia as sick birds are smothered by others and the respiratory mucosal cooling mechanism is compromised.

The diagnosis of avian botulism is based on clinical signs, a lack of specific pathological changes, and the isolation of toxin from serum/tissues of clinically ill birds. Although no pathognomonic changes have been described, postmortem hepatic and renal congestion along with signs of dehydration may be found. The most definitive diagnosis of botulism is the isolation of toxins from the sick bird. Ten mL of blood is the suggested minimum amount for the mouse bioassay; however, if necessary, equal aliquots of blood from individual sick birds may be pooled to accommodate volume requirements of the assay (Dohms, 1987). Following a positive result from the mouse bioassay, the serotype can be identified using the mouse neutralization test. Most outbreaks of avian botulism are due to botulinum toxin/C1; therefore, antiserum for serotype C1 is usually tested first. Isolation of toxins or *C. botulinum* from the bird intestines, cecum, or other tissues may aid in a diagnosis; however, these tests are less valuable because the bacterium can be isolated from the intestinal tract of healthy birds. Furthermore, isolation of toxins or the bacterium from carcass tissues is not definitive because *C. botulinum* may proliferate and spread from the intestinal tract to surrounding tissues of the carcass. The mouse bioassay can be performed on intestinal, cecal, and crop flushes, or samples can be assayed for toxin or bacterium after culture enrichment. In order to identify the source of contamination, feed, water, litter, carcasses, and insects should be assayed for toxin or cultured to isolate the bacterium. Both ELISA and the passive hemagglutination test can be performed to identify serum antibodies to the toxins. However, the levels of toxin that produce illness are usually insufficient to stimulate an immune response in chickens and ducks.

Differential diagnoses for avian botulism in poultry include transient brain paralysis, coccidiostat toxicity, pesticide, or other chemical toxicity, New Castle disease, Marek's disease, avian encephalomyelitis, avian reovirus, fowl tick fever (spirochaetosis), and musculoskeletal problems. Fowl cholera and chemical toxicity, particularly lead poisoning, are the common differentials for botulism in waterfowl. Fowl tick fever is common in poultry in the southern and southwestern United States. However, eyelid paresis and the lack of postmortem lesions are supportive of botulism as the diagnosis.

When possible, clinically ill birds should be isolated and provided fresh water; once these measures are taken, birds often recover fully within a few days. Waterfowl should be herded to uncontaminated shores, and carcasses should be removed daily in poultry operations. Antitoxin therapy may be administered for valuable birds or zoo animals, but it is impractical for most production operations or wildlife. Furthermore, antitoxin protection is transient, and birds may again become susceptible to the toxins. In broiler outbreaks, antimicrobial therapy may be instituted through watering systems or feed. Administration of bacterin (100 g/ton of feed) or streptomycin (500–1000 g/ton of feed or 1 g/L of water for 3 days) was shown to decrease mortality rates in chickens (Schettler, 1979; Sato, 1987). Penicillin may also be administered, but a mixed efficacy has been reported with this treatment. Periodic use of chlortetracycline was reported to reduce botulism outbreaks on one poultry farm. Additives such as sodium selenite (6 g/1000 L of water for 5 days) and vitamins A, D_3, and E may also reduce mortality (Schettler, 1979). Conversely, elevated iron levels in water or feed may promote the intestinal proliferation of *C. botulinum*; therefore, citric acid, an iron chelator, may be added to water as a preventative (Pecelunas et al., 1999). Furthermore, citric acid may lower the pH of the GI tract, inhibiting the growth of *C. botulinum* and promoting the growth of normal flora.

Prevention

Immunization with the toxoid vaccine has been explored in broilers, pheasants, and ducks with mixed results (Shimizu and Kondo, 1978). Protection in broilers between 3 and 8 weeks of age was variable after vaccination at 1 and 14 days of age. Chickens are most susceptible to botulism between 2 and 8 weeks of age, and vaccinations to protect this group may be less efficacious due to interference from maternal antibody and immaturity of the immune system. Routine vaccination further increases production costs, and the toxoid may not provide adequate protection against the high doses of toxin obtained from maggot ingestion. Toxoid immunizations are also impractical for waterfowl. Therefore, preventative measures to minimize outbreaks of avian botulism should be aimed at flock and environmental management in both production birds and waterfowl.

In broiler outbreaks, the goals are to limit further exposure and eliminate *C. botulinum* or toxins from the environment. Unaffected birds should be moved to uncontaminated houses. Carcasses should either be incinerated or buried in a deep hole. Rodents should be eliminated from broiler houses because rodent carcasses may harbor *C. botulinum*. Chicken houses associated with outbreaks should be emptied and cleaned. All litter should be removed. Houses should be washed with high-pressure steam and cleaned with a detergent agent. A surface-active solution should be sprayed on the interior walls. The walls should then be disinfected with an organic iodine solution or an organic iodine and calcium hypochlorite solution. Twenty-four hours later, the interior walls should be sprayed with 10% formalin. Soil in contaminated areas may also be treated with calcium hypochlorite. Houses should also be sprayed with pesticides to limit flies. Iron levels in feed and water sources should be monitored.

Prevention of waterfowl outbreaks is best achieved by reducing the potential for environmental contamination associated with the proliferation of *C. botulinum* in the carcasses of dead vertebrate and invertebrate animals. Carcasses should be collected, and flocks should be herded away from shores associated with outbreaks. Pond management should maintain deep waters, steep banks, and smooth bottoms to prevent deaths of invertebrates and vertebrates. Routine flooding, which may lead to the death of terrestrial invertebrates, should be avoided in areas utilized by waterfowl. Water in wetland areas should be maintained as fresh as possible because oxygen depletion in shallow, stagnant waters leads to aquatic animal die-offs. Any factors that may increase deaths in susceptible wetlands, such as overhead power lines, should be removed or avoided.

The possibility for transmission of botulism from birds to their predators may exist. Coincidence of avian outbreaks with botulism in omnivorous animals has been documented. For instance, Weiss et al. (1982) reported botulism in a fox and a weasel in association with a waterfowl outbreak. In addition, there have been several reports of canine botulism in hunting breeds (Barsanti et al., 1978; Richmond et al., 1978; Jensen and Price, 1987). Farrow et al. (1983) reported the occurrence of botulism in three dogs after the consumption of a rotten duck carcass. Outbreaks of botulism (typically toxins C and D) in cattle and sheep have been associated with the feeding of contaminated poultry litter in silage (Egyed, 1987; McLoughin et al., 1988). No cases of human botulism resulting from the consumption or handling of contaminated birds have been reported, although both scenarios have likely occurred. The risk for the human acquisition of botulism from avian species appears to be limited. Although Smart et al. (1980) reported an outbreak of serotype C in nonhuman primates, humans do not appear to be susceptible to serotypes C or D following oral exposure (Jensen and Price, 1987). Furthermore, proper cooking of poultry should denature any toxin protein and eliminate the possibility of transmission through consumption.

Canine and Feline Botulism

Although carnivores are thought to be more resistant to the development of botulism, cases of canine botulism have been occasionally documented in the United States, Great Britain, continental Europe, and Australia. Most reported cases of botulism in dogs result from the ingestion of botulinum toxin C1-contaminated carrion; however, a few cases of serotype D have been documented in Senegal (Barsanti, 1990, 2006). Barsanti et al. (1978) described an outbreak of type C1 botulism in a hunting colony of American Foxhounds; however, the source of the toxin was not identified. Farrow et al. (1983) described type C1 botulism in three young Australian Cattle Dogs following the ingestion of rotting duck carcasses found in a local Sydney park. Canine botulism has also been associated with the ingestion of contaminated raw meat (Darke et al., 1976).

Until recently, the only documented cases of feline botulism were experimentally induced; however, Elad et al. (2004) described a natural outbreak of botulism in eight cats that ingested parts of a pelican carcass contaminated with botulinum toxin serotype C1. Serotype C1 botulism has also been reported in lions (Critchley, 1991).

Clinical Signs, Diagnosis, and Treatment

The onset of canine botulism can occur within hours or as late as 6 days postexposure. Severe cases are associated with an earlier onset of clinical signs. The course of the disease usually ranges from 12 to 24 days. In the clinical report of an outbreak of feline botulism, clinical symptoms were first noted 3 days postingestion of contaminated pelican muscle (Elad et al., 2004). Although 50% of the exposed cats died, those that survived recovered significantly by 6 days postintoxication.

Lower motor neuron dysfunction and, to a lesser extent, cranial nerve and autonomic nervous system deficits are observed in canine botulism. Paresis begins in the hind limbs and progresses cranially, ultimately resulting in flaccid muscle paralysis and quadriplegia. Interestingly, dogs with botulism maintain the ability to wag their tail. Tremors of the masseter and temporal muscles may be noticed. Muscle atrophy is variable throughout the course of the disease. Mydriasis, decreased pupillary light response, decreased palpebral reflexes, and decreased or weak vocalizations may occur. Hyperemic conjunctiva and decreased Schirmer tear tests may be noted. Heart rates and respiratory patterns are variable; however, as abdominal muscle tone diminishes, diaphragmatic breathing may be noted. Regurgitation, megaesophagus, urinary retention, and constipation are also observed. Secondary complications include aspiration pneumonia, bilateral keratoconjunctivitis sicca, and urinary tract infections. If paralysis progresses to the respiratory muscles, death may occur from respiratory failure; however, death may also result from progressive secondary pneumonia or urinary tract infections. If secondary complications do not arise, the prognosis for canine botulism is good. Recovery occurs in the reverse order from that of the onset of paralysis; cranial nerve function and motor function of the neck and limbs return. In the one case study of natural botulism in cats, clinical signs were similar to those of dogs. Motor deficits and paresis were noted; however, cranial nerve reflexes were normal. Depression, anorexia, mild dehydration, tachycardia, and urinary retention were also noted.

As with EGS in the horse, there has also been speculation of an association between feline dysautonomia (Key–Gaskell disease) and botulinum toxin serotype C. Clinical signs for feline dysautonomia include depression, anorexia, vomiting, regurgitation, mydriasis, constipation, and urinary retention; however, the somatic lower motor neuron paralysis characteristic of classical botulism is not observed. Histological evidence of neuronal degeneration in autonomic ganglia confirms the diagnosis of dysautonomia. Interestingly, botulinum toxin serotype C was detected in feces, ileal contents, and foodstuffs of cats displaying symptoms of dysautonomia (Nunn et al., 2004). Furthermore, affected cats had higher levels of antibotulinum toxin serotype C and *C. botulinum* surface antigen IgA in their feces compared to control cats.

With the exception of dehydration or secondary infection, the CBC count, blood chemistry, urinalysis, and CSF analysis are usually within normal limits in canine and feline botulism. Thoracic radiographs may reveal a megaesophagus and aspiration pneumonia. Electromyographic findings may indicate lower motor neuron disease in clinically ill animals. Decreases in the amplitudes of compound muscle action potentials and motor unit potentials are often detected. Furthermore, fibrillation potentials and decreases in nerve conduction velocity may also be detected. In order to make a definitive diagnosis, toxin must be identified in serum, vomitus or gastric contents, feces, or food samples from animals showing clinical signs. The gold standard MBA appears to have adequate sensitivity for the detection of toxin in canine and feline biological samples or in carrion. Note that the isolation of *C. botulinum* bacteria through cultures of feces, GI contents, or viscera is not a definitive diagnosis because this bacterium can be isolated from the GI tract and viscera of healthy dogs.

Differential diagnoses for canine botulism should include tick paralysis, polyradiculoneuritis (coonhound paralysis), myasthenia gravis, coral snake envenomization, and the dumb form of rabies. Both the lower motor neuron deficits and EMG findings are similar to those of tick paralysis and polyradiculoneuritis; however, due to its action on cholinergic terminals, botulism also causes cranial nerve and autonomic deficits. The nature of botulism outbreaks to affect multiple animals further differentiates the disease from other causes of lower motor neuron dysfunction.

Treatment of canine botulism consists mainly of supportive care (Critchley, 1991; Barsanti, 2006). If the ingestion of toxin-contaminated food has been recent, gastric lavage, cathartics, and enemas may be used to decrease toxin absorption from the GI tract. However, as in other species, magnesium sulfate should be avoided. Supplemental fluids should be administered as needed to maintain hydration. Nutritional support via orogastric or parenteral administration may also be needed. Animals should be monitored for aspiration pneumonia due to megaesophagus and decreased gag reflexes. If constipation develops, enemas and stool softeners may be administered. Manual expression of the bladder may be required to decrease the occurrence of urinary tract infections. Topical ophthalmic ointments should be used to prevent corneal ulcers, which may result from diminished palpebral tone and tear production. Adequate bedding and frequent repositioning are necessary to prevent the development of decubital ulcers. In cases in which respiration is compromised, mechanical ventilation may be necessary. Antimicrobial therapy may be needed for secondary infections; however, as in other species, aminoglycosides, tetracycline, procaine penicillin, metronidazole, aminopyridines, and guanidines should be avoided.

Administration of the equine antitoxin in small animals is controversial. By the time clinical signs are noted, antitoxin is likely to be ineffective because most of the toxin is already bound to the nerve cell or has translocated into the neuron. Only the trivalent antitoxin vaccine for serotypes A, B, and E is available in the United States; this antitoxin is less useful for dogs and cats, which are usually affected by serotype C (Barsanti, 2006). However, the heptavalent antitoxin is available in other countries (Byrne and Smith, 2000; Arnon et al., 2001a,b). Because adverse reactions to antitoxin may occur, and patients with mild disease often recover with supportive care alone, antitoxin administration is usually reserved for severe cases.

CONCLUDING REMARKS AND FUTURE DIRECTIONS

Much of the recent research in to the modes of action of botulinum toxins has been driven by the pharmaceutical development of botulinum toxin serotype A as a pharmaceutical product; however much less research effort has been directed towards the control and treatment of the disease. Control is still heavily based on reducing the risk of exposure via good husbandry techniques and vaccination (where available). Treatment is still heavily based on the use of antitoxins for the neutralization of toxin within the circulation plus basic supportive care. Currently there are no forms of treatment that directly block the effects of the toxins in the presynaptic nerve terminals and/or reduce the persistence of the toxins at these locations. This type of treatment modality, as well as improvements in rapid diagnosis and prevention are the likely areas of future research and development.

REFERENCES

Allison, M.J., Maloy, S.E., Matson, R.R., 1976. Inactivation of *Clostridium botulinum* toxin by ruminal microbes from cattle and sheep. Appl. Environ. Microbiol. 32, 685–688.

Antonucci, F., Rossi, C., Gianfranceschi, L., et al., 2008. Long distance retrograde effects of botulinum neurotoxin A. J. Neurosci. 28, 3689–3696.

Arnon, S.S., Schechter, R., Inglesby, T.V., et al., 2001a. Consensus statement: botulinum toxin as a biological weapon: medical and public health management. J. Am. Med. Assoc. 25, 1059–1070.

Arnon, S.M., Schechter, R., Inglesby, T.V., et al., and Working Group on Civilian Biodefense, 2001b. Botulinum toxin as a biological weapon: medical and public health management. *JAMA* 285: 1059–1070.

Barash, J.R., Arnon, S.S., 2014. A novel strain of *Clostridium botulinum* that produces type B and type H botulinum toxins. J. Infect. Dis. 209, 183–191.

Barsanti, J.A., 1990. Botulism. In: Greene, C.E. (Ed.), Infectious Disease of the Dog and Cat. Saunders, Philadelphia, pp. 515–520.

Barsanti, J.A., 2006. Botulism. In: Greene, C.E. (Ed.), Infectious Disease of the Dog and Cat, third ed. Saunders, Philadelphia, pp. 389–394.

Barsanti, J.A., Walser, M., Hatheway, C.L., et al., 1978. Type C botulism in American foxhounds. J. Am. Vet. Med. Assoc. 172, 809–813.

Bartels, F., Bergel, H., Bigalke, H., et al., 1994. Specific antibodies against the Zn(2 +)-binding domain of clostridial neurotoxins restore exocytosis in chromaffin cells treated with tetanus or botulinum A neurotoxin. J. Biol. Chem. 269, 8122–8127.

Böhnel, H., Schwagerick, B., Gessler, F., 2001. Visceral botulism: a new form of bovine *Clostridium botulinum* toxication. J. Vet. Med. A Physiol. Pathol. Clin. Med. 48, 373–383.

Böhnel, H., Neufeld, B., Gessler, F., 2005. Botulinum neurotoxin type B in milk from a cow affected by visceral botulism. Vet. J. 169, 124–125.

Braun, U., Feige, K., Schweizer, G., et al., 2005. Clinical findings and treatment of 30 cattle with botulism. Vet. Rec. 156, 438–441.

Brook, I., 2007. Infant botulism. J. Perinatol. 27, 175–180.

Byrne, M.P., Smith, L.A., 2000. Development of vaccines for prevention of botulism. Biochimie. 82, 955–966.

Cobb, C.P., Hogg, R.A., et al., 2002. Suspected botulism in dairy cows and its implication for the safety of human food. Vet. Rec. 150, 5–8.

Critchley, E.M., 1991. A comparison of human and animal botulism: a review. J. R. Soc. Med. 84, 295–298.

Darke, P.G.G., Roberts, T.A., Smart, J.L., et al., 1976. Suspected botulism in foxhounds. Vet. Rec. 99, 98–99.

de Paiva, A., Meunier, F.A., Molgo, J., et al., 1999. Functional repair of motor endplates after botulinum neurotoxin type A poisoning: biphasic switch of synaptic activity between nerve sprouts and their parent terminals. Proc. Natl. Acad. Sci. USA. 96, 3200–3205.

Divers, T.J., Bartholomew, R.C., Messick, J.B., et al., 1986. *Clostridium botulinum* type B toxicosis in a herd of cattle and a group of mules. J. Am. Vet. Med. Assoc. 188, 382–386.

Dohms, J.E., 1987. Laboratory investigation of botulism in poultry. In: Eklund, M.W., Dowell, V.R. (Eds.), Avian Botulism: An International Perspective. Charles C Thomas, Springfield, IL, pp. 295–314.

Dohms, J.E., 2003. Botulism. In: Saif, et al., (Eds.), Diseases in Poultry. Iowa State University Press, Ames, IA, pp. 785–791.

Dover, N., Barash, J.R., Hill, K.K., et al., 2014. Molecular characterization of a novel botulinum neurotoxin type H gene. J. Infect. Dis. 209, 192–202.

Egyed, M.N., 1987. Outbreaks of botulism in ruminants associated with ingestion of feed containing poultry waste. In: Eklund, M.W., Dowell, V.R. (Eds.), Avian Botulism: An International Perspective. Charles C Thomas, Springfield, IL, pp. 371–380.

Elad, D., Yas-Natan, E., Aroch, I., et al., 2004. Natural *Clostridium botulism* type C toxicosis in a group of cats. J. Clin. Microbiol. 42, 5406–5408.

Farrow, B.R.H., Murrell, W.G., Revington, M.L., et al., 1983. Type C botulism in young dogs. Aust. Vet. J. 60, 374–377.

Galey, F.D., 2001. Botulism in the horse. Vet. Clin. North Am. Equine Pract. 17, 579–588.

Galey, F.D., Terr, R., Walker, R., et al., 2000. Type C botulism in dairy cattle from feed contaminated with a dead cat. J. Vet. Diagn. Invest. 12, 204–209.

Gill, D.M., 1982. Bacterial toxins: a table of lethal amounts. Microbiol. Rev. 46, 86–94.

Heider, L.C., McClure, J.T., Leger, E.R., 2001. Presumptive diagnosis of *Clostridium botulinum* type D intoxication in a herd of feedlot cattle. Can. Vet. J. 42, 210–212.

Jensen, W.I., Price, J.I., 1987. The global importance of type C botulism in wild birds. In: Eklund, M.W., Dowell, V.R. (Eds.), Avian Botulism: An International Perspective. Charles C Thomas, Springfield, IL, pp. 33–54.

Johnson, A.L., McAdams, S.C., Whitlock, R.H., 2010. Type A botulism in horses in the United States: a review of the past ten years (1998–2008). J. Vet. Diagn. Invest. 22, 165–173.

Kalandakanond, S., Coffield, J., 2001. Cleavage of SNAP-25 by botulinum toxin type A requires receptor-mediated endocytosis, pH-dependent translocation, and zinc. J. Pharmacol. Exp. Ther. 296, 980–986.

Kalb, S.R., Santana, W.I., Geren, I.N., et al., 2011. Extraction and inhibition of enzymatic activity of botulinum neurotoxins /B1, /B2, /B3, /B4, and /B5 by a panel of monoclonal anti-Botulinum toxin/B antibodies. BMC Biochem. 12, 58.

Keller, J.E., Neale, E.A., Oyler, G., et al., 1999. Persistence of botulinum neuro-toxin action in cultured spinal cord cells. FEBS Lett. 456, 137–142.

Kinde, H., Betty, R.L., Ardans, A., et al., 1991. *Clostridium botulinum* type C intoxication associated with consumption of processed alfalfa hay cubes in horses. J. Am. Vet. Med. Assoc. 199 (6), 742–746.

Lamana, C., 1987. The scope of the avian botulism problem. In: Eklund, M.W., Dowell, V.R. (Eds.), Avian Botulism: An International Perspective. Charles C Thomas, Springfield, IL, pp. 5–11.

Lawrence, G.W., Ovsepian, S.V., Wang, J., et al., 2013. Therapeutic effectiveness of botulinum neurotoxin A: potent blockade of autonomic trans-mission by targeted cleavage of only the pertinent SNAP-25. Neuropharmacology. 70, 287–295.

MacKay, R.J., Berkhoff, G.A., 1982. Type C toxicoinfectious botulism in a foal. J. Am. Vet. Med. Assoc. 180 (2), 163–164.

Martin, S., 2003. *Clostridium botulinum* type D intoxication in a dairy herd in Ontario. Can. Vet. J. 44, 493–495.

Matak, I., Lacković, Z., 2014. Botulinum toxin A, brain and pain. Prog. Neurobiol. 119–120, 39–59.

McLoughin, M.F., McIlroy, S.G., Neill, S.D., 1988. A major outbreak of botulism in cattle being fed ensiled poultry litter. Vet. Rec. 122, 579–581.

Mitten, L.A., Hinchcliff, K.W., Holcombe, S.J., et al., 1994. Mechanical ventilation and management of botulism secondary to an injection abscess in an adult horse. Equine Vet. J. 26, 420–423.

Miyazaki, S., Sakaguchi, G., 1978. Experimental botulism in chickens: the cecum as the site of production and absorption of botulinum toxin. Jpn. J. Med. Sci. Biol. 31, 1–15.

Moberg, L.J., Sugiyama, H., 1980. The rat as an animal model for infant botulism. Infect. Immun. 29, 819–821.

Moeller, R.B., Puschner, B., Walker, R.L., et al., 2003. Determination of the median toxic dose of type C botulinum toxin in lactating dairy cows. J. Vet. Diagn. Invest. 15, 523–526.

Nakano, H., Okabe, T., Hashimoto, H., et al., 1990. Incidence of *Clostridium botulinum* in honey of various origins. Jpn. J. Med. Sci. Biol. 43, 183–195.

Nunn, F., Cave, T.A., Knottenbelt, C., et al., 2004. Association between Key–Gaskell syndrome and infection by *Clostridium botulinum* type C/D. Vet. Rec. 155, 111–115.

Ohishi, I., Sakaguchi, G., Riemann, H., et al., 1979. Antibodies to *Clostridium botulinum* toxins in free-living birds and mammals. J. Wildl. Dis. 15, 3–10.

Pearce, L.B., Borodic, G.E., Johnson, E.A., et al., 1995. The median paralysis unit: a more pharmacologically relevant unit of biologic activity for botulinum toxin. Toxicon. 33, 217–227.

Pecelunas, K.S., Wages, D.P., Helm, J.D., 1999. Botulism in chickens associated with elevated iron levels. Avian. Dis. 43, 783–787.

Pirazzini, M., Rossetto, O., Eleopra, R., et al., 2017. Botulinum neurotoxins: biology, pharmacology, and toxicology Pharmacol Rev. 69, 200–235.

Pirie, R.S., Jago, R.C., Hudson, N.P., 2014. Equine grass sickness. Equine Vet. J. 46, 545–553.

Popoff, M.R., Bouvet, P., 2013. Genetic characteristics of toxigenic Clostridia and toxin gene evolution. Toxicon. 75, 63–89.

Richmond, R.N., Hatheway, C.L., Kaufmann, A.F., 1978. Type C botulism in a dog. J. Am. Vet. Med. Assoc. 173, 202–203.

Rooney, J.P., Prickett, M.E., 1967. Shaker foal syndrome. Mod. Vet. Pract. 48, 44–45.

Rossetto, O., Pirazzini, M., Montecucco, C., 2014. Botulinum neurotoxins: genetic, structural and mechanistic insights. Nat. Rev. Microbiol. 12, 535–549.

Sato, S., 1987. Control of botulism in poultry flocks. In: Eklund, M.W., Dowell, V.R. (Eds.), Avian Botulism: An International Perspective. Charles C Thomas, Springfield, IL, pp. 349–356.

Schettler, C.H., 1979. *Clostridium botulinum* type C toxin infection in broiler farms in North West Germany. Berl. Munch Tierarztl Wscr. 92, 50–57.

Schoenbaum, M.A., Hall, S.M., Glock, R.D., et al., 2000. An outbreak of type C botulism in 12 horses and a mule. J. Am. Vet. Med. Assoc. 217, 365–368.

Shimizu, T., Kondo, H., 1978. Preparation and evaluation of botulinal type C toxoid for immunization of pheasants. In: Eklund, M.W., Dowell, V.R. (Eds.), Avian Botulism: An International Perspective. Charles C Thomas, Springfield, IL, pp. 357–369.

Simpson, L., 2013. The life history of a botulinum toxin molecule. Toxicon. 68, 40–59.

Smart, J.L., Robert, T.A., McCullagh, K.G., et al., 1980. An outbreak of type C botulism in captive monkeys. Vet. Rec. 107, 445–446.

Sprayberry, K.A., Carlson, G.P., 1997. Review of equine botulism. AAEP Proc. 43, 379–381.

Swerczek, T.W., 1980. Toxicoinfectious botulism in foals and adult horses. J. Am. Vet. Med. Assoc. 176 (3), 217–220.

Thyssen, A., Hirnet, D., Wolburg, H., et al., 2010. Ectopic vesicular neurotransmitter release along sensory axons mediates neurovascular coupling via glial calcium signaling. Proc. Natl. Acad. Sci. USA. 107, 15258–15263.

Trampel, D.W., Smith, S.R., Rocke, T.E., 2005. Toxicoinfectious botulism in commercial caponized chickens. Avian Dis. 49, 301–303.

Vaala, W.E., 1991. Diagnosis and treatment of *Clostridium botulinum* infection in foals: a review of 53 cases. Proc. 9th Am. Coll. Vet. Med. Forum. 9, 379–381.

Verderio, C., Grumelli, C., Raiteri, L., et al., 2007. Traffic of botulinum toxins A and E in excitatory and inhibitory neurons. Traffic. 8, 142–153.

Weiss, H.E., Wacker, R., Dalchow, W., 1982. Botulismus als ursache eines Massensterbens bei Wassergoveln. Teirarztl. Umschau. 37, 842–846.

Whitlock, R.H., 1996. Botulism, type C: experimental and field cases in horses. Equine Pract. 18, 11–17.

Whitlock, R.H., 2002. Botulism (shaker foals; forage poisoning). In: Smith, B.P. (Ed.), Large Animal Internal Medicine, third ed. Mosby, St. Louis, MO, pp. 1003–1008.

Whitlock, R.H., Buckley, C., 1997. Botulism. Vet. Clin. North Am. Equine Pract. 13, 107–128.

Whitlock, R.H., Buckley, C., Messick, J., 1989. Investigation of herd outbreaks of botulism in cattle and horses. Proc. Am. Assoc. Vet. Lab. Diagn. 40, 38.

Whitlock, R.H., Williams, J.M., 1999. Botulism toxicosis in cattle. Bovine Proc. 32, 44–53.

WHO: World Health Organisation, 2013. Botulism. Fact Sheet N8 270, http://www.who.int/mediacentre/factsheets/fs270/en/ (updated August 2013).

FURTHER READING

Cottrell, D.F., McGorum, B.C., Pearson, G.T., 1999. The neurology and enterology of equine grass sickness: a review of basic mechanisms. Neurogastroenterol. Motil. 11, 79–92.

Dover, N., Barash, J.R., Arnon, S.S., 2009. Novel *Clostridium botulinum* toxin gene arrangement with subtype A5 and partial subtype B3 botulinum neurotoxin genes. J. Clin. Microbiol. 47, 2349–2350.

Garrett, L.A., Brown, R., Poxton, I.R., 2002. A comparative of the intestinal microbiota of healthy horses and those suffering from equine grass sickness. Vet. Microbiol. 87, 81–88.

Hunter, L.C., Miller, J.K., Poxton, I.R., 1999. The association of *Clostridium botulinum* type C with equine grass sickness: a toxicoinfection? Equine Vet. J. 31 (6), 492–499.

McGorum, B.C., Kyles, K.W., Prince, D., et al., 2003. Clinicopathological features consistent with both botulism and grass sickness in a foal. Vet. Rec. 152, 334–336.

Sai, Y.C., Maditz, R., Kuo, C.L., et al., 2010. Targeting botulinum neurotoxin persistence by the ubiquitin-proteasome system. Proc. Natl. Acad. Sci. USA. 107, 16554–16559.

Simpson, L.L., 1981. The origin, structure, and pharmacological activity of botulinum toxin. Pharmacol. Rev. 33, 155–188.

Simpson, L.L., 1989. Peripheral actions of the botulinum toxins. In: Simpson, L.L. (Ed.), Botulinum Neurotoxin and Tetanus Toxin. Academic Press, New York, pp. 153–178.

Wang, Y., Sugiyama, H., 1984. Botulism in metronidazole-treated conventional adult mice challenged orogastrically with spores of *Clostridium botulinum* type A or B. Infect. Immun. 46, 715–719.

Chapter 56

Enterotoxins

Larry J. Thompson

INTRODUCTION

The term food poisoning can be used to describe the result of eating pathogenic organisms or toxins in contaminated food. The list of causative agents for food-borne illness can be quite lengthy, including infectious agents (e.g., bacteria, viruses, and parasites); natural toxins (e.g., bacterial toxins, mycotoxins, shellfish poisons, and plant poisons); and other contaminants (Mead et al., 1999). Veterinarians and owners often use the term garbage intoxication or garbage poisoning to describe the situation in which animals, especially dogs, eat discarded or otherwise poorly preserved foodstuffs and subsequently develop a syndrome composed mainly of severe vomiting and diarrhea. This chapter is focused on the effects of enterotoxins, which are defined as those bacterial exotoxins that are specific for the intestinal tract causing vomiting, diarrhea, and abdominal pain. Although many organisms produce enterotoxins (Vaishnavi, 1996; Fasano, 2002), those produced by *Staphylococcus aureus* and *Bacillus cereus* are stressed in this chapter. In contrast to enterotoxin, the term endotoxin is used to describe a cell-associated bacterial toxin, usually a lipopolysaccharide complex that is found on the outer membrane of Gram-negative bacteria. Endotoxins essentially remain associated with the cell wall until the destruction of the bacteria by autolysis, external lysis, or phagocytic digestion. Although all animals can be affected by endotoxin, horses are especially prone to disease complications due to endotoxemia (Werners et al., 2005).

BACKGROUND

This chapter focuses on the most common situations associated with enterotoxin exposures in veterinary medicine, namely dogs ingesting garbage, carrion, or other spoiled foodstuffs. Dogs readily consume a wide variety of such material, and owners often are unaware when their animal has had access to or has consumed foodstuffs of doubtful origin. Many owners have the mistaken opinion that dogs (and other animals) are not susceptible to food poisoning and thus may feed their pets foods that humans would rather not ingest. Discarded foodstuffs are often high in proteins and carbohydrates and serve as excellent substrates for the rapid growth of bacteria, often with enterotoxin release. Instances of garbage intoxication increase during warm weather and during major holidays when increased food is prepared and discarded. Under conditions of warm temperatures and adequate moisture, these discarded foodstuffs can have an almost explosive growth of bacteria, especially *S. aureus* and *B. cereus*, which are the most common causes of enterotoxin-related food poisonings in humans. Although a great deal of time and energy has been expended by public health officials in the pursuit of the origin and control of food poisonings in humans, there is a paucity of specific information concerning animals.

PHARMACOKINETICS AND MECHANISM OF ACTION

S. aureus is a facultative anaerobic Gram-positive coccus that may be single, paired, or in a grape-like cluster. *S. aureus* does not form spores and thus contamination may be avoided by proper heat treatment of food to kill the bacteria. *S. aureus* is able to grow in a wide range of temperatures (7–48.5°C), with an optimum range from 30°C to 37°C. *S. aureus* can also grow over a wide pH range (4.2–9.3) and can tolerate sodium chloride concentrations of up to 15%. These characteristics allow it to grow in a wide variety of foodstuffs and in situations of discarded food. *S. aureus* is also an important infective pathogen and can easily be found in the nostrils and on the skin of most mammals (Le Loir et al., 2003). A high prevalence of enterotoxigenic *S. aureus* was reported for pet dogs and cats, with the highest incidence of positives (10%) being isolated from the mouths of dogs (Abdel-moein and Samir, 2011). At least 14 different *Staphylococcal* enterotoxin (SE) types have been found,

Veterinary Toxicology. DOI: http://dx.doi.org/10.1016/B978-0-12-811410-0.00056-8

and they are best described as short proteins secreted by the cell into the growth matrix (Balaban and Rasooly, 2000). All SE types are water soluble, very heat resistant, and resist most proteolytic enzymes, such as trypsin and pepsin, which make it possible for them to travel through the digestive tract to their site of action. Thus, all SE types resist the conditions that could easily destroy the bacteria that produced them. SEs are thought to have a direct effect on the intestinal epithelium and on the vagus nerve to cause stimulation of the emetic center as well as increasing peristalsis. Foods that are frequently associated with staphylococcal food poisoning include meat and meat products; poultry and egg products; salads such as egg, tuna, chicken, potato, and macaroni; bakery products such as cream-filled pastries; and milk and other dairy products. An example of a proverbial high-risk food is the potato salad at a summer picnic left out for several hours without refrigeration.

B. cereus is in the family Bacillaceae, which are all Gram-positive rod-shaped bacteria that form endospores. The family has two main divisions: the anaerobic spore-forming bacteria of the genus *Clostridium* and the aerobic or facultatively anaerobic spore-forming bacteria of the genus *Bacillus*. *B. cereus* is a primary inhabitant of soils and contaminates almost all agricultural products. It is also routinely involved in the contamination and spoilage of food products. *B. cereus* can also be involved in wound, eye, or systemic infections. *B. cereus* food poisoning is generally described as having two types of illness caused by different metabolites. The diarrheal type of illness is caused by one or several heat-labile, high-molecular-weight proteins, whereas the vomiting (emetic) type of illness is believed to be caused by a low-molecular-weight, heat-stable peptide that has been named cereulide (Schoeni and Wong, 2005). In humans, the diarrheal syndrome is thought to be the consequence of a food-borne infection with enterotoxic *B. cereus* following the observation that the diarrheal enterotoxins are produced during the vegetative growth of *B. cereus* in the small intestine. *B. cereus* food poisoning has been classically associated with fried rice and other cooked rice dishes because the bacteria is frequently present in uncooked rice and heat-resistant spores may survive cooking. If cooked rice is subsequently held at room temperature, vegetative forms multiply, and a heat-stable toxin is produced that can survive brief heating, such as stir frying. *B. cereus* food poisoning can also be associated with meat- or vegetable-containing foods after cooking where the food was held above room temperature for a prolonged period of time. Dogs have been shown to be susceptible to *B. cereus* food poisoning (Chastain and Harris, 1974) with watery diarrhea reported as the most consistent manifestation.

TOXICITY

The symptoms of staphylococcal food poisoning occur in humans when as little as 100 ng of enterotoxin is ingested (Bennett, 2005). There is a paucity of information on the dose of individual enterotoxins that will cause clinical signs in common domestic animals. The first and most common clinical sign in dogs is vomiting, which usually occurs within 2 or 3 h following ingestion. This can often suffice to remove enough contaminated food from the gastrointestinal tract to prevent the development of more severe clinical signs. However, vomiting can be protracted and lead to fluid and electrolyte abnormalities. Diarrhea can often develop within 2–48 h following ingestion of contaminated food and can be severe, sometimes bloody. The combination of both vomiting and diarrhea in the affected animal can quickly lead to profound fluid and electrolyte abnormalities. The animal may exhibit tenderness to the abdomen or the stomach and the intestinal tract can be distended with gas (Coppock and Mostrom, 1986).

The emetic form of *B. cereus* food poisoning is characterized in humans by an acute attack of nausea and vomiting, which occurs within 1–5 h after consumption of contaminated food. Diarrhea is not a common feature in this type of illness. In humans, the diarrheal syndrome is characterized by abdominal pain, abdominal cramping, and diarrhea that often can be very watery. There is an incubation period of 4–16 h, and clinical signs can persist for 12–24 h. Nausea may accompany the diarrhea, but vomiting rarely occurs.

Testing for enterotoxins requires specialized laboratory techniques and methods of detection have greatly expanded (Wu et al., 2016).

TREATMENT

It is important to remember three factors when a food-borne problem is included in the differential diagnosis: the presenting clinical signs, the possible exposure to foodstuffs not normally included in the animal's diet, and the interval between exposure and onset of clinical problems. Some of these may not be known at the time of initial presentation but should be explored as the case is developed.

In general, treatment of garbage intoxication in animals should be directed at correcting the fluid and electrolyte abnormalities along with considerations of acid–base balance. As mentioned previously, noncomplicated cases will often resolve within hours of presentation with only supportive care. However, because the clinical signs can be similar to those of more serious conditions, a more thorough diagnostic workup (e.g., survey abdominal radiographs) and close observation should always be considered. Because cases most often present following several vomiting episodes, the use of emetics is usually not indicated. In the case of protracted vomiting, the judicious use of antiemetics should be considered. Administration of activated charcoal is not required for known garbage intoxications, but many clinicians will use it as part of a general approach to these cases. Activated charcoal should not be given to dehydrated animals unless fluid administration is also initiated. Antibiotics are not indicated in uncomplicated cases of garbage intoxication.

CONCLUDING REMARKS

This chapter describes garbage intoxication with emphasis on preformed enterotoxins as the causative agents. The great number of other types of food-borne illnesses, including infectious agents and toxins, require other diagnostic and treatment considerations.

REFERENCES

Abdel-moein, K.A., Samir, A., 2011. Isolation of enterotoxigenic *Staphylococcus aureus* from pet dogs and cats: a public health implication. Vector Borne Zoonotic Dis. 11, 627–629.

Balaban, N., Rasooly, A., 2000. Staphylococcal enterotoxins. Int. J. Food Microbiol. 61, 1–10.

Bennett, R.W., 2005. Staphylococcal enterotoxin and its rapid identification in foods by enzyme-linked immunosorbent assay-based methodology. J. Food Protect. 68, 1264–1270.

Chastain, C.B., Harris, D.L., 1974. Association of *Bacillus cereus* with food poisoning in dogs. J. Am. Vet. Med. Assoc. 164, 489–490.

Coppock, R.W., Mostrom, M.S., 1986. Intoxication due to contaminated garbage, food, and water. In: Kirk, R.W. (Ed.), Current Veterinary Therapy IX: Small Animal Practice. Saunders, Philadelphia, PA, pp. 221–225.

Fasano, A., 2002. Toxins and the gut: role in human disease. Gut. 50, 9–14.

Le Loir, Y., Baron, F., Gautier, M., 2003. *Staphylococcus aureus* and food poisoning. Genet. Mol. Res. 2, 63–76.

Mead, P.S., Slutsker, L., Dietz, V., et al., 1999. Food-related illness and death in the United States. Emerg. Infect. Dis. 5, 607–625.

Schoeni, J.L., Wong, A.C.L., 2005. *Bacillus cereus* food poisoning and its toxins. J. Food Protect. 68, 636–648.

Vaishnavi, C., 1996. Bacterial enterotoxins. Trop. Gastroenterol. 17, 160–164.

Werners, A.H., Bull, S., Fink-Gremmels, J., 2005. Endotoxaemia: a review with implications for the horse. Equine Vet. J. 37, 371–383.

Wu, S., Duan, N., Gu, H., et al., 2016. A review of the methods for detection of *Staphylococcus aureus* enterotoxins. Toxins (Basel). 8, 176–196.

Chapter 57

Cyanobacterial (Blue-Green Algae) Toxins

Birgit Puschner

INTRODUCTION

Freshwater cyanobacterial blooms hold the potential to significantly impact the health of both animal and human populations utilizing surface waters for drinking water, daily living, and recreation worldwide. In addition to the often visually stunning nature of these proliferations of cyanobacterial species, the blooms can result in the production of a variety of compounds, from malodorous ones that affect the taste of the water to dermal and gastrointestinal irritants and severe neurotoxicants, gastrointestinal toxicants, and hepatotoxicants. Among the 2000 species identified through morphological criteria, more than 80 are known to be toxigenic, and as assays for detection and toxicity continue to improve, this number will continue to grow. George Francis first reported a toxigenic bloom in the journal *Nature* in 1878. He reported a "poisonous Australian lake" with "a thick scum like green oil paint" and vividly described acute intoxications of sheep, horses, dogs, and pigs. Analysis of archeological evidence coupled with evolving understanding of modern blooms have begun to implicate the role of cyanotoxin poisoning in more widespread mammalian die-offs dating back to the Pleistocene age (i.e., approximately 150,000 years BC; Braun and Pfeiffer, 2002), and even a controversial hypothesis about the role of cyanobacteria in the various mass extinction events has begun to emerge (Castle and Rodgers, 2009).

Since Francis's publication in 1878, numerous case reports describing animal morbidity and mortality after exposure to cyanotoxins have been published (Bautista et al., 2015; Naegeli et al., 1997; Puschner et al., 1998, 2008, 2010; Gugger et al., 2005; Moore et al., 2016; Nasri et al., 2008; Wood et al., 2010). The frequency of cyanotoxins poisoning in animals is likely underreported due to lack of methods to confirm exposure; in addition, geographical distribution of these case reports is likely biased by available resources. Diagnostic confirmation of suspect cyanotoxin poisoning cases of humans and animals requires extensive effort from both toxicologists and clinicians, and resources are often not readily available. New cyanotoxins are continuously being discovered, and oral bioavailability and toxicity data are often unavailable. It is probable that poisonings are more common in animals than in humans due to animals' greater direct dependence and contact with surface waters.

Pursuant to several major human intoxications in Australia, Europe, and Brazil (Falconer and Humpage, 2005), in 1998 the World Health Organization (WHO) proposed a guidance value for the maximum permissible concentration of 1 μg/L free and cell bound MC-LR in potable water sources for microcystin-LR, the most commonly reported cyanotoxin worldwide. Water sanitation agencies in many countries in Europe, North America (Canada), South America (Brazil), and Oceania (Australia and New Zealand) adopted these guidelines. In addition, as a result of a tragedy in 1996 in which more than 100 patients at a hemodialysis clinic received inadequately treated drinking water (Azevedo et al., 2002), most of whom developed acute liver failure as a result of being exposed to cyanotoxins, Brazil has adopted more comprehensive and stringent guidelines to include other cyanotoxins (Burch, 2008). Awareness of imminent health risks for wild and domestic terrestrial vertebrates has increased during approximately the past decade, in part due to veterinary case reports; however, the extent and heterogeneity of the impact are still far from understood. Veterinarians thus have the opportunity to substantially deepen the understanding of the impact of these cyanotoxins on animal and human populations alike.

BACKGROUND

Cyanobacterial blooms are predicted to become more severe and widespread with climate change if land use practices are not altered to minimize nutrient input to

Veterinary Toxicology. DOI: http://dx.doi.org/10.1016/B978-0-12-811410-0.00057-X

surface waters (Pearl et al., 2016). Particularly runoff from nitrogen- and phosphorus-rich fertilizers, soaps, and waste products has led to significant eutrophication worldwide (>40% in Europe, Asia, and America) (Bartram et al., 1999; Smith, 2003). As a major consequence of shifting nutrient additions, previously nutrient-limited photosynthetic microorganisms proliferate. Depending on the limitations of the system and the types of nutrients added, a few species (generally one or two) outcompete the others, thereby considerably reducing the heterogeneity of the phytoplankton community. In such conditions, cyanobacteria often predominate through adaptive processes, and substantial shifts in the microscopic and macroscopic food web may occur. Anoxic conditions can also result in fish kills, and falling debris from blooms can have profound impacts on the invertebrates in the sediment below (Pearl et al., 2001; Havens, 2008).

Among the oldest microorganisms, these oxygenic photosynthetic prokaryotes may be organized as individual cells (e.g., *Synechococcus*), filaments (e.g., *Planktothrix*), or colonies (e.g., *Microcystis*). More than 2000 cyanobacterial species belong to four orders based on morphological and morphometric criteria in botanical code (Anagnostidis and Komarek, 1985); however, classification based on bacterial code defines five sections through combined use of genetic data, morphological criteria, and cellular fission (Rippka et al., 1979).

Both pelagic (suspended in the water column) and benthic (along the bottom) cyanobacteria can proliferate into blooms. Pelagic blooms, which are easier to visually detect because of the evident scum formation at the surface, usually occur in mesotrophic and eutrophic ecosystems (concentrations in phosphorus >30 μg/L), during the summer, in water temperatures greater than 20°C, and in low turbulence. Proliferations of benthic species generally occur during the summer on the surfaces of sediments, stones, or macrophytes in small oligotrophic rivers or in oligotrophic lakes (Mez et al., 1997).

In the past, most cases were diagnosed by positive identification of the algae in the suspect water source along with the occurrence of consistent clinical signs and pathological findings. However, new analytical methods can now be applied to detect toxins in biological specimens of animals or humans with suspect exposure to toxic algal blooms Fig. 57.1illustrates the wide variety in chemical structures of cyanotoxins and the need for specific detection methods (Yuan et al., 2006; Humbert, 2010). These capabilities will allow for in-depth diagnostic investigations and a better estimate of the true frequency of blue-green algae poisonings in livestock, pets, and wildlife. Table 57.1 provides an overview of cyanobacterial species known to produce a large number of toxins. Some species can produce a variety of cyanotoxins and thus it is difficult to predict the nature and the level of the toxin production during a bloom event. This chapter focuses on the several types of cyanotoxins known to have the greatest impact on veterinary species and presents the current understanding of their toxic mechanisms, toxicokinetics, and diagnostic and therapeutic approaches with a focus on veterinary medicine.

MICROCYSTINS

Produced by multiple cyanobacteria, including species within the genera *Microcystis*, *Anabaena*, *Planktothrix*, *Nostoc*, *Oscillatoria*, and *Anabaenopsis*, microcystins have been detected worldwide (Fromme et al., 2000; Hitzfeld et al., 2000; Ballot et al., 2004; Briand et al., 2005; Karlsson et al., 2005a; Ndetei and Muhandiki, 2005; Agrawal et al., 2006; Chatziefthimiou et al., 2014). Not all strains are capable of producing microcystins. Microcystins were responsible for the 2014 drinking water advisory in Toledo, OH (Bullerjahn et al., 2016). In recent years, a useful diagnostic tool to test for the presence of toxin-producing genes has emerged (Hisbergues et al., 2003). Although the reason for production is not understood, environmental factors, such as pH, nutrient concentrations, and water temperature, clearly trigger production, increasing with water temperature, elevated concentrations of phosphorus and nitrogen, iron limitation, and globally with the growth rate (Briand et al., 2005; Downing et al., 2005; Sevilla et al., 2008). Microcystin concentrations may be highest when the growth of the cyanobacteria is high, but toxin concentrations do not necessarily correlate with cell count, and toxins may occur any time of the year. Although predominantly found in freshwater, microcystin-producing blooms have also been described in saline ecosystems (Atkins et al., 2001; Carmichael and Li, 2006). Beyond exposure to microcystin-contaminated water, animals are at risk for microcystin exposure through blue-green algae containing dietary supplements (Bautista et al., 2015; Mittelman et al., 2016).

Potent cyclic heptapeptides causing acute hepatotoxicosis in mammals, microcystins have also been demonstrated to be toxic to reptiles, amphibians, and aquatic species, as well as invertebrates and even plant species (McElhiney et al., 2001; Malbrouck and Kestemont, 2006; Nasri et al., 2008; Amado and Monserrat, 2010). In freshwater, the toxins are retained inside the cyanobacteria and only released upon cell damage, lysis, and death; destruction of algal mats (either naturally or through the application of herbicides) may result in a pulse of microcystin release following destruction of the individual cell walls. After oral exposure to microcystin-containing algae, the acidic environment of the stomach can result in the release of microcystins. Commercially available blue-green algae food supplements also present a potential route of oral exposure (Schaeffer et al., 1999; Dietrich and Hoeger, 2005).

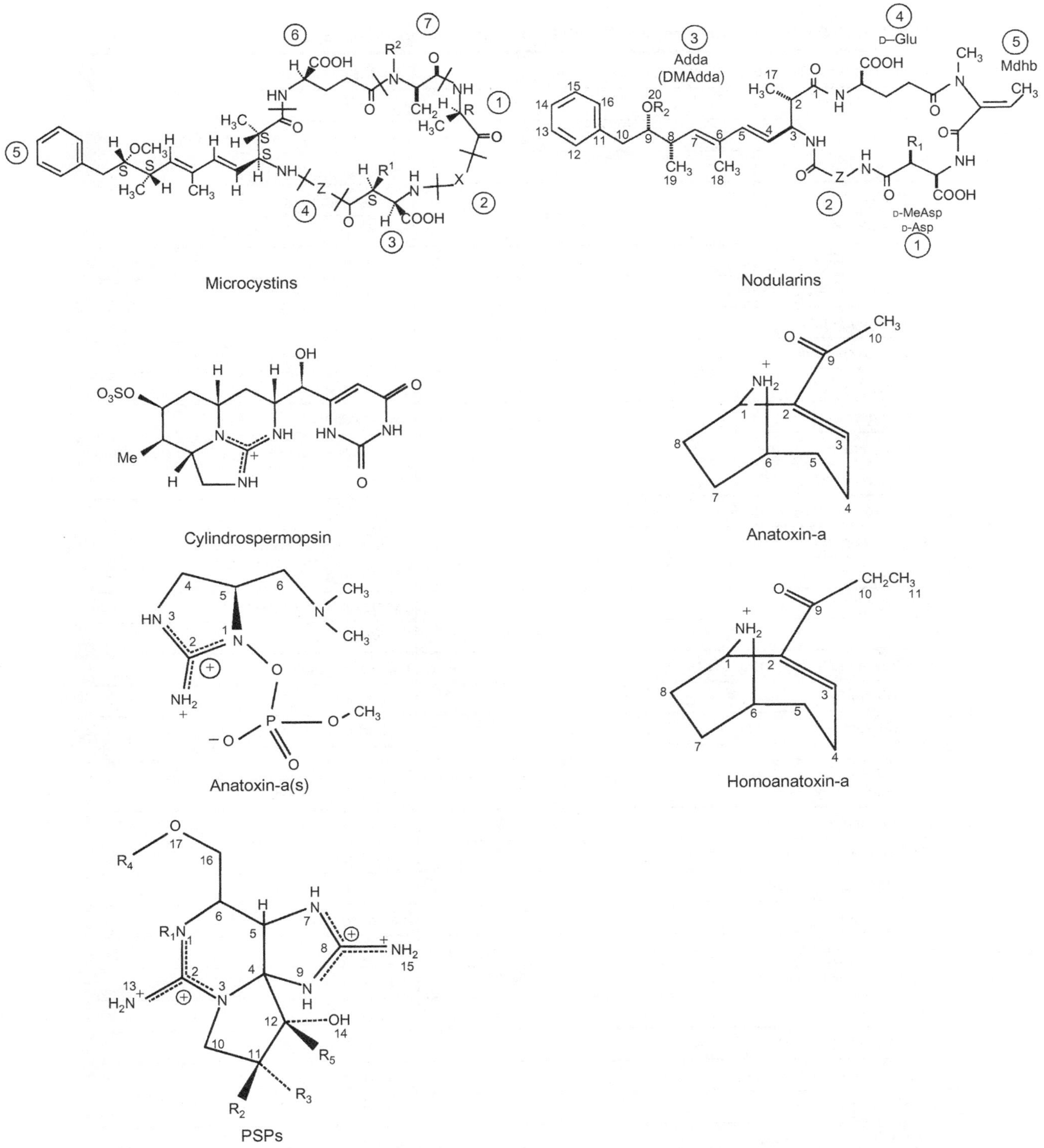
Microcystins
Adda
(DMAdda)
D–Glu
Mdhb
D-MeAsp
D-Asp
Nodularins
Cylindrospermopsin
Anatoxin-a
Anatoxin-a(s)
Homoanatoxin-a
PSPs

FIGURE 57.1 Structural formulas of cyanobacterial toxins.

More than 100 different structural variants of microcystins have been identified from various genera of cyanobacteria (Luukkainen et al., 1994; Lawton et al., 1995; Welker and von Döhren, 2006). The shared structure involves an amino acid called ADDA (3-amino-9-methoxy-2,6,8-trimethyl-10-phenyldeca; 4,6-dienoic acid) and six other amino acids, including two variable positions that designate the congener. The most extensively studied,

TABLE 57.1 Potential Toxins Produced by the Different Cyanobacterial Species

Cyanobacterial Species	Toxins
Anabena bergii	Cylindrospermopsin
Anabaena circinalis	Anatoxin-a, saxitoxins, microcystins
Anabaena flos-aquae	Anatoxins, microcystins
Anabaena lappoinica	Cylindrospermopsin
Anabaena lemmermanni	Microcystins, anatoxin-a(s)
Anabaena macrospora	Anatoxin-a
Anabaena medotae	Anatoxin-a
Anabaena planctonica	Anatoxin-a
Anabaena spiroides	Anatoxin-a, microcystins
Anabaena sp.	Anatoxin-a
Anabaenopsis milleri	Microcystins
Aphanizomenon flos-aquae	Anatoxin-a, saxitoxins, cylindrospermopsin
Aphanizomenon gracile	Saxitoxins
Aphanizomenon issatschenkoi	Saxitoxins, anatoxin-a
Aphanizomenon ovalisporum	Cylindrospermopsin
Aphanizomenon sp.	Anatoxin-a
Arthrospira fusiformis	Anatoxin-a, microcystin-YR
Calothrix crustacean	Aplysiatoxin
Coelosphaerium kuetzingianum	Neuro-/hepatotoxins
Cyanobium bacillare	Microcystins
Cylindrospermopsis raciborskii	Cylindrospermopsin, saxitoxins
Cylindrospermum sp.	Anatoxin-a
Fisherella epiphytica	Neuro-/hepatotoxins
Geitlerinema acutissmum	Dermatotoxins
Geitlerinema pseudacutissimum	Dermatotoxins
Gloeottrichia echinulata	Neuro-/hepatotoxins
Hapalosiphon fontinalis	Neuro-/hepatotoxins
Hapalosiphon hibernicus	Microcystins
Hormothanmnion enteromorphoides	Cytotoxin, hepatotoxins
Limnothrix redekei	Microcystins
Lyngbya gracilis	Debromoaplysiatoxin
Lyngbya majuscula	Lyngbyatoxin-a
Lyngbya wollei	Saxitoxins
Microcystis aeruginosa	Microcystins
Microcystis botrys	Microcystins
Microcystis farlowian	Ichtyotoxin
Microcystis flos-aquae	Microcystins
Microcystis panniformis	Microcystins

(*Continued*)

TABLE 57.1 (Continued)

Cyanobacterial Species	Toxins
Microcystis viridis	Microcystins, microviridin
Microcystis wesenbergii	Microcystins
Microcystis sp.	Anatoxin-a
Nodularia spumigena	Nodularins
Nostoc linckia	Microcystins
Nostoc muscorum	Aplysiatoxin
Nostoc paludosum	Microcystins
Nostoc rivulare	Microcystins
Nostoc zettrstedrii	Microcystins
Nostoc sp.	Microcystins
Oscillatoria formosa	Homoanatoxin-a
Oscillatoria limosa	Microcystins
Oscillatoria perornata	Microcystins
Oscillatoria tenuis	Microcystins
Oscillatoria nigroviridis	Oscillatoxin-a
Oscillatoria sp.	Anatoxin-a
Phormidium favosum	Anatoxin-a
Planktothrix agardhii	Microcystins, anatoxin
Planktothrix isothrix	Microcystins, anatoxin
Planktothrix mougeotii	Microcystins
Planktothrix rubescens	Microcystins
Planktothrix sp.	Anatoxin-a
Pseudanabaena sp.	Neurotoxin
Radiocystis fernandoi	Microcystins
Radiocystis curvata	Cylindrospermopsin
Radphidiopsis curvata	Cylindrospermopsin
Raphidiopsis mediterranea	Homoanatoxin-a
Schizothrix calcicola	Aplysiatoxins
Scytonema mirabile	Antimicrobial
Scytonema ocellatum	Scytophycin
Scytonema pseudohofmannii	Scytophycin
Schizothrix calcicola	Aplysiatoxins
Scytonema hofmanni	Scytophycins a and b
Scytonema pseudohofmanni	Scytophycins a and b
Snowella lacustris	Microcystin
Stigonematales sp.	BMAA
Symploca muscorum	Aplysiatoxin
Synechococcus sp. (marine species)	Hemolysins

(Continued)

TABLE 57.1 (Continued)

Cyanobacterial Species	Toxins
Synechocystis spp.	Anatoxin-a, microcystins
Tolypothix byssoidea	Cytotoxin
Trichodesmium erythraeum	Neurotoxin
Trichodesmium thiebautii	Microcystins, neurotoxins
Trichormus variablis	Anatoxin-a
Umezakia natans	Cylindrospermopsin
Woronichinia naegeliana	Anatoxin-a

microcystin-LR, has been found worldwide and has caused acute, lethal hepatotoxicoses in farm animals (Carbis et al., 1994; Mez et al., 1997; Puschner et al., 1998) and hepatic injury in humans (Azevedo et al., 2002; Rao et al., 2002).

Pharmacokinetics/Toxicokinetics

Despite the abundant literature on microcystins, understanding of pharmacokinetics remains limited, particularly with regard to potential species variations. Most studies have been conducted in mice after intravenous (i.v.) and intraperitoneal (i.p.) administration of cyanobacteria, their filtrates, and, in some instances, purified microcystins. After i.v. and i.p. administration in mice and rats, microcystins are rapidly distributed to the liver (Falconer et al., 1986; Robinson et al., 1991). Plasma half-lives of microcystin-LR in mice after i.v. administration were 0.8 and 6.9 min for the alpha and beta phases of elimination (Robinson et al., 1991). Interestingly, the hepatic concentration of ^{3}H-microcystin-LR remained constant throughout the 6-day study, indicating accumulation in this target organ. This study also demonstrated that approximately 9% and 14% of the dose was excreted in urine and feces, respectively, after 12 h, with 60% of it being excreted unchanged. Additional studies in swine have also indicated that the majority is excreted unchanged, with only two metabolites detected; biliary excretion is also noted after less than 1 h of i.v. administration (Stotts et al., 1997). The exact route of metabolism is yet to be defined, but glutathione and cysteine conjugation have been identified and may represent major detoxification pathways (Kondo et al., 1996; Pflugmacher et al., 1998). Other metabolites have been identified in vivo and in vitro, but further work is needed to define their roles.

Data on bioavailability for microcystins are needed to better evaluate risk from oral ingestion. Absorption occurs in the small intestine (Ito et al., 2000); thus, the integrity of the intestinal mucosa can significantly impact the degree of absorption (Zeller et al., 2011). Altered cell permeability of the small intestine in aged mice lends them more susceptible than young animals (Ito et al., 1997). Once absorbed, microcystins are rapidly distributed to the liver (Runnegar et al., 1981; Fischer et al., 2000), but they can also reach lung, heart, and capillaries (Ito et al., 2000). Based on radiolabeled experiments in which microcystins were administered i.v. in Wistar rats, uptake into the kidney appears to be important for excretion. Results of uptake experiments with radiolabeled dihydro-MC-LR demonstrated that OATP1B1 (organic anion transporter protein) and OATP1B3 are involved in uptake of MC-LR (Seithel et al., 2007). Studies in fish (i.v.) have demonstrated that the liver is the primary target, followed by kidney and gonads, although uptake does occur into muscle tissue and cardiovascular effects are observed (Malbrouck and Kestemont, 2006). Absorption of microcystin via the respiratory route (Ito et al., 2001) has been demonstrated to lead to lethality in mice and also induce damage to nasal epithelium at lower exposures (Benson et al., 2005), thus posing a threat from aerosolization of the compound.

Mechanism of Action

Specifically toxic to liver, microcystins cause severe hepatomegaly macroscopically and progressive centrilobular hepatocyte rounding, dissociation, and necrosis microscopically. Breakdown of the sinusoidal endothelium and intrahepatic hemorrhage ultimately result in death (Hooser et al., 1991a; Falconer and Yeung, 1992). Unable to permeate cell membranes, microcystins enter hepatocytes via the bile acid transporter mechanism (Hooser et al., 1991b). Once inside the hepatocytes, microcystins are potent inhibitors of protein phosphatases

1 and 2A (Falconer and Yeung, 1992; Runnegar et al., 1993). The disruption of the cytoskeletal components and the associated rearrangement of filamentous actin within hepatocytes account for the morphological changes, although other mechanisms play a role in the development of liver lesions. Microcystins induce apoptosis of hepatocytes via induction of free radical formation and mitochondrial alterations (Ding and Ong, 2003). A single-dose i.v. in rats demonstrated an increase in liver sphingolipid levels at higher doses (implicating ceramide-mediated apoptosis), a dose-dependent decreased PP2A expression, and ultimately a dose-dependent decreased expression of Bcl2 family proteins, involved in cell cycle/apoptosis regulation (Billam et al., 2008). The role of oxidative stress has become increasingly apparent, and the ultimate toxic effect may depend on the ability of antioxidant pathways to counter the stressors (Ding and Ong, 2003; Jayaraj et al., 2006; Xiong et al., 2010). In addition, microcystins are classified as tumor-promoting compounds (Humpage and Falconer, 1999). Investigations have indicated the role of protooncogenes in this tumorigenesis, hypothesized to be a sequelae of dysregulation of phosphorylation (Li et al., 2009). Several studies have demonstrated the ability of microcystins to induce DNA damage in liver cells (Zegura et al., 2011).

Clinical signs of microcystin poisoning have been described in a number of reports in livestock, humans, and wildlife in the United States (DeVries et al., 1993; Galey et al., 1987; Puschner et al., 1998) and other countries (Done and Bain, 1993; Van Halderen et al., 1995; Mez et al., 1997; Naegeli et al., 1997; Azevedo et al., 2002; Ballot et al., 2004; Ndetei and Muhandiki, 2005; Handeland and Østensvik, 2010; Wood et al., 2010). Interestingly, laboratory animals select water with microcystin-producing strains of cyanobacteria over a water source with nontoxic strains (Lopez Rodas and Costas, 1999), suggesting an increased risk for toxicosis in animals due to behavioral preferences. Microcystin intoxication should be suspected in cases of acute hepatotoxicosis with clinical signs of diarrhea, vomiting, weakness, pale mucous membranes, and shock. Although most animals die within a few hours of exposure, some animals may live for several hours and develop hyperkalemia, hypoglycemia, nervousness, recumbency, and convulsions. Animals that survive the acute intoxication may develop hepatogenous photosensitization. Nephrotoxic effects have been described in laboratory animals after chronic microcystin exposure (Milutinovic et al., 2003). Evidence suggests potential suppression of immune function at sublethal exposures (Shi et al., 2004). Evidence also suggests MC-LR causing thyroid dysfunction in mice (Zhao et al., 2015). In humans, primary liver cancer as well as colorectal cancer have been associated with microcystin-contaminated drinking water (Ueno et al., 1996; Zhou et al., 2002). In mice, subchronic exposure i. p. of microcystin-LR (20 μg/kg) causes the appearance of hepatic nodules, a characteristic not observed after oral subchronic administration (Ito et al., 1997).

Toxicity

The lethal doses 50 (LD_{50}s) for microcystins vary between 50 μg/kg and 11 mg/kg, depending on the microcystin analog, the species affected, and the route of administration. In mice, the oral LD_{50} value for microcystin-LR is 10.9 mg/kg, whereas the i.p. LD_{50} is 50 μg/kg. Because most blooms contain a number of structural variants of microcystins, it is difficult to estimate the toxicity potential of a bloom. The no-observed-adverse-effect level for orally administered microcystin-LR to mice is 40 μg/kg/day (Fawell et al., 1994). In pigs, the lowest-observed-adverse-effect level for microcystin-LR is 100 μg/kg/day (Falconer et al., 1994), and in rat it is 50 μg/kg/day (Heinze, 1999). WHO set the tolerable daily intake (TDI) for human ingestion of microcystin-LR at 0.04 μg/kg/day (Kuiper-Goodman et al., 1999). The potential risk to humans by ingesting food products derived from animals exposed to microcystins was evaluated in beef (Orr et al., 2003) and dairy cattle (Orr et al., 2001). Based on these studies, it is unlikely that consumption of milk, meat, or liver poses a significant health risk to humans. It might be prudent to establish specific guidelines for nonlethal, chronic microcystin exposure in livestock.

Treatment

No specific antidote for microcystins exists. The rapid onset of acute hepatotoxicosis renders therapeutic intervention quite difficult, and mortality rates are very high. In addition, despite the evaluation of numerous treatment options, no specific therapy has been proven to be effective. The most promising strategy appears to be prevention of uptake into hepatocytes through the administration of compounds that may compete for the specific transporters associated with microcystin uptake; administration of the antibiotic rifampin (i.p.) in mice effectively reduced mortality after exposure (i.p.) to microcystin-LR (Hermansky et al., 1991). By contrast, other compounds, such as glutathione, silymarin, and cyclosporine A, were only beneficial if administered as a prophylactic (Hermansky et al., 1991; Rao et al., 2004). These compounds may help reduce microcystin toxicity in chronic exposure scenarios. Due to the role of oxidative stress, antioxidants such as vitamin E, selenium, and green tea polyphenols also appear to be beneficial prophylactically (Gehringer et al., 2003a,b; Jayaraj et al., 2007; Xu et al., 2007). Although the adsorption of microcystins by activated charcoal was used successfully to decontaminate drinking water (Warhurst et al., 1997), this decontamination procedure was not protective in mice dosed with microcystins (Mereish and Solow, 1989); no data are available for other species.

Diagnosis of microcystin toxicosis is corroborated by identification of microcystin-containing water in the environment of the animal. Identification of algae material in water and gastric contents is an important component of the diagnostic workup but does not confirm intoxication. As described previously, the toxicity of the cyanobacteria is strain specific, and morphological observations alone cannot predict the hazard level, but polymerase chain reaction detection of microcystin-producing genes can help identify a potentially culpable species. Detection of microcystins in gastric contents is confirmatory, but these tests are not routinely available at diagnostic laboratories and are limited to a few structural variants. In the past, the mouse bioassay was used to determine the toxicity of crude algal biomass in suspicious blue-green algae poisonings. Although many assays are available to analyze water samples for microcystins (Maizels and Budde, 2004; McElhiney and Lawton, 2005; Frias et al., 2006), there are only limited methods available to reliably and accurately detect microcystins in biological specimens collected from animals suspected to have died from microcystin intoxication (Bogialli et al., 2005; Karlsson et al., 2005b; Chen et al., 2009). An electrospray ionization liquid chromatography–mass spectrometry method has been developed to determine the bound microcystin concentrations in animal tissues, which provides an estimate of the total microcystin burden in exposed animals (Ott and Carmichael, 2006).

Differential diagnoses in animals with a clinical presentation of liver failure include other toxic ingestions, such as amanitins, cocklebur, cycad palm, aflatoxin, xylitol, certain heavy metals, and acetaminophen overdose. Careful evaluation of the history, feed, and environment of the animal can help eliminate most of the toxicant differentials on the list.

ANATOXINS

Anatoxins are mainly produced by cyanobacteria in the *Anabaena* genus (Beltran and Neilan, 2000) but also by other genera, such as *Plantkothrix*, *Oscillatoria*, *Microcystis*, *Aphanizomenon*, *Cylindrospermum*, and *Phormidium*. Only few data exist about factors resulting in anatoxin-a production (Méjean et al., 2014; Wood et al., 2017) and indicate the impact of multiple physicochemical variables. Reports of anatoxin poisoning are less frequent than those of microcystin toxicosis; however, poisoning has occurred worldwide (Edwards et al., 1992; Gunn et al., 1992; Beltran and Neilan, 2000; Fromme et al., 2000; Gugger et al., 2005; Yang and Boyer, 2005; Wood et al., 2007; Puschner et al., 2008, 2010). Anatoxins are neurotoxins and can generally be divided into anatoxin-a, homoanatoxin-a, and anatoxin-a(s). Anatoxin-a is a secondary amine and has been detected in blooms worldwide. Homoanatoxin-a is a methyl derivative of anatoxin-a and has been identified in blooms in Japan (Namikoshi et al., 2004), Ireland (Furey et al., 2003), Sweden (Skulberg et al., 1992), and New Zealand (Wood et al., 2007). Anatoxin-a(s) is a unique *N*-hydroxyguanidine methyl phosphate ester that has been detected in the Americas (Monserrat et al., 2001) and Europe (Henriksen et al., 1997). Commercially available blue-green algae dietary supplements also represent a potential source (Rellán et al., 2009).

Pharmacokinetics/Toxicokinetics

Definite data on the toxicokinetics of anatoxin-a, homoanatoxin-a, and anatoxin-a(s) have not been established. Based on the rapid onset of clinical signs after oral exposure, rapid absorption of the toxins is suspected. Anatoxin-a has been detected in the urine and bile of a poisoned dog, confirming that anatoxin-a is, at least in part, excreted unchanged in urine and bile (Puschner et al., 2010).

Mechanism of Action

Anatoxin-a is a potent cholinergic agonist at nicotinic acetylcholine receptors (nAChRs) in neurons and at neuromuscular junctions (NMJs) (Thomas et al., 1993). Anatoxin-a has two enantiomers, with (+)anatoxin-a having a higher binding affinity than the (−) form (Spivak et al., 1980; Zhang and Nordberg, 1993). Compared to nicotine, anatoxin-a is approximately 20 times more potent than acetylcholine. After continuous electrical stimulation at the NMJs, a nerve block may follow and result in death due to respiratory paralysis. Furthermore, anatoxin-a has modulatory action at presynaptic nAChRs, which can lead to dopamine as well as noradrenaline release (Barik and Wonnacott, 2006; Campos et al., 2010). Clinical signs of anatoxin-a poisoning include a rapid onset of rigidity and muscle tremors followed by convulsions, paralysis, respiratory failure, cyanosis, and death. Death usually occurs within minutes to a few hours. Anatoxin-a poisonings have been reported in dogs in Europe (Edwards et al., 1992; Gunn et al., 1992; James et al., 1997; Gugger et al., 2005) and the United States (Puschner et al., 2008, 2010). Anatoxin-a is also considered a contributing factor in the deaths of Lesser Flamingos in Kenya (Krienitz et al., 2003). Homoanatoxin-a is a methyl derivate of anatoxin-a with similar pharmacological and toxicological properties (Wonnacott et al., 1992), and it has been implicated in dog deaths in New Zealand (Wood et al., 2007). In addition to being a nicotinic agonist, homoanatoxin-a can increase the release of acetylcholine (ACh) from peripheral cholinergic nerves through opening of endogenous voltage-dependent neuronal L-type Ca^{2+} channels (Aas et al., 1996).

Anatoxin-a(s) is different from anatoxin-a and homoanatoxin-a. This neurotoxin has a unique chemical structure and is a naturally occurring irreversible acetylcholinesterase (AChE) inhibitor. The increased concentrations of ACh in the synapse lead to persistent stimulation, followed by a neuronal muscular block (Cook et al., 1990). The mechanism of toxic action is similar to that of organophosphorus and carbamate insecticides, as well as some chemical warfare nerve agents (Patocka et al., 2011). However, one of the main differences is that anatoxin-a(s) acts only in the periphery, whereas the insecticides inhibit AChE in the brain and retina (Cook et al., 1989). Animals poisoned with anatoxin-a(s) show a rapid onset of excessive salivation ("s" stands for salivation), lacrimation, diarrhea, and urination. Clinical signs of nicotinic receptor overstimulation including tremors, incoordination, convulsions, recumbency, and respiratory arrest are most commonly observed in cases with a lethal outcome. Animals often die within 30 min of exposure. Animals that die from anatoxin-a, homoanatoxin-a, or anatoxin-a(s) toxicosis do not show specific gross or microscopic lesions. Anatoxin-a(s) poisoning has been reported in pigs, birds, dogs, and calves in the United States and Europe (Mahmood et al., 1988; Cook et al., 1989; Onodera et al., 1997). Because of the lack of specific detection methods for anatoxin-a(s), the natural occurrence of this neurotoxin has not been fully evaluated.

Toxicity

In mice, the i.p. LD_{50} of anatoxin-a is 200 μg/kg (Stevens and Krieger, 1991), whereas the i.v. LD_{50} is estimated to be less than 100 μg/kg. The oral toxicity of anatoxin-a is much higher, with an oral LD_{50} in mice reported to be greater than 5 mg/kg. Several studies have shown that there are significant species differences with regard to anatoxin-a toxicity. Whereas an anatoxin-a containing *Aphanizomenon flos-aquae* bloom was toxic to sheep after i.p. administration, oral administration failed to induce toxicity (Runnegar et al., 1988). In contrast, calves developed toxicity after oral administration of an anatoxin-a containing *A. flos-aquae* bloom (Carmichael et al., 1977). The i.p. LD_{50} of homoanatoxin-a in mice is 250 μg/kg (Skulberg et al., 1992). Anatoxin-a(s) is much more toxic than anatoxin-a or homoanatoxin-a, with an i.p. LD_{50} in mice of 20 μg/kg (Briand et al., 2003).

Treatment

There is no specific antidote for anatoxin-a. Because of the rapid onset of clinical signs, emesis is not likely to be useful. Although no studies have evaluated the efficacy of specific decontamination procedures, administration of activated charcoal has been recommended. In addition, artificial respiration may be of benefit along with general supportive care. Specific measures to control seizures include benzodiazepines, phenobarbital, or pentobarbital. If given, they may cause CNS and respiratory depression, and careful monitoring of the animal is necessary. In any seizuring animal, control of body temperature is an important part of the symptomatic care.

Treatment of animals poisoned with anatoxin-a(s) is primarily symptomatic and supportive. Decontamination procedures can be considered but have not been evaluated. It has been shown that 2-PAM is not able to reactivate the inhibited AChE and is therefore not recommended (Hyde and Carmichael, 1991). Atropine should be given at a test dose to determine its efficacy in animals with life-threatening clinical signs. After the test dose, atropine can be given repeatedly until cessation of salivation. It is important to carefully monitor the animal for anticholinergic effects and to reduce or discontinue atropine if adverse effects develop.

As with other cyanobacteria toxins, toxicity is strain specific, and identification of the cyanobacteria alone cannot predict the toxicity level. Therefore, detection of anatoxin-a in biological specimens is confirmatory, but these tests are not routinely available (James et al., 1998; Puschner et al., 2010). Anatoxin-a was confirmed in stomach content, liver, urine, and bile of dogs (Gugger et al., 2005; Puschner et al., 2010). In suspect cases, environmental and biological samples should be saved for toxicological and phylogenetic analysis.

Diagnosis of anatoxin-a(s) toxicosis is aided by the determination of blood AChE activity. However, organophosphorus and carbamate insecticides can also inhibit AChE, and additional diagnostic workup is needed to establish a firm diagnosis. This includes the determination of brain AChE postmortem (unchanged in cases of anatoxin-a(s) poisoning), screening of gastrointestinal contents for insecticides, examination of stomach contents (possible identification of cyanobacteria), and a careful evaluation of the environment (access to freshwater and access to insecticides). Detection methods for anatoxin-a(s) are rare. A biosensor method has been developed that allows the quantitation of anatoxin-a(s) in environmental samples (Devic et al., 2002). New analytical methods for anatoxin-a(s) are necessary to better document the distribution of this neurotoxin in freshwater worldwide. Phylogenetic analysis of 16 S rRNA gene sequences will help in the species identification.

MISCELLANEOUS FRESHWATER CYANOBACTERIAL TOXINS

Although microcystin and anatoxin poisonings comprise the majority of cases reported in animals, other cyanotoxins are of concern. Dermatotoxic cyanobacterial toxins have been reported to cause "swimmers' itch" in Hawaii (Serdula et al., 1982) and have recently been associated with dermatitis in a dog (Puschner et al., 2017). In the documented case a dog developed severe pruritis, urticarial, and malaise after swimming in a freshwater lake in California. Phycological and toxicological evaluation revealed the presence of *Anabaena/Trichormus* sp. and *Lyngbya* sp. and debromoaplysiatoxin. Debromoaplysiatoxin can be produced in the marine and freshwater environment and is a known dermatotoxin (Kaneshima et al., 1983). In addition, debromoaplysiatoxin exposure may occur along with exposure to other cyanotoxins and result in a complex clinical presentation. Saxitoxins and derived forms belong to the group of paralytic shellfish poisoning (PSP) toxins and have been produced by a number of freshwater cyanobacteria, including *A. flos-aquae*, *Cylindrospermopsis raciborskii*, *Anabaena circinalis*, *Lyngbya wollei*, *Planktothrix* sp., and *Aphanizomenon gracile* (Carmichael et al., 1997; Kaas and Henriksen, 2000; Molica et al., 2005; Ballot et al., 2010). All saxitoxin analogs have high toxicity in mammals by blocking voltage-gated sodium channels, leading to respiratory arrest, neuromuscular weakness, and cardiovascular shock. Massive fish mortalities have been linked to saxitoxins produced by both freshwater cyanobacteria and marine dinoflagellates (Pearson et al., 2010; Moustaka-Gouni et al., 2017). Whereas intoxications of birds and cats have been associated with ingestion of PSP contaminated fish and clams (Landsberg, 2002), there is only one confirmed report of PSP toxin-associated mammalian mortality from exposure to contaminated freshwater (Negri et al., 1995). Fourteen sheep showed signs of trembling, recumbency, and death in Australia after exposure to toxic concentrations of PSPs produced by *A. circinalis*. Because PSP toxins are produced by several species of freshwater cyanobacteria, terrestrial animals and humans are at risk of being exposed to these toxins. Thus, it is important to reliably evaluate animals with neurologic signs after access to freshwater for possible PSP exposure because the risk certainly exists.

Another cyanotoxin, the alkaloid cylindrospermopsin, has caused deaths in cattle (Saker et al., 1999) and severe gastrointestinal disease in humans. Cylindrospermopsin is a potent inhibitor of protein synthesis and can lead to various degrees of injury to the liver, kidneys, adrenal gland, intestine, lung, thymus, and heart (Griffiths and Saker, 2003). Furthermore, this cyanotoxin is of particular concern because of its mutagenic and possibly carcinogenic activities. Cylindrospermopsin has been found in Europe, Australia, New Zealand, and Asia (Hawkins et al., 1997; Saker and Griffiths, 2001; Fastner et al., 2003), but it should be considered a potential worldwide problem. Cylindrospermopsin and deoxycylindrospermopsin have been produced by *C. raciborskii* (Ohtani et al., 1992), and 7-epicylindrospermopsin has been produced by *Aphanizomenon ovalisporum* (Banker et al., 1997). After oral exposure, the LD_{50} of cylindrospermopsin obtained with culture extracts of *C. raciborskii* ranged from 4.4 to 6.9 mg/kg in equivalent cylindropsermopsin (Seawright et al., 1999; Shaw et al., 2000).

Nodularins are cyclic pentapeptides that lead to severe hepatotoxicosis in the same way as microcystins (Harding et al., 1995; Ufelmann and Schrenk, 2015). In addition, nodularin is a more potent tumor promoter than microcystin (Sueoka et al., 1997; IARC, 2006; Ufelmann and Schrenk, 2015). The only cyanobacterium species known to produce nodularin is *Nodularia spumigena*. This cyanobacterium can form extensive blooms in the Baltic Sea and in brackish waters in the summer (Francis, 1878; Sivonen et al., 1989). The risk of nodularin intoxication is twofold because toxin exposure can occur not only through recreational or drinking water but also via contamination of seafood (Van Buynder et al., 2001). In cases of acute hepatotoxicity, exposure to microcystins as well as nodularins must be considered.

β-*N*-methylamino-l-alanine (BMAA), a neurotoxic amino acid found globally is thought to be produced by all cyanobacterial taxa and has been implicated in avian vacuolar myelinopathy (Bidigare et al., 2009). BMAA can bioaccumulate in food chains such as fish and seafood and is of considerable human health concern because of its ability to destroy motor neurons in the brain, leading to neurodegenerative diseases likes Parkinson's disease, Alzheimer's, and ALS, commonly referred to as the human amyotrophic lateral sclerosis–parkinsonism–dementia complex of Guam (Guam ALS-PD) and lathyrism (Bradley and Mash, 2009). Birds with avian vacuolar myelinopathy develop ataxia, tilting, weakness, and death, and they have characteristic postmortem lesions of bilateral symmetrical vacuolation of the white matter of the brain and spinal cord (Thomas et al., 1998). Monitoring of water for BMAA is a critical tool to assess nutrient reduction and to develop control strategies.

CONCLUDING REMARKS AND FUTURE DIRECTIONS

The frequency and extent of harmful cyanobacterial blooms appears to increase with the addition of nutrients to surface freshwater ecosystems throughout the world. As demonstrated in Table 57.1, numerous cyanobacterial species have the potential to produce a number of toxins with a range of target organs, but for each cyanobacterial species, it is very difficult to predict the nature and the level of the toxin production for a specific bloom. Although newer detection methods allow for better monitoring of potentially harmful blooms, there is still a need to apply these existing methods spatially and temporally and to develop lower cost, field-ready alternatives accessible to even remote areas. It is also important to develop more sophisticated methods that allow testing for a wider range of cyanotoxins and matrices in order to reliably confirm intoxications and improve overall risk assessment. Some recently developed methods have been useful in analyzing biological specimens in order to confirm a diagnosis of poisoning, but due to lack of availability and high cost, they are rarely pursued in suspect cases. The lack of methods to confirm exposure is most likely responsible for the low number of reported cases in the veterinary literature during the past 20–30 years. The incorporation of new analytical methods into diagnosis should provide insight into the true frequency of cyanotoxin poisoning in animals. For example, in the United States, several dog intoxications due to anatoxin-a have recently been identified in different regions in relation with the development of an analytical method using high-performance liquid chromatograph–mass spectrometry analysis (Puschner et al., 2008, 2010). In addition, information is needed on the efficacy of therapeutic measures. Similar to advisories for human populations, it is advisable to take preventative measures to avoid contact with surface waters containing visible blooms for all veterinary species, particularly when the water is utilized for a drinking source or for bathing.

REFERENCES

Aas, P., Eriksen, S., et al., 1996. Enhancement of acetylcholine release by homoanatoxin-a from Oscillatoria formosa. Environ. Toxicol. Pharmacol. 2, 223–232.

Agrawal, M.K., Ghosh, S.K., et al., 2006. Occurrence of microcystin-containing toxic water blooms in central India. J Microbiol Biotechnol. 16, 212–218.

Amado, L.L., Monserrat, J.M., 2010. Oxidative stress generation in microcystins in aquatic animals: why and how. Environ. Int. 36, 226–235.

Anagnostidis, K., Komarek, J., 1985. Modern approach to the classification system of cyanophytes. Arch. Hydrobiol. Suppl. 7 Algol. Stud. 38–39, 291–302.

Atkins, R., Rose, T., Brown, R.S., Robb, M., 2001. The Microcystis cyanobacteria bloom in the Swan River – February 2000. Water Sci. Technol. 43, 107–114.

Azevedo, S.M., Carmichael, W.W., et al., 2002. Human intoxication by microcystins during renal dialysis treatment in Caruaru-Brazil. Toxicology. 181–182, 441–446.

Ballot, A., Krienitz, L., et al., 2004. Cyanobacteria and cyanobacterial toxins in three alkaline rift valley lakes of Kenya – Lakes Bogoria, Nakuru, and Elmenteita. J. Plankton Res. 26, 925–935.

Ballot, A., Fastner, J., Wiedner, C., 2010. Paralytic shellfish poisoning toxin-producing cyanobacterium *Aphanizomenon gracile* in northeast Germany. Appl. Environ. Microbiol. 76, 1173–1180.

Banker, R., Carmeli, S., et al., 1997. Identification of cylindrospermopsin in *Aphanizomenon ovalisporum* (Cyanophyceae) isolated from lake Kinneret, Israel. J. Phycol. 33, 613–616.

Barik, J., Wonnacott, S., 2006. Indirect modulation by alpha7 nicotinic acetylcholine receptors of noradrenaline release in rat hippocampal slices: interaction with glutamate and GABA systems and effect of nicotine withdrawal. Mol. Pharmacol. 69, 618–628.

Bartram, J., Carmichael, W.W., et al., 1999. Introduction. In: Chorus, I., Bartram, J. (Eds.), Toxic Cyanobacteria in Water: A Guide to Their Public Health Consequences, Monitoring and Management. E & FN Spon, London, pp. 1–14.

Bautista, A.C., Moore, C.E., et al., 2015. Hepatopathy following consumption of a commercially available blue-green algae dietary supplement in a dog. BMC Vet. Res. 11, 136.

Beltran, E.C., Neilan, B.A., 2000. Geographical segregation of the neurotoxin-producing cyanobacterium *Anabaena circinalis*. Appl. Environ. Microbiol. 66, 4468–4474.

Benson, J.M., Hutt, J.A., et al., 2005. The toxicity of microcystin LR in mice following 7 days of inhalation exposure. Toxicon. 45, 691–698.

Bidigare, R.R., Christensen, S.J., Wilde, S.B., et al., 2009. Cyanobacteria and BMAA: possible linkage with avian vacuolar myelinopathy (AVM) in the southeastern United States. Amyotroph. Lateral. Scler. 10 (Suppl. 2), 71–73.

Billam, M., Mukhi, S., et al., 2008. Toxic response indicators of microcystin-LR in F344 rats following a single-dose treatment. Toxicon. 51, 1068–1080.

Bogialli, S., Bruno, M., et al., 2005. Simple assay for analyzing five microcystins and nodularin in fish muscle tissue: hot water extraction followed by liquid chromatography–tandem mass spectrometry. J. Agric. Food Chem. 53, 6586–6592.

Bradley, W.G., Mash, D.C., 2009. Beyond Guam: the cyanobacteria/BMAA hypothesis of the cause of ALS and other neurodegenerative diseases. Amyotroph. Lat. Scler. 10 (Suppl. 2), 7–20.

Braun, A., Pfeiffer, T., 2002. Cyanobacterial blooms as the cause of a Pleistocene large mammal assemblage. Paleobiology. 28, 139–154.

Briand, J.F., Jacquet, S., Bernard, C., et al., 2003. Health hazards for terrestrial vertebrates from toxic cyanobacteria in surface water ecosystems. Vet. Res. 34, 361–377.

Briand, J.F., Jacquet, S., et al., 2005. Variations in the microcystin production of Planktothrix rubescens (Cyanobacteria) assessed from a four-year survey of Lac du Bourget (France) and from laboratory experiments. Microb. Ecol. 50, 418–428.

Bullerjahn, G.S., McKay, R.M., et al., 2016. Global solutions to regional problems: collecting global expertise to address the problem of harmful cyanobacterial blooms. A Lake Erie case study. Harmful. Algae. 54, 223–238.

Burch, M.D., 2008. Effective doses, guidelines and regulations. Adv. Exp. Med. Biol. 619, 831–853.

Campos, F., Alfonso, M., Durán, R., 2010. In vivo modulation of alpha7 nicotinic receptors on striatal glutamate release induced by anatoxin-A. Neurochem. Int. 56, 850–855.

Carbis, C.R., Simons, J.A., et al., 1994. A biochemical profile for predicting the chronic exposure of sheep to Microcystis aeruginosa, an hepatotoxic species of blue-green alga. Res. Vet. Sci. 57, 310–316.

Carmichael, W.W., Li, R., 2006. Cyanobacteria toxins in the Salton Sea. Saline Ecosyst. 2, 5.

Carmichael, W.W., Gorham, P.R., Biggs, D.F., 1977. Two laboratory case studies on oral toxicity to calves of freshwater cyanophyte (blue-green-alga) Anabaena flos-aquae Nrc-44-1. Can. Vet. J. 18, 71–75.

Carmichael, W.W., Evans, W.R., Yin, Q.Q., Bell, P., Moczydlowski, E., 1997. Evidence for paralytic shellfish poisons in the freshwater cyanobacterium *Lyngbya wollei* (Farlow ex Gomont) comb. nov. Appl. Environ. Microbiol. 63, 3104–3110.

Castle, J.W., Rodgers, J.H., 2009. Hypothesis for the role of toxin-producing algae in Phanerozoic mass extinctions based on evidence from the geologic record and modern environments. Environ. Geosci. 16, 1–23.

Chatziefthimiou, A.D., Rowles, H., Powell, J.T., et al., 2014. Cyanotoxins as a potential cause of dog poisonings in desert environments. Vet. Rec. 174, 484–485.

Chen, J., Xie, P., Li, L., Xu, J., 2009. First identification of the hepatotoxic microcystins in the serum of a chronically exposed human population together with indication of hepatocellular damage. Toxicol. Sci. 108, 81–89.

Cook, W.O., Beasley, V.R., et al., 1989. Consistent inhibition of peripheral cholinesterases by neurotoxins from the freshwater cyanobacterium Anabaena flos-aquae: studies of ducks, swine, mice and a steer. Environ. Toxicol. Chem. 8, 915–922.

Cook, W.O., Iwamoto, G.A., et al., 1990. Pathophysiologic effects of anatoxin-a(s) in anaesthetized rats: the influence of atropine and artificial respiration. Pharmacol. Toxicol. 67, 151–155.

Devic, E., Li, D.H., et al., 2002. Detection of anatoxin-a(s) in environmental samples of cyanobacteria by using a biosensor with engineered acetylcholinesterases. Appl. Environ. Microbiol. 68, 4102–4106.

DeVries, S.E., Galey, F.D., Namikoshi, M., Woo, J.C., 1993. Clinical and pathologic findings of blue-green algae (*Microcystis aeruginosa*) intoxication in a dog. J. Vet. Diagn. Invest. 5, 403–408.

Dietrich, D., Hoeger, S., 2005. Guidance values for microcystins in water and cyanobacterial supplement products (blue-green algal supplements): a reasonable or misguided approach? Toxicol. Appl. Pharmacol. 203, 273–289.

Ding, W.X., Ong, N.C., 2003. Role of oxidative stress and mitochondrial changes in cyanobacteria-induced apoptosis and hepatotoxicity. FEMS Microbiol. Lett. 220, 1–7.

Done, S.H., Bain, M., 1993. Hepatic necrosis in sheep associated with ingestion of blue-green algae. Vet. Rec. 133, 600.

Downing, T.G., Sember, C.S., Gehringer, M.M., et al., 2005. Medium N: P ratios and specific growth rate comodulate microcystin and protein content in Microcystis aeruginosa PCC7806 and M. aeruginosa UV027. Microb. Ecol. 49, 468–473.

Edwards, C., Beattie, K.A., Scrimgeour, C.M., et al., 1992. Identification of anatoxin-a in benthic cyanobacteria (blue-green algae) and in associated dog poisonings at Loch Insh, Scotland. Toxicon. 30, 1165–1175.

Falconer, I.R., Humpage, A.R., 2005. Health risk assessment of cyanobacterial (blue-green algal) toxins in drinking water. Int. J. Environ. Res. Public Health. 2, 43–50.

Falconer, I.R., Yeung, D.S., 1992. Cytoskeletal changes in hepatocytes induced by Microcystis toxins and their relation to hyperphosphorylation of cell proteins. Chem. Biol. Interact. 81, 181–196.

Falconer, I.R., Burch, M.D., et al., 1994. Toxicity of the blue-green alga (Cyanobacterium) Microcystis aeruginosa in drinking water to growing pigs, as animal model for human injury and risk assessment. Environ. Toxic. Water. 9, 131–139.

Falconer, I.R., Buckley, T., Runnegar, M.T.C., 1986. Biological half-life, organ distribution and excretion of I-125 labeled toxic peptide from the blue-green-alga Microcystis aeruginosa. Aust. J. Biol. Sci. 39, 17–21.

Fastner, J., Heinze, R., et al., 2003. Cylindrospermopsin occurrence in two German lakes and preliminary assessment of toxicity and toxin production of *Cylindrospermopsis raciborskii* (Cyanobacteria) isolates. Toxicon. 42, 313–321.

Fawell, J.K., James, C.P., James, H.A., 1994. Toxins from Blue-Green Algae: Toxicological Assessment of Microcystin-LR and a Method for Its Determination in Water. Water Research Centre, Medmenham, UK, pp. 1–46.

Fischer, W.J., Hitzfeld, B.C., et al., 2000. Microcystin-LR toxicodynamics, induced pathology, and immunohistochemical localization in livers of blue-green algae exposed rainbow trout (*Oncorhynchus mykiss*). Toxicol. Sci. 54, 365–373.

Francis, G., 1878. Poisonous Australian lake. Nature. 18, 11–12.

Frias, H.V., Mendes, M.A., et al., 2006. Use of electrospray tandem mass spectrometry for identification of microcystins during a cyanobacterial bloom event. Biochem. Biophys. Res. Commun. 344, 741–746.

Fromme, H., Köhler, A., Krause, R., et al., 2000. Occurrence of cyanobacterial toxins – microcystins and anatoxin-a – in Berlin water bodies with implications to human health and regulations. Environ. Toxicol. 15, 120–130.

Furey, A., Crowley, J., et al., 2003. The first identification of the rare cyanobacterial toxin, homoanatoxin-a, in Ireland. Toxicon. 41, 297–303.

Galey, F.D., Beasley, V.R., et al., 1987. Blue-green algae (*Microcystis aeruginosa*) hepatotoxicosis in dairy cows. Am. J. Vet. Res. 48, 1415–1420.

Gehringer, M.M., Downs, K.S., et al., 2003a. An investigation into the effect of selenium supplementation on microcystin hepatotoxicity. Toxicon. 41, 451–458.

Gehringer, M.M., Govender, S., Shah, M., et al., 2003b. An investigation of the role of vitamin E in the protection of mice against microcystin toxicity. Environ. Toxicol. 18, 142–148.

Griffiths, D.J., Saker, M.L., 2003. The palm island mystery disease 20 years on: a review of research on the cyanotoxin cylindrospermopsin. Environ. Toxicol. 18, 78–93.

Gugger, M., Lenoir, S., et al., 2005. First report in a river in France of the benthic cyanobacterium Phormidium favosum producing anatoxin-a associated with dog neurotoxicosis. Toxicon. 45, 919–928.

Gunn, G.J., Rafferty, A.G., et al., 1992. Fatal canine neurotoxicosis attributed to blue-green algae (cyanobacteria). Vet. Rec. 130, 301–302.

Handeland, K., Østensvik, Ø., 2010. Microcystin poisoning in roe deer (*Capreolus capreolus*). Toxicon. 56, 1076–1078.

Harding, W.R., Rowe, N., et al., 1995. Death of a dog attributed to the cyanobacterial (blue-green algal) hepatotoxin nodularin in South Africa. J. South Afr. Vet. Assoc. 66, 256–259.

Havens, K.E., 2008. Cyanobacterial blooms: effects on aquatic ecosystems. Adv. Exp. Med. Biol. 619, 733–747.

Hawkins, P.R., Chandrasena, N.R., et al., 1997. Isolation and toxicity of *Cylindrospermopsis raciborskii* from an ornamental lake. Toxicon. 35, 341–346.

Heinze, R., 1999. Toxicity of the cyanobacterial toxin microcystin-LR to rats after 28 days intake with the drinking water. Environ. Toxicol. 14, 57–60.

Henriksen, P., Carmichael, W.W., An, J.S., et al., 1997. Detection of an anatoxin-a(s)-like anticholinesterase in natural blooms and cultures of cyanobacteria/blue-green algae from Danish lakes and in the stomach contents of poisoned birds. Toxicon. 35, 901–913.

Hermansky, S.J., Stohs, S.J., et al., 1991. Evaluation of potential chemoprotectants against microcystin-LR hepatotoxicity in mice. J. Appl. Toxicol. 11, 65–74.

Hisbergues, M., Christiansen, G., Rouhiainen, L., et al., 2003. PCR-based identification of microcystin-producing genotypes of different cyanobacterial genera. Arch. Microbiol. 180, 402–410.

Hitzfeld, B.C., Lampert, C.S., et al., 2000. Toxin production in cyanobacterial mats from ponds on the McMurdo ice shelf, Antarctica. Toxicon. 38, 1731–1748.

Hooser, S.B., Beasley, V.R., et al., 1991a. Actin filament alterations in rat hepatocytes induced in vivo and in vitro by microcystin-LR, a hepatotoxin from the blue-green alga, Microcystis aeruginosa. Vet. Pathol. 28, 259–266.

Hooser, S.B., Kuhlenschmidt, M.S., et al., 1991b. Uptake and subcellular localization of tritiated dihydro-microcystin-LR in rat liver. Toxicon. 29, 589–601.

Humbert, J.F., 2010. Advances in the detection of phycotoxins and cyanotoxins. Anal. Bioanal. Chem. 397, 1653–1654.

Humpage, A.R., Falconer, I.R., 1999. Microcystin-LR and liver tumor promotion: effects on cytokinesis, ploidy, and apoptosis in cultured hepatocytes. Environ. Toxicol. 14, 61–75.

Hyde, E.G., Carmichael, W.W., 1991. Anatoxin-a(s), a naturally occurring organophosphate, is an irreversible active site-directed inhibitor of acetylcholinesterase (EC 3.1.1.7). J. Biochem. Toxicol. 6, 195–201.

IARC, 2006. Ingested nitrate and nitrite, and cyanobacterial peptide toxins. International Agency for Research on Cancer (IARC) Monographs on the Evaluation of Carcinogenic Risks to Humans. IARC Monograph 94.

Ito, E., Kondo, F., Harada, K., 1997. Hepatic necrosis in aged mice by oral administration of microcystin-LR. Toxicon. 35, 231–239.

Ito, E., Kondo, F., Harada, K., 2000. First report on the distribution of orally administered microcystin-LR in mouse tissue using an immunostaining method. Toxicon. 38, 37–48.

Ito, E., Kondo, F., Harada, K., 2001. Intratracheal administration of microcystin-LR, and its distribution. Toxicon. 39, 265–271.

James, K.J., Sherlock, I.R., Stack, M.A., 1997. Anatoxin-a in Irish freshwater and cyanobacteria, determined using a new fluorimetric liquid chromatographic method. Toxicon. 35, 963–971.

James, K.J., Furey, A., et al., 1998. Sensitive determination of anatoxin-a, homoanatoxin-a and their degradation products by liquid chromatography with fluorimetric detection. J. Chromatogr. A. 798, 147–157.

Jayaraj, R., Anand, T., Rao, P.V., 2006. Activity and gene expression profile of certain antioxidant enzymes to microcystin-LR induced oxidative stress in mice. Toxicology. 220, 136–146.

Jayaraj, R., Deb, U., et al., 2007. Hepatoprotective efficacy of certain flavonoids against microcystin induced toxicity in mice. Environ. Toxicol. 22, 472–479.

Kaas, H., Henriksen, P., 2000. Saxitoxins (PSP toxins) in Danish lakes. Water Res. 34, 2089–2097.

Kaneshima, H., Hiai, H., et al., 1983. Tumor promoter-dependent mouse leukemia cell line. Cancer Res. 43, 4676–4680.

Karlsson, K.M., Kankaanpää, H., Huttunen, M., et al., 2005a. First observation of microcystin-LR in pelagic cyanobacterial blooms in the northern Baltic Sea. Harmful. Algae. 4, 163–166.

Karlsson, K.M., Spoof, L.E., Meriluoto, J.A., 2005b. Quantitative LC-ESI-MS analyses of microcystins and nodularin-R in animal tissue: matrix effects and method validation. Environ. Toxicol. 20, 381–389.

Kondo, F., Matsumoto, H., et al., 1996. Detection and identification of metabolites of microcystins formed in vivo in mouse and rat livers. Chem. Res. Toxicol. 9, 1355–1359.

Krienitz, L., Ballot, A., et al., 2003. Contribution of hot spring cyanobacteria to the mysterious deaths of Lesser Flamingos at Lake Bogoria, Kenya. FEMS Microbiol. Ecol. 43, 141–148.

Kuiper-Goodman, T., Falconer, I., Fitzgerald, J., 1999. Human health aspects. In: Chorus, I., Bartram, J. (Eds.), Toxic Cyanobacteria in Water: A Guide to Their Public Health Consequences, Monitoring and Management. E & FN Spon, London, pp. 113–153.

Landsberg, J.H., 2002. The effects of harmful algal blooms on aquatic organisms. Rev. Fish Sci. 10, 113–390.

Lawton, L.A., Edwards, C., et al., 1995. Isolation and characterization of microcystins from laboratory cultures and environmental samples of Microcystis aeruginosa and from an associated animal toxicosis. Nat. Toxins. 3, 50–57.

Li, H., Xie, P., et al., 2009. In vivo study on the effects of microcystin extracts on the expression profiles of proto-oncogenes (c-fos, c-jun and c-myc) in liver, kidney and testis of male Wistar rats injected i. v. with toxins. Toxicon. 53, 169–175.

Lopez Rodas, V., Costas, E., 1999. Preference of mice to consume Microcystis aeruginosa (toxin-producing cyanobacteria): a possible explanation for numerous fatalities of livestock and wildlife. Res. Vet. Sci. 67, 107–110.

Luukkainen, R., Namikoshi, M., et al., 1994. Isolation and identification of 12 microcystins from four strains and two bloom samples of Microcystis spp.: structure of a new hepatotoxin. Toxicon. 32, 133–139.

Mahmood, N.A., Carmichael, W.W., Pfahler, D., 1988. Anticholinesterase poisonings in dogs from a cyanobacterial (blue-green algae) bloom dominated by Anabaena flos-aquae. Am. J. Vet. Res. 49, 500–503.

Maizels, M., Budde, W.L., 2004. A LC/MS method for the determination of cyanobacteria toxins in water. Anal. Chem. 76, 1342–1351.

Malbrouck, C., Kestemont, P., 2006. Effects of microcystins on fish. Environ. Toxicol. Chem. 25, 72–86.

McElhiney, J., Lawton, L.A., 2005. Detection of the cyanobacterial hepatotoxins microcystins. Toxicol. Appl. Pharmacol. 203, 219–230.

McElhiney, J., Lawton, L.A., Leifert, C., 2001. Investigations into the inhibitory effects of microcystins on plant growth, and the toxicity of plant tissues following exposure. Toxicon. 39, 1411–1420.

Méjean, A., Paci, G., Gatier, V., et al., 2014. Biosynthesis of anatoxin-a and analogues (anatoxins) in cyanobacteria. Toxicon. 91, 15–22.

Mereish, K.A., Solow, R., 1989. Interaction of microcystin-LR with SuperChar: water decontamination and therapy. J. Toxicol. Clin. Toxicol. 27, 271–280.

Mez, K., Beattie, K.A., et al., 1997. Identification of microcystin in benthic cyanobacteria linked to cattle deaths on alpine pastures in Switzerland. Eur. J. Phycol. 32, 111–117.

Milutinovic, A., Zivin, M., et al., 2003. Nephrotoxic effects of chronic administration of microcystins -LR and -YR. Toxicon. 42, 281–288.

Mittelman, N.S., Engiles, J.B., et al., 2016. Presumptive Iatrogenic Microcystin-Associated Liver Failure and Encephalopathy in a Holsteiner Gelding. J. Vet. Intern. Med. 30, 1747–1751.

Molica, R.J.R., Oliveira, E.J.A., et al., 2005. Occurrence of saxitoxins and an anatoxin-a(s)-like anticholinesterase in a Brazilian drinking water supply. Harmful. Algae. 4, 743–753.

Monserrat, J.M., Yunes, J.S., Bianchini, A., 2001. Effects of Anabaena spiroides (cyanobacteria) aqueous extracts on the acetylcholinesterase activity of aquatic species. Environ. Toxicol. Chem. 20, 1228–1235.

Moore, C.E., Juan, J., et al., 2016. Comparison of protein phosphatase inhibition assay with LC-MS/MS for diagnosis of microcystin toxicosis in veterinary cases. Mar. Drugs. 14, 54.

Moustaka-Gouni, M., Hiskia, A., et al., 2017. First report of *Aphanizomenon favaloroi* occurrence in Europe associated with saxitoxins and a massive fish kill in Lake Vistonis, Greece. Mar. Freshwater Res. Available from: http://dx.doi.org/10.4081/aiol.2017.6350

Naegeli, H., Sahin, A., et al., 1997. Sudden deaths of cattle on Alpine pastures in southeastern Switzerland. Schweiz Arch. Tierheilk. 139, 201–209.

Namikoshi, M., Murakami, T., et al., 2004. Biosynthesis and transformation of homoanatoxin-a in the cyanobacterium Raphidiopsis mediterranea Skuja and structures of three new homologues. Chem. Res. Toxicol. 17, 1692–1696.

Nasri, H., El Herry, S., Bouaïcha, N., 2008. First reported case of turtle deaths during a toxic Microcystis spp. bloom in Lake Oubeira, Algeria. Ecotoxicol. Environ. Saf. 71, 535–544.

Ndetei, R., Muhandiki, V.S., 2005. Mortalities of Lesser Flamingos in Kenyan Rift Valley saline lakes and the implications for sustainable management of the lakes. Lakes Reser. Res. Manage. 10, 51–58.

Negri, A.P., Jones, G.J., Hindmarsh, M., 1995. Sheep mortality associated with paralytic shellfish poisons from the cyanobacterium *Anabaena circinalis*. Toxicon. 33, 1321–1329.

Ohtani, I., Moore, R.E., Runnegar, M.T.C., 1992. Cylindrospermopsin: a potent hepatotoxin from the blue-green alga *Cylindrospermopsis raciborskii*. J. Am. Chem. Soc. 114, 7941–7942.

Onodera, H., Oshima, Y., Henriksen, P., et al., 1997. Confirmation of anatoxin-a(s), in the cyanobacterium Anabaena lemmermannii, as the cause of bird kills in Danish lakes. Toxicon. 35, 1645–1648.

Orr, P.T., Jones, G.J., et al., 2001. Ingestion of toxic Microcystis aeruginosa by dairy cattle and the implications for microcystin contamination of milk. Toxicon. 39, 1847–1854.

Orr, P.T., Jones, G.J., Hunter, R.A., Berger, K., 2003. Exposure of beef cattle to sub-clinical doses of Microcystis aeruginosa: toxin bioaccumulation, physiological effects and human health risk assessment. Toxicon. 41, 613–620.

Ott, J.L., Carmichael, W.W., 2006. LC/ESI/MS method development for the analysis of hepatotoxic cyclic peptide microcystins in animal tissues. Toxicon. 47, 734–741.

Patocka, J., Gupta, R.C., Kuca, K., 2011. Anatoxin-A(s): natural organophosphorous anticholinesterase agent. Mil. Med. Sci. Lett. 80, 129–139.

Pearl, H.W., Fulton, R.S., Moisander, P.H., et al., 2001. Harmful freshwater algal blooms with an emphasis on cyanobacteria. Sci. World J. 1, 76–113.

Pearl, H.W., Gardner, W.S., et al., 2016. Mitigating cyanobacterial harmful algal blooms in aquatic ecosystems impacted by climate change and anthropogenic nutrients. Harmful. Algae. 54, 213–222.

Pearson, L., Mihali, T., et al., 2010. On the chemistry, toxicology and genetics of the cyanobacterial toxins, microcystin, nodularin, saxitoxin and cylindrospermopsin. Mar. Drugs. 8, 1650–1680.

Pflugmacher, S., Wiegand, C., et al., 1998. Identification of an enzymatically formed glutathione conjugate of the cyanobacterial hepatotoxin microcystin-LR: the first step of detoxication. BBA-Gen. 1425, 527–533.

Puschner, B., Galey, F.D., et al., 1998. Blue-green algae toxicosis in cattle. J. Am. Vet. Med. Assoc. 213, 1571, 1605–1607.

Puschner, B., Hoff, B., Tor, E.R., 2008. Diagnosis of anatoxin-a poisoning in dogs from North America. J. Vet. Diagn. Invest. 20, 89–92.

Puschner, B., Pratt, C., Tor, E.R., 2010. Treatment and diagnosis of a dog with fulminant neurological deterioration due to anatoxin-a intoxication. J. Vet. Emerg. Crit. Care 20, 518–522.

Puschner, B., Bautista, A.C., Wong, C., 2017. Debromoaplysiatoxin as the Causative Agent of Dermatitis in a Dog after Exposure to Freshwater in California. Front. Vet. Sci. 4, 50. Available from: http://dx.doi.org/10.3389/fvets.2017.00050.

Rao, P.V., Gupta, N., Bhaskar, A.S., et al., 2002. Toxins and bioactive compounds from cyanobacteria and their implications on human health. J. Environ. Biol. 23, 215–224.

Rao, P.V., Jayaraj, R., Bhaskar, A.S., 2004. Protective efficacy and the recovery profile of certain chemoprotectants against lethal poisoning by microcystin-LR in mice. Toxicon. 44, 723–730.

Rellán, S., Osswald, J., et al., 2009. First detection of anatoxin-a in human and animal dietary supplements containing cyanobacteria. Food Chem. Toxicol. 47, 2189–2195.

Rippka, R., Deruelles, J., et al., 1979. Generic assignments, strain histories and properties of pure cultures of cyanobacteria. J. Gen. Microbiol. 111, 1–61.

Robinson, N.A., Pace, J.G., et al., 1991. Tissue distribution, excretion and hepatic biotransformation of microcystin-LR in mice. J. Pharmacol. Exp. Ther. 256, 176–182.

Runnegar, M.T., Kong, S., Berndt, N., 1993. Protein phosphatase inhibition and in vivo hepatotoxicity of microcystins. Am. J. Physiol. 265, G224–G230.

Runnegar, M.T.C., Falconer, I.R., Silver, J., 1981. Deformation of isolated rat hepatocytes by a peptide hepatotoxin from the blue-green alga Microcystis aeruginosa. Naunyn. Schmiedebergs Arch. Pharmacol. 317, 268–272.

Runnegar, M.T.C., Jackson, A.R.B., Falconer, I.R., 1988. Toxicity to mice and sheep of a bloom of the cyanobacterium (blue green-alga) *Anabaena circinalis*. Toxicon. 26, 599–602.

Saker, M.L., Griffiths, D.J., 2001. Occurrence of blooms of the cyanobacterium *Cylindrospermopsis raciborskii* (Woloszynska) Seenayya and Subba Raju in a north Queensland domestic water supply. Mar. Freshwater Res. 52, 907–915.

Saker, M.L., Thomas, A.D., Norton, J.H., 1999. Cattle mortality attributed to the toxic cyanobacterium *Cylindrospermopsis raciborskii* in an outback region of north Queensland. Environ. Toxicol. 14, 179–182.

Schaeffer, D.J., Malpas, P.B., Barton, L.L., 1999. Risk assessment of microcystin in dietary Aphanizomenon flos-aquae. Ecotoxicol. Environ. Saf. 44, 73–80.

Seawright, A.A., Nolan, C.C., et al., 1999. The oral toxicity for mice of the tropical cyanobacterium *Cylindropsermopsis raciborskii* (Woloszynska). Environ. Toxicol. 14, 135–142.

Seithel, A., Eberl, S., et al., 2007. The influence of macrolide antibiotics on the uptake of organic anions and drugs mediated by OATP1B1 and OATP1B3. Drug Metab. Dispos. 35, 779–786.

Serdula, M., Bartolini, G., Moore, R.E., et al., 1982. Seaweed itch on windward Oahu. Hawaii Med. J. 41, 200–201.

Sevilla, E., Martin-Luna, B., et al., 2008. Iron availability affects mcyD expression and microcystin-LR synthesis in Microcystis aeruginosa PCC7806. Environ. Microbiol. 10, 2476–2483.

Shaw, G.R., Seawright, A.A., Moore, M.R., et al., 2000. Cylindrospermopsin, a cyanobacterial alkaloid: evaluation of its toxicologic activity. Ther. Drug. Monit. 22, 89–92.

Shi, Q., Cui, J., et al., 2004. Expression of modulation of multiple cytokines in vivo by cyanobacterial blooms extract from Taihu Lake, China. Toxicon. 44, 871–879.

Sivonen, K., Himberg, K., et al., 1989. Preliminary characterization of neurotoxic cyanobacteria blooms and strains from Finland. Toxic. Assess. 4, 339–352.

Skulberg, O.M., Carmichael, W.W., et al., 1992. Investigations of a neurotoxic oscillatorialean strain (Cyanophyceae) and its toxin: isolation and characterization of homoanatoxin-A. Environ. Toxicol. Chem. 11, 321–329.

Smith, V.H., 2003. Eutrophication of freshwater and coastal marine ecosystems: a global problem. Environ. Sci. Pollut Res. Int. 10, 126–139.

Spivak, C.E., Witkop, B., Albuquerque, E.X., 1980. Anatoxin-a: a novel, potent agonist at the nicotinic receptor. Mol. Pharmacol. 18, 384–394.

Stevens, D.K., Krieger, R.I., 1991. Effect of route of exposure and repeated doses on the acute toxicity in mice of the cyanobacterial nicotinic alkaloid anatoxin-a. Toxicon. 29, 134–138.

Stotts, R.R., Twardock, A.R., et al., 1997. Distribution of tritiated dihydromicrocystin in swine. Toxicon. 35, 937–953.

Sueoka, E., Sueoka, N., et al., 1997. Expression of the tumor necrosis factor alpha gene and early response genes by nodularin, a liver tumor promoter, in primary cultured rat hepatocytes. J. Cancer Res. Clin. Oncol. 123, 413–419.

Thomas, N.J., Meteyer, C.U., Sileo, L., 1998. Epizootic vacuolar myelinopathy of the central nervous system of bald eagles (*Haliaeetus leucocephalus*) and American coots (*Fulica americana*). Vet. Pathol. 35, 479–487.

Thomas, P., Stephens, M., et al., 1993. -Anatoxin-a is a potent agonist at neuronal nicotinic acetylcholine receptors. J. Neurochem. 60, 2308–2311.

Ueno, Y., Nagata, S., et al., 1996. Detection of microcystins, a blue-green algal hepatotoxin, in drinking water sampled in Haimen and Fusui, endemic areas of primary liver cancer in China, by highly sensitive immunoassay. Carcinogenesis. 17, 1317–1321.

Ufelmann, H., Schrenk, D., 2015. Nodularin-triggered apoptosis and hyperphosphorylation of signalling proteins in cultured rat hepatocytes. Toxicol. In Vitro. 29, 16–26.

Van Buynder, P.G., Oughtred, T., et al., 2001. Nodularin uptake by seafood during a cyanobacterial bloom. Environ. Toxicol. 16, 468–471.

Van Halderen, A., Harding, W.R., et al., 1995. Cyanobacterial (blue-green algae) poisoning of livestock in the western Cape Province of South Africa. J S Afr. Vet. Assoc. 66, 260–264.

Warhurst, A.M., Raggett, S.L., et al., 1997. Adsorption of the cyanobacterial hepatotoxin microcystin-LR by a low-cost activated carbon from the seed husks of the pan-tropical tree, Moringa oleifera. Sci. Total Environ. 207, 207–211.

Welker, M., von Döhren, H., 2006. Cyanobacterial peptides: nature's own combinatorial biosynthesis. FEMS Microbiol. Rev. 38, 530–563.

Wonnacott, S., Swanson, K.L., et al., 1992. Homoanatoxin: a potent analogue of anatoxin-A. Biochem. Pharmacol. 43, 419–423.

Wood, S.A., Selwood, A.I., et al., 2007. First report of homoanatoxin-a and associated dog neurotoxicosis in New Zealand. Toxicon. 50, 292–301.

Wood, S.A., Heath, M.W., et al., 2010. Identification of a benthic microcystin-producing filamentous cyanobacterium (Oscillatoriales) associated with a dog poisoning in New Zealand. Toxicon. 55, 897–903.

Wood, S.A., Atalah, J., et al., 2017. Effect of river flow, temperature, and water chemistry on proliferations of the benthic anatoxin-producing cyanobacterium Phormidium. Freshwater Sci. 36, 63–76.

Xiong, Q., Xie, P., et al., 2010. Acute effects of microcystins exposure on the transcription of antioxidant enzyme genes in three organs (liver, kidney, and testis) of male Wistar rats. J. Biochem. Mol. Toxicol. 24, 361–367.

Xu, C., Shu, W.Q., et al., 2007. Protective effects of green tea polyphenols against subacute hepatotoxicity induced by microcystin-LR in mice. Environ. Toxicol. Pharmacol. 24, 140–148.

Yang, X., Boyer, G.L., 2005. Occurrence of the cyanobacterial neurotoxin, anatoxin-a, in lower Great Lakes. IAGLR Conf. Prog. Abst. 48, 203–204.

Yuan, M., Carmichael, W.W., Hilborn, E.D., 2006. Microcystin analysis in human sera and liver from human fatalities in Caruaru, Brazil, 1996. Toxicon. 48, 627–640.

Zegura, B., Straser, A., Filipic, M., 2011. Genotoxicity and potential carcinogenicity of cyanobacterial toxins: a review. Mutat. Res. 727, 16–41.

Zeller, P., Clement, M., Fessard, V., 2011. Similar uptake profiles of microcystin-LR and RR in an in vitro human intestinal mode. Toxicology. 290, 7–13.

Zhang, X., Nordberg, A., 1993. The competition of (−)-[3H]nicotine binding by the enantiomers of nicotine, nornicotine and anatoxin-a in membranes and solubilized preparations of different brain regions of rat. Naunyn. Schmiedebergs Arch. Pharmacol. 348, 28–34.

Zhao, Y., Xue, Q., Su, X., et al., 2015. Microcystin-LR induced thyroid dysfunction and metabolic disorders in mice. Toxicology. 328, 135–141.

Zhou, L., Yu, H., Chen, K., 2002. Relationship between microcystin in drinking water and colorectal cancer. Biomed. Environ. Sci. 15, 166–171.

Section XII

Poisonous and Venomous Organisms

Chapter 58

Terrestrial Zootoxins

Sharon M. Gwaltney-Brant, Eric Dunayer and Hany Youssef

INTRODUCTION

The animal kingdom is populated by a vast variety of creatures whose main focus in life is to live to see tomorrow. To this end, many animals have developed chemical means of defense and/or food procurement. Every phylum within the animal kingdom contains species that produce poisons or venoms. Poisons are compounds produced in nonspecialized tissues as secondary products of metabolism that accumulate in the host animal or that accumulate in predators following ingestion of prey. Poisonous animals, therefore, lack means of actively delivering these chemical compounds to others—exposure generally requires oral contact (rarely dermal) in order for another animal to become poisoned. In contrast, venoms are produced in specialized tissues or glands, and venomous animals have developed a variety of venom apparatuses (stingers, teeth, etc.) to deliver their venom to target animals—a process termed envenomation.

Most venoms and poisons are not composed of a single chemical substance but, rather, are mixtures of a variety of chemical compounds that often act synergistically to produce their toxic effects. Typical constituents include peptides, amines, serotonin, quinones, polypeptides, and enzymes (Russell, 2001). These compounds are collectively termed toxins (the science of the study of toxins is termed toxinology), and toxins produced by members of the animal kingdom are collectively termed zootoxins.

Not every exposure to a poisonous or venomous animal will necessarily result in a toxicosis (Meier, 1995). Within a species, variations in size, age, sex, season, toxin composition, and geographic location can result in zootoxins with relatively more or less toxicity. Similarly, the animal exposed to the zootoxin may be more or less susceptible to toxicosis based on its age, weight, sex, state of health, and degree of exposure.

Compared to other means of injury or illness in animals, envenomation or poisoning from zootoxins is relatively rare in domestic animals, due largely to the protection afforded by animal owners. Wildlife, on the other hand, probably face exposure to potential zootoxins on a frequent basis. Bites and stings from arthropods and snakes certainly can occur in any species, and the potential for oral exposure to animals such as poisonous toads, snakes, or insects will vary with the region and environment. Clinically significant zootoxins can affect various vital organs, such as nervous, cardiovascular, and reproductive and developmental systems (Dorce et al., 2009; Gwaltney-Brant, 2017).

ARTHROPODA

Araneae: Spiders

Introduction

At least 30,000 species of spiders are distributed throughout the world (Goddard, 2003). Spiders have eight segmented legs and bisegmented bodies composed of head/thorax (prosoma or cephalothorax) and abdomen (opisthosoma) (Lucas and Meier, 1995b; Goddard, 2003). Venom is stored in two glands located in the cephalothorax and empties through fangs (chelicerae) located at the rostral end of the prosoma (Lucas and Meier, 1995b). With the exception of spiders in the family Ulobiridae (found in Australia), all spiders are capable of inflicting an envenomating bite via fangs. Most spider envenomations, however, are likely to cause few signs other than local swelling and pain. Anaphylaxis and other allergic reactions to venom components are possible (Goddard, 2003). Although there is disagreement in the literature, it appears that fewer than 100 spider species can inflict a bite of medical significance (Lucas and Meier, 1995b).

*Widow Spiders (*Latrodectus *spp.)*

Background

Latrodectus spp. are found throughout the world. These spiders are identified by a red, yellow, or orange hourglass-shaped marking on the ventral abdomen of the female. Males and immature females are brown; immature females do not have the hourglass marking. The

Veterinary Toxicology. DOI: http://dx.doi.org/10.1016/B978-0-12-811410-0.00058-1

fangs of the male are considered too short to inflict an envenomating bite to humans or other mammals (Lucas and Meier, 1995b). In the United States, there are five major species of widow spiders (Goddard, 2003): *Latrodectus mactans* (black widow spider), *Latrodectus hesperus* (western black widow spider), *Latrodectus variolus* (northern black widow spider), *Latrodectus bishopi* (red widow spider and red-legged widow spider), and *Latrodectus geometricus* (brown widow spider).

Widow spiders are found mostly outside of living spaces, preferring dark secluded areas such as piles of debris and densely growing plants. Inside houses, they prefer dark, rarely disturbed spaces and will often settle under appliances and cabinets. Adult spiders are most active in the warm months and will die during the colder months if not in heated spaces. They build webs to ensnare prey. In general, widow spiders are shy and do not bite larger animals unless provoked (Goddard, 2003).

Mechanism of Action

Widow spider venom is a complex mixture of approximately six neuroactive proteins; there are also some proteolytic enzymes. The principal toxin for mammals is α-latrotoxin, a polypeptide that causes a large release and then depletion of acetylcholine and norepinephrine at postganglionic sympathetic synapses (Lucas and Meier, 1995b).

Toxicity

The venom of widow spiders is extremely potent; the LD_{50} for whole venom of *L. mactans tredecimguttatus* (European black widow) in guinea pigs is 0.0075 mg/kg and for mice is 0.9 mg/kg (White et al., 1995). The syndrome caused by widow venom is called latrodectism. Following a widow spider bite, venom is taken up by lymphatics and then enters the bloodstream (White et al., 1995). Clinically, there may be short-lived, localized pain at the bite site followed in approximately 30–120 min by myalgia and muscle cramps near the site of envenomation. Pain begins to spread to the large muscles groups of the legs, thorax, back, and abdomen, peaking in approximately 2–3 h. Mild to moderate hypertension and tachycardia are common. In most cases, signs resolve in 48–72 h, but signs such as weakness, fatigue, and insomnia may persist for weeks to months (White et al., 1995; Goddard, 2003).

Cats are very sensitive to the effects of widow venom. In one study, 20 of 22 cats died after widow spider bites, with an average survival time of 115 h (Peterson and McNalley, 2006a). Paralysis occurs early in the course; severe pain is evidenced by howling and other vocalizations. Hypersalivation, restlessness, vomiting, and diarrhea were common. Muscle tremors, cramping, ataxia, and inability to stand may precede an atonic paralysis. Cheyne–Stokes respiratory pattern may develop prior to death.

Treatment

Treatment is largely symptomatic, with control of pain by opioids and use of muscle relaxants such as diazepam and methocarbamol to control muscle rigidity. Calcium gluconate, which was once used for treatment of widow envenomation, is no longer recommended because it was found to be less effective at controlling pain than opioids and muscle relaxants (Clarke et al., 1992; Peterson and McNalley, 2006a). An equine-origin antivenin (Lycovac, available in the United States from Merck and Co.) has been used in humans. It is generally administered to high-risk patients (the very young or old) or in those whose signs are progressing despite other medical care. The antivenin is extremely effective; in one study, all 58 patients receiving the agent had resolution of signs within 30 min (Clarke et al., 1992). In one case report (Twedt et al., 1999), a cat with suspected latrodectism was treated with antivenom approximately 26 h after signs began. The cat rapidly recovered neurologic function.

*Recluse or Violin Spiders (*Loxesceles *spp.)*

Background

Although there are at least 50 species of *Loxosceles*, few can inflict the medically significant envenomation known as loxoscelism. In the United States, where several *Loxosceles* species occur, the brown recluse spider (*L. reclusa*) is considered the only one of medical importance. *L. reclusa* is found principally in Missouri, Arkansas, Oklahoma, Kansas, and Tennessee, but its range extends from the southern Gulf states and southern Atlantic states through Indiana and Illinois. Other species of *Loxosceles* are found principally in the southwest United States and California, and the Brazilian native *Loxesceles laeta* appears to have been introduced into the Los Angeles area (Goddard, 2003). Brown recluse spiders (*L. reclusa*) are nocturnal, nonaggressive spiders. They are recognizable by the "fiddle"-shaped marking on the dorsal surface of the cephalothorax.

Mechanism of Action

The venom of recluse spiders contains several necrotizing enzymes, including hyaluronidase, esterases, and alkaline phosphatases. Sphingomyelinase D, a phospholipase, appears to be the most important component; it binds to cell membranes and causes migration and activation of neutrophils in the area of the envenomation. In addition, the venom inactivates serum hemolytic complement, leading to intravascular coagulation, occlusion of small capillaries, and tissue necrosis; systemic depletion of clotting factors (VII, IX, XI, and XII) can also occur (White et al., 1995; Goddard, 2003; Peterson and McNalley, 2006b). Platelet activation can also be seen (Peterson and McNalley, 2006b). In the presence of calcium and C-reactive protein, sphingomyelinase D can cause hemolysis. Finally, lipases can cause free lipids in the blood that may act as inflammatory mediators and/or cause embolization (Peterson and McNalley, 2006b).

Toxicity

Dogs injected intravenously with brown recluse venom developed thrombocytopenia, absence of reticulocytes, and evidence of hemolysis with decreased hematocrit (Denny et al., 1964). Necropsy showed widespread petechial and ecchymotic hemorrhage, dehydration, and hypocellular bone marrow with depression of the erythroid and platelet cell lines. Another study (Futrell et al., 1979) of in vitro hemolysis found that human and pig erythrocytes were far more susceptible to lysis from brown recluse venom than those of dogs.

Initially, the bite may produce little pain or local reaction. Approximately 3–8 h after envenomation, the site becomes red, swollen, and tender and forms a "bull's-eye" lesion. A vesicle may form and be replaced by a black scab or eschar. Tissue around the bite may slough, leaving a 1- to 25-cm ulcer. Venom distribution may occur in areas dependent to the bite due to gravity. Healing is slow and may take months, often leaving a large scar (Goddard, 2003). Diagnosing a brown recluse bite may be difficult if the bite is not witnessed. In many cases, a brown recluse bite is "blamed" for necrotic lesions due to other causes (Mullen, 2002b). Systemic signs, although uncommon, can be seen with a brown recluse bite; they may develop 48–72 h after exposure. Hemolysis with anemia and hematuria, tachycardia, pyrexia, myalgia, vomiting, dyspnea, disseminated intravascular coagulation, and coma have been reported but are rare (Goddard, 2003).

Treatment

For the necrotic lesion, local wound care including chemical debridement with Burrow's solution (aluminum acetate) or hydrogen peroxide and bandaging should be performed. Pruritus may be controlled with diphenhydramine (2.2 mg/kg q8h). Antibiotics, especially if infection is evident, should be administered. Analgesics for pain (nonsteroidal antiinflammatory drugs for mild pain and opioids for severe pain) may be required. Surgical excision, used in the past, is no longer recommended (Peterson and McNalley, 2006b). Dapsone (4,49-diaminodiphenylsulfone) may be helpful in limiting the severity of the necrotic lesion because it inhibits neutrophil migration. In dogs, a dose of 1 mg/kg per day for 14 days has been used experimentally. Dapsone can cause methemoglobinemia as well as hemolysis in individuals with glucose-6-phosphate dehydrogenase deficiency (Peterson and McNalley, 2006b). Antivenins are available for South American *Loxesceles* species. Experimental antivenins for *L. reclusa* have been developed. These have been shown to be effective if given within 4 h of envenomation. However, these antivenins are not currently commercially available (Mullen, 2002b).

*Hobo Spiders (*Tegenaria agrestis*)*

Background

Hobo spiders are native to Europe but were introduced in the Pacific Northwest in the 1930s. They occur mainly in Washington, Oregon, and Idaho, but their range includes central Utah through western Canada to the Alaskan panhandle. In the 1980s, the appearance of necrotic spider bites in the Pacific Northwest was initially blamed on *L. reclusa*, but later the bites were correctly attributed to *T. agrestis* (Goddard, 2003).

Hobo spiders are poor climbers and build a funnel web at ground level or in basements. Males will leave their web at night in search of females and may enter houses while doing so. Males are more venomous than females and are more likely to bite (Mullen, 2002a,b; Goddard, 2003).

Toxicity

In most cases, the bite is initially painless. Within 30 min, a localized expanding area of erythema may occur; the lesion may eventually reach 15 cm in diameter. Then, in approximately 15–35 h, the area ruptures and there is a serous discharge from the wound. The wound may require 3 years to heal, especially if it is in fatty tissue (Goddard, 2003). In humans, systemic signs may occur in approximately 45% of bites, and approximately one-third of these may require hospitalization. Signs may include headache (which can last for days), nausea, weakness, and vision changes. The signs may progress to vomiting (often intractable), watery diarrhea, and bone marrow destruction resulting in anemia, pancytopenia, and thrombocytopenia. Fatalities are rare (Mullen, 2002b).

Treatment

Treatment of the hobo spider bite is supportive and symptomatic.

Tarantulas

Tarantulas of the family Theraphosideae are large, ground-dwelling spiders (Mullen, 2002b). In most cases, the bite of the tarantula causes little more than localized pain that develops slowly but usually resolves within 30 min. Approximately 12 genera of tarantulas that may deliver a potentially life-threatening bite exist in the tropical regions of South America, Africa, and Australia. Their venom contains a neurotoxin; there may also be a necrotoxin and hemolytic toxin. Following envenomation, muscle spasms, edema, hemoglobinuria, jaundice, and circulatory shock may develop (Mullen, 2002b).

Species of tarantula living in the United States are not capable of delivering serious envenomation. However, many of these species have urticating hairs on their abdomen that possess spines and barbs that can penetrate skin. When threatened, these tarantulas can stroke their abdomen and flick the urticating hairs at their attacker. The hairs can cause severe inflammation of the skin, eyes, mouth, and respiratory tract. The effect is purely mechanical because there is no toxin associated with the hairs. Urticaria, edema, and vasodilation may occur in the skin. In the eyes, swelling of the lids and corneal abrasions are common (Mullen, 2002b). Dogs or cats attempting to ingest tarantulas may gag or vomit.

Scorpiones: Scorpions

Background

Scorpions are arachnids with two body divisions: the combined head and thorax, referred to as the prosoma or cephalothorax, and the abdomen or opisthosoma. They possess large paired claws or pincers known as pedipalps and four pairs of legs. At the caudal portion of the abdomen, scorpions have a tail that terminates in the telson—a barbed appendage that houses two venom glands that exit via a stinger at the end of the telson. Scorpions are nocturnal hunters; they may spend the day in burrows or hiding under rocks or vegetation. They may also hide in blankets, shoes, and clothing, which is a common way for humans to be exposed to them (Keegan, 1980).

There are approximately 1400 species of scorpions occurring on all continents except Antarctica (Goddard, 2003). Most occur in tropical or temperate regions (Lucas and Meier, 1995a). Table 58.1 lists locations and species of scorpions capable of inflicting life-threatening envenomations in humans. The main genera of scorpions found in North America are the bark scorpions (*Centruroides* spp.). They are found primarily in Central America, Mexico, and the southern through southwest United States (Mullen and Stockwell, 2002). In the United States, only *Centruroides exilicauda* (Arizona bark scorpion) is considered capable of inflicting a life-threatening sting (Goddard, 2003).

TABLE 58.1 Scorpions of Medical Importance: Species and Location

Location	Species
India	*Hottentotta tamulus*
Mexico and Central America	*Centruroides* spp.
Middle East	*Androctonus* spp. *Buthus* spp. *Hemiscorpion lepturus* *Leiurus quinquestriatus* *Mesobuthus gibbosus*
South Africa	*Parabuthus* spp. *Buthus minax*
South America	*Tityus* spp. *Centruroides gracilis*
United States	*Centruroides sculpturatus*
West Indies (Trinidad)	*Tityus trinitatis*

Source: Adapted from Lucas, S.M., Meier, J., 1995a. Biology and distribution of scorpions of medical importance. In: Meier, J., White, J. (Eds.), Handbook of Clinical Toxicology of Animal Venoms and Poisons. CRC Press, Boca Raton, FL, pp. 239–258 and Keegan, H.L., 1980. Scorpions of Medical Importance. University Press of Mississippi, Jackson, MS.

Mechanism of Action

All scorpions can deliver an envenomating sting (Keegan, 1980). Scorpion venom components vary greatly between genera and may even differ based on geographic location within species (Mullen and Stockwell, 2002). The venom consists of a mixture of low-molecular-weight polypeptides. At least two potent neurotoxins have been identified: α-scorpion toxin found in *Androctonus*, *Leiurus*, and *Buthus* spp. and β-scorpion toxin found in *Centruroides* spp. Both toxins can be found in the venom of *Tityus* spp. These venoms block voltage-sensitive sodium and potassium channels in nerves (Mullen and Stockwell, 2002).

Toxicity

Scorpion stings cause instant, sharp pain at the site of envenomation. Some stings will cause localized pain that resolves over hours. Localized edema and pruritus are common. Regional lymph nodes may enlarge, and there may be an allergic reaction characterized by swelling of the eyelids, tongue, and vomiting. Sloughing of the skin at the site of envenomation can also occur (Mullen and Stockwell, 2002). Signs usually resolve within 24 h (Keegan, 1980). Systemically, signs generally include numbness of face, myalgia, tachycardia or bradycardia, respiratory depression, and seizures; however, there is a lack of evidence that scorpion envenomation in dogs and cats is a serious concern (Mullen and Stockwell, 2002).

Treatment

In most cases, the treatment of scorpion stings consists of analgesics and local wound care. Systemic signs are treated symptomatically with control of hypertension, heart rate changes, and neurologic signs. Some antivenoms in the United States are produced locally; however, because these are not approved by the US Food and Drug Administration, they cannot legally be transported to other states (Goddard, 2003). In addition, their use in veterinary patients is considered controversial (Dalefield and Oehme, 2006).

Ixodida: Ticks

Background

Ticks are well known as being vectors for many human and animal diseases, with the first reports of tick paralysis originating in Australia in 1890 and British Columbia in 1912 (Sonenshine et al., 2002). Worldwide, 43 species of ticks from nine different genera have been associated with tick paralysis: *Amblyomma*, *Argas*, *Dermacentor*, *Haemaphysalis*, *Hyalomma*, *Ixodes*, *Ornithodoros*, *Otobius*, and *Rhipicephalus* (Dipeolu, 1976; Fowler, 1993). Tick paralysis has been reported in North America, Europe, Africa, Australia, and the former Soviet Union.

Mechanism of Action

The exact mechanism(s) of action of tick toxins is not well known, but in most tick species it is suspected that the toxin interferes with the synthesis and/or release of acetylcholine at the neuromuscular junctions, resulting in lower motor neuron paresis and paralysis very similar to that produced by botulinum toxin (Fowler, 1993). The Australian tick, *Ixodes holocyclus*, toxin may differ because it appears to have more of an effect on central nerve centers rather than on peripheral (Fowler, 1993).

Toxicity

Tick paralysis has been reported in a large variety of animal species, including dogs, cats, cattle, sheep, goats, llamas, poultry, wild antelope, bison, foxes, wolves, mice, ground hogs, black-tailed deer, and several species of wild birds (Daly et al., 1992; Fowler, 1993; Beyer and Grossman, 1997; Sonenshine et al., 2002). In North America, most cases of tick paralysis in livestock occur in the Pacific Northwest due to *Dermacentor andersoni*, whereas most cases in dogs are due to *Dermacentor variabilis* (Fowler, 1993; Sonenshine et al., 2002). *Dermacentor occidentalis* occasionally causes tick paralysis in cattle, ponies, and deer but not dogs (Sonenshine et al., 2002). In the southeastern United States, *Ixodes brunneus* has been associated with tick paralysis in wild passerine birds (Luttrell et al., 1996). In Australia, tick paralysis is caused by *I. holocyclus*, whereas *Ixodes rubicundus* and *Rhipicephalus evertsi* are the primary species responsible for tick paralysis in Africa (Sonenshine et al., 2002). Tick paralysis in Europe and Asia has been reported due to bites from *Hyalomma punctata* and *Ixodes ricinus*.

Tick paralysis has occurred following the bite a single tick, and heavily infested animals may succumb quickly (Fowler, 1993). Clinical signs include an ascending ataxia that progresses to paresis and flaccid paralysis. Early in the intoxication, animals remain bright, alert, and able to eat and drink if properly supported. Eventually, paralysis of the respiratory muscles leads to respiratory failure and death. Paralysis produced by *I. holocyclus*, the Australian tick, generally occurs more rapidly and tends to persist following removal of the tick.

Treatment

The main goal of treatment is to remove the ticks and provide supportive care (especially respiratory support) until recovery occurs. Recovery can occur quite rapidly following complete removal of the ticks, or it may take a few days (Fowler, 1993). The use of topical insecticides may aid in the removal of ticks and can be especially helpful in cases in which numerous ticks are embedded. Heavily coated animals may need to be shaved to ensure that all embedded ticks are found and removed. Removal of embedded ticks should be performed carefully to avoid expressing additional toxin into the wound or leaving the head embedded in the skin. Forceps may be used to grasp the tick as close to the skin as possible and gentle traction should be used to remove the tick. In most cases in which ticks are removed before bulbar paralysis has occurred, the prognosis for full recovery is very good. A short-term immunity develops following recovery from tick paralysis.

Myriapoda: Centipedes and Millipedes

Centipedes and millipedes are distantly related to lobsters, crayfish, and shrimp. These arthropods are widely distributed throughout the world, and they are characterized by a long, flat, multisegmented body with one (centipede) or two (millipede) legs emerging from each body segment. Although most centipedes and millipedes are less than 1.5 in. long, centipedes from the genus *Scolopendra* may grow to be 4–6 in. long. All centipedes have a pair of modified front legs (forcipules) that serve as fangs and that are connected to venomous glands directly under the head (Norris, 2004). Larger centipedes can inflict painful bites resulting in local swelling, erythema, and lymphangitis. In addition, the legs of *Scolopendra* spp. are tipped with sharp claws that are capable of penetrating skin, and toxin produced at the attachment point of each leg may drop into these wounds, causing inflammation and irritation due to mast cell degranulation (Tavora et al., 2016).

Centipede venom has been poorly studied, but components identified in various centipedes include a phospholipase A_2, metalloproteases, and hyaluronidase, serotonin, a β-pore-forming compound, a hemolysin (γ-glutamyl transpeptidase), and histamine (Norris, 2004; Undheim et al., 2015). In most cases, systemic toxicosis is not expected, although local necrosis may occur (Russell, 1996); a single case report exists of a human fatality from the bite of *Scolopendra subspinipes* (Norris, 2004). Signs generally subside within 48 h and rarely require more than symptomatic care (e.g., analgesics). Millipedes do not bite but can emit irritating and foul-smelling secretions from repugnatorial glands; some species can spray these fluids over distances of several inches. These secretions are irritating to mucosal surfaces, particularly the eyes, and corticosteroids have been recommended to decrease the inflammatory response (Russell, 1996).

Insecta: Insects

Introduction

Insect and insect-related problems are common in domestic and wild animals. Insects such as lice, fleas, deerflies, horseflies, sand flies, mosquitoes, blackflies, and biting midges may cause severe annoyance to animals because of biting behavior. Members of several groups of insects can inject venom when they bite or sting, most notably bees, wasps, and ants. Bites or stings from insects such as bees, ants, wasps, and chiggers may cause direct effects from venoms or may result in allergic host reactions resulting from overresponsive host immune systems. Contact allergies may occur when certain beetles or caterpillars touch the skin. Other insects, such as blister beetles and certain caterpillars, produce toxins that can cause adverse reactions when they are touched or ingested (Durden and Mullen, 2002). Respiratory allergies can result from inhaling allergic air-borne particles from cockroaches, fleas, or other arthropods (Durden and Mullen, 2002). Some insects invade the body tissues of their host. Various degrees of invasion may occur, ranging from subcutaneous infestations to invasion of organs such as the lungs and intestine (Durden and Mullen, 2002). Insects of veterinary importance are discussed below and outlined in Table 58.2.

Coleoptera: Meloidae (Blister Beetles)

Background

More than 300,000 species of beetles have been described, representing 30%–40% of all known insects. Fewer than 100 species of beetles worldwide are known to be of public health or veterinary importance. Most of these are in the suborder Polyphaga. The species that have the greatest impact on the health of human and domestic animals are in the following families: Meloidae (blister beetles), Oedemeridae (false blister beetles), Staphylinidae (rove beetles), Tenebrionidae (darkling beetles), Dermestidae (larder beetles), and Scarabaeidae (scarab or dung beetles) (Krinsky, 2002).

Blister beetles are elongate, soft-bodied specimens in which the pronotum (section between head and wings) is narrower than the head or wings. Two common blister beetle species are potato beetles, one with orange and black longitudinal stripes and one black with gray wing margins (Goddard, 2003). Members of the genus *Mele* are called oil beetles because they exude an oily substance from their legs when disturbed. Oil beetles are approximately 20–25 mm long and black with no hind wings, giving the appearance that their wings are too short (Goddard, 2003).

Species that pose veterinary problems in the United States include the striped blister beetle (*Epicauta vittata*) (Fig. 58.1), the black blister beetle (*Epicauta pennsylvanica*), the margined blister beetle (*Epicauta pestifera*), and the three-striped blister beetle (*Epicauta lemniscata*), as well as *Epicauta fabricii*, *Epicauta occidentalis*, and *Epicauta temexa*. Of these, the most common species associated with toxicosis are *E. occidentalis* and *E. temexa* (Stair and Plumlee, 2004).

Mechanism of Action

The toxic principle in melioid beetles, cantharidin, is a bicyclic terpenoid (Goddard, 2003; Stair and Plumlee, 2004). The concentration of cantharidin present in beetles varies from 1% to 5% of the dry weight of the beetle. Males always have higher concentrations because the male produces cantharidin and transfers a quantity to the female during copulation (Krinsky, 2002). Cantharidin is present in the hemolymph as well as in the clear, yellow secretion that is exuded at the joints of the legs of these beetles by reflex bleeding (Fig. 58.2).

The mechanism of action of cantharidin may involve interference with enzyme systems responsible for active transport across mitochondrial membranes, resulting in membrane disruption and permeability changes. Mitochondrial damage results in cellular disruption, acantholysis, and vesicle formation. Cantharidin has also been shown to inhibit protein phosphatase 2A, resulting in disruption of signal transduction and cell metabolism (Stair and Plumlee, 2004). Purified, crystalline cantharidin is a potent vesicating agent that is readily absorbed through the gastrointestinal mucosa and, to a lesser degree, the skin. It is eliminated unchanged through the kidneys (Krinsky, 2002).

Toxicity

Adult blister beetles feed on flowering foliage, especially blooming alfalfa (*Medicago sativa*). Blister beetles in alfalfa fields contain enough cantharidin to provide lethal

TABLE 58.2 Miscellaneous Insects of Veterinary Importance

Name	Location	Species Affected	Toxicity, Toxic Principle	Clinical Effects	Lesions	References
Asian ladybeetle (*Harmonia axyridis*)	United States	Dogs	Corrosive, irritating hemolymph	Shock, cyanosis, death; corrosive injury to oral cavity	Irritation, ulceration, hemorrhage of oral cavity and GI tract in association with insect bodies	Hoenerhoff et al. (2002), Stocks and Lindsey (2008)
Caterpillars (many species)	Worldwide	All species	Surface hairs, spines trigger urticarial reactions	Irritation, urticaria, pruritus	Minimal	Mullen (2002a)
Eastern tent caterpillar (ETC) (*Malacosoma americanum*) Processionary caterpillar (PC) (*Ochrogaster lunifer*)	Ohio River Valley (ETC); Australia (PC)	Horses	Setae (hairs) penetrating cornea, GI tract	Early fetal loss, late-term abortions Bacterial placentitis, funisitis, placental edema, fetal death; pericarditis and uveitis in adults	Fibrinous pericarditis, unilateral uveitis, meningitis	McDowell et al. (2010), Caldwell-Smith et al. (2012)
Fireflies (*Photinus* spp.)	North America	Captive reptiles and amphibians	Lucibufagins (cardiac glycosides) in bodies of ingested fireflies	Head shaking, oral gaping, dyspnea, blackening of skin, regurgitation, death	None	Knight et al. (1999)
Monarch butterfly (*Danaus plexippus*)	North, Central, and South Americas	Birds, lizards, small mammals	Cardiotoxic glycosides in bodies of caterpillars and wings of butterflies	Cardiac arrhythmia, cardiac failure, weakness, dyspnea, death	None	Fowler (1993)
Rose chafer (*Macrodactylus subspinosus*)	North America	Immature chickens	Unknown, suspected neurotoxin	Drowsiness, weakness, coma, convulsions, death	Crops may be impacted with beetles	Lamson (1915)
Sawfly (*Arge pullata*, *Lophotoma* spp., *Perreyia flavipes*)	Denmark (*A. pullata*) Australia (*Lophotoma*) Uruguay (*Perreyia*)	Cattle, sheep, goats, pigs	Ingested larvae contain D-amino acid containing peptides: Lophyrotomin: similar to amatoxins Pergidin	Peracute death Cattle: weakness, tremors, depression, agitation, aggression, stupor, icterus, photosensitization Sheep, goats: depression, ataxia, anorexia, recumbency	Hepatocellular necrosis	Fowler (1993), Thamsborg et al. (1996), Dutra et al. (1997), Oelrichs et al. (1999)
Walking sticks (*Anisomorpha* spp.)	Florida, Gulf Coast	All species	Monoterpene dialdehyde sprayed at harasser	Ocular, nasal irritation and pain	None	Brutlag et al. (2011)

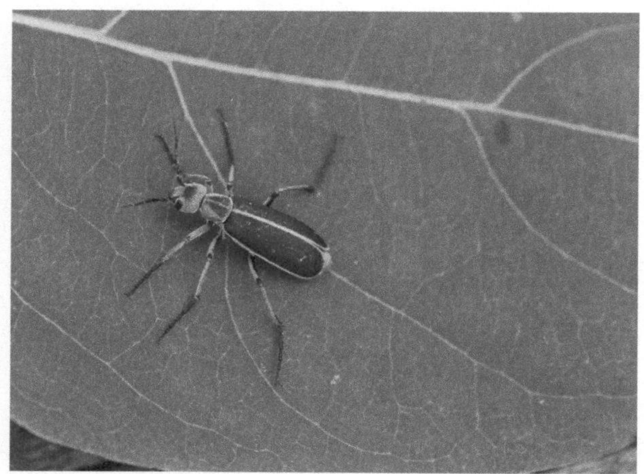

FIGURE 58.1 An adult striped blister beetle (*Epicauta vittata*). *Photo courtesy of James E. Appleby, University of Illinois.*

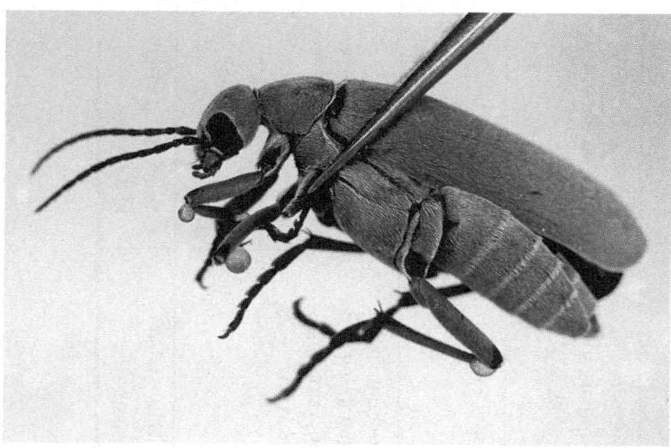

FIGURE 58.2 An adult blister beetle (Epicauta), with hemolymph droplets containing cantharidin. *Photo courtesy of Dr. Maria Eisner, Cornell University.*

doses to livestock that feed on forage when it is used as hay. Modern methods of hay harvesting, especially crimping, decrease the opportunity of blister beetles to vacate the foliage before it is incorporated into hay, thereby increasing the likelihood of blister beetles being trapped in the hay (Stair and Plumlee, 2004). Cantharidin released from crushed adult blister beetles may contaminate hay without visual evidence of insect parts. Cantharidin is very stable and may persist in hay for long periods of time. Because in the United States alfalfa is most widely grown in the South, cantharidin toxicosis is most commonly found in the southern states; however, due to interstate transport of alfalfa hay throughout the country, cantharidin toxicosis can occur in any state.

Horses are the species in which cantharidin toxicosis is most commonly reported. However, the following hosts have also been poisoned in natural or experimental situations: cattle, sheep, goats, rabbits, rats, hedgehogs, dogs, alpacas and emus (Stair and Plumlee, 2004; Simpson et al., 2013). Poisoning in human beings has been noted for decades and is usually the result of either improper medicinal use of cantharides or malicious poisoning (Krinsky, 2002). Horses are particularly susceptible to the effects of cantharidin (Stair and Plumlee, 2004). The estimated lethal dosage of cantharidin for the horse is approximately 0.5−1 mg/kg, and as little as 4 g of dried beetles may be lethal to a horse (Krinsky, 2002). The oral experimental lethal dosage of crystalline cantharidin for dogs and cats was 1.0−1.5 mg/kg, and it was 20 mg/kg for rabbits. It is estimated that the lethal dosage for a human is less than 1.0 mg/kg.

Cantharidin produces an intense, direct irritant effect on the skin and the mucous membranes of the esophagus, stomach, and intestines. Once absorbed, the toxin may affect many different organs. Excretion is via the kidneys, resulting in transfer of the irritant effect to the urinary tract, particularly the bladder and urethra (Krinsky, 2002).

Clinical signs vary with the dose ingested. Massive doses may cause shock and death within 4 h (Krinsky, 2002). Smaller doses may cause gastroenteritis, nephrosis, cystitis, and/or urethritis; thus, signs may include anorexia, soft feces, mucoid to bloody feces, intestinal atony, colic, dysuria (frequent, painful urination, or oliguria to anuria), and hematuria. The body temperature may elevate to 106°F (41.1°C). Other signs observed include depression, weakness, muscle rigidity, collapse, prostration, dehydration, and sweating (Krinsky, 2002). Animals frequently become dyspneic, and rales may be detected on auscultation due to pulmonary edema. Myocarditis may initiate cardiovascular signs including tachycardia, congested mucous membranes, and decreased capillary refill time. Synchronous diaphragmatic flutter and muscle fasciculations have been reported in horses and are thought to be the results of hypocalcemia (Stair and Plumlee, 2004). Ulceration of the oral mucosa membranes may be observed, and animals may be seen dipping their muzzles into water without drinking (Krinsky, 2002). Diarrhea may be observed in animals that live for a few days. The course of the disease may be as short as 4 h, with massive dose ingestion, to 5 days in lethal poisoning. In horses, the mortality rate is approximately 50%, with horses surviving more than 1 week having a favorable prognosis (Krinsky, 2002).

During intoxication, dehydration and shock cause elevations in serum protein and packed cell volume (Stair and Plumlee, 2004). The damaged gastrointestinal mucosa allows rapid invasion of enteric bacteria, resulting in bacteremia and leukocytosis. There may be mild elevation in serum urea nitrogen. Profound hypocalcemia (5.9 mg/dL; normal, 12.8 ± 1.2 mg/dL) and hypomagnesemia (0.7−1.8 mg/dL; normal, 2.5 ± 0.3 mg/dL) have been reported. Specific gravity of urine is low in the early stages of the disease, and erythrocytes are usually present in the urine, yielding a positive occult blood reaction.

Gross lesions may be minimal with massive dose ingestion. In more protracted cases, oral ulcers, vesication and desquamation of patches of the distal esophagus, erosion and ulceration of the gastrointestinal tract, mucus in the renal pelvis, and renal cortical hemorrhages may be seen. Hyperemia and hemorrhages are seen in the urethra and bladder mucosa. Ventricular myocarditis, pulmonary edema, petechial hemorrhages of serosal surfaces, hepatomegaly, and splenomegaly may also be present. The initial microscopic lesion is acantholysis of mucosa of the gastrointestinal tract, epithelium of the urinary tract, and endothelium of vessels (Krinsky, 2002). Other microscopic lesions include myocarditis, renal tubular nephrosis, and degenerative changes in the kidneys and digestive tract.

Cantharidin may be detected in urine, tissues (kidney and blood), gastrointestinal contents, and the dried beetles themselves by high-pressure liquid chromatography or gas chromatography—mass spectrometry. Cantharidin is excreted rapidly and may not be present in detectable amounts after 4 or 5 days following ingestion (Krinsky, 2002).

Treatment

There is no specific treatment. The administration of either activated charcoal or mineral oil via a gastric tube may aid animals that have consumed a small dose or are in the early stages of poisoning. General supportive therapy should include correction of fluid loss and electrolyte imbalances, particularly hypocalcemia and hypomagnesemia (Krinsky, 2002). Broad-spectrum antimicrobial therapy may be necessary to counter secondary bacterial invasion from the gastrointestinal tract avoiding aminoglycosides and other medications that are potentially nephrotoxic or excreted via the kidney.

Hymenoptera: Bees, Wasps, and Hornets

Background

More than 20,000 species of bees are distributed throughout the world (Fowler, 1993). Native honeybees in tropical Southeast Asia were the source of the domestic honeybee, *Apis mellifera*. Africanized honeybees (*Apis mellifera scutellata*) are a subspecies of the common honeybee native to Africa that has spread from South and Central America into south Texas, New Mexico, Arizona, Nevada, California, and Puerto Rico (Akre and Reed, 2002).

Mechanism of Action

There are numerous variations in the venom apparatus of members of Hymenoptera (Fowler, 1993). The stinger is a modification of the ovipositor apparatus and is found only in female bees and wasps. Venom secreted from specialized cells in the acid glands is transported to the venom sac reservoir via small tubules. One-way valves in the bulb of the venom apparatus control the flow of venom during envenomation. At the time of venom injection, the alkaline gland contributes a secretion that enhances the toxicity of the venom. The stinger of the honeybee is covered with retrograde barbs that cause the stinger to remain impaled in thick-skinned victims. When this occurs and the bee attempts to withdraw, the entire stinger apparatus is pulled from the bee, resulting in death of the honeybee.

Honeybee venoms are complex mixtures of proteins, peptides, and small organic molecules (Akre and Reed, 2002). Phospholipases and hyaluronidases present in the venom account for the majority of allergic responses to bee venoms in humans and likely other animals as well. Phospholipase A_2 is one of the most lethal peptides in honeybee venom (Schmidt, 1995). Mellitin is a membrane disruptive compound that increases the susceptibility of cell membranes to the damage caused by phospholipases within the venom (Akre and Reed, 2002). Mellitin can also cause pain, trigger hemolysis, increase capillary blood flow, increase cell permeability, and enhance spread of venom constituents within tissue. Mellitin, in combination with phospholipase and a mast cell degranulating peptide, triggers the release of histamine and serotonin. In mice, mellitin was found to be the primary lethal component of honeybee venom (Schmidt, 1995). Apamin is a neurotoxin that blocks calcium-activated potassium channels and has been associated with transient peripheral nerve effects in humans after bee stings (Saravanan et al., 2004). In cats, bee venom can cause contraction of bronchiolar muscles.

Like honeybees, vespid wasps (including yellow jackets and hornets) produce venoms containing peptides, enzymes, and amines designed to trigger pain (Akre and Reed, 2002). The primary pain-inducing substances are kinins; however, other compounds present in vespid venom, such as serotonin, histamine, tyramine, catecholamines, and acetylcholine, can contribute to the pain as well as local vasoactivity. Several of the constituents of vespid venom can act as allergens and trigger allergic reactions. Some vespid venoms contain neurotoxins or alarm pheromones that alert the swarm to an intruder.

Toxicity

Honeybees can inflict only a single sting, but an animal attacked by a swarm or hive of bees may sustain multiple stings and the cumulative envenomation may be lethal. The Africanized honeybee (*A. mellifera scutellata*) presents a special case. Although its venom is no more toxic than that of the domestic honeybee, the aggressive behavior of the African honeybee increases the likelihood of multiple stings occurring by swarms of these bees (Akre and Reed, 2002). Wasps and hornets either lack a barbed stinger or the barbs are small and do not prevent withdrawal of the stinger. Therefore, a single wasp may inflict multiple stings. Also, because many wasps are highly social, multiple stings are commonplace.

A sting by a single bee or vespid rarely causes more than a transient, painful prick in animals, in contrast to humans where sensitive individuals may die peracutely from a single sting. However, death following a single bee sting has been reported in a dog (Fowler, 1993). Deaths following attacks on livestock by Africanized bees have been reported, although most interactions between livestock and bees or wasps result in only local reactions. Yellow jacket envenomation leading to skin lesions and death has been reported in a group of pigs (Fowler, 1993).

Local reactions to single bee, hornet, or wasp stings consist of swollen, edematous, and erythematous plaques at the site of the sting (Fowler, 1993). Most small animal patients present with facial, periorbital, and/or aural edema. Honeybee stingers will occasionally be located embedded in the area, and a small abscess may form at the site.

Multiple stings may produce numerous wheals, urticaria, and in severe cases may cause severe systemic responses as direct toxic effects of the venom. Systemic effects reported in dogs following multiple stings from bees or vespids include prostration, convulsions, central nervous system (CNS) depression, shock, hyperthermia, bloody diarrhea, bloody vomiting, leukocytosis, intravascular hemolysis, disseminated intravascular coagulopathy, and elevations of blood urea nitrogen and alanine transaminase, suggesting renal and hepatic involvement (Wysoke et al., 1990; Cowell et al., 1991; Fowler, 1993). Hepatic injury in cats has also been reported following exposure to hornet venom. A mare and foal attacked by a swarm of bees experienced urticaria, angioedema, agitation, rhabdomyolysis, hypovolemia, ileus, and renal injury (Lewis and Racklyeft, 2014). Additionally, the mare displayed "almost maniacal behavior" for the first 48 h following envenomation and developed intravascular hemolysis, intrauterine hemorrhage, thrombocytopenia, hypoproteinemia, and recurrent fever; both mare and foal recovered with veterinary care.

The classic anaphylactoid response to bee and vespid venoms that is not uncommon in humans has not been documented in livestock, but anaphylaxis in dogs due to bee stings has been reported (Akre and Reed, 2002). Immune-mediated hemolytic anemia secondary to bee envenomation developed in two dogs (Noble and Armstrong, 1999). Clinical signs included lethargy, hematuria, ataxia, and seizures, and one dog died. Clinicopathologic data included nonregenerative anemia, spherocytosis, positive results for Coomb's test, and occult hematuria. Acute lung injury similar to the human acute respiratory distress syndrome developed in a dog following envenomation by more than 100 bees (Walker et al., 2005), and immune-mediated thrombocytopenia developed in a dog subsequent to massive envenomation by Africanized bees (Nakamura et al., 2013).

Treatment

Ideally, when an insect has stung an animal, identification of the insect should be attempted. Most often, stings occur in areas that are free of hair or have short hair. Retained stingers should be scraped away from the injection site; grasping the stinger with forceps may result in more venom being expressed into the injection site. Cold compresses may be used as first aid to relieve pain and swelling. Antihistamines and corticosteroids are thought to have questionable value once lesions have developed, but they are not contraindicated (Fowler, 1993). Patients should be monitored for development of systemic or anaphylactic reactions, which need to be treated promptly and aggressively. Epinephrine may be used in cases in which anaphylaxis is suspected. In cases of true systemic toxicosis, aggressive intravenous fluid therapy is recommended using balanced fluid solutions. Other treatments that have been recommended include corticosteroids, antihistamines, oxygen for dyspnea, and diazepam as needed for convulsions (Fowler, 1993). Renal and hepatic function should be monitored in animals that develop systemic reactions. In most cases, exposure to single stings from bees and vespids is rarely fatal.

Hymenoptera: Ants

Background

There are more than 10,000 species of ants, some of which bite, some of which sting, and others that both bite and sting. Some ants that lack a sting can spray formic acid, which can cause local irritation to the victim if it gets in the eyes or wounds produced by the ant's mandibles. Multiple stings from venomous ants have resulted in the death of pets, livestock, and wild animals in North, Central, and South America (Fowler, 1993). The red imported fire ant, *Solenopsis invicta*, is the most important species in terms of envenomation of animals. This ant was native to Brazil but entered the United States in the 1940s, where it has become a serious pest in the southeast as far west as Texas.

Mechanism of Action

Ant venoms, like bee venoms, are complex mixtures of compounds that can induce a variety of adverse effects in animals. Fire ant venoms consist largely of alkaloids, with less than 1% proteinaceous component (Akre and Reed, 2002). The alkaloids consist of solenopsins (methyl-*n*-alkylpiperidines) and a piperidine that cause dermal necrosis when injected in skin. These alkaloids have cytotoxic, hemolytic, fungicidal, insecticidal, and bactericidal properties.

Toxicity

Animals most likely to be severely affected by fire ants tend to be those that are unable to move away from a colony, including those that are neonatal, juvenile, or disabled. Attacks of fire ants resulting in deaths of newborn game animals such as rabbits and deer have been reported (Akre and Reed, 2002). Nesting bird chicks and newly hatched quail and poultry have been killed (and often eaten) by fire ants (Fowler, 1993).

Clinical effects of fire ant envenomation include intense pain at the site of the sting. In humans, within minutes of a sting there is formation of an urticarial wheal, which progresses to a vesicle and then a pustule within 24 h (Fowler, 1993). Within a few days, the pustule will rupture, resulting in a crusting lesion. Dogs do not appear to develop the pustules described in humans; instead, they develop erythematous pruritic papules that generally resolve within 24 h (Rakich et al., 1993). There are no reports of anaphylaxis in animals secondary to fire ant stings (Akre and Reed, 2002). Multiple stings may result in systemic signs similar to those of multiple bee or wasp stings.

Treatment

Single bites from fire ants generally require no treatment. Multiple envenomations resulting in severe systemic reactions or anaphylaxis should be managed similarly to systemic reactions to bee stings (i.e., fluids, corticosteroids, and supportive care).

Amphibia, Anura: Toads

Introduction

Poisonous amphibians include frogs, salamanders, and toads, but only toads have been associated with toxicosis in domestic animals. Poisonous frogs belong to the Dendrobatidae family and are popular aquarium pets due to their vivid, gem-like coloration. Poisonous frogs have been found to have nearly 500 different bioactive alkaloids in their skin secretions, most of which are not synthesized by the frogs but originate from insects in the diet; the alkaloids absorbed from the insects are sequestered in skin glands to produce toxic secretions (Daly, 1995a,b). Captive dendrobatids tend to lack these toxic alkaloids in their skin secretions, most likely due to the difference in diets. The remaining discussion focuses on poisonous toads.

Background

Toads are found throughout the world, and all are considered to produce zootoxins capable of causing clinical effects in animals. However, only the larger toads, specifically *Bufo blombergi*, *Bufo alvarius*, *Bufo regularis*, and *Rhinella marinus* (formerly *Bufo marinus*), are generally considered to produce sufficient poison to cause serious toxicosis (Fowler, 1993). *R. marinus* is found in Florida, Texas, Hawaii, the Caribbean, Central and South America, Fiji, Australia, the Philippines, and the Marianas. *B. alvarius* (*Incillus alvarius*) is found in the Imperial Valley of California and the Colorado River basin between Arizona and California. *B. blombergi* (*Rhaebo blombergi*) is found only in Colombia, and *B. regularis* (*Amietophrynus regularis*) is found in Ethiopia (Fowler, 1993). Although smaller toad species are rarely involved in animal intoxications, ingestion of toads by smaller animals or ingestion of multiple toads may result in toxicosis, as occurred with a captive, immature South American fur seal that died after ingesting two adult common toads (*Bufo bufo*) (Toennes et al., 2015).

Toads possess mucous glands that are widely distributed over the skin and that produce slimy secretions that keeps the skin moist and lubricated. The mucus secretions may aid in defense through their objectionable odor and/or taste to predators. Toads produce their toxic secretions from granular glands, modified mucous glands, throughout the head, shoulders, and dorsolateral areas of their skin. The more toxic toad species possess a parotid gland, which is an aggregation of granular glands located caudal and lateral to the ear (Fowler, 1993).

Toxicokinetics

Dogs are the species most commonly involved in toad toxicosis, with smaller dogs at higher risk (Reeves 2004). Mouthing of toads stimulates release of toxins from the parotid gland, with absorption occurring across the mucous membranes in the mouth (Roder, 2004). Toad secretions contain a variety of compounds, including bufogenins, bufotoxins, and bufotenines.

Mechanism of Action

Bufogenins inhibit sodium–potassium ATPase activity in a manner similar to cardiac glycosides such as digitalis, ultimately causing increased intracellular calcium in myocardial cells that results in cardiac arrhythmias (Eubig, 2001). Bufotoxins are bufogenins conjugated with suberyl arginine, and they have a similar mechanism of action as bufogenins. Bufotenines are indolalkylamines such as serotonin and 5-hydroxytryptophan; in combination with catecholamines present in *Bufo and Rhinella* toxins, these agents may be responsible for many of the neurologic and gastrointestinal effects of toad toxins (Eubig, 2001).

Toxicity

The relative potency of toad toxins varies with species of toad, geographic location, and size of the toad (Fowler, 1993). Smaller patients may show more severe signs when exposed to toad secretions (Eubig, 2001). *Rhinella* toads in Florida appear to be more toxic than those in Hawaii and Texas, based on mortality rates of dogs exposed to the toads (Roder, 2004). One hundred milligrams of crude *toad* toxin is said to be toxic for dogs weighing 9–14 kg.

Clinical effects of toad poisoning include hypersalivation, anxiety, and vomiting, which can occur almost immediately following exposure; also, death may occur as rapidly as 15 min following exposure (Eubig, 2001). Other signs, including hyperemic mucous membranes, recumbency, collapse, and tachypnea, may also be present. Neurologic effects are common and include convulsions, ataxia, nystagmus, stupor, or coma (Fowler, 1993; Reeves, 2004; Roder, 2004). A variety of cardiac arrhythmias have been reported, including bradycardia, sinus tachycardia, and sinus arrhythmias (Eubig, 2001). Pulmonary edema, hyperthermia, and hyperkalemia have also been reported (Fowler, 1993).

Treatment

On-the-spot decontamination of the oral cavity by copious water lavage is recommended in cases in which no signs beyond ptyalism and gagging have occurred (Eubig, 2001). Patients displaying more severe signs should be transported to a veterinary facility for stabilization prior to oral lavage. If an entire toad has been ingested, emesis under veterinary supervision is indicated for dogs when no signs beyond hypersalivation have occurred. Endoscopic or surgical removal of the toad from the stomach may be required in cases in which signs have developed, but it is important to stabilize the patient prior to attempts to remove the toad. Alternatively, multiple doses of activated charcoal with a cathartic may be used when entire toads are ingested (Eubig, 2001).

Patients displaying severe signs of toxicosis should be treated symptomatically and aggressively. Seizures may be managed with diazepam or a barbiturate. Intravenous fluid therapy is essential to aid in cardiovascular support. Arrhythmias should be managed as they develop. Bradycardia may be treated using atropine, whereas propranolol or esmolol may be used to treat tachycardia (Eubig, 2001). Correction of potassium imbalances should be performed as needed. Animals experiencing severe hyperkalemia, severe neurologic signs, or severe arrhythmias unresponsive to therapy may be treated with digoxin-specific antigen-binding fragments (digoxin immune Fab); however, the high cost of this product often makes its use in veterinary medicine unfeasible (Eubig, 2001). The prognosis for patients exposed to small toads and/or showing mild clinical signs is good. Animals developing advanced neurologic or cardiac signs have a more guarded prognosis.

REPTILIA

Venomous reptiles come from the order Squamata, which includes the lizards and the snakes. Outbreaks of poisonings from consumption of the flesh of certain turtles and tortoises have occasionally been reported in humans, but the incidence is low; reports in the veterinary literature of chelonitoxism are lacking.

Snakes

Introduction

Approximately 400 of the 35,001 species of snakes in the world are venomous (Russell, 2001). Venomous snakes are widely distributed throughout the world, apart from certain islands, such as Hawaii, Ireland, and New Zealand (Fowler, 1993). Venomous snakes come from the families Colubridae, Crotalidae, Elapidae, Hydrophiidae, Laticaudidae, and Viperidae; only members of the Crotalidae and Elapidae are represented in the Western Hemisphere.

Crotalids

Background

The crotalids are also known as pit vipers, so named for the indented, heat-sensing pits located between the nostrils and eyes. Other features of this family include elliptical pupils, triangular-shaped heads, retractable and hollow front fangs, and a single row of subcaudal scales distal to the anal plate (Peterson, 2004). Rattlesnakes have special keratin "rattles" on the ends of their tails and are members of the genera *Crotalus* and *Sistrus*. Other crotalids native to North America include water moccasins, also known as cottonmouths (*Agkistrodon piscivorus*) and copperheads (*Agkistrodon contortrix*).

At least 29 subspecies of rattlesnakes are found throughout the United States, whereas copperheads and water moccasins are distributed through the eastern and central United States. The approximate distributions of some of the more common species are illustrated in Fig. 58.3. Because of their tendency to associate near areas of human habituation, copperheads are responsible for most human (and likely animal) snakebites in the United States. However, most animal and human deaths in the

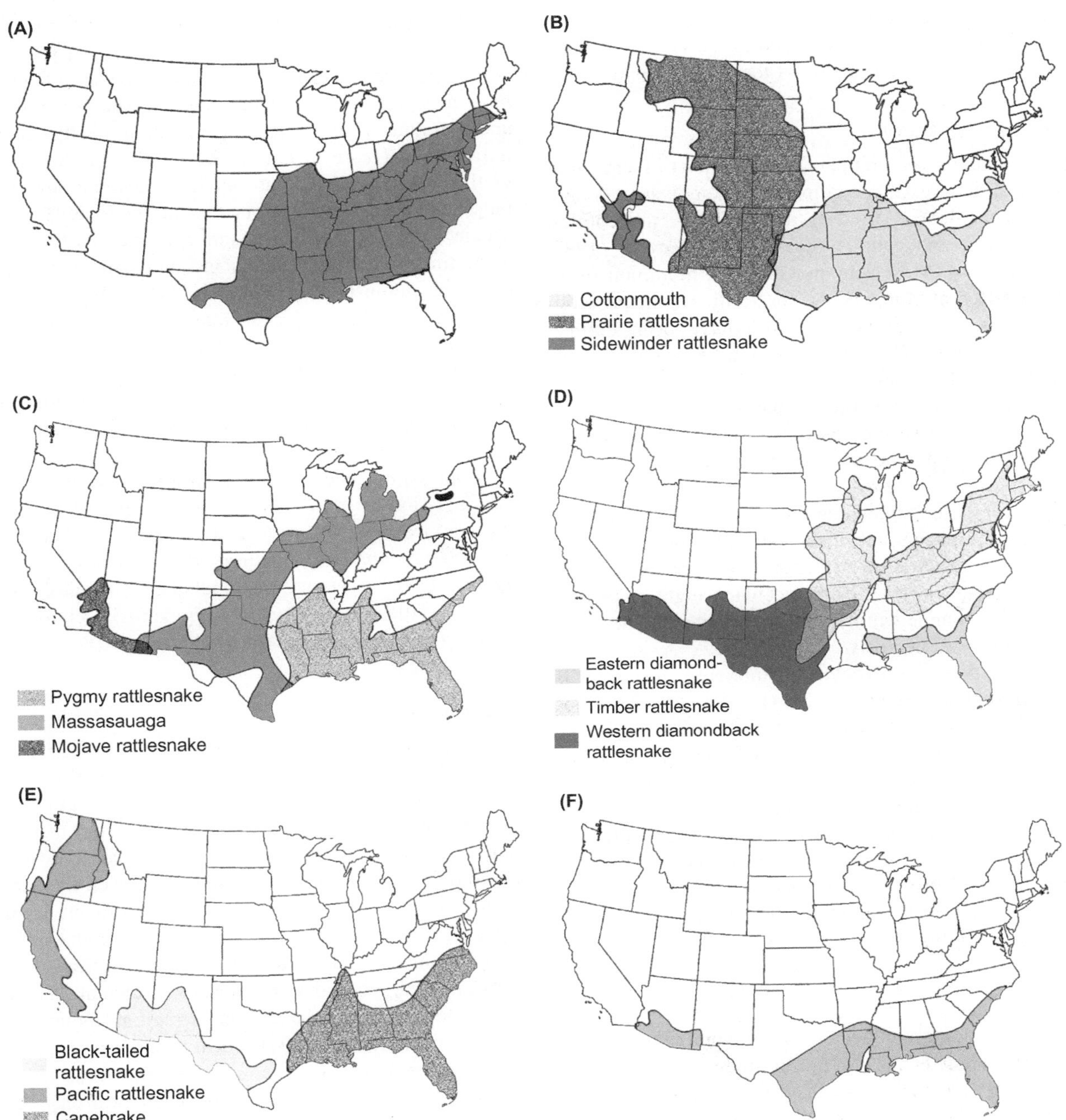

FIGURE 58.3 Distribution of venomous snakes in the United States. (A) Distribution of copperheads (*Agkistrodon contortrix*). (B) Distribution of cottonmouths (*Agkistrodon piscivorus*), prairie rattlesnakes (*Crotalus viridis*), and sidewinder rattlesnakes (*Crotalus cerastes*). (C) Distribution of pygmy rattlesnakes (*Sistrurus miliarius*), massasauga rattlesnake (*Sistrurus catenatus*), and Mojave rattlesnake (*Crotalus scutulatus*). (D) Distribution of the Eastern diamondback rattlesnake (*Crotalus adamanteus*), timber rattlesnake (*Crotalus horridus*), and Western diamondback rattlesnake (*Crotalus atrox*). (E) Distribution of the black-tailed rattlesnake (*Crotalus molossus*), Pacific rattlesnake (*C. atrox*), and canebrake rattlesnake (*C. horridus atricaudatus*). (F) Distribution of coral snakes (*Micruroides euryxanthus* and *Micrurus fulvius*). *Adapted from Fowler,* Veterinary Zootoxicology, *CRC Press, and Professional Pest Control Products website, http://www.pestproducts.com/snakeinfo.htm.*

United States are attributed to rattlesnakes, due to their more potent venoms. It is estimated that from 150,000 to 300,000 animals are bitten every year by pit vipers within the United States (Peterson, 2004; Wallis, 2005).

Pit vipers inject their venom by rotating their retractable fangs downward and forward in a stabbing motion (Peterson, 2004). Contraction of muscles in the venom glands then forces the venom through the hollow fangs and into the tissues of the victim. Snakes can control the amount of venom delivered to the victim by regulating the muscular contraction of the venom glands.

Mechanism of Action

Crotalid venoms are complex combinations of enzymes, cytotoxins, neurotoxins, cardiotoxins, hemolysins, coagulants/anticoagulants, lipids, nucleosides, nucleotides, organic acids, and cations such as zinc (Fowler, 1993; Peterson, 2004). Most venoms contain a minimum of 10 of these different components. In North American rattlesnakes, three general venom types have been defined (Peterson, 2004). "Classic" diamondback venom causes marked tissue destruction, coagulopathy, and hypotension. Mojave A venom causes little tissue destruction or coagulopathy but causes severe neurotoxicosis. The third venom class contains components of both classic and neurotoxic venoms.

Hyaluronidase ("spreading factor") and other enzymes break down collagen and other connective tissues, allowing for rapid penetration of venom components throughout the victim's tissues. Low-molecular-weight myotoxins open sodium channels in the muscle cell membrane, leading to myocyte necrosis. Phospholipase A stimulates hypercontraction of myocyte membranes, resulting in myofibril rupture (Peterson, 2004). Alteration of blood coagulation may lead to either hyper- or hypocoagulation through either direct effects on clotting factors or induction of hyperfibrinolysis, resulting in dissolution of clots as they are forming. Some diamondback rattlesnake venoms contain cardiotoxic agents (myocardial depressant factors) that cause profound hypotension unresponsive to fluid therapy. Neurotoxic components bind the presynaptic nerve membrane, inhibiting neurotransmitter release and causing paralysis (Fowler, 1993).

Toxicity

Dogs are the domestic species most commonly bitten by pit vipers (Witsil et al., 2015). In studies of rattlesnake bites in dogs, most bites occurred in late spring to early fall during the late afternoon (Hackett et al., 2002; Witsil et al., 2015). Most bites involved young dogs (median age, 2.75–3.7 years) and were located on the head. Horses are most commonly bitten on the muzzle, and cattle are more commonly bitten on the tongue or muzzle (Peterson, 2004). Cats are considered more resistant to pit viper venom, but cats are often presented in more severe clinical conditions due to their small body size, tendency to be struck on the torso, and, often, delay in obtaining veterinary care when they run and hide following a bite. Bites to the thoracic wall allow for more rapid and complete venom absorption, whereas bites to the tongue are essentially equivalent to intravenous envenomations.

The toxicity of any given crotalid bite will depend on both victim and snake factors. The species of the victim is an important factor because some species of animals have a degree of natural immunity to snake venoms. In addition, the victim's size, preexisting health, interval until medical care is obtained, and site of the bite are victim-related factors that can influence the severity of the snakebite. Snake factors that affect toxicity include species, size and age of the snake, as well as the time of year, time since the snake's last bite, and whether the bite was defensive or offensive. "Dry" bites, those in which no venom is injected, may occur in up to 25% of snakebites (Peterson, 2004). Snakes that have recently fed may be depleted of venom and thus inject less (Fowler, 1993). Older snakes may have more potent venom, and larger snakes may harbor larger volumes of venom to deliver.

Analysis of venoms from a variety of North American pit vipers indicates that the ranking of relative toxicity of venoms, from highest to lowest, is Mojave A rattlesnake (*Crotalus scutulatus*), eastern diamondback (*Crotalus adamanteus*), western diamondback (*Crotalus atrox*), timber rattlesnake (*Crotalus horridus*), cottonmouth (*A. piscivorus*), and copperhead (*A. contortrix*).

Clinical Effects

In most cases of snakebite, the initial signs are usually local pain and swelling, followed by petechiation, ecchymosis, and discoloration of the skin in the region of the bite. Swelling and/or the haircoat of the victim may mask bite wounds. Bites from snake species that possess only neurotoxic venom may show little local swelling. Several hours may elapse before more significant clinical signs develop. Hypotension, shock, tachycardia or other arrhythmia, vomiting, diarrhea, shallow respiration, lethargy, nausea, obtundation, muscle fasciculations, ptyalism, and pain and enlargement of regional lymph nodes may occur (Peterson, 2004). Local tissue necrosis may be severe, especially in areas with minimal muscle mass. Local swelling from bites to the head or front legs in dogs may result in regional circulatory alterations that reduce venom uptake (Peterson, 2004). Neurotoxic effects, largely attributed to Mojave toxins, reported in dogs and cats following rattlesnake envenomation include ataxia, postural deficits, fasciculation, paresis, paralysis and seizures (Julius et al., 2012). Horses or llamas bitten on the muzzle may succumb to asphyxiation due to occlusion of the nares due to tissue swelling. Horses develop pitting edema that frequently progresses to involve the entire head and neck or limb, but tissue necrosis is uncommon (Fowler, 1993). Hemolysis, rhabdomyolysis, thrombocytopenia, and coagulopathy may occur.

Treatment

Historically, a variety of first aid measures have been described for managing snakebites in humans and animals, including suction, electric shock, ice packs, and tourniquets (Peterson, 2004). However, most of these measures are of questionable value, and they waste precious time that could be used to transport the patient to a veterinary medical facility. Initial first aid should be focused on keeping the animal quiet (exertion will hasten the spread of venom factors into the tissues) and attempting to keep the bitten area below heart level.

The haircoat around the bite area should be clipped to fully visualize the bite. Use of a permanent marker to delineate the margins of local edema and/or circumferential measurements above, at, and below the bite site allows objective evaluation of the progression of local tissue involvement (Fowler, 1993; Peterson, 2004). Vital signs, including blood pressure, should be monitored closely for the first several hours, and all patients should be monitored for a minimum of 24 h before being released (Fowler, 1993). Tracheostomy may be required in cases in which severe swelling in the head or neck region results in respiratory compromise or in cases of obligate nasal breathers (e.g., horses and llamas) that are bitten on the muzzle. Intravenous crystalloid therapy is recommended to manage hypotension or hypovolemia. Coagulopathy and hemolysis should be managed using blood or platelet transfusions. Conditions such as muscle tremors, seizures, cardiac arrhythmias, and pulmonary edema should be managed as they develop using standard medical therapies. Corticosteroid use is controversial in snakebites, with some indicating that corticosteroids have no place in management of snakebite (Peterson, 2004), whereas others suggest that judicious use of corticosteroids may be of benefit (Fowler, 1993). Topical application of dimethyl sulfoxide to the bite site should be avoided because it enhances systemic absorption of venom (Peterson, 2004). Diphenhydramine may be useful for its sedative effect. Broad-spectrum antibiotics are advocated by some to aid in prevention of infection (Peterson, 2004), and horses should receive tetanus antitoxin or toxoid (Fowler, 1993).

The use of intravenous antivenin in crotalid snakebites can result in the reversal of potentially life-threatening problems such as coagulopathy, thrombocytopenia, and paralysis (Peterson et al., 2011). Antivenin cannot reverse tissue necrosis or secondary effects such as renal damage. Currently available antivenins include equine-origin, whole immunoglobulin (IgG), polyvalent antivenin, ovine-derived polyvalent immune Fab fragments (CroFab, BTG, Brentwood TN (formerly Protherics)) and equine-derived $F(ab')_2$ fragments (Anavip, AnovoRx Distribution, Memphis, TN); these have been shown to be effective in management of canine snakebite (Peterson, 2004; Witsil et al., 2015). Advantages of the antibody fragments over whole IgG molecules are decreased antigenicity (and therefore decreased potential for allergic reaction), more rapid elimination, increased stability, and more rapid reconstitution (Gwaltney-Brant and Rumbeiha, 2002; Witsil et al., 2015). Administration of antivenin should begin as early as possible, and patients should be closely monitored for signs of anaphylaxis during antivenin administration. Reported incidences of adverse reactions to antivenin in dogs have ranged from 0.7% to 6% (Peterson et al., 2011; Witsil et al., 2015). Studies in dogs have shown that single vial doses of crotalid Fab antivenin are sufficient to manage most cases of canine snakebite envenomation (Peterson, 2004; Peterson et al., 2011). Coagulation parameters should be monitored, and additional vials of antivenin should be administered if deterioration is noted.

The prognosis for recovery from snake envenomation is dependent on the type of snake involved, the severity of the envenomation, and the rapidity and aggressiveness of veterinary intervention. Mortality rates reported in dogs receiving veterinary care following rattlesnake envenomation have ranged from 3% to 7%; however, a study in dogs and cats displaying neurotoxic effects from rattlesnake envenomation had an overall mortality rate of $\sim$17% for each species (Peterson et al., 2011; Witsil et al., 2015; Julius et al., 2012).

A rattlesnake vaccine (Crotalus Atrox Toxoid, Red Rock Biologics) designed to elicit an immune response to the major protein fractions of *C. atrox* (western diamondback rattlesnake) has been developed for dogs at risk of experiencing crotalid snakebites (Wallis, 2005; Cates et al., 2015). The vaccine may also cross-react to the major protein fractions of some other rattlesnake venoms, but does not induce neutralizing antibodies against Mojave neurotoxin. The vaccine does not eliminate the need to seek veterinary care if a venomous snake bites a vaccinated dog. Clinical trials demonstrated that vaccinated dogs experiencing mild envenomations had more rapid resolution of signs than unvaccinated dogs. Antivenin may still be required, although reduced amounts may be needed (Wallis, 2005). A mouse study showed that vaccination improved survival rate and survival time after exposure to venom from western diamondback rattlesnakes, had limited protection against northern Pacific rattlesnakes and did not provide cross protection against southern Pacific rattlesnake venom (Cates et al., 2015). A study in horses comparing antibody responses to natural snake envenomation and the same rattlesnake vaccine showed that the vaccine yielded lower antibody titers than natural envenomation (Gilliam et al., 2013); no challenge study has been performed to demonstrate efficacy of the vaccine in horses.

Elapids

Background

There are two North American species of venomous elapid snakes: the Sonoran coral snake (*Micruroides euryxanthus*) and several subspecies of *Micrurus fulvius*, including the Texas coral snake (*M. fulvius tenere*), the eastern coral snake (*M. fulvius fulvius*), and the south Florida coral snake (*M. fulvius barbouri*) (Peterson, 2004). The Sonoran coral snake is found in central and southeastern Arizona and southwestern New Mexico. The Texas coral snake is found from eastern and south-central Texas north into Louisiana and southern Arkansas. The eastern coral snake is present from eastern North Carolina south to central Florida and west through Alabama and Mississippi. The south Florida coral snake is restricted to southern Florida.

North American coral snakes tend to be shy, nonaggressive, and nocturnal, making interactions between them and domestic animals less common than interactions with pit vipers (Peterson, 2004). These snakes are brightly colored, with alternating bands of black, red, and yellow, and they have small heads and round pupils. The venom delivery apparatus of coral snakes includes short, fixed (nonhinged) front fangs that are partially covered by a membrane (Fowler, 1993). During the bite, the membrane is pushed away and the venom duct empties at the base of the fang, bathing the fang with venom that runs down grooves within the fang. During the bite, coral snakes hold onto the victim and chew, delivering additional venom to the wound.

Like crotalid venom, coral snake venom is composed of a variety of compounds, mostly small polypeptides and enzymes. Neurologic signs following envenomation may be delayed in onset for up to 12 h, and the duration of effects is prolonged (Peterson, 2004). Total clearance of venom from the body may take up to 14 days.

Mechanism of Action

Neurotoxic peptides in coral snake venom cause a nondepolarizing postsynaptic neuromuscular blockade similar to the effects of curare (Peterson, 2004). Binding of neurotoxins to postsynaptic receptors appears to be irreversible. Enzymes within the venom can cause local tissue necrosis, myoglobinemia in cats, and hemolysis in dogs.

Toxicity

As with crotalid envenomations, the severity of the bite is related to the size of the victim and the amount of venom delivered. The amount of venom injected is related to the duration of the bite, intensity of chewing, and reason for the bite (offensive versus defensive). Clinical signs vary with the species of the victim. Cats develop primarily neurologic signs, including progressive ascending flaccid paralysis, decreased nociperception, CNS depression, and diminished spinal reflexes (Peterson, 2004). Hypotension, respiratory depression, anisocoria, myoglobinemia, and hypothermia have also been described in cats. In dogs, depression of the CNS, decreased spinal reflexes, muscle weakness, and respiratory depression may occur. Vomiting, hypersalivation, hypotension, dyspnea, dysphagia, muscle fasciculation, tachycardia, and hemolysis have also been reported in dogs. Potential complications include dysphagia leading to aspiration pneumonia. Death is due to respiratory paralysis.

Treatment

Management of coral snake envenomations in animals should entail immediate transport for veterinary care. Because onset of clinical signs may be delayed up to 12 h, patients that have been bitten should be closely monitored for a minimum of 24 h. Baseline serum chemistry and complete blood count values should be obtained, and respiratory function should be closely monitored. Ventilatory support may be required if clinical signs progress to the point where respiration is compromised; ventilation may be required for 72 h or more (Peterson, 2004). Administration of specific *Micrurus* antivenin should be considered if neurologic signs begin to develop; early administration is recommended because the antivenin is poorly effective at displacing venom components bound to receptor sites (Peterson, 2004). As with crotalid antivenin, anaphylaxis is a potential complication of *Micrurus* antivenin administration. Broad-spectrum antibiotics and symptomatic wound care may be indicated. Recovery periods of 7–10 days have been reported in cats envenomated by coral snakes (Chrisman et al., 1996). The prognosis for coral snake envenomations in animals is generally good provided prompt and aggressive veterinary care is obtained.

Lizards

Background

Venomous lizards found in North and Central America are members of the genus *Heloderma*. *Heloderma suspectum* and *Heloderma cinctum* are commonly referred to as Gila monsters, whereas *Heloderma horridum* is known as the Mexican beaded lizard. Gila monsters are found in Arizona and areas of Utah, New Mexico, Nevada, and Southern California, whereas the Mexican beaded lizard is found in Mexico from Sonora to the Pacific Coast and into Guatemala (Cantrell, 2003; Peterson, 2004).

Venomous lizards are large and heavily bodied, with blunt, rounded tails, powerful jaws, and short legs with

TABLE 58.3 Contents and Effects of Various *Heloderma* spp. Venom Components

Component	Effects	References
Gilatoxin	"Lethal factor," kallikrein-like activity, pain, hypotension	Fowler (1993), Utaisincharoen et al. (1993)
Helodermin	Vasodilation, hypotension	Grundemar and Hogestatt (1990)
Helospectin I and II	Vasodilation, hypotension	Grundemar and Hogestatt (1990)
Helothermine	Lethargy, paresis, hypothermia	Peterson (2004)
Hyaluronidase	"Spreading factor," degrades connective tissue	Peterson (2004)
Phospholipase A_2	Inhibition of platelet aggregations	Huang and Chiang (1994)

clawed, hand-like feet. The colorful, bead-like scales form a reticular pattern of dark brown to black on a yellow, orange, pink, and/or cream background. Gila monsters, which can reach 55 cm in length, are smaller than Mexican beaded lizards, which can grow up to 1 m in length and weigh up to 2 kg (Cantrell, 2003; Peterson, 2004).

Heloderma spp. possess venom glands in the lower jaw at the base of the teeth, and venom is delivered through grooves in the teeth via capillary action as the lizard masticates. These lizards are generally considered to be docile, but when provoked they can be aggressive biters that can hang on tenaciously to their victim, often requiring prying the jaws open to release the victim (Cantrell, 2003). The teeth are loosely attached and brittle, and they may break off into the wound. The venom is considered a defensive weapon rather than one for procuring food (Peterson, 2004).

Mechanism of Action

Heloderma venom is composed of a complex mixture of proteins and enzymes, many of which are similar to those found in snake venoms, including hyaluronidase, phospholipase A_2, serotonin, and a variety of enzymes (Cantrell, 2003). Hyaluronidase ("spreading factor") catalyzes the cleavage of internal glycoside bonds of acid mucoglycosides, resulting in decreased viscosity of hyaluronic acid, which in turn increases tissue permeability and allows deeper penetration of venom into tissue. Phospholipase A_2 uncouples oxidative phosphorylation, which inhibits cellular respiration, causes cell membrane destruction, and inhibits platelet aggregation (Huang and Chiang, 1994; Peterson, 2004). Various proteolytic enzymes result in local tissue damage as well as aid in the spread of venom through the tissue. In addition, *Heloderma* venoms contain several unique components that have a variety of clinical effects; these are summarized in Table 58.3. Gilatoxin is considered to be the major lethal factor in *Heloderma* venom (Fowler, 1993).

Toxicity

The toxicity of *Heloderma* venoms is dependent on the amount of venom delivered to tissues, which in turn is dependent on the duration and severity of the bite. Due to their inquisitive nature and tendency to harass wildlife that they encounter, dogs are the species most likely to have a significant encounter with *Heloderma* spp. Although rare, *Heloderma* bites to dogs and cats have occurred, and the death of at least one dog has been reported (Fowler, 1993; Peterson, 2004).

The clinical effects of *Heloderma* envenomation include intense local pain, edema, and hemorrhage at the site of the wound (which may contain fractured teeth). Regional lymphangitis and local ecchymoses may occur, although tissue necrosis is not common. Systemic signs described in humans include weakness, dizziness, tinnitus, muscle fasciculations, hypotension, and tachycardia. In dogs and cats, signs may include tachypnea, vomiting, polyuria, salivation, and lacrimation. Aphonia has been reported in cats (Peterson, 2004). Hypotension, tachycardia, and respiratory distress have been reported in dogs and cats injected with boluses of *Heloderma* venom, although reports of these conditions in natural exposures are lacking.

Treatment

Management of *Heloderma* bites in small animals includes initial first aid followed by assessment and monitoring. The first course of action is often disengaging a lizard that is still attached to the victim because these lizards may hold on tenaciously once they bite. Removal should be attempted as quickly as possible because the amount of venom delivered is proportional to the duration of the bite. Suggested means of removal of the lizard include applying a flame from a match or cigarette lighter to the underjaw of the lizard, prying the jaws open with a metal bar, or killing the lizard by incising the jugular vein with a knife. Attempts to pull the lizard off the victim or to strike the lizard in the head may enlarge or deepen the wounds at the site of the bite (Fowler, 1993). Once the lizard is removed, a veterinarian should evaluate the patient. The bite site should be irrigated with 2% lidocaine and the wound probed with a 25-gauge needle to detect any embedded tooth fragments (Peterson, 2006). Benzodiazepines may be helpful in sedating agitated or highly painful animals. Analgesics should be administered as needed, and the patient should be monitored for several hours for the development of hypotension or shock; if either develops, appropriate medical treatment including intravenous fluid therapy is indicated. Broad-spectrum antibiotics should be administered to prevent infection from the myriad of potentially pathogenic bacteria that have been reported to frequent the mouth of reptiles (Peterson, 2006). General wound care should be instituted, and the wound should be examined daily for evidence of infection. Envenomation of pets by *Heloderma* spp. is rare, and in most cases, a favorable outcome can be expected provided prompt and appropriate veterinary care is obtained.

AVES

Two genera of passerine birds native to New Guinea, *Pitohui* ("rubbish bird") and *Ifrita*, ("bitter bird") have poisonous secretions on their feathers, most likely as means of defense against predators (Weldon, 2000; Dumbacher and Fleischer, 2001). The toxins are present in highest concentrations in the contour feathers of the belly, breast, and legs, with lesser amounts on the head, back, tail, and wing feathers (Weldon, 2000). Several steroidal alkaloids have been isolated from the feathers of these birds, including batrachotoxin and homobatrachotoxin as well as derivatives of these compounds; similar compounds are present on the skin of poison dart frogs (Dendrobatidae) from Central and South America (Daly, 1995b).

The toxins found on the birds' feathers are thought to accumulate from insects ingested by the birds rather than by de novo synthesis (Dumbacher et al., 2004). High levels of batrachotoxins have been found in beetles of the genus *Choresine* (family Melyridae) that serve as part of the diet of *Pitohui* species. Batrachotoxins act through the opening of sodium channels in nerve and muscle cells, resulting in depolarization and paralysis (Dumbacher et al., 2004). However, exposure of humans to the feathers of *Pitohui* and *Ifrita* species primarily results in respiratory irritation, allergic-type responses, and burning sensations of the eyes, skin, and oral mucosa (Dumbacher et al., 2000).

MAMMALIA

Only a handful of mammals are poisonous or venomous, and toxicosis from exposure to these animals is uncommon. Poisonous mammals include certain carnivores (e.g., polar bears) and pinnipeds (e.g., walruses and seals), whose livers contain high levels of vitamin A; ingestion of these livers may result in acute or chronic hypervitaminosis A (Cleland and Southcott, 1969; Fishman, 2002). In addition, the meat of marine mammals such as whales may accumulate high levels of organotins, mercury, and other agents that can pose a toxicologic hazard if ingested in sufficient quantity (Endo et al., 2005). Impairment in cell-mediated immunity was found in sled dogs from Greenland that were fed the blubber of minke whales (*Balaenoptera acutorostrata*) (Sonne et al., 2006).

Venomous mammals belong to the orders Monotremata and Insectivora (Fowler, 1993). Venomous monotremes are the platypus and echidna, of which only the platypus is of toxicologic significance because the venom gland in the echidna is nonfunctional. The male platypus possesses a curved, grooved, conical, sharp spur on the medial aspect of the tarsus. The spur is normally kept retracted against the leg, but when stimulated, muscles cause the spur to project perpendicularly to the leg. The venom gland is kidney shaped and located on the medial aspect of the thigh, and venom is first transported to a reservoir near the spur and then moved through a duct to the spur. Envenomation occurs when the platypus kicks the spur into the victim.

Although poorly studied, components identified in platypus venom include a protein similar to natriuretic peptide, a defensin-like peptide, a hyaluronidase, 5-hydroxytryptophan, and histamine (Hodgson, 1997; Torres et al., 2006). Signs of envenomation include intense pain and numbness at the site of the wound and local swelling that may progress proximally (Fowler, 1993). Regional lymph nodes may become enlarged and painful. Humans have reported a feeling of faintness. No reports of human or animal fatality from platypus exist. There are infrequent anecdotal reports of dogs being envenomated by platypus.

Venomous insectivores include various shrews and solenodons and possibly some moles and hedgehogs (Dufton, 1992). The European hedgehog (*Erinaceus europaeus*) has been noted to mix its frothy saliva with toad toxins and smear this mixture over its forward spines. Some moles will store "paralyzed" worms and slugs away, with the paralysis thought to be due to paralytic toxins within the mole's saliva. Studies of the American short-tailed shrew (*Blarina brevicauda*), the Haitian solenodon (*Solenodon paradoxus*), the European water shrew (*Neomys fodiens*), and the Mediterranean shrew (*Neomys anomalus*) have obtained more definitive evidence of the presence of venoms. These mammals possess three pairs of salivary glands: parotid, retrolingual, and submaxillary. The submaxillary glands contribute the bulk of the venom in these species. The Haitian solenodon has grooved incisors that direct the venom to the wound, whereas the shrews have teeth with concave inner surfaces that may play a similar role as grooves.

Envenomation is achieved by biting and chewing the victim, accompanied by copious salivation. Insectivore venoms contain a variety of peptides and enzymes, and a compound isolated from *Blarina* venom has been shown to have kallikrein-like activity (Kita et al., 2005). The venom of *Blarina* appears to be the most toxic, with that of *N. fodiens*, *N. anomalus*, and *Solenodon* being 1/3, 1/6, and 1/20 as toxic, respectively (Dufton, 1992). There is considerable species variation in sensitivity to the venom in shrew and solenodon venom, with voles and rabbits being most sensitive to the effects and mice, cats, and humans being relatively more resistant (Dufton, 1992). In most natural exposures, the primary effects of shrew and solenodon venoms are related to neurotoxicity. Mice bitten by *Blarina* rapidly develop depression and immobility. When submaxillary gland extracts are injected into experimental animals, depression, irregular respiration, dyspnea, ptosis, rear limb paralysis, convulsions, and death occur. Intravenous injection of 7 mg/kg of *Blarina* toxin extract in a cat resulted in decreases in respiratory and heart rates with a concomitant decrease in blood pressure. These effects resolved within 15 min but returned with subsequent doses of 2.5 and 7 mg/kg. Apparent recovery following the final dose was followed by acute respiratory depression and cardiac arrhythmia, and the cat subsequently died. In humans, symptoms of bites from shrews or solenodons result in localized burning sensation surrounding the lower jaw tooth puncture sites and localized swelling. The burning sensation may persist for several days. Systemic toxicosis has not been reported in natural exposures to the bites of shrews or solenodons in humans or domestic animals.

CONCLUDING REMARKS AND FUTURE DIRECTIONS

Every phylum of the animal kingdom contains animals capable of producing toxic effects, either through envenomation or through poisoning. However, only a small number of these animals are sufficiently toxic to be of importance to veterinary clinicians. Arachnids, insects, toads, and snakes cause the most clinically significant problems for domestic and wild animals. Although in some cases specific antidotes (i.e., antivenins) exist for exposures to venomous animals, availability and cost of these antidotes often make their use in veterinary medicine unfeasible. Therefore, most cases of zootoxicosis in animals will be managed with symptomatic and supportive care.

REFERENCES

Akre, R.D., Reed, H.C., 2002. Ants, wasps, and bees (Hymenoptera). In: Mullen, G., Durden, L. (Eds.), Medical and Veterinary Entomology. Academic Press, New York, NY, pp. 383–410.

Beyer, A., Grossman, M., 1997. Tick paralysis in a red wolf. J. Wildl. Dis. 33, 900–902.

Brutlag, A.G., Hovda, L.R., Della Ripa, M.A., 2011. Corneal ulceration in a dog following exposure to the defensive spray of a walkingstick insect (*Anisomorpha* spp.). J. Vet. Emerg. Crit. Care. 21, 382–385.

Caldwell-Smith, A.J., Todhunter, K.H., Anderson, S.T., et al., 2012. Equine amnionitis and fetal loss: mare abortion following experimental exposure to Processionary caterpillars (*Ochrogaster lunifer*). Equine Vet. J. 44, 282–288.

Cantrell, F.L., 2003. Envenomation by the Mexican beaded lizard: a case report. J. Toxicol. Clin. Toxicol. 41, 241–244.

Cates, C.C., Valore, E.V., Couto, M.A., et al., 2015. Comparison of the protective effect of a commercially available western diamondback rattlesnake toxoid vaccine for dogs against envenomation of mice with western diamondback rattlesnake (*Crotalus atrox*), northern Pacific rattlesnake (*Crotalus oreganus oreganus*), and southern Pacific rattlesnake (*Crotalus oreganus helleri*) venom. Am. J. Vet. Res. 3, 272–279.

Chrisman, C.L., Hopkins, A.L., Ford, S.L., et al., 1996. Acute, flaccid quadriplegia in three cats with suspected coral snake envenomation. J. Am. Anim. Hosp. Assoc. 32, 343–349.

Clarke, R.F., Wethern-Kestner, S., Vance, M.V., et al., 1992. Clinical presentation and treatment of black widow spider envenomation: a review of 163 cases. Ann. Emerg. Med. 7, 782–787.

Cleland, J.B., Southcott, R.V., 1969. Illnesses following the eating of seal liver in Australian waters. Med. J. Aust. 1, 760–763.

Cowell, A.K., Cowell, R.L., Tyler, R.D., et al., 1991. Severe systemic reactions to Hymenoptera stings in three dogs. J. Am. Vet. Med. Assoc. 198, 1014–1016.

Dalefield, R.R., Oehme, F.W., 2006. Antidotes for specific poisons. In: Peterson, M.E., Talcott, P.A. (Eds.), Small Animal Toxicology, second ed. Saunders, St. Louis, MO, pp. 459–474.

Daly, J.W., 1995a. Alkaloids from frog skins: selective probes for ion channels and nicotinic receptors. Braz. J. Med. Biol. Res. 28, 1033–1042.

Daly, J.W., 1995b. The chemistry of poisons in amphibian skin. Proc. Natl. Acad. Sci. U.S.A. 92, 9–13.

Daly, J.W., Kaneko, T., Wilhalm, J., et al., 1992. Diseases diagnosed in gray foxes (*Urocyon cinereoargenteus*) from the southeastern United States. J. Wildl. Dis. 28, 28–33.

Denny, W.F., Dillaha, C.J., Morgan, P.N., 1964. Hemotoxic effect of *Loxesceles reclusus* venom: in vivo and in vitro studies. J. Lab. Clin. Med. 64, 291–298.

Dipeolu, O.O., 1976. Tick paralysis in a sheep caused by nymphs of *Amblyomma variegatum*: a preliminary report. Z. Parasitenkd. 10, 293–295.

Dorce, A.L.C., Bellot, R.G., Dorce, V.A.C., et al., 2009. Effects of prenatal exposure to *Tityus bahiensis* scorpion on rat offspring development. Reprod. Toxicol. 28, 365–370.

Dufton, M.J., 1992. Venomous mammals. Pharmacol. Ther. 53, 199–215.

Dumbacher, J.P., Fleischer, R.C., 2001. Phylogenetic evidence for color pattern convergence in toxic pitohuis: Mullerian mimicry in birds? Proc. Biol. Sci. 268, 1971–1976.

Dumbacher, J.P., Spande, T.F., Daly, J.W., 2000. Batrachotoxin alkaloids from passerine birds: a second toxic bird genus (*Ifrita kowaldi*) from New Guinea. Proc. Natl. Acad. Sci. U.S.A. 97, 12970–12975.

Dumbacher, J.P., Wako, A., Derrickson, S.R., et al., 2004. Melyrid beetles (Choresine): a putative source for the batrachotoxin alkaloids found in poison-dart frogs and toxic passerine birds. Proc. Natl. Acad. Sci. U.S.A. 101, 15857–15860.

Durden, L.A., Mullen, G.R., 2002. Introduction. In: Mullen, G., Durden, L. (Eds.), Medical and Veterinary Entomology. Academic Press, New York, NY, pp. 1–8.

Dutra, F., Riet-Correa, F., Mendez, M.C., et al., 1997. Poisoning of cattle and sheep in Uruguay by sawfly (*Perreyia flavipes*) larvae. Vet. Hum. Toxicol. 39, 281–286.

Endo, T., Hotta, Y., Haraguchi, K., et al., 2005. Distribution and toxicity of mercury in rats after oral administration of mercury-contaminated whale red meat marketed for human consumption. Chemosphere. 61, 1069–1073.

Eubig, P.A., 2001. Bufo species toxicosis: big toad, big problem. Vet. Med. 96, 594–599.

Fishman, R.A., 2002. Polar bear liver, vitamin A, aquaporins, and pseudotumor cerebri. Ann. Neurol. 52, 531–533.

Fowler, M.E., 1993. Veterinary Zootoxicology. CRC Press, Boca Raton, FL.

Futrell, J.M., Morgan, B.B., Morgan, P.N., 1979. An in vitro model for studying hemolysis associated with venom from the brown recluse spider (*Loxesceles reclusa*). Toxicon. 17, 355–362.

Gilliam, L.L., Carmichael, R.C., Holbrook, T.C., et al., 2013. Antibody responses to natural rattlesnake envenomation and a rattlesnake toxoid vaccine in horses. Clin. Vaccine Immunol. 20, 732–737.

Goddard, J., 2003. Physician's Guide to Arthropods of Medical Importance. fourth ed. CRC Press, Boca Raton, FL.

Grundemar, L., Hogestatt, E.D., 1990. Vascular effects of helodermin, helospectin I and helospectin II: a comparison with vasoactive intestinal peptide. Br. J. Pharmacol. 99, 526–528.

Gwaltney-Brant, S.M., 2017. Zootoxins. In: Gupta, R.C. (Ed.), Reproductive and Developmental Toxicology. Academic Press/ Elsevier, Amsterdam, pp. 963–972.

Gwaltney-Brant, S.M., Rumbeiha, W.K., 2002. Newer antidotal therapies. Vet. Clin. Small Anim. 32, 323–339.

Hackett, T.B., Wingfield, W.E., Mazzaferro, E.M., et al., 2002. Clinical findings associated with prairie rattlesnake bites in dogs: 100 cases (1989–1998). J. Am. Vet. Med. Assoc. 220, 1675–1680.

Hodgson, W.C., 1997. Pharmacological action of Australian animal venoms. Clin. Exp. Pharmacol. Physiol. 24, 10–17.

Hoenerhoff, M., Rumbeiha, W.K., Patterson, J.S., et al., 2002. Small intestinal hemorrhage associated with *Harmonia axyridis* (Asian ladybeetle) ingestion in a dog. In: Proc Am Ass Vet Lab Diagn, 45th Annual Conf, St. Louis, MO. Davis, CA.

Huang, T.F., Chiang, H.S., 1994. Effect on human platelet aggregation of phospholipase A2 purified from *Heloderma horridum* (beaded lizard) venom. Biochem. Biophys. Acta. 1211, 61–68.

Julius, T.M., Kaelble, M.K., Leech, E.B., et al., 2012. Retrospective evaluation of neurotoxic rattlesnake envenomation in dogs and cats: 34 cases (2005–2010). J. Vet. Emerg. Crit. Care. 22, 460–469.

Keegan, H.L., 1980. Scorpions of Medical Importance. University Press of Mississippi, Jackson, MS.

Kita, M., Okumura, Y., Ohdachi, S.D., et al., 2005. Purification and characterisation of blarinasin, a new tissue kallikrein-like protease from the short-tailed shrew *Blarina brevicauda*: comparative studies with blarina toxin. Biol. Chem. 386, 177–182.

Knight, M., Glor, R., Smedley, S.R., et al., 1999. Firefly toxicosis in lizards. J. Chem. Ecol. 62, 378–380.

Krinsky, W.L., 2002. Beetles (Coleoptera). In: Mullen, G., Durden, L. (Eds.), Medical and Veterinary Entomology. Academic Press, New York, NY, pp. 87–100.

Lamson, G.H., 1915. The poisonous effect of the rose chafer upon chickens. J. Econ. Entomol. 8, 547–548.

Lewis, N., Racklyeft, D.J., 2014. Mass envenomation of a mare and foal by bees. Aust. Vet. J. 92, 141–148.

Lucas, S.M., Meier, J., 1995a. Biology and distribution of scorpions of medical importance. In: Meier, J., White, J. (Eds.), Handbook of Clinical Toxicology of Animal Venoms and Poisons. CRC Press, Boca Raton, FL, pp. 239–258.

Lucas, S.M., Meier, J., 1995b. Biology and distribution of spiders of medical importance. In: Meier, J., White, J. (Eds.), Handbook of Clinical Toxicology of Animal Venoms and Poisons. CRC Press, Boca Raton, FL, pp. 205–220.

Luttrell, M.P., Creekmore, L.H., Mertins, J.W., 1996. Avian tick paralysis caused by *Ixodes brunneus* in the southeastern United States. J. Wildl. Dis. 32, 133–136.

McDowell, K.J., Webb, B.A., Williams, N.M., et al., 2010. Invited review: the role of caterpillars in mare reproductive loss syndrome: a model for environmental causes of abortion. J. Anim. Sci. 88, 1379–1387.

Meier, J., 1995. Venomous and poisonous animals: a biologist's view. In: Meier, J., White, J. (Eds.), Handbook of Clinical Toxicology of Animal Venoms and Poisons. CRC Press, Boca Raton, FL, pp. 1–8.

Mullen, G.R., 2002a. Moths and butterflies (Lepidoptera). In: Mullen, G., Durden, L. (Eds.), Medical and Veterinary Entomology. Academic Press, New York, NY, pp. 363–381.

Mullen, G.R., 2002b. Spiders (Araneae). In: Mullen, G., Durden, L. (Eds.), Medical and Veterinary Entomology. Academic Press, New York, NY, pp. 427–448.

Mullen, G.R., Stockwell, S.A., 2002. Scorpions (Scorpiones). In: Mullen, G., Durden, L. (Eds.), Medical and Veterinary Entomology. Academic Press, New York, NY, pp. 411–423.

Nakamura, R.K., Fenty, R.K., Bianco, D., 2013. Presumptive immune-mediated thrombocytopenia secondary to massive Africanized bee envenomation in a dog. J. Vet. Emerg. Crit. Care. 23, 652–656.

Noble, S.J., Armstrong, P.J., 1999. Bee sting envenomation resulting in secondary immune-mediated hemolytic anemia in two dogs. J. Am. Vet. Med. Assoc. 214 (1021), 1026–1027.

Norris, R., 2004. Centipede Envenomations. Available at: <http://www.emedicine.com/EMERG/topic89.htm>.

Oelrichs, P.B., MacLeod, J.K., Seawright, A.A., et al., 1999. Unique toxic peptides isolated from sawfly larvae in three continents. Toxicon. 37, 537–544.

Peterson, M.E., 2004. Reptiles. In: Plumlee, K.H. (Ed.), Clinical Veterinary Toxicology. Mosby, St. Louis, MO, pp. 104–111.

Peterson, M.E., 2006. Poisonous lizards. In: Peterson, M.E., Talcott, P.A. (Eds.), Small Animal Toxicology, second ed. Saunders, St. Louis, MO, pp. 812–816.

Peterson, M.E., McNalley, J., 2006a. Spider envenomation: black widow. In: Peterson, M.E., Talcott, P.A. (Eds.), Small Animal Toxicology, second ed. Saunders, St. Louis, MO, pp. 1063–1069.

Peterson, M.E., McNalley, J., 2006b. Spider envenomation: brown recluse. In: Peterson, M.E., Talcott, P.A. (Eds.), Small Animal Toxicology, second ed. Saunders, St. Louis, MO, pp. 1070–1075.

Peterson, M.E., Matz, M., Seibold, K., et al., 2011. A randomized multicenter trial of Crotalidae polyvalent immune Fab antivenomfor the treatment of rattlesnake envenomation in dogs. J. Vet. Emerg. Crit. Care. 21, 335–345.

Rakich, P.M., Latimer, K.S., Mispagel, M.E., et al., 1993. Clinical and histologic characterization of cutaneous reactions to stings of the imported fire ant (*Solenopsis invicta*). Vet. Pathol. 30, 555–559.

Reeves, M.P., 2004. A retrospective report of 90 dogs with suspected cane toad (*Bufo marinus*) toxicity. Aust. Vet. J. 82, 608–611.

Roder, J.D., 2004. Toads. In: Plumlee, K.H. (Ed.), Clinical Veterinary Toxicology. Mosby, St. Louis, MO, p. 113.

Russell, F.E., 1996. Toxic effects of animal toxins. In: Klassen, C.D. (Ed.), Casarett and Doull's Toxicology: The Basic Science of Poisons, fifth ed. McGraw-Hill, New York, NY, pp. 801–839.

Russell, F.E., 2001. Toxic effects of terrestrial animal venoms and poisons. In: Klassen, C.D. (Ed.), Casarett and Doull's Toxicology: The Basic Science of Poisons, sixth ed. McGraw-Hill, New York, pp. 945–964.

Saravanan, R., King, R., White, J., 2004. Transient claw hand owing to a bee sting: a report of two cases. J. Bone Joint Surg. Br. 86, 404–405.

Schmidt, J.O., 1995. Toxinology of venoms from the honeybee genus Apis. Toxicon. 33, 917–927.

Simpson, K.M., Streeter, R.N., De Souza, P., et al., 2013. Cantharadin toxicosis in 2 alpacas. Can. Vet. J. 54, 456–462.

Sonenshine, D.E., Lane, R.S., Nicholson, W.L., 2002. Ticks (Ixodida). In: Mullen, G., Durden, L. (Eds.), Medical and Veterinary Entomology. Academic Press, New York, NY, pp. 517–558.

Sonne, C., Dietz, R., Larsen, H.J., et al., 2006. Impairment of cellular immunity in West Greenland sledge dogs (*Canis familiaris*) dietary exposed to polluted minke whale (*Balaenoptera acutorostrata*) blubber. Environ. Sci. Technol. 40, 2056–2062.

Stair, E.L., Plumlee, K.H., 2004. Blister beetles. In: Plumlee, K.H. (Ed.), Clinical Veterinary Toxicology. Mosby, St. Louis, MO, pp. 101–103.

Stocks, I.C., Lindsey, D.E., 2008. Acute corrosion of the oral mucosa in a dog due to ingestion of multicolored Asian lady beetles (*Harmonia axyridis*: Coccinellidae). Toxicon. 52, 389–391.

Tavora, B.C., Kimura, Antoniazzi, M.M., et al., 2016. Involvement of mast cells and histamine in edema induced in mice by *Scolopendra viridicornis* centipede venom. Toxicon. 121, 51–60.

Thamsborg, S.M., Jorgensen, R.J., Brummerstedt, E., et al., 1996. Putative effect of silymarin on sawfly (*Arge pullata*)-induced hepatotoxicosis in sheep. Vet. Hum. Toxicol. 38, 89–91.

Toennes, S.W., Peters, M., Osman, C., et al., 2015. Death of a South American fur seal (*Arctocephalus australis*) after the ingestion of toads—evaluation of toad poisoning by toxicological analysis. Berl. Munch. Tierarztl. Wochenschr. 128, 252–256.

Torres, A.M., Tsampazi, M., Tsampazi, C., et al., 2006. Mammalian l-to-d-amino-acid-residue isomerase from platypus venom. FEBS Lett. 580, 1587–1591.

Twedt, D.C., Cuddon, P.A., Horn, T.W., 1999. Black widow spider envenomation in a cat. J. Vet. Int. Med. 13, 613–616.

Undheim, E.A., Fry, B.G., King, G.F., 2015. Centipede venom: recent discoveries and current state of knowledge. Toxins (Basel). 7, 679–704.

Utaisincharoen, P., Mackessy, S.P., Miller, R.A., et al., 1993. Complete primary structure and biochemical properties of gilatoxin, a serine protease with kallikrein-like and angiotensin-degrading activities. J. Biol. Chem. 268, 21973–21975.

Walker, T., Tidwell, A.S., Rozanski, E.A., et al., 2005. Imaging diagnosis: acute lung injury following massive bee envenomation in a dog. Vet. Radiol. Ultrasound. 46, 300–303.

Wallis, D.M., 2005. Rattlesnake vaccine to prevent envenomation toxicity in dogs. In: Proc 77th Ann West Vet Conf, Las Vegas. West Vet Conf, Las Vegas.

Weldon, P.J., 2000. Avian chemical defense: toxic birds not of a feather. Proc. Natl. Acad. Sci. U.S.A. 97, 12948–12949.

White, J.W., Cardoso, J.L., Fan, H.W., 1995. Clinical toxicology of spider bites. In: Meier, J., White, J. (Eds.), Handbook of Clinical Toxicology of Animal Venoms and Poisons. CRC Press, Boca Raton, FL, pp. 259–329.

Witsil, A.J., Wells, R.J., Woods, C., Sangeeta, R., 2015. 272 cases of rattlesnake envenomation in dogs: demographics and treatment including safety of F(ab')2 antivenom use in 236 patients. Toxicon. 105, 19–26.

Wysoke, J.M., Bland, V.D.B.P., Marshall, C., 1990. Bee sting-induced haemolysis, spherocytosis and neural dysfunction in three dogs. J. South Afr. Vet. Assoc. 61, 29–32.

FURTHER READING

Daly, J.W., Kaneko, T., Wilhalm, J., et al., 2002. Bioactive alkaloids of frog skin: combinatorial bioprospecting reveals that pumiliotoxins have an arthropod source. Proc. Natl. Acad. Sci. U.S.A. 99, 13996–14001.

Hoggan, S.R., Carr, A., Sausman, K.A., 2011. Mojave toxin-type ascending flaccid paralysis after an envenomation by a Southern Pacific Rattlesnake in a dog. J. Vet. Emerg. Crit. Care. 21, 558–564.

Isbister, G.K., Seymour, J.E., Gray, M.R., et al., 2003. Bite by spiders of the family Theraphosidae in humans and canines. Toxicon. 41, 519–524.

Koch, R.L., 2003. The multicolored Asian lady beetle, *Harmonia axyridis*: a review of its biology, uses in biological control, and nontarget impacts. J. Insect Sci. 3, 32.

Oelrichs, P.B., MacLeod, J.K., Seawright, A.A., et al., 2001. Isolation and identification of the toxic peptides from *Lophyrotoma zonalis* (Pergidae) sawfly larvae. Toxicon. 39, 1933–1936.

Roberts, B.K., Aronsohn, M.G., Moses, B.L., et al., 2000. *Bufo marinus* intoxication in dogs: 94 cases (1997–1998). J. Am. Vet. Med. Assoc. 216, 1941–1944.

Sutherland, S.K., Tibballs, J., 2001. Australian Animal Toxins: The Creatures, Their Toxins and Care of the Poisoned Patient. Oxford University Press, Oxford.

Thamsborg, S.M., Jorgensen, R.J., Brummerstedt, E., 1987. Sawfly poisoning in sheep and goats. Vet. Rec. 121, 253–255.

Section XIII

Estrogenic Toxicants

Chapter 59

Chemical-Induced Estrogenicity

Stephen Safe, Un Ho Jin and Xi Li

INTRODUCTION

17β-Estradiol (E2) and related steroidal hormones play an important role in multiple physiological processes. However, these hormones are risk factors for hormone-dependent diseases including breast and endometrial cancer. Inappropriate exposures (high or low) to estrogens can also lead to adverse health effects. The identification of estrogenic compounds in the environment, coupled with human exposures to these compounds has generated public, regulatory and scientific concern regarding their potential hormonal toxicity to humans and wildlife due to their endocrine disruptor-like activity. This chapter is focused on chemical-induced estrogenicity and the potential toxicological impacts of these compounds. The genesis of the endocrine disruptor hypothesis was due to a few key papers and hypotheses. Carlsen and coworkers (1992) published a meta-analysis of sperm count studies from various clinics and reported that between 1938 and 1991, there was a 40% global decline in sperm counts, and this was soon followed by a hypothesis suggesting that decreasing sperm counts were due to in utero exposure to estrogenic compounds (Sharpe and Skakkebaek, 1993). At about the same time, it was hypothesized that the increased incidence of breast cancer was due to environmental estrogens (Davis et al., 1993) and this was supported by two small studies showing higher levels of polychlorinated biphenyls (PCBs) or 1,1-bis(*p*-chlorophenyl)-2,2-dichloroethylene (DDE) in breast cancer patients versus controls (Falck et al., 1992; Wolff et al., 1993). The initial hypothesis on decreased male reproductive capacity was expanded to include a host of male reproductive tract diseases (Skakkebaek et al., 2001) including cryptorchidism, fertility, hypospadias, prostate and testicular cancer. More recently, some scientists hypothesize that in utero exposure to "environmental estrogens" and other endocrine disruptors also contribute to a multitude of diseases including obesity and related diseases, diabetes, attention deficit disorders, multiple cancers, decreased fertility and reproductive capacity, and neurodevelopment disorders (Gore et al., 2015; Heindel et al., 2015).

These hypotheses and their validity have been challenged (Autrup et al., 2015; Safe, 2000; Sharpe, 2010; Sharpe and Drake, 2010) and some studies, particularly those on breast cancer, suggest that some of these hypotheses are highly unlikely. Nevertheless, this is an area of extensive ongoing research in the laboratory and with human populations, and at least some of the unanswered questions with regards to the effects of endocrine disruptors on human health need to be resolved.

ESTROGENIC CHEMICALS OF CONCERN

Introduction and Background

The hypothesis that environmental/dietary estrogens may play a role in male reproductive tract problems and the increased incidence of breast cancer is controversial and the significance of these compounds on human health is not resolved. Nevertheless this resulted in legislation in the United States requiring the Environmental Protection Agency to develop testing procedures for examining industrial compounds for their activity as estrogens/antiestrogens, androgens/antiandrogens, and thyroid hormone mimics. Initial screening studies for estrogens used the MCF−7 cell proliferation assay (E-screen) (Sonnenschein and Soto, 1998), and this was complemented by development of receptor binding and transactivation studies in various cell lines. All of these assays have advantages and disadvantages and for the most part give complementary results on the estrogenic activity of individual compounds.

Steroidal and nonsteroidal estrogens and antiestrogens have been developed as pharmacologic agents and Fig. 59.1 illustrates the structures of 17β-estradiol, the endogenous hormone, diethylstilbestrol (DES) and three clinically used antiestrogens, tamoxifen, ICI 182780 (fulvestrant) and raloxifene (Jordan, 2003). It is well known that phytoestrogenic compounds in the diet also constitute a major source of exposure to estrogens and these

Veterinary Toxicology. DOI: http://dx.doi.org/10.1016/B978-0-12-811410-0.00059-3

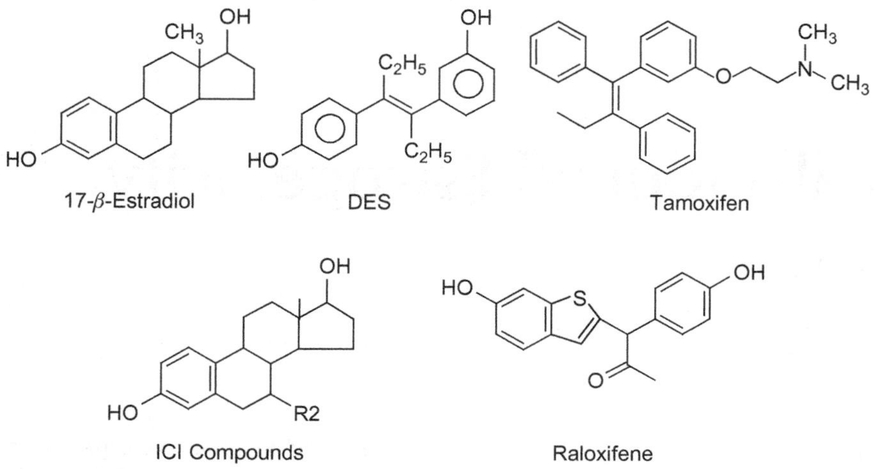

FIGURE 59.1 Structures of 17β-estradiol, DES and the clinically used SERMs tamoxifen, ICI compounds ($R = C_{14}H_{24}F_5OS$, fulvestrant), and raloxifene.

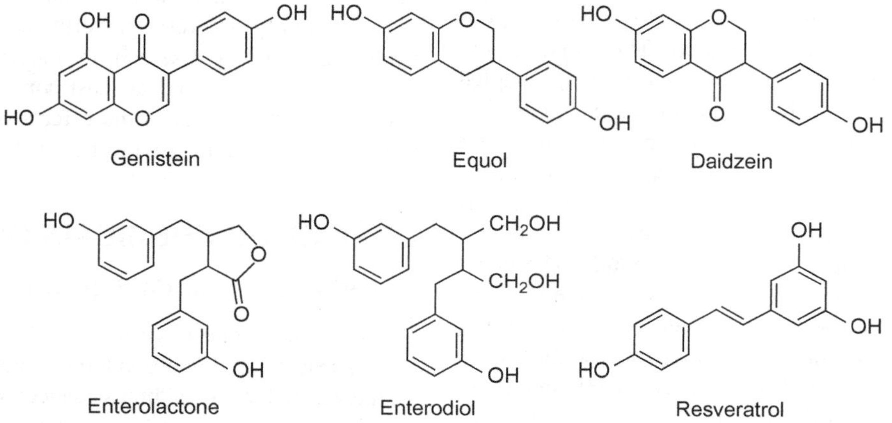

FIGURE 59.2 Structures of the phytoestrogenic flavonoids (genistein, equol, and daidzein), lignans (enterolactone and enterodiol), and resveratrol.

compounds are present in fruits, nuts and vegetables and are particularly high in many soy products that are enriched in isoflavonoids (Havsteen, 2002). Fig. 59.2 shows the structures of genistein, a major isoflavonoid in soy; equol, a genistein metabolite; and naringenin, a flavonoid found in grapefruit. Genistein and equol can be detected in human serum and urine along with the estrogenic lignans enterodiol and enterolactone and these compounds are used as biomarkers of exposure to dietary phytoestrogenic compounds. Resveratrol is an estrogenic polyphenolic stilbene analog found in grapes and wine.

The list of synthetic estrogenic compounds continues to grow as testing of current and new synthetic industrial chemicals progresses and expands through the auspices of EPA and the ToxCast program (Janesick et al., 2016; Rotroff et al., 2013). A major class of xenoestrogens of concern are the alkylphenols such as nonylphenol, which are widely used in industry as ethoxylates. These compounds are surfactants and are used in detergents, paints, herbicide/pesticide formulation and plastics. Alkyl hydroxybenzoates (parabens) (Fig. 59.3) used as preservative agents and cosmetic UV filters such as 4-methylbenzylidene camphor that are used in homecare products also exhibit estrogenic activity (Schreurs et al., 2005). Bisphenol A (BPA) is perhaps one of the most controversial xenoestrogens since it is extensively used in plastic production and plastic liners for cans in which trace levels of BPA have leached directly into food products. This estrogenic compound has also been identified in the environment. Other estrogens of concern include PCBs and hydroxy-PCBs, have been identified in the environment and in humans, the pesticide metabolite DDE and kepone. These compounds are persistent environmental contaminants, and kepone induced estrogenic poisoning in a group of exposed production workers. The compounds illustrated in Fig. 59.4 exhibit relatively weak binding to the ER and induce reporter gene expression in transactivation assays in cell culture systems and some of these compounds exhibit uterotrophic effects in female rodents. The important toxicological question concerning these chemical estrogens is whether they differ only in potency that's governed by their intrinsic estrogenicity and bioavailability based on their metabolism and pharmacokinetics. However, since the estrogenic activity of these compounds is receptor dependent, it is also possible that the estrogenic activity of structurally diverse xenoestrogens is unique and not strictly governed by intrinsic ER binding affinities and pharmacodynamic factors.

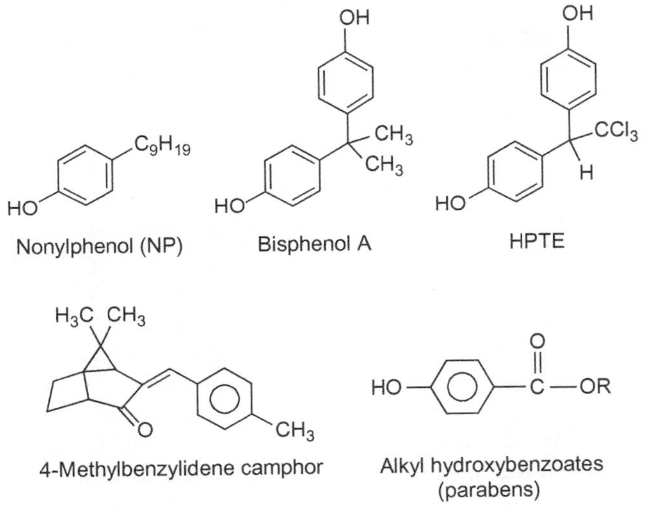

Nonylphenol (NP) Bisphenol A HPTE

4-Methylbenzylidene camphor Alkyl hydroxybenzoates (parabens)

FIGURE 59.3 Structures of the aromatic xenoestrogens nonylphenol, bisphenol A, HPTE, 4-methylbenzylidene camphor, and parabens.

MECHANISMS OF ESTROGEN-INDUCED TRANSACTIVATION: ERα AND ERβ DOMAIN STRUCTURE

The estrogen receptor (ER) is a member of the nuclear receptor superfamily of transcription factors, which exhibit modular structures and similar mechanisms of action. For example, the transactivation function of ER is mediated by two separate but not mutually exclusive transactivation domains namely, ligand-independent activation function (AF) 1 (within the A/B) and ligand-dependent AF-2 (within the ligand binding domain, LBD) (Tora et al., 1989) (Fig. 59.5). The A/B domain is the least conserved region between ERα and ERβ with only 30% similarity at the amino acid level. The activity of AF-1 in ERβ is negligible on estrogen-responsive element (ERE) reporter constructs compared to the AF-1 of ERα in several different cell lines (Cowley and Parker, 1999).

ERα and ERβ also exhibit distinctive responses to the synthetic antiestrogens such as tamoxifen and raloxifene, which act as partial ER agonists for ERα and as pure ER antagonists for ERβ (Barkhem et al., 1998). The functional differences between the respective A/B regions of ERα and ERβ may explain their differences in ligand-dependent activation (Matthews and Gustafsson, 2003). The AF-1 region of ERα interacts with different transcriptional regulators and coactivators that affect ligand-independent transactivation. The activity of AF-1 is also regulated through kinase-dependent phosphorylation and the individual pathways involved vary with cell and promoter context. In most cell lines, both AFs act synergistically to attain maximum transcriptional activity while in other cells only one AF may be activated (Benecke et al., 2000).

The DNA binding domain (DBD) (region C) is highly conserved between ERα and ERβ and exhibits 96% identity. This domain contains two zinc finger (CI and CII) as observed for other nuclear receptors. The DBD of both

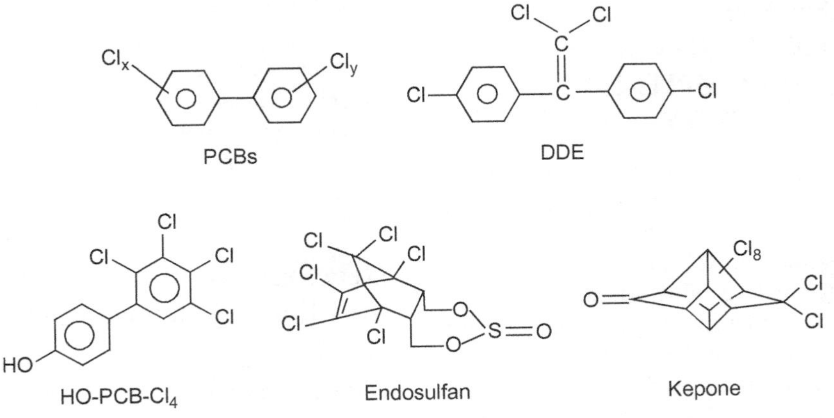

PCBs DDE

HO-PCB-Cl_4 Endosulfan Kepone

FIGURE 59.4 Structures of the organochlorine xenoestrogens PCBs, DDE, hydroxyl-PCB, endosulfan, and kepone.

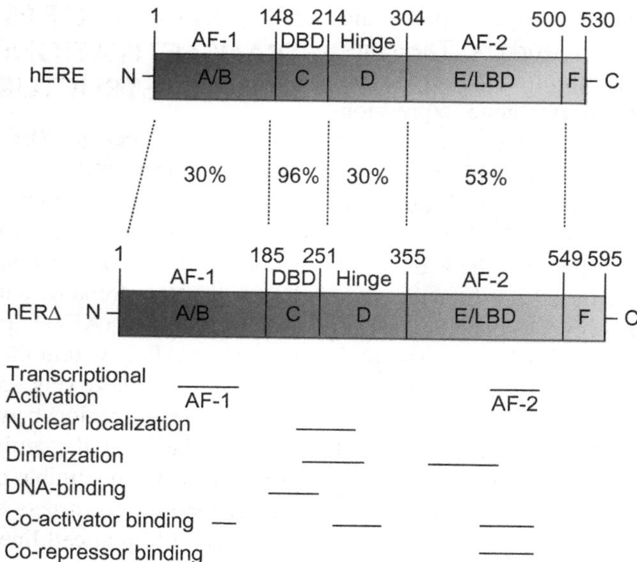

FIGURE 59.5 Structural domains of human ERα and ERβ. The percent identity between the individual domains at the amino acid level is indicated. *Modified from Koehler, D.F., Helguero, L.A., Haldosen, L.A., et al., 2005. Reflections on the discovery and significance of estrogen receptor beta. Endocr. Rev. 26, 465-478.*

ERα and ERβ bind with high affinity to EREs. The C-terminal E/F region encompasses the LBD, a coregulator binding surface, a dimerization domain, another nuclear localization signal and AF-2 (Nilsson et al., 2001). Significant homology between the two receptors exists in the E/F region and both proteins display essentially the same binding affinity for E2 and many other estrogenic compounds (Kuiper et al., 1997). However, the two receptors differ in their binding affinities for only a few ligands including antiestrogens and phytoestrogens. For example, the phytoestrogen genistein binds with approximately a 30-fold higher affinity for ERβ than ERα (Barkhem, et al., 1998).

XENOESTROGENS AND PHYTOESTROGENS AS SELECTIVE ER MODULATORS: COMPLEXITY OF ESTROGENIC ACTIVITY

Results of X-ray crystallographic analysis clearly demonstrates that both ER agonists differentially bind the ER and induce compound-specific changes in the bound complex. Although tamoxifen and E2 induce distinct conformations of the ER and exhibit antiestrogenic and estrogenic activity in breast cancer, these compounds both induce ER-dependent activity in the uterus and prolonged treatment with tamoxifen increases the risk for endometrial cancer (Bernstein, 2002). Tamoxifen is also an ER agonist in the bone and vascular system and there are tissue- and species-specific ER agonist or antagonist activities in animal models where tamoxifen is an ER antagonist in chicks, a partial ER agonist/antagonist in rats and an ER agonist in several short-term assays in mice (MacGregor and Jordan, 1998). Studies on tamoxifen and other ER agonists has led to the development of the acronym selective ER modulators (SERMs), which exhibit a complex pharmacology and induce tissue-specific ER agonist or antagonist activities. These structure-dependent differences are related to differential activation of estrogen-responsive genes/pathways and due to several factors, including:

1. structure of the estrogenic compound;
2. tissue-specific expression of ER subtype (ERα and ERβ) or variant;
3. tissue-specific expression of critical coactivators and other coregulatory proteins; and
4. promoter context and chromatin state, which is dependent on histone methylation or acetylation, promoter methylation, and expression of critical modulating trans-acting factors.

Development of Bioassays for Clinically Relevant SERMs

SERMs were primarily developed for treatment of hormone-dependent diseases or conditions and define the increasing complexity of ER action. If xenoestrogens and phytoestrogens are SERMs, then their estrogenic and

TABLE 59.1 The SERMs Tamoxifen, Raloxifene, ICI 164384 and E2 Differentially Activate ERα and Also Exhibit Unique in Vivo Biologies (Tzukerman et al., 1994)

SERM	ERα	ERα-AF-1	ERα-AF-2	In Vivo ER Activity		
	A/B C/D E F	A/B C/D E***F	C/D E F	Bone	Breast	Uterus
Estradiol	+++[a]	+++	+++	Ag[b]	Ag	Ag
Tamoxifen	+	+	ND	Ag	Ant	Ag
Raloxifene	ND	+	ND	Ag	Ant	–
ICI 164,384	ND	ND	ND	–	Ant	Ant

[a]E2 induced maximal responses in all assays (+++), and responses. 40% (11) or, 40% (+) of that observed for E2 are indicated. ND indicates no significant induction or inhibition of activity.
[b]Ag and Ant indicate ER agonist and antagonist, respectively; (–) indicates no agonist activity.

antiestrogenic activities will also be tissue-specific and their role in causation or protection from hormone-dependent problems will depend on the structure of the individual compound, the amount of exposure (assuming a threshold) and the time of exposure where critical modifications of hormone-responsiveness are induced. The structurally diverse SERMs, E2, tamoxifen, raloxifene, and ICI 164,384 have unique in vivo biologies and were used as model compounds to develop an in vitro bioassay that would distinguish between these compounds (McDonnell et al., 1995). This bioassay utilizes the modular structure of ERα and ERβ in which the various domains (E–F) exhibit both separable and overlapping functions that govern their interactions with other coregulatory proteins and promoter DNA. AF-1 and AF-2 are located in the A/B and E domains, respectively, and are particularly important for this assay system. Results in Table 59.1 show that these four compounds differentially induce transactivation in human hepatoma HepG2 cells transfected with the E2-responsive pC3 construct (human complement C3 promoter linked to the luciferase gene) and expression plasmids for wild-type ERα, ERα-AF-2 in which the AF-1 domain has been deleted, or ERα-AF-1 in which the critical amino acids in AF-2 have been mutated (aa D538N, E542Q and D545N). E2 induces transactivation in HepG2 cells transfected with wild-type/variant ERα; in contrast raloxifene activates ERαAF-1, tamoxifen activates ERα and ERα-AF-1, and ICI 164,384 does not induce or inhibits transactivation.

XENOESTROGENS AND PHYTOESTROGENS AS SERMS

The assay developed by McDonnell and coworkers (1995) has been used for distinguishing between different structural classes of xenoestrogens and phytoestrogens including BPA (2′,4′,6′-tricholo-4-biphenylol (Cl_3–PCB–OH), 2′,3′,4′,5′-tetrachloro-4-biphenylol (Cl_4–PCB–OH), *p-t*-octylphenol (OP), *o*-nonylphenol (NP), naringenin, kepone, resveratrol and 2,2-bis(*p*-hydroxyphenyl)-1,1,1-trichloroethane (HPTE). E2, ICI 182,780, and 4-hydroxytamoxifen were used as positive controls (Gould et al., 1998; Yoon et al., 2000, 2001). Results obtained in several cell lines using the E2-responsive complement pC3-luc construct or a construct ($pERE_3$) containing three EREs linked to luciferase demonstrate that xenoestrogens/phytoestrogens also differentially induce transactivation.

Results summarized in Table 59.2 compare the maximal induced responses observed for these compounds using human hepatoma HepG2 and human U2 osteogenic cancer cell lines transfected with $pERE_3$ and ERα, ERα-AF-1 or ERα-AF-2 (Yoon et al., 2001). Even among structurally-related compounds, such as the hydroxy-PCBs, alkylphenols, and bisphenolics HPTE and BPA, there were some significant differences in their induction of transactivation. Moreover, using a similar approach in HepG2, U2 and MDA-MB-231 cancer cell lines transfected with a pC3-luc construct similar differences were observed (Yoon et al., 2000). For example, the two bisphenolic compounds HPTE and BPA exhibit a similar pattern of transactivation in many assays except that in U2 cells BPA but not HPTE induces transactivation in cells transfected with ERα-AF-1. It was also apparent from other in vivo and in vitro studies that BPA and HPTE exhibit difference in their estrogenic activities. For example, HPTE was a more potent estrogen than BPA in the female rat uterus; however in combination with E2, lower doses of BPA inhibited E2-induced uterine progesterone receptor (PR) binding and peroxidase activity (Gould et al., 1998). HPTE versus BPA also exhibited other differences in HepG2 cells where both HPTE and BPA are ERα agonists, whereas HPTE is an ERβ and androgen receptor (AR) antagonist and BPA is an ERβ agonist and did not affect AR in this cell line (Gaido et al., 1999). These activities can also vary in other cell contexts but clearly demonstrate significant in vitro and

TABLE 59.2 Different Structural Classes of Xenoestrogens, Phytoestrogens, E2 and 4-Hydroxytamoxifen Differentially Induce Transactivation in HepG2 and U2 Cells Transfected With pERE$_3$, Wild-Type and Variant Forms of ERα (Yoon et al., 2001)

	ERα		ERα-AF-1		ERα-AF-2	
	A/B C/D E F		A/B C/D E***F		C/D E F	
	HepG2	U2	HepG2	U2	HepG2	U2
17β-estradiol	+++[a]	+++	+++	+++	+++	+++
4-Hydroxytamoxifen	+	ND	ND	ND	ND	ND
NP	+	+	++	ND	++	ND
OP	+	+	+	+	ND	ND
HO–PCB–Cl$_4$	++	++	+	ND	++	+++
HO–PCB–Cl$_3$	++	++	+	++	+++	+++
HPTE	+++	+	+	ND	+++	++
BPA	++	++	+	++	++	+++
Kepone	ND	ND	+	ND	+	ND
Naringenin	ND	ND	ND	ND	ND	ND
Resveratrol	ND	ND	ND	ND	ND	ND

[a]*E2 induced a maximal response (+++) in all assays. A significant induction response of 0.40% (+++) or 0.40% (+) of that observed for E2, and no significant induction (ND) are indicated. ICI 182,780 gave an ND for all responses. The doses used were 10 nM and 1 μM for E2 and 4′-hydroxytamoxifen, respectively, 100 μM for BPA, and 10 μM for the remaining compounds.*

in vivo biological differences between HPTE and BPA, suggesting that structurally diverse estrogenic compounds are SERMs and this has recently been confirmed in a study examining different regions of ERα-AF-2 (Arao et al., 2015).

Several other in vitro studies have demonstrated significant differences among different structural classes of estrogenic compounds and the planar phytoestrogens coumestrol and genistein. For example, an ERα mutant (D351G) is activated by E2 and DES but not by 4′-hydroxytamoxifen or the nonplanar HPTE and related compounds (Jordan et al., 2001). It was also reported that isoflavones, daidzein, biochanin, and genistein are ERβ-selective and this is due to their preferential induction of coactivator interactions with AF-2 of ERβ compared to AF-2 of ERα (An et al., 2001). Other reports also show that activation of gene expression in in vitro assays by structurally diverse xenoestrogens/phytoestrogens depends on the promoter context (i.e., different consensus versus nonconsensus EREs) and on coactivator interactions (Hall et al., 2002). Recent studies have also demonstrated structure-dependent activation of nongenomic kinase pathways by xenoestrogens/phytoestrogens (Li et al., 2006). Moreover it has also been shown that some estrogenic compounds activate kinases via ER-independent pathways by directly binding to a G-protein coupled receptor (GPR30) (Revankar et al., 2005). The structure dependence on this ER-dependent pathway has yet to be determined. These results clearly imply that xenoestrogens/phytoestrogens are SERMs.

SERMS: IMPLICATIONS FOR RISK ASSESSMENT

Xenoestrogens and phytoestrogens differentially activate wild-type and variant ERα in vitro suggesting that these compounds are SERMs. This implies that their estrogenic activity and potency cannot be determined by simple ER binding or gene expression assays. Thus, in order to fully understand the estrogenic or antiestrogenic activities of phytoestrogens and xenoestrogens studies will have to focus on their tissue-specific impacts at various critical periods of exposure. Risk assessment of these compounds will be complex and dependent on all the variables indicated in a previous section. Moreover, since individual SERMs exhibit unique biologies, the overall impact of mixtures of these compounds may not be additive. Another complication associated with the mechanisms of action and risk assessment of many xenoestrogens is due to their multiple tissue-/species-activities and this is illustrated by BPA and its interaction with receptors (Fig. 59.6). As indicated above, BPA activates ERα and ERβ (Kuiper et al., 1997) and also binds and activates GPR30 (Dong et al., 2011). BPA also induces

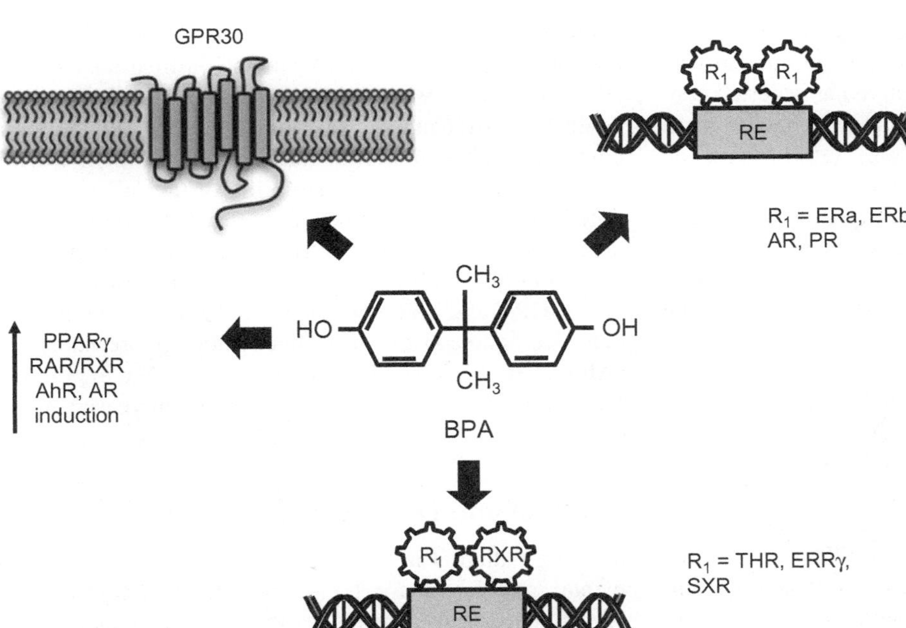

FIGURE 59.6 BPA exhibits tissue-specific agonist or antagonist activities for multiple receptors and also induces expression of some receptors.

CaBP-9k, a progestin-responsive gene in the mouse uterus (Jung et al., 2005), and induces neuronal PR mRNA levels in rats (Funabashi et al., 2004). BPA also acts as an AR agonist and antagonist in different assays (Kruger et al., 2008) and exhibits thyroid hormone receptor antagonist activity (Moriyama et al., 2002). BPA also binds and/or activates estrogen-related receptor γ (Matsushima et al., 2007) and the steroid and xenobiotic receptor and induces NR4A1 in mouse testicular Leydig cells (Song et al., 2002). Moreover, it has also been reported that BPA induces the aryl hydrocarbon receptor, AR, retinoid receptors, and peroxisome proliferator-activated receptor γ and this can also result in modulation of receptor-mediated responses (Kruger et al., 2008; Kwintkiewicz et al., 2010; Nishizawa et al., 2005). These factors highlight the challenges faced by scientists and regulators in addressing the health risks and benefits of estrogenic compounds.

Although high throughput screening assays continue to identify estrogenic compounds through ER binding or transactivation studies, it is likely that most of these compounds will be SERMs. Although subclasses of structurally-related compounds may exhibit similar/overlapping estrogenic activities as SERMs, the only way to confirm the response-specific ER activity is to test the compounds individually. Thus, results of high throughput assays must be used with caution in terms of risk assessment.

ROLE OF ENVIRONMENTAL ESTROGENS IN DISEASES

Background

Estrogens regulate the development and function of the female reproductive system and their effects are mediated through ERα and ERβ. However, estrogens are by no means only female hormones. In both males and females, estrogens play crucial physiological roles, including sex differentiation, bone development and maintenance, central nervous system and cardiovascular function. The ER is important for mammary gland development and ERα knockout (αERKO) mice are viable but sterile and are estrogen-insensitive in several estrogen target organs, including mammary glands, reproductive tracts and gonads. The well-recognized estrogenic responses, such as uterine weight increase and vaginal cornification, are all absent in αERKO mice (Korach, 1994). In αERKO mice, mammary glands undergo normal development in the prenatal period, but fail to develop terminal end buds and are severely undertropic during adulthood (Korach, 1994). Surprisingly, adult male αERKO mice are also infertile because of impaired spermatogenesis (Eddy et al., 1996). In contrast to the extensive reproductive tract abnormalities in αERKO mice, ERβ knockout (βERKO) mice are fertile but exhibit reduced fertility (Korach, 1994).

Estrogens and Women's Health

Women have significantly lower risk of cardiovascular disease than men and this has been putatively attributed to the beneficial effects of estrogen on cardiovascular function. Estrogen decreases low-density lipoprotein level and increases high-density lipoprotein levels. Estrogen exhibits vasodilatory effects and protects against vascular injury (Pare et al., 2002) and also induces COX-2-dependent upregulation of atheroprotective prostacyclin PGI_2 (Egan et al., 2004). In epidemiological studies, estrogen has been linked with improved cardiovascular functions and. Bilateral ovariectomy before menopause elevates the risk for coronary heart disease and the increased risk is eliminated by estrogen-replacement therapy (Colditz et al., 1987). However, a large clinical trial conducted by Women's Health Initiative has reported contradictory results on the effects of estrogens since women taking hormone replacement therapies (HRT) have an increased risk for heart diseases and stroke (Rossouw et al., 2002). The relationships between estrogen and cardiovascular diseases require further assessment.

Estrogen is also important for bone development, maintenance (Cutler, 1997), and sexual differentiation in the brain and reproductive behavior (Bakker et al., 2003), and sustained estrogen treatment improves learning ability, memory and fine motor skills in animal models (Lacreuse and Herndon, 2003). However, results of the Women's Health Initiative show that the use of HRT can lead to increased risks for heart disease and stroke. There is concern that these estrogens may induce some adverse neurological responses (Espeland et al., 2004). The most well-characterized adverse responses of endogenous and exogenous estrogens is associated with their effects on both breast and endometrial cancer in women (Hilakivi-Clarke, 2000) and there is also concern that fetal or early postnatal exposure of males to estrogens will affect the male reproductive tract functions in adults (Skakkebaek et al., 2001).

Risks for Breast Cancer Genetic Factors

There are several different risk factors for breast cancer and there is a strong interplay of genetic and environmental factors. Five to ten percent of all breast cancers are associated with the inheritance of mutations in one of the two major breast cancer susceptibility genes, BRCA1 and BRCA2 (Venkitaraman, 2002). There is an 80% chance of developing breast cancer during a lifetime in women with an inherited BRCA1 or BRCA2 mutation. BRCA1 and BRCA2 are tumor suppressor genes and their proteins have been implicated in a multitude of different processes including DNA repair and recombination, cell cycle control and transcription (Venkitaraman, 2002). Several other genetic mutations also contribute to the risk in breast cancer and these include genes such as p53, which also increase the risk for multiple cancers.

Hormonal Risk Factors for Breast Cancer

Several studies have shown that prolonged exposure to the hormone estrogen increases the risk of breast cancer. Epidemiological studies have established a strong link between higher risk of breast cancer and reproductive factors that increase the overall number of menstrual cycles such as early menarche (before age 12), late menopause (after age 55), age of women at first birth (over 30–35), and nulliparity (Russo et al., 1992). Breast cancer risk is lower in women with multiple pregnancies and women with a pregnancy prior to age 24 (Lambe et al., 1996). Women who are above 30–35 years of age at first birth are at higher risk compared to nulliparous women (Rosner et al., 1994). The protective effects of pregnancy against breast cancer is explained by the induction of complete differentiation of the breast that may markedly reduce the carcinogen susceptibility of the fully differentiated mammary gland due, at least in part, to the decreased proliferative activity of parous epithelium (Russo et al., 2000). Recent studies have shown that the use of HRT and oral contraceptives for long time periods can also increase the risk of developing breast cancer (Althuis et al., 2003). In some studies women exposed to DES were also found to be at slightly increased breast cancer risk (Titus-Ernstoff et al., 2001).

Lifestyle and Dietary Risk Factors

Ionizing radiation is the most well-characterized environmental risk factor for breast cancer. Radiation-induced breast cancer risk depends on the various factors including age at exposure (highest before age 30 years), the status of hormone levels, parity and other genetic disorders (Coyle, 2004). Other risk factors include solar radiation, light and chemicals. Solar radiation creates an active form of vitamin D that may lower the risk of breast cancer and studies show that women who work at nights are at higher breast cancer risk. This may be due to decreased vitamin D synthesis and suppression of normal nocturnal production of melatonin by the pineal gland, increases the estrogen release by the ovaries thereby disrupting circadian patterns (Schernhammer et al., 2001).

Various lifestyle factors, such as poor diet, limited exercise, smoking, and alcohol consumption, are related to an increased risk of developing breast cancer (Key et al., 2003). Confirmation of the risk of dietary fat intake and breast cancer has not been substantiated in large epidemiology studies. However, a dietary pattern of high fiber and low fat intakes is associated with a lower risk of breast cancer in postmenopausal women (Mattisson et al., 2004). In some studies protective effects of some vegetable fats, vitamin E, selenium, and other antioxidants have been observed (Gerber et al., 2003). Decreased ovarian hormone levels decreased the risk of breast cancer in populations in Asia and is related to their high consumption of soy products containing significant amount of the isoflavones, daidzein, and genistein that act as weak estrogens (Mezzetti et al., 1998).

Environmental Estrogens and Breast Cancer

The hypothesis linking environmental estrogens to the increased incidence of breast cancer was due primarily to studies of a small number of breast cancer patients in Connecticut and New York showing higher levels of PCBs and DDE, respectively, in patients versus controls (Falck et al., 1992; Wolff et al., 1993). It was hypothesized that these compounds and possibly other environmental estrogens were risk factors for breast cancer (Davis et al., 1993); however, this hypothesis was initially challenged (Safe, 2000) based on the fact that there was minimal evidence for the estrogenicity of either PCBs or DDE (Mayes et al., 1998; Silinskas and Okey, 1975). Nevertheless, the putative linkage between PCBs, DDE and breast cancer was investigated worldwide and the results showed that levels of DDE and PCBs were similar in breast cancer patients versus controls, although there were some inconsistent differences in levels of specific PCB congeners. A meta-analysis of the studies on levels of DDE in breast cancer patients versus controls showed no differences, although overall levels of DDE decreased by over 95% from 1965 to 1995 (Lopez-Cervantes et al., 2004). In a study of women on Long Island, it was concluded by Gammon and coworkers (2002), these findings, based on the largest number of samples analyzed to date among primarily white women, do not support the hypothesis that organochlorines increase breast cancer risk among Long Island women. Reports on PCBs, PCB congeners, DDE, and other organochlorine pesticides and their differential expression in breast cancer patients continue to be published with variable results and only occasionally are some significant differences observed. Two recent studies suggest that in utero exposure to DDT may enhance breast cancer in offspring (Cohn et al., 2015) and DDT levels may be associated with increased mortality from breast cancer (Parada et al., 2016) and these are areas that require further confirmatory studies.

ESTROGENS AS RISK FACTORS FOR MALE REPRODUCTIVE TRACT PROBLEMS

Although estrogens are female steroid hormones and influence normal physiology and disease in women, there has been increasing concern on the potential adverse effect of estrogenic compounds on development of the male reproductive tract (Sharpe and Skakkebaek, 1993). Support for the hypothesis that "environmental estrogens" (xenoestrogens) and other endocrine disrupting compounds are responsible for an increase in male reproductive tract problems is derived from laboratory animal, wildlife and human studies. For example, there are numerous reports of feminized fish in river systems, particularly those in the United Kingdom and this has been linked to their exposures to endogenous estrogens (17β-estradiol/estrone), synthetic contraceptives (17-ethinylestradiol) and industrial byproducts such as alkylphenols (Routledge et al., 1998). There is some evidence that nonylphenol and alkylphenols may contribute to estrogenization of fish near sewage outflows.

It has also been suggested that the major concern regarding environmental/dietary estrogens is in utero or early postnatal exposures during the important initial periods of male reproductive tract development (Skakkebaek et al., 2001). The potent estrogenic drug DES was extensively used by pregnant women with disastrous consequences for their male and female offspring (Giusti et al., 1995). Females exposed in utero develop a high incidence of a rare vaginal adenocarcinoma, whereas male offspring developed a range of responses including deformed genitalia. The adverse effects of DES form one of the bases of the endocrine disruption hypothesis and the opinion that a testicular dysgenesis syndrome, which includes low sperm counts, increased hypospadias and cryptorchidism and testicular cancer may be linked to in utero exposure to estrogenic compounds and other endocrine disrupting compounds (Skakkebaek et al., 2001). This opinion and hypothesis have been challenged (Handelsman, 2001; Safe, 2000).

Meta-analysis of sperm bank donors initially demonstrated a nearly 40% decrease in sperm counts over the 1938–91 period (Carlsen et al., 1992) and this stimulated research worldwide on time-dependent changes in sperm counts (rev. in Fisch and Braun, 2013) and implications for fertility. In addition, there has also been extensive research on various factors that affect sperm counts that were not known (or corrected for) at the time of the meta-analysis. It was demonstrated that in Europe, France and North America, sperm counts varied with respect to region/location (Fisch et al., 1996; Jorgensen et al., 2002; Younglai et al., 1998). Subsequent research has demonstrated that multiple factors affect sperm counts and these include population selection (i.e., random or self-selected) (Handelsman, 1997), seasonal and age variability (Chen et al., 2003), age of sampling (Perheentupa et al., 2016), body mass index (Guo et al., 2017), dietary components including fruits and vegetables, fat and sweeteners (Chiu et al., 2014, 2016; Karayiannis et al., 2017; Olsen and Ramlau-Hansen, 2012), alcohol consumption (Jensen et al., 2014), sleep disturbances (Jensen et al., 2013) physical activity (Gaskins et al., 2015), and even earthquakes (Chen et al., 2016). There is also evidence that high levels of air pollutants affect (decrease) sperm quality (Deng et al., 2016) and a recent meta-analysis of 20 studies showed that smoking also reduced sperm counts (Sharma et al., 2016). These are just a sampling of studies showing that many factors affect sperm counts and sperm quality. A recent analysis reported that the evidence for correlations between endocrine disruptor exposure and adverse male reproductive tract disorders "is limited" (Bonde et al., 2016). In contrast, a review of all studies on sperm count changes over the period between 1980 and 2015 indicates a "significant decline in North America, Europe, Asia and Africa" but an increase in Australia (Sengupta et al., 2016). The reason for these declines is not known, but the authors point out the inverse correlation between decreasing sperm counts and quality with increasing obesity and it is possible that this could be a contributing factor to global declines in sperm quality. Moreover, the worldwide epidemic of obesity, which has been primarily linked to increased caloric intake and decreased physical activity, may also be the major underlying cause of several claimed endocrine disruptor-induced responses. Hopefully, this will be resolved in the near future.

CONCLUDING REMARKS AND FUTURE DIRECTIONS

The list of endocrine disrupting chemicals with estrogenic activity is long and will continue to grow as EPA-sponsored screening activities identify new estrogenic compounds. The role of environmental estrogens as causal agents for breast cancer or for decreased sperm counts is unlikely based on currently available data. There have been many hypotheses that attempt to link estrogenic EDCs to health issues such as obesity, diabetes, heart disease, neurological diseases, and cancer; however, their association with these health issues is not well established. There is evidence that in developed countries early onset of puberty is being observed and this is a bona fide endocrine problem with disease implications. The role of "environmental factors" (including diet) on early onset of puberty should be further investigated.

ACKNOWLEDGMENTS

Financial support for preparation of this chapter has been provided by the National Institutes of Health (P30-ES023512), Texas AgriLife Research, and Sid Kyle endowment.

REFERENCES

Althuis, M.D., Brogan, D.R., Coates, R.J., et al., 2003. Hormonal content and potency of oral contraceptives and breast cancer risk among young women. Br. J. Cancer. 88, 50–57.

An, J., Tzagarakis-Foster, C., Scharschmidt, T.C., et al., 2001. Estrogen receptor beta-selective transcriptional activity and recruitment of coregulators by phytoestrogens. J. Biol. Chem. 276, 17808–17814.

Arao, Y., Coons, L.A., Zuercher, W.J., et al., 2015. Transactivation function-2 of estrogen receptor alpha contains transactivation function-1-regulating element. J. Biol. Chem. 290, 17611–17627.

Autrup, H., Barile, F.A., Blaauboer, B.J., et al., 2015. Principles of pharmacology and toxicology also govern effects of chemicals on the endocrine system. Toxicol. Sci. 146, 11–15.

Bakker, J., Honda, S., Harada, N., et al., 2003. The aromatase knockout (arko) mouse provides new evidence that estrogens are required for the development of the female brain. Ann. N. Y. Acad. Sci. 1007, 251–262.

Barkhem, T., Carlsson, B., Nilsson, Y., et al., 1998. Differential response of estrogen receptor alpha and estrogen receptor beta to partial estrogen agonists/antagonists. Mol. Pharmacol. 54, 105–112.

Benecke, A., Chambon, P., Gronemeyer, H., 2000. Synergy between estrogen receptor alpha activation functions af1 and af2 mediated by transcription intermediary factor tif2. EMBO Rep. 1, 151–157.

Bernstein, L., 2002. Epidemiology of endocrine-related risk factors for breast cancer. J. Mammary Gland. Biol. Neoplasia. 7, 3–15.

Bonde, J.P., Flachs, E.M., Rimborg, S., et al., 2016. The epidemiologic evidence linking prenatal and postnatal exposure to endocrine disrupting chemicals with male reproductive disorders: a systematic review and meta-analysis. Hum. Reprod. Update. 23, 104–125.

Carlsen, E., Giwercman, A., Keiding, N., et al., 1992. Evidence for decreasing quality of semen during past 50 years. BMJ. 305, 609–613.

Chen, X.M., Chen, S.M., Yue, H.X., et al., 2016. Semen quality in adult male survivors 5 years after the 2008 wenchuan earthquake. Andrologia. 48, 1274–1280.

Chen, Z., Toth, T., Godfrey-Bailey, L., et al., 2003. Seasonal variation and age-related changes in human semen parameters. J. Androl. 24, 226–231.

Chiu, Y.H., Afeiche, M.C., Gaskins, A.J., et al., 2014. Sugar-sweetened beverage intake in relation to semen quality and reproductive hormone levels in young men. Hum. Reprod. 29, 1575–1584.

Chiu, Y.H., Gaskins, A.J., Williams, P.L., et al., 2016. Intake of fruits and vegetables with low-to-moderate pesticide residues is positively associated with semen-quality parameters among young healthy men. J. Nutr. 146, 1084–1092.

Cohn, B.A., La Merrill, M., Krigbaum, N.Y., et al., 2015. Ddt exposure in utero and breast cancer. J. Clin. Endocrinol. Metab. 100, 2865–2872.

Colditz, G.A., Willett, W.C., Stampfer, M.J., et al., 1987. Menopause and the risk of coronary heart disease in women. N. Engl. J. Med. 316, 1105–1110.

Cowley, S.M., Parker, M.G., 1999. A comparison of transcriptional activation by er alpha and er beta. J. Steroid Biochem. Mol. Biol. 69, 165–175.

Coyle, Y.M., 2004. The effect of environment on breast cancer risk. Breast Cancer Res. Treat. 84, 273–288.

Cutler Jr., G.B., 1997. The role of estrogen in bone growth and maturation during childhood and adolescence. J. Steroid Biochem. Mol. Biol. 61, 141–144.

Davis, D.L., Bradlow, H.L., Wolff, M., et al., 1993. Medical hypothesis: xenoestrogens as preventable causes of breast cancer. Environ. Health Perspect. 101, 372–377.

Deng, Z., Chen, F., Zhang, M., et al., 2016. Association between air pollution and sperm quality: a systematic review and meta-analysis. Environ. Pollut. 208, 663–669.

Dong, S., Terasaka, S., Kiyama, R., 2011. Bisphenol a induces a rapid activation of erk1/2 through gpr30 in human breast cancer cells. Environ. Pollut. 159, 212–218.

Eddy, E.M., Washburn, T.F., Bunch, D.O., et al., 1996. Targeted disruption of the estrogen receptor gene in male mice causes alteration of spermatogenesis and infertility. Endocrinology. 137, 4796–4805.

Egan, K.M., Lawson, J.A., Fries, S., et al., 2004. Cox-2-derived prostacyclin confers atheroprotection on female mice. Science. 306, 1954–1957.

Espeland, M.A., Rapp, S.R., Shumaker, S.A., et al., 2004. Conjugated equine estrogens and global cognitive function in postmenopausal women: women's health initiative memory study. JAMA. 291, 2959–2968.

Falck Jr., F., Ricci Jr., A., Wolff, M.S., et al., 1992. Pesticides and polychlorinated biphenyl residues in human breast lipids and their relation to breast cancer. Arch. Environ. Health. 47, 143–146.

Fisch, H., Braun, S.R., 2013. Trends in global semen parameter values. Asian J. Androl. 15, 169–173.

Fisch, H., Goluboff, E.T., Olson, J.H., et al., 1996. Semen analyses in 1,283 men from the united states over a 25-year period: no decline in quality. Fertil. Steril. 65, 1009–1014.

Funabashi, T., Nakamura, T.J., Kimura, F., 2004. P-nonylphenol, 4-tert-octylphenol and bisphenol a increase the expression of progesterone receptor mrna in the frontal cortex of adult ovariectomized rats. J. Neuroendocrinol. 16, 99–104.

Gaido, K.W., Leonard, L.S., Maness, S.C., et al., 1999. Differential interaction of the methoxychlor metabolite 2,2-bis-(p-hydroxyphenyl)-1,1,1-trichloroethane with estrogen receptors alpha and beta. Endocrinology. 140, 5746–5753.

Gammon, M.D., Wolff, M.S., Neugut, A.I., et al., 2002. Environmental toxins and breast cancer on long island. Ii. Organochlorine compound levels in blood. Cancer Epidemiol. Biomarkers Prev. 11, 686–697.

Gaskins, A.J., Mendiola, J., Afeiche, M., et al., 2015. Physical activity and television watching in relation to semen quality in young men. Br. J. Sports Med. 49, 265–270.

Gerber, B., Muller, H., Reimer, T., et al., 2003. Nutrition and lifestyle factors on the risk of developing breast cancer. Breast Cancer Res. Treat. 79, 265–276.

Giusti, R.M., Iwamoto, K., Hatch, E.E., 1995. Diethylstilbestrol revisited: a review of the long-term health effects. Ann. Intern. Med. 122, 778–788.

Gore, A.C., Chappell, V.A., Fenton, S.E., et al., 2015. Executive summary to edc-2: the endocrine society's second scientific statement on endocrine-disrupting chemicals. Endocr. Rev. 36, 593–602.

Gould, J.C., Leonard, L.S., Maness, S.C., et al., 1998. Bisphenol a interacts with the estrogen receptor alpha in a distinct manner from estradiol. Mol. Cell. Endocrinol. 142, 203–214.

Guo, D., Wu, W., Tang, Q., et al., 2017. The impact of bmi on sperm parameters and the metabolite changes of seminal plasma concomitantly. Oncotarget. Available from: http://dx.doi.org/10.18632/oncotarget.14950.

Hall, J.M., McDonnell, D.P., Korach, K.S., 2002. Allosteric regulation of estrogen receptor structure, function, and coactivator recruitment by different estrogen response elements. Mol. Endocrinol. 16, 469–486.

Handelsman, D.J., 1997. Sperm output of healthy men in australia: magnitude of bias due to self-selected volunteers. Hum. Reprod. 12, 2701–2705.

Handelsman, D.J., 2001. Estrogens and falling sperm counts. Reprod. Fertil. Dev. 13, 317–324.

Havsteen, B.H., 2002. The biochemistry and medical significance of the flavonoids. Pharmacol. Ther. 96, 67–202.

Heindel, J.J., vom Saal, F.S., Blumberg, B., et al., 2015. Parma consensus statement on metabolic disruptors. Environ. Health. 14, 54.

Hilakivi-Clarke, L., 2000. Estrogens, brca1, and breast cancer. Cancer Res. 60, 4993–5001.

Janesick, A.S., Dimastrogiovanni, G., Vanek, L., et al., 2016. On the utility of toxcast and toxpi as methods for identifying new obesogens. Environ. Health Perspect. 124, 1214–1226.

Jensen, T.K., Andersson, A.M., Skakkebaek, N.E., et al., 2013. Association of sleep disturbances with reduced semen quality: a cross-sectional study among 953 healthy young danish men. Am. J. Epidemiol. 177, 1027–1037.

Jensen, T.K., Gottschau, M., Madsen, J.O., et al., 2014. Habitual alcohol consumption associated with reduced semen quality and changes in reproductive hormones; a cross-sectional study among 1221 young danish men. BMJ Open. 4, e005462.

Jordan, V.C., 2003. Antiestrogens and selective estrogen receptor modulators as multifunctional medicines. 2. Clinical considerations and new agents. J. Med. Chem. 46, 1081–1111.

Jordan, V.C., Schafer, J.M., Levenson, A.S., et al., 2001. Molecular classification of estrogens. Cancer Res. 61, 6619–6623.

Jorgensen, N., Carlsen, E., Nermoen, I., et al., 2002. East-west gradient in semen quality in the nordic-baltic area: a study of men from the general population in denmark, norway, estonia and finland. Hum. Reprod. 17, 2199–2208.

Jung, Y.W., Hong, E.J., Choi, K.C., et al., 2005. Novel progestogenic activity of environmental endocrine disruptors in the upregulation of calbindin-d9k in an immature mouse model. Toxicol. Sci. 83, 78–88.

Karayiannis, D., Kontogianni, M.D., Mendorou, C., et al., 2017. Association between adherence to the mediterranean diet and semen quality parameters in male partners of couples attempting fertility. Hum. Reprod. 32, 215–222.

Key, T.J., Allen, N.E., Spencer, E.A., et al., 2003. Nutrition and breast cancer. Breast. 12, 412–416.

Korach, K.S., 1994. Insights from the study of animals lacking functional estrogen receptor. Science. 266, 1524–1527.

Koehler, D.F., Helguero, L.A., Haldosen, L.A., et al., 2005. Reflections on the discovery and significance of estrogen receptor beta. Endocr. Rev. 26, 465–478.

Kruger, T., Long, M., Bonefeld-Jorgensen, E.C., 2008. Plastic components affect the activation of the aryl hydrocarbon and the androgen receptor. Toxicology. 246, 112–123.

Kuiper, G.G., Carlsson, B., Grandien, K., et al., 1997. Comparison of the ligand binding specificity and transcript tissue distribution of estrogen receptors alpha and beta. Endocrinology. 138, 863–870.

Kwintkiewicz, J., Nishi, Y., Yanase, T., et al., 2010. Peroxisome proliferator-activated receptor-gamma mediates bisphenol a inhibition of fsh-stimulated igf-1, aromatase, and estradiol in human granulosa cells. Environ. Health Perspect. 118, 400–406.

Lacreuse, A., Herndon, J.G., 2003. Effects of estradiol and aging on fine manual performance in female rhesus monkeys. Horm. Behav. 43, 359–366.

Lambe, M., Hsieh, C.C., Chan, H.W., et al., 1996. Parity, age at first and last birth, and risk of breast cancer: a population-based study in sweden. Breast Cancer Res. Treat. 38, 305–311.

Li, X., Zhang, S., Safe, S., 2006. Activation of kinase pathways in mcf-7 cells by 17beta-estradiol and structurally diverse estrogenic compounds. J. Steroid Biochem. Mol. Biol. 98, 122–132.

Lopez-Cervantes, M., Torres-Sanchez, L., Tobias, A., et al., 2004. Dichlorodiphenyldichloroethane burden and breast cancer risk: a meta-analysis of the epidemiologic evidence. Environ. Health Perspect. 112, 207–214.

MacGregor, J.I., Jordan, V.C., 1998. Basic guide to the mechanisms of antiestrogen action. Pharmacol. Rev. 50, 151–196.

Matsushima, A., Kakuta, Y., Teramoto, T., et al., 2007. Structural evidence for endocrine disruptor bisphenol a binding to human nuclear receptor err gamma. J. Biochem. 142, 517–524.

Matthews, J., Gustafsson, J.A., 2003. Estrogen signaling: a subtle balance between er alpha and er beta. Mol. Interv. 3, 281–292.

Mattisson, I., Wirfalt, E., Johansson, U., et al., 2004. Intakes of plant foods, fibre and fat and risk of breast cancer--a prospective study in the malmo diet and cancer cohort. Br. J. Cancer. 90, 122–127.

Mayes, B.A., McConnell, E.E., Neal, B.H., et al., 1998. Comparative carcinogenicity in sprague-dawley rats of the polychlorinated biphenyl mixtures aroclors 1016, 1242, 1254, and 1260. Toxicol. Sci. 41, 62–76.

McDonnell, D.P., Clemm, D.L., Hermann, T., et al., 1995. Analysis of estrogen receptor function in vitro reveals three distinct classes of antiestrogens. Mol. Endocrinol. 9, 659–669.

Mezzetti, M., La Vecchia, C., Decarli, A., et al., 1998. Population attributable risk for breast cancer: diet, nutrition, and physical exercise. J. Natl. Cancer Inst. 90, 389–394.

Moriyama, K., Tagami, T., Akamizu, T., et al., 2002. Thyroid hormone action is disrupted by bisphenol a as an antagonist. J. Clin. Endocrinol. Metab. 87, 5185–5190.

Nilsson, S., Makela, S., Treuter, E., et al., 2001. Mechanisms of estrogen action. Physiol. Rev. 81, 1535–1565.

Nishizawa, H., Morita, M., Sugimoto, M., et al., 2005. Effects of in utero exposure to bisphenol a on mrna expression of arylhydrocarbon and retinoid receptors in murine embryos. J. Reprod. Dev. 51, 315–324.

Olsen, J., Ramlau-Hansen, C.H., 2012. Dietary fats may impact semen quantity and quality. Asian J. Androl. 14, 511–512.

Parada Jr., H., Wolff, M.S., Engel, L.S., et al., 2016. Organochlorine insecticides ddt and chlordane in relation to survival following breast cancer. Int. J. Cancer. 138, 565–575.

Pare, G., Krust, A., Karas, R.H., et al., 2002. Estrogen receptor-alpha mediates the protective effects of estrogen against vascular injury. Circ. Res. 90, 1087–1092.

Perheentupa, A., Sadov, S., Ronka, R., et al., 2016. Semen quality improves marginally during young adulthood: a longitudinal follow-up study. Hum. Reprod. 31, 502–510.

Revankar, C.M., Cimino, D.F., Sklar, L.A., et al., 2005. A transmembrane intracellular estrogen receptor mediates rapid cell signaling. Science. 307, 1625–1630.

Rosner, B., Colditz, G.A., Willett, W.C., 1994. Reproductive risk factors in a prospective study of breast cancer: the nurses' health study. Am. J. Epidemiol. 139, 819–835.

Rossouw, J.E., Anderson, G.L., Prentice, R.L., et al., 2002. Risks and benefits of estrogen plus progestin in healthy postmenopausal women: principal results from the women's health initiative randomized controlled trial. JAMA. 288, 321–333.

Rotroff, D.M., Dix, D.J., Houck, K.A., et al., 2013. Using in vitro high throughput screening assays to identify potential endocrine-disrupting chemicals. Environ. Health Perspect. 121, 7–14.

Routledge, E.J., Sheahan, D., Desbrow, C., et al., 1998. Identification of estrogenic chemicals in stw effluent. 2. *In vivo* responses in trout and roach. Environ. Sci. Technol. 32, 1559–1565.

Russo, J., Rivera, R., Russo, I.H., 1992. Influence of age and parity on the development of the human breast. Breast Cancer Res. Treat. 23, 211–218.

Russo, J., Hu, Y.F., Yang, X., et al., 2000. Developmental, cellular, and molecular basis of human breast cancer. J. Natl. Cancer Inst. Monogr. 27, 17–37.

Safe, S.H., 2000. Endocrine disruptors and human health--is there a problem? An update. Environ. Health Perspect. 108, 487–493.

Schernhammer, E.S., Laden, F., Speizer, F.E., et al., 2001. Rotating night shifts and risk of breast cancer in women participating in the nurses' health study. J. Natl. Cancer Inst. 93, 1563–1568.

Schreurs, R.H., Sonneveld, E., Jansen, J.H., et al., 2005. Interaction of polycyclic musks and uv filters with the estrogen receptor (er), androgen receptor (ar), and progesterone receptor (pr) in reporter gene bioassays. Toxicol. Sci. 83, 264–272.

Sengupta, P., Dutta, S., Krajewska-Kulak, E., 2016. The disappearing sperms: analysis of reports published between 1980 and 2015. Am. J. Mens. Health. 11 (4), 1279–1304.

Sharma, R., Harlev, A., Agarwal, A., et al., 2016. Cigarette smoking and semen quality: a new meta-analysis examining the effect of the 2010 world health organization laboratory methods for the examination of human semen. Eur. Urol. 70, 635–645.

Sharpe, R.M., 2010. Is it time to end concerns over the estrogenic effects of bisphenol a? Toxicol. Sci. 114, 1–4.

Sharpe, R.M., Drake, A.J., 2010. Bisphenol a and metabolic syndrome. Endocrinology. 151, 2404–2407.

Sharpe, R.M., Skakkebaek, N.E., 1993. Are oestrogens involved in falling sperm counts and disorders of the male reproductive tract? Lancet. 341, 1392–1395.

Silinskas, K.C., Okey, A.B., 1975. Protection by 1,1,1-trichloro-2,2-bis (p-chlorophenyl)ethane (ddt) against mammary tumors and leukemia during prolonged feeding of 7,12-dimethylbenz(a)anthracene to female rats. J. Natl. Cancer Inst. 55, 653–657.

Skakkebaek, N.E., Rajpert-De Meyts, E., Main, K.M., 2001. Testicular dysgenesis syndrome: an increasingly common developmental disorder with environmental aspects. Hum. Reprod. 16, 972–978.

Song, K.H., Lee, K., Choi, H.S., 2002. Endocrine disrupter bisphenol a induces orphan nuclear receptor nur77 gene expression and steroidogenesis in mouse testicular leydig cells. Endocrinology. 143, 2208–2215.

Sonnenschein, C., Soto, A.M., 1998. An updated review of environmental estrogen and androgen mimics and antagonists. J. Steroid Biochem. Mol. Biol. 65, 143–150.

Titus-Ernstoff, L., Hatch, E.E., Hoover, R.N., et al., 2001. Long-term cancer risk in women given diethylstilbestrol (des) during pregnancy. Br. J. Cancer. 84, 126–133.

Tora, L., White, J., Brou, C., et al., 1989. The human estrogen receptor has two independent nonacidic transcriptional activation functions. Cell. 59, 477–487.

Tzukerman, M.T., Esty, A., Santiso-Mere, D., et al., 1994. Human estrogen receptor transactivational capacity is determined by both cellular and promoter context and mediated by two functionally distinct intramolecular regions. Mol. Endocrinol. 8, 21–30.

Venkitaraman, A.R., 2002. Cancer susceptibility and the functions of brca1 and brca2. Cell. 108, 171–182.

Wolff, M.S., Toniolo, P.G., Lee, E.W., et al., 1993. Blood levels of organochlorine residues and risk of breast cancer. J. Natl. Cancer Inst. 85, 648–652.

Yoon, K., Pellaroni, L., Ramamoorthy, K., et al., 2000. Ligand structure-dependent differences in activation of estrogen receptor alpha in human hepg2 liver and u2 osteogenic cancer cell lines. Mol. Cell. Endocrinol. 162, 211–220.

Yoon, K., Pallaroni, L., Stoner, M., et al., 2001. Differential activation of wild-type and variant forms of estrogen receptor alpha by synthetic and natural estrogenic compounds using a promoter containing three estrogen-responsive elements. J. Steroid Biochem. Mol. Biol. 78, 25–32.

Younglai, E.V., Collins, J.A., Foster, W.G., 1998. Canadian semen quality: an analysis of sperm density among eleven academic fertility centers. Fertil. Steril. 70, 76–80.

Chapter 60

Phytoestrogens

Michelle Mostrom and Tim J. Evans

INTRODUCTION

Phytoestrogens are nonsteroidal, natural plant compounds that are structurally or functionally similar to mammalian estrogens, particularly 17β-estradiol (Fig. 60.1). Typically, phytoestrogens or their active metabolites exert their estrogenic effect on the central nervous system and on the reproductive system of males and females, inducing estrus and stimulating growth of the genital tract and mammary glands in females. The classic test for estrogenicity of compounds is proliferation of the female reproductive tract. Phytoestrogens may bind to estrogen receptors, mimicking the conformational structure of estradiol (Kuiper et al., 1997, 1998), and act as agonists, partial agonists, or antagonists inducing estrogen-responsive gene products and may exert metabolic effects not related to estrogen receptors. Phytoestrogens are considered endocrine disruptors because these chemicals may interfere with the body's endocrine system and produce adverse developmental, reproductive, and neurological effects in both humans and animals. A large volume of literature has been published on phytoestrogens with regard to their beneficial effects in humans related to reducing atherosclerosis, osteoporosis, angiogenesis, diabetes, and vasomotor effects (hot flushes) at menopause and acting as antioxidants, antineoplastics, anti-inflammatories, and probiotics. Fewer publications discuss adverse effects of phytoestrogens causing infertility in livestock and possible impaired reproductive processes in humans. This chapter focuses on the most extensively studied phytoestrogens found in legumes and beans, such as the isoflavones and coumestans, which may affect reproduction.

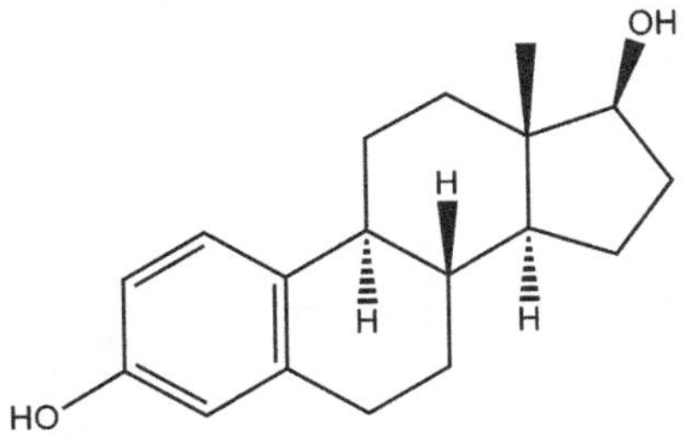

17BETA-ESTRADIOL

(8*R*,9*S*,13*S*,14*S*,17*S*)-13-methyl-7,8,9,11,12,13,14,15,16,17-decahydro-6*H*-cyclopenta[*a*]phenanthrene-3,17-diol

FIGURE 60.1 Chemical structure of the estrogen found in animals or 17β-estradiol.

Description

Phytoestrogens are polyphenolic compounds that can be divided into several broad categories (Table 60.1). Many phytoestrogens are grouped into flavonoids and isoflavonoids, including the isoflavone compounds found in soybeans (*Glycine max* L.), red clover (*Trifolium pretense* L.), and white clover (*Trifolium repens* L.). These compounds include daidzein, genistein, formononetin, biochanin A, and glycitein. The normal isoflavone concentration in red clover is between 0.5 and 2.5% of dry matter, which can be 2–10 times greater than the isoflavone concentration found in soybeans. Hops and beer may contain a very potent phytoestrogen, the flavanone 8-prenylnaringenin. β-Sitosterol is one of several plant sterols widely distributed in the plant kingdom, with a chemical structure similar to that of cholesterol. It is found in corn, soybeans, sugar beets, avocados, pistachios, pecans, almonds, and saw palmetto. Coumestrol is a potent estrogenic phytoestrogen in the coumestan group. Coumestrol may be found in alfalfa (*Medicago sativa* L.), white clover, spinach, and soybean sprouts. The stilbenes, such as *trans*-resveratrol, are found in red wine (grape skin) and peanuts. Lignans are compounds found in plant cell walls and fiber-rich foods, seeds (flax and sesame seeds), berries, cereals, nuts, and fruits. Typically, a mixture of phytoestrogens can be found in plants and processed food. An excellent database for foods and flavanoid contents can be found online at the U.S. Department of Agriculture (www.ars.usda.gov). In addition to phytoestrogen exposure through plant products, the environmental distribution of phytoestrogens in streams in the United States has been evaluated (Kolpin et al., 2010). Phytoestrogens (particularly

Veterinary Toxicology. DOI: http://dx.doi.org/10.1016/B978-0-12-811410-0.00060-X

TABLE 60.1 Categories of Phytoestrogens and Selected Compounds

Category	Phytoestrogen Examples	Dietary Sources	Basic Chemical Structure
Isoflavones	Daidzein Genistein Fomononetin Biochanin A Glycitein	Clovers (red and white) Soybeans Beans Split peas	ISOFLAVONE
Flavanones	Naringenin	Hops (8-prenylnaringenin) Apples, red onions	FLAVANONE
Flavonoids	Apigenin Leteolin	Parsley Capsicum pepper Alfalfa	FLAVONE
	Quercetin Kaempferol	Tomatoes Broccoli Apples Onions	FLAVONOL
Plant sterols	B-sitosterol	Corn Soybeans Sugar beet forage Saw palmetto (*Serenoa repens*) Avocados Pistachios and almonds Wood	BETA-SITOSTEROL
Coumestans	Coumestrol	Legumes (alfalfa, clover) Spinach Split peas, lima beans Soybean sprouts	COUMESTROL
Stilbenes	*Trans*-resveratrol (*trans*-3,5,4′ trihydroxystilbene)	Grape skin (red wine) Peanuts	RESVERATROL
Lignans	Secoisolariciresinol, matairesinol	Flaxseed (linseed) Squash, pumpkin seeds Tea (black and green) Sunflower seeds Strawberries Cranberries Brans	SECOISOLARICIRESINOL

Adapted from Patisaul and Jefferson (2010).

formononetin) were commonly detected in several rivers and streams throughout Iowa, but the concentrations were generally less than 50 ng/L and not considered to contribute to an estrogenic effect, although the impact of long-term, low-level exposures of contaminants in streams is unknown.

This chapter does not include the estrogenic *Fusarium* spp. mycotoxins, zearalenone, zearalanols, and zearalenols, which are resorcyclic acid lactones produced as secondary fungal metabolites in plants and grasses. Additional information on phytoestrogens can be found elsewhere with regard to mechanistic effects (Rosselli et al., 2000; Bhavnani et al., 2008), physiology (Kurzer and Xu, 1997; Tham et al., 1998; Benassayag et al., 2002; Patisaul and Jefferson, 2010; Pilšáková et al., 2010), and reproductive functions (Whitten and Patisaul, 2001; Dusza et al., 2006; Cederroth et al., 2009; Baber, 2010).

HISTORICAL BACKGROUND

More than 55 years ago in Australia, a syndrome of temporary or permanent infertility occurred in female sheep grazing subterranean clover (*Trifolium subterraneneum* L.) containing high concentrations of isoflavone phytoestrogens, particularly formononetin (Adams, 1995). Temporary infertility was related to direct effects of phytoestrogen on the ovarian follicle decreasing ovulation and increasing embryo mortality and was associated with abnormalities of ovum transport and uterine function. Prolonged exposure to growing, green subterranean clover caused permanent infertility in ewes that was associated with morphological changes in the cervix, including thick, fused cervical folds and the appearance of cystic tubular glands. Changes in the uterus included development of cystic uterine glands and mild endometritis. The cervical mucus became watery and lost viscoelasticity, allowing loss of spermatozoa from the cervix and reducing the chances for conception. External genitalia of some ewes underwent masculinization, with fusion of the vulvar lips at the lower commissure and hypertrophy of the clitoris. The permanent changes in cervical structure were analogous to the organizational effects of estrogen reported in mice treated with estrogen neonatally and in women exposed to diethylstilbestrol during fetal development. Unlike sheep, cattle apparently are not permanently affected by phytoestrogens. However, elevated concentrations of phytoestrogens can negatively impact cattle reproduction and induce estrogenic clinical signs. For example, concentrations of coumestrol greater than 25–30 ppm in a ration (on a dry weight basis), or even lower coumestrol concentrations when feedstuffs are fed at high proportions of a ration to dairy cows, can cause ovarian dysfunction, early embryonic death, and repeat breeding in cattle. The potential health benefits and adverse effects of phytoestrogens in humans and animals related to reproduction are described in this chapter.

PHARMACOKINECTICS/TOXICOKINETICS

Plant Impact

The concentration of phytoestrogens in plant material varies widely. In addition to participating in plant defense, these compounds play a role in attraction of pollinators and seed-dispersing organisms. Phytoestrogens are not translocated within the vascular pathways of a plant but are synthesized and degraded in localized areas that vary with the specific tissue. For example, coumestrol concentrations are found in higher concentrations near the top segment of the alfalfa plant canopy compared to the lower part of the plant (Seguin et al., 2004).

A number of factors affect production of phytoestrogens. Plant fungal infections, animal predation, or insect invasions may increase phytoestrogen production. Growing conditions, particularly temperature and rainfall, can dramatically affect phytoestrogen concentrations in legumes. In cool, wet spring and fall conditions, legumes may contain high concentrations of phytoestrogens (isoflavones and coumestrol). Generally, the concentrations of phytoestrogens decrease with successive cuttings of legumes in a season, with coumestrol at higher concentrations in early and late maturity of the alfalfa crop. Seguin and Zheng (2006) reported that coumestrol concentrations in alfalfa were lower in harvests of first-year seeding than in harvests of the postseeding years. The variety of alfalfa cultivar had little impact on coumestrol concentrations. Coumestrol may also be found in alfalfa cubes, extracts, and powders, which can be incorporated into nutraceuticals or livestock and pet feeds.

Fresh herbage tends to have higher concentrations of phytoestrogens than silage or hay (Sivesind and Seguin, 2005). Sivesind and Seguin reported that the red clover cultivar "Start" was consistently lower in detectable isoflavones during multiyear and multisite trials. Lundh (1995) estimated the daily consumption of phytoestrogens by dairy cows on red clover forage to be 50–100 g. Table 60.2 lists typical concentrations of phytoestrogens in legume feeds and soy foods.

In soy foods, boiling, milling, or processing of the commodity does not appear to destroy daidzein or genistein, but roasting soybeans can reduce these isoflavones by 15% (Franke et al., 1995). Three estrogenic isoflavones – daidzein, genistein, and glycitein – were found in soy foods in four chemical forms: aglycone, glucoside, acetylglucoside, and malonylglucoside. Fermentation and processing of soy foods increased the aglycone and glycoside forms of the isoflavone, respectively. Soy processing appears to influence isoflavone bioavailability; the unconjugated isoflavones infermented soy food may be more bioavailable than glucosides. The total isoflavone content of raw soy beans ranges widely from 18 to greater than 500 mg/100 g.

TABLE 60.2 Typical Phytoestrogen Concentrations in Plants used for Livestock Forage and Soy Food

Plant	Phytoestrogen	Concentration (mg/kg or ppm dry weight)
Alfalfa	Coumestrol	25–65[a]
Red clover	Formononetin and biochanin A	3,000–15,000[b]
	Genistein	300–1,500
	Daidzein	<300
White clover	Isoflavonoids	100–600
	Coumestrol	<10
Soy foods	Daidzein and genistein	~1,000–3,500

[a]*Concentrations from 18 to >180 mg/kg coumestrol have been associated with infertility in cattle (Mostrom, 2010).*
[b]*Concentrations >500 to 750 mg/kg have been associated with infertility in cattle (Mostrom, 2010).*
From Saloniemi *et al.* (1995) and Franke *et al.* (1995).

Animal Biotransformation

Similar to any drug or toxin, the dose or intake of phytoestrogens is not equivalent to the dose at the active site or receptor in tissue. Dietary phytoestrogens undergo the processes of absorption in the gastrointestinal tract, biotransformation, distribution, and excretion in urine, bile, feces, and milk. Effects of phytoestrogens may vary with the individual phytoestrogen; species exposed; sex; the route, dose, and duration of exposure; and the timing of exposure during reproductive development and cycling. Most phytoestrogens occur in plants as biologically inactive glycoside conjugates with glucose or carbohydrate moieties. Plant glycosides can be hydrolyzed by plant enzymes, or after consumption the glycosides are hydrolyzed and further demethylated in the acidic gut or rumen by microbes and the heterocyclic phenols (aglycones) are free in the gastrointestinal tract. Gut flora may become adapted over a matter of days to the diet and expand their populations for enhanced metabolism. Microbial metabolism of isoflavones can vary greatly between individuals. Isoflavone absorption and bioavailability in humans can vary with intestinal microbial population, gut transit time, fecal digestion rates, and fiber content in the diet (Neilsen and Williamson, 2007).

Absorption

In ruminants, a majority of the metabolic transformations of phytoestrogens occur in the rumen by microbial action. Complete metabolic pathways have not been defined (Lundh, 1995). Basically, in ruminants, biochanin A is demethylated to genistein and via ring cleavage to *para*-ethyl phenol and organic acids (Fig. 60.2). *Para*-ethyl phenol is considered a non-estrogenic compound. Formononetin is primarily demethylated to daidzein and further

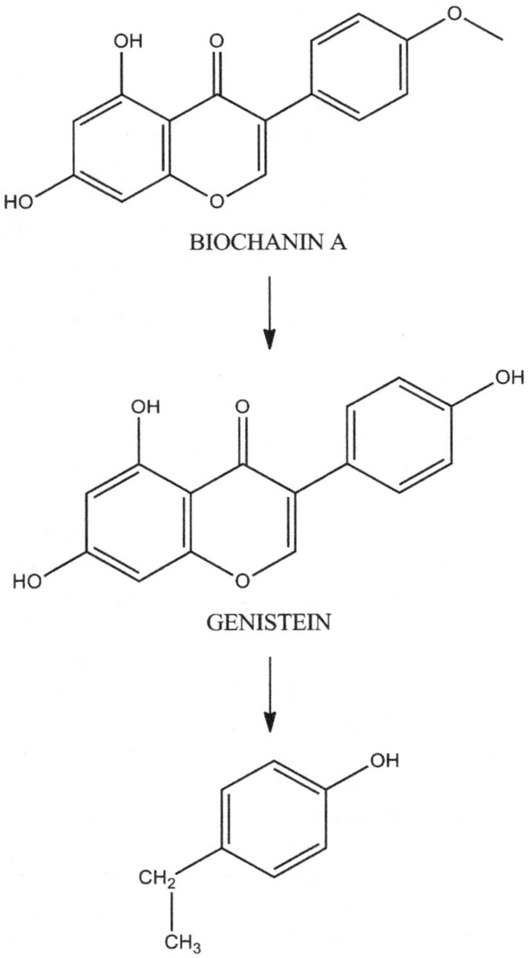

OH O HO O O
BIOCHANIN A

OH O HO O OH
GENISTEIN

OH CH_2 CH_3
P-ETHYL PHENOL

FIGURE 60.2 Schematic of rumen metabolism of biochanin A to genistein (Cox and Davies, 1988).

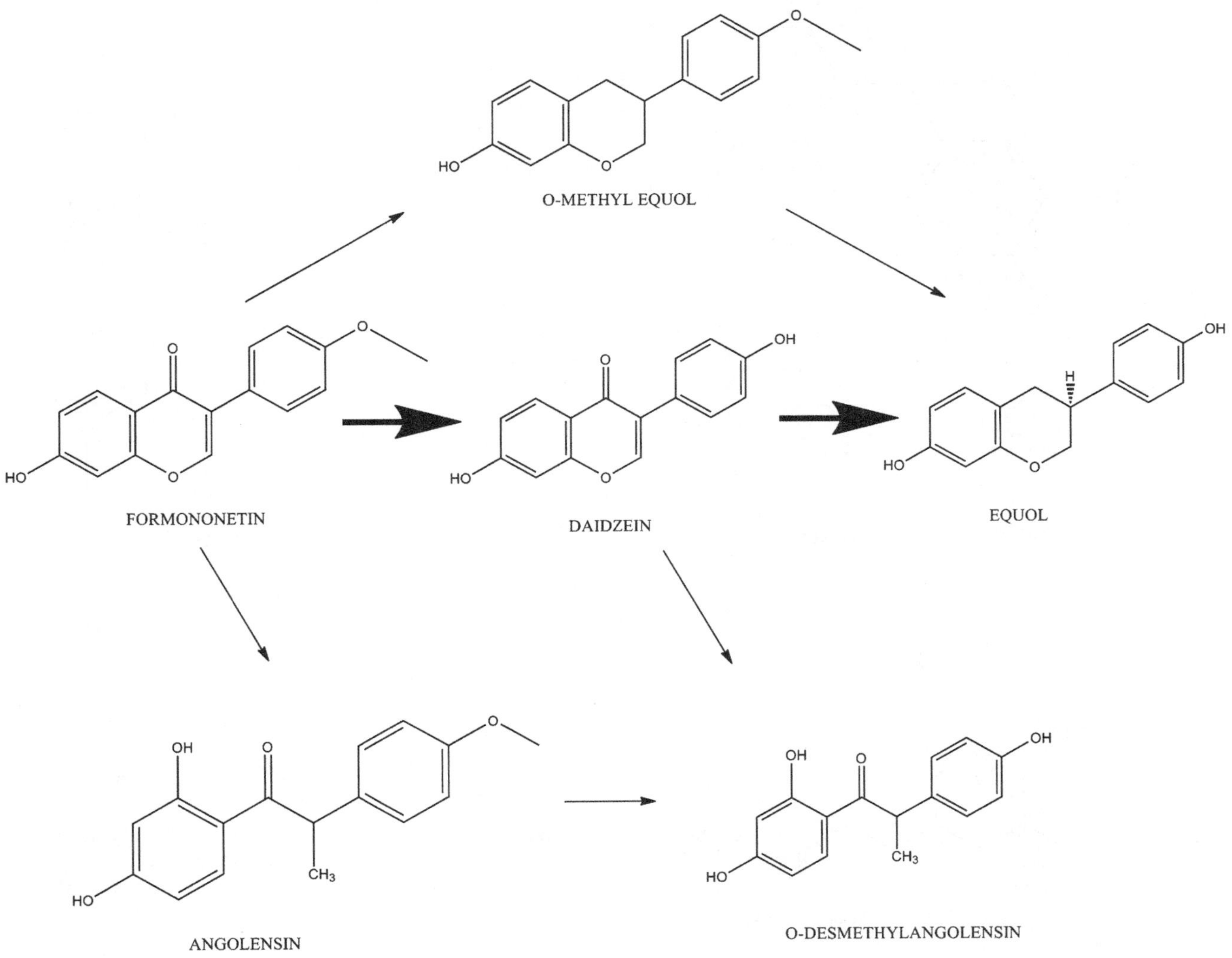

FIGURE 60.3 Metabolic pathway of formononetin via daidzein to equol in the rumen (Cox and Davies, 1988).

metabolized via hydrogenation and ring fission to equol (Fig. 60.3). Equol contains a chiral center and occurs as two distinct diastereoisomers with R-(+)equol and S-(−)equol; intestinal bacteria synthesize exclusively the S-(−)equol enantiomer that has selective affinity for the estrogen receptor-β (Setchell and Clerici, 2010a,b). Formononetin can also undergo reduction to *O*-methyl equol or can be metabolized to *O*-desmethylangolensin. In ruminants, daily consumption of phytoestrogens in the diet can lead to adaption and a larger population of rumen microbes capable of phytoestrogen metabolism. Therefore, estrogenic activity of biochanin A and genistein in ruminants is generally limited to a few initial days of exposure when the unadapted rumen microbes have slower metabolism to non-estrogenic metabolites *para*-ethylphenol and phenolic acid. With the ingestion of formononetin and daidzein, metabolism may lead to compounds with less or greater estrogenic activity (i.e., equol).

Enterodiol and enterolactone are the active, estrogenic mammalian lignans formed by microbes in the intestinal tract from plant lignans matairesinol and secoisolariciresinol and their glycosides (Wang, 2002) (Fig. 60.4).

Only the unconjugated forms (aglycones) and active metabolites appear to exert estrogen-like activity in animals. Most hydrolyzed phytoestrogens are conjugated by glucuronic acid (a minor fraction is conjugated with sulfate) in the gut epithelium, which is a major mechanism for detoxification of phytoestrogens. A small portion of the free, hydrolyzed compounds are absorbed through the gut or rumen mucosa and reach the blood circulation unconjugated. Absorption of phytoestrogens is fairly rapid. In cattle, formononetin and daidzein (free and conjugated) reached a maximum level in plasma within 1 h after feeding (Lundh, 1995). The unconjugated phytoestrogens reaching the circulation are conjugated by liver (hepatic UDP-glucuronosyltransferases and sulfotransferases) and

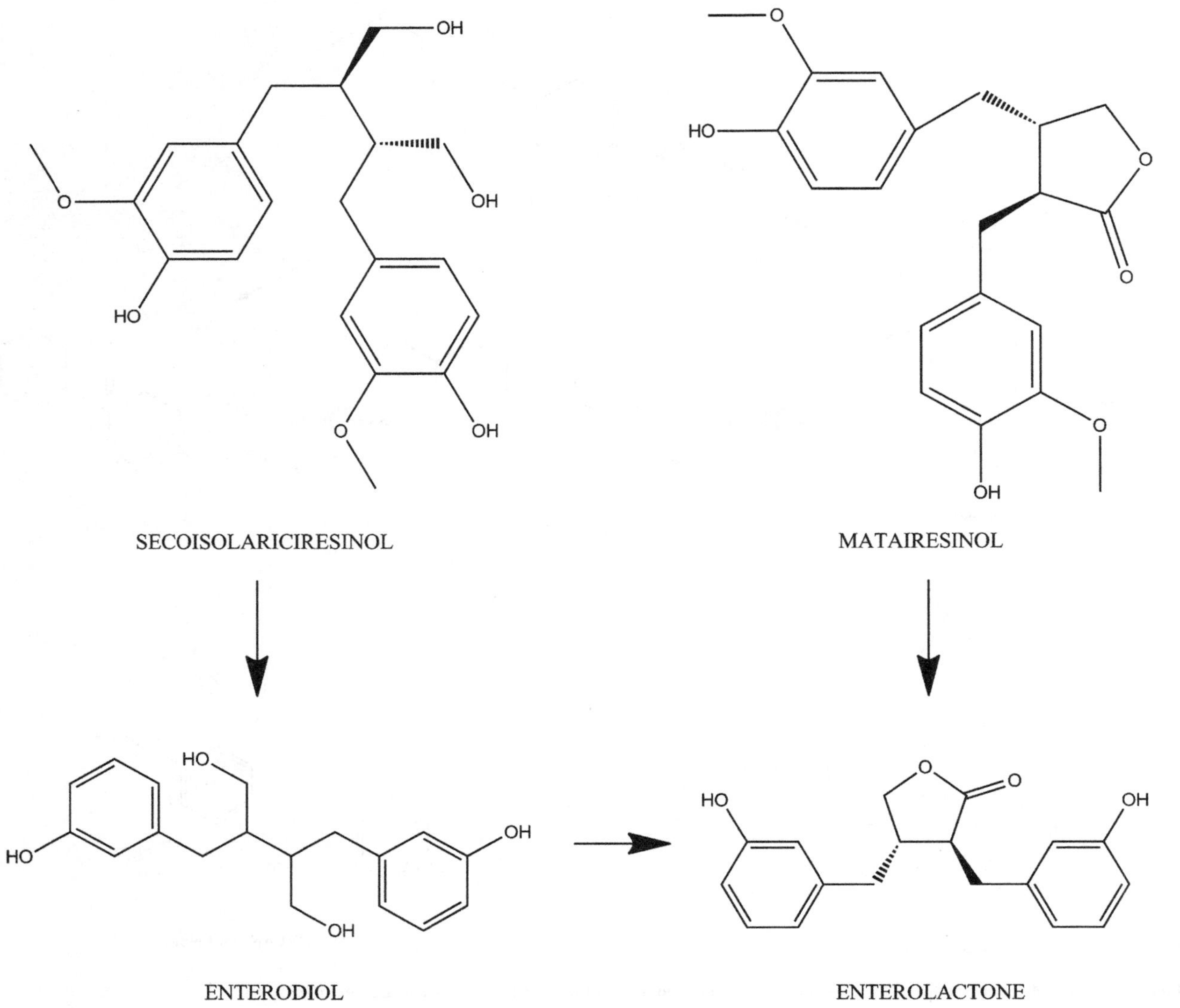

SECOISOLARICIRESINOL

MATAIRESINOL

ENTERODIOL

ENTEROLACTONE

FIGURE 60.4 Schematic diagram of metabolism of plant lignans.

other tissues, including kidney. Glucuronide conjugated compounds and free phytoestrogens circulate throughout the body. Mammalian lignans and isoflavones can be detected in serum, bile, and urine following phytoestrogen consumption. Like endogenous estrogens, these conjugated phytoestrogens undergo enterohepatic circulation. The metabolism of coumestrol has not been characterized.

Conjugated equol in the plasma of cattle or sheep is approximately 95–99% of total equol, whereas in pigs approximately 50–70% of total equol is conjugated (Lundh, 1995). The estrogenic effects are related to free compounds and active metabolites, such as equol, which is suggested to have 0.061% of the potency compared to 17β-estradiol (Markiewicz et al., 1993). Equol was considered the primary chemical responsible for infertility in sheep consuming isoflavones in subterranean clover. Ingestion of high concentrations of red clover silage by ruminants can lead to extremely high concentrations of unconjugated equol in plasma and potency 100 times higher than the 17β-estradiol activity during estrus. Following consumption of mixed red clover–grass silage, the concentration of free equol was approximately 10 times greater in bovine plasma compared with ovine plasma, suggesting that the difference in isoflavone sensitivity between cattle and sheep was not caused by differences in metabolism or detoxification of formononetin and daidzein (Lundh et al., 1990).

Tissue Distribution

Data are limited on the tissue distribution of phytoestrogens. Following an intravenous injection of daidzein in rats (40 mg/kg body weight), daidzein was detected at high concentrations in plasma, liver, lung, and kidney and at lower concentrations in spleen, heart, and skeletal muscle (Yueh and Chu, 1977). Tissue distribution of isoflavones was determined in two lactating ewes after being fed red clover silage for 1 month (Urpi-Sarda et al., 2008). The fermented silage contained only aglycones and provided a daily intake of approximately 157 mg/kg body weight of isoflavones, with an average of 82 mg/kg body weight formononetin, 65 mg/kg body weight biochanin A, 7 mg/kg body weight genistein, and 3 mg/kg body weight daidzein. The major compounds recovered in tissues were equol, generally in the largest concentration, and daidzein as glucuronides. The highest concentrations of equol and daidzein were found in kidney – 10-fold higher than in other tissues – and in decreasing order of concentrations in tissues liver, plasma, aorta, suprarenal glands, uterus, thyroid, and mammary gland. Lower isoflavone concentrations were detected in lung, pituitary gland, thymus, heart, muscle, olfactory lobe of brain, cerebellum, and cerebral hemisphere. The penetration into the brain was very limited. Interestingly, isoflavones were found in the thyroid. Red clover silage ingestion has been documented to stimulate thyroid hormone secretion (total and free triiodothyronine) and increase thyroid follicle size and the ERα immune reactivity of thyroid glands in ovariectomized ewes (Madej et al., 2002). The two major isoflavones found in red clover, formononetin and biochanin A, were not recovered in tissues, which is consistent with extensive rumen metabolism of methylated isoflavones.

Excretion

Conjugated and free metabolites are excreted in urine. A variable amount of phytoestrogens are excreted into bile and feces; for example, a greater fraction of genistein compared with daidzein is eliminated in bile and feces in rats (reviewed by Manach et al., 2005). Phytoestrogens are also excreted into milk, with animal diet playing a major role in detectable concentrations.

Data indicate that animal feeds, such as soy meals, clovers, and grass/alfalfa feedstuffs, may influence milk phytoestrogen content. In a dairy cow ration of mixed red clover–grass silage, formononetin (0.3–0.5%) and biochanin A (0.2%) were the predominant isoflavones. Dairy cows fed a mixed red clover silage produced milk with high concentrations of equol (272 and 364 μg/L or parts per billion (ppb)) and enterolactone (21 and 27 μg/L), metabolites of formononetin and the plant lignans (secoisolariciresinol and matairesinol), respectively (Steinshamn et al., 2008). Higher equol concentrations were determined in milk from cows fed red clover silage compared with those fed white clover silage. Skimmed milk originating from organically managed Finnish dairy operations contained higher concentrations of isoflavonoids, with equol concentrations of 411 ± 65 μg/L, compared to that from conventionally managed dairy operations (Hoikkala et al., 2007). The presence of equol and enterolactone at elevated concentrations in dairy milk, from 14.1 to 293 μg/L and 14.3 to 94 μg/L, respectively, could be considered a health concern in children (Antignac et al., 2004). Trace concentrations of methoxylated formononetin and biochanin A and hydroxylated daidzein and genistein (0.1–5.0 μg/L) were detected in bovine milk. Antignac et al. found that phytoestrogen concentrations in skimmed and full cream milk were similar, indicating that phytoestrogens are not very lipophilic compounds. For comparison purposes, the total isoflavone content of soy milk has been reported to be 6–10 mg aglucone equivalents/100 g wet weight (Chan et al., 2009).

MECHANISM OF ACTION

Reproduction is under hormonal regulation. Abnormalities in the dynamics of hormone production, metabolism, target molecule binding, and elimination can lead to alterations in the structure and/or function of the reproductive system. Estrogens influence cell growth and differentiation of both female and male reproductive tissue. They regulate the ovaries and testes, uterus, vagina, mammary glands, epididymis, and prostate gland. Phytoestrogens have been reported to affect physiological responses related to reproduction through numerous mechanisms (Table 60.3). Phytoestrogens are considered weak estrogens, with an activity on the order of 10^{-2} to 10^{-3} of 17β-estradiol, but may be present in the body at concentrations 100-fold higher than those of endogenous estrogens (Adlercreutz and Mazur, 1997). A number of phytoestrogens have been shown to stimulate uterine growth in laboratory and farm animals. However, not all mouse strains were susceptible to isoflavone-induced uterine hypertrophy. The Swiss albino CD-1 mouse and ICR mouse showed no or only a slight response to phytoestrogens, respectively, which may be related to metabolism (reviewed by Kurzer and Xu, 1997). In addition, the isoflavone genistein has been demonstrated to inhibit important pathways for cellular growth and proliferation in multiple tissues.

Estrogen Receptors

Estrogens play an important role in physiological functions via a genomic mechanism. Phytoestrogens can mediate their effects by diffusing through the cell membrane and binding to specific estrogen receptors (ERs) in the target cell. After binding, the phytoestrogens do not act like typical estrogen agonists but, rather, more like selective estrogen receptor modulators (SERMS) that have differential actions as agonists or antagonists in

TABLE 60.3 Several Proposed Mechanisms of Phytoestrogen Actions on Reproduction and Development

Genomic effects through binding to estrogen receptors α and β causing endocrine disruption
Non-genomic effects through binding to steroid membrane receptors
Affects metabolism through inhibition of enzymes in steroidogenesis (3βand 17β-hydroxysteroid dehydrogenase, aromatase, 5α-reductase, 17β-hydroxysteroid oxidoreductase type 1)
Stimulation of sex hormone-binding globulin (SHBG)
Inhibition of protein tyrosine kinase involved with signal transduction and cell proliferation
Inhibition of DNA topoisomerases I and II required for DNA replication
Inhibits matrix metalloproteinase 9 (MMP9) involved in cell growth
Down-regulates expression of vascular endothelial growth factor (VEGF) involved with growth factorgenes and angiogenesis
Inhibits prostaglandin synthesis via lipoxygenase or cyclooxygenase-2 and exert antioxidant activity

different tissue potentially causing endocrine disruption. The differential action occurs partly from ER ligand conformational changes and the influence of coregulator proteins (reviewed by Patisaul and Jefferson, 2010). Following phytoestrogen−receptor complex conformation changes, the complex translocates to the nucleus. Within the nucleus, the complex binds to selective regions of the DNA, the estrogen response element (ERE), and stimulates or inhibits specific genes that may result in the production of messenger RNA and subsequently new specific proteins. Numerous studies have focused on the direct effects of phytoestrogen receptor binding *in vitro*. Binding affinities to the ERs, whose subtypes are ERα and ERβ, vary greatly with phytoestrogens and the various cell lines used in studies and chosen endpoints of estrogenic potency (Kuiper et al., 1997, 1998). Compared to any phytoestrogen tested, the most potent activator of binding to ERs was the endogenous hormone 17β-estradiol. Daidzein, genistein, coumestrol, equol, and *O*-desmethylangolensin apparently bind to ERs from sheep uterine cytosol, suggesting estrogenic effects. Formononetin at physiological concentrations did not bind to the ER but could be metabolized to daidzein and eventually to equol, both of which have estrogenic properties (Kuiper et al., 1998). Daidzein preferentially activated binding of ERβ, but with metabolism of daidzein to equol, both ERβ and ERα can be activated (Kostelac et al., 2003). Phytoestrogens appear to have a predilection for greater affinity to ERβ. Studies have shown that coumestrol has a 2-fold higher affinity for ERβ than for ERα, and genistein has a pronounced affinity (30-fold) for ERβ (Kuiper et al., 1997).

Although coumestrol may bind to both ERα and ERβ, it is an atypical estrogen because it does not stimulate uterine cellular hyperplasia. Coumestrol significantly increased uterine wet and dry weights in ovariectomized rats, but it did not stimulate cytosolic ER depletion or nuclear ER accumulation (Markaverich et al., 1995). These findings suggest that the estrogenic effects of coumestrol may be mediated by increased sensitivity of the tissue to endogenous estradiol. An antiestrogenic effect of phytoestrogens has been proposed when high concentrations of phytoestrogens compete with endogenous estrogens and bind the ER, which blocks endogenous estrogen actions and reduces cellular growth (Rosselli et al., 2000).

Differential expression of ERs has been reported in tissues, and several physiological roles have been associated with the ER subtypes (Table 60.4). Both subtypes have been found in blood vessels and in breast, uterus, and ovaries of women, but the proportions of α and β subtypes appear to vary with estrogen target tissues, physiological and pathological status, and age of the individual. Each of these ERs may influence the function of the other, creating a complex process of estrogenic effects in tissues in which both subtypes are co-expressed (Benassayag et al., 2002). The resulting changes in physiological functions can be difficult to interpret.

Estradiol can bind with high affinity to plasma membrane forms of steroid receptors and may mediate nongenomic actions with a variety of short-term estrogen effects (Pietras and Szego, 1975; Swego, 1984). Estradiol has been shown to induce rapid changes in intracellular calcium concentrations/flux, potassium conductance, and cyclic AMP levels (reviewed by Rosselli et al., 2000). The direct effects of phytoestrogens and membrane ERs have not been fully defined. Resveratrol, a stilbene phytoestrogen found in red wine, apparently binds to and increases the transcriptional activity of ERα and ERβ. Klinge and co-workers (2005) reported that resveratrol, at nanomolar concentrations achieved by reasonable red wine consumption, can activate membrane-initiated (nongenomic) ER signaling in endothelial cells that activate mitogen-activated protein kinases (MAPKs) involved in signaling pathways and endothelial nitric oxide synthase. Resveratrol increased nitric oxide levels in human umbilical vein endothelial cells after short-term exposure, suggesting a potential cardioprotective effect.

Impact on Steroidogenesis

Certain phytoestrogens may alter key steroidal enzymes in tissues, although most studies have used in vitro cell

TABLE 60.4 Estrogen Receptor α and β Proposed Actions and Distribution[a]

ERα and ERβ function in:	Normal ovarian follicular development
	Vascular endothelial cells
	Myocardial cells
	Smooth muscle cells
	Breast cells
ERα associated with:	Bone maturation in males and females
	Important role maintaining follicle-stimulating hormone and luteinizing hormone in blood
	More predominant in kidney, adrenal, nonpregnant human myometrium
ERβ associated with:	Bone maintenance
	Frontal lobe-mediated memory and learning
	Coumestrol and genistein bind with higher estrogenic potential
	Equol has modest affinity for binding
	More predominant in human brain, thymus, bladder, ovarian granulosa cells, testis Sertoli and germ cells, lung, bone, and pregnant term human myometrium

[a]*Distribution of estrogen receptors in tissues can change over a life span and is sexually dimorphic.*
Based on Kuiper et al. (1997, 1998) and Patisaul and Jefferson (2010).

lines or purified microsomal or enzyme preparation (Lacey et al., 2005). Phytoestrogens may interfere with the synthesis or metabolism of steroid hormones, such as cytochrome P450arom (aromatase), an enzyme that can catalyze the conversion of testosterone to 17β-estradiol and Δ4-androstenedial to estrone. The enzyme aromatase has a critical role in the ovary (in premenopausal women) and peripheral tissues, which are sites for estradiol synthesis in postmenopausal women and men. Using an *in vitro* assay with human breast cancer MCF-7 cells, Almstrup and co-workers (2002) reported that phytoestrogens, but not genistein, were aromatase inhibitors at low concentrations ($<1\ \mu M$) but at higher concentrations ($>1\ \mu M$) were estrogenic. The aromatase inhibition at low doses of phytoestrogens may provide antiestrogenic properties that play a role in protection against breast cancer.

Phytoestrogens may decrease endogenous estrogen concentrations through effects on the sex (or serum) hormone-binding globulin (SHBG). This binding protein has specific affinity for estrogens and androgens. Minor changes in the amount or availability of SHBG, caused by phytoestrogens, may change the free fraction of endogenous hormones in circulation either locally or systemically. The phytoestrogen enterolactone ($1-10\ \mu M$) stimulated SHBG in vitro with HepG2 cells (Adlercreutz et al., 1992). Equol, genistein, daidzein, enterolactone, and enterodiol appear to exert a dose-dependent inhibitory effect on binding of steroids to SHBG, displacing 17β-estradiol or testosterone (Benassayag et al., 2002). Additional mechanisms of action may affect steroid hormones. Coumestrol and, to a lesser degree, genistein have been shown to inhibit the enzyme 17β-hydroxysteroid oxidoreductase type 1, which converts [^{3}H]-estrone to [^{3}H]-estradiol in a dose-dependent manner (Mäkelä et al., 1995). *In vitro* studies have reported that phytoestrogens inhibit 17β-hydroxysteroid dehydrogenase, converting androstenedione to testosterone, and 5α-reductase, converting testosterone to the more potent dihydrotestosterone (reviewed by Whitten and Patisaul, 2001). Biochanin A displayed dose-dependent inhibition of 3β-hydroxysteroid dehydrogenase, an enzyme that catalyzes the conversion of pregnenolone to progesterone and androstenediol to testosterone, in primary cultures of human granulosa luteal cells (Lacey et al., 2005).

Additional Impact on Cell Functions

Angiogenesis is essential for ovarian follicle development and for tumor growth, invasion, and metastasis. Several studies have reported that phytoestrogens inhibited vascular endothelial growth factor (VEGF)-induced endothelial cell functions and signaling pathways. The flavonoid quercetin at 5 and 50 μg/mL (concentrations higher than physiological range) inhibited VEGF production by porcine granulosa cells *in vitro* (Santini et al., 2009). Santini et al. determined that quercetin inhibited steroidogenesis, specifically progesterone production, but not granulosa cell growth.

Genistein has been reported to inhibit ethoxyresorufin-*O*-deethylase (EROD) activity, part of the enzyme cytochrome P450 family (CYP1A) that is critical in the metabolism of 17β-estradiol to hydroxylated estrogen, in mammalian cell culture lines (Shon et al., 2006). In addition, the activity of ornithine decarboxylase, a critical enzyme in polyamine biosynthesis and normal cell growth and proliferation, was markedly reduced after genistein treatment of MCF-7 breast cancer cells, suggesting that genistein might be of therapeutic value in preventing human breast cancer.

Altered Signal Transduction and Cell Proliferation

Genistein may alter cell growth at several signal transduction pathways, inhibiting protein tyrosine kinase activity and down-regulating epidermal growth factor receptor autophosphorylation, which phosphorylates tyrosyl residues of membrane-bound receptors (Akiyama et al., 1987), and MAPK activity and mitogen proliferation in human aortic smooth muscle cells (Dubey et al., 1999). Inhibition of protein tyrosine kinases and MAPK by isoflavones may play a role in improving heart function. Genistein can inhibit DNA replication enzymes associated with cancer growth, including DNA topoisomerases I and II (required for DNA replication) and matrix metalloproteinase 9 (a matrix enzyme that can degrade a number of structural components) (Kurzer and Xu, 1997). Although inhibition of these pathways may lead to inhibited cell growth and a protective effect, a number of phytoestrogens, including coumestrol, genistein, biochanin A, daidzein, and enterolactone, can stimulate cellular proliferation of the estrogen-dependent MCF-7 human breast cancer cells at concentrations less than 1–10 μM (reviewed by Kurzer and Xu, 1997). The influence of genistein on cells in vitro appears to be biphasic in nature, inducing cell growth of MCF-7 cells at low concentrations and inhibiting cell growth at higher concentrations (reviewed by Rosselli et al., 2000). Genistein, which shows a high affinity to ER, has been shown to inhibit growth in both ER-positive and ER-negative cell lines in vitro.

The antioxidant activity of phytoestrogens has been reported both in vitro and in vivo. Isoflavones inhibit lipoxygenase action and prevent sheep erythrocyte hemolysis in vitro and inhibit production of hydrogen peroxide in HL60 cells (reviewed by Benassayag et al., 2002). Inhibition of lipoxygenase and possibly cyclooxygenase may modulate production of prostaglandins and leukotrienes involved in inflammation, carcinogenesis, and reproduction.

ADVERSE HEALTH EFFECTS

Developmental Effects

The effects of preand neonatal exposure to phytoestrogens on development in laboratory animals have been studied, with variable effects observed. Preand neonatal treatment of rodents with phytoestrogens has resulted in altered prepubertal or adult morphology and possible function of the uterus, vagina, ovary, breast, pituitary, and hypothalamus (reviewed by Whitten and Patisaul, 2001). *In utero* exposure to several estrogens, including genistein, down-regulated the expression of several testicular genes in the rat and mouse (reviewed by Phillips and Tanphaichitr, 2008). Both male and female rat offspring from dams treated with high levels of genistein (5000 μg) had shorter anogenital distances at birth, and females in this treatment group had a later onset of vaginal opening or puberty (Levy et al., 1995). High levels of dietary coumestrol (100 mg/kg) fed to weanling female rats on days 21–24 or 22–60 caused earlier vaginal opening and irregular vaginal cycles (Whitten and Naftolin, 1992). Coumestrol treatment of neonatal female rats, given a 100 μM dose, resulted in premature uterine gland development and increased uterine weights on postnatal days 1–5, and at later ages the uterine weights and ER levels were reduced; however, if coumestrol was administered on postnatal days 10–14, the uterine gland growth was inhibited (Benassayag et al., 2002).

Female neonatal rats given a subcutaneous injection of 10 μg of genistein showed an increased pituitary response to gonadotropin-releasing hormone, with higher genistein doses causing a decreased luteinizing hormone secretion on postnatal days 1–10 (Faber and Hughes, 1993). The effects of the higher doses were similar to the typical effects of estrogens in masculinizing the brain and decreasing pituitary response. Oral exposure of female CD-1 mice to genistin, the glycosylated form of genistein found in soy-based infant formulas, treated on postnatal days 1–5 caused estrogenic responses, including altered ovarian differentiation (multi-oocyte follicles), delayed vaginal opening, and, subsequently in the adult mouse, abnormal estrous cycles, decreased fertility, and delayed parturition (Jefferson et al., 2009a). Jefferson et al. noted that the glucoside forms of isoflavones were quickly hydrolyzed to produce the aglycone forms and subsequently absorbed. The glycosylated form can be passively transported across the intestinal membrane and enter circulation by the sodium-dependent glucose transporter, unlike passive diffusion by the aglycone form. Major contributions to infertility in genistein-treated neonatal mice were determined to be (1) delay in fertilization by an undetermined mechanism that could lead to altered developmental timing (lack of development between the twoand four-cell stage), (2) adverse oviductal environment because more than half of the embryos were lost in early embryo development, and (3) the reproductive tract (uterus not responsive to hormonal cues) was not capable of sustaining pregnancy (Jefferson et al., 2009b).

Estrogen receptors are located in numerous areas of the brain, and phytoestrogens can have extensive effects.

The paraventricular nucleus of the hypothalamus (PVN) is a region coordinating reproductive, social, and stress behaviors that primarily expresses ERβ (reviewed by Patisaul and Jefferson, 2010). ERβ is expressed at higher levels than ERα in the basal forebrain, hippocampus, and cerebral cortex (areas important for memory) in the adult. Notably, ERα is primarily expressed in the ventromedial nucleus (VMN) of the brain, which along with the PVN nucleus is important for initiation and regulation of sexual behavior. Patisaul and Jefferson noted that the PVN is the main site for oxytocin production, involved with social behavior and facilitation of sexual behavior. Estrogen binding to ERβ may stimulate oxytocin production from the PVN, which subsequently binds to the oxytocin receptor in the VMN, a nucleus involved in mediating the lordosis response in females. Up-regulation of oxytocin receptors involves binding to ERα.

The central nervous system–gonadal axis and male sexual behavior of the rat appear to be sensitive to phytoestrogens in the rat (Santti et al., 1998). Altering the isoflavone dietary concentrations significantly affected both the sexually dimorphic nucleus of the preoptic area and the anteroventral periventricular nucleus in the brain of rodents (Lephart et al., 2005).

Phytoestrogens may be incorporated as an alternative protein source for aquatic nutrition and have been found in discharged kraft mill effluent and sewage treatment plant effluent, with low concentrations of genistein detected that could impact fish populations. Phytoestrogens may alter sex differentiation in early development, causing a paradoxical sex reversal with increased male phenotypic sex resulting from the administration of an estrogen mimic in the diet. Increased concentrations of genistein, from 0 to 8 mg/g in the diet, fed chronically to sexually undifferentiated channel catfish (*Ictalurus punctatus*) altered gonadal sex differentiation, with increasing proportions of intersex fish and phenotypically male individuals (Green and Kelly, 2009).

Preliminary evidence indicates that soy infant formulas may exert estrogenic activity in the developing human reproductive tract. Phytoestrogens can cross the placenta and are capable of crossing the blood–brain barrier to a limited extent. The human myometrium primarily expresses ERβ in late pregnancy and may be a target for genistein, which preferentially binds to this receptor subtype. A pilot study of female infants fed soy formula, cow milk formula, and breast milk revealed that soy milk-fed infants had re-estrogenization of vaginal cells at 6 months of age (Bernbaum et al., 2008). However, an expert panel report from the National Toxicology Program and the National Institute of Environmental Health Sciences concluded in 2006 that there was insufficient human or experimental animal data to permit determination of the toxicity of soy infant formula on development or reproduction (Rozman et al., 2006).

Hormones and Estrous Cycles

Following adult exposures, phytoestrogens may suppress the adult hypothalamic–pituitary–gonadal axis. Data from studies of ovariectomized rodents and of humans suggest that ingestion of isoflavone-rich soy food may suppress circulating estrogen and progesterone concentrations and can attenuate the preovulatory surge of luteinizing hormone (LH) and follicle-stimulating hormone (FSH) (reviewed by Patisaul and Jefferson, 2010). Several studies have reported on the effects of soy isoflavones in premenopausal women. In a limited study during one menstrual cycle in six premenopausal women given 45 mg of isoflavones daily, the follicular phase length was increased and delayed menstruation (Cassidy et al., 1994). Follicular estradiol concentrations were increased and mid-cycle surges of LH and FSH were significantly suppressed. One case report on three women described adverse effects of abnormal uterine bleeding, leiomyomas, and endometriosis related to high intakes of soy products; all of the women improved after withdrawal of soy from their diet (Chandrareddy et al., 2008). A prospective cohort study of almost 20,000 non-Hispanic white women between 35 and 59 years of age, who were enrolled in the National Institute of Environmental Health Sciences Sister Study, evaluated associations of in utero and early life exposures and selfreporting of physician-diagnosed fibroids (D'Aloisio et al., 2010). Fibroids are benign smooth muscle tumors (uterine leiomyomata) associated with reproductive problems in women. Increased risk for fibroids in early adulthood was associated with being fed soy formula during infancy, having a mother with pre-pregnancy diabetes, being born at least 1 month early, and growing up in lower socioeconomic conditions. The authors suggested that exposure of infants to soy formula within the first 2 months of life is a sensitive time period and can result in infant isoflavone levels more than five times higher than typical levels found in adults consuming soy-based foods.

Infertility

Phytoestrogens have the capability to affect reproduction at many levels, from the hypothalamic–pituitary level to local levels of the ovary and uterus and testis and prostate gland (see Chapter 19, Fig. 19.4). In laboratory animals, intravenous infusion of coumestrol, but not genistein, affected control of LH secretion at both pituitary and hypothalamic levels (McGarvey et al., 2001). At the pituitary level, coumestrol inhibited gonadotropin-releasing hormone–LH release in vivo, and at the hypothalamic level, coumestrol reduced the frequency of the gonadotropin-releasing hormone pulse generator. The inhibitory effects of coumestrol on LH at the pituitary level occurred via an ER-mediated process. Additional evidence that phytoestrogens immediately affect pituitary responsiveness was found in ewes when genistein was administered directly into the central nervous system (Romanowicz et al., 2004). Lower plasma LH concentrations were detected in ovariectomized ewes infused intracerebroventricularly for 6 h with two different levels of genistein at 1 and 10 μg/100 μL/h. In addition, the plasma prolactin concentrations were significantly higher in treated ewes compared with control ewes. Estrogen has been shown to be a potent stimulator of prolactin release in the pituitary lactotropes.

Initial cases of temporary and permanent infertility in animals related to phytoestrogens occurred in sheep ingesting subterranean clover in Australia (Adams, 1995). Red clover, a livestock forage supplement, caused adverse effects in reproductive organs of ovariectomized sheep, with increased teat length (a relatively sensitive parameter), mammary gland development, and milky fluid secretions (galactorrhea) from the teats. Nwannenna and co-workers (1995) described clinical effects of edema and mucous discharge from the vulva, fluid accumulation in the uterus, elongated teats, and the presence of milky fluid in the mammary glands in ovariectomized heifers fed 20 kg of 100% red cl2over silage (daily intake of 35 g phytoestrogens, primarily formononetin and biochanin A) per day for 14 days. The magnitude of the pituitary response to gonadotropinreleasing hormone injections was diminished with lower LH release. The authors noted that the abnormal mounting behavior in one of the heifers was similar to the sexual behavior of cattle treated with estradiol.

Cattle seem to be less sensitive than sheep to clover forage, with temporary estrogenic signs and infertility occurring following ingestion of clover or alfalfa forages, although coumestrol is thought to have a cumulative effect. Concentrations of coumestrol of approximately 25 mg/kg (dry matter) in forage may have adverse effects on reproduction in livestock and reduce fertility (Saloniemi et al., 1995), whereas dietary coumestrol concentrations of 50 mg/kg provided for more than 180 h induced uterine enlargement in rats (Whitten et al., 1992). There is marked variability in the effects of phytoestrogens for different species. High concentrations of daidzein and genistein from soybeans in captive cheetah diets, with an approximate consumption of 50 mg isoflavones/day, may have been a major contributor to the decreased fertility and the veno-occlusive liver disease in the cheetah population (Setchell et al., 1987).

Physiology, particularly the stage of pregnancy or cycling, appears to influence the concentrations of isoflavones (daidzein and genistein) in the plasma of heifers fed 2.5 kg soybeans (Woclawek-Potocka et al., 2008). Pregnancy influenced the kinetics of the isoflavones; plasma concentrations of daidzein and genistein were significantly higher in cycling heifers than in early or late pregnant heifers. In addition, heifers that were 2 months pregnant had higher concentrations of the active metabolite equol compared to heifers that were 8 months pregnant or heifers at the mid-luteal phase of the estrous cycle. Piotrowska and co-workers (2006) found elevated concentrations of equol and *para*-ethylphenol in corpus luteal tissue and plasma of cows fed a soy diet (2.5 kg soybean/animal/day) compared with a standard diet. Metabolites of isoflavone phytoestrogens, such as equol, appear to disturb bovine corpus luteum function in vitro by inhibiting LH (needed for a preovulatory surge) and prostaglandin-stimulated progesterone secretion.

Uterine endometrial release of prostaglandin F2α is under regulation by oxytocin, progesterone (P4) and estradiol (E2) in ruminants and causes luteolysis and regression of the corpus luteum. In cattle and sheep, an increase in oxytocin receptors on endometrial epithelial cells is a primary initiator of luteolysis (Goff, 2004). Oxytocin has a functional role in the regulation of ovarian function in ruminants. Mlynarczuk and co-workers (2011a,b) determined that coumestrol, daidzein, and genistein stimulated the expression of several genes that are responsible for synthesis of the oxytocin precursor, neurophysin-I/OT, and post-translation synthesis of oxytocin, peptidyl-glycine-α-amidating monooxygenase or PGA, in granulosa and luteal cells in cattle. These phytoestrogens stimulated the secretion of oxytocin stored in bovine ovarian follicles and corpora lutea, which in cattle may result in premature luteolysis, the formation of persistent corpus lutea, and impair pregnancy maintenance in the cow.

Higher concentrations of active estrogenic metabolites (i.e., equol) in early pregnancy could lead to increased insemination rates (number of breedings) and decreased number of successful pregnancies in cattle fed soybeans at 2.5 kg/head/day (Woclawek-Potocka et al., 2005a,b). The concentrations of a metabolite of prostaglandin PGF2α or PGFM were significantly higher in the soybean-fed cattle plasma through the first 21 days after ovulation and artificial insemination; the high concentrations of PGFM were correlated with isoflavone metabolites in the plasma. Woclawek-Potocka et al. concluded that the soy-derived phytoestrogens and their metabolites disrupt reproduction and uterine function by modulating the ratio of $PGF_{2\alpha}$ to PGE_2, leading to elevated, nonphysiological production of luteolytic $PGF_{2\alpha}$ by the bovine endometrium during the estrous cycle and early pregnancy in cattle. In ruminants, $PF_{2\alpha}$ is the major luteolytic agent, whereas PGE_2 is considered luteoprotective with anti-luteolytic properties; the ratio of $PGF_{2\alpha}$ to PGE_2 is important for the development and maintenance of the corpus luteum and establishment of pregnancy.

Male Infertility

There are a limited number of reports of adverse effect of phytoestrogens on male reproductive function. In a review on soy and male reproductive function, Cederroth et al. (2009) stated that overall there are some indications that phytoestrogens may alter reproductive hormones, spermatogenesis, sperm capacitation, and fertility; however, there is lack of consistency in human and animal studies examining these effects. Adult male mice fed a soy-rich diet from conception to adulthood exhibited normal male behavior and were fertile but had a 25% reduction in epididymal sperm counts and a 21% reduction in litter size (Cederroth et al., 2010). Irrigated red clover, containing higher estrogenic activity than non-irrigated clover, was fed with non-irrigated red clover in diets to Japanese quail chicks for 2 weeks (Rochester et al., 2009). Both irrigated and non-irrigated red clover reduced chick growth compared with that of control chicks, but irrigated red clover reduced both absolute and relative testes and ovary weights and increased the relative oviduct weighs, suggesting isoflavones affect avian reproductive development. Bilgoraj ganders were fed diets containing high concentrations of phytoestrogens ($\sim 140\,\mu g/g$ of diet) from soy and alfalfa meal during growth, photorefractoriness, and laying periods (reviewed by Dusza et al., 2006). Semen samples analyzed from phytoestrogen-fed ganders had decreased volume of ejaculates and increased number of abnormal spermatozoa, but fertility of eggs and the percentage of normal hatching were not different in males and females fed the control and phytoestrogen diets during the breeding season.

Male goat kids fed a conventional diet supplement with red clover isoflavones (60% biochanin A), at approximately 3 or 4 mg/kg/day for 3 months, exhibited a rise in plasma-free and total triiodothyronine (T_3) followed by a significant increase in plasma testosterone concentrations during puberty compared with those of control goats (Gunnarsson et al., 2009). The increased concentration of T_3 had a direct effect on pubertal Leydig cell steroidogenesis leading to increased testosterone. In an *in vitro* experiment with pubertal rat Leydig cells, Maran and co-workers (2000) reported that T_3 modulated LH-mediated secretion of testosterone and estradiol in a dose-dependent manner. Additional phytoestrogen studies have not found an effect on thyroid hormones.

Phytoestrogens have been evaluated with normal sperm to determine altered cell signaling through inhibition of tyrosine kinase. Protein tyrosine kinase is believed to have a major role in sperm function in humans and other animals through phosphorylation of tyrosine proteins on the spermatozoa and subsequent capacitation, followed by the zona pellucida-induced acrosomal reaction and penetration of zona pellucida-intact oocytes (Pukazhenthi et al., 1998). Utilizing in vitro genistein exposure and cat spermatozoa, no effect was detected in sperm motility, but genistein inhibited the zona pellucida-induced acrosome reaction and reduced sperm penetration into the inner zona pellucida. Menzel and coworkers (2007) reported similar findings in cryopreserved bovine spermatozoa incubated with a range of genistein concentrations, from 0.74 to 7.4 μmol/L. Genistein did not affect tyrosine phosphorylation in cryopreserved spermatozoa, but it inhibited the progesterone and ZP3-6 peptide-induced acrosomal exocytotic event or reaction and decreased sperm–zona pellucida binding, probably by a process independent of protein tyrosine kinase inhibition.

Data from castrated rats treated with 5α-dihydrotestosterone (DHT) and equol showed that equol bound and sequestered DHT from the androgen receptor, resulting in increased plasma concentrations of DHT (Lund et al., 2004). Lund et al. reported that equol administration to intact male rats somewhat blocked the negative feedback effects of DHT on pituitary LH regulation, increasing circulating LH levels and reducing ventral prostate and epididymal weights, acting as an anti-androgen. Tan and co-workers (2006) used seven marmoset monkey twins to evaluate potential adverse effects of feeding human male infants soy milk formula. Male co-twin marmoset monkeys were fed soy milk formula from age 4 or 5 days for approximately 5 or 6 weeks, which resulted in normal body weights, penis length, and fertility. However, the soy-fed monkeys had significantly increased testis weights and Sertoli and Leydig cell numbers per testis. Additional studies are needed on the influence of phytoestrogens on male development and subsequent adult male reproductive and endocrine functions.

RISK ASSESSMENT

Phytoestrogens may result in marked adverse effects on reproduction in livestock. This risk has been recognized for years in livestock, particularly in sheep and cattle production. With regard to sheep grazing subterranean clover in Australia, temporary and permanent fertility are recognized reproductive conditions. The occurrence of adverse reproductive effects from clover or alfalfa forage consumption in livestock cannot be reliably predicted, nor can most of the factors affecting enhanced phytoestrogen concentration be controlled (e.g., weather and insect or fungal invasion). Elevated phytoestrogen concentrations in soybeans and forages can be analyzed in rations. Producers can mitigate most of the adverse effects by diluting or eliminating the forage from the ration.

In subchronic and chronic studies of oral genistein dosing in beagle dogs, the no-observed-adverseeffect level (NOAEL) was considered to be greater than

500 mg/kg/day for the 4-week and 52-week studies (McClain et al., 2005). The primary effects reported were in reproductive organs and included (1) increased uterine weights in female dogs in the 4-week study, (2) atrophy of the testes and prostate gland and absent spermatozoa in the epididymis in males in the 52-week study, and (3) small decreases in ovarian weights in female dogs in the 52-week study. The no-observedeffect level (NOEL) was considered to be 150 mg/ kg/day for the 4-week study and 50 mg/kg/day for the 52-week study. A 4-week recovery period, after the 52-week study at 500 mg/kg/day of genistein, resulted in no observed changes in the dogs. To assess teratogenic and fetal toxic potential of genistein in rats, McClain and co-workers (2007) conducted several in vivo embryo–fetal developmental safety studies using genistein by gavage, with dosages of 0–1000 mg/kg/ day from days 6 to 20 of gestation, and dietary admix, with dosages of 0–500 mg/kg/day from days 5 to 21 of gestation, and an in vitro rat whole embryo culture assay (preliminary screen) using 1–100 μg/mL genistein. In vitro genistein exposure in the embryo culture at 10 μg/mL or greater resulted in anomalies that were not predictive of in vivo findings. A slight maternal toxicity was reported at 1000 mg genistein/kg/day by gavage doses and included decreased maternal body weights and food consumption, with adverse effects in pups reported as increased pup mortality and reduced pup body weights and milk uptake. No external malformations were noted in pups, with minor visceral and skeletal variations observed at the high dose. At the high dietary admix dose of 500 mg/kg/day, maternal body weight and feed consumption were reduced, and the incidence of fetal resorptions increased with a corresponding decrease in the number of live fetuses per dam. Fetal body weights were reduced, but no treatment-related teratogenic effects were detected during external, visceral, and skeletal examinations of fetuses or in body weight normalized anogenital distance. The authors concluded that on the basis of the definitive prenatal developmental safety study (oral dietary admix exposure), the NOAEL for maternal toxicity and adverse effects on embryonic development was 100 mg genistein/kg/day when given orally by dietary admix.

TREATMENT

The focus of phytoestrogens is on both beneficial and adverse effects. Regarding the adverse impact of phytoestrogens on livestock fertility, the current recommendation is to either delete or dilute the estrogenic component of the diet. Typically, problems with fertility (irregular cycling) or mammary gland hypertrophy in cattle or horses are related to using specific cuttings of alfalfa or clover forages. Forages and soybeans can be analyzed for isoflavones and coumestrol concentrations, and nondetectable or low phytoestrogen feeds can be substituted into rations. A washout period of several weeks (4 to 6 or more weeks) will usually result in a return to normal reproductive cycling. The current phytoestrogen data for humans do not substantiate any treatment recommendations for humans.

CONCLUDING REMARKS AND FUTURE DIRECTIONS

Because of the variability in multiple parameters of exposure (dose, timing, and duration of exposure) of numerous phytoestrogens to experimental animals and humans, there are not adequate data to determine the developmental and reproductive toxicity in animals. Laboratory and livestock research should focus on the dose–response relationship of phytoestrogens (particularly isoflavones and coumestrol) on ovarian follicular development, ovarian follicle counts, and ovarian failure. The dose–response relationship for isoflavones and coumestrol in forages and potential for adverse effects of ovarian dysfunction and early embryonic death in livestock, particularly in dairy, need to be determined. Further research on the mechanisms that underlie the impact – detrimental or beneficial – of phytoestrogens on reproductive processes in humans and farm animals is necessary.

REFERENCES

Adams, N.R., 1995. Organizational and activational effects of phytoestrogens on the reproductive tract of the ewe. Proc Soc Exp Biol Med. 208, 87–91.

Adlercreutz, H., Mazur, W., 1997. Phyto-oestrogens and Western diseases. Ann Med. 29, 95–120.

Adlercreutz, H., Mousavi, Y., Clark, J., Höckersted, K., Hämäläinen, E.K., Wähälä, K., et al., 1992. Dietary phytoestrogens and cancer: *in vitro* and *in vivo* studies. J Steroid Biochem Mol Biol. 41, 331–337.

Akiyama, T., Ishida, J., Nakagawa, S., Ogawara, H., Watanabe, S.-I., Itoh, N., et al., 1987. Genistein, a specific inhibitor of tyrosine-specific protein kinases. J Biol Chem. 262, 5592–5595.

Almstrup, K., Fernández, M.F., Petersen, J., Olea, N., Skakkebæk, N.E., Leffers, H., 2002. Dual effects of phytoestrogens result in U-shaped dose–response curves. Environ Health Perspect. 110, 743–748.

Antignac, J.-P., Cariou, R., LeBizec, R., André, F., 2004. New data regarding phytoestrogens content in bovine milk. Food Chem. 87, 275–281.

Baber, R., 2010. Phytoestrogens and post reproductive health. Maturitas. 66, 344–349.

Benassayag, C., Perrot-Applanat, M., Ferre, F., 2002. Phytoestrogens as modulators of steroid action in target cells. J Chromatogr B. 777, 233–248.

Bernbaum, J.C., Umbach, D.M., Ragan, N.B., Ballard, J.L., Archer, J.I., Schmidt-Davis, H., et al., 2008. Pilot studies of estrogenrelated physical findings in infant. Environ Health Perspect. 116, 416–420.

Bhavnani, B.R., Tam, S.-P., Lu, X., 2008. Structure–activity relationships and differential interactions and functional activity of various equine estrogens mediated via estrogen receptors (ERs) ERα and ERβ. Endocrinology. 149, 4857–4870.

Cassidy, A., Bingham, S., Setchell, K.D.R., 1994. Biological effects of a diet of soy protein rich in isoflavones on the menstrual cycle of premenopausal women. Am J Clin Nutr. 60, 333–340.

Cederroth, C., Zimmermann, C., Beny, J.-L., Schaad, O., Combepine, C., Descombes, P., et al., 2010. Potential detrimental effects of a phytoestrogen-rich diet on male fertility in mice. Mol Cell Endrocrinol. 321, 152–160.

Cederroth, C.R., Auger, J., Zimmermann, C., Eustache, F., Nef, S., 2009. Soy, phyto-oestrogens and male reproductive function: a review. Int J Androl. 33, 304–316.

Chan, S.G., Murphy, P.A., Ho, S.C., Kreiger, N., Darlington, G., So, E. K.F., et al., 2009. Isoflavonoid content of Hong Kong soy foods. J Agric Food Chem. 57, 5390–5836.

Chandrareddy, A., Muneyyirci-Delale, O., McFarlane, S.I., Murad, O.M., 2008. Adverse effects of phytoestrogens on reproductive health: a report of three cases. Complement Ther Clin Pract. 14, 132–135.

Cox, R.I., Davies, L.H., 1988. Modification of pasture oestrogens in the gastrointestinal tract of ruminants. Proc Nutr Soc Aust. 13, 61–67.

D'Aloisio, A.A., Baird, D.D., DeRoo, L.A., Sandler, D.P., 2010. Association of intrauterine and early-life exposures with diagnosis of uterine leiomyomata by 35 years of age in the sister study. Environ Health Perspect. 118, 375–381.

Dubey, R.K., Gillespie, D.G., Imthurn, B., 1999. Phytoestrogens inhibit growth and MAP kinase activity in human aortic smooth muscle cells. Hypertension. 33, 177–182.

Dusza, L., Ciereszko, R., Skarzyki, D.J., Nogowski, L., Opalka, M., Kamiska, B., et al., 2006. Mechanism of phytoestrogen action in reproductive processes of mammals and birds. Reprod Biol 6. Suppl 1, 151–174.

Faber, K.A., Hughes Jr, C.L., 1993. Dose–response characteristics of neonatal exposure to genistein on pituitary responsiveness to gonadotropin releasing hormone and volume of the sexually dimorphic nucleus of the preoptic area (SDN-POA) in postpubertal castrated female rats. Reprod Toxicol. 7, 35–39.

Franke, A.A., Custer, L.J., Cerna, C.M., Narala, K., 1995. Rapid HPLC analysis of dietary phytoestrogens from legumes and from human urine. Proc Soc Exp Biol Med. 208, 18–26.

Goff, A.K., 2004. Steroid hormone modulation of prostaglandin secretion in the ruminant endometrium during the estrous cycle. Biol Reprod. 71, 11–16.

Green, C.C., Kelly, A.M., 2009. Effects of the estrogen mimic genistein as a dietary component on sex differentiation and ethoxyresorufin-O-deethylase (EROD) activity in channel catfish (*Ictalurus punctatus*). Fish Physiol Biochem. 35, 377–384.

Gunnarsson, D., Selstam, G., Ridderstråle, Y., Holm, L., Ekstedt, E., Madej, A., 2009. Effects of dietary phytoestrogens on plasma testosterone and triiodothyronine (T3) levels in male goat kids. Acta Vet Scand. 51, 51.

Hoikkala, A., Mustonen, E., Saastamoinen, I., Joekla, T., Taponen, J., Saloniemi, H., et al., 2007. High levels of equol in organic skimmed Finnish cow milk. Mol Nutr Food Res. 51, 782–786.

Jefferson, W.N., Doerge, D., Padilla-Banks, E., Woodling, K.A., Kissling, G.E., Newbold, R., 2009a. Oral exposure to genistin, the glycosylated form of genistein, during neonatal life adversely affects the female reproductive system. Environ Health Perspect. 117, 1883–1889.

Jefferson, W.N., Padilla-Banks, E., Goulding, E.H., Lao, S.-P., Newbold, R.R., Williams, C.J., 2009b. Neonatal exposure to genistein disrupts ability of female mouse reproductive tract to support preimplantation embryo development and implantation. Biol Reprod. 80, 425–431.

Klinge, C.M., Blankenship, K.A., Risinger, K.E., Bhatnagar, S., Noisin, E.L., Sumanasekera, W.K., et al., 2005. Reseveratrol and estradiol rapidly activate MAPK signaling through estrogen receptors α and β in endothelial cells. J Biol Chem. 280, 7460–7468.

Kolpin, D.W., Hoerger, C.C., Meyer, M.T., Wettstein, F.E., Hubbard, L. E., Bucheli, T.D., 2010. Phytoestrogens and mycotoxins in Iowa streams: an examination of underinvestigated compounds in agricultural basis. J Environ Qual. 39, 2089–2099.

Kostelac, D., Rechkemmer, G., Briviba, K., 2003. Phytoestrogens modulate binding response of estrogen receptors alpha and beta to the estrogen response element. J Agric Food Chem. 51, 7632–7635.

Kuiper, G.G., Carlsson, B., Grandien, K., Enmark, E., Haggblad, J., Nilsson, S., et al., 1997. Comparison of the ligand binding specificity and transcript tissue distribution of estrogen receptors alpha and beta. Endocrinology. 138, 863–870.

Kuiper, G.G., Lemmen, J.G., Carlsson, B., Corton, J.C., Safe, S.H., van der Saag, P.T., et al., 1998. Interaction of estrogenic chemicals and phytoestrogens with estrogen receptor β. Endocrinology. 139, 4252–4263.

Kurzer, M.S., Xu, X., 1997. Dietary phytoestrogens. Annu Rev Nutr. 17, 353–381.

Lacey, M., Bohday, J., Fonseka, S.M.R., Ullah, A.I., Whitehead, S.A., 2005. Dose–response effects of phytoestrogens on the activity and expression of 3 β-hydroxysteroid dehydrogenase and aromatase in human granulosa-luteal cells. J Steroid Biochem Mol Biol. 96, 279–286.

Lephart, E.D., Setchell, K.D., Lund, T.D., 2005. Phytoestrogens: hormonal action and brain plasticity. Brain Res Bull. 65, 193–198.

Levy, J.R., Faber, K.A., Ayyash, L., Hughrs Jr, C.L., 1995. The effect of prenatal exposure to the phytoestrogen genistein on sexual differentiation in rats. Proc Soc Exp Biol Med. 208, 60–66.

Lundh, T., 1995. Metabolism of estrogenic isoflavones in domestic animals. Proc Soc Exp Biol Med. 208, 33–39.

Lundh, T., Pettersson, H.I., Martinsson, K.A., 1990. Comparative levels of free and conjugated plant estrogens in blood plasma of sheep and cattle fed estrogenic silage. J Agric Food Chem. 38, 1530–1534.

Lund, T.D., Munson, D.J., Haldy, M.E., Setchell, K.D.R., Lephart, E.D., Handa, R.J., 2004. Equol is a novel anti-androgen that inhibits prostate growth and hormone feedback. Biol Reprod. 70, 1188–1195.

Madej, A., Persson, E., Lundh, T., Ridderstråle, Y., 2002. Thyroid gland function in ovariectomized ewes exposed to phytoestrogens. J Chromatogr B. 777, 281–287.

Mäkelä, S., Poutanen, M., Lehtimäki, J., Kostian, M.L., Santti, R., Vihko, R., 1995. Estrogen-specific 17beta-hydroxysteroid oxidoreductase type 1 (E.C.1.1.1.62) as a possible target for the action of phytoestrogens. Proc Soc Exp Biol Med. 208, 51–59.

Manach, C., Williamson, G., Morand, C., Scalbert, A., Rémésy, C., 2005. Bioavailability and bioefficacy of polyphenols in humans: I. Review of 97 bioavailability studies. Am J Clin Nutr. 81 (Suppl), 230S–242S.

Maran, R.R.M., Arunakaran, J., Aruldhas, M.M., 2000. T3 directly stimulate basal and modulates LH induced testosterone and oestradiol production by rat Leydig cells *in vitro*. Endocr J. 47, 417–428.

Markaverich, B.M., Webb, B., Densvore, C.L., Gregory, R.R., 1995. Effects of coumestrol on estrogen receptor function and uterine growth in ovariectomized rats. Environ Health Perspect. 103, 574–581.

Markiewicz, L., Garey, J., Adlercreutz, H., Gurpide, E., 1993. *In vitro* bioassay of non-steroidal phytoestrogens. J Steroid Biochem Mol Biol. 45, 399–405.

McClain, R.M., Wolz, E., Davidovich, A., Pfannkuch, F., Bausch, J., 2005. Subchronic and chronic safety studies with genistein in dogs. Food Chem Toxicol. 43, 1461–1482.

McClain, R.M., Wolz, E., Davidovich, A., Edwards, J., Bausch, J., 2007. Reproductive safety studies with genistein in rats. Food Chem Toxicol. 45, 1319–1332.

McGarvey, C., Cates, P.S., Brooks, N., Swanson, I.A., Milligan, S.R., Coen, C.W., et al., 2001. Phytoestrogens and gonadotropinreleasing hormone pulse generator activity and pituitary luteinizing hormone release in the rat. Endocrinology. 142, 1202–1208.

Menzel, V.A., Hinsch, E., Hägele, W., Hinsch, K.-D., 2007. Effect of genistein on acrosome reaction and zona pellucid binding independent of protein tyrosine kinase inhibition in bull. Asian J Androl. 9, 650–658.

Mlynarczuk, J., Wrobel, M.H., Kotwica, J., 2011a. The adverse effect of phytoestrogens on the synthesis and secretion of ovarian oxytocin in cattle. Reprod Domest Anim. 46, 21–28.

Mlynarczuk, J., Wrobel, M.H., Kotwica, J., 2011b. Adverse influence of coumestrol on secretory function of bovine luteal cells in the first trimester of pregnancy. Environ Toxicol. 28, 411–418. [e-pub ahead of print]. http://dx.doi.org/10.1002/tox.20735.

Mostrom MS (2010) Unpublished data. North Dakota Veterinary Diagnostic Laboratory, Fargo, North Dakota.

Neilsen, I.L., Williamson, G., 2007. Review of the factors affecting bioavailability of soy isoflavones in humans. Nutr Cancer. 57, 1–10.

Nwannenna, A.I., Lundh, T., Madej, A., Fredriksson, G., Björnhag, G., 1995. Clinical changes in ovariectomized ewes exposed to phytoestrogens and 17β-estradiol implants. Proc Soc Exp Biol Med. 208, 92–97.

Patisaul, H.B., Jefferson, W., 2010. The pros and cons of phytoestrogens. Front Neuroendocrinol. 31, 400–419.

Phillips, K.P., Tanphaichitr, N., 2008. Human exposure to endocrine disrupters and semen quality. J Toxicol Environ Health B. 11, 188–220.

Pietras, R.J., Szego, C.M., 1975. Endometrial cell calcium and oestradiol action. Nature. 253, 357–359.

Pilšáková, L., Rieanský, I., Jagla, F., 2010. The physiological actions of isoflavone phytoestrogens. Physiol Rev. 59, 651–664.

Piotrowska, K., Woclawek-Potocka, I., Bah, M.M., Piskula, M., Pilawski, W., Bober, A., et al., 2006. Phytoestrogens and their metabolites inhibit the sensitivity of the bovine corpus luteum on luteotropic factors. J Reprod Dev. 52, 33–41.

Pukazhenthi, B.S., Wildt, D.E., Ottinger, M.A., Howard, J., 1998. Inhibition of domestic cat spermatozoa acrosome reaction and zona pellucid penetration by tyrosine kinase inhibitors. Mol Reprod Dev. 49, 48–57.

Rochester, J.R., Klasing, K.C., Stevenson, L., Denison, M.S., Berry, W., Millam, J.R., 2009. Dietary red clover (*Trifolium pretense*) induces oviduct growth and decreases ovary and testes growth in Japanese quail chicks. Reprod Toxicol. 27, 63–71.

Romanowicz, K., Misztal, T., Barcikowski, B., 2004. Genistein, a phytoestrogen, effectively modulated luteinizing hormone and prolactin secretion in ovariectomized ewes during seasonal anestrus. Neuroendocrinology. 79, 73–81.

Rosselli, M., Reinhart, K., Imthurn, B., Keller, P.J., Dubey, R.K., 2000. Cellular and biochemical mechanisms by which environmental oestrogens influence reproductive function. Hum Reprod Update. 6, 332–350.

Rozman, K.K., Bhatia, J., Calafat, A.M., Chambers, C., Culty, M., Etzel, R.A., et al., 2006. NTP-CERHR expert panel report on the reproductive and developmental toxicity of soy formula. Birth Defects Res B. 77, 280–397.

Saloniemi, H., Wähälä, K., Nykänen-Kurki, P., Kallela, K., Saastamoinen, I., 1995. Phytoestrogen content and estrogenic effect of legume fodder. Proc Soc Exp Biol Med. 208, 13–17.

Santini, S.E., Basini, G.B., Bussolati, S., Grasselli, F., 2009. The phytoestrogen quercetin impairs steroidogenesis and angiogenesis in swine granulosa cells*in vitro*. J Biomed Biotech. pp. 1–8. http://dx.doi.org/10.1155/2009/419891.

Santti, R., Mäkelä, S., Strauss, L., Korkman, J., Kostian, M.-L., 1998. Phytoestrogens: potential endocrine disruptors in males. Toxicol Ind Health. 14, 223–237.

Seguin, P., Zheng, W., 2006. Phytoestrogen content of alfalfa cultivars grown in eastern Canada. J Sci Food Agric. 86, 765–771.

Seguin, P., Zheng, W., Souleimanov, A., 2004. Alfalfa phytoestrogen content: impact of plant maturity and herbage components. J Agron Crop Sci. 190, 211–217.

Setchell, K.D.R., Clerici, C., 2010a. Equol: history, chemistry, and formation. J Nutr. 140, 1355S–1362S.

Setchell, K.D.R., Clerici, C., 2010b. Equol: pharmacokinetics and biological actions. J Nutr. 140, 1363S–1368S.

Setchell, K.D.R., Gosselin, S.J., Welsh, M.B., Johnston, J.O., Balistreri, W.F., Kramer, L.W., et al., 1987. Dietary estrogens: a probable cause of infertility and liver disease in captive cheetahs. Gastroenterology. 93, 225–233.

Shon, Y.H., Park, S.D., Nam, K.S., 2006. Effective chemopreventive activity of genistein against human breast cancer cells. J Biochem Mol Biol. 39, 448–451.

Sivesind, E., Seguin, P., 2005. Effects of the environment, cultivar, maturity, and preservation method on red clover isoflavone concentration. J Agric Food Chem. 53, 6397–6402.

Steinshamn, H., Purup, S., Thuen, D., Hansen-Møller, J., 2008. Effects of clover–grass silages and concentrate supplementation on the content of phytoestrogens in dairy cow milk. J Dairy Sci. 91, 2715–2725.

Swego, C.M., 1984. Mechanisms of hormone action: parallels in receptor-mediated signal propagation for steroid peptide effectors. Life Sci. 35, 2381–2396.

Tan, K.A., Walker, M., Morris, K., Greig, I., Mason, J.I., Sharpe, R.M., 2006. Infant feeding with soy formula milk: effect in puberty progression, reproductive function and testicular cell numbers in marmoset monkeys in adulthood. Hum Reprod. 21, 896–904.

Tham, D.M., Gardner, C.D., Haskell, W.I., 1998. Potential health benefits of dietary phytoestrogens: a review of the clinical, epidemiological, and mechanistic evidence. J Clin Endocrinol Metab. 83, 2223–2235.

Urpi-Sarda, M., Morand, C., Besson, C., Kraft, G., Viala, D., Scalbert, A., et al., 2008. Tissue distribution if isoflavones in ewes after consumption of red clover silage. Arch Biochem Biophys. 476, 205–210.

Wang, L.-Q., 2002. Mammalian phytoestrogens: enerodiol and enterolactone. J Chromatogr B. 777, 289–309.

Whitten, P.L., Naftolin, F., 1992. Effects of a phytoestrogen diet on estrogen-dependent reproductive processes in immature female rats. Steroids. 57, 56–61.

Whitten, P.L., Patisaul, H.B., 2001. Cross-species and interassay comparisons of phytoestrogen action. Environ Health Perspect. 109 (Suppl 1), 5–20.

Whitten, P.L., Russell, E., Naftolin, F., 1992. Effects of a normal human concentration phytoestrogen diet on rat uterine growth. Steroids. 57, 98–106.

Woclawek-Potocka, I., Acosta, T.J., Korzekwa, A., Bah, M.M., Shibaya, M., Okuda, K., et al., 2005a. Phytoestrogens modulate prostaglandins production in bovine endometrium: cell type specificity and intracellular mechanism. Exp Biol Med. 230, 326–333.

Woclawek-Potocka, I., Bah, M., Korzekwa, A., Piskula, M., Wiczkowski, W., Depta, A., et al., 2005b. Soybean-derived phytoestrogens regulate prostaglandin secretion in endometrium during cattle estrous cycle and early pregnancy. Exp Biol Med. 230, 189–199.

Woclawek-Potocka, I., Piskula, M.K., Bah, M.M., Siemieniuch, M.J., Korzekwa, A., Brzezicka, E., et al., 2008. Concentrations of isoflavones and their metabolites in the blood of pregnant and non-pregnant heifers fed soy bean. J Reprod Dev. 54, 358–363.

Yueh, T.L., Chu, H.Y., 1977. The metabolic fate of daidzein. Sci Sin. 20, 513–522.

Section XIV

Poisonous Plants

Chapter 61

Poisonous Plants of the United States

Kip E. Panter, Kevin D. Welch, Dale R. Gardner, Steven T. Lee, Ben T. Green, James A. Pfister, Daniel Cook, Thomas Z. Davis and Bryan L. Stegelmeier

INTRODUCTION

Poisonous plants and the secondary compounds they produce cause major economic losses to the livestock industries throughout the world. Based on 1989 data, it was determined that poisonous plants cause losses of more than $340 million annually to the livestock industry in the 17 western states of the United States (Nielsen et al., 1988; Nielsen and James, 1992). This cost only considered death losses and specific reproductive losses in cattle and sheep, and only the 17 western states were included. Less obvious costs such as lost grazing opportunities, additional feed costs, increased health care costs, management changes, increased culling costs, lost weight gains, delayed or failed reproduction, and the emotional stress accompanying many poisonous plant cases were not included in the Nielsen and James analysis. When one considers these other costs, inflation, and current animal values, and when all pastures and ranges in the United States are factored in, the economic cost of poisonous plants to the livestock industry is very high. In addition, an often ignored cost is the lost biodiversity frequently resulting from invasive species, many of which are poisonous. These invasive and poisonous species are often aggressive invaders and reduce optimum utilization of private, federal, and state managed forest, range, and pasture lands. This aspect alone has far-reaching implications, not only for livestock producers but also for many other segments of society.

A frequently asked question is why do animals consume plants that may harm them or their offspring? In some cases, it is a matter of survival. For example, in the arid livestock-producing regions of the world, such as the western United States, regions of South Africa, Australia, China, and others, browsing or grazing animals may have limited access to high-quality forage at certain times of the year and are forced to survive by grazing some poisonous species. In other instances, hay or forages harvested in areas where poisonous plants are abundant may be contaminated with a high percentage of poisonous plants, and when animals are fed contaminated hay, they may be poisoned. Poisonous plant problems are often exacerbated during periods of below normal rainfall when the abundance of grasses is reduced. Frequently, the animal's diet shifts during the season as grasses and palatable forbs mature and senesce; for example, the consumption of some poisonous plants such as lupines, locoweeds, or larkspurs, which stay green longer into the season, may increase as the season progresses. In other instances, poisoning occurs early in the season before grasses begin to grow but poisonous plants have emerged and are usually very toxic. Poisoning by plants only occurs when animals eat too much too fast or graze it over a prolonged period of time. Therefore, management strategies to control these factors can minimize losses from poisonous plants.

At the Poisonous Plant Research Laboratory in Logan, Utah, poisonous plant problems are dealt with using a multidisciplinary approach. Veterinary medicine, chemistry, toxicology, pathology, animal and plant physiology, and range management are all key in the approach to reduce losses to the livestock industry. The plants discussed in this chapter are some of the most important poisonous plants in the United States, and considerable research has been conducted to reduce their incidence of poisoning.

This chapter is not intended to be all-inclusive but focuses on some of the most economically important and geographically widespread poisonous plants to livestock producers in the United States. There are excellent comprehensive texts available with a more general and broad coverage of specific poisonous plants (Burrows and Tyrl, 2001; Knight and Walter, 2001; Keeler et al., 1978 (ISOPP1); Seawright et al., 1985 (ISOPP2); James et al., 1992 (ISOPP3); Colegate and Dorling, 1994 (ISOPP4); Garland and Barr, 1998 (ISOPP5); Acamovic et al., 2004 (ISOPP6); Panter et al., 2007 (ISOPP7); Riet-Correa et al., 2011 (ISOPP8)). The ISOPP series, 1–8, 1978–2011 (Proceedings of the International Symposium on Poisonous Plants), provides a worldwide view of poisonous plant research. In 2013, the ninth international symposium

Veterinary Toxicology. DOI: http://dx.doi.org/10.1016/B978-0-12-811410-0.00061-1

(ISOPP 9) will be held in Ho Hot, Inner Mongolia, China. In addition, current research information on poisonous plants from throughout the world is available in the online peer-reviewed journal, the *International Journal of Poisonous Plant Research*, by the Poisonous Plant Research Laboratory, U.S. Department of Agriculture – Agricultural Research Service. International research, both basic and applied, as well as case reports of plant poisonings and short communications are published in a spring and a fall issue each year.

ASTRAGALUS AND *OXYTROPIS* SPECIES (LOCOWEEDS, NITRO SPP., AND SELENIUM SPP.)

Locoweeds

Of all the poisonous plants in the United States, the *Astragalus* and *Oxytropis* genera cause the most losses to the livestock industry in the western states (Graham et al., 2009; Cook et al., 2009c). The locoweeds are those species of the *Astragalus* and *Oxytropis* genera that contain the "loco" toxin (swainsonine) and induce the classic neurological and pathological signs of "locoism." Swainsonine is also present in other *Astragalus* species not usually considered locoweeds, such as some selenium and nitro-containing *Astragalus*. There are three toxic syndromes associated with these species: (1) locoism, caused by the indolizidine alkaloid swainsonine **(1)** (24 species); (2) nitrotoxins (356 taxa); and (3) species that accumulate selenium at high levels (22 species).

Description

These species are members of the Fabaceae (Leguminosae) or pea family. This family is distinguished by its papilionaceous flower (butterfly-like) having a single large banner petal, two side petals or wings, and two lower petals fused together to form a keel. Flowers are leguminous (pea-like), few or many, in axillary racemes, and they may be blue, purple, yellow, or white in color; fruit is a legume pod of various shapes, sizes, and surfaces among the species containing one or more kidney-shaped seeds. The distinguishing feature in *Oxytropis* is the porrect beak on the keel petal, whereas the *Astragalus* have a blunt keel petal (Figure 61.1). Some *Astragalus* species have extensions of the keel forming points, but they are not turned upward as in *Oxytropis*. In addition, *Oxytropis* species are acaulescent (without a stem, all leaves basal) with leafless flowering stalks originating from the crown, whereas leaflets of *Astragalus* species grow from the multibranched stems with the flowering head on top (Figure 61.1). Leaflets are opposite and pinnately compound. Pod shape, size, and chambers are very diverse and are a principal means of distinguishing between species (Figure 61.1).

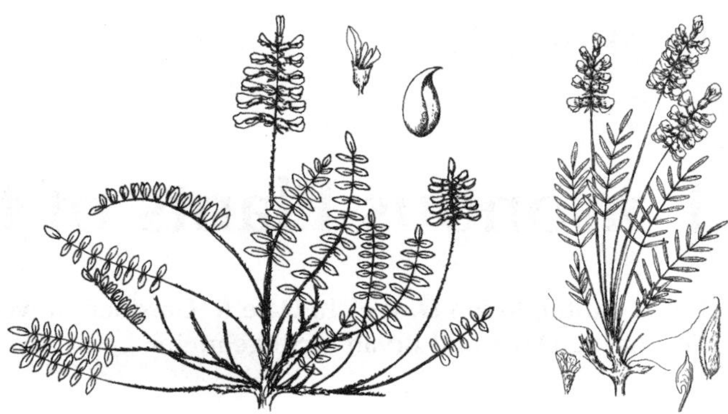

FIGURE 61.1 Comparison of *Astragalus* and *Oxytropis*. *Astragalus mollissimus* (purple loco) is on the left, and *Oxytropis lambertii* is on the right.

Astragalus is a very large and complex genus, with 354 species and 198 varieties of *Astragalus* (552 taxa) in the United States and Canada (Welsh et al., 2007). *Oxytropis* is much smaller, with 22 species and 35 varieties (57 taxa). Barneby (1964) earlier described and classified 368 species and 184 varieties of *Astragalus* and 35 species of *Oxytropis* in North America. Regardless, the *Astragalus* genus is the largest of the Leguminosae family. Species and variety identification are difficult even for trained botanists. Because of obvious similarities between *Oxytropis* and *Astragalus*, some botanists treat them together as *Astragalus*. Certainly, from a toxicology perspective, both can contain swainsonine and induce the same condition in livestock; therefore, both genera are treated the same in this discussion.

Distribution and ecology

The *Astragalus* and *Oxytropis* are worldwide in their distribution and toxic effects on livestock. Table 61.1 lists those species in the western United States suspected of field cases of poisoning or that have been shown by chemical analysis to contain swainsonine (Molyneux et al., 1991).

Species of *Astragalus* and *Oxytropis* occur in every major plant community. However, livestock poisoning is erratic due to the cyclic nature of the locoweed populations. Locoweeds have different survival strategies that allow perpetuation of the species through long-term climatic cycles and short-term weather conditions (Ralphs et al., 2003). Climate controls the establishment and growth of these plants by the amount and timing of precipitation. The following are the three main survival strategies:

1. Annual plants avoid drought by seed dormancy through dry cycles and germinate in years when sufficient moisture is available (winter annuals such as *wootonii* and *A. emoryanus*).

TABLE 61.1 Locoweed (*Astragalus* and *Oxytropis*) Species, Habitat, and Distribution and *Astragalus* Species Containing nitro-toxins or Accumulating Selenium[a]

Species	Common Name	Habitat	Distribution
A. allochrous	Rattleweed	Desert grassland	AZ, NM
A. asymmertricus	Horse loco	Annual grasslands	CA
A. bisulcatus[b]	Two-grooved milkvetch	Limestone, shale, high in Se	MT, ND, WY, CO, NM, UT
A. didymocarpus		Creosote deserts	CA, AZ, NV
A. drummondii[b]	Drummond milkvetch	Prairies, sage, oak, P/J	MT, WY, CO, NM, UT
A. emoryanus[c]	Red stem peavine	Creosote, mesquite, P/J	NM, TX
A. humistratus	Ground cover milkvetch	P/J woodlands	AZ, NM
A. lentiginosus	Spotted locoweed	Salt-desert shrub, sage, P/J	AZ, UT, NV, ID
A. lonchocarpus	Great rushy milkvetch	P/J woodlands	CO, UT, AZ, NV
A. missouriensis	Missouri milkvetch	Shortgrass prairies	Canada to TX
A. mollissimus	Woolly loco	Shortgrass prairies	CO, KA, OK, TX, NM
A. nothoxys	Beaked milkvetch	Oakbrush, P/J woodlands	AZ
A. oxyphysus	Diablo loco	Desert grasslands	CA
A. praelongus[b]	Stinking milkvetch	Sandstone, shale high in Se	UT, NM, AZ
A. pubentissimus	Green river milkvetch	Salt-desert shrub	CO, WY, UT
A. purshii	Pursh loco	Sagebrush, P/J woodlands	WY, MT, ID, NV
A. pycnostachyus	Brine milkvetch	Salt marshes and beaches	CA
A. tephrodes	Ashen milkvetch	Oakbrush, P/J woodlands	AZ, NM
A. thurberi	Thurber milkvetch	Creosote, oak, P/J woodlands	AZ, NM
A. wootoni	Garbancillo	Creosote desert	AZ, NM, TX
O. besseyi	Red loco	Gravely hill tops	MT, WY
O. campestris	Yellow loco	Prairies, mountain meadows	MT, Canada
O. lambertii	Lambert locoweed	Short- and mid-grass prairies	MT, ND, SD, WY, CO, NM
O. sericea	White locoweed	Rocky soils, foothills, and mountains	MT, SD, WY, CO, NM, UT
Nitro-toxins			
A. atropubescens	Kelsey milkvetch	Gravelly benches	ID, MT
A. Canadensis	Canada milkvetch	Introduced	Throughout U.S.
A. convallarius	Rushy milkvetch	Sagebrush	ID, NV, UT, WY
A. emoryanus	Red-stem peavine	Shortgrass prairies	AZ, NM, TX
A. falcatus		Introduced	
A. miser	Timber milkvetch		
var. *serotinus*	Columbia milkvetch	Rough fescue grasslands	BC Canada
var. *hylophilas*	Yellowstone milkvetch	Sagebrush/timber	WY, MT
var. *oblongifolius*	Wasatch milkvetch	Mountains, sagebrush	UT, CO
A. pterocarpus	Winged milkvetch	Sagebrush	CA, NV
A. tetrapterus	Four-winged milkvetch	Sagebrush	CA, NV
A. toanus[d]	Toano milkvetch	Salt-desert shrub	Great Basin
A. whitneyi		Sierra Mountains	CA, NV

(*Continued*)

TABLE 61.1 (Continued)

Species	Common Name	Habitat	Distribution
Selenium Accumulators			
A. albulus[d]	Cibola milkvetch	Salt-desert shrub	Northwestern NM, AZ
A. beathii[c]	Beath's milkvetch	Badlands	AZ, NV, UT
A. bisulcatus	Two-grooved milkvetch	Sagebrush	MT, WY, ND, SD, CO,UT, NM
A. crotalariae[d]	Rattle box milkvetch	Desert	AZ, CA
A. cutleri[d]			
A. debequaeus[d]			
A. eastwoodiae[d]	Eastwood's milkvetch	Badlands	Four Corners
A. flavus	Yellow milkvetch	Alkaline soils	Colorado Plateau
A. grayii[d]	Gray's milkvetch	Badlands	WY, MT
A. moencoppenis	Moenkopi milkvetch	Badlands	UT, AZ
A. nelsonianus[d]		Alkaline flats	WY
A. oocalycis[d]		Sagebrush	CO, NM
A. osterhouti	Osterhout milkvetch	Clay hills	Grand Co., CO
A. pattersoni	Patterson milkvetch	Oakbrush	Rocky Mountains
A. pectinatus	Tine-leaved milkvetch	Northern prairies	MT, ND, WY, CO, KA
A. praelongus	Stinking milkvetch	Badlands	Four Corners
A. racemosus	Alkali milkvetch	Badlands	Plains states
A. sabolosus	Cisco milkvetch	Badlands	Eastern UT
A. saurinus[d]	Dinosaur milkvetch	Badlands	Eastern UT
A. sophoroides[d]	Painted desert milkvetch		AZ
A. toanus[d]	Toano milkvetch	Salt-desert shrub	Great Basin

P/J, pinyon–juniper.
[a]*Many varieties, especially of* A. lentiginosus, A. mollissimus, *and* O. sericea, *have been referred to as separate species in the past.*
[b]*Also contains selenium.*
[c]*Also contains nitro-toxins.*
[d]*Minor species.*
From Ralphs et al. (2003) and Welsh et al. (2007).

2. Biennial or short-lived perennial plants exhibit opportunistic survival strategies by relying on both timely and adequate moisture for germination, growth, flowering, and seed set. Seeds germinate in fall following autumn rains, persist over winter, and flower in spring. If sufficient moisture is available, they will remain for 2 or 3 years until the next drought occurs (*A. mollissimus*, *A. lentiginosus*, and *A. pubentissimus*).
3. Long-lived perennial plants exhibit a stress-tolerant survival strategy. They have deep taproots that can access deep stored water. They grow where moisture is more abundant and more regularly available. The plants flower and produce seed for many years following initial establishment, although they too may die out during extended droughts (*O. sericea* and *O. lambertii*).

The seed bank in the soil supports these cycles. The seeds have hard coats and remain viable for many years, thus providing an ecological advantage to exploit environmental conditions and maintain the "boom and bust" population cycles (Ralphs et al., 2003). Livestock poisonings follow these cycles, often in catastrophic proportions.

Toxicology

Locoweed poisoning was one of the first poisonous plant problems recognized by stockmen and reported as early as 1873. Extensive stock losses in the western United States eventually led to the establishment of a field station in Hugo, Colorado, in 1905 to study the problem. Research from 1905 to 1907 determined that certain species of the *Astragalus* and *Oxytropis* genera were responsible, and this research was published in 1909 as a U.S. Department of Agriculture bulletin titled "The Locoweed Disease of the Plains" by C.D. Marsh.

There are numerous effects of locoweed on animals, but the classic syndrome from which the term "locoism" derived is one of neurological dysfunction. The disease is a chronic one developing after weeks of ingesting locoweeds and beginning with depression, dull-appearing eyes, incoordination progressing to aberrant behavior including aggression, staggering, solitary behavior, and emaciation and ending in death if continued consumption is allowed. Other problems associated with locoweed ingestion include reproductive failure, abortion, birth defects, weight loss, and enhanced susceptibility to brisket disease at high elevations (Panter et al., 1999b).

Locoweed poisoning affects all animals, but because of the transient nature of the poisoning, animals removed from the locoweed early in the toxicosis will recover most of their function and may be productive animals. In the final stages of locoism, central nervous system tissue shows swelling of axonal hillocks (meganeurites) and growth of new dendrites and synapses. This altered synaptic formation in nervous tissue in severely affected animals is permanent and may be the cause of some irreversible neurological signs. Because of neurological dys-function and apparent permanence of some lesions in the nervous system, horses are believed to be unpredictable and therefore unsafe to use for riding, but they may remain reproductively sound once they have recovered from the poisoning.

Toxin

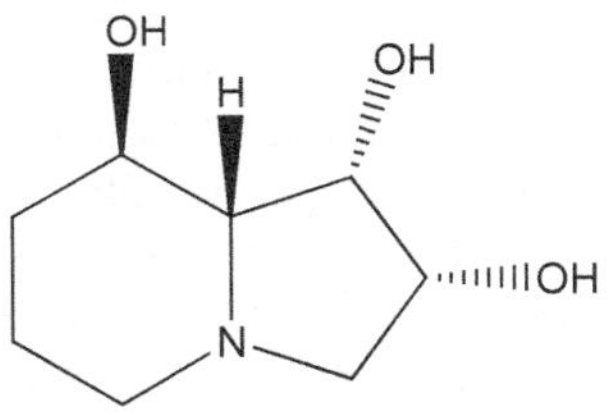

OH H OH OH N

(1)
Swainsonine

The toxin in locoweeds is the indolizidine alkaloid swainsonine **(1)**. First isolated from the Australian plant *Swainsona canescens* (Colegate et al., 1979), swainsonine and its N-oxide were isolated and identified soon thereafter from the locoweeds (Molyneux and James, 1982). Remarkably, in 1909, C.D. Marsh made the connection between the clinical and pathological syndrome of locoweed poisoning and a similar condition reported in Australian livestock called "peastruck." Confirmation feeding trials in New South Wales with Darling pea (*Swainsona* spp.) were reported a few years before Marsh reported the details of locoweed poisoning. Ironically, the toxin (swainsonine) was isolated and characterized from *S. canescens* and reported in Australia in 1979 (Colegate et al., 1979) and subsequently identified and isolated from locoweeds (*Astragalus* and *Oxytropis*) in the United States and reported in 1982 (Molyneux and James, 1982).

The isolation and characterization of swainsonine from *S. canescens* resulted from investigations by a multidisciplinary research team in Australia whose members were experienced in various aspects of lysosomal storage diseases in domestic animals (Dorling et al., 1989). This investigation concentrated on the details of the pathogenesis of the toxicosis enabling the research team to elucidate the mechanism of action, which provided the bioassay method for toxin isolation and identification. A review of the historical aspects can be found in Dorling et al. (1989). In essence, the locoism syndrome is a lysosomal storage disease in which α-mannosidase is inhibited, resulting in prevention of hydrolysis of mannose-rich oligosaccharides in cells and accumulation of these oligosaccharides resulting in cellular dysfunction. Swainsonine has also been identified with mixtures of other glycosidase-inhibiting polyhydroxy alkaloids in toxic species of *Ipomoea*, *Sida*, *Solanum*, *Physalis*, and *Convolvulus* (Asano et al., 1995; Haraguchi et al., 2003). Most organ systems are affected, but some are more susceptible, such as glandular and neurological tissues. Comparative pathology of the glycosidase inhibitors swainsonine, castanospermine, and calystegines A3, B2, and C1 in mice was reported (Stegelmeier et al., 2008). Although there were similar vacuolar changes, there were differences in the organ systems involved and minor changes in protein glycosylation, and it was determined that in mice calystegines and castanospermine are less toxic than swainsonine.

It has been discovered that swainsonine in *Astragalus* and *Oxytropis* species is produced by a fungal endophyte, *Undifilum oxytropis* (formerly called *Embellesia oxytropis*). A positive correlation was shown to exist between swainsonine concentrations found in the plant and concentrations of swainsonine produced by the endophytic fungus cultured from the same plant (Pryor et al., 2009; Cook et al., 2009a). This same correlation was demonstrated for *Oxytropis glabra*, an important poisonous plant in Inner Mongolia steppe (Ping et al., 2009). Major locoweeds were screened for the presence of endophyte and swainsonine content using both culture methods and polymerase chain reaction (PCR; Ralphs et al., 2008). PCR was demonstrated to be the most sensitive method of detecting the endophyte because the endophyte in plants with very low levels of swainsonine ($<0.01\%$) was not detected by culture methods, only PCR. Oldrup et al. (2010) demonstrated that *U. oxytropis* is transferred by seed and the endopyte resides in the parenchymal layers of the seeds. Seedlings of *Astragalus lentiginosus* produced in embryo culture without seed coats did not contain swainsonine or the fungus. Plants produced from whole seed contained *Undifilum* in both foliage and root tissues. Simulated environmental stresses, including high temperature, low and high pH media, nutrient-deficient media, and polyethylene glycol-amended media, impacted both dry mass and swainsonine levels.

Research results have shown that inhibition of α-mannosidase is relatively transient and quickly reversible once animals stop eating locoweed (Stegelmeier et al., 1994). Blood serum clearance of swainsonine is rapid (half-life of 20 h); thus, the effects of locoweed should be reversible if tissue damage has not become extensive and permanent. This suggests that intermittent grazing of locoweed should be an effective means of reducing locoweed poisoning. There is also an apparent threshold dosage where severity of cell damage is more time dependent than dosage dependent. Once the threshold dosage is reached, which appears to be relatively low (0.35 mg/kg in the rat), eating more locoweed does not accelerate the toxicosis. Therefore, increasing animal numbers on loco pastures and reducing time of grazing is also a logical method to reduce adverse effects.

Many locoweeds are biennials or perennials that flourish periodically under optimum environmental conditions. Historically, losses are regional and sporadic, with large regional economic impact. Individual cases of significant losses are frequent and reported in James and Nielsen (1988). In a single case, 25% of more than 500 mother cows of a university foundation herd either aborted or apparently resorbed their fetuses after grazing pastures with *O. sericea*. Necropsy of aborted fetuses showed pathological lesions characteristic of locoweed poisoning, and 50 calves born alive showed out-ward signs of toxicity (James, personal communication, 1994). Follow-up communication indicated that locoed calves were immunologically compromised, and 3 or 4% of these calves died after weaning. The remainder of the loco calves remained approximately 200 pounds less than calves not exposed to locoweed even though after the first 28 days in the feedlot, the rate of gain was approximately the same.

Conditions of Grazing

The early literature suggested that locoweeds were distasteful and animals were forced to start eating them because of hunger. However, once started, animals seemed to become addicted to locoweeds. Recent research showed that locoweeds are not addicting but, rather, are relatively more palatable than associated forages during various seasons of the year.

Preference for locoweed is relative to what other forage is available. Many locoweeds are cool-season species that green up and start growth early in the spring, flower, set seed and go dormant in summer, and then resume growth in fall. Livestock generally prefer the green, growing locoweeds to dormant grass. Sheep preferred the regrowth foliage of Green River milkvetch to dormant grasses during late fall and early winter on desert range in eastern Utah. Horses selected green spotted locoweed instead of dormant grasses in spring in Arizona (Pfister et al., 2003). Cattle readily grazed Wahweap milkvetch in proportion to its availability on desert winter range in southeastern Utah. In a series of grazing studies in northeast New Mexico, cattle readily grazed white locoweed in March–May but stopped grazing it in June as warm-season grasses became abundant and white locoweed matured and became coarse and rank. Stocker cattle grazed white locoweed on short-grass prairies in May and early June, but the weight loss continued throughout the summer, even though they were not eating locoweed. On mixed-grass prairies on the eastern foothills of the Rocky Mountains in northern Colorado, cattle ceased grazing white locoweed when it matured following flowering in mid-June and became rank and unpalatable. However, they continued to graze it throughout the subsequent summer when abundant summer precipitation caused locoweed leaves to remain succulent (Ralphs et al., 2001).

Prevention of Poisoning and Management Recommendations

Prevention of poisoning remains a matter of management strategy adapted to individual grazing programs to minimize grazing of locoweed plants (Graham et al., 2009). Currently, no broad management schemes or methods of treatment are known to generally prevent locoweed poisoning. Management strategies for individual operations have been developed once the grazing practices and options are identified, allowing utilization of the particular range and yet minimizing losses. It was determined that cattle generally rejected woolly loco even under extreme grazing conditions, but once they were forced to start eating it, they continued to graze it and became intoxicated. Ranchers should watch for these "loco eaters" and remove them to clean pastures. Shortage of feed with high grazing pressure, social facilitation (loco eaters teaching non-loco eaters to eat loco), or supplementing with alfalfa hay or cubes may compel cattle to start grazing woolly locoweed. White locoweed is more palatable than woolly locoweed and is green before spring grasses begin to grow in northeastern New Mexico. Therefore, cattle readily graze white loco in early spring while grasses are dormant, and once green grass starts to grow, cattle switch off of loco. Recommendations include creating loco-free pastures through spraying, fencing, or selection of low loco-infested pastures for early spring grazing and also to provide a place to move the identified loco-eaters. This practice appears to reduce the impact of locoweed on these ranges.

Many minerals, feed additives, and clay minerals have been investigated to prevent poisoning, but none have been effective. The poisonous plant literature is filled with statements that native livestock are less likely to be poisoned than new, inexperienced livestock. Locoweed poisoning does not follow this general trend. Cattle that are familiar with locoweed will likely select it first. Early observations by C.D. Marsh as early as 1909 suggested that black cattle and black-faced sheep were more inclined to be poisoned by locoweed than were white-faced cattle and sheep. In a grazing study comparing breeds, Brangus steers consumed more locoweed than did Hereford and Charolais steers. The gregarious nature of Brangus cattle may have facilitated the social acceptance of locoweed among the steers.

Livestock should be denied access to locoweeds during critical periods when they are relatively more palatable than associated forages. On short-grass prairies of northeastern New Mexico, stocker cattle should not be turned onto locoweed-infested rangelands until warm season grasses start growth in late May or early June. Cattle on rangeland year-round should be removed from locoweed-infested areas in the spring when it is green and growing and warm-season grasses remain dormant. They can be returned to locoweed-infested pastures in summer when warm-season grasses are abundant.

Most locoweed species are endemic, growing only in certain habitats or on specific soils. Fences could be constructed on soil or vegetation boundaries to provide seasonal control of grazing. Reserving locoweed-free pastures for grazing during critical periods in spring and fall can prevent locoweed poisoning.

Locoweed-free areas can be created by strategic herbicide use. White locoweed is most susceptible to Clopyralid, but Picloram and Escort are also effective. However, natural population cycles should be considered to determine the practicality of spraying large areas and the potential lifetime of control. With the abundant seed bank in the soil, locoweeds are sure to germinate and reestablish when environmental conditions are favorable.

Animals that start eating locoweed may influence others to start. Social facilitation or peer pressure is a very strong influence inducing others to start eating locoweed (Ralphs et al., 1994). Graham developed the "eat and pull" management strategy, whereby livestock should be watched closely and removed if they start eating locoweed to prevent poisoning and prevent them from influencing others to start.

Grazing pressure can also force cattle to begin grazing locoweed when they run short of desirable forage (Ralphs et al., 1994). Ranchers should not overstock locoweed-infested ranges but, rather, should ensure adequate forage is always available. Improper use of some grazing systems can cause livestock to graze locoweed. Rest-rotation grazing systems are designed to force livestock to uniformly graze all forage in a pasture. This caused cattle and horses to start grazing spotted locoweed in western Utah. Changing to a three-herd, four-pasture deferred rotation grazing system stopped locoweed poisoning by reducing the grazing pressure and allowing the cattle to select alternative forages in preference to white locoweed. The heavy grazing pressure associated with short-duration grazing systems may also induce poisoning problems.

Conditioned food aversion can be used as a management tool to train animals to avoid grazing locoweed. In the conditioning protocol, animals are brought into a pen and fed fresh-picked locoweed, and then lithium chloride (an emetic that causes gastrointestinal distress) is administered by stomach tube. The animals associate the induced illness with the taste of the plant and subsequently avoid eating it. Naive animals that are unfamiliar with the target plant form strong and lasting ($>$3 years) aversions following a single dose. Averted animals must be kept separate from nonaverted animals on locoweed areas to prevent social facilitation from extinguishing the aversions. Aversion conditioning may be feasible where losses are heavy and persist year after year.

Summary

Locoweed is the most widespread poisonous plant problem in the western United States. Knowledge of sites where locoweeds grow and environmental conditions when they cause problems is necessary to manage livestock and prevent poisoning. Locoweeds are relatively palatable, and many locoweeds are the first plants to start growing in the spring and they may also regrow in the fall. Livestock generally prefer the green-growing locoweeds to other forage that is dormant in the fall, winter, and spring. The most effective management strategy is to deny livestock access to locoweeds during critical periods when they are more palatable than associated forage. Reserving locoweed-free pastures or controlling existing locoweed populations with herbicides can provide "safe" pastures for critical periods. Watching animals closely and removing those that begin eating locoweed can prevent further intoxication and prevent them from influencing others to start. Finally, conditioned food aversion is an effective practice to train animals to avoid eating locoweeds, and it may be economical where losses are large and persistent. Good range management and wise grazing strategies can provide adequate forage for livestock and avoid critical periods of the year when locoweed is relatively more palatable than associated forages.

Nitro-containing *Astragalus* (milkvetches)

There are more than 260 species and varieties (356 taxa) of nitro-containing *Astragalus* in North America (Barneby, 1964; Welsh et al., 2007). They are frequently referred to as milkvetches, as are some of the other *Astragalus* species. Nitro-toxins are therefore the most common toxin in the *Astragalus*, followed by swainsonine (loco) and selenium. Major livestock losses occur in many regions of the western United States. These plants are very diverse and concentrated on the deserts, foothills, and mountains of the west.

Description

The description of these plants is the same as that of the locoweeds. The milkvetches emerge from late April to June depending on elevation and snow cover. After seed dispersal in July or August, the stems and leaves become dry and less dangerous as toxicity and palatability are reduced.

Distribution

The aliphatic nitro-containing *Astragalus* are distributed throughout North America, with substantial livestock losses occurring in the 17 western states where cattle or sheep are concentrated in areas of milkvetch infestation (Table 61.1). There are examples of a number of *Astragalus* spp. such as *A. cicer* that are good forages and apparently contain low levels of the toxins discussed. Because of the extent of this group of *Astragalus*, only a few of those implicated in poisonings are mentioned here. For a more comprehensive review of the nitro-containing *Astragalus*, the reader is referred to Williams and Barneby (1977). Examples of these include *A. emoryanus* (emory milkvetch) in New Mexico, Texas, and Arizona (*A. emoryanus* also contains swainsonine); *A. tetrapterus* (four-winged milkvetch) in Oregon, Utah, Nevada, and Arizona; *A. pterocarpus* (winged milkvetch) in Nevada; and *A. miser* var. *serotinus*, *A. miser* var. *oblongifolius*, and *A. miser* var. *hylophylus* (collectively referred to as timber milkvetch) in western Canada, Montana, Idaho, Utah, Colorado, and Wyoming.

Toxicology

The nitro-containing *Astragalus* species cause an acute and chronic type of poisoning in sheep and cattle. The acute form results in weakness, increased heart rate, respiratory distress, coma, and death. Although blood methemoglobin is high (induced from nitro-toxin metabolism to nitrites) and a contributing factor to the respiratory difficulties, administration of methylene blue in cattle does not prevent death. Therefore, the methemoglobinemia is apparently not the primary cause of death. The chronic form is the most frequent form of poisoning observed and follows a course of general weakness, incoordination, central nervous system involvement resulting in knuckling of the fetlocks, goose stepping, clicking of the hooves, "cracker heels" progressing to paralysis, and death. A respiratory syndrome is also present in the chronic and acute forms, with emphysema-like signs causing the animals to force respiration: "roaring disease." Sheep manifest the respiratory syndrome more than the central nervous syndrome and are more resistant to poisoning compared to cattle.

The toxic principles are β-D-glycosides of 3-nitro-1-propanol (NPOH) or 3-nitropropionic acid (NPA). The glycoside conversion occurs more readily in the ruminant because of the microflora and is apparently the reason for increased toxicity in ruminants. The glycoside (miserotoxin) is metabolized to the highly toxic NPOH in the gastrointestinal (GI) tract of ruminants (Williams et al., 1970). Thus, NPOH is absorbed in the gut and apparently converted to NPA by the liver. Further metabolism yields inorganic nitrite and an unidentified metabolite that may be involved in toxicity. It appears that NPOH is more rapidly absorbed from the gut than is NPA; therefore, forage containing the alcohol form is the most toxic.

Prevention and Treatment

There is no preferred treatment for milkvetch poisoning, although treatment with methylene blue appears to reverse the methemoglobinemia but does not prevent death in cattle. Oxidation of NPOH to NPA was prevented if alcohol dehydrogenase was saturated with ethanol or inhibited with 4-methylpyrazole before NPOH was given. This suggests that NPOH is a good substrate for the enzyme alcohol dehydrogenase. This information could be useful in acute cases; however, its value in treatment of poisoning in the field is unknown.

Livestock losses can be reduced by decreasing the density of the *Astragalus* species with herbicides or avoiding grazing livestock on infested areas when the plant is most poisonous. Wasatch milkvetch contains the highest concentration of miserotoxin from bloom to immature pod stage of growth. Nitro compounds are found in all parts of the plant, but the leaves contain the highest concentration. Once the leaves begin to dry and lose their green color, the nitro levels drop very rapidly and the plant is relatively nontoxic. However, the toxins in plants pressed green and preserved in herbaria appear to remain stable for years (Williams and Barneby, 1977). Herbicide treatment decreases the density of plants and also decreases the toxicity of the plants once they start to dry; therefore, spraying milkvetch appears to be the best method to reduce losses and still utilize infested ranges.

Seleniferous *Astragalus*

Approximately 22–24 species of *Astragalus* known to accumulate selenium (Se) have been identified (Rosenfeld and Beath, 1964; Welsh et al., 2007). These are less numerous and more geographically restricted than the nitro-containing species. Many of these species are referred to as Se-indicator plants because they only grow on soils high in bioavailable selenium; therefore, they are helpful in locating and identifying areas or soils high in selenium. The *Astragalus* are generally deep rooted plants and may bring selenium from deeper soil profiles unavailable to other plants so that it is available and can subsequently be taken up by grasses and other forbs. It is these facultative accumulators that create most of the subacute or chronic toxicity problems for livestock.

Description

The selenium-containing *Astragalus* species appear similar to those of locoweed and nitro-containing species as discussed previously. One identifying feature of the selenium-containing *Astragalus* species is an unpleasant garlic-like odor of the volatile selenium compound dimethyl diselenide, especially if picked and allowed to sit in a warm car or window. The Se-indicator plants are generally considered to be unpalatable to livestock because of their high selenium content. Some *Astragalus* species have been shown to accumulate selenium at concentrations of up to 10 mg Se/g (dry weight) while growing on soils containing 2–10 μg Se/g. The majority of selenium in accumulator plants is found as organic methylselenocysteine and selenocystathionine or as inorganic selenate. Many selenium-containing *Astragalus* may also contain other toxins; for example, *A. praelongus* and *A. bisulcatus* contain swainsonine (the loco toxin), and *A. toanus* contains nitro-toxins and swainsonine in addition to selenium.

Distribution

The selenium-containing *Astragalus* species are limited in their distribution to geographical locations and soil sites of high selenium (Table 61.1), of which most are alkaline in nature, causing selenium to be oxidized and making it soluble and available to plants. Major seleniferous areas of the west are in North and South Dakota, Montana, Wyoming, Colorado, and Utah, with minor isolated pockets of seleniferous soils in most of the other western states.

The *Astragalus* species most associated with selenium poisoning include *A. bisulcatus* (two-grooved milkvetch), *A. praelongus* (stinking milkvetch), *A. pattersonii* (Patterson milkvetch), *A. pectinatus* (tiny-leaved milkvetch), and *A. racemosus* (alkali milkvetch).

Toxicity

With selenium poisonings, one may observe acute, subacute, or chronic selenosis depending on the daily dose and duration of exposure. Acute cases of selenium poisoning are rare and usually involve animals that have been exposed by one of three methods. First, livestock graze forages that have accumulated selenium from seleniferous soils. Second, selenium toxicosis occurs from environmental contamination from agricultural drain water, reclaimed soils from phosphate or ore mining, or from fly ash. Third, acute selenosis can be caused by accidental overdosing with organic selenium or Bo-Se in the treatment of white muscle disease or by misformulated feed mixes. The signs of acute selenium poisoning include diarrhea, unusual postures, increased temperature and heart rate, dyspnea, tachypnea, respiratory distress, prostration, and death (Tiwary et al., 2006). Gross pathological findings are usually limited to pulmonary congestion and hemorrhage and pulmonary edema. Histologically, multifocal myocardial necrosis and pulmonary alveolar vasculitis are common (Tiwary et al., 2006).

Chronic selenium poisoning is common and referred to as alkali disease because most areas with high concentrations of available selenium are alkaline in nature. Chronic selenosis occurs from prolonged ingestion of seleniferous forages containing 5–40 ppm Se. Clinical signs include rough coat, hair or wool loss, poor growth, emaciation, abnormal hoof growth and lameness, dermatitis, and depressed reproduction (Rosenfeld and Beath, 1964; Raisbeck, 2000). In swine, a condition of paralysis (poliomyelomalacia or polioencephalomalacia) often occurs with cervical or lumbar involvement (Panter et al., 1996b). The description of a second chronic syndrome in cattle called "blind staggers" has been redefined and is now believed to be polioencephalomalacia induced by high sulfate water or high sulfate forage sources.

Selenium is found in plants in both inorganic and organic forms. The organic forms are more bioavailable than the inorganic forms, resulting in higher tissue concentrations when administered at equivalent doses (Tiwary et al., 2006; Davis et al. 2011). Although a dramatic difference in tissue selenium uptake between organic (selenomethionine) and plant (*A. bisulcatus*) forms and inorganic (sodium selenate) forms occurs, the clinical and pathological syndromes are similar – that is, poliomyelomalacia in pigs (Panter et al., 1996b) and pulmonary edema and hemorrhage in sheep (Tiwary et al., 2006, Davis et al. 2011).

Prevention of Poisoning

There is no treatment for selenium poisoning except removal of the source, allowing spontaneous recovery in chronic cases. Monitoring soils in a particular area and understanding the plant communities can provide the management information to avoid poisoning. In areas where selenium is a problem, many ranchers have switched to grazing steers because of decreased reproductive efficiency in cows. Sheep appear to be more resistant to chronic selenosis compared to cattle and are better adapted for some of these ranges. However, sheep are sensitive to acute selenium poisoning, as was observed when a large number of sheep died within days after grazing on mine reclamation sites that contained very high soil and plant selenium concentrations (Panter, personal communications, 2004). Monitoring for selenium concentrations and forms in soil, vegetation, as well as animal tissues and hair can help avoid poisoning incidences. Likewise, deficiency problems can be rapidly resolved with frequent monitoring and supplementation.

LARKSPURS (*DELPHINIUM* SPP.)

There are more than 80 wild species of larkspurs in North America, and there are a larger number of domestic horticultural varieties. Wild larkspurs are classified into three general categories based primarily on mature plant height and distribution: low, tall, and plains larkspurs (Figure 61.2). The dominant larkspur species in the western United States are shown in Table 61.2. The larkspurs are a major cause of cattle losses on western ranges. As early as 1913, C.D. Marsh reported that more cattle deaths on western ranges are caused by *Delphinium* spp. than by any other poisonous plant except locoweed.

Description

Most of the wild larkspurs have flowers of blue or purple, bilaterally symmetrical, in erect terminal racemes or panicles: five sepals, the upper prolonged backwards in a prominent spur; petals smaller and variable among species, usually four and sometimes two, with the upper pair projecting back inside the spur; and carpals one to five, sometimes fused, ripening into many-seeded follicles.

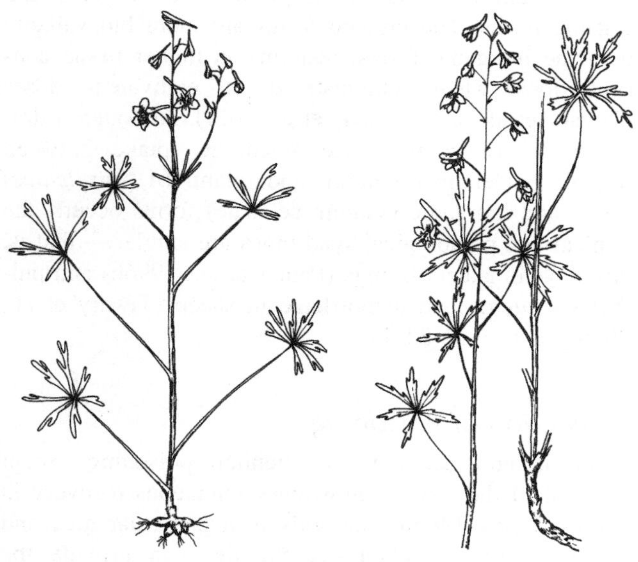

FIGURE 61.2 Low larkspur (*Delphinium bicolor*) is on the left and tall larkspur (*D. barbeyi*) is on the right.

The tall larkspurs (Figure 61.2) are 1 or 2 m tall or more, flower in summer, and set seed in late summer, subsequently senescing in the fall. In the west, the tall larkspurs typically inhabit higher mountain elevations in the more open moist areas of canyons, draws, and meadows. *Delphiniums* are frequently confused with *Aconitum*, but certain features distinguish them. As implied by the common names, *Delphiniums* have a distinct spur (hence larkspur), whereas *Aconitum* has no spur but a hood (hence monkshood). Tall larkspurs have hollow stems, and their leaves are relatively long petioled, whereas monkshood has stems that are solid and pithy and leaves are short petioled.

Low larkspurs (Figure 61.2) appear similar to tall larkspurs except they grow in different habitats and locations – that is, lower elevations in drier habitats, on foothills and flats. They appear first as a rosette-like clump in early spring, soon producing an erect flowering stem, usually not more than 1 m in height, and then die back in early summer.

Plains larkspur falls between the low and tall larkspur classifications. Plants range from 0.3 to 2 m tall. It grows on the short-grass plains of Wyoming into Nebraska and in the sagebrush and juniper woodlands of the Colorado Plateau.

Distribution and Habitat

Low larkspur

D. nelsonii – Idaho, South Dakota, Wyoming, Colorado, and Utah
D. bicolor – North Dakota, Montana, Wyoming, Oregon, and Washington
D. andersonii–Oregon, California, Nevada, Utah, and Idaho
D. tricorne – Nebraska and Oklahoma eastward
D. virescens – Great Plains, east of the Rockies

Intermediate larkspur

D. geyeri – Colorado, Wyoming, Nebraska, and Utah

Tall larkspur

D. barbeyi – Utah, Wyoming, Colorado, and New Mexico
D. occidentale – Washington, Idaho, Wyoming, Nevada, Utah, and Colorado
D. glaucescens – Idaho and Montana
D. glaucum – Washington, Oregon, California, Nevada, Idaho, and Montana
D. trolliifolium – Washington, Oregon, and California
D. robustum – Colorado and New Mexico

TABLE 61.2 Characteristics of the Dominant Larkspur Species in Western North America

Class/species	Height at Maturity (cm)	Elevation (m)	Associated Plant Communities	Toxicity Ranking[a]	Typical Risk of Losses[b]
Tall Larkspurs					
D. glaucum[c]	90–200	>2000	Aspen, conifers, alpine meadows	1	Low
D. barbeyi	90–180	>2200	Aspen, conifers, alpine meadows, mountain brush, alpine tundra	2	Moderate to severe
D. glaucescens	76–90	>2000	Mountain meadows, sagebrush	3	Low to moderate
D. occidentale	90–180	>2000	Mountain brush, sagebrush, conifer, aspen	4	Low to severe
Low Larkspurs					
D. nuttallianum	20–60	>1200	Mountain brush, sagebrush, aspen, conifer, mountain and foothill meadows	2	–
D. bicolor	20–40	>800	Mountain brush, sagebrush	–	–
D. andersonii	10–60	>1200	Desert shrub, mountain brush, sagebrush, pinyon–juniper	1	–
Plains Larkspur					
D. geyeri	40–80	>1500	Desert shrub, mountain brush, sagebrush, short-grass prairie	–	–

[a] *Tall larkspur and low larkspur species are each ranked according to the concentration of toxic alkaloids, from greatest (1) to least (4).*
[b] *The risk of losing cattle to tall larkspur species is a subjective evaluation based on plant toxicity, numbers of grazing cattle threatened during the growing season, and the geographical distribution of the larkspur species.* Delphinium glaucescens *is relatively more toxic late in the growing season compared to mature plants of the other tall larkspur species. Spatial and temporal variability in plant density and toxicity preclude making such a risk assessment ranking for low larkspurs and plains larkspur.*
[c] D. glaucum = D. brownii *in Canada; livestock losses to* D. brownii *in Canada may greatly exceed those of* D. glaucum *in the United States.*

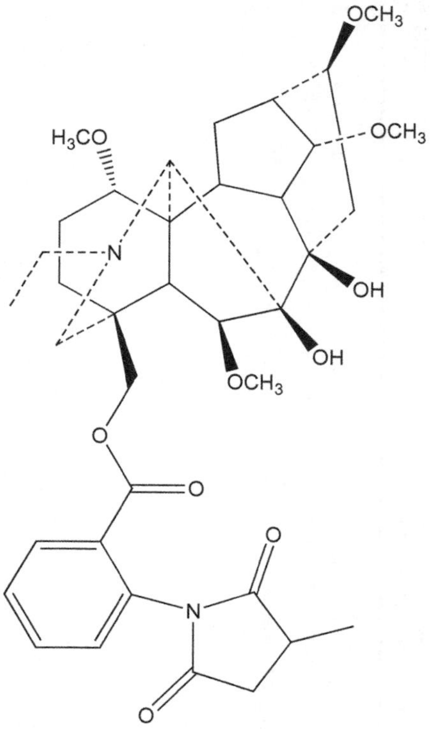

(2)
Methyllycaconitine (MLA)

Toxicology

Larkspurs (*Delphinium* spp.) are a serious toxic problem for cattle on foothill and mountain rangelands in western North America. The toxicity of larkspur plants is due to norditerpenoid alkaloids, which occur as one of two chemical structural types – the 7,8-methylenedioxylycoctonine (MDL) type and the *N*-(methylsuccinimido) anthranoyllycoctonine (MSAL) type. Although the MSAL-type alkaloids are much more toxic (typically >20 ×) (Panter et al., 2002), the MDL-type alkaloids are generally more abundant in *D. barbeyi* and *D. occidentale* populations (Gardner et al., 2002). Three MSAL-type alkaloids that are of primary concern are methyllycaconitine (MLA **(2)**), 14-deacetylnudicauline (DAN), and nudicauline (NUD). MLA and DAN occur to some extent in all classes of larkspurs, whereas NUD occurs only in low and plains larkspurs. The LD_{50} for NUD, MLA, and DAN in mice is 2.7, 4.8, and 4.0 mg/ kg intravenously (i.v.), respectively (Table 61.3; Panter et al., 2002). The toxic alkaloid concentration of the tall larkspur (*D. barbeyi*) dosed to cattle in a lethality study was not determined. However, data from a pen study in which Hereford cattle were dosed via oral gavage with ground plant material indicate that a lethal dose of *D. glaucum* is approximately 2.5 g dried plant material/kg body weight (BW) (unpublished observations). The lethal dose in a grazing situation, however, may be quite different due to the fact that tall larkspur is often ingested repeatedly over 2–4 days.

There are two primary structural features necessary for toxicity: (1) an *N*-ethyl bicyclo tertiary alkaloid nitrogen atom and (2) a C-18 anthranilic acid ester. Other studies have also shown that MLA's aromatic ester function is a significant haptophore and that the succinimide group imparts significant toxicity to alkaloids. Two other structural features also enhance toxicity: (1) functionality at the anthranilic acid amine nitrogen and (2) functionality at C-14 (Panter et al., 2002).

Tall larkspur species vary substantially in toxicity, with a relative ranking (most to least toxic, based on the MSAL alkaloid content) of *D. glaucum* (*D. brownii* in Canada), *D. barbeyi*, *D. glaucescens*, and *D. occidentale*. Generally in tall larkspurs, the concentration of MLA and DAN is highest in immature plant tissue. MLA concentrations in immature tall larkspurs may exceed 20 mg/g. Before shattering, tall larkspur pods are relatively high in toxicity (MLA + DAN = 7–12 mg/g). Toxicity declines rapidly in tall larkspurs once pods begin to shatter. Measuring plant toxicity early in the growing season may allow prediction of season-long toxicity and risk (Ralphs et al., 2002).

Due to the fact that the MSAL-type alkaloids are much more toxic than the MDL-type alkaloids, management recommendations for grazing cattle on larkspur-containing ranges are based primarily on the concentration of MSAL-type alkaloids in larkspur (Pfister et al., 2002; Ralphs et al., 2002). However, in many species of tall larkspur, the MDL-type alkaloids are generally more abundant (Pfister et al., 1999; Gardner et al., 2002). Research using a mouse model suggested that MDL-type alkaloids enhance the overall acute toxicity of MLA in an additive manner (Welch et al., 2008). In subsequent studies with cattle, the MSAL-type alkaloids such as MLA were the primary factors responsible for the toxicity of larkspur plants (Welch et al., 2010). However, populations of larkspur plants that contained large amounts of MDL-type alkaloids, in addition to high MSAL-type alkaloid content, were found to be more dangerous to cattle than plants with only high MSAL-type alkaloids. Consequently, for a larkspur plant to be toxic to livestock, a sufficient quantity of MSAL-type alkaloids is required. However, MDL-type alkaloids appear to potentiate the overall toxicity of the MSAL-type alkaloids and should be considered when predicting potential toxicity of larkspur populations. Therefore, when chemical analyses are performed on larkspur plants to assess their toxic potential, the concentration of both the MSAL-type and the total alkaloids should be determined, with more weight given to the MSAL-type alkaloids.

MLA and NUD are the dominant toxic alkaloids in low larkspurs, with concentration ranges of 0.8–4.5 and 1–4 mg/g, respectively, for MLA and NUD in low

TABLE 61.3 Relative Toxicity of Individual Larkspur Alkaloids in Order of Toxicity According to Alkaloid Class and Determined by Mouse Bioassay

MSAL class	Lycoctonine class	MDL class
Alkaloid; LD_{50} (mg/kg)	Alkaloid; LD_{50} (mg/kg)	Alkaloid; LD50 (mg/kg)
Nudicauline; 2.5 i.v.	Anthronyllycoctonine; <365 s.c.	Deltaline; 720 s.c., 133 i.v.
14-Deacetylnudicauline; 4.5 i.v.	Lycoctonine; 75 i.v.	14-*O*-acetyldictyocarpine; 110 i.v.
Methyllycaconitine (MLA); 7.5 i.v.	14-Dehydrobrownine; >254 s.c.	Dictyocarpine; >2000 s.c
Barbinine; >115.5 i.v.	Brownine; >720 s.c.	

i.v., intravenous; MDL, 7,8-methylene dioxyllycoctonine (least toxic); MSAL, methylsuccinimido anthranoyllycoctonine (most toxic); s.c., sub-cutaneous. From Panter et al. (2002) and Welch et al. (2008).

larkspur populations (*D. nuttallianum* and *D. andersonii*) in Utah, Colorado, and Arizona (Gardner, unpublished data). Reports of very high concentrations of MLA (up to 8.7 mg/g) in vegetative low larkspur (*D. nuttallianum*) from Canada were contrasted with a concentration of 2 mg/g in flowering plants (Bai et al., 1994). Unlike tall larkspurs, concentrations of toxic alkaloids in low larkspurs do not decline precipitously after senescence (Gardner, unpublished data). MLA is the major toxic alkaloid in plains larkspur (*D. geyeri*), with concentrations ranging from 1 to 4 mg/g in Wyoming and Colorado. We emphasize that NUD is more toxic than MLA, and both alkaloids are frequently found together in low larkspurs (Gardner, unpublished data). Thus, the potential lethality of low larkspurs can be highly variable depending on alkaloid concentrations and plant density.

The primary result of larkspur toxicosis is neuromuscular paralysis from blockage at the postsynaptic neuromuscular junction (Benn and Jacyno, 1983). MLA also elicits central effects in mice and rats (Stegelmeier et al., 1998). Larkspur alkaloids compete as postsynaptic inhibitors of acetylcholine particularly at α_1 nicotinic sites (Dobelis et al., 1999). MLA strongly competes with α-bungarotoxin at nicotinic acetylcholine receptors (nAChRs). Larkspur alkaloid binding to nAChRs appears to be correlated with toxicity in various tissues and may explain sheep tolerance to larkspur if larkspur toxins bind less avidly to nAChRs in sheep (Stegelmeier et al., 1998).

Clinical signs of intoxication include muscular weakness and trembling, straddled stance, periodic collapse into sternal recumbency, respiratory difficulty, and death while in lateral recumbency. An effective dose of larkspur causes labored breathing, rapid and irregular heartbeat, and collapse but not death. The effective i.v. dose for purified MLA is 2 mg/kg BW in calves versus 10 mg/kg in sheep given a single injection (Panter, unpublished data). Nation et al. (1982) reported that an effective dose of MLA in cattle receiving two i.v. injections was 1.1 mg/kg. Conversely, the effective i.v. dose for deltaline in both calves and sheep is 50 mg/kg (Panter, unpublished data). Cattle typically show clinical signs (i.e., tremors and periodic collapse) when given an MLA DAN dose (i.e., via ground plant) of 20 ± 3 mg/ kg BW (Pfister et al., 1994). Stress and/or exertion will reduce the effective dose. Assuming an MLA + DAN concentration of 5 mg/g (dry wt), a 450-kg cow may show clinical signs after rapidly eating 1.8 kg (dry wt) of tall larkspur ($\approx$7.2 kg wet wt).

Key factors in larkspur intoxication are the amount eaten and the rate of ingestion. Studies utilizing direct observations of grazing animals have provided a number of insights into the amount and timing of tall larkspur ingestion. More than 10 such studies have been conducted since 1986 and have led to two major conclusions: (1) cattle eat little or no tall larkspur before the plant has elongated flowering racemes, and (2) weather patterns are very important determinants of larkspur consumption (Pfister et al., 1999). Cattle often eat more tall larkspur during summer storms and reduce larkspur consumption during drought for reasons that are not clear. Another variable that may play a role in the susceptibility of cattle to larkspur toxicosis is breed differences. Anecdotal observations of differences in the susceptibility of different breeds of cattle to larkspur toxicosis have been supported using a rodent model in which different strains of mice had up to a twofold difference in LD_{50} to MLA (Welch et al., 2009a).

Cattle generally begin consuming tall larkspur after flowering racemes are elongated, and consumption increases as larkspur matures. Consumption usually peaks during the pod stage of growth in late summer, when cattle may eat large quantities (25–30% of diet as herd average; >60% on some days by individual animals). Because larkspur toxicity generally declines throughout the growing season and cattle tend to eat more larkspur after flowering, the period of greatest danger has been termed a "toxic window" (Pfister et al., 2002). This toxic window extends from the flower stage into the pod stage, or approximately 5 weeks depending on temperature and elevation (Figure 61.3). Many ranchers typically defer grazing on tall larkspur-infested ranges until the flower stage to avoid death losses. This approach wastes much valuable forage and often places cattle into larkspur-infested pastures when risk of losses is high. An

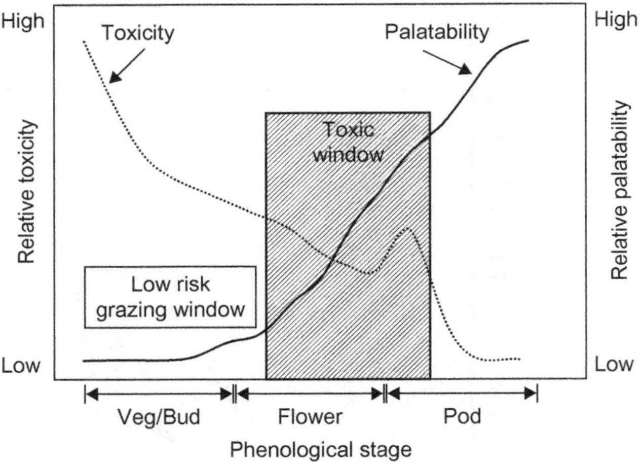

FIGURE 61.3 Relationship between toxicity and palatability in tall larkspurs. Most cattle deaths are predicted to occur during the toxic window when the concentration of toxic alkaloids is relatively high and consumption by cattle begins to increase after flowering racemes elongate. There is a low-risk grazing window early in the season before flowering when larkspur is generally very toxic but risk is low because cattle typically eat little tall larkspur during this phenological stage. There is also a low-risk grazing window in late summer after pods shatter.

additional 4–6 weeks of grazing may be obtained by grazing these ranges early, before larkspur elongates flowering racemes. The risk of losing cattle is low when grazing before flowering, even though larkspur is very toxic, because larkspur consumption is typically very low. Once pods are mature and begin to shatter, larkspur ranges can usually be grazed with impunity because pod toxicity declines rapidly, and leaf toxicity is low. Based on limited study, cattle increase consumption of low larkspur after flowering, and increases in grazing pressure increase amounts of low larkspur eaten by cattle. No consistent consumption patterns of plains larkspur (*D. geyeri*) by cattle were found; thus, management recommendations need to be tailored to each specific year and location (Pfister et al., 2002).

Studies have been performed to characterize the kinetic profile of larkspur alkaloids in cattle (Green et al., 2009b, 2011). In these studies, the elimination half-life of MLA from cattle dosed once with dried and finely ground larkspur via oral gavage was approximately 20 h. In addition, the T_{max}, or time to maximal toxin concentration, was approximately 10 h. These data suggest that cattle that have consumed larkspur will be most susceptible to poisoning 10 h after consumption, and that after the cattle have stopped consuming larkspur, greater than 99% of the toxins will be eliminated after 6 days.

Prevention and Management of Poisoning

Grazing Management

A simple and low-risk grazing management scheme can often be used based simply on tall larkspur growth and phenology: (1) graze during early summer when sufficient forage is available until larkspur elongates flowering racemes (4–6 weeks depending on elevation and weather); (2) remove livestock, or contend with potentially high risk from flowering to early pod stages of growth (4 or 5 weeks); and (3) graze with low risk during the late season when larkspur pods begin to shatter (4–6 weeks). This scheme can be refined substantially if livestock producers periodically obtain an estimate of the toxicity of tall larkspur, and if ranchers spend time periodically observing and documenting larkspur consumption by grazing cattle.

Management to reduce losses to low larkspur begins with recognition of the plant during spring. Vegetative low larkspur plants will typically begin growth before the major forage grasses. Low larkspur populations fluctuate with environmental conditions (Pfister, unpublished data). Risk of losing cattle is much higher during years with dense populations. During those years, recognizing the plant, and finding alternative pasture or waiting to graze infested pastures for 4–6 weeks until the low larkspur has dried up, will reduce losses. In addition, it is recommended that animals not be watered or provided mineral supplementation in areas that have high densities of larkspurs.

Graze Sheep Before Cattle

Sheep can be herded into or bedded on the patches to reduce larkspur availability or acceptability to cattle on tall larkspur-infested ranges where larkspur grows as discrete patches. In those areas in which larkspur is uniformly spaced over a pasture, sheep must eat immature larkspur and leave sufficient feed for subsequent grazing by cattle. This can be problematic because early growth tall larkspur may not be palatable to sheep. Our observations (Pfister, unpublished data) indicate that sheep eat little low larkspur (*D. nuttallianum*) unless a high stock density is used.

Drug Intervention

A variety of remedies have been applied in the field when ranchers find intoxicated animals (e.g., bleeding by cutting the tail), but most are without a solid scientific rationale. Any imagined success with these treatments was probably related to the dose. If less than a lethal dose were ingested, the animal would likely recover despite any treatment, unless bloat or aspiration pneumonia occurred during recumbency. Treatment for overt poisoning is usually symptomatic, and recovery is often spontaneous if animals are not stressed further by driving. Once the animal is observed showing muscular tremors, it should be allowed to drop back and proceed at its own pace. Poisoned animals should never be forced to continue moving because this will exacerbate the clinical effects and can result in death. Drugs that increase acetylcholine effectiveness at the neuromuscular junction have potential for reversing larkspur toxicosis or reducing susceptibility. The cholinergic drug physostigmine (0.08 mg/kg i.v.) has been successfully used under field and pen conditions to reverse clinical larkspur intoxication (Nation et al., 1982; Pfister et al., 1994). Similarly, i.v. administration of neostigmine (0.04 mg/kg) significantly reduced clinical signs in cattle (Green et al., 2009a), and neostigmine administered intramuscularly at 0.02 mg/kg can be used as a rescue treatment for cattle in recumbency. This reversal lasts approximately 2 h, and repeated injections of physostigmine are sometimes required. Under field conditions, physostigmine temporarily abates clinical signs and animals quickly (~15 min) become ambulatory. Depending on the larkspur dose, the intoxication may recur. The use of physostigmine-based treatments may aggravate losses in the absence of further treatment if suddenly ambulatory animals later develop increased muscular fatigue, dyspnea, and death.

Herbicidal Control

Larkspur losses can be greatly reduced if dense larkspur populations are reduced by herbicides. Picloram, metsulfuron, and glyphosate have proven to be effective in killing tall larkspurs when applied at specific growth stages (Ralphs et al., 1991). These herbicides do not reduce toxic alkaloid concentrations in treated larkspur plants, and metsulfuron may increase toxicity. Therefore, sprayed areas should not be grazed until the following growing season.

LUPINES (*LUPINUS* SPP.)

The *Lupinus* genus contains more than 150 species of annual, perennial, or soft woody shrub lupines. More than 95 species occur in California alone. The lupines are rich in alkaloids, responsible for most of the toxic and teratogenic properties. There are domestic lupines that through plant breeding are low in alkaloid content and have been selected for ornamental purposes or for animal and human food. Only those range lupines known to cause poisoning or birth defects are discussed here.

Stockmen have long recognized the toxicity of lupines when livestock, particularly sheep, were poisoned in the fall by the pods and seeds of lupine. Major losses in sheep were reported in the 1950s, and individual flock losses of hundreds and even thousands were reported. Lupines are also poisonous to other livestock, and field cases of poisoning in cattle, horses, and goats have been reported. However, the most recognized condition of lupine ingestion is the "crooked calf syndrome," a congenital condition in calves resulting in skeletal contracture-type malformations and cleft palate after their mothers have grazed lupines during sensitive periods of pregnancy (Panter et al., 1999a,b). The condition was first reported in 1959 and experimentally confirmed after large outbreaks in Oregon and Montana in 1967.

Description

Lupines belong to the Leguminosae family, with alternate palmately compound leaves with 5–17 oblong to lanceolate leaflets (Figure 61.4). Flowers are terminal legume-like and can be blue, purple, white, yellow, or reddish. The seeds are flattened in legume-like pods. Range lupines are generally low, perennial or annual forbs, and species and varieties are taxonomically difficult because extensive hybridization occurs and the literature may be somewhat confusing in this regard.

The plant grows early in spring, flowering in early to mid-summer, and forms pods in late summer or early fall. Seedlings may germinate in fall if temperature and moisture are conducive for seed germination. Some lupines are annuals and others are woody and shrub-like; however, neither the annual nor the woody species have been reported in livestock poisoning.

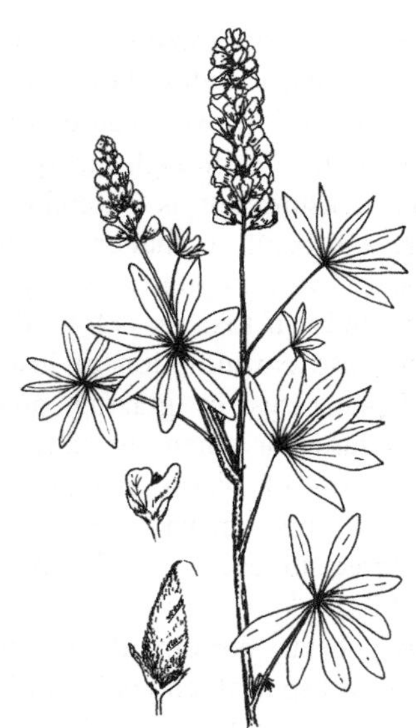

FIGURE 61.4 Lupinus leucophyllus.

Chemical profiles (chemo-taxonomy) can support or contradict taxonomic identification, and this is a valuable resource if included in a voucher specimen, especially if the identified species is implicated in toxicoses or teratogenicity and is identified by geographical location. Cook et al. (2009b) demonstrated this variability in a single species, *Lupinus sulphureus*, which is yellow lupine species, selected from herbaria or collected from different geographical regions of Oregon, Washington, and British Columbia. A total of seven distinct alkaloid profiles were reported, and each alkaloid profile was unique in its geographical distribution and its potential risk to livestock. A collection near Pendleton, Oregon, came from a population that was responsible for a significant outbreak of crooked calf syndrome in a herd of cattle (56% loss) and the alkaloid profile showed high levels of the teratogen anagyrine (Panter et al., 1997). Therefore, taxonomic classification without chemical support is of little value in predicting risk of crooked calf syndrome.

Distribution

Most species of lupines grow in states and provinces from the Rocky Mountains westward. They are classified as increaser species; that is, they increase in abundance following disturbance from overgrazing or fire, to the point that they may dominate the plant community at times. Their populations also cycle, increasing in wet years and dying back during drought. Table 61.4 lists species involved in toxicity and their common names, habitats, and geographical distribution.

TABLE 61.4 Lupine Species Known to be Toxic or Teratogenic

Scientific Name	Common Name	Habitat	Distribution
L. alpestris	Mountain silvery lupine	Dry rocky soils	CA to MT, CO and AZ
L. arcticus			AK, British Columbia
L. andersonii	Anderson's lupine	Mountain meadows and clearings	Sierra Nevada, CA to 2900 m elevation
L. arbustus	Spur lupine	Dry open hillsides	NV, CA to CO, western MT
L. argenteus	Silvery lupine	1200–1500 m elevation; dry flats, slopes, woods, open hillsides	CA to MT, NM, OR, ID, UT, NV
L. caudatus	Tail cup lupine		CA, OR, ID to UT, NV
L. cyaneus			MT
L. formosus	Lunara lupine	Dry flats	CA
L. greenei		Plains and hills	WY, NV, CO, AZ
L. latifolius	Broad-leaved lupine	Mountain meadows, stream banks	Pacific states
L. laxiflorus	Spurred lupine	Hillsides, dry soils	WA, OR, ID
L. leucophyllus	White-leaved lupine, poison lupine	Dry soils	WA, MT, UT, CA
L. nootkatensis	Nootka lupine		AK
L. onustus	Plumes lupine	Open pine wood	CA
L. polyphyllus (five varieties)	Meadow lupine	Mountain meadows, banks	WA, British Columbia
L. pusillus	Rusty lupine, small lupine	Dry plains	British Columbia to KS, NM, AZ
L. sericeus	Silky lupine	Dry hills, valleys	UT, WY to MT, British Columbia
L. sulphureus	Yellow lupine	Open hillsides	OR

Toxicology

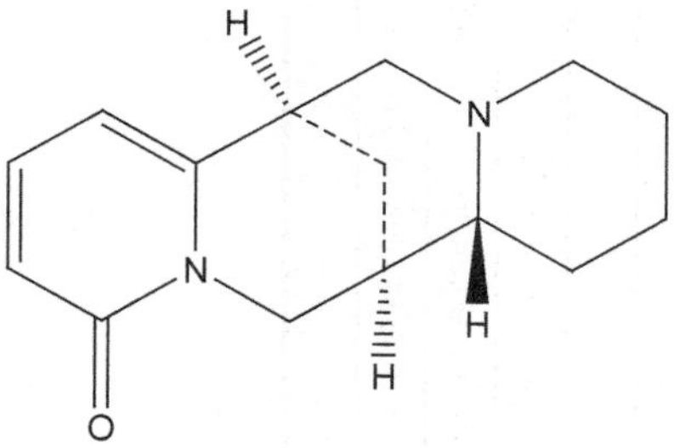

(3)
Anagyrine

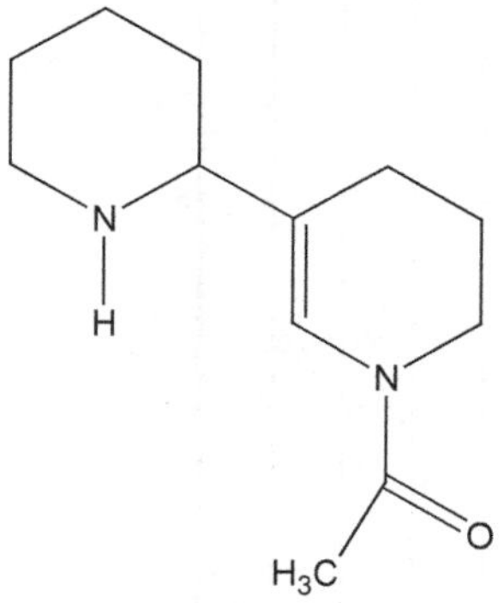

(4)
Ammodendrine

Most lupine species contain quinolizidine alkaloids, a few contain piperidine alkaloids, and some contain both. The specific alkaloids responsible for crooked calf syndrome are anagyrine (**3**), ammodendrine (**4**), and *N*-methyl ammodendrine. Hence, risk is based on chemical profile and the presence and concentration of these teratogenic alkaloids. It is known that chemical profile and concentration differ, resulting in changing levels of toxicity within and between species and populations. The chemical phenology has been studied in *L. caudatus* and *L. leucophyllus* (Lee et al., 2007b). Total alkaloid concentration is high in the new early growth but diluted as the plant biomass increases. Pools of total alkaloids increase during the phenological growth stages and peak at the pod stage, concentrating in the pods. The teratogenic alkaloid anagyrine appears to be an end product in the biosynthetic pathway and accumulates in the floral parts and is stored in the seed. Following seed shatter, both concentration and pools of all alkaloids decline precipitously, leaving the senescent plant relatively nontoxic.

Stockmen recognize the toxicity of lupines in the fall when the pods and seeds are ripe. Historically, lupines were responsible for more sheep deaths than any other single plant in Montana, Idaho, and Utah. Most losses occurred from hungry sheep grazing seed pods. Poisoning occurred following trucking or trailing bands in late summer or fall or after getting caught in early snowstorms that covered herbaceous vegetation. Hungry sheep nonselectively grazed lupine pods, which are highest in alkaloids, and were poisoned. Large losses have also occurred when lupine hay harvested in the seed pod stage was fed in winter. Seeds alone can be toxic to sheep at 0.25–1.5% of their body weight depending on alkaloid composition. A few cases of poisoning occurred on young plants. Losses of 80–100 sheep in multiple bands have been reported during the past 5 years in Idaho and Wyoming (Panter, personal communication, 2005).

Poisoning by lupine plants should not be confused with lupinosis reported in Australia. This condition is entirely different and is a mycotoxicosis of livestock caused by toxins produced by the fungus *Phomopsis leptostromiformis*, which colonizes domestic lupine stubble. It affects livestock that graze lupine stubble and limits the use of this animal feed in Australia.

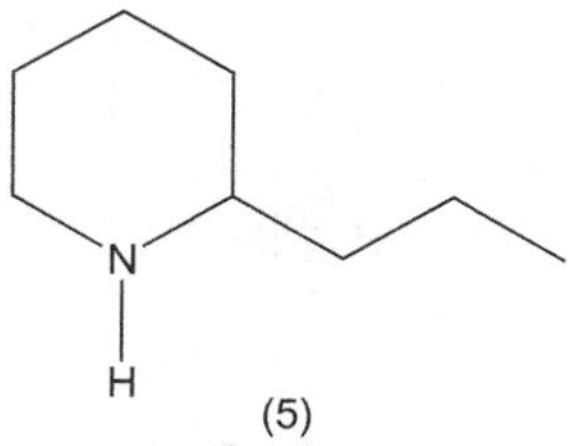

(5)
Coniine

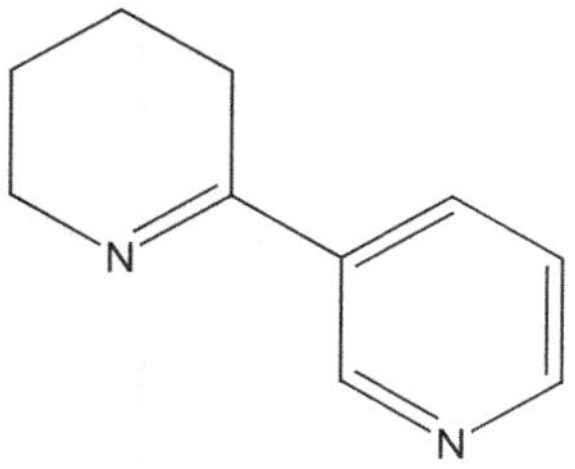

(6)
Anabasine

The lupine-induced crooked calf syndrome was first reported in 1959 and 1960 and experimentally confirmed in 1967 (Panter et al., 1999a). Crooked calf disease includes various skeletal contracture-type birth defects and occasionally cleft palate. The skeletal defects are similar to an inherited genetic condition reported in Charolais cattle. Based on epidemiologic evidence and chemical comparison of teratogenic and nonteratogenic lupines, the quinolizidine alkaloid anagyrine was determined to be the teratogen (Keeler, 1973). A second teratogen, a piperidine alkaloid called ammodendrine found in *Lupinus formosus*, was also demonstrated to cause the condition (Keeler and Panter, 1989). Further research determined that the anagyrine-containing lupines only caused birth defects in cattle and did not affect sheep or goats; however, the piperidine-containing lupine *L. formosus* induced similar birth defects in cattle and goats (Keeler and Panter, 1989). This led to interesting speculation about possible metabolism or absorption differences between cattle and small ruminants. Keeler and Panter (1989) hypothesized that perhaps the cow was metabolizing the anagyrine to a complex piperidine, meeting the structural characteristics determined for a teratogenic piperidine. This was supported by feeding trials with other piperidine-containing plants, extracts, and pure compounds. Coniine (**5**), a simple piperidine from poison hemlock, and anabasine (**6**), a simple piperidine from tree tobacco (*Nicotiana glauca*), induced the same defects in cattle, sheep, and goats. Although comparative studies support the hypothesis that the cow may metabolize the quinolizidine anagyrine to a complex piperidine, evidence regarding the absorption and elimination patterns of many of the quinolizidine alkaloids, including anagyrine, in cattle, sheep, and goats does not support the metabolism theory (Gardner and Panter, 1993). This research is currently ongoing at the Poisonous Plant Research Laboratory. A review of lupine-induced cases of crooked calf syndrome reported to the Poisonous Plant Research Lab during the past 20 years can be found in Lee et al. (2007a).

Different lupines produce varying toxic syndromes in a given species of livestock, apparently because the alkaloid profile varies remarkably among species. Season and environment influence alkaloid concentration in a given species of lupine. Generally, alkaloid content is highest in young plants and in mature seeds. Alkaloids are not lost upon drying, so wild hay may be highly toxic if young lupine plants or especially seed pods are present. For many lupines, the time and degree of seeding vary from year to year. Most losses occur under conditions in which animals consume large amounts of pods in a brief period, such as when they are being driven through an area of heavy lupine growth, unloaded into such an area, trailed through an area where the grass is covered by snow but the lupine is not, or when feeding lupine hay when lupine is in the pod stage, which apparently is palatable. Most serious poisonings may occur in the late summer or early fall because lupine remains green after other forage has dried and seed pods are present. Once the poisonings were understood, the practice of harvesting lupine hay for winter sheep feed was discontinued.

Cattle Grazing

Lupine is not very palatable to cattle, although it has been considered fair to good quality feed on some ranges that are heavily utilized. Its palatability or acceptability depends on availability and maturity of other forage. In a grazing study of velvet lupine (*L. leucophyllus*) on annual cheatgrass ranges in eastern Washington (Ralphs et al., 2006), cows selected lupine in July and August after cheatgrass dried and other forbs were depleted or matured and became rank. The deep-rooted lupine remained green and succulent longer into the summer than the other forage. Lupine was higher in crude protein and lower in fiber (NDF) than the other forages throughout the season (the crude protein level in foliage was 15%, and in seeds it was 36%). However, the thick, velvety pubescence was believed to be partially responsible for its lack of palatability. The high alkaloid concentration in the floral parts

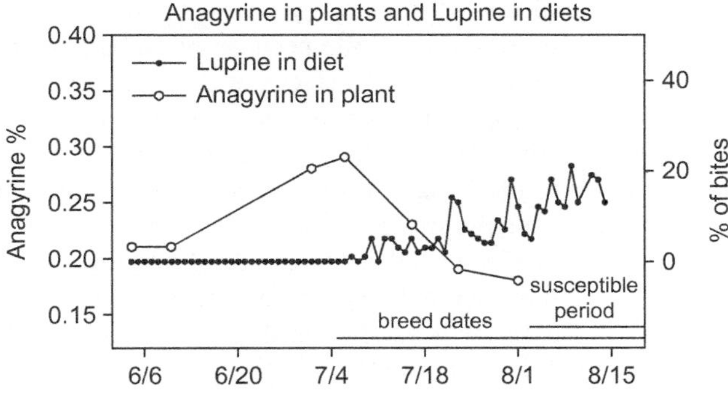

FIGURE 61.5 The relationship between the concentration of the teratogen anagyrine in the plant and the amount of lupine in the diets of cattle during breeding and susceptible gestational stages.

and seed pods may also have contributed to its lack of palatability. Once the seeds shattered in early July, the alkaloid concentration declined, and the cows began selecting lupine. Figure 61.5 shows the overlap of lupine consumption with the susceptible period of gestation, in relation to the anagyrine concentration in the lupine plants. Cattle selected velvet lupine in July after cheatgrass and other forbs matured.

The abundance of lupine is another factor influencing the amount of lupine consumed. Lupine population cycles are influenced by weather patterns. Catastrophic losses from lupine-induced crooked calves occurred in the Channel Scabland region of eastern Washington in 1997. Annual precipitation from 1995 to 1997 was 33% above average, initiating an outbreak of lupine throughout the region. The density of velvet lupine plants has declined since then (Ralphs, unpublished data), and the incidence of crooked calves has returned to what has become an acceptable tolerance of 1–5% incidence.

Clinical signs of poisoning are those of muscular weakness (neuromuscular blockade) beginning with nervousness, frequent urination and defecation, depression, frothing at the mouth, relaxation of the nictitating membrane, ataxia, muscular fasciculations, weakness, lethargy, collapse, sternal recumbency followed by lateral recumbency, respiratory failure, and death. Signs may appear within 15 min to 1 h after ingestion or as late as 24 h depending on the amount and rate of ingestion. Death usually results from respiratory paralysis.

The incidence of crooked calves is variable geographically and from year to year within a given herd. Up to 100% of a given calf crop may be affected, and individuals may be more severely affected than others. Affected calves are generally born alive at full term. Dystocia may occur when calves are severely deformed and assistance is required, often by cesarean section.

Arthrogryposis is the most common malformation observed and is often accompanied by one or more of the following: scoliosis, torticollis, kyphosis, or cleft palate. Elbow joints are often immobile because of malalignment of the ulna with the articular surfaces of the distal extremity of the humerus. The part of the limb distal to the elbow joint is often rotated laterally. In crooked calf disease, the osseous changes observed are permanent and generally become progressively worse as the calf grows and its limbs are subjected to greater load-bearing stress. Frequently, minor contractions such as "buck knees" often attributed to lupine will resolve on their own and the calf will appear relatively normal.

No breed predilection or genetic susceptibility to the lupine-induced condition has been determined. Likewise, lactation or age did not influence the propensity for cattle to graze lupine (Pfister et al., 2008a). However, body condition was shown to affect the absorption and elimination half-life of anagyrine in sheep (Lopez-Ortiz et al., 2004). Research on cattle has demonstrated that body condition impacts absorption, distribution, and elimination of the alkaloids and therefore could impact the risk of toxicity or teratogenic outcome of lupines (Lee et al., 2008d). This difference in toxicokinetics was significant for two teratogenic alkaloids – anagyrine and ammodendrine. The disposition of teratogenic alkaloids in the fetal compartment is unknown and will require further research.

The sensitive gestational period in the pregnant cow for exposure is 40–70 days with suspicious periods extending to day 100 (Panter et al., 1997). The condition has been experimentally induced with dried ground lupine at 1 g/kg BW and with semi-purified preparations of anagyrine (the apparent teratogen) at 30 mg anagyrine/kg BW fed daily from 30 to 70 days of gestation. The dose range of anagyrine to cause crooked calves is 6.5–11.9 mg/kg BW/day for 3 or 4 weeks during gestation days 40–70. Crooked calf disease has also been induced by feeding the piperidine alkaloid-containing lupine, *L. formosus* (Keeler and Panter, 1989). The teratogenic piperidines, ammodendrine, *N*-acetylhystrine, and *N*-methyl ammodendrine, are absorbed quickly after ingestion and can be detected in blood plasma by 0.5 h, with peak levels maintained for more than 24 h (Gardner and Panter, 1993). The mechanism of action has been determined to be an alkaloid-induced reduction in fetal movement by a neuromuscular blocking effect during the critical stages of gestation (Panter et al., 1990a). This inhibition of fetal movement is due to stimulation followed by desensitization of skeletal muscle-type nAChR (Lee et al., 2006). This mechanism is a common factor for multiple alkaloids found in many species of lupines, poison hemlock (*Conium*), and wild tree tobacco (*N. glauca*), and research using TE-671 cells that express human fetal muscle-type nAChR and SH-SY5Y cells that express human autonomic-type nAChR supports this mechanism (Green et al., 2010). Interestingly, many of these teratogenic alkaloids are produced in the plants as enantiomeric pairs and exhibit differences in activity using these specialized cells and when compared using a mouse bioassay (Lee et al., 2006, 2008a–c). This inhibited fetal activity is responsible for the skeletal contracture malformations and cleft palates (Panter et al., 1990a), and a goat model developed in the 1990s using anabasine as the teratogen and ultrasound imaging to evaluate fetotoxicity has been utilized for biomedical research to improve treatments and potential fetal intervention for cleft palate in children (Panter and Keeler, 1992; Weinzweig et al., 1999, 2008).

Prevention, Management, and Treatment

Keeler et al. (1977) proposed a simple management solution to prevent crooked calves: stagger grazing of lupine-infested pastures so that the susceptible period of gestation (40–70 days) does not overlap the flower and pod stage of growth when anagyrine is highest. Ralphs et al. (2006) refined Keeler's recommendations to restrict access during the susceptible period of gestation, when anagyrine concentration is still high in the flower and pod stage, only when cattle are likely to eat lupine, and in years when it is abundant. Panter (unpublished data) suggested that intermittent grazing between lupine pastures and clean pastures would allow the fetus to regain normal movement for a few days during the sensitive stage of gestation. It has been hypothesized that inhibited fetal movement over a prolonged period of time is required for severe malformations to occur (Panter et al., 1999a).

Lupines are easily controlled with 2,4-D-type broadleaf herbicides (Ralphs et al., 1991); however, herbicide treatment alone rarely provides long-term solutions to poisonous plant problems. Seed reserves in the soil will rapidly reestablish the stands if grazing management practices are not implemented.

Death losses in sheep can be reduced by recognizing the variability in lupine toxicity with stage of growth and the conditions under which animals graze the plant. Providing a choice of other quality forages usually prevents excess lupine grazing. The dangerous period of plant growth for sheep exists mainly with plants in the pod stage. The hazard increases if sheep are hungry, as is often the case with crowding, hauling, driving, or overgrazed conditions. The hazard is reduced or eliminated when lupine is in post-seed stage.

Treatment for overt poisoning is usually symptomatic, and recovery is often spontaneous if animals are not stressed further by driving. Once the animal is observed showing muscular tremors, it should be allowed to drop back and proceed at its own pace. Poisoned animals should never be forced to continue moving because this will exacerbate the clinical effects and can result in death.

The elimination of the toxic alkaloids in the urine is quite rapid ($t_{½} = 6.32–6.88$ h) and begins within hours of ingestion (Lopez-Ortiz et al., 2004). Therefore, allowing the animal to rest and move slowly will often result in full recovery within 24 h. There is no treatment for the malformations, and euthanasia is recommended for the serious skeletal defects and cleft palate. However, less severe contracture defects, particularly of the front legs (buck knees), will often resolve if the knee joint can be locked within 1 week after birth. If not, the defect generally becomes worse with growth and size, and although the animal will continue to grow, the front legs will break down and the animal will not be adequate for the feedlot.

Summary

A reduction in incidence can be expected and has been achieved by using one or more of the following: (1) coordinating grazing periods according to plant growth stage, (2) changing time of breeding by either advancing or delaying or changing from spring to fall calving, (3) reducing lupine populations through herbicide treatment, and (4) intermittent grazing between clean pastures and lupine pastures to break the cycle of lupine ingestion.

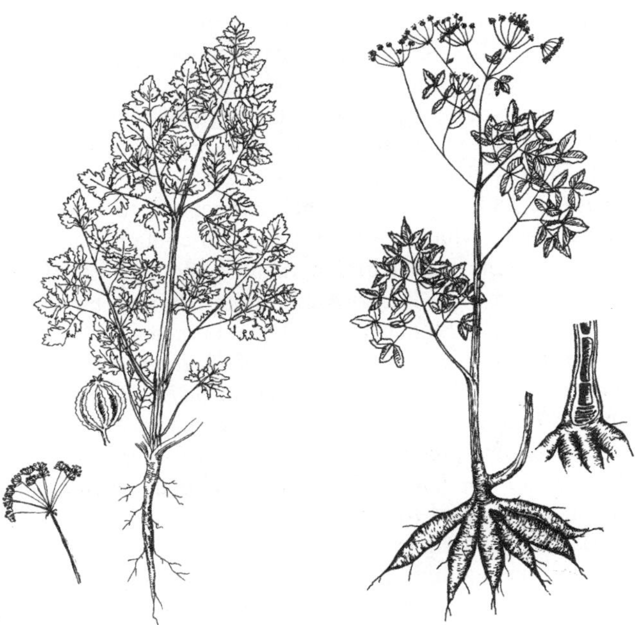

FIGURE 61.6 The hemlocks – poison hemlock (*Conium maculatum*) on the left and water hemlock (*Cicuta douglassii*) on the right. Note the tubers and partitioned stalk on water hemlock versus the single taproot on poison hemlock. Leaf structure is different, and poison hemlock has purple spots on the stems.

POISON HEMLOCK (*CONIUM MACULATUM*)

Poison hemlock was introduced into the United States as an ornamental herb and grows throughout the country. Generally, poison hemlock grows in waste areas where adequate moisture will sustain the biennial stands. Four species are recognized worldwide, but only one (*Conium maculatum*) is found in the United States. Historically, poison hemlock has been associated with human poisoning more than livestock and is believed to be the tea used to execute Socrates.

Description

Unlike the lupines, locoweeds, etc., multiple *Conium* species are few worldwide, and only one species, *C. maculatum*, is described in the United States. *Conium maculatum* is a biennial plant 1–2.5 m tall (Figure 61.6). The stems are stout, rigid, smooth, and hollow except at the nodes. A distinguishing characteristic of the plant is the purple spots found up and down the main stem and a single carrot-like taproot. The leaves are large, triangular, fern-like, and alternate on the erect stem. The stem grows the second year from a rosette and taproot established from seed. Frequently, seeds will germinate in the fall before winter and then complete their reproductive cycle the following year. The flowers are small, white or cream colored, and in umbellate clusters. The fruits are grayish brown with conspicuous wavy, knotted ridges. The plant has a fleshy, usually unbranched, white taproot that looks like parsnips. Roots have been mistaken for parsnip, seeds for anise, and leaves for parsley.

The geographical distribution of poison hemlock is throughout the United States, restricted only by cultivation and adequate moisture to sustain stands of the plant from year to year. The plant usually grows in waste places where moisture may accumulate and protect it from cultivation.

Toxicology

N

(7)
γ-coniceine

Eight piperidine alkaloids are known in poison hemlock, five of which are commonly discussed in the literature. Two alkaloids (coniine **(5)** and γ-coniceine **(7)**) are prevalent and likely responsible for toxicity and teratogenicity of the plant. γ-Coniceine is the predominant alkaloid in the early vegetative stage of plant growth and is a bio-chemical precursor to the other *Conium* alkaloids

(Panter and Keeler, 1989). Coniine predominates in late growth and is found mainly in the seeds. γ-Coniceine is seven or eight times more toxic than coniine in mice. This makes the early growth plant most dangerous in the early spring and the seedlings and regrowth again in the fall. This is also the time when green feed is limited to livestock and may impact their propensity to graze this plant. Seeds, which are very toxic, can contaminate poultry and swine cereal grains (Panter and Keeler, 1989). Plants often lose their toxicity upon drying, but seeds remain toxic as long as the seed coat is intact.

An analysis of a single plant of *Conium*, second-year rosette, revealed γ-coniceine levels of 387, 326, 198, 176, and 850 mg/g fresh plant for whole plant, root crown, stem, leaf, and green seed, respectively. Coniine was only detected in the leaf at 12 mg/g fresh plant (Panter and Gardner, unpublished data, 1994).

The clinical signs of toxicity are the same in all species and include initial stimulation (nervousness) resulting in frequent urination and defecation (no diarrhea), rapid pulse, temporarily impaired vision from the nictitating membrane covering the eyes, muscular weakness, muscle fasciculations, ataxia, incoordination followed by depression, recumbency, collapse, and death from respiratory failure (Panter et al., 1988).

Conium plant and seed are teratogenic, causing contracture-type skeletal defects and cleft palate like those of lupine. Field cases of teratogenesis have been reported in cattle and swine and experimentally induced in cattle, swine, sheep, and goats (Panter et al., 1999a). Birth defects include arthrogryposis (twisting of front legs), scoliosis (deviation of spine), torticollis (twisted neck), and cleft palate. Field cases of skeletal defects and cleft palate in swine and cattle have been confirmed experimentally.

In cattle, the susceptible period for *Conium*-induced terata is the same as that described for lupine and is between day 40 and day 70 of gestation. The defects, susceptible period of pregnancy, and probable mechanism of action are the same as those of crooked calf disease induced by lupines (Panter et al., 1999a). In brief, these alkaloids and their enantiomers in poison hemlock, lupines, and *N. glauca* were more effective in depolarizing the specialized cells TE-671, which express human fetal muscle-type nAChR, relative to SH-SY5Y, which predominantly express autonomic nAChRs, in a structure–activity relationship (Panter et al., 1990a; Lee et al., 2006, 2008b; Green et al., 2010). In swine, sheep, and goats, the susceptible period of gestation is 30–60 days. Cleft palate has been induced in goats only when plant or toxins were fed from 35 to 41 days of gestation (Panter and Keeler, 1992).

Field cases of poisoning have been reported in cattle, swine, horses, goats, elk, turkeys, quail, chickens, and Canadian geese (Panter et al., 1999a). Poisoning in wild geese eating small seedlings in early spring was most recently reported (Panter, personal communication). Human cases of poisoning are frequently reported in the literature, and a case of a child and his father mistakenly ingesting the plant has been reported. Field cases of teratogenesis have been reported in cattle and swine and experimentally induced in cattle, sheep, goats, and swine (Panter et al., 1990a). Pigs become habituated to poison hemlock, and if access to the plant is not limited, they will eat lethal amounts within a short time.

There are no diagnostic lesions in poisoned animals, and diagnosis is based on clinical history of exposure and/or alkaloid detection in liver, urine, or blood. At necropsy, the presence of plant in the stomach and a characteristic pungent odor in the contents with chemical confirmation of the alkaloids may be diagnostic.

Prevention and Treatment

Prevention of poisoning is based on recognizing the plant and its toxicity and avoidance of livestock exposure when hungry. If a lethal dose has not been ingested, the clinical signs will pass spontaneously, and a full recovery can be expected. Avoidance of stressing animals poisoned on *Conium* is recommended. However, if lethal doses have been ingested, supporting respiration, gastric lavage, and activated charcoal are recommended. Control of plants is easily accomplished using broadleaf herbicides; however, persistent control measures are recommended because seed reserves in the soil will quickly reestablish a population.

The mechanism of action of the *Conium* alkaloids is twofold. The most serious effect occurs at the neuromuscular junction, where they act as nondepolarizing blockers like curare. Systemically, the toxins cause biphasic nicotinic effects, including salivation, mydriasis, and tachycardia, followed by bradycardia as a result of their action at the autonomic ganglia. The teratogenic effects are undoubtedly related to the neuromuscular effects on the fetus and have been shown to be related to reduction in fetal movement (Panter et al., 1990a). Likewise, cleft palate is caused by the tongue interfering in palate closure during the reduced fetal movement and occurs during days 30–40 of gestation in swine, days 32–41 in goats, and days 40–50 in cattle (Panter and Keeler, 1992).

WATER HEMLOCK (*CICUTA* SPP.)

Water hemlock (*Cicuta* spp.) is among the most violently poisonous plants known to humans. It is often confused with poison hemlock because of its name, growth patterns, and appearance. There are distinct differences in appearance, as shown in Figure 61.6.

TABLE 61.5 Water Hemlock Species and Geographical Distribution

Species	Geographical Distribution
C. bulbifera	Northern U.S., southern Canada
C. bolanderi	Central to western CA
C. californica	Central to western CA
C. douglasii	Throughout U.S.
C. machenziana	Southeastern AK north to the Brooks Range
C. occidentalis	Rocky Mountains, Black Hills, WA; south into NV and NM
C. vagans	Pacific Northwest U.S. and Canada

Distribution

There are approximately 20 species of *Cicuta* throughout the world, and all are poisonous. Most of these species are found in North America; nine are common in the United States, and seven are found in the western United States (Table 61.5).

Description

Water hemlock is often confused with poison hemlock; in fact, there are similar plant characteristics and both belong to the Umbelliferae family (Figure 61.6). However, their toxic effects are dramatically different, and when toxicoses occur, differentiation between the two genera is important.

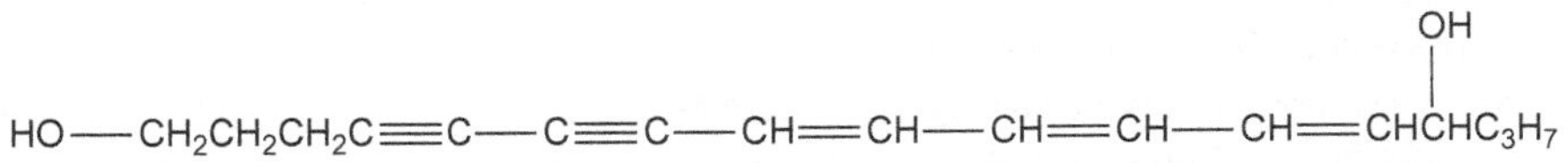

$$HO{-}CH_2CH_2CH_2C{\equiv}C{-}C{\equiv}C{-}CH{=}CH{-}CH{=}CH{-}CH{=}CH\underset{}{C}H(OH)C_3H_7$$

(8)
Cicutoxin

Water hemlock (*Cicuta*) is a biennial, 1 or 2 m tall, with thickened tubers possessing long, slender parsnip-like roots radiating out from the main tuber. Water hemlock frequently grows directly in streambeds or water sources and is limited to wet habitats. The tubers are bulbous and exhibit several chambers or cavities separated by cross-partitions as seen in a vertical cut through the tuber at the base of the stem. The cut surface of the stem or tuber exudes a yellowish, thick, oily liquid believed to be predominantly cicutoxin (**8**). This oily substance has a parsnip-like odor. The chambered tuber is a distinguishing feature of this plant (Figure 61.6). The roots extending from the tuber may be solid, white, and fleshy, closely resembling a parsnip. The stems are hollow except at the nodes, hairless, and occasionally have purple stripes up the stem. Leaf stalks alternate up the stem and leaves two or three pinnately divided may be 30–60 cm long. Flowers are small, white or cream colored, and in terminal umbrella-shaped clusters. The fruits are small, with prominent ribs, and encased in a hard brownish shell very similar to those of poison hemlock. The primary distinguishing feature separating water and poison hemlock is the tuberous roots with the very distinct partitions in water hemlock (Figure 61.6). Poison hemlock lacks the large tubers, although occasionally there are very small partitions observed in the area where the root and stem connect if the plant is cut vertically. The parsnip-like root is a single taproot in poison hemlock, whereas there are often multiple white parsnip-like roots radiating off the main tubers in water hemlock (Figure 61.6).

Toxicology

The toxic principle in water hemlock is a long-chain, highly unsaturated alcohol called cicutoxin. Water hemlock acts on the central nervous system as a stimulant, inducing violent grand mal seizures and death from respiratory failure.

Tubers are the most toxic part of the plant, especially in early spring. The parsnip-like roots extending from the tuber are two to four times less toxic, and as the vegetative parts of the plant grow and mature, they become less toxic. Preliminary studies suggest that mature leaves and stems are much less toxic and after drying are non-toxic (Panter et al., 1988). Historically, water hemlock was believed to be most dangerous in early spring, and poisoning usually occurred when animals milled around in streambeds or sloughs and exposed tubers, which were then ingested. Although this is true, a recent case of poisoning and death in cattle after ingesting flower and green seed heads implicates this phenological stage as dangerous also (Panter et al., 2011). Chemical comparison of green seed and tubers and mouse bioassay studies showed that green seed was equally as toxic as tubers. Like tubers, the more mature vegetation, including leaves, flowers, and green seed heads, was very palatable. Free choice exposure of hamsters to the white parsnip-like roots suggests that they are quite palatable and are less toxic than the tuber. Observations of cattle grazing early in spring suggest that the young shoots of water hemlock are very palatable because young plants growing in streambeds were frequently and extensively grazed (Panter, personal observation).

Clinical signs of poisoning appear within 10–15 min after ingestion and progress from nervousness, frothing, ataxia, dyspnea, muscular tremors, and weakness to involuntary, spastic head and neck movements accompanied by rapid eye blinking and partial occlusion of the eyes from the nictitating membranes. This is quickly followed by collapse and intermittent grand mal seizures lasting 1 or 2 min each followed by relaxation periods of 8–10 min. Depending on the dosage, recovery may occur or seizures continue until death from exhaustion or respiratory failure. There appears to be a threshold response in which very small increases in dosage will induce an apparently normal animal into grand mal seizures (Panter et al., 1996a).

Upon necropsy, gross lesions are confined to pale areas in heart muscle and skeletal muscles, particularly the long digital extensor muscle groups (Panter et al., 1996a). Microscopic lesions include multifocal, sub-acute to chronic myocardial degeneration characterized by granular degeneration of myofiber cytoplasm necrosis and replacement fibrosis in the heart. These areas correspond to the pale areas observed grossly. There is bilateral symmetrical, subacute to chronic myofiber degeneration and necrosis of the long digital extensor muscle groups. Clinical serum chemistry changes of elevated lactic dehydrogenase, aspartate aminotransferase, and creatine kinase occur in relation to severity of seizures. The extent of gross and microscopic lesions and clinical chemistries are a result of the severity of the seizures. Experimentally, barbiturates prevented seizures, death, and lesions in sheep, and a 3× lethal dose of water hemlock could be reversed with pentobarbital and no death occurred (Panter et al., 1996a). In animals in which seizures were prevented by barbiturates, there were no lesions observed even though doses of two and three times the lethal dose were administered.

Prevention and Treatment

Prevention of poisoning is accomplished by recognizing the plant and avoiding exposing animals to it early in the spring or when in flower/seed stage. Water hemlock is easily controlled with herbicides (2,4-D per manufacturer's specification); however, herbicide use is often restricted near natural water sources. If few plants are present, hand pulling may be accomplished using caution to discard tubers away from possible exposure to animals or humans.

Successful treatment with barbiturates or perhaps tranquilizers prevents death and the lesions and serum chemistry changes; however, treatment must be prompt (Panter et al., 1996a). This treatment has been successful in humans, but in animals it has never been demonstrated in the field and would require a veterinarian to be on sight soon after the ingestion of this plant.

PONDEROSA PINE NEEDLES (*PINUS* SPP.)

The needles of ponderosa pine have been known for years to induce abortion in pregnant cows when grazed, particularly during the last trimester of pregnancy (Gardner et al., 1999). Occasional toxicosis in pregnant cows occurs; however, cases of toxicosis in nonpregnant cows, steers, or bulls are not reported.

Description

Ponderosa pine (*Pinus ponderosa*) is one of the most prevalent species of *Pinus* in the western United States. Under ideal conditions, it grows to heights of more than 60 m and 1.5–2.5 m in diameter. It is extensively harvested for lumber. During early growth, the bark is dark brown to black, hence the name "black jack" pine. Older trees have a bark of cinnamon brown to yellow, hence the name "yellow" pine. Ponderosa pine is a three-needled pine, although groups of two and three can be found on the same tree. The needles are approximately 8–20 cm long growing in clusters. They are soft and quite palatable, especially in the winter, when green feed is limited. The cones are brown, 7–15 cm long, and frequently grow in clusters. Two varieties of ponderosa pine have been identified, var. *ponderosa* and var. *scopulorum*, along with a separate five-needled species *Pinus arizonica*.

Distribution

Ponderosa pine grows in every state west of the Great Plains and in western Canada. It has a total stand greater than any native tree in the western United States except Douglas fir. It grows at elevations between 1500 and 2500 m, although populations in California do extend almost to sea level. Ponderosa pine is drought resistant and is extensively harvested for lumber. Gardner and James (1999) surveyed numerous other *Pinus*, *Juniperus*, *Abies* species, etc. for isocupressic acid content, and Table 61.6 lists common name, location, and isocupressic acid concentration of many species of trees or shrubs. The bark from both Utah juniper and western juniper trees has also been found to be abortifacient to cattle (Gardner et al., 2010; Welch et al., 2011a).

TABLE 61.6 Concentration of Isocupressic Acid (ICA) and Related Metabolic Compounds from Selected Species and Locations

Species	Common Name	Location	ICA Concentration (%DW)
Abies concolor	White fir	Arizona	n.d.
		California	n.d.
		Colorado	0.04
		Utah	n.d.
Abies grandis	Grand fir	Idaho	n.d.
		Oregon	n.d.
Abies lasiocarpa	Subalpine fir	Oregon	n.d.
		Colorado	n.d.
		Idaho	0.04
		Utah	n.d.
Abies magnifica	Red fir	California	0.05
Cupressus macrocarpa	Monterey cypress	California	n.d.–0.06
		New Zealand	0.89–1.24
Cupressus X ovensii	Ovens cypress	New Zealand	0.81
Juniperus californica	California juniper	California	0.93 needles
			0.05 bark
Juniperus communis	Mountain common juniper	Colorado	2.05–2.88
		Utah	1.50–5.0
Juniperus monosperma	One seed juniper	Arizona	0.14
		New Mexico	n.d.
Juniperus occidentalis	Western juniper	Oregon	0.10
			Imbricatoloic acid = 1.0
		California	0.10
			Imbricatoloic acid = 1.0
			1.83 stems = total labdane acids
Juniperus osteosperma	Utah juniper	Utah	n.d.
		Nevada	0.07
		Arizona	n.d.
		Colorado	n.d.
		Utah	Agathic acid 1.50
Juniperus scopulorum	Rocky mountain juniper	Utah	0.84
		New Mexico	0.33
		Arizona	0.42
Juniperus virginiana	Eastern red cedar	Nebraska	Needles, low bark, <0.10 – high
Larix occidentalis	Western larch	Oregon	n.d.
Libocedrus decurrens	Incense cedar	Oregon	0.07
Picea engelmannii	Engelmann spruce	California	0.27
		Colorado	n.d.

(Continued)

TABLE 61.6 (Continued)

Species	Common Name	Location	ICA Concentration (%DW)
		Idaho	0.04
		Montana	0.31
		Oregon	n.d.
		Utah	n.d.
Picea pungens	Colorado blue spruce	Utah	0.17
		Colorado	n.d.
Pinus aristata	Bristle cone pine	Colorado	0.01–0.05
Pinus arizonica	Arizona pine	California	n.d.
		Arizona	n.d.
Pinus contorta	Lodgepole pine	Oregon	0.28
		Idaho	0.11
		Colorado	0.29–0.47
		Utah	0.66
		Canada (British Columbia)	0.45
Pinus densiflora	Japanese red pine	Korea	n.d.
Pinus echinata	Short leaf pine	Arkansas	n.d.
Pinus edulis	Pinyon pine	Arizona	n.d.
		Colorado	0.12
		New Mexico	0.10
		Utah	0.45
Pinus elliottii	Slash pine	Arkansas	n.d.
Pinus flexilis	Limber pine	Colorado	n.d.–0.06
		Utah	n.d.
Pinus halepensis	Aleppo pine	California	n.d.
Pinus jeffreyi	Jeffrey pine	California	0.04–0.54
Pinus koraiensis	Korean pine	Utah	Positive
		Korea	0.02
Pinus monophylla	Single-leaf pinyon	Nevada	0.32
Pinus montezumae	Montezuma pine	California	n.d.
Pinus palustris	Long-leaf pine	Arkansas	n.d.
Pinus patula	Patula pine	South Africa	<0.10
Pinus ponderosa	Ponderosa pine	Oregon	0.74–1.30
		Arizona	0.49
		California	0.08–1.35
		Utah	0.51
		Colorado	0.49–0.58
		South Dakota	0.10–1.30
		Wyoming	0.58–1.11
		Germany	0.62

(*Continued*)

TABLE 61.6 (Continued)

Species	Common Name	Location	ICA Concentration (%DW)
Pinus radiata	Radiata pine	New Zealand	n.d.–0.26
Pinus strobus	White pine		n.d.
Pinus taeda	Loblolly pine	Arizona	n.d.
		Arkansas	n.d.
Pseudotsuga menziesii	Douglas fir	Utah	0.04
		Colorado	0.05
		California	n.d.
		Idaho	n.d.
		Arizona	n.d.
		Oregon	n.d.
Thuja plicata	Western red cedar	Arizona	0.42
		New Mexico	0.33
		Utah	0.84
		Germany	n.d.
Tsuga mertensiana	Mountain hemlock	Oregon	n.d.

n.d., not detected (<0.01%).

Pinus ponderosa var. *ponderosa* (western variety) extends from the mountains of southern California northward on the western and eastern sides of the Sierra Nevada–Cascade crest to Canada. The eastern variety *P. ponderosa* var. *scopulorum* meets the western variety near the Continental Divide in west-central Montana and extends southward throughout mountains, plains, and basins to scattered stands in the Sierra Madre Occidental and Sierra Madre Oriental of northern Mexico. *Pinus arizonica* (once considered a third variety) has scattered populations in southern Arizona and New Mexico.

Toxicology

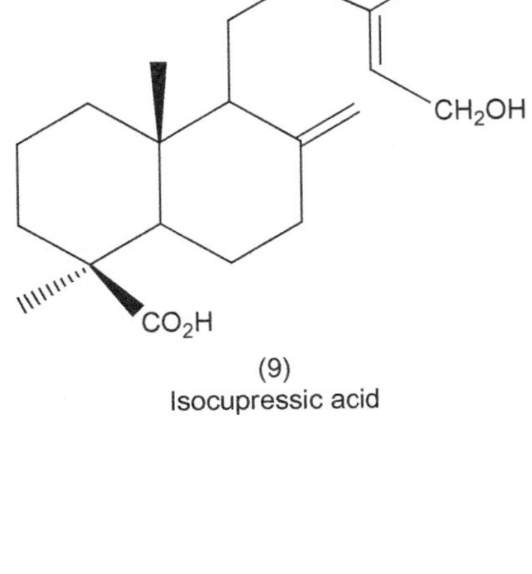

CH_2OH

CO_2H

(9)
Isocupressic acid

The toxin in ponderosa pine that induces abortion in cattle is the labdane resin acid isocuppressic acid **(9)** (ICA; Gardner et al., 1994). Two related derivatives (succinyl ICA and acetyl ICA) also contribute to the induction of abortion after hydrolytic conversion to ICA in the rumen (Gardner et al., 1996). Other related labdane acids (agathic acid, imbricatoloic acid, and dihydroagathic acid) that are found in ponderosa pine needles at low levels may also contain abortifacient properties based on their similar chemical structure to ICA. Other genera and species have also been implicated in abortions, such as Monterey cypress (Parton et al., 1996), Korean pine (Kim et al., 2003), and California juniper and lodgepole pine (Panter, personal communications). Table 61.6 summarizes current information on plant species analyzed for ICA and/or ICA derivatives believed to contribute to abortions. Current research indicates that the concentration of ICA in ponderosa pine needles is not uniform throughout the same tree, the concentration of ICA in ponderosa pine needles can vary from location to location, and there is evidence for seasonal fluctuations as well (Cook et al., 2010).

The primary toxicological effects of ponderosa pine needles in cattle are abortion and complications associated with abortion, such as retained fetal membranes, metritis, and occasional overt toxicosis and death (Gardner et al., 1999). The abortions generally occur in the last trimester of pregnancy in the late fall, winter, or early spring. Abortions have been induced as early as 3 months of gestation and have been reported by ranchers to occur any time; however, the closer to the time of normal parturition that ingestion of pine needles occurs, the higher the risk of abortion. Abortions may occur following a single exposure to the needles, but results from controlled experiments indicate the highest incidence of abortion is in cows eating the needles over a period of days. Abortions have been associated with grazing of green needles from trees, slash from the lumber industry, and dead, dry needles from the ground.

Abortions are generally characterized by weak uterine contractions, uterine bleeding, incomplete cervical dilation, dystocia, birth of weak but viable calves, agalactia, and retained fetal membranes (Gardner et al., 1999). Two syndromes seem to occur depending on the amount of pine needles eaten. In the first syndrome, abortion occurs relatively quickly (3–6 days) with no signs of pending abortion, such as udder filling, vulvar swelling, or pelvic relaxation, but a small weak calf is quickly delivered. In the second syndrome, abortion occurs after 6–14 days, and all the previously mentioned signs occur before the calf is born. Unless complications occur, most calves are born alive, and the closer to normal parturition, the higher the survival rate. Calves born Isocupressic acid after 255 days of gestation will often survive with extra care but need to be supplemented with colostrum and milk from other sources until the dam begins to lactate. Cows with retained fetal membranes may need antibiotic therapy to avoid uterine infections.

Pine needles will induce abortion in buffalo, but sheep, elk, and goats do not abort. Pine needles, pine bark, and new growth tips of branches are all abortifacient and new growth tips are also toxic (Panter et al., 1990b).

A separate toxic syndrome has been described in addition to abortion in which the abietane-type diterpene resin acids cause depression, feed refusal, weakness, neurological problems, and, eventually, death. Specific compounds include abietic acid, dehydroabietic acid, and other related compounds (Stegelmeier et al., 1996). At 15–30% of the diet, pine needles have been shown to alter rumen microflora and affect the rumen fermentation (Pfister et al., 1992). Rumen stasis is part of the toxic syndrome (Stegelmeier et al., 1996).

Pine needle-induced abortion appears to mimic normal parturition except it is premature. The mechanism of action appears to be a reduction in blood flow to the caruncular vascular bed stimulating the fetal parturition mechanism (Ford et al., 1992). ICA has not been found to be directly vasoactive, and it is unclear if ICA metabolites are vasoactive or if the vasoconstriction is a secondary response to ICA or ICA metabolites. Further research is needed to determine the cellular or biochemical mechanism and whether metabolic alteration of the ICA occurs.

Extensive vasoconstriction of the caruncular vascular bed with accompanying necrosis and hemorrhage are the only reported pathological changes in maternal tissues. These findings are supported by Ford et al. (1992), who reported that serum from pregnant cows fed pine needles showed vaso (vasoconstriction) activity *in vitro*.

Prevention and Treatment

The only recommendation to prevent pine needle abortion is to avoid grazing pregnant cows around pine trees, especially in the third trimester. There is no known treatment for cattle once ingestion of pine needles has occurred. Open cows, steers, or bulls are apparently unaffected by pine needles; likewise, sheep, goats (pregnant or not), and horses can graze pine needles with impunity and experience no adverse effects. Supportive therapy (antibiotic treatment or uterine infusion for retained fetal membranes) is recommended for cows that have aborted, and intensive care of the calf may save its life. Grazing of pine needles intensifies during cold inclement weather and if other forage is in short supply. In spring, before green grass is available, cows will leave feeding grounds in search of new green grass and frequently graze old, dry needles from surrounding trees where the snow has melted. These cows are at risk and should be kept away from the pines. Research has also determined that low body conditioned cows are more likely to eat pine needles than cattle in adequate body condition (Pfister et al., 2008b). Consequently, it is recommended that pregnant cattle grazing in ponderosa pine areas be maintained in good body condition (Pfister et al., 2008b). Anecdotal information suggests that pregnant llamas may be at risk from pine needles, but no experimental support has been presented (Panter, personal communications).

BROOM SNAKEWEED (*GUTIERREZIA* SPP.)

Broom snakeweed causes significant loss to cattle, sheep, and goat producers in Texas and New Mexico from abortions and toxicoses. There are some similarities with ponderosa pine needles, except pine needles apparently affect only cattle.

Description and Distribution

There are two major species of broom snakeweed, *Gutierrezia sarothrae* (perennial snakeweed or turpentine weed) and *G. microcephala* (threadleaf broomweed). Snakeweeds are short-lived perennial half shrubs ranging from 15 to 60 cm tall (Ralphs and McDaniel, 2011). Many unbranched erect stems originate from a woody base and die back when the plant enters dormancy. They have a suffrutescent growth form, with new stems originating from the crown each year without becoming woody. The stems originate from the crown and are unbranched, giving rise to the common name of broom snakeweed, with the stems resembling the straight straws of a broom. Leaves are narrow and linear and alternately arranged on stems. These species are of the Composite family; thus, they have two types of flowers. Disc flowers are tightly clustered in the center of the head, whereas long yellow petal ray flowers radiate out from the head (Lane, 1985).

Broom Snakeweed (Gutierrezia sarothrae (Pursh) Britt. & Rusby)

Broom snakeweed has more than three florets (usually seven) per involucre or flowering cluster. Broom snakeweed is one of the most ubiquitous range plants and is widely distributed throughout North America, ranging from the cold temperate climate of Canada to sub-tropical areas of Mexico and from the subhumid Great Plains to the montane Rocky Mountains and Sierras and the arid Great Basin. It ranges in elevation from 50 to 2900 m, rainfall from 20 to 50 cm, and temperatures from 4 to 21 °C. It is a principal component of the following plant communities: desert creosote, desert grassland, short-grass prairie, salt-desert shrub, sagebrush, pinyon–juniper, and mountain brush. Its wide tolerance limits allow it to inhabit a broad range of environments, and it can dominate and cause significant problems as both a noxious and a poisonous weed in the short-grass prairies and sagebrush plant communities.

*Threadleaf snakeweed (*G. microcephala* (DC) Gray)*

Threadleaf snakeweed has one floret per flowering cluster. Threadleaf snakeweed is restricted to the Mojave, Sonoran, and Chihuahuan deserts of the southwestern United States and northern Mexico. It grows in dry, desert habitat and favors sandy soils, and it has a greater tolerance for arid climates than does broom snakeweed.

Ecology

Broom snakeweed is a native range shrub found throughout semiarid rangelands of the western United States. Although a minor component of pristine plant communities, it can predominate on rocky ridges, gravely slopes, and immature infertile soils. Ralphs and McDaniel (2011) provide an up-to-date review of broom snakeweed ecology, including seed ecology, population cycles, toxicology, and management. Broom snakeweed increases and may dominate rangelands following disturbances such as overgrazing, fire, and drought (Ralphs and Banks, 2009). Broom snakeweed will increase where it is established and will invade deeper soils and more productive habitats. It is very competitive with desirable grasses and greatly suppresses forage production.

A two-tier root system allows the deep taproot to extract deep-stored water, and the extensive adventitious roots near the surface take advantage of the light sporadic rain showers. It has little leaf stomatal control; thus, it is a luxuriant water user for maximum growth. It grows early in the spring and depletes moisture from the entire soil profile before warm-season grasses break dormancy. Broom snakeweed is one of the most undesirable plants in the various regions of the west. On many localized rangelands of the southwest, it is the most significant problem limiting forage and livestock production.

Broom snakeweed is short-lived and experiences dramatic population cycles, which appear to be related to climatic patterns. Although it is very competitive for soil moisture, it is not particularly drought tolerant. Broom snakeweed populations die off in drought and from insect depredation, but it is one of the first plants to germinate and establish when rains resume, forming wide-spread monospecific stands (Ralphs and Sanders, 2002).

Toxicology

The snakeweeds are toxic and abortifacient to cattle, sheep, and goats. Abortions and retained fetal membranes in cattle are among the most serious problems in livestock. In 1985, McGinty estimated losses in excess of $15 million annually to the cattle industry in Texas alone and more than $30 million when losses in New Mexico and Arizona were included. This does not account for indirect losses, such as loss of usable forage, management changes, increased calving intervals, or added veterinary care.

Snakeweed contains toxic and abortifacient compounds. Extracts of a saponin fraction from threadleaf snakeweed caused abortions in rabbits, goats, and cattle at low doses and caused death at high doses. Molyneux et al. (1980) identified some major monoterpenes and sesquiterpenes in the essential oil fraction of snake-weed, including α-pinene, myrcene, linalool, *cis*-verbenol, *trans*-verbenol, verbenone, geraniol, caryophyllene, and γ-humulene. Several furanoditerpene acids and flavones from the resinous exudate in trichomes on leaves of broom snakeweed have been identified. These diterpene acids were structurally similar to ICA, the abortifacient compound in ponderosa pine (*P. ponderosa* Laws) needles. Gardner et al. (1999) speculated that some of the furanoditerpene acids may be abortifacient, whereas others may be toxic, and the relative concentrations determine whether animals are poisoned or abort. The crude resin content of broom snakeweed, which includes the diterpene acids along with other monoterpenes, increased from 5% in early growth up to 13% at flowering in August (Ralphs et al., 2007).

Snakeweeds are both abortifacient and toxic. In west Texas in the 1930s, 10–60% of cattle ranches experienced abortions, and cows retained placentas, which led to infection and death of the cows. Many calves were born small and weak. Threadleaf snakeweed was fed to cattle, sheep, and goats, causing damage to the liver and kidneys, but no abortions were produced. Dollahite and Anthony (1957) and others found that threadleaf snakeweed did cause abortions, retained placenta, and weak calves, and it was more toxic on sandy soils. Low levels of snakeweed cause abortions and high levels are toxic. Clinical signs of poisoning include anorexia, mucopurulent nasal discharge, loss of appetite and listlessness, diarrhea, and then constipation and rumen stasis, which may lead to death.

There appears to be a relationship between nutrition and fertility problems caused by broom snakeweed. Smith et al. (1991) summarized research in rats at New Mexico State University and concluded that increasing amounts of snakeweed in rat diets reduced intake, which led to malnutrition and contributed to diminished fertility and increased fetal mortality. Edrington et al. (1993) confirmed that increasing amounts of snakeweed in rat diets reduced intake and contributed to problems of malnutrition and toxicity. However, they determined that the overriding factor in reducing fertility and reproduction was the impaired hormone balance and disruption of blood flow to the uterus and developing embryos. Ewes on a high-quality alfalfa diet (18% crude protein) consumed snakeweed for up to 25% of the ration with no adverse effects on estrus; whereas ewes fed blue grama hay (11% crude protein) would not consume rations containing more than 10% snakeweed, and 43% of these ewes did not show estrus and did not breed. In heifers fed snakeweed as 15% of a balanced diet before breeding and during early gestation, there was no effect on progesterone levels or conception rates. During the last trimester of gestation, snakeweed added up to 30% of this same diet did not cause abortion or lower calf birth weight. In a grazing trial on snakeweed-infested crested wheatgrass, cows in the last trimester of gestation were forced to graze snakeweed as a biological control. Snakeweed consumption averaged 10% of bites over the day and peaked at 20% of bites in the evening grazing periods. There were no signs of toxicity or abortions, even though their feed intake was severely restricted (Ralphs et al., 2007).

Management and Treatment

Broom snakeweed is usually not palatable to most large ungulates; cattle will not graze snakeweed unless all other vegetation is depleted (Ralphs et al., 2007). Thus, the management strategy to prevent grazing of broom snakeweed and prevent toxicosis is simple: ensure adequate feed is available. This can be accomplished by maintaining range in good condition and moving animals when proper utilization is reached. Although this sounds relatively simple, there are thousands of acres of rangeland on which broom snakeweed is dominant; thus, how can these ranges be restored or utilized by livestock or wildlife?

Thacker et al. (2008) studied the invasion of broom snakeweed in two plant communities during a 5-year period following disturbance and evaluated vegetation change in a state-and-transition model. In a sagebrush/bunchgrass community that burned, bluebunch wheatgrass became the dominant species, and in the sagebrush-only dominated community that burned, broom snakeweed quickly established and dominated the community. Snakeweed cover increased from 2 to 31% during the 5-year period.

Broom snakeweed can be controlled by the common rangeland herbicides: Tordon® (0.25–0.5 lb/ac) is most consistent, Escort (3–6 oz./ac) is a promising herbicide, and 2,4-D (1–2 lb/ac) can be applied for two successive years when soil moisture is not limiting growth (Whitson and Freeburn, 1990). Better control is obtained in fall after flowering, when the carbohydrate stream is going down and carries the herbicide to the roots.

Ralphs and Banks (2009) used intense short-duration grazing pressure and high stocking rates to force cattle to graze snakeweed in an attempt to reduce snakeweed dominance. This intense targeted grazing pressure actually reduced snakeweed plants, but this method of snakeweed control has yet to be recommended, especially considering the health of the animals and the potential for reestablishment of snakeweed. Although the long-term success of targeted grazing to control snakeweed is yet to be determined, one should strongly consider seeding with cool-season grasses following episodes of overgrazing or targeted grazing such as reported by Ralphs and Banks. Defoliation studies to mimic grazing suggested that spring treatments put snakeweed at a disadvantage compared to fall clipping (Ralphs, 2009). Although there was little difference in the effect of clipping cool-season grasses in the spring versus the fall, there was a distinct effect on snakeweed.

Snakeweed is readily killed by fire, and prescribed burning is an effective control in the early stages of the population cycle while there is sufficient grass to carry a fire and respond to the released resources. In the latter part of the population cycle, grasses will be crowded out, and spraying with herbicides may be the only alternative. In this case, spraying must be followed by seeding to ensure a weed-resistant plant community is established that will resist reinvasion of snakeweed. Cool-season grasses such as crested, pubescent, and bluebunch wheatgrass will compete with snakeweed seedlings. Following drought, wildfires, or herbicide control, it was recommended that cool-season grasses should be seeded in an attempt to establish a solid stand that will prevent snakeweed establishment and subsequent domination in the plant community. If this approach is not successful, downy brome will likely fill in, which will also often suppress the establishment of broom snakeweed.

Insects may play a role in snakeweed population die-off. Many insects are associated with snakeweed: defoliators (leaf tyers, grasshoppers, and weevils), sap suckers (scale insects and mealybugs), and root-boring weevils and gall formers. Individually and collectively, they contribute to the demise of mature snakeweed populations. However, it is unlikely that they will contribute to preventing a population buildup because of the time lag of their populations in relation to that of snakeweed.

Treatment of sick animals is only symptomatic, providing supplementation to weak calves and antibiotic therapy to cows with retained fetal membranes to avoid infection.

RAYLESS GOLDENROD *(HAPLOPAPPUS HETEROPHYLLUS)*

Rayless goldenrod (*Haplopappus heterophyllus*) is a toxic range plant of the southwestern United States. The disease associated with toxicity has been referred to as "alkali disease" because originally it was associated with drinking of alkali water. Currently, it is referred to as "milk sickness" or "trembles" (the same as white snake-root in the Midwest) because the toxin tremetone **(10)** is excreted in the milk and subsequently results in poisoning of humans and nursing offspring. *Haplopappus acradenius* was implicated in poisoning in cattle in southern California (Galey et al., 1991).

CH_3 C O CH_3 C CH_2

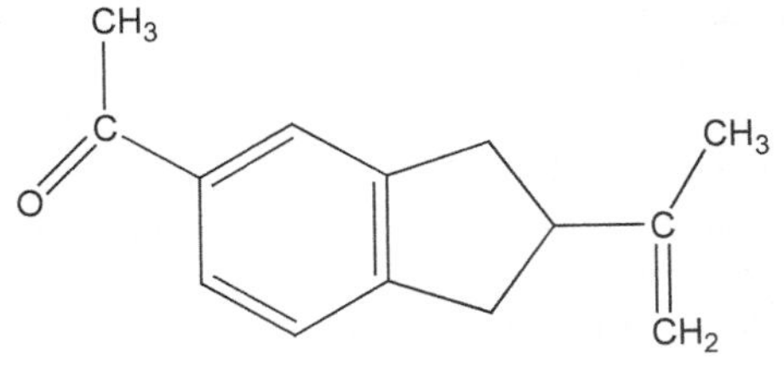

(10)
Tremetone

Description

Rayless goldenrod is an erect, bushy, unbranched Peromial shrub that grows 0.5–1.5 m tall. The base is woody, and leaves alternate linearly up the stem. Heads are numerous, small, and clustered at the top of the stem, with 7–15 yellow flowers on each head.

Distribution

Rayless goldenrod grows in the desert rangelands of the southwestern United States from southern Colorado into Texas, New Mexico, Arizona, and California into Mexico. The plant grows abundantly on alkaline and gypsic soils in western Texas and the Pecos River Valley.

Toxicology

The toxic constituents of rayless goldenrod are similar to those found in white snakeroot, and the original term, tremetol, is a mixture of ketones and alcohols. Tremetone (5-acetyl-2,3-dihydro-2-isopropenyl-benzofuran) was thought to be the principle toxic factor; however, 11 different compounds have now been isolated and identified (Lee et al., 2010). This elucidation of different chemotypes of white snakeroot partially explains the sporadic and unpredictable toxicoses reported in livestock throughout the midwestern United States.

The toxicity of rayless goldenrod mimics that of white snakeroot. Clinical signs of poisoning may occur after ingestion of 1–15% BW during a 1- to 3-week period. Signs begin with depression or inactivity, followed by noticeable trembling of the fine muscles of the nose and legs. Most cases of poisoning reported constipation, nausea, vomition, rapid labored respiration, progressive muscular weakness, stiff gait, standing in a humped-up position, dribbling urine, inability to stand, coma, and death. Signs are similar in cattle, sheep, and goats. The disease is often more acute and severe in horses than in cattle, and horses may die of heart failure after subacute ingestion of white snakeroot and presumably rayless goldenrod. Cattle have also been poisoned on a related plant (*Haplopappus acradenius*) in southern California (Galey et al., 1991). In this case, 21 of 60 cattle died and 15 of 60 were affected but recovered. Creatine phosphokinase and ketones were elevated, and severe myonecrosis was described in the dead animals.

Prevention and Treatment

Rayless goldenrod is not readily palatable, and toxicity results from animals being forced to graze the plant due to lack of good quality forage. Avoiding overgrazing will usually minimize poisoning in livestock.

Control of rayless goldenrod can be accomplished with herbicide applications. Late summer and early fall application of picloram or 2,4-D ester is successful in reducing plant populations.

Treatment is generally symptomatic and supportive, providing dry bedding, good shelter, and fresh feed and water. Activated charcoal and saline cathartic may be beneficial. Treatment may include fluids, B vitamins, ketosis therapy, and tube feeding. Hay and water should be placed within reach if the animal is recumbent. In lactating cows, frequent milking may facilitate a more rapid elimination of the toxins. In horses, monitoring of cardiac arrhythmias and electrocardiogram will provide information concerning heart damage and associated circulatory dysfunction. Treatment is the same for rayless goldenrod and white snakeroot because the toxins are the same.

HALOGETON (*HALOGETON GLOMERATUS*)

Halogeton is an alien, invasive, noxious, and poisonous weed introduced from central Asia in the early 20th century. It was first collected along a railroad spur near Wells, Nevada, in 1934 and rapidly invaded 11.2 million acres of the cold deserts of the western United States (Young, 1999). There has been no appreciable spread since the 1980s because halogeton has filled all the suitable niches within its tolerance limits. It currently infests disturbed areas within the salt-desert shrub and sage-brush plant communities in the Great Basin, Colorado Plateau, and Wyoming's Red Desert physiographic provinces, which have 3–15 in. of annual precipitation.

Halogeton's infamy began in the 1940s and 1950s by causing large, catastrophic sheep losses. There were many instances of large dramatic losses; sometimes entire bands of sheep died overnight from halogeton poisoning. *Life* magazine ran a cover story titled "Stock Killing Weed" that focused national attention on halogeton. Congress passed the Halogeton Act in 1952 with the intent to

- detect the presence of halogeton;
- determine its effects on livestock; and
- control, suppress, and eradicate this stock-killing weed.

Federal research was reallocated from the Forest Service Experiment Stations to the Bureau of Plant Industries, creating the Range Research unit devoted specifically to "solving" the halogeton problem. It was realized that halogeton was not the problem but a symptom of a larger problem – that of degradation of desert rangelands (Young, 1999). It invaded disturbed sites where sheep congregated – around railroad loading sites, trail heads, stock drive ways, and water holes. When hungry sheep were turned loose to graze, halogeton was the only feed available, and they consumed too much, too rapidly, and were poisoned.

Description and Ecology

Halogeton is an annual plant germinating from seed each year. Its stems are branched from the base and tinged with red and purple. Its leaves are fleshy and "hot dog" shaped, with the distinguishing feature of a single spine on its tip. It can be distinguished from Russian thistle and pigweed (with which it grows) by the tubular, spine-tipped leaf. It does not have flowers but, rather, bracteoles formed in the axils of leaves from which seed clusters develop. These seed clusters occur throughout the length of its stems. A robust plant may have 1500 linear inches of stem, with 75 seeds/in., producing 200–400 lb seed/acre. The seeds are winged and are spread by wind and rodents.

Its seeds are dimorphic, which is key to its successful survival strategy. The majority of its seeds are black and readily germinate anytime when temperature and soil moisture are favorable. However, the black seeds are viable for less than 1 year. A small percentage of the seeds are hard and brown with low germination rates, but they survive for long periods in the soil and germinate when favorable conditions return. The dimorphic seed provided abundant seed for germination each year but also a reserve if drought killed its populations over successive years.

Although halogeton will germinate whenever conditions are favorable, it remains as a seedling until May, at which time lateral branches develop and ascend. It reaches its reproductive stage by mid-summer, or when soil moisture becomes limiting. When mature, the winged fruits are blown by wind or carried and deposited by rodents.

Halogeton is not competitive with perennial shrubs and grasses. It will not invade healthy desert plant communities. When a site is disturbed, halogeton will invade and establish, and its allelopathic properties provide an added advantage to its invasive nature. It takes up sodium and potassium from saline soils, forming the respective oxalates. These oxalates provide an important metabolic function to maintain high cell sap osmotic potential to allow the plant to take up saline water. Oxalates accumulate during the growing season, reaching peak concentration in the fall (20–36% of plant dry weight). Soluble oxalates leach out of the senescent foliage during the winter and accumulate on the soil surface, increasing its salinity. Thus, halogeton modifies its environment, making it more saline to meet its requirements, while exceeding the tolerance limits of associated species.

Toxicology

The toxins are sodium and potassium oxalates, and plants are high in these oxalates in the fall and early winter when sheep enter the desert winter ranges. Poisoning occurs when sheep consume more oxalates than the body can detoxify (James, 1999). Rumen microbes can detoxify the oxalates, and their populations can be induced to accommodate increasing levels of oxalates. Furthermore, calcium in the native plants or Ca supplements will rapidly combine with the oxalates in the rumen to form Ca oxalates that cannot be absorbed and are excreted in feces. If the Na oxalates are absorbed, they can be flushed out in urine. If they reach the blood-stream, they precipitate the Ca from the blood, creating Ca oxalate crystals, causing hypocalcemia resulting in shock and death. The Ca oxalate crystals physically damage the tubules of the kidney. The Na oxalates interfere with two key enzymes (succinic dehydrogenase and lactic dehydrogenase) in the Krebs cycle, disrupting energy metabolism. Combined, they cause rapid and acute death.

Clinical signs of poisoning include depression, anorexia, weakness, incoordination, recumbency, blood-tinged nasal discharge, coma, and rapid death. Gross pathologic changes include hemorrhage and edema of the rumen wall, hyperemia of the abomasal wall, and intestinal mucosa and ascites. Morphologic changes include hemorrhage and calcium oxalate crystal formation in the rumen wall and oxalate crystals with accompanying cellular damage in the renal tubules of the kidney.

Treatment of Poisoned Animals

Animals can be drenched with water to flush oxalates out in the urine, or including dicalcium phosphate in the drench provides Ca that will combine with oxalates in the rumen and can be excreted. Intravenous injection of calcium gluconate can maintain blood Ca levels, but the forming Ca oxalate crystals will continue to damage kidneys (James, 1999). However, it is generally impractical to treat a severely poisoned animal. Prevention is the key to avoid poisoning. Only hungry sheep are poisoned. Research has demonstrated that as little as 1 oz. of soluble oxalates can be lethal to fasted, hungry sheep. Well-fed sheep grazing nutritious forage throughout the day can tolerate more than 4 oz. of soluble oxalate. Sheep grazed in a desert plant community infested with halogeton consumed it from 5 to 25% of their diets without ill effect. If other forage is available, they will likely not get a lethal dose.

Management to Prevent Poisoning

Never turn hungry sheep onto dense halogeton-infested sites. Provide good feed following trucking or trailing. Ensure there is good feed available following watering. Introduce sheep gradually to halogeton to allow rumen microbes to adjust. Some sheep producers graze their sheep on shadscale ranges (which contain low oxalate levels) before going into halogeton areas. Do not over-graze; maintain desert range in good condition. This prevents halogeton invasion as well as provides an alternative food source.

Herbicide control is not recommended because the waxy surface of halogeton's leaves hinders absorption of most herbicides. More important, however, desirable desert shrubs are killed, leaving the site open for further invasion and degradation by halogeton and other invasive weeds.

OAK POISONING

Toxicoses in cattle from ingestion of oak buds, leaves, and acorns occurs in many areas of the United States and Europe. Poisoning is usually seasonal, with ingestion of buds and leaves in spring and acorns in fall.

All oaks should be considered potentially toxic (Table 61.7). Oaks are perennial trees or woody shrubs. They grow in all areas of the United States, especially in the southwestern states of Texas, Arizona, and Utah, and they also grow in Europe and New Zealand.

Conditions of Poisoning

The most dangerous period for oak poisoning is during March and April when new foliage is sprouting. Poisoning of cattle and, less frequently, sheep and goats occurs on ranges of the southwest and especially during drought years when the forage is limited. Supplemental feeding so that oak ingestion is below 50% of their diet will usually prevent poisoning. Acorn poisoning occurs in the fall, particularly when an acorn crop is heavy. Cattle, sheep, horses, and swine have been involved, and craving

TABLE 61.7 Oak Species Believed to Contribute to Poisoning

Species	Common Name
Quercus gambelii	Gambel's oak
Q. harvardii	Shin or shinnery oak
Q. marilandica	Jack oak
Q. stellata	Post oak
Q. breviloba or *durandii*	
Q. coccinea	Scarlet oak
Q. pedunculata or *robur*	European oak
Q. prinus	Chestnut oak
Q. xubra	Northern red oak
Q. velutina	Yellow-barked oak

for acorns has been observed in which animals appear to seek them out.

Swine seem to be somewhat resistant, and goats apparently utilize oak browse and are used to control oakbrush. Feeding high levels of immature gambel oak to goats did not induce any toxicosis.

The toxins in oak are tannins, particularly tannic acid and the phenolic acid gallic acid, and these are highest in new spring growth. Clinical signs of poisoning begin with depression, nasal discharge, abdominal pain, constipation, thirst, frequent urination, and rapid pulse, progressing over 1–3 days to rumen atony, anorexia, emaciation, weakness, prostration, rough coat, dry muzzle, subnormal temperature, bloody diarrhea, and death. Diagnosis is based on history of ingestion; clinical signs; elevated serum glutamic oxaloacetic transaminase, blood urea nitrogen, creatinine, and serum potassium; and lower urine specific gravity. Death may occur within 24 h of the onset of clinical signs.

Gross and microscopic lesions include gastritis, nephritis, increased peritoneal and pleural fluids, perirenal edema, and hemorrhages with pale swollen kidneys. The proximal convoluted tubules of the kidneys may be damaged, and abundant hyaline or granular casts may be evident. Mucous and blood are common in voided feces.

Prevention and Treatment

The best method of prevention is to provide adequate feed to reduce oak ingestion to less than 50% of the diet. Supplemental high-energy feed at 0.5–1 kg/head/day of a 54% cottonseed or soybean meal with 30% alfalfa meal, 6% vegetable oil, and 10% calcium hydroxide may be beneficial. Treatment includes blood transfusions if anemic, fluid therapy, rumenotomy if warranted, activated charcoal, plenty of fresh water, and avoiding stressing animals as much as possible.

PYRROLIZIDINE ALKALOID CONTAINING PLANTS

Pyrrolizidine alkaloid (PA)-containing plants are numerous and worldwide in distribution and in toxic significance (Cheeke and Shull, 1985). Three plant families predominate in PA-producing genera and species: Compositeae (*Senecio* spp.), Leguminosae (*Crotalaria* spp.), and Boraginaceae (*Heliotropium*, *Cynoglossum*, *Amsinckia*, *Echium*, and *Symphytum* spp.). All of these do not occur in the western United States. For plant descriptions, readers are referred to those species that cause losses in the western United States, which are listed in Table 61.8 with common names and distribution.

Toxicology

More than 150 PAs have been identified and structural characteristics elucidated. The PAs contain the pyrrolizidine nucleus and can be represented by the basic structures of senecionine and heliotrine. The toxic effects of

TABLE 61.8 PA-containing Plants in the Western United States: Common Names, Habitat, and Distribution

Scientific Name	Common Name	Habitat	Distribution
Amsinckia intermedia	Tarweed, fiddleneck	Dry, open cultivated fields	Pacific Coast; CA, WA, OR, ID
Cynoglossum officinale	Houndstongue	Dry, open areas; cultivated fields	Throughout West
Echium vulgare	Vipers bugloss		CA
Symphytum officinale	Comfrey		
Senecio brasiliensis			
Senecio cineraria	Dusty miller		Ornamental
Senecio glabellus	Bitterweed	Wet soils	TX and east
Senecio integerrimus			MT; Rocky Mountains, CA,
Senecio jacobaea	Stinking willy, tansy ragwort	Open fields and woods	Pacific Northwest
Senecio longilobus	Woody or groundleaf groundsel	Deserts	WY to NE, south to AZ and TX
Senecio spartioides	Broom groundsel		CO, UT south to TX, AZ, NM
Senecio riddellii	Riddell groundsel	Deserts	CO, UT south to TX, AZ, NM
Senecio vulgaris	Common groundsel		CA, OR
Crotalaria sagittalis			Pacific Northwest

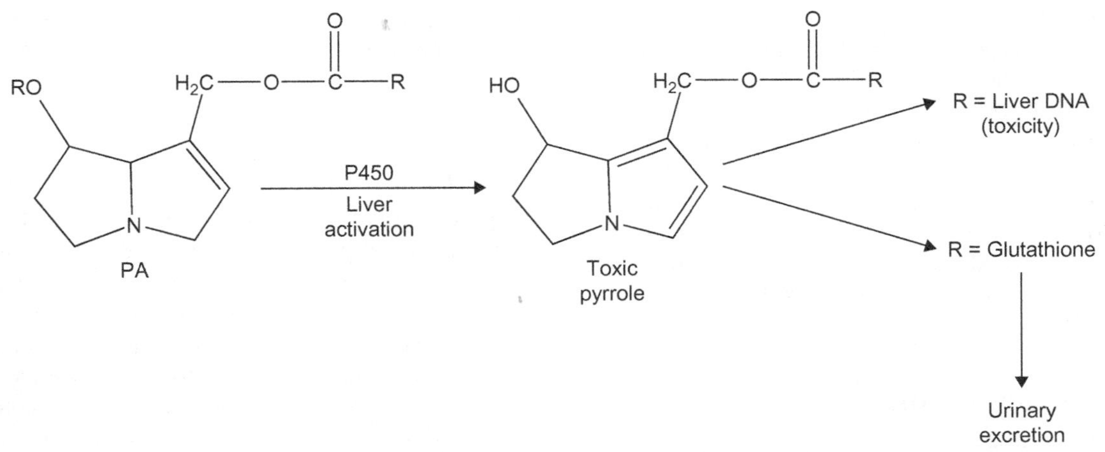

FIGURE 61.7 Metabolic pathway of pyrrolizidine alkaloids showing the toxic pyrrole pathway and glutathione conjugate pathway for excretion.

all PAs are somewhat similar, although their potency varies due to their bioactivation in the liver to toxic metabolites called pyrroles (Figure 61.7). These pyrroles are powerful alkylating agents that react with cellular proteins and cross-link DNA, resulting in cellular dysfunction, abnormal mitosis, and tissue necrosis. The primary effect is hepatic damage; however, many alkaloid and species-specific extrahepatic lesions have been described. Small amounts of pyrrole may enter the blood and be transported to other tissues, but there is debate on this issue because most pyrroles are super-reactive and not likely to make it into the circulation (Stegelmeier et al., 1999). When PA metabolites circulate, they are probably protein adducts that may be recycled. Some alkaloids (monocrotaline) may come off their carrier blood proteins and damage other tissues such as lung. Pigs seem more prone to develop extrahepatic lesions.

Toxicity of *Senecio*, *Heliotropium*, and *Echium* is largely confined to the liver, whereas *Crotalaria* will also cause significant lung damage. Typical histologic lesions are swelling of hepatocytes, hepatocyte necrosis, periportal necrosis, megalocytosis (enlarged parenchymal cells), karyomegaly (enlarged nuclei) fibrosis, bile duct proliferation, and vascular fibrosis and occlusion. Hepatic cells may be 10–30 times normal size, and DNA content may be 200 times normal.

In most species affected by PA poisoning, the liver becomes hard, fibrotic, and smaller. Because of decreased bile secretion, bilirubin levels in the blood rise, causing jaundice. Common clinical signs include ill thrift, depression, diarrhea, prolapsed rectum, ascites, edema in the GI tract, photosensitization, and aberrant behavior. In horses, "head pressing" or walking in straight lines regardless of obstacles in the path may occur. These neurological signs in horses are due to elevated blood ammonia from reduced liver function. PA poisoning may cause elevated blood ammonia, resulting in spongy degeneration of the central nervous system.

Elevated levels of serum enzymes such as alanine aminotransferase, aspartate aminotransferase, γ-glutamyl transferase, and alkaline phosphatase are reported (Stegelmeier et al., 1999). Use of these tests for diagnosis is supportive but should not be relied on exclusively because they vary with animal species and other conditions. They may also be in the normal range even though liver damage has occurred, and they tend to be transient. Liver function tests such as bilirubin, bile acids, or sulfobromophthalein (BSP) clearance may be useful estimates of the extent of liver damage.

There are marked differences in susceptibility of livestock and laboratory animals to PA toxicosis. Cows are most sensitive, followed by horses, goats, and sheep, respectively. In small laboratory animals, rats are most sensitive, followed by rabbits, hamsters, guinea pigs, and gerbils, respectively. Among avian species, chickens and turkeys are highly susceptible, whereas Japanese quail are resistant (Cheeke and Shull, 1985).

Detoxification mechanisms of PAs generally involve the liver and GI tract. Evidence of ruminal detoxification in sheep suggests this contributes to the reduced toxicity in that species. There are also substantial species-specific differences in the rate of PA metabolism. Both probably contribute to species susceptibility. For example, *Echium* and *Heliotropium* PAs are easily degraded by certain rumen microflora, but there is little evidence of ruminal degradation of *Senecio* PAs. The PAs in *Senecio* are macrocyclic closed esters of retronecine as opposed to the open esters found in heliotridine. Therefore, the reason for the difference in *Senecio* toxicity between sheep and cattle is unlikely to be the rumen detoxification but more likely differences in species-specific enzymatic activation of *Senecio* PAs. For example, in *in vitro* studies, retrorsine metabolism has been shown to be high in those species that are most susceptible and lowest in animals of least susceptibility. In addition, in *in vivo* studies, it was demonstrated that a higher pyrrole production rate occurred in cattle compared to sheep. Simple induction of liver microsomal enzymes by phenobarbitone increased pyrrole production and increased PA toxicity (LD_{50} in guinea pigs from >800 to 216 mg/kg). PA toxicity may disrupt other hepatic functions. Abnormal copper metabolism coagulation, NH_3 metabolism, protein metabolism, etc. may be affected in PA poisoning.

Prevention and Treatment

Because there are no proven effective methods of prevention or treatment, avoidance of the plant and controlling plant populations with herbicides or biological control is essential. Resistance to PA toxicosis in some species suggests that the possibility may exist to increase resistance to PAs. Dietary factors such as increased protein, particularly those high in sulfur amino acids, had minor protective effects in some species. Antioxidants such as BHT and ethoxyquin induced increased detoxifying enzymes such as glutathione *S*-transferase and epoxide hydrolase. Zinc salts have been shown to provide some protection against hepatotoxicosis from sporidesmin or lupinosis in New Zealand and Australia, and zinc supplementation reduced toxicity in rats from *Senecio* alkaloids (Burrows and Tyrl, 2001; Knight and Walter, 2001).

Many of these plants were introduced either inadvertently or intentionally. Without natural predators to keep populations in check, they experienced explosive growth and distribution followed by epidemic proportions of toxicity. Introduction of biological controls and natural population controls have reduced many of the plant populations and thus toxicoses have declined. Sheep, a resistant species, have been used to graze plants, particularly *S. jacobaea.*

PHOTOSENSITIZING PLANTS

Numerous plants cause photosensitization resulting in losses to the livestock industry. Photosensitization is the development of abnormally high reactivity to ultra-violet radiation or natural sunlight in the skin or mucous membranes. Primarily induced in livestock by various poisonous plants, the syndrome in livestock has been defined as primary and secondary photosensitization.

Description and Distribution

Photosensitizing plants are too numerous to describe individually, and readers are referred to taxonomic texts for plant description. Photosensitizing plants occur throughout the world and are common in the diets of livestock and people. Their distribution in the western United States, common names, and toxins are listed in Table 61.9.

Toxicology

Primary

In primary photosensitization, the photoreactive agent is absorbed directly from the plant and reaches the peripheral circulation and skin, where it reacts with the ultraviolet rays of the sun and results in sunburn, particularly of unprotected areas of the body. Hypericin and fagopyrin are polyphenolic derivatives from St. John's wort and buckwheat, respectively, and are primary photodynamic agents (Cheeke and Shull, 1985). By definition, primary photosensitization does not induce hepatic damage. Most agents are ingested, but some may induce lesions through skin contact. Several of these plants are weedy in nature and can contaminate pastures and feed. Exposure to some plants is increasing as they are becoming widely used as herbal remedies and holistic medicines. In most cases, the photodynamic agent is absorbed from the digestive tract unchanged and reaches the skin in its "native" form (Stegelmeier, 2002).

There are drugs and other toxins known to cause primary photosensitization, and these should be considered in the differential diagnosis. Phenothiazine-induced photosensitization is most common in ruminants because the photodynamic agent is phenothiazine sulfoxide, a rumen metabolite. Clinical signs in addition to photosensitivity include corneal edema and kerato conjunctivitis from the phenothiazine sulfoxide excreted in tears and the aqueous humor. Other toxins associated with primary photosensitivity include thiazides, acriflavins, sulfonamides, tetracyclines, methylene blue, coal-tar derivatives, furosemide, promazine, chlorpromazine, quinindine, and some antimicrobial soaps (Stegelmeier, 2002).

Secondary

In secondary or hepatogenous photosensitization, the photoreactive agent is phylloerythrin, a degradation product of chlorophyll. Phylloerythrin is produced in the stomach of animals, especially ruminants, and absorbed into the bloodstream. In normal animals, the hepatocytes conjugate phylloerythrin and excrete it in the bile. However, if the liver is damaged or bile secretion is impaired, phylloerythrin accumulates in the liver, the blood, and subsequently the skin, causing photosensitivity. This is the most common cause of photosensitization in livestock and horses (Knight and Walter, 2001). Because chlorophyll is almost always present in the diet of livestock, the etiologic agent of secondary photosensitization is the hepatotoxic agent.

The dermatologic signs of photosensitization in livestock are similar regardless of the plant or toxicant involved. Degree of severity varies, depending on the

TABLE 61.9 Photosensitizing Plants of the Western United States, Listed as Primary and Secondary Photosensitizers

Scientific Name	Common Name	Distribution	Toxin
Primary Photosensitizers			
Hypericum perforatum	St. John's wort, Klamath weed	Pacific Coast states	Hypericin
Fagopyrum sagittatum	Buckwheat	Northwestern U.S.	Fagopyrin
Cymopterus watsoni	Spring parsley	Southwestern U.S.	Furocoumarins
Ammi majus	Bishop's weed	Southwestern U.S.	Furocoumarins
Secondary Photosensitizers			
Artemesia	Sagebrush	Western U.S.	
Tetradymia glabrata	Spineless horsebrush	Western U.S.	
Tetradymia canescens	Gray horsebrush	Western U.S.	
Agave lecheguilla	Lechuguilla	Southwest	Saponins
Nolina texana	Sacahuiste	Southwest	Saponins
Tribulus terrestris	Puncture vine	Southwest	Saponins
Trifolium hybridum	Alsike clover	North, Midwest	
Lantana spp.	Lantana	Southwest	Saponins
Panicum spp.	Panic grass, Kleingrass	Western U.S.	
Brassica napus	Rape	Western U.S.	
Senecio spp.	Senecios	Western U.S.	PAs
Cynoglossum officinale	Houndstongue	Western U.S.	PAs
Cooperia pedunculata	Amaryllis family	Southwest U.S.	
Thamnosma texana	Dutchmans breeches	Southwest U.S.	Psoralens
Kochia scoparia	Kochia, burning bush		Saponins
Descurania pinnata	Tansymustard		Unknown

PAs, pyrrolizidine alkaloids.

amount of toxin or reactive phylloerythrin in the skin, degree of exposure to sunlight, and amount of normal physical photoprotection (hair and pigmentation). First signs in most animals are restlessness or discomfort from irritated skin, followed by photophobia, squinting, tearing, erythema, itching, and sloughing of skin in exposed areas (i.e., lips, ears, eyelids, udder, external genitalia, or white pigmented areas) (Burrows and Tyrl, 2001). Swelling in the head and ears (edema) of sheep after ingestion of *Tetradymia* has been referred to as big head. It was determined that sheep grazing black sagebrush (*Artemesia nova*) before *Tetradymia* were three times more likely to develop this photosensitization. Tissue sloughing and serum leakage may occur where tissue damage is extensive. Primary photosensitization rarely results in death. However, in secondary or hepatogenic photosensitization, the severity of liver damage and secondary metabolic and neurologic changes of hepatic failure may ultimately result in death. Recovery may leave sun-burned animals debilitated from scar tissue formation and wool or hair loss.

Prevention and Treatment

Prevention of poisoning lies in controlling plants with photosensitizing potential and providing adequate quality forage to animals. Treatment after poisoning involves removing animals from sun exposure, treating areas of necrosis and sunburn, antibiotic therapy, and supplementing young animals when access to sunburned udders is prevented because of nursing discomfort to dams. Identifying chronic hepatic disease is complicated because many of the serum markers for hepatic disease have returned to normal. As normal hepatocytes become replaced with fibrous connective tissue, there are fewer damaged cells to elevate serum enzymes. Percutaneous liver biopsies are invaluable in identifying and diagnosing these cases (Stegelmeier et al., 1999).

Plant-induced hepatopathy generally results in characteristic histologic lesions. For example, pyrrolizidine alkaloids generally cause bridging portal fibrosis with hepatocellular necrosis, biliary proliferation, and megalocytosis. *Panicum* and *Tribulus* species generally produce a crystalline cholangiohepatitis. Liver biopsy also provides prognostic information. The degree of damage is correlated directly with the animal's ability to compensate, recover, and provide useful production. Note that the liver reacts to insult in a limited number of ways, and most histologic changes are not pathognomonic. Hepatic cirrhosis (necrosis, fibrosis, and biliary proliferation) involves nonspecific changes that can be initiated by a variety of toxic and infectious agents (Stegelmeier et al., 1999).

DEATH CAMAS

All death camas species are assumed to be toxic; however, variation in toxicity exists between species and even within species depending on season, climate, soils, and geographical locations. Poisoning in sheep, cattle, horses, pigs, fowl, and humans has been reported. The largest losses generally occur in sheep. Sheep are primarily affected because of their tendency to select forbs, particularly in early spring when they are turned onto range before grasses have emerged.

Death camas is generally not palatable to livestock but is one of the earliest species to emerge in the spring. Poisoning most frequently occurs in spring when other more palatable forage is not available, or on overgrazed ranges where there is a lack of more desirable forage. Poisonings have resulted due to management errors in which hungry animals were placed in death camas-infested areas (Panter et al., 1987).

Description, Habitat, and Geographical Distribution

Foothill death camas is typical of the 15–20 species of *Zigadenus* in North America and Asia (Figure 61.8). A list of death camas species and their habitats, distributions, and growth periods is provided in Table 61.10. It is difficult to distinguish between species because they are taxonomically similar. A member of the lily family, death camas is a perennial, glabrous herb with basal V-shaped grass-like leaves growing from an onion-like bulb with a dark-colored outer coat. Stems produced at flowering are single, unbranched, sparingly leafed, and terminated by a terminal raceme of greenish-white, cream-colored, or pink inflorescence. The perianth is six-membered, consisting of three lanceolate or ovate sepals and three petals separate or united below, with one or two glands just above the base; six stamens; and three styles. Floral parts are persistent as the fruits develop. The seed is a three-cavitied capsule, separating into three members and opening inwardly at maturity. Death camas is easily confused with wild onion, mariposa lily, or common camas particularly before flowering. Wild onions are distinguished by tubular leaves and their onion-like odor. The leaves of mariposa lilies are more U-shaped in cross section, and common camas has a blue flower. Death camas is prevalent in western North America and is native to the open plains and foothills of the United States.

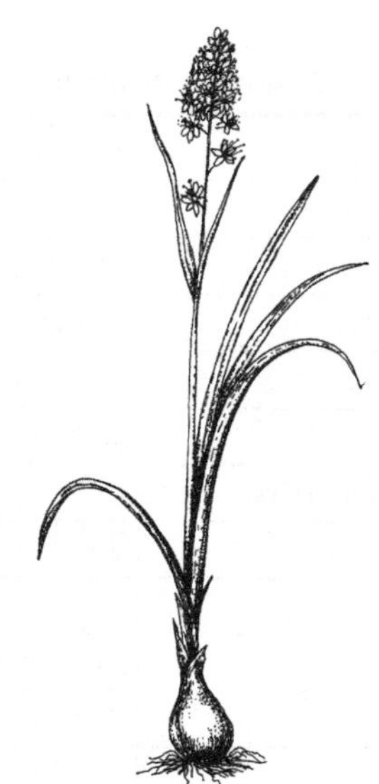

FIGURE 61.8 Foothill death camas with leaf structure, flower head, and bulb.

Toxicity of Death Camas to Livestock

The toxins in death camas are of the cevanine steroidal alkaloid type – that is, zigacine **(11)**. Zigacine is a very

(11)
Zigacine

TABLE 61.10 *Zigadenus* spp.: Common Name, Distribution, Habitat, and Growth Periods

Species	Common Name	Distribution	Habitat	Growth Period
Z. paniculatus S. Watson	Foothill death camas; sand-corn; panicled death camas	Eastern WA, OR, ID, UT, WY, NV, eastern CA, northern AZ and NM	Foothills and benches	May–July
Z. venenosus S. Watson =	Meadow death camas; grassy death camas	WA, OR, ID, MT, ND; south to NE, UT, CO, NV, CA; north to western Canada	Plains, prairies, meadows and open coniferous woods	May–July
Z. gramineus Rydb. =				
Z. intermedium Rydb. =				
Z. salinus Rydb.				
Z. nuttallii A. Gray	Nuttall's death camas; poison camas	TN, AR, OK, KS, and northern TX	Prairies and rocky sites	April–June
Z. gramineus Rydb.	Grassy death camas	Southwestern Canada, MT, ID, WA; south through WY, CO, UT, NV, AZ, NM	Open hills and plains	April–July
Z. elegans Pursh =	White camas, elegant death camas, mountain death camas	AK, western Canada, MT, south into AZ and east into MN and IA	Prairies and meadows	June–August
Z. glaucus Nutt.				
Z. leimanthoides A. Grey	–	Southwestern U.S. and coastal plains of DE, NJ, and RI	Sandy pine lands and bogs of the coastal plains	June–August
Z. fremontii Torr.	–	Southwestern OR and western CA	Dry grassy or brushy slopes	May–July
Z. glaberrimus Michx.	–	Southeastern U.S.	Savannas and wet pine lands	July–Sept.
Z. densus Desr.	Black snakeroot, crow poison, St. Agnes' feather, black death camas	Southeastern U.S.	Damp soils, pine woods and bogs	May–June
Z. exaltatus Eastw.	–	Central CA		May–June
Z. micranthus Eastw.	–	Northwestern CA, southwestern OR		
Z. vaginatus Rydb.	Alcove death camas	Northwestern CA, southwestern OR		
Z. virescens Kunth.	AZ, NM, and northern Mexico			

potent compound with an i.v. LD_{50} of 2 mg/kg and an oral LD_{50} of 130 mg/kg in mice (Welch et al., 2011b). Clinical signs of toxicosis are similar in all livestock poisoned by *Zigadenus*, irrespective of the species of plant Zigacine involved. Excessive salivation is noted first, with foamy froth around the nose and muzzle that persists, followed by nausea and occasionally vomition in ruminants (Panter et al., 1987). Intestinal peristalsis is dramatically increased, accompanied by frequent defecation and urination. Muscular weakness with accompanying ataxia, muscular fasciculations, prostration, and eventual death may follow. The pulse becomes rapid and weak, and the respiration rate increases but the amplitude is reduced. Some animals become cyanotic, and the spasmodic struggling for breath may be confused with convulsions. The heart fails before respiration, and at necropsy the heart is usually found in diastole. A comatose period may range from a few hours to a few days before death.

Pathological lesions are those of pulmonary congestion. Gross lesions of sheep include severe pulmonary congestion, hemorrhage, edema, and subcutaneous hemorrhage in the thoracic regions. Microscopic lesions include severe pulmonary congestion with infiltration of red blood cells in the alveolar spaces and edema. Diagnosis of poisoning may be established by clinical signs of toxicosis, evidence of death camas being grazed, histopathological analysis of tissues from necropsied animals, and identification of death camas in the rumen or stomach contents (Panter et al., 1987).

Similarity in clinical signs of toxicosis between certain species of these plants suggests that the same alkaloids are present; however, differences in concentrations can explain the differences in relative toxicity of different species (Table 61.11).

Management and Prevention

Conditions conducive to poisoning by death camas include driving animals through death camas-infested ranges; not allowing animals to graze selectively; unloading hungry animals in infested areas; lambing, bedding, watering, or salting livestock in death camas-infested areas; or placing animals on range where little forage is available. Poisoning generally occurs in the early spring when death camas is the first green forage available and the young immature foliage is the most toxic. Single losses of 300–500 sheep have been reported (Panter et al., 1987). In the 1987 case, 80% of the dead sheep were 80- to 90-lb lambs. Three key factors contributed to the losses: (1) ewes with lambs were driven through a heavily infested area of death camas when the sheep were hungry; (2) the sheep were bedded down for the night near the death camas area, providing immediate access to death camas the following morning; and (3) the herder panicked and rapidly forced the sheep out of the area, contributing to the stress and probably exacerbating the toxic effects and increasing the losses.

VERATRUM SPP.

Veratrum belongs to the Liliaceae (Lily) family and is composed of at least five species in North America. During the mid-20th century, up to 25% of pregnant ewes that grazed on pastures infested with *Veratrum californicum* in the mountains of central Idaho gave birth to lambs with serious craniofacial malformations. These malformations ranged from the gross anomaly of cyclops to less severe deformities of the upper and lower jaws. The Basque shepherds called the cyclopic defect "chatto," which translated as "monkey faced" lamb disease. Although losses from *Veratrum* have long been reduced or eliminated on these ranges due to the application of research findings and recommended management strategies, biomedical research using the alkaloids, isolated and identified at the Poisonous Plant Research Laboratory, as molecular probes has opened a new frontier for human medical research (James et al., 2004).

TABLE 61.11 Relative Toxicity in Sheep of Five *Zigadenus* spp.

Zigadenus Species	Average Minimum Toxic Dose[a]	Average Minimum Lethal Dose[a]
Z. gramineus	4	6
Z. paniculatus	10	25
Z. venenosus	4	20
Z. elegans	20	60
Z. nuttallii	2	5

[a]Grams of green plant per kilogram body weight.

Distribution

Veratrum californicum grows primarily in the high mountain ranges of the western United States (Knight and Walter, 2001). *Veratrum viride* is the most widespread species and grows in the northwestern United States north through western Canada into Alaska and is also widespread in the northeastern United States. *Veratrum insolitum* grows in a relatively small region of northwestern California and southwestern Oregon; *V. parviflorum* grows in the central southeastern states; and *V. woodii* grows from Ohio to Missouri, Oklahoma, and Arkansas. Two other species have been reported to cause poisoning in other countries: *V. japonicum* in Korea and *V. album* in Europe. Common names include western false hellebore, hellebore, skunk cabbage, corn lily, Indian poke, and wolfsbane. Caution should be used with common names because they may be used interchangeably within this genera but also in unrelated genera. For example, the name hellebore is also used for the genus *Helleborus* in the buttercup family.

Habitat and Description

Most *Veratrum* spp. are found in similar habitats of moist, open alpine meadows or open woodlands, marshes, along waterways, in swamps or bogs, and along lake edges in high mountain ranges. Most species grow at higher elevations. All species are similar, with coarse, erect plants approximately 1–2.5 m tall with short perennial rootstalks. The leaves are smooth, alternate, parallel veined, broadly oval to lanceolate, up to 30 cm long, 15 cm wide, in three ranks, and sheathed at the base. The inflorescence is panicle flowers; the lower ones often staminate and the upper ones perfect. The flowers of *V. viride* are distinctly green, and the fruit is three-chambered with several seeds.

Toxicology

More than 50 complex steroidal alkaloids have been identified from the *Veratrum* spp. Five classes of steroidal alkaloids have been characterized: veratrines, cevanines, jervanines, solanidines, and cholestanes. The veratrines and cevanines are of considerable interest in toxicology because they are neurological toxins and hypotensive agents that bind to sodium channels, delaying closure and causing cardiotoxic and respiratory effects. The cevanine alkaloids, such as zigacine, are also found in *Zigadenus* spp., which are also members of the Lily family. The jervanines are most significant for their teratogenic effects; the most notable alkaloids were named cyclopamine **(12)** and jervine, both potent inducers of the congenital cyclopia monkey faced lamb syndrome reported in many flocks of sheep in the late 1950s in central Idaho. This cyclopic defect is induced in the sheep embryo during the blastocyst stage of development when the pregnant mother ingests the plant during the 14th day of gestation. Early embryonic death up to day 19 of gestation and other defects, such as limb defects and tracheal stenosis, occur when maternal ingestion includes days 28–33 of gestation (Keeler and Stuart, 1987). The solanidine alkaloids are also found in many *Solanum* spp. and are toxic and teratogenic. The cholestanes have been used as hypotensive drugs but are much less likely to induce birth defects. The structure–activity relationship is very important in potency to produce birth defects. It is now known that this structure–activity relationship is key in the mechanism of action, which is the inhibition of the sonic hedgehog signaling pathway (Gaffield and Keeler, 1996). This sonic hedgehog gene pathway and the subsequent downstream regulation of other genes' expression have been implicated in numerous cancers, birth defects, and other anomalies. The toxin cyclopamine has become a significant tool in the study of this very complex sonic hedgehog pathway. Clinical trials have been proposed and studies are ongoing to further identify the hedgehog complex of genes and to understand its mechanism and function in formation and growth of numerous cancers, childhood birth defects, and manipulation of regulatory pathways.

Clinical signs of poisoning are most likely caused by the neurotoxic cevanine alkaloids present in most species of *Veratrum*. Typical signs begin with excess salivation with froth around the mouth, slobbering, and vomiting progressing to ataxia, collapse, and death. The elimination half-life of cyclopamine in sheep is approximately 1.1 h (Welch et al., 2009b). Consequently, 8 h after consuming *Veratrum*, greater than 99% of the toxins should be eliminated from the animal.

Prevention and Treatment

Control of *Veratrum* is relatively easy with herbicides such as broad-leaf herbicides, and long-term control has been demonstrated. The teratogenic effects of *Veratrum* can be avoided by keeping sheep and other livestock species off pastures containing the plants during the first trimester of pregnancy. Observation of toxicoses in the field is rare unless herders move the animals soon after exposure. The neurological signs, which are likely produced by the cevanine alkaloids (both *Veratrum* and *Zigadenus* spp.), can be treated with atropine to improve the cardiovascular output. Activated charcoal to adsorb toxins and administration of picrotoxin to improve respiration have been recommended (Burrows and Tyrl, 2001).

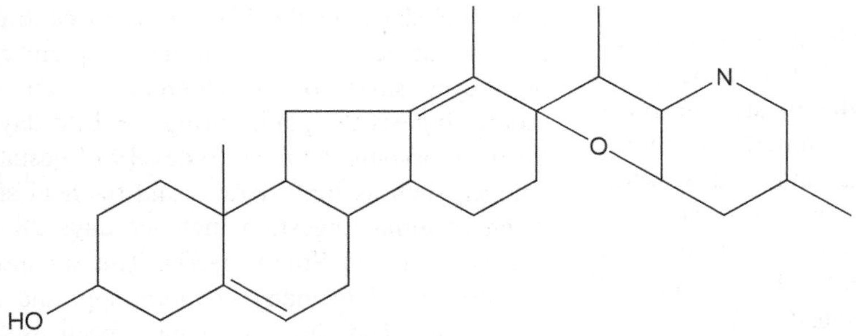

HO

(12)
Cyclopamine

BRACKEN FERN (*PTERIDIUM* AND *AQUILINUM*)

Distribution and Habitat

The bracken fern family is worldwide in distribution and includes approximately 20 genera and more than 400 species. Although most species described are found in the tropics, there are 4 genera and 6 species described in North America (Burrows and Tyrl, 2001). The bracken fern most associated with toxicoses in the United States is *Pteridium aquilinum* (Kuhn), which is distributed throughout North America. It is reported to be one of the most widespread species of vascular plants, only exceeded in geographical range by a few annual weeds. Four varieties of *P. aquilinum* have been described: var. *pubescens* (western bracken fern), found throughout the western United States; var. *caudatum* (lacy bracken), restricted to southern Florida; var. *latiusculum* (eastern bracken), distributed throughout the eastern United States; and var. *pseudocaudatum* (tailed bracken), located mostly in the southeastern quarter of the United States.

Western bracken grows best in rocky, gravelly, well-drained soils in dry, open woodlands to semishaded habitats. Extensive stands frequently grow along pasture edges, in logged areas, or where fires have opened up the canopy. Moisture needs are modest in comparison with those of many of the ferns, and good soil drainage is important.

Description

Bracken plants are deciduous and grow from brown to black woody rhizomes, forming large, often dense patches. The leaves emerge from erect fronds and are pinnately compound, scattered, erect, coarse, narrowly or broadly triangular, to 2 m in height. Fronds (leaves) are pinnules (ultimate segments), oblong, entire in the apices of the pinnae, and lobed toward the stalk. Reproduction is by spores produced in sporangia lining the undersurface margins of the photosynthetic fronds; when reproductive, they are covered by the narrow recurved edge of the leaf (Burrows and Tyrl, 2001).

Toxicology

Toxicity of bracken fern was first recognized in the 1800s and described in horses as a neurological condition. Contaminated hay was believed to be the cause, and the condition was described in the United Kingdom and Pacific Coast states of the United States (Taylor, 1990). Early research determined that 20–25% bracken for 3 or 4 weeks would induce a neurological disease followed soon after by death. Although the neurological condition is mostly described in horses, low hematocrits and reddish-brown urine have also been described in suspected cases of bracken poisoning.

Bracken causes a wide range of syndromes that have been described in livestock, including thiamine deficiency in monogastrics, acute hemorrhagic disease associated with bone marrow aplasia and ulceration of the upper GI tract, "bright blindness" progressive retinal degeneration, and neoplasia of the urinary bladder and upper digestive tract. The major toxin is the sesquiterpene glucoside, ptaquiloside **(13)**. Other toxins, carcinogens, and mutagens may also be implicated in the disease conditions.

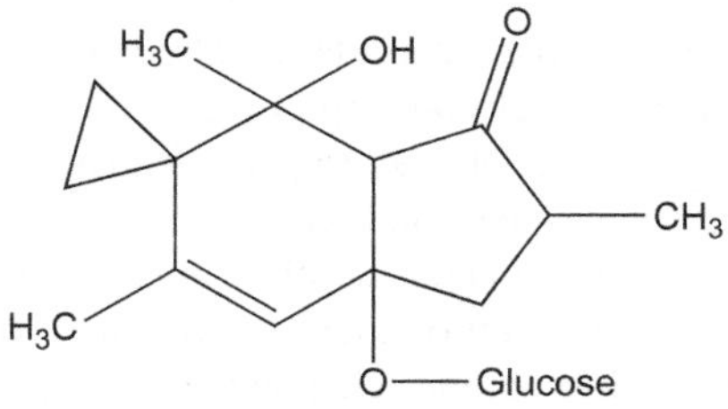

H_3C OH O CH_3 H_3C O—Glucose

(13)
Ptaquiloside

People have consumed the rhizomes or croziers of bracken fern as a traditional food or out of necessity, and the toxin is transferred through milk of cows grazing the plant. Epidemiological evidence suggests that some cancers in humans probably result from primary or secondary consumption of the carcinogens. Ptaquilosides form adducts with DNA, binding to certain base sequences, resulting in mutated codons associated with known oncogenes. This hypothesis has been proposed in the pathogenesis of the disease.

Syndromes of bracken poisoning are well recognized in livestock. Many factors must be considered in the genesis of the disease, such as quantity consumed, phenological stage of the plant, time of year, consumption rate and length of time consumption occurs, animal species, age, and sex of the animal. The disease conditions described include thiamine deficiency in monogastrics, acute hemorrhagic disease, bright blindness, enzootic hematuria, and small intestine carcinoma. These conditions have been experimentally produced by feeding bracken fern and ptaquiloside to livestock species and rodent models. Bracken fern feeding studies in rodents have produced neoplasms in the ileum, urinary bladder, mammary glands, and lungs of rodents.

The toxin ptaquiloside was isolated, characterized, and the structure published in the early 1980s (Saito et al., 1990). Different species and varieties of *Pteridium* have been compared for ptaquiloside concentration, and all examined to date contained ptaquiloside. Large variations in concentration were demonstrated between locations, altitude, season, etc., suggesting a genetic component or another factor, such as endophyte-produced compounds. These differences were maintained when bracken fern rhizomes were transferred to a greenhouse and soils were changed; thus, the ptaquiloside differences were still evident for the next 3 years. Ptaquiloside concentrations are highest in young growing parts (i.e., the tips of the croziers and immature fronds), whereas concentrations diminish as the plant matures and as samples are taken from more mature pinnae and toward the base of the lamina. In all samples of rhizome, the apices of the fronds or primordia taken from below the soil surface had no ptaquiloside; however, very immature croziers only a few centimeters above the surface showed the presence of the toxin. The emergence of the crozier apices and exposure to light apparently influence the bio-synthesis of the toxin. The spores have not been shown to contain ptaquiloside, but they have caused cancer and formed DNA adducts, suggesting that carcinogenic or mutagenic derivatives are present. Ptaquiloside and other ptaquiloside-like compounds with carcinogenic activity have been isolated from other ferns from the genera *Histiopteris*, *Cheilanthes*, *Cibotium*, *Dennstadtia*, *Hypolepis*, *Pteris*, and *Pityrogramma* (Saito et al., 1990).

Although bracken fern poisoning occurs in the United States, the most serious risk is in countries such as Australia, New Zealand, Japan, and the United Kingdom, where bracken is more prevalent and utilized for human food or animal feed. Epidemiology studies have associated increased esophageal and gastric cancers with direct ingestion, secondary ingestion (i.e., milk from cows grazing bracken), or living in bracken fern-infested areas. Bracken fronds steeped in water or treated with wood ash or sodium bicarbonate have reduced toxicity, but this process only reduces the concentration and does not eliminate the toxins.

Lesions in horses poisoned by bracken fern are indicative of thiamine deficiency and include congestion of the brain, a swollen and edematous cerebrum grossly, and necrosis of some neurons microscopically. Acute hemorrhagic disease in cattle is characterized by extensive hemorrhage of the mucous membranes and subcutaneous hemorrhage and edema.

Pathology of the bracken-induced enzootic hematuria includes desquamated and proliferative bladder epithelium, and areas of vascularized epithelial proliferation appear as polyploid, papillary, or fungoid reddened foci. Microscopically, columns of transitional epithelium infiltrate into the lamina propria along with mononuclear cells. Neoplasia, when it occurs, is most commonly the noninvasive papillomatous type, but other papillary types of transitional cell carcinoma, squamous cell carcinoma, adenocarcinoma, or hemangiomas may also develop (Burrows and Tyrl, 2001).

Treatment

Bracken-induced thiamine deficiency in horses is treatable with administration of thiamine parenterally at 0.5–1 g, followed by decreasing doses during the next few days. Symptomatic care with good feed and fresh water accompanied by administration of a laxative but not mineral oil is helpful. In ruminants, the bone marrow suppression and deficiency of blood platelets and neutrophils is best treated with antimicrobials to counteract any bacterial infection that might occur because of diminished immune function. Good veterinary care, symptomatic treatment, clean water, and quality feed in a quiet, clean environment are recommended.

MILKWEEDS (*ASCLEPIAS* SPP.)

Description

Milkweeds are classified into two broad groups: (1) narrow-leaved, with narrow, linear, lanceolate leaves, and (2) broad-leaved, with leaves approximately 4 cm wide throughout much of their length (Figure 61.9). There are more than 150 species of *Asclepias*, of which 108 occur in North America. Milkweeds are perennial, summer or early autumn flowering herbs with a milky latex-like cream in the stems. Of the many species found in North America, several are important toxicologically and are

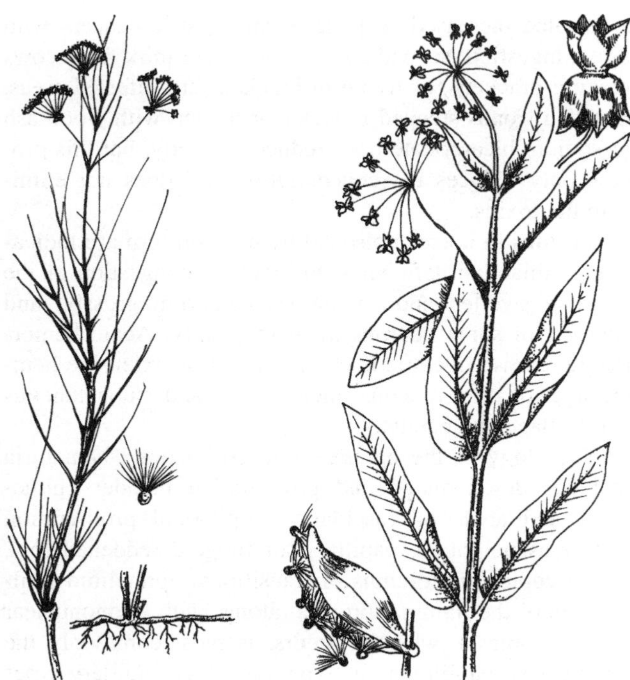

FIGURE 61.9 Narrow leaf (left) and broad leaf (right) milk-weeds (*Asclepias* spp.) represented.

represented in Table 61.12. The stems of the plants are erect and range from 4 to 150 cm tall; leaves are opposite or whorled. Flowers are of various colors, umbellate clusters or solitary, and terminal or extra-axillary. Numerous seeds are contained in an inflated milkweed-type pod and are flat and large, with each bearing a tuft of long, silk-like hairs for wind distribution.

Distribution and Habitat

Milkweeds are adapted to a broad range of habitats and environmental conditions and are found in most plant communities. Occupied habitats include prairies, woodlands, open areas, rocky plains, sand dunes, swamps, marshes, seeps, canyon bottoms, dry washes, desert lands, and waste lands. Most species are weedy and form small to large patches often along roadsides, in disturbed areas, or in overgrazed pastures.

Toxicology

Some species of milkweeds have been used as medicines, food, or a source of poison. Most species contain a mixture of steroidal glycosidic cardenolides **(14)** that are toxic and induce two syndromes – one with GI/cardio-toxic effects and the other with neurological effects. The early literature suggested that the broad-leaved group was cardiotoxic, whereas the narrow-leaved type was neurotoxic. However, most narrow-leaved species have now been shown to also contain cardiotoxins (Ogden et al., 1992).

Historically, naturalists observed as early as the mid- 1800s that birds avoided eating certain butterflies, such as the monarchs, whose larvae fed on milkweeds. It was later learned that the feeding larvae were able to concentrate some of the cardenolides that were potent emetics and thus created an effective defense against herbivory. As of the late 1980s, 27 species of milkweed were recognized as common feed for butterfly larvae, and the most toxic species were often preferred. Milkweeds are also host to many other insect species.

(14)
Cardenolide

The basic structure of the series of identified cardenolides is a 23-C steroidal backbone with a five-membered, singly unsaturated lactone ring at the C-17 position, a hydroxyl group at C-14, and methyl groups at C-10 and C-13. Glycosidic linkage usually occurs at the C-3 or C-2 positions and may include glucose, rhamnose, or thevetose as the sugars. Additional functionalities attached to the backbone further influence solubility and binding, thus increasing or decreasing toxicity. The cardenolides inhibit Na^{+}/K^{+}-ATPase, and the structure–activity relationship is believed to reside in the unsaturated lactone ring at C-17 and the hydroxyl group at C-14 (Joubert, 1989).

Sheep, goats, cattle, horses, and domestic fowl have been poisoned with milkweeds. Clinical signs usually begin with depression, weakness, and labored breathing accompanied by ataxia and loss of balance, progressing to recumbency, seizures, and death. The order of clinical signs is dependent on the type of animal affected, the toxicity of the plant, the time of ingestion, and the amount of the toxin consumed. Clinical effects appear within a few hours of ingestion, and death may follow within 1 to a few days later in fatal cases.

TABLE 61.12 Milkweeds: *Asclepias* spp., Common Name, Distribution, Habitat, and Toxin

Species	Common Name	Distribution	Habitat	Toxin; Content[a]
Narrow-leaved Milkweeds				
A. labriformis Jones	Labriform milkweed	Southeastern UT	Along old streambeds in sandy soils	Cardiac glycosides, digitoxin; very high
A. verticillata L.	Eastern whorled milkweed, spider milkweed	From TX to MI, east to FL and MA	Dry open areas	Cardenolides; very low
A. subverticillata Vail	Western whorled milkweed, horsetail milkweed	Western KS and OK, UT, AZ, TX and into Mexico	Dry plains and foothills, spreads rapidly along waterways and canals	Cardenolides; very low
A. pumila Vail	Low whorled milkweed, plains whorled milkweed	East of the Rockies from TX and NM north to southeast	Small patches in draws and ravines	Cardenolides; very low
A. mexicana Cav.	Mexican whorled milkweed	MT and southwest ND Southern TX to central Mexico	Open areas and dry soils	Cardenolides; unknown
A. asperula Woodson	Antelope horn milkweed	KS, AR to NV and AZ	Open areas and dry soils	Cardenolides; very high
A. fascicularis Decne.	Mexican milkweed	CA, western OR through eastern WA, ID and NV		Cardenolides; very low
A. brachystephana Engelm.	Short-crown milkweed	West central TX, southern AZ into NM and Mexico		Cardenolides; very high
A. subulata Decne.	Desert milkweed, yamate, ajamete	Southern CA, AZ, west coastal region of Mexico		Cardenolides; very high
Broad-leaved Milkweeds				
A. eriocarpa Benth.	Woolly pod milkweed	CA	Dry soils	Cardenolides; very high
A. latifolia Brit.	Broadleaf milkweed	KS, CO to TX and AZ	Dry plains	Cardenolides; high
A. speciosa Torr.	Showy milkweed	MN south to MI and TX; west to CA	Prairies and open spaces	Cardenolides; intermediate
A. syriaca L.	Common milkweed	Widely distributed in central and eastern U.S.	Open areas and along roadsides	Cardenolides; intermediate
A. incarnata L.	Swamp milkweed	IN	Cool damp soils	Cardenolides; very low
A. vestita Hook and Am.	Woolly milkweed	Central and south western CA		Cardenolides; very high
A. virdis Walter	Green milkweed, spider milkweed	South-central states, FL		Cardenolides; high

[a]*Cardenolide content mg/g plant from <0.25 (very low) to >4 (very high).*
Adapted from Burrows and Tyrl (2001) and Knight and Walter (2001).

Treatment and Control

There are two syndromes of milkweed poisoning – a neurological one and a cardiac one. Treatment for the cardiotoxic signs is approached similar to that of digitalis glycoside toxicity – that is, activated charcoal, atropine for atrioventricular block, and/or antiarrhythmic drugs. There is no specific treatment for the neurological syndrome except symptomatic treatment to control seizures and supportive therapy. A field test with a detection threshold of 0.057% is available for detecting cardenolides in the latex of milkweeds (Sady and Seiber, 1991). Knowledge of the milkweed species in the pasture, stage of plant growth when consumed, and history of grazing and clinical effects are all important in developing a diagnosis and eliminating other causes.

In most cases, knowledge that the plant exists in one's pasture and prevention of ingestion is the best way to avoid poisoning. Purchase of weed-free hay to avoid poisoning via contamination is also important. Know where the hay comes from, and always be alert as to the content of the hay. Control of milkweeds can be accomplished with herbicides such as 2,4-D, picloram, amitrole, or gyphosate, depending on the other forage it has infested and the circumstances. Always follow the manufacturer's recommendations.

NIGHTSHADES

The nightshade family comprises more than 80–90 genera and more than 2300 species worldwide. Some of the more common poisonous genera are *Brugmansia*, *Brunfelsia*, *Capsicum*, *Cestrum*, *Datura*, *Hyoscyamus*, *Lycium*, *Lycopersicon* (tomato), *Nicotiana* (tobacco), *Solandra*, *Solanum*, *Nicandra*, and *Physalis*. Some common nightshade species are listed in Table 61.13. In the United States and Canada, the nightshades can be annual, perennial, or shrubs with alternate, simple or compound leaves, axillary inflorescences, radially symmetrical flowers composed of five free sepals, five free petals, and usually five stamens with anthers grouped conically about the stigma and berry-like fruits of variable colors.

Toxins

The nightshades have a variety of toxins known to affect people and animals, including the tropane alkaloids, which affect the autonomic nervous system by blocking the action of cholinesterase (Knight and Walter, 2001). This results in accumulation of acetylcholine and subsequent inhibition of the parasympathetic nervous system, causing dry mouth, decreased intestinal motility, dilated pupils, and tachycardia. The tropane alkaloids also affect the GI tract, causing colic in horses, constipation, and/or hemorrhagic diarrhea. The *Nicotiana* spp. contain neurological toxins including the pyridine and piperidine alkaloids that are responsible for toxicoses and teratogenesis. Some species of *Solanum* cause a neurological disease in cattle, sheep, and goats characterized by loss of equilibrium, tremors, ataxia, collapse, opisthotonus, seizures, and death. *Solanum malacoxylon* and *Cestrum* spp. contain vitamin D-like compounds that cause abnormal calcium absorption and metabolism resulting in calcified tissues, lameness, and weight loss. Green potatoes, sprouts, and vines contain steroidal glycoalkaloids that are both toxic and teratogenic. Table 61.13 provides a limited overview of selected species, their distributions, and their toxins (Burrows and Tyrl, 2001; Knight and Walter, 2001).

Clinical Signs

The toxins in the Solanaceae family contribute to various clinical effects depending on the amount of plant/toxin ingested, the plant species eaten, and the animal species consuming the plant. Signs range from mild digestive upset to severe colic in horses when contaminated hay is fed; neurological dysfunction, seizures, and death in sheep and cattle; big head and calcification of the blood vessels; and teratogenesis.

Treatment

Animals showing severe neurological signs, such as tremors, ataxia, and dilated pupils, may be treated with physostigmine. Oral activated charcoal as an adsorbent may be effective if administered in a timely manner. However, most animals will recover if treated symptomatically and if the animals are not overly stressed.

KNAPWEEDS (*CENTAUREA* SPP.)

The knapweeds are a large group with primarily noxious, invasive characteristics. Although this genus is not a great risk for livestock producers, a serious disease of horses called nigropallidal encephalomalacia warrants its inclusion in this chapter. There are 450–500 species of *Centaurea*, and 29 species have been described in North America (Burrows and Tyrl, 2001). Most of these have been introduced and have had a huge negative impact on rangelands in the western United States. Although most species are opportunists and will aggressively invade rangelands, especially those that have been over-grazed, burned, or disturbed, only 2 species are of any toxicologic significance – *Centaurea repens* (Russian knapweed) and *C. solstitialis* (yellow star thistle).

TABLE 61.13 Nightshade Species with Known Links to Toxicosis in Humans or Animals: Common Names, Distribution, and Toxins

Species	Common Name	Distribution	Toxins
Solanum elaeagnifolium	Silverleaf nightshade	Southern U.S.	Solanine and solanidine
S. nigrum	Black nightshade	Throughout North America	Tropane and glycoalkaloids
S. dulcamara	Bittersweet; climbing nightshade	Eastern half of U.S.; areas of OR, WA, NV, CA, UT and WY	Glycoalkaloids
S. rostratum	Buffalo bur	Central U.S. to north and south borders	Glycoalkaloids
S. triflorum	Cutleaf nightshade	Central U.S. to north border	Glycoalkaloids
S. americanum	Huckleberry; wonderberry	Southern U.S.	Glycoalkaloids
S. physalifolium	Tropical soda apple	Throughout U.S.	Glycoalkaloids
S. sarrachoides	Hairy nightshade		Glycoalkaloids
S. carolinense	Horse or bull nettle	Eastern half of U.S.; west coast	Tropane alkaloid solanine
S. tuberosum	White or Irish potato	Worldwide	Glycoalkaloids
Datura wrightii	Sacred datura	Southwestern U.S.	Tropane alkaloids
D. stramonium	Jimson weed; thorn apple	Southeastern half of U.S.; west coast	Tropane alkaloids
Nicotiana tabacum	Cultivated or burley tobacco	Southern U.S.	Pyridine alkaloids (nicotine)
N. glauca	Tree tobacco	Southern U.S.	Piperidine alkaloids
Capsicum annum	Green or chili pepper	Cultivated in U.S.	Capsaicinoids
Cestrum parqui	Willow-leaved jessamine	Southern Gulf states	Glycoside of vitamin D
Atropa belladonna	Deadly nightshade; belladonna	Cultivated as an ornamental	Tropane alkaloids
Hyoscyamus niger	Black henbane	Northern U.S.	Tropane alkaloids, calystegins
Physalis virginiana	Ground cherry	Plains states and eastern U.S.	Glycoalkaloids, calystegins
P. lobota	Chinese lantern	Southern regions; cultivated throughout U.S.	Glycoalkaloids
Lycopersicon esculentum	Tomato	Worldwide	Glycoalkaloids

Adapted from Burrows and Tyrl (2001) and Knight and Walter (2001).

Habitat and Distribution

Yellow star thistle is most abundant in the western United States from central California north through Oregon, Washington, and Idaho. Smaller invasions are reported in many states east of the intermountain region, and although these have not received the attention of the larger invasions in the west, they have the potential to rapidly spread under the right environmental conditions (Panter, 1991; Burrows and Tyrl, 2001; Knight and Walter, 2001). Russian knapweed has invaded very large areas of the intermountain region of the western United States and the Great Plains. Again, smaller populations have invaded areas of the Midwest and northeastern United States and have the potential to expand rapidly. Although the aggressive nature of these species threatens rangelands and prohibits optimum utilization, a greater threat is the risk to sensitive or threatened native plant species and the balance of plant biodiversity.

Toxicology

The compounds isolated from knapweeds include a large class called sesquiterpene lactones. Although the putative toxin causing the neurological disease in horses has not been specifically identified, six of these compounds have been screened for cytotoxicity in an *in vitro* neuronal cell bioassay. The rank order of activity is repen > subluteolide > janerin > cynaropicrin > acroptilin > solstitialin (Riopelle and Stevens, 1993). Toxicity of solstitialin A-13 acetate and cynaropicrin to primary cultures of fetal rat substantia nigra cells has been demonstrated. These sesquiterpene lactones are quite unstable, and it has been hypothesized that they are precursors to the ultimate neurotoxin. Also, there are aspartic and glutamic acids present in these plants, and they possess neuroexcitatory properties.

Clinical Signs

Thus far, only yellow star thistle and Russian knapweed have been implicated in toxicoses in the United States and only in horses. Apparently, ruminants are not affected, and the *Centaurea* spp. may be useful forage for sheep and goats. However, in other countries, toxicoses in ruminants have been reported. For example, in South Africa, *C. repens* fed to sheep at 600 g dosages for 2 days caused an acute digestive upset and pulmonary edema and ascites. In Azerbaijan, *C. repens* is reported to cause a neurological disease in buffalo similar to that which has been described in horses. However, no neuropathology similar to that seen in horses was observed in the buffalo.

Toxicity generally occurs in summer and fall when forage is depleted and horses are forced to graze less palatable species. Ingestion often occurs for several months or more before an abrupt onset of neurological dysfunction is observed. Impaired eating and drinking are often the first observable signs. Depression and hypertonicity of the lips and tongue follow, and a constant chewing may be observed, hence the name "chewing disease." Abnormal tongue and lip postures may be observed, and other neurological signs include locomotor difficulties such as aimless walking, drowsy appearance, and inactivity with the head held low. The neurological disease is considered permanent, and although some improvement may be seen, difficulty eating and drinking may preclude long-term recovery. Often, the disease progresses to dehydration, starvation, and bizarre behavior including submergence of the head in water to allow water to flow into the esophagus or lapping water like a dog. *Centaurea repens* appears to be more toxic than *C. solstitialis*, but prolonged ingestion is required by both before disease appears. The amount of plant ingested to induce the clinical effects is reported to be 60% or more of body weight for *C. repens* and 100% or more of body weight for *C. solstitialis*. Intermittent grazing can prevent disease, indicating that there is not a cumulative effect but, rather, a threshold must be exceeded before neurological signs are observed (Cordy, 1978). Once neurological signs are observed in horses, prognosis for recovery is poor and euthanasia should be considered.

Pathology

The lesions are very specific and limited to the globus pallidus and the substantia nigra (nigropallidal encephalomalacia), where distinct pale yellowish to buff-colored foci or softening and cavitation are seen (Cordy, 1978). The lesions are typically bilateral and symmetrical. This specificity of the lesions for the basal ganglia has prompted more investigations into unraveling the mysteries of human diseases associated with dopaminergic pathways, such as Parkinson's or Huntington's disease, and tardive dyskinesia. This disease in horses is often called equine parkinsonism. This unusual disease is manifest by an almost immediate onset after prolonged ingestion, suggesting an all-or-none type of acute neurological crisis. The lesions develop quickly and completely, and progressive stages of degeneration rarely occur except for some changes in the adjoining neurons adjacent to the necrotic foci in the globus pallidus and the pars reticularis of the substantia nigra (Cordy, 1978). Microscopically, there is extensive necrosis of neurons, glia, and capillaries within sharply defined margins of the involved brain centers. Occasionally, lesions may be observed in the gray and white matter of the brain.

Prevention and Treatment

Good veterinary care and supportive therapy including good feed, easy access to water, supplemental vitamins, and good nursing care is essential for survival. Treatment of the disease once it is manifest is not generally successful. However, in Argentina, affected horses have been treated with glutamine synthetase and a bovine brain ganglioside extract given daily intramuscularly for 1 month with some success. When animals are first observed grazing *Centaurea* spp., they should be immediately removed to better pastures. Prevention of the disease is easily accomplished by knowing the plants that exist in one's pastures, by providing good quality and adequate amounts of forages and feed, and by frequent observation of one's animal's grazing patterns and behavior.

Control of plant invasion by good range/pasture management to prevent overgrazing and loss of other competitive grasses and forbs is important. Herbicide control is quite easily accomplished with broadleaf products including 2,4-D, dicamba, and picloram applied according to label. These plants are prolific seed producers, and follow-up treatment is required to eliminate the populations. Seeds are often distributed through contaminated hay or other feed sources, and initial populations often start near feed bunks and spread from there. Because of their morphology, size, and parachute-like structures, seeds are easily spread by wind and water. Understanding one's weeds and close monitoring of populations will help in the control of these highly invasive species.

CONCLUSIONS

Even with our ever-increasing knowledge about poisonous plants and their toxins, poisonings continue to occur, some catastrophic, on livestock operations. Poisoning in humans and companion animals from toxic plants also continues to be a significant risk, especially to pets and children. As the influx of small-acreage farmers onto native rangelands increases and ranchettes become more common, the potential risk for poisonous plant problems increases. Lack of understanding and increased grazing pressure on these small acreages often contribute to the consumption of toxic plants by animals. In some cases, novel or unusual animal species are exposed to unfamiliar forages, further contributing to potential poisonings. Plant poisonings will undoubtedly also increase in wild-life populations as humans continue to encroach on their native ranges and interrupt their migratory pathways.

The following basic concepts can help reduce risk of poisoning:

1. Understand and recognize the plants on your range or pastures and know the potential hazards of grazing where poisonous plants grow. Know the conditions under which poisoning may occur.
2. Do not introduce unfamiliar animals onto ranges where poisonous plants may present a hazard.
3. Avoid introducing animals to poisonous plant-infested ranges when adequate, good-quality forage is not available.
4. Do not throw grass, shrub, or tree clippings into paddocks where animals reside (yew clippings are a common cause of poisoning in many animals).
5. Provide free access to fresh water and minerals/salt.
6. Do not overstock the range or pastures.
7. Avoid bedding, lambing/calving, watering, salting, or unloading hungry animals near poisonous plant populations.
8. Avoid excess stress to those animals showing clinical signs of poisoning, and contact your veterinarian.
9. If economically feasible, control poisonous plants through hand grubbing, mechanical clipping, or herbicide treatment.

ACKNOWLEDGMENTS

We thank Ms. Terrie Wierenga for technical assistance in preparing the manuscript and Holly Broome Hyer for artistic representation of selected poisonous plants.

REFERENCES

Acamovic, T., Stewart, C.S., Pennycott, T.W. (Eds.), 2004. *Poisonous Plants and Related Toxins (ISOPP6)*. CAB International, New York.

Asano, N., Kato, A., Oseki, K., Kizu, H., Matsui, K., 1995. Calystegins of *Physalis alkekengi* var. *francheti* (Solanaceae): structure determination and their glycosidase inhibitory activities. Eur. J. Biochem. 229, 369–376.

Bai, Y., Sun, F., Benn, M., Majak, W., 1994. Diterpenoid and norditerpenoid alkaloids from *Delphinium nuttallianum*. Phytochemistry. 37, 1717–1724.

Barneby, R.C., 1964. Atlas of North American Astragalus: Parts I and II, Vol. 13. Memoirs New York Botanical Garden, New York.

Benn, M.H., Jacyno, J.M., 1983. The toxicology and pharmacology of the diterpenoid alkaloids. In: Pelletier, S.W. (Ed.), Alkaloids: Chemical and Biological Perspectives. Wiley, New York, pp. 153–210.

Burrows, G.E., Tyrl, R.J., 2001. Toxic Plants of North America. Iowa State University Press, Ames, IA.

Cheeke, P.R., Shull, L.R., 1985. Natural Toxicants in Feeds and Poisonous Plants. AVI, Westport, CT.

Colegate, S.M., Dorling, P.R. (Eds.), 1994. Plant-Associated Toxins, Agricultural, Phytochemical and Ecological Aspects (ISOPP4). CAB International, Wallingford, UK.

Colegate, S.M., Dorling, P.R., Huxtable, C.R., 1979. A spectroscopic investigation of swainsonine: an α-mannosidase inhibitor isolated from *Swainsona canescens*. Aust J. Chem. 32, 2257–2264.

Cook, D., Gardner, D.R., Welch, K.D., Roper, J.M., Ralphs, M.H., Green, B.T., 2009a. Quantitative PCR method to measure the fungal endophyte in locoweeds. J. Agric. Food Chem. 57, 6050–6054.

Cook, D., Lee, S.T., Gardner, D.R., Pfister, J.A., Welch, K.D., Green, B. T., et al., 2009b. The alkaloid profiles of *Lupinus sulphureus*. J. Agric. Food Chem. 25, 1646–1653.

Cook, D., Ralphs, M.H., Welch, K.D., Stegelmeier, B.L., 2009c. Locoweed poisoning in livestock. Rangelands. 31 (1), 16–21.

Cook, D., Gardner, D.R., Pfister, J.A., Panter, K.E., Stegelmeier, B.L., Lee, S.T., et al., 2010. Differences in ponderosa pine isocupressic acid concentrations across space and time. Rangelands. 32, 14–17.

Cordy, D.R., 1978. Centaurea species and equine nigropallidal encephalomalacia. In: Keeler, R.F., Van Kampen, K.R., James, L.F. (Eds.), Effects of Poisonous Plants on Livestock. Academic Press, New York, pp. 327–336.

Davis, T.Z., Stegelmeier, B.L., Green, B.T., Welch, K.D., Panter, K.E., Hall, J.O., 2011. Acute toxicity of selenium compounds commonly found in selenium-accumulator plants. In: Riet-Correa, F., Pfister, J., Schild, A.L., Wierenga, T.L. (Eds.), Poisoning by Plants, Mycotoxins, and Related Toxins. CAB International, Wallingford, UK, pp. 525–531.

Dobelis, P., Madl, J.E., Pfister, J.A., Manners, G.D., Walrond, J.P., 1999. Effects of *Delphinium* alkaloids on neuromuscular transmission. J. Pharmacol. Exp. Ther. 291, 538–546.

Dollahite, J.W., Anthony, W.V., 1957. Poisoning of cattle with *Gutierrizia microcephala*, a perennial broomweed. J. Am. Vet. Med Assoc. 130, 525–530.

Dorling, P.R., Coelgate, S.M., Huxtable, C.R., 1989. Toxic species of the plant genus *Swainsona*. In: James, L.F., Elbein, A.D., Molyneux, R.J., Warren, C.D. (Eds.), Swainsonine and Related Grycosidase Inhibitors. Iowa State University Press, Ames, IA, pp. 14–22.

Edrington, T.S., Smith, G.S., Ross, T.T., Hallford, D.M., Samford, M.D., Tilsted, J.P., 1993. Embryonic mortality in Sprague–Dawley rats induced by snakeweed. J. Anim. Sci. 71, 2193–2198.

Ford, S.P., Christenson, L.K., Rosazza, J.P., Short, R.E., 1992. Effects of ponderosa pine needle ingestion on uterine vascular function in late-gestation beef cows. J. Anim. Sci. 70, 1609–1614.

Gaffield, W., Keeler, R.F., 1996. Steroidal alkaloid teratogens: molecular probes for investigation of craniofacial malformations. J. Toxicol. Toxin Rev. 15, 303–326.

Galey FD, Hoffman R, Maas J, Barr B, Holstege D, Giacomazzi R (1991) *Suspected Haplopappus acradenius toxicosis in beef heifers*. Paper presented at the 34th annual meeting of the American Association of Veterinary Laboratory Diagnosticians, October, San Diego.

Gardner, D.R., James, L.F., 1999. Pine needle abortion in cattle: analysis of isocupressic acid in North American gymnosperms. Phytochem Anal. 10, 1–5.

Gardner, D.R., Panter, K.E., 1993. Comparison of blood plasma alkaloid levels in cattle, sheep and goats fed *Lupinus caudatus*. J. Nat. Toxins. 2, 1–11.

Gardner, D.R., James, L.F., Molyneux, R.J., Panter, K.E., Stegelmeier, B.L., 1994. Ponderosa pine needle-induced abortion in beef cattle: identification of isocupressic acid as the principal active compound. J. Agric. Food Chem. 42, 756–761.

Gardner, D.R., Panter, K.E., Molyneux, R.J., James, L.F., Stegelmeier, B.L., 1996. Abortifacient activity in beef cattle of acetyl- and succinylisocupressic acid from ponderosa pine. J. Agric. Food Chem. 44, 3257–3261.

Gardner, D.R., James, L.F., Panter, K.E., Pfister, J.A., Ralphs, M.H., Stegelmeier, B.L., 1999. Ponderosa pine and broom snakeweed: poisonous plants that affect livestock. J. Nat. Toxins. 8, 27–34.

Gardner, D.R., Ralphs, M.H., Turner, D.L., Welsh, S.L., 2002. Taxonomic implications of diterpene alkaloids in three toxic tall larkspur species (*Delphinium* spp.). Biochem. Syst. Ecol. 30, 77–90.

Gardner, D.R., Panter, K.E., Stegelmeier, B.L., 2010. Implication of agathic acid from Utah juniper bark as an abortifacient compound in cattle. J. Appl. Toxicol. 30, 115–119.

Garland, T., Barr, C.A. (Eds.), 1998. Toxic Plants and Other Natural Toxicants (ISOPP5). CAB International, New York.

Graham, D., Creamer, R., Cook, D., Stegelmeier, B., Welch, K., Pfister, J., et al., 2009. Solutions to locoweed poisoning in New Mexico and the western United States. Rangelands. 31 (6), 3–8.

Green, B.T., Pfister, J.A., Cook, D., Welch, K.D., Stegelmeier, B.L., Lee, S.T., et al., 2009a. Effects of larkspur (*Delphinium barbeyi*) on heart rate and electrically evoked electromyographic response of the external anal sphincter in cattle. Am. J. Vet. Res. 70, 539–546.

Green, B.T., Welch, K.D., Gardner, D.R., Stegelmeier, B.L., Davis, T.Z., Cook, D., et al., 2009b. Serum elimination profiles of methyllycaconitine and deltaline in cattle following oral administration of larkspur (*Delphinium barbeyi*). Am J. Vet. Res. 70, 926–931.

Green, B.T., Lee, S.T., Panter, K.E., Welch, K.D., Cook, D., Pfister, J. A., et al., 2010. Actions of piperidine alkaloid teratogens at fetal nicotinic acetylcholine receptors. Neurotoxicol Teratol. 32, 383–390.

Green, B.T., Welch, K.D., Gardner, D.R., Stegelmeier, B.L., Pfister, J. A., Cook, D., et al., 2011. A toxicokinetic comparison of norditerpenoid alkaloids from *Delphinium barbeyi* and *D. glaucescens* in cattle. J. Appl. Toxicol. 31, 20–26.

Haraguchi, M., Gorinak, S.L., Ikeda, K., Minami, Y., Kato, A., Watson, A.A., et al., 2003. Alkaloidal components in the poisonous plant, *Ipomoea carnea* (Convolculaceae). J. Agric. Food Chem. 51, 4995–5000.

James, L.F., 1999. Halogeton poisoning in livestock. J. Nat. Toxins. 8, 395–403.

James, L.F., Nielsen, D.B., 1988. Locoweeds: assessment of the problem on western U.S. rangelands. In: James, L.F., Ralphs, M.H., Nielsen, D.B. (Eds.), The Ecology and Economic Impact of Poisonous Plants on Livestock Production. Westview, Boulder, CO, pp. 119–129.

James, L.F., Keeler, R.F., Bailey Jr, E.M., Cheeke, P.R., Hegarty, M.P., 1992. Poisonous Plants: Proceedings of the Third International Symposium (ISOPP3). Iowa State University Press, Ames, IA.

James, L.F., Panter, K.E., Gaffield, W., Molyneux, R.J., 2004. Biomedical applications of poisonous plant research. J. Agric. Food Chem. 52, 3211–3230.

Joubert, J.P.J., 1989. Cardiac glycosides. In: Cheeke, P.R. (Ed.), Toxicants of Plant Origin, Vol. 2. CRC Press, Boca Raton, FL, pp. 61–96.

Keeler, R.F., 1973. Lupin alkaloids from teratogenic and nonteratogenic lupines: 2. Identification of the major alkaloids by tandem gas chromatography–mass spectrometry in plants producing crooked calf disease. Teratology. 7, 31–36.

Keeler, R.F., Panter, K.E., 1989. Piperidine alkaloid composition and relation to crooked calf disease-inducing potential of *Lupinus formosus*. Teratology. 40, 423–432.

Keeler, R.F., Stuart, L.D., 1987. The nature of congenital limb defects induced in lambs by maternal ingestion of *Veratrum californicum*. Clin. Toxicol. 25, 273–286.

Keeler, R.F., James, L.F., Shupe, J.L., Van Kampen, K.R., 1977. Lupine-induced crooked calf disease and a management method to reduce incidence. J. Range Manage. 30, 97–102.

Keeler, R.F., Van Kampen, K.R., James, L.F. (Eds.), 1978. Effects of Poisonous Plants on Livestock (ISOPP1). Academic Press, New York.

Kim, I.-H., Choi, K.-C., An, B.-S., Choi, I.-G., Kim, B.-K., Oh, Y.-K., et al., 2003. Effect on abortion of feeding Korean pine needles to pregnant Korean native cows. Can J. Vet. Res. 67, 194–197.

Knight, A.P., Walter, R.G., 2001. A Guide to Plant Poisoning of Animals in North America. Teton New Media, Jackson, WY.

Lane, M., 1985. Taxonomy of *Gutierrezia* Lag. (Compositeae: Astereae) in North America. Systemic Bot. 10, 7–28.

Lee, S.T., Panter, K.E., Gardner, D.R., Molyneux, R.J., Kem, W.R., Chang, W.R., et al., 2006. Relative toxicities and neuromuscular nicotinic receptor agonistic potencies of anabasine enantiomers and anabaseine. Neurotoxicol Teratol. 28, 220–228.

Lee, S.T., Cook, D., Panter, K.E., Gardner, D.R., Ralphs, M.H., Motteram, E.S., et al., 2007a. Lupine induced "crooked calf disease" in Washington and Oregon: identification of the alkaloid profiles in *Lupinus sulfureus*, *Lupinus leucophyllus*, and *Lupinus sericeus*. J. Agric. Food Chem. 55, 10649–10655.

Lee, S.T., Ralphs, M.H., Panter, K.E., Cook, D.C., Gardner, D.R., 2007b. Alkaloid profiles, concentration and pools in velvet lupine (*Lupinus leucophyllus*) over the growing season. J. Chem. Ecol. 33, 75–84.

Lee, S.T., Gardner, D.R., Change, C.W., Panter, K.E., Molyneux, R.J., 2008a. Separation and measurement of plant alkaloid enantiomers by RP-HPLC analysis of their Fmoc–Alanine analogs. Phytochem Anal. 19, 395–402.

Lee, S.T., Green, B.T., Welch, K.D., Pfister, J.A., Panter, K.E., 2008b. Stereoselective potencies and relative toxicities of coniine enantiomers. Chem. Res. Toxicol. 21, 2061–2064.

Lee, S.T., Molyneux, R.J., Panter, K.E., 2008c. Separation of enantiomeric mixtures of alkaloids and their biological evaluation. Bioactive Natural Products Detection, Isolation Struct Determination. 7, 209–219.

Lee, S.T., Panter, K.E., Pfister, J.A., Gardner, D.R., Welch, K.D., 2008d. The effect of body condition on serum concentrations of two teratogenic alkaloids (anagyrine and ammodendrine) from lupines (*Lupinus* species) that cause crooked calf disease. J. Anim. Sci. 86, 2771–2778.

Lee, S.T., Davis, T.Z., Gardner, D.R., Colegate, S.M., Cook, D., Green, B.T., et al., 2010. Tremetone and structurally related compounds in white snake-root (*Ageratina altissima*): a plant associated with trembles and milk sickness. J. Agric. Food. Chem. 58, 8560–8565.

Lopez-Ortiz, S.L., Panter, K.E., Pfister, J.A., Launchbaugh, K.L., 2004. The effect of body condition on disposition of alkaloids from silvery lupine (*Lupinus argenteus* Pursh) in sheep. J. Anim. Sci. 82, 2798–2895.

McGinty, A., 1985. Survey suggests broomweed costs far more than previously thought. Livestock Weekly. September 5–6.

Molyneux, R.J., James, L.F., 1982. Loco intoxication: indolizidine alkaloids of spotted locoweed (*Astragalus lentiginosus*). Science. 216, 190–191.

Molyneux, R.J., Stevens, K.L., James, L.F., 1980. Chemistry of toxic range plants: volatile constituents of broomweed (*Gutierrezia sarothrae*). J. Agric. Food Chem. 28, 1332–1333.

Molyneux, R.J., James, L.F., Panter, K.E., Ralphs, M.H., 1991. Analysis and distribution of swainsonine and related polyhydroxyindolizidine alkaloids by thin-layer chromatography. Phytochem. Anal. 2, 125–129.

Nation, P.N., Benn, M.H., Roth, S.H., Wilkens, J.L., 1982. Clinical signs and studies of the site of action of purified larkspur alkaloid, methyllycaconitine, administered parenterally to calves. Can. Vet. J. 23, 264–266.

Nielsen, D.B., James, L.F., 1992. The economic impacts of livestock poisonings by plants. In: James, L.F., Keeler, R.F., Bailey, E.M., Cheeke, P.R., Hegarty, M.P. (Eds.), The Ecology and Economic Impact of Poisonous Plants on Livestock Production. Iowa State University Press, Ames, IA, pp. 3–10.

Nielsen, D.B., Rimbey, N.R., James, L.F., 1988. Economic considerations of poisonous plants on livestock. In: James, L.F., Keeler, R.F., Bailey, E.M., Cheeke, P.R., Hegarty, M.P. (Eds.), The Ecology and Economic Impact of Poisonous Plants on Livestock Production. Westview, Boulder, CO, pp. 5–15.

Ogden, L., Burrows, G.E., Tyrl, R.J., Ely, R.W., 1992. Experimental intoxication in sheep by *Asclepias*. In: James, L.F., Keeler, R.F., Bailey, E.M., Cheeke, P.R., Hegarty, M.P. (Eds.), Poisonous Plants: Proceedings of the Third International Symposium on Poisonous Plants (ISOPP3). Iowa State University Press, Ames, IA, pp. 495–499.

Oldrup, E., McLain-Romero, J., Padilla, A., Moya, A., Gardner, D., Creamer, R., 2010. Localization of endophytic *Undifilum* fungi in locoweed seed and influence of environmental parameters on a locoweed *in vitro* culture system. Botany. 88, 512–521.

Panter, K.E., 1991. Neurotoxicity of the knapweeds (*Centaurea* spp.) in horses. In: James, L.F., Evans, J.O., Ralphs, M.H., Child, R.D. (Eds.), Noxious Range Weeds. Westview, Boulder, CO, pp. 495–499.

Panter, K.E., Keeler, R.F., 1989. Piperidine alkaloids of poison hemlock (*Conium maculatum*). In: Cheeke, P.R. (Ed.), Toxicants of Plant Origin, Vol. I: Alkaloids. CRC Press, Boca Raton, FL, pp. 109–132.

Panter, K.E., Keeler, R.F., 1992. Induction of cleft palate in goats by *Nicotiana glauca* during a narrow gestational period and the relation to reduction in fetal movement. J Nat Toxins. 1, 25–32.

Panter, K.E., Ralphs, M.H., Smart, R.A., Duelke, B., 1987. Death camas poisoning in sheep: a case report. Vet Hum Toxicol. 29, 45–48.

Panter, K.E., Keeler, R.F., Baker, D.C., 1988. Toxicoses in livestock from the hemlocks (*Conium* and *Cicuta* spp.). J Anim Sci. 66, 2407–2413.

Panter, K.E., Bunch, T.D., Keeler, R.F., Sisson, D.V., Callan, R.J., 1990a. Multiple congenital contractures (MCC) and cleft palate induced in goats by ingestion of piperidine alkaloid-containing plants: reduction in fetal movement as the probable cause. Clin. Toxicol. 28, 69–83.

Panter, K.E., James, L.F., Short, R.E., Molyneux, R.J., Sisson, D.V., 1990b. Premature bovine parturition induced by ponderosa pine: effects of pine needles, bark, and branch tips. Cornell Vet. 80, 329–333.

Panter, K.E., Baker, D.C., Kechele, P.O., 1996a. Water hemlock (*Cicuta douglasii*) toxicoses in sheep: pathologic description and prevention of lesions and death. J. Vet. Diagn. Invest. 8, 474–480.

Panter, K.E., Hartley, W.J., James, L.F., Mayland, H.F., Stegelmeier, B. L., Kechele, P.O., 1996b. Comparative toxicity of selenium from seleno-DL-methionine, sodium selenate, and *Astragalus bisulcatus* in pigs. Fundam Appl. Toxicol. 32, 217–223.

Panter, K.E., Gardner, D.R., Gay, C.C., James, L.F., Mills, R., Gay, J. M., et al., 1997. Observations of *Lupinus sulphureus*-induced crooked calf disease. J. Range Manage. 50, 587–592.

Panter, K.E., James, L.F., Gardner, D.R., 1999a. Lupines, poison-hemlock and *Nicotiana* spp.: toxicity and teratogenicity in livestock. J. Nat. Toxins. 8, 117–134.

Panter, K.E., James, L.F., Stegelmeier, B.L., Ralphs, M.H., Pfister, J.A., 1999b. Locoweeds: effects on reproduction in livestock. J. Nat. Toxins. 8, 53–62.

Panter, K.E., Manners, G.D., Stegelmeier, B.L., Lee, S.T., Gardner, D. R., Ralphs, M.H., et al., 2002. Larkspur poisoning: toxicology and alkaloid structure-activity relationships. Biochem Syst Ecol. 30, 113–128.

Panter, K.E., Wierenga, T.L., Pfister, J.A. (Eds.), 2007. Poisonous Plants: Global Research and Solutions (ISOPP7). CAB International, Wallingford, UK.

Panter, K.E., Gardner, D.R., Stegelmeier, B.L., Welch, K.D., Holstege, D., 2011. Water hemlock poisoning in cattle: ingestion of immature *Cicuta maculata* seed as the probable cause. Toxicon. 57, 157–161.

Parton, K., Gardner, D., William, N.B., 1996. Isocupressic acid, an abortifacient component of *Cupressus macrocarpa*. N Z Vet. J. 44, 109–111.

Pfister, J.A., Adams, D.C., Wiedmeier, R.D., Cates, R.G., 1992. Adverse effects of pine needles on aspects of digestive performance in cattle. J Range Manage. 45, 528–533.

Pfister, J.A., Panter, K.E., Manners, G.D., 1994. Effective dose in cattle of toxic alkaloids from tall larkspur (*Delphinium barbeyi*). Vet Hum Toxicol. 36, 10–11.

Pfister, J.A., Gardner, D.R., Panter, K.E., Ralphs, M.H., Manners, G.D., Stegelmeier, B.L., et al., 1999. Larkspur (*Delphinium* spp.) toxicity to livestock. J. Nat. Toxins. 8, 81–94.

Pfister, J.A., Ralphs, M.H., Gardner, D.R., Stegelmeier, B.L., Manners, G.D., Panter, K.E., et al., 2002. Management of three toxic *Delphinium* species based on alkaloid concentration. Biochem Syst Ecol. 30, 129–138.

Pfister, J.A., Stegelmeier, B.L., Gardner, D.R., James, L.F., 2003. Grazing of spotted locoweed (*Astragalus lentiginosus*) by cattle and horses in Arizona. J. Anim Sci. 81, 2285–2293.

Pfister, J.A., Lee, S.T., Panter, K.E., Motteram, E.S., Gay, C.C., 2008a. Effects of experience and lactation on lupine consumption by cattle. Rangeland Ecol Manage. 61, 240–244.

Pfister, J.A., Panter, K.E., Gardner, D.R., Cook, D., Welch, K.D., 2008b. Effect of body condition on consumption of pine needles (*Pinus ponderosa*) by beef cows. J. Anim Sci. 86, 3608–3616.

Ping, L., Child, D., Meng-Li, Z., Gardner, D.R., Gui-Fen, L., Guo-Dong, H., 2009. Culture and identification of endophytic fungi from *Oxytropis glabra* DC. ACTA Ecol Sinica. 20 (1), 53–58.

Pryor, B.M., Creamer, R., Shoemaker, R.A., McClain-Romero, J., Hambleton, S., 2009. *Undifilum*, a new genus for endophytic *Embellesia oxytropis* and parasitic *Helminthosporium bornmuelleri* on legumes. Botany. 87, 178–194.

Raisbeck, M.F., 2000. Selenosis. Vet Clin North Am Food Anim Pract. 16, 465–480.

Ralphs, M.H., 2009. Response of broom snakeweed (*Gutierrezia sarothrae*) and cool-season grasses to defoliation. Invasive Plant Sci. Manage. 2, 28–35.

Ralphs, M.H., Banks, J.E., 2009. Cattle grazing as a biological control for broom snakeweed: vegetation response. Rangeland Ecol Manage. 62, 38–43.

Ralphs, M.H., McDaniel, K.C., 2011. Broom snakeweed (*Gutierrezia sarothrae*): toxicology, ecology, control, and management. Invasive Plant Sci. Manage. 4, 125–132.

Ralphs, M.H., Sanders, K.D., 2002. Population cycles of broom snakeweed in the Colorado Plateau and Snake River plains. J. Range Manage. 55, 406–411.

Ralphs, M.H., Whitson, T.D., Ueckert, D.N., 1991. Herbicide control of poisonous plants. Rangelands. 13 (2), 73–77.

Ralphs, M.H., Graham, D., James, L.F., 1994. Social facilitation influences cattle to graze locoweed. J. Range Manage. 47, 123–126.

Ralphs, M.H., Greathouse, G., Knight, A.P., James, L.F., 2001. Cattle preference for Lambert locoweed over white locoweed throughout their phenological stages. J. Range Manage. 54, 265–268.

Ralphs, M.H., Gardner, D.R., Turner, D.L., Pfister, J.A., Thacker, E., 2002. Predicting toxicity of tall larkspur (*Delphinium barbeyi*): measurement of the variation in alkaloid concentration among plants and among years. J. Chem. Ecol. 28, 2327–2341.

Ralphs, M.H., Pfister, J.A., Welsh, S.L., Graham, D., Purvines, J., Jensen, D.T., et al., 2003. Locoweed population cycles. Rangelands. 25, 14–18.

Ralphs, M.H., Panter, K.E., Gay, C.C., Motteram, E., Lee, S.T., 2006. Cattle consumption of velvet lupine (*Lupinus leucophyllus*) in the channel scablands of eastern Washington. J. Range Ecol Manage. 59, 204–207.

Ralphs, M.H., Wiedmeier, R.D., Banks, J.E., 2007. Decreasing forage allowance can force cattle to graze broom snakeweed (*Gutierrezia sarothrae*) as a potential biological control. Rangeland Ecol. Manage. 60, 487–497.

Ralphs, M.H., Creamer, R., Baucom, D., Gardner, D.R., Welsh, S.L., Graham, J.D., et al., 2008. Relationship between the endophyte *Embellisia* spp. and the toxic alkaloid swainsonine in major locoweed species (*Astagalus* and *Oxytropis*). J. Chem. Ecol. 34, 32–38.

Riet-Correa, F., Pfister, J.A., Schild, A.L., Wierenga, T.L. (Eds.), 2011. Poisoning by Plants, Mycotoxins, and Related Toxins (ISOPP 8). CAB International, Wallingford, UK.

Riopelle, R.J., Stevens, K.L., 1993. *In vitro* neurotoxicity bioassay: neurotoxicity of sesquiterpene lactones. In: Colegate, S.M., Molyneux, R.J. (Eds.), Bioactive Natural Products: Detection, Isolation, and Structural Determination. CRC Press, Boca Raton, FL, pp. 457–463.

Rosenfeld, I., Beath, O.A., 1964. *Selenium: Geobotany, Biochemistry, Toxicity and Nutrition*. Academic Press, New York.

Sady, M.B., Seiber, J.N., 1991. Field test for screening milkweed latex for cardenolides. J. Nat. Prod. 54, 1105–1107.

Saito, K., Nagao, T., Takasuki, S., Koyama, K., Natori, S., 1990. The sesquiterpenoid carcinogen of bracken fern, and some analogs, from the Pteridaceae. Phytochemistry. 29, 1475.

Seawright, A.A., Hegarty, M.P., James, L.F., Keeler, R.F., 1985. Plant Toxicology: Proceedings of the Australia–USA Poisonous Plants Symposium (ISOPP2). Queensland Poisonous Plant Committee, Yeerongpilly, Australia.

Smith, G.S., Ross, T.T., Flores-Rodriguez, G.I., Oetting, B.C., Edrington, T.S., 1991. Toxicology of snakeweeds *Gutierrezia microcephala* and *G. sarothrae*. In: James, L.F., Evans, J.O., Ralphs, M.H., Child, R.D. (Eds.), Noxious Range Weeds. Westview, Boulder, CO, pp. 236–246.

Stegelmeier, B.L., 2002. Equine photosensitization. Clin Tech Equine Pract. 1 (2), 81–88.

Stegelmeier, B.L., Ralphs, M.H., Gardner, D.R., Molyneux, R.J., James, L.F., 1994. Serum α-mannosidase and the clinicopathologic alterations of locoweed (*Astragalus mollissimus*) intoxication in range cattle. J. Vet. Diagn. Invest. 6, 473–479.

Stegelmeier, B.L., Gardner, D.R., James, L.F., Panter, K.E., Molyneux, R.J., 1996. The toxic and abortifacient effects of ponderosa pine. Vet. Pathol. 33, 22–28.

Stegelmeier, B.L., Panter, K.E., Pfister, J.A., James, L.F., Manners, G. D., Gardner, D.R., et al., 1998. Experimental modification of larkspur (*Delphinium* spp.) toxicity. In: Garland, T., Barr, C. (Eds.), Toxic Plants and Other Natural Toxicants. CAB International, New York, pp. 205–210.

Stegelmeier, B.L., Edgar, J.A., Colegate, S.M., Gardner, D.R., Schoch, T.K., Coulombe, R.A., et al., 1999. Pyrrolizidine alkaloid plants, metabolism and toxicity. J. Nat. Toxins. 8, 95–116.

Stegelmeier, B.L., Molyneux, R., Asano, N., Watson, A., Nash, R., 2008. The comparative pathology of the glycosidase inhibitors: swainsonine, castanospermine, and calystegines A3, B2 and C1 in mice. Toxicol. Pathol. 36 (5), 651–659.

Taylor, J.A., 1990. The bracken problem: a global perspective. In: Thomson, J.A., Smith, B.L. (Eds.), Bracken Biology and Management. Australian Institute of Agricultural Science, Sydney, Australia, pp. 3–19. , No. 40.

Thacker, E., Ralphs, M.H., Call, A., Benson, B., Green, S., 2008. Invasion of broom snakeweed (*Gutierrezia sarothrae*) following disturbance: evaluating change in a state-and-transition model. Rangeland Ecol. Manage. 61, 263–268.

Tiwary, A.K., Stegelmeier, B.L., Panter, K.E., James, L.F., Hall, J.O., 2006. Comparative toxicosis of sodium selenite and selenomethionine in lambs. J. Vet. Diagn Invest. 18, 61–70.

Weinzweig, J., Panter, K.E., Marcello, P., Spangenberger, A., Harper, J. S., Lui, F., et al., 1999. The fetal cleft palate: I. Characterization of a congenital model. Plastic Reconstr. Surg. 103 (2), 419–428.

Weinzweig, J., Panter, K.E., Patel, J., Smith, D.M., Spangenberger, A., Freeman, M.B., 2008. The fetal cleft palate: V. Elucidation of the mechanism of palatal clefting in the congenital caprine model. Plastic Reconstr. Surg. 121 (4), 1328–1334.

Welch, K.D., Panter, K.E., Gardner, D.R., Green, B.T., Pfister, J.A., Cook, D., et al., 2008. The effect of 7,8-methylenedioxylycoctonine-type diterpenoid alkaloids on the toxicity of methyllycaconitine in mice. J. Anim. Sci. 86, 2761–2770.

Welch, K.D., Green, B.T., Panter, K.E., Gardner, D.R., Pfister, J.A., Cook, D., et al., 2009a. Investigation of the susceptibility of various strains of mice to methyllycaconitine toxicosis. J. Anim. Sci. 87, 1558–1564.

Welch, K.D., Panter, K.E., Lee, S.T., Gardner, D.R., Stegelmeier, B.L., Cook, D., 2009b. Cyclopamine-induced synophthalmia in sheep: defining a critical window and toxicokinetic evaluation. J. Appl. Toxicol. 29, 414–421.

Welch, K.D., Green, B.T., Gardner, D.R., Cook, D., Pfister, J.A., Stegelmeier, B.L., et al., 2010. Influence of 7,8-methylenedioxylycoctonine-type alkaloids on the toxic effects associated with ingestion of tall larkspur (*Delphinium* spp.) in cattle. Am J. Vet. Res. 71, 487–492.

Welch, K.D., Gardner, D.R., Panter, K.E., Stegelmeier, B.L., Parsons, C., Pfister, J.A., et al., 2011a. Western juniper-induced abortions in beef cattle. Int J. Poisonous Plant Res. 1, 72–79.

Welch, K.D., Panter, K.E., Gardner, D.R., Stegelmeier, B.L., Green, B. T., Pfister, J.A., et al., 2011b. The acute toxicity of the death camas (*Zigadenus* spp.) alkaloid zygacine in mice, including the effect of methyllycaconitine co-administration on zygacine toxicity. J. Anim. Sci. 89, 1650–1657.

Welsh, S.L., Ralphs, M.H., Panter, K.E., Pfister, J.A., James, L.F., 2007. Locoweeds of North America. In: Panter, K.E., Wierenga, T.L., Pfister, J.A. (Eds.), Poisonous Plants: Global Research and Solutions. USDA Forest Service, Rocky Mountain Research Station, Ogden, UT.

Whitson, T.D., Freeburn, J.W., 1990. Broom Snakeweed Control Two Years Following Herbicide Treatments, Progress Report. Western Society of Weed Science, Las Cruces, NM, pp. 54–55.

Williams, M.C., Barneby, R.C., 1977. The occurrence of nitro-toxins in North American *Astragalus* (Fabaceae). Brittonia. 29, 310–326.

Williams, M.C., Norris, F.A., Van Kampen, K.R., 1970. Metabolism of miserotoxin to 3-nitro-1-propanol in bovine and ovine ruminal fluids. Am. J. Vet. Res. 31, 259–262.

Young, J.A., 1999. Halogeton: a History of Mid-20th Century Range Conservation in the Intermountain Area. U.S. Department of Agriculture, Agricultural Research Service, Washington, DC.

Chapter 62

Poisonous Plants of the Europe

Arturo Anadón, María R. Martínez-Larrañaga, Irma Ares and Maria A. Martínez

INTRODUCTION

European flora is much less rich in dangerous species than those found in the American and African flora; however, the number of plant poisons is considerable. Poisoning of livestock and companion animals by plants is a sporadically occurring clinical problem, and the possibility of plant poisoning is usually neglected in a differential diagnosis. In intensive rearing of animals like swine or poultry, contact of the animal with the toxic plant is unlikely. Also, the maintenance in confinement of some semipermanent stall dairy cattle and young beef cattle minimizes this risk. The common use of herbicides destroys some poisonous plant species. However, in many cases, it must be determined whether animals have come in contact with toxic plants either in the pasture or by means of poisonous plants mixed with forage and distributed in conserved forage.

Plant poisoning in small animals is usually accidental. Accidents can be prevented by understanding the conditions under which poisoning may be expected to occur and then taking positive steps to prevent its occurrence. Moreover, problems can occur with animals in ornamental, garden and natural environments and homes. Pets are usually the victims of this type of accident. A considerable numbers of veterinarians are not familiar with plants found in and around the home that may be potentially harmful if ingested; therefore they are responsible for being prepared to deal with plant poisoning should it occur. Many house and garden plants grown in Europe contain chemical substances in sufficient quantities that lead to toxic effects in animals. Dogs and cats are not herbivores and infrequently consume large quantities of plant materials. It is recognized, however, that they do occasionally ingest plant materials, especially grass. When conditions are favorable, both dogs and cats will consume other herbaceous materials that cause toxicity. Although plant poisoning of adult dogs and cats is unlikely, puppies often taste anything they encounter and are the principal candidates for the accidental ingestion of toxic plant materials.

Occasionally, a client may observe a pet consuming a fruit or leafy material. A frantic call to the veterinarian may prove fruitless if the plant cannot be identified by visual description. The amount consumed is also of importance. Rarely will a single bite of any plant prove to be lethal. Fortunately, most plants do not cause toxicity, and may only cause mild to moderate gastrointestinal irritation. A few plants in certain localities, regions or countries can produce serious toxicity, including oleander (*Nerium oleander*) and castor beans (*Ricinus communis*).

Household pets are exposed to the same harmful substances as young children. Puppies and kittens, like children, seem to have a predilection to ingest attractive foreign materials, such as parts of house and garden plants (berries, fruits, seeds, leaves). Both older and immature animals may suffer from boredom or behavioral abnormalities or may simply be investigating a new addition to the environment, all of which may lead to ingestion of poisonous plant material.

Small pets are at greatest risk with exotic plants. They are usually not herbivores, and as a result, they never develop detoxification mechanisms for plants. By contrast, most herbivores have coevolved elaborate detoxification mechanisms to cope with the thousands of alkaloids, glycosides, amines, and resinoids found in plants that they typically consume. When animals and plants evolve together, a commensal relationship often develops. Such relations are interrupted when plants are introduced into new environments exposing the resident animals to substances for which they lack detoxification mechanisms.

Finally, many poisonous substances found in plants are also used medicinally. Cardioactive glycosides, atropine, and acetylcholine are three examples. Poisoning from plant material presupposes consumption of sufficient quantities of one or several active ingredients that in turn

Veterinary Toxicology. DOI: http://dx.doi.org/10.1016/B978-0-12-811410-0.00062-3

can act synergistically. The toxic dosage varies with the species of the plant, the stage of plant growth, the part of the plant consumed (i.e., leaves, roots, etc.), the type of soil, and other environmental factors.

Plants can be roughly classified depending on which body system they affect. The pharmacology and toxicology of commonly found plants are known. However, even if a plant is suspected of causing an adverse outcome, without information about similar cases, toxicological analysis of biofluids, or pharmacological or toxicological effects of the plant, further investigation might prove difficult or impossible.

Plant Identification

Plant toxicity occurs consistently at the genus level, although species variation may alter toxicity. Consequently, accurate identification of the plant and its toxic compounds, is necessary (genus and species), which often requires recognition of the scientific name and the plant parts by a qualified person. Usually, a family member knows the common names of household and garden plants, but the problem is that the same common names are used for many different plants (e.g., milk plant and milk-weed). Some are hazardous to livestock, and other ornamentals may be hazardous to small animals. Still others are edible or innocuous (Fowler, 1981). For this reason, therapeutic decisions are sometimes based on imprecise common names. Currently, plant toxicology is changing; knowledge of poisonous plant names is important to ensure that the same name is universally applied. Both common names and scientific names are needed for communication with the public and for scientific exchange.

Ornamental plants are not easily identified botanically and standard botanical keys are not very helpful. If the species of an ornamental plant is in question, it should be taken to a qualified person for identification. Botany or horticultural herbaria in museums, colleges, or universities are helpful resources for plant identification (Forsyth, 1968).

TABLE 62.1 Diagnosis of Plant Poisoning

General approach
History: After stabilization of vital signs, the questions addressed to the animal owner should be accurate
Animal species, breed, sex, age, pregnancy, number of animals/ current size of groups (for herds), weight (loss, gain, stable), condition, vaccination status, mineral supplements, feeding or pasture changes, and other treatments
Plant identification: Accurate identification of the plant is needed (genus and species) as well as recognition of the scientific name, common name and the plant parts
Relevant circumstances: breed, sex, age, number, condition, vaccination status, mineral supplements, feeding or pasture changes, and other treatment
Clinical signs: Number of affected animals, signs, clinical course and progression of signs (sudden death; acute onset moving to less severe; gradual onset becoming more severe), lesions, mortality, and suspicious odors
Postmortem examination: Animal condition and lesions
Laboratory tests: Toxicant isolation, search for toxic plants (in the meadow or forage) and search of toxicant in animals (rumen and stomach; gastrointestinal tissues and contents). Blood tests to evaluate inflammation, organ function, and evaluate immunological response to infectious agents (complete blood cell counts and serum element, metabolites and clinical chemistry analysis, and serological tests). Hay, silage, or concentrated feed samples; water, salt, and mineral supplements (location and use) (samples frozen for analysis)
Treatment
Decontamination, especially gastrointestinal: emesis, gastric lavage, activated charcoal, enemas, laxatives/cathartics
Elimination enhancement: Diuresis, urine acidification, urine alkalinization
Antidotes

Diagnosis of Plant Poisoning

The following information is usually required for diagnosis: region, location, time and amount of exposure, type of plant, part of plant ingested, onset and progression of symptoms, type of symptoms, and the presence of insecticides or herbicides. A formal diagnosis of poisoning must be made using a thorough history of the poisoning incident, clinical signs and laboratory analysis of samples (Table 62.1). Clinical signs are of primary importance to the clinician. The owner may be able to provide data on what toxicants may be in the environment in which animals are living. However, many times owners are not aware of potential toxic plants that are present. Field information can also help in the diagnosis, particularly: (1) general conditions of affected animals, unusual behaviors, clinical signs, and lesions; (2) forage availability, plant species composition, and evidence of grazing patterns; collection of potential problem plants or unidentified plants (dried samples for identification, frozen samples for chemical analysis); and (3) physical location, weather conditions at the time of the poisoning and their effect on forage and forage availability (Welch et al., 2012).

Many infectious, degenerative, and immunological diseases produce clinical signs, biochemical changes, and lesions identical to those caused by poisonous plants and thus must be ruled out. Therefore, an extensive differential diagnosis must be initiated embracing physical examination, blood biochemical or serological evaluations, possible *postmortem* evaluation and chemical or microscopic evaluations of plants and/or animal tissues (Welch et al., 2012). A thorough *postmortem* examination, or necropsy, provides the most information needed to formulate a definitive diagnosis.

Clinical signs are of prime importance to the clinician and toxicologist. Both the nature of the signs and their sequence of occurrence may be important. Loss of one or more animals in a herd or a single animal at risk provides an invaluable opportunity to increase diagnostic information for toxicology. Lesions are often absent in certain toxicosis, and lack of lesions should correlate with the indicated clinical signs (Osweiler, 2011).

Pets

The diagnosis of plant poisoning in dogs is not always easy because symptoms are rarely characteristic and treatment is often disappointing. The clinical signs of poisoning produced by ornamental plants certainly were not noticed in the past, either because the clinical examination was lacking or because symptoms that presented in the poisoned animal were not sufficiently alarming to consult or notify veterinarians. The frequency and severity of poisoning are extremely variable. The toxicity of a given ornamental plant varies from one variety to another and from one organ to another, and it also depends on the state of maturity. Animals react differently depending on the species, age, health status before the poisoning, their sensitivity to the plant and the amount ingested, and whether the plant has been macerated or not. It is difficult to make a diagnosis of poisoning by an ornamental plant in view of the few symptoms and lesions presented by a sick animal. It is essential to identify the plant in the stool or vomitus to make a diagnosis by the symptoms correspond with those observed in similar cases previously. The symptoms and lesions are varied; they predominantly affect the digestive tract when the poisoning is benign and the nervous and cardiovascular systems when poisoning is serious. At necropsy of the intoxicated animal, gastroenteritis lesions are often observed. For the previous reasons, prevention must play an essential role. It is first necessary to know the plants that are poisonous to pets and avoid planting them in kennel areas or maintaining them in the home. It is also necessary to ensure that animals receive a sufficient and balanced diet, corresponding to their specific needs, and that they have regular daily exercise.

Generally, *Liliaceae* spp. and *Araceae* spp. are the major plant families involved in poisoning; most of the cases are related to accidental ingestion of ornamental plants rather that wild plants, particularly at certain times of the year. Cats appear to be more sensitive than dogs probably due to the tendency to chew on plant leaves. *Convallaria majalis* and *N. oleander* have also been commonly reported to cause severe and potentially lethal cardiac disorders, and *R. communis* and *Datura stramonium* cases were also frequently observed (Gault et al., 1995).

Small animal veterinarians must deal with a number of potentially poisonous, commonly occurring, household and garden plants (Table 62.2). In many cases, the client does not know name of the plant that the animal encountered. As indicated, veterinarians should familiarize themselves with the most potentially toxic plants and their clinical signs (in clinic, farm, or field situations) and any naturally occurring dangerous plants in their area (Flood and Fitzgerald et al., 2006).

The seasonal houseplants, such as poinsettia (Euphorbia pulcherrima) (Euphorbiaceae family), mistletoe and holly bring a greater potential for plant poisoning with the many beautiful live decorative plants brought into the home.

Mistletoe (*Viscum album* L) (Viscaceae family) has a long medicinal use history. All parts of the plant are poisonous. The concentration of viscotoxins (polypeptides) in European mistletoe varies with individual strains, but the concentration of these compounds is relatively stable during the harvesting season (Schaller et al., 1998). In high doses, viscotoxins are cardiotoxic as a result of the inhibition of papillary muscle function. Blood pressure is increased as are pulse and respiratory rates. Ingestion of high amounts of mistletoe may cause nausea, vomiting, and gastroenteritis.

English Holly (*Ilex aquifolium* L.) (Aquifoliaceae family) plants are grown as ornamental plants. The red or black berries (Christmas holly) are attractive decorations, especially for pets. Polyphenols, saponins, triterpenes, steroids and alkaloids have been extracted from *Ilex opaca*. The compounds found in Holly are digitalis-like cardiotonic and a saponin, which has hemolytic activity. The symptoms of poisoning are nonspecific and they consist of abdominal pain, vomiting, and diarrhea. These appear when large amounts of the fruit are ingested.

Livestock

Livestock can be poisoned by many different plant species, but an analytically confirmed diagnosis is not always easy, and most cases are only suspected following necropsy and identification of leaves, stems, or pods in the rumen. A diagnosis of plant poisoning can rarely be made by the clinical syndrome alone. Signs accompanied by a history of exposure to the plant are usually necessary.

TABLE 62.2 Household Plants

Family	Genus/Species	Clinical Presentation
Amaryllidaceaes	*Amaryllis, Clivia, Crinium, Hippeastrum*	Vomiting and diarrhea
Apocynaceae	*Allamanda cathartica, Dipladenia sanderi*	Skin (dermatitis) and digestive disorders
Araceae:		
Dieffenbachia	*Dieffenbachia sanguine, D. picta*	Keratoconjunctivitis, edema of the eyelids, and corneal ulceration; reactions on the lips, tongue, palate and pharynx, esophagus, and vomiting and diarrhea. The cat is particularly sensitive
Other dangerous Araceae	*Alocasia* spp., *Anthurium* spp., *Arisaema* spp., *Caladium* spp., *Monster* spp., *Philodendron* spp., *Xanthosoma* spp., *Zantedeschia aethiopica*	They can cause similar disorders to *Dieffenbachia* and sometimes dermatitis as a result of animal contact with the plant
Ericaceae	*Rhododendron obtusum, R. simsii*	Vomiting, diarrhea, violent equilibrium changes and convulsions, paralysis, and dyspnea; coma and death (at high doses)
Euphorbiaceae	*Euphorbia pulcherrima*	Irritating to skin and projected into the cornea; local disorders, vesicular dermatitis, conjunctivitis, stomatitis, vomiting and diarrhea
Liliaceae	*Tulipa* sp., *Hyacinthus* spp.	Vomiting with gastroenteritis
Moraceae	*Ficus elastic, Ficus lyrata*	Similar to those caused by *Euphorbiaceae* and also urinary signs

Judicious questioning of the client may be necessary when plant poisoning is suspected. The client may not know the plants in the home or garden if a spouse or other family member is the gardener, and further inquiry is necessary to establish the presence of a suspected plant in or around the home.

Conditions Conducive to Plant Poisoning

Cross-breeding, environmental conditions and seasonal variation in toxin content may also alter toxicity outcome. Although plant poisoning of adult dogs and cats is possible, puppies often eat anything they encounter and are prime candidates for accidental ingestion of toxic plant materials. Kittens are less likely than puppies to ingest such foreign material but occasionally will do so (Fowler, 1981).

Caged birds present special problems. Psittacines (budgerigars, cockatiels, parrots, and macaws) are generally seed-eaters. As a rule, they are fed seeds from a commercial source, and the likelihood of poisoning is remote. Sometimes a well-meaning owner collects and feeds wild seeds, which can pose a slight hazard if the person is unable to identify all of the plants from which the seeds are collected (Fowler, 1981).

Higher concentrations of many poisonous substances are found in the seeds than in the rest of the plant. Thus, seed-eaters, such as psittacine birds are at particular risk when such plants are the source of food. Birds that are allowed to fly free in the home or that escape from a cage may peck at and ingest poisonous houseplants.

Predictive and Toxicity Factors

Age

By nature, puppies and kittens continually explore with their mouths. Teething irritation may be relieved by chewing on objects in the environment. Any available plant materials, such as seeds, pits, bulbs, branches, and even leaves, may be chewed and ingested. Puppies and kittens have low activities of the hepatic biotransformation enzymes as well as low levels of conjugating moieties. Newborn animals are generally deficient in drug metabolizing enzymes (e.g., cytochrome P450), and this lack may persist for 1–2 months after birth. Both phase I (e.g., oxidative) and phase II (e.g., glucuronidation) reactions are reduced. Poisonous plants whose toxicity is generated from toxic metabolites may be less toxic because there is decreased formation of active components. A poorly developed blood-brain barrier, weak biotransformation activity, and immature mechanisms for excretion combine to make puppies very vulnerable to toxic effects of poisonous plants. Owners should be informed of the necessity to "pet proof" the surroundings of young animals by removing or preventing access to hazardous substances, including toxic plants (Fowler, 1981). Very old animals, with depressed protein synthesis due to increased organ dysfunction may also suffer the same deficit. Interactions with hormones at various ages may also be involved. Significant changes in the body composition and regional blood flow occur as aging progresses, and there is a steady decline in physiological function.

Sex

There is differential toxicity for certain toxic plants between sexes. The sex differences in metabolism are mainly observed after puberty and are probably largely related to hormonal influences.

Species

Some species are very susceptible to toxic plants, whereas other are not. For example, rabbits are insensitive to the effects of *Galega officinalis*, and certain species of birds can consume *Cicuta* spp. without toxicity occurring. Marked differences among species metabolism of the same chemical compound exist. For example, cats lacking adequate glucuronyl transferase form glucuronides poorly and are therefore more susceptible to poisoning by certain toxic plants. The cat is unable to synthesize adequate amounts of taurine because of low activity of the decarboxylase enzymes involved in taurine formation; the particular sensitivity of the cat is heightened by its total dependence on taurine for bile acid conjugation.

In ruminants, after a toxic plant is consumed, it will depend on the balance of many factors whether toxicity will be expressed. Some plant poisons are rapidly inactivated in the rumen by the microbiota, while other (potentially toxic) compounds may be activated by the microbes faster than they will be detoxified in the gut. Among the toxic compounds that may be degraded in the rumen are oxalates, pyrrolizidine alkaloids, essential oils, but also cyanides, seleniferous amino acids, digitalis alkaloids and caffeic acid among others.

Genetics and Strain

Within animal species, certain breeds or strains vary in ability to detoxify toxic plants. For example, the Dalmatian breed lacking uricase is less able to carry out purine metabolism.

Boredom

Both older animals and immature animals may suffer from apathy. Dogs, in particular, have problems resigning themselves to continuous confinement compared to others that have unlimited freedom. A dog with nothing to do may resort to aberrant behavior, such as ingestion of any available plant material(s). If these plants are poisonous, toxicity may result. Clay (1977) describes three instances of dogs poisoned by plants within their confined space.

Changes in Surroundings

New objects placed within the environment of a pet are novel and subject to a thorough investigation. During the holiday season, new plants are often brought into the home, and some of them are potentially dangerous. When a family moves into a new home or goes on vacation with its pet(s), new plants are often encountered.

Pets used to "star billing" in a household may feel neglected when a new baby arrives and receives all the attention. In such circumstances, many pets resort to pica. Illness of an owner may require "pet sitting" by others and thus initiate the same response (Fowler, 1981).

Behavioral Abnormalities

Behavioral abnormalities are increasingly being recognized as specific clinical entities. A few behaviorist-trained veterinarians are beginning to unravel some of the complex interrelationships of pet behavior and disease. Ingestion of foreign materials is one such manifestation of deranged behavior. Plant poisoning may be a consequence of such behavior. The veterinary profession needs to distinguish the many minor exposures from the few serious ones and to treat those toxic exposures appropriately. Such a task may be difficult because the plant involved is not easily identified. Even when it is known, predicting toxicity is difficult because of variation in plant toxicity, amount ingested, and animal/species susceptibility (Fowler, 1981).

Plants

The following factors of plants are linked to toxicity:

- The concentration of active ingredient varies among different species of plants.
- The entire plant can be toxic, but in some cases, parts of the plant are responsible for toxicity (e.g., grain, leaves, and fruit).
- The active ingredient content can vary depending on the state of plant development (e.g., *G. officinalis* becomes toxic only after flowering).
- Preservation procedures can destroy the active ingredients; e.g., drying can reduce toxicity (e.g., *Cicuta* spp.)
- Herbicide treatments may increase the toxic principle content and can make animals crave plants more.

AMIANTHIUM MUSCAETOXICUM (LILIACEAE FAMILY)

Common Names: Fly Poison, Stagger Grass, and Crow Poison

This *Amianthium muscaetoxicum* plant is found in open woods, fence rows, old fields, roadsides, and pinelands, particularly in clay soils, although it can also be found in sandy soils. These plants are perennial, subscapose, and bulbous herbs. Leaves are mostly basal and linear. Flowers are white, turning greenish in age; they are borne in dense racemes. Plants are found mostly in moist, wooded slopes, meadows, open fields, and bogs.

Toxicity

The highest concentration of the toxin, an alkaloid, is found in the bulb of the plant. The alkaloid is also found in the fruit and leaves. Animals consume the plant only when other forage is unavailable. Cases of toxicity occur in the spring, summer, and fall. Cattle and sheep are most commonly affected.

Clinical Presentation

Animals exhibit vomiting, frothing at the mouth, salivation, staggering, dyspnea, subnormal temperature, and weakness. Death is caused by respiratory failure.

CANNABIS SATIVA (CANNABINACEAE FAMILY)

Common Names: Marijuana, Marihuana, Bhang, Hashish, Ganja, and Sinsemilla

The term marijuana refers to the dried leaves and flowers of the Indian hemp plant, which is cultivated illicitly for its psychological effects. It is an illicit drug plant and its leaves, flowers, and seeds contain several cannabinoids that are favored by some people for their psychoactive properties. Originally, the plant *Cannabis sativa* was an annual herb that was native to Asia, but it has spread throughout the world. Marijuana hemp both come from the same cannabis species, but are genetically distinct and are further distinguished by use, chemical makeup, and cultivation methods; have been employed for thousands of years as a source of fiber to make rope in Asia and in the Middle East as a medicinal and recreational drug. Only since the 1960s and 1970s has the recreational use of marijuana become common in the Eastern world. It is currently sold in the illicit drug trade and can be found growing in European countries in out-of-the-way places, in flower beds, or in pots within homes or vacant lots. Marijuana is the term used to describe the dried leaves and flowering heads of the cannabis plant.

Active Principle

The main psychoactive ingredient in the plant is the complex chemical delta-9-tetrahydrocannabinol (THC). This accounts for 3%–4% of the dry weight of the herbal material, although modern strains of the plant grown indoors under intensive cultivation conditions may contain as much as 15%–20%. The pharmacological effect of this agent is to produce central nervous system (CNS) depression and derangement. THC is absorbed when taken by mouth, having a low oral bioavailability resulting from a large first-pass effect because of extensive liver metabolism (taking as long as 3 or 4 h to reach peak blood levels).

Conditions of Poisoning

The quantity of the active ingredient exposed varies markedly according to the variety of the plant, the sex of the plant, the geographical location (pasture, woods, dry lot, near river or pond, confined indoors), the stage of growth, and the nature of the growing season. The greatest concentration of the active ingredient is in the flowering tops of the female plant, whereas leaves are less potent and seeds contain little of the active ingredient (Osweiler, 2011).

Individuals involved in the use of illicit drugs frequently keep pets that have access to the plants, or to products made from the plants, and this can potentially cause marijuana poisoning. Some individuals delight in involving their pets in the drug experience with them. In other cases, accidental ingestion results in toxicity to the pet.

Clinical Presentation

Clinical signs seen in man with high doses of marijuana include hallucinations and strange fantasies, and the user can no longer hold a coherent conversation. There is commonly a sudden stimulation of appetite, particularly for sweet foods. These effects may be followed by tiredness and sleep.

Animals show behavioral abnormalities and hyperexcitability. The animal most affected is the dog. The main clinical signs in the poisoned dog are vomiting, salivation, incoordination, alternating somnolence and hyperactivity, muscular weakness, and hyperthermia. Moreover, CNS and respiratory depression is another important sign in the dog. This is followed by coma and possibly death.

COLCHICUM AUTUMNALE L (LILIACEAE OR COLCHICACEAE FAMILY)

Common Names: Colchium, Meadow Saffron, Autumn Crocus, Wonder Bulb, and Naked Ladies

Colchium autumnale is locally abundant in meadows (meadow saffron; autumn crocus) throughout most European countries. It is a perennial herb, ovoid underground corm covered with brown membrane or scales. Large leaves, lanceolate, basal, ovate, smooth, ribbed, appear in spring and die back before flowering (Kahn, 2010).

Toxicity

All parts of the plant *C. autumnale* contain the alkaloids colchicine and colchiceine, of which the former is more toxic. The colchicine exists in all parts of the plant, but its highest concentration is in the bulb (~0.8% by weight). The pale purple flowers contain approximately 0.1% colchicine by weight. Both alkaloids withstand storage, drying (persist in contaminated hay), and boiling. At doses of 0.25 mg/kg body weight (BW), colchicine has a purgative effect. At higher doses, colchicine is a potent gastrointestinal toxin and causes intractable multiorgan failure. The European native is located in wet meadows with poisoning occurring during the spring. Poisoning of animals in the spring involves ingestion of the young leaves, whereas in the autumn the flowers of plants growing wild in pastures are implicated (Humphreys, 1988).

Clinical Presentation

Poisoning primarily affects cattle but can affect horses and pigs raised on pasture. Clinical signs appear approximately 48 h after ingestion. In cattle, the clinical signs of intoxication are predominantly related to the digestive tract and are characterized by salivation, dysphagia, colic, abdominal pain, diarrhea, and fetid feces that are green or black with tenesmus. Death occurs from cardiorespiratory failure and may be delayed for several days depending of the amount of plant ingested. The visible *postmortem* finding is gastroenteritis. Lesions that appear are edema and intestinal bleeding. In the horse, abdominal and thoracic serous effusions also occur.

CONIUM MACULATUM (APIACEAE (FORMALLY UMBILLIFERAE) FAMILY)

Common Name: Hemlock

Hemlock (*Conium maculatum*) is a glabrous, branching biennial herbaceous plant, with hollow purple-spotted stems arising from a thick taproot. It is a tall, branched plant with white flowers. This biennial plant is most often noticed during its second year of growth when it bolts and can reach heights of less than two meters. The poison hemlock usually has only one fleshy taproot, there are no pithy partitions in a hollow area at the juncture of stem and root, and stem and upper stem leaves are divided. Leaves resemble parsley, and they have a parsnip odor when crushed. Many small white flowers are arranged in an umbel in florescence. Poison hemlock stems have purple blotches, a characteristic that distinguishes it from wild carrot. Also, poison hemlock's leaves are more angular that those of wild carrot. This is probably more common that spotted water hemlock and found in drier, more upland habitats. It is found in roadside ditches and in damp waste areas.

Toxicity

Poison hemlock is one of the most toxic members of the plant kingdom. The concentrations and the relative ratio of different *Conium* alkaloids appear to depend on different factors such as temperature, moisture, time and age of the plant. It contains piperidine alkaloids (coniine and cyanapine) and other compounds that are capable of poisoning livestock, poultry, and humans. The consumption of varying parts of the plants (leaves, fruits) can cause different degrees of clinical effects. The stems, leaves, and mature fruits are toxic. All parts contain the toxin, especially in young plants. The leaves are more dangerous in spring, and the fruit is the most dangerous in fall. There appears to be different susceptibility to toxicity between species.

Clinical Presentation

Symptoms are gastrointestinal irritation and neurological effects (nervousness, trembling, loss of coordination, staggering, and coldness of the extremities), hyperpnea, and tachycardia (Lorgue et al., 1996). Eventually, depression, coma and death occur from respiratory failure. Birth defects may also occur. In general, animals can recover within hours.

Hemlock is more toxic to cattle than to other animals. Fresh plants collected at the same site were lethal to cows at the dosage of 5.3 g plant/kg bw. The general symptoms of poisoning in cattle are: arthrogryposis, depression, diarrhea, gait incoordination, lateral rotation of limbs, muscle spasms, salivation, teeth grinding, torticollis, trembling, coffee-colored urine and vomiting. Congenital skeletal malformations in calves from ingestion of hemlock have been reported (Keeler and Balls, 1978). Sheep and goat are also affected when fresh plant material is ingested.

The ingestion of hemlock by pigs leads to the following clinical signs: ataxia, tremors, severe lacrimation, mydriasis, tachycardia, polypnea, and fever (Widmer, 1984).

CONVALLARIA MAJALIS (LILIACEAE FAMILY)

Common Names: Lily of the Valley, May Lily, Jacob's Lily and Our Lady's Tears

This is a native European perennial plant of garden or wood that contains poisonous substances in the roots and stems. The leaves are long and broad, typical of the Liliaceae family. It is an ornamental houseplant. The animals most affected are dogs, cats and poultry. Dogs and cat usually chew and/or swallow the flowers and birds (poultry, duck, and geese) usually ingest the fresh plants.

Toxicity

The plant *Convallaria majalis* contains cardiotoxicants and convallatoxins.

Clinical Presentation

Poisoned animals are often found dead. Occasionally, terminal seizures are evidenced. Symptoms vary from mild gastrointestinal perturbation (vomiting, diarrhea) to terminal cardiac dysfunction (arrhythmias, bradycardia).

CORIARIA MYRTIFOLIA (CORIARIACEAE FAMILY)

Common Names: Tanner's Herb, Mediterranean Coriaria, and Redoul

This is an ornamental plant that grows in the Mediterranean countries of Europe.

Toxicity

Coriaria myrtifolia contains coriamyrtine, which can cause convulsions similar to those produced by strychnine or picrotoxin. The entire plant is toxic, and poisoning occurs via ingestion of the stems, branches, and fruits.

Clinical Presentation

The frequency of poisoning is high in goats and low in cattle and horses. Goats of all ages are very sensitive in regions in which redoul (imported breeds) is present. The number of affected individuals in herds varies from 10% to 50%. The lag time is short, 20 min (sometimes <5 min) to 2 h after ingestion of the plant (Faliu et al., 1985).

Mild symptoms are characterized by drunkenness, ptyalism, mydriasis, sometimes chills, loss of appetite, and bloating. These symptoms are followed by a severe form characterized by nervous signs such as retching, trembling, violent seizures that last 10–15 min, muscular contractions, ataxia, anorexia, tachycardia, intense tachypnea and dyspnea, nystagmus, mydriasis, ptyalism, and bloating. Death can occur within 20 min to 2 h after a crisis by respiratory arrest (20%–50% of cases), or there may be a progressive cure. The lesions are not specific and are characterized by severe and generalized congestion, edema and cyanosis of the mucous membranes (Faliu et al., 1985; Lorgue et al., 1996).

DATURA SPP. (SOLANACEAE FAMILY)

Common Name: Thorn Apple

All species of *Datura* are poisonous. The following species may be found where pets may be exposed:

- *Datura stramonium* (jimsonweed or Jamestown weed)
- *Datura metaloides* (thorn apple, apple of Peru, and tolguacha),
- *Datura arborea* (trumpet vine and angel's trumpet).

These species and others are grown as ornamentals, such as trumpet vine, or occur as weeds. The plants vary in appearance, but all have large, tubular flowers ranging in color from white to lavender. The fruit is an ovoid spiny capsule, giving rise to the common name, thorn apple. Most of the plants emit an objectionable odor.

Toxicity

Poisonous substances found in *Datura* are tropane alkaloids (atropine, hyoscine, and scopolamine) and hyoscyamine in all parts of the plant, particular in the seeds. The foliage may contain as much as 0.25%–0.7% alkaloids. The seeds are likely to be the source of toxicity for pets.

Conditions of Poisoning

In the illicit drug culture, *Datura* seeds are circulated to produce hallucinations. As with other plants involved in the illicit drug trade, pets are likely to consume toxic material accidentally if their owners are careless in handling the plant. Occasionally, a person may deliberately give the material to his or her animals.

Clinical Presentation

Clinical signs associated with *Datura* poisoning are similar to those caused by an overdose of atropine. The signs may occur a few moments after ingestion or may not appear for several hours. The poisoning has an acute course in which there is a weak, rapid pulse and heartbeat; disturbances of vision (dilated pupils due to mydriatic effects of *Datura*); dry mouth; incoordination; convulsions; and coma.

DATURA STRAMONIUM (SOLANACEAE FAMILY)

Common Name: Datura, Jimson Weed, False Castor Oil Plant, Stramonium, Spiny Apple, or Mad Apple

A coarse, foul-smelling, glabrous annual, with green or purple-tinged stems. Leaves alternate, and are coarsely and irregularly toothed. Leaves are ovate in outline, but coarsely toothed. *Datura stramonium contains flowers* are large, white to lavender in color, long and funnel ("tubular") form. Fruit are distinctive round, erect, dry, spiny capsules, with many black brown seeds. This plant is a greater problem in row crop agriculture than pastures. However, it is occasionally found in neglected or unused pastures; is abundant in fertile fields, gardens, and barn lots. There are rare incidences when animals ingest fresh plants because of the unpleasant odor (most animals avoid it).

One quick identifier is to rub the leaves, then smell your fingers. Jimson weed's unique scent makes it easy to confirm identification. Jimson weed can grow up to five feet tall. Its stems are green to purple. Leaves are ovate in outline, but coarsely toothed. Flowers are tubular and white or violet. The fruit is a capsule armed with prickles.

Toxicity

The toxic principles of this common hog lot and barnyard plant are the alkaloids atropine, L-hyoscyamine, and scopolamine (hyoscine). All parts of the plant, including seeds, are considered poisonous, whether green or dry. However, the seeds are particularly poisonous. Usually, this plant is not eaten except when other forage is unavailable. Cattle and swine are primarily affected, but horses, poultry, dogs, and humans have been affected. The toxin is not destroyed by drying. Plants may also take up nitrates.

Clinical Presentation

Symptoms can appear quickly. Early symptoms include a weak and rapid pulse and heartbeat, widely dilated eyes, and dryness of mouth and other mucous membranes. As the pulse increases, respiration can slow. Animals can appear blind and develop digestive problems such as nausea and diarrhea. Later symptoms include slow breathing, lowered temperature, convulsions, or coma. After eating the plants, sheep may have abnormal leg movements, disturbed vision, and intense thirst; they may bite at imaginary objects in the air. Pupils will often dilate. Pregnant sows consuming *D. stramonium* during their second and third months of gestation have produced deformed pigs. Some pigs may be born alive but exhibit varying degrees of flexed hips, stifles, and forelegs. The hocks may be overextended. In horses the incidence is rare, however the symptoms are anorexia, depression, narcosis, tachycardia, tachypnea, mydriasis, polyuria and polydipsia (Lorgue et al., 1996).

EQUISETUM SPP. (HORSETAIL FAMILY)

Common Names: Horsetail, Monkey Grass, Snake Grass, Scouting Rush

Plants of *Equisetum* species are generally found in wetter portions of a field. often moves into fields from drainage ditches or creeks along the fields' edges. Well maintained pastures can compete with horsetail, and moving can suppress growth. Parts of the plant sometimes find their way into baled hay. This weed most often affects horses, but equisetosis (the condition horsetail causes) typically occurs only after prolonged feeding.

Grows in colonies that appear like green straws. Its stems are hollow, can be separated into segments, and are rough to the touch. Its leaves are scale-like and inconspicuous. There are two primary stem types: one is a reproductive stem that generally does not branch, the other is a vegetative stem that has smaller stems radiating from the segmented stem.

Toxicity

Clinical Presentation

Poisoning from prolonged horsetail feeding can lead to breathing and heart problems as well as digestive problems. In some cases, animals may have convulsions. Young animals are more susceptible than older ones.

GALEGA OFFICINALIS L (PAPILIONACEAE FAMILY)

Common Name: Goat's Rue

Galega officinalis is a perennial European legume with a lush alfalfa-like appearance in early growth, but it becomes very rank when mature. It is a perennial herbaceous plant with a hollow stem and elliptical or lanceolate leaves. The flowers are light blue to violet in color. The plant is unpalatable to livestock, particularly when mature, and its use as forage is advocated only for very young plants.

Toxicity

This leguminous plant contains two nitrogen guanidine components, galegin (isoamylene guanidine) and hydroxygalegine, that are present in all parts during flowering and fruit formation. These substances have pharmacological properties as hypoglycemic and galactogenic agents.

Galegin decreases blood pressure and paralyzes the CNS. This plant appears in summer, especially during the months of July and August when the plant is in flower or producing pods, and it is found in the southern part of France. Accidental poisoning affects mainly sheep, but some cases have also been seen in cattle (Bezard et al., 2002). *G. officinalis* L. is generally rejected by cattle, probably due to its foul odor and bitter taste, especially when freshly cut. In case reports describing cattle and sheep fed the same hay, only sheep ate the toxic plant and were poisoned. Poisoning is usually related to feeding dry hay or freshly cut fodder contaminated by *Galega*, and it is assumed that fodder containing no more than 10% *Galega* will be toxic to sheep (Puyt et al., 1981).

Clinical Presentation

The latency period is usually 12–24 h after ingestion of the plant. It is characterized by an asphyxic syndrome caused by hydrothorax, which leads to death within hours. A voluminous hydrotorax is observed during postmortem examination.

HYPERICUM PERFORATUM (HYPERICACEAE FAMILY)

Common Names: St. John's Wort, Goat Weed, and Klamath Weed

There are various species of *Hypericum*, but the only species of importance in Europe is *Hypericum perforatum*. This perennial plant has a habitat and distribution in dry soil, wood, pastures, ranges, and along roadsides.

Toxicity

The photodynamic pigment (hypericin), a red fluorescent found in the black dots that are scattered over the surface of the leaves, stems, and petals, can be absorbed and is capable of sensitizing the pigment of animals to sunlight.

Clinical Presentation

The clinical signs occur from 48 h to 21 days of grazing the plant or as a result of ingesting contaminated hay or fodder. This delay depends on the time required for hypericin to reach a critical concentration in the skin and also the intensity and duration of sunlight to which animals are exposed (Faliu et al., 1986).

The animals most affected are cattle, horses, sheep, and goats; pigs are rarely affected. Poisoning occurs when the animals are exposed to sunlight and is characterized by photosensensitization, severe pruritus (head, ears, face, and extremities) and dermatitis with ulceration, erythema, blindness, convulsions, diarrhea, and extreme hypersensitivity to touch and to contact with cold water. The lesions observed are mainly cutaneous (dermatitis), degeneration of liver, and inflammation of gallbladder. For example, in cattle, the affected skin peels off in patches resembling leather. Deaths have been described. In horses, the white areas or mucous membranes are the site of depigmented erythema, pruritis, followed by edema (Faliu et al., 1986).

LUPINUS SPP.

Common Names: Lupines, Bluebonnet

The habitat and distribution of Lupinus is from dry to moist soils, roadsides, fields, and mountains. *Lupinus* spp. have alternate, palmately compound leaves and a variety of colored flowers (red, yellow, blue, white, purple). There are more than 500 species of annual, perennial, and soft woody lupines worldwide with about 12 species in Europe. *Lupinus* are cultivated in the Eastern Europe and Mediterranean regions as supplemental feed for livestock with regulatory limitations of 100 μg alkaloids/g material. The concentrations of major alkaloids are highest in the stems and leaves early in the growth phase, and these alkaloids decrease as the plant matures.

Toxicity

Many species of *Lupinus* contain teratogenic quinolizidine (anagyrine) and piperidine (ammodendrine) alkaloids. Quinolizidine alkaloids (20 known) and piperidine alkaloids concentrate in seeds (fresh and dry).

Clinical Presentation

All grazing animals, particularly ruminants (i.e., sheep, cattle, goats), are affected by *Lupinus* spp. Horses and pigs are also affected. Acute course is characterized by inappetence, dyspnea, struggle, convulsions, and death from respiratory paralysis. Some species are teratogenic in cattle (Kahn, 2010). They produced congenital birth defects (cleft palate, multiple congenital contractures, bowed limbs, scoliosis, kyphosis, and torticollis) in pregnant goats gavaged with plant material during gestation days 30–60 (Panter et al., 1990). The mechanism of action for *Lupinus*-induced malformations and cleft palate has been attributed to reduction in fetal movement. The mechanism of action of the teratogenic effects of *Lupinus*, *Conium* and *Nicotiana* spp. is believed to be identical (Panter et al., 1990).

Lupinosis is an animal disease characterized by hepatic steatosis, anorexia, weight loss, jaundice, and stupor that occurs in animals grazing on *Lupinus* species infected by a saprophytic fungus, mycotoxin-producing *Diaporthe toxica* (formerly *Phomopsis leptostromiformis*). Ingestion of the fungal metabolites, the hexapeptide phomopsis, can lead to liver disease in sheep called lupinosis.

NERIUM OLEANDER (APOCYNACEAE FAMILY)

Common Name: Oleander

Nerium oleander is a very common ornamental plant in Mediterranean areas of Europe; it is also grown in temperate climates in conservatories and greenhouses. *N. oleander* is a large ornamental evergreen shrub. The long, pointed leaves are oblong and contain a prominent midrib. Large clusters of white, pink, or red flowers appear at the end of the branches in summer. It is particularly abundant on sandy soils near the coast. It is widely cultivated and used as landscaping along roadsides and edges of woods and in lawns and gardens.

Toxicity

All parts of *N. oleander* contain very toxic cardiac glycosides (oleandrin, digitoxigenin, neriin, folinerin, and rosagenin) that apparently exert a digitoxin-like effect (cardiotoxic potential) (Langford and Boor, 1996). Toxins may also be inhaled in smoke when plants are burned. Human poisoning occasionally occurs from eating hot dogs roasted on sticks from nearby oleander plants. This extremely toxic plant can poison livestock and humans at any time of the year. The lethal dose in horses, donkeys, and calves is 30–50 mg/kg BW (Oryan et al., 1996).

Clinical Presentation

Severe gastroenteritis, diarrhea, abdominal pain, sweating, and weakness are the usual symptoms. These signs appear within a few hours after eating the leaves. Cardiac irregularities are common, often characterized by increased heart rate. However, a slower heart rate is often detected in the later stages. In comparison with other species, turkey poults have not been found to be very sensitive to *Oleander*.

POISONOUS PLANTS AFFECTING THE ANIMALS

Aconitum napellus (Ranunculaceae Family)

Common Names: Aconite, Monkshood, and Wolfsbane

Aconitum napellus has blue or white flowers bilateraly symmetrical with a prominent upper hood, which gives the genus its name. The perennial herb has palmate leaves and a tuberous root. Several species are common garden plants, but cases of poisoning in European countries are not common. However, it should be remembered that these plants are potentially poisonous.

Toxicity

All parts of the plant contain the toxic alkaloid aconitine, with the highest concentration in the tubers (roots) and seeds and lower amounts in the leaves and stems. Alkaloid content and composition varies throughout the year. The alkaloid content is highest when plants are flowering (June and July). Horses, donkeys, and goats are more sensitive to aconitum than sheep. The plant is not usually eaten (acrid test), and field poisoning is uncommon. Aconitine may also be present when forage or hay are contaminated by it.

Clinical Presentation

The clinical signs produced by this plant include vomiting, colic, bradypnea and dyspnea, muscular weakness, paralysis, pupillary dilatation (mydriasis), and death. Death is due to asphyxia, and the *postmortem* findings are those associated with suffocation. The lesions are not specific, usually appearing to be gastric and renal congestion (Lorgue et al., 1996).

PTERIDIUM AQUILINUM L OR *PTERIS AQUILINA* L (POLYPODIACEAE FAMILY)

Common Name: Bracken Fern

Pteridium aquilinum is also classified by some authorities as three separate species, *P. aquilinum*, *P. esculentum*, and *P. yarrabense*.

It is distributed throughout all European countries and on every continent of the world. Bracken fern is most common in woods, old fields, waste places, and roadsides, particularly on relatively dry sites. *P. aquilinum* is regarded as a potentially serious threat to the health of both animals and man. Poisoning is common in places where *P. aquilinum* grows naturally.

Toxicity

In poisoning by *P. aquilinum*, a polioencephalomalacia occurs because these plants contain the enzyme thiaminase, which inactivates thiamine (Vitamin B_1) in cattle, sheep, and horses; this is called "pteridism". The thiaminase hydrolyzes vitamin B_1, leading to a depletion of vitamin B_1 and produces a clinical syndrome of thiamin deficiency primarily in horses.

Ingestion of the green plant during periods of food shortage or when dried plant material (dryness does not reduce toxicity) is mixed in with hay or straw over a prolonged period (15–30 days) is toxic. Toxic effects from the plant appear to be cumulative, and symptoms may not appear until several weeks or months later (1–3 months), depending on the species of the animal, the amount ingested, the time of the year, and other factors. Clinical cases are most often seen in the spring or late summer or fall, especially after periods of drought when other forage is short or not available. Animals have shown toxicity from consuming hay containing the dried plants.

In ruminants, an aplastic anemia causes depression of the bone marrow; this effect is cumulative but appears over a short period of time. Sheep are less susceptible than cattle and horses to the toxic effects.

Clinical Presentation

P. aquilinum causes poisoning in several unique ways. First, ingestion by ruminants over a short period causes depression of bone marrow activity leading to pancytopenia manifested mainly as ecchymotic hemorrhages in mucosa, septicemia, and severe diarrhea. Second, ingestion over a long period causes proliferative lesions in and bleeding from the urinary bladder mucosa.

Cattle may exhibit two types of symptoms. The laryngeal form is often seen in younger animals and is characterized by edema of the throat region, resulting in difficult and loud breathing. The enteric form may be preceded by the laryngeal form and is characterized by bloody feces and urine and excessive bleeding from fly bites. The blood is slow to clot because platelets are deficient. Death usually occurs within a few days after symptoms appear. Sheep have shown blindness due to progressive retinal atrophy after grazing bracken fern; affected animals are permanently blind and adopt a characteristic alert attitude.

Horses exhibit muscular weakness and tremor, motor incoordination, and a crouching stance with arched neck and feet placed wide apart. Occasionally, a fever up to 48°C is present. Before death, horses may "head press" objects and have spasms with the head and neck drawn backwards. Death is preceded by tonic-clonic spams and opisthotonus. The disease is almost always fatal, and the lesions in cattle are indicative of a general hemorrhagic syndrome. Necropsy reveals multiple hemorrhages throughout the carcass; necrotic ulcers may be present in the gastrointestinal tract (abomasum and intestine).

In differential diagnosis, other plants, such as *Equisetum arvense* (horsetail) and *Beta vulgaris* (turnip), should be taken into account as these plants also induce thiamine deficiency. In horses, the condition must be distinguished from other neurological disorders produced by other poisonous plants such as *Crotalaria* spp. or *Senecio jacobea* (ragwort).

QUERCUS SPP. (FAGACEAE FAMILY)

Common Names: Live Oaks (Evergreens), and Acorns

Different species of oaks are responsible for poisoning. Acorns are the fruits of different species of oak, which have a detachable cap covering a hard oval body. Common in England and Northern Europe are: *Quercus ilex* (holm oak, evergreen oak), *Quercus pedunculata* (pedunculate oak), *Quercus robur* (common oak or English oak), and *Quercus petraea* syn *sessiliflora* (sessile oak or durmast oak).

Toxicity

Most animals are susceptible, although cattle and sheep are most often affected. Acorns and oak leaves contain large amounts of tannic acid along with small amounts of a volatile oil. The toxic principle, which appears to be gallotannins or their metabolites, causes gastrointestinal toxicity and renal damage. The incidence of poisoning is often associated with weather conditions, such as during hot dry summer, when the forage is scarce and an abundant acorns in the fall, or wind causing acorns to fall while still green. Pigs are resistant to pyrogallic and tannic acids (Lorgue et al., 1996).

Clinical Presentation

Consumption of large quantities of young oak leaves in the spring or green acorns in the fall produces clinical signs approximately 4 weeks after ingestion. The toxic syndrome is characterized by a gastrointestinal toxicity and renal dysfunction (Barbier, 2005).

Green and unripe acorns are more toxic than brown acorns and contain the highest levels of pyrogallic acids (up to 8%). In addition, certain species of oak (e.g., the pedunculate oak) are more toxic than others. The age of the tree is significant, with youngest trees having the highest levels of pyrogallic acids and tannins (Lorgue et al., 1996). The tannin content decreases with maturity. Cattle are most affected, especially young animals (1−3 years); sheep are not sensitive, and goats are rarely affected.

It is considered that the high tannic acid content is responsible for toxicity. Tannins have a direct action by decreasing digestive secretions and have a constipating effect as an indirect action after hydrolysis in the rumen. The metabolites gallic acid and pyrogallol are water soluble, and they are well absorbed in the gut. The metabolites are responsible for liver and kidney damage as well as necrotic lesions in the intestine.

Clinical signs in cattle include anorexia, prostration often accompanied by low temperature, depression, emaciation, rumen stasis, serous nasal discharge, polydipsia, polyuria, and constipation followed by mucoid to hemorrhagic diarrhea, dark fetid diarrhea, and sometimes blood clots. Nephrosis is another sign of toxicity. In sheep, the clinical signs are characterized by somnolence, leading to staggering and going down (Humphreys, 1988). In horses, the signs observed included dullness, hypothermia, weakness, inability to walk, incoordination, mouth ulcers, mucosa discoloration, patchy sweating but no colic, passage of hard or sloppy feces, and red or brown urine

(Warren and Waughan, 1985). The rumen contains acorns in large numbers. Evolution is frequently fatal. Hemorrhagic lesions of the gastrointestinal tract, nephritis, and perirenal edema may be important.

ROBINIA PSEUDOACACIA (PAPILIONACEAE FAMILY)

Common Names: False Acacia, Locust Tree and Black Locust Tree

Robinia pseudoacacia is a large ornamental tree with alternate, compound leaves and unbranched spines resembling rose thorns. It is often used in landscaping and grows wild. Black locusts growing near pastutes can hang over fences and drop seedpods into a pasture that may be bundled in hay. This plant has been cultivated and is a common tree in dry woodlands, old fields, roadsides, fence rows, and pinelands, particularly in clay soils, although it can be found in sandy soils.

Toxicity

Toxic principles include the phytotoxin robinin and the glycoside robitin (emetic and purgative) found throughout the plant, although the flowers have been suggested to contain the toxic principles. The toxic parts are leaves particularly wilted ones, young shoots, pods, seeds, and inner bark. Apparently, the toxin is heat labile, and it produces gastrointestinal distress. Horses, cattle, sheep, goats, poultry, and humans may be poisoned by ingesting roots, bark, sprouts, seed pods, or trimmings during periods of drought or food shortage. Horses are most susceptible to the effects of *Robinia pseudoacacia*.

Clinical Presentation

Symptoms include diarrhea, anorexia, weakness, posterior paralysis, depression, mydriasis, loss of appetite, irregular pulse, and difficult breathing. Intestinal problems can lead to bloody diarrhea. Death is not frequent. *Postmortem* lesions are restricted to the gastrointestinal tract. Symptoms can appear 1–2 h after ingestion. Mucous membranes turn yellow, appendages become cold and pupils dilate.

RICINUS COMMUNIS (EUPHORBIACEAE FAMILY)

Common Name: Castor Bean

The plant *Ricinus communis* has large, palmately lobed leaves, and it is a robust annual (in southern regions) or perennial (in tropics and subtropics regions) woody herb. It is cultivated and occasionally escapes and persists in pinelands, waste places, and roadsides.

Flowers are green and inconspicuous; staminate flowers near the base, and pistillate flowers are mostly near the top of a small panicle. The fruit is a three-lobed capsule with a soft, spiny exterior, 1.5–2 cm long. There are three seeds per capsule. Seeds are shiny, grayish brown mottled with reddish brown, and 10 mm long and 6 or 7 mm wide. Seeds resemble engorged ticks and usually tree in a somewhat spiny pod.

Toxicity

The poisonous principle is a phytotoxin called ricin. In Europe, the plant is commonly planted not only as an ornamental but also in vegetable gardens to repel moles. Horses are most susceptible to poisoning, but all livestock and humans can be affected. All parts of the plant are toxic, especially the seeds. Toxicity is seen most often in spring and summer.

Clinical Presentation

Animals are most often poisoned when feed grains have become contaminated with the castor bean seeds. Depending on the amount consumed, symptoms appear from several hours to days after animals consume the toxin. Violent purgation in the form of straining and bloody diarrhea is the classical sign. Other signs are dullness, abdominal pain, weakness, trembling, and incoordination.

SENECIO SPP. (COMPOSITEAE FAMILY)

Common Names: Ragwort and Groundsel

This plant is very common in pastures and agricultural lands. Ragwort appears to be less common and is perennial, while groundsel is an annual and has a hollow stem. These plants maintain toxicity after drying, so they are still toxic in baled hay. Plants in this group start as basal rosettes. The genus of this family contains more than 1200 species, of which 25 are known to be toxic and causes seneciosis. Members of the plant family include *Senecio aquaticus* (marsh ragwort), *S. jacobea* (ragwort or tansy ragwort), *S. squalidus* (Oxford ragwort) and *S. vulgaris* (groundsel). In the United Kingdom, there have been many reported incidents involving exposure to ragwort. Ragwort (*S. jacobea*) is a highly toxic plant that grows widely in pastures, as well as on many areas of waste land, and like the buttercup (*Ranunculus* spp.), it often remains ungrazed so long as there is an alternative supply of feed. However, there is a crucial difference between these two plants that renders buttercups relatively harmless (the toxic principle is an unstable chemical that is not found in hay made from such meadows) while ragwort continues to be a major problem to both ruminants and horses.

Toxicity

The toxic parts are the seeds, flowers, and leaves. Young plants are more toxic than older plants. These plants contain hepatotoxic pyrrolizidine alkaloids including: jacobine, jacidine, jaconine, and retrorsine. Retrorsine is the most widely distributed pryrrolizidine alkaloids.

Not all animal species are equally susceptible, since some species can activate, detoxify and eliminate pyrrolizidine alkaloids. While cattle and horses are quite susceptible, needing, e.g., a dry-mass intake of *Senecio jacobea* of only about 5% of their BW to be lethal, sheep and goats are more resistant, requiring intakes of several hundred percent of their BWs (Cheeke and Shull, 1985). Susceptibility is influenced by species-specific metabolism, age, sex and other temporary factors (i.e., biochemical, physiological, and nutritional status). Young animals are generally more susceptible to pyrrolizidine alkaloids than aged animals (Colegate and Molyneux, 2008).

Clinical Presentation

Seneciosis is an acute and chronic hepatic insufficiency caused by the ingestion of plants containing senecio. Poisoning occurs when the fresh plant is ingested (in pastures) or when it contaminates hay or silage (Vos et al., 2002). All animals can be affected, but cattle and horses are especially sensitive.

Poisoning can present after a latent period of weeks to months. The clinical picture is characterized by a syndrome of photosensitization, jaundice and CNS derangement. Clinical signs are extremely diverse and include anorexia, weight loss, poor hair coat, constipation, mild jaundice of the mucosa, reduction in vision followed by blindness, ataxia with trembling, weakness, and drowsiness. Generally, poisoning results in liver failure, jaundice, and death. The lesions are characterized by enlargement and congestion of the liver, hepatitis (a cirrhotic form) with ascites, nephritis, and edema of the abomasum (Lorgue et al., 1996). Dose-dependent swelling of hepatocytes is the first cellular indication of pyrrolizidine alkaloid intoxication. Acute intoxication often produces pan-lobular hepatocellular necrosis accompanied by hemorrhage and minimal inflammation. Serum biochemical changes include massive elevations in AST, SDH, ALK and GGT activities with increased amounts of bilirubin and bile acids (Colegate and Molyneux, 2008).

Most outbreaks occur in animals on pasture, but can occur in housed animals, fed hay contaminated by the foliage or seeds. In horses, photosensitization may develop following plant ingestion. Pyrrolizidine alkaloids can be passed into the milk of lactating animals (Goeger et al., 1982).

TAXUS BACCATA L. (TAXACEAE FAMILY)

Common Name: Yew

The yew (*Taxus baccata*) has been noted as the most poisonous plant in all of Europe. The yew is a tree or shrub of the family *Taxaceae* that will accommodate all types of soils and grows in shade and sun. It is planted in parks, gardens, and cemeteries, especially for ornamental fences. Other yew species are also toxic; *T. cuspidala* (Japanese yew) and *T. canadensis* (Canada yew) are widely planted in gardens. Poisoning occurs in animals located in pastures, woods, or gardens or as a result of careless disposal of yew clippings or leaves. All parts of the tree are poisonous, and all species of animals are susceptible. The leaves are harmful at all stages of plant growth, and drying and storage do not lessen their toxicity. The sexes are separate, and the pistillate plants bear bright scarlet fruit in the fall. The red flesh covers a hard seed, and although the flesh is not poisonous, the seed is extremely poisonous. The sap of the tree contains volatile oils that are irritants, and the leaves contain the alkaloid taxine (taxine A and taxine B) and ephedrine and cyanide (hydrocyanic acid). Taxine is found in all parts of the tree except the fleshy red part of the berry. These compounds are capable of causing hypotension, bradycardia, and depressed myocardial contractility and conduction delay, similar to digitalis poisoning (Alexander et al., 1946).

Toxicity

Chewing seeds has proven fatal to animals and humans. The foliage is even more toxic, and it is this that proves so poisonous to cattle, sheep, goats, pigs and horses. There are probably more problems with children eating these berries than any other, except possibly pokeweed. Chewing these seeds and then swallowing can cause serious poisoning. The relatively greater resistance of ruminants is probably due to the dilution of the ingested material by the rumen contents. This effect may also account for the individual variation in susceptibility of different animals and for the delay, sometimes seen in cattle, before clinical signs of yew poisoning become apparent (Humphreys, 1988).

Clinical Presentation

The conditions of poisoning are by consumption of leafy branches or lying in situ (fall) in the soil after harvest or a thunderstorm. The most common feature of yew poisoning is sudden death (1–48 h depending of the amount ingested). The clinical signs observed are nervousness, trembling, ataxia, dyspnea, and collapse (Barbier, 2005). Bradycardia progressing to cardiac standstill and death ensues without struggle. Death occurs within approximately 5 min. Empty right heart, dark tarry blood in left heart, and limited nonspecific postmortem lesions such as congestion of the kidneys, liver, spleen, and lungs are seen (Ogden, 1988). The presence of yew leaves in the rumen contents may help in making the diagnosis of yew poisoning.

THUJA OCCIDENTALIS L. (CUPRESSACEAE FAMILY)

Common Name: Thuja

Thuja (*Thuja occidentalis* L.) shrubs are found throughout Europe. They are frequently planted in parks and gardens for ornamental purposes, especially in enclosures. Animal species affected are cattle and sheep, and, rarely, goats. Poisoning occurs by consumption of branches or branches dropped on the ground after being cut down or following a storm.

Clinical Presentation

Peracute intoxication is within a few minutes, especially in sheep. Clinical signs of acute or subacute intoxication are essentially related to the digestive tract (hypersalivation, colics, bloating, and bloody diarrhea) (Jean-Blain and Grisvard, 1973). Toxicity progresses to dyspnea and paralysis, accompanied by a cooling of the extremities. Death can occur between 1 and 48 h depending on the amount of plant parts ingested. The lesions are characterized by discrete congestive gastroenteritis, which is not specific. The presence of thuja leaves in the rumen contents confirms poisoning.

TREATMENT

Management of poisoning by toxic plants is complicated by the lack of antidotes to most plant toxins. However, general treatment is intended to induce emesis, reduce absorption, or enhance elimination of toxin. The effect of treatment may be difficult to determine because of the wide variability in toxic reactions to the same plant. Table 62.3 describes some of the systemic effects of poisonous plants.

TABLE 62.3 Systemic Effects of Plant Poisoning

Gastrointestinal irritants	*Ricinus Communis*, Araceae Family
Cardiovascular abnormalities	*Convallaria majalis*, *Digitalis purpurea*, *Aconitum* spp.
Renal dysfunction	*Datura stramonium*, *Cicuta* spp.
Hepatic dysfunction	*Senecio* (pyrrolizidine alkaloids)
Convulsions	*Cicuta* spp., *Coriaria myrtifolia*, *Aconitum*, *Taxus*, and *Veratrum* plant species (*Veratrum calcifornicum*)
Nicotine symptoms	*Conium maculatum*
Atropine symptoms	*Datura stramonium*

Nonspecific Treatment

The most important aspect of emergency medicine treatment is to ensure adequate physiologic functioning. Treatment generally requires stabilization of vital signs. Most plant poisoning cases respond to supportive care. Frequently, the veterinarian must treat the animal before plant identification is done. The recognition of certain syndromes characteristic of specific plants is of importance.

Many plant poisonings will not be diagnosed at the onset of the disease. Therapy will, of necessity, be symptomatic. Even when a positive diagnosis can be made, there are rarely any specific antidotes. The most important step in therapy for any plant poisoning case is to remove any residual plant materials from the digestive tract as quickly as possible.

Removal of unabsorbed poison from the gut can be achieved by several means, including induction of emesis, gastric lavage, and use of activated charcoal, tannins, and cathartics. Tannins and activated charcoal may be administered in water slurry via oral route.

In emergency medicine and for critical patients, begin resuscitation with the airways and then breathing and circulation in an overdose scenario. Therapeutic management strategies can be summarized as follows: establishment of a patent airway, artificial respiration, cardiac massage, and perhaps the application of defibrillation techniques. Following stabilization of vital signs, the clinician may proceed with subsequent therapeutic measures. Treatment involves enhancing the removal of the absorbed poison and providing supportive therapy to combat the effects of the poison already absorbed.

Decontamination Procedures

Ingestion is the most common route of poisoning in large and small animals. Decisions about gastric emptying depend on an accurate identification of the plant responsible for poisoning because the majority of casual ingestions require no specific therapy. Once identified, decontamination is based on plant toxicity, symptoms, and time since ingestion. Unless contraindicated, emesis is preferred to lavage because plant pieces are difficult to remove by gastric tube in some animal species, in particular those that are small.

Gastric Decontamination

Many methods have been used to prevent the absorption of toxic substances from the gastrointestinal tract, with varying success.

Vomiting can be induced in the conscious patient by the administration of apomorphine, (0.04 mg/kg BW intravenously (i.v.), or 0.08 mg/kg BW intramuscularly (i.m.) or subcutaneously (s.c.). Apomorphine, a morphine derivative, may cause respiratory and CNS depression and may induce protracted emesis, ultimately resulting in a severely debilitated animal. These effects can be controlled by using a narcotic antagonist such as naloxone (0.04 mg/kg BW i.v.). When naloxone hydrochloride is given i.v., the dosage may be repeated at 2- to 3-min intervals as necessary (Bright et al., 2011).

Gastric lavage may be used to enhance removal of toxins still present in the stomach. There are two decontamination procedures-gastric lavage or irrigation. When it is ascertained that an animal has ingested a potentially poisonous substance within less than 2 h, efforts should be made to remove it from the upper gastrointestinal tract. If the animal has not vomited and can swallow, an emetic should be given promptly. In the case of an irritating toxin, rinsing of the mouth with sodium gluconate for at least 2 h can be performed.

Gastric lavage is an important emergency procedure, but it is relatively ineffective in suspected poisoning cases in which significant time has elapsed. Changes in techniques (e.g., using a larger tube, more volume, and more frequent lavages) have proven to be a useful procedure when undertaken within 2 h of ingestion of a toxicant (Hanna, 1986). Gastric lavage is recommended if the animal is presented within 60 min of a potentially lethal ingestion of a plant. Proper placement of the patient may help prevent aspiration and improve the yield of the procedure. If more than 2 h has passed since ingestion of the plant material, it is likely that the stomach will have already emptied into the intestine. In such cases, subjecting the pet to further stress through induced emesis is unwise. The patient should be sedate and as large a gastric tube as possible should be inserted to facilitate aspiration of the ingesta back out through the tube.

The use of activated charcoal has revolutionized the treatment of poisoning. Charcoal for medicinal use is created by the controlled pyrolytic decomposition of carbon-based compounds. Activation with gases at high temperature removes previously absorbed substances and further reduces particle size, resulting in an exceptionally porous final product. Due to its small particle size and enormous surface area, it can adsorb a large amount of toxicant. Some "superactivated" charcoal preparations have a surface area of up to 3500 m^2/g or about 175,000 m^2 per 50-g bottle. This allows the adsorption of toxins through weak intermolecular forces, with nonionized, organic compounds binding more avidly than dissociated, inorganic ones (Olson, 2010). The usual dose is 1 g/kg BW or 10 parts of activated charcoal for every one part of toxin, whichever is greater (large animals: 250–250 g; small animals: 5–50 g). Activated charcoal is effective in preventing absorption of toxicant when it is properly utilized. Most toxicologists recommend single-dose activated charcoal at 1 h following a significant ingestion. Charcoal as a "universal antidote" has a wide spectrum of activity and when properly used is probably the most valuable single agent known (Juurlink, 2015). It can be administered after vomiting has occurred or can be used in the gastric lavage solution. Decontamination with a single-dose of activated charcoal is conceptually different from the use of multiple-dose activated charcoal, a less commonly deployed intervention involving the administration of multiple (typically, two to six) doses (Juurlink, 2015). The single-dose activated charcoal can be associated not only with altered toxicokinetics (influence the area under the curve of toxic concentration versus time, enhancing the total body clearance, and reducing systemic absorption) when given shortly after dosing, but also with improvements in clinical outcomes. The "universal antidote" should be avoided because magnesium oxide and tannic acid interfere with the adsorption capacity of activated charcoal. Activated charcoal adsorbs most alkaloids well and should be administered in almost all symptomatic cases. Although generally safe, the single-dose activated charcoal is not free of risk. The most widely cited concern associated with the single-dose activated charcoal is pulmonary aspiration, although the risk of this complication is low. GI complications represent another potential risk of single-dose activated charcoal administration such as bowel obstruction, bezoars, and stercoliths.

Other adsorbents, such as magnesium oxide and kaolin, are less effective than activated charcoal. Soap and water are often used dermally to remove a toxin from the skin and/or reduce toxin absorption.

Ipecac syrup and cathartics have not been shown to be of benefit in cases of ingestion of poisonous plants. However, the use of emetics such as syrup of ipecac is recommended if the animal is conscious (i.e., the poisonous plant does not cause rapid onset of coma and convulsions) and the absorption time is less than 2 h. Apomorphine can be injected subcutaneously at a dose of 0.2 mg/kg, but it is effective only in dogs. Ipecac syrup up to 10% at a dose of 1 or 2 mL/kg BW can be used in cats and dogs. Xylazine is also an effective emetic, particularly in cats (0.05–1 mg/kg BW i.m.) but it is less effective in dogs.

Some veterinarians prefer gastric lavage or activated charcoal as the major gastrointestinal measures. Gastric lavage is practical and effective if ingestion of the poison is recent (<2 h). Gastric lavage is performed with 5–10 mL/kg of isotonic sodium chloride and activated charcoal in suspension. After lavage, a laxative agent may be placed into the stomach to further evacuate the intestine. Mineral oil is a suitable laxative. The dosage for small animals is 5–30 mL in dogs and 2–6 mL in cats. An oral saline cathartic of sodium sulfate (0.5 g/kg BW) is an efficient agent for evacuation of the bowel and may be used in an emergency in small animals. Magnesium sulfate (1 g/kg BW) and castor oil (10–60 g per animal) can also be used; either can be used instead of mineral oil if desired. A high colonic enema is indicated to evacuate the toxicants from the lower gastrointestinal tract. Warm water with castile soap makes an excellent enema solution. Other enema preparations can be useful. The entire digestive tract of a dog can be emptied by a judicious combination of a gastric lavage and a high colonic enema. Care should be taken to avoid the induction of dehydration and electrolyte and acid-base imbalances once the gastrointestinal tract has been evacuated.

Gastric aspiration and serial activated charcoal are useful in nicotine and related poisoning because of the secretion of nicotine into the acid milieu of the stomach of carnivores.

Enemas

This is a technique very useful for removing toxins from the lower gastrointestinal tract. The best enema solution is lukewarm water that is infused into the rectum of a patient. The enemas should be repeated after 2 h.

Laxatives and Purgatives (Cathartics)

Mineral oil, sodium sulfate, and other laxatives are used to enhance elimination of toxins still present in the gastrointestinal tract. Laxatives promote the elimination of soft, formed feces, whereas purgatives produce a more fluid evacuation. The following substances may be used for these purposes:

- Lubricant and emollient laxatives (fecal softeners): mineral oil (liquid paraffin)(cattle, 250–500 mL; horses, 250–1000 mL; pigs, 25–300 mL; dogs, 5–30 mL; cats, 2–6 mL).
- Bulk laxatives: methylcellulose (dogs, 0.5–5 g, and cats, 0.5–1 g, per os; carboxymethylcellulose sodium, psyllium, or plantago seed (dogs, 3–10 g, and cats, 3 g per os); agar; wheat bran.
- Osmotic cathartics (saline purgative)-these are not absorbed and retain water in the intestinal lumen: magnesium sulfate (cattle, 250–500 g; horses, 30–100 g; pigs, 25–125 g; dogs, 5–25 g; cats, 2–5 g), sodium sulfate (cattle, 500–750 g; horses, 250–375 g; pigs, 30–60 g; dogs, 5–25 g; cats, 2–5 g), sugar alcohols (mannitol and sorbitol), lactulose (dogs, 5–15 mL, t.i.d., per os).
- Irritant cathartics: In this context, purgatives can be included with diphenylmethane or anthraquinone.

Enhanced Removal and Elimination

This procedure includes pH manipulation of urine or blood, or both and other adjunct therapeutic modalities that may be useful in toxic situations. Administration of fluids and diuretics may enhance the glomerular filtration rate. Fluids may be given to treat dehydration. Fluids such as saline lactated Ringer's solution are administered to promote urine production. Bicarbonate may be given to treat acidosis.

Osmotic diuresis may be induced by infusion of mannitol 10% solution or hypertonic glucose from 10% to 30% at 20–40 mL/kg BW. The application of diuretics such as furosemide (3–5 mg/kg BW) i.m. or i.v. may enhance urine production. Furosemide may also be used to treat edema.

The theory of ion trapping is that reabsorption of basic poisons that are excreted renally may be prevented by acidification of the urine, and reabsorption of acid poisons that are excreted renally may be prevented by alkalinization of the urine (Dalefield and Oehme, 2006).

So, forced acid diuresis to eliminate weak bases can be reached with ammonium chloride orally (20–40 g in large animals, 100–200 mg/kg BW in dogs, and 20 mg/kg BW in cats) to maintain a urine pH of 5.5–6.5, with arginine choride i.m. or i.v. (7–10 g in large animals, and 100–200 mg/kg BW in small animals), or with ascorbic acid i.v. (40 mg/kg BW in all animal species). Ammonium chloride should not be used in acidotic animals; overuse may result in ammonia toxicosis (Dalefield and Oehme, 2006).

Forced alkaline diuresis to eliminate weak acids can be done with sodium bicarbonate 1.4% by i.v. infusion to maintain a urine pH higher than 7 (2–4 mL/kg BW during 24 h in large animals or given by slow, continuous administration for best results in small animals) and with lactated Ringer's by i.v. infusion (5–10 mL/kg BW per hour in all species).

Specific Treatment

Specific treatment is possible only in rare cases. For instance, in the case of intoxication by *Pteridium aquilinum*, horses can be treated with thiamine intramuscularly at a dosage of 100–200 mg per day for 7–14 days, or the anticyanide treatment can be used with sodium thiosulfate

(20% solution), 4 mL/kg BW, strictly intravenously, and sodium nitrite (10% solution), 2 mL/kg BW, strictly intravenously.

SUPPORTIVE THERAPY

Treatment of most cases of poisoning is largely supportive. The aim of the supportive measures is to preserve the vital organ function until the poison is eliminated from the body and the patient resumes normal physiological functions, including control of body temperature, maintenance of cardiopulmonary function and renal system, control of acid-base status, alleviation of pain and control of CNS effects with proper care for coma, seizures, hypotension, arrhythmias, hypoxia, and acute renal failure. If seizures occur, diazepam, phenobarbital or pentobarbital may be used; an initial diazepam dose of 0.5 mg/kg BW i.v. may be repeated every 20 min up to three times. If diazepam is not sufficiently effective in small animals, use pentobarbital at 6 mg/kg BW i.v. or pentobarbital at 24–29 mg/kg BW i.v. (Dalefield and Oehme, 2006). Body temperature should be monitored. Hypothermia can be controlled with a circulating hot water blanket and by keeping the animal in a warm and draft-free cage. Hyperthermia is treated with ice bags, cold water baths, and enemas. It is vitally important that the animal's body temperature be constantly monitored to prevent overcorrection.

Respiratory support requires an adequate patent airway, using a cuffed endotracheal tube in an unconscious animal or by performing a tracheostomy under local anesthesia. A respirator is of great value, or an anesthesia machine may be utilized with manual compression of the bag. Administer supplemental 100% oxygen.

It is more appropriate to insert an endotracheal tube and provide positive pressure ventilation if needed. A patient that is depressed sufficiently to require respiratory assistance must be continuously monitored. All unconscious or shock patients require intubation.

Be prepared to supply respiratory support. Although analeptic agents such as doxapram used in respiratory depression may provide immediate support, the effect is transient and cannot be relied on to sustain a pet free from poisoning. Doxapram 1–10 mg/kg BW intravenously may cause seizures if administered in overdoses (70–75 times the therapeutic dose in healthy animals) (Dalefield and Oehme, 2006).

Cardiovascular support requires the presence of adequate circulating blood volume, cardiac function, tissue perfusion, and acid-base balance. Blood volume and cardiac activity are of most immediate concern.

In the presence of hypovolemia due to loss of both cells and volume, whole blood is needed. A sufficient quantity of whole blood should be given to raise the packed volume to 75% of the animal's estimated normal level. Hypovolemia due to fluid loss alone can be treated with the administration of lactated Ringer's solution or plasma expanders.

Cardiac activity can be aided by the application of closed-chest cardiac massage for immediate cardiovascular support, but the administration of calcium gluconate, infused slowly intravenously, can stimulate cardiac activity in most instances. This agent is also a good nonspecific treatment of many toxicities.

Control of acid-base balance problems is primarily a matter of physiologically maintaining an animal in a homeostatic condition. The most common acid-base disturbance seen is metabolic acidosis, but alkalosis may also occur in cases of poisoning. In correcting acidosis not of respiratory origin, sodium bicarbonate intravenously is the drug of choice. Caution must be exercised with alkalinizing agents to avoid the induction of alkalosis. For initial therapy, it is usually sufficient to administer 0.9% NaCl (physiologic saline) intravenously, followed by oral administration of divided doses of ammonium chloride.

Control of pain with a minimal dose of morphine or meperidine is used in animals. Management of CNS disorders in cases of intoxication is complex. Therapy depends on the presence of CNS depression or hyperactivity. Either disorder can easily be reversed to the extreme by overzealous treatment. CNS depression can also be considered with respiratory depression because the management of the two conditions is very similar. Although the intravenous administration of analeptic agents, such as doxapram, is reported to be efficacious, their actions are short-lived, and CNS depression returns if the animal is not monitored continuously. Bemegride is also occasionally used to stimulate the respiratory centers in the medulla. Analeptics may also induce convulsions.

Cases of CNS hyperactivity, including convulsions, can be managed by the administration of CNS depressants or tranquilizers. Pentobarbital sodium, phenobarbital, phenytoin, and primidone are the agents of choice for convulsions and hyperactivity; care must be taken, however, because a respiratory depressing dose may be required to alleviate all adverse signs. Inhalant anesthetics are excellent for long-term management of CNS hyperactivity. Central acting skeletal muscle relaxants and minor tranquilizers (methocarbamol, glyceryl guaiacolate, and diazepam) are also used for convulsant intoxicants. The animal should be placed in a quiet, dark room to reduce excitation due to auditory or visual stimuli.

CONCLUDING REMARKS AND FUTURE DIRECTIONS

Compared to North American and African flora, European flora have fewer dangerous species; however the number of plant poisonings is considerable. Local veterinarians are familiar with regional livestock management practices, livestock diseases, and many endemic plants, and are frequently called upon to treat known or suspected animal toxicosis in clinic, farm, or field conditions; thus, they should play a key role in diagnosing plant poisoning. Plant identification, the accurate diagnosis of plant poisoning, the conditions conducive to plant poisoning, and predictive and toxicity factors are relevant in the field of plant toxicology; these are a valuable guide to avoiding future losses and ensuring safe and high-quality animal food products. In general, plants cause poisoning only when eaten and affect livestock and companion animals. Many wild plants, houseplants, or illicit drug plants grown in Europe contain chemical substances in sufficient quantities to cause toxic effects in animals. *Liliaceae* spp. and *Araceae* spp. are the major plant families involved in poisoning of companion animals. Most cases are related to accidental ingestion of ornamental plants rather that wild plants, particularly at certain times of the year. In addition to the previously mentioned poisonous plants for dogs, the following plant families are also implicated: Euphorbiaceae, Apocynaceae, Solanaceae, Ericaceae, and Amaryllidaceae. Both specific and nonspecific treatments, including decontamination procedures, used in animal poisoning by plants are considered essential in veterinary toxicology.

REFERENCES

Alexander Jr., E., Morris, D.P., Eslick, R.L., 1946. Atropine poisoning: report of a case with recovery after ingestion of one gram. N. Engl. J. Med. 234, 258–259.

Barbier, N., 2005. Bilan d'activité du Centre National d'Informations Toxicologiques Véterinaires pour l'2003. Thèse de Doctorat Vétérinaire, Lyon, France.

Bezard, M., Grancher, D., Vialard, J., et al., 2002. Un troupeau ovin intoxiqué par le *Galéga officinal*. Le Point Vétérinaire. 227, 66–67.

Bright, S.J., Murphy, M.J., Steinschneider, J.C., et al., 2011. Treatment of animal toxoses: a regulatory perspective. Vet. Clin. Food Anim. 27, 481–512.

Cheeke, P.R., Shull, L.R., 1985. Alkaloids. Natural Toxicants in Feeds and Poisonous Plants. AVI Publ Co, Inc, Westport, CT, pp. 92–172.

Clay, B.R., 1977. Poisoning and injury by plants. In: Kirk, R.W. (Ed.), Current Veterinary Therapy VI, vol. 6. Saunders, Philadelphia, pp. 179–184.

Colegate, S.M., Molyneux, R.J., 2008. Bioactive Natural Products: Detection, Isolation and Structural Determination. second ed. CRC Press/Taylor & Francis, Boca Raton, FL.

Dalefield, R.R., Oehme, F.W., 2006. Antidotes for specific poisons. In: Peterson, M.E., Talcott, P.A. (Eds.), Small Animal Toxicology. Saunders-Elsevier, Saint Louis, pp. 459–474.

Faliu, L., Puyt, J.D., Jean-Blain, C., 1985. Intoxication végétale: Redoul. Le Point Vétérinaire. 17 (92), 531–532.

Faliu, L., Dorchies, P.H., Puyt, J.D., 1986. Intoxication végétale: Millepertuis. Le Point *Vétérinaire*. 18 (98), 299–301.

Flood, A.A., Fitzgerald, K.T., 2006. The poison-proof practice. Clin. Tech. Small Anim. Pract. 21, 164–173.

Forsyth, S.S., 1968. British Poisonous Plants. Bulletin 161 of the Ministry of Agriculture, Fisheries and Food. Her Majesty's Stationery Office, London.

Fowler, M.E., 1981. Plant Poisoning in Small Companion Animals. Raston Purina, St. Louis, MO.

Gault, G., Berny, P., Lorgue, G., 1995. Plantes toxiques pour les animaux de compagnie. Rec. Méd. Vét. 171, 171–176.

Goeger, D.E., Cheeke, P.R., Schmitz, J.A., et al., 1982. Effect of feeding milk from goats fed tansy ragwort (*Senecio jacobaea*) to rats and calves. Am. J. Vet. Res. 43, 1631–1633.

Hanna, G., 1986. Plant poisoning in canines and felines. Vet. Hum. Toxicol. 28 (1), 38–40.

Humphreys, D.J., 1988. Veterinary Toxicology. third ed. Bailliere Tindall, London.

Jean-Blain, C., Grisvard, M., 1973. Genévrier sabine, Thuya. Plantes Vénéneuses: Toxicology. La Maison Rustique, Paris, pp. 24–25.

Juurlink, D.N., 2015. Activated charcoal for acute overdose: a reappraisal. Br. J. Clin. Pharmacol. 81 (3), 482–487.

Kahn, C.M. (Ed.), 2010. The Merck Veterinary Manual. tenth ed. Merck & Co, Inc., Whitehouse Station, NJ.

Keeler, F., Balls, D., 1978. Teratogenic effects in cattle of *Conium maculatum* and *Conium* alkaloids and analogues. Clin. Toxicol. 12, 49–64.

Langford, S., Boor, P., 1996. Oleander toxicity: an examination of human and animal toxic exposures. Toxicology. 109, 1–13.

Lorgue, G., Lechenet, J., Rivière, A., 1996. Clinical Veterinary Toxicology. Blackwell Science Ltd, Oxford, UK.

Ogden, L., 1988. Taxus (yews): a highly toxic plant. Vet. Hum. Tox. 30 (6), 563–564.

Olson, K.R., 2010. Activated charcoal for acute poisoning: one toxicologist's journey. J. Med. Toxicol. 6, 190–198.

Oryan, A., Maham, M., Rezakhani, A., et al., 1996. Morphological studies on experimental oleander poisoning in cattle. J. Vet. Med. A. 43, 625–634.

Osweiler, G.D., 2011. Diagnostic guidelines for ruminant toxicosis. Vet. Clin. Food Anim. 27, 247–254.

Panter, K.E., Keeler, R.F., Bunch, T.D., et al., 1990. Congenital skeletal malformations and cleft palate induced in goats by ingestion of *Lupinus*, *Conium* and *Nicotiana* species. Toxicon. 28, 1377–1385.

Puyt, J.D., Faliu, L., Keck, G., et al., 1981. Fatal poisoning of sheep by *Galega officinalis* (French honeysuckle). Vet. Hum. Toxicol. 23 (6), 410–412.

Schaller, G., Urech, K., Grazi, G., et al., 1998. Viscotoxin composition of the three European subspecies of *Viscum album*. Planta Med. 64, 677–678.

Vos, J.H., Geerts, A.A.J., Borgers, J.W., et al., 2002. Jacobskruiskruid: bedrieglijke schoonheid. Vergiftiging met *Senecio jacobea*. Tijdschrift voor Diergeneskunde. 127, 753–756.

Warren, C.G.B., Waughan, S.M., 1985. Acorn poisoning. Vet. Rec. 116 (3), 82.

Welch, K.D., Panter, K.E., Gardner, D.R., et al., 2012. The good and the bad of poisonous plants: an introduction to the USDA-ARS poisonous plant research laboratory. J. Med. Toxicol. 8, 153–159.

Widmer, R., 1984. Poison hemlock toxicosis in swine. Vet. Med. 79, 405–408.

Chapter 63

Poisonous Plants of Australia and New Zealand

Rhian Cope and Selina Ossedryver

INTRODUCTION

Due to space constraints, this chapter largely focuses on the indigenous flora of Australia and New Zealand that has been noted to produce substantial livestock losses and some of the major problematic introduced plants. It is not possible to cover all of the poisonous plants in Australia and New Zealand that are known to have caused livestock losses in a single chapter, and the reader is referred to more authoritative references for this. To allow for reasonable coverage of the most important species, the information is presented in tabular form.

The climate of Australia is unique compared with those of the other continents, and this has a substantial impact upon plant poisonings in grazing livestock. Australia is easily the driest of all continents: most of Australia is desert or semiarid, and 40% of the landmass is covered by sand dunes. Eighty percent of Australia's landmass has an average annual rainfall of less than 600 mm, with 50% of the landmass having less than 300 mm. Rainfall for much of the continent is highly variable, and droughts, which may last several years, are a regular feature over much of the agriculturally productive areas of Australia. Accordingly, many of the toxicologically problematic indigenous plants are well adapted to this climate: they are extremely drought resistant (or their seeds are resilient), and they are able to grow very rapidly during the short periods of relatively suitable conditions. In these circumstances, poisonous indigenous flora often outcompete introduced fodder plants or they emerge earlier after the onset of ideal conditions or they persist longer than introduced fodder plants when less than ideal conditions set it. Poisonings often occur under such conditions. Another common circumstance of poisoning is when indigenous plants are the last remaining plants and they are cut and fed to livestock during drought as survival feed (drought lotting). A summary of the characteristics of important plant species used in drought lotting in Australia is provided as Table 63.1. Common and important plants that are hazardous to live stock are described in Table 63.2.

The long biogeographic isolation of the Zealandia continent and the islands of New Zealand has also resulted in a unique variety of native flora and associated unique toxicological concerns (Table 63.3).

REDUCING LIVESTOCK LOSSES ASSOCIATED WITH POISONOUS PLANTS IN AUSTRALIA AND NEW ZEALAND

The key factors in reducing losses due to plant toxicoses are an awareness of the types of potentially toxic plants relevant to the geographical area of production, an understanding of both the plant and the animal factors that influence the risk of poisoning, and an understanding of what indigenous plants can and cannot be used as feed for livestock under drought conditions.

A common, important plant-related factor in Australia is the ability of indigenous plants in the semiarid and arid areas of the country to outgrow and outcompete introduced fodder plants, particularly following the breaking of a drought or under poor environmental conditions. In such circumstances, the new plant growth may contain relatively high amounts of relevant toxins. This situation, combined with cold, stressed, hungry and/or inexperienced stock is a recipe for significant stock losses. This type of scenario has been classically associated with the rangeland northern cattle industry and the arid zone and semiarid zone sheep industries in Australia. The following are approaches known to reduce the risks associated with these circumstances:

- Mechanical methods of plant removal: Because of the sheer physical size of livestock properties in the semiarid and arid regions of Australia, such methods are often impractical. However, on a small scale, such

Veterinary Toxicology. DOI: http://dx.doi.org/10.1016/B978-0-12-811410-0.00063-5

TABLE 63.1 Common Fodder Trees Used for Scrub Feeding/Drought Lotting in Australia

Common Name	Scientific Name	Palatability (A-D With A+ Being the Most Palatable)	Nutritional Value (A-D with A+ Being the Highest Nutritional Value)	Comments
Athel pine	*Tamarix aphylla*	A	A	Well eaten, short supply
Bauhinia	*Lysiphyllum carroni*	B	A	Deciduous, of little value in winter and spring
Beefwood	*Grevillea striata*	B	C	Leaves eaten by sheep
Belah	*Casuarina cristata*	C	C	Eaten readily; twigs can be a problem
Bendee	*Acacia catenulata*	B	B	Generally grows in the poorest quality land areas in the Pilbara region, not particularly palatable, can be toxic at some stages
Boonaree, Dogwood, Rosewood	*Alectryon oleifolius*	A	A	Can cause cyanide poisoning particularly at flowering or young growth stages
Boree, weeping myall, true myall, silver-leaf boree, balaar, nilyah	*Acacia pendula*	A–B	B	Readily eaten by sheep, very fibrous. Weeping myall woodlands are threatened habitats in Queensland.
Bottle tree leaves	*Brachychiton austral*	A+	A+	Some individual trees may be toxic to hungry cattle, potential cause of nitrate poisoning; has laxative effect. Very palatable and one of the best scrub feeds
Bottle tree pith		B	C	
Brigalow (>15 cm high)	*Acacia harpophylla*	C	C	A last resort feed. Brigalow woodland is a threatened habitat in Queensland
Brigalow (<15 cm high)		B	A	
Budda sandalwood, false sandalwood	*Eremophila mitchellii*	D	C	Not readily eaten, claimed to reduce the risk of impaction if mixed with fibrous scrub
Bulloak	*Allocasuarina luehmannii*	D	D	Eaten fairly readily, very fibrous
Bumble tree, native orange, wild lemon, native pomegranate, native capers	*Capparis mitchellii, C. arborea* and other *Capparis* sp.	A	A	Excellent fodder but short supply. The fruits are considered as a delicacy. These trees are also important native butterfly habitat and the narrow leafed bumble (*Capparis loranthifolia*) is endangered and should not be used
Coolibah	*Eucalyptus coolabah*	B	C	Leaves of young trees eaten when half dry. Adult trees have been fed with urea/molasses. Coolibah-black box woodland is a threatened habitat in Queensland
Currant bush	*Scaevola spinescens*	C	B	Not readily eaten
Desert gum, cabbage gum	*Eucalyptus amplifolia*	B	B	Eaten fairly readily
Doolan	*Acacia salicina*	B	B	May be toxic to hungry stock
Gidyea, gidgee	*Acacia cambagei*	C	B	Best to feed after a fire; good results if animals can be induced to eat it

Green wattle	*Acacia decurrens*	–	–	Not eaten by cattle
Ironbark tree	*Eucalyptus* sp.	B	C	Eaten fairly readily when supplemented with urea/molasses. Should not be mistaken for the ironwood tree (*Erythrophleum chlorostachys*, Leguminous Ironwood; Red Ironwood; Black Bean; Cooktown Ironwood; Camel Poison; Ironwood, Cooktown; Ironwood; Ironwood, Leguminous; Ironwood), which is highly poisonous to livestock (diterpinoid alkaloids)
Leopard wood	*Flindersia maculosa*	A	A	Member of the citrus family. Often conserved/encouraged because of the usefulness of the wood for fence posts and pick handles
Lime bush, desert limes	*Citrus glauca*	C	B	Young plants are unpalatable. Readily hybridizes with many common citrus species. Fruit are a highly prized bushfood that have a strong lime-like flavor. Plant is under threat due to agricultural clearing
Mimosa bush	*Acacia farnesiana*	B	A	Grazed by sheep. South American plant that has become naturalized in Australia, widespread in Queensland. Often controlled as an invasive plant in many areas
Mulga	*Acacia aneura*	A	B	Well eaten and a plentiful supply in southwest Queensland. Dense stands make easy pushing and cutting. Causes black livers (nutritional melanosis)
Myrtle tree, myrtle wattle	*Acacia myrtifolia*	B	B	Readily eaten by sheep and cattle
Old man saltbush	*Atriplex nummularia*	A+	A+	One of the most common and important native forage shrubs in southern Australia
Plumwood, pinkwood, eastern leatherwood tree	*Eucryphia moorei*	A +	A+	Limited supplies available. Other *Eucryphia sp.* on mainland Australia are either rare or endangered. They should not be used.
Popla box, bimble box	*Eucalyptus populnea*	C	C	Only eaten if no other fodder is available
Vine tree, supplejack, whip vine	*Ventilago viminalis*	A+	A+	Limited supply
Wilga	*Geijera parviflora*	A	A	Good fodder, palatability variable from year to year
Weeping willow and other willows	*Salix* sp.	A	A	Regarded as a weed of national significance. They are among the worst weeds in Australia because of their invasiveness, potential for spread, and economic and environmental impacts. Should be destroyed on sight. Cannot transported, sold or given away without a permit. Should be cut down, used for stock feed and then the stumps and any fragments of stems or twigs should be killed
Whitewood	*Atalaya hemiglauca*	A	A	Fruits and seeds are poisonous to horses, sheep and cattle and are avoided by stock (toxic principle is unknown). Extremely drought tolerant. The gum from the tree was used by indigenous Australians as a chewing gum
Yapunyah	*Eucalyptus ochrophloia*	C	C	Limited consumption of leaves occurs. Regionally important tree for honey production although pollen substitutes must be fed to the bees

TABLE 63.2 Summary of Major Australian Plants That are Hazardous to Livestock

Common Name of Disease	Species and Identification	Diseases	Toxins	Distribution	Risk Factors	Toxidrome	Association with Other Diseases
Paterson's curse poisoning	*Echium plantagineum* (Paterson's curse; salvation Jane) Winter growing annual; grows initially as a rosette; flowering stems are produced in early spring; seeds in late spring; dies after flowering; rosettes have green to light green hairy egg-shaped leaves up to 30 cm long; flowers are generally purple; 2–3 cm long and shaped like curved trumpets; a stout taproot with numerous lateral roots is present	Hepatogenous pyrrolizidine alkaloid (PA) toxicosis	Pyrrolizidine alkaloids; plant often has a high copper:molybdenum ratio; all parts and stages of the plant are toxic	Widespread; highly invasive; introduced; high economic losses in sheep and cattle; significant infestations in temperate, winter rainfall areas of VIC and NSW, as well as the southwestern parts of WA, southern QLD, and the eastern half of TAS	Overgrazing, drought and fire increase the pasture dominance of the plant; PA content is highest when flowering; not particularly palatable; pasture dominance of the plant in combination with reduced availability of alternative forages increases the risk; pigs, poultry, and horses (monogastric animals) are regarded as highly susceptible, cattle moderately susceptible, and sheep and goats the least susceptible; merino sheep and wethers relatively resistant compared with British breeds and Merino/British breed crosses; large variability in individual animal susceptibility	Acute, subacute or chronic megalocytic hepatopathy. Horses: characterized clinically food refusal; depression; irritability; ill-thrift; evidence of hepatic insufficiency (icterus, secondary photosensitization, repeated yawning, head pressing, aimless wandering, compulsive walking, dyspnea secondary to recurrent laryngeal nerve dysfunction, and other signs of hepatic encephalopathy). Pigs: rarely seen except in grazed animals. Cattle: general ill-thrift; chronic weight loss and/or failure to thrive; unpredictable bouts of aggression; evidence of persistent diarrhea with tenesmus and secondary photosensitization of sheep: deaths directly related to Paterson's curse are uncommon; PAs cause decreased productive life span; most common clinical issue found in sheep is copper toxicity rather than PA toxicity per se; PAs do not enhance copper accumulation per se, but they modulate the disease; *E. plantagineum* often contains a high copper:molybdenum ratio, which can induce copper toxicity in sheep; no effective treatment	Relative copper excess/ relative molybdenum deficiency toxidrome ("copper toxicity") in sheep due to high copper: molybdenum ratio in the plant; increased risk of ammonia poisoning (particularly when using nonprotein nitrogen dietary sources in ruminants); increased risk of pregnancy toxemia in sheep

Viper's bugloss poisoning	*E. vulgaris* Similar to *E. plantagineum*; perennial or biennial rather than annual; unlike *E. plantagineum*; flowers are not arranged in a violin neck	Hepatogenous PA toxicosis	Pyrrolizidine alkaloids; all parts and stages of the plant are toxic	Less common than *E. plantagineum*; mostly confined to the temperate tablelands of southeastern Australia	As per *E. plantagineum*	As per *E. plantagineum*	May influence relative copper excess/relative molybdenum deficiency toxidrome ("copper toxicity") in sheep; increased risk of ammonia poisoning (particularly when using nonprotein nitrogen dietary sources in ruminants); increased risk of pregnancy toxemia in sheep
Blue heliotrope poisoning	*Heliotropium amplexicaule* Summer growing perennial; many hairy, branched stems radiating from a woody rootstock with a sender taproot; highly aromatic; extends over 1–2 m in diameter; leaves are alternate, dull green, and tapered at both ends; flowers are bluish-purple with yellow centers and are arranged in dense clusters along one side of a coiled stalk that resembles a violin neck; drought resistant	Hepatogenous PA toxicosis	Pyrrolizidine alkaloids; all parts and stages of the plant are toxic	Widespread in southeastern QLD and northern NSW; scattered colonies can be found in central and southern NSW, near Adelaide, in the Flinders ranges, and around Victor Harbor in SA	As per *E. plantagineum*	As per *E. plantagineum*. Significant causes of loss of young cattle; not a source of high copper:molybdenum ratio fodder, but like most PA-containing plants, can influence copper toxicity in sheep	May influence relative copper excess/relative molybdenum deficiency toxidrome ("copper toxicity") in sheep; increased risk of ammonia poisoning (particularly when using nonprotein nitrogen dietary sources in ruminants); increased risk of pregnancy toxemia in sheep
European heliotrope poisoning; European turnsole poisoning	*H. europaeum* Summer-growing annual; prostrate to ascending up to 60 cm high; well-developed root system; emits a foul odor when crushed; leaves 1.5–9 cm long, 0.8–3 cm wide; ovate; paler below; leaf stalk to 4 cm long; flowers are arranged in	Hepatogenous PA toxicosis	Pyrrolizidine alkaloids; all parts and stages of the plant are toxic; PA content is generally lower than *H. amplexicaule*	Major noxious weed of temperate Australia; common in overgrazed or fallow land; recorded in all states except NT and TAS; greatest concentration is	As per *E. plantagineum*	As per *E. plantagineum*. Significant cause of loss of young cattle; not a source of high copper:molybdenum ratio fodder, but like most PA-containing plants, can influence copper toxicity in sheep	May influence relative copper excess/relative molybdenum deficiency toxidrome ("copper toxicity") in sheep; increased risk of ammonia poisoning (particularly when using nonprotein nitrogen dietary sources in ruminants); increased

(*Continued*)

TABLE 63.2 (Continued)

Common Name of Disease	Species and Identification	Diseases	Toxins	Distribution	Risk Factors	Toxidrome	Association with Other Diseases
	two rows on either side of a caterpillar-like cyme; flowers are white with yellow throats; drought resistant			west of the Great Dividing Range in NSW and Victoria			risk of pregnancy toxemia in sheep
Heliotrope poisoning	*Heliotropium ovalifolium* Native to Australia; ascending to spreading perennial or annual (in adverse conditions) herb; 0.15–0.8 m high; flowers are white	Hepatogenous PA toxicosis	Pyrrolizidine alkaloids; all parts and stages of the plant are toxic	Kimberley region of WA	As per *E. plantagineum*	As per *E. plantagineum*. Primarily associated with disease in horses, but other species are likely to be susceptible	As per *E. plantagineum*
Tansy ragwort poisoning Fireweed poisoning Groundsel poisoning Cotton fireweed poisoning African daisy poisoning	*Senecio jacobaea, S. linearifolius, S. lautus, S. madagascariensis, S. quadrientatus, S. pterophorus* Daisy-like; flower heads are normally rayed; completely yellow; the heads are borne in branched clusters	Hepatogenous PA toxicosis	Pyrrolizidine alkaloids; all parts and stages of the plant are toxic	Humid temperate regions with annual rainfall >750 mm; generally occur on heavy soils of moderate fertility; commonly found in areas cleared for pasture but never on properly developed or on poorly managed and/or; degraded pastures	As per *E. plantagineum*. Somewhat less important in Australia compared with Paterson's curse and heliotropes	As per *E. plantagineum*	May influence relative copper excess/relative molybdenum deficiency toxidrome ("copper toxicity") in sheep; increased risk of ammonia poisoning (particularly when using nonprotein nitrogen dietary sources in ruminants); increased risk of pregnancy toxemia in sheep
Fiddleneck poisoning	*Amsinckia calycina, A. lycopsoides, A. intermedia, A. menziesii* Short-lived autumn/winter perennials; 20–70 cm tall; grow as a rosette from which a flowering stem is produced; flowers are tube-shaped, yellow	Hepatogenous PA toxicosis	Pyrrolizidine alkaloids; all parts and stages of the plant are toxic	All of NSW and VIC; southern QLD; southeastern SA	As per *E. plantagineum*. Plants are unpalatable and poisoning occurs mostly when there are few or no other food sources	As per *E. plantagineum*	As per *E. plantagineum*

	or orange, and are arranged along a curved flower spike (a fiddleneck)						
Kimberley horse poison Kimberly horse disease Crotalism Walkabout disease	*Crotalaria crispate*, *C. ramosissima*, *C. dissitiflora*, *C. linifolia*, *C. mitchellii*, *C. spectabilis*, *C. verrucosa*, *C. pallida*, *C. juncea*, *C. montana*, *C. novae-hollandiae*, *C. brevis*, *C. eremaea*, *C. retusa* Herbaceous plants and woody shrubs; commonly known as rattlepods due to the fact that the seeds become loose in the pod as they mature and rattle when the pod is shaken; flowers are typically yellow and have the classical legume "pea-like" flower form	Hepatogenous PA toxicosis; monocrotaline-induced proliferative pulmonary vasculitis; pulmonary hypertension and pneumotoxicity	Pyrrolizidine alkaloids; monocrotaline	Most areas of Australia with the exception of TAS	Kimberley horse disease/walkabout disease is a major cause of mortality in horses in northern Australia; in general, all Australian *Crotalaria* species regarded as toxic to horses until proven otherwise; the plants are not palatable; poisoning usually occurs when there is a shortage of feed, which causes horses to graze indiscriminately; poisoning may occur when toxic plants are accidentally incorporated with conserved fodder such as hay; horses are 30–40 times more susceptible to the disease than are sheep and goats	Clinical signs in horses relate to PA hepatopathy/hepatic encephalopathy and include dull and depressed; often stand with their heads held down; anorexia; weight loss; icterus; muscle tremors (especially of the head and neck); frequent yawning; head pressing; copper-colored or red urine; episodes of frenzy and violent, uncontrollable galloping; difficulty swallowing (stop eating halfway through a mouthful of hay or grass); may appear to be blind; may aimlessly wander (walking in circles or bumping into objects); drag their hind legs (hooves have worn tips). Disease is untreatable; occasionally, horses develop pulmonary toxicity following ingestion of some *Crotalaria* sp.; the introduced plant *C. spectabilis* is most noted for this effect; pigs tend to develop nephrosis rather than a hepatopathy; disease in cattle often resembles that of *E. plantagineum*, although pulmonary disease can occur if monocrotaline is present	Death from misadventure; increased risk of ammonia poisoning (particularly when using nonprotein nitrogen dietary sources in ruminants); increased risk of pregnancy toxemia in sheep

(*Continued*)

TABLE 63.2 (Continued)

Common Name of Disease	Species and Identification	Diseases	Toxins	Distribution	Risk Factors	Toxidrome	Association with Other Diseases
Yellow wood poisoning McKenzie River disease	*Terminalia oblongata* Bushy tree 12 m high; branching close to the ground; bark is dark gray and furrowed; leaves alternate, pale green to yellow green, with rounded tips; deciduous; flowers are tiny; fruits have a wing on both sides	Hepatogenous photosensitization; nephrosis	Hydrolyzable tannins	McKenzie River Basin of QLD	Used as drought fodder will keep the sheep alive, but produces chronic kidney disease; cattle should be kept away from fallen leaves in winter if possible	Nervous symptoms in sheep; acute disease in cattle (McKenzie River disease): abdominal pain; photosensitization; dehydration; dark brown urine, depression, limb stiffness, tremor; icterus, collapse; nephrosis; chronic disease in cattle is characterized by liver disease, nephrosis, and long-term ill-thrift	
Poison peach	*Trema* sp.	Hepatotoxic	Unknown	Coastal and inland north and eastern Australia	Potentially poisonous at all times	Liver damage (periacinar hepatocyte coagulation necrosis); most animals die; death is usually rapid	Resembles yellow daisy poisoning
Yellow daisy poisoning	*Wedelia asperrima* Erect herb; yellow daisy-like flowers		Kaurene (diterpenoid glycoside)	Northern Australian grasslands		Liver damage (periacinar hepatocyte coagulation necrosis)	Resembles poison peach
Swainsona poisoning Darling or Swainson Pea poisoning	*Swainsona galegifolia, S. canescens, S. luteola, S. greyana, S. procumbens* Stout-stemmed; erect plant; 30 + cm tall with numerous hairy leaflets; large purple, blue, pink, or red pea-shaped flowers; long woolly seed pods; plants tend to grow from August to October especially after winter rains	Swainsonism	Swainsonine (indolizidine alkaloid)	Subtropical and temperate regions of all states	Individual animals may develop a craving for the plants; horses especially selectively graze Swainson pea; there are approximately 85 native *Swainsona* sp. in Australia; all should be regarded as poisonous until proven otherwise	Swainsonine, which acts in two ways: blocks the enzyme mannosidase, which produces an acquired mannose lysosomal storage disease and interferes in the normal production of enzymes, hormones and immunoglobulins. Cattle: can graze the plant for several weeks before development of clinical signs; signs after ~6 weeks of grazing include paddling gait, hyperexcitability, loss of condition, charge when approached; clinical signs progress to depression, incoordination, some deaths; animals that survive are poor in condition; long-term	Toxidrome in horses resembles Birdsville disease (*Indigofera linnaei* poisoning); animals may have concurrent access to both plants; Birdsville disease occurs only in horses, whereas swainsona poisoning occurs in both horses and cattle; swainsona poisoning is mostly a disease of late winter to early summer, whereas Birdsville disease occurs primarily in summer, particularly after the first summer rains; mannose lysosomal storage disease is histologically identifiable in swainsona

						effects include infertility and abortion. Toxidrome is reversible if exposure is up to 4 weeks. Horses develop clinical signs after ~2 weeks of grazing; initial signs include paddling gait, hypersensitivity to touch, tremor, forced respiration; these progress to depression, incoordination, head pressing, hind leg dragging, front leg high-stepping, recumbency, death; long-term effects include emaciation, difficulty eating, lowered head, ventral swelling, apparent blindness, walking in circles	poisoning, whereas there are no specific anatomic pathology changes associated with Birdsville disease
Weir vine poisoning	*Ipomea calobra* Slender vine with heart-shaped leaves and trumpet-shaped pink flowers	Swainsonism	Swainsonine (indolizidine alkaloid)	Maranoa district of QLD	As per swainsona poisoning	As per swainsona poisoning	As per swainsona poisoning
Birdsville disease Birdsville indigo poisoning	*Indigofera linnaei* Low; spreading plant; thick taproot; numerous thin woody stems forming a mat up to 1.5 m across; leaves fern-like; flowers are very small and occur in dense clusters in the forks of the leaves; flowers are red turning blue as the leaves dry out; seed pods are gray, very narrow, sharply pointed at the tip, and contain two cube-shaped seeds	3-Nitropropionic acid toxicity in horses; indospicine poisoning in dogs fed raw or cooked meat from poisoned horses or from camels grazing *I. linnaei*	Indospicine (hepatotoxin); 3-nitropropionic acid (neurotoxin); horses are resistant to the hepatotoxic effects of indospicine; toxins are present in the leaves and seeds of the plant at all times (green or dry)	Widespread in subtropical and arid regions of WA; NT and QLD	Drought resistant and responds rapidly to rain; disease outbreaks commonly occur in spring or summer after rains because of the rapid response of the plant to moisture; up to 100% mortality in horses; under normal conditions, the plant does not cause clinical disease in cattle; raw and cooked meat from poisoned horses is toxic to dogs because of the indospicine—	In horses, clinical signs can develop after 10 days of feeding; clinical signs include general weakness, nervousness, depression, incoordination, shivering, twitching, and swaying; neuromotor signs are more evident when the animal is, or has been, under physical stress; bad breath; toe dragging (tracks are characteristic) and excessive wear on the front of the hoof; continuous ingestion will result in death; neurological signs are irreversible; secondary indospicine poisoning in dogs is characterized by acute	Can be confused with swainsona poisoning, and it is possible for the two diseases to occur concurrently; see swainsona poisoning

(*Continued*)

TABLE 63.2 (Continued)

Common Name of Disease	Species and Identification	Diseases	Toxins	Distribution	Risk Factors	Toxidrome	Association with Other Diseases
					secondary poisoning may occur	fulminant and sometimes fatal hepatic failure	
Bitter bark poisoning Quinine tree poisoning Quinine bush poisoning	*Alstonia constricta* Tree to 12 m height; suckers from the roots producing thickets; leaves are narrow, lanceolate, 5–20 cm in length; flowers white to cream, 2–4 cm diameter; bark has a corky textured; white sap	Indole alkaloid poisoning in ruminants and dogs fed meat from poisoned animals	Indole alkaloids (alstonine; altonidine; reserpine); does not contain quinine (common name derived from the bitter taste of the bark); alstonine and reserpine are used as antipsychotic drugs	Eastern Australia from the Tropic of Capricorn southward to northern NSW	Leaves and fruit are poisonous; poisoning usually occurs when there is a shortage of feed; meat from poisoned animals is toxic to dogs	Tetanus-like toxidrome: excitability, nervousness, stiff legs, saw horse gait, staggers, redness of the ocular mucous membranes	
Wax flower poisoning Waxvine poisoning	*Hoya australis* Evergreen climbing vine; shiny round succulent leaves; milky sap; clusters of white flowers 1.5–2.5 cm in diameter, with five thick, waxy, triangular petals; strong sweet scent and produce copious nectar	Tetanus-like toxidrome	Unknown neurotoxin	Popular garden plant; natural distribution is from Grafton in northern NSW to Cape York; grows on the edges of rain forest and in rocky exposed habitat	Unpalatable; poisoning usually occurs when there is a shortage of feed	Tetanus-like toxidrome: incoordination, knuckling of fetlocks, tremoring, collapse of either fore- or hindquarters, recumbency, tetanic spasms; no effective treatment, although mildly effected animals may recover	
Poison morning glory Australian morning glory poisoning	*Ipomoea muelleri* Slender vine with heart-shaped leaves and trumpet-shaped pink flowers	Neurological toxidrome in ruminants and horses	Calystegines implicated	Northern Australia; found in open forest; margins of monsoon forest and vine thicket; garden plant	Often the only green feed at the start of the wet season and the end of the dry season	Animals appear inebriated and develop hindquarters ataxia that may be permanent in cattle; associated with transient staggering toxidrome in sheep; affected animals appear during the wet season and die by the following dry season	
Floodplain staggers Stewart Range syndrome	*Agrostis avenacea* Native to Australia and New Zealand; invasive weed in California, Texas, and Hawaii; tufted perennial grass to 65 cm	Corynetoxin poisoning in ruminants, pigs, horses	Corynetoxins (tunicaminyluracils) produced by *Rathayibacter toxicus* in nematode (*Anguina funesta*) induced galls	Southeastern SA, northern NSW	Toxin production is greatest when the grass is haying off; most outbreaks occur ~1 week after the start of haying	Resembles annual ryegrass toxicity: onset of toxidrome delayed up to 4–5 days; reluctant to move; uncoordinated gait; limb weakness; muscle	Resembles annual ryegrass toxicity; Identical to annual beard grass (*Polypogon monspeliensis*) toxicity

Pacific bent grass poisoning Blown grass poisoning	tall; inflorescence is a panicle of wispy strands terminated by 2–3 mm long fuzzy spikelets; grass is most commonly found in flat low-lying areas that are flooded up to 30 cm during winter and in channels and depression where water collects		in the seed heads and crowns of the plant		off; bacteria is identifiable as a yellow slime on the seed heads that dries to an orange-colored material; nematode galls can be identified in the seed heads; unlike annual ryegrass toxicity, the plant can become infected two times per year; outbreaks occur with favorable weather conditions; hay from affected pastures is poisonous	fasciculations; stand with a backwards and forwards rocking motion; individual muscle movements rigid; irregular and abrupt; whole limb movements excessively pronounced; high stepping or "rocking horse" gaits; loss of hind limb control; sudden collapse while running; intermittent episodic convulsions; movement or exercise exacerbates the clinical signs; high mortality (up to 90%); triggers abortion; lambing and calving losses to 30%	
Caustic bush poisoning Caustic vine poisoning Milk vine poisoning	*Sarcostemma australis* Leafless succulent scrambler or bush; with smooth, jointed, succulent stems; flowers are pale green to cream-white, star shaped and waxy; in clusters at the stem joints; sap is corrosive to skin and eyes	Neurological toxidrome in sheep, cattle; toxic to horses	Unidentified neurotoxin; may resemble cynanchoside	Northern Australia extending southwards to northern NSW	Moderately palatable; rarely grazed except in very dry seasons when fodder is scarce; fresh shoots may be more toxic than the old shoots	Toxidrome consists of restlessness, staggering and collapse, rapid breathing, paddling legs, jaws may be clamped shut, excessive salivation, seizures, convulsions, limb paddling	Plant can be confused with *Euphorbia sarcostemmoides*; *Euphorbia* sp. in Australia produce acute GI irritation (and cyanogenic glycoside toxicity in some species)
Grass tree poisoning Called "wamps" in NT (after the sound that cattle make when they collapse and hit the ground)	*Xanthorrhoea johnsonii*, *Xanthorrhoea fulva* grass trees	Neurological toxidrome in cattle	Unidentified	Coastal and subcoastal eastern Australia	Flower spikes are the most toxic parts, but leaves have caused problems	Toxidrome consists of transient spinal cord dysfunction with associated posterior ataxia and urinary incontinence; delayed onset after access may be up to 10 weeks; clinical signs: constant sideways lurching of hindquarters, fall easily, have difficulty rising, urinary incontinence, weight loss; toxidrome is reversible within 2–3 weeks after cessation of exposure in most cases	

(Continued)

TABLE 63.2 (Continued)

Common Name of Disease	Species and Identification	Diseases	Toxins	Distribution	Risk Factors	Toxidrome	Association with Other Diseases
Byfield fern poisoning Zamia fern poisoning Zamia staggers	*Bowenia serrulata*, *Bowenia spectabilis* Fern-like cycad; distinctive among cycads because they have bipinnate leaves	Neurological toxidrome in cattle is most common disease observed	Unidentified neurotoxin (neurotoxin possibly related to β-methylamino-L-alanine and/or β-oxalylamino-L-alanine); cycasin (a protoxin that is transformed by plants and intestinal flora to methylazoxymethanol, an inhibitor of protein synthesis)	QLD rain forest; located on protected slopes; usually near a stream	Leaves are toxic and remain neurotoxic even when dried; *B. spectabilis* is a cultivated ornamental plant; cycasin is destroyed by drying of the plant, but the dried plant remains neurotoxic	Clinical signs consist of hindquarters ataxia consisting of an unusual swaying motion of the hind limbs, flexion of the hock and fetlock, wobbling and malpositioning of the hind legs	Resembles poisoning by other members of the cycadales order (cycads); i.e., zamia poisoning, lepidozamia poisoning, cycad poisoning; possibly similar to human amyotrophic lateral sclerosis/ parkinsonism–dementia complex (Guam disease, lytico-bodig disease)
Zamia staggers Burrawang staggers	*Macrozamia* sp. Palm-like cycad with slender leaves; seeds red to yellow in male or female cones *Lepidozamia* sp. Unbranched tall tree-like cycads with persistent leaf bases	Neurological disease in cattle and liver disease in sheep are the most common presentations; horses and pigs are also susceptible	As per *Bowenia* sp.	*Macrozamia* sp.: QLD and NSW; mainly in coastal areas; Bega to Macleay River; and westward toward Goulburn *Lepidozamia* sp.: rain forests of QLD and NSW	As per *Bowenia* sp.; may be found as a contaminant in chaff; cultivated as ornamental plants; all species are regarded as toxic unless proven otherwise	A slowly developing, irreversible nervous paralysis of the hind legs similar to *Bowenia* sp. or clinical signs relate to chronic liver damage: loss of appetite, ill-thrift, diarrhea, chronic weight loss, eventual death due to hepatic insufficiency. Poisoning may eventually be irreversible	As per *Bowenia* sp.: seed cones from *Macrozamia* sp. were used as a food source by indigenous Australians (notably the Cadigal) but require extensive processing to render them safe
Corkwood poisoning	*Duboisia myoporoides*, *D. leichhardtii* Small tree members of the nightshade family; cork-like bark; simple leaves; white tubular flowers in bunches at the branch ends; fruits are black and berry-like	Deliriant anticholinergic tropane alkaloid poisoning	Tropane alkaloids including hyoscyamine and scopolamine	Coast and tablelands of NSW; central and coastal QLD; found in high rainfall areas near rain forests; up to 1000 m altitude; and also in rain forest regrowth areas	Toxic to cattle, sheep, horses, camels, pigs, dogs, and cats; generally unpalatable; rarely grazed except in very dry seasons when fodder is scarce; may be grazed by animals inexperienced with the plant; sheep somewhat resistant compared with other species; used in herbal remedies	Classical deliriant anticholinergic toxidrome: that is, hyperthermia, tachycardia, bizarre and possibly violent behavior, severe mydriasis, photophobia, muscle trembling, muscular weakness, staggers, colic and scours, death within 12 h but may recover with no long-term effects; can be treated using physostigmine; mnemonic for the toxidrome: "blind as a bat; mad as a hatter; red as a beet; hot as hell; dry as a bone; the bowel and bladder lose their tone; and the heart runs alone"	Resembles atropine and *Datura* sp. (e.g., jimson weed or Jamestown weed) poisoning; leaves are harvested commercially for production of scopolamine and hyoscyamine; workers handling the leaves have been affected with dry throat, headache, and loss of visual acuity; plant is a target for recreational drug users

Pituri poisoning Pitchuri thorn apple poisoning Pitcheri poisoning	*D. hopwoodii* Erect shrub; 1–3 m high; long, narrow leaves; flowers are white, bell-shaped with violet-striped throats; flowers June to November; berries are black, 3–6 mm in diameter	Nicotine poisoning	Nicotine; nornicotine	Arid interior regions of Australia	Toxic to cattle, sheep, horses, camels, pigs, dogs, and cats; generally unpalatable; rarely grazed except in very dry seasons when fodder is scarce; may be grazed by animals inexperienced with the plant; plants with high nornicotine: nicotine ratios are generally more poisonous	Classical nicotine poisoning (depolarizing neuromuscular block): tremoring, weakness, stumbling and/or incoordination, depression or hyperactivity, tachypnea, respiratory insufficiency, excessive salivation, dilated pupils, apparent blindness, vomiting, diarrhea, colic, seizures, collapse, bradycardia or tachycardia; ruminants may bloat; some animals may be found dead with no history of neurological signs (presumably from lethal cardiac arrhythmias)	Dried leaves from plants in the Mulligan River area (high nicotine and low nornicotine content) were mixed with *Acacia* sp. ash and used by indigenous Australians as a form of chewing tobacco; in areas where the plants have a high nornicotine:nicotine ratio, the plants were used as an animal poison for food gathering
Finger cherry poisoning	*Rhodomyrtus macrocarpa* Small tree; opposite broad leaves with oil glands; white flowers with five petals; red fruit	Blindness	Unidentified	Northern QLD rain forest	Also cultivated as a garden plant	Produces permanent blindness within ~24 h of consumption due to optic nerve degeneration	Native guava causes a similar disease
Native guava poisoning	*R. psidioide* Resembles *R. macrocarpa* except leaves are narrow, lance-shaped, and 25 cm long	Blindness	Unidentified	Northern QLD rain forest		Produces permanent blindness within ~24 h of consumption due to optic nerve degeneration	Finger cherry produces a similar disease
Blind grass poisoning	*Stypandra* sp. Tufted perennial herb, with rhizome and fibrous roots; up to 1 m diameter; erect aerial stems with opposite leaves; small blue to white flowers, in spring	Neuromotor disease plus blindness	Stypandrol	WA; eastern NSW, QLD, VIC, and TAS; forest and woodland	Plants vary in their toxic content; most toxic times seem to be when shoots are young and green and when plants are flowering	High-stepping gait; rapidly developing hind leg weakness; difficulty in raising head; progresses to total paralysis; depression; permanent blindness, death; some animals may recover if exposure stopped	*Dianella* sp. (blue flax lily) and *Hemerocallis* sp. (day lilies) cause similar problems

(*Continued*)

TABLE 63.2 (Continued)

Common Name of Disease	Species and Identification	Diseases	Toxins	Distribution	Risk Factors	Toxidrome	Association with Other Diseases
Austral bracken fern poisoning; bright blindness in sheep; chronic hematuria syndrome in ruminants	*Pteridium esculentum*	Thiamine deficiency polioencephalomalacia; bright blindness in sheep; chronic hematuria syndrome in ruminants; immunodeficiency; chronic anemia/neutropenia; mutagenic and carcinogenic	Thiaminase; ptaquiloside; norsequiterpene glucocides	All states; particularly in wet areas with well-drained soils	Rhizomes are very toxic; poisoning develops after protracted feeding; often symptoms do not appear until days or weeks later; cattle and horses most affected, sheep less so; 2–4 weeks of intake required for toxicity	Depressed bone marrow functions in cattle and sheep resulting in anemia, thrombocytopenia, neutropenia, and immunotoxicity; polioencephalomalacia; bladder cancer in sheep and cattle (chronic hematuria syndrome); progressive retinopathy in sheep (bright blindness)	Similar disease with mulga (rock) fern
Mulga fern poisoning Rock fern poisoning; blindness in sheep	*Cheilanthes* sp.	As per bracken fern	Thiaminase; norsequiterpine glucocides (particularly ptaquiloside)	Throughout Australia	Generally avoided but eaten in drought periods when there is little else available; low-level ingestion is safe, but too much is dangerous; fern-infested paddocks can be grazed safely if animals are moved after ~10 days and rested in fern-free areas for ~3 weeks	Resembles bracken fern toxicity	Bracken fern toxicity
Nardoo poisoning	*Marsilea drummondii* A water fern, or herb; short creeping rhizome; leaves have a slender stalk tipped with four wedge-shaped leaflets that float on the surface, or spread on dry land and look like a four-leaf clover	Thiamine deficiency polioencephalomalacia; chronic nonresponsive anemia due to bone marrow depletion; immunotoxic; mutagenic/carcinogenic; beriberi (human)	Thiaminase; norsequiterpine glucosides	Inland areas; in depressions or river flats subject to flooding; different *Marsilea* sp. found in all mainland states; all species should be considered potentially toxic; sporocarps are very drought resistant, surviving up to 100 years in dry conditions	Toxin levels highest in summer, lowest in winter; often grazed without ill effect, but if they are the only plants available, there will be overdosing and stock losses; mainly sheep and horses are affected; good fodder plant under normal conditions	Typical polioencephalomalacia toxidrome in ruminants; chronic anemia/neutropenia/thrombocytopenia; chronic hematuria/bladder neoplasia syndrome in cattle; was an important food source for indigenous Australians (Cooper Creek and the Yandruwandha peoples), who rendered the plant safe by cooking it into "cakes" called "padlu"; famous as a potential cause of death of the explorers Burke and Wills	Other causes of polioencephalomalacia (e.g., dietary sulfur); other sources of thiaminase (e.g., bracken ferns)

Stinging tree Gympie stinger	*Dendrocnide* sp. Five species in Australia; large trees, but early stages and low, new growth are common sources of exposure; leaves are large, heart-shaped, with two rounded lobes at the base, margins may be toothed, and young leaves are covered with large, stiff, stinging hairs	Extreme pain	Hemolytic saponins; morodoin; stinging hairs contain acetylcholine, histamine and 5-hydroxytryptomine	Cape York to Kiama and Nepean area in NSW; grows on the edges of rain forests and in clearings	Generally not palatable, except for goats; simple contact with skin is extremely painful; horses are particularly vulnerable to the skin effects; leaves still dangerous when dried (remain dangerous for at least 40 years)	Contact with leaves of the plant is extremely painful; irritant toxins are injected through the skin by hollow plant hairs; pain is often intolerable, long-lasting, and recurrent for many weeks; horses often display a frenzied agony after skin contact with the plant; pain is difficult to control or treat, particularly in horses	
Georgina gidgee poisoning	*Acacia georginae*	Fluoroacetate poisoning	Organic fluoroacetates	Northwest QLD and adjacent eastern NT	Toxic to most animals (with the exception of some native Australian marsupials); most deaths occur during the dry season; most dominant animals are most likely to be affected; meat from poisoned livestock is poisonous to dogs and cats	Death within minutes of first clinical signs; animals often found dead; tachypnea; trembling; sudden heart failure; cardiac arrhythmias; bloat; frequent urination	1080 poisoning; 1080 is the sodium salt of monofluoroacetate; the number "1080" was the original catalog number for the substance; identical toxidrome to poison pea (*Gastrolobium* sp.) toxicity; several other Australian native plant genera contain the toxin: *Gompholobium* sp., *Oxylobium* sp., *Nemcia* sp.
Poison pea toxicity; desert poison bush; heart-leaf poisoning; wallflower poisoning; and numerous other species and/or location-specific names	*Gastrolobium* sp. More than 100 Australian native species; leafy shrub to 2 m high; dull-green opposite leaves, notched at the tip; leaves are thick and stiff; several stems arising from lignotubers; flowers are pea-shaped, dark red to purple	Fluoroacetate poisoning	Organic fluoroacetates; one of the most toxic plants in Australia	Southwest region of WA	As per Georgina gidgee poisoning; mostly affects sheep; plants are most toxic when flowering; flowers and seeds are highly toxic; suckers are very poisonous; leaves are less palatable and less toxic; most species	As per Georgina gidgee poisoning	As per Georgina gidgee poisoning

(*Continued*)

TABLE 63.2 (Continued)

Common Name of Disease	Species and Identification	Diseases	Toxins	Distribution	Risk Factors	Toxidrome	Association with Other Diseases
					are potentially toxic, although toxicity is often intermittent and seasonal; goats have been used to control the plant, but with some animal losses		
Billy button poisoning Plains plover daisy poisoning	*Leiocarpa* (*Ixiolaena*) *brevicompta* Low growing, branched, annual or short-lived perennial; woody base; woody stems with white cottony hairs; green narrow leaves with no stalk; circular single yellow flower head with basal bristles; multiple angular hairless seeds	Striated muscle myopathy	Crepenynic acid and other toxic unsaturated fatty acids	Common in inland Australia, from central QLD to central NSW to SA	Mostly affects sheep; lambs are usually the first affected; only mature dried seed heads are poisonous; toxins are concentrated in the seeds	Toxidrome occurs within 2 weeks after start of grazing; sudden collapse and death during herding, exercise intolerance, muscle weakness; short strides; staggering; hind limb collapse; cardiac arrhythmias; hyperthermia, tachypnea; movement and mustering exacerbate the toxidrome; treatment with selenium may be helpful in some cases	Can be confused with white muscle disease (nutritional muscular dystrophy, vitamin E/ selenium deficiency)
Cyanogenic glycoside poisoning	*Brachyachne* sp. (native couches), *Eremophila maculate* (spotted emu bush), *Eucalyptus cladocalyx* (sugar gum), *Euphorbia* sp. (some species), *Heterodendron oleifolium* (rosewood), *Lotus* sp. (birdsfoot trefoils)	Acute cyanide poisoning	Cyanogenic glycosides	Most areas of Australia contain a cyanogenic glycoside-containing plant species	Ruminants generally more susceptible; consumption of water following ingestion of plants increases the hydrolysis of cyanogenic glycosides to cyanide; the following generally increase the cyanide content of the plants: damage to plant, young rapid growth, seeds, regrowth after cutting, cool moist growing conditions, nitrate fertilization	Sudden death with few clinical signs is the most common toxidrome; animals may have "cherry red" venous blood due to high venous pO_2; "cherry red" venous blood is often a necropsy finding, hence "cherry-red equals dead"	

Nitrate poisoning	*Dactyloctenium radulans* (button grass)	Acute nitrate poisoning	Nitrate	Widespread native pasture grass in all states	Dangerous only when heavily fertilized	Classical nitrate poisoning	
Pimelea poisoning	*Pimelea trichostachya*, *P. simplex*, *P. elongate* Annual herbs; opposite leaves on multiple branches; branches end in a flower spike with many flask-shaped yellow-green flowers	Chronic right-sided heart failure, anemia and persistent diarrhea in cattle only	Simplexin (diterpenoid)	Inland northeastern regions; often in disturbed areas	Unpalatable; poisoning usually after the plants die and contaminate other pasture plants or hay; poisoning more likely after winter rains	In cattle only, produces chronic right-sided heart failure, anemia, and chronic diarrhea; produces only diarrhea in other species	
Cardiac glycoside poisoning	*Adonis microcarpa*, *Asclepias curassavica*, *Thevetia peruviana*, *Cryptostegia gandiflora*, *Glyceria maxima*, *Gomphocarpus* sp., *Homeria flaccid*, *H. miniata*, *Bryophyllum* sp.	Cardiac glycoside poisoning	Cardiac glycosides	Most regions of Australia have at least one cardiac glycoside-producing plant; many are introduced plants that have been important causes of stock losses	Generally not palatable; often only grazed during dry seasons when fodder is scarce; may be grazed by animals inexperienced with the plants; potential contaminants of hay	Typical cardiac glycoside poisoning; may show signs of GI distress (e.g., scouring) due to other irritants present in the plant	Camel poisoning
Camel poison	*Erythrophleum chlorostachys* (Cooktown ironwood) Large tree; smooth white or yellow-brown bark; discolorous leaves; white flowers; barrel-like fruit	Cardiac glycoside-like poisoning	Diterpenoid alkaloids and cinnamic acid derivatives	Northern Australia; open woodland	All parts of the plant are toxic; aggressively suckers and suckers are toxic and accessible to grazing animals; affects ruminants and horses	Resembles cardiac glycoside poisoning	
Cattle bush poisoning Whitewood poisoning	*Atalaya hemiglauca* Small- to medium-sized tree; gray bark; leaves alternate, varying shape, dull gray, or bluish green; flowers are cream green, in large panicles; very hardy and drought resistant	Cardiac failure syndrome particularly in horses and to lesser degree in ruminants	Unknown	Inland WA, QLD, NT, western NSW	Young shoots and fruit are toxic; poisoning occurs when plant forms a large part of the diet; high palatability; used as a drought fodder for cattle but should not be fed to horses	Either no effects or death; in horses: vague signs of distress, staggers, severe swelling of the head, muscle weakness, myoglobinuria, followed by fairly rapid death; staggers in cattle	
Poison sedge	*Schoenus asperocarpus* Tufted perennial; grass-like or herb (sedge); 0.15–1 m high	Pneumotoxin	An isoprenyl guanidine: galegine	Southwestern WA		Toxin affects pulmonary vascular permeability; acute massive pulmonary edema and thoracic effusion	

(Continued)

TABLE 63.2 (Continued)

Common Name of Disease	Species and Identification	Diseases	Toxins	Distribution	Risk Factors	Toxidrome	Association with Other Diseases
Stinkwood poisoning; panting disease	*Zieria arborescens* Tall shrub or small tree; to 4 m high, 3 m across; branches covered with star-shaped hairs; highly aromatic; fast growing; leaves have unpleasant odor when crushed	Pneumotoxin	Unknown	TAS, VIC, southeast NSW, wet forest areas		Acute massive pulmonary edema and emphysema	
Soluble oxalate poisoning	*Neobassia proceriflora* (soda bush), *Portulaca oleracea* (inland pig weed, munyeroo) *Salsola kali* (soft roly-poly), *Setaria sphacelata*, *Cenchrus ciliaris* (buffel grass) *Oxalis* sp., *Rumex* sp., *Acetosella vulgaris*, *Trianthema* sp.	Calcium oxalate tubular nephrosis; hypocalcemia; *C. ciliaris* is noted for producing secondary nutritional hyperparathyroidism in horses ("big head")	Soluble and absorbable oxalates	Most areas of Australia have at least one soluble oxalate-containing plant	Typically, the plants are more palatable when young	Typical soluble oxalate acute hypocalcemia + crystalline tubular nephrosis toxidrome; chronic renal nephrosis toxidrome	Milk fever (post-parturient hypocalcemia)
Alkali disease; blind staggers	*Morinda reticulate* (mapoon, adaa), *Neptunia amplexicaulis* (selenium weed)	Selenium toxicity: alkali disease and blind staggers	Selenoamino acids in *M. reticulate*; ethanol-soluble selenium compounds in *N. amplexicaulis*	*M. reticulate*, Cape York; *N. amplexicaulis*, central QLD	Cases often occur after burning back of scrub and in the spring	Classical alkali disease and blind staggers; alkali disease is more common	
Poison sage; lamb poison	*Isotropis* sp. Shrubs or herbs; pea-type flowers; flowers are purple, yellow, or orange	Irreversible nephrosis	Iforrestine	Not found in VIC or QLD	Most toxic when flowering	Anorexia; anuria; renal failure; gastroenteritis; sudden death can occur	
Gastroenteritis (partial list)	*Castanospermum austral* (black bean tree), *Euphorbia* sp., *Stemodia kingii*	Acute and severe gastroenteritis	Cucurbitacins in *Stemodia kingii*	Most areas of Australia contain plants capable of triggering acute gastroenteritis		Acute, often severe, diarrhea	

NSW, New South Wales; *NT*, Northern Territory; *QLD*, Queensland; *SA*, South Australia; *TAS*, Tasmania; *VIC*, Victoria; *WA*, Western Australia.

TABLE 63.3 Summary of Major New Zealand Plants That Are Hazardous to Livestock

Common Name of Disease	Species and Identification	Diseases	Toxins	Distribution	Risk Factors	Toxidrome	Association with Other Diseases
Strathmore or Pimelea or New Zealand Daphne poisoning	*Pimelea prostrate* Small, prostrate, branched woody shrub; to 50 cm in diameter; branches are scarred, dark brown to black; leaves pointed oval, greenish-gray, ~5 mm long; waxy white flowers, 3–4 mm long, red or white ovoid berries	Irritant (mucous membranes and skin); hypersensitivity; strong effect on cardiovascular function	Prostratin (dipterpene acetate) in the leaves and bark	North and south islands; grasslands; open shrubland; along river terraces; up to an altitude of 1500 m	Poisonings more common in winter when feed is restricted. Formerly a toxicity of primarily horses, it is now reported more often in cattle; sheep are resistant to poisoning	Horses: profuse watery diarrhea, blistering and irritation of oral mucous membranes and eyes, depression, loss of appetite, muscular pain, strong disinclination to move; necropsy features include gastric ulceration and gastroenteritis, fatty degeneration of liver; toxidrome in cattle resembles that of horses	Differentials include *Pieris japonica* poisoning, causes of jaundice (e.g., facial eczema), allergic hypersensitivity reactions, bacterial or viral enteritis, systemic bacteremias, and viremias including foot and mouth disease
Tutu toxicity	*Coriaria arborea* Leaves opposed, vary from narrow or filiform to ovate to lanceolate; flowers axillary or terminal racemes; fruit usually black or purple	Tetanus-like with CNS excitation (blocking of spinal glycine and CNS $GABA_A$ receptors)	Tutin (lactone from the picrotoxin group); localizes in the CNS, causing medullary excitatory poisoning	Throughout New Zealand; often found in stony areas	Toxicity usually in hungry or starved cattle and occasionally sheep; all parts are poisonous except the petals surrounding the seeds and the roots; toxin is concentrated in leaves (particularly young seeds); horses are not attracted to tutu; circus elephants have been poisoned	Picrotoxin-like: salivation, nausea, excitement, convulsions, coma, and death; sudden onset 24–48 h after ingestion; cattle may exhibit blind charging, muscle twitching, extreme excitement, epileptiform convulsions, bloating, and regurgitation; produces amnesia in humans; stock losses of 5%–10% of beef herds in the South Island high country; honey produced from tutu is toxic	
Ngaio toxicity	*Myoporum laetum*	Hepatogenous damage and photosensitization	Ngaione and several other furanosesquiterpenoid essential oils. Ngaione is a protoxin that requires hepatic metabolic activation	Common in coastal areas and lowland forests as far south as Otago; common in gardens	Toxicity of individual plants varies; leaves normally most toxic part; serious losses in cattle, sheep, pigs, and horses; most poisonings occur after storms blow down tree branches or when clippings are thrown out	Hepatogenous secondary photosensitization; recovery among survivors is very slow; severe constipation, abdominal pain, dullness, loss of appetite, no rumination; occasionally icterus	Exposure to sporidesmin (facial eczema), ragwort, microcystis or nodularin (algal blooms), and other hepatotoxic compounds may exacerbate Ngaio toxicity

(*Continued*)

TABLE 63.3 (Continued)

Common Name of Disease	Species and Identification	Diseases	Toxins	Distribution	Risk Factors	Toxidrome	Association with Other Diseases
					where stock have access to them		
Karaka poisoning	*Corynocarpus laevigatus* Tree to 15 m tall; leaves oblong, 10–15 cm long, dark green, thick, and glossy; flowers are small, yellow green; orange fruit, 25–40 mm long with three layers (outer skin, fleshy layer, and hard inner layer enclosing the seed)	Neurological problems; paralysis	Karakin (glucose ester of 3-nitropropionic acid)	Lowlands, especially the coasts; abundant in the North Island; found in Nelson, Marlborough, and Banks Peninsula in the South Island	Risk of ingestion is higher in autumn; fruit and seeds are main toxic parts; fruits remain toxic for months; fruit used as food by the Maori but require extensive processing to render them safe; nectar is toxic to bees	In cattle, paralysis of the hind limbs and an end to lactations may occur. In dogs, convulsions and spasms may precede paralysis of the hind limbs and muscle incoordination. Death may occur. A goat that ate karaka berries showed pain, depression, and diarrhea	
Kowhai toxicity	*Sophora* sp. 27 (very similar) species; trees or shrubs to 20 m tall; leaves are ≥15 cm in length, with each bearing 20–40 pairs of leaflets; flowers ostentatious yellow in drooping racemes or panicles in spring; pods are long and winged; seeds yellow	Stimulation of respiration; excitation of muscle; paralysis of peripheral sympathetic ganglia	Cytisine (acts like nicotine); also anagyrine, matrine, *N*-methyl-cytisinesophoramine, and sophochrysine	Throughout New Zealand in open forests, along forest margins, riverbanks, and in open damp or rocky places; commonly grown as an ornamental	All parts are poisonous; most poisonings are caused by seeds; children, livestock, and bees have been poisoned by seeds, plant material, or nectar, respectively; all species are toxic until proven otherwise	Resembles nicotine poisoning; recumbency, ataxia, tachycardia, increased respirations, abdominal pain, and hypomotility have been reported; death is due to nicotinic stimulation of the nervous system	
Tree nettle toxicity Ongaonga poisoning	*Urtica ferox* Bush to 2 m tall; plants are much branched; stinging hairs up to 6 mm long covering the	Nervous and gastrointestinal signs as well as local irritation	Histamine, serotonin; acetylcholine, and other unidentified pain-producing agents; toxins are	Throughout New Zealand and abundant; particularly on waste and neglected land;	Contact with plant causes toxicity; all species susceptible	Horses: excitable and restless; lesions can be seen in sheep on the udder and hairless parts. Dogs: trembling, vomiting, difficulty breathing, and	

	stalks and margins of the leaves; flowers are small and green		concentrated in the stinging hairs	extend south to Otago		general pain; convulsions and death may follow in severe cases; temporary loss of scenting ability in dogs; survivors have muscle pain for several days	
Poroporo toxicity Bullibul; Bullibulli; large kangaroo apple (Australia)	*Solanum laciniatum* and *S. aviculare* Soft wooded shrub to 3 m tall; leaves narrow, lanceolate, 15–30 cm long; flowers blue-purple; fruit pale yellow or orange berry	Irritant, hemolytic, CNS depression with cardiac and respiratory failure	Solasonine, solamargine, and β-solamargine	Lowland forest margins and shrublands throughout New Zealand	Not normally palatable; all parts are poisonous; toxins concentrated in unripe berries; fully ripe fruit are probably not toxic; poisoning associated with ingestion of green fruit and plant material by hungry or naive stock	Profuse diarrhea with abdominal pain, depression, weakness and incoordination, trembling, rapid respiration and heart rate, dyspnea, excessive salivation, nasal discharge, and jaundice; sudden death	
Bushman's friend Rangiora toxicity	*Brachyglottis repanda* Shrub or small tree; to 6 m height; branches are covered in soft white hairs; leaves ovate, 10–25 cm long, obvious veins; dull gray/green above and covered with white hairs on the underside; flowers white to creamy white in large drooping panicles	Hepatogenous pyrrolizidine alkaloid (PA) toxicosis	Senkirkine and other PAs	Abundant in the North Island and found as far south as Kaikoura and Greymouth in the South Island	PAs most concentrated in young growing tips, leaf petioles, and in the cortex of thin stems; PAs not present in the flowers and only in low concentrations in the mature leaves; all species susceptible, although sheep somewhat resistant	Senkirkine causes irreversible hepatic damage and altered vitamin A metabolism; typical PA toxidrome	Other liver toxicants, such as sporidesmin, copper, phosphorous, iron, and phenolics, increase the risk of toxicity by PAs
Buttercup poisoning Waoriki poisoning	*Ranunculus rivularis* (syn. *amphitrichus*) Perennial, creeping, hairless buttercup; it prefers wet places	Gastrointestinal tract irritant	Ranunculin (protoanemonin)	Ubiquitous; most poisonings in the North Island	Most toxic during flowering; hay containing the plant is safe when dried	Severe gastroenteritis; milk has taste taint	

techniques may be valuable. A notable use of physical removal of poisonous plants over relatively large land areas is the use of "scalping" in the wheat belt of Western Australia. "Scalping" involves the removal of all topsoil that may contain *Gastrolobium* sp. seeds and replacing the topsoil with new poison pea-free soils sourced from elsewhere. This extreme and expensive technique has been historically used with some success.

- Use of herbicides: Again, because of the sheer physical size of livestock properties in the semiarid and arid regions of Australia, such methods are often uneconomic. Herbicide use may, in fact, increase the toxicity (and in some cases the palatability) of some plants.
- Use of biocontrol agents: A number of biocontrol agents are being developed in Australia for the control of introduced poisonous plants, notably for Paterson's curse. Biocontrol agents are unlikely to be developed for indigenous plants.
- Sheep, cattle, and goats are somewhat more tolerant of some poisonous plants than are other livestock. The use of goats to control *Gastrolobium* sp. and the use of sheep on pastures containing heavy growths of Paterson's curse and heliotrope are common examples. However, some stock losses are often encountered in these types of enterprises, and they require careful management.
- Supplementary feeding (including the use of safe, but not normally consumed native plants) during drought is also commonly and successfully used to avoid the effects of drought and poisonous plants on livestock. This has led to the common practices of drought lotting and scrub feeding—the creation of temporary feedlots utilizing native plants in order to maintain key livestock. Various relevant state government departments commonly maintain registers of safe native plants that can be used for drought feeding. The leaves of *Acacia aneura* (mulga) have historically been extensively used as drought feed for sheep in the arid, central zone of Australia. Although the plant is effective for this purpose, consumption results in nutritional melanosis of the liver and kidneys of sheep (commonly called "black liver" or "mulga liver" or "bore water liver"). The pigment accumulation is benign and the animals suffer no adverse effects, but the liver and kidneys from affected animals cannot be sold for human consumption for aesthetic reasons, resulting in some financial loss. Another known problem with this system is gastric impaction, which often results from cutting too little of the leaf material (i.e., forcing the animals to eat twigs and branches) and/or allowing the plant material to dry out and/or the animals not drinking enough water. Current recommendations for scrub feeding include: (1) cut only one species at a time, (2) provide sufficient leafy material to minimize the eating of twigs and branches, (3) follow a set feeding routine; it is common to cut two to three day's supply, but daily cutting may be necessary in summer to avoid leaves withering; as the drought progresses, the foliage on uncut scrub dries out and fresh scrub may need to be cut daily, (4) while stocks are strong, cut the scrub most distant from water; then cut closer scrub, (5) if acceptance is poor, spraying with a molasses-water mixture may increase intakes, but some trees in every stand of scrub are unpalatable; generally, older mulga (*A. aneura* and related *Acacia* sp.) trees are preferred to young ones, (6) pulling with a chain or bulldozing can reduce acceptance because of high dust levels, (7) supplementation with protein nitrogen (e.g., cottonseed meal), nonprotein nitrogen (e.g., urea), sulfur (e.g., sulfate of ammonia) and phosphorus (e.g., dicalcium phosphate) has been found to be beneficial during scrub feeding, particularly during pregnancy and lactation (stimulate the rumen function and increase feed intakes); irregular supplementation with molasses appears to reduce the risk of impaction, (8) consider the long-term environmental effects of pulling scrub; leave strips of trees for regeneration, wildlife protection and the like, (9) often sheep and cattle will lose their appetite for scrub after a couple of months, so other sources of feed must be available, (10) stock will eat some trees, but will leave others of the same species, on the same soil type; seek local knowledge in determining which trees and shrubs are suitable for feed in your district; observing the scrub that stock regularly eat and trees that have a clear browse line can also aid in determining palatable species; (11) when toxicity has occurred, it has often involved young, newly emerged leaves, and (12) heavy stock losses can occur when weak cattle "chase the green pick" following drought breaking rain; if possible, confine weak cattle and continue to feed scrub until sufficient grass has grown for them to get their fill without expending valuable energy. Notably, "mulga apples," the common wasp-induced galls on mulga trees (*A. aneura*), are edible (a well-known bushfood traditionally used by the Arrente language peoples of Central Australia), sweet tasting, and highly nutritious. Feeding information on common fodder trees is provided in Table 63.1. These plants should be preserved and encouraged in drought prone areas of Australia (except for those that have been declared as noxious weeds/invasive plants).
- A long-standing and well-proven strategy to reduce the risk of stock losses due to drought conditions and/or when poisonous plants are present has been to physically relocate livestock from properties/regions that are entering into drought conditions to geographic

areas where there are better prevailing conditions. This technique was pioneered by the implementation in the early 1900s of traveling stock routes (TSRs; authorized thoroughfares for the walking of domestic livestock such as sheep or cattle from one location to another) stretching across northern Australia, Queensland, and New South Wales to South Australia near the Flinders Ranges and also across New South Wales. TSRs remain an often critical source of feed for livestock during drought conditions. Traveling stock on a TSR must travel 6 miles a day (by law) in order to avoid the grazing off of all fodder within a particular TSR area. However, the use of TSRs under drought conditions is not foolproof and there have been many notable large-scale stock losses on TSRs due to movement of stock into areas where there are unfamiliar local poisonous plants. Knowledge of the likely poisonous plants in different geographical areas remains critical to the success of these methods.

- Another long-standing and well-proven strategy to reduce the risk of stock losses due to the rapid emergence of indigenous poisonous plants following a break in a drought is to not allow livestock into a grazing area until safe fodder plants dominate the pasture. Again, the ability to geographically relocate stock into safe areas and hold them there until the pastures return to a good and safe condition, as well as knowledge of the local flora and physical inspection of the pastures, is critical to the success of such a strategy.
- Good pasture management is often a key factor in reducing the impact of many poisonous plants. Critical factors include not overgrazing pastures, not overstocking pastures, and pasture spelling/rotation.
- Another common problem in Australia has been the introduction of toxic weeds into a hitherto clean area. Effective integrated weed management programs are critical to reducing risks of this nature.

One of the important animal-related factors that are amenable to human intervention is to ensure that livestock are familiar with the local fauna. Large-scale stock losses that have occurred when naive stock are moved or released into a new geographic area are commonplace in the history of poisonous plants in Australia. Limited, staged, and well-controlled introduction of naive livestock into a new geographic area may reduce the risk of such events. It is also critical to ensure that the new geographic area has plenty of safe forage and that relevant poisonous plants do not dominate the edible local flora. Particular care should be taken to ensure livestock are not hungry when they are introduced into a new area.

Another animal-related factor that is amenable to human intervention is boredom in horses. Horses that are not active or have low levels of environmental stimulation may indiscriminately graze on plants simply due to boredom.

CONCLUDING REMARKS AND FUTURE DIRECTIONS

Poisonous plants continue to be an important cause of financial loss within the livestock industries in Australia. Compounding the pure financial losses is the fact that "outbreaks" of plant poisonings are often tied to climatic conditions, such as droughts and floods, when producers are focused primarily on maintaining the minimal core herds of livestock that will allow them to rapidly restock and take advantage of good climatic and pasture conditions when they return. Currently available practical techniques are partially successful in reducing livestock losses, although well-proven techniques such as geographic relocation of livestock are economically expensive and capital intensive.

Historically, the investigation of plant poisoning in the Australian and New Zealand livestock industries has generally focused on death or severe acute events as key endpoints. There is little doubt that within these contexts, there is still much to learn regarding the poisonous plant flora of Australia and New Zealand. However, subclinical losses (e.g., diminished growth rates rather than outright stock losses) and the use of indigenous plants as safe sources of fodder (particularly during adverse climatic conditions) are also likely to be areas of future investigation.

REFERENCES

Australian Plants

ABARE, Australian Bureau of Agricultural and Resource Economics, 2006. Gross value of farm and fisheries production. Aust. Commodities. 13 (2), 438–439.

Covacevich, J., Davie, P., Pearn, J., 1987. Toxic Plants and Animals: A Guide for Australia. Queensland Museum, Brisbane.

Dowling, R.M., McKenzie, R.A., 1993. Poisonous Plants: A Field Guide. Queensland Department of Primary Industries, Brisbane.

Everest, S.L., 1974. Poisonous Plants of Australia. Angus & Robertson, Sydney.

Gardner, C.A., 1956. The Toxic Plants of Western Australia. West Australian Newspapers, Periodicals Division, Perth.

House, J., 2007 New South Wales Department of Primary Industry. PRIME FACTS. Scrub Feeding. PRIMEFACT 348.

Lowry, J.B., 1995. Deciduous trees: a dry season feed resource in Australian tropical woodlands. Trop. Grassl. 29, 13–17.

McBarron, E.J., 1983. Poisonous Plants: Handbook for Farmers and Graziers. Inkata Press, Melbourne.

Offord, M., 2006. Plants Poisonous to Horses. An Australian Field Guide. Australian Government Rural Industries Research and Development Corporation, Barton.

Queensland Department of Agriculture and Fisheries, 2012. Fodder Trees for Beef Cattle Feeding. <https://www.daf.qld.gov.au/environment/drought/managing-drought/drought-strategies/fodder-trees-for-survival-feeding-of-beef-cattle>.

Seawright, A.A., 1982. Animal Health in Australia: Volume 2. Chemical and Plant Poisons. Australian Government Publishing Service, Canberra.

Shepherd, R.C.H., 2010. Is That Plant Poisonous? An Australian Field Guide for Livestock. Pets and People. RG and FJ Richardson, Melbourne.

New Zealand Plants

Conner, H.E., 1992. The Poisonous Plants in New Zealand. GP Publications, Wellington.

Fuentealba, J., Guzmán, L., Manríquez-Navarro, P., Pérez, C., Silva, M., Becerra, J., et al., 2007. Inhibitory effects of tutin on glycine receptors in spinal neurons. Eur. J. Pharmacol. 559 (1), 61–64.

Holloway, I., 2002. Sudden death in hoggets while grazing a crop. Proc. Sheep Beef Cattle Veterinarians NZVA. 32, 31–35.

Chapter 64

Cyanogenic Glycoside–Containing Plants

Kip E. Panter

INTRODUCTION

Plants containing cyanogenic glycosides are widespread in nature and are responsible for multiple disease conditions in animals and people. The ubiquitous nature of plants containing cyanogenic glycosides is represented by more than 2500 species found within most plant families including the Rosaceae, Leguminoseae, Gramineae, Araceae, Poaceae, Compositeae, Euphorbiaceae, and Passifloraceae (Kingsbury, 1964; Knight and Walter, 2001; Burrows and Tyrl, 2013). Some of the more common plant genera reported to cause poisoning and represented in the literature include the *Prunus* spp. (wild cherry, black cherry, choke cherry); *Sambucus* spp. (elderberry, *Linum* (flax)); *Sorghum* spp. (sorghum, sudan grass, Johnson grass); *Triglochin* spp. (arrow grass); *Manihot* (cassava) and *Bambusa* (bamboo) to name a few (Table 64.1). More than 50 cyanogenic glycosides have been identified and some of the more common ones include amygdalin and prunasin found in wild cherries, mountain mahogany, Saskatoon service berries, and the kernels of almonds, apricots, peaches, and apples, dhurrin found in *Sorghum* spp., and linamarin and lotaustralin found in cassava and lima beans (Seigler, 1975; Conn, 1980; Majak et al., 1981; Knight and Walter, 2001; Minunni and Bilia, 2008; Kudtak et al., 2017). While cyanide is usually sequestered in plants in a relatively nontoxic form (glycoside) there are a few plants that contain cyanolipids (Kudtak et al., 2017). These are usually oil seed plants and pose less risk for toxicity compared to the cyanogenic glycosides. Cyanide poisoning in animals from plants may be acute with rapid death or a more chronic form with debilitating neurological effects as occurs after repeated long-term exposure. When ingestion occurs at a high enough rate to overwhelm the detoxification and excretion mechanisms then death may occur very rapidly. Readers are referred to Knight and Walter (2001) and Burrows and Tyrl (2013) for a more comprehensive review of cyanide-containing plants.

TABLE 64.1 Common Plants Associated with Cyanogenic Glycosides and Poisoning in Animals and People[a]

Common Name	Taxonomic Name
Sorghum, Johnson grass, Sudan grass	*Sorghum* spp.
Choke cherry/Black cherry	*Prunus* spp.
Elder berry	*Sambuccus* spp.
Arrow grass	*Triglochin* spp.
Common vetch	*Vicia sativa*
White clover	*Trifolium repens*
Bracken fern	*Pteridium aquilinum*
Bamboo	*Bambusa* spp.
Peaches, apricots, (pits)	*Prunus* spp.
Apple (seeds)	*Malus* spp.
Birds foot trefoil	*Lotus* spp.
Cassava, tapioca, manioc	*Manihot esculenta*
Catclaw, acacia	*Acacia* spp.
Service or Saskatoon berry	*Amelanchier*
Mountain mahogany	*Cercocarpus montanum*
Eucalyptus, gum tree	*Eucalyptus* spp.
Flax	*Linium* spp.
Corn, maize	*Zea mays*
Lima beans	*Phaseolus lunatus*
Almonds	*Prunus dulcis*

[a]*This table reports some of the most common cyanogenic plants associated with animal and human poisoning. However, this is far from a complete list.*
Source: Adapted from multiple sources: Kingsbury, J.M., 1964. Poisonous Plants of the United States and Canada. Prentice Hall, Englewood Cliffs, NJ, pp. 23–26; Knight, A.P., Walter, R.G., 2001. A Guide to Plant Poisoning of Animals. Teton Press; Burrows, G.E., Tyrl, R. J., 2013. Toxic Plants of North America. John Wiley and Sons Publishing, Ames, IA, 1381 pp.

Veterinary Toxicology. DOI: http://dx.doi.org/10.1016/B978-0-12-811410-0.00064-7

CLINICAL DISEASE

Clinical manifestation of cyanide poisoning may be acute or chronic depending on the amount of glycoside in the plant, the amount and rate of ingestion, and the animal species involved. Acute poisoning occurs when hydrogen cyanide (HCN = prussic acid) is liberated from the glycoside through enzymatic interactions and the detoxification mechanism in the animal is overwhelmed (Cheeke and Shull, 1985). There are major animal species difference in ability to utilize plants containing cyanogenic glycosides (Ballhorn, 2011; Ballhorn et al., 2016). For example, ruminants are generally more susceptible than nonruminants because the rumen pH is more neutral in supporting the glucosidases and lyases required to liberate the HCN from the glycoside, and these enzymes are readily available in the rumen soup due to microbial activity (Majak et al., 1990). Poisoning in sheep, cattle, goats, and wild ruminants have all been reported (Gibb et al., 1974; Burrows and Way, 1979; Burrows, 1981; Quinton, 1985; Knight and Walter, 2001; Soto-Blanco et al., 2008). Conversely, simple stomached animals such as pigs, dogs, and humans with relatively high acidic pH in the stomach have a reduced rate of glycoside hydrolysis and acute cyanide poisoning from plant origin is less common (Ballantyne, 1983). Horses have a large cecum to digest plant material but respond similar to simple stomached animals when compared to ruminants. Most plant-induced cyanide poisoning in people is chronic and associated with consumption of high starch diets consisting of cassava tubers. If the plant material containing cyanogenic glycosides is eaten in toxic amounts or over a prolonged period of time multiple disease conditions may be manifest from acute toxicoses and rapid death to a more protracted chronic neurological disease.

An interesting example of co-evolutionary adaptation to cyanide-containing plants is the giant panda bear, bamboo lemurs of Madagascar, and mountain gorillas of Rwanda (Ballhorn et al., 2016). Bamboo is a grass and the new growth bamboo shoots contain the highest levels of cyanogenic glycosides of any plant species (Table 64.2). While the panda lives almost exclusively on bamboo, consuming large quantities of leaves, stems, and shoots (up to 25% of their body weight daily), the lemurs and gorillas forage on bamboo during certain times of the year when the shoots are succulent and tender. Interestingly, this is when the bamboo contains the highest levels of cyanide. Thus, the panda, lemurs, and gorillas have a unique ability to utilize this high CN-containing forage without any acute or chronic deleterious effects (Ballhorn et al., 2016). Lemurs and gorillas only eat the bamboo at certain times and only as a part of their diet whereas the panda subsists almost exclusively on bamboo. The mechanism associated with the panda's ability to utilize this high CN-containing forage is being studied but is yet unknown (Ballhorn et al., 2016). Obviously the panda's evolutionary niche involves some metabolic advantage to utilize this plant as a major nutritional source. In a general statement, this evolutionary

TABLE 64.2 Common Plants Sources and Reported Cyanide Levels

Plant Source	HCN (mg/100 g Plant)
Sorghum	
Seeds	<10
Young plant tips	240
Green leaves	60
Arrow grass	77
Almonds[a]	
Bitter seeds	290
Young leaves	20
Choke cherry	140–370
Peach	
Pits	160
Leaves	125
Bamboo	
Stems	300
New shoots	800
Cassava	
Leaves	100–200
Bitter tubers	80–400
Sweet tubers	<50
Linseed meal	53
Service berry	200–400
Lima beans[b]	
Black beans	300–400
Colored beans	17–312
White beans	10–210

[a]*Fifty bitter almonds may be lethal in adults or 5–10 in children (Chaouali et al., 2013).*
[b]*Levels of HCN varied depending on which country reporting.*
Source: Adapted from multiple sources: Montgomery, R.D., 1965. The medical significance of cyanogen in plant foodstuffs. Am. J. Clin. Nutr. 17, 103–113 (Montgomery, 1965); Montgomery, R.D., 1980. Cyanogens. In: Liener, I.E. (Ed.), Toxic Constituents of Plant Foodstuffs. Academic Press, New York, NY, pp. 143–160 (Montgomery, 1980); Baumeister, R.G.H., Schievelbein, H., Zickgraf-Rudel, G., 1975. Toxicological and clinical aspects of cyanide metabolism. Drug Res. 25, 1056–1064 (Baumeister et al., 1975); Kingsbury, J.M., 1964. Poisonous Plants of the United States and Canada. Prentice Hall, Englewood Cliffs, NJ, pp. 23–26 (Kingsbury, 1964); Cheeke, P.R., Shull, L.R., 1985. Natural Toxicants in Feeds and Poisonous Plants. AVI Publishing, Westport, CN, pp. 173–234 (Cheeke and Shull, 1985).

advantage to utilize toxins from poisonous plants is not unique to the panda. There are many examples in the literature reporting animal, insect or microbial adaptation to certain toxins providing some level of protection against predators or a novel nutritional advantage.

ACUTE POISONING

As a glycoside, the cyanogenic glycosides in plants are relatively nontoxic to plants or animals. Cyanogenic glycosides only become toxic when the free hydrogen cyanide (HCN) is cleaved from the glycoside through a two-step enzymatic process (Cheeke and Shull, 1985). In the plant the glycosides and enzymes are in different plant compartments, thus protecting the plant cells from HCN toxicity. The glycosides are usually contained within cellular vacuoles whereas the enzymes (glycosidases, lyases) are found in the plant cytosol. When plant cells are damaged or stressed through crushing, chewing, frost, drought etc., the glycoside comes in direct contact with the enzymes and the HCN levels increase quickly, and if ingestion occurs, poisoning may result (Wattenbarger et al., 1968; Burrows and Tyrl, 2013). Drying or curing over time will reduce cyanide levels and ensiling of cyanide-containing plants is reported to reduce cyanide content by more than 50% (Pickrell et al., 1991). It is important to allow sufficient time for these processes to reduce HCN levels before feeding to livestock. Cyanide poisoning is a factor of multiple events such as ingestion rate, HCN liberation rate from the plants, animal species involved, health status of the animals and detoxification and excretion rates. As previously mentioned animal species differ in response to cyanide toxicity and this is especially true for acute cyanide toxicity.

Acute cyanide poisoning may occur in people also and reports of poisoning from eating bitter almonds, apricot pits or seeds from other stone fruits or bamboo shoots can be found in the literature (Burrows and Tyrl, 2013). Bamboo shoots are a popular food item with some Asian cultures, and bitter cassava is still an important source of food in tropical countries. Both can lead to acute poisoning if not properly prepared.

CHRONIC POISONING

On a worldwide basis chronic cyanide poisoning in humans is a serious health issue especially in tropical regions. Cassava is a primary nutritional staple for more than 300 million people throughout the tropics (Balagopalan et al., 1988). In people a permanent chronic neurological condition associated with cassava ingestion is referred to as "Tropical Ataxic Neuropathy" (Salkowski and Penney, 1994). The disease is manifest as paralysis of the lower extremities resulting in ataxia and other neurological effects of the central nervous system involving the optic and auditory nerves. In the tropics and in West Africa cassava is an important source of starch in diets of many people and animals. While low cyanide cultivars of cassava have been developed the tubers still must be prepared properly to avoid the disease. Cassavas are classified into two main types: sweet cassava and bitter cassava. Sweet cassava tubers usually contain fewer than 50 mg HCN/kg on fresh weight basis, whereas bitter cassava may contain up to 400 mg HCN/kg (Table 64.2). Sweet cassava can generally be made safe to eat by peeling and thoroughly cooking the tubers (Kwok, 2008). Bitter cassava requires more extensive preparation. Usually the tubers are peeled, grated and soaked in water to allow leaching of CN. The water is discarded then the cassava is thoroughly cooked. Likewise, for safe human consumption, bamboo shoots must be boiled before eating (Kwok, 2008).

Livestock species ingesting low levels of cyanide (Sudan grass hay, silage or sorghum) over prolonged periods develop a similar neurological disease including posterior paralysis, ataxia, urinary incontinence and cystitis (Smith et al., 1963; McKenzie and McMicking, 1977). This is especially severe in horses and the disease has been called "Equine Sorghum Cystitis-Ataxia Syndrome" (Adams et al., 1969; Van Kampen, 1970). Mares exhibiting theses clinical signs are sometimes called "dribblers" because the mares rear legs and tail are dirty and un-kept from constant urine dribbling down both back legs. This also happens in male horses with obvious different gross observations. In mares the CN-induced cystitis is further complicated by an ascending infection of the urinary tract and kidneys. While some improvement may occur if the forage source is removed, the demyelination of the nerve tracts leaves some permanent irreversible debilitation (Van Kampen, 1970). In pregnant sheep ingestion of forage containing low levels of CN has been associated with goiters in lambs (Cheeke and Shull, 1985). Ultimately, this thyroid enlargement in the neonate results from one step in the detoxification mechanism producing a thiocyanate intermediate that inhibits the metabolism of iodine and elevates the concentration of thyroid stimulating hormone (Tewe and Iyayi, 1989; Soto-Blanco et al., 2008).

Teratogenic effects in foals and piglets have been reported when cyanogenic glycosides were ingested during certain times of gestation (Burrows and Tyrl, 2013). Skeletal malformations in pigs were reported in Missouri when pregnant sows ate wild black cherry leaves (Selby et al., 1971). Piglets were born with limb deformities and other malformations, while foals from mares grazing in Sudan grass pastures exhibited arthrogryposis and ankylosis of the joints (Prichard and Voss, 1967). Seaman et al. (1981) reported limb deformities in calves from pregnant heifers grazing Sudan grass pastures. Keeler (1984) suggested the skeletal deformities could be mediated through a hypoxic mechanism induced by the chronic ingestion of cyanide.

FACTORS AFFECTING CYANIDE LEVELS IN PLANTS

Cool moist growing conditions enhance conversion of nitrates to amino acids increasing the production of cyanogenic glycosides instead of the N-containing proteins (Pickrell et al., 1991; McMahon and Sayre, 1995). Nitrate fertilization of cyanogenic glycoside-containing plants has the potential to increase content of cyanogenic glycosides in plants. Similarly, environmental stresses such as cold or heat stress and drought will increase glycoside levels. Young plants, new shoots and regrowth after cutting contain higher levels of CN-glycoside content thus increasing the risk of poisoning (Nass, 1972; Haskens et al., 1987). Herbicide treatment will also increase CN content and sprayed plants should not be grazed until they are completely desiccated (Grossman, 2003).

Leaves and seeds usually contain the highest concentrations of the cyanogenic glycosides, however the glycosides are found in all plant tissues (Table 64.2). Generally speaking, young growth and new shoots are the most dangerous. Other factors may also influence the levels of glycosides and it's important to recognize these factors when scheduling harvesting or grazing. Glycoside levels present in plant tissues are influenced by diurnal cycles, season of the year, environmental factors and genetics (Majak et al., 1980; Haskens et al., 1987). Plant tissue damage from frost, drought, mechanical damage, etc. will contribute to increased toxicity of cyanide-containing plants. Genetic selection of low cyanide cultivars of sudan grass, almonds, cassava, lima beans and others over the last several years has led to safer forages for animals and better quality foods for humans. While low CN-containing cultivars are available and reduce the potential toxicity there is a cost to the plant and diseases and insect herbivory maybe higher on these low CN varieties requiring additional management.

MECHANISM AND CONDITIONS OF POISONING

HCN or prussic acid as it is frequently called, is highly poisonous to all animals because of its ability to block cellular respiration (Way, 1984; Panter, 2005). The free HCN is readily absorbed through the gut and lungs and the cyanide ion has a strong affinity to bind with the trivalent iron component of the cytochrome oxidase molecule preventing cellular respiration. A pathognomonic characteristic of cyanide poisoning in animals is the cherry red venous blood (Panter, 2005). This occurs when oxygen-saturated hemoglobin cannot release O_2 at the tissue level because the cytochrome oxidase is inhibited, thus super-oxygenated venous blood appears cherry red. Acute cyanide poisoning is a function of the plant source, forage quality, animal species, rate of ingestion and other available nontoxic forage. In most animal species (the panda is an exception) the acute lethal dose of HCN ranges between 2 and 2.5 mg/kg body weight (Salkowski and Penney, 1994; Knight and Walter, 2001).

Under normal growing conditions the cyanide in the plant is bound as a relatively nontoxic glycoside and no free HCN occurs in plant tissues. In fact free HCN is toxic to plant cells as well as animal cells. Presumably, that is why the cyanide is in a glycoside form in the vacuoles of the plant. Poisoning occurs when plant tissue is damaged or crushed allowing the catabolic enzymes found in the cytosol to mix with the glycosides in the vacuoles liberating the HCN. To reiterate, there is a two-step process whereby the enzymes (glucosidases) cleave the sugar from the aglycone (Cheeke and Shull, 1985). Then in the second step a lyase cleaves the HCN from the aglycone and the free HCN is quickly liberated in the crushed plant material. If the rate of ingestion is high enough death can occur very quickly. Ruminants also have these enzymes in the rumen soup and because of this and grazing habits, ruminants are more likely to be poisoned on these plants (Majak et al., 1990). To better illustrate, anecdotal reports from ranchers suggest that sheep and cattle often graze on choke cherry or elderberry leaves when being trailed but move to fresh pastures when rounded up. The browsing of these cyanogenic glycoside-containing forages and the chewing and grazing process provides the tissue damage mentioned above necessary to bring the enzymes in contact with the glycosides. Ranchers then report that once these animals go to water they die rapidly. This is because the water increases the enzyme/substrate mixing increasing the rapid release of HCN that overwhelms the detoxification mechanism resulting in acute poisoning and death. Therefore, animals are often found dead near a water source (Panter, unpublished information).

DETOXIFICATION MECHANISM

Cyanide is readily detoxified in the mammalian system via a thiosulfate sulfur transferase enzyme called rhodanese (Way, 1984). In brief, the CN is catalyzed to thiocyanate, which is excreted in the urine. In a poisoned animal or human this reaction is the essence of the recommended treatment method. Sodium thiosulfate and sodium nitrate can be injected (iv) in a controlled environment. While the nitrate serves to slow the process by converting hemoglobin to methemoglobin, which has a greater affinity for the cyanide than does the cytochrome oxidase (site of cellular toxicity). The thiosulfate provides the sulfur source by which the cyanide becomes bound and then excreted. In acutely poisoned animals and humans treatment must be readily available and quickly administered soon after exposure to prevent death. In the case of animals it is very difficult to prevent death if a lethal dose has been ingested unless all the necessary tools and antidotes are readily available and someone experienced with treatment is present.

DIAGNOSIS AND PATHOLOGY OF CYANIDE POISONING

Diagnosis of acute versus chronic CN poisoning involve multiple and different diagnostic techniques or histopathological analysis. Characteristic cherry red venous blood and bright pink mucous membranes is strongly indicative of acute HCN exposure. Upon necropsy the blood clotting time is prolonged, muscle tissues are dark and congested and internal organs are congested and cyanotic. Hemorrhage is often observed in lungs, heart and other organs. A characteristic "bitter almond" smell in rumen contents upon opening the gastro intestinal tract is another important clue of CN poisoning (Burrows and Tyrl, 2013).

If CN is suspected, rumen content, liver, and blood samples should be collected immediately and frozen as CN is rapidly lost from animal tissues. Plant material from the location where poisoning occurs should also be collected and frozen. Suspected plant material containing 200 ppm HCN is potentially toxic and liver or blood levels greater than 1 ppm HCN is highly suggestive of cyanide poisoning. The most diagnostically significant tissues for CN confirmation is brain and ventricular myocardium and levels of 100 μg/100 g wet tissue are diagnostic (Ballantyne, 1983). CN-containing plant identification, evidence of grazing these plants and positive CN analysis of tissues is conclusive evidence that CN poisoning occurred.

PREVENTION AND TREATMENT OF CN POISONING

Understanding the potential threat of plants containing cyanogenic glycosides provides a significant advantage for producers to avoid animal losses or clinical disease. New cultivars for animal forages and human foods have been developed over the last several years. However, low level cyanide ingestion is still a threat for chronic disease. Selection of low CN-containing cultivars is a method to reduce disease but cassava still needs to be properly prepared. Forage samples submitted for CN analysis can reduce risk, however time of sample collection and methods of preparation for analysis may influence CN content and should be noted. Allowing sudan grasses to grow to at least 2 ft tall before grazing or harvesting will reduce risk of poisoning (Knight and Walter, 2001). Proper curing of hay and silage and allowing adequate time before feeding will reduce toxic levels of CN.

Treatment in animals is often futile and involves the rapid inactivation and removal of CN by metabolizing to a nontoxic product or complexing it with other compounds to facilitate urinary excretion (Burrows and Tyrl, 2013). Intravenous administration of sodium nitrite (10–20 mg/kg) and sodium thiosulfate (250–500 mg/kg) is an antidote but should be administered slowly to prevent secondary toxicosis. The mechanism associated with this treatment involves sodium nitrite conversion of hemoglobin to methemoglobin, which has a greater affinity for CN subsequently producing cyanmethemoglobin. This reaction restores the cytochrome oxidase system critical for cellular respiration. The sodium thiosulfate in the presence of the rhodanese enzyme rapidly complexes the CN molecule cleaved from the cyanmethemoglobin to a form relatively nontoxic sodium thiocyanate, which is excreted in the urine (Salkowski and Penney, 1994). However, this sodium thiocyanate is the intermediate that interferes with iodine metabolism potential causing goiter. However, goiter is easily resolved with iodine supplementation.

CONCLUDING REMARKS AND FUTURE DIRECTIONS

Appropriate management of grazing systems to avoid introducing livestock to potentially toxic plants will help prevent or reduce animal losses. Knowledge and understanding what plants are in pastures and what conditions and risks are associated with forages. For example, timing when livestock are introduced to sudan grass pastures is important. Allowing sudan to grow to at least 2 ft tall before grazing, avoid grazing frozen or damaged crops, and proper curing of hay or ensiling of cut forages will reduce risk. Selection of low CN cultivars will further reduce risk. Long-term maintenance of horses on sudan grass hay or other forages with low levels of CN is discouraged. In people, proper preparation of cassava and other CN-containing foods and avoidance of daily, long-term ingestion of these foods will reduce the risk of neurological effects. Cyanide-containing plants are ubiquitous and with knowledge of the potential risk of poisoning one should be able to avoid poisoning of animals and people.

REFERENCES

Adams, L.G., Dollahite, J.W., Romane, W.M., 1969. Cystitis and ataxia associated with sorghum ingestion in horses. J. Am. Vet. Med. Assoc. 155, 518–524.

Balagopalan, C., Padmaja, G., Nanda, S., et al., 1988. Cassava in Food, Feed and Industry. CRC Press, Boca Raton, FL, pp. 224.

Ballantyne, B., 1983. Artifacts in the definition of toxicity by cyanides and cyanogens. Fundam. Appl. Toxicol. 3, 400–408.

Ballhorn, D.J., 2011. Cyanogenic glycosides in nuts and seeds. In: Preedy, V.R., Watson, R.R., Patel, V.B. (Eds.), Nuts and Seeds in Health and Disease Prevention, first ed. Academic Press, New York, NY, pp. 129–136.

Ballhorn, D.J., Rakotoarivelo, F.P., Kautz, S., 2016. Co-evolution of cyanogenic bamboos and bamboo lemurs on Madagascar. PLoS One. 11 (8), e0158935.

Baumeister, R.G.H., Schievelbein, H., Zickgraf-Rudel, G., 1975. Toxicological and clinical aspects of cyanide metabolism. Drug Res. 25, 1056–1064.

Burrows, G.E., 1981. Cyanide intoxication in sheep: therapeutics. Vet. Human Toxicol. 23, 22–28.

Burrows, G.E., Tyrl, R.J., 2013. Toxic Plants of North America. John Wiley and Sons Publishing, Ames, IA, pp.1381.

Burrows, G.E., Way, J.L., 1979. Cyanide intoxication in sheep: enhancement of efficacy of sodium nitrite, sodium thiosulfate and cobaltous chloride. Am. J. Vet. Res. 40, 613–617.

Chaouali, N., Gana, I., Dorra, A., et al., 2013. Potential toxic levels of cyanide in almonds (*Prunus amygdalus*), apricot kernels (*Prunus armeniaca*), and almond syrup. ISRN Toxicol. Online September 19. http://dx.doi.org/10.1155/2013/610648.

Cheeke, P.R., Shull, L.R., 1985. Natural Toxicants in Feeds and Poisonous Plants. AVI Publishing, Westport, CN, pp. 173–234.

Conn, E.E., 1980. Cyanogenic compounds. Annu. Rev. Plant Physiol. 31, 433–451.

Gibb, M.C., Carberry, J.T., Carter, R.G., et al., 1974. Hydrocyanic acid poisoning of cattle associated with sudan grass. NZ Vet. J. 22, 127.

Grossman, K., 2003. Mediation of herbicide effects by hormone interactions. J Plant Growth Regul. 22, 109–122.

Haskens, F.A., Gorz, H.J., Johnson, B.E., 1987. Seasonal variation in leaf hydrocyanic potential of low and high-dhurrin sorghums. Crop Sci. 27, 903–906.

Keeler, R.F., 1984. Teratogens in plants. J. Anim. Sci. 58, 1029–1039.

Kingsbury, J.M., 1964. Poisonous Plants of the United States and Canada. Prentice Hall, Englewood Cliffs, NJ, pp. 23–26.

Knight, A.P., Walter, R.G., 2001. A Guide to Plant Poisoning of Animals. Teton Press, Jackson, Wyoming.

Kudtak, B., Wieczerzak, M., Namiesnik, J., 2017. Cyanogenic compounds and estrogen disruptors. In: Witczak, A., Sikorski, Z.E. (Eds.), Toxins and Other Harmful Compounds in Foods. CRC Press, Boca Raton, FL, pp. 243–251.

Kwok, J., 2008. Cyanide Poisoning and Cassava. Centre for Food Safety. <http://www.cfs.hk/english/multimedia/multimedia_pub/multimedia_pub_fsf_19_01.html>.

Majak, W., McDiarmid, R.E., Hall, J.W., et al., 1980. Seasonal variation in the cyanide potential of arrow grass (*Triglochin maritima*). Can. J. Plant Sci. 60, 1235–1241.

Majak, W., McDiarmid, R.E., Hall, W.J., 1981. The cyanide potential of Saskatoon service berry (*Amelanchier alnifolia*) and choke cherry (*Prunus virginiana*). Can. J. Anim. Sci. 61, 681.

Majak, W., McDiarmid, R.E., Hall, J.W., et al., 1990. Factors that determine rates of cyanogenesis in bovine ruminal fluid in vitro. J. Anim. Sci. 68, 1648–1655.

McKenzie, R.A., McMicking, L.I., 1977. Ataxia and urinary incontinence in cattle grazing sorghum. Aust. Vet. J. 53, 496–497.

McMahon, J.M., Sayre, R.T., 1995. Cyanogenic glycosides: physiology and regulation of synthesis. In: Gustine, D.L., Flores, H.E. (Eds.), Phytochemicals and Health. American Society of Plant Physiologists, Penn State, pp. 112–121.

Minunni, M., Bilia, A.R., 2008. Biosensing approach in natural product research. In: Colegate, S.M., Molyneux, R.J. (Eds.), Bioactive Natural Products. CRC Press, Boca Raton, FL, pp. 299–321.

Montgomery, R.D., 1965. The medical significance of cyanogen in plant foodstuffs. Am. J. Clin. Nutr. 17, 103–113.

Montgomery, R.D., 1980. Cyanogens. In: Liener, I.E. (Ed.), Toxic Constituents of Plant Foodstuffs. Academic Press, New York, NY, pp. 143–160.

Nass, H.G., 1972. Cyanogenesis: it's inheritance in *Sorghum bicolor*, *Sorghum sudanese*, lotus, and *Trifolium repens*-a review. Crop Sci. 12, 503–506.

Panter, K.E., 2005. Natural toxins of plant origin. In: Dabrowski, W.M., Sikorski, Z.E. (Eds.), Toxin in Foods. CRC Press, Boca Raton, FL, pp. 11–63.

Pickrell, J.A., Oehme, F.W., Hichman, S.R., 1991. Drought increases forage nitrate and cyanide. Vet. Human Toxicol. 33, 247–251.

Prichard, J.T., Voss, J.L., 1967. Fetal ankylosis in horses associated with hybrid sudan pasture. J. Am. Vet. Med. Assoc. 150, 871–873.

Quinton, D.A., 1985. Saskatoon service berry toxicity to deer. J. Wild Life Manage. 49, 362–364.

Salkowski, A.A., Penney, D.G., 1994. Cyanide poisoning in animals and humans: a review. Vet. Human Toxicol. 36, 455–466.

Seaman, J.T., Smeal, M.G., Wright, J.C., 1981. The possible association of a sorghum (*Sorghum Sudanese*) hybrid as a cause of developmental defects in calves. Aust. Vet. J. 57, 351–352.

Seigler, D.S., 1975. Isolation and characterization of naturally occurring cyanogenic compounds. Phytochemistry. 14 (1), 107–114.

Selby, L.A., Menges, R.W., Houser, E.C., et al., 1971. An outbreak of swine malformations associated with black cherry, Prunus serotina. Arch. Environ. Health. 22, 496–501.

Smith, A.D.M., Duckett, S., Waters, A.H., 1963. Neuropathological changes in chronic cyanide intoxication. Nature. 4902, 179–181.

Soto-Blanco, B., Stegelmeier, B.L., Pfister, J.A., et al., 2008. Comparative effects of prolonged administration of cyanide, thiocyanate and choke cherry (*Prunus virginiana*) to goats. J. Appl. Toxicol. 28, 356–363.

Tewe, O.O., Iyayi, E.A., 1989. Cyanogenic glycosides. In: Cheek, P.R. (Ed.), Toxicants of Plant Origin, Volume II: Glycosides. CRC Press, Boca Raton, FL, pp. 44–60.

Van Kampen, K.R., 1970. Sudan grass and sorghum poisoning in horses: a possible lathyrogen disease. J. Am. Vet. Med. Assoc. 156, 629–630.

Wattenbarger, D.W., Gray, E., Rice, J.S., et al., 1968. Effects of frost and freezing on hydrocyanic potential of sorghum plants. Crop Sci. 8, 526–528.

Way, J.L., 1984. Cyanide intoxication and its mechanism of antagonism. Ann. Rev. Pharmacol. Toxicol. 24, 451–481.

Chapter 65

Nitrate- and Nitrite-Accumulating Plants

Jeffery O. Hall

INTRODUCTION

Nitrate poisoning is a commonly encountered disease state in herbivores. Ruminants are the most susceptible to acute nitrate poisoning. Microflora in the rumen reduce nitrates to nitrites and then ammonia for microbial growth. Excess intake of nitrates may overwhelm further reduction capacity, allowing toxic amounts of nitrite to accumulate and be absorbed into the blood, where it causes the formation of methemoglobin. Thus, even though the clinical syndrome is referred to as nitrate poisoning, it is actually poisoning by the nitrite ion. Goats browse leafy portions of plants and may not ingest toxic amounts of nitrates as readily as sheep and cattle since higher concentrations of nitrate occur in stalks and stems of accumulating forages. Sheep are not as commonly poisoned as cattle, which may be due to the fact that they eat slower than cattle. Ruminants have the potential to graze or be fed a variety of grasses and weeds that can accumulate large amounts of nitrate that may prove toxic if eaten in a sufficient dose. Excessive nitrate may be present in grazed forages and weeds, hay, or fresh cut forage fed to animals as green-chop. Excessive fertilization, drought, herbicides, hail damage, or reduced sunlight can enhance plant accumulation of nitrates via increased uptake or diminished metabolism and utilization for plant protein synthesis. Forages and weeds growing in soil rich in manure waste or in holding pens are a potential source of poisoning. It should be noted that ensiling may reduce forage nitrate by 30% or more over 30–60 days, but silage can still contain toxic amounts of nitrates if the original materials were very high. Nitrate fertilizers are commonly used around livestock and accidental ingestion or feed contamination occasionally occurs. For example, water hauled in tanks previously used to transport nitrate-based fertilizer can be a source of exposure. When evaluating the potential for nitrate/nitrite poisoning, one must include both forages and water sources, as nitrates and nitrites are soluble and may contaminate available water sources.

Monogastric animals are less susceptible to the toxic effects of nitrate ingestion. Horses and rabbits can convert some nitrate to nitrite in the large bowel (Bruning-Fann and Kaneene, 1993), but are much less sensitive than ruminants, with nitrate toxicosis in horses being rarely reported (Hintz and Thompson, 1998; Oruc et al., 2010). Other monogastric species are susceptible to the systemic toxic effects of nitrites, when ingested as nitrites from nonplant sources (Worth et al., 1997).

BACKGROUND

When evaluating the potential for nitrate poisoning, forage and water can be reported in several ways. For clarity, this chapter will use nitrate ion concentrations. Other means of expressing nitrates can be conversion to the nitrate ion via the following calculations:

Potassium nitrate X 0.61 = Nitrate ion
Sodium nitrate X 0.72 = Nitrate ion
Nitrate-Nitrogen X 4.4 = Nitrate ion

Plants take up nitrogen from the soil primarily in the form of the nitrate ion. Excessive accumulation of nitrates can be associated with excessive uptake or hindered utilization of the nitrates for protein and other nitrogen containing chemicals. Numerous plant species have the potential to accumulate toxic amounts of nitrates, but certain ones are more commonly found to have high nitrate concentrations (Table 65.1). Nitrate accumulation in the stems and leaves of plants may be associated with excessive concentrations of nitrogen (nitrates or ammonia) in the soil. Young plants are more likely to have high nitrates than are more mature plants. For example, nitrate concentrations decline considerably in all parts of sudangrasses (*Sorghum* spp.) following maturation or heading (Whitehead and Moxon, 1952; Mizukami et al., 1997). Plants growing in highly fertilized soil, where large amounts of livestock manure/urine are applied as

Veterinary Toxicology. DOI: http://dx.doi.org/10.1016/B978-0-12-811410-0.00065-9

TABLE 65.1 Common Nitrate Accumulating Plants

Amaranthus spp.	Pigweed
Amskinckia spp.	Tarweed
Ambrosia spp.	Ragweed
Avena sativa	Oats
Beta vulgaris	Beets
Brassica spp.	Rutabaga, rape, broccoli, turnip
Chenopodium spp.	Lamb's quarters
Cirsium arvense	Canada thistle
Convolvulus spp.	Bindweed
Datura spp.	Jimsonweed
Daucus carota	Wild carrot, Queen Anne's lace
Eleusine indica	Goose grass
Eupatorium purpureum	Thoroughwort
Glycine max	Soybean
Gnaphalium purpureum	Purple cudweed
Helianthus annuus	Sunflower
Hordeum vulgare	Barley
Ipomoea batatas	Sweet potato
Kochia spp.	Firebush
Lactuca serriola	Prickly lettuce
Linum spp.	Flax
Malva parviflora	Small mallow
Melilotus officinalis	Sweet clover
Panicum capillare	Panic grass
Polygonum spp.	Smartweed
Rumex spp.	Dock
Salsola iberica	Russian thistle
Secale cereale	Rye
Solanum spp.	Nightshades, potato
Solidago spp.	Goldenrods
Sorghum spp.	Johnson grass, milo, sudangrass
Stellaria media	Chickweed
Tribulus terrestris	Puncture vine
Triticum sativum	Wheat
Urtica dioica	Stinging nettle
Verbesina encelioides	Golden crownbeard
Zea Mays	Corn

fertilizer, or where waste accumulations occur in holding pens may accumulate excessive nitrates. A variety of factors that diminish plant growth or photosynthesis can inhibit utilization of accumulating nitrates, such as damage to leaves by disease, wind, hail, or herbicides, as well as drought, decreased sunlight, or nutritional inadequacies in plants (Whitehead and Moxon, 1952; Hicks and Peterson, 1976). For example, molybdenum is a component in enzymatic reactions of nitrate reductase in plants, so molybdenum deficient plants can accumulate nitrates due to poorer utilization. These factors can decrease the further processing of the nitrates into plant proteins, resulting in a build-up of potentially toxic concentrations.

A major reason plants accumulate nitrates is drought. During periods of drought, the growth of forages and weeds is reduced, but the roots can continue to collect nitrate resulting in high nitrate in plant materials. This is particularly true of well-fertilized sorghum hybrid (*Sorghum* spp.) and millet (*Pennisetum* spp.) forages grown for temporary summer grazing and for hay production (Clay et al., 1976). Corn, oats, sorghum, millet and a variety of weeds are well known to accumulate nitrates during drought. Shortages of forage caused by a 2-year drought in Kansas were further exacerbated by increases of nitrate and cyanide in those forages based on analyses of samples submitted to a diagnostic laboratory (Pickrell et al., 1991).

Plants may accumulate nitrates during periods of reduced sunlight. Sunlight is needed to drive photosynthesis and the energy-dependent nitrate reductase system in plants. Forage or weeds growing in the shade of trees may be subject to nitrate accumulation. Nitrate poisoning is occasionally a problem in areas of the United States where winter grazing for cattle consists of fertilized pastures of ryegrass (*Lolium multiflorum*), oats (*Avena* spp.), turnips (*Brassica rapa*), or wheat (*Triticum* spp.). During extended periods of overcast weather, perhaps several days, the nitrate content of the forage may increase to potentially toxic concentrations. Accumulation is more likely when temperatures are mild, or where growth slows or stops but the roots continue uptake of nitrate, which is stored in the stems until there is adequate sunlight for growth to resume. Generally, a day or two of sunlight with temperatures above 55°F allows plant growth to continue, converting excess stored nitrate into plant protein.

Within a given field or pasture, forage nitrates may vary considerably, requiring multiple forage samples for testing to achieve accurate assessment of the risk of nitrate–nitrite intoxication. Determining the nitrate status of bales of stored hay can be a challenge because only the forage growing in a portion of a hayfield may have been affected. Obtaining a representative sample requires using a hollow handheld commercial tool that cuts through to the center of the bale and recovers a core sample. At least two samples from each bale should be collected. An individual investigation might reveal, e.g., that part of the bales have low nitrate content, while some may contain toxic amounts. Thus, extreme care should be emphasized in the interpretation of relative risk, since there is always the potential for localized toxic concentrations to be missed in the testing.

Nitrate content is not reduced by drying and baling as hay. High nitrate hay fed to cattle months after baling can cause deaths and abortions. Mortality can be striking, as in a case in Nebraska in which *Amaranthus/Kochia* hay with 2.99% nitrate and sudangrass with 4.88% nitrate were fed to 390 cattle, resulting in the deaths of 226 and 42 abortions (Hibbs et al., 1978). High nitrate summer hay fed during the winter of 1977–78 killed cattle in Oklahoma (Haliburton and Edwards, 1978).

Risks from high nitrate content forages can be reduced by some management strategies. As nitrate is water soluble, high nitrate forages that are senescent can have some of the nitrate leached from the forage by precipitation. However, if high concentrations were present, there may still be toxic amounts present after leaching. Corn stalks left in a field had an average decrease of only 30% after 90 days (Johnson et al., 1992). Properly ensiled forages can have a significant amount of nitrate utilized by the fermenting microbes, but ensiled, high nitrate forages should always be tested prior to feeding to determine whether adequate nitrate has been lost or if additional dilution is required to ensure safe feed concentrations. Since nitrates are soluble, drained silage fluids could have a significant nitrate content and pose a potential hazard.

It has been understood that rumen microorganisms can adapt to and utilize increasing amounts of nitrate in the diet. The period of maximum acclimation occurs within 6 days (Allison and Reddy, 1984). However, adaptation can be lost within a few days. The ability of rumen microorganisms to safely reduce nitrate and further reduce nitrite can be increased by feeding corn-based supplements to cattle (Burrows et al., 1987; Nolan et al., 2016). In addition, it has been shown that adaptation to increased nitrate may also have some systemic effects, as induction of methemoglobin reductase activity was observed in cattle (Godwin et al., 2014).

It has been stated that rate of intake for nitrate containing forages is a major factor in the potential for toxic effects (Burrows and Tyrl, 2001). Ingestion of dry forage containing high nitrate may have greater risk than green forages, as the rate of intake on a total dry matter basis and the rate of microbial exposure to nitrates is much faster (Geurink et al, 1979). To reduce forage trampling, farm management may employ limited grazing periods, allowing hungry cattle to consume a large amount of forage for short periods. This increases risk because of the time–dose relationship that exists when excess nitrate is present and conversion of nitrate to nitrite exceeds the ability of the rumen flora to convert nitrite to ammonia. Hungry cattle and sheep introduced to stockyards containing a dominant or pure growth of button grass (*Dactyloctenium radulans*) suffered acute nitrate–nitrite toxicity in four incidents in inland Queensland between 1993 and 2001 (McKenzie et al., 2004b). The nitrate content of the button grass from within the stockyards ranged from 2.44% to 7.87% nitrate in dry matter and from outside the stockyards ranged from less than 0.12% to 0.24%.

PHARMACOKINETICS/TOXICOKINETICS

Action of the rumen flora reduces nitrate to the much more toxic nitrite relatively rapidly, which is normally further reduced to ammonia and utilized by the microorganisms. Nitrite is absorbed into the blood when the intake of nitrates and the production of nitrite exceed the capacity of the rumen flora to further metabolize the nitrite. In some cases, preformed nitrite in hay may shorten the period from ingestion to onset of signs. Both nitrates and nitrites are absorbed into the blood but the absorbed nitrite is the proximate cause of methemoglobin formation that results in poisoning. With IV administration of nitrite, peak methemoglobin formation was observed at 1.5 h after the onset of the infusion (van't Klooster et al., 1990), which likely is due to peak nitrite accumulation and not due to a delay in the formation of the methemoglobin.

The nitrate ion is primarily eliminated in the urine of monogastrics and preruminant calves, but ruminants eliminate much smaller amounts (Casteel and Evans, 2004). This is likely due to ruminants readily recycling nitrogen through the rumen to enhance overall utilization. The half-life of nitrate is estimated to be 9 h in adult cattle and more than 24 h in the bovine fetus (Johnson et al., 1992). The half-lives of nitrate and nitrite in the blood of sheep are 4.2 and 0.5 h, respectively (Schneider and Yeary, 1975). In comparison, the elimination half-life for nitrate is reported to be 44.7 h in dogs and 4.8 h in ponies (Bruning-Fann and Kaneene, 1993), while elimination half-life for nitrites is reported to be 0.5 h in dogs and 0.57 h in ponies.

MECHANISM OF ACTION

The nitrite anion causes vasodilation and oxidizes ferrous iron (Fe^{2+}) in hemoglobin to the ferric iron (Fe^{3+}) state forming methemoglobin, which then cannot accept molecular oxygen. The formation of methemoglobin is likely rapid with the cumulative development occurring as nitrite is absorbed. As the percentage of methemoglobinemia rises, oxygen starvation of tissues increases and blood becomes chocolate brown in color. In sheep, the half-life of methemoglobinemia is approximately 1.5 h (Schneider and Yeary, 1975). Clinical signs such as exercise intolerance appear at 30%–40% methemoglobinemia, with death from hypoxia likely when concentrations exceed 80% (Burrows, 1980). In nonfatal cases, a red blood cell intrinsic NADH-dependent diaphorase or reductase system gradually reduces methemoglobin to hemoglobin, which then is able to accept molecular oxygen and carry it to the tissues.

TOXICITY

Total dietary intake of nitrate should be considered in the evaluation of toxic risk. Nitrate in drinking water adds to dietary intake. Nitrate concentrations in water in excess of 1000 ppm may cause nitrate poisoning in livestock. Nitrate level <100 ppm in drinking water is considered safe (Puls, 1994). Water source nitrate can be more toxic than forage source, as forage nitrate must first leach from the plant material, allowing for more gradual increases that rumen microbes could more efficiently handle. This was found when nitrate salt was compared to nitrate in forage, with the toxic dose of the salt form in cattle being half that of the forage nitrate (Crawford et al., 1966).

The nitrate content of plant material that is generally accepted as safe for all classes of livestock is less than 0.5% on a dry weight basis. Nitrate content greater than 1.0% on a dry weight basis is most likely to cause lethal nitrate poisoning in ruminants, with cattle appearing to be the most susceptible, due to feeding behavior. It is recommended that pregnant animals not be fed forage or hay with a nitrate content greater than 0.5% on a dry weight basis, but due to known potential error in testing, some recommendations are to not feed pregnant animals greater than 0.2% nitrate forage on a dry weight basis. The rate of conversion of nitrate to nitrite and then to ammonia is a limiting factor in safe utilization of nitrates by ruminants. Hungry animals are at greater risk, and intake of dry matter from hay may be faster than from grazing.

The rumen flora can safely utilize higher amounts of nitrate if sufficient dietary energy is present to promote reductive activity. Feeding corn-based supplements to cattle reduced nitrite accumulation (Burrows et al., 1987). In this study, the feeding of 3.2 kg of corn protected against nitrate poisoning by reducing intraruminal nitrite and blood methemoglobin ($P < .05$).

Clinical signs of nitrate–nitrite toxicosis in cattle include weakness, cyanosis of mucous membranes, tremors, ataxia, collapse, tachypnea, dyspnea, abortions, and death. Affected animals may remain standing but then collapse and die within minutes. Dead animals may be found in sternal recumbency or lying on their side. Blood is generally dark and may have an obvious brown color when drawn into a syringe or spread on a white cloth. However, this color change may not be as apparent with necropsy of animals that have been dead several hours.

Three cows fed *Chenopodium album* hay died 30 min after showing ataxia, bluish-brown mucous membranes, rapid and difficult breathing, increased heart rates, tremors, and coma. Brown-colored and badly coagulated blood was the prominent necropsy finding. Slight pulmonary edema was prominent, and all visceral organs were hyperemic. The hay contained 1.1% nitrate and 33 ppm nitrite (Ozmen et al., 2003). Nitrate–nitrite poisoning killed four adult alpacas and induced the abortion of a full-term fetus after access to oat hay (*Avena sativa*) containing 1.95% nitrate on a dry matter basis (McKenzie et al., 2004a). Necropsy findings were cyanosis, dark-colored blood, and pulmonary congestion and edema.

In cattle, abortions may occur in the herd 2–10 days after acute nitrate toxicosis. Less oxygen is available to the fetus because of decreased vascular perfusion (decreased arterial pressure) and methemoglobinemia in the cow, and nitrite induces methemoglobinemia in fetal blood (Bruning-Fann and Kaneene, 1993). Bovine abortion has been reported to occur with forages containing 0.61%–1% nitrate (van't Klooster et al., 1990).

DIAGNOSTIC TESTING

Differential diagnoses to consider include acute toxicoses caused by insecticides, carbohydrate overload, hypomagnesemia in cattle, cyanide, blue-green algae, urea (ammonia), and potent oxidizing agents such as sodium chlorate herbicide and aniline dyes. Lesions are not diagnostic. Blood and tissues may appear brown at time of death, but this becomes less obvious as autolysis proceeds. Dark blood may also suggest septicemia. Agonal hemorrhages in the epicardium or mild pulmonary congestion/edema may be present.

Ocular fluid is an excellent postmortem sample for nitrate analysis and is stable at room temperatures for 24 h and for a week when refrigerated (Boermans, 1990). Because of continued microbial metabolism after death, rumen content analysis is not recommended for suspected nitrate poisoning cases. Plasma and serum are also acceptable samples. Ocular fluid nitrate concentrations are 35% lower than serum (Boermans, 1990). The diphenylamine blue test is widely used for testing fluids and plant tissues (Burrows, 1980; Bhikane and Singh, 1990). The diazotization test has also been used (Bhikane and Singh, 1991). Nitrate test strips and ion- specific electrodes are also being utilized.

Normal background ocular nitrate content is generally <5.0 ppm. Nitrate concentrations in ocular fluid of 10–20 ppm are indicative of excessive nitrate exposure, and concentrations greater than 20 ppm are considered diagnostic of poisoning (Burrows and Tyrl, 2001). In abortion and stillbirth situations, interpreting bovine fetal ocular fluid nitrate levels is more problematic because normal concentrations may approach 20 ppm in weak or stillborn calves (Johnson et al., 1994). A content of greater than 30 ppm or content greater than 20 ppm with additional diagnostic information such as high forage nitrates may be needed to confirm nitrate abortion (Casteel and Evans, 2004). In an alpaca nitrate poisoning case, aqueous humor from two adults contained 25 ppm nitrate and that from the fetus contained 10 ppm (McKenzie et al., 2004a).

Clinical history may be suggestive of nitrate poisoning. However, identification of diagnostic concentrations of nitrate in the ocular fluid, serum, or plasma is needed for confirmation. Since nitrite is short lived in biologic samples, nitrate analysis is much more reliable. All sources of forages, weeds, water, feed supplements, and fertilizers to which the animals had access should be determined and sampled for nitrate analysis.

TREATMENT

Care must be taken to minimize stresses to nitrate poisoned animals. These animals will be clinically hypoxic and subject to sudden death.

Treatment is with intravenous methylene blue in a 1% or 2% aqueous solution at a rate of 4–15 mg/kg body wt (Burrows, 1980). Risk of toxic effect from this treatment are low. The response to intravenous treatment of a 2% solution of methylene blue at a dosage of 20 mL/100 kg body wt is rapid, with reversal of the clinical signs within several minutes (Burrows and Tyrl, 2001). In severe cases, treatment at a lower dose can be repeated. Methylene blue has a serum elimination half-life of about 1.5 h, but some tissue accumulation has a much longer elimination time. Methylene blue serves as an electron carrier for an NADPH-dependent system to reduce methemoglobin to hemoglobin. Methylene blue is most effective in humans and ruminants (Burrows and Tyrl, 2001). Tissues in the treated animals are stained, and the urine becomes dark green. Treated animals should not be sold for slaughter for 180 days. Other dyes, such as tolonium chloride (tolonium blue), are effective in reducing methemoglobin to hemoglobin but have a narrow therapeutic index (Gupta et al., 1992; Cudd et al., 1996).

CONCLUDING REMARKS AND FUTURE DIRECTIONS

Safe use and storage of nitrate containing fertilizers is essential if accidental poisoning of livestock, especially ruminants, is to be avoided. Use of liquid fertilizer tanks to deliver water to livestock is a documented hazard for toxicoses. The potential for nitrate accumulation as well as the factors that can predispose to nitrate accumulation in weeds and forages intended for feeding or grazing and the risks this poses to ruminants, especially cattle, should be pointed out to farmers and ranchers. Cutter blades can be raised to reduce the amount of edible stalk in harvested forages if conditions suggest the possibility of high nitrate in the stalks and stems. Prefeeding testing of potentially high-nitrate forages is very important, especially when environmental conditions predispose to accumulation. Feeding cattle an energy source such as corn can increase the rate of nitrite reduction by rumen flora and decrease the potential for poisoning. Other management strategies, such as ensiling or allowing weathering of stalks, can be beneficial, but it is still essential to test prior to utilizing the forage materials.

REFERENCES

Allison, M.J., Reddy, C.A., 1984. Adaptations of gastrointestinal bacteria in response to changes in dietary oxalate and nitrate. In: Klug, M.J., Reddy, C.A. (Eds.), Current Perspectives in Microbial Ecology. American Society for Microbiology, Washington, DC, pp. 248–256.

Bhikane, A.U., Singh, B., 1990. Diphenylamine blue test for diagnosis of experimental nitrite poisoning in crossbred calves. Indian Vet. J. 67, 808–812.

Bhikane, A.U., Singh, B., 1991. Diazotization test for diagnosis of experimental nitrite poisoning in cross bred cattle. Indian J. Anim. Sci. 61, 61–62.

Boermans, H.J., 1990. Diagnosis of nitrate toxicosis in cattle, using biological fluids and a rapid ion chromatographic method. Am. J. Vet. Res. 51, 491–495.

Bruning-Fann, C.S., Kaneene, J.F., 1993. The effects of nitrate, nitrite, and N-nitroso compounds on animal health. Vet. Hum. Toxicol. 35 (3), 237–253.

Burrows, G.E., 1980. Nitrate intoxication. J. Am. Vet. Med. Assoc. 177, 82–83.

Burrows, G.E., Tyrl, R.L., 2001. Toxic Plants of North America. Iowa State University Press, Ames, IA, pp. 934–941.

Burrows, G.E., Horn, G.W., McNew, R.W., et al., 1987. The prophylactic effect of corn supplementation on experimental nitrate intoxication in cattle. J. Anim. Sci. 64, 1682–1689.

Casteel, S.W., Evans, T.J., 2004. Feed associated toxicants: nitrate. In: Plumlee, K.H. (Ed.), Clinical Veterinary Toxicology. Mosby, St. Louis, MO, pp. 127–130.

Clay, B.R., Edwards, W.C., Peterson, D.R., 1976. Toxic nitrate accumulation in sorghums. Bovine. Pract. 11, 28–32.

Crawford, R.F., Kennedy, W.K., Davidson, K.L., 1966. Factors influencing the toxicity of forages that contain nitrate when fed to cattle. Cornell. Vet. 56, 3–17.

Cudd, L.A., Burrows, G.E., Clarke, C.R., 1996. Pharmacokinetics and toxicity of tolonium chloride in sheep. Vet. Hum. Toxicol. 38, 329–332.

Geurink, J.H., Malestein, A., Kemp, A., et al., 1979. Nitrate poisoning in cattle. 3. The relationship between nitrate intake with hay or fresh roughage and the speed of intake on the formation of methemoglobin. Neth. J. Agric. Sci. 27, 268–276.

Godwin, I., Li, L., Luijben, K., et al., 2014. The effects of chronic nitrate supplementation on erythrocytic methaemoglobin reductase in cattle. Anim. Prod. Sci. 55 (5), 611–616.

Gupta, D., Singh, B., Bhikane, A.U., et al., 1992. Treatment of experimental nitrate poisoning with tolonium chloride in buffalo calves. Indian J. Anim. Sci. 62, 1180–1182.

Haliburton, J.C., Edwards, W.C., 1978. Nitrate poisoning in Oklahoma cattle during the winter of 1977–1978. Vet. Hum. Toxicol. 20, 401–403.

Hibbs, C.M., Stencel, E.L., Hill, R.M., 1978. Nitrate toxicosis in cattle. Vet. Hum. Toxicol. 20, 1–2.

Hicks, D.R., Peterson, R.H., 1976. Defoliation and fertilizer nitrogen effects on nitrate-nitrogen profile in maize. Agron. J. 68, 476–478.

Hintz, H.F., Thompson, L.J., 1998. Nitrate toxicosis in horses. Equine Pract. 20, 5.

Johnson, J.L., Hergert, G.W., Schneider, N.R., et al., 1992. Post-harvest change in cornstalk nitrate and its relationship to bovine fetal nitrite/nitrate exposure. In: James, L.F., Keeler, R.F., Bailey Jr., E.M., Cheeke, P.R., Hegarty, M.P. (Eds.), Poisonous Plants: Proceedings of the Third International Symposium. pp. 423–430.

Johnson, J.L., Grotelueschen, D.M., Knott, M., 1994. Evaluation of bovine perinatal nitrate accumulation in western Nebraska. Vet. Hum. Toxicol. 36, 467–471.

McKenzie, R., Gordon, A., Burren, B., et al., 2004a. Alpaca plant poisonings: nitrate–nitrite and possible cyanide. Aust. Vet. J. 82 (10), 630–634.

McKenzie, R.A., Rayner, A.C., Thompson, G.K., et al., 2004b. Nitrate–nitrite toxicity in cattle and sheep grazing *Dactyloctenium radulans* (button grass) in stockyards. Aust. Vet. J. 82 (10), 630–634.

Mizukami, Y., Kanbe, M., Inami, S., et al., 1997. Changes in the nitrate content of millets and sudangrass. Res. Bull. Aichi-ken Agric. Res. Cent. 29, 71–76.

Nolan, J.V., Godwin, I.R., de Raphelis-Soissan, V., et al., 2016. Managing the rumen to limit the incidence and severity of nitrite poisoning in nitrate-supplemented ruminants. Anim. Prod. Sci. 56 (8), 1317–1329.

Oruc, H.H., Akkoc, A., Uzunoglu, I., et al., 2010. Nitrate poisoning in horses associated with ingestion of forage and alfalfa. J. Eq. Vet. Sci. 30 (3), 159–162.

Ozmen, O., Mor, F., Ayhan, U., 2003. Nitrate poisoning in cattle fed *Chenopodium album* hay. Vet. Hum. Toxicol. 45 (2), 83–84.

Pickrell, J.A., Oehme, F.W., Hickman, S.R., 1991. Drought increases forage nitrate and cyanide. Vet. Hum. Toxicol. 33 (3), 247–251.

Puls, R., 1994. Mineral Levels in Animal Health. second ed. Sherpa Int Publ., Clearbrook, Canada, p. 306.

Schneider, N.R., Yeary, R.A., 1975. Nitrate and nitrite pharmacokinetics in the dog, sheep, and pony. Am. J. Vet. Res. 36, 941–947.

van't Klooster, A.Th, Malestein, A., Akkersdijk, E.M., 1990. On the pathogenesis of abortion in acute nitrite toxicosis of pregnant dairy cows. Theriogenology. 33, 1075–1089.

Whitehead, E.I., Moxon, A.L., 1952. Nitrate poisoning. SD Agric. Exp. Stat. Bull. Paper.424.

Worth, A.J., Ainsworth, S.J., Brocklehurst, B.J., et al., 1997. Nitrite poisoning in cats and dogs fed a commercial pet food. NZ Vet. J. 45 (5), 193–195.

Chapter 66

Toxicity of Yew (*Taxus* spp.) Alkaloids

Christina R. Wilson and Stephen B. Hooser

INTRODUCTION

Yews (*Taxus* spp., *Taxaceae*) are evergreen plants often used for ornamental landscaping in many areas of the United States, Europe, and elsewhere throughout the world. Common varieties in the United States are English yew (*Taxus baccata*), American yew (*Taxus canadensis*), Japanese yew (*Taxus cuspidata*), and Pacific or Western yew (*Taxus brevifolia*) (Kingsbury, 1964). These plants can be highly toxic and have been implicated in numerous human and animal poisonings. The poisonous taxine alkaloids are present in the foliage, bark, and seeds of the plants but not in the fleshy scarlet aril (berry) (Bryan-Brown, 1932; Kingsbury, 1964).

Historical Background

References to yew toxicity date back more than two millennia (Bryan-Brown, 1932). In the first century BCE, Julius Caesar (102–44 BCE) wrote of Catuvolcus, the king of Eburones, who poisoned himself with yew "juice" (Fröhne and Pfänder, 1984). Ancient Celts often committed ritual suicides by drinking extracts from yew plants and applied the poisonous sap to the tips of their arrows during the Gaelic Wars (Foster and Duke, 1990; Hartzell, 1995). Some primitive cultures are reported to have used yew extracts as hunting and fishing aids (Watt and Breyer-Brandwijk, 1962; Hartzell, 1995). During the 18th and 19th centuries, concoctions brewed from yew leaves were documented as having been used as an abortifacient or an emmenagogue by women in Europe and India (Bryan-Brown, 1932; Watt and Breyer-Brandwijk, 1962).

Chemical Characterization

The first preparation of an amorphous, white, noncrystalline powder called "taxine" originated from an analysis of alkaloid content from yew foliage (*T. baccata* L.) in 1856 by Lucas. It was isolated in crystalline form approximately 20 years later by Marmé, a French scientist (Hilger and Brande, 1890). However, it was not until 1956 that Graf and Boeddeker discovered that taxine was a mixture of heterogeneous compounds. Further investigations using electrophoretic analyses of taxine extracts revealed two major bands, thus recognizing the presence of two major types of taxine alkaloids: taxine A and taxine B (Graf, 1956). The farthest migrating electrophoretic band was designated taxine A, which comprised approximately 1.3% of the total alkaloid extract. The other electrophoretic band, taxine B, represented approximately 30% of the total alkaloid fraction extracted from *T. baccata* L. (Graf, 1956; Graf and Bertholdt, 1957). Subsequent analyses elucidated the molecular and structural formula of taxine A as well as its basic physical and chemical properties (Graf and Bertholdt, 1957; Graf et al., 1982). A structural analog of taxine A, 2-deacetyltaxine A ($C_{33}H_{45}NO_9$), was isolated from the leaves of *T. baccata* in 1994 (Poupat et al., 1994). The chemical and structural properties of taxine A and 2-deacetyltaxine A are given in Table 66.1 and Fig. 66.1. Although the preliminary structure of taxine B was first reported in 1986 (Graf et al., 1986), the molecular and structural formulas were not completely elucidated until 1991 (Ettouati et al., 1991). Purified taxine fractions from various *Taxus* spp. revealed the presence of several taxine B-related compounds. Isotaxine B ($C_{33}H_{45}NO_8$), a structural isomer of taxine B, is present as a major constituent in the alkaloid fractions (Poupat et al., 1994; Jenniskens et al., 1996; Potier et al., 1997; Adeline et al., 1997). Present as minor constituents in *Taxus* spp. are 1-deoxytaxine B and 1-deoxyisotaxine B (Fig. 66.2) (Jenniskens et al., 1996; Potier et al., 1997). The physical properties and chemical structures for taxine B and isoforms of taxine B are detailed in Table 66.1 and Fig. 66.2. Other minor constituents, comprising approximately 2% of the total concentration, are the taxine B pseudoalkaloids 13-deoxo-13α-acetyloxytaxine B ($C_{35}H_{49}NO_9$), 13-deoxo-13α-acetyloxy-1-deoxytaxine B ($C_{35}H_{49}NO_8$), and 13-deoxo-13α-acetyloxy-1-deoxy-nortaxine B ($C_{34}H_{47}NO_8$) (Appendino et al., 1997).

Veterinary Toxicology. DOI: http://dx.doi.org/10.1016/B978-0-12-811410-0.00066-0

TABLE 66.1 Physical and Chemical Properties of Taxine Alkaloids

Taxine	Molecular Formula	Melting Point (°C)	UV Maximum (nm)	IR Maximum (cm^{-1})
Taxine A	$C_{35}H_{47}NO_{10}$	204–206	220, 255	1780, 1250
2-Deacetyltaxine A	$C_{33}H_{45}NO_9$	–	224, 264	1734, 1691
Taxine B	$C_{33}H_{45}NO_8$	115	210, 277	3578, 1730
Isotaxine B	$C_{33}H_{45}NO_8$	–	282	–

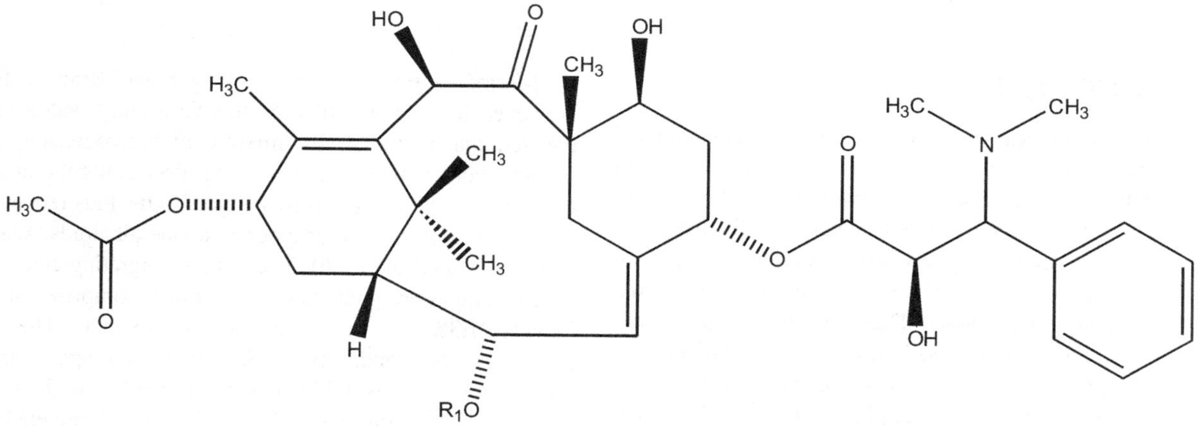

Taxine alkaloids	R_1
Taxine A	Ac
2-Deacetyltaxine A	H

FIGURE 66.1 Structural formulas for taxines A.

PHARMACOKINETICS/TOXICOKINETICS

For reasons likely related to their acute toxicity and lack of pharmaceutical uses, pharmacokinetic studies on taxine alkaloids have not been well characterized. However, extensive pharmacokinetic studies have been reported for the widely used antineoplastic drugs paclitaxel (isolated from *T. brevifolia*) and docetaxel (synthesized via a taxane precursor from *T. baccata*), which are also members of the taxane diterpenoid family. These studies revealed that both compounds are highly protein bound (>95%) in the serum and are metabolized by hepatic P450 enzymes. One differentiating characteristic noted was that paclitaxel exhibits nonlinear kinetics at therapeutic doses, whereas the kinetics of docetaxel are linear. The linear kinetics of docetaxel is thought to be the result of metabolism by CYP 3A4 to pharmacologically inactive oxidation products that are excreted in the bile through a p-glycoprotein–dependent mechanism (Gustafson et al., 2003; Baker et al., 2006). Tissue distribution is extensive, except for the central nervous system (CNS) and testes. The elimination half-life for paclitaxel is 5–7 h (two-compartment model) or 20 h (three-compartment model), whereas the elimination half-life for docetaxel is 12 h (two-compartment model) or 13 h (three-compartment model). Liver insufficiency or coadministration of compounds that modulate P450 activity may influence the activity of these antineoplastic drugs and, presumably, the activity of more acutely toxic members of the family, such as taxines A and B (Brown, 2003).

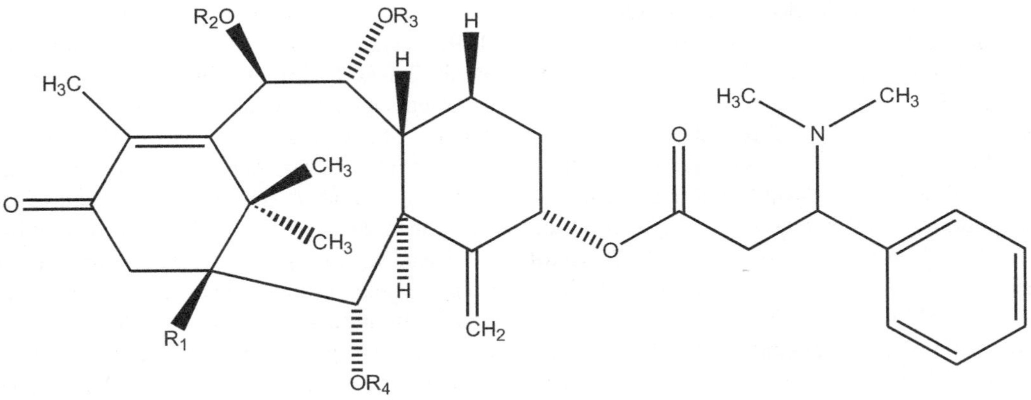

Taxine alkaloids	R_1	R_2	R_3	R_4
Taxine B	OH	Ac	H	H
Isotaxine B	OH	H	Ac	H
1-Deoxytaxine B	H	Ac	H	H
1-Deoxyisotaxine B	H	H	Ac	H

FIGURE 66.2 Structural formulas for taxines B.

PHYSIOLOGY/MECHANISM OF ACTION

Due to their instability and the lack of highly purified taxines A and B for experimental use, research delving into the mechanism of action of taxines frequently involved the use of crude extracts of taxines from yew. The earliest investigations were published in 1921 and described cardiovascular effects upon administration of crude extracts of yew. When administered by intraperitoneal or intravenous routes in rabbits and dogs, hypotension and cardiac arrest occurred in both species (Bryan-Brown, 1932). In addition, when toxicity was severe enough to result in cardiac abnormalities, it was noted that peristaltic contractions in the gastrointestinal tract ceased. Electrocardiographs conducted on isolated, perfused hearts from rabbits and frogs revealed that crude taxine extracts gradually induced bradycardia, resulting in diastolic cardiac arrest. Further investigations have indicated that taxines depress atrioventricular conduction in a dose-dependent manner in isolated frog heart, having the greatest effect on ventricular rate (Smythies et al., 1975; Tekol and Kameyama, 1987). In those studies, the cardiotoxic effect could not be inhibited by the administration of atropine, performing a vagotomy, or through ganglionic/adrenergic blockade (Bryan-Brown, 1932; Vohora, 1972). It was thus concluded that the hypotension induced by taxine extracts was not mediated via the sympathetic or parasympathetic nervous systems but, rather, by a direct action on myocardium (Vohora, 1972).

Significant differences in the cardiotoxicity of taxine A and taxine B have been reported (Bauereis and Steiert, 1959; Alloatti et al., 1996). Through administration of taxine B either in vivo or in vitro, it was shown that taxine B is more cardiotoxic than taxine A, causing inotropic effects while eliciting marked changes in atrioventricular conduction. In isolated, perfused guinea pig hearts, a 5 μM concentration of taxine B markedly increased atrioventricular conduction time and widening of the QRS interval, whereas a 1 μM concentration (the lowest concentration used) significantly reduced heart rate (Alloatti et al., 1996). These changes led to atrioventricular conduction blocks and complete diastolic cardiac arrest. The marked increase in QRS duration has also been reported one human case of yew poisoning and also in intravenous administrations of yew extracts to pigs (Matthew et al., 1993; Ruha et al., 2002). Taxine B has been shown to cause a marked reduction in the maximum rate of depolarization of the action potential in isolated papillary muscle, which thus resembles the action of class I antiarrhythmic drugs (e.g., flecainide, procainamide, and quinidine) (Bauereis and Steiert, 1959; Tekol, 1985; Alloatti et al., 1996). In contrast, taxine A had a minimal effect on atrioventricular conduction time and QRS duration. Even at the highest concentration used (10 μM), taxine A induced only mild reductions in heart rate (Alloatti et al., 1996).

More detailed investigations of the effects of taxine extracts on cardiomyocytes and axons indicated that taxines cause an increase in cytoplasmic calcium, acting as calcium and sodium channel antagonists (Smythies et al., 1975; Tekol, 1985; Tekol and Kameyama, 1987; Tekol and Gögüsten, 1999). In addition, isolated aorta, atrium, and jejunum from rabbits were used to compare the cardioselectivity of taxines to verapamil, a known calcium channel antagonist. From these experiments, Tekol and Gögüsten concluded that the mechanism of action of taxines is primarily based on calcium channel antagonistic properties. Therefore, it is likely that the toxicity of taxines in animals and humans also occurs through the same mechanism.

Taxine alkaloids have minimal toxic effects on other organs. In the few studies reported, crude taxine extracts have some adverse effects on involuntary muscle, but not on voluntary muscle. Uterine contractions, relaxation of the intestines, and contraction of the duodenum and ileum have been noted in experimental animals dosed with yew extracts (Bryan-Brown, 1932; Vohora, 1972). Tekol and Gögüsten (1999) reported that taxine sulfate inhibited peristaltic movement in rabbit jejunum, with a median inhibitory concentration (IC_{50}) of 1.86×10^{-5} g/mL.

TOXICITY

With the exception of the fleshy aril that surrounds the seed, all parts of the yew plant contain taxine alkaloids and are extremely poisonous. One study in laboratory rodents indicated that higher toxicity was found in the stems compared to the needles (leaves) (Shanker et al., 2002). Although maximal concentrations occur during the winter (Watt and Breyer-Brandwijk, 1962), toxic amounts of taxines remain in the plants throughout the year and are not appreciably decreased by drying (Alden et al., 1977). It has been reported that the cardiotoxic taxines A and B are relatively abundant in English yew (*T. baccata*) and Japanese yew (*T. cuspidata*), but only minimal amounts are found in Pacific yew (*T. brevifolia*) (Tyler, 1960; Suffness, 1995; Brown, 2003).

Clinical cases resulting in poisoning are often accidental and are frequently a result of livestock or animals being unwittingly fed clippings from yew bushes. Yew intoxication has been reported in cattle (Casteel and Cook, 1985; Panter et al., 1993), horses (Tiwary et al., 2005), sheep (Rae and Binnington, 1995) and goats (Coenen and Bahrs, 1994), dogs (Evans and Cook, 1991; Taksdal, 1994), a bear (Bacciarini et al., 1999), fallow deer (Wacker, 1983), a moose (Handeland, 2008), emus (Fiedler and Perron, 1994), budgies (Shropshire et al., 1992), canaries (Arai et al., 1992), and monkeys (Lacasse et al., 2007). It is interesting to note that yew (*T. baccata*) is often eaten by white-tailed deer and roe deer in the United States without apparent adverse effects (Weaver and Brown, 2004; Angus, 2010). This may be due, in part, to increased ruminal detoxification of the taxines present in the yew (Weaver and Brown, 2004).

Because of the difficulties in obtaining purified, stable taxines in quantities sufficient for mammalian studies, in the past, minimum lethal dose (LD_{min}) values were assessed through the oral administration of yew leaves and branches (Watt and Breyer-Brandwijk, 1962; Clarke and Clarke, 1988). Estimating that 1 g of yew leaves contains approximately 5 mg of taxines (Smythies et al., 1975; Tekol, 1985; Jenniskens et al., 1996; Tekol and Gögüsten, 1999), minimal toxic doses of taxines (mg/kg body weight) in animals can be estimated and are summarized in Table 66.2. The body weights of the animals listed are average values for adult animals only (Spector, 1956). From Table 66.2, it is evident that the minimal toxic dose of taxines varies among species. Comparatively, horses are more sensitive (LD_{min} of 1.0–2.0 mg/kg) and chickens are least sensitive (LD_{min} of 82.5 mg/kg) to yew toxins.

Adverse clinical signs in animals can vary depending on the amount of yew ingested. However, in most cases of acute poisoning, animals are often found dead within 24 h or fewer after ingestion without demonstrating abnormal behavior or adverse signs of toxicity. In subacute poisonings, which have been reported infrequently, clinical signs may include ataxia, bradycardia, dyspnea, muscle tremors, recumbency, and convulsions leading to collapse and death (Evers and Link, 1972; Casteel and Cook, 1985; Veatch et al., 1988; Evans and Cook, 1991; Tekol, 1991; Arai et al., 1992).

In cases of deliberate yew poisoning in humans, adverse symptoms of toxicity are similar to those reported in animals. Documented clinical signs in humans include dizziness, mydriasis, nausea, vomiting, diffuse abdominal pain, tachycardia (initially), severe right ventricular dilatation with biventricular dysfunction, muscle weakness, and convulsions (Blyth, 1884; Czerwek and Fischer, 1960; Fröhne and Pribilla, 1965; Schulte, 1975; Wilson et al., 2001; Panzeri et al., 2010). In some cases, these symptoms proceed to bradycardia, bradypnea, diastolic cardiac standstill, or death (Blyth, 1884; Fröhne and Pribilla, 1965; Schulte, 1975; Sinn and Porterfield, 1991).

DIAGNOSIS

Diagnosis of yew poisoning in animals is frequently based on history of exposure. Frequently, poisoning is associated with pruning bushes and then feeding the trimmings to the livestock. In some cases, yew fragments (sometimes

TABLE 66.2 Oral Lethal Doses of Yew Leaves in Animals

Animal	Estimated Average Body Weight (kg)[a]	LD_{min} of Yew Leaves (g)	LD_{min} (g Yew Leaves/kg Body Weight)	Estimated LD_{min} of Taxines (mg/kg Body Weight)[b,c,d]
Chicken	1.82	30	16.5	82.5
Cow	250	500	2.0	10.0
Dog	13	30	2.3	11.5
Goat	40	480	12.0	60.0
Horse	500	100–200	0.2–0.4	1.0–2.0
Pig	102	75	0.7	3.5
Sheep	40	100	2.5	12.5
Mouse	0.025	Not reported	Not reported	0.5 (s.c.)[e]
Rat	0.25	Not reported	Not reported	5.0 (s.c.)[e]
Human	80	50–100	0.6–1.3	3.0–6.5
Rabbit	2.5	1.75	0.7	3.5

[a]*Estimated average body weights of adult animals in this table referenced in Spector (1956).*
[b]*Clarke and Clarke (1988).*
[c]*Tekol (1991), Tekol and Gögüsten (1999).*
[d]*Watt and Breyer-Brandwijk (1962).*
[e]*Mose and rat LD_{min}s are based on subcutaneous (s.c.) dose.*

visible only by microscopic examination) are found in the mouth, stomach content, rumen content, and/or small intestine (Frommherz et al., 2006; Lacasse et al., 2007; Handeland, 2008; Panzeri et al., 2010). Occasionally, exposure may be indicated in the history but gross identification of intact plant material is not observed. This can be especially true in species, such as horses, that masticate their food more thoroughly. In these cases, diagnosis of taxine poisoning often requires a more detailed microscopic and/or chemical evaluation of the gastrointestinal contents (Karns, 1983; Tiwary et al., 2005).

Chemical analysis of biological samples using gas chromatography/mass spectroscopy (GC/MS) or liquid chromatography/mass spectroscopy (LC/MS) has been successful in diagnosing some cases of yew poisoning in mammals (Stahr et al., 1977; Kite et al., 2000; Tiwary et al., 2005). LC/MS has been used to detect taxine B and isotaxine B in blood (Beike et al., 2003; Frommherz et al., 2006) and taxines A and B from yew plant fragments (Hough et al., 2010). GC/MS and LC/MS detection of 3,5-dimethoxyphenol, an aglycone metabolite of taxicatine, has been used as a unique marker for yew exposure in mammals. 3,5-Dimethoxyphenol has been detected in blood, serum, urine, bile, and gastric contents from mammals exposed to yew plants (Froldi et al., 2010; Panzeri et al., 2010; Kobusiak-Prokopowicz et al., 2016).

At postmortem examination, there are no lesions that are pathognomonic in animals that have died due to yew toxicosis. Indeed, neither gross nor microscopic abnormalities (with the exception of large pieces of yew leaves and stems, if they are present in the gastrointestinal tract) are observed (Kingsbury, 1964; Alden et al., 1977; Ogden, 1988; Rooks, 1994). An exception to this is one case of yew poisoning in a horse in which ecchymotic hemorrhages were visible grossly along the endocardial surfaces of the ventricles, and microscopically, mild multifocal necrosis of the myocardium was identified in the ventricular wall and papillary muscles of the heart (Tiwary et al., 2005). In subacute poisonings, gastroenteritis may be evident; however, the inflammation is probably due to irritant oils present in the yew and not due to taxine alkaloids (Watt and Breyer-Brandwijk, 1962; Kingsbury, 1964; Evans and Cook, 1991). Rarely, other gross changes have been reported at necropsy, including moderate to severe rumenitis, superficial hemorrhages in the right ventricular myocardium and right atrium, and mild focal interstitial myocarditis (Ogden, 1988; Panter et al., 1993). There have been two reports of presumptive, chronic toxicity in cattle in which, histologically, areas of the myocardium were observed to be replaced with fibrous connective tissue consistent with myocardial necrosis (Burcham et al., 2013; Sula et al., 2013).

In cases of yew poisoning in humans, the gross anatomic observations documented include acute congestion of internal organs, cerebral edema, and hemorrhagic pulmonary edema (Beike et al., 2003; Wehner and Gawatz, 2003). In these cases, histology of the myocardium revealed interstitial edema, positive staining for troponin C with depletion in areas of the left ventricle, and alveolar hemorrhagic edema.

TREATMENT

Death is frequently the first adverse clinical sign in animals that have eaten toxic amounts of yew; therefore, opportunities to treat exposed animals are rare. However, in instances in which known ingestion has recently occurred, it is important to remove the plant material from the gastrointestinal tract and limit absorption. Rumenotomy, followed by replacement therapy with a mixture of mineral oil, electrolytes, activated charcoal, and alfalfa pellets, has been effective in treating some cases of yew poisoning in ruminants (Casteel and Cook, 1985). There is no specific antidote for taxine poisoning; however, atropine or lidocaine have been suggested to be beneficial in alleviating the cardiotoxicity (Kingsbury, 1964; Schulte, 1975). In experimental animal studies (Bryan-Brown, 1932; Vohora, 1972) and in human cases in which the cardiac responses to attempted treatment were closely monitored via electrocardiography, classic antiarrhythmic therapy proved ineffective (Willaert et al., 2002). Extreme extracorporeal life-support measures, in combination with antiarrhythmic therapy, were warranted for complete recovery in one case of yew intoxication (Panzeri et al., 2010).

CONCLUDING REMARKS AND FUTURE DIRECTIONS

Although advances in analytical toxicology are progressively improving detection of taxine alkaloids and other markers for diagnosis of yew poisoning, toxicoses in animals and humans still occur frequently and are usually fatal. The potent cardiotoxic effects of taxine alkaloids in the yew plant, combined with the absence of an efficacious treatment for poisoning cases, reemphasizes the need to prevent or limit exposure of animals and livestock to these toxic plants.

REFERENCES

Adeline, M.T., Wang, X.P., Poupat, C., et al., 1997. Evaluation of taxoids from *Taxus* sp. crude extracts by high performance liquid chromatography. J. Liq. Chromatogr. Rel. Technol. 20 (19), 3135–3145.

Alden, C.L., Fosnaugh, C.J., Smith, J.B., Mohan, R., 1977. Japanese yew poisoning in large domestic animals in the Midwest. J. Am. Vet. Med. Assoc. 170 (3), 314–316.

Alloatti, G., Penna, C., Levi, R.C., et al., 1996. Effects of yew alkaloids and related compounds on guinea-pig isolated perfused heart and papillary muscle. Life Sci. 58 (10), 845–854.

Angus, K.W., 2010. Apparent low toxicity of yew for roe deer (*Capreolus capreolus*). Vet. Rec. 166 (7), 216.

Appendino, G., Özen, H., Fenoglio, I., et al., 1997. Pseudoalkaloid taxanes from *Taxus baccata*. Phytochemistry. 33 (6), 1521–1523.

Arai, M., Stauber, E., Shropshire, C.M., 1992. Evaluation of selected plants for their toxic effects in canaries. J. Am. Vet. Med. Assoc. 200 (9), 1329–1331.

Bacciarini, L.N., Wenker, C.J., Muller, M., Iten, P., 1999. Yew (*Taxus baccata*) intoxication in a captive brown bear (*Ursus arctos*). Eur. J. Vet. Pathool. 5 (1), 29–32.

Baker, S.D., Sparreboom, A., Verweij, J., 2006. Clinical pharmacokinetics of docetaxel: recent developments. Clin. Pharmacokin. 45 (3), 235–252.

Bauereis, V.R., Steiert, W., 1959. Pharmakologische eigenschaften von taxin A und B. Arzneim. Forschung. 9, 77–79.

Beike, J., Karger, B., Meiners, T., et al., 2003. LC-MS determination of *Taxus* alkaloids in biological specimens. Int. J. Legal Med. 117, 335–339.

Blyth, A.W., 1884. Taxine. Poisons: Their Effects and Detection. Charles Griffin, London, pp. 383–384.

Brown, D.T., 2003. Preclinical and clinical studies of the taxanes. In: Itokawa, H., Lee, K.-H. (Eds.), Taxus: The Genus Taxus. Taylor & Francis, New York, NY, pp. 387–435.

Bryan-Brown, T., 1932. The pharmacological actions of taxine. Quart. J. Pharm. Pharmacol. 5, 205–219.

Burcham, G.N., Becker, K.J., Tahara, J.M., et al., 2013. Myocarcial fibrosis associated with previous ingestion of yew (*Taxus* sp.) in an Holstein heifer: evidence for chronic yew toxicity. J. Vet. Diagn. Invest. 25 (1), 147–152.

Casteel, S.W., Cook, W.O., 1985. Japanese yew poisoning in ruminants. Modern Vet. Pract. 66, 875–876.

Clarke, E.G.C., Clarke, M.L., 1988. Poisonous plants, Taxaceae, Veterinary Toxicology. third ed. Baillière, Tindall & Cassell, London, pp. 276–277.

Coenen, M., Bahrs, F., 1994. Fatal yew poisoning in goats as a result of ingestion of foliage from garden prunings. Deut. Tier. Wochen. 101 (9), 364–367.

Czerwek, H., Fischer, W., 1960. Tödlicher vergiftungsfall mit *Taxus baccata*. Arch. Toxikol. 18, 88–92.

Ettouati, B., Ahond, A., Poupat, C., Potier, P., 1991. Révision structurale de la taxine B, alcaloïde majoritaire des feuilles de L'if d'Europe, *Taxus baccata*. J. Nat. Prod. 54 (5), 1455–1458.

Evans, K.L., Cook, J.R., 1991. Japanese yew poisoning in a dog. J. Am. Anim. Hosp. Assoc. 27, 300–302.

Evers, R.A., Link, R.P., 1972. Yews, *Taxus* species. Poisonous Plants of the Midwest and Their Effects on Livestock. University of Illinois, Champaign, IL, pp. 81–82.

Fiedler, H.H., Perron, R.M., 1994. Yew poisoning in Australian emus (*Dromarius novaehollandiae* LATHAM). Berl. Munch. Tierarzl. Wochenschr. 107 (2), 50–52.

Foster, S., Duke, J., 1990. American yew. Eastern/Central Medicinal Plants. Houghton Mifflin, Boston, MA, p. 226.

Fröhne, D., Pfänder, J., 1984. Taxaceae, *Taxus baccata* L., yew, A Colour Atlas of Poisonous Plants. second ed. Wolfe, London, pp. 223–225.

Fröhne, D., Pribilla, O., 1965. Tödliche Vergiftung mit *Taxus baccata*. Arch. Toxikol. 21, 150–162.

Froldi, R., Croci, P.F., Dell'Acqua, L., et al., 2010. Preliminary gas chromatography with mass spectrometry determination of 3,5-dimethoxyphenol in biological specimens as evidence of *Taxus* poisoning. J. Anal. Toxicol. 34, 53–56.

Frommherz, L., Kintz, P., Kijewski, H., et al., 2006. Quantitative determination of taxine B in body fluids by LC-MS-MS. Int. J. Legal Med. 120, 346–351.

Graf, E., 1956. Zur chemie des taxins. Angew. Chem. 68, 249–250.

Graf, E., Bertholdt, H., 1957. Das amorphe taxin und das kristallisierte taxin A. Pharm. Zentralhalle. 96, 385–395.

Graf, E., Boeddeker, H., 1956. Zur kenntnis der -dimethylamino-hydrozimtsäure. Arch. Pharm. Ber. Deutsch. Pharm. Ges. 289, 364–370.

Graf, E., Kirkel, A., Wolf, G.J., Breitmaier, E., 1982. Die aufklärung von taxin A aus *Taxus baccata* L. Liebigs Annal. Chem.376–381.

Graf, E., Weinandy, S., Koch, B., Breitmaier, E., 1986. ^{13}C-NMR-untersuchung von taxin B aus *Taxus baccata* L. Liebigs Annal. Chem.1147–1151.

Gustafson, D.L., Long, M.E., Zirrolli, J.A., et al., 2003. Analysis of docetaxel pharmacokinetics in humans with the inclusion of later sampling time-points afforded by the use of a sensitive tandem LCMS assay. Cancer Chemother. Pharmacol. 52, 159–166.

Handeland, K., 2008. Acute yew (*Taxus*) poisoning in a moose (*Alces alces*). Toxicon. 52 (7), 829–832.

Hartzell, H., 1995. Yew and us: a brief history of the yew tree. In: Suffness, M. (Ed.), Taxol: Science and Applications. CRC Press, Boca Raton, FL, pp. 27–34.

Hilger, A., Brande, F., 1890. Ueber taxin, das alkaloïd des eibenbaumes (*Taxus baccata*). Ber. Deutsch. Chem. Ges. 23, 464–468.

Hough, R.L., Crews, C., White, D., et al., 2010. Degradation of yew, ragwort, and rhododendron toxins during composting. Sci. Total Environ. 408, 4128–4137.

Jenniskens, L.H.D., van Rozendaal, E.L.M., van Beek, T.A., 1996. Identification of six taxine alkaloids from *Taxus baccata* needles. J. Nat. Prod. 5, 117–123.

Karns, P.A., 1983. Intoxication in horses due to ingestion of Japanese yew (*Taxus cuspidata*). Eq. Pract. 5 (1), 12–14.

Kingsbury, J.M., 1964. Taxaceae. Poisonous Plants of the United States and Canada. Prentice-Hall, New Jersey, pp. 121–123.

Kite, G.C., Lawrence, T.J., Dauncey, E.A., 2000. Detecting Taxus poisoning in horses using liquid chromatography/mass spectrometry. Vet. Human Toxicol. 42 (3), 151–154.

Kobusiak-Prokopowicz, M., Marciniak, A., Slusarczyk, S., et al., 2016. A suicide attempt by intoxication with *Taxus baccata* leaves with ultra-fast liquid chromatography-electrospray ionization-tandem mass spectrometry, analysis of patient serum and different plants samples: case report. BMC Pharmacol. Toxicol. 17 (41), 1–8.

Lacasse, C., Gamble, K.C., Poppenga, R.H., et al., 2007. *Taxus* sp. intoxication in three Fracois' langurs (*Trachypithecus francoisi*). J. Vet. Diagn. Invest. 19, 221–224.

Lucas, H., 1856. Ueber ein in den blätter von *Taxus baccata* L. enhaltenes alkaloid (das taxin). Arch. Pharm. 135, 145–149.

Matthew, N., Elsner, G., Purdy, C., Zipes, D.P., 1993. Wide QRS rhythm due to taxine toxicity. J. Cardiovasc. Electrophysiol. 3, 59–61.

Ogden, L., 1988. *Taxus* (yews): a highly toxic plant. Vet. Human Toxicol. 30 (6), 563–564.

Panter, K.E., Molyneux, R.J., Smart, R.A., et al., 1993. English yew poisoning in 43 cattle. J. Am. Vet. Med. Assoc. 202 (9), 1476–1477.

Panzeri, C., Bacis, G., Ferri, F., et al., 2010. Extracorporeal life support in a severe *Taxus baccata* poisoning. Clin. Toxicol. 48, 463–465.

Potier, C.R., Poujol, H., Ahond, A., et al., 1997. Taxoïdes: Nouveaux analogues du 7-déshydroxydocétaxel préparés à partir des alcaloïdes de I'lf. Tetrahedron. 53 (14), 5169–5184.

Poupat, C., Ahond, A., Potier, P., 1994. Nouveau taxoïde basique isolé des feuilles d'if, *Taxus baccata*: La 2-désacétyltaxine A. J. Nat. Prod. 57 (10), 1468–1469.

Rae, C.A., Binnington, B.D., 1995. Yew poisoning in sheep. Can. Vet. J. 36 (7), 446.

Rooks, J.S., 1994. Japanese yew toxicity. Vet. Med. 89, 950–951.

Ruha, A.M., Tanen, D.A., Graeme, K.A., et al., 2002. Hypertonic sodium bicarbonate for *Taxus* media-induced cardiac toxicity in swine. Acad. Emer. Med. 9 (3), 179–185.

Schulte, T., 1975. Tödliche vergiftung mit eibennadeln (*Taxus baccata*). Arch. Toxikol. 34, 153–158.

Shanker, K., Pathak, N.K.R., Trivedi, V.P., et al., 2002. An evaluation of toxicity of *Taxus baccata* Linn. (Talispatra) in experimental animals. J. Ethnopharmacol. 79, 69–73.

Shropshire, C.M., Stauber, E., Arai, M., 1992. Evaluation of selected plants for acute toxicosis in budgerigars. J. Am. Vet. Med. Assoc. 200 (7), 936–939.

Sinn, L.E., Porterfield, J.F., 1991. Fatal taxine poisoning from yew leaf ingestion. J. Forensic Sci. 36 (2), 599–601.

Smythies, J.R., Benington, F., Morin, R.D., et al., 1975. The action of the alkaloids from yew (*Taxus baccata*) on the action potential in the *Xenopus* medullated axon. Experentia. 31, 337–338.

Spector, W.S., 1956. Handbook of Biological Data. Wright–Patterson Air Force Base, OH.

Stahr, H.M., Hyde, W., Kiesey, J., Ross, P.F., 1977. Alkaloids: extraction and qualitative identification. Analytical Methods in Toxicology. Iowa State University Press, Iowa, pp. 178–183.

Suffness, M., 1995. Taxol: Science and Applications. CRC Press, Florida, pp. 7-8, 311–312.

Sula, M.J.M., Morgan, S., Bailey, K.L., et al., 2013. Characterization of cardiac lesions in calves after ingestion of Japanese yew (Taxus cuspidata). J. Vet. Diagn. Invest. 25, 522–526.

Taksdal, T., 1994. Diagnoses from the Norwegian State Veterinary Laboratory. Norsk Vet. 106 (4), 305–306.

Tekol, Y., 1985. Negative chronotopic and atrioventricular blocking effects of taxine on isolated frog heart and its acute toxicity in mice. Planta Med. 5, 357–360.

Tekol, Y., 1991. Acute toxicity of taxine in mice and rats. Vet. Human Toxicol. 33 (4), 337–338.

Tekol, Y., Gögüsten, B., 1999. Comparative determination of the cardioselectivity of taxine and verapamil in the isolated aorta, atrium, and jejunum preparations of rabbits. Arzneim. Forschung. 49 (8), 673–678.

Tekol, Y., Kameyama, M., 1987. Elektrophysiologische untersuchungen über den wirkungsmechanisms des eibentoxins taxin auf das herz. Arzneim. Forschung. 37 (4), 428–431.

Tiwary, A.K., Puschner, B., Kinde, H., Tor, E.R., 2005. Diagnosis of Taxus (yew) poisoning in a horse. J. Vet. Diagn. Invest. 17 (3), 252–255.

Tyler, V.E., 1960. Note on the occurrence of taxine in *Taxus brevifolia*. J. Am. Pharm. Assoc.683–684.

Veatch, J.K., Reid, F.M., Kennedy, G.A., 1988. Differentiating yew poisoning from other toxicoses. Vet. Med. 83, 298–300.

Vohora, S.B., 1972. Studies on *Taxus baccata*. Planta Med. 22 (1), 59–65.

Wacker, R., 1983. Yew poisoning in fallow deer. Tierarztliche Umschau. 38 (4), 267–268.

Watt, J.M., Breyer-Brandwijk, M.G., 1962. Taxaceae. The Medicinal and Poisonous Plants of Southern and Eastern Africa. Livingstone, Edinburgh, pp. 1019–1022.

Weaver, J.D., Brown, D.L., 2004. Incubation of European yew (*Taxus baccata*) with white-tailed deer (*Odocoileus virginianus*) rumen fluid reduces taxine A concentrations. Vet. Human Toxicol. 46 (6), 300–302.

Wehner, F., Gawatz, O., 2003. Suicidal yew poisoning: From Caesar to today – or suicide instructions on the Internet. Arch. Kriminol. 211 (1–2), 19–26.

Willaert, W., Claessens, P., Vankelecom, B., Vanderheyden, M., 2002. Intoxication with *Taxus baccata*: cardiac arrhythmias following yew leaves ingestion. Pacing Clin. Electrophysiol. 25 (4), 511–512.

Wilson, C.R., Sauer, J.M., Hooser, S.B., 2001. Taxines: a review of the mechanism and toxicity of yew (*Taxus* spp.) alkaloids. Toxicon. 39, 175–185.

Chapter 67

Mushroom Toxins

Birgit Puschner

INTRODUCTION

Management of mushroom poisonings of humans and animals can demand extensive effort from clinicians and toxicologists and often involves emotion and publicity. The public expects the toxicology profession to provide guidance and a coherent approach regarding these cases. Although it is estimated that very few species are lethal, it is not clear how many of the mushrooms worldwide contain potentially toxic compounds. New species are being discovered continuously, and for many species, toxicity data are unavailable. It is very difficult to establish a confirmed diagnosis of mushroom poisoning in animals; thus, clinical reports of mushroom poisoning are uncommon. In fact, because animals are at much greater risk of exposure to toxic mushrooms than are humans, mushroom poisonings in animals are most likely underreported.

BACKGROUND

The reported frequency of mushroom poisonings in veterinary medicine is low because routine diagnostic methods to confirm exposure are lacking. Most cases are diagnosed by positive identification of the suspect mushroom along with the occurrence of consistent clinical signs and clinicopathological changes. Animals are often left unattended, and a history of mushroom ingestion is not available. An estimated 200–300 calls related to mushroom ingestions have been registered each year by animal poison control centers in the United States. California accounts for more than 10% of these cases, the highest among all states. California also leads the United States in the number of reported cases of mushroom ingestions in humans; 894 cases were reported in 2008. Many factors influence the toxicity of mushroom toxins, such as genus and species of mushroom, the season and geographic location, preparation of mushroom prior to ingestion, and the individual's susceptibility. Although not inclusive of all mushroom toxins, this chapter is organized by the various types of toxins, providing detailed information on their toxic mechanisms, toxicokinetics, and diagnostic and therapeutic approaches, with a focus on veterinary medicine.

HEPATOTOXIC CYCLOPEPTIDES

Worldwide, most fatalities are caused by exposure to cyclopeptides. Three genera—*Amanita*, *Galerina*, and *Lepiota* (Lincoff and Mitchel, 1977a)—are known to contain hepatotoxic cyclopeptides, with *Amanita phalloides*, the ubiquitous death cap or death angel, and *Galerina sulpices* being considered the most toxic worldwide. *A. phalloides* (Fig. 67.1) is found throughout North America, commonly in association with oaks, birch, and pine, and it is the species most frequently resulting in fatalities in humans (Mitchel, 1980; Barbato, 1993) and probably dogs. It can also be found in open pastures. *A. phalloides* is particularly common in the San Francisco Bay area, the Pacific Northwest, and the Northeast, and it is most abundant in warm, wet years. The large fruiting bodies appear in the late summer and fall, and they have

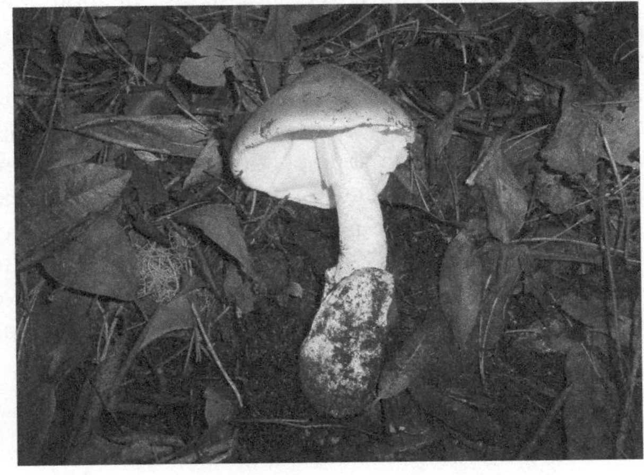

FIGURE 67.1 *Amanita phalloides. Courtesy of Dr. R. Michael Davis, University of California at Davis.*

Veterinary Toxicology. DOI: http://dx.doi.org/10.1016/B978-0-12-811410-0.00067-2

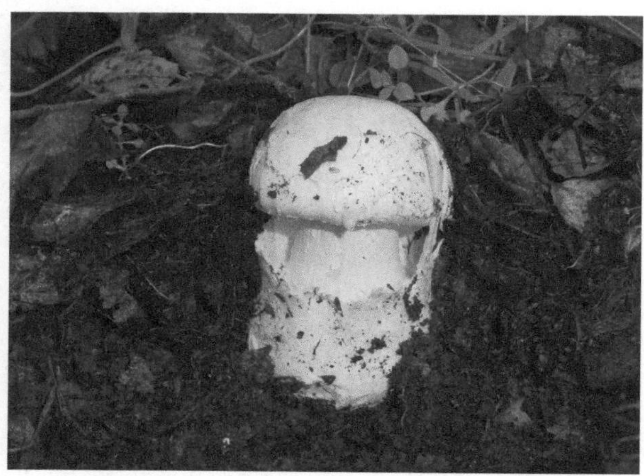

FIGURE 67.2 *Amanita ocreata. Courtesy of Dr. R. Michael Davis, University of California at Davis.*

several characteristics: a smooth, yellowish-green to yellowish-brown cap; white gills; a white ring around the upper part of the stem (veil); and a white cuplike structure (volva) around the base of the stem. *Amanita ocreata* (Fig. 67.2) is commonly known as western North American destroying angel and grows from Baja California, Mexico, along the Pacific Coast to Washington. *A. ocreata* is most commonly found in sandy soils under oak or pine and has caused fatalities in dogs (B. Puschner, unpublished data). The fruiting bodies are usually found in late winter and spring. *A. ocreata* has a white or cream-colored cap; white, short gills; a white stem with a white, thin, broken, partial veil (annulus); and a white, thin volva. *Amanita bisporigera*, *Galerina autumnalis*, and *Lepiota josserandii* have also been attributed to animal and human deaths in North America (Beug, 2009). In Eastern Europe, *G. sulpices* is considered the species most commonly associated with human fatalities, followed by *A. phalloides* (Klan, 1993). There are three groups of cyclopeptides: the amatoxins, phallotoxins, and virotoxins. Amatoxins are bicyclic octapeptides and include the amanitins (α-, β-, γ-, and ε-amanitins), amanin, amanullin, and proamanullin (Vetter, 1998). Severe poisonings and lethality are mainly attributable to the amanitins. The bicyclic heptapeptides phallotoxins were once thought to be the cause of gastrointestinal clinical signs; however, they are no longer believed to exert any acute toxicity. Although research is limited, bicyclic heptapeptides virotoxins are not considered to have toxic effects after oral exposure. Therefore, phallotoxins and virotoxins are not discussed further.

PHARMACOKINETICS/TOXICOKINETICS

Exact data on the bioavailability for amanitins are lacking, although there are known species differences (Faulstich and Fauser, 1980). The bioavailability of amanitins appears to be much greater in humans than in rodents, dogs, and rabbits. Within animal species, the absorption rate of amanitins is estimated to be much greater in dogs than in mice and rabbits, and rats appear resistant to the toxic effects of amanitins. α-Amanitin is taken up by cells in the gastrointestinal tract, where the first damaging effects are seen (Gundala et al., 2004). Following systemic absorption, α-amanitin is taken up by hepatocytes via OATP1B3, an organic anion-transporting polypeptide (Letschert et al., 2006). The α-amanitin has a low volume of distribution. Renal clearance is high and rapid, and similar to the creatinine clearance (Faulstich et al., 1985). Following intravenous (i.v.) administration in dogs, it was shown that plasma half-life of amanitins is short, ranging from 25 to 50 min, and that amanitins are not detectable in plasma after 4–6 h. In pigs following intraportal administration of α-amanitin, systemic plasma and portal plasma amanitin concentrations declined to baseline levels within 24 h (Thiel et al., 2011). There is no known metabolism or plasma protein binding of the α-amanitin. Between 80% and 90% of the administered dose of amanitins is eliminated in urine, and up to 7% is eliminated in bile (Faulstich et al., 1985). After oral ingestion of *A. phalloides* in humans, α- and β-amanitins were detected in plasma up to 36 h after ingestion and in urine up to 72 h postexposure (Jaeger et al., 1993). This may partly be due to slow intestinal absorption, enterohepatic circulation, and reduced renal elimination resulting from nephrotoxicity. Plasma and urine amanitin concentrations do not seem to correlate with the clinical severity or outcome.

Amanitins can be detected in serum and urine well before any clinical sign of poisoning, whereas routine laboratory tests such as complete blood count and serum chemistry profiles are unremarkable until liver or kidney damage has occurred. Early recognition of exposure is critical because survival rates are greatly improved with timely therapeutic intervention. Amanitin concentrations in kidneys and livers of people ingesting *A. phalloides* have been detected up to 22 days postingestion. The kidneys contain higher concentrations than the liver, indicating that toxins are bound to renal tissue.

MECHANISM OF ACTION

Amanitins are of greatest significance because, unlike phalloidins, they are heat stable and are not degraded by the acid environment of the stomach or by freezing (Himmelmann et al., 2001). Therefore, amanitins are toxic by ingestion, whereas phalloidins have only been shown to be toxic when experimentally administered by parenteral routes. Amanitins exert their toxicity by inhibiting nuclear RNA polymerase II (Lindell et al., 1970;

Wieland, 1983). The decrease in mRNA and associated decrease in protein synthesis result in hepatocyte necrosis. Cells with a high metabolic rate, such as hepatocytes, crypt cells, and proximal convoluted tubules of the kidneys, are most commonly affected. Although this mechanism is well established, research has confirmed additional cellular effects that contribute to pathogenesis. In mice and cultured dog hepatocytes, apoptosis contributed to amanitin-induced liver failure (Leist et al., 1997; Magdalan et al., 2010b), and in pancreatic rat islets α-amanitin resulted in a dose-dependent insulin-releasing and a β-cytotoxic effect (De Carlo et al., 2003). Acute tubular necrosis in the kidneys is believed to be a result of reabsorption of amanitins by renal tubules after glomerular filtration.

The clinical course is divided into four phases, with the initial phase being the latency period of approximately 6–12 h. The second phase is characterized by severe gastrointestinal signs, such as nausea, vomiting, bloody diarrhea, and severe abdominal pain. In dogs, the onset of clinical signs is generally 6–24 h after mushroom ingestion. Beagles experimentally given an oral sublethal dose of amanitins developed vomiting and diarrhea at 16 h. Gastrointestinal signs improved after 60 h (Vogel et al., 1984). The gastroenteric phase is often followed by a lag period of several hours to a few days during which the human or animal will appear to have recovered. During this third phase, close monitoring of liver and kidney function is essential in order to prevent misdiagnosis. The final stage begins approximately 36–84 h after exposure to amanitins. In this stage, fulminant hepatic failure with subsequent coagulation disorders, encephalopathy, and renal failure may occur. In dogs, significant elevations in serum of aspartate aminotransferase (AST), alanine aminotransferase (ALT), alkaline phosphatase, and bilirubin are commonly observed (Vogel et al., 1984; Kallet et al., 1988). In humans, a combination of the prothrombin (PT) index along with serum creatinine concentrations determined between three and 10 days after ingestion was most useful as a predictor of death (Ganzert et al., 2005). Although no controlled study exists in dogs, PT and partial thromboplastin may provide critical information for case assessment (Tegzes and Puschner, 2002). In pigs, decreased albumin and total plasma protein concentrations in the first 24 to 24 h indicated a lethal outcome (Thiel et al., 2014). Clinical signs of renal failure include polyuria, polydypsia, vomiting, and anorexia. Severe hypoglycemia can occur in dogs after the gastrointestinal phase, and it is associated with the breakdown of liver glycogen (Puschner et al., 2007). In a study in which dogs were given lethal doses of amanitin toxins or pieces of *A. phalloides*, 50% of dogs died from hypoglycemia 1 or 2 days after exposure (Faulstich and Fauser, 1980). In clinical cases, dogs must be monitored closely for hypoglycemia, and treatment may be necessary. Clinical signs of hypoglycemia in dogs and cats include seizures, coma, and death. Finally, it is important to note that not all cases present with the classic four stages. In cases of large exposure to amanitins, or ingestion by puppies, the animal may die within 24 h (Cole, 1993).

TOXICITY

Amanitins are extremely toxic, and poisonings have been confirmed in dogs, horses (Beug, 2009), and cattle (Yee et al., 2012). The i.v. LD_{50} of α-amanitin in dogs is 0.1 mg/kg body weight (Faulstich et al., 1985). Based on an oral dosing study in dogs, the oral LD_{50} for methyl-γ-amanitin was estimated to be 0.5 mg/kg body weight. In mice and rats, the i.v. LD_{50} of α-amanitin is 0.35 and 3 or 4 mg/kg body weight, respectively, illustrating significant species differences. Guinea pigs and rabbits are considered to be approximately equally sensitive as dogs to amanitins, with i.v. LD_{50}s of α-amanitin of 0.1 and 0.2 mg/kg, respectively. In humans, the estimated oral LD_{50} of α-amanitin is 0.1 mg/kg body weight. Considering the average concentration of amanitins per mushroom, one *A. phalloides* has the potential to kill a dog or horse.

TREATMENT

No specific antidote for amanitins exists, and thus there is wide variability in treatment and overall response rate. Prompt measures, including decontamination and supportive care, are required to improve prognosis. Even with supportive measures, the reported mortality rate from *Amanita* poisoning in humans is 15%–20%, and it is often higher in children (Enjalbert et al., 2002). In humans with amanitin poisoning, silibinin, penicillin, and *N*-acetylcysteine (NAC) are most commonly recommended, although clinical efficacy data are ambiguous. Similar treatment approaches have been used with variable success rates in dogs suffering from amanitin poisoning (Tegzes and Puschner, 2002).

Silibinin and penicillin reduce the uptake of amanitins into hepatocytes. Silibinin (also known as silybin) is the main component of silymarin, which is extracted from the common milk thistle (*Silybum marianum*). Silibinin is also a free radical scavenger, and it has immunostimulatory and iron binding properties (Mayer et al., 2005). In Europe, a silibinin-contained product (Legalon-Sil) is a well-established and approved treatment for amanitin poisonings in humans. Treatment consists of a 5 mg/kg loading dose i.v. followed by 20 mg/kg/day via continuous infusion (Karlson-Stiber and Persson, 2003) until coagulopathy is no longer present and liver function tests have returned significantly toward normal. In 2009, an open clinical trial was sanctioned by the U.S. Food and Drug Administration and is currently being conducted in northern California (http://clinicaltrials.gov/ct2/show/NCT00915681). In dogs, silibinin was shown to be effective when given twice at a dose of 50 mg/kg i.v. 5 and 24 h after exposure to *A. phalloides* (Vogel et al., 1984). Dosed dogs had better indices of liver function as assessed by serum elevations of AST, ALT, bilirubin, and prolonged PT time. On histopathology, no hepatic lesions were found. Side effects of silibinin administration are rare but include anaphylactic reactions, mild laxative effects, and interactions with certain phase I and phase II metabolism enzymes (Venkataramanan et al., 2000). Oral administration of milk thistle preparations is not recommended because they are poorly absorbed.

Penicillin G was shown to protect against amanitin-induced cell damage in cultured human hepatocytes (Magdalan et al., 2010a). Mice given 1000 mg/kg of penicillin G intraperitoneally 8 h after exposure to a lethal dose 95 (LD_{95}) of amanitin had less morbidity and mortality than did control mice (Floersheim, 1972). In dogs, i. v. administration of 1000 mg/kg of penicillin G at 5 h post *A. phalloides* exposure was considered an effective treatment (Floersheim, 1978).

The benefits of several antioxidants in amanitin intoxications have been evaluated in humans. Most information is available for NAC, which was shown to be as effective as silibinin in reducing mortality (Enjalbert et al., 2002) and protecting against cell damage (Magdalan et al., 2010a). In mice, NAC administration was not effective (Schneider et al., 1992). Although efficacy data of NAC administration in dogs with amanitin poisoning are lacking, there is no reason not to include the glutathione precursor in the treatment regimen. Ascorbic acid may also be of benefit when managing amanitin poisoning in dogs, but specific data are not available. In contrast, cimetidine, thioctic acid, and steroids are no longer recommended because of poor clinical efficacy.

With the identification of OATP1B3 as the primary hepatic uptake transporter for amatoxins in humans, high-affinity substrates and inhibitors of OATB1B3 provide excellent candidates for antidotes (Letschert et al., 2006). Silibinin and penicillin G are in this category, but rifampicin, cyclosporine A, and montelukast must be further evaluated because they may be superior in preventing amanitin uptake into hepatocytes.

Hemodialysis, hemoperfusion, activated charcoal, plasmapharesis, forced diuresis, and nasoduodenal suctioning have been used to treat amanitin poisonings. Controversy remains with regard to the efficacy of decontamination procedures because specific efficacy data do not exist. Recent studies assessing the kinetics and enterohepatic circulation of α-amanitin in pigs demonstrated that clinically relevant systemic plasma and portal plasma toxin concentrations and intestinal reuptake of α-amanitin do not exist beyond 24 h after poisoning (Thiel et al., 2011). Therefore, decontamination and interruption of enterohepatic circulation is most effective within 24 h after poisoning. In addition, external drainage of the bile through as a more invasive approach for detoxification is likely only beneficial within the first 24 h and remains controversial due to lack of data and risk of procedure in veterinary patients. In general, activated charcoal is considered beneficial and recommended to be given every 2–6 h until 2 or 3 days postingestion. Close monitoring, fluid replacement, and supportive care are the essential components of intensive care therapy. Intravenous fluids, correction of hypoglycemia and electrolyte imbalances, vitamin K_1, and plasma transfusions should be considered. In humans, liver transplantation has been used successfully in patients with fulminant liver failure. Currently, liver transplantation is not an option for animals poisoned with amanitins.

Diagnosis of amanitin toxicosis is aided by identification of amanitin-containing mushrooms in the environment of the animal. Mushroom pieces found in gastric contents can confirm exposure. Accurate mushroom identification will require consultation with an experienced mycologist. Detection of amanitins in biological specimens is confirmatory, but these tests are not routinely available at diagnostic laboratories. A liquid chromatography–mass spectrometry method was developed and successfully applied to confirm amanitin poisonings in animals and humans (Filigenzi et al., 2007). A competitive enzyme-linked immunosorbent assay was constructed that allows for the detection of β-amanitin in human serum and urine, but this assay is not available in clinical settings (Abuknesha and Maragkou, 2004). Rapid confirmation of amanitins in suspect exposures assists in the early recognition of exposure, whereas a negative result can prevent unnecessary hospitalization. The well-known reported newspaper test of Wieland or the Meixner test should not be used alone to identify amanitin-containing mushrooms (Beuhler et al., 2004). In suspect cases of aminitin poisoning, serum and urine samples should be collected at various time points beginning as early after exposure as possible. In postmortem presentations, liver and kidney samples are suitable for testing to confirm exposure. The suspect mushroom or vomited gastrointestinal contents should also be saved for further analysis.

Differential diagnoses in dogs and cats with a clinical presentation that involves gastroenteritis and hepatic failure include other toxic ingestions, such as microcystins, cocklebur, cycad palm, aflatoxin, xylitol, ricin, abrin, gyromitrin, and acetaminophen overdose. The history and geographic environment of the animal can help to eliminate most of the toxicant differentials on the list.

HYDRAZINES

Gyromitra species are members of the false morel family, and Helvellaceae are usually found under conifers, aspens, and sometimes around melting snow banks. The species most commonly associated with poisoning and studied in most detail is Gyromitra *esculenta*, but the toxins have been found in other species of Helvellaceae (Viernstein et al., 1980), including Gyromitra *gigas*, Gyromitra *fastigiata*, Gyromitra *infula*, *Helvella crispa*, and *Helvella lacunose*. The toxins associated with false morel poisoning are hydrazine analogs. The toxins are heat labile, volatile, and water soluble (Michelot and Toth, 1991). The process of boiling and drying decreases, but does not completely eliminate, the toxin concentrations (Pyysalo, 1976). People who eat only a few of the cooked mushrooms may ingest sufficiently detoxified amounts so as to remain symptom free. This has caused misunderstandings among people with regard to the potential lethality of these mushrooms. Animals generally eat raw mushrooms; therefore, any exposure to these mushrooms can result in serious morbidity and mortality. Poisoning by some species of *Helvella*, *Verpa*, *Morchella*, *Peziza*, *Disciotis*, and *Sarcosphaera* closely resembles the syndrome caused by gyromitrin. It has been speculated that these mushrooms also contain hydrazines, although analysis has yet to confirm the presence of these toxins (Lincoff and Mitchel, 1977b).

Pharmacokinetics/Toxicokinetics

There is very limited information available. Toxicosis can result after oral and inhalation exposure. Ingestion of gyromitrin (acetaldehyde *N*-methyl *N*-formylhydrazone)-containing mushrooms results in the hydrolysis of gyromitrin to *N*-methyl-*N*-formylhydrazine, which is further metabolized to monomethylhydrazine. The degree of hydrolysis is dependent on the pH in the stomach, but it is not complete (Wright et al., 1978). Inhalation of the fumes during the cooking process can also result in poisoning. Once hydrazines reach the liver, they are further metabolized to reactive intermediates, such as methyl cations and free methyl radicals (Gannett et al., 1991).

Mechanism of Action

Gyromitrin is considered a gastrointestinal irritant leading to vomiting, abdominal pain, and diarrhea 6–12 h after ingestion (Coulet and Guillot, 1982). The principal toxin responsible for convulsions seen in severe cases is monomethylhydrazine, which inhibits pyridoxal phosphokinase resulting in decreased pyridoxal 5′-phosphate concentrations (Lheureux et al., 2005). Depletion of pyridoxal 5′-phosphate leads to decreased γ-aminobutyric acid (GABA) synthesis and an increase in glutamic acid concentrations. Based on a study of mice in which GABA concentrations in the brain were not significantly decreased after methylhydrazine exposure (Maynert and Kaji, 1962), other mechanisms have been proposed. In addition to the gastrointestinal irritation and neurotoxicity, liver and renal failure as well as hemolysis has been described. *N*-methyl-*N*-formylhydrazine inhibits cytochrome P450 and glutathione-metabolizing enzymes (Braun et al., 1979), and it can cause liver necrosis. However, the highly reactive metabolites, such as methyl cations, generated in the liver may significantly contribute to the hepatic injury. Furthermore, the hydrazine analogs present in false morels are carcinogenic in laboratory animals (Toth and Gannett, 1994). Only one case report exists in the veterinary literature. A 10-week-old dog vomited 2 or 3 h after chewing on a mushroom later identified as *G. esculenta* (Bernard, 1979). Six hours postingestion, the dog was lethargic, became comatose, and died 30 min later. Histopathological findings included renal tubulonephrosis, periascinar hepatic degeneration, and erythrophagocytosis.

Toxicity

In humans, there seems to be great individual variability with regard to the toxicity of false morel. In mice, the oral LD_{50}s of gyromitrin, *N*-methyl-*N*-formylhydrazine, and monomethylhydrazine are 344, 118, and 33 mg/kg, respectively (Wright et al., 1978). In humans, the estimated lethal dose of gyromitrin is 20–50 mg/kg for adults and 10–30 mg/kg for children (Schmidlin-Meszaros, 1974). Toxicity information for dogs or cats does not exist. Gyromitrin concentrations in fresh *G. esculenta* are estimated to be 0.12%–0.16%.

Treatment

Most humans only develop mild gastrointestinal symptoms and recover fully within several days after exposure. Management is principally supportive. Early decontamination is often not possible because of the delayed onset of clinical signs. Administration of activated charcoal has been recommended, although efficacy data do not exist. Correction of fluid and electrolytes is an important measure along with the administration of pyridoxine. The recommended dose in humans is 25 mg/kg i.v. over 15–30 min. The dosing can be repeated but should not exceed more than 20 g/day. Although pyridoxine can successfully control seizure activity, it has no benefit in preventing liver injury. In dogs, pyridoxine has been used successfully for nonmushroom toxin–induced seizure activity. It can be used alone or in combination with diazepam, but combination therapy has better efficacy than pyridoxine alone (Villar et al., 1995). The dose for dogs is 75–150 mg/kg body weight, given i.v., during acute phases of seizure activity. Diazepam is given to dogs and cats at 0.5–1.0 mg/kg i.v. to effect. Phenobarbital is not recommended for seizure control because of its cytochrome P450-inducing capability. Administration of folinic acid has been recommended in humans, but controlled studies have not been performed. NAC can be considered. The dosing is the same as that given in acetaminophen-induced hepatic injury. Hemodialysis has been reported in the literature, but its role in removing gyromitrin or its toxic metabolites is not known.

Diagnosis of gyromitrin toxicosis is aided by identification of gyromitrin-containing mushrooms in the environment of the animal. Identification by a mycologist is important to distinguish between the true and the false morels. Detection of gyromitrin, hydrazine analogs, or metabolites in mushrooms or biological specimens is not routinely available (Arshadi et al., 2006). Diagnosis is mainly based on clinical and clinicopathological findings and also mushroom identification.

MUSCARINIC AGENTS

Inocybe and *Clitocybe* spp. contain the highest concentrations of muscarine, but lower concentrations are found in many other genera, including *Entoloma* and *Mycena* (Young, 1994). Muscarine was first discovered and characterized in *A. muscaria*, but concentrations of muscarine are only approximately 0.0003% (Eugster and Schleusener, 1969). In comparison, *Inocybe* and *Clitocybe* species have muscarine concentrations between 0.1 and 0.33%. *Inocybe* and *Clitocybe* species have worldwide distributions and are relatively common. *Inocybe* species grow in association with either conifers or broad-leaved trees. *Clitocybe* species grow on forest litter or grassland humus. The risk of poisoning remains after cooking because of the heat stability of muscarine. There are very few published reports of *Inocybe spp.* poisonings in dogs (Yam et al., 1993; Seljetun and von Krogh, 2017) and only one reported death of a dog presumably from *Inocybe* sp. exposure (Beug, 2009).

Pharmacokinetics/Toxicokinetics

Limited data are available. The naturally occurring form of muscarine is the (L)+ form. In general, quarternary ammonium compounds are poorly absorbed after oral exposure. Once absorbed, muscarine is quickly distributed throughout the body, and clinical signs develop within 30 min to 2 h. Because of its quaternary configuration, muscarine does not cross the blood–brain barrier, and its cholinergic effects are entirely peripheral. A portion of the ingested muscarine is eliminated unchanged in urine, but detailed toxicokinetic studies have not been performed.

Mechanism of Action

Muscarine acts in the peripheral nervous system, where it competes with acetylcholine at its receptor binding sites. The muscarinic cholinergic receptors are found in the heart in both its nodes and its muscle fibers, in smooth muscles, and in glands. They do not occur in skeletal muscles. Once bound to the receptor, muscarine mimics the effect of acetylcholine. Muscarine is unable to inactivate acetylcholinesterase (Young, 1994), and uncontrolled overstimulation of receptors occurs. Clinical signs appear within a few hours and include salivation, lacrimation, vomiting, diarrhea, abdominal pain, miosis, and bradycardia (Lurie et al., 2009). Clinical signs in the dog eating *I. phaecocomics* were observed 3 h after exposure and included salivation, diarrhea, vomiting, depression, and collapse (Yam et al., 1993).

Toxicity

The i.v. LD_{50} of muscarine in mice is 0.23 mg/kg (Waser, 1961). The lethal dose of muscarine in humans is estimated to be between 180 and 300 mg. Ingestion of a single mushroom containing 0.33% muscarine on a dry weight basis can be lethal (Bresinsky and Besl, 1990a).

Treatment

Treatment includes induction of emesis and administration of activated charcoal in asymptomatic animals. Fluid rehydration to restore fluid balance and electrolytes is a key component of treatment. If life-threatening clinical signs are present, atropine should be administered. After giving a test dose of 0.04 mg/kg (1/4 i.v. and 3/4 i.m. or s.c.) to determine its efficacy, atropine can be given repeatedly until symptoms are abolished or until cessation of salivation. Doses in dogs and cats given to effect range from 0.2 to 2.0 mg/kg (1/4 i.v. and 3/4 i.m. or s.c.). Other criteria for therapeutic endpoint with atropine include ease of respiration and lack of respiratory secretions. Mydriasis is not an indicator of its effectiveness. Because atropine also competes with acetylcholine at the receptors, ongoing treatment must be carefully monitored for its anticholinergic effects, including tachycardia, gastrointestinal stasis, severe behavioral changes (e.g., delirium), and hyperthermia. The dose of atropine should be reduced or discontinued with these adverse effects.

ISOXAZOLES

Poisoning in this group is attributed to the heat-stable isoxazoles derivatives, ibotenic acid, and muscimol. *Amanita pantherina* (panther cap or panther agaric) and *A. muscaria* (fly agaric) are most commonly associated with poisonings in humans in this group (Hall and Hall, 1994). The mushrooms grow from summer to autumn in coniferous and deciduous forests, and they are abundant in the Pacific Northwest, where they are often found under Douglas fir trees. Other species containing these toxins include *Amanita gemmata*, *Amanita smithiana*, *Amanita strobiliformis*, and *Tricholoma muscarium* (Lincoff and Mitchel, 1977c). There are a few reports of poisoning in dogs (Naude and Berry, 1997; Beug, 2009) and cats (Ridgway, 1978) after ingesting *A. pantherina*. Ingestion of *A. muscaria* presumably resulted in clinical signs in a horse (Beug, 2009).

Pharmacokinetics/Toxicokinetics

Definitive data on the toxicokinetics of muscimol and ibotenic acid have not been established. Based on the rapid onset of clinical signs after oral exposure, rapid absorption of toxins is suspected. Once absorbed, muscimol and ibotenic acid appear to cross the blood–brain barrier by an active transport system. Ibotenic acid decarboxylates to form muscimol in the stomach, liver, and brain (Nielsen et al., 1985). Muscimol and ibotenic acid can be detected in urine within 1 h of exposure (Ott et al., 1975; Merova et al., 2008).

Mechanism of Action

The major toxins are muscimol and ibotenic acid, but other active substances have been identified, although with minor pharmacological activates. Ibotenic acid is known to act on glutamic acid receptors in the central nervous system (CNS) and produces an excitatory action (Cleland, 1996), whereas muscimol is a potent agonist at $GABA_A$ receptors (Chebib and Johnston, 1999). Although both muscimol and ibotenic acid are present in mushrooms, muscimol is produced by spontaneous decarboxylation of ibotenic acid that can occur during dehydration of the mushroom, digestion in the stomach, or after absorption in a variety of tissues. Therefore, muscimol is mainly responsible for the clinical signs. On activation by muscimol, the membrane permeability for anions increases, usually resulting in a slight, short-lasting hyperpolarization and associated decreased excitability of the receptive neuron. Effects on the CNS are similar to those produced by therapeutic doses of diazepam.

Clinical signs of muscimol toxicosis begin within 30 min to 2 h after ingestion and have been termed the "pantherine–muscaria" syndrome in humans, which is characterized by mydriasis, dryness of mouth, ataxia, confusion, euphoria, dizziness, and tiredness. Gastrointestinal signs are not consistently seen in cases of isoxazole poisoning. Full recovery is expected within 1 or 2 days. In cats, clinical signs have been observed within 15–30 min after ingestion of *A. pantherina* (Ridgway, 1978). After a brief period of sedation, cats experienced a 4-h-long state of excitement with pronounced muscle spasms, followed by a deep sleep. Cats are expected to fully recover within 24 h after ingestion, especially if decontamination measures are taken. In dogs, clinical signs observed after ingestion of *A. pantherina* include disorientation, opisthotonus, paresis, seizures, paddling, chewing movements, miosis, vestibular signs, respiratory depression, coma, and death (Hunt and Funk, 1977; Naude and Berry, 1997). Recoveries are recorded within 12–24 h after aggressive supportive care measures, including mechanical ventilation during periods of respiratory depression; however, death was reported in several dogs. Similar clinical signs were reported in a dog that survived *A. muscaria* poisoning (Martin, 1956).

Toxicity

In mice, the oral LD_{50} is 22 mg/kg for muscimol and 38 mg/kg for ibotenic acid (Hall and Hall, 1994). In rats, the oral LD_{50} is 45 mg/kg for muscimol and 129 mg/kg for ibotenic acid. The intraperitoneal LD_{50} of muscimol is 2.5 mg/kg in mice and 3.5 mg/kg in rats. In humans, the toxic threshold is estimated to be 6 mg of muscimol and 30–60 mg of ibotenic acid (Halpern, 2004). The concentration of ibotenic acid in *A. muscaria* was estimated at 100 mg/kg fresh weight, whereas the concentration of muscimol was less than 3 mg/kg fresh weight. Thus, an average-sized fruit body of *A. muscaria* weighing 60–70 g can contain a toxic concentration. Toxicity data for dogs are not available. However, postmortem examination of puppies indicated that the ingestion of a single *A. pantherina* can be lethal (Hunt and Funk, 1977).

Treatment

Treatment of exposed animals is mainly symptomatic and supportive. Decontamination measures should be considered in recent exposures, although emetics are only recommended in animals that are not at risk for developing aspiration pneumonia. Specific measures to control seizures are not without complication. Benzodiazepines, as GABA agonists, may potentiate any CNS depression. Therefore, when diazepam is used, CNS and respiratory depression may be severe and prolonged, necessitating the use of mechanical ventilation. As long as ventilation is maintained adequately, the prognosis for recovery is good. Diazepam can be given to dogs and cats at 0.5 mg/kg i.v. to effect and can be repeated as needed every 10 min for up to three doses. Other drugs used to control seizures include phenobarbital and pentobarbital. Phenobarbital is dosed at 6 mg/kg i.v. Pentobarbital is given at 5–15 mg/kg i.v. to effect to dogs and cats. These, too, are agonists at the GABA receptors, and they can potentiate CNS and respiratory depression. Careful monitoring of the animal's oxygenation status is vital until the animal is fully awake and alert. Supplemental oxygen can be used if necessary. General supportive measures of unconscious animals include maintaining hydration with i.v. fluids, maintaining the airway free of respiratory secretions, and frequent position changes to prevent decubitus skin ulcerations. In humans, the use of atropine is contraindicated because of the atropine-like clinical presentation in poisonings.

PSILOCIN AND PSILOCYBIN

Mushrooms that contain psilocybin are commonly referred to as hallucinogenic or magic mushrooms. *Psilocybe*, *Panaeolus*, *Conocybe*, and *Gymnopilus* are the four genera in North America that contain psilocybin (Smolinske, 1994). Many of these mushrooms are coprophilic and grow in fields and animal pastures, particularly in the northwestern and southeastern United States. The majority of mushrooms contain only psilocybin, but some, such as *Psilocybe cyanescens*, contain both psilocybin and psilocin. The concentrations of psilocybin and psilocin are influenced by growth conditions, geographic location, storage conditions, and species. Species commonly found in the Pacific Northwest contain between 1.2 and 16.8 mg/kg psilocybin on a dry weight basis. If psilocin is present, concentrations may reach up to 9.6 mg/kg on a dry weight basis (Smolinske, 1994). Psilocin and psilocybin are sensitive to heat. Some mushrooms in this group also contain other pharmacologically active substances, such as serotonin and tryptophan. There is only one published report of hallucinogenic mushroom ingestion in a dog (Kirwan, 1990).

Pharmacokinetics/Toxicokinetics

Psilocybin is a prodrug and is rapidly dephosphorylated to psilocin. Dephosphorylation can take place in a variety of tissues, but high activity has been identified in kidney and liver of rodents (Horita and Weber, 1961) and in plasma of humans (Grieshaber et al., 2001). However, the general assumption is that complete conversion of psilocybin to psilocin occurs prior to absorption into the systemic circulation (Laatsch, 1996). In humans, the absolute bioavailability of psilocin liberated from orally administered psilocybin was estimated to be 52.7% ± 20% (Hasler et al., 1997). Absorption is rapid with maximum concentrations reached in 1–1.5 h. In plasma, psilocin is further metabolized to 4-hydroxytryptophole (4HT) and 4-hydroxyindole-3-acetic acid (4HIAA). Psilocin crosses the blood–brain barrier and concentrates in brain tissue (Horita and Weber, 1961). Psilocin is excreted unchanged or as psilocin–glucuronide in urine and to some extent unchanged via the bile (Hasler et al., 2002).

Mechanism of Action

Psilocin is the pharmacologically active metabolite of psilocybin. Because of its structural similarity to serotonin, psilocin stimulates serotonin receptors in the CNS (McKenna et al., 1990). Psilocin has affinity for 5-HT_{1A}, 5-HT_{2A}, and 5-HT_{2C} receptors (Halberstadt et al., 2010). Activation of 5-HT_{2A} receptors leads to increased cortical activity via glutamatergic excitatory postsynaptic potentials (Aghajanian and Marek, 1997). Activation of 5-HT_{1A} receptors results in the inhibition of pyramidal cell activity (Puig et al., 2005). In addition, psilocin may have peripheral effects that involve serotonergic receptors. In humans, psilocin's psychoactive effects are similar to those produced by LSD, are observed within 20–30 min of ingestion, and include visual hallucinations, intensified hearing, and incoordination. Other autonomic-mediated effects include increased heart rate, increased blood pressure, mydriasis, tremors, and increased temperature. The effects can last up to 8 h, but hallucinogenic activity rarely exceeds 1 h. Clinical signs in dogs include ataxia, vocalization, overt aggression, nystagmus, and increased body temperature (Kirwan, 1990). In contrast to the CNS effects after exposure to isoxazoles, there is no subsequent coma. Sedation may be necessary until behavioral signs resolve.

Toxicity

In many countries (e.g., the United States, Great Britain, and Germany), psilocybin and psilocin are classified as controlled substances. In humans, oral exposure to 10–20 mg of psilocybin can cause mood changes and hallucinations. Information regarding lethal doses in animals is not found in the literature.

Treatment

The management of hallucinogenic mushroom poisonings is primarily supportive, and in most cases treatment is not necessary. Gastric emptying procedures have not proven beneficial and are not recommended. The effect of activated charcoal in poisonings is not known, but activated charcoal administration can be considered. If severe neurologic signs such as seizures occur, diazepam is considered the first-line medication. Diazepam can be given to effect to dogs and cats at 0.5–1.0 mg/kg i.v. in increments of 5–10 mg. If diazepam is unsuccessful, subsequent seizures can be controlled with phenobarbital at 6 mg/kg to effect. In addition, control of body temperature is an important factor in symptomatic care.

Diagnosis of psilocybin exposure is confirmed by the detection of psilocin and psilocin–glucuronide in urine, serum, and blood. A number of methodologies are available and are routinely used in forensic investigations (Kamata et al., 2003; Albers et al., 2004; Laussmann and Meier-Giebing, 2010). Because of the infrequent presentation of hallucinogenic mushroom poisoning in animals, these methodologies are not routinely available at veterinary diagnostic laboratories.

GASTROINTESTINAL IRRITANTS

This group includes mushrooms that result in gastroenteritis as the primary clinical sign. There are very few reports in the veterinary literature. Genera included are *Agaricus*, *Boletus*, *Chlorophyllum*, *Entoloma*, *Lactarius*, *Omphalotus*, *Rhodophyllus*, *Scleroderma*, and *Tricholoma*. The specific toxins in most have not been identified (Spoerke, 1994).

One of the mushrooms in this group commonly reported to cause poisoning is *Chlorophyllum molybdites*. This mushroom is commonly found in the United States except in the colder, northern areas, and the principal toxin has not been clearly identified. Clinical signs of nausea, vomiting, and diarrhea appear 1–6 h after ingestion in humans, and there is complete recovery within 24–48 h (Blayney et al., 1980). A dog with *C. molybdites* poisoning had clinical signs of drooling and diarrhea, whereas a horse that had presumably eaten several bites of *C. molybdites* died (Beug, 2009). *Omphalotus olearius*, *Omphalotus subilludens*, and *Lampteromyces japonicus* contain illudin S (Bresinsky and Besl, 1990b).

Illudin S is a sesquiterpene with a unique chemical structure. In humans, vomiting and diarrhea occur 1–2.5 h after ingestion (French and Garrettson, 1988). In a pot-bellied pig, death was reported 5 h after it ingested a fruiting body of *Scleroderma citrinum* (Galey et al., 1990). The pig vomited and collapsed 20 min after exposure and remained weak and recumbent until death. The toxins in *S. citrinum* have not been characterized. In *Boletus satanas*, lectins may contribute to serious gastroenteritis in humans. Lectins, which are storage proteins that may play a role in plant defense, are widely distributed in many species of mushrooms (Wang et al., 1998).

Poisonings by mushrooms of this group are rarely fatal; hence, they are likely to be underreported by owners and seldom recorded in the literature. After a usually short latent period of 15 min to 2 h after ingestion, an animal may present with vomiting, diarrhea, and abdominal pain. Usually, these clinical signs resolve spontaneously within a few hours, but they may last 1 or 2 days. The clinical signs may resemble any other common cause of gastroenteritis in small or large animals, including bacterial and viral infections, sudden diet changes or eating spoiled foods, and inflammatory mediated syndromes such as acute pancreatitis. The diagnostic challenge is that many of the more toxic mushrooms cause initial gastrointestinal signs. Cyclopeptides cause vomiting and diarrhea after a lag period similar to that seen with the gastrointestinal irritants. Therefore, any animal presenting with gastrointestinal signs after a known history of mushroom ingestion must be carefully assessed.

Treatment is entirely nonspecific and supportive. Vomiting is a hallmark of poisoning by gastrointestinal irritant mushrooms. Thus, in most cases, the stomach has already been emptied, and emetics are not necessary. Activated charcoal is thought to adsorb most of the toxins in this group and should be administered orally unless there is protracted vomiting. There are no specific antidotes for the toxins in this group. Treatment is aimed at rehydration and correction of serum electrolyte abnormalities.

RENAL TOXIC MUSHROOMS

Orellanine-containing mushrooms cause acute renal failure without any hepatic insult. Mushrooms of the genus *Cortinarius* contain the highly potent nephrotoxin orellanine (Frank et al., 2009), which is similar in chemical structure to paraquat. *Cortinarius rubellus* and *Cortinarius orellanosus* exist in North America; *C. rubellus* is found in northern areas of both the east and west coasts while *C. orellanosus* is reported in Michigan but its entire geographic distribution is currently unknown. In North America, there are only a few reported cases in humans, but poisonings occur with much greater frequency in western and central Europe. In humans, symptoms gradually develop over 2–20 days after ingestion. In general, gastrointestinal signs occur a few days after exposure, and renal failure develops 4–15 days after ingestion. Hemodialysis may be necessary until renal function gradually improves. There are no reports of orellanine poisoning in pets; however, poisoning was documented in grazing sheep in Norway (Overås et al., 1979).

A. smithiana has resulted in delayed renal failure in humans without evidence of hepatic dysfunction (West et al., 2009). The toxin is allenic norleucine. Key clinical features are vomiting and abdominal pain with little or no diarrhea within a few hours of ingestion. Renal failure develops 1–4 days after exposure and may require several weeks of hemodialysis before recovery. There are no reports of *A. smithiana* poisoning in animals, but it is a common mushroom in the Pacific Northwest.

RAMARIA FLAVO-BRUNNESCENS

This mushroom is found in North America, Australia, China, Brazil, and Uruguay and has caused poisoning in cattle and sheep (Kommers and Santos, 1995). *Ramaria flavo-brunnescens* is exclusively found in eucalyptus woods, and thus the poisoning has been termed "eucalyptus sickness." Clinical signs have been observed as early as 3 days after exposure but may be delayed until 6 days postexposure. Typically, animals develop anorexia, salivation, diarrhea, and recumbency. This is followed by alteration in keratinization, which becomes apparent by loss of hair and hooves, similar to what is seen in chronic selenosis. The toxins have not been identified but are most likely volatile and interfere with the incorporation of sulfur-containing amino acids.

CONCLUDING REMARKS AND FUTURE DIRECTIONS

Overall, the number of reported mushroom poisonings in animals is low, although this is likely a result of the lack of methods to confirm exposure and a lack of national clearing house mechanisms. In humans, most cases are diagnosed by positive identification of the suspect mushroom, which is often impossible in veterinary medicine. The chances of obtaining an intact and representative mushroom are slim because animals are often left unattended and a history of ingestion is not available. The development of new analytical techniques to identify mushroom toxins in biological samples of poisoned animals will provide insight into the true frequency of mushroom poisonings. Currently, therapeutic measures are primarily based on both mechanisms of toxicity and clinical signs. Rapid toxin identification would allow for a confirmed, early diagnosis, which is especially important in cases in which intensive care is indicated. To develop analytical techniques for specific mushroom toxins, further research is necessary in the area of toxin characterization and toxicokinetics. Although thousands of mushrooms exist worldwide, only a few have been researched in-depth. It is also important to improve our knowledge of the efficacy of commonly recommended, but poorly evaluated, therapeutic procedures.

REFERENCES

Abuknesha, R.A., Maragkou, A., 2004. A highly sensitive and specific enzyme immunoassay for detection of beta-amanitin in biological fluids. Anal. Bioanal. Chem. 379, 853–860.

Aghajanian, G.K., Marek, G.J., 1997. Serotonin induces excitatory postsynaptic potentials in apical dendrites of neocortical pyramidal cells. Neuropharmacology. 36, 589–599.

Albers, C., Kohler, H., Lehr, M., et al., 2004. Development of a psilocin immunoassay for serum and blood samples. Int. J. Legal Med. 118, 326–331.

Arshadi, M., Nilsson, C., Magnusson, B., 2006. Gas chromatography–mass spectrometry determination of the pentafluorobenzoyl derivative of methylhydrazine in false morel (*Gyromitra esculenta*) as a monitor for the content of the toxin gyromitrin. J. Chromatogr. A. 1125, 229–233.

Barbato, M.P., 1993. Poisoning from accidental ingestion of mushrooms. Med. J. Aust. 158, 842–847.

Bernard, M.A., 1979. Mushroom poisoning in a dog. Can. Vet. J. 20, 82–83.

Beug, M., 2009. NAMA Toxicology Committee Report for 2009: North American mushroom poisonings. McIlvainea. 19, 1–5.

Beuhler, M., Lee, D.C., Gerkin, R., 2004. The Meixner test in the detection of ⟨-amanitin and false positive reactions caused by psilocin and 5-substituted tryptamines. Ann. Emerg. Med. 44, 114–120.

Blayney, D., Rosenkranz, E., Zettner, A., 1980. Mushroom poisoning from *Chlorophyllum molybdites*. West J. Med. 132, 74–77.

Braun, R., Greeff, U., Netter, K.J., 1979. Liver injury by the false morel poison gyromitrin. Toxicology. 12, 155–163.

Bresinsky, A., Besl, H., 1990a. Muscarine syndrome. In: Bresinsky, A., Besl, H. (Eds.), A Colour Atlas of Poisonous Fungi. Wolfe, London, pp. 71–73.

Bresinsky, A., Besl, H., 1990b. Gastrointestinal syndrome. In: Bresinsky, A., Besl, H. (Eds.), A Colour Atlas of Poisonous Fungi. Wolfe, London, pp. 130–176.

Chebib, M., Johnston, G.A., 1999. The "ABC" of GABA receptors: a brief review. Clin. Exp. Pharmacol. Physiol. 26, 937–940.

Cleland, T.A., 1996. Inhibitory glutamate receptor channels. Mol. Neurobiol. 13, 97–136.

Cole, F.M., 1993. A puppy death and *Amanita phalloides*. Aust Vet. Assoc. 70, 271–272.

Coulet, M., Guillot, J., 1982. Poisoning by Gyromitra: a possible mechanism. Med. Hypotheses. 8, 325–334.

De Carlo, E., Milanesi, A., Martini, C., et al., 2003. Effects of *Amanita phalloides* toxins on insulin release: *in vivo* and *in vitro* studies. Arch. Toxicol. 77, 441–445.

Enjalbert, F., Rapior, S., Nouguier-Soule, J., et al., 2002. Treatment of amatoxin poisoning: 20-year retrospective analysis. J. Toxicol. Clin. Toxicol. 40, 715–757.

Eugster, C.H., Schleusener, E., 1969. Stereomere Muscarine kommen in der Natur vor. Gas-chromatographische Trennung der Norbasen 30: Mitteilung über Inhaltsstoffe von Fliegenpilzen. Helv. Chim. Acta. 52, 708–715.

Faulstich, H., Fauser, U., 1980. The course of *Amanita* intoxication in beagle dogs. In: Faulstich, H., Kommerell, B., Wieland, T. (Eds.), Amanita Toxins and Poisoning. Verlag Gerhard Witzstrock, Baden-Baden, Germany, pp. 115–123.

Faulstich, H., Talas, A., Wellhoner, H.H., 1985. Toxicokinetics of labeled amatoxins in the dog. Arch. Toxicol. 56, 190–194.

Filigenzi, M.S., Poppenga, R.H., Tiwari, A.K., Puschner, B., 2007. Determination of alpha-amanitin in serum and liver by multistage linear ion trap mass spectrometry. J. Agric. Food Chem. 55, 784–790.

Floersheim, G.L., 1972. Antidotes to experimental ⟨-amanitin poisoning. Nat. New Biol. 236, 115–117.

Floersheim, G.L., 1978. Experimental basis for the therapy of *Amanita phalloides* poisoning. Schweiz. Med. Wochenschr. 108, 185–197.

Frank, H., ZilkerKirchmair, M., Kirchmair, M., et al., 2009. Acute renal failure by ingestion of *Cortinarius* species confounded with psychoactive mushrooms: a case series and literature survey. Clin. Nephrol. 71, 557–562.

French, A.L., Garrettson, L.K., 1988. Poisoning with the North American Jack O'Lantern mushroom, *Omphalotus illudens*. J. Toxicol. Clin. Toxicol. 26, 81–88.

Galey, F.D., Rutherford, J.J., Wells, K., 1990. A case of *Scleroderma citrinum* poisoning in a miniature Chinese pot-bellied pig. Vet. Hum. Toxicol. 32, 329–330.

Gannett, P.M., Garrett, C., Lawson, T., et al., 1991. Chemical oxidation and metabolism of *N*-methyl-*N*-formylhydrazine: evidence for diazenium and radical intermediates. Food Chem. Toxicol. 29, 49–56.

Ganzert, M., Felgenhauer, N., Zilker, T., 2005. Indication of liver transplantation following amatoxin intoxication. J. Hepatol. 42, 202–209.

Grieshaber, A.F., Moore, K.A., Levine, B., 2001. The detection of psilocin in human urine. J. Forensic. Sci. 46, 627–630.

Gundala, S., Wells, L.D., Milliano, M.T., et al., 2004. The hepatocellular bile acid transporter Ntcp facilitates uptake of the lethal mushroom toxin alpha-amanitin. Arch. Toxicol. 78, 68–73.

Halberstadt, A.L., Koedood, L., Powell, S.B., et al., 2010. Differential contributions of serotonin receptors to the behavioral effects of indoleamine hallucinogens in mice. J. Psychopharmacol. 25, 1548–1561.

Hall, A.H., Hall, P.K., 1994. Ibotenic acid/muscimol-containing mushrooms. In: Spoerke, D.G., Rumack, B.H. (Eds.), Handbook of Mushroom Poisoning: Diagnosis and Treatment. CRC Press, Boca Raton, FL, pp. 265–278.

Halpern, J.H., 2004. Hallucinogens and dissociative agents naturally growing in the United States. Pharmacol. Ther. 102, 131–138.

Hasler, F., Bourquin, D., Brenneisen, R., et al., 1997. Determination of psilocin and 4-hydroxyindole-3-acetic acid in plasma by HPLC-ECD and pharmacokinetic profiles of oral and intravenous psilocybin in man. Pharm. Acta Helv. 72, 175–184.

Hasler, F., Bourquin, D., Brenneisen, R., et al., 2002. Renal excretion profiles of psilocin following oral administration of psilocybin: a controlled study in man. J. Pharm. Biomed. Anal. 30, 331–339.

Himmelmann, A., Mang, G., Schnorf-Huber, S., 2001. Lethal ingestion of stored *Amanita phalloides* mushrooms. Swiss Med. Wkly. 131, 616–617.

Horita, A., Weber, L.J., 1961. The enzymic dephosphorylation and oxidation of psilocybin and psilocin by mammalian tissue homogenisates. Biochem. Pharmacol. 7, 47–54.

Hunt, R.S., Funk, A., 1977. Mushrooms fatal to dogs. Mycologia. 69, 432–433.

Jaeger, A., Jehl, F., Flesch, F., et al., 1993. Kinetics of amatoxins in human poisoning: therapeutic implications. J. Toxicol. Clin. Toxicol. 31, 63–80.

Kallet, A., Sousa, C., Spangler, W., 1988. Mushroom (*Amanita phalloides*) toxicity in dogs. Calif. Vet. 42, 1, 9–11, 22, 47.

Kamata, T., Nishikawa, M., Katagi, M., et al., 2003. Optimized glucuronide hydrolysis for the detection of psilocin in human urine samples. J. Chromatogr. B Analyt Technol. Biomed. Life. 796, 421–427.

Karlson-Stiber, C., Persson, H., 2003. Cytotoxic fungi: an overview. Toxicon. 42, 339–349.

Kirwan, A.P., 1990. "Magic mushroom" poisoning in a dog. Vet. Rec. 126, 149.

Klan, J., 1993. A review of mushrooms containing amanitins and phalloidines. Cas. Lek Cesk. 132, 449–451.

Kommers, G.D., Santos, M.N., 1995. Experimental poisoning of cattle by the mushroom *Ramaria flavo-brunnescens* (Clavariaceae): a study of the morphology and pathogenesis of lesions in hooves, tail, horns and tongue. Vet. Hum. Toxicol. 37, 297–302.

Laatsch, H., 1996. Zur Pharmakologie von Psilocybin und Psilocin. In: Liggenstorfer, R., Rätsch, C. (Eds.), Maria Sabina, Botin der heiligen Pilze. Vomtraditionellen Schamanentum zur weltweiten Pilzkultur. Nachtschatten Verlag, Solothum, Switzerland, pp. 192–202.

Laussmann, T., Meier-Giebing, S., 2010. Forensic analysis of hallucinogenic mushrooms and khat (Catha edulis Forsk) using cation-exchange liquid chromatography. Forensic. Sci. Int. 195, 160–164.

Leist, M., Gantner, F., Naumann, H., et al., 1997. Tumor necrosis factor-induced apoptosis during the poisoning of mice with hepatotoxins. Gastroenterology. 112, 923–934.

Letschert, K., Faulstich, H., Keller, D., et al., 2006. Molecular characterization and inhibition of amanitin uptake into human hepatocytes. Toxicol. Sci. 91, 140–149.

Lheureux, P., Penaloza, A., Gris, M., 2005. Pyridoxine in clinical toxicology: a review. Eur. J. Emerg. Med. 12, 78–85.

Lincoff, G., Mitchel, D.H., 1977a. Cyclopeptide poisoning. Toxic and Hallucinogenic Mushroom Poisoning: A Handbook for Physicians and Mushroom Hunters. Van Nostrand Reinhold, New York, pp. 25–48.

Lincoff, G., Mitchel, D.H., 1977b. Monomethylhydrazine poisoning. Toxic and Hallucinogenic Mushroom Poisoning: A Handbook for Physicians and Mushroom Hunters. Van Nostrand Reinhold, New York, pp. 49–61.

Lincoff, G., Mitchel, D.H., 1977c. Ibotenic acid–muscimol poisoning. Toxic and Hallucinogenic Mushroom Poisoning: A Handbook for Physicians and Mushroom Hunters. Van Nostrand Reinhold, New York, pp. 77–99.

Lindell, T.J., Weinberg, F., Morris, P.W., et al., 1970. Specific inhibition of nuclear RNA polymerase II by alpha-amanitin. Science. 170, 447–449.

Lurie, Y., Wasser, S.P., Taha, M., et al., 2009. Mushroom poisoning from species of genus *Inocybe* (fiber head mushroom): a case series with exact species identification. Clin. Toxicol. 47, 562–565.

Magdalan, J., Ostrowska, A., Piotrowska, A., et al., 2010a. Benzylpenicillin, acetylcysteine and silibinin as antidotes in human hepatocytes intoxicated with ⟨-amanitin. Exp. Toxicol. Pathol. 62, 367–373.

Magdalan, J., Ostrowska, A., Piotrowska, A., et al., 2010b. ⟨-Amanitin induced apoptosis in primary cultured dog hepatocytes. Folia Histochem. Cytobiol. 48, 58–62.

Martin, J.G., 1956. Mycetism (mushroom poisoning) in a dog: case report. Vet. Med. 51, 227–228.

Mayer, K.E., Myers, R.P., Lee, S.S., 2005. Silymarin treatment of viral hepatitis: a systematic review. J. Viral. Hepat. 12, 559–567.

Maynert, E.W., Kaji, H.K., 1962. On the relationship of brain gamma-aminobutyric acid to convulsions. J. Pharmacol. Exp. Ther. 137, 114–121.

McKenna, D.J., Repke, D.B., Lo, L., et al., 1990. Differential interactions of indolealkylamines with 5-hydroxytryptamine receptor subtypes. Neuropharmacology. 29, 193–198.

Merova, B., Ondra, P., Stankova, M., et al., 2008. Isolation and identification of the *Amanita muscaria* and *Amanita pantherina* toxins in human urine. Neuro Endocrinol. Lett. 29, 744–748.

Michelot, D., Toth, B., 1991. Poisoning by *Gyromitra esculenta*: a review. J. Appl. Toxicol. 11, 235–243.

Mitchel, D.H., 1980. *Amanita* mushroom poisoning. Annu. Rev. Med. 31, 51–57.

Naude, T.W., Berry, W.L., 1997. Suspected poisoning of puppies by the mushroom *Amanita pantherina*. J. S. Afr. Vet. Assoc. 68, 154–158.

Nielsen, E.O., Schousboe, A., Hansen, S.H., et al., 1985. Excitatory amino acids: studies on the biochemical and chemical stability of ibotenic acid and related compounds. J. Neurochem. 45, 725–731.

Ott, J., Wheaton, P.S., Chilton, W.S., 1975. Fate of muscimol in the mouse. Physiol. Chem. Phys. 7, 381–384.

Overås, J., Ulvund, M.J., Bakkevig, S., et al., 1979. Poisoning in sheep induced by the mushroom *Cortinarius speciosissimus*. Acta Vet. Scan. 20, 148–150.

Puig, M.V., Artigas, F., Celada, P., 2005. Modulation of the activity of pyramidal neurons in rat prefrontal cortex by raphe stimulation *in vivo*: involvement of serotonin and GABA. Cereb. Cortex. 15, 1–14.

Puschner, B., Rose, H.H., Filigenzi, M.S., 2007. Diagnosis of *Amanita* toxicosis in a dog with acute hepatic necrosis. J. Vet. Diagn. Invest. 19, 312–317.

Pyysalo, H., 1976. Tests for gyromitrin, a poisonous compound in false morel *Gyromitra esculenta*. Z Lebensm. Unters Forsch. 160, 325–330.

Ridgway, R.L., 1978. Mushroom (*Amanita pantherina*) poisoning. J. Vet. Med. Assoc. 172, 681–682.

Schmidlin-Meszaros, J., 1974. Gyromitrin in Trockenlorcheln (*Gyromitra esculenta sicc.*). Mitt. Geb. Lebensm. Hyg. 65, 453–465.

Schneider, S.M., Michelson, E.A., Vanscoy, G., 1992. Failure of N-acetylcysteine to reduce alpha amanitin toxicity. J. Appl. Toxicol. 12, 141–142.

Seljetun, K.O., von Krogh, A., 2017. Acute *Inocybe* mushroom toxicosis in dogs: 5 cases (2010–2014). J. Vet. Emerg. Crit. Care.http://dx.doi.org/10.1111/vec.12567.

Smolinske, S.C., 1994. Psilocybin-containing mushrooms. In: Spoerke, D. G., Rumack, B.H. (Eds.), Handbook of Mushroom Poisoning: Diagnosis and Treatment. CRC Press, Boca Raton, FL, pp. 309–324.

Spoerke, D.G., 1994. Gastrointestinal irritant mushrooms. In: Spoerke, D. G., Rumack, B.H. (Eds.), Handbook of Mushroom Poisoning: Diagnosis and Treatment. CRC Press, Boca Raton, FL, pp. 347–366.

Tegzes, J.H., Puschner, B., 2002. *Amanita* mushroom poisoning: efficacy of aggressive treatment of two dogs. Vet. Hum. Toxicol. 44, 96–99.

Thiel, C., Thiel, K., Klingert, W., et al., 2011. The enterohepatic circulation of amanitin: kinetics and therapeutical implications. Toxicol. Lett. 203, 42–146.

Thiel, K., Schenk, M., Sipos, B., Sperveslage, J., Peter, A., Morgalla, M. H., et al., 2014. Hepatol. Int. 8, 128–136.

Toth, B., Gannett, P., 1994. *Gyromitra esculenta* mushroom: a comparative assessment of its carcinogenic potency. In Vivo. 8, 999–1002.

Venkataramanan, R., Ramachandran, V., Komoroski, B.J., et al., 2000. Milk thistle, a herbal supplement, decreases the activity of CYP3A4 and uridine diphosphoglucuronosyl transferase in human hepatocyte cultures. Drug Metab. Dispos. 28, 1270–1273.

Vetter, J., 1998. Toxins of *Amanita phalloides*. Toxicon. 36, 13–24.

Viernstein, H., Jurenitsch, J., Kubelka, W., 1980. Vergleich des Giftgehaltes der Lorchelarten *Gyromitra gigas, Gyromitra fastigiata* und *Gyromitra esculenta*. Ernährung/Nutrition. 4, 392–395.

Villar, D., Knight, M.K., Holding, J., et al., 1995. Treatment of acute isoniazid overdose in dogs. Vet. Hum. Toxicol. 37, 473–477.

Vogel, G., Tuchweber, B., Trost, W., et al., 1984. Protection by silibinin against *Amanita phalloides* intoxication in beagles. Toxicol. Appl. Pharmacol. 73, 355–362.

Wang, H.X., Ng, T.B., Ooi, V.E., 1998. Lectin activity in fruiting bodies of the edible mushroom Tricholoma mongolicum. Biochem. Mol. Biol. Int. 44, 135–141.

Waser, P.G., 1961. Chemistry and pharmacology of muscarine, muscarone, and some related compounds. Pharmacol. Rev. 13, 465–515.

West, P.L., Lindgren, J., Horowitz, B.Z., 2009. *Amanita smithiana* mushroom ingestion: a case of delayed renal failure and literature review. J. Med. Toxicol. 5, 32–38.

Wieland, T., 1983. The toxic peptides from *Amanita* mushrooms. Int. J. Pept. Protein Res. 22, 257–276.

Wright, A.V., Niskanen, A., Pyysalo, H., et al., 1978. The toxicity of some *N*-methyl-*N*-formylhydrazones from *Gyromitra esculenta* and related compounds in mouse and microbial tests. Toxicol. Appl. Pharmacol. 45, 429–434.

Yam, P., Helfer, S., Watling, R., 1993. Mushroom poisoning in a dog. Vet. Rec. 133, 24.

Young, A., 1994. Muscarine-containing mushrooms. In: Spoerke, D.G., Rumack, B.H. (Eds.), Handbook of Mushroom Poisoning: Diagnosis and Treatment. CRC Press, Boca Raton, FL, pp. 289–301.

Yee, M.M., Woods, L.W., Poppenga, R.H., Puschner, B., 2012. Amanitin intoxication in two beef calves in California. J. Vet. Diagn. Invest. 24, 241–244.

Chapter 68

Cottonseed Toxicity

Rhian B. Cope

INTRODUCTION

Cotton (*Gossypium* spp.; tribe *Gossypieae*, family Malvaceae) is one of the oldest groups of cultivated plants having been used as a textile raw material for at least 7000 years. The genus *Gossypium* consists of more than 50 species of plants found in arid and semiarid regions of the tropics and subtropics. Only four species (*Gossypium hirsutum* (>90% of world production), *G. barbadense* (3%–4% of world production), *G. arboreum* and *G. herbaceum* (about 2% of world production, combined)) are used for almost all global cotton production. Transgenic cottons that incorporate one or several *Bacillus thuringiensis* genes (Bt Cotton) coding for insecticidal proteins currently dominate world production. Attempts at breeding cotton that is low in gossypol or free of it have been scientifically successful but have been commercially unviable because the absence of the pigment strips the plant of one of its major mechanisms of insect defense. Transgenic techniques have also produced strains that produce small interfering RNAs that disrupt gossypol synthesis. These transgenic plants produce seeds with approximately 0.2 g/kg of gossypol.

A byproduct of fiber production is cotton seeds, cottonseed meals, and cottonseed oil. These materials are commonly used in animal feeds mostly as a cheaper source of protein, energy and/or fiber (Table 68.1; Blasi and Drouillard, 2002). All of these feed products are notably low in lysine. The basic processing of cotton to cottonseed meals consists of: (1) ginning, (2) cleaning to remove leaves, stems and dirt, (3) delinting, (4) hull removal, (5) flaking, (6) oil extraction either by solvent (usually hexane) extraction and desolventing or by pressing, (7) refining byproducts (usually the oil-rich material) may be added back to the flakes to increase energy content/energy density, and (h) drying to 10%–12% moisture.

The nutrient content of cotton byproducts varies depending on the oil-extraction methods employed. As a general rule, mechanically extracted cottonseed meals have higher oil contents than prepressed solvent or solvent extracted products. However this is not always the case since refinery byproducts, such as fatty acid sodium salts, may be returned back into the meal stream immediately before the desolventizer-toaster process. The nutritional content of these products has also changed over time in association with genetic selection and changes in production methods. Current cottonseed meals tend to have higher levels of crude protein, lower levels of ether extract, lower levels of magnesium, potassium, and sulfur, and lower levels of crude fiber, copper, and manganese compared with similar products produced 20–30 years ago (Blasi and Drouillard, 2002).

Although cottonseed meals are bulky and present handling challenges (i.e., may require hand feeding and may not flow well through self-feeders), dietary levels up to 50% of intake been used with success (Blasi and Drouillard, 2002). However, a slow incremental increase in the dietary level is recommended to avoid scouring. Notably cottonseed meals may not mix well with salt or other intake limiters. Cottonseed meals also need to be free of foreign debris. Cotton seeds and cottonseed meals stored at >10% moisture are prone to fungal growth, increasing the risk of aflatoxicosis and other mycotoxin-induced diseases.

GOSSYPOL

Introduction

All cotton (*Gossypium*) species as well as okra (*Abelmoschus esculentus*) contain gossypol (Blasi and Drouillard, 2002, Gadelha et al., 2014). Gossypol (Fig. 68.1) is a stereoisomeric (+ or *S* configuration, − or *R* configuration), yellow-green, hexaphenolic dicarbonylnaphthalene pigment produced by pigment glands found throughout the plants (Fig. 68.2). The cotton pigment glands are especially concentrated in cotton seeds

Veterinary Toxicology. DOI: http://dx.doi.org/10.1016/B978-0-12-811410-0.00068-4

TABLE 68.1 Some Characteristics of Common Cotton Byproducts Used as Animal Feed

Name	Crude Protein	Comments
IFN 5-01-625 Cottonseeds meal mechanical extracted 36% protein	Not less than 36% (wt/wt)	The product is obtained by finely grinding the cake that remains after removal of most of the oil from cottonseed by a mechanical extraction process. It must contain not less than 36% crude protein. It may contain an inert, nontoxic conditioning agent either nutritive or nonnutritive or any combination thereof, to reduce caking and improve flowability in an amount not to exceed that necessary to accomplish its intended effect and in no case exceed 0.5%. The name of the conditioning agent must be shown as an added ingredient
IFN 5-01-632 Cottonseeds meal solvent extracted 36% protein	Not less than 36% (wt/wt)	The product is obtained by finely grinding the flakes, which remain after removal of most of the oil from cottonseed by a solvent extraction process. It must contain not less than 36% crude protein. It may contain an inert, nontoxic conditioning agent either nutritive or nonnutritive or any combination thereof, to reduce caking and improve flowability in an amount not to exceed that necessary to accomplish its intended effect and in no case exceed 0.5%. The name of the conditioning agent must be shown as an added ingredient
Ammoniated Cottonseed Meal	See comments	Obtained by the treatment of cottonseed meal with anhydrous ammonia until a pressure of 50 pounds per square inch gauge is reached. It is to be used in the feed of ruminants as a source of protein and/or as the sole source of nonprotein nitrogen in an amount not to exceed 20% of the total ration
IFN 5-01-609 Cottonseeds meal mechanical extracted	23%	The product is composed of sound, mature, clean, delinted, and unhulled cottonseed, from which most of the oil has been removed by mechanical pressure. It must be designated and sold by its crude protein content. If ground, it must be so designated
IFN 5-01-633 Low Gossypol Cottonseed Meal, Solvent Extracted	Not less than 36% (wt/wt)	The product must contain not more than 0.04% free gossypol
IFN 1-01-599 Cotton hulls	4.1%–5%	The product consists primarily of the outer covering of the cottonseed. Primarily used as a fiber supplement
IFN 1-08-413 Cotton gin byproduct	No data	The product consists of the residue from the ginning of cotton. It contains cotton burrs, leaves, stems, lint, immature seeds, and sand and/or dirt. It shall not contain more than 38% crude fiber, nor more than 15% ash. It must be labeled with minimum guarantees for crude protein and crude fat and maximum guarantees for crude fiber and ash. If it contains more than 15% ash, the words "sand and/or dirt" must appear in the product name

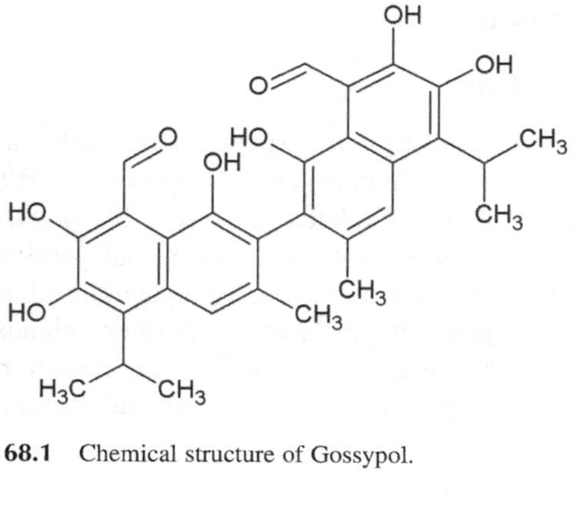

FIGURE 68.1 Chemical structure of Gossypol.

(Fig. 68.2; Boatner et al., 1947). Related purple (gossypurpurin) and orange (gossyfulvin) derivatives of gossypol are also typically present in the glands (Boatner et al., 1947). Notably, the pigment glands are very resistant to mechanical rupture as well as to solvent extraction (Boatner et al., 1947). The pigment gland contents (including unbound gossypol) can be extracted from the glands by water (rupture of the gland) and low molecular weight polar organic solvents. Storage of moist cottonseed may increase release of the pigments (including gossypol) from the pigment glands (Boatner et al., 1947).

In experimental studies, a racemate (+/ −)-gossypol, or an acetic acid complex is usually used. Gossypol exhibits complex tautomerism due to the presence of its

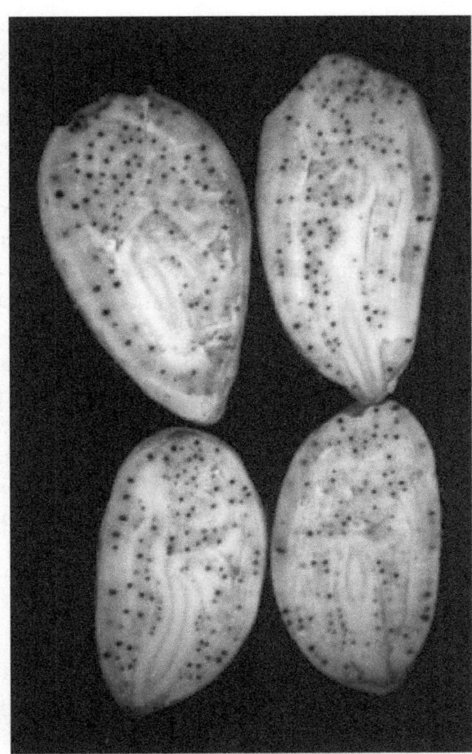

FIGURE 68.2 Sections of cottonseed showing darkly colored pigment glands. *Courtesy, Prof. K. S Rathore, Professor, Department of Soil & Crop Sciences, IPGB Laboratory for Crop Transformation, Texas A&M University.*

polyhydroxylated aromatic aldehyde moieties. The two halves of the molecule may have different tautomeric forms resulting in multiple molecular species. This influences its chemical reactions. The gossypol molecule is hindered around the bond connecting the two halves of the molecule thus the molecule is nonplanar and has a twofold axial dissymmetry.

Both gossypol stereoisomers typically both occur in the plant, often with a slight predominance of the (+)-isomer. However, upland cottons may have a 3:2 (+):(−) isomer ratio and some *Gossypium* sp. and commercial cotton varieties produce high levels (+) of isomer gossypol (e.g., *G. hirsutum* var. *marie* produces about 82% (+)-gossypol). As a crude generalization, the (−) gossypol isomer is reputedly more toxic than the (+) isomer (it is more cytotoxic, binds more strongly to proteins, it is the active antispermatogenic agent, and it is generally more toxic; Alexander et al., 2008, Blasi and Drouillard, 2002). However, the (+) isomer is more slowly eliminated.

Cottonseeds contain about 0.4%−2% unbound gossypol (wt/wt) depending on species, variety, plant growth conditions and level of insect predation (Blasi and Drouillard, 2002; Gadelha et al., 2014). Seeds from upland cotton (*G. hirsutum*) typically contain lower levels of gossypol than PIMA varieties. Seeds from PIMA varieties typically contain higher levels of the more toxic (−) isomer ($\approx$ 50%) compared with upland cotton varieties ($\approx$ 40% (−)).

Dietary Bioavailability and Level of Exposure

Gossypol isomers exist in 2 states: bound and unbound (covalent protein adducts, typically with lysine residues) with the unbound form being the most toxicologically active and the unbound form being mostly biologically unavailable (Blasi and Drouillard, 2002; Gadelha et al., 2014). Bound gossypol can be partially released by heating with acids. Maceration and rumen microflora actions typically decrease the unbound bioavailable fraction due to protein binding to ε-amino nitrogen, attaching to microbial cell walls, and binding with iron (all forms of presystemic detoxification).

Extruding, grinding and cracking of whole cotton seeds to improve digestibility may also increase the level of unbound gossypol, particularly with PIMA varieties (Blasi and Drouillard, 2002). These processes expose more of the seed pigment glands to the rumen environment more quickly plus PIMA variety seeds typically have fewer residual lint fibers and this tends to reduce their rumen residency time. This combination of effects reduces rumen presystemic detoxification, thus increasing toxic potential.

Heating during the cottonseed meal manufacturing process tends to increase the level of bound gossypol (Blasi and Drouillard, 2002), typically reducing the level of free gossypol to 0.1%−0.2%. The introduction of expander-solvent technology (currently used in about 97% of cottonseed meal manufactured in the United States) in the manufacturing process has also resulted in a reduction of free gossypol levels by $\approx$50% compared with typical levels in the 1960s and 1970s. Currently, cottonseed hulls typically have less than 0.049% free gossypol content (Blasi and Drouillard, 2002). Improvements in mechanical and air separation techniques have reduced the residual oil and protein levels in the hulls that are important sources of gossypol. Pelleting can further reduce cottonseed hull gossypol levels.

TOXICOKINETICS

Dietary interactions with iron and rumen microfloral fermentation can substantially reduce the systemic bioavailability of free gossypol. In rats, oral bioavailability is about 60% (Othman and Abou-Donia, 1988). Gossypol is often highly protein-bound to amino acids, particularly to those rich in lysine. In rats, the volume of distribution is small following IV dosing, implying limited distribution beyond the plasma. The major sites of concentration are in the liver and kidneys and the major route of excretion is biliary following glucuronidation and/or sulfation and/or complexation with iron (Gadelha et al., 2014). Small amounts are excreted in urine. In rats, elimination is biphasic. Repeated daily PO dosing is associated with an approximate doubling of the apparent elimination half-life (to 101.89 h) compared with single dosing and plasmatic/whole body accumulation is apparent (Othman and Abou-Donia, 1988). This is consistent with gossypol usually behaving as a cumulative toxin. Studies on individuals isomers have reported conflicting results: one study demonstrated no effect of isomeric form on pharmacokinetic parameters in rats (Othman and Abou-Donia, 1988). However, a separate single IV dose study in rats demonstrated that the terminal half-life of the (+) isomer was approximately double that of the (−) isomer (Chen et al., 1987). Single IV dose studies in dogs demonstrated that the elimination and volume of distribution of (+)-gossypol were five and six times those of (−)-gossypol whereas total body clearance and the AUC of the two enantiomers were similar (Wu et al., 1986). In humans the elimination half-life of (+)-gossypol was 29 times that of (−)-gossypol (Wu et al., 1986). In mid-lactation Brown Swiss dairy cows, repeated daily PO dosing for 7 days was associated with a terminal elimination half-life of ≈ 40–68 h (Lin et al., 1991).

Interspecies pharmacokinetic differences are also apparent among rodents: compared with mice, rats have a much lower volume of distribution and a substantially lower AUC for a given dose. The volume of distribution in mice is much higher than 1 L/kg, implying substantial tissue sequestration (consistent with accumulation in liver and kidney). Mice also eliminate gossypol approximately seven times faster compared with rats. These pharmacokinetic differences may contribute to the resistance of mice (compared with rats) to the contraceptive action of (+/−)-gossypol (Abou-Donia et al., 1989).

Excretion of gossypol in milk is usually regarded as being extremely low (negligible). However, gossypol was detected in milk following 30 and 60 days of feeding of whole cotton seeds containing 385.43–611.2 mg/kg of free gossypol (but not cottonseed meal containing 91.15–117.32 mg/kg free gossypol) to dairy cattle (Wang et al., 2012).

SUSCEPTIBILITY TO TOXICITY

Gossypol toxicity has been reported in poultry, pigs, dogs, cats, guinea pigs, sheep, goats, cattle, rabbits, rodents, monkeys, fish, and humans (Table 68.2). As a rule of thumb, all species should be regarded as being susceptible

TABLE 68.2 Dietary Gossypol and Disease

Species	Dietary Level	Effects	Reference
Horse (yearling)	115 ppm	No adverse effects noted	Potter G.D. (1981) Use of cottonseed meal in rations for young horses. *Feedstuffs* (53): 29
Horse (foal)	348 ppm	No adverse effects noted	McCall M.A. (1982) *Cottonseed Meal Supplement in Weanling and Suckling Foal Diets.* Texas A&M University, College Station, TX. MS thesis
Cattle (calves, dairy)	400 mg/kg BW/day Free gossypol	Centrilobular hepatic necrosis, cardiocyte vacuolation	Velasquez-Pereira J., Risco C.A., McDowell L.R., et al. (1999) Long-term effects of feeding gossypol and vitamin E to dairy calves. J Dairy Sci. 82: 1240–1251
Cattle (calves, dairy)	250–380 ppm	Fed during first 10 weeks of age. High mortality; developed ascites, diarrhea, weakness after consuming for 70–180 days	Holmberg C.A., Weaver L.D., Guterbock W.M., et al. (1988) Pathological and toxicological studies of calves fed a high concentration cottonseed meal diet. Vet Pathol 25: 147–153
Cattle (adult, dairy)	6.2 mg/kg BW/day Free gossypol	No adverse effects	Lindsey T.O., Hawkins G.E., Guthrie L.D. (1980) Physiological responses of lactating cows to gossypol from cottonseed meal rations. *J Dairy Sci* 63: 562–573
	8.8 mg/kg BW/day	Fed for 100 days.	

(Continued)

TABLE 68.2 (Continued)

Species	Dietary Level	Effects	Reference
		Increased erythrocyte fragility, decreased hemoglobin levels, increased respiratory rate	
Cattle (adult)	900–1200 ppm Free gossypol Dietary source was whole cottonseed (gossypol is extensively bound during digestion and is less bioavailable)	No adverse effects	Rogers G.M., Moore M.H. (1995) Optimal feeding management of gossypol-containing diets for beef cattle. *Vet Med* 90: 994–1005
	200–600 ppm Dietary source was cottonseed meal	No adverse effects	
Cattle (adult, dairy)	17.8–36.8 mg/kg BW/day Free gossypol	Fed for 70 days. Increased number of low quality embryos (fewer live cells, smaller in diameter, decreased blastocyst development, increased time to reach blastocyst stage) at 36.8 mg/kg BW/day (corresponded to plasma gossypol concentrations of >7 μg/mL)	Villaseñor M., Coscioni A.C., Galvão K.N., et al. (2008) Gossypol disrupts embryo development in heifers. J Dairy Sci. 91: 3015–3024
Cattle (adult, dairy)	≥28.43 mg/kg BW/day Free gossypol	Increased erythrocyte fragility	Mena H., Santos J.E., Huber J.T., Tarazon M., Calhoun M.C. (2004) The effects of varying gossypol intake from whole cottonseed and cottonseed meal on lactation and blood parameters in lactating dairy cows. J Dairy Sci. 87: 2506–2518
Cattle (adult, dairy)	951 mg/kg BW/day Free gossypol	Fed for 170 days. Reduced conception rates, lower pregnancy rates	Santos J.E., Villasenor M., Robinson P.H., et al. (2003) Type of cottonseed and level of gossypol in diets of lactating dairy cows: plasma gossypol, health, and reproductive performance. J Dairy Sci. 86: 892–905
Cattle (Angus, bulls)	8 mg/kg BW/day Free gossypol	Fed for ≥28 days. Increase in primary and secondary sperm abnormalities (effects slowly reversible after cessation of exposure)	Hassan M.E, Smith G.W., Ott R.S., et al. (2004) Reversibility of the reproductive toxicity of gossypol in peripubertal bulls. Theriogenology. 61: 1171–1179
Sheep (lambs)	900 ppm Free gossypol	Died from acute cardiac failure after 3 weeks of feeding	Morgan S., Stair E.L., Martin T., et al. (1988) Clinical, clinicopathologic, and toxicologic alterations associated with gossypol toxicosis in feeder lambs. *Am J Vet Res* 49: 439–493
Sheep	47 mg/kg BW/day Free gossypol	Reduced number of viable ovarian follicles (particularly primary and transition follicles), increased number of atretic ovarian follicles	Câmara A.C., Gadelha I.C., Borges P.A., et al. (2015) Toxicity of gossypol from cottonseed cake to sheep ovarian follicles. PLoS One. 10: e0143708
Sheep	≥9 mg/kg BW/day Free gossypol	Decreased ejaculate volume, increased percentage dead sperm, decreased total functional sperm fraction, decreased percentage	El-Mokadem M.Y., Taha T.A., Samak M.A., et al. (2012) Alleviation of reproductive toxicity of gossypol

(*Continued*)

TABLE 68.2 (Continued)

Species	Dietary Level	Effects	Reference
		forward motility, sperm abnormalities	using selenium supplementation in rams. J Anim Sci. 90: 3274–3285
Goats (adult, dairy)	250–300 ppm 348–414 mg/animal/day Free gossypol Fed for several months	Congestive heart failure	East N.E., Anderson M., Lowenstine I.J. (1989) Apparent gossypol-induced toxicosis in adult dairy goats. *J Am Vet Assoc* 204: 642–643
Swine	200–300 ppm Free gossypol	Cardiac insufficiency, respiratory distress, mortality > 50%	Haschek W.M., Beasley V.R., Buck W.B., Finnell J.H. (1989) Cottonseed meal (gossypol) toxicosis in a swine herd. *J Am Vet Assoc* 195: 613–615
	100 ppm Free gossypol	Considered "safe"	
Dog	5.4–5.7 mg/kg BW/day Free gossypol Duration of feeding unknown	Severe congestive heart failure, abnormalities in myocardial contractility	Patton C.S., Legendre A.M., Gompf R.E., Walker M.A. (1985) Heart failure caused by gossypol poisoning in two dogs. *J Am Vet Med Assoc* 187: 625–627
Dog	20 mg/kg/day Gossypol acetic acid	Reduced serum testosterone and estradiol-17 beta	Chang W.Y., Shidaifat F., Chang C. J., et al. (1996) Experimentally induced prostatic hyperplasia in young beagles: a model to evaluate the chemotherapeutic effects of gossypol. Res Commun Mol Pathol Pharmacol. 92: 341–360
Monkey (cynomolgus)	1.5–5 mg/kg BW/day (–)-free gossypol 25 mg/kg BW/day (+/–) free gossypol	Dosing for 4 weeks (1.5–5 mg/kg BW/day): Gastrointestinal distress, adverse effects on body weight gain, negative effect on serum protein, serum ion disturbances (including hypokalemia), adverse effects on reproduction. 13 weeks (25 mg/kg BW/day): Cardiotoxicity, hepatotoxicity, renal toxicity, and testicular damage	Heywood R. (1988) The toxicology of gossypol acetic acid and (–)-gossypol. Contraception. 37: 185–190
Monkey (rhesus)	4–8 mg/kg BW/day Free gossypol	Gastrointestinal toxicity and adverse effects on body weight after 4 weeks following dosing at 8 mg/kg BW/day	Sang G.W., Zhang Y.G., Shi Q.X., et al. (1980) Chronic toxicity of gossypol and the relationship to its metabolic fate in dogs and monkeys. Zhongguo Yao Li Xue Bao. 1:39–43
Chicken (broiler chicks)	1600 mg/kg BW/day Purified gossypol	Fed for 1–23 days. Weight loss, 28.1% mortality, increased feed conversion, decreased plasma iron, decreased hematocrit, enlarged gall bladders, Severe perivascular lymphoid aggregate formation, biliary hyperplasia, and hepatic cholestasis	Henry M.H., Pesti G.M., Brown T.P. (2001) Pathology and histopathology of gossypol toxicity in broiler chicks. *Avian Dis* 45: 598–604
	800 mg/kg BW/day Purified gossypol	Fed for 1–23 days. Weight loss, 28.1% mortality, increased feed conversion, decreased plasma iron, decreased hematocrit, enlarged gall bladders, Severe perivascular lymphoid aggregate formation, biliary hyperplasia, and hepatic cholestasis	
	400 mg/kg BW/day Purified gossypol	Fed for 1–23 days. Poor feed conversion, mild perivascular	

(Continued)

TABLE 68.2 (Continued)

Species	Dietary Level	Effects	Reference
		lymphoid aggregate formations and biliary hyperplasia	
Chicken (broiler)	≤ 186 mg/kg/day	Fed for 42 days. No adverse effects	Özdoğan M., Wellmann K., Paksuz E. (2012) Effect of gossypol on blood serum parameters and small intestinal morphology of male broilers. J Anim Physiol Anim Nutr (Berl). 96: 95–101
Chicken	1000 mg/kg BW/day Purified gossypol	Fed for 21 days. Reduced weight gain, weight loss, hepatotoxicity	Blevins S., Siegel P.B., Blodgett D.J., et al. (2010) Effects of silymarin on gossypol toxicosis in divergent lines of chickens. Poult Sci. 89: 1878–1886
Ducks	The threshold for adverse effect on growth of gossypol after 7 and 14 days of exposure were 32.20 (total gossypol) and 2.64 mg/day (free gossypol), and 92.12 (total gossypol) and 9.62 mg/day (free gossypol), respectively	Fed for up to 21 days. Effects included hepatotoxicity, reduced weight gain	Zeng Q.F., Yang G.L., Liu G.N., et al. (2014) Effects of dietary gossypol concentration on growth performance, blood profiles, and hepatic histopathology in meat ducks. Poult Sci. 93:2000–2009
Fish (tilapia)	0.11%–0.44% in the diet Total gossypol	Fed for 16 weeks. Decreased hematocrit, decreased hemoglobin, increased reticulocytes, increased abnormal erythroctyes (keratocytes, dacrocytes, schizocytes, knizocytes, segmentation), spleen abnormalities at the higher dose levels (hemosiderosis, melanosis, lymphoid depletion, necrosis, splenic vacuolation)	Garcia-Abiado M.A., Mbahinzireki G., Rinchard J., et al. (2004) Effect of diets containing gossypol on blood parameters and spleen structure in tilapia, *Oreochromis* sp., reared in a recirculating system. J Fish Dis. 27: 359–368
Fish (rainbow trout; juvenile)	0.11%–0.16% in the diet Total gossypol	Fed for 16 weeks. Decreased body weight, decreased body weight gain, decreased feed conversion, decreased protein efficiency ratio, decreased hematocrit	Lee K.J., Dabrowski K., Blom J.H., et al. (2002) A mixture of cottonseed meal, soybean meal and animal byproduct mixture as a fish meal substitute: growth and tissue gossypol enantiomer in juvenile rainbow trout (*Oncorhynchus mykiss*). J Anim Physiol Anim Nutr (Berl). 86: 201–213
Fish (rainbow trout)	142–619 ppm in the diet Free gossypol	Fed for 9 months. Decreased hematocrit and hemoglobin, decreased fecundity of females, decreased egg weight, decreased eye stage embryo survival, increased early embryonic loss, gossypol transferred to the eggs	Blom J.H., Lee K.J., Rinchard J., et al. (2001) Reproductive efficiency and maternal-offspring transfer of gossypol in rainbow trout (*Oncorhynchus mykiss*) fed diets containing cottonseed meal. J Anim Sci. 79: 1533–1539
Fish (rainbow trout)	0.013%–0.059% in the diet Free gossypol	Fed for up to 131 days. Reduced hematocrit and hemoglobin, reduced plasma protein, reduced seminal plasma protein	Dabrowski K., Rinchard J., Lee K.J., et al. (2000) Effects of diets containing gossypol on reproductive capacity of rainbow trout (*Oncorhynchus mykiss*). Biol Reprod. 62: 227–234

to gossypol toxicity until proven otherwise. In general, monogastric animals and preruminant stage sheep, goats and cattle are more susceptible than adult ruminants due to the lack of rumen presystemic detoxification. Critically, poisoning can still occur among adult ruminants if the intake is sufficiently high. Goats appear to be more sensitive than sheep and cattle. Among monogastric animals, guinea pigs and rabbits appear to be the most sensitive species. Horses are relatively resistant to toxicity, but caution is still required.

It should be noted that ammoniation of cottonseed meals (a procedure used to reduced aflatoxin content) may increase the risk of gossypol toxicity (Smalley and Bicknell, 1982).

MECHANISM OF ACTION

The mechanisms of action of gossypol are complex and incompletely understood: (1) gossypol has six phenolic hydroxyl groups and two aldehyde groups that allow covalent binding to epsilon-amino acids via Schiff's base condensation reactions (Fig. 68.3); this mechanism may explain the disruptive effects of gossypol on a large range of enzymes and proteins; (2) it uncouples mitochondrial oxidative phosphorylation; (3) it chelates iron, copper, aluminum and zinc resulting in mineral deficiencies (commonly iron deficiency); (4) it has complex oxidant and antioxidant activities; (5) it alters biological membrane potential, fluidity and permeability; (6) it binds to tubulin and inhibits microtubule assembly; (7) it disrupts gap junctions and cell to cell communication; (8) it induces renal leakage of potassium (most likely due to a direct effect on renal tubular epithelia) resulting in hypokalemia; (9) it increases erythrocyte osmotic fragility; (10) it stimulates eryptosis by increasing erythrocyte cytolsolic Ca^{2+}; (11) it decreases myocardial contractility resulting in congestive heart failure; (12) it disrupts cardiac conduction; and (13) it alters DNA synthesis and cell cycle progression. Gossypol poisoning can (rarely) occur acutely, but more typically the toxidrome develops slowly after weeks to months of exposure. Critically, because of its long elimination half-life and tissue sequestration, gossypol is generally regarded as a cumulative toxin.

Important features of gossypol-induced overt toxidromes, apart from negative effects on growth and production, include: (1) gossypol poisoning (acute/subacute/subchronic); (2) anemia; (3) hepatotoxicity; (4) disruption of reproduction; (5) immunotoxicity; and (6) effects on eggs.

TOXICITY

The gossypol dose-response has been poorly explored in most species. Much of the available information derives from small research studies utilizing a limited dose range and anecdotal clinical information (Table 68.2). Notably, gossypol toxicity has been associated with the use of cottonseed bedding for dogs (Uzal et al., 2005).

Acute Gossypol Poisoning

Acute poisoning is rare, but may occur if free gossypol intake levels are sufficiently high. Gossypol has only moderate acute lethality in most species (oral LD_{50}s of 2400–3340 mg/kg for rats, 500–950 mg/kg for mice, 350–600 mg/kg for rabbits, 550 mg/kg for pigs and 280–300 mg/kg for guinea pigs) with monogastric species being more susceptible than ruminants. The clinical signs of acute toxicity are similar across species and are relatively nonspecific: respiratory distress, impaired body weight gain, anorexia, weakness, apathy, and death after several days (Alexander et al., 2008; Kerr, 1989; Morgan et al., 1988; Rogers et al., 1975; Holmberg et al., 1988; Risco et al., 1992; Zelski et al., 1995; Fombad and Bryant, 2004). Heart failure is a feature of acute toxicity in calves, lambs, and dogs (Holmberg et al., 1988; East et al., 1994; Patton et al., 1985). Necropsy findings in ruminants include cardiogenic pulmonary edema, yellowish pleural effusions and ascites, gastroenteritis, centrilobular liver necrosis, and hypertrophic cardiac fiber degenerations, sometimes with evidence of acute congestive heart failure and cardiac dilation. An increased

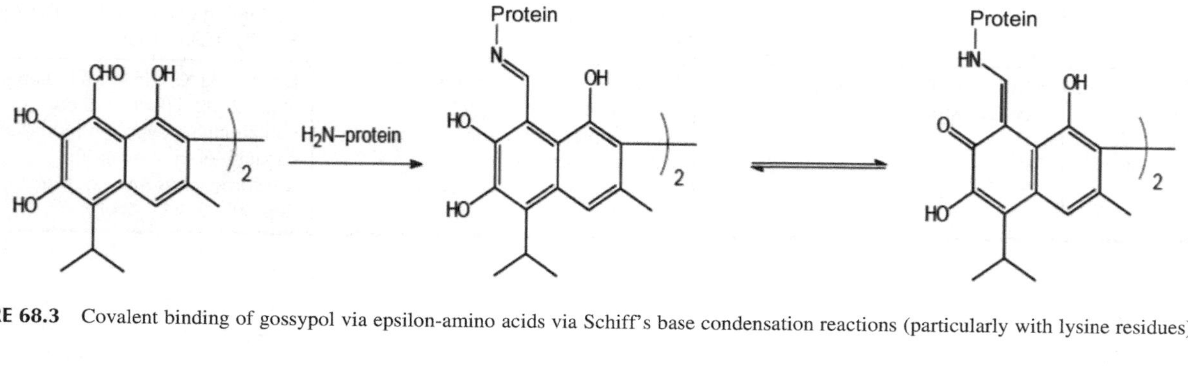

FIGURE 68.3 Covalent binding of gossypol via epsilon-amino acids via Schiff's base condensation reactions (particularly with lysine residues).

incidence of pneumonia is also associated with acute gossypol disease. Poisoning in pigs may result in reduced weight gain, anorexia, respiratory distress/thumping, cardiac insufficiency, coughing, exercise intolerance, fluid accumulation in body cavities, edema and congestion in liver, lung, and spleen and cardiomyopathy and cardiac hypertrophy (Fombad and Bryant, 2004).

Anemia

Reduced hematocrit and hemoglobin are sensitive markers of excessive dietary gossypol (Table 68.2). The effects may be due to iron deficient anemia due to gossypol complexation of iron in the gut and alterations in iron utilization (Braham et al., 1967; Clawson et al., 1975; Randel et al., 1996; Lindsey et al., 1980; Zhang et al., 2007; Mena et al., 2004; Skutches et al., 1973). However, gossypol also increases erythrocyte fragility and stimulates eryptosis via a calcium-dependent mechanism (Zbidah et al., 2012).

Hepatotoxicity

Hepatotoxicity is a noted effect in ruminants, pigs, rabbits, dogs, cats, monkeys, poultry, and fish. A number of species (notably sheep, swine, broiler chickens, rainbow trout, and catfish) display preferential accumulation of gossypol in the liver (Alexander et al., 2008). Gossypol feeding of juvenile turbot (*Scophthalmus maximus*) was associated with a proinflammatory cytokine state, activation of the endoplasmic reticulum unfolded protein cellular stress response and hepatic fibrosis (Bian et al., 2016). Diffuse hepatocyte fatty change (severity was dose-related), individual hepatocyte necrosis, perivascular lymphoid aggregates were notable features in meat ducks exposed to dietary gossypol for up 14 days at levels that resulted in impaired growth performance (Zeng et al., 2014). Dose-related hepatotoxicity, characterized by perivascular lymphoid aggregate formation, biliary hyperplasia, and hepatic cholestasis, occurred in chicks fed ≥ 400 mg of gossypol/kg (Henry et al., 2001). In calves, gossypol-induced hepatotoxicity is characterized by centrilobular hepatocellular necrosis (Holmberg et al., 1988; Velasquez-Pereira et al., 1999). However, in preruminant calves, hepatotoxicity was characterized by periacinar necrosis in acute cases and periacinar fibrosis in chronic cases (Zelski et al., 1995). Gossypol poisoning of dairy goats was associated with acute centrilobular necrosis of the liver (East et al., 1994). Toxicity in pigs following ingestion of 1300 mg/kg of free gossypol featured marked centrilobular congestion, loss of hepatocytes, and fatty degeneration (Haschek et al., 1989).

Disruption of Reproduction

Gossypol exposure adversely affects both male and female fertility as well as embryogenesis. In males, the undoubted adverse effects of gossypol on the testis and spermatogenesis have been mostly explored in rats, mice, hamsters, rabbits, monkeys, and humans (selected studies summarized in Table 68.3). Gossypol has antifertility effects in male rats at about 30 mg/kg where has humans are approximately 100 times more sensitive with antifertility effects being noted at 0.3 mg/kg (Coutinho, 2002). Antifertility effects in humans are compounded by hypokalemia and possibly irreversible sterilization or a slow recovery pattern. The modes of action of gossypol's effect on male fertility are incompletely understood. Known effects include: (1) inhibition of release and utilization of ATP by spermatocytes; (2) effects on microtubular function; (3) inhibition of calcium influx; (4) ultrastructural damage to the nuclear membrane, endoplasmic reticulum and mitochondria; (5) DNA damage in Sertoli cells; and (6) reduction in androgen receptors in Leydig cells, Sertoli cells, and myoid cells.

Selected studies on the effects of gossypol on female reproduction are summarized in Table 68.4 Key effects on female reproduction include: (1) disruption of the estrus cycle; (2) disruption of granulosa cell function; (3) disruption of ovarian follicle development; (4) inhibition of ovarian steroidogenesis; and (5) disruption of oocyte cumulus expansion and nuclear maturation.

Gossypol is known to disrupt embryonic development and embryonic implantation (Gadelha et al., 2014). The mode of action of these effects is assumed to be direct cytotoxicity, possibly in combination with oxidative stress, disruption of intercellular communication, and increased intracellular calcium. In vitro data demonstrates that in cattle, the critical window for gossypol exposure is at the one-cell stage of embryonic development (Hernández-Cerón et al., 2005). Selected studies on the effects of gossypol on embryonic development are summarized in Table 68.5.

Undesirable Effects of Cottonseed Meals on Eggs

In general, cottonseed products should be used with caution in laying hens during egg production. There are two main concerns, both of which involve egg discoloration. The first problem is that free gossypol is transferred from the hen to the eggs where it can combine with iron in the egg yolk resulting in discoloration ranging from olive green to brown to black. The yolk discoloration can be extensive or focal (i.e., yolk mottling consisting of spots or blotches ranging in color from transparent to brownish orange to almost black). The yolk color taint typically

TABLE 68.3 Summary of Selected Studies on the Effects of Gossypol on Male Reproduction

Species	Gossypol Dose	Effects	Reference
Hamster	10 mg/kg/day	Spermatocyte degeneration	Hahn D.W., Rusticus C., Probst A. (1981) Antifertility and endocrine activities of gossypol in rodents. *Contraception*. 24: 97–105
Rat	20 mg/kg/day	Spermatocyte degeneration	
Rat	25 mg/kg/day	Reduced spermatogenesis + Sertoli cell and seminiferous tubule damage	Heywood R., Lloyd G.K., Majeed S.K., Gopinath C. (1986) The toxicity of gossypol to the male rat. *Toxicology*. 40: 279–284
Rat	10 mg/kg/day	Seminiferous tubule damage, reduced serum testosterone, prostatic and seminal vesicle involution	Gåfvels M., Wang J., Bergh A., et al. (1984) Toxic effects of the antifertility agent gossypol in male rats. *Toxicology*. 32: 325–333
Rat	5–20 mg/kg/day	Decreased sperm count, decreased sperm motility, increased abnormal sperm count, reduced serum testosterone, LH and FSH	El-Sharaky A.S., Newairy AA, Elguindy NM, Elwafa AA. (2010) Spermatotoxicity, biochemical changes, and histological alteration induced by gossypol in testicular and hepatic tissues of male rats. *Fd Chem Toxicol*. 48: 3354–3361
Sheep	0.5 mg/kg/day for 20 days	No adverse effects on semen volume, sperm concentration, motility and morphology	Nunes F.D.C.R., de Araujo D.A.F.V., Bezerra M.B., Soto-Blanco B. (2010) Effects of gossypol present in cottonseed cake on the spermatogenesis of goats. *f Anim Vet Adv*. 9: 75–78
Goat			Guedes F.C.B., Soto-Blanco B. (2010) Sperm quality of sheep fed cottonseed cake. *Acta Scientiae Veterinariae*. 38: 415–418
Cattle	16.4 mg/kg/day	Decreased sperm production, reduced sperm motility, increased sperm mid-piece abnormalities	Chenoweth P.J., Risco C.A., Larsen R.E., et al. (1994) Effects of dietary gossypol on aspects of semen quality, sperm morphology and sperm production in young Brahman bulls. *Theriogenology*. 42:1–13
Cattle	8 mg/kg/day	Primary and secondary sperm abnormalities, increased number of sperm with proximal droplets	Hassan M.E., Smith G.W., Ott R.S., et al. (2004) Reversibility of the reproductive toxicity of gossypol in peripubertal bulls. *Theriogenology*. 61: 1171–1179

intensifies with increasing gossypol intake and with egg cold storage.

The second concern is associated with cottonseed meals containing more than 0.5%–1% residual oil. These meals typically contain cyclopropenoid fatty acids result in a pink discoloration of the albumen, particularly in stored eggs.

Immunotoxicity

Immunotoxicity has been demonstrated in several species. In rodents, gossypol inhibits lymphocyte mitogenesis and induces lymphocyte apoptosis (Quintana et al., 2000; Xu et al., 2009). Lymphoid depletion in thymus, mesenteric lymph nodes, and spleen has been noted in mice and these effects correlated with reduced humoral responses to T-cell–dependent antigens (Sein, 1986; Sijun et al., 2012). After inoculation with *Brucella abortus* smooth strain 99 (S99), specific anti-*Brucella* antibody production was impaired in lambs (Nagalakshmi et al., 2001) and calves (Pattanaik et al., 2003) fed cottonseed meal.

DIAGNOSIS

Diagnosis of gossypol poisoning is typically based on a history of long-term exposure to cottonseed products, the presence of the clinical toxidromes, and determination of free gossypol levels in food. Reduction in plasma iron has been used as a biomarker of possible gossypol toxicity in broiler chicks fed extruded cottonseed meal (Henry et al., 2001).

Feed gossypol levels of concern are: (1) >100 mg/kg (100 ppm) of feed in the diet of pigs or young ruminants <4 mo old; (2) >1000 ppm for adult ruminants; (3)

TABLE 68.4 Summary of Selected Studies on the Effects of Gossypol on Female Reproduction

Species	Gossypol Dose	Effects	Reference
Rat	5 mg/kg/day	Longer diestrus	Gu Y., Anderson N.O. (1985) Effects of gossypol on the estrous cycle and ovarian weight in the rat. *Contraception*. 32: 491–496
Rat	25 mg/kg/day	Lower levels of estradiol-17β	Lin Y.C., Fukaya T., Rikihisa Y., Walton A. (1985) Gossypol in female fertility control: ovum implantation and early pregnancy inhibited in rats. *Life Sci*. 37: 39–47
Rat	20 mg/kg/day	Irregular and longer estrous cycles, prolonged time for mating, decreased pregnancy rate, and reduced number of viable embryos	Lagerlöf R.K., Tone J.N. (1985) The effect of gossypol acetic acid on female reproduction. Drug Chem Toxicol. 8: 469–482
Cattle	≈51 mg/kg/day	No interference on cycling, first service conception rate, and ovarian morphology	Gambill M.D., Humphrey W.D. (1993) Effects of diets containing gossypol on ovarian histology, function and fertility in prepubertal beef heifers. *Theriogenology*. 40:585–593
Cattle	5 g free gossypol/animal/day	Reduced number of ovarian follicles >5 mm	Randel R.D., Willard S.T., Wyse S.J., French L.N. (1996) Effects of diets containing free gossypol on follicular development, embryo recovery and corpus luteum function in brangus heifers treated with bFSH. *Theriogenology*. 45: 911–922

TABLE 68.5 Summary of Selected Studies on the Effects of Gossypol on Embryonic Development and Embryonic Implantation

Species	Gossypol Dose	Effects	Reference
Cattle (superovulated)	36.8 mg/kg/day free gossypol for 70 days (gossypol plasma concentrations >7 μg/mL)	Increased number of low quality embryos, fewer number of live cells per embryo, smaller embryo diameter	Villaseñor M., Coscioni A.C., Galvão K.N., et al. (2008) Gossypol disrupts embryo development in heifers. J Dairy Sci. 91:3015–3024
Cattle	12 g/day free gossypol for 76 days	Lower pregnancy rates were associated with harvested embryos	Galvão K.N., Santos J.E., Coscioni A.C., et al. (2006) Embryo survival from gossypol-fed heifers after transfer to lactating cows treated with human chorionic gonadotropin. J Dairy Sci. 89:2056–2064
Cattle (superovulated)	43.5 g/day total gossypol	No adverse effects	Velasquez-Pereira J., Aréchiga C.F., McDowell L.R., et al. (2002) Effects of gossypol from cottonseed meal and dietary vitamin E on the reproductive characteristics of superovulated beef heifers. J Anim Sci. 80:2485–2492
Rat	5.30 μg/uterine horn	Complete inhibition of embryo implantation	Lin Y.C., Rajamahendran P., Rikihisa Y. (1991) Inhibition of rat embryo implantation in the gossypol-treated uterine horn. Theriogenology. 35: 769–7677
Rat		Delayed egg transport and retarded early development of the embryo in the oviduct	Lei H.Q., Xu Y.X. (1990) Effects of gossypol acetic acid on transport and development of fertilized eggs in rats. Yao Xue Xue Bao. 25: 561–565

≥350–400 ppm in mature dairy goats; (4) ≤6 mg/kg/day free gossypol for dogs. However, dietary gossypol intake alone is insufficient for a definitive diagnosis.

Tissue gossypol levels are supportive of gossypol exposure. Liver and kidney samples are typically the most diagnostically useful. However, definitive levels associated with toxicity have not been systematically established in domestic animals.

Differential Diagnosis

Important differential diagnoses include: (1) cardiotoxic ionophoric antibiotics (e.g., monensin, lasalocid, salinomycin, narasin) and ammonia; nutritional or metabolic disorders (e.g., selenium, vitamin E, or copper deficiency); infectious diseases; noninfectious diseases (e.g., pulmonary adenomatosis, emphysema); mycotoxicoses caused by *Fusarium*-contaminated grain; and toxicoses caused by plants with cardiotoxic and other effects (English yew *Taxus baccata*, Japanese yew *Taxus cuspidata*, laurel *Kalmia* spp., azalea *Rhododendron* spp., oleander *Nerium oleander*, yellow oleander or yellow-be-still tree *Thevetia peruviana*, purple foxglove *Digitalis purpurea*, lily-of-the-valley *Convallaria majalis*, dogbane *Apocynum* spp., coffee senna *Senna occidentalis*, bracken fern *Pteridium aquilinum*, white snakeroot *Eupatorium rugosum*, death camas *Zygadenus* spp., lantana *Lantana camara*, monkshood *Aconitum napellum*, and milkweed *Asclepias* spp.).

PREVENTION

The single best method of prevention is to accurately measure concentrations in feed and limit the dietary intake. The US FDA and the European Union have established maximum acceptable levels of gossypol in feeds. US 21CFR172.894 states that cottonseed products intended for human consumption must contain not more than 450 ppm of free gossypol. The European Union directive 2002/32 states that the maximum free gossypol concentrations for cottonseed meal is 5000 ppm and for cake is 1200 ppm. For complete feedstuffs, the maximum permissible level for laying hens is 20 ppm, for piglets is 60 ppm, for adult pigs is 60 ppm, for rabbits is 60 ppm, for other poultry is 100 ppm and is 500 ppm for cattle, sheep, and goats.

A selected summary of techniques used to reduce gossypol exposure is shown in Table 68.6. Critically, ammoniation of cottonseed meals should be avoided since it increases gossypol bioavailability. Immunoprotection via vaccination of a bovine serum albumin-gossypol conjugate has been attempted. Despite being immunogenic, the procedure increased the susceptibility to gossypol-induced hepatotoxicity (Fonseca et al., 2013).

TABLE 68.6 Selected Methods of Reducing the Risk of Gossypol Poisoning

Method	Comments
Heat treatments Roasting Extrusion	Heat treatment likely increases protein binding. However there is limited evidence that the conjugates that are formed can be broken down in the ruminant and chicken digestive tract, releasing free gossypol
Irradiation Gamma irradiation Electron beam irradiation	Mechanism of the effect is unknown. It is assumed that irradiation results in gossypol molecule aggregation, or cross-linking, fragmentation or oxidation
Fungal fermentation *Aspergillus niger* *oryzae* *Candida tropicalis* *Saccharomyces cerevisiae* *Geotrichum candidum*	These techniques are largely experimental and appear to be safe. However these products are not yet commercially available
Nutritional supplementation Ferric sulfate Sodium selenite Vitamin E	Dietary iron supplementation is a classic technique that relies upon complexation of gossypol and iron in the gut. The recommended rate of supplementation is 1 mol of iron for each mol of gossypol in the feed
	Supplementation of sheep with 1 mg of sodium selenite/day reduced the effects of gossypol on male fertility parameters
	Supplementation of cattle with 4000 IU/day reversed the effects of gossypol on male fertility parameters and the effects on the erythron

Since cottonseed products are notably low in lysine, supplementation (2% lysine) has been recommended when cottonseed constitutes a significant part of the diet of growing horses and broiler chicks (Henry et al., 2001). Iron supplementation may also be required (Henry et al., 2001).

CONCLUDING REMARKS AND FUTURE DIRECTIONS

Due to the advances in feed technology that have resulted in lower levels of gossypol in feed and greater awareness acute gossypol poisoning is now very low. However, the more chronic effects of impaired reproduction and immunotoxicity (particularly the potential effects on vaccine efficacy) remain a cause of substantial economic losses to the livestock industries. While cottonseed products are potentially useful feed sources for laying hens during molting, the effects of gossypol and cyclopropenoid fatty acids on eggs reduces the usefulness of this relatively cheap feed source during egg production.

Due to the fact that removing gossypol from the plants via genetic/biotechnological means strips them of their major defenses against insect predation, current efforts have focused on reducing the level of gossypol in cottonseed products after harvesting and on reducing the oral bioavailability of gossypol in feeds.

REFERENCES

Abou-Donia, M.B., Othman, M.A., Obih, P., 1989. Interspecies comparison of pharmacokinetic profile and bioavailability of (+/−)-gossypol in male Fischer-344 rats and male B6C3F mice. Toxicology. 55, 37−51.

Alexander, J., Benford, D., Cockburn, A., et al., 2008. Gossypol as undesirable substance in animal feed. EFSA J. 908, 1−55.

Bian, F., Jiang, H., Man, M., et al., 2016. Dietary gossypol suppressed postprandial TOR signaling and elevated ER stress pathways in Turbot (*Scophthalmus maximus* L.). Am. J. Physiol. Endocrinol. Metab. 312, E37−E47.

Blasi, D.A., Drouillard, J., 2002. Composition and Feeding Value of Cottonseed Feed Products for Beef Cattle. Kansas State University Agricultural Experiment Station and Cooperative Extension Service, MF-2538. pp1−20.

Boatner, C.H., Hall, C.M., Rollins, M.L., Castillon, L.E., 1947. Pigment Glands of Cottonseed. II. Nature and Properties of Gland Walls. Bot. Gazette. 108, 484−494.

Braham, J.E., Jarquín, R., Bressani, R., et al., 1967. Effect of gossypol on the iron-binding capacity of serum in swine. J. Nutr. 93, 241−248.

Chen, Q.Q., Chen, H., Lei, H.P., 1987. Comparative study on the metabolism of optical gossypol in rats. J. Ethnopharmacol. 20, 31−37.

Clawson, A.J., Maner, J.H., Gomez, G., et al., 1975. Unextracted cottonseed in diets for monogastric animals. I. The effect of ferrous sulfate and calcium hydroxide in reducing gossypol toxicity. J. Anim. Sci. 40, 640−647.

Coutinho, E.M., 2002. Gossypol: a contraceptive for men. Contraception. 65, 259−263.

East, E., Anderson, M., Lowenstine, L.J., 1994. Apparent gossypol-induced toxicosis in adult dairy goats. J. Am. Vet. Med. A. 204, 642−643.

Fombad, R.B., Bryant, M.J., 2004. An evaluation of the use of cottonseed cake in the diet of growing pigs. Trop. Anim. Health Product. 36, 295−305.

Fonseca, N.B.S., Gadelha, I.C.N., Oloris, S.C.S., Soto-Blanco, B., 2013. Effectiveness of albumin-conjugated gossypol as an immunogen to prevent gossypol-associated acute hepatotoxicity in rats. Food Chem. Toxicol. 56, 149−153.

Gadelha, I.C., Fonseca, N.B., Oloris, S.C., et al., 2014. Gossypol toxicity from cottonseed products. Sci. World J. 2014, 231635.

Haschek, W.M., Beasley, V.R., Buck, W.B., Finnell, J.H., 1989. Cottonseed meal (gossypol) toxicosis in a swine herd. J. Am. Vet. Med. Assoc. 195, 613−615.

Henry, M.H., Pesti, G.M., Bakalli, R., et al., 2001. The performance of broiler chicks fed diets containing extruded cottonseed meal supplemented with lysine. Poult Sci. 80, 762−768.

Hernández-Cerón, J., Jousan, F.D., Soto, P., Hansen, P.J., 2005. Timing of inhibitory actions of gossypol on cultured bovine embryos. J. Dairy Sci. 88, 922−928.

Holmberg, C.A., Weaver, L.D., Gutterbock, W.M., et al., 1988. Pathological and toxicological studies of calves fed a high concentration cotton seed meal diet. Vet. Pathol. 25, 147−153.

Kerr, L.A., 1989. Gossypol toxicosis in cattle. Compendium on Continuing Education for the Practising. Veterinarian. 11, 1139−1146.

Lin, Y.C., Nuber, D.C., Gu, Y., et al., 1991. Gossypolpharmacokinetics in mid-lactation Brown Swiss dairy cows. Vet. Res. Commun. 15, 379−385.

Lindsey, T.O., Hawkins, G.E., Guthrie, L.D., 1980. Physiological responses of lactating cows to gossypol from cottonseed meal rations. J. Dairy Sci. 63, 562−573.

Mena, H., Santos, J.E.P., Huber, T.J., et al., 2004. The effects of varying gossypol intake from whole cottonseed and cottonseed meal on lactation and blood parameters in lactating dairy cows. J. Dairy Sci. 87, 2506−2518.

Morgan, S., Stair, E.L., Martin, T., et al., 1988. Clinical, clinicopathologic, pathologic, and toxicologic alterations associated with gossypol toxicosis in feeder lambs. Am. J. Vet. Res. 49, 493−499.

Nagalakshmi, D., Sastry, V.R.B., Agrawal, D.K., Katiyar, R.C., 2001. Haematological and immunological response in lambs fed on raw and variously processed cottonseed meal. Asian-Aust. J. Anim. Sci. 14, 21−29.

Othman, M.A., Abou-Donia, M.B., 1988. Pharmacokinetic profile of (+/−)-gossypol in male Sprague-Dawley rats following single intravenous and oral and subchronic oral administration. Proc. Soc. Exp. Biol. Med. 188, 17−22.

Pattanaik, A.K., Sastry, V.R.B., Singh, D.K., et al., 2003. Effect of gossypol from cottonseed meal diets on some clinico-biochemical parameters and humoral immune response of crossbred calves fed barley or sorghum. Asian-Aust. J. Anim. Sci. 16, 1291−1296.

Patton, C.S., Legendre, A.M., Gompf, R.E., Walker, M.A., 1985. Heart failure caused by gossypol poisoning in two dogs. J. Am. Vet. Med. A. 187, 625−627.

Quintana, P.J.E., de Peyster, A., Klatzke, S., Park, H.J., 2000. Gossypol-induced DNA breaks in rat lymphocytes are secondary to cytotoxicity. Toxicol. Lett. 117, 85−94.

Randel, R.D., Willard, S.T., Wyse, S.J., French, L.N., 1996. Effects of diets containing free gossypol on follicular development, embryo recovery and corpus luteum function in brangus heifers treated with bFSH. Theriogenology. 45, 911–922.

Risco, C.A., Holmberg, C.A., Kutches, A., 1992. Effect of graded concentrations of gossypol on calf performance: toxicological and pathological considerations. J. Dairy Sci. 75, 2787–2798.

Rogers, P.A.M., Henaghan, T.P., Wheeler, B., 1975. Gossypol poisoning in young calves. Irish Vet. J. 29, 9–13.

Sein, G.M., 1986. The embryotoxic and immunodepressive effects of gossypol. Am. J. Chinese Med. 14, 110–115.

Sijun, D., Pawlak, A., Poźniak, B., et al., 2012. Effects of gossypol acetic acid on cellular and humoral immune response in non-immunized and SRBC-immunized mice. Central-Eur. J. Immunol. 37, 11–19.

Skutches, C.L., Herman, D.L., Smith, F.H., 1973. Effect of intravenous gossypol injection on iron ultilization in swine. J. Nutr. 103, 851–855.

Smalley, S.A., Bicknell, E.J., 1982. Gossypol toxicity in dairy cattle. Compend. Cont. Educat. Pract. Vet. 4, S378–S381, 1982.

Uzal, F.A., Puschner, B., Tahara, J.M., Nordhausen, R.W., 2005. Gossypol toxicosis in a dog consequent to ingestion of cottonseed bedding. J. Vet. Diagn. Invest. 17, 626–629.

Velasquez-Pereira, J., Risco, C.A., McDowell, L.R., et al., 1999. Long-term effects of feeding gossypol and vitamin E to dairy calves. J. Dairy Sci. 82, 1240–1251.

Wang, A.P., Zhang, J.M., Meng, Y.L., 2012. Effects of different sources and levels of dietary gossypol on gossypol residues in plasma and milk of lactating cows. J. Dairy Sci. 95, 5127–5132.

Wu, D.-F., Yu, Y.-W., Tang, Z.-M., Wang, M.-Z., 1986. Pharmacokinetics of (±)-, (+)-, and (−)-gossypol in humans and dogs. Clin. Pharmacol. Ther. 39, 613–618.

Xu, W.-B., Xu, L.-H., Lu, H.-S., et al., 2009. The immunosuppressive effect of gossypol in mice is mediated by inhibition of lymphocyte proliferation and by induction of cell apoptosis. Acta Pharmacol. Sinica. 30, 597–604.

Zbidah, M., Lupescu, A., Shaik, N., Lang, F., 2012. Gossypol-induced suicidal erythrocyte death. Toxicology. 302, 101–105.

Zelski, R.Z., Rothwell, J.T., Moore, R.E., Kennedy, D.J., 1995. Gossypol toxicity in preruminant calves. Aust. Vet. J. 72, 394–398.

Zeng, Q.F., Yang, G.L., Liu, G.N., et al., 2014. Effects of dietary gossypol concentration on growth performance, blood profiles, and hepatic histopathology in meat ducks. Poult Sci. 93, 2000–2009.

Zhang, W.-J., Xu, Z.-R., Pan, X.-L., et al., 2007. Advances in gossypol toxicity and processing effects of whole cottonseed in dairy cows feeding. Livestock Sci. 111, 1–9.

FURTHER READING

Waites, G.M., Wang, C., Griffin, P.D., 1998. Gossypol: reasons for its failure to be accepted as a safe, reversible male antifertility drug. Int. J. Androl. 21, 8–12.

Wang, X., Howell, C.P., Chen, F., et al., 2009. Gossypol - a polyphenolic compound from cotton plant. Adv. Food Nutr. Res. 58, 215–263.

Section XV

Mycotoxins

Chapter 69

Aflatoxins

Robert W. Coppock, Ralph G. Christian and Barry J. Jacobsen

INTRODUCTION

Aflatoxins (AFs), on a worldwide scale, are considered the most important mycotoxins in human foods and animal feedstuffs because of their hepatotoxicity and carcinogenicity. In the late 1950s and early 1960s, AFs were identified as the cause of the mysterious turkey "X" disease in Great Britain (Allcroft and Lewis, 1963). In the U.S., studies incriminated AFs as the cause of epizootic hepatitis in dogs, as the cause of moldy corn poisoning in pigs and as a potent carcinogen in rainbow trout (Newberne et al., 1966a, b; Newberne and Butler, 1969). AF linkages to human liver disease were made in the 1960s. Since these early discoveries, intensive research has shown and continues to show that the risk of exposure to AFs is a worldwide animal and human health issue. Many authors believe other fungal metabolites produced by aflatoxigenic and other fungi contribute to the toxicology observed under field exposure conditions (Coppock and Jacobsen, 2009).

AF-linked adverse health effects occur in companion animals, livestock, poultry, aquatic animals, humans, and other species because AFs are potent hepatotoxins, mutagens, carcinogens immunosuppressants, teratogens, have adverse epigenetic effects, and are linked with reproductive dysfunctions, and stunted growth (Allcroft and Lewis, 1963; Eaton and Gallagher, 1994; Shuaib et al., 2010a). AFs are the most potent naturally occurring hepatic carcinogens. AF contamination causes economic losses of corn, cottonseed, peanuts, sorghum, wheat, rice, nuts and spices, condiments, other commodities and processed foods. Because of their prevalence and toxicity, AFs are important worldwide in public health, with concerns centered on both primary poisoning from AFs in commodities, food, and feedstuffs, and relay poisoning from AFs in milk and other animal products. Aflatoxicosis in the human population, especially in areas stricken by poverty, drought, and other adverse growing conditions for plants, is an important public health problem and may be worsening by increasing climate stressors on plants. Another public health concern is that plant-source illicit drugs may contain AFs, and the interactions between AFs and infectious diseases can contribute to spread of infectious diseases in populations consuming these drugs.

Most governmental jurisdictions regulate the levels of AFs allowed in animal feedstuffs and human foods because of their toxicity. The allowable levels of AFs in animal feedstuffs and human foods vary with governmental jurisdictions and the perceived risk. For example, the regulated level for AFs in feedstuffs for dairy animals is lower than AFs in feedstuffs fed to beef cattle because of AFs being excreted in milk for human consumption. Commodities considered unsafe for human foodstuffs are often incorporated into animal feedstuffs, and most governments have regulations allowing this diversion. Grain and other seeds used for feeding wildlife can be high in AFs and these feedstuffs are generally under-regulated. Regulatory information for AFs is generally posted on government and WHO websites.

AFLATOXIGENIC FUNGI

Varga et al. (2009) have reviewed aflatoxigenic species. Three sections likely account for all the aflatoxigenic species of *Aspergillus*, namely *Flavi*, *Ochraceorosei*, and *Nidulantes* (Table 69.1). The most commonly recognized aflatoxigenic fungi are *Aspergillus flavus*, *Aspergillus parasiticus,* and *Aspergillus nomius*; other species of *Aspergillus* have been reported to produce AFs and are given in Table 69.1. Aflatoxigenic species of *Aspergillus* commonly grow in plant-source debris on the soil and can also grow in feedlot manure. Insects and wind currents spread the spores of aflatoxigenic fungi to plants and these fungi commonly colonize floral organs and areas of insect damage. Management of insect pests in the order Lepidoptera is a key to reducing AF contamination in corn, cotton and some tree nuts. In corn, infection can take place via silks and the subterranean flowers of peanuts can also be infected without insect injury. In addition

Veterinary Toxicology. DOI: http://dx.doi.org/10.1016/B978-0-12-811410-0.00069-6

TABLE 69.1 Species of *Aspergillus* Identified as Producers of Aflatoxins (AFs)

Species[a]	Country	Mycotoxins Identified[b]
A. bombycis (F)	Japan, Indonesia	AFB, AFG, KA
A. flavus (F)	Ubiquitous	AFB_1, AFB_2, KA, CPA, others
A. nomius (F)	United States, Thailand, S. America	AFB, AFG, KA, others
A. parasiticus (F)	Likely ubiquitous	AFB, AFG, KA, others
A. parvisclerotigenus (F)	Africa	AFB, AFG, CPA, KA
A. pseudocaelatus (F)	Argentina	AFB, AFG, CPA, KA
A. minisclerotigenes (F)	United States, Africa, Australia, S. America	AFB, AFG, KA, CPA, other
A. arachidicola (F)	S. America	AFB, AFG, KA, CPA, others
A. pseudonomius (F)	United States	AFB1, KA, other
A. pseudotamarii (F)	Japan, S. America	AFB_1, KA CPA
A. ochraceoroseus (O)	Africa	AFB_1, AFB_2, ST, others
A. rambellii (O)	Africa	AFB_1, AFB_2, ST, others
E. astellata (N)	S. America	AFB_1, ST, others
E. olivicola (N)	S. Europe	AFB_1, ST, others
E. venezuelensis (N)	S. America	AFB_1, ST, others

[a]*Section and F, Flavi; O, Ochraceorosei; and N, Nidulantes.*
[b]*AFB, aflatoxin B; AFG, aflatoxin G; CPA, cyclopiazonic acid; ST, sterigmatocystin; KA, kojic acid (not mycotoxins). For others see Varga et al. (2009, 2011).*
Source: Adapted with permission from Varga, J., Frisvad, J.C., Samson, R.A., 2009. A reappraisal of fungi producing aflatoxins. World Mycotoxin. J. 2, 263–277.

to plant residues, spores, mycelia, or sclerotia of aflatoxigenic fungi are commonly found in soil, commodity storage areas, processing facilities, and in the distribution systems for manufactured products. Strains of *A. flavus* can vary in AF capability from nontoxic to highly toxigenic and are more likely to produce more aflatoxin B_1 (AFB_1) than aflatoxin G_1 (AFG_1). *A. flavus* and other species can also produce cyclopiazonic acid. Strains of *A. parasiticus* generally have less variation in toxigenicity and generally produce AFB_1 and varying amounts of AFB_2, AFG_1, and AFG_2. The AF profile produced by *A. nomius* is like *A. parasiticus*, and like *A. parasiticus*, is not known to produce cyclopiazonic acid. Aflatoxigenic strains of *Aspergillus* can also produce sterigmatocystin (Table 69.1).

CONDITIONS FOR AFLATOXIN PRODUCTION

The fungi associated with AF production are *A. flavus*, *A. parasiticus*, and *A. nomius*, and these fungi are common in most soils and are usually involved in decay of plant materials (Jacobsen et al., 2007). The general growth conditions for aflatoxigenic species are described as requiring moisture contents in equilibrium with 80%–85% or more and temperatures of 13–42°C with optimum growth at 25–37°C. For example, the critical moisture content for growth of *A. flavus* in starchy cereal grains is 17%–18%, soybeans 17%–17.5% and for peanuts is 9%–10.5%. The upper limit of moisture for growth of *A. flavus* and production of AFs is about 30%. *A. flavus* will grow slowly below 13°C, and most rapidly at 37°C, but does not produce AFs at temperatures below 13°C or above 42°C. In addition to temperature and equilibrium relative humidity, other factors that influence AF production are carbon, nitrogen, plant metabolites, and sugars in substrates. High maximum and high minimum temperatures with high net evaporation are more important triggers than temperature and humidity alone. High AF production generally occurs when the fungus grows in the seed embryo. Both epigenetic and genetic factors affect AF production and the interactions are not well understood. Aflatoxigenic *A. flavus* isolates vary from 40% to >70% of the total *A. flavus* population. The percent of aflatoxigenic isolates can vary between ingredients and finished feeds, and finished feeds that have spoiled can have high primary production of AFs. Seeds damaged during harvest and damaged during handling in the commodity systems are more susceptible to invasion by species of *Aspergillus* and other fungi. Growth of aflatoxigenic fungi and AF production can rapidly occur especially in damaged high-moisture seeds. Experimental study on maize with 57% damaged kernels had 25 ppm AFB_1 at 6.5 days (Seitz et al., 1982). High levels of AF production can occur in maize before a 0.5% loss in dry matter occurs. High levels of AFs in corn are not linked to the production of kojic acid (black light fluorescence).

Moisture Management of Grain

The most common methods of preventing the growth of aflatoxigenic fungi in dry-stored commodities are by controlling the moisture level and temperature. Water available for aflatoxigenic fungi in stored grain is best indicated by equilibrium relative humidity or water activity (a_w, percent relative humidity/100) in the air around the grain. Temperature of the grain is important as the a_w increases with temperature. In cereal grains, aflatoxigenic fungi generally cannot grow when the a_w is below 0.80. A lower a_w is required for protection of oilseeds. Oilseeds have more available water on the seed surface because the seed absorbs less moisture. For most cereal grains, storage moisture of 12% is recommended for a wide range of grain temperatures, and for oilseeds the storage moisture from <8% to 9% is recommended for a wide range of temperatures inside the storage unit since other species of *Aspergillus* can grow in commodities at lower a_w than *A. flavus*. The growth of other fungi produce both heat and metabolic water creating a favorable moisture and temperature for *A. flavus* to grow rapidly.

Measuring moisture with a grain tester provides the average moisture of the kernels being tested, and the average value can misinterpret the storability of grain and oilseeds. If the moisture is heterogeneously distributed among the seeds or finished feed pellets, hot spots can occur. This phenomenon occurs because a microbial microcosm exists around each high-moisture seed and that microcosm can meet the requirements for fungal growth and mycotoxin production. This is the reason why high- and low-moisture grain and finished feeds should not be blended to give a lower average moisture test. In the microcosm with a favorable a_w level, growth of aflatoxigenic fungi can occur around each seed and the microcosm created by other organisms. The metabolism of microorganisms in the microcosms produce moisture and some microorganisms can also produce heat. Insects and other pests in grain also produce moisture, and hot spots can form because of insect and other pests in stored grain. Monitoring multiple areas of a storage unit and controlling insects are essential for preventing the production of mycotoxins. Samples for AF analyses and culture colonization should be placed in moisture-proof bags to prevent desiccation. As soon as possible after sampling, the individual moisture content of at least 100 seeds or pellets should be determined to identify moisture distribution in the kernels or pellets. This test result provides valuable insights into the storability of the commodity. Culture colonization can subsequently be done on each surface sterilized seed to determine infection with mycotoxigenic fungi.

Aflatoxigenic fungi prefer minimum temperatures of >25°C, with the abiotic and biotic microclimate of a geographic region having major effects on the genera and species of aflatoxigenic *Aspergillus* present and on production of AFs. Contamination of commodities in the field with AFs can be divided into two distinct phases. Growth of aflatoxigenic fungi and mycotoxin production occurring preharvest in the developing crop and postharvest mycotoxin production after the crop has matured and has been harvested. In the preharvest phase, wounds in the developing crop including those caused by insects, birds, mammals, and hail provide entry points for aflatoxigenic fungi. Insect damage to ears, bolls, pods, or nuts has been shown to dramatically increase the risk of AF production in maize, cotton, peanuts, almonds, and pistachios. Controlling insect damage reduces the risk of fungal infection and mycotoxin production. Excessive heat and drought generally decrease the native resistance of plants to aflatoxigenic fungi by physiological and anatomical mechanisms. Delayed irrigation and resulting drought stress at silking can increase the risk for AF production in maize. The postharvest fungal invasion and AF production can occur from maturation in the field to the point of human and animal consumption. Postharvest AF contamination can occur when the commodity is suitable for growth of aflatoxigenic fungi at harvest, and during transport, storage, and manufacturing. AF contamination in wheat is principally a postharvest phenomenon (Jacobsen, 2010), whereas maize contamination can be either preharvest or postharvest. Delayed harvest due to wet conditions with sufficient heat to support growth of aflatoxigenic fungi can result in high levels of AFs being produced. In some tree nuts, such as walnut, almond, and pistachio and in cotton, a natural opening in the nut hull or boll combined with delayed harvest and warm, humid conditions can result in significant fungal invasion and AF contamination. Damage to kernels or nuts during harvest, cleaning, and general grain handling weakens the mature seeds to fungal invasion. The suitability of grain for storage at harvest is adversely affected by moisture content, physical damage to the kernels, and the extent to which fungi have invaded the seed before storage. Moisture level is a risk factor for mycotoxins in stored commodities (Jacobsen et al., 2007). Blending grain of high moisture levels with grain of lower moisture levels can produce microcosms favoring mold growth and mycotoxin production because moisture equilibrium occurs at a slow rate. The high-moisture seeds provide a niche with a high a_w around the seed that is favorable for the growth of toxigenic and other fungi, which if allowed to grow, produces additional moisture and heat via microbial metabolic activity. The probability of fungal infection in seeds increases when the moisture content and temperature of the seed is increased. AF formation can rapidly occur (Coppock et al., 1989, 2012). High-moisture corn and sorghum lightly inoculated with *A. flavus* produces ppm levels of AFs within 48 h. Over-mature sweet corn was shown to contain 2.36 ppm AFB_1 and 0.21 mg of AFB_2 (Hall et al., 1989). Sweet corn may be more hazardous than field corn because of its higher free sugar content. Prevention of AF contamination before harvest strategies are being investigated and used. These include timing of irrigation, breeding maize, and other plants to increase resistance to fungal infection, and use of nonaflatoxigenic strains of *Aspergillus* spp. to displace toxigenic strains of *Aspergillus* spp. (Dorner, 2008; Ehrlich, 2014; Warburton and Williams, 2014).

In Vivo Production of Aflatoxins

A. flavus and *A. fumigatus* have also been identified as pathogens in animals and humans. AFs can be produced in tissues by toxigenic fungi. Assays of cultured *A. flavus* and *A. fumigatus* isolated from tissues have shown these fungi can produce AFs, and chemical analyses of infected tissues have shown AFs to be present (Pepeljnjak et al., 2004). Typically, aflatoxigenic fungi infect animals and humans that are immunocompromised. *A. nomius* has been identified as an etiology of keratitis.

PREVENANCE OF AFLATOXINS IN FEEDSTUFFS AND FOODS

Sources and Occurrences of Aflatoxicosis

Almost any food or feedstuffs that can support the growth of aflatoxigenic fungi can contain AFs. AFs and their metabolites can be transferred from the feed to edible animal products. Occurrences of contaminated cows', goats', and human milk with AFM_1 (animal metabolite of AFB_1) for human consumption have been identified (Fig. 69.1). Under field conditions, essentially all species of domestic animals have been poisoned with AFs. Outbreaks of aflatoxicosis linked to foods, birdseed, and other wildlife feeds have occurred and likely are under-reported. The sources of the AFs in pet foods have been primarily maize and maize byproducts, rice, millet, and peanut byproducts. Food garbage, moldy bread, and other diverted foods to animal feeds can be a source of AFs. Tree nuts, peanuts, figs, oilseeds, tobacco, coconut, condiments and spices,

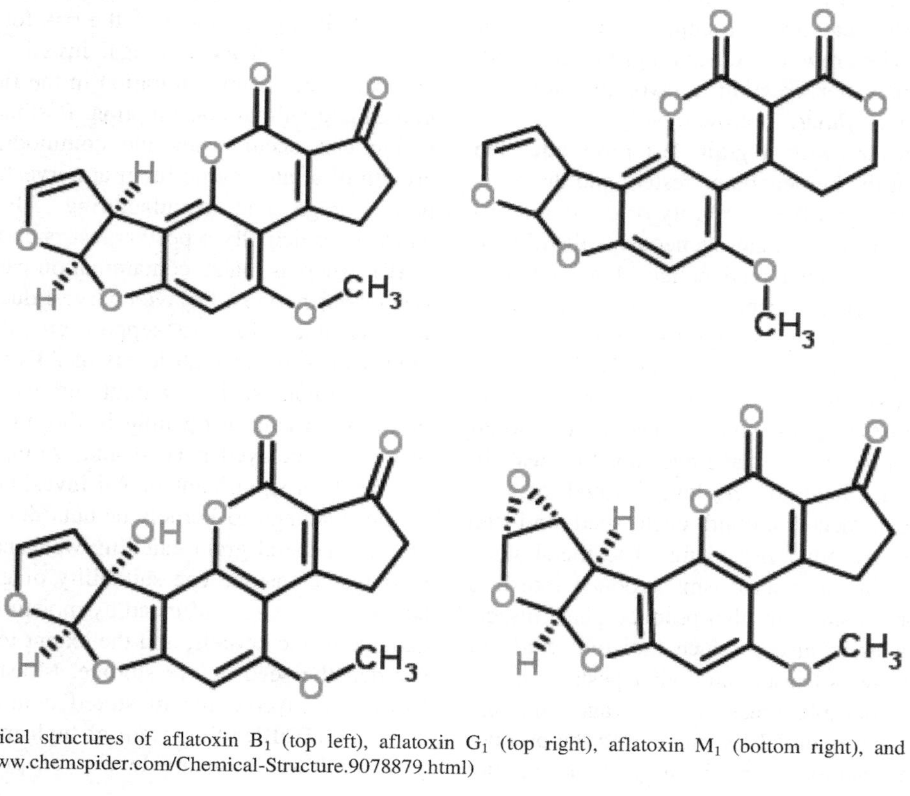

FIGURE 69.1 Chemical structures of aflatoxin B_1 (top left), aflatoxin G_1 (top right), aflatoxin M_1 (bottom right), and aflatoxin B_1 epoxide (bottom left). (http://www.chemspider.com/Chemical-Structure.9078879.html)

cereal grains, egg products, cheese and many other commodities, feedstuffs and foodstuffs have been shown to contain AFs. Cottonseed and other oilseeds can be a source of AFs in animal diets. Preharvest contamination of cottonseed with AFs occurs. In storage, growth of aflatoxigenic fungi may occur in cottonseeds when the average moisture level is greater than 7%–8%. The lipids and protein in cottonseeds enhances production of AFs. Peanut hay, peanuts, and peanut byproducts are an important source of AFs.

In stored peanuts, the growth of aflatoxigenic fungi can occur when moisture exceeds 8% and ambient temperature is above 25°C. *A. flavus* can grow in soybeans at a_w of 0.77. Distiller's byproducts can be a source of AFs. Fermentation does not destroy AFs. On a dry matter basis, the concentration of AFs in the stillage, compared to AFs in the feedstock, is increased by a factor of 3–4 due to the loss of starch. Approximately 40% of the AFs are in the syrup (distiller's solubles) fraction and 60% are in the solids fraction. AFs generally are not found in the alcohol fraction.

CHEMISTRY AND SAMPLING AND ANALYSIS

AFs have a difuranocoumarin chemical structure (Fig. 69.1). Approximately 18 AFs have been chemically characterized. AFs are in two chemical groups, the difurocoumarocyclopentenone series (includes AFB_1, AFB_2, AFB_{2A}, AFM_1, AFM_2, AFM_{2A}, and aflatoxicol) and the difurocoumarolactone series (includes AFG_1 and AFG_2). The "B" Group fluoresce blue in long wavelength ultraviolet light and the "G" Group fluoresce green. The primary concern in foodstuffs and feedstuffs are AFB_1, AFB_2, AFG_1, and AFG_2. Analytical results generally are the sum of the concentrations of these four toxins. AFB_1 is the most potent AF, a carcinogen, and this chemical form is generally the most abundant in feedstuffs and foodstuffs. The order of toxicity is $AFB_1 > AFG_1 > AFB_2 > AFG_2$. Hydroxylated aflatoxin metabolites are excreted in milk, and the important metabolites are AFM_1 and AFM_2, from AFB_1 and AFB_2, respectively. Although AFM_1 and AFM_2 are commonly associated with milk and other edible animal products, aflatoxigenic fungi can also release these metabolites into the substrate.

The analytical methods for AFs have recently been reviewed and will not be discussed in this chapter (Xie et al., 2016). In assaying for AFs, the assumption is the analytical results can be applied to the matrix samples. A representative sample may be difficult to obtain because the distribution of AFs in the suspect feedstuff or foodstuff can be highly heterogeneous inclusive of feeds and foods "thoroughly" mixed during manufacturing (Shephard, 2016). Heterogenous distribution of AFs often occurs in storage-transport because of the infinite number of microcosms that can be formed around each seed. A small percentage of the kernels in a lot of wheat, barley, corn, cottonseed, peanuts, and other feedstuffs and foodstuffs may be contaminated with very high concentrations of AFs. Sampling error can occur even with a well-designed sampling protocol. Accurate sampling is essential and can be overlooked when using AF test kits in the field. Interpretations of analytical findings must be done in context of the sampling procedure, and aflatoxicosis cannot be ruled out based on negative chemical analyses of feedstuffs. Lumps of feedstuffs can be very high in AFs and these lumps can be consumed.

PHARMACOKINETICS/TOXICOKINETICS

Absorption

AFs are efficiently absorbed by passive diffusion from the gastrointestinal tract and are primarily transferred from the intestine into the hepatic portal blood. The rate of absorption of AFB_1 in rats is dependent on concentration providing evidence that AFs are absorbed by passive diffusion. Young animals absorb AFs more efficiently than older animals. For example, rats at 2.5 weeks of age absorbed AFB_1 at a rate ~15 times greater than rats 4–5 weeks of age. Rats absorb AFB_1 most efficiently from the duodenum and jejunum. Lactation can affect AF absorption. The rate of AFB_1 absorption from the duodenum of rats in diestrus was greater than the rate of absorption of AFB_1 from the duodenum in rats in mid-lactation. Cattle were given a single oral dose of AFs from rice culture (42% AFB_1 and 27% AFB_2) in gelatin capsules (Cook et al., 1986). AFB_1 and AFM_1 were observed in venous blood 30 min after dosing and reached maximal levels 4–8 h after dosing. The maximal levels of AFM_1 occurred before AFB_1 and the maximal blood levels of AFB_1 generally were higher than AFM_1. These findings suggest that AFs are rapidly absorbed from the rumen.

Metabolism and Excretion

Biotransformation of AFs in the liver is important in the toxicology of AFs. The biotransformation of AFs can also occur in the kidney and intestinal tract. Research has focused on the biotransformation of AFB_1. Except for the AFB_1-8,9-epoxide, the biotransformation products are less toxic than AFB_1. Cytochrome P450s (CYP enzymes) have a key role in the biotransformation of AFB_1 to AFB_1-8,9-epoxide. The formation of AFB_1-8,9-epoxide is the most significant biotransformation pathway because the AFB_1-8,9-epoxide forms adducts with DNA, RNA, and proteins. Conjugation of AFB_1-8,9-epoxide with glutathione (GSH) is an important detoxification pathway.

Other biotransformation products of AFB_1 are AFQ_1, which can be metabolized to AFH_1. AFB_1 is also metabolized to AFP_1, AFM_1, aflatoxicol and other metabolites. The AFP_1, AFM_1, AFQ_1 and aflatoxicol form glucuronide and sulfate conjugates.

Turkeys are a sensitive species and they activate AFB_1 3.5 times more than chickens by hepatic enzymes homologs to human CYP1A2, CYP1A5 and other CYPs to form AFB_1-8,9-epoxide. Younger birds activate AFB_1 at a greater rate than older birds. Conjugation of the AFB_1-8,9-epoxide by GSH is generally considered to be the rate-limited determinant in species susceptibility to AFB_1 rather than the rate at which AFB_1-8,9-epoxide is formed. The affinity of the glutathione S-transferases for AFB_1-8,9-epoxide is also important. Cattle were given single oral doses (ranging from 0.2 mg, 0.4 mg, 0.6 mg, and 0.8 mg/kg body weight) of AFs from rice culture (42% AFB_1 and 27% AFB_2) in gelatin capsules (Cook et al., 1986). AFM_1 was identified in rumen contents 2 h after dosing. This observation suggests that AFM_1 is formed by the flora and fauna in the rumen. Urine from these cattle contained AFB_1 and AFM_1. Bovine hepatocytes metabolized AFB_1 to AFM_1, AFB_1 dihydrodiol and minor levels of AFB_1 glutathione conjugate. Pretreatment of goats with phenylbutazone and benzoflavones increased the toxicity of AFB_1. Hepatic Kupffer and endothelial cells in the rat have been shown to have upregulated activity of enzymes that convert AFB_1 to AFM_1 (Gemechu-Hatewu et al., 1996). The P450 inducers used were phenobarbitol, isosafrole, Aroclor 1254, and 3-methylcholanthrene.

AFs are excreted in milk, eggs, urine, semen, bile, and feces. Bingham et al. (2004) identified AFM_1 and AFP_1 in dog urine. AFB_1, AFM_1, and aflatoxicol are transferred to the egg. Humans exposed to dietary AFs excrete ABM_1, AFP_1, and AFB_1-N^7-Guanine in urine. AFs have been shown to be excreted in boar semen. Rats excrete AFB_1 into the intestinal tract via bile and the intestinal mucosa also excretes AFs. Cattle excrete AFB_1 predominately in the feces and AFM1 predominately in the urine (Stubblefield et al., 1983).

Aflatoxins in Milk

AFs can be present in milk and processed milk products (Becker-Algeri et al., 2016). Milk products such as cheese and dried milk also can become directly contaminated with AFs by fungal growth in these substrates. AFs appear in cows' milk within 12–48 h after ingestion. The percentage of dietary AFs being excreted in milk varies from 0.17% to 3%. Veldman et al. (1992) derived the formula for excretion of AFM_1 in milk as (ng AFM_1/kg milk = 1.19 × dietary intake of μg AFB_1/day/ cow + 1.9). Alternatively, herd-specific analytical data can be used to calculate the dietary:milk ratio for AFs and is an accurate predictor. To compare with other mammalian species, humans excrete 0.09%–0.43% of dietary AFB_1 intake as AFM_1 in breast milk, sheep excrete 0.26%–0.33% of the dietary AFB_1 as AFM_1 in the milk, and AFs in sows' milk have been shown to be ~1000-fold less that the AFs in the diet (Zarba et al., 1992; Silvotti et al., 1997; Battacone et al., 2009). The dietary threshold for AF excretion in cows' milk appears to be ~15 ppb dietary level or 230 μg AFB_1/cow/day. AFs in milk generally disappear within 24–72 h after all the AFs have been removed from the diet. The percentage of AFs in milk increases with increasing milk yields. Cows in early lactation can excrete from 3.8% to 6.2% of the dietary AFB_1 as AFM_1 in the milk, and cows in late lactation can excrete 1.8% to 2.5% of dietary AFB_1 as AFM_1. This phenomenon appears to be linked to cows having upregulation of AFB_1 metabolism during early lactation. Sheep and swine excrete AFs in milk. Sheep excreted 0.26% to 0.33% of the dose of AFB_1 as AFM_1 in milk. AF level in curds is two times higher than whole milk (Battacone et al., 2005). AFs are excreted in sows' milk (Silvotti et al., 1997). The levels of AFs in sows' milk increased over a 25-day lactation period. The sows were fed diets containing 800 ppb AFB_1 or a diet containing 400 ppb AFB_1 + 400 ppb AFG_1 for the entire gestation and lactation period. The average ratio of AFs in the diet to AFs in milk was ~1000:1. Sows fed diets containing 800 ppb AFB_1 or 400 ppb AFB_1 + 400 ppb AFG_1 excreted AFB_1 or AFB_1 + AFG_1, respectively. Sows fed AFB_1 excreted AFM_1 and sows fed AFB_1 + AFG_1 excreted AFM_1 + AFM_2 metabolites. The consensus in the scientific literature is that AFs are stable in milk (Becker-Algeri et al., 2016). Approximately 75% of AFs in milk are found in the casein (protein) fraction and 25% in the whey fraction of milk. AFs are also found in butter and the division is ~84% in butter milk and ~16% in butter. AFs are concentrated in cheese, and the concentration factor varies with the type of cheese and cheese-making procedures.

Residues in Meat and Eggs

Chickens were fed a diet containing rice culture that AGB_1 produced by *A. parasiticus* (Pandey and Chauhan, 2007). At 2 weeks of age groups of birds were placed on diets containing 0.0, 2.5, 3.13, and 3.91 ppm AFB_1, respectively. These diets were fed for 40 weeks. Tissues and eggs were collected on day 40 for AF analyses. AFB_1 in eggs increased with feed levels, the mean levels were 1.43, 1.39, and 1.63 ppb, respectively, for the different treatment groups. AFB_1 levels in breast meat were 18, 26, and 26 ppb, respectively, for the chickens in the different treatment groups. The levels of AF metabolites were not reported. Young birds require longer to clear AFB_1 from tissues. Laying hens (Hy-Line Brown) were feed a diet for 6 weeks containing peanut meal naturally contaminated with AFs (Jia et al., 2016). The mixed diets averaged 89.5, 20.2, 9.6, and 3.7 mg/kg of AFB_1, AFB_2, AFG_1, and AFG_2, respectively. The average egg weighed 39.9 g and the mean AFB_1, AFB_2, and AFM_1 were 0.02, 0.11 and 0.02 μg/kg of egg, respectively. No AFG_1 and AFG_2 were identified in the eggs.

The translocation of AFs into edible tissues of pigs has been studied. Jacobson et al. (1978) fed feeder pigs (54–72 kg body mass) diets containing pure AFB_1 at 100, 200, and 400 ppb. The basal diet contained 0.1 ppb AFB_1 and 0.1 ppb AFB_2. These diets were fed for 4 weeks. Liver, kidney, and skeletal muscle contained levels of AFB_1 that were correlated with the feeding level. In decreasing dietary level, AFB_1 levels in liver were 1.5, ~0.5, and ~0.2 ppb; levels in skeletal muscle were ~1, ~0.5 and ~0.2 ppm; and levels in kidney were 4.4, ~0.7, and ~0.2 ppb.

Steers were fed rations containing 0, 60, 300, and 600 ppb AFB_1 (Helferich et al., 1986). FB_1 and AFM_1 were detected in the liver in the animal receiving the 300 and 600 ppb AFB_1 and these residues cleared in 7 days.

TOXICODYNAMICS

Mechanisms of Action

The metabolism of AFs is linked with toxication (Eaton and Gallagher, 1994). AFB_1 is metabolized in a CYP-dependent reaction to AFB_1-8,9-epoxide that forms adducts with macromolecules in the cell. The affinity of AFB_1-8,9-epoxide in decreasing order for macromolecules is DNA > RNA > protein. The DNA adduct is formed with N^7-guanine and this adduct is relatively resistant to DNA repair processes. Upregulation of the CYP system increases the toxicity of AFs. AFB_1 alters genetic expression in the immune system, liver and likely all organ systems in the body. Species sensitivity to AFs is linked to the rate of bioactivation and the rate of detoxification. AFB_1-8,9-epoxide is primarily detoxified in Phase II synthetic reactions by GSH. In mammals, glutathione S-transferase mediated conjugation is an important detoxification pathway, and species differences in enzyme activity in part account for differences in species susceptibility. Other Phase II pathways that decrease the toxicity of AFs include formation of glucuronide and sulfates.

Immunotoxic Effects

AFs are immunotoxic and reduce the native resistance to disease and vaccine protection is also impaired. The apparent clinical signs of aflatoxicosis may be limited to increased occurrences and severity of common infectious disease. Recovery from infectious disease may be prolonged and require additional treatments. A clue to immune dysfunction can be infections caused by organisms that are not generally considered to be hard hitting pathogens. Studies have shown that the immunotoxicity of AFs could be a teratogenic effect of prenatal or pre-hatching exposure to AFs. As a general summary, AFB_1 lowers lymphoid cell populations especially circulating activated lymphocytes, suppresses lymphoblastogenesis and decreases both cutaneous delayed-type hypersensitivity, and graft versus host reaction and suppresses innate immunity. AFB_1 reduces natural killer cytolysis and macrophage functions including phagocytic activity and production of oxidative radicals. AFB_1 alters genetic expression of immune responses of innate and acquired immunity. A brief literature review is provided for the immunotoxic effects of AFs in different species. The immunotoxic effects of AFs have been studied in pigs. Treatment with AFB_1 has been shown to shorten the incubation period of *Serpulina* (*Treponema*) *hyodysenteriae* in pigs (Joens et al., 1981). Pigs given AFB_1 and infected with *S. hyodysenteriae* also had a longer period of diarrhea. Feeding weanling piglets a diet containing 140 or 280 ppb AFs (~70% AFB_1) for 4 weeks caused an increase in serum γ-globulin (Marin et al., 2002). At the 280 ppb level, a reduced immune response to vaccination for *Mycoplasma agalactiae* was observed. There were indications that expression of interleukin-1β and tissue necrosis factor-α was decreased by exposure at the 280 ppb level. The white blood cell numbers responded by a decrease at the 140 ppb level and increased at the 280 ppb level. Sows were fed diets containing 800 ppb AFB_1 or a diet containing 400 ppb AFB_1 + 400 ppb AFG_1 for the entire gestation and lactation period (Silvotti et al., 1997). At 25 days of age the piglets born to the sows were found to have decreased immune functions in lymphoproliferative response to mitogens, monocyte-derived macrophages failed to have induced oxygen bursts and granulocytes had reduced chemotactic response. AFs have been shown to be immunotoxic in ruminants. Feeding a diet containing 2 ppm AFs (83.4% AFB_1, 12.3% AFB_2 and AFG_1 and AFG_2) to lambs for 37 days increased serum γ-globulin, decreased bacteriostatic activity in serum and decreased cellular immunity (Fernandez et al., 2000). AF inhibits thymidine uptake by phytohemagglutinin-stimulated lymphocytes. Holstein steers (183 kg), fed a diet containing ~375 ppb AF for 17.5 weeks, were observed to have a decrease in delayed cutaneous hypersensitivity (Richard et al., 1983). Changes were not observed in antibody production (*Brucella abortus* antigen) and lymphoblastogenesis. AFs reduce the native resistance of the mammary gland to disease. The immunotoxic effects of AFs on native resistance of poultry to infectious diseases have been studied. Immunotoxic effects in poultry are lymphocytopenia, reduced T cell counts, and reduced native resistance to disease. Exposure to AFs can increase or decrease the immune response to vaccinations. The more constant finding is a decreased response to vaccination to Newcastle virus, fowl adenovirus serotype-4, and dinitrochlorobenzene-induced hypersensitization. Exposure of hens can cause immune dysfunction in chicks.

Reproductive and Teratogenic Effects

AFs can impair reproductive performance and prenatal exposure can have adverse in utero/in ovum effects. The observed effects of AFs in mature roosters are testicular degeneration, a reduction in plasma testosterone, reduction in testicular mass and altered hormonal response. In hens, exposure to AFs reduces egg production and egg hatchability. Pregnant rats (P_1) were administered AFB_1 intramuscularly from day 12 to day 19 of pregnancy (Supriya and Reddy, 2015; Supriya et al., 2016). The offspring (F_1) were evaluated for anatomical morphology and tested to determine developmental, behavior and response to physical stress. The birth weight of the F_1 pups exposed to AFB_1 in utero was significantly less than controls. For the F_1 offspring in both studies, the behavioral evaluations (cliff avoidance, negative geotaxis, righting from supine position and ascending wire mesh, and locomotor and exploratory activities) were impaired. For the F_1 females, there was a delay in sexual maturity (vaginal opening), prolonged corticosterone response to stress, irregular estrus, and at maturity, decreased fertility. For the F_1 males, body weights, and the relative weights of the testis, cauda epididymis, prostate, seminal vesicles, and liver were decreased on postpartum day 100. Spermatozoa parameters were reduced in the F_1 males. The numbers of viable and mobile sperm were reduced and the numbers of abnormal sperm were increased. Exposure to AFB_1 in utero also decreased serum testosterone and fertility indices. In F_1 males, testosterone, and activity of testicular hydroxysteroid dehydrogenases were significantly decreased in a dose-dependent manner with a significant increase in the serum follicle-stimulating hormone and luteinizing hormone. Deterioration in the testicular and cauda epididymal architecture was observed in the F_1 generation rats from exposed P_1 females. Fertility studies on the exposed F_1 generation revealed a significant decrease in the mating index rats with an increase in the pre- and postimplantation losses in rats mated with prenatal AFB_1-exposed males. In pigs, sows exposed to AFs are at risk for increased fetal loss, birthing piglets with reduced birth weight. Harvested porcine oocytes exposed in vitro to AFB_1 have impaired maturity. The effects of AFs on human reproduction have been reviewed (Shuaib et al., 2010b). There is evidence that dietary AFs decrease male fertility (Ibeh et al., 1994). A study at an infertility clinic showed that there is a correlation between dietary levels and serum levels of AFs. The mean AF levels in serum were 1.660 ± 0.04 μg/mL (infertile men) and 1.041 ± 0.01 μg/mL (fertile men). The infertile men had a higher percentage (50%) of abnormal spermatozoa and AF in their semen. Exposure to AFs increases fetal loss. Women with high serum levels of AFB_1-lysine adduct ($\geq$11.34 pg/mg of albumen) are at greater risk for delivering a child with low birth weight. Women with increased blood levels of AFM_1 have increased risk to give birth to a baby with abnormally low birth weight.

TOXICOPATHOLOGY OF AFLATOXINS

Clinicopathology

Acute aflatoxicosis causes changes in clinicopathology parameters and these changes can occur before the onset of clinical signs. The activities of liver enzymes in serum are increased and the increased activity is indicative of hepatic damage. Increased activity of hepatic enzymes in serum includes γ-glutamyl transpeptidase (transferase) (GGT), aspartate aminotransferase (AST), alkaline phosphates (ALP), sorbitol dehydrogenase (SDH), ornithine carbamyl transferase (OCT), and isocitrate dehydrogenase (ICD). Once released into serum the activities of hepatic enzymes decrease as metabolic processes remove the hepatic enzyme from serum. The activities of hepatic enzymes in serum that have been reported to be the most consistently elevated in aflatoxicosis are GGT, AST, ALT (nonruminants), and SDH. Serum bilirubin levels are also increased and in ruminants, photosensitization can occur. Serum proteins can decrease in aflatoxicosis, or albumin and β-globulins decrease and γ-globulins increase. Elevated serum bilirubin and ALT, low cholesterol, may be a predictor of a fatal outcome of aflatoxicosis in dogs (Bruchim et al., 2012). Prolonged prothrombin and activated partial thromboplastin times also are a guarded prognosis. A leukocytosis may or may not occur. Thrombocytopenia increases the likelihood of concurrent diffuse intravascular coagulation. In poultry, a decrease in erythrocyte numbers, hemoglobin, and leukopenia consisting of heteropenia and lymphopenia can occur. The timing of hepatic enzyme determinations in terms of the pathogenesis of aflatoxicosis is important. The rate of enzyme release from hepatic cells and the half-life of the enzyme in serum must be considered in interpretation of laboratory findings as well as nonhepatic sources of the enzymes. The activity of GGT in serum has a slower temporal decrease than AST. Dehydration must be considered in interpretation of serum proteins and in advanced aflatoxicosis, multiorgan shutdown can occur. Hemorrhage can alter the hematology parameters. Thus, the expression of clinical signs and pathology can vary with each incidence and this may be due to exposure, under field conditions, to multiple mycotoxins. Animals infected with aflatoxicosis can have concurrent infectious diseases. The clinicopathology of aflatoxicosis have been presented in more detail in the second edition of *Veterinary Toxicology: Basic and Clinical Principles* (Coppock et al., 2012).

Macroscopic and Microscopic Pathology

Edema and Hemorrhage

The pathology of aflatoxicosis has been described in several species. Edema including anasarca and edema fluid in the peritoneal and thoracic cavities can be observed (Osweiler and Trampel, 1985; Bastianello et al., 1987; Coppock et al., 1989; Hall et al., 1989). The gall bladder, bile duct, abomasal wall, and colonic mesentery may be edematous. There may be edema of the omentum near the stomach or abomasum and in the colonic mesentery. Gall bladder and perirenal edema may be marked in cattle and pigs. Edema of the brain has been reported for horses (Angsubhakorn et al., 1981). Hemorrhage into the gastrointestinal tract, into body cavities and on body organs has been reported. Hemorrhage is due to decreased production of clotting factors by the liver. Acute aflatoxicosis in cattle, horses, pigs, and dogs may result in serious hemorrhages in the gastrointestinal tract, on serosal surfaces, on the epicardium and endocardium, in skeletal muscle, perirenal and in the urinary bladder (McKenzie et al., 1981; Bortell et al., 1983; Jakhar and Sadana, 2004; Bruchim et al., 2012). Pigs can also have hemorrhage occurring in the pleural and peritoneal cavity. The urine may be dark red colored.

Hepatic Lesions

Histopathology includes bile duct proliferation, hepatocyte necrosis, and early fibrosis of the liver (Newberne and Butler, 1969). Regeneration of hepatocytes may be found in dogs, and nodular hyperplasia may be present in turkeys, trout, and ducklings (Newberne et al., 1966b; Newberne and Butler, 1969; Bastianello et al., 1987). Variation in the size of hepatocytes, with some megalocytes and binucleate cells, is recorded in many reports. Chronic liver lesions are characterized by firm, fibrous pale livers, by nodular hyperplasia, and in some cases, neoplasia. Icterus is present. The liver may be swollen, friable, and congested. Histologically, the liver may have necrosis in variable patterns. In the rat, monkey, and duckling, the necrosis is reported to be periportal, while in cattle, pigs, horses, goats, and sheep, the pattern is recorded to be centrilobular (Butler, 1964; Newberne et al., 1966a; Samarajeewa et al., 1975; Carlton and Szczech, 1978; Abdelsalam et al., 1989; Coppock et al., 1989; Mathur et al., 1991). In the dog the pattern may be either or both periportal and centrilobular, while in the rabbit the pattern is reported to be midzonal (Newberne et al., 1966a; Chaffee et al., 1969; Clark et al., 1980). Hyperplasia of the bile duct cells occurs rapidly in ducklings and may be present in horses, dogs, and chickens, and mild bile duct cell hyperplasia may be seen in cattle and pigs (Newberne and Butler, 1969; Ketterer et al., 1975; Coppock et al., 1989). Multinucleated hepatocytes have been observed in dogs, cattle, and other species. Reactive fibroblasts have been observed in dogs. Humans infected with hepatitis B virus appear to be at greater risk for hepatic neoplasia when they are exposed to AFs. Chronic liver injury and regenerative hyperplasia are considered critical for the development of liver neoplasia. Dividing liver cells are more likely to form DNA adducts. In sub-Saharan Africa, consumption of corn is associated with increased HIV and consumption of rice is associated with increased liver cancer (Williams et al., 2010).

Other Lesions

Renal lesions of protein in proximal tubules and glomerular spaces are recorded in horses and rats (Butler, 1964; Newberne and Butler, 1969; Bortell et al., 1983). Hemosiderin deposition in tubule cells occurs in horses (Angsubhakorn et al., 1981). Cardiac myofiber degeneration is recorded in horses and rats (Butler, 1964; Angsubhakorn et al., 1981). Brain lesions described as focal malacia in the cerebral hemispheres in horses were reported and for other species (Angsubhakorn et al., 1981). Hepatic encephalopathy can occur because of liver damage. Subacute lesions observed at necropsy include firm, pale livers in all species and clear yellow ascites and pleural fluid accumulation especially in pigs and dogs (Newberne and Butler, 1969). Icterus is usually present. Pneumonia is reported in calves as likely secondary to edema and the effects of AF on the immune system. Lesions of photosensitization have been reported in cattle.

Differential Diagnosis

The lesions of aflatoxicosis and those of pyrrolizidine alkaloid toxicosis have been observed to be very similar especially in cattle (Loosmore and Markson, 1961). Cattle are generally considered to be more susceptible to pyrrolizidine alkaloids. When AFs and pyrrolizidine alkaloid are at issue, it is important to examine pasture, forage, concentrate feeds, and gastrointestinal contents to determine the presence of poisonous plants that may contain pyrrolizidine alkaloids. In some geographic areas seeds containing pyrrolizidine alkaloids can be present in grain screenings, and their identity lost in the grinding and pelleting processes. Finished feeds and screenings can be assayed for pyrrolizidine alkaloids.

TREATMENT AND PREVENTATIVE ANTIDOTES

A specific treatment for aflatoxicosis has not been identified. AFs from all sources should be removed from the diet. Symptomatic care of the affected animals is recommended. Animals on a low protein diet are more susceptible to AFs (Cullen and Newberne, 1994). Supplementing poultry diets with choline and methionine and N-acetylcystine is probably beneficial (Cullen and Newberne, 1994). Adding vitamin E to swine diets containing 2.5 ppm AFs does not ameliorate the severity of aflatoxicosis, but can reduce the clinical expression of aflatoxicosis while not changing the pathology. Changing mineral supplementation in cattle generally is not beneficial in aflatoxicosis. It is the experience of the authors that domestic animals with signs of aflatoxicosis never fully recover.

The best prevention of AFs is to avoid the conditions under human control for formation, and if possible, avoid the consumption of AFs. Different materials have been shown to reduce the toxic effects of AFs. One approach is to use natural products and drugs to alter the biotransformation of AFs. For example, green tea reduces or blocks initiation of AFB_1-induced hepatocarcinogenesis likely by the polyphenols reducing the activity of CYP1A1 (Coppock and Dziwenka, 2016). Enteric binding of AFs has been studied. Briefly, these products adsorb AFs and thereby make them unavailable for absorption. Studies have shown that clays in the smectite group, including hydrated sodium calcium aluminosilicate (calcium montmorillonite), reduce the clinical expression of toxicity of dietary AFs in several species. The surface activity of the smectite clay for AFs can be enhanced by manufacturing processes. The oxymoron in some studies is liver pathology was not changed by the addition of adsorbents to the diet and performance parameters were improved. It is of interest to point out that clay eating has been observed to be a long-standing practice in some African societies where aflatoxicosis is endemic. Modified yeast cell wall *Saccharomyces cerevisiae* can decrease absorption of AFs in some species and not in others.

AFLATOXIN INTERACTIONS

The presence of AFs in feeds and foods greatly increases the probability of other mycotoxins being present. The most plausible explanations for multiple mycotoxins being present are: conditions exist for food-feed stuffs and their ingredients to support the growth of differing fungi, often in rapid succession; some species of fungi can produce multiple mycotoxins; and ingredients in foods and feeds can have differing geographic and storage conditions that supported fungal growth. The presence of multiple mycotoxins can alter the dose–response curve of each mycotoxin present. The toxic interactions of AFB_1, zearalenone, and deoxynivalenol (DON) were studied in mice (Sun et al., 2014). AFB_1 + DON displayed synergistic effects, while AFB_1 + zearalenone displayed antagonistic effects. Parameters used were liver weights, serum ALT, AST, albumin, total protein, hepatic total antioxidant capacity, and elevated hepatic malondialdehyde. The level of a mycotoxin that is generally considered to be safe can be altered by the presence of other mycotoxins. The interactions of mycotoxins may vary between the indicators of effect. AFB_1 and FB_1 combination were shown to decrease feed conversion and feed consumption in feeder pigs (Dilkin et al., 2003). The dietary levels were 30 ppm FB_1 and 50 ppb AFB_1. Pigs were fed a diet containing AFs produced in rice culture, a diet containing FB_1 produced in corn culture and a diet containing both the rice and corn cultures (Harvey et al., 1995). The interactions of AFs and FB_1 for immunologic and liver disease parameters were essentially additive. Cultures containing AFs and T_2 toxin when fed in combination to Japanese quail showed interactions appeared to be additive (Madheswaran et al., 2004). Ochratoxin A (2.0 μg) and AFB_1 (0.5 μg) injected into eggs on day 3 of incubation increases the number of abnormal fetuses. The interactions of AFs and DON in naturally contaminated maize were studied in pigs (Chaytor et al., 2011). This study showed that diets containing both AFs and DON greater than 60 and 300 μg/kg, respectively, may diminish growth and reduce feed intake. Diets containing 120 μg of AFs/kg and 600 μg of DON/kg may reduce native resistance to disease, alter systemic inflammation and cause liver damage. Ethanol was found to potentiate AFB_1-induced hepatocarcinogenesis (Tanaka et al., 1989). There are interactions between AFs and infectious agents. Henry et al. (2002) estimated that the presence of hepatitis B surface antigen in serum increased the human susceptibility to AFs by a factor of 30. Shivachandra (2003) showed the immunosuppression of AFs was additive with fowl adenovirus serotype-4. Exposure to AFs is a risk factor for mammary tumors in dogs (Frehse et al., 2015).

CONCLUDING REMARKS AND FUTURE DIRECTIONS

Worldwide, AFs are an important group of mycotoxins. Human and animal populations are exposed to AFs in foodstuffs and feedstuffs, respectively. Fungal growth and AF production can occur before harvest and during transportation and storage. The distribution of AFs in substrate being sampled can have a huge influence on analytical findings. Contamination of foodstuffs and feedstuffs with AFs is an important economic loss. The parent AF and its toxic metabolites can be present in edible animal products, especially milk. AFB_1 is the most potent known naturally occurring carcinogen. AFs target the liver, the immune system, reproduction, and have teratogenic and epigenetic effects. The differences between species in the toxication of AFs, especially AFB_1, likely explain species differences in toxicity. The reaction of AFB_1 epoxide with DNA, RNA, and proteins are important mechanisms of intoxication. Agronomic practices, pest control, and ensuring that stored commodities cannot support growth of fungi are the best control for prevention of AF contamination of foods and feeds. For future direction, there is a need to investigate the excretion of AFB_1-adducts by domestic and companion animals for use as a diagnostic test for exposure. The interactions of mycotoxins are important considerations in terms of predicting safe exposure of humans and animals to mycotoxins.

REFERENCES

Abdelsalam, E.B., el-Tayeb, A.E., Nor Eldin, A.A., et al., 1989. Aflatoxicosis in fattening sheep. Vet. Rec. 124, 487–488.

Allcroft, R., Lewis, G., 1963. Groundnut toxicity in cattle: experimental poisoning of calves and a report on clinical effects in older cattle. Vet. Rec. 75, 487–493.

Angsubhakorn, S., Poomvises, P., Romruen, K., et al., 1981. Aflatoxicosis in horses. J. Am. Vet. Med. Assoc. 178, 274–278.

Bastianello, S.S., Nesbit, J.W., Williams, M.C., et al., 1987. Pathological findings in natural outbreak of aflatoxicosis in dogs. Onderstepoort J. Vet. Res. 54, 635–640.

Battacone, G.A., Nudda, M., Palomba, M., et al., 2005. Transfer of aflatoxin B_1 from feed to milk and from milk to curd and whey in dairy sheep fed artificially contaminated concentrates. J. Dairy Sci. 88, 3063–3069.

Battacone, G.A., Nudda, M., Palomba, M., et al., 2009. The transfer of aflatoxin M_1 in milk of ewes fed diet naturally contaminated by aflatoxins and effect of inclusion of dried yeast culture in the diet. J. Dairy Sci. 92, 4997–5004.

Becker-Algeri, T.A., Castagnaro, D., de Bortoli, K., et al., 2016. Mycotoxins in bovine milk and dairy products: a review. J. Food Sci. 81, R544–552.

Bingham, A.K., Huebner, H.J., Phillips, T.D., et al., 2004. Identification and reduction of urinary aflatoxin metabolites in dogs. Food Chem. Toxicol. 42, 1851–1858.

Bortell, R., Asquith, R.L., Edds, G.T., et al., 1983. Acute experimentally induced aflatoxicosis in the weanling pony. Am. J. Vet. Res. 44, 2110–2114.

Bruchim, Y., Segev, G., Sela, U., et al., 2012. Accidental fatal aflatoxicosis due to contaminated commercial diet in 50 dogs. Res. Vet. Sci. 93, 279–287.

Butler, W.H., 1964. Acute toxicity of aflatoxin B_1 in rats. Br. J. Cancer. 18, 756–758.

Carlton, W.W., Szczech, G.M., 1978. Mycotoxicosis in laboratory animals. In: Wyllie, T.W., Morehouse, L.G. (Eds.), Mycotoxic Fungi. Mycotoxins, Mycotoxicoses. An Encyclopedic Handbook, vol. 2. Marcel Dekker, New York, New York.

Chaffee, V.W., Edds, G.T., Himes, J.A., et al., 1969. Aflatoxicosis in dogs. Am. J. Vet. Res. 30, 1737–1748.

Chaytor, A.C., See, M.T., Hansen, J.A., et al., 2011. Effects of chronic exposure of diets with reduced concentrations of aflatoxin and deoxynivalenol on growth and immune status of pigs. J. Anim. Sci. 89, 124–135.

Clark, J.D., Mahaffey, E.A., Hatch, R.C., et al., 1980. Experimentally induced chronic aflatoxicosis in rabbits. Am. J. Vet. Res. 41, 1841–1845.

Cook, W.O., Richard, J.L., Osweiler, G.D., et al., 1986. Clinical and pathologic changes in acute bovine aflatoxicosis: rumen motility and tissue and fluid concentrations of aflatoxins B_1 and M_1. Am. J. Vet. Res. 47, 1187–1825.

Coppock, R.W., Dziwenka, M., 2016. Green tea extract. In: Gupta, R.C. (Ed.), Nutraceuticals. Efficacy, Safety and Toxicity. Academic Press/Elsevier, Amsterdam, pp. 633–652.

Coppock, R.W., Jacobsen, B.J., 2009. Mycotoxins in animal and human patients. Toxicol. Ind. Health. 25, 637–655.

Coppock, R.W., Reynolds, R.D., Buck, W.B., et al., 1989. Acute aflatoxicosis in feeder pigs, resulting from improper storage of corn. J. Am. Vet. Med. Assoc. 195, 1380–1381.

Coppock, R.W., Christian, R.G., Jacobsen, B.J., 2012. Aflatoxins. In: Gupta, R.C. (Ed.), Veterinary Toxicology Basic and Clinical Principles, second ed. Elsevier, Toronto.

Cullen, J.M., Newberne, P.M., 1994. Acute hepatotoxicity of aflatoxins. In: Eaton, D.L., Groopman, J.D. (Eds.), The Toxicology of Aflatoxins. Human Health, Veterinary, and Agricultural Significance. Academic Press, Toronto.

Dilkin, P., Zorzete, P., Simas, M.M., et al., 2003. Toxicological effects of chronic low doses of aflatoxin B_1 and fumonisin B_1-containing *Fusarium moniliforme* culture material in weaned piglets. Food Chem. Toxicol. 41, 1345–1353.

Dorner, J.W., 2008. Management and prevention of mycotoxins in peanuts. Food Addit. Contam. 25, 203–208.

Eaton, D.L., Gallagher, E.P., 1994. Mechanisms of aflatoxin carcinogenesis. Annu. Rev. Pharmacol. Toxicol. 34, 135–172.

Ehrlich, K.C., 2014. Non-aflatoxigenic *Aspergillus flavus* to prevent aflatoxin contamination in crops: advantages and limitations. Front. Microbiol. 5, 50.

Fernandez, A., Hernandez, M., Verde, M.T., et al., 2000. Effect of aflatoxin on performance, hematology, and clinical immunology in lambs. Can. J. Vet. Res. 64, 53–58.

Frehse, M.S., Martins, M.I., Ono, E.Y., et al., 2015. Aflatoxins ingestion and canine mammary tumors: there is an association? Food Chem. Toxicol. 84, 74–78.

Gemechu-Hatewu, M., Platt, K.L., Oesch, F., et al., 1996. Distribution and induction of aflatoxin B_1-9a-hydroxylase activity in rat liver parenchymal and non-parenchymal cells. Arch. Toxicol. 70, 553–558.

Hall, R.F., Harrison, L.R., Colvin, B.M., 1989. Aflatoxicosis in cattle pastured in a field of sweet corn. J. Am. Vet. Med. Assoc. 194, 938.

Harvey, R.B., Edrington, T.S., Kubena, L.F., et al., 1995. Influence of aflatoxin and fumonisin B_1-containing culture material on growing barrows. Am. J. Vet. Res. 56, 1668–1672.

Helferich, W.G., Garrett, W.N., Hsieh, D.P., et al., 1986. Feedlot performance and tissue residues of cattle consuming diets containing aflatoxins. J. Anim. Sci. 62, 691–696.

Henry, S.H., Bosch, F.X., Bowers, J.C., et al., 2002. Aflatoxin, hepatitis and worldwide liver cancer risks. Adv. Exp. Med. Biol. 504, 229–233.

Ibeh, I.N., Uraih, N., Ogonar, J.I., et al., 1994. Dietary exposure to aflatoxin in human male infertility in Benin City, Nigeria. Int. J. Fertil. Menopausal. Stud. 39, 208–214.

Jacobsen, B.J., 2010. Mycotoxins. In: Bockus, W.W., Bowden, R.L., Hunger, R.M., et al., Compendium of Wheat Diseases and Pests, third ed. APS Press, St. Paul, MN.

Jacobsen, B.J., Coppock, R.W., Mostrom, M.S., 2007. Mycotoxins and Mycotoxicoses (Extension Publication EBO174). Montana State University, Bozeman, MT.

Jacobson, W.C., Harmeyer, W.C., Jackson, J.E., et al., 1978. Transmission of aflatoxin B into the tissues of growing pigs. Bull. Environ. Contam. Toxicol. 19, 156–161.

Jakhar, K.K., Sadana, J.R., 2004. Sequential pathology of experimental aflatoxicosis in quail and the effect of selenium supplementation in modifying the disease process. Mycopathologia. 157, 99–109.

Jia, R., Ma, Q., Fan, Y., et al., 2016. The toxic effects of combined aflatoxins and zearalenone in naturally contaminated diets on laying performance, egg quality and mycotoxins residues in eggs of layers and the protective effect of *Bacillus subtilis* biodegradation product. Food Chem. Toxicol. 90, 142–150.

Joens, L.A., Pier, A.C., Cutlip, R.C., 1981. Effects of aflatoxin consumption on the clinical course of swine dysentery. Am. J. Vet. Res. 42, 1170–1172.

Ketterer, P.J., Williams, E.S., Blaney, B.J., et al., 1975. Canine aflatoxicosis. Aust. Vet. J. 51, 355–357.

Loosmore, R.M., Markson, L.M., 1961. Poisoning of cattle by Brazilian groundnut meal. Vet. Rec. 73, 813–814.

Madheswaran, R., Balachandran, C., Murali Manohar, B., et al., 2004. Influence of dietary cultural material containing aflatoxin and T2 toxin on certain serum biochemical constituents in Japanese quail. Mycopathologia. 158, 337–341.

Marin, D.E., Cureu, I., Sarca, M., et al., 2002. Changes in performance, blood parameters, humoral and cellular immune responses in weanling piglets exposed to low doses of aflatoxin. J. Anim. Sci. 80, 1250–1257.

Mathur, M., Rizvi, T.A., Nayak, N.C., 1991. Effect of low protein diet on chromic aflatoxin B_1-induced liver injury in rhesus monkey. Mycopathologia. 113, 175–179.

McKenzie, R.A., Blaney, B.J., Connole, M.D., et al., 1981. Acute aflatoxicosis in calves fed peanut hay. Aust. Vet. J. 57, 284–286.

Newberne, P.M., Butler, W.H., 1969. Acute and chronic effects of aflatoxin on the liver of domestic and laboratory animals: a review. Cancer Res. 29, 236–250.

Newberne, P.M., Russo, R., Hall, A., 1966a. Acute toxicity of aflatoxin B_1 in the dog. Path. Vet. 3, 331–340.

Newberne, P.M., Wogan, G.N., Hall 3rd., A., et al., 1966b. Effects of dietary modifications on response of the duckling to aflatoxin. J. Nutr. 90, 123–130.

Osweiler, G.D., Trampel, D.W., 1985. Aflatoxicosis in feedlot cattle. J. Am. Vet. Med. Assoc. 187, 636–637.

Pandey, I., Chauhan, S.S., 2007. Studies on production performance and toxin residues in tissues and eggs of layer chickens fed on diets with various concentrations of aflatoxin AFB_1. Br. Poult. Sci. 48, 713–723.

Pepeljnjak, S., Slobodnjak, Z., Segvic, M., et al., 2004. The ability of fungal isolates from human lung aspergilloma to produce mycotoxins. Hum. Exp. Toxicol. 23, 15–19.

Richard, J.L., Pier, A.C., Stubblefield, R.D., et al., 1983. Effect of feeding corn naturally contaminated with aflatoxin on feed efficiency, on physiologic, immunologic, and pathologic changes, and on tissue residues in steers. Am. J. Vet. Res. 44, 1294–1299.

Samarajeewa, U., Arseculeratne, S.N., Tennekoon, G.E., et al., 1975. Spontaneous and experimental aflatoxicosis in goats. Res. Vet. Sci. 19, 269–277.

Seitz, L.M., Mohr, H.E., Sauer, D.B., 1982. Storage of high-moisture corn: fungal growth and dry matter loss. Cereal Chem. 59, 100–105.

Shephard, G.S., 2016. Current status of mycotoxin analysis: a critical review. J. AOAC Int. 99, 842–848.

Shivachandra, S.B., Sah, R.L., Snigh, S.D., et al., 2003. Immunosuppression in broiler chicks fed aflatoxin and inoculated with fowl adenovirus serotype-4 (FAV-4) associated with hydropericardium syndrome. Vet. Res. Commun. 27, 39–51.

Shuaib, F.M., Ehiri, J., Abdullahi, A., et al., 2010a. Reproductive health effects of aflatoxins: a review of the literature. Reprod. Toxicol. 29, 262–270.

Shuaib, F.M., Jolly, P.E., Ehiri, J.E., et al., 2010b. Association between birth outcomes and aflatoxin B_1 biomarker blood levels in pregnant women in Kumasi, Ghana. Trop. Med. Int. Health. 15, 160–167.

Silvotti, L., Petterino, C., Bonomi, A., et al., 1997. Immunotoxicological effects on piglets of feeding sows diets containing aflatoxins. Vet. Rec. 141, 469–472.

Stubblefield, R.D., Pier, A.C., Richard, J.L., et al., 1983. Fate of aflatoxins in tissues, fluids and excrements from cows dosed orally with aflatoxin B_1. Am. J. Vet. Res. 44, 1750–1752.

Sun, L.H., Lei, M.Y., Zhang, N.Y., et al., 2014. Hepatotoxic effects of mycotoxin combinations in mice. Food Chem. Toxicol. 74, 289–293.

Supriya, Ch, Reddy, P.S., 2015. Prenatal exposure to aflatoxin B_1: developmental, behavioral, and reproductive alterations in male rats. Naturwissenschaften. 102, 26.

Supriya, Ch, Akhila, B., Pratap Reddy, K., et al., 2016. Effects of maternal exposure to aflatoxin B_1 during pregnancy on fertility output of dams and developmental, behavioral and reproductive consequences in female offspring using a rat model. Toxicol. Mech. Methods. 26, 202–210.

Tanaka, T., Nishikawa, A., Iwata, H., et al., 1989. Enhancing effect of ethanol on aflatoxin B_1-induced hepatocarcinogenesis in male ACI/N rats. Jpn. J. Cancer Res. 80, 526–530.

Varga, J., Frisvad, J.C., Samson, R.A., 2009. A reappraisal of fungi producing aflatoxins. World Mycotoxin. J. 2, 263–277.

Varga, J., Frisvad, J.C., Samson, R.A., 2011. Two new aflatoxin producing species, and an overview of *Aspergillus* section Flavi. Stud. Mycol. 69, 57–80.

Veldman, A., Meijs, J.A., Borggreve, G.J., et al., 1992. Carry-over of aflatoxin from cows' food to milk. Anim. Prod. 55, 163–168.

Warburton, M.L., Williams, W.P., 2014. Aflatoxin resistance in maize: what have we learned lately? Adv. Botany. 14, Article ID 352831. http://dx.doi.org/10.1155/2014/352831.

Williams, J.H., Grubb, J.A., Davis, J.W., et al., 2010. HIV and hepatocellular and esophageal carcinomas related to consumption of mycotoxin-prone foods in sub-Saharan Africa. Am. J. Clin. Nutr. 92, 154–160.

Xie, L., Chen, M., Ying, Y., 2016. Development of methods for determination of aflatoxins. Crit. Rev. Food Sci. Nutr. 56, 2642–2664.

Zarba, A., Wild, C.P., Hall, A.J., et al., 1992. Aflatoxin M_1 in breast milk from the Gambia West Africa quantified by combined monoclonal antibody immunoaffinity chromatography and HPLC. Carcinogenesis. 13, 891–894.

Chapter 70

Ergot and Fescue Toxicoses

Ramesh C. Gupta, Tim J. Evans and Steven S. Nicholson

INTRODUCTION

Ergot is a general term that applies to all species of the fungus *Claviceps*. Ergotism refers to the disease conditions associated with long-term ingestion of toxic levels of ergot by animals and humans. Ergot contaminated rye (*Secale cereale*) used as flour was responsible for episodes of human ergotism in Europe during the Middle Ages. Significance, chemistry, and determination of ergot alkaloids were reviewed by Krska and Crews (2008). The genus *Claviceps* includes very specialized fungi that parasitize the flowers of grasses and cereal grains with no other part of the plant infected. Ergot alkaloids produced by *Claviceps cyperi* in nutsedge was described as a toxicant in dairy cattle (Naude et al., 2005). *Claviceps africana* ergot in sorghum produced dihydroergosine (DHES) and related alkaloids, which caused hyperthermia in cattle but dilution in ensilage reduced average concentrations of DHES to approximately 1 mg/kg, a relatively safe level for cattle (Blaney et al., 2010). This chapter primarily addresses alkaloids produced by *Claviceps purpurea* and the various toxic effects, called ergotism, that are produced in animals and humans. The source of exposure for animals includes ergot-infected grains in feeds such as barley, rye, wheat, and oats as well as infected seeds in forages consumed while grazing or in hay and silage. Removal of ergotized seeds along with broken grain kernels and debris by the process of mechanical screening of harvested and stored grain concentrates the ergot in the screenings. Utilizing such contaminated grain screenings for human food or animal feed would create a distinct hazard.

Clinical syndromes include gangrene of the extremities of cattle and horses; hyperthermia and production loss in cattle; agalactia and abortion in swine; and agalactia and other reproductive effects in mares. Most countries have a regulatory limit of 0.1%–0.2% ergot in flour. The suggested maximum level for safety is 0.05%. In the United States, wheat and rye with 0.3% sclerotia are considered unsafe, and oats, triticale, or barley having more than 0.1% sclerotia are deemed unfit for human consumption.

Clinical disease associated with *Claviceps* has a parallel in fescue grass toxicosis where gangrenous ergotism, hyperthermia, production loss in cattle, and adverse effects on reproduction and lactation in horses are similar (Evans et al., 2004a,b, 2012). The seeds of fescue grass can be infected with *C. purpurea* but the ergot alkaloids of fescue grass toxicosis are produced by the endophyte (endo = within; phyte = plant) fungus *Neotyphodium coenophialum*.

Today, it is believed that greater than 95% of fescue pastures containing mostly Kentucky 31 variety are infected by the endophyte, *N. coenophialum*. The tall fescue plant and its endophyte enjoy a symbiotic relationship, each benefits from the survival of the other. The plant supplies required nutrients to the endophyte. The endophyte generates multiple toxins that are distributed throughout the plant, thereby making the plant more resistant to drought, insects, parasitic nematodes, fungi, and herbivores (Evans et al., 2012). Ergot alkaloid induced fescue toxicosis has been studied in much more detail than has ergotism from ingested *C. purpurea* sclerotia. A similar endophyte fungus (*N. lolli*), containing ergovaline, has been found in perennial and annual rye grass and has been associated with clinical toxicosis (Bourke, 2003; Schneider et al., 1996). This chapter describes ergot and fescue poisoning in animals.

BACKGROUND

C. purpurea has a host range exceeding 200 species of grasses. It is distributed worldwide in temperate climatic zones. During infection by *C. purpurea*, the ovary of the grass seed or cereal grain is replaced by fungal mycelia. A sticky exudate known as honeydew is produced that contains conidia, which can be transferred to infect other seeds. The honeydew hardens to form a hard brown, purple or black compact mass of fungal tissue called a sclerotium (Fig. 70.1). The ergot bodies or sclerotia contain up to 1.2% dry weight of toxic alkaloids (Burrows and Tyrl, 2001). Sclerotia of most *Claviceps* species are one to four times larger than the host seed and are readily

Veterinary Toxicology. DOI: http://dx.doi.org/10.1016/B978-0-12-811410-0.00070-2

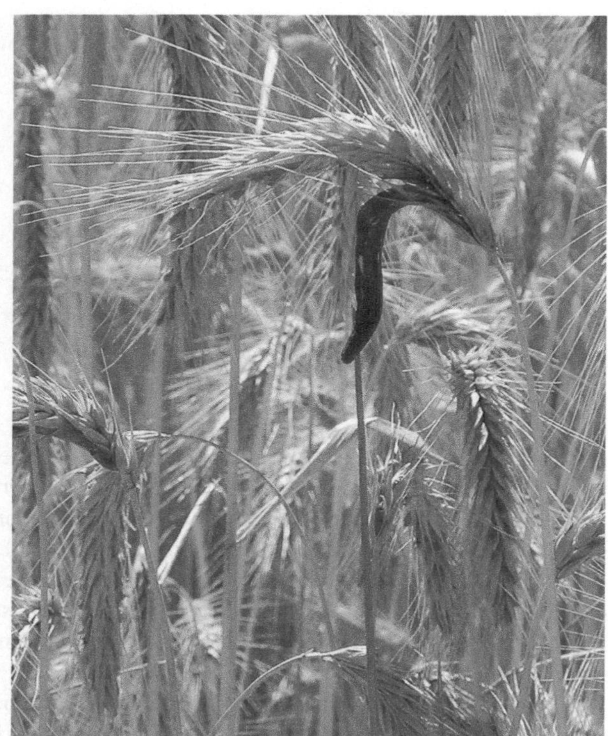

FIGURE 70.1 *Claviceps purpurea* fungal sclerotia growing on barley. *Wikipedia.Com.*

identified in cereal grains. Compared to sclerotia in oats or barley, the sclerotia are quite small in grass seeds such as Bahia grass (*Paspalum notatum*). Sclerotia fall to the ground to over winter and later complete the fungal life cycle by germinating and producing ascospores capable of infecting the ovary of developing seeds.

Alkaloids from *C. purpurea* are among the most important natural products used by the pharmaceutical industry. Prior to the industrial cultivation of *C. purpurea* in the pure culture, ergot was grown as a crop on rye under field conditions for use in the manufacture of important medicinal drugs. Synthesized ergot alkaloids have a variety of uses in human and veterinary medicine. Chemical structures of some of the ergot alkaloids are shown in Fig. 70.2. Unlike *C. purpurea*, *N. coenophialum* produces multiple classes of toxins, including ergot alkaloids, loline alkaloids, and peramine.

PHARMACOKINETICS/TOXICOKINETICS

Ergot alkaloids responsible for most clinical signs and lesions are of the ergopeptine class including ergotamine, ergocristine, ergosine, ergocornine, ergocryptine, and ergovaline (Burrows and Tyrl, 2001; Cheeke, 1998; Carson, 1999, Evans et al., 2004a,b). The rumen and small intestine are most likely the principal sites of ergot alkaloid uptake, which, depending on pH, animal species, and physiological state, can involve both passive and active processes. Strickland et al., 2011) reported that most of the gastrointestinal absorption of the ergopeptine alkaloids takes place in the small intestine. Concentrations of ergovaline are very low in endophytes (parts per billion or low parts per million), so they are rarely detected in animal tissue or fluids. Ergovaline is difficult to detect in rumen fluid and is metabolized by rumen microbes to lysergic acid. Oliver (1997) found that 50%–60% of ingested ergovaline is in the abomasal contents, and minimal amounts of ergovaline remain in the ileal contents or feces. Ergovaline is also believed to be metabolized in the liver by cytochrome P450 3A4. Intravenous injection of several ergopeptides in calves documented a distribution and tissue equilibrium phase in serum lasting approximately 1 h (Moubarak et al., 1996), followed by an elimination phase with a half-life of approximately 20–30 min.

Urine, bile, feces, and to a much lesser extent milk are the primary routes of elimination and excretion for ergot alkaloids (Evans et al., 2004a, 2012; Strickland et al., 2011). In cattle, 96% of the ergot metabolites are found in urine. Ergot alkaloids are detected in urine within 12 h of exposure to fescue endophytes and are maximal within 24 h. After removal from a fescue pasture, ergot metabolites are gone within 48 h from the urine of cattle. Injected intravenously, ergopeptine alkaloids are rapidly cleared from the blood by the liver (Cheeke, 1998) and excreted in the bile.

MECHANISM OF ACTION

Ergot alkaloids have structures similar to the biogenic amines norepinephrine, serotonin, and dopamine. Vasoconstriction is produced by an agonist activity, and this effect varies with different vascular beds. Other effects include hyperthermia and uterine stimulation. The alkaloids are antagonistic to dopamime at D_1 vasodilatory receptors (Cross et al., 1995). Dopaminergic activity at D_2 receptors causes inhibition of prolactin secretion (Goldstein et al., 1980). Ergovaline is a dopamine D_2 receptor agonist (Oliver, 1997). Ergopeptine alkaloids have a 10-fold greater affinity for dopamine D_2 receptor binding than do ergoline alkaloids (Larson, 1997). Dopamine agonists mimic the endogenous tonic inhibition of pituitary lactotropes by dopamine and inhibit prolactin secretion by the anterior pituitary. Prolactin inhibition is one of the most consistent problems observed in multiple species exposed experimentally to ergopeptine alkaloids and/or those experiencing clinical fescue toxicosis. In essence, this effect of ergovaline and other ergot alkaloids is an exquisite, naturally occurring example of "endocrine disruption" and is a sensitive biomarker for exposure to these compounds (Evans et al., 2012). Lower prolactin

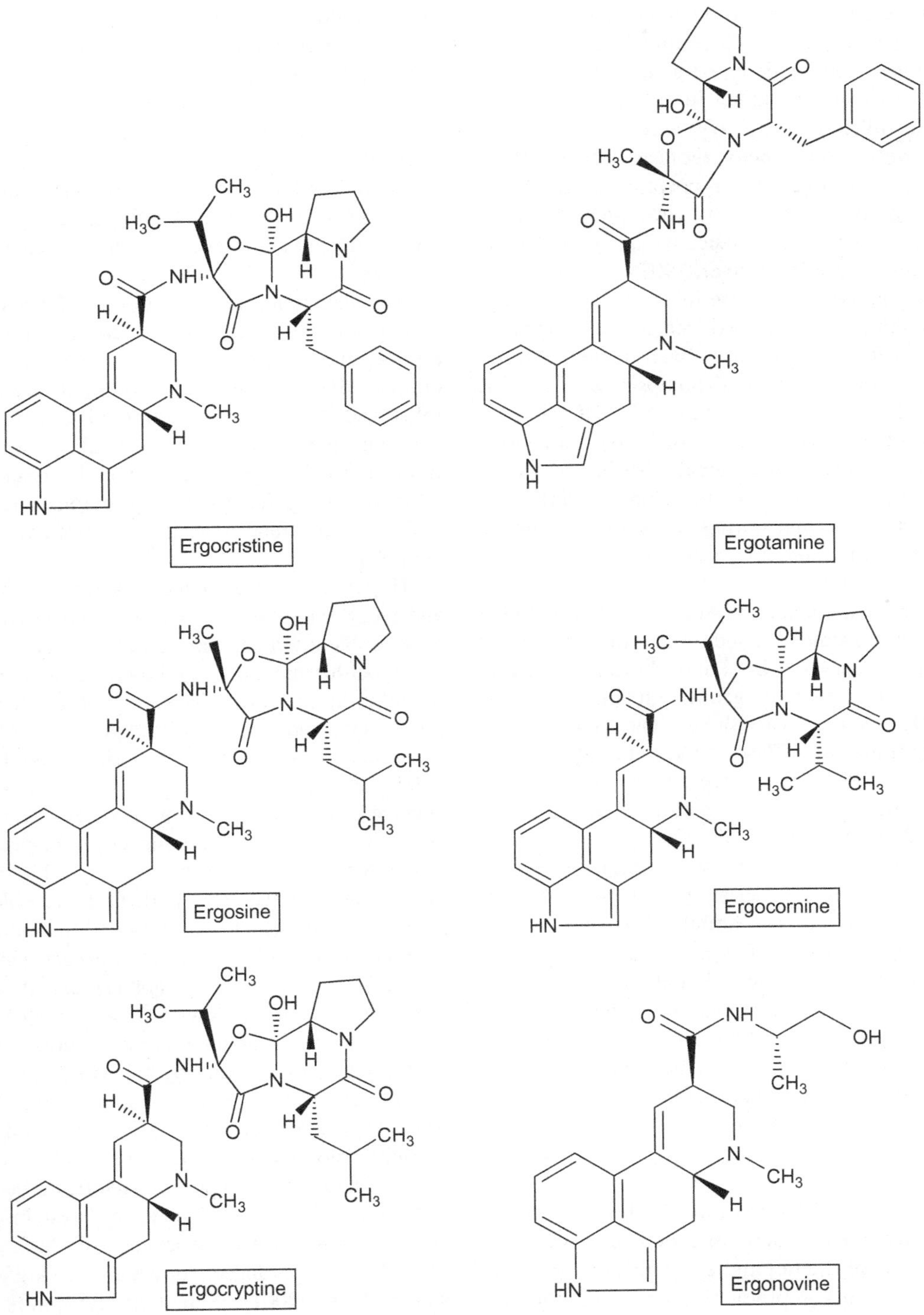

Ergocristine

Ergotamine

Ergosine

Ergocornine

Ergocryptine

Ergonovine

FIGURE 70.2 Chemical structures of some ergot alkaloids.

concentrations in dairy and beef cows consuming endophyte infected fescue as well as diminished feed intake associated with ingestion of endophyte infected fescue can be reflected by decreased milk production (up to 50%) observed after the perinatal period (Evans et al., 2004b, 2012). Effects of ergovaline and other ergot alkaloids on other reproductive hormones include low progesterone production in both cows and mares, diminished progestagens in late-gestational mares, suppressed relaxin associated with possible impaired placental function, and alterations in estrogen concentrations in pregnant mares (Evans, 2011). These imbalances of reproductive hormones lead to early pregnancy problems in cattle and late pregnancy problems in mares.

Ergopeptine alkaloids are α_1 adrenergic receptor antagonists as well as α_2 receptor agonists (Oliver, 1997). Many of the clinical effects of ergopeptine alkaloids are easily described in terms of α_2 receptor agonism. Ergovaline acts as a potent α_2 receptor agonist on blood vessels, especially arterioles (Oliver, 1997). The persistent vasoconstriction of peripheral arterioles in the back legs of cattle consuming fescue is believed to be responsible for thickening of the smooth muscle wall of the arterioles seen with fescue foot problems (Thompson et al., 2001; Strickland et al., 2011). Chronic exposure of cattle to endophyte infected fescue makes their α_2 adrenergic receptors more reactive to ergot alkaloids (Oliver, 1997). Constriction of blood vessels in the skin of cattle also contributes to hyperthermia during the summer months, by decreasing dissipation of heat through the skin (Thompson et al., 2001).

Some biochemical changes associated with ergovaline and other ergot alkaloids include inhibition of cyclic AMP production, decreases in serum cholesterol, triglycerides, alkaline phosphatase, gamma-glutamyl transferase, GOT, GPT, creatine kinase, lipase, and LDH (Oliver, 1997), and inhibition of ATPase in the brain and kidneys (Moubarak et al., 1993). Oxidative stress occurs due to depletion of glutathione and antioxidative proteins (Lakritz et al., 2002; Settivari et al., 2008).

Ergot alkaloids also act at the serotonergic$_2$ receptors (Oliver, 2005). Ergovaline is an agonist at the serotonergic$_2$ receptors of uterine and umbilical arteries (Dyer, 1993). Serotonergic activity of ergot alkaloids may also be important in the enhanced mitogenesis of vascular smooth muscle, hypothalamic thermoregulatory center effects, pulmonary vasoconstriction and bronchoconstriction, and more importantly, the appetite suppression seen with fescue toxicosis (Oliver, 1997, 2005).

TOXICITY

Clinical toxicosis caused by ergot alkaloids can occur in four forms in livestock. These include: cutaneous and gangrenous lesions of the tail and extremities, hyperthermia and production loss, reproductive failure, and a convulsive or nervous form. The latter form is apparently uncommon, not well documented, and is perhaps caused by acute ingestion of a large dose of sclerotia. Muscle tremors and hyperexcitability are signs in cattle caused by nonergot compounds produced by *Claviceps paspali* in seeds of paspalum grasses (Cole et al., 1977). Staggers in horses grazing paspalum grass seeds infected with *C. paspali* occurs as well (Cawdell-Smith et al., 2010). Indole-diterpenes and ergot alkaloids were confirmed in Bermuda grass *(Cynodon dactylon)* infected with *Claviceps cynodontis* from an outbreak of tremors in cattle in South Africa (Uhlig et al., 2009). In countries where cereal grains in commerce are subject to regulatory oversight, the presence of ergotized seed at significant levels in food and feedstuffs is not common. Ergotism in cattle caused by sclerotia ingested while grazing remains a sporadic problem in the United States (Burrows and Tyrl, 2001).

The cutaneous and gangrenous form of ergotism is associated with subacute or chronic ingestion of the ergopeptine alkaloids. Cold temperatures enhance the clinical effects. Constriction of small arteries and arterioles leads to necrosis affecting all four limbs, tips of the ears, and the distal third of the tail. Distinct lines separating normal tissue from nonviable tissues appear. The odor of rotting flesh may be obvious and affected animals may continue to walk until sloughing of the digits occurs.

Hyperthermia was noted in steers exposed to sunlight and fed 180 mg/kg body wt of *C. purpurea* even at moderate ambient temperatures and humidity (Bourke, 2003).

Hyperthermia induced by high ambient temperature and humidity in lactating dairy cattle reduced feed intake, milk production, and increased embryonic losses. Ingestion of ergot alkaloids enhances this effect (Al-Tamimi et al., 2003). Hyperthermia and a 30% drop in milk yield occurred in succession in two Holstein dairy herds ($n = 240$ and $n = 150$ milking cows, respectively) on the South African Highveld (Naude et al., 2005). Examination of the maize silage from both farms revealed that it was heavily contaminated with nutsedge that contained minute sclerotia, identified as those of *C. cyperi*. This was the first report of bovine ergotism not associated with the grass family Poaceae infected with *C. purpurea* or *N. coenophialum*. High levels of total ergot alkaloids, predominantly ergocryptine, were found by LC-MS in the silage as well as in the total mixed ration (115–975 ppb and 65–300 ppb, respectively). The ergot alkaloid content (mainly ergocryptine) of the maize silage on the second affected farm was 875 ppb. A significant decrease in milk (4.6 L) production in a herd of Holstein-Friesian dairy cows in Australia was associated with high concentrations of endophyte produced ergovaline (1.6 μg/g) in ryegrass silage (Lean, 2001). Simultaneously, milk somatic cell counts increased significantly over a comparable period and reproductive performance declined. Body condition score and coat condition of cows were adversely affected. In a study to determine if ergot alkaloids from *C. purpurea* were carried over to the milk, Holstein cows were fed a contaminated diet (concentrate contained 2.25% ergot, which caused an alkaloid concentration of the daily ration between 504.9 and 619.5 μg/kg DM) over a period of 4 weeks. Daily feed amounts were adjusted to the current performance, which resulted in a dry matter intake variation between 6.0 and 18.5 kg/day. The actual alkaloid exposure varied between 4.1 and 16.3 μg/kg body wt when the ergot contaminated concentrate was fed. Approximately 67% of the alkaloids fed were recovered in the duodenal ingesta, and approximately 24% were excreted with the feces. No alkaloid residues could be detected in the blood or milk samples (Schumann et al., 2009).

Diminished prolactin and/or dopamine receptor perturbation causes the thermoregulatory center to deregulate and contributes to the development of hypothermia or hyperthermia observed in endophyte/ergot alkaloid exposed animals. Deregulation is more likely when environmental temperatures are outside of the thermoneutral range of the animal (Spiers et al., 2005a,b). Fescue foot problems are more likely at temperatures less than 8°C (Tor-Agbidye et al., 2001), whereas summer slump problems are more apparent when temperatures exceed 31°C (Spiers et al., 2005a,b). Other potential clinical signs include nervousness, increased salivation, increased respiratory rate, delayed puberty, and reduced conception rates, possibly arising from adverse effects on the male as well as the female (Strickland et al., 2011; Evans et al., 2012). Although sudden deaths during hot summer months have been reported, negligible mortality is associated with summer slump arising from ingestion of endophytic toxins alone, without concurrent exposure to ergopeptine alkaloids produced by *C. purpurea*.

There are reports of small ruminants affected by ergotism. Sheep are susceptible to the vasoconstrictive effects of ergopeptine alkaloids but ergot toxicosis is described as typically mild and not accompanied by gangrenous lesions (Greatorex and Mantle, 1973). Sloughing of the tip of the tongue is said to occur (Burrows and Tyrl, 2001). Another major effect in ewes is infertility (Thompson et al., 2001). Sheep may be affected by fescue and have a syndrome very similar to summer slump in cattle (Evans et al., 2012). Ewes grazing fescue have decreased milk production and increased early embryonic mortality (Schmidt and Osborn, 1993; Thompson et al., 2001). Fescue foot problems are possible in sheep with threshold dietary concentrations of 500 ppb ergovaline at environmental temperatures equal to 7.8°C (Tor-Agbidye et al., 2001). There are also reports of goats and deer experiencing lipomatosis (Evans et al., 2004a,b).

Pregnant mares are most susceptible to the adverse effects of endophyte infected fescue after day 300 of gestation (average gestational length of 335–345 days). Lack of prolactin in the late-gestational mare, along with decreased progestagens and higher or lower than normal estrogen concentrations, can cause problems in the mare and/or foal (Evans, 2011; Evans et al., 2012). Failure to remove mares from fescue pasture or hay during the last month of gestation might result in foal abnormalities, prolongation of pregnancy by 20–27 days and agalactia. "Fescue foals" can be smaller than average and are predisposed to dysmaturity (birth of dysmature or "dummy" foals). Due to endophyte toxin-induced prolonged gestation, foals overmature, and the consequences may include dystocia, uterine, cervical, and/or vaginal trauma. In addition, the chorioallantois might detach prematurely and precede the foal through the birth canal, presenting as a "red bag." In these unfortunate circumstances, the mare and/or foal can die, and if the mare survives, she frequently experiences rebreeding problems. Retained fetal membranes are also more common with fescue toxicosis. Endophyte toxins can predispose horses to laminitis or painful inflammation of the dermal laminae within the hoof, a condition that can result in potentially life-threatening lameness (Rohrbach et al., 1995).

The effects of ergot alkaloids in swine are primarily those of agalactia, production loss, and an impact on reproduction. Diets containing 0, 1 and 10 g ergot (*C. purpurea*)/kg were fed to 12 pigs in the body weight range of 30–115 kg. Tendencies toward reduced feed intake and low rate of weight gain were observed at a feeding level of 4.66 mg total alkaloids/kg diet. At that level, protein digestibility was significantly reduced (Mainka et al., 2005). Birth weight in pigs is reduced, stillbirths increased and neonatal mortality increased due to agalactia in the sow (Lopez et al., 1997).

Agalactia, small, weak foals, stillborn foals, and placental edema occur in pregnant mares ingesting ergot alkaloids in the last month of gestation. This is a common occurrence in mares grazing endophyte infected tall fescue grass in the United States. Similar effects caused by ingestion of *C. purpurea* sclerotia are seldom reported perhaps because heavily infected ergot cereal grains are generally kept out of feed grain commerce. There remains the situation where heavily contaminated cereal grain screenings could be fed to horses. Twelve pregnant mares fed black oat (*Avena strigosa*) during the predelivery period experienced agalactia and delivered weak and unviable foals, which showed no suckling reflex and died within a few hours of birth. *C. purpurea* sclerotia were identified in 0.22% of the examined oat seeds (Copetti et al., 2002). Chickens develop gangrene involving the comb, beak and toes, weight loss, and debilitation. Rabbits are extremely sensitive to the hyperthermic effects caused by ergot alkaloids (Burrows and Tyrl, 2001). Ergot alkaloids are embryocidal and abortifacient in laboratory animals (Mantle, 1969).

In dogs and rodents corporea lutea are essential to maintain pregnancy. In these animals, ergot alkaloids inhibit prolactin secretion causing loss of corpora lutea and abortion.

Ergot alkaloids in oats fed to female mink bred to untreated males caused reduced numbers of kits born compared to controls (Sharma et al., 2002). There was a significant effect on kit survivability with no kits surviving in the 12 ppm group. Serum prolactin was significantly depressed in the three ergot alkaloid groups compared to the control group. This study indicated that ingestion of ergot alkaloids at 3 ppm or higher resulted in reproductive toxicity in mink.

TREATMENT

Removing the source of ergot sclerotia in grain/endophyte infected fescue or other grasses from the animals' diet is an obvious first step in treatment. Removal of the mare from endophyte infested pasture and hay beginning on gestational day 300 will prevent agalactia, prolonged gestation, and foaling problems associated with endophytic toxin exposure. The hyperthermic effect in dairy cattle should abate within 1–2 weeks. Animals that have developed gangrene of the extremities would not be expected to recover and should be euthanized.

The D_2 dopamine receptor antagonist domperidone can be given once a day to mares kept on fescue during the final 10–14 days before expected parturition (Cross, 1997; Cross et al., 1995). This is an effective treatment in mares to prevent agalactia and uterine effects induced by ergot alkaloids in endophyte infected tall fescue grass (Redmond et al., 1993, 1995). Also, the D_2 dopamine receptor antagonist fluphenazine (25 mg IM) in pony mares on day 320 of gestation) has been used to prevent decreases in relaxin related to ergopeptine alkaloid-induced placental dysfunction (Evans, 2011).

CONCLUDING REMARKS AND FUTURE DIRECTIONS

Ergot infection in cereal grains and grasses remains a concern for livestock and horses. Commercial cereal grain screenings and cereal grains produced and fed on the farm, and not inspected, are potential sources of ergotized grain. Exposure while grazing infected grasses may go unnoticed initially, especially if management is not aware of the risk. The major disease syndromes associated with fescue toxicosis arise from the prolactin-inhibiting and vasoconstrictive properties of endophytic ergot alkaloids. Newer analytical procedures are being developed, which might help elucidate the precise role of ergovaline and other ergot alkaloids, and their metabolites in the pathogenesis of toxicosis in various livestock species (Strickland et al., 2011; Evans et al., 2012).

REFERENCES

Al-Tamimi, H.J., Rottinghaus, G.E., Spiers, D.E., et al., 2003. Thermoregulatory response of dairy cows fed ergotized barley during summer heat stress. J. Vet. Diagn. Invest. 15, 355–360.

Blaney, B.J., Ryley, M.J., Boucher, B.D., 2010. Early harvest and ensilage of forage sorghum infected with ergot (*Claviceps africana*) reduces the risk of livestock poisoning. Aust. Vet. J. 88 (8), 311–312.

Bourke, C.A., 2003. Evidence that enforced sunlight exposure can cause hyperthermia in cattle ingesting low levels of ergot of rye (*Claviceps purpurea*), when air temperature and humidity conditions are only moderate. Aust. Vet. J. 81, 553–558.

Burrows, G.E., Tyrl, R.J., 2001. Toxic Plants of North America. Iowa State University Press, Ames, IA.

Carson, T.L., 1999. In: Howard, J.L., Smith, R.A. (Eds.), Current Veterinary Therapy 4: Food Animal Practice. W. B. Saunders, Philadelphia.

Cawdell-Smith, A.J., Scrivener, C.J., Bryden, W.L., 2010. Staggers in horses grazing paspalum infected with *Claviceps paspali*. Aust. Vet. J. 88 (10), 393–395.

Cheeke, P.R., 1998. Natural Toxicants in Feeds, Forages, and Poisonous Plants. Interstate Publishers, Danville, IL.

Cole, R.J., Dorner, J.W., Lansden, J.A., et al., 1977. Paspalum staggers: isolation and identification of tremorgenic metabolites from sclerotia of *Claviceps paspali*. J. Agric. Food Chem. 25 (5), 1197–1201.

Copetti, M.V., Santurio, J.M., Boeck, A.A., et al., 2002. Agalactia in mares fed with grain contaminated with *Claviceps purpurea*. Mycopathologia 154, 199–200.

Cross, D.L., 1997. Fescue toxicosis in horses. In: Bacon, C.W., Hill, N.S. (Eds.), Neotyphodium/Grass Interactions. Plenum, New York, pp. 289–309.

Cross, D.L., Redmond, L.M., Strickland, J.R., 1995. Equine fescue toxicosis: signs and solutions. J. Anim. Sci. 73, 899–908.

Dyer, D.C., 1993. Evidence that ergovaline acts on serotonin receptors. Life Sci. 53, PL223–PL228.

Evans, T.J., 2011. The endocrine disruptive effects of ergopeptine alkaloids on pregnant mares. Vet. Clin. North Am. Equine Pract. 27, 165–173.

Evans, T.J., Rottinghaus, G.E., Casteel, S.W., 2004a. Ergot. In: Plumlee, K.H. (Ed.), Clinical Veterinary Toxicology. Mosby Inc, St. Louis, pp. 239–243.

Evans, T.J., Rottinghaus, G.E., Casteel, S.W., 2004b. Fescue. In: Plumlee, K.H. (Ed.), Clinical Veterinary Toxicology. Mosby Inc, St. Louis, pp. 243–250.

Evans, T.J., Blodgett, D.J., Rottinghaus, G.E., 2012. Fescue toxicosis. In: Gupta, R.C. (Ed.), Veterinary Toxicology: Basic and Clinical Principles, second ed. Academic Press/Elsevier, Amsterdam, pp. 1166–1177.

Goldstein, M.J., Lew, J.Y., Sauter, A., et al., 1980. Affinities of ergot compounds for dopamine agonist and dopamine antagonist receptor sites. Advances in Biochemical Psychopharmacology. Raven Press, New York, pp. 75–82.

Greatorex, J.C., Mantle, P.G., 1973. Experimental ergotism in sheep. Res. Vet. Sci. 15, 337–346.

Krska, R., Crews, C., 2008. Food Addit Contam Part A Chem Anal Control Expo Risk Assess. 25 (6), 722–731.

Lakritz, J., Leonard, M.J., Eichen, P.A., et al., 2002. Whole blood concentrations of glutathione in cattle exposed to heat stress or a combination of heat stress and endophyte-infected tall fescue toxins in controlled environmental conditions. Am. J. Vet. Res. 63, 799–803.

Larson, B., 1997. *Neotyphodium* toxicosis: an animal cellular/molecular research technique perspective. In: Bacon, C.W., Hill, N.S. (Eds.), Neotyphodium/Grass Interactions. Plenum, New York, pp. 347–360.

Lean, I.J., 2001. Association between feeding perennial ryegrass (Lolium perenne cultivar Grasslands Impact) containing high levels of ergovaline, and health and productivity in a herd of lactating dairy cows. Aust. Vet. J. 79, 262–264.

Lopez, T.A., Campero, C.M., Chayer, R., et al., 1997. Ergotism and photosensitization in swine produced by combined ingestion of *Claviceps purpurea* sclerotia and *Ammi majus* seeds. J. Vet. Diagn. Invest. 9, 68–71.

Mainka, S., Danike, S., Boehme, H., et al., 2005. The influence of ergot-contaminated feed on growth and slaughtering performance, nutrient digestibility and carry-over of ergot alkaloids in growing-finishing pigs. Arch. Anim. Nutr. 59, 377–395.

Mantle, P.G., 1969. The role of alkaloids in the poisoning of mammals by sclerotia of Claviceps spp. J. Stored Prod. Res. 5, 237.

Moubarak, A.S., Piper, E.L., West, C.P., et al., 1993. Interactions of purified ergovaline from endophyte-infected tall fescue with synaptosomal ATPase enzyme system. J. Agric. Food Chem. 41, 407–409.

Moubarak, A.S., Piper, E.L., Johnson, Z.B., et al., 1996. HPLC method for detection of ergotamine, ergosine, and ergine after intravenous injection of a single dose. J. Agric. Food Chem. 44, 146–148.

Naude, T.W., Botha, C.J., Vorster, J.H., et al., 2005. *Claviceps cyperi*, a new cause of severe ergotism in dairy cattle consuming maize silage and teff hay contaminated with ergotised *Cyperus esculentus* (nut sedge) on the Highveld of South Africa. Onderstepoort J. Vet. Res. 72, 23–37.

Oliver, J.W., 1997. Physiological manifestations of endophyte toxicosis in ruminant and laboratory species. In: Bacon, C.W., Hill, N.S. (Eds.), Neotyphodium/Grass Interactions. Plenum, New York, pp. 311–346.

Oliver, J.W., 2005. Pathophysiologic response to endophyte toxins. In: Roberts, C.A., West, C.P., Spiers, D.E. (Eds.), Neotyphodium n Cool Season Grasses. Blackwell, Ames, pp. 291–304.

Redmond, L.M., Cross, D.L., Kennedy, S.W., 1993. Effect of three levels of domperidone on gravid mares grazing endophyte (*Acremonium coenophialum*) infected tall fescue. J. Anim. Sci. 71 (Suppl. 1), 16 (Abstr).

Redmond, L.M., Cross, D.L., Strickland, J.E., et al., 1995. Efficacy of domperidone and sulipride as treatments for fescue toxicosis in horses. Am. J. Vet. Res. 55, 772.

Rohrbach, B.W., Green, E.M., Oliver, J.W., et al., 1995. Aggregate risk study of exposure to endophyte-infected (*Acremonium coenophialum*) tall fescue as a risk factor for laminitis in horses. Am. J. Vet. Res. 56, 22–26.

Schmidt, S.P., Osborn, T.G., 1993. Effects of endophyte-infected tall fescue on animal performance. Agric. Ecosyst. Env. 44, 233–262.

Schneider, D.J., Miles, C.O., Garthwaite, I., et al., 1996. First report of field outbreaks of ergot-alkaloid toxicity in South Africa. Onderstepoort J. Vet. Res. 2, 97–108.

Schumann, B., Lebzien, P., Ueberschär, K.H., et al., 2009. Effects of the level of feed intake and ergot contaminated concentrate on ergot alkaloid metabolism and carry over into milk. Mol. Nutr. Food Res. 53 (7), 931–938.

Settivari, R.S., Evans, T.J., Rucker, E., et al., 2008. Effect of ergot alkaloids associated with fescue toxicosis on hepatic cytochrome P450 and antioxidant properties. Toxicol. Appl. Pharmacol. 227, 347–356.

Sharma, C., Aulerich, R.J., Render, J.A., et al., 2002. Reproductive toxicity of ergot alkaloids in mink. Vet. Hum. Toxicol. 44, 324–327.

Spiers, D.E., Eichen, P.A., Rottinghaus, G.E., 2005a. A model of fescue toxicosis: responses of rats to intake of endophyte-infected tall fescue. J. Anim. Sci. 83, 1423–1434.

Spiers, D.E., Evans, T.J., Rottinghaus, G.E., 2005b. Interactions between thermal stress and fescue toxicosis: animal models and new perspectives. In: Roberts, C.A., West, C.P., Spiers, D.E. (Eds.), Neotyphodium in Cool Season Grasses. Blackwell, Ames, pp. 243–270.

Strickland, J.R., Looper, M.L., Matthews, J.C., et al., 2011. Board-invited review: St. Anthony's fire in livestock: causes, mechanisms, and potential solutions. J. Anim. Sci. 89, 1603–1626.

Thompson, F.N., Stuedemann, J.A., Hill, N.S., 2001. Anti-quality factors associated with alkaloids in eastern temperate pasture. J. Range. Manage. 54, 474–489.

Tor-Agbidye, J., Blythe, L.L., Craig, A.M., 2001. Correlation of endophyte toxins (ergovaline and lolitrem B) with clinical disease: fescue foot and perennial ryegrass staggers. Vet. Hum. Toxicol. 43, 140–146.

Uhlig, S., Botha, C.J., Vralstad, T., et al., 2009. Indole-diterpenes and ergot alkaloids in *Cynodon dactylon* (Bermuda grass) infected with *Claviceps cynodontis* from an outbreak of tremors in cattle. J. Agric. Food Chem. 57 (23), 11112–11119.

Chapter 71

Fumonisins

Geof W. Smith

INTRODUCTION

Fumonisins are a group of naturally occurring mycotoxins produced by the fungi *Fusarium verticillioides* (formerly *F. moniliforme*), *Fusarium proliferatum* and other *Fusarium* species. These toxic metabolites of corn have been implicated in field cases of porcine pulmonary edema (PPE) (Colvin et al., 1993; Harrison et al., 1990; Osweiler et al., 1992) and equine leukoencephalomalacia (ELEM) (Jovanović et al., 2015; Wilson et al., 1990a). Experimentally, fumonisin has been shown to cause liver damage in multiple species including pigs, horses, cattle, rabbits, and primates (Gumprecht et al., 1995; Haschek et al., 1992; Jaskiewicz et al., 1987; Osweiler et al., 1993; Ross et al., 1993; Voss et al., 1989) as well as species-specific target organ toxicity, such as lung in pigs (Haschek et al., 1992), brain in horses (Ross et al., 1993), kidney in rats, rabbits, and sheep (Edrington et al., 1995; Gumprecht et al., 1995; Voss et al., 1989), and esophagus in rats and pigs (Casteel et al., 1993; Lim et al., 1996). Many grain-based human foods have been shown to be contaminated with fumonisin metabolites (Scott, 2012) and epidemiologic data has linked ingestion of corn contaminated with *F. verticillioides* to human esophageal cancer (Rheeder et al., 1992) and infant neural tube defects (Voss et al., 2011). Fumonisins have been shown to be hepatocarcinogenic in rats and mice (Gelderblom et al., 1988; Howard et al., 2001) and the International Agency for Research on Cancer (IARC) has designated fumonisin B1 in Group 2B meaning "possibly carcinogenic to humans." More recently the fungus *Aspergillus niger* has also been shown to produce some fumonisin metabolites, which have been found in grapes, raisins, wine, and coffee (Scott, 2012).

BACKGROUND

Chemical Structure

First isolated in 1988, the fumonisins are a group of structurally related compounds with the terminal carboxy group composed of propane-1,2,3-tricarboxylic acid involved in ester formation with the C-14 and C-15 hydroxy groups. The 20C chain base carries either 2-acetylamino or 2-amino-12,16-dimethyl-3,5,10,14,15, pentahydroxyicosane (Fig. 71.1). The structures of FB_1 and FB_2 have been shown to have the empirical formulas of $C_{34}H_{59}NO_{15}$ and $C_{34}H_{59}NO_{14}$, respectively, with the only difference being the hydroxyl group present at the C-10 position in FB_1 (Bezuidenhout et al., 1988). Additional fumonisin metabolites have been isolated (including B_3, B_4, B_5, B_6, A_1, and A_2), but appear to occur in much lower concentrations than FB_1 or FB_2, and are considered less important at this time (Gelderblom et al., 1992).

Occurrence and Distribution

Although fumonisin metabolites have been found in many different grains including barley, millet, oats, and wheat (Scott, 2012), they are most commonly detected in corn and corn-based foods. ELEM has long been associated with the consumption of moldy corn, and has been reported in most of the world's continents. Specific cases of ELEM that were directly associated with fumonisin-contaminated feed have been reported in South Africa and Egypt (Thiel et al., 1991), the United States (Ross et al., 1991; Wilson et al., 1990a), Brazil (Sydenham et al., 1992), Hungary (Bela and Endre, 1996), Spain (Cerrillo et al., 1996), New Caldonia (Bailly et al., 1996), Mexico (Rosiles et al., 1998), Iran (Raoofi et al., 2003),

Veterinary Toxicology. DOI: http://dx.doi.org/10.1016/B978-0-12-811410-0.00071-4

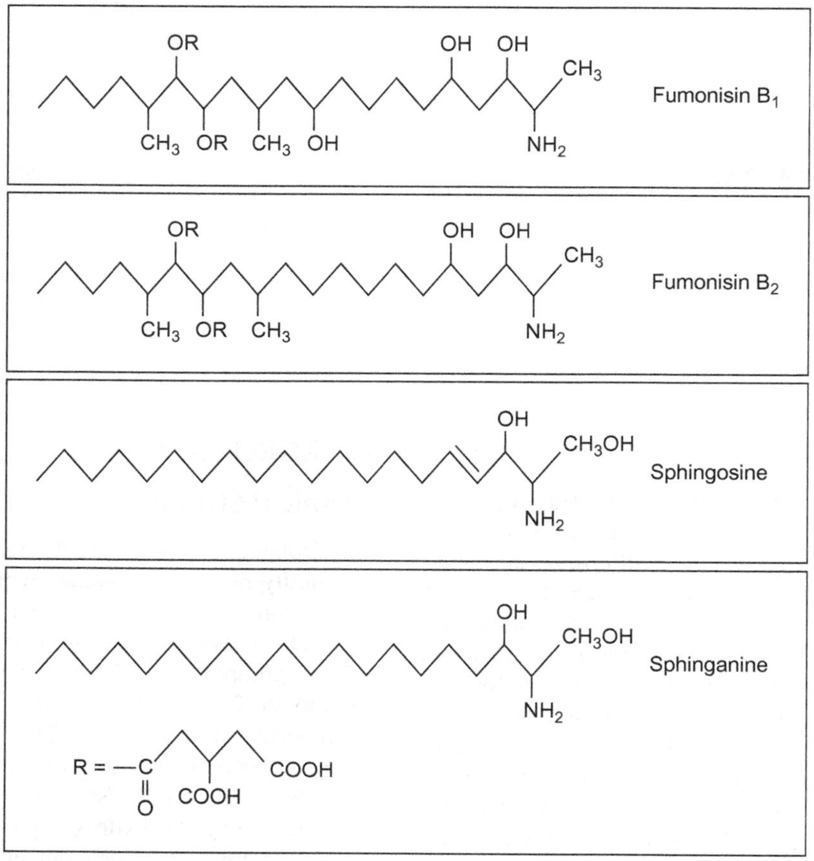

FIGURE 71.1 The structure of fumonisin B_1, fumonisin B_2, sphingosine, and sphinganine.

Argentina (Giannitti et al., 2011) and Serbia (Jovanović et al., 2015). Additionally cases of PPE have been associated with fumonisin-contaminated feeds in the United States (Harrison et al., 1990; Osweiler et al., 1992), Brazil (Sydenham et al., 1992), Hungary (Fazekas et al., 1998), and Thailand (Patchimasiri et al., 1998).

PHARMCOKINETICS/TOXICOKINETICS

The pharmacokinetics of fumonisin B_1 have been examined in several species including rats, pigs, cattle, laying hens, and primates (Martinez-Larranaga et al., 1999; Prelusky et al., 1994; Prelusky et al., 1995; Richard et al., 1996; Shephard et al., 1995; Vudathala et al., 1994). In general, fumonisin is rapidly absorbed following intravenous or intraperitoneal administration and is eliminated in both the feces and urine. Levels are undetectable by 24 h after dosing in virtually all species and significant concentrations (residues) have not been found in muscle, milk, or eggs. Following oral dosing, very little fumonisin B_1 is typically found in the serum of animals indicating low bioavailability.

More specifically, the toxicokinetics of radiolabeled fumonisin B_1 were examined after intragastric (0.5 mg fumonisin B_1/kg) or intravenous (0.4 mg fumonisin B_1/kg) administration to bile-cannulated and noncannulated pigs (Prelusky et al., 1994). Fumonisin-derived radioactivity was not detected in the plasma of pigs dosed intravenously after 180 min in the noncannulated group, or after 90 min in the cannulated group. Urinary excretion began within 3 h of administration and virtually ended after 8 h, accounting for only a small amount of administered toxin. Fecal excretion of fumonisin persisted for 48 h. The excretion in the intravenously dosed group occurred primarily via the bile, with biliary excretion greatest during the first 4 h, but persisting for 24–36 h.

Plasma radioactivity in intragastrically dosed pigs was first detected 30–45 min after dosing, with maximal activity present between 60 and 90 min. As reflected in plasma and elimination data, systemic bioavailability of the dose ranged from 3% to 6%. Excretion of the fumonisin occurred primarily via feces, with only trace amounts excreted via urine or bile.

At 72 h after administration, tissue radioactivity was highest in the liver, kidney, and large intestine in all groups. Intragastrically dosed groups had 10–20 fold lower tissue concentrations than did intravenously dosed groups, and only intravenously dosed groups had measurable radioactivity in brain, lung, and adrenal. Thus, it seems that liver and kidney are the primary organs of fumonisin metabolism and excretion in the pig, and that enterohepatic circulation prolongs the persistence of fumonisin in the body. The toxicokinetics of fumonisin B_1 in horses has not been evaluated.

When pigs were fed fumonisin at daily concentrations between 50 and 500 μg of fumonisin B_1 per kg of body weight for the last 5 months before slaughter, no muscle or kidney residues were detected (Liguoro et al., 2004). Fumonisin B_1 was not detected in the eggs from laying hens following either intravenous or oral administration (Vudathala et al., 1994). Although negligible concentrations have been shown to cross the mammary barrier (Spotti et al., 2001), the toxin was not detected in milk from cattle that consumed a diet containing fumonisins (Richard et al., 1996). Therefore, it appears that fumonisin residues in meat, milk, or eggs do not represent a hazard or food safety concern for humans consuming these products.

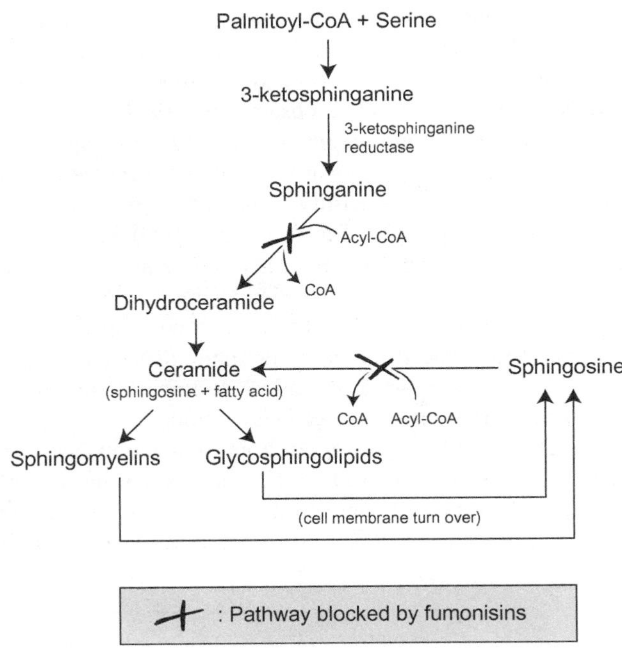

FIGURE 71.2 The effects of fumonisin on the sphingolipid biosynthetic pathway.

MECHANISM OF ACTION

Sphingolipid Alterations

Fumonisins are structurally related to sphingosine, the major long-chain base backbone of cellular sphingolipids (Fig. 71.1). They are competitive inhibitors of sphinganine and sphingosine *N*-acyltransferase (also known as ceramide synthase), key enzymes in the de novo sphingolipid biosynthetic pathway (Fig. 71.2). These *N*-acyltransferase enzymes are responsible for catalyzing the acylation of sphinganine and the reutilization of sphingosine derived from sphingolipid turnover. This inhibition by fumonisin has been characterized in vitro using liver and brain microsomes, as well as in intact mammalian cells in culture (hepatocytes, neurons, renal cells, and macrophages) (Merrill et al., 1995). Fumonisin B_1 blocks the incorporation of radiolabeled serine into the sphingoid base backbone of ceramides and complex sphingolipids and prevents the conversion of sphinganine to sphingosine via addition of the 4,5 *trans* double bond, which occurs after acylation of sphinganine. Fumonisin also blocks reacylation of sphingoid bases (primarily sphingosine) released by hydrolysis of more complex sphingolipids (Merrill et al., 1995).

Sphingolipids are located in cellular membranes, lipoproteins (especially low-density lipoproteins), and other lipid-rich structures. Complex sphingolipids are critical for the maintenance of membrane structure, particularly microdomains such as caveolae. They also serve as binding sites for extracellular matrix proteins as well as for some microorganisms, microbial toxins, and viruses, and regulate the behavior of growth factor receptors (Merrill and Sweeley, 1996). Complex sphingolipids function as precursors for second messengers that mediate cell responses to growth factors, cytokines (including tumor necrosis factor-α), differentiation factors, and 1,25-dihydroxy-vitamin D_3. Therefore, sphingolipids are involved in the regulation of cell growth, cell to cell communication, differentiation, and neoplastic transformation (Hannun and Bell, 1989).

This enzyme inhibition by fumonisin produces a disruption of sphingolipid metabolism resulting in increased sphinganine and sphingosine along with a decrease in complex sphingolipids in the serum and tissues of animals (Wang et al., 1991). These elevations in concentrations of sphinganine and sphingosine have also been observed in vivo in several species including pigs, horses, and calves (Goel et al., 1996; Mathur et al., 2001; Riley et al., 1993; Smith et al., 1999; Smith et al., 2000). This disruption of sphingolipid metabolism is generally accepted as the probably mechanism of fumonisin toxicity; however, only in pigs has the pathophysiology been definitively determined.

PPE has been shown to be a direct result of acute left-sided heart failure related to an increase in plasma and myocardial sphinganine and sphingosine concentrations (Constable et al., 2000; Smith et al., 1999, 2000). Sphingosine is an important intracellular second messenger that inhibits L-type calcium channels in myocardial cells, thereby decreasing sarcoplasmic reticulum Ca^{2+}-induced Ca^{2+}-release and cardiac contractility (McDonough et al., 1994; Webster et al., 1994). As sphingosine concentrations begin to increase in pigs that consume fumonisin, myocardial calcium channels are blocked and contractility begins to decrease (Constable et al., 2000; Smith et al., 2000). Ultimately this decrease in cardiac contractility causes acute left ventricular failure and pulmonary edema (Fig. 71.3).

The mechanism of ELEM may also be a direct result of fumonisin-induced increases in sphingosine concentrations. Cardiovascular dysfunction following fumonisin administration in horses has been demonstrated (Smith et al., 2002). This study reported an association between neurologic signs, increased serum and myocardial sphingosine concentrations, and cardiovascular depression in fumonisin-treated horses. At necropsy, horses with leukoencephalomalacia have histologic evidence of cerebral edema in the brain. Another study reported that fumonisin-treated horses also have elevated protein, albumin, and IgG levels in cerebrospinal fluid samples (Foreman et al., 2004). Taken together, these findings indicate that fumonisin toxicity in horses is associated with the development of vasogenic cerebral edema as a direct result of increased blood–brain barrier permeability. Horses are dependent on autoregulation of cerebral blood flow when they lower their head to graze. Because of gravitational forces, distal carotid artery pressure can increase tremendously when the animal bends to eat or drink. However, this rise in carotid pressure does not create a significant increase in cerebral blood flow due the constriction and dilation of cerebral arterioles, which maintain normal cerebral blood pressures (Faraci and Heistad, 1990). It has been shown that L-type calcium channels are the primary mediators of vascular tone in these cerebral arterioles (Michelakis et al., 1994). Therefore, it has been hypothesized that fumonisin-induced increases in sphingosine concentrations inhibit the calcium channels in cerebral arterioles leading to the inability to maintain normal cerebral blood pressure and vasogenic cerebral edema. This hypothesis requires further research to be proven definitively.

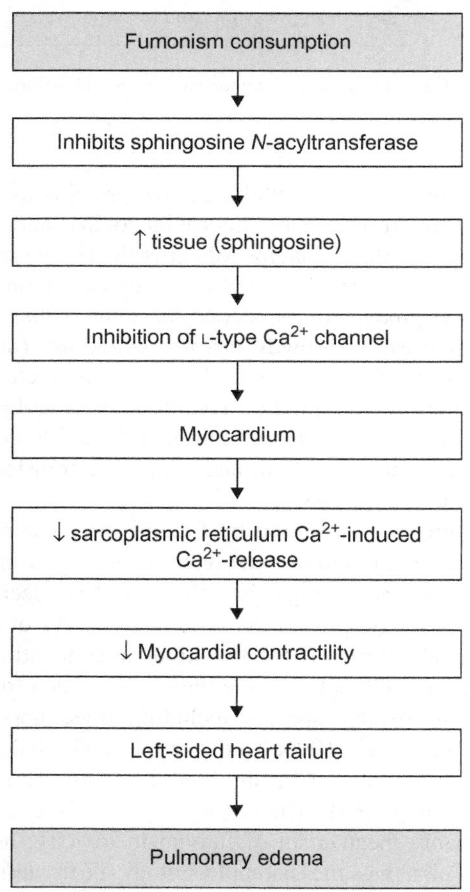

FIGURE 71.3 Mechanism of fumonisin-induced pulmonary edema in swine. Fumonisin inhibition results in increased tissue sphingosine and sphinganine concentrations. The increased sphingosine concentrations inhibit the L-type Ca^{2+} channels of cardiac myocytes resulting in decreased myocardial contractility. This decrease in contractility results in acute left-sided heart failure and pulmonary edema.

TOXICITY

Fumonisin has been shown to cause liver damage in multiple species including pigs, horses, cattle, rabbits, and primates (Gumprecht et al., 1995; Haschek et al., 1992; Jaskiewicz et al., 1987; Osweiler et al., 1993; Ross et al., 1993; Voss et al., 1989) as well as species-specific target organ toxicity, such as lung in pigs (Haschek et al., 1992), brain in horses (Ross et al., 1993), kidney in rats, rabbits, and sheep (Edrington et al., 1995; Gumprecht et al., 1995; Voss et al., 1989), and esophagus in rats and pigs (Casteel et al., 1993; Lim et al., 1996). This chapter will focus on fumonisin toxicity in pigs and horses since they exhibit the most common clinical poisonings dealt with in veterinary medicine, however cattle and poultry will be briefly discussed.

Spontaneous and Experimental Fumonisin Toxicosis in Swine

In early research prior to the initial isolation and characterization of fumonisins, *F. verticillioides* culture material was reported toxic to swine (Kriek et al., 1981). In that experiment, three pigs were fed *F. verticillioides* culture material grown on corn. Two of the three pigs fed the culture material in this study died within 5 days of pulmonary edema. The third pig was fed culture material for 89 days and was then killed following a period of feed refusal.

The 1989, corn crop in many Midwestern and Southeastern parts of the United States was heavily infected with *F. verticillioides*, and contaminated screenings fed to animals led to fatal outbreaks of PPE (Harrison et al., 1990; Osweiler et al., 1992). This syndrome was also reproduced experimentally with contaminated corn screenings and purified fumonisin B_1 (Harrison et al., 1990; Osweiler et al., 1992).

Lung and liver are the major target organs of fumonisin toxicosis in pigs; however, other organs have been reported to be affected. Pigs that ingest fumonisin at concentrations high enough to cause pulmonary edema usually die after about 4 days in field cases (Osweiler, 1992) and after 3–6 days of fumonisin exposure experimentally (Gumprecht et al., 1998; Haschek et al., 1992; Motelin et al., 1994). Pigs that survive chronic exposure to high doses of fumonisin without developing pulmonary edema typically demonstrate hepatic disease with anorexia, weight loss, and generalized icterus (Colvin et al., 1993; Osweiler et al., 1992). Hepatic toxicity occurs at doses significantly lower than those necessary to cause pulmonary edema (Colvin et al., 1993; Motelin et al., 1994).

Fumonisins in Swine-Pulmonary Effects

Pulmonary edema (Fig. 71.4) has been reported in pigs fed naturally contaminated fumonisins-containing food, fumonisin-containing culture material or following IV administration of fumonisin (Harrison et al., 1990; Haschek et al., 1992; Motelin et al., 1994; Osweiler et al., 1992). Reported concentrations of fumonisin required to produce pulmonary edema have been variable, presumably due to variability in susceptibility among exposed animals (Table 71.1). However, other constituents in the diet and analytical detection related to the ability to extract fumonisin from different matrices could account for some of the variability. In addition, some reports have reported only the concentration of fumonisin B_1 associated with the development of pulmonary edema, while others have reported both fumonisin B_1 and fumonisin B_2. Fumonisin B_2 usually occurs at about 30% of fumonisin B_1 in naturally-contaminated corn, and is generally considered to be equitoxic to fumonisin B_1 (Ross et al., 1994). Reported doses that induced pulmonary edema in swine include 100 ppm of fumonisin B_1 and fumonisin B_2 in naturally-contaminated corn (Motelin et al., 1994), 16 mg fumonisin B_1/kg/day as fumonisin-containing culture material (Colvin et al., 1993), and 20 mg fumonisin B_1/kg/day as culture material (Gumprecht et al., 1998). Fumonisin-induced pulmonary edema has also been reported with naturally-contaminated corn (330 mg of fumonisin B_1 per kg of feed) in Hungary (Fazekas et al., 1998), Brazil (Sydenham et al., 1992), and Thailand (Patchimasiri et al., 1998).

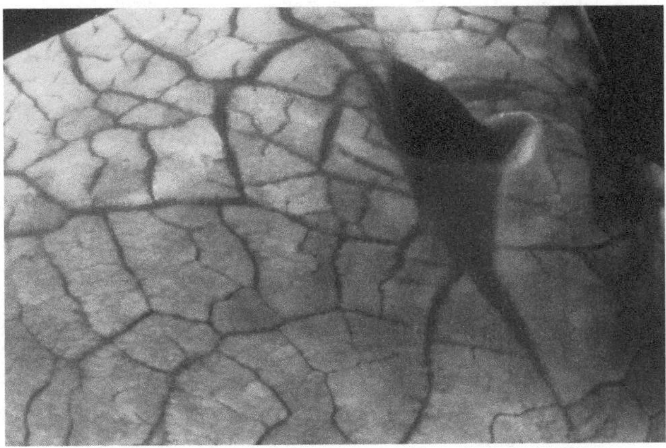

FIGURE 71.4 Lung from a pig fed fumonisin-containing culture material at a dose of 20 mg fumonisin B_1 per kg of body weight for 4 days. Pulmonary edema is characterized by severe widening of the interlobular septa.

Another study has suggested that even lower concentrations of fumonisins may be able to induce pulmonary edema in swine (Zomborszky et al., 2000). Fumonisin B_1 was fed added to the feed of weaned pigs at doses of 0, 10, 20, and 40 ppm for 4 weeks as fumonisin-containing culture material (five pigs per group). Computed tomography (CT) of the lungs and magnetic resonance imaging of the brains were performed prior to the study and at 2 and 4 weeks of fumonisin feeding. Histopathology was also done at the time of necropsy (4 weeks). The results of this study showed that all five pigs fed fumonisin B_1 at 40 ppm developed "severe" pulmonary edema as assessed by CT and histopathology. Two of the five pigs fed fumonisin B_1 at 20 ppm had "severe" pulmonary edema while two other pigs in the group had "mild" edema. In the 10 ppm group, three of the five pigs were reported to have "mild" pulmonary edema. Magnetic resonance studies of the brain were not able to identify any significant changes during the course of the study in any group.

Clinical signs associated with the development of pulmonary edema consistently begin 3–6 days after initiation of exposure to a high concentration of fumonisins. These include dyspnea and open mouthed breathing, increased respiratory rate, cyanosis of skin and mucous membranes, inactivity and sudden death (Osweiler et al., 1992). Pigs usually die within a few hours after the onset of definitive respiratory distress. Histologically, pulmonary edema is present by day three of fumonisin exposure (Gumprecht et al., 1998) and is characterized by interstitial edema around airways and vessels, in interlobular and subpleural connective tissues, and in alveolar interstitium (Gumprecht et al., 1998; Harrison et al., 1990; Haschek et al., 1992; Osweiler et al., 1992). Lymphatics are dilated and alveolar edema is often present. Fluid is also present within the thoracic cavity.

TABLE 71.1 Effect of Fumonisin in Pigs

Number of Animals	Dose & Route	Duration	Toxic Effects	Reference
Experimental Studies Using Purified Fumonisin				
4 pigs	0.174–0.4 mg FB_1 per kg of BW/day, IV	4–8 days	2 high dose pigs developed pulmonary edema	Harrison et al. (1990)
2 pigs	0.88–1.15 mg FB_1 per kg of BW/day, IV	1 pig for 4 days (0.88 mg/kg/day)—2nd pig for 9 days (1.15 mg/kg/day)	Mild interstitial pulmonary edema histologically in 1 pig; hepatic lesions; pancreatic lesions	Haschek et al. (1992)
3 pigs	4.5–6.6 mg FB_1 per kg of BW/day in feed	5–15 days	2 of the 3 pigs developed severe pulmonary edema; hepatic lesions and mild pancreatic lesions noted	Haschek et al. (1992)
2 pigs	0.4 mg FB_1 per kg of BW/day, IV	12–14 days	Elevated AST, GGT, bilirubin; liver lesions	Osweiler et al. (1992)
8 pigs	10 ppm FB_1 added to the diet-fed ad libitum	8 weeks	Decreased weight gain	Rotter et al. (1996)
			Elevated cholesterol	
6 pigs	1 mg FB_1 per kg of BW/day, IV	4 days	Decrease in left ventricular contractility and mild pulmonary edema	Smith et al. (2000)
Experimental Studies Using Fumonisin-Containing Culture Material				
6 pigs	Feeds containing 100 and 190 ppm FB_1 fed ad libitum	100 ppm diet-fed ad libitum for 7 days followed by 190 ppm diet for 83 days	Elevated AST, ALP, GGT; nodular hyperplasia of the liver; histologic esophageal lesions	Casteel et al., 1993
4 pigs	Feed containing 200 ppm of FB_1 fed ad libitum	Up to 43 days	Elevated bilirubin, AST, cholesterol; hepatic lesions; decreased weight gain	Colvin et al. (1993)
7 pigs	16–64 mg FB_1 per kg of BW/day as oral gavage	3–5 days	All pigs developed pulmonary edema within 5 days	Colvin et al. (1993)
3 pigs	4–16 mg FB_1 per kg of BW/day as oral gavage	up to 45 days	Severe hepatic disease; icterus; elevated liver enzymes; no pulmonary edema	Colvin et al. (1993)
11 pigs	Feeds containing 100, 160, and 190 ppm FB_1 fed ad libitum	6 pigs were fed 100 ppm for 10 days then 190 ppm for up to 83 days; 5 pigs were fed 100 ppm for 5 days and then 160 ppm for up to 205 days	Nodular hyperplasia of the liver; Elevated AST, ALP, GGT, bilirubin	Casteel et al. (1994)
			Right ventricular hypertrophy; medial hypertrophy of the small pulmonary arteries	
6 pigs	feed containing 47 ppm FB_1 fed ad libitum	28 days	Decreased feed consumption; Elevated AST, GGT, ALP, and creatinine; hepatic and renal lesions; medial hypertrophy of the pulmonary arteries	Harvey et al. (1996)
10 pigs	20 mg of FB_1 per kg of BW/day, in feed	7 days	Pulmonary edema and cardiovascular abnormalities	Smith et al. (1996a,b)
2 pigs	14.5 and 16 mg of FB_1 per kg of BW/day, in feed	4 days	Severe pulmonary edema; renal lesions	

(Continued)

TABLE 71.1 (Continued)

Number of Animals	Dose & Route	Duration	Toxic Effects	Reference
24 pigs	20 mg of FB_1 per kg of BW/day, in feed	Up to 5 days-some pigs were euthanized each day of the study	All 12 pigs euthanized on days 0, 1 and 2 had no lesions	Gumprecht et al. (1998)
			2/5 day 3 pigs and all of the day 4 and 5 pigs had pulmonary edema	
			Elevations in liver enzymes and hepatic lesions seen on day 2—bile acids first liver parameter to increase	
6 pigs	20 mg of FB_1 per kg of BW/day, in feed	5–6 days – pigs were euthanized as they developed pulmonary edema	Increased pulmonary artery pressure, pulmonary artery wedge pressure and decreased cardiac output, heart rate, and mean arterial pressure	Smith et al. (1999)
5 pigs	Feed containing 40 ppm FB_1 fed ad libitum	4 weeks	No clinical signs-gross pulmonary edema evident at necropsy	Zomborszky et al. (2000)
5 pigs	Feed containing 20 ppm FB_1 fed ad libitum	4 weeks	2 of the 5 pigs had gross pulmonary edema—2 additional pigs had mild evidence of edema present histologically	Zomborszky et al. (2000)
4 pigs	Feed containing 20 ppm FB_1 fed ad libitum	28 days	3 of the 4 pigs had mild pulmonary edema evident histologically	Zomborszky et al. (2000)
7 pigs	20 mg of FB_1 per kg of BW/day, in feed	3 days	Decreased left ventricular contractility; heart rate, cardiac output, and mechanical efficiency of the left ventricle	Constable et al. (2000)
Experimental Studies Using Naturally-Contaminated Corn Screenings				
6 pigs	105–155 ppm FB_1 in corn screenings fed ad libitum	Up to 28 days	3 of 6 pigs developed pulmonary edema; liver and pancreatic lesions	Harrison et al. (1990)
8 pigs	92 ppm FB_1 in corn screenings fed ad libitum	Up to 21 days	6 of 8 pigs developed pulmonary edema; the remaining 2 pigs were icteric with increased liver enzymes	Osweiler et al. (1992)
5 pigs	175 ppm ($FB_1 + FB_2$) as corn screenings mixed in a complete ration	Up to 14 days	3 of 5 pigs developed pulmonary edema; hepatotoxicity; decreased weight gain	Motelin et al. (1994)
5 pigs	101 ppm ($FB_1 + FB_2$) as corn screenings mixed in a complete ration	Up to 14 days	Elevated GGT, ALT, AST, ALP, and bilirubin; liver lesions; decreased weight gain	Motelin et al. (1994)
5 pigs	39 ppm ($FB_1 + FB_2$) as corn screenings mixed in a complete ration	14 days	Histologic liver lesions	Motelin et al. (1994)
5 pigs	39 ppm ($FB_1 + FB_2$) as corn screenings mixed in a complete ration	14 days	Histologic liver lesions	Motelin et al. (1994)

(Continued)

TABLE 71.1 (Continued)

Number of Animals	Dose & Route	Duration	Toxic Effects	Reference
Reported Fumonisin Concentrations From Naturally-Occurring Outbreaks				
34 pigs from 2 farms	105–155 ppm FB_1	Unknown	Lethal pulmonary edema	Harrison et al. (1990)
16 pigs from 9 farms	All feed samples associated with pulmonary edema contained ≥20 ppm FB_1 to a maximum of 330 ppm FB_1	Unknown	Lethal pulmonary edema	Osweiler et al. (1992)

In ultrastructural studies using immersion fixed lungs, the endothelium was found to be swollen, vacuolated, and sometimes missing in pigs with pulmonary edema (Haschek et al., 1992). Additional studies using intravascularly perfused lungs (to allow better examination of the vascular system) demonstrated accumulations of fragmented membranous material in the cytocavitary region of endothelial cells (Gumprecht et al., 1998).

Fumonisins in Swine-Hepatic Effects

Hepatic changes in pigs exposed to fumonisins include elevation of liver associated enzyme activities, altered clinical chemistries, changes in sphingolipid parameters, and morphological alterations. In pigs, hepatic toxicity occurs prior to the development of pulmonary edema, and alterations are time and dose-dependent (Motelin et al., 1994). Increased activities of serum enzymes such as alkaline phosphatase (ALP), aspartate aminotransferase (AST) and gamma glutamyl transpeptidase (GGT) and concentrations of total bilirubin, bile acids, and cholesterol have been reported as early as 1 day after the initiation of fumonisin exposure (Colvin et al., 1993; Gumprecht et al., 1998; Harrison et al., 1990; Haschek et al., 1992; Motelin et al., 1994; Osweiler et al., 1992). These alterations reflect hepatocyte damage as well as altered hepatic function.

Morphologic alterations are dose related and progressive with continued ingestion of fumonisins. Following short term exposure, changes include hepatic cord disorganization, cytoplasmic vacuolation, apoptosis, scattered necrosis, and increased cell proliferation (Gumprecht et al., 1998; Harrison et al., 1990; Motelin et al., 1994; Osweiler et al., 1992). Histologic alterations were observed as early as 2 days after the initiation of treatment with a lethal dose (Gumprecht et al., 1998), and at a concentration as low as 23 ppm when fed for 14 days (Motelin et al., 1994). Long-term fumonisin exposure can result in fibrosis or development of hyperplastic nodules in the liver (Casteel et al., 1993; Harrison et al., 1990). Ultrastructurally, large accumulations of proteinaceous and membranous material were observed in the space of Disse in pigs that developed fumonisin-induced pulmonary edema (Haschek et al., 1992). Hepatocytes lost microvilli from their sinusoidal face while numerous Kupffer cells contained multilamellar bodies.

Fumonisins in Swine-Cardiovascular Effects

Fumonisins have been shown to decrease left ventricular contractility, heart rate, cardiac output, mean arterial pressure, arterial and mixed venous blood O_2 tensions, and systemic oxygen delivery, while increasing mean pulmonary artery pressure, oxygen consumption, and oxygen extraction ratio in swine (Constable et al., 2000; Smith et al., 1996a,b, 1999, 2000). The decrease in cardiac contractility leads to acute left ventricular failure and pulmonary edema in pigs exposed to high concentrations of fumonisin in feed. Chronic exposure to lower levels of fumonisin leads to the development of right ventricular hypertrophy and medial hypertrophy of the small pulmonary arteries in pigs, likely a result of pulmonary hypertension (Casteel et al., 1994).

Fumonisins in Swine-Immunologic Effects

Fumonisins have also been shown to predispose pigs to respiratory disease. In one case-control study, swine farms with ≥20 ppm of fumonisin in the feed were at significantly greater risk for pneumonia as compared to farms with low fumonisin concentrations (Bane et al., 1992). As the concentration of fumonisin in the feed increased, the risk of respiratory disease continued to increase. Later it was shown that exposure to fumonisins depressed pulmonary intravascular macrophage function, and pigs exposed to this toxin had decreased pulmonary clearance of blood–borne particulates and bacteria when compared to control animals (Smith et al., 1996c). In a more recent study, exposure to fumonisin exacerbated respiratory disease in a *Pasteurella multocida* challenge model (Halloy et al., 2005). Pigs that were fed 0.5 mg of FB_1 per kg of body weight/day for 7 days had delayed growth, increased coughing and more severe lung lesions that control pigs. In another study, pigs fed FB_1 at 20 ppm and exposed to *Mycoplasma hyopneumoniae* had more severe lung lesions as assessed by CT and histopathology as compared to pigs exposed to Mycoplasma but diets without FB_1 (Pósa et al., 2013). Therefore at levels well below those needed to cause hepatic lesions or pulmonary edema, fumonisins are likely to reduce growth rates and increase disease in pigs.

Fumonisin Toxicosis in Horses-Historical

Several outbreaks of a neurologic disease in horses occurred in the United States in the early 1900s with thousands of deaths reported in several states. The earliest citation of neurologic deaths associated with the feeding of contaminated corn was from Maryland (MacCallum and Buckley, 1902). The condition was commonly referred to as "cerebrospinal meningitis" and presented with fairly characteristic signs. The duration of disease varied from a few hours to a week, and the brains from affected horses had "softened" areas in the cerebrum involving only the white matter. Additional outbreaks were subsequently reported from Kansas, Iowa, Mississippi, and North Carolina. A similar disease, described as "epizootic cerebritis" had been encountered in 1891, however it is not known whether this was associated with corn (Butler, 1902). When feed from an outbreak of "leucoencephalitis" in Kansas was fed to a horse, it died after developing neurologic signs (Butler, 1902). At necropsy, the left cerebral hemisphere was "soft to the touch, and when cut through, the white matter was broken down extensively, nearly the entire hemisphere being involved." Several attempts were made to identify an infectious agent in the brain of affected horses and all were negative (MacCallum and Buckley, 1902). The authors concluded that a toxic etiology was likely.

In Central Illinois, more than 5,000 horses died during the winter of 1934–35 from a syndrome referred to as "cornstalk disease" (Graham, 1935). Brain tissue suspensions and filtrates were inoculated into laboratory animals, however no infectious etiology could be identified. Graham then placed 8 horses into a field containing cornstalks in Rantoul, Illinois. Two of these animals died, 23 and 26 days after being placed in the field (Graham, 1936). These outbreaks were similar to those reported in 1893 and 1914, which had occurred following a summer drought (Graham, 1936). Neurologic deaths with similar lesions were also reported in Iowa during the winter of 1914 and in the spring of 1935 (Schwarte et al., 1937). Histologic examination of the brain revealed no evidence of infectious agents. This "syndrome" was then subsequently reproduced by feeding moldy corn and corn fodder to five horses (Schwarte et al., 1937). A similar disease syndrome was identified and confirmed by feeding trials in Egypt (Badiali et al., 1968; Wilson and Maronpot, 1971) and in South Africa (Marasas et al., 1976). At necropsy, these studies were able to consistently demonstrate swelling of the cerebral hemispheres and flattening of the overlying gyri. On coronal sections, there were cavities of varying sizes with liquefactive necrosis of subcortical white matter in one or both cerebral hemispheres (Fig. 71.5). There was also scattered multifocal hemorrhages in the surrounding white matter (Marasas et al., 1976; Haliburton et al., 1979). Based on these findings, Marasas et al. (1976) coined the term "ELEM" as a distinct clinical and morphologic syndrome in horses associated with the feeding of corn.

F. verticillioides was later isolated from corn collected from field outbreaks in Egypt, and leukoencephalomalacia was subsequently reproduced in donkeys fed corn inoculated with the fungus (Wilson and Maronpot, 1971). In South Africa however, samples of corn inoculated with *F. verticillioides* produced liver damage and icterus in several horses and donkeys, but not brain lesions

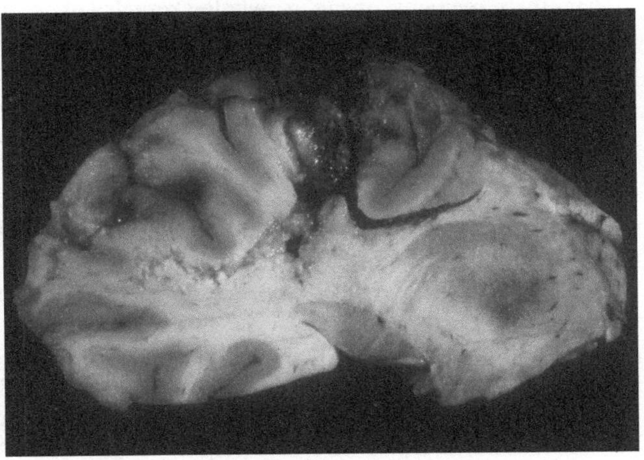

FIGURE 71.5 A cross section of a cerebral hemisphere from a horse demonstrating liquefactive necrosis of the white matter typical of equine leukoencephalomalacia.

(Kellerman et al., 1972). Marasas et al. (1976) then produced a batch of culture material using a strain of *F. verticillioides* from an outbreak of leukoencephalomalacia to produce liver damage and neurologic disease in a horse. It was then concluded that both hepatic disease and ELEM were manifestations of the same toxicosis, with different clinical syndromes occurring depending on toxin dose and length of exposure. Following the isolation and purification of FB_1 in the late 1980s, ELEM was experimentally induced by the administration of purified toxin (Kellerman et al., 1990; Marasas et al., 1988).

Spontaneous and Experimental Fumonisin Toxicosis in Horses

Since the discovery of fumonisin as the causative agent of ELEM, many more disease outbreaks associated with the feeding of corn have been reported on virtually all continents of the world (Bailly et al., 1996; Bela and Endre, 1996; Binkerd et al., 1993; Cerrillo et al., 1996; Christley et al., 1993; Giannitti et al., 2011; Jovanović et al., 2015; Rosiles et al., 1998; Ross et al., 1991, 1993; Uhlinger, 1991; Wilkins et al., 1994; Wilson et al., 1990a). Purified fumonisin B_1 has induced ELEM when administered orally (Kellerman et al., 1990) and intravenously (Foreman et al., 2004; Marasas et al., 1988; Laurent et al., 1989). Purified fumonisin B_2 has also induced ELEM when given orally (Ross et al., 1994). Fumonisin B_1 is considered to be the primary cause of ELEM however, as fumonisin B_2 is usually present in concentrations that are 20%–40% of fumonisin B_1 (Ross et al., 1991). Although ELEM has occurred in horses eating commercial feedstuffs (Ross et al., 1991; Wilson et al., 1990b), the feeding of corn screenings has been more frequently associated with ELEM, because fumonisin concentrations are much higher in screenings than in whole kernels of corn (Binkerd et al., 1993). Fumonisin B_1 also appears to survive the pelleting process for equine feeds (Ross et al., 1991).

Leukoencephalomalacia has been reproduced with intravenous administration of fumonisin B_1 in three separate studies (Foreman et al., 2004; Laurent et al., 1989; Marasas et al., 1988). Marasas et al. (1988) administered 0.125 mg fumonisin B_1/kg of body weight, IV, q24h, which produced ELEM in 9 days. Laurent et al. (1989) administered 0.1 mg fumonisin B_1/kg of body weight, IV, q24h for 16 days followed by 0.2 mg/kg/day for 2 additional days. Leukoencephalomalacia was induced in 18 days. Foreman et al. (2004) administered 0.05, 0.1 or 0.2 mg fumonisin B_1/kg of body weight IV q24h to 10 horses and all developed neurologic signs and were euthanized between days 4 and 12 of the study. In contrast, horses dosed with 0.01 mg fumonisin B_1/kg of body weight for 28 days in this study did not develop neurologic signs. Purified fumonisin B_1 has also been administered orally in other studies (1.25 or 2.5 mg fumonisin B_1/kg of body weight, PO, q24h), producing mild edema of the brain stem and hepatic disease in 11–12 days in two horses. In a subsequent study, animals were fed 0.6–4.0 mg fumonisin B_1/kg of body weight, PO, q 24 h for 33 or 35 days, producing hepatotoxicity and neurologic signs starting on days 22 and 24 in two weanling horses (Kellerman et al., 1990).

Doses of fumonisin reported from naturally occurring cases of fumonisin have varied (Table 71.2). One field report calculated that the ingestion of 0.6–2.1 mg fumonisin B_1/kg of body weight would induced ELEM in 24–28 days (Wilson et al., 1990b). Another study found that leukoencephalomalacia was associated with ingestion of feed containing fumonisin B_1 concentrations greater than 10 ppm, and concluded that feed with fumonisin B_1 concentrations greater than 10 ppm was not safe to be fed to horses (Ross et al., 1991).

Neurologic and Hepatic Effects in Horses

Several reports have considered ELEM and hepatotoxicity to be two separate syndromes associated with fumonisin toxicity in horses, with the terms "classic neurotoxic syndrome" and "hepatic syndrome" being used (McCue, 1989). However it appears more likely these are not true "distinct" syndromes but are related to the concentration of fumonisin in the feed, the duration of toxin consumption, and the tolerance of the individual horse to fumonisin. In some outbreaks, horses have died from ELEM while other horses have died from hepatotoxicity, and occasionally individual horses exhibiting both neurologic and hepatic signs have been described. Reported clinical signs associated with hepatic disease include icterus, mucous membrane petechiae, and swelling of the lips or muzzle (Ross et al., 1993; Uhlinger, 1991).

Ross et al. (1993) described an experimental study where one horse died acutely with "mild encephalopathy and hepatic necrosis" after 9 days of fumonisin exposure whereas two other horses died after 75 and 78 days of ELEM. The horse that died on day 9 showed neurologic signs prior to death ("visual impairment, mild ataxia, and slight head tremors") and had histologic evidence of leukoencephalomalacia at necropsy, however his death was primarily attributed to hepatotoxicity. This study lead to a common generalization that high doses of fumonisin were likely to induce hepatotoxicity, whereas lower doses of toxin over a longer period of time were necessary to induce ELEM (McCue, 1989; Plumlee and Galey, 1994). However in other experimental studies, intravenous administration of fumonisin B_1 induced ELEM in 9 days (Marasas et al., 1988) and 18 days (Laurent et al., 1989).

TABLE 71.2 Effect of Fumonisin in Horses

Number of Animals	Dose & Route	Duration	Toxic Effects	Reference
Experimental Studies Using Purified Fumonisin				
One horse	0.125 mg/kg/day, IV	7 treatments over 9 days	Leukoencephalomalacia	Marasas et al. (1988)
			Elevated AST, GGT	
One horse	2.5 mg/kg/day, PO (by gavage)	6 doses over 11 days	Severe hepatosis	Marasas et al. (1988)
			Elevated AST, GGT	
One horse	1.25 mg/kg/day, PO (by gavage)	6 doses over 11 days	Mild hepatosis	Marasas et al. (1988)
			Elevated AST, GGT	
One horse	0.1 mg/kg/day, IV and 0.2 mg/kg/day, IV	0.1 mg/kg dose given for 16 days then 0.2 mg/kg dose given for 2 additional days	Leukoencephalomalacia	Laurent et al. (1989)
One horse	1.25 mg/kg to 4.0 mg/kg, PO	20 doses given over 35 days	Leukoencephalomalacia	Kellerman et al. (1990)
			Elevated AST	
One horse	1.0 mg/kg to 4.0 mg/kg, PO	20 doses given over 33 days	Leukoencephalomalacia	Kellerman et al. (1990)
			Elevated AST, GGT	
13 horses	0.01 to 0.20 mg/kg, IV	Up to 10 days	Leukoencephalomalacia at 0.10 and 0.20 mg/kg—hepatic toxicity only at lower doses	Smith et al. (2002); Foreman et al. (2004)
Experimental Studies Using Fumonisin-Containing Culture Material				
2 horses	Diet contained 19 ppm FB_1 and was fed ad libitum	27 days	None	Schumacher et al. (1995)
2 horses	Diet contained 200 ppm FB_1 and was fed ad libitum	12 and 16 days	Leukoencephalomalacia	Schumacher et al. (1995)
			Increased GGT	
2 horses	2 diets containing 65 and 130 ppm FB_1 and was fed ad libitum	−65 ppm fed for 10 days	Leukoencephalomalacia	Schumacher et al. (1995)
		−130 ppm fed for an additional 17 days	Increased GGT	
Experimental Studies Using Naturally-Contaminated Corn Screenings				
4 ponies	Diet contained 44 ppm FB_1 and was fed ad libitum	10–97 days	2 horses died with ELEM on days 10 and 45–2 horses were normal after 97 days	Wang et al. (1992)
4 ponies	Diets contained between 1 and 22 ppm FB_1 and were fed ad libitum	238–326 days	ELEM in 2 of 5 horses	Wilson et al. (1992)
			Moderate to mild hepatosis in all 5 horses	
5 ponies	Diet contained 8 ppm FB_1 and was fed ad libitum	180 days	Mild histologic lesions in the brain and liver at necropsy	Wilson et al. (1992)
4 ponies	Diets contained between 1 and 88 ppm FB_1 and were fed ad libitum	9–120 days	ELEM in all 4 ponies (day 9–120)—also severe hepatosis in 2 ponies	Ross et al. (1993)

(Continued)

TABLE 71.2 (Continued)

Number of Animals	Dose & Route	Duration	Toxic Effects	Reference
Reported Fumonisin Concentrations From Naturally-Occurring Outbreaks				
18 horses	37−122 ppm FB_1	Unknown	ELEM confirmed in 14 horses	Wilson et al. (1990)
45 horses	8−126 ppm FB_1	7−35 days	All cases had confirmed leukoencephalomalacia	Ross et al. (1991)
6 horses	370 ppm FB_1 & 105 ppm FB_2	Unknown	4 horses died with ELEM; 2 horses with neurologic signs apparently recovered	Wilkins et al. (1994)
100^+ donkeys	4−29 ppm FB_1	Unknown	many donkeys died of neurologic disease-ELEM confirmed in 3 cases	Rosiles et al. (1998)
7 horses	12.5 ppm FB_1 and 5.3 ppm FB_2	10 days	At least 7 horses died with ELEM—at least one other horse with neurologic signs recovered with feed was removed	Giannitti et al. (2011)
100^+ horses	6.0 ppm FB_1 and 2.4 ppm FB_2	<30 days	21 horses developed neurologic signs—15 died within a month period	Jovanović et al. (2015)

In a large study with varying doses of fumonisin, horses treated with higher doses developed leukoencephalomalacia (in 5−8 days), whereas horses that received lower concentrations developed primarily hepatic lesions without any evidence of neurotoxicity (Foreman et al., 2004). Therefore it can be concluded ELEM results from an acute exposure to feed containing high concentrations of fumonisin B_1, while hepatotoxicity occurs with chronic ingestion of lower levels.

Serum biochemical changes associated with fumonisin toxicity in horses have been predominantly related to hepatotoxicity (increased AST, Wang et al., 1992; increased AST and GGT, Laurent et al., 1989; Kellerman et al., 1990; increased GGT and SDH, Schumacher et al., 1995; increased AST, GGT, and ALP, Ross et al., 1993; increased AST, GGT, ALP, total bilirubin, and bile acids, Wilson et al., 1992; and "elevated liver enzymes," Ross et al., 1994).

The neurologic signs are usually summarized as sudden onset of one or more of the following: frenzy, aimless circling, head pressing, paresis, ataxia, blindness, depression, and hyperexcitability (Ross et al., 1991; Wilson et al., 1992). Other reports have stated that "the disease started with lack of appetite, followed by the disturbance of swallowing and chewing indicating the paralysis of cephalic and pharyngeal muscles. Paralysis of cephalic and cervical muscles spread to the muscles of the extremities and trunk. The animals moved with difficulties, tottering and ataxia developed. Signs of 'blindness' developed in one animal. At the final stage of disease, the affected animals lied down and died. In a comprehensive study, early neurologic signs included mild proprioceptive abnormalities, including hindlimb ataxia, delayed forelimb placing reactions, and decreased tongue tone and movement (Foreman et al., 2004). These signs progressed over 12−48 h to become more readily apparent. Hindlimb and trunkal ataxia in particular became more apparent with time. A variety of behavioral changes were observed including depression, hyperesthesia, and intermittent dementia. All horses had intact menace and pupillary light responses at the time of death.

Cerebrospinal fluid findings from horses with ELEM include elevations in protein concentration, albumin, and IgG concentrations and increased albumin quotients (Foreman et al., 2004). Cerebrospinal fluid red blood cell, leukocyte, and glucose concentrations along with creatine kinase activity are not altered in horses with neurologic disease. Along with the histopathologic findings, these cerebrospinal fluid changes indicate the presence of a vasogenic cerebral edema in horses with leukoencephalomalacia.

Fumonisin Toxicity in Cattle

Adult beef cattle appear relatively resistant to fumonisin. Feeder calves fed a diet containing fumonisin concentrations up to 148 ppm for 31 days had only mild hepatotoxicity (Osweiler et al., 1993). Although it is tempting to speculate that cattle are able to break down the toxin, it has been shown that fumonisin is poorly metabolized by the rumen. Instead it is though that cattle have an increased tolerance to fumonisin because of differences in the mechanism of action. In milk-fed calves treated with purified fumonisin B_1, the kidney was the target organ of toxicity (Mathur et al., 2001). However this study also demonstrated that sphingosine and sphinganine concentrations did not increase in the serum and tissues of calves to the same degree that has been shown in pigs and horses.

When a group of 26 dairy cattle were fed a ration containing 100 ppm of fumonisin for the first 70 days of their lactation period, they had a significant decrease in dry matter intake and a lower milk yield as compared to the control group (Diaz et al., 2000). Milk production averaged 7 kg lower in the group fed the ration containing fumonisin and there was a 13% decrease in feed intake over the duration of the study period. Therefore it has been recommended to avoid fumonisin concentrations higher than 30 ppm in the total ration of dairy cattle.

Fumonisin Toxicity in Poultry

Fumonisins can be toxic to both chickens and turkeys with concentrations in the feed as low as 100 mg/kg causing decreased body weight gain, diarrhea, and hepatotoxicity (Bermudez et al., 1997; Ledoux et al., 1992). There has also been an association between *F. verticillioides* (the fungus that produces fumonisin) and an acute death syndrome recognized in young chicks called spiking mortality syndrome. It was initially hypothesized that fumonisins were directly cardiotoxic to poultry and were the cause of this syndrome; however, more recent research has suggested moniliformin (another *F. verticillioides* produced mycotoxin) is primarily responsible.

DIAGNOSIS AND TREATMENT

In addition to pathologic findings in animals, diagnosis of fumonisin toxicosis typically relies on detecting the actual toxin in feed samples. Fungal culture of feeds has little value in diagnosing fumonisin toxicosis because some corn samples contain very high concentrations of toxin with low levels of fungus, while others samples have heavy growths of *Fusarium* fungus with little to no detectable fumonisin. This is partly because the fungus that produced fumonisin also produces other mycotoxins. Therefore, the definitive diagnosis of fumonisin toxicosis in animals must involve analyzing the feed for the presence of the actual toxin. Many diagnostic laboratories across the world offer assays to detect both fumonisin B_1 and B_2 in corn and feed samples. The two most commonly used methods for toxin detection are chromatography (HPLC) and immunologic (ELISA) assays. To date, there are no commercially available assays that detect fumonisin in serum or tissues of animals.

Another assay that may be used more commonly in the future to diagnose fumonisin toxicosis in animals is the sphinganine-to-sphingosine ratio (Sa:So ratio). Because of the fumonisin-induced disruption of sphingolipid biosynthesis (Wang et al., 1992), the Sa:So ratio increases in the serum and tissues of pigs and horses exposed to fumonisin. It has been suggested that this assay could be used to diagnose fumonisin toxicosis when feed analysis is not possible. Sphinganine and sphingosine data may be available from enough pigs and horses in the near future to provide values for normal and affected animals.

To date there have been no treatments described for either ELEM or PPE. Generally the onset of clinical signs is acute and the progression of disease is rapid for both syndromes. The most important treatment is to identify and remove the source of contaminated feed to prevent other animals from developing clinical signs.

Guidelines for the maximum recommended levels of fumonisins in animal feeds have been published by the FDA Center for Veterinary Medicine (Table 71.3). It is

TABLE 71.3 Recommended Levels for Total Fumonisins (B_1 and B_2) in Animal Feeds

Animal	Recommended Maximum Level of Total Fumonisins in Corn to be Used for Feed (ppm)	Recommended Maximum Level of Total Fumonisin in the Ration (ppm)
Horse[a]	5	1
Swine	20	10
Ruminants[b]	60	30
Poultry[c]	100	50
Ruminant and poultry breeding stock[d]	30	15
Catfish	20	10
Other animals[e]	10	5

[a]*Includes donkeys, asses, and zebras.*
[b]*Cattle, sheep, goats, and other ruminants that are >3 months of age and are being fed for slaughter.*
[c]*Turkeys, chickens, ducklings, and other poultry being fed for slaughter.*
[d]*Includes lactating dairy cows, bulls, laying hens, and roosters.*
[e]*Includes dogs and cats.*
Source: From the United States Food and Drug Administration, Center for Veterinary Medicine.

important that livestock producers be aware of these guidelines and have their corn periodically tested for mycotoxins. Research has not yet found effective ways to decrease fumonisin concentrations in animal feedstuffs through processing or feed additives (i.e., binding agents). Corn containing significant levels of fumonisin should be discarded, diluted with corn containing lower concentrations of fumonisin, or fed to a less-sensitive species (i.e., ruminants or poultry interested for slaughter).

CONCLUDING REMARKS AND FUTURE DIRECTIONS

Fumonisins remain an active research topic however most studies in the last few years have focused on the potential effects of this mycotoxin in humans. More animal studies are needed to further define the mechanism of neurotoxicity in horses. Studies also need to be done examining the long-term cardiovascular effects associated with lower doses of fumonisin exposure in swine and humans. High fumonisin concentrations seem to appear in the corn crop from the United States every 3–4 years depending on weather, so they will continue to be a toxin of high regulatory concern in the future. Veterinarians and toxicologists must be familiar with this mycotoxin and should be able to quickly recognize clinical signs and gross lesions associated with fumonisin toxicity in animals.

REFERENCES

Badiali, L., Abou-Youssef, M.H., Radwan, A.I., et al., 1968. Moldy corn poisoning as the major cause of an encephalomalacia syndrome in Egyptian equidae. Am. J. Vet. Res. 29, 2029–2035.

Bailly, J.D., Raymond, I., Le Bars, P., et al., 1996. Leucoencephalomalacie des equides cas rapportes au CNITV. Rev. Med. Vet. 147, 787–796.

Bane, D.P., Neumann, E.J., Hall, W.F., et al., 1992. Relationship between fumonisin contamination of feed and mystery swine disease. Mycopathology 117, 121–124.

Bela, F., Endre, B., 1996. Occurrence of the equine leukoencephalomalacia (ELEM) caused by fumonisin-B_1 mycotoxin in Hungary. Magyar Allatorvosok Lapja 8, 484–487.

Bermudez, A.J., Ledoux, D.R., Rottinghaus, G.E., Bennett, G.A., 1997. The individual and combined effects of the Fusarium mycotoxins moniliformin and fumonisin B_1 in turkeys. Avian Dis. 41, 304–311.

Bezuidenhout, S.C., Gelderblom, W.C.A., Gorst-Allman, C.P., et al., 1988. Structure elucidation of the fumonisins, mycotoxins from Fusarium moniliforme. J. Chem. Soc. Chem. Commun.743–745.

Binkerd, K.A., Scott, D.H., Everson, R.J., et al., 1993. Fumonisin contamination of the 1991 Indiana corn crop and its effects on horses. J. Vet. Diagn. Invest. 5, 653–655.

Butler, T., 1902. Notes on a feeding experiment to produce leucoencephalitis in a horse, with positive results. Am. Vet. Rev. 26, 748–751.

Casteel, S.W., Turk, J.R., Cowart, R.P., Rottinghaus, G.E., 1993. Chronic toxicity of fumonisin in weanling pigs. J. Vet. Diagn. Invest. 5, 413–417.

Casteel, S.W., Turk, J.R., Rottinghaus, G.E., 1994. Chronic effects of dietary fumonisin on the heart and pulmonary vasculature of swine. Fundam. Appl. Toxicol. 23, 518–524.

Cerrillo, G.N., Rodriguez, F.S., Gordo, L.G., et al., 1996. Clinical and pathological aspects of an outbreak of equine leukoencephalomalacia in Spain. J. Vet. Med. A. 43, 467–472.

Christley, R.M., Begg, A.P., Hutchins, D.R., Hodgson, D.R., 1993. Leukoencephalomalacia in horses. Aust. Vet. J. 70, 225–226.

Colvin, B.M., Cooley, A.J., Beaver, R.W., 1993. Fumonisin toxicosis in swine: clinical and pathological findings. J. Vet. Diagn. Invest. 5, 232–241.

Constable, P.D., Smith, G.W., Rottinghaus, G.E., Haschek, W.M., 2000. Ingestion of fumonisin B_1-containing culture material decreases cardiac contractility and mechanical efficiency in swine. Toxicol. Appl. Pharmacol. 162, 151–160.

Diaz, D.E., Hopkins, B.A., Leonard, L.M., et al., 2000. Effect of fumonisin on lactating dairy cattle. J. Dairy Sci. 83, 1171.

Edrington, T.S., Kamps-Holtzapple, C.A., Harvey, R.B., et al., 1995. Acute hepatic and renal toxicity in lambs dosed with fumonisin-containing culture material. J. Anim. Sci. 72, 508–515.

Faraci, F.M., Heistad, D.D., 1990. Regulation of large cerebral arteries and cerebral microvascular pressure. Circ. Res. 66, 8–17.

Fazekas, B., Bajmocy, E., Glavits, R., et al., 1998. Fumonisin B_1 contamination of maize and experimental acute fumonisin toxicosis in pigs. J. Vet. Med. B. 45, 171–181.

Foreman, J.H., Constable, P.D., Waggoner, A.L., et al., 2004. Neurologic abnormalities and cerebrospinal fluid changes in horses administered fumonisin B1 intravenously. J. Vet. Int. Med. 18, 223–230.

Gelderblom, W.C.A., Jaskiewicz, K., Marasas, W.F.O., et al., 1988. Fumonisins-novel mycotoxins with cancer-promoting activity produced by *Fusarium moniliforme*. Appl. Environ. Micro. 54, 1806–1811.

Gelderblom, W.C.A., Marasas, W.F.O., Vleggaar, R., et al., 1992. Fumonisins: isolation, chemical characterization and biological effects. Mycopathology 117, 11–16.

Giannitti, F., Diab, S.S., Pacin, A.M., et al., 2011. Equine leukoencephalomalacia (ELEM) due to fumonisins B1 and B2 in Argentina. Pesq. Vet. Bras. 31, 407–412.

Goel, S., Schumacher, J., Lenz, S.D., Kemppainen, B.W., 1996. Effects of *Fusarium moniliforme* isolates on tissue and serum sphingolipid concentrations in horses. Vet. Hum. Toxicol. 38, 265–270.

Graham, R., 1935. Results of inoculating laboratory animals with equine brain-tissue suspensions and equine brain-tissue filtrates from spontaneous cases of so-called cornstalk disease. J. Am. Vet. Med. Assoc. 39, 778–780.

Graham, R., 1936. Cornstalk disease investigations: toxic encephalitis or non-virus encephalomyelitis of horses. Vet. Med. 31, 46–50.

Gumprecht, L.A., Marcucci, A., Vesonder, R.F., et al., 1995. Effects of intravenous fumonisin B_1 in rabbits: nephrotoxicity and sphingolipid alterations. Nat. Toxins 3, 395–403.

Gumprecht, L.A., Beasley, V.R., Weigel, R.M., et al., 1998. Development of fumonisin-induced hepatotoxicity and pulmonary edema in orally dosed swine: morphological and biochemical alterations. Toxicol. Pathol. 26, 777–788.

Haliburton, J.C., Vesonder, R.F., Lock, T.F., Buck, W.B., 1979. Equine leukoencephalomalacia (ELEM): a study of *Fusarium moniliforme* as an etiologic agent. Vet. Hum. Toxicol. 21, 348–351.

Halloy, D.J., Gustin, P.G., Bouhet, S., Oswald, I.P., 2005. Oral exposure to culture material extract containing fumonisins predisposes to the development of pneumonitis caused by *Pasteurella multocida*. Toxicology. 213, 34–44.

Hannun, Y.A., Bell, R.M., 1989. Functions of sphingolipids and sphingolipid breakdown products in cellular regulation. Science 243, 500–507.

Harrison, L.R., Colvin, B.M., Greene, J.T., et al., 1990. Pulmonary edema and hydrothorax in swine produced by fumonisin B_1, a toxic metabolite of *Fusarium moniliforme*. J. Vet. Diagn. Invest. 2, 217–221.

Harvey, R.B., Edrington, T.S., Kubena, L.F., et al., 1996. Effects of dietary fumonisin B_1-containing culture material, deoxynivalenol-contaminated wheat, or their combination on growing barrows. Am. J. Vet. Res. 57, 1790–1794.

Haschek, W.M., Motelin, G., Ness, D.K., et al., 1992. Characterization of fumonisin toxicity in orally and intravenously dosed swine. Mycopathology 117, 83–96.

Howard, P.C., Eppley, R.M., Stack, M.E., et al., 2001. Fumonisin B_1 carcinogenicity in a two-year feeding study using F344 rats and $B6C3F_1$ mice. Environ. Health Perspec. 109 (Suppl. 2), 277–282.

Jaskiewicz, K., Marasas, W.F.O., Taljaard, J.J.F., 1987. Hepatitis in vervet monkeys caused by *Fusarium monliforme*. J. Comp. Path. 97, 281–291.

Jovanović, M., Trailovic, D., Kukolj, V., et al., 2015. An outbreak of fumonisin toxicosis in horses in Serbia. World Mycotoxin J. 8, 387–391.

Kellerman, T.S., Marasas, W.F.O., Pienaar, J.G., Naude, T.W., 1972. A mycotoxicosis of equidae caused by *Fusarium moniliforme* sheldon: a preliminary communication. Onderstepoort J. Vet. Res. 39, 205–208.

Kellerman, T.S., Marasas, W.F.O., Thiel, P.G., et al., 1990. Leukoencephalomalacia in two horses induced by oral dosing of fumonisin B_1. Onderstepoort J. Vet. Res. 57, 269–275.

Kriek, N.P.J., Kellerman, T.S., Marasas, W.F.O., 1981. A comparative study of the toxicity of *Fusarium verticillioides* (=*F. moniliforme*) to horses, primates, pigs, sheep and rats. Onderstepoort J. Vet. Res. 48, 129–131.

Laurent, D., Pellegrin, F., Kohler, F., et al., 1989. Fumonisin B_1 in equine leucoencephalomalacia pathogenesis. Microbiologie Aliments Nutr. 7, 285–291.

Ledoux, D.R., Brown, T.P., Weibking, T.S., Rottinghaus, G.E., 1992. Fumonisin toxicity in broiler chicks. J. Vet. Diagn. Invest. 4, 330–333.

Liguoro, M., Petterino, C., Mezzalira, G., et al., 2004. Vet. Hum. Toxicol. 46, 303–305.

Lim, C.W., Parker, H.M., Vesonder, R.F., Haschek, W.M., 1996. Intravenous fumonisin B_1 induces cell proliferation and apoptosis in the rat. Nat. Toxins 4, 33–41.

MacCallum, W.G., Buckley, S.S., 1902. Acute epizootic leucoencephalitis in horses. Am. Vet. Rev. 26, 21–36.

Marasas, W.F.O., Kellerman, T.S., Pienaar, J.G., Naude, T.W., 1976. Leukoencephalomalacia: a mycotoxicosis of equidae caused by *Fusarium moniliforme* sheldon. Onderstepoort J. Vet. Res. 43, 113–122.

Marasas, W.F.O., Kellerman, T.S., Gelderblom, W.C.A., et al., 1988. Leukoencepalomalacia in a horse induced by fumonisin B_1 isolated from *Fusarium moniliforme*. Onderstepoort J. Vet. Res. 55, 197–203.

Martinez-Larranaga, M.R., Anadon, A., Diaz, M.J., et al., 1999. Toxicokinetics and oral bioavailability of fumonisin B_1. Vet. Hum. Toxicol. 41, 357–362.

Mathur, S., Constable, P.D., Eppley, R.M., et al., 2001. Fumonisin B_1 increases serum sphinganine concentration but does not alter serum sphingosine concentration or induced cardiovascular changes in milk-fed calves. Toxicol. Sci. 60, 379–384.

McCue, P.M., 1989. Equine leukoencephalomalacia. Comp. Contin. Educ. Pract. Vet. 11, 646–651.

McDonough, P.M., Yasui, K., Betto, R., et al., 1994. Control of cardiac Ca^{2+} levels: inhibitory actions on sphingosine on Ca^{2+} transients and L-type Ca^{2+} channel conductance. Circ. Res. 75, 981–989.

Merrill Jr., A.H., Sweeley, C.C., 1996. Sphingolipids metabolism and cell signaling. In: Vance, D.E., Vance, J.E. (Eds.), Biochemistry of Lipids, Lipoproteins, and Membranes. Elsevier, New York, pp. 43–73.

Merrill Jr., A.H., Wang, E., Schroeder, J.J., et al., 1995. In: Elklund, M., Richards, M., Mise, K. (Eds.), Molecular Approaches to Food Safety. Issues Involving Toxic Microorganisms. Alaken Press, Fort Collins CO, pp. 429–443.

Michelakis, E., Tewari, K., Simard, J.M., 1994. Calcium channels in smooth muscle cells from cerebral precapillary arterioles activate at more negative potentials than those from basilar artery. Pflugers Arch. 426, 459–461.

Motelin, G.K., Haschek, W.M., Ness, D.K., et al., 1994. Temporal and dose-response features in swine fed corn screenings contaminated with fumonisin mycotoxins. Mycopathology 126, 27–40.

Osweiler, G.D., Ross, P.F., Wilson, T.M., et al., 1992. Characterization of an epizootic of pulmonary edema in swine associated with fumonisins in corn screenings. J. Vet. Diagn. Invest. 4, 53–59.

Osweiler, G.D., Kehrli, M.E., Stabel, J.R., et al., 1993. Effects of fumonisin-contaminated corn screenings on growth and health of feeder calves. J. Anim. Sci. 71, 459–466.

Patchimasiri, T., Sailasuta, A., Kawtheerakul, K., 1998. Pathological findings in swine in association with fumonisin contaminated feed. Thai J. Vet. Med. 28, 71–82.

Plumlee, K.H., Galey, F.G., 1994. Neurotoxic mycotoxins: a review of fungal toxins that cause neurological disease in large animals. J. Vet. Int. Med. 8, 49–54.

Pósa, R., Magyar, T., Stoev, S.D., et al., 2013. Use of computed tomography and histopathologic review for lung lesions produced by the interaction between *Mycoplasma hyopneumoniae* and fumonisin mycotoxins in pigs. Vet. Pathol. 50, 971–979.

Prelusky, D.B., Trenholm, H.L., Savard, M.E., 1994. Pharmacokinetic fate of ^{14}C-labelled fumonisin B_1 in swine. Nat. Toxins 2, 73–80.

Prelusky, D.B., Savard, M.E., Trenholm, H.L., 1995. Pilot study on the plasma pharmacokinetics of fumonisin B_1 in cows following a single dose by oral gavage or intravenous administration. Nat. Toxins 3, 384–394.

Raoofi, A., Mardjanmehr, S.H., Khosravi, A.R., et al., 2003. J. Eq. Vet. Sci. 23, 469–470.

Rheeder, J.P., Marasas, W.F.O., Thiel, P.G., et al., 1992. *Fusarium moniliforme* and fumonisins in corn in relation to human esophageal cancer in Transkei. Phytopathology 82, 353–357.

Richard, J.L., Meerdink, G., Maragos, C.M., et al., 1996. Absence of detectable fumonisins in the milk of cows fed *Fusarium proliferatum* (Matusushima) Nirenberg culture material. Mycopathology 133, 123–126.

Riley, R.T., An, N.H., Showker, J.L., et al., 1993. Alteration of tissue and serum sphinganine to sphingosine ratio: an early biomarker of exposure to fumonisin-containing feeds in pigs. Toxicol. Appl. Pharmacol. 118, 105–112.

Rosiles, M.R., Bautista, J., Fuentes, V.O., Ross, F., 1998. An outbreak of equine leukoencephalomalacia at Oaxaca, Mexico, associated with fumonisin B_1. J. Vet. Med. A. 45, 299–302.

Ross, P.F., Rice, L.G., Reagor, J.C., et al., 1991. Fumonisin B_1 concentrations in feeds from 45 confirmed equine leukoencephalomalacia cases. J. Vet. Diagn. Invest. 3, 238–241.

Ross, P.F., Ledet, A.E., Owens, D.L., et al., 1993. Experimental equine leukoencephalomalacia, toxic hepatitis, and encephalopathy caused by corn naturally contaminated with fumonisins. J. Vet. Diagn. Invest. 5, 69–74.

Ross, P.F., Nelson, P.E., Owens, D.L., et al., 1994. Fumonisin B_2 in cultured *Fusarium proliferatum*, M-6104, causes equine leukoencephalomalacia. J. Vet. Diagn. Invest. 6, 263–265.

Rotter, B.A., Prelusky, D.B., Fortin, A., et al., 1996. Response of growing swine to dietary exposure to fumonisin B_1 during an eight-week period: growth and clinical parameters. Nat. Toxins 4, 42–50.

Schumacher, J., Mullen, J., Shelby, R., et al., 1995. An investigation of the role of *Fusarium moniliforme* in duodenitis/proximal jejunitis of horses. Vet. Human Toxicol. 37, 39–45.

Schwarte, L.H., Biester, H.E., Murray, C., 1937. A disease of horses caused by feeding moldy corn. J. Am. Vet. Med. Assoc. 43, 76–85.

Shephard, G.S., Thiel, P.G., Sydenham, E.W., Savard, M.E., 1995. Fate of a single dose of ^{14}C-labelled fumonisin B_1 in Vervet monkeys. Nat. Toxins 3, 145–150.

Scott, P.M., 2012. Recent research on fumonisins: a review. Food Addit. Contam. 29, 242–248.

Smith, G.W., Constable, P.D., Bacon, C.W., et al., 1996a. Cardiovascular effects of fumonisins in swine. Fundam. Appl. Toxicol. 31, 169–172.

Smith, G.W., Constable, P.D., Haschek, W.M., 1996b. Cardiovascular responses to short-term fumonisin exposure in swine. Fundam. Appl. Toxicol. 33, 140–148.

Smith, G.W., Constable, P.D., Smith, A.R., et al., 1996c. Effects of fumonisin-containing culture material on pulmonary clearance in swine. Am. J. Vet. Res. 57, 1233–1238.

Smith, G.W., Constable, P.D., Tumbleson, M.E., et al., 1999. Sequence of cardiovascular changes leading to pulmonary edema in swine fed culture material containing fumonisin. Am. J. Vet. Res. 60, 1292–1299.

Smith, G.W., Constable, P.D., Eppley, R.M., et al., 2000. Purified fumonisin B_1 decreases cardiovascular function but does not alter pulmonary capillary permeablity in swine. Toxicol. Sci. 56, 240–249.

Smith, G.W., Constable, P.D., Foreman, J.H., et al., 2002. Cardiovascular changes associated with intravenous administration of fumonisin B_1 in horses. Am. J. Vet. Res. 63, 538–545.

Spotti, M., Caloni, F., Fracchiolla, L., et al., 2001. Fumonisin B_1 carry-over into milk in the isolated perfused bovine udder. Vet. Hum. Toxicol. 43, 109–111.

Sydenham, E.W., Marasas, W.F.O., Shephard, G.S., et al., 1992. Fumonisin concentrations in Brazilian feeds associated with field outbreaks of confirmed and suspected animal mycotoxicoses. J. Agric. Food Chem. 40, 994–997.

Thiel, P.G., Shephard, G.S., Sydenham, E.W., et al., 1991. Levels of fumonisin B_1 and B_2 in feeds associated with confirmed cases of equine leukoencephalomalacia. J. Agric. Food Chem. 39, 109–111.

Uhlinger, C., 1991. Clinical and epidemiologic features of an epizootic of equine leukoencephalomalacia. J. Am. Vet. Med. Assoc. 198, 126–128.

Voss, K.A., Norred, W.P., Plattner, R.D., Bacon, C.W., 1989. Hepatotoxicity and renal toxicity of corn samples associated with field cases of equine leukoencephalomalacia. Fd. Chem. Toxicol. 27, 89–96.

Voss, K.A., Riley, R.T., Gelineau-van, W.J., 2011. Fumonisins. In: Gupta, R.C. (Ed.), Reproductive and Developmental Toxicology. Academic Press/Elsevier, Amsterdam, pp. 725–737.

Vudathala, D.K., Prelusky, D.B., Ayroud, M., et al., 1994. Pharmacokinetic fate and pathological effects of 14C-fumonisin B_1 in laying hens. Nat. Toxins 2, 81–88.

Wang, E., Norred, W.P., Bacon, C.W., et al., 1991. Inhibition of sphingosine biosynthesis by fumonisins. J. Biol. Chem. 266, 14486–14490.

Wang, E., Ross, P.F., Wilson, T.M., et al., 1992. Increases in serum sphingosine and sphinganine and decreases in complex sphingolipids in ponies given feed containing fumonisins, mycotoxins produced by *Fusarium moniliforme*. J. Nutr. 122, 1706–1716.

Webster, R., Sabbadini, R.A., Paolini, P., 1994. Sphingosine effects on the contractile behavior of skinned cardiac myocytes. J. Mol. Cell Cardiol. 26, 1273–1290.

Wilkins, P.A., Vaala, W.E., Zivotofsky, D., Twitchell, E., 1994. A herd outbreak of equine leukoencephalomalacia. Cornell Vet. 84, 53–59.

Wilson, B.J., Maronpot, R.R., 1971. Causative fungus agent of leucoencephalomalacia in equine animals. Vet. Rec. 88, 484–486.

Wilson, T.M., Ross, P.F., Rice, L.G., et al., 1990a. Fumonisin B_1 levels associated with an epizootic of equine leukoencephalomalacia. J. Vet. Diagn. Invest. 2, 213–221.

Wilson, T.M., Nelson, P.E., Marasas, W.F.O., et al., 1990b. A mycological evaluation and in vivo toxicity evaluation of feed from 41 farms with equine leukoencephalomalacia. J. Vet. Diagn. Invest. 2, 352–354.

Wilson, T.M., Ross, P.F., Owens, D.L., et al., 1992. Experimental reproduction of ELEM. A study to determine the minimum toxic dose in ponies. Mycopathology. 117, 115–120.

Zomborszky, M.K., Vetesi, F., Repa, I., et al., 2000. Experiment to determine limits of tolerance for fumonisins B_1 in weaned piglets. J. Vet. Med. B. 47, 277–286.

FURTHER READING

Diaz, G.J., Boermans, H.J., 1994. Fumonisin toxicosis in domestic animals: a review. Vet. Human Toxicol. 36, 548–555.

Smith, G.W., Constable, P.D., 2004. Fumonisin. In: Plumlee, K.H. (Ed.), Clinical Veterinary Toxicology. Mosby, St. Louis, MO, pp. 250–254.

Chapter 72

Ochratoxins and Citrinin

Ramesh C. Gupta, Ajay Srivastava and Rajiv Lall

INTRODUCTION

Ochratoxins and citrinin are produced by several species of the genera *Aspergillus* and *Penicillium*. The two most common species that produce ochratoxin A (OTA) are *Aspergillus ochraceus* and *Penicillium verrucosum*. These fungi are ubiquitous, and the potential for contamination of animal feed and human food is widespread. *Aspergillus* spp. appears to produce ochratoxins under conditions of high humidity and temperature, whereas some *Penicillium* spp. may produce ochratoxins at temperatures as low as 5°C. OTA has been found in a variety of food/feed, with levels in commodities used as feed ranging up to 27 ppm, and with levels in foodstuffs for human consumption in the range of trace to about 100 ppb. OTA is a pentaketide-derived dihydroisocoumarin moiety coupled with a 12-carboxy group by a peptide bond to *L*-phenylalanine. There are two commonly recognized OTA analogs, ochratoxin B (OTB) and ochratoxin C (OTC), and, of course, alkyl esters of ochratoxins. Unlike OTA, the occurrence of OTB and OTC is rare. Chemical structures of ochratoxins are shown in Fig. 72.1 and the order of their toxicity is OTA > OTB > OTC. All metabolites of OTA are less toxic than the parent compound.

Citrinin was first isolated as a pure compound from a culture of *Penicillium citrinum* in 1931. Later, it was also isolated from *A. ochraceus*, *P. verrucosum* and related species that contaminate grain. In 1951, yellowish colored rice imported from Thailand to Japan was found to be contaminated with *P. citrinum*, which contained citrinin. Synthesized citrinin is also used in molecular biological research, as it induces mitochondrial permeability pore opening and inhibits respiration by interfering with complex I of the respiratory chain. The chemical structure of citrinin is shown in Fig. 72.2.

Both OTA and citrinin cause nephropathy in animals and they have also been implicated as the cause of Balkan Endemic Nephropathy (BEN) in humans. Literature reveals that OTA has been studied to a greater extent than citrinin, because OTA is at least ten times more toxic than citrinin. This chapter describes in detail the toxicity of ochratoxins and citrinin in animals.

BACKGROUND

The fungi producing ochratoxins and citrinin are commonly encountered in animal feed and human food around the world. They are encountered with great frequencies in the Balkan and Scandinavian countries. There are three major ochratoxins (OTA, OTB and OTC), but OTA occurs naturally with a greater frequency in a variety of cereal grains (barley, wheat, oats, corn and beans), peanuts, dried fruits, grapes/raisins, cheese, and other food products. OTA accumulates in the food chain because of its long half-life. Citrinin usually cooccurs with OTA, and commonly contaminates cereal grains, including wheat, barley, oats, corn, and rice. Citrinin also contaminates peanuts and fruits. Levels of OTA and citrinin have been found far lower in human food than in raw animal feed, because during the processing and baking of human food, citrinin is almost eliminated and OTA is significantly reduced. Compared to OTA, OTB, and OTC are rarely found and are much less toxic.

Both OTA and citrinin are well-known nephrotoxins. OTA is also known to possess genotoxic (Meisner et al., 1983), carcinogenic (Creppy et al., 1985), reproductive, developmental and teratogenic (Arora et al., 1983; Minervini et al., 2013; Gupta et al., 2017), immunotoxic (Stormer and Lea, 1995), neurotoxic (Bruinink and Sidler, 1997; Sava et al., 2006), mutagenic (Stetina and Votava, 1986) properties. In humans, exposure to OTA and citrinin has been linked with BEN, a chronic kidney disease associated with tumors of the renal system, which can be fatal. However, some researchers have doubted OTA as the etiological factor in BEN (Mally et al., 2007). A recent molecular epidemiological study provided a strong relationship between chronic dietary exposure to aristolochic acid (AA), a principal component of *Aristolochia*

Veterinary Toxicology. DOI: http://dx.doi.org/10.1016/B978-0-12-811410-0.00072-6

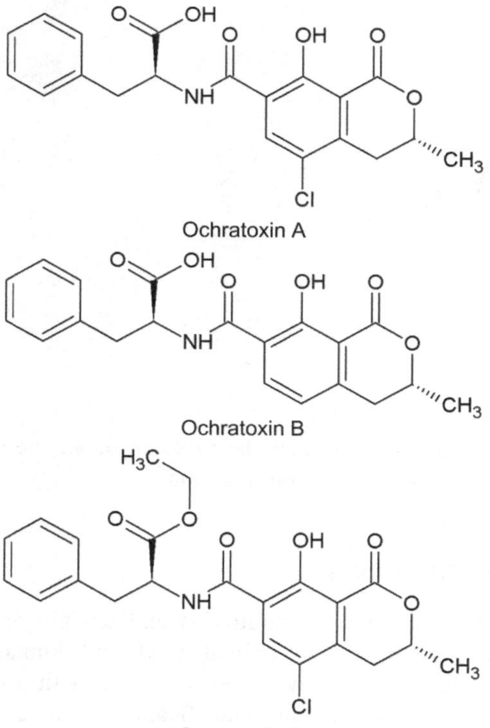

Ochratoxin A

Ochratoxin B

Ochratoxin C

FIGURE 72.1 Chemical structures of ochratoxins.

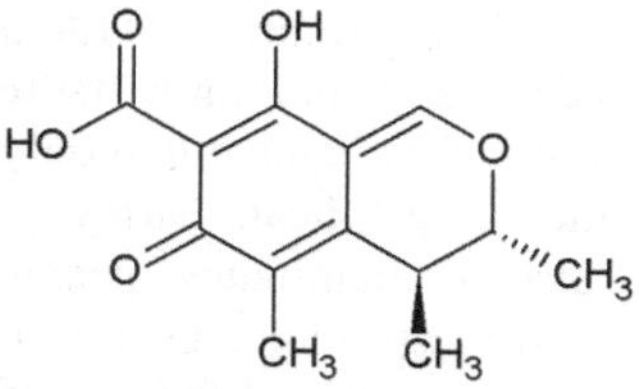

FIGURE 72.2 Chemical structure of citrinin.

clematitis, which grows as a weed in the wheat fields of the BEN region, and nephropathy (Stiborová et al., 2016). Co-occurrence of citrinin with OTA has been implicated in nephropathy of pigs in Denmark, Sweden, Norway and Ireland. Citrinin and OTA are also involved in avian nephropathies. Residues of OTA have been detected in the tissues of pigs in slaughterhouses, and it has been shown, under experimental conditions, that residues can still be detected in tissues 1 month after the end of exposure. Due to the long half-life of OTA in feed and biological systems, serious concerns have been raised about animal health as well as the human consumption of meat.

TOXICOKINETICS

OTA is absorbed from the stomach because of its lipid soluble, nonionized and acidic properties ($pK_a = 7.1$) (reviewed in Gupta et al., 2017). Absorption of OTA also takes place in the duodenum and jejunum, is involved in enterohepatic circulation and its biliary excretion is very efficient (Kumagai and Aibara, 1982; Kumagai, 1988). OTA is distributed to various organs, mainly to the kidneys. Liver, muscle and fat contain lower concentrations. Following oral administration, the overall percentage of OTA absorption is found to be 66% in pigs, 56% in rats, 56% in rabbits and 40% in chickens (Suzuki et al., 1977; Galtier et al., 1981). After a single oral dose, the maximum concentrations of OTA are found within 10–48 h in pigs and rats (Galtier et al., 1979, 1981), 2–4 h in calves (Sreemannarayana et al., 1988), after 1 h in rabbits and after 0.33 h in chickens (Galtier et al., 1981). Maximum tissue concentrations in rat tissues occur within 48 h.

OTA has shown a high binding affinity for plasma proteins. Vettorazzi et al. (2009) demonstrated that male rats had lower OTA bioavailability than females due to the male-specific protein alpha-2u-globulin. OTA was found in decreasing order of concentrations in kidney < liver < fat < muscle. The serum half-life of OTA is long and varies widely among species, e.g., 24–39 h in mice, 55–120 h in rats, 6.7 h in quail, 510 h in *Macaca mulata* monkeys (Hagelberg et al., 1989), 72–120 h in pigs, 4.1 h in chicken (Galtier et al., 1981) and 840 h in a human (Benford et al., 2001). Fasting has been shown to increase the rate of OTA absorption and its maximum plasma concentrations in rats (Vettorazzi et al., 2009).

Toxicokinetics of OTA in pigs revealed that the kidney is generally the most heavily contaminated tissue and that levels in the blood are about fivefold greater than in the kidney. Krog et al. (1976) illustrated that if the level of OTA in swine kidney is 12.1 ng/g (resulting from about 1000 ng/g in the feed), its levels would be 7.8 ng/g in the liver, 4.2 ng/g in the muscle and 2.8 ng/g in adipose tissue. OTA in ruminants is usually hydrolyzed in the forestomach by protozoans and bacterial enzymes, and consequently little OTA is found in the tissues (Hult et al., 1976).

In the context of metabolism, various tissues of all species that are examined, OTA is hydrolyzed to ochratoxin *alpha*, which is the major metabolite (reviewed in Gupta et al., 2017). This detoxication process also takes place in the cecum of rats and is facilitated by bacterial microflora (Galtier, 1978). The enzymes responsible for hydrolysis to ochratoxin *alpha* in cows, sheep and rodents are carboxypeptidase A and chymotrypsin. Suzuki et al. (1977) demonstrated that the rat tissue homogenate of the duodenum, ileum and pancreas also has a high activity of these enzymes to catalyze this reaction. Activity of these enzymes in liver and kidney are low. Studies in mice suggest that OTA circulates from the liver into the bile and into the intestine, where it is hydrolyzed to ochratoxin *alpha* (Moroi et al., 1985). About 25%–27% of OTA, given either i.p. or orally to rats, was found as ochratoxin *alpha* in the urine. Its presence in the urine can be explained by reabsorption from the intestine. A similar mechanism of intestinal reabsorption of ochratoxin *alpha* has been suggested to occur in ruminant calves (Sreemannarayana et al., 1988). In sheep, Höhler et al. (1999) demonstrated that OTA hydrolysis in the gastrointestinal tract was substantially less than previously described, especially if OTA was ingested in combination with concentrate-rich diets. For further details on metabolism of OTA, readers are referred to Wu et al. (2012) and Malir et al. (2013).

OTA and its metabolites excrete in the urine and feces in all species (Höhler et al., 1999; Ringot et al., 2006; Coronel et al., 2011; Klapec et al., 2012). OTA also passes in the milk in animal species (such as rats and rabbits) and humans (Munoz et al., 2014), but very little is excreted in cows' milk because of its metabolism by the ruminal microflora (Breitholtz-Emanuelsson et al., 1993; Signorini et al., 2012). This route is of importance because the milk is consumed by the offspring. Subsequent to its urinary excretion, OTA is reabsorbed in all nephron segments. Excretion of OTA can be influenced by the route of administration, the dose and the gender, age and weight of the animal (Vettorazzi et al., 2009, 2014). Excretion of OTA is also impacted by the extent of enterohepatic circulation and binding to serum albumin and other macromolecules (Galtier et al., 1980; Hult and Fuchs, 1986). The association constant for the binding of OTA to serum albumin is 7.1×10^4 per mol for pigs, 5.1×10^4 per mol for chickens and 4.0×10^4 per mol for rats (Galtier et al., 1981).

Placental transfer of OTA in mammalian species like mice, rat and swine is well known. However, in ruminants the placental transfer of OTA is very little. After intravenous administration of a high dose of OTA (1 mg/kg body weight) to pregnant ewes, Munro et al. (1973) did not detect OTA in the amniotic fluid and fetal tissue levels were 400–1000 times lower than in the maternal blood. The exact mechanism involved in placental transfer of OTA is yet to be elucidated. OTA can be present in eggs due to its biliary excretion if the laying hens are exposed to this mycotoxin at high doses (Armorini et al., 2015).

By now, it is clear from several animal studies that OTA has a high degree of bioavailability, a low plasma clearance rate and a long tissue half-life. Because of the differences in animal physiology, wide variations are seen in the toxicokinetic patterns of OTA. For further details on biotransformation, toxicokinetics, and toxicodynamics of OTA, readers are referred to recent publications elsewhere (Ringot et al., 2006; Vettorazzi et al., 2014; Gupta et al., 2017).

Toxicokinetic data of citrinin in animals are scarce due to lack of a validated method to determine the concentrations of citrinin and its major metabolite dihydrocitrinone (HO-CIT) in body fluids and tissues. In recent human studies, LC-MS/MS has been used to determine the concentrations of citrinin and HO-CIT in urine (Ali et al., 2015; Huybrechts et al., 2015; Föllmann et al., 2016).

MECHANISM OF ACTION

Both OTA and citrinin are well-known nephrotoxicants. In addition to nephrotoxicity, OTA is known to exert neurotoxic, immunotoxic, teratogenic and carcinogenic effects in mammalian species. OTA also disrupts blood coagulation and glucose metabolism. In general, the mechanisms associated with OTA toxicity include inhibition of protein synthesis, ROS formation, lipid peroxidation, disturbance of calcium homeostasis and impairment of mitochondrial oxidation reactions. A brief description of the mechanisms involved in common toxic effects is given below.

Nephrotoxicity

Both OTA and citrinin produce nephrotoxicity involving multiple mechanisms. At high doses, OTA affects both renal function and morphology, as indicated by increased weight, urine volume, blood urea nitrogen, urinary glucose, and proteinuria. The last two findings indicate that the site of reabsorption (i.e., the proximal convoluted tubules) is damaged. OTA specifically causes defect of the organic anion transport mechanism located on the brush border of the proximal convoluted tubules and basolateral membranes. OTA also adversely affects the organic ion transport system by which OTA enters the proximal tubular cells. The middle (S2) and terminal (S3) segments of the proximal tubule of the isolated nephron are the most sensitive to the toxic effects of OTA, as evidenced by marked decreases in cellular and mitochondrial ATP contents.

Studies suggest that both OTA and citrinin cause mitochondrial dysfunction in renal and hepatic tissues (Aleo et al., 1991; Chagas et al., 1995). OTA toxicity is associated with inhibition of both protein and RNA synthesis (Dirheimer and Creppy, 1991). OTA is known to interfere with the charging of tRNA with amino acids. OTA treatment can increase oxidative stress in peripheral organs. Administration of OTA to rats (1 mg/kg) resulted in a 22% decrease in α-tocopherol plasma levels and a fivefold increase in the expression of the oxidative stress responsive protein heme oxygenase-1, specifically in the kidney (Gautier et al., 2001). Cell death occurs by apoptosis (Ramyaa and Padma, 2013).

Neurotoxicity

Evidence strongly suggests that OTA affects selected structures of the brain and it has the potential for neuroinflammation and neurotoxicity (Belmadani et al., 1998; Bruinink et al., 1998; Von Tobel et al., 2014). This mycotoxin has multiple mechanisms of action, including oxidative stress, bioenergetic compromise, inhibition of protein synthesis, production of DNA single-stranded breaks, and formation of OTA-DNA adducts (Sava et al., 2006; González-Arias et al., 2014). Sava et al. (2006) reported that administration of OTA in mice, at a single dose (3.5 mg/kg) that is approximately 10% of the reported LD_{50}, caused widespread oxidative injury in six discrete brain regions.

Immunotoxicity

There is ample evidence from studies conducted in several animal species that under certain conditions of treatment, OTA can produce defects in the structure and/or function of elements comprising the immune system (Pohland et al., 1992; Khatoon et al., 2013; Marin and Taranu, 2014; Kupski et al., 2016). The size of the mouse thymus was reduced to 33% of that of controls after four i.p. injections of OTA at 20 mg/kg body weight on alternate days, a dose that caused minimal nephrotoxicity. Bone marrow depression was dose related, and changes included decreased marrow cellularity, a reduction in bone marrow macrophage-granulocyte progenitors, a decreased number of hematopoietic stem cells, a significant decrease in erythropoiesis and increased phagocytosis by macrophages (Boorman et al., 1984). The effects of OTA on the bone marrow and lymphatic cell population may reflect the sensitivity of these cells to the inhibition of protein synthesis. These effects on the structural components of the immune system indicated that OTA adversely affects immune function.

In chickens fed diets containing OTA at a concentration of 2–4 mg/kg for 20 days, the lymphoid cell population of immune organs was decreased, and IgA and IgM in lymphoid tissues and serum were decreased (Dwivedi and Burns, 1984a,b). Complement activity was slightly affected in birds fed diets containing 2 mg/kg for 5–6 weeks (Campbell et al., 1983). Immune suppression was observed in chickens fed diets containing OTA at 0.05 or 2 mg/kg for 21 days. Treated animals showed reduced total serum protein, lymphocyte counts and weights of the thymus, bursa of fabricus and spleen (Singh et al., 1990).

Carcinogenicity

The exact mechanism by which OTA induces nephrocarcinogenicity is yet to be established, although both genotoxic and nongenotoxic modes of action seem to be involved (Pfohl-Leszkowicz and Manderville, 2007; Marin-Kuan et al., 2008; Golli-Bennour et al., 2010; Stoev, 2010a, b). Cavin et al. (2007) suggested that the reduction of antioxidant defense appears to be involved in OTA toxicity and carcinogenicity. Interestingly, Taniai et al. (2014) reported that OTA induces karyomegaly and cell cycle aberrations in renal tubular cells without inducing oxidative stress.

TOXICITY

The toxic effects of OTA have been studied extensively in a number of domestic, companion and experimental animals. All evidence suggests that OTA continues to be a huge problem to animal health worldwide (O'Brien and Dietrich, 2005; Gupta et al., 2017). Overall toxicity of OTA is greatly influenced by species, sex and route of administration. Based on acute toxicity data, dogs, pigs, and chickens are the most sensitive species and rats and mice the least sensitive. Oral LD_{50} values (expressed as mg/kg body weight) of OTA are reported to be 46–58 in mouse, 20–30 in rat, 3.9 in neonate rat, 0.2 in dog, 1 in pig, and 3.3 in chicken (Harwig et al., 1983). LD_{50} values via i.p. route are reported to be 22–40 in mouse and 20–30 in rat; and with i.v. route, 26–34 in mouse and 13 mg/kg in rat. OTA causes renal toxicity, nephropathy, neurotoxicity, immunotoxicity, carcinogenicity and developmental/reproductive toxicity in several animal species (reviewed in Gupta et al., 2017).

The acute LD_{50} (expressed as mg/kg body weight) of citrinin is reported to be 50 (oral) and 67 (s.c. or i.p.) in rat, 35–58 in mouse and 19 (i.p. or i.v.) in rabbit. Citrinin toxicity, especially in terms of nephropathy, has been reported in various animal species, including rats, hamsters, dogs and poultry. Citrinin causes kidney damage and mild liver damage in the form of fatty infiltration. Other toxic effects include vasodilatation, constriction of the bronchi and increased muscular tone.

All animals studied so far have been found susceptible to orally administered OTA with a varying degree of response. It is important to mention that at higher doses, OTA causes alterations in kidneys and also in other organs and tissue, but renal lesions can be found at an exposure level that is identical to those occurring environmentally. OTB is rarely found as a natural contaminant and is much less toxic than OTA. The other ochratoxins have never been encountered in natural products.

Weanling Fischer 344/*N* rats of both sexes receiving OTA by gavage in maize oil at a dose of 0.06, 0.12, 0.25, 0.5 or 1 mg/kg body weight/day for 5 days/week for 91 days, showed growth retardation and a reduced relative kidney weight in males at the two higher doses. Karyomegaly of dose-related severity was observed in the proximal tubules at all doses. Milder renal changes consisting of tubular atrophy were seen at a dose of 1, 4, or 16 mg/kg body weight/day on 5 days/week for a total of 12 doses over 16 days. Rats receiving the highest dose had diarrhea and nasal discharge and died before the end of the study. Increased relative weights of kidneys, heart and brain, thymus atrophy, forestomach necrosis, and/or hyperplasia, and hemorrhage of adrenal glands were seen at the two higher doses. Bone marrow hyperplasia and nephropathy were seen at all doses, involving renal tubular degenerative and regenerative changes (NTP, 1989).

OTA has been shown to produce nephrotoxic effects in all animal species examined, with the exception of adult ruminants (Pohland et al., 1992). The nephrotoxic potential of OTA is well documented from all experimental studies, with a feed level of 200 ppb causing nephropathy in pigs and rats. Evidence strongly supports that OTA is involved in porcine nephropathy, which is characterized by degeneration of the proximal tubules, atrophy of the tubular epithelium, interstitial fibrosis in the renal cortex and hyalinized glomeruli. Field cases of OTA-induced nephropathy in farm animals have long been recognized. Benford et al. (2001) suggested that the adverse effect at the lowest effective dose in several mammalian species is nephrotoxicity. Citrinin is also nephrotoxic, but it is ten times less toxic than OTA.

In a series of experiments, sows were given feed containing OTA at a concentration of 0.2, 1, or 5 mg/kg (equivalent to 0.008, 0.04 and 0.2 mg/kg body weight/day), for a period of 5 days, 8 or 12 weeks, or up to 2 years. Decreased renal function, nephropathy and reduced renal enzyme activity were observed. Progressive nephropathy but no renal failure was seen in pigs given feed containing 1 mg/kg for 2 years (Krog et al., 1976; Elling et al., 1985).

Beagle dogs receiving OTA in capsule form at a dose of 0.1 or 0.2 mg/kg body weight/day for 14 days showed tubular necrosis and ultrastructural changes in the proximal tubules at all doses. Necrosis of lymphoid tissues of the thymus and tonsils was also seen at all doses (Kitchen et al., 1977a,b,c). In another set of experiments, young beagle dogs were given OTA and citrinin separately and combined for 14 days (Kitchen et al., 1977b). OTA was administered by capsule at 0.1 and 0.2 mg/kg; and citrinin (5 and 10 mg/kg) dissolved in ethanol was given by i.p. injection. Clinical signs of toxicosis with 10 mg/kg citrinin and the higher combined doses included anorexia, retching, tenesmus, weight loss, prostration and death. Severity of the clinical disease and mortality were increased when the mycotoxins were combined, which indicated synergism. The clinicopathological abnormalities reflected renal damage, cellular and granular casts, and ketones as well as protein and glucose in the urine of dogs given large doses of citrinin alone or combination with OTA. In pathological studies, these authors found gross lesions, such as focal peritonitis and intestinal intussusceptions with citrinin. Changes in the kidneys of dogs given OTA were degeneration and necrosis with desquamation of tubular epithelial cells, primarily in the straight segment of the proximal tubules. Dogs given 10 mg/kg citrinin had similar changes in the distal tubules and collecting ducts. Dogs given combined doses of citrinin and OTA had degeneration and necrosis in proximal and distal tubules, and in thin segments and the collecting ducts and ulceration of the mucosa of the intestine.

In experimental studies, dogs given citrinin showed serous nasal discharge and lacrimation (Carlton et al., 1974; Kitchen et al., 1977a,b). It is important to mention that citrinin is a very strong emetic in dogs, which is a protective mechanism in this species. Therefore, it is very unlikely that dogs will be poisoned by citrinin alone because high amounts of this mycotoxin will induce emesis and feed refusal.

Chickens, turkeys and ducklings are all susceptible to OTA and it appears that OTA-contaminated feed has a major economic impact on the poultry industry (Stoev, 2010a,b). Field cases of OTA-induced nephropathy are regularly encountered in poultry. Clinical signs of ochratoxicosis include retarded growth rate, reduction in weight gain, poor feed conversion, reduced egg production, poor egg shell quality, nephrotoxicity/nephropathy, and mortality. Feed refusal has been observed in turkeys.

In chickens, OTA at a dose rate of 3.6 mg/kg can cause 5% mortality. OTB at a dose rate of 54 mg/kg causes lowered growth rate, edema of visceral organs, and accumulation of uric acid in kidneys, liver, heart and spleen. These mycotoxins induce suppression of blood formation in bone marrow, and lymph formation in spleen and bursa of fabricus. The highest toxicity of OTA is found to be in broiler chickens. OTA given to broiler chickens at a dietary concentration of 4 mg/kg for 2 months caused a 42% mortality (Gibson et al., 1990). This toxin is involved in reduced growth rate at 5 ppm, high mortality rate at 4–8 ppm and cessation of egg production at 4 ppm. In a recent study, Stoev (2010b) demonstrated that OTA-induced suppressive effect on egg production in laying hens, and this effect was partially protected by some feed additives (sesame seed and water extract of artichoke).

In chickens, nephrotoxicity and hepatotoxicity occur at dietary levels of 250 μg/g of citrinin with liver and kidney enlargements of 11% and 22%, respectively. Necropsy of affected birds revealed the presence of pale and swollen kidneys (Wyatt, 1979). Citrinin is at least ten times less nephrotoxic than OTA.

Griffiths and Done (1991) described an outbreak of citrinin toxicosis in a herd of cows that ingested citrus pulp (visibly moldy) pellets that contained 30–40 ppb citrinin. Affected cows showed signs of pruritis, pyrexia, and hemorrhagic syndrome. Signs of the syndrome occurred within 3 days of ingesting the citrus pulp, which was fed for 21 days. Five calves whose dams had been fed citrus pulp were subsequently born with superior prognathism. Older animals were more susceptible to citrinin. The clinical signs, gross pathology and histology were suggestive of citrinin involvement. OTA has been well tested for carcinogenicity by oral administration in mice and rats. When OTA was administered in the diet, hepatocellular tumors (designated as well-differentiated trabecular adenomas), renal cell tumors (renal cystadenomas and solid renal-cell tumors), hepatomas (some exhibiting the trabecular structure) and hyperplastic hepatic nodules were observed in male mice (IARC, 1993).

In another study, administration of OTA in the diet-induced hepatocellular carcinomas and adenomas in female mice. Gavage administration of OTA to male and female rats resulted in a dose-related increase in the incidence of renal cell adenomas and adenocarcinomas. Furthermore, metastasis of the renal-cell tumors was also observed in male and female rats. OTA also increased the incidence and multiplicity of fibroadenomas of the mammary gland in female rats (NTP, 1989; IARC, 1993). In essence, these data suggest that OTA increases the incidence of hepatocellular tumors in mice of each sex and produces renal-cell adenomas in male mice and in rats of each sex. Based on sufficient evidence of carcinogenicity in experimental animals, OTA is classified as a possible carcinogen in humans (Group 2B) (IARC, 1993). Citrinin has been demonstrated to be mutagenic in hepatocytes (Bailly et al., 2002). There is limited evidence for the carcinogenicity of citrinin to animals.

It is well established that OTA and citrinin are reproductive and developmental toxicants (Qingqing et al., 2012; Gupta et al., 2017). OTA is known to induce teratogenicity in mice, rats, hamsters, chicken and pigs. In the rodent fetus, OTA targets the CNS, but skeletal deformities are also observed. While the mechanism involved in OTA or citrinin-induced teratogenesis remains unclear, it seems to directly affect both the progenitor cells and the embryos (Chan, 2008; Wu et al., 2013). Details of reproductive and developmental effects of citrinin and OTA can be found in other publications elsewhere (Singh et al., 2007; Gupta, 2009; Gupta et al., 2017).

In an in vitro study, the mixture of OTA and citrinin exerted additive effects in cytotoxicity assays (Föllmann et al., 2014). Currently, in vivo studies are not available to describe.

DIAGNOSIS

Diagnosis is usually based on the determination of OTA/citrinin levels in feed samples. In urine samples, OTA and its metabolite OTα can be detected using HPLC coupled with fluorescence detector, and citrinin and its metabolite dihydrocitrinone can be detected using LC-MS/MS.

TREATMENT

There is no specific antidote for ochratoxin(s) or citrinin toxicity. Recovery is usually slow. Immediate removal of the suspected feed and replacement with clean feed supplemented with increased vitamin levels can be rewarding. Growth of *A. ochraceus* in a common food, such as cereals, can be controlled or minimized by drying them rapidly and thoroughly. Effective approaches to grain storage include fumigation, aeration and cooling, sealed storage, and controlled atmosphere in tropical and subtropical regions where insect damage is a major problem. Citrinin is less of a problem because it is heat unstable. Citrinin is also likely to be destroyed during brewing. Propionic acid, added as a preservative to protect barley in the feed from fungi, destroys citrinin during storage. Currently, highly sophisticated methods are available to detect these mycotoxins at ppb or lower levels in food/feed or their products, so as to prevent animal health from toxicosis and economic loss.

CONCLUDING REMARKS AND FUTURE DIRECTIONS

OTA and citrinin both contaminate a wide range of animal feed and human food. Human risk is lower because the levels of these mycotoxins are minimized during processing and baking, but the raw feed remains a potential source for animal poisoning. Because of its long half-life, OTA accumulates in the body. These mycotoxins have a serious impact on the health of animals, especially pigs, dogs, and poultry. Pigs and dogs are most sensitive, while rats and mice are least sensitive. In general, females are more sensitive than males. The kidney is a major target organ (as evidenced by functional and morphological changes) for both mycotoxins, but other organs are affected as well. OTA and its analogs can produce a variety of toxic effects, referred to as "ochratoxicosis," including mutagenesis, carcinogenesis, embryotoxicity, reproductive and developmental toxicity, and immune suppression, by damaging mitochondria, DNA, protein, and RNA by lipid peroxidation and oxidative injury. Cell death occurs by apoptosis and/or necrosis. Citrinin produces toxic effects similar to OTA, but the severity is at least ten times less. Profiling of circulatory microRNA will aid in identifying the target organs, other than kidney, for the toxicity of OTA and citrinin.

ACKNOWLEDGMENT

Authors would like to thank Mrs. Robin B. Doss for her technical assistance in the preparation of this chapter.

REFERENCES

Aleo, M.D., Wyatt, R.D., Schnellman, R.G., 1991. Mitochondrial dysfunction is an early event in ochratoxin A but not oosporein toxicity to rats' renal proximal tubules. Toxicol. Appl. Pharmacol. 107, 73–80.

Ali, N., Blaszkewicz, M., Degen, G.H., 2015. Occurrence of the mycotoxin citrinin and its metabolite dihydrocitrinone in urines of German adults. Arch. Toxicol. 89, 573–578.

Armorini, S., Al-Qudah, K.M., Altafini, A., et al., 2015. Biliary ochratoxin A as a biomarker of ochratoxin exposure in laying hens: an experimental study after administration of contaminated diets. Res. Vet. Sci. 100, 265–270.

Arora, R.G., Froler, H., Fellner-Feldegg, H., 1983. Inhibition of ochratoxin A teratogenesis by zearalenone and diethylstilbestrol. Food Chem. Toxicol. 21, 779–783.

Bailly, J.D., Querin, A., Bars-Bailly, S.L., et al., 2002. Citrinin production and stability in cheese. J. Food Protect. 65, 1317–1321.

Belmadani, A., Tramu, G., Betbeder, A.M., et al., 1998. Regional selectivity to ochratoxin A, distribution and cytotoxicity in rat brain. Arch. Toxicol. 72, 656–662.

Benford, D., Boyle, C., Decant, W., et al., 2001. Ochratoxin A. Joint Exp. Comm. Food Addit. 47, 1–125.

Boorman, G.A., Hong, H.L., Dieter, M.P., et al., 1984. Myelotoxicity and macrophage alteration in mice exposed to ochratoxin A. Toxicol. Appl. Pharmacol. 72, 304–312.

Breitholtz-Emanuelsson, A., Olsen, M., Oskarson, A., et al., 1993. Ochratoxin A in cow's milk and in human milk with corresponding human blood samples. J. AOAC Intl. 76, 842–846.

Bruinink, A., Sidler, C., 1997. The neurotoxic effects of ochratoxin-A are reduced by protein binding but are not affected by l-phenylalanine. Toxicol. Appl. Pharmacol. 146, 173–179.

Bruinink, A., Rasonyi, T., Sidler, C., 1998. Differences in neurotoxic effects of ochratoxin A, ochracin and ochratoxin alpha in vitro. Nat. Toxins. 6, 173–177.

Campbell Jr, M.L., May, J.D., Huff, W.E., Doerr, J.A., 1983. Evaluation of immunity of young broiler chickens during simultaneous aflatoxicosis and ochratoxicosis. Poult Sci. 62, 2138–2144.

Cavin, C., Delatour, T., Martin-Kuan, M., et al., 2007. Reduction in antioxidant defenses may contribute to ochratoxin A toxicity and carcinogenicity. Toxicol. Sci. 96, 30–39.

Carlton, W.W., Sansing, G., Szczech, G.M., Tuite, J., 1974. Citrinin mycotoxicosis in beagle dogs. Food Cosmet. Toxicol. 12, 479–490.

Chagas, G.M., Oliveira, M.B.M., Campello, A.P., et al., 1995. Mechanism of citrinin-induced dysfunction of mitochondria III. Effects on renal cortical and liver mitochondrial swelling. J. Appl. Toxicol. 15, 91–95.

Chan, W.-H., 2008. Citrinin induces apoptosis in mouse embryonic stem cells. IUBMB Life 60, 171–179.

Coronel, M.B., Marin, S., Tarragó, M., et al., 2011. Ochratoxin A and its metabolite ochratoxin alpha in urine and assessment of the exposure of inhabitants of Lleida, Spain. Food Chem. Toxicol. 45, 1436–1442.

Creppy, E.E., Kane, A., Dirheimer, G., et al., 1985. Genotoxicity of ochratoxin A in mice: DNA single-strand break evaluation in spleen, liver, and kidney. Toxicol. Lett. 28, 29–35.

Dirheimer, G., Creppy, E.E., 1991. Mechanism of action of ochratoxin A. IARC Sci. Publ. 115, 171–186.

Dwivedi, P., Burns, R.B., 1984a. Pathology of ochratoxicosis A in young broiler chicks. Res. Vet. Sci. 36, 92–103.

Dwivedi, P., Burns, R.B., 1984b. Effect of ochratoxin A on immunoglobulins in broiler chicks. Res. Vet. Sci. 36, 117–121.

Elling, F., Nielsen, J.P., Lillehoj, E.B., et al., 1985. Ochratoxin A-induced porcine nephropathy: enzyme and ultrastructure changes after short-term exposure. Toxicology. 23, 247–254.

Föllmann, W., Behm, C., Degen, G.H., 2014. Toxicity of the mycotoxin citrinin and its metabolite dihydrocitrinone and the mixtures of citrinin and ochratoxin A *in vitro*. Arch. Toxicol. 88, 1097–1107.

Föllmann, W., Ali, N., Blaszkewicz, M., Degen, G.H., 2016. Biomonitoring of mycotoxins in urine: pilot study in mill workers. J. Toxicol. Environ. Health Part A. 79, 1015–1025.

Gautier, J.C., Holzhaeuser, D., Marcovic, J., et al., 2001. Oxidative damage and stress response from ochratoxin A exposure in rats. Free Radic. Biol. Med. 30, 1089–1098.

Galtier, P., 1978. Contribution of pharmacokinetic studies to mycotoxicology-ochratoxin A. Vet. Sci. Commun. 1, 349–358.

Galtier, P., Charpenteau, J.L., Alvinerie, M., Labouche, C., 1979. The pharmacokinetic profile of ochratoxin A in the rat after oral and intravenous administration. Drug Metabol. Disposit. 7, 429–434.

Galtier, P., Camguilhem, R., Bodin, G., 1980. Evidence for in vitro and in vivo interaction between ochratoxin A and three acidic drugs. Food Cosmet. Toxicol. 18, 493–496.

Galtier, P., Alvinerie, M., Charpenteau, J.L., 1981. The pharmacokinetic profile of ochratoxin A in pigs, rabbits, and chickens. Food Cosmet. Toxicol. 19, 735–738.

Gibson, R., Baily, C., Kubena, L., et al., 1990. Impact of L-phenylalanine supplementation on the performance of three-week-old broiler fed diets containing ochratoxin A. I. Effects on body weight, feed conversion, relative organ weight, and mortality. Poult. Sci. 69, 414–419.

Golli-Bennour, E.E., Kouidhi, B., Bouslimi, A., et al., 2010. Cytotoxicity and genotoxicity induced by aflatoxin B1, ochratoxin A, and their combination in cultured vero cells. J. Biochem. Mol. Toxicol. 24, 42–50.

González-Arias, C.A., Benitez-Trinidad, A.B., Sordo, M., et al., 2014. Low doses of ochratoxin A induce micronucleus formation and delay DNA repair in human lymphocytes. Food Chem. Toxicol. 74, 249–254.

Griffiths, I.R., Done, S.H., 1991. Citrinin as a possible cause of the pruritis, pyrexia, hemorrhagic syndrome in cattle. Vet. Rec. 129, 113–117.

Gupta, R.C., 2009. Toxicology of the placenta. In: Ballantine, B., Marrs, T.C., Syversen, T. (Eds.), General and Applied Toxicology, third ended. John Wiley and Sons, West Sussex, UK, pp. 2003–2039.

Gupta, R.C., Lasher, M.A., Miller Mukherjee, I.R., Srivastava, A., Lall, R., 2017. Aflatoxins, ochratoxins, and citrinin. In: Gupta, R.C. (Ed.), Reproductive and Developmental Toxicology, second edn. Academic Press/Elsevier, Amsterdam, pp. 945–962.

Hagelberg, S., Hult, K., Fuchs, R., 1989. Toxicokinetics of ochratoxin A in several species and its plasma-binding properties. J. Appl. Toxicol. 9, 91–96.

Harwig, J., Kuiper-Goodman, T., Scott, P.M., 1983. Microbial food toxicants: ochratoxins. In: Richcigl, M. (Ed.), Handbook of Foodborne Diseases of Biological Origin. CRC Press, Boca Raton, FL, pp. 193–238.

Höhler, D., Südekum, K.H., Wolffram, S., Frohlich, A.A., Marquardt, R. R., 1999. Metabolism and excretion of ochratoxin A fed to sheep. J. Aim. Sci. 77, 1217–1223.

Hult, K., Fuchs, R., 1986. Analysis and dynamics of ochratoxin A in biological systems. In: Steyn, P.S., Vleggaar, R. (Eds.), Mycotoxins and Phycotoxins. Elsevier Sci. Publ. BV, Amsterdam, pp. 365–367.

Hult, K., Teiling, A., Gatenbeck, S., 1976. Degradation of ochratoxin A by a ruminant. Appl. Environ. Microbiol. 32, 443–444.

Huybrechts, B., Martins, J.C., Debongnei, P., et al., 2015. Fast and sensitive LC-MS/MS method measuring human mycotoxin exposure using biomarkers in urine. Arch. Toxicol. 89, 1993–2005.

IARC, 1993. Ochratoxin A. IARC Monographs on the Evaluation of Carcinogenic Risks to Humans. 56, 489–521.

Khatoon, A., Zargham Khan, M., Khan, A., et al., 2013. Amelioration of ochratoxin A-induced immunotoxic effects by silymarin and vitamin E in White Leghorn cockerels. J. Immunotoxicol. 10, 25–31.

Kitchen, D.N., Carlton, W.W., Hinsman, E.J., 1977a. Ochratoxin A and citrinin induced nephrosis in beagle dogs. III. Terminal renal ultrastructural alterations. Vet. Pathol. 14, 392–406.

Kitchen, D.N., Carlton, W.W., Tuite, J., 1977b. Ochratoxin A and citrinin induced nephrosis in beagle dogs: I. Clinical and clinicopathological features. Vet. Pathol. 14, 154–172.

Kitchen, D.N., Carlton, W.W., Tuite, J., 1977c. Ochratoxin A and citrinin induced nephrosis in beagle dogs. II. Pathology. Vet. Pathol. 14, 261–272.

Klapec, T., Šarkanj, B., Banjari, I., Strelec, I., 2012. Urinary ochratoxin A and ochratoxin alpha in pregnant woman. Food Chem. Toxicol. 50, 4487–4492.

Krog, P., Elling, F., Hald, B., et al., 1976. Experimental avian nephropathy. Acta Pathol. Microbiol. Scand. A. 84, 215–221.

Kumagai, S., 1988. Effects of plasma ochratoxin A and luminal pH on the jejunal absorption of ochratoxin A in rats. Food Chem. Toxicol. 26, 753–758.

Kumagai, S., Aibara, K., 1982. Intestinal absorption and secretion of ochratoxin A in the rat. Toxicol. Appl. Pharmacol. 64, 94–102.

Kupski, L., Freitas, M., Ribeiro, D., et al., 2016. Ochratoxin A activates neutrophils and kills these cells through necrosis, an effect eliminated through its conversion into ochratoxin α. Toxicology 268-269, 91–102.

Malir, F., Ostry, V., Novotna, E., 2013. Toxicity of the mycotoxin ochratoxin A in the light of recent data. Toxin. Rev. 32, 19–33.

Mally, A., Hard, G.C., Dekant, W., 2007. Ochratoxin A as a potential etiologic factor in endemic nephropathy: lessons from toxicity studies in rats. Food Chem. Toxicol. 45, 2254–2260.

Marin, D.E., Taranu, I., 2014. Ochratoxin A and its effects on immunity. Toxin Rev. 34, 11–20.

Marin-Kuan, M., Cavin, C., Delatour, T., Schilter, B., 2008. Ochratoxin A carcinogenicity involves a complex network of epigenetic mechanisms. Toxicon. 52, 195–202.

Meisner, H., Cimbala, M.A., Hanson, R.W., 1983. Decrease of renal phosphoenolpyruvate carboxykinase RNA and poly(A)RNA level by ochratoxin A. Arch. Biochem. Biophys. 223, 264–270.

Minervini, F., Giannoccaro, A., Nicassio, M., et al., 2013. First evidence of placental transfer of ochratoxin A in horses. Toxins. 5, 84–92.

Munoz, K., Blaszkewicz, M., Campos, V., et al., 2014. Exposure of infants to ochratoxin A with breast milk. Arch. Toxicol. 88, 837–846.

Moroi, K., Suzuki, S., Kuga, T., et al., 1985. Reduction of ochratoxin A toxicity in mice treated with phenylalanine and phenobarbital. Toxicol. Lett. 25, 1–5.

Munro, I.C., Scott, P.M., Moodie, C.A., Willes, R.F., 1973. Ochratoxin A – occurrence and toxicity. J. Am. Vet. Med. Assoc. 163, 1269–1278.

National Toxicology Program, 1989. Technical Report on the toxicology and carcinogenesis studies of ochratoxin A in F344 rats (Gavage studies) (NIH Publication No. 89–2813). National Institutes of Health, Bethesda, MD.

O'Brien, E., Dietrich, D.R., 2005. Ochratoxin A: the continuing enigma. Crit. Rev. Toxicol. 35, 33–60.

Pfohl-Leszkowicz, A., Manderville, R.A., 2007. Ochratoxin A: an overview on toxicity and carcinogenicity in animals and humans. Mol. Nutr. Food Res. 51, 61–99.

Pohland, A.E., Nesheem, S., Friedman, L., 1992. Ochratoxin A: a review. Pure Appl. Chem. 64, 1029–1046.

Qingqing, H., Linbo, Y., Yunqian, G., et al., 2012. Toxic effects of citrinin on the male reproductive system in mice. Exp. Toxicol. Pathol. 64, 465–469.

Ramyaa, P., Padma, V.V., 2013. Ochratoxin-induced toxicity, oxidative stress and apoptosis ameliorated by quercetin-Modulated by Nrf2. Food Chem. Toxicol. 62, 205–216.

Ringot, D., Chango, A., Schneider, Y.-J., Larondelle, Y., 2006. Toxicokinetics and toxicodynamics of ochratoxin A, an update. Chem. Biol. Interact. 159, 18–46.

Sava, V., Reunova, O., Velazquez, A., et al., 2006. Acute neurotoxic effects of the fungal metabolite ochratoxin A. Neurotoxicology 27, 82–92.

Signorini, M.L., Gaggiotti, M., Molineri, A., et al., 2012. Exposure assessment of mycotoxins in cow's milk in Argentina. Food Chem. Toxicol. 50, 250–257.

Singh, G.S., Chanhan, H.V., Jha, G.J., Singh, K.K., 1990. Immunosuppression due to chronic ochratoxicosis in broiler chicks. J. Comp. Pathol. 103, 389–410.

Singh, N.D., Sharma, A.K., Dwivedi, P., et al., 2007. Citrinin and endosulfan induced maternal toxicity in pregnant Wistar rats: pathomorphological study. J. Appl. Toxicol. 27, 589–601.

Sreemannarayana, O., Frohlich, A.A., Vitti, T.G., 1988. Studies of the tolerance and disposition of ochratoxin A in young calves. Aim. Sci. 66, 1703–1711.

Stetina, R., Votava, M., 1986. Induction of DNA single-stranded breaks and DNA synthesis inhibition by patulin, ochratoxin A, citrinin, and aflatoxin B, in cell lines CHO and AWRF. Folia Biol. 32, 128–144.

Stiborová, M., Arlt, V.M., Schmeiser, H.H., 2016. Balkan endemic nephropathy: an update on its etiology. Arch. Toxicol. 90, 2595–2615.

Stormer, F.C., Lea, T., 1995. Effects of ochratoxin A upon early and late events in human T-cell proliferation. Toxicology 95, 45–50.

Stoev, S.D., 2010a. Studies on carcinogenic and toxic effects of ochratoxin A in chicks. Toxins 2, 649–664.

Stoev, S.D., 2010b. Studies on some feed additives and materials giving partial protection against the suppressive effect of ochratoxin A on egg production of laying hens. Res. Vet. Sci. 88, 486–491.

Suzuki, S., Satoh, T., Yamazaki, M., 1977. The pharmacokinetics of ochratoxin A in rats. Jpn. J. Pharmacol. 27, 735–744.

Taniai, E., Yafune, A., Nakajima, M., et al., 2014. Ochratoxin A induces karyomegaly and cell cycle aberrations in renal tubular cells without relation to induction of oxidative stress response in rats. Toxicol. Lett. 224, 64–72.

Vettorazzi, A., Gonzalez-Penas, E., Troconiz, I.F., et al., 2009. A different kinetic profile of ochratoxin A in mature male rats. Food Chem. Toxicol. 47, 1921–1927.

Vettorazzi, A., Gonzalez-Penas, E., deCerain, A.L., 2014. Ochratoxin A kinetics: a review of analytical methods and studies in rat model. Food Chem. Toxicol. 72, 273–288.

Von Tobel, J.S., Antinori, P., Zurich, M.-Z., et al., 2014. Repeated exposure to ochratoxin A generates a neuroinflammatory response, characterized by neurodegenerative M1 microglial phenotype. Neurotoxicology 44, 61–70.

Wu, Q., Dohnal, V., Huang, L., et al., 2012. Metabolic pathways of ochratoxin A. Curr. Drug Met. 12, 1–10.

Wu, T.-S., Yang, J.-J., Yu, F.-Y., et al., 2013. Cardiotoxicity of mycotoxin citrinin and involvement of microRNA-138 in zebrafish embryos. Toxicol. Sci. 136, 402–412.

Wyatt, R.D., 1979. Biological effects of mycotoxins (other than ochratoxin) on poultry. Interaction of mycotoxins in animal production. Nat. Acad. Sci., Washington, DC, pp. 87–95.

Chapter 73

Slaframine

Geof W. Smith

INTRODUCTION

Slaframine is an alkaloidal mycotoxin produced by the fungus *Rhizoctonia leguminicola* that causes profuse salivation ("slobbers") in animals. *R. leguminicola* is a common fungal pathogen of red clover (*Trifolium pratense*) and causes a syndrome known as black patch disease in the plant. Ingestion of clover hay containing slaframine causes salivary episodes that last from several hours to over 3 days in ruminants and horses. Although the disease is short term and animals generally recover without treatment, the dramatic clinical signs associated with slaframine ingestion make it readily apparent to livestock owners. Diagnosis can be made by identification of *R. leguminicola* in suspect forage or by the detection of slaframine in plasma samples from exposed animals.

BACKGROUND

Outbreaks of profuse salivation in cattle were initially reported in the late 1940s and 1950s from agricultural experiment stations in the Midwestern United States (O'Dell et al., 1959). Most of these cases were associated with the feeding of second-cutting red clover hay. In 1956 it was first reported that fungal contamination of red clover with *R. leguminicola* was associated with a pasture disease called black patch, which derives its name from the appearance of affected areas in the field and not the characteristic black lesions on the leaves of affected plants (Croom et al., 1995). Although its primary host is red clover, black patch disease has been reported in other legumes including white clover, soybeans, kudzu, cowpea, blue lupine, alsike clover, alfalfa, lespedeza, and milk vetch (Smalley and Sanderson, 1993). However, in most of these cases, infected red clover plants were present in the same areas of the field. Fungal infestations are usually associated with periods of wet weather and high humidity (Croom et al., 1995). Transmission is thought to be primarily seedborne as the fungus overwinters on contaminated hay and can survive at least 2 years on contaminated seed.

CHEMISTRY AND TOXICOKINETICS

Several laboratories were able to isolate the "slobber-causing" agent in *R. leguminicola* contaminated red clover (Aust and Broquist, 1965; Rainey et al., 1965) and in 1968 the chemical structure was described as 1-acetoxy-6-aminooctohydroindolizine (Gardiner et al., 1968). The term slaframine became the most commonly used word for describing this compound (Aust et al., 1966). Slaframine is a piperidine or indolizidine alkaloid with the empirical formula $C_{10}H_{10}N_2O_2$ which gives it a molecular weight of 198 Da (Croom et al., 1995).

Slaframine is activated by hepatic microsomal enzymes into a ketoimine that is required to produce clinical signs (Fig. 73.1). In cattle, the onset of salivation is shorter with more direct routes of administration, with intravenous injections producing salivation faster than intraperitoneal or intramuscular routes, which, in turn, are faster than the subcutaneous route (Croom et al., 1995). It has been suggested that slaframine is metabolized in the liver by a microsomal flavoprotein oxidase to the ketoimine metabolite (Guengerich and Aust, 1977) consisting of a quaternary nitrogen separated from an acetate ester by two carbon atoms (Fig. 73.1). This structure is very similar to that of acetylcholine (ACh), a parasympathetic neurotransmitter.

MECHANISM OF ACTION

Pharmacologically, slaframine would be classified as a cholinergic agonist and/or a parasympathomimetic chemical. The majority of the available data indicate that the clinical signs produced by slaframine are due to its high affinity for the M_3 muscarinic receptor subtype which are believed to be important in the control of exocrine and endocrine glands (Croom et al., 1995). Early studies

Veterinary Toxicology. DOI: http://dx.doi.org/10.1016/B978-0-12-811410-0.00073-8

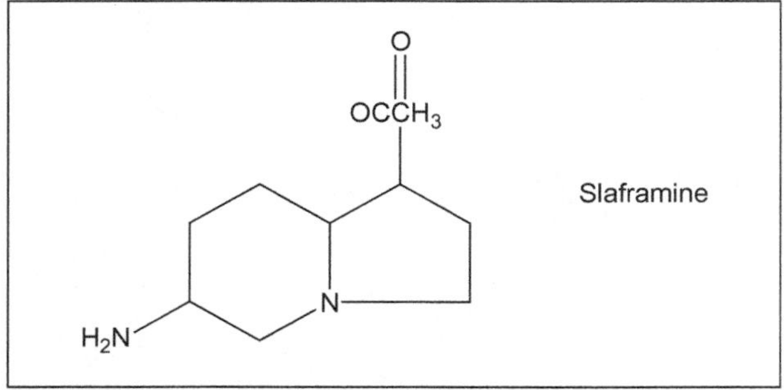

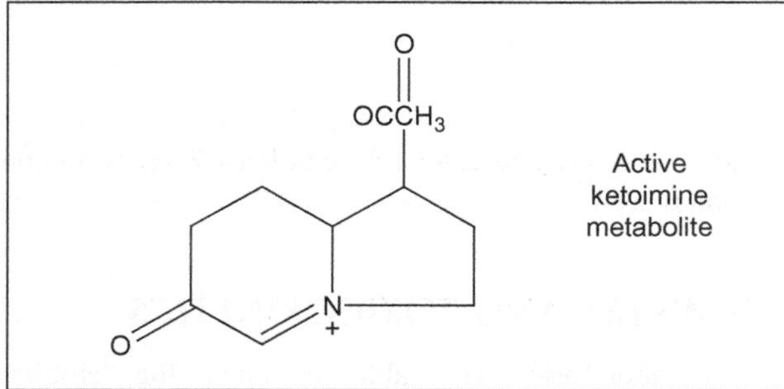

FIGURE 73.1 The structure of slaframine and the active ketoimine metabolite.

demonstrated that the increased salivation associated with slaframine toxicity could be blocked with preadministration of atropine (Aust, 1970). Additionally, mortality in broiler chicks when slaframine is dosed at the LD_{50} can be significantly decreased by the preadministration of the muscarinic receptor antagonists atropine (which has affinity for M_1, M_2, and M_3 receptors), and pirenzepine (M_1 and M_2 selective), but not gallamine, which is M_2 selective (Croom et al., 1995). The preadministration of the M_3 selective antagonist 4-diphenylacetoxy-*N*-methylpiperidine methiodide (4DAMP) can also block the increase in pancreatic fluid output induced by slaframine (Walker et al., 1994). Furthermore, slaframine has no effect on the cardiovascular system or arterial pressure at doses stimulatory to exocrine glands (Aust et al., 1968), nor does it inhibit blood cholinesterase activity (Crump et al., 1967; Hagler and Croom, 1989).

The stimulation of M_3 muscarinic receptors by slaframine produces a profound stimulation of exocrine glands, particularly the salivary gland and pancreas. Steers given an intramuscular administration of purified slaframine had resting salivary flow rates 50%–70% greater than saline treated controls (Froetschel et al., 1986). Similar findings documenting increases in saliva production both in cattle and sheep have been reported in other studies as well (Bird et al., 1993; Hibbard et al., 1995). Additional reported physiological effects of slaframine include increased pancreatic enzyme secretion (Aust et al., 1968, Aust, 1970), increased rumen pH and rate of nutrient passage, and decreased ruminal motility in cattle (Croom et al., 1995).

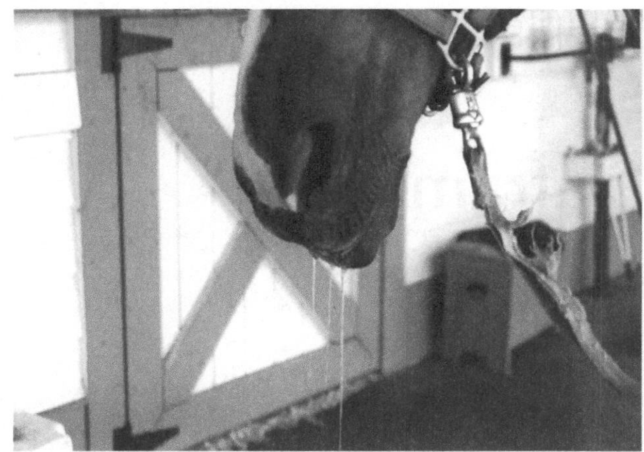

FIGURE 73.2 A horse showing profuse salivation from ingesting slaframine-contaminated red clover hay.

TOXICITY

Clinical signs of slaframine toxicity are similar in all species. Following exposure to contaminated forages, animals begin to salivate profusely. Experimentally, a single dose of slaframine produces salivation for 6–10 h. However, clinically affected animals can "slobber" for several days, presumably because they have continued access to slaframine-contaminated forages. Other clinical signs can include anorexia, diarrhea, frequent urination, and bloat. Decreased milk production can be expected in dairy cattle, likely related to a decrease in feed intake (Crump, 1973). Although slaframine toxicosis has been experimentally induced in a variety of species including swine, poultry, cats, dogs, guinea pigs, and rodents; naturally occurring cases are primarily reported in horses and ruminants (Borges et al., 2012; Croom et al., 1995; Crump et al., 1967; Sockett et al., 1982; Wijnberg et al., 2009) (Fig. 73.2).

Cyanosis and open-mouth breathing have been reported under experimental conditions in sheep, swine, and guinea pigs. Pigs also were observed to vomit, became dyspneic, and collapse with stiffened pelvic limbs (Crump et al., 1967). Only mild salivation was noted in a small chicken fed slaframine and clinical signs resolved within a few hours. The LD_{50} in day-old broiler chicks was estimated at approximately 81.6 mg/kg of body weight (Croom et al., 1995), but higher doses (250–300 mg/kg) were required to produce death in guinea pigs (Crump et al., 1967). Gross lesions in these animals consisted of vascular congestion of the thoracic and abdominal cavities. Pulmonary edema, disruption of the alveolar structure, emphysema, and hepatic centrilobular necrosis were noted histologically. Death in these animals was attributed to suffocation from pulmonary edema and/or emphysema.

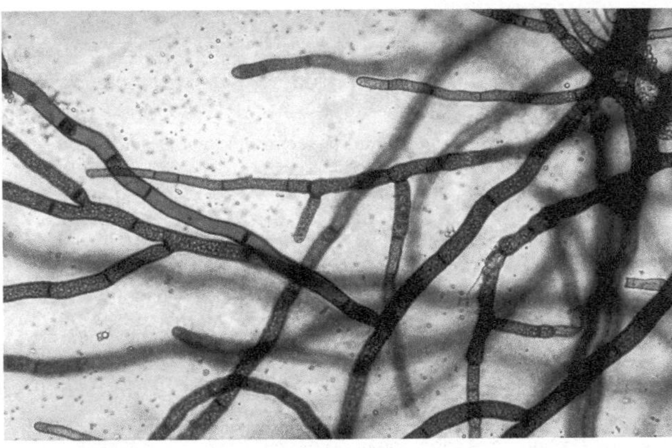
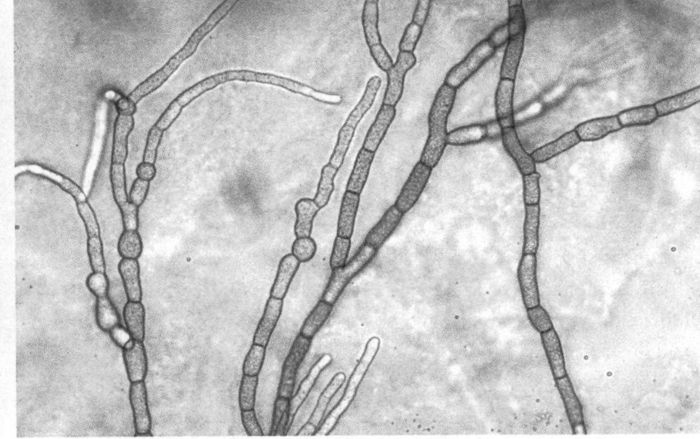

FIGURE 73.3 Two photomicrographs of *Rhizoctonia leguminicola* mycelia growing in culture—200 × magnification—note the normal difference in pigment color between the two isolates.

The clinical signs associated with the "slobbers syndrome" as described under field conditions include salivation, lacrimation, feed refusal, bloating, stiff joints, diarrhea, and weight loss. However, very few of these signs have been seen following the administration of purified slaframine under experimental conditions. That has led to speculation that the alkaloid swainsonine might also be involved in producing clinical signs in classic slaframine toxicity (Croom et al., 1995). Swainsonine is another alkaloid produced by *R. leguminicola* and has a similar structure to slaframine. Although it is better known for its association with locoweed toxicity, it is possible swainsonine is partially responsible for some of the clinical signs classically observed with the "slobbers syndrome."

DIAGNOSIS AND TREATMENT

Diagnosis of slaframine toxicity is generally made by observation of clinical signs (salivation) in animals consuming legume forage, particularly red clover hay. Further tests can identify the fungus *R. leguminicola* in the hay, which usually can be easily isolated in culture. Although chemical analysis for slaframine is not usually necessary, chromatographic methods for detecting the toxin in hay, plasma, or milk have been described (Hagler and Croom, 1989; Imerman and Stahr, 1998) (Fig. 73.3).

Treatment is not usually indicated, as animals usually recover spontaneously when the contaminated hay is removed. However, clinical signs may persist for 1–2 days following removal of the toxic forage. In severe cases, atropine may be of benefit to reverse the parasympathomimetic effects of slaframine. However, it is unlikely for the clinical signs to be completely resolved. In guinea pigs, simultaneous administration of atropine and a lethal dose of slaframine prevented clinical signs for 5 h, after which mild salivation was observed. When atropine was given 2–4 h after slaframine administration, profuse salivation was observed. However, there was no mortality (Crump et al., 1967). Atropine should be used with caution in ruminants and horses because of possible gastrointestinal side effects. Therefore treatments other than removing the contaminated hay are not usually recommended in affected animals.

Control of black patch disease remains a major problem for agronomists. Fungicides applied before flowering do not reduce seed infection, and ground sprays at the time of plant growth in the spring and/or immediately after the first hay cutting have not been shown to reduce fungal contamination. Prevention requires selecting *R. leguminicola* varieties that are less susceptible to fungal infection and chemically treating seed prior to planting. Feasible mechanisms to detoxify or degrade the toxin in pasture and/or hay have not been found. Therefore control of slaframine outbreaks rely on completely replacing contaminated forages.

CONCLUDING REMARKS AND FUTURE DIRECTIONS

There has not been any active research on slaframine in the last 20 years. However, clinical cases still occur relatively frequently. It is important for veterinarians and toxicologists to be familiar with this mycotoxin, to recognize the likely cause of profuse salivation in horses and cattle consuming red clover hay and to be able to make appropriate recommendations for treatment and control.

REFERENCES

Aust, S.D., 1970. Effect of slaframine on exocrine gland function. Biochem. Pharmacol. 19, 427–433.

Aust, S.D., Broquist, H.P., 1965. Isolation of a parasympathomimetic alkaloid of fungal origin. Nature 205, 204.

Aust, S.D., Broquist, H.P., Rinehart Jr., K.L., 1966. Slaframine. Structural studies of a parasympathomimetic alkaloid of fungal origin. J. Am. Chem. Soc. 88, 2879–2880.

Aust, S.D., Broquist, H.P., Rinehart Jr., K.L., 1968. Slaframine: a parasympathomimetic from *Rhizoctonia leguminicola*. Biotech. Bioeng. 10, 403–412.

Borges, A., Oliveira-Fiho, J., Palumbo, M.I., Imerman, P., 2012. Slaframine toxicosis in Brazilian horses causing excessive salivation. Equine Vet. Educ. 24, 279–283.

Bird, A.R., Croom Jr., W.J., Bailey, J.V., et al., 1993. Tropical pasture hay utilization with slaframine and cottonseed meal: ruminal characteristics and digesta passage in wethers. J. Anim. Sci. 71, 1634–1640.

Croom Jr., W.J., Hagler Jr., W.M., Froetschel, M.A., Johnson, A.D., 1995. The involvement of slaframine and swainsonine in slobbers syndrome: a review. J. Anim. Sci. 73, 1499–1505.

Crump, M.H., 1973. Slaframine (slobber factor) toxicosis. J. Am. Vet. Med. Assoc. 163, 1300–1302.

Crump, M.H., Smalley, E.B., Nichols, R.E., Rainey, D.P., 1967. Pharmacologic properties of a slobber-inducing mycotoxin from *Rhizoctonia leguminicola*. Am. J. Vet. Res. 28, 865–874.

Froetschel, M.A., Croom Jr., W.J., Hagler Jr., W.M., et al., 1986. Effects of slaframine on ruminant digestive function: resting salivary flow and composition in cattle. J. Anim. Sci. 62, 1404–1411.

Gardiner, R.A., Rinehart Jr., K.L., Snyder, J.J., Broquist, H.P., 1968. Slaframine. Absolute stereochemistry and a revised structure. J. Am. Chem. Soc. 90, 5639–5640.

Guengerich, F.P., Aust, S.D., 1977. Activation of the parasympathomimetic alkaloid slaframine by microsomal and photochemical oxidation. Mol. Pharmacol. 13, 185–195.

Hagler Jr., W.M., Croom Jr., W.J., 1989. Slaframine: occurrence, chemistry, and physiological activity. In: Cheeke, P.R. (Ed.), Toxicants of Plant Origin, vol. 1. CRC Press, Boca Raton, FL, pp. 257–279.

Hibbard, B., Peters, J.P., Chester, S.T., et al., 1995. The effect of slaframine on salivary output and subacute and acute acidosis in growing beef steers. J. Anim. Sci. 73, 516–525.

Imerman, P.M., Stahr, H.M., 1998. New, sensitive high-performance liquid chromatography method for the determination of slaframine in plasma and milk. J. Chromatogr. A. 815, 141–145.

O'Dell, B.L., Reagan, W.O., Beach, T.J., 1959. A study of the toxic principle in red clover. Univ. of Missouri Agric. Exp. Sta. Bull. 702, 1–12.

Rainey, D.P., Smalley, E.B., Crump, M.H., Strong, F.M., 1965. Isolation of salivation factor from *Rhizoctonia leguminicola* on red clover hay. Nature 205, 203–204.

Smalley, E.B., Sanderson, J.M., 1993. Slaframine (slobber factor). In: Howard, J.L. (Ed.), Current Veterinary Therapy 3: Food Animal Practice. W.B. Saunders Company, Philadelphia, PA, pp. 338–339.

Sockett, D.C., Baker, J.C., Stowe, C.M., 1982. Slaframine (*Rhizoctonia leguminicola*) intoxication in horses. J. Am. Vet. Med. Assoc. 181, 606.

Walker, J.A., Krehbiel, C.R., Harmon, D.L., et al., 1994. Effects of slaframine and 4-diphenylacetoxy-N-methylpiperidine methiodide (4DAMP) on pancreatic exocrine secretion in the bovine. Can. J. Physiol. Pharmacol. 72, 39–44.

Wijnberg, I.D., van der Ven, P.J., Fink-Gremmels, G.J., 2009. Outbreak of salivary syndrome on several hore farms in the Netherlands. Vet. Rec. 164, 595–597.

Chapter 74

Tremorgenic Mycotoxins

Tim J. Evans and Ramesh C. Gupta

INTRODUCTION

Fungi belonging to the genera *Penicillium*, *Aspergillus*, *Claviceps*, and *Neotyphodium* can produce tremorgenic mycotoxins, which are secondary fungal metabolites that elicit either intermittent or sustained tremors in vertebrate species (Cole and Cox, 1981; Selala et al., 1989; Burrows and Tyrl, 2001). Over 20 mycotoxins containing a tryptophan-derived indole moiety, including: penitrems, roquefortine A, verruculogen, tryptoquivaline, aflatrem, paspalinine, and paxilline as well as the paspalitrems and lolitrems (Table 74.1 and Fig. 74.1), have demonstrated tremorgenic potential in animals and humans (Selala et al., 1989; Burrows and Tyrl, 2001). Several other fungal metabolites, such as roquefortine C, paspaline, paspalacine, and cyclopiazonic, are chemically related to these mycotoxins but have been shown to not be tremorgenic (Knaus et al., 1994; Tiwary et al., 2009). With increased analytical capabilities, particularly the emergence of advanced NMR, HPLC-MS, and LC-MS/MS spectroscopic methodologies, other "known" mycotoxins, with both related and unrelated structures, such as ergonovine (ergometrine), ergine (lysergic acid amide), and patulin, as well as "new" secondary fungal metabolites, like secopenitrem D, have been detected in samples associated with clinical cases of tremorgenic syndromes and their associated neurotoxicities (Sabater-Vilar et al., 2004; Tor et al., 2006; Uhlig et al., 2009; Moldes-Anaya et al., 2011). However, the precise roles of these detected fungal metabolites in the pathogenesis of the observed tremorgenic syndromes are yet to be determined, and this task is complicated by the diversity of fungal matrices, the propensity for myco- and phytotoxins to be present in complex mixtures, and difficulties inherent to relating xenobiotic structure to function and concentration to biological relevance.

Tremorgen-producing fungi grow on a wide variety of foodstuffs, including dairy or grain-containing products intended for human consumption (e.g., cheeses and pastas), stored grains and nuts (e.g., peanuts and walnuts) and a number of forages (e.g., legumes and grasses) consumed by livestock species, and even food or beverage manufacturing byproducts, garbage and compost piles can be sources of tremorgenic mycotoxins (Burrows and Tyrl, 2001; Boysen et al., 2002; Young et al., 2003). Although there have been several human cases in which tremors and convulsions were attributed to consumption of mold-contaminated food containing penitrem A (Gordon et al., 1993; Lewis et al., 2005), this chapter focuses on the toxicity of tremorgenic mycotoxins in animal species. Dogs, because of their relatively indiscriminate appetite and frequently unsupervised roaming behavior, appear to be very susceptible to intoxication by penitrem A, as well as roquefortines (Boysen et al., 2002; Young et al., 2003; Eriksen et al., 2010). Mycotoxin-associated stagger syndromes in livestock, also described in the literature as "grass staggers" (not to be confused with "grass staggers" or "grass tetany" related to hypomagnesemia), have most frequently occurred following the ingestion of endophyte (*Neotyphodium lolii*) infected perennial ryegrass (*Lolium perenne*) or consumption of Dallisgrass (*Paspalum dilatatum*) or Bahiagrass (*Paspalum notatum*) contaminated by sclerotia of *Claviceps paspali*.

BACKGROUND

Penicillium-Associated Tremorgenic Mycotoxins

Although a variety of different fungi synthesize indole–diterpene mycotoxins having specific tremorgenic effects on the central nervous system (CNS), tremorgens produced by *Penicillium* spp. (especially penitrem A and roquefortines) are the most commonly encountered of these mycotoxins. Penitrem A is a potent neurotoxin which causes a syndrome characterized by sustained tremors and, at high doses, convulsions and death in laboratory and farm animals (Wilson, 1971; Arp and Richard, 1981; Peterson and Penny, 1982; Shreeve et al., 1983;

Veterinary Toxicology. DOI: http://dx.doi.org/10.1016/B978-0-12-811410-0.00074-X

TABLE 74.1 Representative Tremorgenic Mycotoxins, Associated Fungi and Substrates

Tremorgenic Mycotoxin	Associated Fungi	Common Substrates
Penitrem A	*Penicillium crustosum*	Meat, cereals, nuts, cheeses, eggs, fruits, processed/refrigerated foods, refuse, compost
	Penicillium cyclopium	
	Penicillium commune	
	Penicillium spp.	
Roquefortines[a]	*Penicillium roqueforti*	Same as penitrem A
	Same as penitrem A and sometimes concurrently with penitrem A	
Janthitrems A, B, and C	*Penicillium janthinellum*	Perennial ryegrass
Verruculogen	*Penicillium* spp.	Soil, seeds, cereal crops
	Aspergillus spp.	
Tryptoquivaline tremorgens[b]	*Penicillium* spp.	Soil, seeds, cereal crops
	Aspergillus clavatus	Sprouting cereal grains, malting byproducts
Territrems A and B	*Aspergillus terreus*	Cereal grains
Aflatrem	*Aspergillus flavus*	Corn
Lolitrems A, B, C and D	*Neotyphodium lolii*	Perennial ryegrass
Paxilline	*Neotyphodium lolii*	Perennial ryegrass
Lolitriol	*Neotyphodium lolii*	Perennial ryegrass
Paspalitrems A, B and C	*Claviceps paspali*	Dallisgrass
	Claviceps cinerea	Bahiagrass
		Hilaria spp.
	Claviceps cynodontis	Bermudagrass
Paspalinine	Same as paspalitrems	Same as paspalitrems

[a]*Roquefortine C has actually been associated with paralysis in several species.*
[b]*Includes quinazoline ring-containing indole alkaloids with structures similar to tryptoquivaline.*

Hocking et al., 1988; Breton et al., 1998; Cavanagh et al., 1998). Dogs can be poisoned by eating walnuts and a variety of other unused or discarded foodstuffs infected with *Penicillium* spp. (Richard et al., 1981; Boysen et al., 2002; Young et al., 2003; Munday et al., 2008), and field cases of poisoning have also been documented in cattle, sheep, and horses (Cavanagh et al., 1998; Hocking et al., 1988; Boysen et al., 2002; Walter, 2002; Young et al., 2003). *Penicillium crustosum* is an especially common foodborne fungus that causes spoilage in a wide variety of foods, including meat, cereals, nuts, cheese, eggs, fruits, and processed and refrigerated food, and almost all *P. crustosum* isolates produce the mycotoxin penitrem A (Hocking and Pitt, 2003; Rundberget et al., 2004). Roquefortines can also be synthesized by *Penicillium* spp. (Hooser and Talcott, 2006), and, interestingly, *P. crustosum*, as well as several other *Penicillium* spp., can produce penitrem A and roquefortines concurrently following growth and sporulation (Vesonder et al., 1980; Wagener et al., 1980; Kyriakidis et al., 1981; Mantle et al., 1983; Boysen et al., 2002; Young et al., 2003). In fact, roquefortine C, which has itself been associated with anorexia and paralysis, has been found to be a reliable biomarker for the tremorgenic mycotoxin penitrem A, in instances where that tremorgen was present in lower concentrations, at or slightly below its level of detection (Tiwary et al., 2009). Additionally, three other tremorgenic mycotoxins, janthitrem A, B, and C (molecular weight 601, 585, and 565, respectively) can also be produced

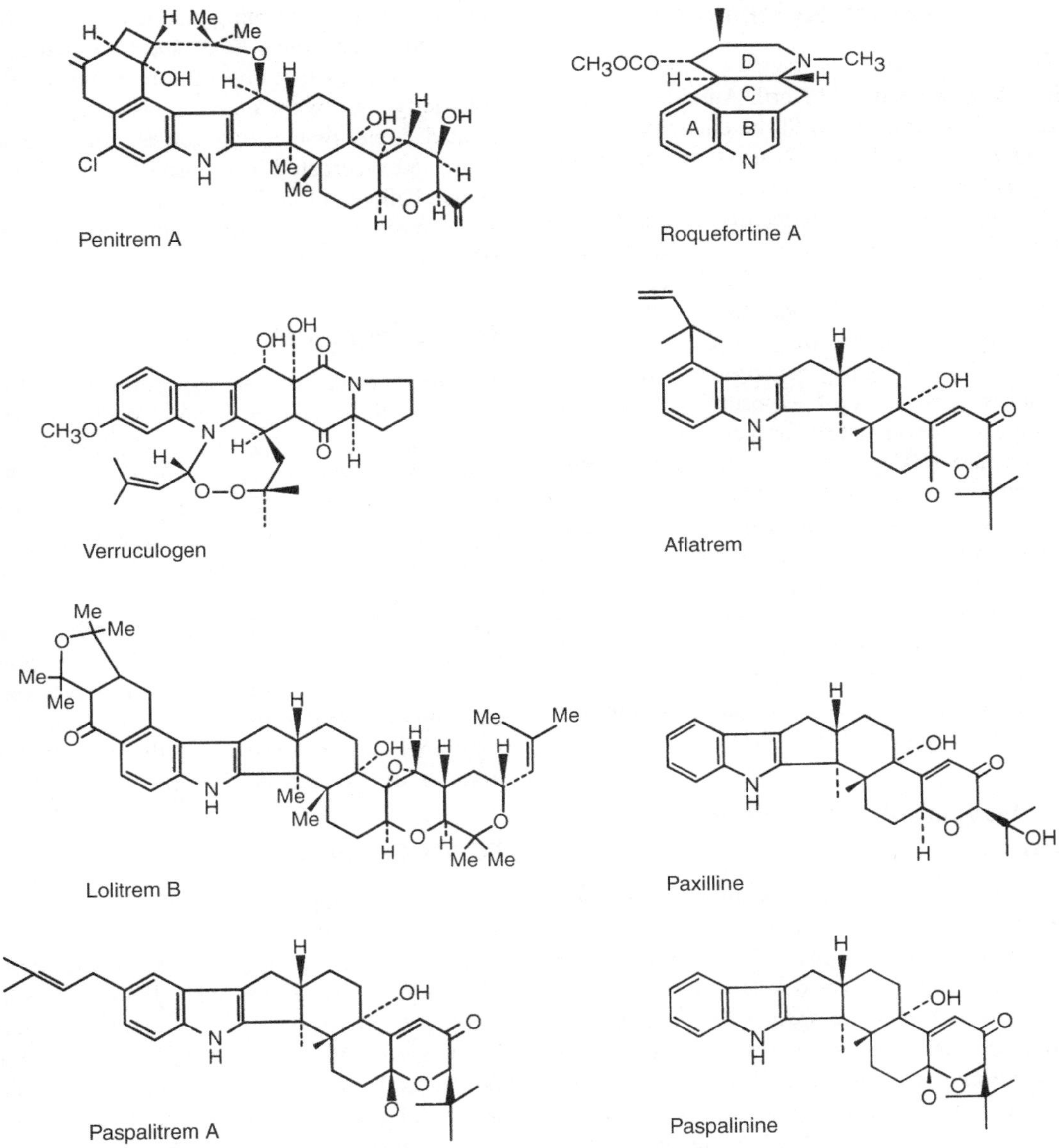

Penitrem A

Roquefortine A

Verruculogen

Aflatrem

Lolitrem B

Paxilline

Paspalitrem A

Paspalinine

FIGURE 74.1 The structures of selected indole–diterpene tremorgenic mycotoxins are shown. *This figure was adapted, with permission, from Council for Agricultural Science and Technology (CAST), 2003. Mycotoxins: Risks in Plant, Animal, and Human Systems. Task Force Report 139. CAST, Ames, Iowa and from Cole, R.J., Cox, R.H., 1981. Handbook of Toxic Fungal Metabolites. Academic Press, New York, NY. Modifications courtesy of Don Connor and Howard Wilson.*

by a species of *Penicillium* (i.e., *Penicillium janthinellum*), and these tremorgens have been associated with staggers outbreaks in sheep grazing ryegrass (Gallagher et al., 1980; Burrows and Tyrl, 2001).

Aspergillus-Associated Tremorgenic Mycotoxins

Verruculogen, another tremorgenic mycotoxin containing the indole moiety and associated with tremors in mice, rats, and farm animals, is produced by species of *Aspergillus* as well as *Penicillium* (Gallagher and Latch, 1977). Likewise, tryptoquivaline and related quinazoline ring-containing indole alkaloids are also produced by *Aspergillus* and *Penicillium* spp. (Gao et al., 2011). Tremorgenic mycotoxins isolated from *Aspergillus terreus* include territrem A and B, which were previously designated as C_1 and C_2, respectively (Ling et al., 1979), and *Aspergillus flavus* can, in addition to aflatoxins, also produce tremorgenic aflatrem and other indole–diterpene mycotoxins (e.g., paspalinine) in contaminated corn (Burrows and Tyrl, 2001).

Neotyphodium-Associated Tremorgenic Mycotoxins

In Australia, New Zealand, and North America, perennial ryegrass (*L. perenne*) infected with the endophyte *N. lolii* (formerly *Acremonium lolii*) has been associated with a "grass staggers" syndrome in horses, deer, cattle and, especially, sheep, which is frequently referred to as "perennial ryegrass staggers" and is distinct from annual ryegrass toxicosis (Galey et al., 1991; Cheeke, 1998; Burrows and Tyrl, 2001). *N. lolii* concentrates in the caryopsis/seed and the outer, lower leaf sheaths of perennial ryegrass, and the "staggers" syndrome is most often observed after several days of exposure to endophyte-infected ryegrass during late summer when there is shortage of pasture (Galey et al., 1991; Cheeke, 1998). Ergovaline and other ergot alkaloids associated with "fescue toxicosis" are also produced by *N. lolii* (Cheeke, 1998), but the classic neurological signs of perennial ryegrass staggers are indistinguishable from those associated with *Penicillium* and *Aspergillus* species and the adverse effects of neurotoxic indole–diterpene tremorgens, including lolitrems A, C, and D, lolitrem precursors (e.g., paxilline and lolitriol) and, especially, lolitrem B (Cheeke, 1998; Burrows and Tyrl, 2001).

Claviceps-Associated Tremorgenic Mycotoxins

While *Claviceps purpurea* is notoriously associated with "classic" ergotism in human and animals and, historically, occasional tremors or convulsions (i.e., nervous ergotism or convulsive ergotism) in livestock (Burrows and Tyrl, 2001; Evans et al., 2004), other species of *Claviceps* produce toxicoses primarily characterized by a tremorgenic "staggers" syndrome (Burrows and Tyrl, 2001). Sheep, horses, and cattle, in particular, can develop a "grass staggers" syndrome several days following the ingestion of mature Dallisgrass (*P. dilatatum*) or Bahiagrass (*P. notatum*) infected with the sclerotia of *C. paspali* (Cheeke, 1998; Burrows and Tyrl, 2001). "Dallisgrass staggers" and "Bahiagrass staggers" have most frequently been observed in the southeastern United States, Central and South America, parts of Europe and South Africa, as well as Australia and New Zealand. Traditionally, the ergot alkaloids produced in large quantities by *C. purpurea* and in much smaller quantities by *C. paspali* were thought to be responsible for the tremors observed in conjunction with exposure to both species of *Claviceps* (Cheeke, 1998). However, it is now understood, at least with respect to the "staggers" syndromes associated with *C. paspali* and, less commonly, *Claviceps cinerea* (fungal infections of *Hilaria* spp. (curly mesquite, curly-grass, galleta, etc.)), that the large concentrations of indole–diterpene tremorgenic mycotoxins (i.e., paspalinine and paspalitrems A, B, and C) found in the sclerotia of these species of *Claviceps* are responsible for the neurotoxicity. As with other "grass staggers," *Claviceps*-related tremorgenic syndromes are characterized by exercise-exacerbated nervousness, "wild" facial expressions, belligerent attitude, tremors, ataxia, convulsions, and occasional deaths attributed primarily to misadventure (Burrows and Tyrl, 2001).

Bermudagrass Staggers

Periodic episodes of tremors have been observed in cattle in the southern United States and Oklahoma and Texas, as well as horses in California, which have been ingesting mature Bermudagrass (*Cynodon dactylon*) (Cheeke, 1998; Burrows and Tyrl, 2001). Ergot-type alkaloids (ergine, ergonovine and ergonovinine) are produced by several species of *Claviceps*, including *Claviceps cynodontis*, and have been isolated in several instances of "Bermudagrass staggers" (Cheeke, 1998; Burrows and Tyrl, 2001; Uhlig et al., 2009). However, higher concentrations of paspalitrem-type indole alkaloids have recently been detected in samples from a clinical case of this disease syndrome and are most likely the primary Bermudagrass tremorgens (Uhlig et al., 2009).

TOXICOKINETICS

It should be kept in mind that, while the onset and duration of the various "staggers" syndromes might vary somewhat, the tremorgenic neurotoxicities associated with the various grasses and aflatoxin-infected corn are essentially identical to one another (Cheeke, 1998). Tremorgenic indole-containing mycotoxins are lipophilic molecules that easily cross the blood–brain barrier (BBB) and rapidly gain access to the CNS (Patterson et al., 1981). Although there might be some subtle differences between compounds and species of animals, tremorgenic indole–diterpene alkaloids are generally rapidly absorbed from the gastrointestinal tract, and the toxic signs, depending on the specific toxins and the exposed species, are usually seen within several hours (especially penitrem A and roquefortines in dogs) to a few days (frequently lolitrems and paspalitrems in ruminants) following ingestion of contaminated foodstuffs (Burrows and Tyrl, 2001; Hooser and Talcott, 2006). As evidenced by the lack of a cumulative effect following repeated doses, these particular mycotoxins do not appear to accumulate in the body (Peterson and Penny, 1982). Despite some hepatic metabolism, these mycotoxins are usually eliminated mainly through biliary excretion into the feces (Burrows and Tyrl, 2001; Hooser and Talcott, 2006). Young animals are more sensitive than adults to the toxicity of tremorgenic mycotoxins, with 5-month-old lambs being more susceptible than 15-month-old sheep to verruculogen toxicity (Patterson et al., 1981).

MECHANISM OF ACTION

It should be pointed out that, although related in structure, tremorgenic mycotoxins do not exert toxicity by a single common mechanism, and the exact mechanisms involved in neurotoxicity induced by these tremorgens are yet to be fully elucidated. These mycotoxins work at a different functional level of the nervous system than other mycotoxins having more widespread targets for toxicity associated with the inhibition of basic cellular functions, such as protein synthesis. Several pharmacological/toxicological mechanisms of tremorgenic action have been proposed, and, in general, tremorgenic mycotoxins interfere with inhibitory neuroreceptors and enhance excitatory amino acid neurotransmitter release mechanisms (Wilson, 1971; Norris et al., 1980; Selala et al., 1989). In experimental studies, the inhibitory action of this type of mycotoxins at gamma aminobutyric acid (GABA) receptors was demonstrated (Stern, 1971; Hotujac and Stern, 1974; Hotujac et al., 1976; Selala et al., 1989; Abramson, 1997). Gant et al. (1987) studied the effects of four fungal tremorgens and one nontremorgenic mycotoxin on $GABA_A$ receptor-binding in the rat's brain, and, in high concentrations, the tremorgenic action of these mycotoxins was, in part, most likely due to inhibition of $GABA_A$ receptor function. Conversely, other studies have shown how tremorgenic mycotoxins increase the release of excitatory neurotransmitters (Norris et al., 1980).

Among the tremorgenic mycotoxins, penitrem A has been studied the most for the elucidation of its mechanism of action and toxicity. There is convincing evidence suggesting that penitrem A acts on the CNS to induce seizures (Sobotka et al., 1978; Arp and Richard, 1981). Penitrem A was shown to increase the spontaneous release of aspartate and glutamate, as well as, interestingly, GABA (Norris et al., 1980). Glutamate and aspartate are the neurotransmitters of the parallel and climbing fibers, respectively, which are two major excitatory inputs to Purkinje cells. There is also evidence for a penitrem A-induced partial decrease in glycine levels in the brain in association with pathology related to penitrem A exposure (Catovic et al., 1975). Cavanagh et al. (1998) demonstrated that, in rats, penitrem A can cause widespread degeneration of Purkinje cells and foci of necrosis in the cerebellar granular cell layers. These striking lesions are confined to the cerebellum, with no lesions found elsewhere in the brain. Cerebellar Purkinje cells are the primary targets cells for the adverse effects of penitrem A. Penitrem A-induced tremors might also be partly explained by a presynaptic inhibition of inhibitory interneurons.

Similar mechanisms of action have been demonstrated for other tremorgenic mycotoxins. Verruculogen-induced tremors in rats have been associated with an increased level of excitatory neurotransmitters (glutamate and aspartate) in the lateral ventricle, suggesting subcortical, verruculogen-induced tremorgenic activity. Selala et al. (1989) demonstrated that tremorgenic mycotoxins can be partial agonists of GABA. Verruculogen increases spontaneous glutamate and aspartate release in vivo in guinea pig ileum preparations and also causes an increase in contractile responses to electrical field stimulation, which has been attributed to the enhanced release of acetylcholine from presynaptic nerve terminals. Although paxilline blocks high-conductance Ca^{2+}-activated K^+ channels, some related nontremorgenic fungal metabolites, such as paspaline, have also been shown to inhibit these particular ion channels (Burrows and Tyrl, 2001). Paxilline also inhibits the cerebellar inositol 1,4,5-triphosphate receptor. Paspalinine and the paspalitrems are thought to impair GABA- and glycine-mediated inhibitory pathways (Burrows and Tyrl, 2001).

TOXICODYNAMICS

Central Effects

Tremorgenic mycotoxins are known to act on the CNS, causing sustained tremors, convulsions, and, occasionally, deaths in animals. In general, the clinical signs and symptoms typically observed during tremorgenic mycotoxicoses include diminished activity and immobility, followed by hyperexcitability, muscle tremor, ataxia, tetanic seizures, and convulsions (Cole and Cox, 1981; Valdes et al., 1985; Barker et al., 2013). These clinical signs are reversible if the affected animal is removed from tremorgen-contaminated source. Death is limited by the emetic effect of these tremorgens. In dogs, the clinical disease involves the development of muscle tremors and seizures, vomiting, alterations in behavior, hyperthermia, depression, coma, and pulmonary edema.

Depending on the level of tremorgenic mycotoxin exposure, death can occur in some instances within 2–4 h and is usually secondary to respiratory compromise, metabolic acidosis, and/or hyperthermia. In severe cases, clinical signs of toxicosis can persist for several days, and fine tremors can be seen for a week or more. The tremors produced by penitrem A are very similar in most species and begin within a few minutes of intraperitoneal (IP) injection and even sooner with IV injection. The tremors can be sustained and lead to both ataxia and episodic spasms (Cavanagh et al., 1998). Larger doses of penitrem A can cause seizures, massive liver necrosis, and death

(Hocking et al., 1988). In a histopathological study in rats, Breton et al. (1998) revealed that penitrem A–induced dose-related injuries in the cerebellum with massive degeneration of Purkinje cells and a significant vacuolization within the molecular layer. In one instance of neurological disorders in dairy cattle associated with *Aspergillus clavatus*-contaminated beer residues, neuronal degeneration was observed within the brainstem and ventral spinal cord, but no analyses for tremorgenic mycotoxins were performed in order to confirm a causal relationship between any tremorgens and the observed pathology (Loretti et al., 2003).

Peripheral Effects

Tremorgenic mycotoxins have also been studied for peripheral effects (Cotton et al., 1997; McLeay et al., 1999; Dalziel et al., 2005). The tremorgenic mycotoxins, such as penitrem A, paxilline, and lolitrem B can have profound effects on electromyographic (EMG) activity of smooth muscle of the reticulorumen in conscious sheep, with a time course of action similar to their respective characteristic effects on the induction (1–2, 15–20, and 20–30 min) and the duration (1–2, 1–2, and 8–12 h) of tremors. Response to penitrem A revealed a greater sensitivity of smooth muscle than skeletal muscle. The excitatory local effects were partially blocked by atropine, indicating that stimulation of muscarinic cholinergic receptors was involved. Increased local activity may mediate a reflex inhibition of cyclical contractions. However, a nontremorgenic isomer of lolitrem B (31-epi-lolitrem B) had no effect on the reticulorumen. The intensity and duration of the effects of lolitrem B (up to 12 h) indicate that severe disruption of digestion may occur in animals grazing *N. lolii*-infected pasture. Moderately severe muscle contractions, traumatic events secondary to ataxia, and prolonged recumbency, especially in large animals, can potentially result in muscle damage following suspected exposure to tremogenic mycotoxins, but directly myotoxic effects of some mycotoxins cannot be ruled out (Loretti et al., 2003).

Genotoxicity

Five tremorgenic mycotoxins (fumitremorgen B, paxilline, penitrem A, verruculogen, and verrucosidin), which have been associated with molds found in fermented meats, were assessed for genotoxicity (Sabater-Vilar et al., 2003). The mycotoxins were tested in two short-term in vitro assays using different genotoxic end points, in different phylogenetic systems, with the use of mammalian-microsome assay and the single-cell gel electrophoresis assay of human lymphocytes. The findings revealed that all of the tested mycotoxins, with the exception of penitrem A, exhibited a certain degree of genotoxicity. Verrucosidin appeared to have the highest toxic potential, testing positive in both assays. Verruculogen tested positive in the *Salmonella*/mammalian-microsome assay, and paxilline and fumitremorgen B caused DNA damage in human lymphocytes.

Acute Toxicity

Acute toxicity data are available for only few of the tremorgenic mycotoxins. It should be noted that the relative doses resulting in lethality in different species might not necessarily be reflective of the relative tremorgenic potentials of these mycotoxins. The LD_{50} of penitrem A in mice is 15–19 mg/kg, IP (Ling et al., 1979). The LD_{50} of verruculogen is reported to be 15.2 mg/kg, IP, and 266 mg/kg, following oral exposure, in the chicken, with the corresponding LD_{50} values in mice being 2.4 mg/kg, IP, and 127 mg/kg, following oral exposure. The LD_{50} value of penitrem A in mice is 15–19 mg/kg, IP (Ling et al., 1979). Dogs receiving penitrem A (0.5 mg/kg, IP) showed tremors within 10 min, followed by clonic or tonic convulsions (Hayes et al., 1976). Dose-related liver damage varied from massive necrosis in dogs receiving 2.5–5.0 mg/kg of penitrem A to no pathologic alterations in dogs given 0.125 mg/kg.

Potential Interactions

In previous studies, concurrent production of roquefortines and penitrem A by various species of *Penicillium* (e.g., *P. crustosum*, *P. cyclopium* Westling, and *P. commune*) was demonstrated in culture extracts (Vesonder et al., 1980; Wagener et al., 1980; Kyriakidis et al., 1981; Mantle et al., 1983). Braselton and Rumler (1996) first reported the concurrent presence of both tremorgenic mycotoxins in naturally occurring field cases of canine intoxication and raised the issue of the potential synergistic interactions between these tremorgens. In two recent cases, both Boysen et al. (2002) and Young et al. (2003) diagnosed concurrent intoxication with penitrem A and roquefortines in several dogs. Given that roquefortines and penitrem A can have similar mechanisms of action, there might be the potential for some synergism between the two tremorgenic mycotoxins or at least a reduction in the amount of ingested contaminated material required for the onset of clinical signs. Likewise, it would seem logical in instances of "grass staggers" that a greater concentration of multiple, potential tremorgenic mycotoxins in contaminated forages would increase the likelihood and, potentially, the severity of observed intoxications. However, the behavior of mycotoxins, especially those interacting with specific receptors, might not be predictable in mixtures, and the paralytic tremorgen, roquefortine C, might actually be a reliable biomarker for penitrem A in some tremorgenic syndromes (Tiwary et al., 2009).

CLINICAL ASPECTS OF TREMORGENIC MYCOTOXICOSES

Diagnosis

Diagnosis of tremorgenic mycotoxin-related intoxication is based on clinical circumstances, a history of exposure to or consumption of moldy foodstuffs, clinical signs of tremors and seizures, and, ideally, detection of tremorgenic mycotoxin(s) in the suspected source material, vomitus, gastrointestinal tract contents, urine or bile. Detection of molds without detection of tremorgenic mycotoxins suggests the possibility but does not confirm the occurrence of a tremogenic mycotoxicosis. Differential diagnoses should rule out ethylene glycol, strychnine, metaldehyde, methylxanthines, pyrethroids, nicotine, organochlorine insecticides, bromethalin, acetylcholinesterase-inhibiting insecticides (organophosphates and carbamates), other potential neurotoxicants, and eclampsia in pregnant animals (Hooser and Talcott, 2006; Puschner, 2009; Barker et al., 2013). It needs to be pointed out that in field cases of perennial ryegrass staggers, as well as Dallisgrass and Bahiagrass staggers, the onset of clinical signs is most likely related to the intake of lolitrem B and paspalinine and/or paspalitrems, respectively. The effects of these tremorgenic mycotoxins could potentially be more insidious and longer lasting than those of penitrem A (Burrows and Tyrl, 2001; Hooser and Talcott, 2006). Depending on the laboratory, tremorgenic mycotoxins can generally be quantified using LC-MS/MS (Tiwary et al., 2009), HPLC-MS (Rundberget and Wilkins, 2002), GC-MS/MS (Braselton and Rumler, 1996), or TLC (Hooser and Talcott, 2006). Analyses for roquefortines and penitrem A are generally more likely to be available to clinicians than analytical procedures for the other tremorgenic mycotoxins. Detection of roquefortine C in samples from a tremogenic syndrome, especially in dogs, where penitrem A is not detected, might serve as a biomarker for exposure to this common tremorgen (Tiwary et al., 2009).

Treatment

In a small animal setting the minimum initial database should include a complete blood count, serum biochemical profile, and assessment of acid–base status and urinalysis (Hooser and Talcott, 2006; Barker et al., 2013). Depending on the species, the time period since exposure and the presence and severity of clinical signs, suspected poisoned animals should be stabilized then decontaminated by emesis, gastric lavage, activated charcoal, and/or administration of cathartics. Given that intoxications with tremorgenic mycotoxins can be characterized by convulsions or, conversely, severe depression and coma, care should be taken to not induce vomiting when contraindicated by an increased risk for aspiration pneumonia. Especially in companion animals, tremors and convulsions might be controlled by diazepam or methocarbamol, but animals unresponsive to these medications can be treated with barbiturates (Hayes et al., 1976; Shell, 2000). The animal should be periodically assessed for metabolic acidosis, hyperthermia, pulmonary edema, and aspiration pneumonia. With proper initial and ongoing assessment and in the absence of complications, affected animals should recover relatively uneventfully following removal from the source and appropriate decontamination and other therapeutic procedures. Animals with mild clinical signs or progression of clinical abnormalities following discharge should be reassessed to evaluate the potential for neuronal damage.

Prevention

Care should be taken to avoid the presence of moldy feedstuffs in areas where animals have unsupervised and unrestricted access, and potentially contaminated materials should be disposed of properly. Trash receptacles should have securely fitting lids, and animals should not be free to roam in areas where discarded foodstuffs or refuse are stored or in the vicinity of compost piles. Livestock should not be fed overtly mold-contaminated forages or concentrates, and care should be taken when feeding food- or beverage-manufacturing byproducts. With respect to "grass staggers," appropriate stocking rates should be maintained, and management practices should be instituted, which ensure that animals have access to young growing plants, especially in pastures dominated by perennial ryegrass, dallisgrass, bahiagrass, or Bermudagrass (Burrows and Tyrl, 2001).

CONCLUDING REMARKS AND FUTURE DIRECTIONS

Tremorgenic mycotoxins containing a tryptophan-derived indole moiety affect many mammalian species, especially sheep, cattle, and dogs. Improved analytical techniques are likely to increase the likelihood of detection of "known" or, even, "new" tremorgenic mycotoxins in foodstuffs or biological samples associated with clinical neurological syndromes characterized by tremors and/or convulsions. Roquefortines and penitrem A are produced by several species of *Penicillium*, and dogs exposed to these potent tremorgens exhibit tremors and, potentially, severe convulsive episodes and seizures. Several common forages, especially perennial ryegrass, are susceptible to infection by fungi capable of producing indole–diterpene tremorgenic mycotoxins, such as lolitrems and paspalitrems, which cause "grass staggers" in susceptible species. Although multiple mechanisms are involved in the neurotoxicity of tremorgenic mycotoxins, impaired GABA- and glycine-mediated inhibitory pathways and enhanced excitatory neurotransmitter (i.e., glutamate and aspartate) release appear to play major roles in the onset of clinical signs. Removal of the animal from contaminated foodstuffs usually results in recovery, but severely poisoned animals should be properly assessed; their tremors and/or convulsions treated; and appropriate steps taken to avoid complications, such as aspiration pneumonia. Whenever possible, animals should not have unrestricted and unsupervised access to mold-contaminated foodstuffs.

REFERENCES

Abramson, D., 1997. Toxicants of the Genus *Penicillium*. In: Felix, J.P. (Ed.), Handbook of Plant and Fungal Toxicants. CRC Press, Boca Raton, FL, pp. 303–317.

Arp, L.H., Richard, J.L., 1981. Experimental intoxication of guinea pigs with multiple doses of the mycotoxin, Penitrem A. Mycopathologia. 73, 109–113.

Barker, A.K., Stahl, C., Ensley, S.M., et al., 2013. Tremorgenic mycotoxins. Compend. Contin. Educ. Vet. VetLearn. Com. E1–E6.

Boysen, S.R., Rozanski, E.A., Chan, D.L., et al., 2002. Tremorgenic mycotoxicosis in four dogs from a single household. J. Am. Vet. Med. Assoc. 221, 1441–1444.

Braselton, W.E., Rumler, P.C., 1996. MS/MS screen for the tremorgenic mycotoxins roquefortine and penitrem A. J. Vet. Diagn. Invest. 8, 515–518.

Breton, P., Bizot, J.C., Bull, J., et al., 1998. Brain neurotoxicity of penitrem A: electrophysiological, behavioral and histopathological study. Toxicon. 36, 645–655.

Burrows, G.E., Tyrl, R.J., 2001. Toxic Plants of North America. Iowa State University Press, Ames, IA, pp. 1–1342.

Catovic, S., Filipovic, N., Stern, P., 1975. The effect of Penitrem A upon the level of glycine in the CNS. Bull. Sci. Sect A Yugoslavia. 20, 284–285.

Cavanagh, J.B., Holton, J.L., Nolan, C.C., et al., 1998. The effects of the tremorgenic mycotoxin penitrem A on the rat cerebellum. Vet. Pathol. 35, 53–63.

Cheeke, P.R., 1998. Natural Toxicants in Feeds. second ed. Interstate Publishers, Inc, Danville, IL, pp. 1–479.

Cole, R.A., Cox, R.H., 1981. Handbook of Toxic Fungal Metabolites. Academic Press, New York, NY.

Cotton, K.D., Hollywood, M.A., McHale, N.G., et al., 1997. Outward currents in smooth muscle cells isolated from sheep mesenteric lymphatics. J. Physiol. 503, 1–11.

Dalziel, J.E., Finch, S.C., Dunlop, J., 2005. The fungal neurotoxin lolitrem B inhibits the function of human large conductance calcium-activated potassium channels. Toxicol. Lett. 155, 421–426.

Eriksen, G.S., Jäderlund, K.H., Moldes-Anaya, A., et al., 2010. Poisoning of dogs with tremorgenic *Penicillium* toxins. Med. Mycol. 48 (1), 188–196.

Evans, T.J., Rottinghaus, G.E., Casteel, S.W., 2004. Ergot. In: Plumlee, K.H. (Ed.), Clinical Veterinary Toxicology. Mosby, Inc, St. Louis, MO, pp. 239–243.

Galey, F.D., Tracy, M.L., Craigmill, A.L., et al., 1991. Staggers induced by consumption of perennial ryegrass in cattle and sheep from northern California. J. Am. Med. Assoc. 199, 466–470.

Gallagher, R.T., Latch, G.C.M., 1977. Production of the tremorgenic mycotoxins verruculogen and fumitremorgen B by *Penicillium piscarium* Westling. Appl. Environ. Microbiol. 33, 730–731.

Gallagher, R.T., Latch, G.C., Keogh, R.G., 1980. The janthitrems: fluorescent tremorgenic toxins produced by *Penicillium janthinellum* isolates from ryegrass pastures. Appl. Environ. Microbiol. 39, 272–273.

Gant, D.B., Cole, R.J., Valdes, J.J., et al., 1987. Action of tremorgenic mycotoxins on GABA/subA/receptor. Life Sci. 41, 2207–2214.

Gao, X., Chooi, Y.-H., Ames, B.D., et al., 2011. Fungal indole alkaloid biosynthesis: genetic and biochemical investigation of the tryptoquialanine pathway in *Penicillium aethiopicum*. J. Am. Chem. Soc. 133, 2729–2741.

Gordon, K.E., Masotti, R.E., Waddell, W.R., 1993. Tremorgenic encephalopathy: a role of mycotoxins in the production of CNS disease in humans? Can. J. Neurol. Sci. 20, 237–239.

Hayes, A.W., Presley, D.B., Neville, J.A., 1976. Acute toxicity of penitrem A in dogs. Toxicol. Appl. Pharmacol. 35 (2), 311–320.

Hocking, A.D., Pitt, J.I., 2003. In: Hocking, A.D. (Ed.), Foodborne Microorganisms of Public Health Significance. AIFST Food Microbiology Group, Sydney, pp. 641–674.

Hocking, A.D., Holds, K., Tobin, N.F., 1988. Intoxication by tremorgenic mycotoxin (Penitrem A) in a dog. Aust. Vet. J. 65, 82–85.

Hooser, S.B., Talcott, P.A., 2006. Mycotoxins. In: Peterson, M.E., Talcott, P.A. (Eds.), Small Animal Toxicology, second ed. Elsevier Saunders, St. Louis, MO, pp. 888–897.

Hotujac, L.J., Stern, P., 1974. Pharmacological examination of verruculogen induced tremor. Acta Med. Iugosl. 28, 223–229.

Hotujac, L.J., Muftic, R.H., Filipovic, N., 1976. Verruculogen: a new substance for decreasing of GABA levels in CNS. Pharmacology 14, 297–300.

Knaus, H.-G., McManus, O.B., Lee, S.H., et al., 1994. Tremorgenic indole alkaloids potently inhibit smooth muscle high-conductance calcium-activated potassium channels. Biochemistry 33, 5819–5828.

Kyriakidis, N., Waight, E.S., Day, J.B., et al., 1981. Novel metabolites from *Penicillium crustosum*, including penitrem E, a tremorgenic mycotoxin. Appl. Environ. Microbiol. 42, 61–62.

Lewis, P.R., Donohue, M.B., Hocking, A.D., et al., 2005. Tremor syndrome associated with a fungal toxins sequelae of food contamination. Med. J. Aust. 182, 582–584.

Ling, K.H., Yang, C.K., Peng, F.T., 1979. Territrems, tremorgenic mycotoxins of *Aspergillus terreus*. Appl. Environ. Microbiol. 37, 355–357.

Loretti, A.P., Colodel, E.M., Driemeier, D., et al., 2003. Neurological disorder in dairy cattle associated with consumption of beer residues contaminated with *Aspergillus clavatus*. J. Vet. Diagn. Invest. 15, 123–132.

Mantle, P.G., Perera, K.P.W.C., Maishman, N.J., et al., 1983. Biosynthesis of penitrems and roquefortine by *Penicillium crustosum*. Appl. Environ. Microbiol. 45, 1486–1490.

McLeay, L.M., Smith, B.L., Munday-Finch, S.C., 1999. Tremorgenic mycotoxins paxilline, penitrem, and lolitrem B, the non-tremorgenic 31-epilolitrem B and electromyographic activity of the reticulum and rumen of sheep. Res. Vet. Sci. 66, 119–127.

Moldes-Anaya, A., Rundberget, T., Uhlig, S., et al., 2011. Isolation and structure elucidation of secopenitrem D, an indole alkaloid from *Penicillium crustosum* Thom. Toxicon. 57, 259–265.

Munday, J.S., Thompson, D., Finch, S.C., et al., 2008. Presumptive tremorgenic mycotoxicosis in a dog in New Zealand, after eating mouldy walnuts. N. Z. Vet. J. 56 (3), 145–147.

Norris, P.J., Smith, C.C.T., De Belleroche, J., et al., 1980. Actions of tremorgenic fungal toxins on neurotransmitters release. J. Neurochem. 34, 33–42.

Patterson, D.S., Shreeve, B.J., Roberts, B.A., et al., 1981. Verruculogen produced by soil fungi in E. Wales. Appl. Environ. Microbiol. 42, 916–917.

Peterson, D.W., Penny, R.H.C., 1982. A comparative study of sheep and pigs given the tremorgenic mycotoxins verruculogen and Penitrem A. Res. Vet. Sci. 33, 1983–1987.

Puschner, B., 2009. Penitrem A and roquefortine. In: Plumlee, K.H. (Ed.), Clinical Veterinary Toxicology. Mosby, St. Louis, MO, pp. 258–259.

Richard, J.L., Bacchetti, P., Arp, L.H., 1981. Moldy walnut toxicosis in a dog caused by the mycotoxin, penitrem A. Mycopathologia 76, 55–58.

Rundberget, T., Wilkins, A.L., 2002. Determination of Penicillium mycotoxins in foods and feeds using liquid chromatography-mass spectrometry. J. Chromatogr. A. 964, 189–197.

Rundberget, T., Skaar, I., Flaoyen, A., 2004. The presence of Penicillium and Penicillium mycotoxins in food wastes. Intl. J. Food Microbiol. 90, 181–188.

Sabater-Vilar, M., Mijmeijer, S., Fink-Gremmels, J., 2003. Genotoxicity assessment of five tremorgenic mycotoxins (fumitremorgen B, paxilline, penitrem A, verruculogen, and verrucosidin) produced by molds isolated from fermented meats. J. Food Prot. 66, 2123–2129.

Sabater-Vilar, M., Maas, R.F.M., De Bosschere, H., et al., 2004. Patulin produced by an *Aspergillus clavatus* isolated from feed containing malting residues associated with a lethal neurotoxicosis in cattle. Mycopathologia 158, 419–426.

Selala, M.I., Daelemans, F., Schepens, P.J.C., 1989. Fungal tremorgens: the mechanism of action of single nitrogen containing toxin. A hypothesis. Drug Chem. Toxicol. 12, 237–257.

Shell, M., 2000. Tremorgenic mycotoxin ingestion. Vet. Med. 95, 285–286.

Shreeve, B.J., Patterson, D.S.P., Roberts, B.A., et al., 1983. Tremorgenic fungal toxins. Vet. Res. Commun. 7, 155–160.

Sobotka, T.J., Brodie, R.E., Spaid, S.L., 1978. Neurobehavioral studies of tremorgenic mycotoxins, verruculogen and penitrem A. Pharmacology 16, 287–294.

Stern, P., 1971. Pharmacological analysis of the tremor induced by cyclopium toxin. Jugoslav Physiol. Pharmacol. 7, 187–196.

Tiwary, A.K., Puschner, B., Poppenga, R.H., 2009. Using roquefortine C as a biomarker for penitrem A intoxication. J. Vet. Diagn. Invest. 21, 237–239.

Tor, E.R., Puschner, B., Filigenzi, M.S., et al., 2006. LC-MS/MS screen for penitrem A and roquefortine C in serum and urine samples. Anal. Chem. 78, 4624–4629.

Uhlig, S., Botha, C.J., Vrålstad, T., Rolén, E., et al., 2009. Indole-diterpenes and ergot alkaloids in *Cynodon dactylon* (bermuda grass) infected with *Claviceps cynodontis* from an outbreak of tremors in cattle. J. Agric. Food Chem. 57, 11112–11119.

Valdes, J.J., Cameron, J.E., Cole, R.J., 1985. Aflatrem: a tremorgenic mycotoxin with acute neurotoxic effects. Environ. Health Perspect. 62, 459–463.

Vesonder, R.F., Tjarks, L., Rohwedder, W., et al., 1980. Indole metabolites of *Penicillium cyclopium.* Experiencia 36, 308.

Wagener, R.E., Davis, N.D., Diener, U.L., 1980. Penitrem A and roquefortine production by *Penicillium commune*. Appl. Environ. Microbiol. 39, 882–887.

Walter, S.L., 2002. Acute penitrem A and roquefortine poisoning in a dog. Can. Vet. J. 43, 372–374.

Wilson, B.J., 1971. Miscellaneous penicillium toxins. In: Ciegler, A., Kadis, S., Ajil, S.J. (Eds.), Microbial Toxin, vol. 6. Academic Press, New York, NY, pp. 459–521.

Young, K.L., Villar, D., Carson, T.L., et al., 2003. Tremorgenic mycotoxin with penitrem A and roquefortine in two dogs. J. Am. Med. Assoc. 222, 52–53.

Chapter 75

Trichothecenes

Rhian B. Cope

INTRODUCTION

The foci of this chapter are on: (1) the general toxicological characteristics of the trichothecene mycotoxins; and (2) the more common problematic trichothecenes encountered in veterinary medicine, i.e., T-2 toxin (a type A trichothecene), dexoxynivalenol (DON; a type B trichothecene), stachybotryotoxicosis, myrotheciotoxicosis, and dendrodochiotoxicosis. Of the trichothecenes, DON is probably the most commonly detected in cereal grains throughout the world (Rotter et al., 1996; CAST, 2003). It is important to remember: (1) all of the 180-plus members of the trichothecene family should be regarded as toxic to domestic animals until proven otherwise; (2) the most common presentation in veterinary medicine is feed refusal and associated effects on performance and reproduction; and (3) site of first contact irritancy (mouth, eyes, perioral area in the case of ingestion; skin in the case of bedding) and ulceration are common.

General Toxicological Characteristics

Trichothecenes are a family of sesquiterpene mycotoxins with the common core chemical structure as shown in Fig. 75.1. The 12, 13-epoxy ring structure is important for biological activity and toxicity. The presence of hydroxyl groups and the structure and position of side chains influence the biological activity. Trichothecenes can be chemically classified into four types based on substitutions at five positions of the trichothecene skeleton, including Type A, which includes T-2 toxin and HT-2 toxin; Type B including nivalenol and DON; Type C including crotocin; and Type D or macrocyclics. Type A trichothecenes include some of the most toxic trichothecenes: T-2 toxin, its deacetylated metabolite, HT-2 toxin, and DAS (or anguidine). The plant synthesis pathways for trichothecenes resemble the metabolic pathways for amino acid synthesis and fatty acid metabolism. While some of the toxins, particularly the macrocyclics, can become airborne and are associated with "sick building syndromes," the most important source of veterinary exposure is ingestion in food.

Sources of the toxins: Trichothecenes are produced by several genera of fungi, including *Fusarium*, *Stachybotrys*, *Myrothecium*, *Trichothecium*, *Trichoderma*, *Cephalosporium*, *Cylindrocarpon*, *Verticimonosporium*, and *Phomopsis* (Scott, 1989). The fruiting bodies of *Podostroma cornu-damae*, a poisonous mushroom species found in Japan and China, also contains trichothecenes (slatratoxins, verrucarin) and the toxins are also produced by the Brazillian plant genus *Baccharis* spp. However, the most medically and economically important source of trichothecene mycotoxins in North America is from *Fusarium* spp. fungi. *Fusarium* spp. are important plant pathogens and grain contaminants in temperate regions (fusarium head blight in wheat, barley, triticale, and other grains).

Factors affecting trichothecene production: The ecological factors likely to increase the level of trichothecene contamination include: ideal temperatures for fungal growth (0–50°C depending on species), humidity (≥70%), moisture level of the growth medium (10%–20%; optimum water activity is >0.88), oxygen level in the growth medium (fungal growth is heavily oxygen dependent), substrate type (nutrient composition), monsoonal weather, unseasonal rains during harvest times, flash flooding, insect interactions and methods of grain handling and storage (Adhikari et al., 2017; Smalley and Strong, 1974). Unusually cool weather conditions in late summer and early fall, coupled with heavy rainfall in the upper Midwest of the United States, can result in widespread, severe *Fusarium* infestation and mycotoxin production (Bamburg et al., 1968; Jacobsen et al., 1995; Park et al., 1996). *Fusarium* species vary in toxigenic potential by strain, which in turn varies with geographic location. Environmental conditions can substantially influence the types of mycotoxins produced by *Fusarium* fungi, e.g., DON is produced under conditions of low oxygen tension, whereas zearalenone (a nontrichothecene, estrogenic

Veterinary Toxicology. DOI: http://dx.doi.org/10.1016/B978-0-12-811410-0.00075-1

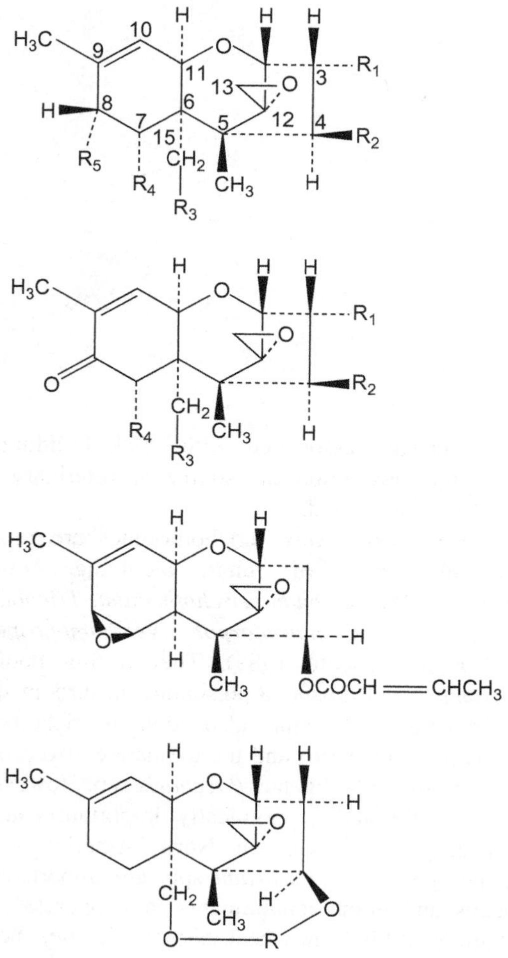

FIGURE 75.1 Core chemical structure of trichothecenes.

mycotoxin) production by the same fungi requires high oxygen levels (Miller, 2002). *Fusarium* occurrence has increased with the practice of no-till farming and utilizing corn in crop rotations.

Trichothecenes also occur in hay, green feed, straw and silage, particularly when hay is baled wet or stored under high moisture conditions (>20%; Mostrom et al., 2005). Fungal growth in silage usually takes place on the front edges of silage in bunker silos or where silage is not adequately packed allowing aerobic conditions to exist. Under these conditions, hay, straw, or silage from *Fusarium*-contaminated wheat, barley, oats and corn can contain high levels of trichothecenes, particularly DON and its acetylated metabolites.

Factors allowing the persistence of trichothecenes in the food chain: Trichothecenes are stable when exposed to air, light or both (Wannemacher and Wiener, 1997). They are not inactivated by normal autoclaving and thermal inactivation requires heating at high temperatures for relatively long periods of time (e.g., 482°C for 10 min). Trichothecenes can be inactivated by strongly acidic and alkaline conditions. Because of their chemical stability, trichothecenes are resistant to milling and food processing and readily enter the animal feed and human food chains (JECFA, 2001). Foodborne trichothecene contamination, in particular DON, has been linked to acute human toxicoses in China, India and Japan, however little information is available regarding potential health effects from chronic exposure (Bhat et al., 1989; Kuiper-Goodman, 1994).

Key features of mammalian and avian toxicokinetics: In general, trichothecenes are lipophilic and are readily absorbed across the gastrointestinal tract, and respiratory mucosae (Wannemacher and Wiener, 1997). Absorption through the skin occurs (particularly with T-2 toxin) but is slow. Distribution is wide, rapid and usually without tissue accumulation. The liver is the major site of metabolism. Phase I hydrolysis and oxidation and phase II glucuronide conjugation occur in the body tissues; however, reduction of the 12,13-epoxide (deepoxidation) is generally due to gut microfloral metabolism. The exception is T-2 toxin where the four basic reactions or pathways occur simultaneously in the same animal (Swanson and Corley, 1989). Deepoxidation is critical step in detoxification of trichothecenes. Acetylation and/or hydrolysis reactions catalyzed by hepatic nonspecific microsomal carboxyl esterase are usually rapid.

Orally administered trichothecenes do not accumulate to a significant extent in the body. Elimination is rapid (plasma $T_{1/2}$ 2–4 h with elimination mostly completed within 48–72 h) (Swanson and Corley, 1989). Biliary and renal excretion are the most important elimination pathways.

Poultry have a greater tolerance to trichothecenes than monogastric mammals because of poor absorption following oral exposure, extensive metabolism, and rapid elimination from the body (Prelusky et al., 1986b).

All trichothecenes are cytotoxic and do not require metabolic activation for toxicity to occur.

Excretion into milk and eggs: Lactating cows or laying hens consuming elevated concentrations of DON transfer low to minimal concentrations of DON to the milk or eggs (Charmley et al., 1993; Côté et al., 1986; El-Banna et al., 1983; Prelusky et al., 1984; Valenta and Dänicke, 2005). Excretion of T-2 toxin into cow's milk is also usually low (Robison et al., 1979). Glávits and Ványi (1995) described a "perinatal form of T-2 toxicosis" in swine in Hungary. T-2 toxin excretion in milk was associated with characteristic T-2 lesions and mortality in the suckling piglets.

Microbial metabolism: Substantial rumen microflora-mediated rumen metabolism (predominantly detoxification by deepoxidation) occurs (Côté et al., 1986; Dänicke et al., 2005; He et al., 1992; Kiessling et al., 1984; King et al., 1984; Prelusky et al., 1986a; Westlake et al.,

1987a,b). Intestinal microflora-mediated deepoxidation is also an important factor influencing toxicity in swine and poultry (He et al., 1992; Hedman and Pettersson, 1997). Induction of microbial trichothecene deepoxidation (and other largely protective detoxifying reactions) may account for the time course of toxidrome and is potentially influenced by the time needed for this microbial adaptation. Microbial adaption may require several weeks of trichothecene exposure. Microbial deepoxidation is reduced by lower pH levels (He et al., 1992). This implies that low rumen pH in ruminants may increase the risk of toxicity in these normally relatively resistant species.

Key overall toxicological modes of action: In broad mechanistic terms the major effect of the trichothecenes is polyribosomal disaggregation and inhibition of protein synthesis with a variety of secondary effects including a complex ribotoxic stress response, and inhibition of RNA and DNA synthesis (Wannemacher and Wiener, 1997). Most of the other effects of trichothecenes are secondary to the disruption of protein, RNA and DNA synthesis. The most intensively researched secondary effects are disruption of reproduction, dysregulation of energy balance and disruption of intestinal barrier integrity (Pinton et al., 2009; Lessard et al., 2015). The most important nonribosomal effect is oxidative stress—associated damage to biological membranes (Pestka, 2010; Chaudhary and Rao, 2010; Yang et al., 2014).

Inhibition of protein synthesis and the ribotoxic stress response: Trichothecenes bind to ribosomes in eukaryotic cells (ribosomal 60S) and interfere with peptidyl transferase activity (McLaughlin et al., 1977). This effect requires an intact 9,10 double bond and a C-12,13 epoxide thus explaining why deepoxidation is an important detoxification reaction. Trichothecenes can be divided into two groups based on their site of action on protein synthesis, either preferential inhibition of initiation or inhibition of elongation or termination. Trichothecenes with hydroxyl and acetyl substitutions at both C-3 and C-4, such as T-2 toxin, DAS, scirpentriol and verrucarin A, predominantly inhibit initiation, and compounds such as trichodermin, crotocol, crotocin, and verrucarol inhibit elongation or termination (McLaughlin et al., 1977). The cytotoxicity of DON, a trichothecene with a keto group at C-8 and a hydroxyl group at C-7, results from protein synthesis inhibition at the ribosomal level during the elongation and termination step in mammalian cells (Ehrlich and Daigle, 1987). Inhibition of RNA and DNA synthesis by trichothecenes is most likely secondary to their effects on protein synthesis.

The binding of trichothecene mycotoxins to the 60S ribosomal subunit also triggers the ribotoxic stress response (Lebrun et al., 2015). This response consists of the activation of several mitogen activated protein kinases (MAP kinases) including p38, c-Jun, JUNK, ERK-1 and ERK-2. Mononuclear leukocytes are particularly susceptible to the trichothecene-induced, ribotoxic-stress response and two paradoxical competing signaling pathways are activated: (1) the p38 mediated pathway is a proapoptosis pathway; and (2) the ERK-1/ERK-2 pathway favors survival and a surge in proinflammatory cytokine expression mediated by the double-stranded RNA-activated protein kinase (PKR) and hematopoietic cell kinase (Hck). PKR and Hck are associated with ribosomes and may act as sensors for trichothecene-induced changes in ribosome structure. The overall net cell fate is dependent on the level and duration of trichothecene exposure.

Trichothecene-induced reactive oxygen production: Trichothecenes likely increase production of oxygen radicals, overwhelming the scavenging system for oxygen radicals and resulting in biological membrane lipid peroxidation and cell injury (Rizzo et al., 1994; Vila et al., 2002). The effect has been best evaluated with T-2 and DON. Inhibition of protein synthesis, coupled with inhibition of DNA and RNA synthesis, likely compounds these effects due to suppression of cellular antioxidant responses.

Trichothecene neurotransmitter effects: DON produces two main clinical signs in monogastric animals: (1) vomiting or emesis at higher concentrations; and (2) reduced food consumption or feed refusal at lower concentrations (Forsyth et al., 1977). The exact mechanism(s) of these effects are largely unknown. DON could act directly via a central mechanism controlling hunger or satiety or possibly peripherally through nonspecific mechanisms inducing lethargy or depression. However, DON is known to affect norepinephrine, and serotonin (5-hydroxytryptamine) homeostasis in brain (Prelusky et al., 1992; Swamy et al., 2004). However, these effects do not definitively correlate with the known neurochemical profile of chemically induced anorexia. The observed effects may also be simply secondary to emesis. At the end of a study in broilers, chicks on mycotoxin-contaminated diets had linear increases of serotonin in the pons and cortex, and norepinephrine and dopamine concentrations in the pons.

Trichothecene-induced emesis likely involves effects at the chemoreceptor trigger zone in the area prostrema and delayed effects that act independently of this system (Borison and Goodheart, 1989; Wang et al., 2014).

Trichothecene immunotoxicity: Trichothecene immunotoxicity is likely mostly secondary to the inhibition of protein synthesis. The most potent immunosuppressive trichothecenes are T-2 toxin, DAS, DON, and fusarenon X, which are the most potent protein synthesis inhibitors (Corrier, 1991). T-2 immunosuppression is also likely to be associated with lymphoid system depletion and necrosis (Friend et al., 1983; Hayes et al., 1980; Hoerr et al., 1981; Osweiler et al., 1981; Taylor et al., 1989; Ueno, 1977;

Weaver et al., 1978a). Neonatal animals are likely more susceptible than adults (Holladay et al., 1993). However, the effects of trichothecenes on humoral responses are complex and contradictory. They both stimulate and impair humoral immunity, cell-mediated immunity and host resistance in experimental and food animals (Bottex et al., 1990; Corrier, 1991; Pestka and Bondy, 1994; Rotter et al., 1996; Bondy and Pestka, 2000; Pestka and Smolinski, 2005). The effect observed depends on dose, duration of exposure and time of measurement. Immunostimulation after small doses of trichothecenes is likely due to the initial inflammatory responses at the genomic and cytokine levels (Azcona-Olivera et al., 1995; Zhou et al., 1997; Ji et al., 1998; Moon and Pestka, 2002; Pestka et al., 2005).

The effect of DON on susceptibility to infection and vaccination responses is an important area of research. The observed effects have been contradictory depending on dose, species and the particular vaccine used (Accensi et al., 2006; Chowdhury et al., 2005; Harvey et al., 1991; Øvernes et al., 1997; Rotter et al., 1994; Tryphonas et al., 1986).

Reproductive toxicity: There is currently no evidence of DON-induced reproductive toxicity under natural exposure conditions. However, T-2 is a known reproductive toxin in pigs (Glávits et al., 1983). This effect is associated with cystic degeneration of the ovaries and uterine atrophy. Rumen acidification combined with T-2 toxin exposure may delay maturation of the dominant ovarian follicle and ovulation and shorten corpora lutea lifespan in sheep and cattle (Huszenicza et al., 2000).

Based on rat data, T-2 toxin crosses the placenta and is distributed to fetal tissues (Lafarge-Frayssinet et al., 1990). Maternotoxic doses of T-2 toxin were associated with fetal mortality and effects on the CNS and skeletal system in rats (Rousseaux and Schiefer, 1987). T-2 toxin can trigger abortion and small litters in sows (Weaver et al., 1978b). Trichothecene toxin exposure of poultry is classically associated with reduced egg production. Embryofetal development studies in mice have demonstrated that DON is teratogenic (effects on nervous and skeletal systems) at submaternotoxic doses (Khera et al., 1982).

Genotoxicity and carcinogenesis: Based on classical in vitro tests, trichothecenes generally do not induce reverse mutations in bacteria. However, they are clastenogenic in vitro (Hsia et al., 1988). DON was not carcinogenic in a near life-time exposure study in mice (Iverson et al., 1995). It was not teratogenic in rabbit studies at submaternotoxic doses (Khera et al., 1986). Minor malformations described as delayed ossification and un-withdrawn yolk sac were reported in chick embryos from hens fed rations containing DON at 2.5 and 3.1 mg DON/kg diet (Bergsjo et al., 1993).

Dysregulation of energy balance: Trichothecene-induced dysregulation of energy balance is a complex multisystem response that consists of at least the following components (Lebrun et al., 2015): (1) gastrointestinal malaise/satiation and food refusal; (2) centrally driven sickness behavior and anorexia; (3) targeting of the liver; and (4) and alteration of somatotropic axis.

Type B trichothecenes, including DON, 15-ADON, 3-ADON, FUS-X, and NIV, and the Type A trichothecene T2 are all potent emetics, and DON and T2 are potent triggers of conditioned taste aversion (Lebrun et al., 2015). However, IV dosing DON at 10 mg/kg (but not at 1 or 2 mg/kg) triggered a gastrointestinal motor pattern reminiscent of the typical fed (i.e., satiated) pattern in rats (Lebrun et al., 2015). The effect was mediated from outside of the gut, i.e., via peripheral autonomic ganglia or by vagal efferents. Several patents have been filed regarding the potential use of natural and synthetic trichothecenes based on the concept that they trigger satiation. Other findings of potential trichothecene anorexigenic effects include DON (IV 0.3–3 mg/kg or 150–570 ng/kg injected into the central pattern generator of swallowing) induced inhibition of the swallowing reflex in a manner that resembles the anorexigenic effects of agents like leptin and brain-derived neurotrophic factor (Lebrun et al., 2015). Furthermore, dosing with DON (12.5 mg/kg PO, gavage) resulted in a reduction in meal frequency and size in rats that had free access to feed, triggered the release of anorexigenic gut hormones (CCK, peptide YY 3-36), and induced pica in rats. Similar effects have been noted with T2. The effects were not associated with a nauseagenic response.

A hallmark of trichothecene toxicosis is the activation of the innate immune system resulting in a surge of proinflammatory cytokines (IL-1β, IL-6, TNF-α, TGF-β) that resembles an acute phase response (both peripherally and centrally within the hypothalamus and dorsal vagal complex). The proinflammatory cytokine surge triggers a set of clinical signs referred to as sickness behaviors (anorexia, changes in core body temperature, decreased motor activity, social withdrawal). Sickness behaviors are generally regarded as an adaptive response to an infection. Acute oral exposure to DON or T-2 toxin triggers classical acute phase initiated sickness behaviors in mice (Lebrun et al., 2015). This response is associated with c-Fos activation in brain structures associated with sickness behaviors (nucleus tractus solitaries, area prostrema, ventrolateral medulla, lateral parabrachial nucleus, locus coeruleus, and various locations within the hypothalamus). These changes are markers of induction of centrally mediated taste aversion, feed refusal, anorexia, and hypothermia.

Oral dosing of mice with DON upregulates liver suppressor of cytokine signaling 3 (SOC3) which, in turn, restricts weight gain by interfering with growth hormone signaling, i.e., alteration of the somatotropic axis (Lebrun et al., 2015).

Alteration of the intestinal barrier: T-2 toxin causes an impairment of the barrier function of porcine intestinal epithelial cells (IPEC-J2 cells) and increased bacterial translocation in vitro (Akbari et al., 2016). T-2 toxin, DON, 3-acetyl-DON and 15-acetyl-DON also decrease the transepithelial electrical resistance (a marker of barrier integrity) of IPEC-J2 and human epithelial colorectal adenocarcinoma cell (Caco-2) monolayers. DON also adversely alters the expression and/or distribution of enterothelial tight junction proteins in porcine jejunal explants ex vivo and in vivo in pigs, mice, and broiler chickens.

T-2 Toxin

T-2 toxin, a member of the Type A trichothecene family, is predominantly associated with *Fusarium* spp. growth on wheat and corn (Adhikari et al., 2017). T-2 toxin and its metabolite HT-2 has also been reported in barley, rice, soy beans, oats, and products produced from these grains. The chemical weapon potential of T-2 toxin was recognized in World War II following an outbreak of T-2 toxin alimentary toxic aleukia (ATA) in Orenburg, in the Russian Urals. The outbreak was due to consumption of *Fusarium* spp. infected, overwintered wheat and millet. From 1942 to 1947 ATA was responsible for the death of about 10% of the population of Oregnburg (100,000 human fatalities) (Wannemacher and Wiener, 1997). A similar, ATA like disease called Akakabibyo (called "bean-hulls poisoning" in the equine cases) was subsequently reported in Japan (Ueno et al., 1973). In this outbreak neosolaniol (a metabolite of T-2 toxin) and T-2 toxin were detected in bean hulls contaminated with *Fusarium solani*. This outbreak demonstrated an important feature of T-2 toxin: it often cooccurs with its metabolites (e.g., HT-2 toxin, neosolaniol, etc.) and other trichothecenes such as diacetoxyscirpenol. When T-2 toxin contaminated products are blended with different batches of grain, multiple different mycotoxins can cooccur resulting in mixed mycotoxin poisonings.

Controversy remains regarding weaponization of T-2 toxin by the Soviet Union and the possible use of such weapons by its client states in Laos, Cambodia ("yellow rain" incidents from 1975 to 1981) and Afghanistan (Wannemacher and Wiener, 1997). In these cases T-2 toxin may have been mixed with various combinations of phosgene, phosgene oxide, sarin, soman, mustard gas, alpha-chlorbenzylidene malonitrile (CS), or 3-quinuclidinyl benzilate (BZ). Unambiguous identification of these weapons was difficult because many different chemical weapon combinations prepared by the Soviet Union used the same yellow dye. In fact, T-2 may have been desirable chemical weapon because it has been very difficult to definitively detect its use after the fact. T-2 may have also been used in the 1964 Egyptian attacks against Yemeni Royalists and during the Iran-Iraq war of 1983–84 (Wannemacher and Wiener, 1997).

Critically in relation to the chemical weapon potential of T-2 toxin, it is the only member of the trichothecene family that can be absorbed through the skin in sufficient amounts to results in serious systemic toxicity (Wannemacher and Wiener, 1997).

Toxicokinetics: The toxicokinetics of T-2 toxin conforms to the general trichothecene pattern, i.e., rapid bioavailability following ingestion and inhalation. Importantly, T-2 toxin undergoes various combinations of deacylation, C-12/13 deepoxidation, and oxidization by ruminal microflora, intestinal bacteria and by many different cell types. Metabolism is generally detoxifying: T-2 toxin is about 1.5–1.7 times as toxic as HT-2, which is 4.8 times as toxic as T-2 tetraol (Ueno et al., 1973). Ruminal and intestinal microflora metabolism is generally detoxifying and is an important protective effect (Adhikari et al., 2017; Wannemacher and Wiener, 1997).

Because of ruminal detoxification, monogastric animals are generally more susceptible than ruminant species. Tissue distribution studies demonstrate that the liver is the quantitatively most important organ for trichothecene metabolism (Wannemacher and Wiener, 1997). The major metabolites are HT-2 toxin and its hydroxyl and glucuronide metabolites and T-2 tetraol and its glucuronide. Hepatic microsomal carboxyl esterase is an important catalyst of T-2 toxin metabolism. Metabolite excretion occurs via the urine and bile. Very little T-2 toxin is excreted intact.

Modes of action: Like all of the important trichothecenes, T-2 toxin is a site of first contact irritant. This results in serious hemorrhagic ulceration and necrosis of the gastrointestinal tract (GIT) following ingestion. Disruption of the intestinal microflora and associated secondary effects can occur. Cytotoxic damage in the liver, heart, kidneys, lymphoid tissues, bone marrow, and peripheral ganglia occurs as the toxin undergoes distribution in the circulation. The key toxicological modes of action of T-2 toxin are inhibition of protein synthesis and increasing oxidative stress. The secondary consequences of these are widespread and include: DNA/RNA damage, reduced DNA/RNA synthesis, impaired amino acid metabolism, cytotoxicity, impaired energy metabolism due to disruption of the TCA cycle, and severe immunosuppression.

Acute toxicity: T-2 toxin is amongst the most toxic of the trichothecene mycotoxins. As with all of the trichothecenes, the most commonly observed phenomenon in veterinary medicine is feed refusal and associated secondary effects. The oral acute LD_{50} range for mammals and poultry is in the 4–10 mg/kg range (Wannemacher and Wiener, 1997). The hallmark features of acute oral toxicity resemble ATA (Wannemacher and Wiener, 1997):

- First (gastrointestinal distress) stage:
  - Oral pain
  - Oral and perioral inflammation, gum bleeding, oral and perioral bullae, mucosal ulceration, mucosal sloughing, excessive salivation, aphonia, or dysphonia (due to laryngeal damage and pain)
  - Possible corneal and skin injuries at sites of contact with the suspect material
  - Lethargy, loss of coordination, epistaxis, hematemesis, abdominal pain (often severe), tachycardia
  - Evidence of acute liver injury may be present
  - Coagulation deficits may be present
  - Onset of watery diarrhea progressing to frankly bloody diarrhea within minutes to hours of ingestion; deaths may occur at this stage due to hypotension, fluid disturbances, ion disturbances, or suffocation due to airway/laryngeal injury, and edema
- Second (leukopenic or latent) stage
  - Survivors of the first stage develop the hallmark effects of profound leukopenia, granulocytopenia, progressive lymphocytosis and radiomimetic effects in bone marrow
  - Apparent clinical improvement may occur at this stage
- Third (recrudescence) stage
  - This stage is characterized by intensive ulceration, gangrenous processes and severe nasal, oral, gastric, and intestinal hemorrhagic diathesis
- Fourth (recovery) stage
  - The hallmarks of this stage are slow clinical improvement and high susceptibility to secondary infections (particularly pneumonia)
  - Recovery is often very slow; up to 2 months may be required for full bone marrow recovery and multiple transfusions may be required to maintain red cell mass

Chronic toxicity: The most common effects observed in veterinary medicine relate to feed refusal and decreased food production. This is most likely to be seen in swine and poultry. A more chronic, low dose toxicity most commonly results in weight loss, reduced weight gain and reduction in production parameters. Skin, oral, and perioral irritation may be present due to site of first contact effects. Feather alterations have been reported in chickens (Adhikari et al., 2017). Other effects include immune alterations, decreased erythrocyte mass, leukopenias, opportunistic infections, chronic gastric ulceration, and hepatotoxicity. Effects on reproduction (likely secondary to feed refusal and nutritional effects) have been reported.

Chronic toxicity is poorly described in horses. Oral ulceration and necrosis and muscle tremor has been described (Adhikari et al., 2017).

It is important to remember that adult ruminants will usually be more resistant to the systemic effects of T-2 toxin. However, local site of first contact effects in the gastrointestinal tract and on the skin, may still occur. Gastritis, abomasal hemorrhages, intestinal hemorrhage and ulceration may occur. The toxidrome in preruminant stage sheep and cattle resembles the monogastric syndrome.

Effects in poultry: Poultry are reputedly less susceptible to T-2 toxin compared with pigs. However, T-2 toxin is a well-known cause of hemorrhagic gastrointestinal inflammation, necrohemorrhagic dermatitis, impaired immunity, destruction of the hematopoietic system, organ damage, declining egg production, egg shell thinning, feed refusal, weight loss, altered feather patterns, neural disturbance, and hysteroid seizures (Sokolović et al., 2008). Common histopathology findings include fatty change and strong granular degeneration in the liver, kidneys and, more rarely, in the heart. It is a major cause of loss in the poultry industry where *Fusarium* sp. contamination of feeds is common.

Diagnosis: While toxicity may be suspected on the basis of clinical signs and performance data a definitive diagnosis relies on detection of T-2 toxin in feed.

Treatment: The key treatment action is to stop exposure. With the more common veterinary scenarios, clinical signs of feed refusal will usually disappear within 7 days after removal of the contaminated feed. No specific therapies for trichothecene mycotoxicoses are available. Some trichothecenes undergo enterohepatic recirculation and are excreted in the feces. Gastrointestinal decontamination with repeat dose activated charcoal in combination with magnesium sulfate was reputed to have some beneficial effects in acute T-2 poisoning in swine (Poppenga et al., 1987). Metoclopramide, given intravenously immediately prior to and following T-2 toxin administration, was only partially successful as an antiemetic (Poppenga et al., 1987).

Prevention: The most effective preventative measure is measurement of T-2 toxin in feeds and appropriate drying and storage of hays and grains. Measurement is potentially challenging because of the risk of the sampling method missing hot spots in bulk materials. Chemical oxidation, and bentonite have been used in an attempt to reduce feed levels and bioavailability.

Deoxynivalenol (DON, Vomitoxin)

DON is currently the most prevalent food-associated mycotoxin in the United States (Payros et al., 2016). In

North America, 73% of wheat crops and 92% of corn crops are contaminated with DON. DON is a major feed hazard for livestock and humans in the United States.

The most important source of DON in North America is *Fusarium* spp. infection of grains, which produces two main other acetylated forms (3-acetyl-DON and 15-acetyl-DON). Biologically modified forms are commonly also present in foodstuffs (plant-derived dexoxynivalenol-3-β-D-glycopyronoside and the bacterial metabolites deepoxy-DON, 3-epi-DON, 3-keto-DON). Chemically modified forms (norDON A-C due to heating and DON sulfonates) are also common in foodstuffs.

Toxicokinetics: The extent of absorption from the gastrointestinal tract depends on species, age and sex. Gastrointestinal absorption is highest in pigs following chronic exposure (89%) but is lowest in ruminants (about 7%) and in poultry (Payros et al., 2016). Oral bioavailability correlates with species susceptibility. DON absorption is higher in younger animals.

DON is rapidly and widely distributed and crosses the placenta. In animals, DON does not undergo Phase I metabolism. It is neither bioactivated to more toxic substances or detoxified by phase I metabolism in vivo. Phase II reactions consist of glucuronide, sulfate and sulfonate conjugates. The pattern of glucuronidation of DON varies across species. Sulfate and sulfonate conjugation is mostly observed in rats and chickens.

Like T-2 toxin, gastrointestinal microflora generally detoxify DON by deepoxidation and acetylation. As would be expected, adult ruminants are less susceptible to DON poisoning due to rumen-mediated presystemic detoxification.

Excretion is predominantly by the renal and biliary routes. Plasma elimination is biphasic with a rapid α phase ($T_{½} \approx 0.36$ h) and a slower β phase ($T_{½} \approx 7.62$ h). Residues in edible tissues, milk and eggs are generally regarded as being negligible (Wang et al., 2014).

Modes of action: Like other trichothecenes, DON primarily acts by binding to ribosomal 60S, blocking protein synthesis and inducing a ribotoxic stress response. Induction of oxidative stress and lipid peroxidation have also been noted. DON induces cell-cycle arrest and apoptosis, particularly in hematopoietic and enterothelial cells. These effects are likely secondary to the ribotoxic stress response and oxidative stress effects. DON also triggers substantial remodeling of the cell cytoskeleton due to effects on actin.

The intestinal enterothelium is one of the first toxicological targets for DON, particularly in rodents, swine, and chickens (Payros et al., 2016). The key effects are shortening, edema and fusion of intestinal villi and enterothelial apoptosis and necrosis. DON adversely affects the balance between enterothelial stem cell in the intestinal crypts and enterothelial maturation, migration, and eventual apoptosis. DON is a notable inhibitor of enterothelial cell proliferation. DON also disrupts the affects the absorption of amino acids and sugars due to inhibition of enterothelial transporters (notably SGLT1, GLUT5). DON also induces enterothelial barrier disruption due to disruption of tight junction formation (Payros et al., 2016). This results in increased commensal and pathogenic bacterial leakage across the intestinal barrier. The sum total overall effect of DON in the gut is to produce chronic intestinal disease, reduce the intestinal surface area for absorption, reduce nutrient bioavailability, reduce feed efficiency, and reduce growth and production values.

DON is reputed to cause a transient intestinal microflora dysbiosis in swine (Payros et al., 2016). The effect is associated with a reduction in *Clostridium perfringens* without effects on the *Enterobacteria* sp. population. DON also modulates the pathogenicity of gut *Salmonella* sp.

Exacerbation of the proinflammatory cytokine response of the intestine (notably IL-8 production) is a hallmark of DON's effects on the intestine (Payros et al., 2016). DON ingestion also triggers a substantial increase in serum IgA and serum IgA-immune complexes (Payros et al., 2016). This is accompanied by increases in serum IgE and decreases in serum IgG and IgM. The IgA effect is due to clonal expansion of polyclonal IgA-secreting cells in Peyer's patches. The effect may be secondary to intestinal barrier disruption, i.e., increased antigenic exposure, or it may be due to intestinal microflora dysbiosis. As with other trichothecenes, DON induces systemic lymphoid depletion and is likely immunomodulatory. DON inhibits Th1 immune responses and stimulates Th2 cytokine responses (Payros et al., 2016).

Consistent with the actions of other trichothecenes, DON is hematotoxic and myelotoxic resulting in dysfunction in both the blood and bone marrow compartments.

DON rapidly crosses the blood–brain barrier (BBB), particularly in pigs. This has direct effects on neurons, the glia and the neurotransmitter milieu (Payros et al., 2016). DON activates a number of central anorexigenic neuronal pathways and may influences the central neuronal pathways involved in food intake. However, the definitive anorexigenic mechanism of DON remains unknown.

DON is potentially genotoxic based on comet assay studies in intestinal cell lines, lymphocytes and hepatocytes (Payros et al., 2016). The observed effects may have been secondary to oxidative damage. The carcinogenic potential of DON has been poorly studied. Currently, it is classified as an IARC 3 human carcinogen (i.e., not classifiable as to its carcinogenicity to humans).

The reproductive toxicity of DON has mostly been examined in rodents. DON is a male reproductive toxin in rats (Payros et al., 2016). Treatment is associated with reduced fertility, reduced sperm counts, increased sperm abnormalities, and effects on testosterone, FSH and LH. DON adversely affects development in mice (embryotoxicity, skeletal malformations, increased postnatal mortality) and is a teratogen in rats. There is little evidence that DON affects reproduction in pigs and other domestic species.

Key effects in domestic animals: The commonly encountered veterinary toxidromes associated with DON are: (1) emesis, anorexia and growth effects; and (2) increased susceptibility to infections and impaired vaccine responses.

Acute poisoning with DON classically induces abdominal pain, excessive salivation, diarrhea and emesis. DON was originally called vomitoxin due to its potent emetic effects in humans, pigs, dogs, and mink. More chronic, lower level, exposure is classically associated with centrally mediated anorexia, feed refusal, weight loss, impaired performance, hypoproteinemia, and weakness.

Increased susceptibility to infection may occur due to effects on intestinal barrier function. However, the effects of DON on immune responses and resistance to infection have been shown to be somewhat paradoxical, e.g., exacerbation of the early immune response to *Salmonella typhimurium* while simultaneously enhancing *S. typhimurium* invasion and translocation in the ileum of pigs. DON is reputedly a predisposing factor for *C. perfringens* necrotic enteritis in chickens due to its capacity to disrupt the enterothelial barrier. DON also impairs the immune response of chickens to *Eimeria* sp., reduces the efficacy of coccidiostats and delays intestinal repair after *Eimeria* sp. infection. DON-mediated immunomodulation causing a Th1 to Th2 shift has been associated with impaired immune responses to reovirus in mice. Exposure to DON in feed is associated with increased susceptibility of pigs to porcine reproductive and respiratory syndrome virus. This effect is associated with impaired humoral responses to this virus. DON exposure also increases the replication of porcine circovirus type 2.

Feed exposure to DON also impairs humoral immune responses to infectious bronchitis virus and Newcastle disease virus in chickens. Impaired immune responses to an experimental ovalbumin vaccine have also been demonstrated in pigs.

Diagnosis: Feed analysis is the only definitive method of diagnosis. A change of feed source can be suggestive of exposure, particularly in pigs. Appetite recovery in pigs is often relatively quick following a change to an uncontaminated feed source.

Treatment: The only effective treatment is cessation of exposure and basic supportive care (antibiotic coverage, glucocorticoid antiinflammatory treatment).

Prevention: As per other trichothecenes, various attempts to use DON feed binders (e.g., calcium aluminosilicates, bentonite, sodium bisulfite, and yeast-based glucomannans) have been largely unsuccessful.

STACHYBOTRYOTOXICOSIS, MYROTHECIOTOXICOSIS, AND DENDRODOCHIOTOXICOSIS

Stachybotryotoxicosis was first reported as a syndrome amongst human farm workers in Russia, Yugoslavia and Hungary and was caused by *Stachybotrys atra* (syn *Stachybotrys alternans*) infection of hay (Wannemacher and Wiener, 1997). The syndrome, which consisted of a sore throat, bloody nasal discharge and dyspnea, was likely caused by satratoxin. Similar syndromes in horses, cattle, sheep, pigs, and poultry have been reported from the Ukraine, Europe and South Africa. In domestic animals, the toxidrome resembles ATA, i.e., cutaneous and mucocutaneous lesions, panleukopenia, nervous signs, abortion, and death in 2–12 days.

Myrotheciotoxicosis in ruminants and horses has been reported in New Zealand and India. The trichothecenes of concern are verrucarins and roridins produced by molds of the genus *Myrothecium* sp. The acute form of the disease is associated with gastroenteritis, diarrhea, abomasal hemorrhage, hepatitis, and pulmonary congestion.

Dendrodochiotoxicosis is a similar disease of horses and humans reported from Russia. It is due to trichothecenes produced by *Dendrodochium toxicum* and is associated with acute gastroenterocolitis.

CONCLUDING REMARKS AND FUTURE DIRECTIONS

Trichothecenes remain an ever-present mycotoxicological challenge in terms of safety of the food supply. While overt acute toxicity has now become relatively rare in veterinary medicine, subclinical production loss associated with feed refusal and reduced feed intake are ongoing challenges. Current research is heavily focused on the search for ways of binding the trichothecenes in feeds so as to reduce their bioavailability. The potential for T-2 toxin as a bioweapon remains an ongoing threat.

REFERENCES

Accensi, F., Pinton, P., Callu, P., et al., 2006. Ingestion of low doses of deoxynivalenol does not affect hematological, biochemical, or immune responses of piglets. J. Anim. Sci. 84, 1935–1942.

Adhikari, M., Negi, B., Kaushik, N., et al., 2017. T-2 mycotoxin: toxicological effects and decontamination strategies. Oncotarget 8, 33933–33952.

Akbari, P., Braber, S., Varasteh, S., et al., 2016. The intestinal barrier as an emerging target in the toxicological assessment of mycotoxins. Arch. Toxicol. 91 (3), 1007–1029.

Azcona-Olivera, J.I., Ouyang, Y., Warner, R.L., et al., 1995. Induction of cytokine mRNAs in mice after oral exposure to the trichothecene vomitoxin (deoxynivalenol):relationship to toxin distribution and protein synthesis inhibition. Toxicol. Appl. Pharmacol. 133, 109–120.

Bamburg, J.R., Riggs, N.V., Strong, F.M., 1968. The structures of toxins from two strains of *Fusarium tricinctum*. Tetrahedron 24, 3329–3336.

Bergsjo, B., Herstad, O., Nafstad, I., 1993. Effects of feeding deoxynivalenol-contaminated oats on reproductive performance in White Leghorn hens. Br. Poult. Sci. 34, 147–159.

Bhat, R.V., Beedu, S.R., Ramakrishna, Y., et al., 1989. Outbreak of trichothecene mycotoxicosis associated with consumption of mould-damages wheat production in Kashmir Valley, India. Lancet 8628, 35–37.

Bondy, G.S., Pestka, J.J., 2000. Immunomodulation by fungal toxins. J. Toxicol. Environ. Health B. 3, 109–143.

Borison, H.L., Goodheart, M.L., 1989. Neural factors in acute emetic, cardiovascular, and respiratory effects of T-2 toxin in cats. Toxicol. Appl. Pharmacol. 101, 399–413.

Bottex, C., Martin, A., Fontanges, R., 1990. Action of a mycotoxin (diacetoxyscirpenol) on the immune response of the mouse – interaction with an immunomodulator (OM-89). Immunopharmacol. Immunotoxicol. 12, 311–325.

CAST, 2003. Mycotoxins. Risks in Plant, Animal, and Human Systems. Council for Agriculture, Science and Technology, Ames, IA, Task Force Report No. 139.

Charmley, E., Trenholm, H.L., Thompson, B.K., et al., 1993. Influence of level of deoxynivalenol in the diet of dairy cows on feed intake, milk production, and its composition. J. Dairy Sci. 76, 3580–3587.

Chaudhary, M., Rao, L., 2010. Brain oxidative stress after dermal and subcutaneous exposure to T-2 toxin in mice. Food Chem. Toxicol. 48, 3436–3442.

Chowdhury, S.R., Smith, T.K., Boermans, H.J., et al., 2005. Effects of feed-borne *Fusarium* mycotoxins on hematology and immunology of turkeys. Poultry Sci. 84, 1698–1706.

Corrier, D.E., 1991. Mycotoxins: mechanisms of immunosuppression. Vet. Immunol. Immunopathol. 30, 73–87.

Côté, L.-M., Dahlem, A.M., Yoshizaa, T., et al., 1986. Excretion of deoxynivalenol and its metabolite in milk, urine and feces of lactating dairy cows. J. Dairy Sci. 69, 2416–2423.

Dänicke, S., Matthaus, K., Lebzien, P., et al., 2005. Effects of *Fusarium* toxin-contaminated wheat grain on nutrient turnover, microbial protein synthesis and metabolism of deoxynivalenol and zearalenone in the rumen of dairy cows. J. Anim. Physiol. Anim. Nutr. (Berlin). 89, 303–315.

Ehrlich, K.C., Daigle, K.W., 1987. Protein synthesis inhibition by 8-oxo-12,13-epoxytrichothecenes. Biochim. Biophys. Acta 923, 206–213.

El-Banna, A.A., Hamilton, R.M.G., Scott, P.M., et al., 1983. Nontransmission of deoxynivalenol (vomitoxin) to eggs and meat in chickens fed deoxynivalenol-contaminated diets. J. Agric. Food Chem. 31, 1381–1384.

Forsyth, D.M., Yoshizawa, T., Morooka, N., et al., 1977. Emetic and refusal activity of deoxynivalenol to swine. Appl. Environ. Microbiol. 34, 547–552.

Friend, S.C.E., Hancock, D.S., Schiefer, H.B., et al., 1983. Experimental T-2 toxicosis in sheep. Can. J. Comp. Med. 47, 291–297.

Glávits, R., Ványi, A., 1995. More important mycotoxicoses in pigs. Comprehensive clinico-pathological communication. Magy Állatorvosok Lapja 50, 407–420.

Glávits, R., Gabriella, S., Sándor, S., et al., 1983. Reproductive disorders caused by trichothecene mycotoxins in a large-scale pig herd. Acta Vet. Hung. 31, 173–180.

Harvey, R.B., Kubena, L.F., Huff, W.E., et al., 1991. Hematologic and immunologic toxicity of deoxynivalenol (DON)-contaminated diets to growing chickens. Bull. Environ. Contam. Toxicol. 46, 410–416.

Hayes, M.A., Bellamy, J.E.C., Schiefer, H.B., 1980. Subacute toxicity of dietary T-2 toxin in mice, morphological and hematological effects. Can. J. Comp. Med. 44, 203–218.

He, P., Young, L.G., Forsberg, C., 1992. Microbial transformation of deoxynivalenol (vomitoxin). Appl. Environ. Microbiol. 58, 3857–3863.

Hedman, R., Pettersson, H., 1997. Transformation of nivalenol by gastrointestinal microbes. Arch. Anim. Nutr. 50, 321–329.

Hoerr, F.J., Carlton, W.W., Yagen, B., 1981. Mycotoxicosis caused by a single dose of T-2 toxin or diacetoxyscirpenol in broiler chickens. Vet. Pathol. 5, 652–664.

Holladay, S.D., Blaylock, B.L., Comment, C.E., et al., 1993. Fetal thymic atrophy after exposure to T-2 toxin: selectivity for lymphoid progenitor cells. Toxicol. Appl. Pharmacol. 121, 8–14.

Hsia, C.C., Wu, J.L., Lu, X.Q., et al., 1988. Natural occurrence and clastogenic effects of nivalenol, deoxynivalenol, 3-acetyl-deoxynivalenol, 15-acetyl-deoxynivalenol, and zearalenone in corn from a high-risk area of esophageal cancer. Cancer Detect. Prev. 13, 79–86.

Huszenicza, G., Fekete, S., Szigeti, G., et al., 2000. Ovarian consequences of low dose peroral *Fusarium* (T-2) toxin in a ewe and heifer model. Theriogenology 53, 1631–1639.

Iverson, F., Armstrong, C., Nera, E., et al., 1995. Chronic feeding study of deoxynivalenol in B6C3F1 male and female mice. Teratog. Carcinog. Mutag. 15, 283–306.

Jacobsen, B.J., Harlin, K.S., Swanson, S.P., et al., 1995. Occurrence of fungi and mycotoxins associated with field mold damaged soybeans in the Midwest. Plant Dis. 79, 86–88.

JECFA, 2001. Trichothecenes. Safety Evaluation of Certain Mycotoxins in Food. Joint FAO/WHO Expert Committee on Food Additives, FAO Food and Nutrition Paper 74/WHO Food Additives Series 47. World Health Organization, Geneva, pp. 419–680.

Ji, G.E., Park, S.Y., Wong, S.S., et al., 1998. Modulation of nitric oxide, hydrogen peroxide and cytokine production in a clonal macrophage model by the trichothecene vomitoxin (deoxynivalenol). Toxicology. 125, 203–214.

Khera, K.S., Whalen, C., Angers, G., et al., 1982. Embryotoxicity of 4-deoxynivalenol (vomitoxin) in mice. Bull. Environ. Contam. Toxicol. 29, 487–491.

Khera, K.S., Whalen, C., Angers, G., 1986. A teratology study on vomitoxin (4-deoxynivalenol) in rabbits. Food Chem. Toxicol. 5, 421–424.

Kiessling, K.-H., Pettersson, H., Sandholm, K., et al., 1984. Metabolism of aflatoxin, ochratoxin, zearalenone, and three trichothecenes by intact rumen fluid, rumen protozoa, and rumen bacteria. Appl. Environ. Microbiol. 47, 1070–1073.

King, R.R., McQueen, R.E., Levesque, D., et al., 1984. Transformation of deoxynivalenol (vomitoxin) by rumen microorganisms. J. Agric. Food Chem. 32, 1181–1183.

Kuiper-Goodman, T., 1994. Prevention of human mycotoxicoses through risk assessment and risk management. In: Miller, J.D., Trenholm, H.L. (Eds.), Mycotoxins in Grain: Compounds Other than Aflatoxin. Eagan Press, St. Paul, pp. 439–469.

Lafarge-Frayssinet, D., Chakor, K., Lafont, P., et al., 1990. Transplacental transfer of T2-toxin: pathological effect. J. Environ. Pathol. Toxicol. Oncol. 10, 64–68.

Lebrun, B., Tardivel, C., Félix, B., et al., 2015. Dysregulation of energy balance by trichothecene mycotoxins: mechanisms and prospects. Neurotoxicology 49, 15–27.

Lessard, M., Savard, C., Deschene, K., et al., 2015. Impact of deoxynivalenol (DON) contaminated feed on intestinal integrity and immune response in swine. Food Chem. Toxicol. 80, 7–16.

McLaughlin, C.S., Vaughan, M.H., Campbell, I.M., et al., 1977. Inhibition of protein synthesis by trichothecenes. In: Rodricks, J.V., Hesseltine, C.W., Mehlman, M.A. (Eds.), Mycotoxins in Human and Animal Health. Pathotox Publishers, Inc., Park Forest South, IL, pp. 263–275.

Miller, J.D., 2002. Aspects of the ecology of *Fusarium* toxins in cereals. In: DeVries, J.W., Trucksess, M.W., Jackson, L.S. (Eds.), Mycotoxins and Food Safety. Kluwer Academic/Plenum Publishers, New York, NY, Adv. Exp. Med. Biol. 54, 19–27.

Moon, Y., Pestka, J.J., 2002. Vomitoxin-induced cyclooxygenase-2 gene expression in macrophages mediated by activation of ERK and p38 but not JNK mitogen-activated protein kinases. Toxicol. Sci. 69, 373–382.

Mostrom, M.S., Tacke, B., Lardy, G., 2005 Field corn, hail, and mycotoxins. In: Proceedings of the North Central Conference of the American Association of Veterinary Laboratory Diagnosticians, Fargo, ND.

Osweiler, G.D., Hook, B.S., Mann, D.D., et al., 1981. Effects of T-2 toxin in cattle. In: Proc US Anim Health Assoc. 85th Ann Meet, St. Louis, MO, pp. 214–231.

Øvernes, G., Matre, T., Sivertsen, T., et al., 1997. Effects of diets with graded levels of naturally deoxynivalenol-contaminated oats on immune response in growing pigs. J. Vet. Med. A. 44, 539–550.

Park, J.J., Smalley, E.B., Chu, F.S., 1996. Natural occurrence of *Fusarium* mycotoxins in field samples from the 1992 Wisconsin corn crop. Appl. Environ. Microbiol. 62, 1642–1648.

Payros, D., Alassane-Kpembi, I., Pierron, A., et al., 2016. Toxicology of deoxynivalenol and its acetylated and modified forms. Arch. Toxicol. 90 (12), 2931–2957.

Pestka, J.J., Bondy, G.S., 1994. Immunotoxic effects of mycotoxins. In: Miller, J.D., Trenholm, H.L. (Eds.), Mycotoxins in Grain. Compounds Other than Aflatoxin. Eagan Press, St. Paul, pp. 339–358.

Pestka, J.J., Smolinski, A.T., 2005. Deoxynivalenol: toxicology and potential effects on humans. J. Toxicol. Environ. Health B. 8, 39–69.

Pestka, J.J., Uzarski, R.L., Islam, J., 2005. Induction of apoptosis and cytokine production in the Jurkat human T cells by deoxynivalenol: role of mitogen-activated protein kinases and comparison to other 8-ketotrichothecenes. Toxicology 206, 207–219.

Pestka, J.L., 2010. Deoxynivalenol: mechanisms of action, human exposure, and toxicological relevance. Arch. Toxicol. 84, 663–679.

Pinton, P., Nougayrède, J.-P., Del-Rio, J.-C., et al., 2009. The food contaminant deoxynivalenol, decreases intestinal barrier permeability and reduces claudin expression. Toxicol. Appl. Pharmacol. 237, 41–48.

Poppenga, R.H., Lundeen, G.R., Beasley, V.R., 1987. Assessment of a general therapeutic protocol for the treatment of acute T-2 toxicosis in swine. Vet. Hum. Toxicol. 29, 237–239.

Prelusky, D.B., Trenholm, H.L., Lawrence, G.A., et al., 1984. Nontransmission of deoxynivalenol (vomitoxin) to milk following oral administration to dairy cows. J. Environ. Sci. Health B. 19, 593–609.

Prelusky, D.B., Veira, D.M., Trenholm, H.L., et al., 1986a. Excretion profiles of the mycotoxin deoxynivalenol, following oral and intravenous administration to sheep. Fundam. Appl. Toxicol. 6, 356–363.

Prelusky, D.B., Hamilton, R.M.G., Trenholm, H.L., et al., 1986b. Tissue distribution and excretion of radioactivity following administration of 14C-labelled deoxynivalenol to White Leghorn hens. Fundam. Appl. Toxicol. 7, 635–645.

Prelusky, D.B., Yeun, J.M., Thompson, B.K., et al., 1992. Effect of deoxynivalenol on neurotransmitters in discrete regions of swine brain. Arch. Environ. Contam. Toxicol. 22, 36–40.

Rizzo, A.F., Atroshi, F., Ahotupa, M., et al., 1994. Protective effect of antioxidants against free radical-mediated lipid peroxidation induced by DON or T-2 toxin. Zentralbl. Veterinarmed. A. 41, 81–90.

Robison, T.S., Mirocha, C.J., Kurtz, H.J., et al., 1979. Transmission of T-2 toxin into bovine and porcine milk. J. Dairy Sci. 62, 637–641.

Rotter, B.A., Thompson, B.K., Lessard, M., et al., 1994. Influence of low-level exposure to *Fusarium* mycotoxins on selected immunological and hematological parameters in young swine. Fundam. Appl. Toxicol. 23, 117–124.

Rotter, B.A., Prelusky, D.B., Pestka, J.J., 1996. Toxicology of deoxynivalenol (vomitoxin). J. Toxicol. Environ. Health. 48, 1–34.

Rousseaux, C.G., Schiefer, H.B., 1987. Maternal toxicity, embryolethality and abnormal fetal development in CD-1 mice following one oral dose of T-2 toxin. J. Appl. Toxicol. 7, 281–288.

Scott, P.M., 1989. The natural occurrence of trichothecenes. In: Beasley, V.R. (Ed.), Trichothecene Mycotoxicosis: Pathophysiologic Effects, vol. I. CRC Press, Inc., Boca Raton, FL, pp. 1–26.

Sokolović, M., Garaj-Vrhovac, V., Simpraga, B., 2008. T-2 toxin: incidence and toxicity in poultry. Arh. Hig. Rada Toksikol. 59 (1), 43–52, http://dx.doi.org/10.2478/10004-1254-59-2008-1843.

Smalley, E.B., Strong, F.M., 1974. Toxic trichothecenes. In: Purchase, I.F.H. (Ed.), Mycotoxins. Elsevier, New York, NY, pp. 199–228.

Swamy, H.V.L.N., Smith, T.K., MacDonald, E.J., 2004. Effects of feeding blends of grains naturally contaminated with *Fusarium* mycotoxins on brain regional neurochemistry of starter pigs and broiler chickens. J. Anim. Sci. 82, 2131–2139.

Swanson, S.P., Corley, R.A., 1989. The distribution, metabolism, and excretion of trichothecene mycotoxins. In: Beasley, V.R. (Ed.), Trichothecene Mycotoxicosis: Pathophysiologic Effects, vol. I. CRC Press, Inc., Boca Raton, FL, pp. 37–61.

Taylor, M.J., Pang, V.F., Beasley, V.R., 1989. The immunotoxicity of trichothecene mycotoxins. In: Beasley, V.R. (Ed.), Trichothecene Mycotoxicosis: Pathophysiologic Effects, vol. II. CRC Press, Inc., Boca Raton, FL, pp. 1–37.

Tryphonas, H., Iverson, F., So, Y., et al., 1986. Effects of deoxynivalenol (vomitoxin) on the humoral and cellular immunity of mice. Toxicol. Lett. 30, 137–150.

Ueno, Y., 1977. Mode of action of trichothecenes. Pure Appl. Chem. 49, 1737–1745.

Ueno, Y., Sato, N., Ishii, K., et al., 1973. Biological and chemical detection of trichothecene mycotoxins in *Fusarium* species. Appl. Microbiol. 25, 699–704.

Ueno Y. General toxicology. In Ueno Y (Ed). Trichothecenes-Chemical, Biological, and Toxicological Aspects. Elsevier, New York, pp. 135–146.

Valenta, H., Dänicke, S., 2005. Study on the transmission of deoxynivalenol and de-epoxy-deoxynivalenol into eggs of laying hens using a high-performance liquid chromatography–ultraviolet method with clean-up by immunoaffinity columns. Mol. Nutr. Food Res. 49, 779–785.

Vila, B., Jaradat, Z.W., Marquardt, R.R., et al., 2002. Effect of T-2 toxin on *in vivo* lipid peroxidation and vitamin E status in mice. Food Chem. Toxicol. 40, 479–486.

Wang, Z., Wu, Q., Kuča, K., 2014. Deoxynilvalenol: signalling pathways and human exposure risk assessment-an update. Arch. Toxicol. 88, 1915–1928.

Wannemacher, R.W., Wiener, S.L., 1997. Trichothecene mycotoxins (Chapter 34). In: Sidell, F.R., Takafuji, E.D., Franz, D.R. (Eds.), Medical Aspects of Chemical and Biological Warfare. Textbook of Military Medicine Series, Office of The Surgeon General, Department of the Army, United States of America.

Weaver, G.A., Kurtz, H.J., Bates, F.Y., et al., 1978a. Acute and chronic toxicity of T-2 mycotoxin in swine. Vet. Rec. 103, 531–535.

Weaver, G.A., Kurtz, H.J., Mirocha, C.J., et al., 1978b. Mycotoxin-induced abortions in swine. Can. Vet. J. 19, 72–74.

Westlake, K., Mackie, R.I., Dutton, M.F., 1987a. T-2 metabolism by ruminal bacteria and its effect on their growth. Appl. Environ. Microbiol. 53, 587–592.

Westlake, K., Mackie, R.I., Dutton, M.F., 1987b. Effects of several mycotoxins on specific growth rate of *Butyrivibrio fibrisolvens* and toxin degradation in vitro. Appl. Environ. Microbiol. 53, 613–614.

Yang, W., Yu, M., Fu, J., et al., 2014. Deoxynivalenol induced oxidative stress and genotoxicity in human peripheral blood lymphocytes. Food Chem. Toxicol. 64, 383–396.

Zhou, H.-R., Yan, D., Pestka, J.J., 1997. Differential cytokine mRNA expression in mice after oral exposure to the trichothecene vomitoxin (deoxynivalenol): dose response and time course. Toxicol. Appl. Pharmacol. 144, 294–305.

FURTHER READING

Ueno, Y., Ishii, K., Sakai, K., Kanaeda, S., et al., 1972. Toxicological approaches to the metabolites of Fusaria. IV. Microbial survey on "bean-hulls poisoning of horses" with the isolation of toxic trichothecenes, neosolaniol and T-2 toxin of *Fusarium solani* M-1-1. Japanese J. Exp. Med. 42, 187–203.

Chapter 76

Zearalenone

Ramesh C. Gupta, Michelle S. Mostrom and Tim J. Evans

INTRODUCTION

Zearalenone is a nonsteroidal estrogenic mycotoxin produced by several species of *Fusarium* fungi. The primary producer of zearalenone is *Fusarium graminearum* (teleomorph *Gibberella zeae*). Additional *Fusarium* fungi capable of producing zearalenone include *F. culmorum*, *F. verticillioides* (*F. moniliforme*), *F. sporotrichioides*, *F. semitectum*, *F. equiseti*, and *F. oxysporum*. Contamination of cereal grains by zearalenone has been reported worldwide, primarily in temperate climates. Typically, zearalenone concentrations are low in grain contaminated in the field, but increase under storage conditions with moisture greater than 30%–40%. Zearalenone has major effects on reproduction in females (as evidenced by hyperestrogenism), but it affects the male reproductive system as well. Prepubertal swine are the most sensitive species. Typical clinical signs of hyperestrogenism are swelling of the vulva, increase in uterine size and secretions, mammary gland hyperplasia and secretion, prolonged estrus, anestrus, increased incidence of pseudopregnancy, infertility, decreased libido, and secondary complications of rectal and vaginal prolapses, stillbirths, and small litters. Recent reports suggest that zearalenone is also a significant human health concern (EFSA, 2011; Belhassen et al., 2014; Mally et al., 2016). This chapter describes toxicity of zearalenone and its major metabolites in animals.

BACKGROUND

Estrogenism in swine was reported in the mid-1920s in the Midwestern United States (McNutt et al., 1928). A condition of swelling and eversion of the vagina in young gilts and swelling of the prepuce in males was associated with consuming moldy corn. Prolapse of the vagina and occasionally the rectum were noted as secondary effects. With replacement of the moldy corn with clean corn, the animals recovered to normal, but if exposure to moldy corn continued, eversion of the uterus, secondary infections, and death occurred. Mirocha et al. (1971) noted high death losses in some herds and hypothesized that mortality was related to vaginal and rectal prolapses and subsequent septicemias; however, the presence of additional mycotoxins could not be excluded in causing death. Stob et al. (1962) isolated an active metabolite with uterotrophic and anabolic activities from culture of *G. zeae* (*F. graminearum*).

The *Fusarium* compound found in corn with uterotrophic activity was named zearalenone, previously known as F-2, and is chemically described as 6-(10-hydroxy-6-oxo-*trans*-1-undecenyl)-β-resorcylic acid lactone (Fig. 76.1). At least seven derivatives of zearalenone have been found that naturally occur in corn. Zearalenone and uterotrophic active derivatives were classified as estrogens in the sense that they produce estrus or cornification of the vagina of adult mice (Mirocha and Christensen, 1974). Zearalenone can be produced on numerous substrates, including wheat, barley, corn, corn silage, rice, rye, sorghum, and occasionally in forages. Production in soybeans is uncommon. Moisture content and the presence of oxygen are critical factors for zearalenone production. In laboratory cultures, *Fusarium* growth occurs during a 3-week period at moisture levels over 20% and temperature between 20°C and 25°C. If the fungus is stressed by cool temperatures of 8–15°C for several weeks, zearalenone can be produced. Production of zearalenone in the field is similar to that in the laboratory, with alternating moderate and low temperature weather capable of stimulating zearalenone production. Zearalenone can be produced fairly quickly in the field during wet weather in the late summer or early fall following hail damage to corn. Very high concentrations of zearalenone, which can occur naturally in some field samples, generally result from improper storage at high moisture rather than production in the field. Corn stored in a crib and exposed to winter weather was particularly prone to fungal invasion and production of zearalenone. In addition to the cooccurrence of other estrogenic metabolites,

Veterinary Toxicology. DOI: http://dx.doi.org/10.1016/B978-0-12-811410-0.00076-3

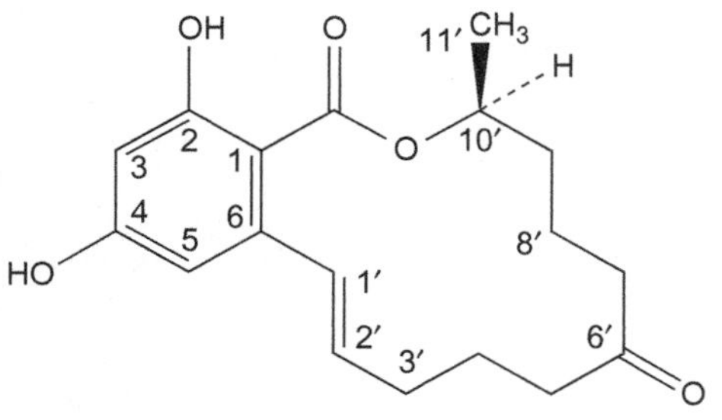

FIGURE 76.1 Chemical structure of zearalenone.

such as α- and β-zearalenols, zearalenone is commonly detected in grains with another *Fusarium* mycotoxin deoxynivalenol. Zearalenone is heat stable, but can be partially destroyed during extrusion cooking of cereals (Castells et al., 2005).

TOXICOKINETICS

The toxicokinetics of zearalenone have been reported in several species following different routes of its administration (Prelusky et al., 1989; Mallis et al., 2003; Dänicke et al., 2005; Shin et al., 2009a,b,c; Devreese et al., 2015). Studies in animals indicate rapid absorption of zearalenone from the gastrointestinal tract (GIT) following oral exposure (Dailey et al., 1980). Oral bioavailability is very low in poultry and rats (<10%) due to extensive metabolism (Fitzpatrick et al., 1988; Zimedine et al., 2007; Shin et al., 2009a; Devreese et al., 2015). Following a single oral dose of 10 mg zearalenone/kg body wt to 15–25 kg pigs, the absorption was approximated to be 80%–85% (Biehl et al., 1993). Once entered in the body, zearalenone is mainly metabolized in the liver, which seems to be one of the main targets of the toxin (Zimedine et al., 2007; Jiang et al., 2012; Koraichi et al., 2012). In liver, zearalenone could impact maternal and fetal liver to ABC transporters substrates, and influence fetal development through nuclear receptor modulation (Koraichi et al., 2012). Zearalenone is also distributed to various other tissues including, kidney, adipose tissue, and estrogen target tissues, such as the uterus, testes, and ovarian follicles (Liang et al., 2015; Mally et al., 2016). In pigs, zearalenone and its metabolites were found in the plasma of a pig in less than 30 min after initiating feeding with the parent compound. Once administered, zearalenone can be localized in reproductive tissues (ovary and uterus) (Gajecka et al., 2012), adipose tissue, and interstitial cells of the testes (Ueno et al., 1977; Kuiper-Goodman et al., 1987). The reported biological half-life of total plasma zearalenone radioactivity following oral dosage in pigs is 86 h (Biehl et al., 1993). Species differences in zearalenone susceptibility might be related to hepatic biotransformation, with the highest amount of α-zearalenol, which has increased estrogenic activity compared to α-zearalanol and zearalenone produced by pig hepatic microsomes, whereas chicken microsomes produced the highest amounts of β-zearalenol, which has lower estrogenic activity (Malekinejad et al., 2006; Zimedine et al., 2007). Zearalenone and its metabolites are conjugated with glucuronic acid (Malekinejad et al., 2006; Pfeiffer et al., 2010). Pigs readily conjugated almost all absorbed zearalenone and α-zearalenol through glucuronidation. While the liver plays a major role in glucuronidation, the intestinal mucosa is also active. Zearalenone was reduced to α- and β-zearalenol in sow intestinal mucosa homogenates (duodenum and jejunum) in vitro (Olsen et al., 1987). Cytochrome P450 may also be involved in zearalenone metabolism (EFSA, 2011). Gastrointestinal flora can aid in the metabolism of zearalenone. Zearalenone can undergo rumen metabolism, with reduction to mostly α-zearalenol and to a lower amount of β-zearalenol (Kiessling et al., 1984). Whether rumen metabolism will increase or decrease zearalenone toxicity depends on absorption by the GIT, liver metabolism by hydroxysteroid dehydrogenase, and competition at the cytosolic receptor sites in the animal species.

Zearalenone undergoes extensive enterohepatic circulation and biliary excretion in most species (Biehl et al., 1993; Shin et al., 2009a,b). The major route of excretion for most species is through the feces, although rabbits primarily excrete zearalenone in the urine. Most zearalenone administered in a dose is excreted within a 72-h period. Approximately 94% of radiolabeled zearalenone, given orally to White Leghorn laying hens at 10 mg/kg body wt, was eliminated through the excreta within 72 h postdosing (Dailey et al., 1980). No major retention of radiolabeled activity was found in edible muscle tissue, but lipophilic metabolite(s) were reported in egg yolk (at about 2 mg/kg concentration) 72 h postdosing.

Concern has focused on potential residue of zearalenone and its metabolites in milk, eggs, and foods and precocious development of sexual characteristics in young female girls (Kuiper-Goodman et al., 1987; JECFA, 2000; Massart et al., 2008). Zearalenone and α- and β-zearalenols can be transmitted into the milk of sheep, cows, and pigs administered high doses of zearalenone (Hagler et al., 1980; Mirocha et al., 1981). Hyperestrogenism has been reported in lambs and pigs nursing dams dosed with zearalenone (Hagler et al., 1980; Palyusik et al., 1980; Smith et al., 1990). Dairy cows fed rations with purified zearalenone at 50 mg zearalenone/day and 165 mg zearalenone/day for 21 days had no detectable concentrations of zearalenone or α- and β-zearalenol in the milk or plasma (Prelusky et al., 1990). One cow dosed with 544.5 mg zearalenone/day for 21 days had maximum concentrations of 2.5 ng zearalenone/mL and 3.0 ng α-zearalanol/mL in the milk. Cows dosed orally with a 1-day dose of 1.8 or 6 g zearalenone had maximum milk levels on day 2 of 4.0 and 6.1 ng zearalenone/mL, respectively. This study indicates a minimal transmission of zearalenone into the milk and only for a short period of time after exposure to high concentrations of zearalenone. Because only minimal amounts of zearalenone and its metabolites could be transmitted to the milk (Prelusky et al., 1990), most animals and humans start to be exposed to zearalenone directly from food, which is the main route for zearalenone exposure.

Following intubations of tritiated-zearalenone into the crops of 7-week-old broiler chickens, the greatest accumulation of radioactivity occurred in the liver 30 min postadministration, which became a trace of radioactivity by 48 h postadministration (Mirocha et al., 1982). Only zearalenone was detected in muscle tissue at approximately 4 ppb at 48-h postadministration, indicating the zearalenone residues in edible tissue are minimal.

MECHANISM OF ACTION

Zearalenone undergoes reduction of the 6′ ketone to a secondary alcohol, which leads to two diastereoisomeric zearalenols (α and β), which are naturally occurring fungal metabolites. The α-zearalenol metabolite is three times more estrogenic than zearalenone, is an anabolic growth-promoting compound, zeeranol or Ralgro, used in both cattle and sheep commercially.

Zearalenone and metabolites can interact directly with the cytoplasmic receptor that binds to 17β-estradiol and translocate receptor sites to the nucleus (Katzenellenbogen et al., 1979). In the nucleus, stimulation of RNA leads to protein synthesis and clinical signs of estrogenism. Following subcutaneous injection of the compounds, the zearalenols and zearalenone stimulated production of a specific uterine protein and increased uterine weights. Within the resorcylic acids, α-zearalenol exhibited the greatest binding affinity for cytosolic estrogen receptors, while zearalenone and β-zearalanol displayed much lower binding affinities (Fitzpatrick et al., 1989). The hydroxylation of zearalenone to α-zearalenol apparently is an activation process, whereas the production of β-zearalenol would be a deactivation process. The relative binding affinity of α-zearalenol was greater in the pig than in the rat or chicken. Interspecies variations and age-related differences in sensitivity to zearalenone in the feed could be related to different metabolites produced and the relative binding affinities of zearalenone and metabolites formed (Malekinejad et al., 2006; Haneweer et al., 2007; Parveen et al., 2009).

Zearalenone can also act on the hypothalamic–hypophysial axis. Using 70-day-old Yorkshire gilts (20–27 kg) fed 1.5–2 mg zearalenone/kg feed for 45–90 days, Rainey et al. (1990) determined that prepubertal exposure to zearalenone affected the hypothalamic–hypophysial axis and the luteinizing hormone (LH) surges that lasted for at least 44 days postexposure. However, zearalenone consumption did not delay the onset of pubertal estrus nor impair conception rates, ovulation rates, or number of fetuses. Slightly older prepubertal gilts (178 days of age and 94 kg) fed 10 mg zearalenone daily for 2 weeks had suppressed mean serum concentrations of LH, but the onset of puberty and subsequent reproduction were not adversely affected (Green et al., 1990). Gilts treated daily with zearalenone in feed (at a corresponding dose of 200 μg/kg body wt) for 8 days revealed disturbances in the development and maturation of the largest ovarian follicles through the activation of an apoptotic-like process in the granular cells (Zwierzchowski et al., 2005). These authors further suggested that α-zearalenol was the chief factor evoking changes in the ovarian follicles in the first days of intoxication. In a transgenerational toxicity study in pigs, Schoevers et al. (2012) demonstrated that zearalenone reduced the quantity of healthy follicles, which may have led to premature oocyte depletion in adulthood. In this study, expression of estrogen receptor β mRNA increased following zearalenone exposure, whereas expression of genes coding for estrogen converting enzymes remained unchanged.

Zhao et al. (2013) emphasized that peripubertal and early pregnancy are two sensitive periods that can be influenced by zearalenone exposure, which affects not only puberty and estrous cyclicity but also early pregnancy events, including fertilization, embryo development, embryo transport, and embryo implantation.

Male rats, 70 days old, dosed orally with zearalenone at 20 mg/kg body wt for 35 days had elevated serum prolactin concentrations but showed no changes in serum LH and follicle stimulating hormone concentrations, body and testes weights, or in spermatogonia, spermatocytes, and spermatids (Milano et al., 1995). In a recent study, Zheng et al. (2016) reported that zearalenone may affect the secretory function of Sertoli cells by disrupting cytoskeletal structure (α-tubulin filaments and F-actin bundles) and by damaging the nucleus of Sertoli cells, and these effects may be an underlying cause of zearalenone-induced male reproductive toxicity. At relatively high concentrations in vitro, approximately 400 μM, zearalenone appeared to act directly on interstitial cells of the testes inhibiting steroidogenesis (Fenske and Fink-Gremmels, 1990). In a recent in vitro study, Liu et al. (2014) demonstrated that zearalenone interferes with testosterone biosynthesis in mouse Leydig cells via the crosstalk of estrogen receptor signaling and orphan nuclear receptor Nur77 expression.

While zearalenone primarily affects reproduction, it appears to have additional effects (such as oxidative stress and inflammation) targeting liver, kidney, spleen and blood in weanling piglets (Tiemann and Danicke, 2007;

Marin et al., 2013; Liang et al., 2015). During exposure of in vitro cell lines, zearalenone acted as a ligand for human pregnene X receptor (hPXR), which can activate a transcription factor regulating the expression of numerous hepatic drug-metabolizing enzymes, including expression of cytochrome P450 enzymes (Ding et al., 2006). This suggests a potential for zearalenone to induce metabolism of drugs.

At natural contamination levels in feeds, zearalenone does not appear to impact the immune response. Results from in vitro studies of zearalenone and metabolites α- and β-zearalenol and α- and β-zearalanol and mitogen testing with leukoagglutinin, concanavalin A, and pokeweed revealed that these mycotoxins inhibited mitogen-induced proliferation of both B and T lymphocytes (Forsell and Pestka, 1985). No treatment differences were observed in B6C3F1 mice fed a diet with 10 mg zearalenone/kg diet for 8 weeks and control mice that were tested with a splenic plaque-forming response to sheep erythrocytes and a delayed hypersensitivity response to keyhole hemocyanin (Pestka et al., 1987).

It needs to be mentioned that in addition to estrogenic activity, zearalenone and its metabolites exert antiandrogenic activity (Molina-Molina et al., 2014). These investigators, in an in vitro study, confirmed that zearalenone and its metabolites are full agonists for human estrogen receptor alpha (hERα) in MCF-7 cells, and possess human androgen receptor (hAR)-mediated antagonistic activity in PALM cells.

TOXICITY

Zearalenone has low acute toxicity in most species, including farm animals (Minervini and Dell' Aquila, 2008). In most natural conditions, concentrations of zearalenone in feed ingredients are less than 20 mg/kg (ppm) and generally less than 5 mg zearalenone/kg feed (Sundlof and Strickland, 1986). Prepubertal swine are most sensitive to zearalenone, ruminants may exhibit some adverse effects, and poultry appear to be the least sensitive species. Females are more sensitive than males, and cycling female pigs may be more sensitive than pregnant sows. Pregnant swine may abort. Abortions have been associated in field cases with natural *Fusarium* mold exposure, but have not been reproduced with purified zearalenone (Mirocha and Christensen, 1974). Younger male pigs appear to be more sensitive than older males and can undergo atrophy of the testes and enlargement of mammary glands (Jakimiuk et al., 2009).

Swine

Gilts fed rations with 0, 3, 6, or 9 mg purified zearalenone/kg feed that started the day after they showed the first estrus were bred at subsequent heat periods (Young and King, 1986a). A majority of gilts fed 6 or 9 mg zearalenone/kg feed became pseudopregnant based on examination of their reproductive tracts or plasma progesterone levels. Gilts fed rations with 3 mg zearalenone/kg feed had no reproductive effects. After removal of zearalenone from the diet, approximately half of the gilts fed 6 or 9 mg zearalenone/kg feed returned to estrus spontaneously. Edwards et al. (1987a) reported luteal maintenance and extended inter-estrous intervals in sexually mature gilts fed purified zearalenone at concentrations of 5–10 mg/kg feed from days 5–20 of the estrous cycle. Approximately 86% of the retained corpora lutea underwent spontaneous regression and most gilts came into estrus within the next 30 days. In a subsequent study, Edwards et al. (1987b) fed prepubertal gilts a diet with 0 or 10 mg zearalenone/kg feed for 30 days from 145 to 193 days of age, switched the gilts to a control diet, and then exposed the gilts to a mature boar. While treated gilts displayed vulvar swelling during the 30-day feeding period and were delayed in showing first estrus, the proportion of gilts showing estrus with exposure to the boar was similar between treatment and control gilts, and subsequent cycling was not affected when the treated feed was removed. Young et al. (1990) reported an increased weaning-to-estrus interval and embryonic mortality (measured as a decreased ratio of fetuses to corpora lutea) and a decreased number of fetuses per sow in second parity sows fed 10 mg zearalenone/kg diet. No reproductive effects were observed in prepubertal gilts fed a ration with 0.5 mg zearalenone/kg feed (Friend et al., 1990).

Young gilts (30–35 kg) administered 5 mg of purified zearalenone *per os* daily developed swelling of the vulva on the fourth day of treatment, an approximate daily dose of 0.143–0.167 mg zearalenone/kg body wt (Mirocha and Christensen, 1974). Gilts dosed with 1 mg of purified zearalenone daily for 8 days developed pronounced vulvar swelling. Gilts exposed to higher concentrations of zearalenone may show atrophy of the ovaries along with edema and cellular proliferation of all layers in the uterus. Kuiper-Goodman et al. (1987) noted a no adverse effects level for zearalenone in pigs reaching puberty at 0.06 mg zearalenone/kg body wt/day.

Male swine fed a high concentration of zearalenone (30 mg/kg feed) appeared to initially have accelerated maturation of spermatogenesis, which occurred 1.5–2 months earlier than control animals (Ványi and Széky, 1980). Although germinal epithelium damage was limited to several foci initially, with continued zearalenone exposure the damage became widespread, with proliferation of the interstitium around seminiferous tubules. Young and King (1986b) fed lower levels of zearalenone in the diet (0, 3, 6, and 9 mg zearalenone/kg feed) to boars from 32 days of age up to 145 or 312 days of age. Feeding up to 9 mg zearalenone/kg feed to the boars did not affect libido, but boars fed the highest dose of zearalenone produced lower total and gel-free volumes of semen with lower total motile sperm. Zearalenone does not appear to affect mature boars. No adverse effects in reproductive parameters, including testicular size, libido, sperm motility and morphology, plasma testosterone and 17β-estradiol concentrations, were reported in mature Yorkshire boars fed increasing concentrations of purified zearalenone at 0, 2, 20, and 200 mg/kg ration for 8 weeks (Ruhr et al., 1983).

The European Union (2006) guidance values for zearalenone in feedstuff (with a moisture content of 12%) for piglets and gilts is 0.1 mg/kg or ppm, for sows and fattening pigs is 0.25 mg/kg, and for calves, dairy cattle, sheep, and goats is 0.5 mg/kg.

Ruminants

Several case reports have associated dairy herd health problems and zearalenone in moldy feed. Young dairy heifers, 6–14 months of age, developed slight enlargement of at least one mammary gland quarter while fed moldy corn in a ration (Bloomquist et al., 1982). Following a change in the ration, the heifers returned to normal 7 weeks later. Zearalenone contamination of the moldy ration was detected by thin-layer chromatography. Roine et al. (1971) reported turbid discharge from the vulva, obvious estrous behavior lasting for 1–2 weeks, and infertility in dairy cows and heifers. Strains of *F. graminearum* and *F. culmorum* were isolated from the feed that caused an increase in uterine weight in rats and were capable of producing between 3 and 9.5 mg zearalenone/kg feed. Ványi et al. (1974) reported a drop in milk production, feed intake, and swelling of the vulva in dairy cows exposed to varying concentrations of zearalenone, ranging from 5 to 75 mg zearalenone/kg feed. In an experimental study, 18 cycling heifers were dosed with 0 or 250 mg of purified zearalenone daily through one nonbreeding estrous cycle and the next two consecutive estrous cycles during which the heifers were bred (Weaver et al., 1986a). The authors calculated that treated heifers were given an average of 250 mg zearalenone/364 kg body wt/day or 0.69 mg zearalenone/kg body wt/day. The control and treated heifers had conception rates of 87% and 62%, respectively, at a statistical probability of $P = .065$. Eighteen dairy cows (three cows per group) dosed orally with 0, 31.25, 62.5, 125, 250, and 500 mg of purified zearalenone daily for two consecutive estrous cycles had no changes in serum progesterone concentration, erythrocyte and leukocyte blood counts, packed cell volume, estrous cycle length, clinical health, or sexual behavior (Weaver et al., 1986b).

Zearalenone can affect ewe reproduction when ewes are exposed to the mycotoxin prior to mating. Zearalenone, administered orally at concentrations greater than 3 mg/animal/day, given to ewes prior to mating depressed ovulation rates and reduced lambing percentages (Smith et al., 1990). Ewes administered a similar range of oral doses of zearalenone (0, 1.5, 3, 6, 12, and 24 mg/ewe/day) for 10 days, starting 5 days after mating, showed no effect of zearalenone exposure after mating on pregnancy rate or embryonic loss. Breeding rams fed a diet containing 12 mg zearalenone/kg feed for 8 weeks had no significant adverse effects on semen volume, concentration, motility, or morphology during the trial and for 6 weeks after zearalenone feeding was ceased (Milano et al., 1991).

Equine

Gimeno and Quintanilla (1983) reported estrogenic signs of edematous vulvas, prolapsed vaginas, oversized uteruses, and internal hemorrhage in mares and severe flaccidity of genitals in two male horses fed corn screenings for 30 days in a field exposure. All sick animals collapsed with respiratory paralysis and sudden blindness, and died quickly. Analysis for zearalenone in the feed detected 2–3 mg zearalenone/kg diet. While the authors tested for a variety of mycotoxins by thin-layer chromatography, fumonisins in the corn screenings were not determined because they had not yet been recognized as mycotoxins and a cause of death in horses. Fumonisins would have to be considered as a primary cause of some of the adverse effects, particularly blindness and death, in these horses.

In a study of six cycling trotter mares, Juhász et al. (2001) determined that daily oral administration of 7 mg purified zearalenone starting 10 days after ovulation until the subsequent ovulation had no adverse effect on reproduction. Zearalenone had no effect on the length of the interovulatory intervals, luteal and follicular phases of the ovary, and did not significantly affect uterine edema. The authors noted that zearalenone exposure started 10 days after ovulation and the exposure period to zearalenone was short in this study. The dose of purified zearalenone represented a natural contamination of feed of about 1 mg zearalenone/kg feed and ranged between 0.013 and 0.010 mg zearalenone/kg body wt/day for approximately 8–10 days.

Poultry

Growing female White Leghorn chickens dosed once orally with 15 g zearalenone/kg body wt showed no adverse effects in reproductive tissues (Chi et al., 1980). In a second experiment, chickens dosed orally or intramuscularly with increasing concentrations of zearalenone

(0–800 mg/kg body wt) for 7 consecutive days had increased oviduct weights with increasing zearalenone doses. Poultry appear to be fairly resistant to the effects of zearalenone.

TREATMENT

Quick removal of zearalenone contaminated feed from the ration and replacement with clean feed is essential. Generally, 3–7 weeks following removal of the contaminated feed, animals will return to normal reproductive status. No zearalenone mycotoxin binder has been proven to be efficacious in any species of livestock by the US Food and Drug Administration.

BIOMONITORING AND RISK ASSESSMENT

Biomonitoring is an integrative approach to assess animal or human exposure to toxicants/toxins from various sources and by all routes, using appropriate and validated biomarkers (Gupta, 2014; Föllmann et al., 2016). Multiple state-of-the art validated methods are available for quantification and confirmation of zearalenone and its metabolites for toxicokinetics, biomonitoring and risk assessment (Shin et al., 2009c; Gambacorta et al., 2013; Belhassen et al., 2014: Föllmann et al., 2016; Mally et al., 2016). Urinary concentrations of zearalenone and its metabolites from humans and pigs support biomonitoring as a viable approach to assess human exposure to zearalenone (Njumbe Ediage et al., 2013; Wallin et al., 2015). Measurement of α- and β-zearalenols is as important as zearalenone, since both metabolites are endocrine disrupting compounds (Metzler et al., 2010; Frizzell et al., 2011; Zhao et al., 2013; Molina-Molina et al., 2014). Based on animal and human toxicokinetic data, and validated PBPK models, human exposure to zearalenone and modified forms of zearalenone may be close to or even exceed the tolerable daily intake (TDI) derived by the European Food Safety Authority (EFSA) for some consumer groups (Mally et al., 2016). While zearalenone exhibits low acute toxicity, long-term exposure to zearalenone may present a health risk due to its high estrogenic activity. The maximum allowable amount of zearalenone in foods and feeds ranges from 50 to 1000 μg/kg in various countries (FAO, 2004), and a TDI of 0.1 μg/kg was proposed as a margin of safety in humans (Kuiper-Goodman et al., 1987). The EFSA Panel on Contaminants in the Food Chain derived a TDI for zearalenone of 0.25 μg/kg body wt based on a NOEL of 10 μg/kg body wt/day for estrogenic effects in female pigs (reddened/swollen vulva and cervix, increased uterus weight) as the most sensitive endpoint of zearalenone toxicity with an uncertainty factor of 40 (4 for interspecies differences in toxicokinetics and 10 for interhuman variability) (JECFA, 2000; EFSA, 2011, 2014; Mally et al., 2016).

CONCLUDING REMARKS AND FUTURE DIRECTIONS

Maintaining moisture concentrations less than 15%–16% in feeds should adequately prevent zearalenone production during storage. When naturally contaminated feed must be used, incorporation into rations for less susceptible species, such as feedlot animals or poultry, should be considered. At naturally occurring concentrations of zearalenone in grains, residues in meat, milk, and eggs are probably not significant. The effects of zearalenone have been widely investigated, especially in sensitive animal species such as swine. Sows are more sensitive than boars, and immature gilts are more sensitive than adults. Future studies are needed to identify novel biomarkers for detecting early effects of zearalenone and its metabolites on reproductive and developmental, and other organs.

REFERENCES

Belhassen, H., Jiménez-Díaz, I., Ghali, R., et al., 2014. Validation of a UHPLC-MS/MS method for quantification of zearalenone, α-zearalenol, β-zearalenol and zearalenone in human urine. J. Chromatogr. B. 962, 68–74.

Biehl, M.L., Prelusky, D.B., Koritz, G.D., et al., 1993. Biliary excretion and enterohepatic cycling of zearalenone in immature pigs. Toxicol. Appl. Pharmacol. 121, 152–159.

Bloomquist, C., Davidson, J.N., Pearson, E.G., 1982. Zearalenone toxicosis in prepubertal dairy heifers. J. Am. Vet. Med. Assoc. 189, 164–165.

Castells, M., Marin, S., Sanchis, V., Ramos, A.J., 2005. Fate of mycotoxins in cereals during extrusion cooking: a review. Food Addit. Contam. 22, 150–157.

Chi, M.S., Mirocha, C.J., Weaver, G.A., et al., 1980. Effect of zearalenone on female White Leghorn chickens. Appl. Environ. Microbiol. 39, 1026–1030.

Dailey, R.E., Reese, R.E., Brouwer, E.A., 1980. Metabolism of [14C] zearalenone in laying hens. J. Agric. Food Chem. 28, 286–291.

Dänicke, S., Swiech, E., Buraczewska, L., et al., 2005. Kinetics and metabolism of Zearalenone in young female pig. J. Anim. Physiol. Anim. Nutr. 89, 268–276.

Devreese, M., Antonissen, G., Broekaert, N., et al., 2015. Comparative toxicokinetics, absolute oral bioavailability, and biotransformation of zearalenone in different poultry species. J. Agric. Food Chem. 63, 5092–5098.

Ding, X., Lichti, K., Staudiner, J.L., 2006. The mycoestrogen zearalenone induces CYP3A through activation of the pregnene X receptor. Toxicol. Sci. 91, 448–455.

Edwards, S., Cantley, T.C., Rottinghaus, G.E., et al., 1987a. The effects of zearalenone on reproduction in swine. I. The relationship between ingested zearalenone dose and anestrus in non-pregnant, sexually mature gilts. Theriogenology 28, 43–49.

Edwards, S., Cantley, T.C., Day, B.N., 1987b. The effects of zearalenone on reproduction in swine. II. The effect on puberty attainment and post weaning rebreeding performance. Theriogenology 28, 51–58.

EFSA, 2011. Scientific opinion on the risks for public health related to the presence of zearalenone in food. EFSA J. 9, 2197.

EFSA, 2014. Evaluation of the increase of risk for public health related to a possible temporary derogation from the maximum level of deoxynivalenol, zearalenone and fumonisins for maize and maize products. EFSA J. 12, 3699.

EU Commit. Official Journal of the European Union Commission Recommendation of 17 August 2006. The Commission of European Communities 23.8.2006. Brussels.

FAO, 2004. Worldwide Regulations for Mycotoxin in Food and Feed in 2003. FAO Food and Nutrition Paper No. 81. Food and Agriculture Organization of the United Nations, Rome.

Fenske, M., Fink-Gremmels, J., 1990. Effects of fungal metabolites on testosterone secretion *in vitro*. Arch. Toxicol. 64, 72–75.

Fitzpatrick, D.W., Arbuckle, L.D., Hassen, A.M., 1988. Zearalenone metabolism and excretion in the rat: effect of different doses. J. Environ. Sci. Health B. 23, 343–354.

Fitzpatrick, D.W., Picken, C.A., Murphy, L.C., et al., 1989. Measurement of the relative binding affinity of zearalenone, α-zearalenol and β-zearalenol for uterine and oviduct estrogen receptors in swine, rats and chickens: an indicator of estrogenic potencies. Comp. Biochem. Physiol. 94C, 691–694.

Föllmann, W., Ali, N., Blaszkewicz, M., et al., 2016. Biomonitoring of mycotoxins in urine: pilot study in mill workers. J. Toxicol. Environ. Health Part A. 79, 1015–1025.

Forsell, J.H., Pestka, J.J., 1985. Relation of 8-ketotrichothecene and zearalenone analog structure to inhibition of mitogen-induced human lymphocyte blastogenesis. Appl. Environ. Microbiol. 50, 1304–1307.

Friend, D.W., Trenholm, H.L., Thompson, B.K., et al., 1990. The reproductive efficiency of gilts feds very low levels of zearalenone. Can. J. Anim. Sci. 70, 635–645.

Frizzell, C., Ndossi, D., Verhaegen, S., et al., 2011. Endocrine disrupting effects of zearalenone, alpha- and beta-zearalenone at the level of nuclear receptor binding and steroidogenesis. Toxicol. Lett. 206, 210–217.

Gajecka, M., Rybarczyk, L., Jakimiuk, E., et al., 2012. The effect of experimental long-term exposure to low-dose zearalenone on uterine histology in sexually immature gilts. Exp. Toxicol. Pathol. 64, 537–542.

Gambacorta, I., Solfrizzo, M., Visconti, A., et al., 2013. Validation study on urinary biomarkers of exposure for aflatoxin B_1, ochratoxin A, fumonisin B_1, deoxynivalenol and zearalenone in piglets. World Mycotoxin J. 6, 299–308.

Gimeno, A., Quintanilla, J.A., 1983. Analytical and mycological study of a natural outbreak of zearalenone mycotoxicosis in horses. Proceedings of International Symposium on Mycotoxins. National Research Centre, Cairo, Egypt, pp. 387–392.

Green, M.L., Diekman, M.A., Malayer, J.R., et al., 1990. Effect of prepubertal consumption of zearalenone on puberty and subsequent reproduction of gilts. J. Anim. Sci. 68, 171–178.

Gupta, R.C. (Ed.), 2014. Biomarkers in Toxicology. Academic Press/ Elsevier, Amsterdam, 1128 pp.

Hagler, W.M., Dankó, G., Horvath, L., et al., 1980. Transmission of zearalenone and its metabolite into ruminant milk. Acta Vet. Acad. Sci. Hung. 28, 209–216.

Haneweer, M., Houtman, R., Poortman, J., et al., 2007. Estrogenic effects in the immature rat uterus after dietary exposure to ethinylestradiol and zearalenone using a system biology approach. Toxicol. Sci. 99 (1), 303–314.

Jakimiuk, E., Gajecka, M., Jana, B., et al., 2009. Factors determining sensitivity of prepubertal gilts to hormonal influence of zearalenone. Pol. J. Vet. Sci. 12, 149–158.

JECFA, Joint FAO/WHO Expert Committee on Food Additives, 2000. Zearalenone. In: Safety Evaluation of Certain Food Additives and Contaminants, WHO Food Additives Series, vol. 44, pp. 393–482.

Jiang, S.Z., Yang, Z.B., Yang, W.R., et al., 2012. Effect on hepatonephric organs, serum metabolites, and oxidative stress in postweaning piglets fed purified zearalenone-contaminated diets with or without Calibrin-Z. J. Anim. Physiol. Anim. Nutr. (Berlin). 96, 1147–1156.

Juhász, J., Nagy, P., Kulcsár, M., et al., 2001. Effect of low-dose zearalenone exposure on luteal function, follicular activity, and uterine oedema in cycling mares. Acta Vet. Hung. 49, 211–222.

Katzenellenbogen, B.S., Katzenellenbogen, J.A., Mordecai, D., 1979. Zearalenones: characterization of the estrogenic potencies and receptor interactions of a series of fungal È-resorcylic acid lactones. Endocrinology 105, 33–40.

Kiessling, K.H., Pettersson, H., Sandholm, K., et al., 1984. Metabolism of aflatoxin, ochratoxin, zearalenone, and three trichothecenes by intact rumen fluid, rumen protozoa, and bacteria. Appl. Environ. Microbiol. 47, 1070–1073.

Koraichi, F., Videmann, B., Mazallon, M., et al., 2012. Zearalenone exposure modulates the expression of ABT transporters and nuclear receptors in pregnant rats and fetal liver. Toxicol. Lett. 211, 246–256.

Kuiper-Goodman, T., Scott, P.M., Watanabe, H., 1987. Risk assessment of the mycotoxin zearalenone. Regul. Toxicol. Pharmacol. 7, 253–306.

Liang, Z., Ren, Z.H., Gao, S., et al., 2015. Individual and combined effects of deoxynivalenol and zearalenone on mouse kidney. Environ. Toxicol. Pharmacol. 40 (3), 686–691.

Liu, Q., Wang, Y., Gu, J., et al., 2014. Zearalenone inhibits testosterone biosynthesis in mouse Leydig cells via the crosstalk of estrogen receptor signalling and orphan nuclear receptor Nur77 expression. Toxicol. In Vitro 28 (4), 647–656.

Malekinejad, H., Maas-Bakker, R., Fink-Gremmels, J., 2006. Species differences in the hepatic biotransformation of zearalenone. Vet. J. 172, 96–102.

Mallis, L.M., Sarkahian, A.B., Harris, H.A., et al., 2003. Determination of rat oral bioavailability of soy-derived phytoestrogens using an automated on-column extraction procedure and electrospray tendem mass spectrometry. J. Chromatogr. B. 796, 71–86.

Mally, A., Solfrizzo, M., Degen, G.H., 2016. Biomonitoring of the mycotoxin zearalenone: current state-of the art and application to human exposure assessment. Arch. Toxicol. 90 (6), 1281–1292.

Marin, D.E., Pistol, G.C., Neagoe, I.V., et al., 2013. Effects of zearalenone on oxidative stress and inflammation in weanling piglets. Food Chem. Toxicol. 58, 408–415.

Massart, F., Meucci, V., Saggese, G., et al., 2008. High-growth rate of girls with precocious puberty exposed to estrogenic mycotoxins. J. Pediatr. 152 (5), 690–695.

McNutt, S.H., Purwin, P., Murray, C., 1928. Vulvovaginitis in swine. J. Am. Vet. Med. Assoc. 26, 484–492.

Metzler, M., Pfeiffer, E., Hildebrand, A., 2010. Zearalenone and its metabolites as endocrine disrupting chemicals (EDC). World Mycotoxin J. 3, 385–401.

Milano, G.D., Odriozola, E., Lopez, T.A., 1991. Lack of effect of a diet containing zearalenone on spermatogenesis in rams. Vet. Rec. 129, 33–35.

Milano, G.D., Becu-Villalobos, D., Tapia, O., 1995. Effects of long-term zearalenone administration on spermatogenesis and serum luteinizing hormone, follicle-stimulating hormone, and prolactin values in male rats. Am. J. Vet. Res. 56, 954–958.

Minervini, F., Dell' Aquila, M.E., 2008. Zearalenone and reproductive function in farm animals. Int. J. Mol. Sci. 9, 2570–2584.

Mirocha, C.J., Christensen, C.M., 1974. Oestrogenic mycotoxins synthesized by *Fusarium*. In: Purchase, I.F.H. (Ed.), Mycotoxins. Elsevier, New York, NY, pp. 129–148.

Mirocha, C.J., Christensen, C.M., Nelson, G.H., 1971. F-2 (zearalenone) estrogenic mycotoxin from *Fusarium*. In: Kadis, S., Ciegler, A., Ajl, S.J. (Eds.), Microbial Toxins, vol. VII. Academic Press, New York, NY, pp. 107–138.

Mirocha, C.J., Pathre, S.V., Robison, T.S., 1981. Comparative metabolism of zearalenone and transmission into bovine milk. Food Cosmet. Toxicol. 19, 25–30.

Mirocha, C.J., Robison, T.S., Pawlosky, R.J., et al., 1982. Distribution and residue determination of [3H]zearalenone in broilers. Toxicol. Appl. Pharmacol. 66, 77–87.

Molina-Molina, J.-M., Real, M., Jimenez-Diaz, I., et al., 2014. Assessment of estrogenic and anti-androgenic activities of the mycotoxin zearalenone and its metabolites using *in vitro* receptor-specific bioassays. Food Chem. Toxicol. 74, 233–239.

Njumbe Ediage, E., Mavungu, D.D.J., Song, S., et al., 2013. Multimycotoxin analysis in urines to assess infant exposure: a case study in Cameroon. Environ. Int. 57-58, 50–59.

Olsen, M., Pettersson, H., Sandholm, K., et al., 1987. Metabolism of zearalenone by sow intestinal mucosa *in vitro*. Food Chem. Toxicol. 25, 681–683.

Palyusik, M., Harrach, B., Mirocha, C.J., et al., 1980. Transmission of zearalenone and zearalenol into porcine milk. Acta Vet. Acad. Sci. Hung. 28, 217–222.

Parveen, M., Zhu, Y., Kiyama, R., 2009. Expression profiling of the genes responding to zearalenone and its analogues using estrogen-responsive genes. FEBS Lett. 583 (14), 2377–2384.

Pestka, J.J., Tai, J.H., Witt, M.F., et al., 1987. Suppression of immune response in the B6C3F1 mouse after dietary exposure to the *Fusarium* mycotoxins deoxynivalenol (vomitoxin) and zearalenone. Food Chem. Toxicol. 25, 297–304.

Pfeiffer, E., Hildebrand, A., Mikula, H., et al., 2010. Glucuronidation of zearalenone, zeranol, and four metabolites *in vitro*: formation of glucuronides by various microsomes and human UDP-glucuronosyltransferase isoforms. Mol. Nutr. Food Res. 54, 1468–1476.

Prelusky, D.B., Warner, R.M., Trenholm, H.L., 1989. Sensitive analysis of the mycotoxin zearalenone and its metabolites in biological fluids by high-performance liquid chromatography. J. Chromatogr. 494, 267–277.

Prelusky, D.B., Scott, P.M., Trenholm, H.L., et al., 1990. Minimal transmission of zearalenone to milk of dairy cows. J. Environ. Sci. Health. B25, 87–103.

Rainey, M.R., Tubbs, R.C., Bennett, L.W., et al., 1990. Prepubertal exposure to dietary zearalenone alters hypothalamo-hypophysial function but does not impair postpubertal reproductive function of gilts. J. Anim. Sci. 68, 2015–2022.

Roine, K., Korpinen, E.L., Kallela, K., 1971. Mycotoxicosis as a probable cause of infertility in dairy cows. Nord. Vet. Med. 23, 628–633.

Ruhr, L.P., Osweiler, G.D., Foley, C.W., 1983. Effect of the estrogenic mycotoxin zearalenone on reproductive potential in the boar. Am. J. Vet. Res. 44, 483–485.

Schoevers, E.J., Santos, R.R., Colenbrander, B., et al., 2012. Transgenerational toxicity of zearalenone in pigs. Reprod. Toxicol. 34, 110–119.

Shin, B.S., Hong, S.H., Bulitta, J.B., et al., 2009a. Disposition, oral bioavailability, and tissue distribution of zearalenone in rats at various dose levels. J. Toxicol. Environ. Health Part A. 72, 1406–1411.

Shin, B.S., Hong, S.H., Bulitta, J.B., et al., 2009b. Physiologically based pharmacokinetics of zearalenone. J. Toxicol. Environ. Health Part A. 72, 1395–1405.

Shin, B.S., Hong, S.H., Hwang, S.W., et al., 2009c. Determination of zearalenone by liquid chromatography/tandem mass spectrometry and application to a pharmacokinetic study. Biomed. Chromatogr. 23, 1014–1021.

Smith, J.E., di Menna, M.E., McGowan, L.T., 1990. Reproductive performance of Coopworth ewes following oral doses of zearalenone before and after mating. J. Reprod. Fert. 89, 99–106.

Stob, M., Baldwin, R.S., Tuite, J., et al., 1962. Isolation of an anabolic, uterotrophic compound from corn infected with *Gibberella zeae*. Nature 29, 1318.

Sundlof, S.F., Strickland, C., 1986. Zearalenone and zearanol: potential residue problems in livestock. Vet. Hum. Toxicol. 28, 242–250.

Tiemann, U., Danicke, S., 2007. *In vivo* and *in vitro* effects of the mycotoxins zearalenone and deoxynivalenol on different non-reproductive and reproductive organs in female pigs: a review. Food Addit. Contam. 243 (3), 306–314.

Ueno, Y., Ayaki, S., Sato, N., et al., 1977. Fate and mode of action of zearalenone. Ann. Nutr. Aliment. 31, 935–948.

Ványi, A., Széky, A., 1980. Fusariotoxicoses. VI. The effect of F-2 toxin (zearalenone) on the spermatogenesis of male swine. Magy Állatorv Lapja. 35, 242–246.

Ványi, A., Szemerédi, G., Szailer, E.R., 1974. Fusariotoxicoses on a cattle farm. Magy Állatorv Lapja. 29, 544–546.

Wallin, S., Gambacorta, L., Kotova, N., et al., 2015. Biomonitoring of concurrent mycotoxin exposure among adults in Sweden through urine multibiomarker analysis. Food Chem. Toxicol. 83, 133–139.

Weaver, G.A., Kurtz, H.J., Behrens, J.C., et al., 1986a. Effect of zearalenone on the fertility of virgin heifers. Am. J. Vet. Res. 47, 1395–1397.

Weaver, G.A., Kurtz, H.J., Behrens, J.C., et al., 1986b. Effect of zearalenone on dairy cows. Am. J. Vet. Res. 47, 1826–1828.

Young, L.G., King, G.J., 1986a. Low concentrations of zearalenone in diets of mature gilts. J. Anim. Sci. 63, 1191–1196.

Young, L.G., King, G.J., 1986b. Low concentrations of zearalenone in diets of boars for a prolonged period of time. J. Anim. Sci. 63, 1197–1200.

Young, L.G., Ping, H., King, G.J., 1990. Effects of feeding zearalenone to sows on rebreeding and pregnancy. J. Anim. Sci. 68, 15–20.

Zhao, F., Li, R., Xiao, S., et al., 2013. Preweaning exposure to dietary zearalenone, a mycotoxin, promotes premature onset of puberty and disrupts early pregnancy events in female mice. Toxicol. Sci. 132 (2), 431–442.

Zheng, W., Pan, S.Y., Wang, G., et al., 2016. Zearalenone impairs the male reproductive system functions via inducing structural and functional alterations of sertoli cells. Environ. Toxicol. Pharmacol. 42, 146–155.

Zimedine, A., Soriano, J.M., Moltó, J.C., et al., 2007. Review on the toxicity, occurrence, metabolism, detoxification, regulations and intake of zearalenone: an estrogen mycotoxin. Food Chem. Toxicol. 45, 1–18.

Zwierzchowski, W., Przybylowicz, M., Obremski, K., et al., 2005. Level of zearalenone in blood serum and lesions in ovarian follicles of sexually immature gilts in the course of zearalenone micotoxicosis. Pol. J. Vet. Sci. 8 (3), 209–218.

Section XVI

Feed and Water Contaminants

Chapter 77

Melamine and Cyanuric Acid

Karyn Bischoff

INTRODUCTION

Melamine, or 1,3,5-triazine-2,4,6-triamine, is a small, nitrogen-rich molecule used in the manufacture of plastics, adhesives, cleaners, and yellow dye. Though once considered practically nontoxic based on early laboratory animal studies, significant morbidity and mortality related to crystalluria, nephrolithiasis, and renal tubular necrosis have resulted from pet food contamination.

Beginning in early 2007, reports of renal failure in cats and dogs fed various commercial pet foods led to concerns about possible contamination, and a widespread recall of suspect foods was initiated prior to identification of the toxin. Eventually, >150 pet food products were identified as containing contaminated ingredients and were recalled. Analysis revealed that these products contained up to approximately 3200 ppm melamine and 600 ppm cyanuric acid (Cianciolo et al., 2008; Skinner et al., 2010). Samples of imported wheat gluten used in the pet food manufacture contained 8.4% melamine as well as the following melamine breakdown products: 5.3% cyanuric acid, 2.3% ammelide, and 1.7% ammeline (Rumbeiha et al., 2010). Melamine had been added to pet food ingredients to fraudulently increase the apparent protein concentration (McEvoy, 2016). Because melamine is 67% nitrogen, based on molecular weight, and protein is commonly estimated based on the nitrogen content of a feed or food measured via the Kjeldahl or similar method, the addition of melamine increased the apparent protein content.

It was later determined that similar episodes of pet food contamination had occurred in Asia and South Africa. An incident in 2004 was estimated to have affected more than 6000 dogs and cats in the Republic of Korea, Japan, Thailand, Malaysia, Singapore, Taiwan, and the Philippines. Earlier in 2007, there was a melamine-associated pet food recall in South Africa (Osborne et al., 2008; Yhee et al., 2009). Aside from pet food, feeds intended for chickens, hogs, and fish were also contaminated (Reimschuessel et al., 2008, 2009). Melamine-contaminated pet food scraps were fed on hog farms in seven US states and contaminated feeds were traced to 38 poultry farms and at 197 fish hatcheries (Acheson, 2007; FDA, 2010). Contamination of agricultural feeds had also happened previously, and investigation of renal failure in piglets in Spain between 2003 and 2006 found that the kidneys contained melamine, cyanuric acid, and relatively high concentrations of ammelide and ammeline (Gonzalez et al., 2009). Later, hundreds of fur-bearing raccoon dogs in China died after being fed melamine-contaminated feeds in 2008 (Bhalla et al., 2009).

The 2007 pet food recall was considered a sentinel event by some (Osborne et al., 2008; Lewin-Smith et al., 2009; McEvoy, 2016). Indeed, 1 year later, melamine contamination of milk-based products, particularly baby formula, was detected in China. Chinese authorities detected melamine concentrations between 2.5 and 2563 ppm in 13 commercial brands of milk powder and trace contamination of 9 others (Bhalla et al., 2009). Approximately 300,000 children could have been affected, more than 52,000 were hospitalized, and, unfortunately, 6 died. Children in Taiwan, Hong Kong, and Macau could also have been affected (Hau et al., 2009; Reimschuessel et al., 2009; Skinner et al., 2010; McEvoy, 2016). Due to global marketing of products and ingredients, melamine-contaminated products were found in almost 70 countries, including the United States.

SOURCE

Melamine, or 1,3,5-triazine-2,4,6-triamine (Fig. 77.1), which contains three carbon atoms, six nitrogen atoms, and six hydrogen atoms, was first synthesized in the 1830s and has found numerous uses in manufacturing. Melamine is polymerized with formaldehyde to produce a variety of durable resins, adhesives, cleansers, and flame retardants. Melamine is also a major ingredient in the pigment Yellow 150, used in textile dyes and inks. China,

Veterinary Toxicology. DOI: http://dx.doi.org/10.1016/B978-0-12-811410-0.00077-5

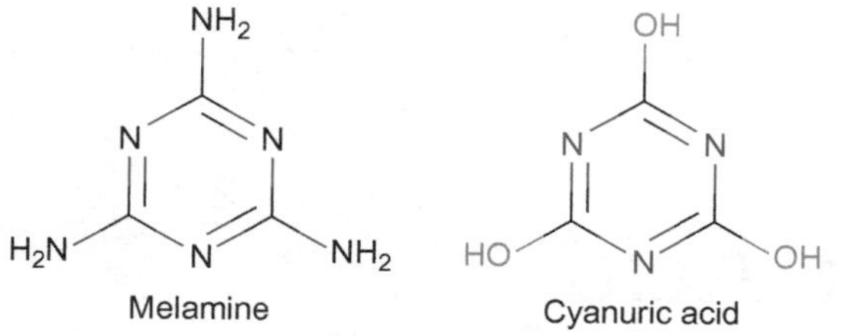

FIGURE 77.1 Structural formulas of melamine and cyanuric acid.

the largest melamine producer, produces a quarter of the melamine used in the world.

Cyanuric acid, often found as a cocontaminant with melamine, is an intermediate produced during melamine manufacture and degradation. It is commonly used to stabilize chlorine in swimming pools and in the manufacture of bleach, disinfectants, and herbicides (Dalal and Goldfarb, 2011).

PHARMACOKINETICS/TOXICOKINETICS

Melamine is minimally, if at all, metabolized in most monogastric mammals, but could be partially metabolized in the rumen of cattle and small ruminants. There is some evidence of metabolism of melamine to cyanuric acid in poultry (Suchý et al., 2014). Approximately 90%–95% of ingested melamine is absorbed in chickens and ducks (Poapolathep et al., 2015; Suknikom et al., 2016). Melamine does not accumulate over time in the animal body. The half-life for urinary elimination of melamine is given as 6 h in dogs and approximately 4 h in swine (Lipschitz and Stokey, 1945; Yang et al., 2011). Renal elimination of unchanged melamine is almost complete after 32 h in poultry (Poapolathep et al., 2015). Therefore, melamine should be almost completely excreted within 2 days of the last exposure in these monogastric mammals and birds; however, crystals were seen microscopically in feline kidneys 8 weeks after dietary exposure to melamine and cyanuric acid (Cianciolo et al., 2008). The elimination half-life of melamine in small ruminants is three- to sixfold slower than in monogastrics, possibly due to prolonged sequestration in the rumen (Baynes et al., 2010). Urinary excretion accounted for 54.1% of melamine administered to sheep, and 23.7% was found in the feces (Cruywagen et al., 2011).

Detectable melamine concentrations have been reported in edible tissues from animals. It was estimated that 3.6% of melamine fed to sheep partitioned to muscle (Cruywagen et al., 2011). Melamine concentrations in the kidney were higher than concentrations in the skeletal muscle or liver in lambs, and these concentrations decreased below 20 ppb 4 days after cessation of exposure, but addition of cyanuric acid to the diet did not affect melamine deposition (Lv et al., 2010). The highest tissue melamine concentrations in chickens fed melamine-containing diets were found in the kidneys, with lower concentrations in the liver and muscle (Bai et al., 2010; Suknikom et al., 2016; Zapletal et al., 2016). Tissue residues were depleted 10–20 days after exposure ceased (Bai et al., 2010). Melamine administered to pregnant rats was detected in the placenta and fetuses (Jingbin et al., 2010).

Melamine concentrations were detected in catfish and trout within 1 day of dosing, and the half-life of melamine in skeletal muscle of fish ranged from 1.5 to 4 days (Reimschuessel et al., 2009). Due to the longer elimination half-life of melamine and cyanuric acid in fish, these compounds do not need to be given together. Melamine can be given 1–3 days after cyanuric acid (dependent on fish species) and produce crystals, and cyanuric acid can be given 7–14 days (dependent on species) after melamine and produce crystals (Reimschuessel et al., 2010).

Melamine is excreted by dairy cattle into milk, particularly in high-producing cattle, though milk yield and composition are otherwise unaffected. Melamine can be detected in milk within 8 h of exposure and remains detectable until 4 days after cessation of exposure. Transfer efficiency from feed to cows' milk was calculated to be between 0.66% and 0.95% and was not dependent on melamine dose (Shen et al., 2010). Approximately 0.3% of a melamine dose was excreted in milk in dairy goats, and milk melamine concentrations remained above the level of concern (1.0 μg/mL) until 3 days after cessation of dosing (Baynes et al., 2010).

Melamine fed to chickens is deposited within eggs within a day or 2 days postexposure (Chen et al., 2010; Bai et al., 2010). The melamine concentration in eggs is proportional to the dietary concentration; a dietary concentration of 164 ppm could produce an actionable melamine concentration in eggs of 2.5 ppm (Chen et al., 2010). A 4-day withdrawal period has been recommended for eggs from melamine-exposed chickens, though trace concentrations of melamine remain detectable in eggs for about 9 days after exposure ceases (Yang et al., 2011).

MECHANISM OF ACTION

Though previous animal studies found that both melamine and cyanuric acid were relatively nontoxic when given individually, they caused crystal formation in renal tubules of mammals when given together (Puschner and Reimschuessel, 2011). Melamine and cyanuric acid crystallize, forming a molecular lattice structure, at a pH of 5.8 (Osborne et al., 2008; Bhalla et al., 2009). Crystals recovered from kidneys and urine of cats that ingested melamine-contaminated food contained 70% cyanuric acid and 30% melamine, based on infrared spectra results (Osborne et al., 2008; Thompson et al., 2008).

Renal pathology is believed to result from intratubular obstruction causing increased intrarenal pressure. This may be the explanation of the renal hemorrhage and inflammation reported in affected cats and dogs. Since melamine has diuretic properties, pre-renal azotemia could contribute to the renal pathology (Bhalla et al., 2009).

Cyanuric acid did not contribute to the formation of urinary calculi in children as it did in companion animals (Gao, 2010). However, calculi in children were produced by a similar interaction between melamine and uric acid. This interaction has also been reported in poultry (Bai et al., 2010). Humans and most other primates lack the enzyme uricase, which converts uric acid to allantoin (Reimschuessel et al., 2008). Compared to adults, human infants excrete between five and eight times more uric acid, which increases their susceptibility to melamine toxicosis (Skinner et al., 2010). Urinary pH <5.5 is associated with the formation of urate crystals and low pH is believed to be involved in melamine/urate crystal formation (Gao, 2010). Crystals associated with nephrotoxicosis in infants contained melamine and uric acid at a molar ratio of 1:1–2, respectively (Skinner et al., 2010; Wen et al., 2010). Birds and reptiles also excrete uric acid; therefore, susceptibility in these species could be similar to those seen in human neonates. Dalmatian dogs, too, have reduced uric acid metabolism, and thus excrete uric acid.

TOXICITY

Melamine, by itself, has relatively low toxicity based on animal studies. The oral LD_{50} of melamine is 3200 mg/kg in male rats, 3800 mg/kg in female rats, 3300 mg/kg in male mice and 7000 mg/kg in female mice. Long-term administration of melamine to laboratory rodents at concentrations ranging from 0.225% to 0.9% of the diet produces urolithiasis. Lesions in the urinary bladder, including transitional cell carcinoma, were observed in rats fed diets containing 0.45% melamine (Melnick et al., 1984). The mechanism of carcinogenesis was most likely secondary to epithelial hyperplasia caused by mechanical irritation (Melnick et al., 1984; Hau et al., 2009). Urolithiasis was consistently identified in rats fed diets containing 0.3%–3.0% melamine (Okumura et al., 1992). Renal cortical fibrosis and lymphoplasmacytic nephritis were reported in female rats fed diets containing 0.45% melamine (Melnick et al., 1984). Among domestic animals, sheep given single (217 mg/kg) or multiple (200–1351 mg/kg/day) doses of melamine had dose-dependent clinical signs of anorexia, anuria, and uremia after 5–31 days (Clark, 1966). Dogs fed 125 mg/kg melamine had crystalluria but no other adverse effects were identified (Lipschitz and Stokey, 1945). Poultry fed diets containing >1% melamine had decreased feed intake and weight gain, and mortality increased at a dietary melamine concentration >2% (Brand et al., 2012).

Cyanuric acid has similarly low toxicity when given alone. It produces degenerative renal changes in guinea pigs when given at 30 mg/kg body weight for 6 months, in rats fed a diet containing 8% monosodium cyanurate for 20 weeks, and in dogs fed a diet containing 8% monosodium cyanurate. Lesions included ectasia of the distal collecting tubules and multifocal epithelial cell proliferation (Canelli, 1974).

The combination of melamine and cyanuric acid is markedly more toxic to most domestic animals than either compound when given alone. Administration of 50 mg/kg melamine or cyanuric acid to rats did not result in adverse effects, but when both were given together at the dose of 50 mg/kg, evidence of nephropathy was observed (Puschner and Reimschuessel, 2011). Cats fed diets containing up to 1% melamine or cyanuric acid alone had no evidence of clinical abnormalities. However, cats fed diets containing 0.2% each of both melamine and cyanuric acid had evidence of acute renal failure and crystaluria within 48 h due to renal tubular necrosis. Lesions typical of those associated with the pet food recall were observed (Puschner et al., 2007). A pig fed 400 mg/kg melamine and 400 mg/kg cyanuric acid daily had bloody diarrhea within 24 h, which resolved. Necropsy revealed perirenal edema and round golden-brown crystals with radiating striations in the kidneys. Similar lesions were present in tilapia, rainbow trout and catfish dosed with 400 mg/kg each of melamine and cyanuric acid per day for 3 days, though most of the fish survived the renal damage (Reimschuessel et al., 2008).

CLINICAL SIGNS

Early clinical signs of vomiting and inappetence were apparent in cats and dogs ingesting contaminated food, followed later by evidence of renal failure. The most common clinical signs in cats and dogs were inappetence, vomiting, polyuria, polydipsia, and lethargy (Cianciolo et al., 2008). The most common symptoms described in children were increased or reduced frequency of urination or anuria, hematuria, stranguria, and unexplained crying, but many children were asymptomatic (Hau et al., 2009; Wen et al., 2010; Hu et al., 2010).

CLINICAL PATHOLOGY

Affected cats had urine specific gravities <1.035, elevated serum urea nitrogen and creatinine concentrations within 36 h, and hyperkalemia and hyperphosphatemia (Cianciolo et al., 2008; Puschner and Reimschuessel, 2011). Urinalysis revealed the presence of circular green-brown crystals in urine sediment (Cianciolo et al., 2008).

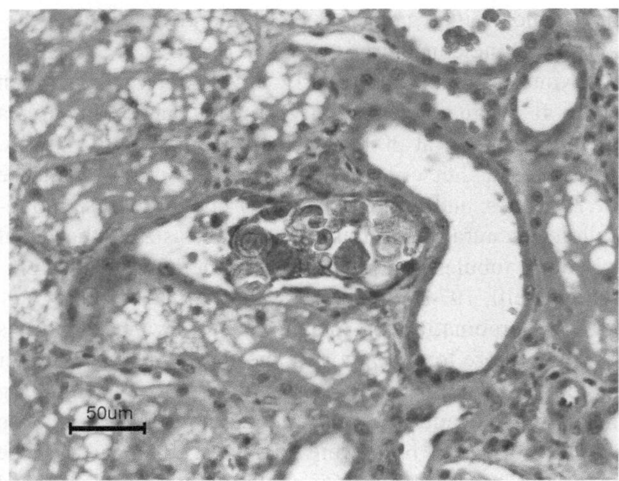

FIGURE 77.2 Renal histology from a cat that ingested melamine and cyanuric acid contaminated food. Typical crystals are present within the renal tubule at the center. *Courtesy of Dr. R. Cianciolo.*

Serum chemistry findings included elevated serum urea nitrogen and creatinine concentrations.

Serum chemistry findings in affected infants included elevated serum potassium, urea nitrogen, and creatinine concentrations (Sun et al., 2010). Hematuria and the presence of fan-shaped crystals was reported in urine samples and urine pH ranged from 5.0 to 7.5 (Hau et al., 2009).

PATHOLOGY

Postmortem findings from animals that died typically included bilateral renomegaly and evidence of uremia (Thompson et al., 2008; Cianciolo et al., 2008).

Microscopic lesions were found primarily in the kidneys. Renal tubular necrosis with evidence of rupture and regeneration were present. Distal convoluted tubules contained large golden-brown birefringent crystals (15–80 μm in diameter; Fig. 77.2) with centrally radiating striations, sometimes in concentric rings, and smaller amorphous crystals (Cianciolo et al., 2008; Thompson et al., 2008). Crystals were spherical with a hedgehog-like appearance on images from scanning electron microscopy (Fig. 77.3). Crystals were still present in distal convoluted tubules 8 weeks after cessation of exposure to contaminated feed (Cianciolo et al., 2008). Perivascular inflammation of subcapsular veins was also reported.

Melamine/cyanuric acid crystals could be differentiated from more common types of urinary crystals based on morphology and histochemistry or special staining. Von Kossa stains calcium oxalate and calcium phosphate crystals and Alizarin red S at pH between 4.1 and 4.3 stains calcium phosphate crystals only, but neither stains melamine/cyanuric acid crystals. Oil red O, usually used to identify lipids, stains melamine/cyanuric acid crystals but not calcium

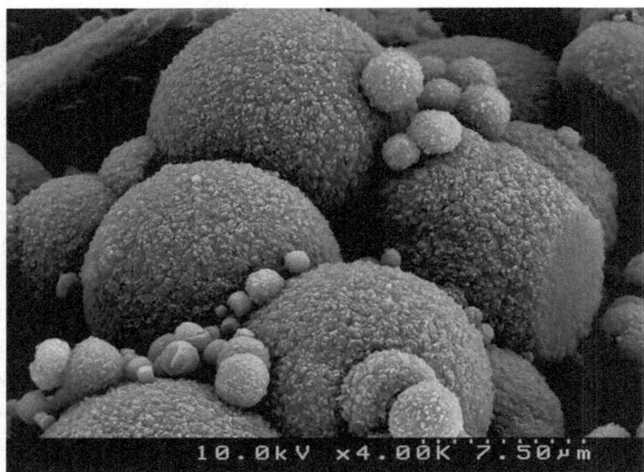

FIGURE 77.3 Scanning electron micrograph of melamine/cyanuric acid crystals from the urine of a cat. *Courtesy of Dr. B. Hoff.*

oxalate or calcium phosphate crystals (Cianciolo et al., 2008). Melamine/cyanuric acid crystals dissolve over time when kidney sections are stored in formalin (Puschner and Reimschuessel, 2011).

A cat that was euthanized 8 weeks after exposure had moderate tubular necrosis with regeneration and severe crystalluria. The finding of severe perivenous fibrosis and venous luminal stenosis in this cat was of concern because it suggests that cats that survived melamine-induced acute renal failure may have been predisposed to chronic renal ischemia leading to chronic renal disease (Cianciolo et al., 2008).

Lesions secondary to uremia were sometimes observed in affected cats and included bilateral white plaques on the ventral surface of the tongue and gastric mineralization (Cianciolo et al., 2008).

Glomerular sclerosis, swelling and necrosis of renal tubular epithelium, tubular dilation with tubular dilation with lumenal crystals, and an interstitial lymphoplasmacytic infiltrate were noted in a renal biopsy from a melamine-affected child. These changes were hypothesized to be due to urinary tract obstruction (Sun et al., 2010). Stones found in the urinary tract of affected children ranged in size from 2 to 18 mm in diameter, and approximately half were <5 mm in diameter. Diameter of the stone correlated with concentration of melamine in the diet, but not the duration of exposure (Hu et al., 2010). Renal calculi were usually bilateral, and calculi were sometimes found in the ureter, unilaterally or bilaterally, and in the urinary bladder (Hau et al., 2009; Gao, 2010; Wen et al., 2010).

Fish may be more susceptible to melamine toxicosis than mammals, and feeding a melamine-contaminated diet to tilapia was associated with prominent lesions affecting the liver and gills as well as the kidneys (Phromkunthong et al., 2013).

DIAGNOSIS

Diagnosis of melamine poisoning is based on the presence of melamine and cyanuric acid in samples of urine or kidney from affected animals, or the contaminated food or feed. Gas chromatograph/mass spectroscopy (GC/MS) and liquid chromatography/tandem MS are used to analyze for melamine and cyanuric acid (Cianciolo et al., 2008; Hon et al., 2011; Puschner and Reimschuessel, 2011). Infrared spectroscopy or Raman spectroscopy can be used to determine the composition of the urine crystals (Puschner and Reimschuessel, 2011). Identification of crystals on histopathology or urinalysis is also helpful in the diagnosis.

TREATMENT AND PROGNOSIS

The basic treatment regimens for crystalluria and urolithiasis related to melamine ingestion include fluid therapy and supportive care in both veterinary and pediatric patients (Anonymous, 2007; Wen et al., 2010). Increased water intake and fluid therapy were used to increase urine output. Because low urinary pH is associated with crystal formation in infants, alkalization of the urine was used to maintain urine pH between 6.0 and 7.8 in affected children. Sodium bicarbonate or potassium citrate was added to intravenous fluids for this purpose (Gao, 2010; Wen et al., 2010).

Antispasmodic drugs, such as anisodamine or atropine, were given to facilitate excretion of uroliths in children, and pain management was instituted (Bhalla et al., 2009; Wen et al., 2010). Most children recovered with this conservative management (Gao, 2010; Wen et al., 2010). However, hemodialysis was required in some patients, as was surgical intervention (Wen et al., 2010). Most children recovered fully, but 12% were found to have renal abnormalities 6 months after treatment (Liu et al., 2010).

Analysis of 586 cases reported during the pet food recall of 2007 by veterinarians and accredited veterinary diagnostic laboratories found 451 cases matching the case definition of melamine toxicosis, of which 65.5% were cats and 34.4% were dogs. Older animals and animals with preexisting conditions were less likely to survive, and 73.3% of affected dogs and 61.5% of affected cats died (Rumbeiha et al., 2010). However, >80% of exposed cats during the original feeding trials survived, suggesting that not all exposed cats became severely affected (Cianciolo et al., 2008).

CONCLUDING REMARKS AND FUTURE DIRECTIONS

Melamine poisoning in small animals and infants was associated with intentional, fraudulent contamination of pet food and milk products to increase the apparent protein concentration. Although there are some data on the number of infants affected, there is no way to determine the number of cats and dogs affected by the pet food recalls in 2007 because of a lack of veterinary care for many animals and a lack of central reporting of morbidity and mortality for companion animals. Estimates vary depending on the source and have ranged from 571 to 39,000 cats and dogs (Osborne et al., 2008; Puschner and Reimschuessel, 2011). Although many cats and dogs succumbed to melamine toxicosis, others survived with supportive and symptomatic care. There are few data on the long-term effects of melamine on cats and dogs.

REFERENCES

Acheson, D., 2007. Importation of Contaminated Animal Feed Ingredients. Statement Before the House Committee on Agriculture. Washington DC, United States, May 9, 2007.

Anonymous, 2007. Specialists confer about the pet food recall. J. Am. Vet. Med. Assoc. 233, 1603.

Bai, X., Bai, F., Zhang, K., et al., 2010. Tissue deposition and residue depletion in laying hens exposed to melamine-contaminated diets. J. Agric. Food Chem. 58, 5414–5420.

Baynes, R.E., Barlow, B., Mason, S.E., Riviere, J.E., 2010. Disposition of melamine residues in blood and milk from dairy goats exposed to an oral bolus of melamine. Food Chem. Toxicol. 48, 2542–2546.

Bhalla, V., Grimm, P., Chertow, G.M., Pao, A.C., 2009. Melamine nephrotoxicity: an emerging epidemic in an era of globalization. Kidney Int. 7, 774–779.

Brand, L.M., Murarolli, R.A., Gelven, R.E., et al., 2012. Effects of melamine in young broiler chickens. Poultry Sci. 91, 2022–2029.

Canelli, E., 1974. Chemical, bacteriological, and toxicological properties of cyanuric acid and chlorinated isocyanurates as applied to swimming pool disinfection, a review. Am. J. Pub. Health. 64, 155–162.

Chen, Y., Wenjun, Y., Wang, Z., et al., 2010. Deposition of melamine in eggs from laying hens exposed to melamine contaminated feed. J. Agric. Food Chem. 58, 3512–3516.

Cianciolo, R.E., Bischoff, K., Ebel, J., et al., 2008. Clinicopathologic, histologic, and toxicologic findings in 70 cats inadvertently exposed to pet food contaminated with melamine and cyanuric acid. J. Am. Vet. Med. Assoc. 333, 729–737.

Clark, R., 1966. Melamine crystalluria in sheep. J. S. Afr. Vet. Med. Assoc. 37, 349–351.

Cruywagen, C.W., van de Vyer, W.F.J., Stander, M.A., 2011. Quantification of melamine absorption, distribution to tissues and excretion by sheep. J. Anim. Sci. 89, 2164–2169.

Dalal, R.P., Goldfarb, D.S., 2011. Melamine-related kidney stones and renal toxicity. Nat. Rev. Nephrol. 7, 267–274.

FDA, 2010. Melamine Pet Food Recall – Frequently Asked Questions February 2, 2010. Retrieved July 3, 2010, from United States Food and Drug Administration Department of Health and Human Services: <http://www.fda.gov/animalveterinary/safety-health/RecallsWithdrawals/ucm129932.htm#AnimalFeed>.

Gao, J.Y.S., 2010. Therapeutic effects of potassium sodium, hydrogen citrate on melamine-induced urinary calculi in China. Chin. Med. J. 123, 1112–1116.

Gonzalez, J., Puschner, B., Pérez, V., et al., 2009. Nephrotoxicosis in Iberian piglets subsequent to exposure to melamine and derivatives in Spain between 2003 and 2006. J. Vet. Diagn. Invest. 21, 536–558.

Hau, A.K., Kwan, T.H., Kam-tao, P., 2009. Melamine toxicity in the kidney. J. Am. Soc. Nephrol. 20, 245–250.

Hon, P.Y.T., Chu, P.W.S., Cheng, C.H., et al., 2011. Development of melamine certified reference material in milk using two different isotope dilution mass spectrometry techniques. J. Chromatogr. A. 1218, 6907–6913.

Hu, P., Ling, L., Hu, B., Zhang, C.R., 2010. The size of melamine-induced stones is dependent on the melamine content of the formula fed, but not the duration of exposure. Ped. Nephrol. 25, 565–566.

Jingbin, W., Ndong, M., Kai, H., et al., 2010. Placental transfer of melamine and its effects on rat dams and fetuses. Food Chem. Toxicol. 48, 1791–1795.

Lewin-Smith, M.R., Kalasinsky, V., Mullick, F.G., Thompson, M.E., 2009. Melamine-containing crystals in the urinary tracts of domestic animals: sentinel event? Arch. Pathol. Lab. Med. 133, 341–342.

Lipschitz, W.L., Stokey, E., 1945. The mode of action of three new diuretics: melamine, adenine, and formoguanamine. J. Pharmacol. Exp. Ther. 82, 235–348.

Liu, J.M., Ren, A., Yang, L., et al., 2010. Urinary tract abnormalities in Chinese rural children who consumed melamine-contaminated dairy products: a population-based screening and follow-up study. Can. Med. Assoc. J. 182, 439–443.

Lv, X., Wang, J., Wu, L., et al., 2010. Tissue deposition and residue depletion in lambs exposed to melamine and cyanuric acid-contaminated diets. J. Agric. Food Chem. 58, 943–948.

McEvoy, J.D.G., 2016. Emerging food safety issues: an EU perspective. Drug Test Anal. 8, 511–520.

Melnick, R.L., Boorman, G.A., Haseman, J.K., et al., 1984. Urolithiasis and bladder carcinogenicity of melamine in rodents. Toxicol. Appl. Pharmacol. 72, 292–303.

Okumura, M., Hasegawa, R., Shirai, T., Ito, M., Yamada, S., Fukushima, S., 1992. Relationship between calculus formation and carcinogenesis in the urinary bladder of rats administered the non-genotoxic agents, thymine or melamine. Carcinogenesis 13, 1043–1045.

Osborne, C.A., Lulich, J.P., Ulrich, L.K., 2008. Melamine and cyanuric acid-induced crystaluria, uroliths, and nephrotoxicity in dogs and cats. Vet. Clin. N. Am. Small Anim. 39, 1–14.

Phromkunthong W., Nuntapong N., Boonyaratpalin M., Kiron V., Toxicity of melamine, an adulterant in fish feeds: experimental assessment of its effects on tilapia, J. Fish Diseases 36, 2013, 555–568.

Poapolathep, S., Klangkaew, N., Arreesrisom, P., et al., 2015. Toxicokinetics and absolute oral bioavailability of melamine in broiler chickens. J. Vet. Pharmacol. Ther. 38, 101–104.

Puschner, B., Reimschuessel, R., 2011. Toxicosis caused by melamine and cyanuric acid in dogs and cats: uncovering the mystery and subsequent global implications. Clin. Lab. Med. 31, 181–199.

Puschner, B., Poppenga, R., Lowenstine, L., et al., 2007. Assessment of melamine and cyanuric acid toxicity in cats. J. Vet. Diagn. Invest. 19, 616–624.

Reimschuessel, R., Gieseker, C.M., Miller, R.A., et al., 2008. Evaluation of the renal effects of experimental feeding of melamine and cyanuric acid to fish and pigs. Am. J. Vet. Res. 69, 1217–1228.

Reimschuessel, R., Evans, E., Andersen, W.C., et al., 2009. Residue depletion of melamine and cyanuric acid in catfish and rainbow trout following oral administration. Vet. Pharmacol. Ther. 33, 172–182.

Reimschuessel, R., Evans, E., Stine, C.B., et al., 2010. Renal crystal formation after combined or sequential oral administration of melamine and cyanuric acid. Food Chem. Toxicol. 48, 2898–2906.

Rumbeiha, W.K., Agnew, D., Maxie, G., et al., 2010. Analysis of a survey database of pet food-induced poisoning in North America. J. Med. Toxicol. 6, 172–184.

Shen, J.S., Wang, J.Q., Wei, H.Y., et al., 2010. Transfer efficiency of melamine from feed to milk in lactating dairy cows fed with different doses of melamine. J. Dairy Sci. 93, 2060–2066.

Skinner, C.G., Thomas, J.D., Osterloh, J.D., 2010. Melamine toxicity. J. Med. Toxicol. 6, 50–55.

Suchý, P., Novák, P., Zapletal, D., Straková, E., 2014. Effect of melamine-contaminated diet on tissue distribution of melamine and cyanuric acid, blood, variables, and egg quality in laying hens. Br. Poult. Sci. 55, 375–379.

Suknikom, P., Jermnak, U., Poapolathep, S., et al., 2016. Dipositions and tissue depletion of melamine in ducks. J. Vet. Pharmacol. Ther. 39, 90–94.

Sun, N., Shen, Y., He, L.J., 2010. Histopathological features of the kidney after acute renal failure from melamine. N. Engl. J. Med. 362, 662.

Thompson, M.E., Lewin-Smith, M.R., Kalasinsky, K., et al., 2008. Characterization of melamine-containing and calcium oxalate crystals in three dogs with suspected pet food-induced nephrotoxicosis. Vet. Pathol. 55, 417–426.

Wen, J.G., Li, Z.Z., Zhang, H., et al., 2010. Melamine related bilateral renal calculi in 50 children: single center experience in clinical diagnosis and treatment. J. Urol. 183, 1533–1538.

Yang, T., Huangfu, W.G., Wu, Y.L., 2011. Melamine residues in eggs of laying hens exposed to melamine-contaminated feed. Poultry Sci. 90, 701–704.

Yhee, J.Y., Brown, C.A., Yu, C.H., et al., 2009. Retrospective study of melamine/cyanuric acid-induced renal failure in dogs in Korea between 2003 and 2004. Vet. Pathol. 46, 348–354.

Zapletal, D., Strakova, E., Novak, P., Suchy, P., 2016. Broiler chickens exposed to melamine and cyanuric acid-contaminated diets. Hum. Exp. Toxicol. 35, 760–766.

FURTHER READING

Bischoff, K., 2011. Melamine and cyanuric acid. In: Gupta, R.C. (Ed.), Reproductive and Developmental Toxicology. Academic Press/ Elsevier, Amsterdam.

Chapter 78

Ionophores

Meliton N. Novilla

INTRODUCTION

Ionophores are compounds that form lipid soluble, dynamically reversible complexes with cations and by this means facilitate specific ionic transport across biologic membranes (Pressman, 1976; Reed, 1982; Taylor et al., 1982). There are two major subclasses of ionophores, (1) neutral ionophores, which are highly toxic because they form charged complexes that are capable of perturbing biologic membranes and action potentials, and (2) carboxylic ionophores, which form zwitterionic complexes with cations and promote electrically neutral cation exchange diffusion that is tolerated better in intact organisms. The ionophoric activity may alter normal concentration gradients resulting in cellular ion imbalance, pH change, calcium overload, lipid peroxidation, and disruption of plasma membranes. The alteration in the membrane transport of ions is the basis for the metabolic, organic, and functional effects of this class of compounds. Since their pharmacologic activity is dose related, the usefulness of carboxylic ionophores is based on selective toxicity to protozoan parasites and bacteria and margins of safety in the approved target species. Desirable effects occur when animals are provided feed containing approved dosage ranges, but higher levels may result in adverse effects.

This chapter attempts to provide an overview of ionophores as they relate to veterinary medicine, with emphasis on ionophore-induced toxicity. Large numbers of ionophore safety and toxicity studies have been conducted in support of marketing approval, but results of many studies are unpublished. For this reason, information presented was gleaned from published laboratory and field reports of toxicoses in various species of animals, available reviews and Freedom of Information summaries obtained from the US FDA. However, due to space limitations, not all information can be included, hence apologies are extended to laboratory scientists and field researchers whose work has been omitted or inadvertently missed.

BACKGROUND

Presently, seven carboxylic ionophores are approved for the control of coccidiosis and promotion of growth and feed efficiency in several animals of economic importance. Since their introduction carboxylic ionophores have played significant roles in livestock and poultry production systems throughout the world. Monensin, first introduced as Coban in the United States for the control of coccidiosis in chickens in 1971, was later marketed in 1975 as Rumensin to promote growth and/or increase feed efficiency in cattle. Similarly, lasalocid has been marketed since 1977 as Avatec for chickens and since 1982 as Bovatec for cattle. Later, laidlomycin (Cattlyst) was used in cattle and salinomycin (Bio-cox, Sacox), narasin (Monteban, Maxiban), maduramicin (Cygro), and semduramycin (Aviax) were used in chickens respectively (Fig. 78.1).

Other benefits of ionophore use include (1) reduction of coccidial oocyst discharge in ruminants, (2) prevention of acute bovine pulmonary edema and emphysema, (3) decreased incidence of bloat, (4) prevention of ruminal lactic acidosis, and (5) amelioration of ketosis in lactating dairy cows (Duffield et al., 2002; Heuer et al., 2001; Parker et al., 1986; Nocerini et al., 1985). The reduction of deaths in some cattle herds has been hypothetically related to the reduction of indigestion, metabolic stress, bloat and enterotoxemia associated with monensin feeding.

Potential uses of the ionophores are under experimental investigation in many parts of the world and off-label uses of some ionophores are known to occur. Monensin has been used for the control of toxoplasmosis in pregnant sheep (Buxton et al., 1988), disseminated visceral

Veterinary Toxicology. DOI: http://dx.doi.org/10.1016/B978-0-12-811410-0.00078-7

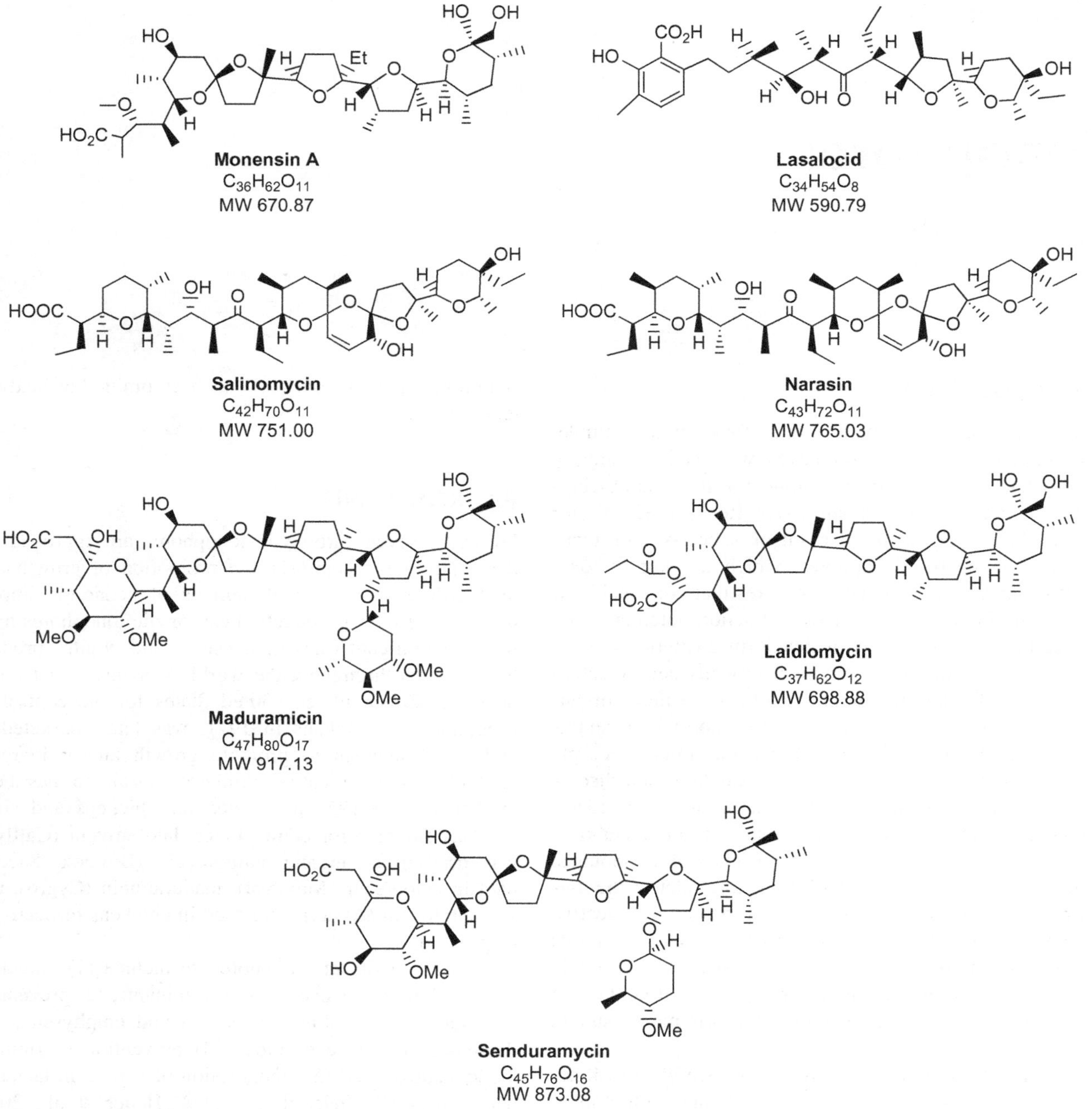

Monensin A
$C_{36}H_{62}O_{11}$
MW 670.87

Lasalocid
$C_{34}H_{54}O_8$
MW 590.79

Salinomycin
$C_{42}H_{70}O_{11}$
MW 751.00

Narasin
$C_{43}H_{72}O_{11}$
MW 765.03

Maduramicin
$C_{47}H_{80}O_{17}$
MW 917.13

Laidlomycin
$C_{37}H_{62}O_{12}$
MW 698.88

Semduramycin
$C_{45}H_{76}O_{16}$
MW 873.08

FIGURE 78.1 Structures of carboxylic ionophores.

coccidiosis in cranes (Carpenter and Novilla, 1992), diarrheal disease in swine (Kyriakis et al., 1993), gregarine infections in shrimp (Jones et al., 1994; Fajer-Avila et al., 2005), and microsporidial gill disease in fish (Becker et al., 2002). Experimental studies on the use of ionophores for the treatment of malaria (Adovelande and Schrevel, 1996; Gumila et al., 1997), mycobacteriosis (Brumbaugh et al., 2004; Greenstein et al., 2009), lead poisoning (Hamidinia et al., 2002) and as an aid in the potentiation of anticancer therapies (Griffin et al., 1993; Shaik et al., 2001) have been conducted. Salinomycin has been shown to selectively kill breast cancer stem cells and apoptotic resistant cancer cells and is considered to be a potential anticancer drug for the prevention and treatment of cancer (Huczynski, 2012). These studies were conducted in cell culture or as challenge studies in laboratory animals and have shown some degree of efficacy. In spite of these encouraging results, there have been no reports of investigational use of ionophores in humans.

PHARMACOLOGY/PHARMACOKINETICS

Pharmacology

Investigational studies were conducted to determine if ionophores had any undesirable pharmacological properties. A series of general pharmacology studies was conducted with monensin (Novilla, 2004). The studies with monensin assessed its effects on the central, peripheral and autonomic nervous systems and the digestive, respiratory and cardiovascular systems. The test systems with doses and route of administration and no-observed-effect-level (NOEL) are shown in Table 78.1.

In mice, an oral dose of 10 mg monensin/kg produced no significant effects on general behaviors, coordinating activity in skeletal muscles, electroshock seizures and acetic acid writhing. However, slight sedation, decreased sensitivity to tactile stimulation, slight depression of muscular coordination and depressed acetic acid writhing occurred at 30 mg/kg. In cats, immobilized by D-tubocurarine or anaesthetized with urethane and α-chloralose, an oral dose of 30 mg/kg produced no effect on the electroencephalogram and the spinal reflex. At the same dose in anaesthetized cats, the heart rate, electrocardiogram, respiration and blood pressure responses to epinephrine, acetylcholine (ACh), histamine and contractions of the nictitating membrane in response to electrical stimulation of the cervical sympathetic ganglion were not affected. Charcoal meal transit in mice was not affected by an oral dose of 10 mg/kg while 30 mg/kg significantly depressed the transit rate. Gastric secretion was not affected by an oral dose of 30 mg/kg in rats. In isolated guinea pig illegal preparations, monensin in a bath concentration of 10^{-5} g/mL had no antagonistic effects on contractures induced by ACh, histamine and barium chloride. In the rat anticarrageenan edema test, monensin given orally at 30 mg/kg did not significantly inhibit carrageenan-induced edema of the hind paw.

The studies targeting specific organ systems of laboratory animals indicated that monensin at a dose of 10 mg/kg

TABLE 78.1 General Pharmacology Studies on Monensin

Test System	Species	Monensin Dose (mg/kg)	Route	NOEL (mg/kg)
General behavior	Mouse	0, 10 and 30	Oral	10
Coordinating activity of skeletal muscles	Mouse	0, 10 and 30	Oral	10
Antielectroshock seizures	Mouse	0 and 30	Oral	30
Analgesic effect	Mouse	0, 10 and 30	Oral	10
Spinal reflex	Cat	0 and 30	Oral	30
Electroencephalogram (D-tubocurarine immobilized)	Cat	0 and 30	Oral	30
Circulatory, respiratory and autonomic effects	Cat	0 and 30	Oral	30
Charcoal meal transit	Mouse	0, 10 and 30	Oral	10
Gastric secretion	Rat	0 and 30	Oral	30
Isolated ileum	Guinea pig	1×10^{-5} g/mL	In vitro	1×10^{-5} g/mL
Carrageenan-induced edema	Rat	0 and 30	Oral	30
Cardiovascular study	Dog (conscious)	0, 0.0069, 0.0138, 0.0345, 0.0690 and 0.138	Intravenous	0.0345
		0, 0.138, 0.345, 0.690 and 1.38	Oral	0.345[a]
Cardiovascular and respiratory effects	Dog (anesthetized)	0, 0.00069, 0.0014, 0.0035, 0.0069, 0.014, 0.035, 0.069, 0.14, 0.35, 0.69 and 1.4	Intravenous	0.0035
Cardiovascular and respiratory effects	Pig (anesthetized)	0, 0.00069, 0.0014, 0.0035, 0.0069, 0.014, 0.035, 0.069, 0.14, 0.35 and 0.69	Intravenous	0.0035

[a]*Based on transient increases in coronary blood flow at doses ≥ 0.69 mg/kg.*

orally produced no effect on the central, peripheral and autonomic nervous systems or the respiratory and digestive systems. However, striated (heart and skeletal) muscle has been identified as the primary targets of toxicity in laboratory animals and domestic livestock given large doses of monensin and other ionophores by oral or parenteral routes (Todd et al., 1984; Novilla and Folkerts, 1986; Van Vleet et al., 1991; Novilla and Todd, 1991; Dowling, 1992).

The cardiovascular effects of oral and intravenous administration of monensin were evaluated in conscious dogs (Holland, 1978). In the oral study, doses of 0, 0.138, 0.345, 0.69, or 1.38 mg monensin/kg body weight in 15 mL of 10% acacia were given by gavage to four or six dogs. Effects were limited to increased coronary blood flow at doses $\geq$0.69 mg monensin/kg. At the 0.69 mg/kg dose, coronary flow increased from 24 mL/min before dosing to a maximum of 40 mL/min 17.5 min after dosing. At the 1.38 mg/kg dose, coronary flow increased from 18 mL/min predosing to a maximum of 49 mL/min 13 min after dosing. In both cases, coronary blood flow had returned to normal levels by 30 min after dosing. Heart rate and mean blood pressure of monensin-treated dogs did not change significantly from the controls at any dose level. Coronary artery flow did not increase following doses of 0.138 and 0.345 mg monensin/kg. In the intravenous (IV) study, coronary blood flow, blood pressure and heart rate were measured in each of six dogs given total cumulative doses of 0.0069, 0.0138, 0.0345, 0.069 and 0.138 mg monensin/kg body weight. Four control dogs were given dextrose alone. Coronary artery flow significantly increased at 0.069 and 0.138 mg/kg and mean blood pressure increased significantly at 0.138 mg/kg. Coronary artery flow did not change significantly following doses of 0.0345 mg/kg while heart rate did not change significantly from the controls at any dose level. Mean blood pressure also did not change significantly at dose levels of 0.0069, 0.0345 and 0.069 mg/kg. Based on the transient increases in coronary blood flow observed in these studies, the NOELs were 0.345 and 0.0345 mg monensin/kg following oral and intravenous dosing, respectively.

The cardiovascular effects of monensin are similar to those observed for lasalocid. Hypothetically, based on their inotropic and chronotropic properties, ionophores were considered as potential therapies for human cardiac disease (Pressman, 1976; Hanley and Slack, 1982).

These pharmacological studies are considered relevant to the overall safety of ionophores as they provide insight into the secondary pharmacological actions and support the margins of safety for exposure in humans during the manufacturing processes or in the mixing or handling of the premixes in preparing feeds for the target species. In regard to the dog cardiovascular studies, monensin-induced increases in coronary blood flow observed at oral doses of 0.69 and 1.38 mg/kg were transient and considered not to be toxicologically important. At these doses, the respective increases of 67% and 172% in blood flow are in the physiologic range by virtue of the autoregulatory coronary flow reserve. Further, the phenomenon was not considered to be deleterious because recognized indicators of cardiovascular toxicity, such as increased blood pressure and/or heart rate, were not observed concurrently in the oral study. If it can be assumed that the relative potency of IV dosing to produce increased blood pressure is 11 times greater than by oral dosing (Holland, 1978), then the equivalent dose of 1.52 mg monensin/kg given orally by capsule would be expected to produce this change. According to Pressman and Fahim (1983), a single oral dose of 2.0 mg/kg in dogs produced increased heart rate and arterial pressure for up to 2 h after dosing, hence the lower dose of 1.38 mg monensin/kg may be considered as the no observed adverse effect level. If one takes 0.69 mg monensin/kg as a pharmacologically significant oral dose and 0.345 mg/kg as a NOEL for humans, then a 60 kg person would require 41.4 mg of monensin to manifest a transient effect on coronary blood flow while 20.7 mg monensin will have no effect (Donoho, 1984).

Human exposure to systemic levels of monensin and other ionophores high enough to produce any toxicological effects is very unlikely. With the use of safety equipment and close adherence to good manufacturing practices and label instructions, personnel manufacturing and handling ionophore products should not be subjected to undue risk. Furthermore, it is highly unlikely for these exposures to occur in humans consuming meat and milk products from animals fed a complete feed formulated with ionophores because residues are extremely low (Novilla, 2004).

Pharmacokinetics

Tissue residue and metabolism studies were required to be conducted on all marketed ionophores to support human safety. For monensin, several studies with both ^{14}C-monensin and unlabeled compound have shown that following oral administration in cattle and other species, monensin is rapidly absorbed and extensively metabolized by the liver and that most of the administered monensin and its metabolites are excreted in the bile. Results of biochemical studies on the metabolic fate of monensin in animals have been published (Davison, 1984; Donoho, 1984; Atef et al., 1993; Nebbia et al., 2001). The metabolite pattern for monensin is similar in cattle, chickens, rats, turkeys, sheep and pigs. Metabolite characterization studies indicated that hydroxylation (o-demethylation and oxidation) is the primary metabolic pathway of monensin resulting in low concentrations of a large number of polar metabolites in the feces of ^{14}C-monensin-dosed animals.

The pattern of metabolites in cattle and rats is similar. Based on radiolabeled studies in steers and dairy cows, the liver had the highest total monensin residue following zero withdrawal (Davison, 1984; Donoho, 1984; Kennington et al., 1995). Parent monensin and five metabolites were identified in liver, bile and/or feces from monensin-treated steers and dairy cows. Studies have shown that metabolite M-1 (o-desmethyl monensin) was 20 times less active than parent monensin, the marker residue. Hence, the suspected first step in monensin metabolism appears to eliminate most of the biological activity. Plasma levels of monensin are low and decline rapidly in cattle treated with monensin. In cattle administered ^{14}C-monensin, residues of radioactivity depleted rapidly from the tissues. In a recent tissue residue study, no monensin was detected in extracted fat, liver, kidney and muscle tissues from cattle given feed containing 100 ppm to provide a dose of 0.9 mg monensin/kg body weight/day for 28 days (Coyle and Walker, 2005). Feeding of muscle, liver and other viscera from cattle provided dietary levels of 165 ppm monensin (five times the approved use level) to rats and dogs for 3 months produced no adverse effects. Moreover, monensin does not accumulate in tissues of animals even when given intoxicating doses (Donoho, 1984; Atef et al., 1993). Thus, exposure of humans to residues of monensin in meat or milk from animals treated according to the label instructions will be very limited and will be due primarily to the parent compound. Furthermore, when residues, primarily the parent compound, are present in animal products intended for human consumption, they will be at minimal levels for which a sufficient margin of safety has been demonstrated in the toxicology studies (Novilla, 2004).

Pharmacokinetic studies with other marketed ionophores generated data similar to that of monensin. Results of these studies in the FOI summaries facilitated determination of the safe residue concentration, acceptable daily intake, marker residue and tolerance, and withdrawal time by the US FDA.

MECHANISM OF ACTION

Carboxylic ionophores are known to form cationic (Na^+, K^+, Ca^{++}) complexes that enhance their transport across bimolecular lipid membranes (Pressman, 1976; Pressman and Fahim, 1982, 1983; Taylor et al., 1982; Reed, 1982; Mollenhauer et al., 1990). However, ion proclivities differ and evidence gathered in various laboratories indicates that carboxylic ionophores may have multiple effects at the cellular level (Fig. 78.2).

In this diagram, monensin, classified as an Na^+ selective ionophore, binds to Na^+ outside the cell, carries it into the cell and produces higher intracellular concentrations of Na^+. Influx of Na^+ is counterbalanced by an

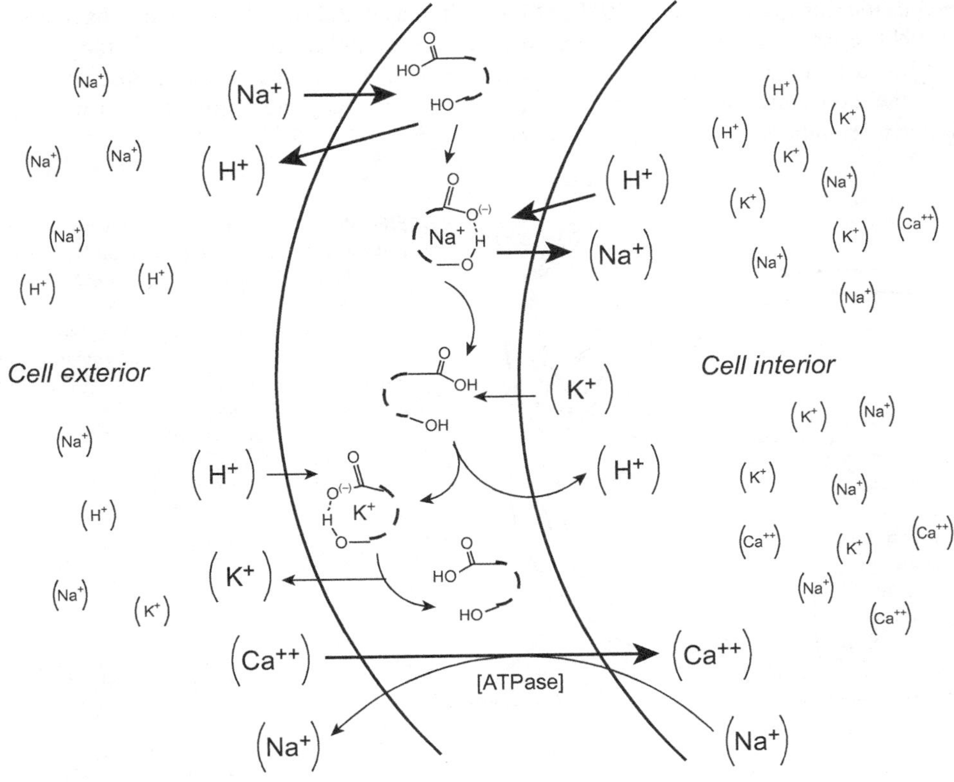

FIGURE 78.2 Diagram of cation ion exchange diffusion across plasma membranes facilitated by monensin. *Large arrows* indicate major transport activity.

efflux of K^+ but, since K^+ efflux is slow, an initial efflux of proton (H^+) occurs, which may result in intracellular alkalosis. With salinomycin and narasin and others that show K^+ selectivity, the K^+ egress is countered by an initial H^+ ingress, which could result in intracellular acidification. Salinomycin and narasin preferentially complex with K^+ over Na^+ at a ratio of 4:1. An ionophore-mediated rise in intracellular Na^+ is known to increase the intracellular levels of Ca^{++} due to an ATPase-driven exchange mechanism at the cell membrane. Monensin was reported to shorten the duration of the action potential and suppressed the pacemaker potential in cardiac tissue (Novilla, 2004). These membrane current effects were related to transmembrane alterations in the gradients of Na^+ and K^+ ions and to increased intracellular Ca^{++} following the increase in cytoplasmic Na^+ concentration, probably via an Na^+/Ca^{++} exchange mechanism. Lasalocid directly translocates Ca^{++} because it forms complexes with divalent cations with a range of complexing and transport capabilities including primary amines, e.g., catecholamines (Hanley and Slack, 1982). Monensin also causes release of catecholamines from cultured adrenal chromaffin cells, and salinomycin causes a multifold augmentation of plasma catecholamines in animals. Catecholamines and toxic oxidation products have been implicated in myocardial necrosis through greater influx of Ca^{++} and formation of free radicals.

By special immunohistochemistry staining, monensin treatment was shown to increase Na^+K^+-ATPase and Ca^{++}-ATPase and NO synthase activities in the heart of chickens (Calo et al., 2002, 2003). Nitric oxide, the product of NO synthases, is recognized as a regulator of calcium homeostasis. Alterations in the concentrations of Ca^{++} and other cations extracellularly as well as changes in their intracellular distribution have been associated with changes in subcellular organelles and cell damage (Shier and DuBourdieu, 1992; Calo et al., 2002, 2003; Sandercock and Mitchell, 2004).

Carboxylic ionophores directly affect the asexual and sexual developmental stages of *Eimerian* coccidia by causing the normal transport of Na^+ and K^+ ions to fail (Smith and Galloway, 1983). In studies with free *Eimerian* sporozoites, monensin causes increased Na^+ levels in the parasite, increased activity of the sodium pump, decreased intrasporozoite ATP and stimulation of glycolysis (Smith et al., 1981). Continuous exposure to monensin results in an increased osmotic gradient within the developing sporozoan parasite. Water follows and the organisms utilize energy to maintain intracellular homeostasis. When energy is exhausted the parasite swells with damage to organelles and death ensues (Smith et al., 1981; Mehlhorn et al., 1983). While most ionophores target free coccidial stages in the intestinal lumen (sporozoites and merozoites), the first intracellular generation (trophozoites) was most sensitive to lasalocid (Long and Jeffers, 1982) (Fig. 78.3).

Similar events occur in susceptible bacteria. By reducing acetic and butyric acid–producing (Gram-positive) bacteria and promoting growth of propionic acid–producing (Gram-negative) bacteria, ionophores improve the efficiency of rumen fermentation resulting in a greater retention of feed energy in metabolizable nutrients (Bergen and Bates, 1984; Russell and Strobel, 1989). Monensin, lasalocid and laidlomycin have been shown to alter the molar ratios of volatile fatty acids (VFAs) such that there is increased propionate and decreased acetate and butyrate without altering total VFA concentration.

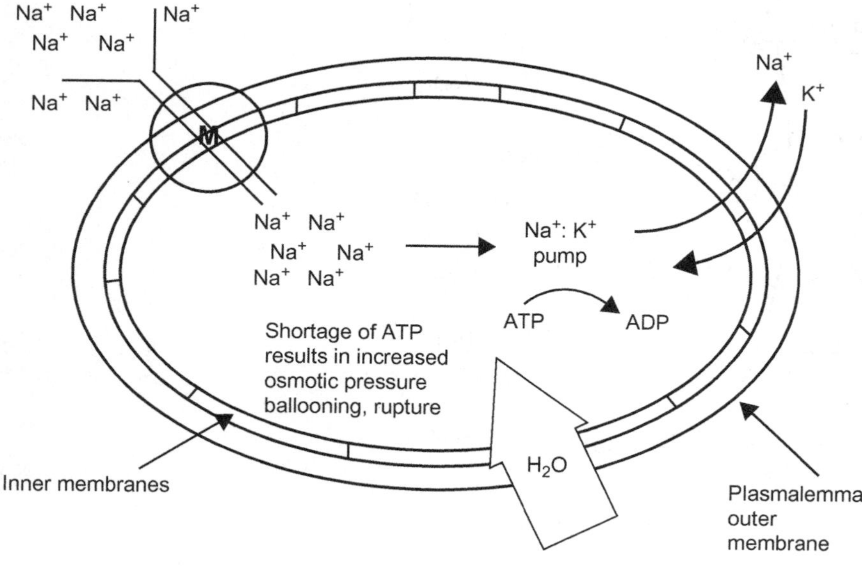

FIGURE 78.3 Effect of ionophores on ion and water dynamics in the coccidia. *M*, monensin. *From Thomas, E.E., Smith, C.K., McGuffey, R.F., Quin, M.E., 1985. Monensin Provides Coccidiosis Control: Site and Mode of Action. Tech Talk Scientific Update from Elanco Animal Health, Division of Eli Lilly and Company, Indianapolis, IN (Thomas et al., 1985) Elanco Animal Health.*

TOXICITY

Pathogenesis

The exact mechanism of the toxicity induced by ionophores is not known. However, reasonable hypotheses have been generated based on their inherent ionophoric activity (Van Vleet et al., 1983c, 1991; Novilla and Folkerts, 1986). All ionophores facilitate transmembrane ion fluxes and dissipation of ion gradients, which are exaggerated at toxic levels. Cells respond to the metabolic insult by expending energy to maintain homeostasis. When homeostatic mechanisms are exceeded, toxicity ensues from excessive influxes of Na^+ and Ca^{++} leading to degeneration and necrosis of cardiac and skeletal muscle cells. Although the ionophore mode of action is simple, four biochemical changes, including intracellular pH effects, calcium overloading, catecholamine release and lipid peroxidation, probably occur during ionophore toxicosis (Fig. 78.4).

In the diagram, monensin facilitates cation exchange diffusion as it intercalates with plasma membranes (Pressman, 1976; Reed, 1982). The exaggerated pharmacologic activity at toxic levels disrupts not only osmotic gradients but the intracellular pH as well. Since drastic changes in acid–base balance are incompatible with life, the pH shifts may be responsible for the peracute deaths observed with very high toxic levels of ionophores (Novilla and Folkerts, 1986). The monensin-induced entry of Na^+ is followed by entry of calcium, due to an ATPase-driven exchange mechanism at the cell membrane. A calcium ionophore like lasalocid or A23817 promotes Ca^{++} entry directly. Ionophores are known to trigger the release of Ca^{++} from intracellular stores further increasing Ca^{++} levels in the cytoplasm.

Two other mechanisms contribute to calcium overloading: exaggerated release of neurotransmitters like catecholamines and increased peroxidation of lipids. Monensin, lasalocid, and salinomycin have been reported, respectively, to release catecholamines from adrenal chromaffin cells, transport catecholamines directly, or augment catecholamine plasma levels. The degradation products of catecholamines have been implicated in myocardial necrosis, through the formation of free radicals and calcium influx (Reichenback and Benditt, 1982). Since ionophores are lipophilic and have detergent properties, dose-related perturbations of plasma membranes can promote increased lipid peroxidation. It is known that lipid peroxidation promotes membrane damage, and consequently increases Ca^{++} influx.

Since they are not mutually exclusive, one or more of the above pathogenic mechanisms may increase calcium concentrations in the cell. The rise in intracellular calcium can be buffered by calcium pumps in the plasma membrane, mitochondria and sarcoplasmic reticulum. However, toxicity overwhelms this buffering mechanism and a vicious cycle ensues, resulting in calcium overloading. Elevated calcium levels then activate muscle proteases and phospholipases which initiate degradative processes (disassembly of myofilaments and membrane damage) in striated muscle and ultimately cell death (Van Vleet et al., 1983c, 1991; Sandercock and Mitchell, 2004).

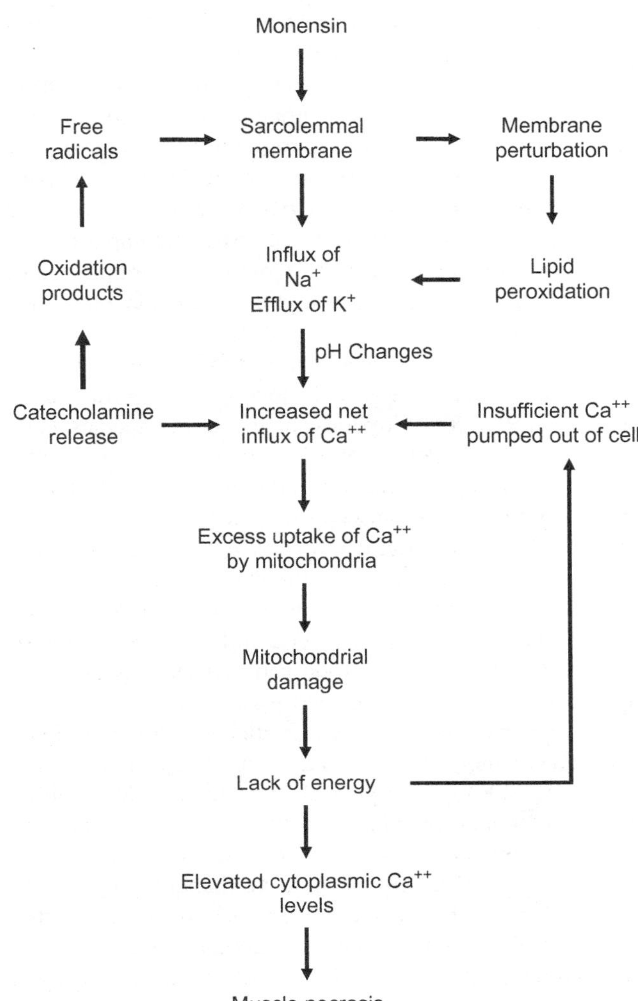

FIGURE 78.4 Probable sequence of events induced by monensin in muscle cells. *Adapted from Novilla, M.N., Folkerts, T.M., 1986. Ionophores: monensin, lasalocid, salinomycin, narasin. In: Howard, J.L. (Ed.), Current Veterinary Therapy-Food Animal Practice. Academic Press, New York, NY, pp. 359–363.*

Occurrence

Generally, the marketed ionophore products have been found to be safe and effective in the target species provided the approved dosage ranges. However, excessive ionophore feed concentrations have resulted in the ionophore toxic syndrome (Novilla, 1992). Toxic syndromes have occurred from the following: (1) feed mixing errors or ingestion of premix concentrates with unsafe amounts of ionophores; (2) extra label use, either accidental or intentional, have resulted in adverse reactions in horses, dogs, rabbits, adult poultry, ostriches, camels, deer, water buffaloes, and humans; and (3) drug incompatibilities with other compounds such as tiamulin, chloramphenicol and macrolides such as triacetyloleandomycin have also resulted in toxicity.

Feed mixing errors have caused the most toxicity problems in animals for which ionophore use has been approved. Reports of toxicity in the target species have been reviewed (Potter et al., 1984; Dowling, 1992; Novilla, 2004). Among the nontarget species, horses appear to be the most susceptible and fish the most tolerant to high levels of ionophores. Except for a direct exposure to a monensin premix following a barn break-in, horse toxicity cases have resulted from feed contamination at the mill. Similarly, feed mill contamination of commercial dog food, cat food and concentrate ration for ostriches have resulted in toxicoses.

In humans, there are two publications of intentional exposure to monensin. According to Kouyoumdjian and associates (2001), a 17-year-old Brazilian male admitted ingesting monensin premix (Rumensin, exact amount unknown), probably to develop muscle. Instead he fell ill, was hospitalized and died from acute rhabdomyolysis with renal failure. Although the amount of monensin ingested in this case was not estimated, in another case cited, two deaths among six people that consumed baked goods made with premix were attributed to monensin exposure of at least 10 times the optimum daily dose fed to cattle. In another report from Brazil, a 16-year-old farm worker who ingested approximately 500 mg of monensin (5 g of Rumensin 100 premix) “to become stronger” developed an early and severe rhabdomyolysis followed by acute renal failure, heart failure and death (Caldeira et al., 2001).

In target species, culprit feeds usually contained five times the maximum approved ionophore use level in the total mix ration provided to the affected animals, with two exceptions. Toxic episodes have occurred from amending cattle and sheep rations with poultry litter (30% or above) containing maduramicin residues and incompatibilities with drugs concurrently administered via feed or drinking water (Van Vleet, 1986; Dowling, 1992). Poultry litter contained levels of maduramicin that proved to be toxic to cattle and sheep. Various antibiotics, including tiamulin, chloramphenicol, macrolides and sulfa drugs, such as sulfachlorpyrazine, have been reported to potentiate ionophore toxicity. Among drug combinations that resulted in adverse effects in cattle, chickens (Frigg et al., 1983), turkeys (Weisman et al., 1983) and swine (Van Vleet, 1986), the most frequently reported drug interaction is with the pleuromotilin derivative, tiamulin. According to Meingassner et al. (1979), tiamulin interferes with the metabolic degradation of monensin in the liver, causing the ionophore to accumulate to toxic levels. The primary step in monensin metabolism is o-demethylation (Donoho, 1984) which is catalyzed by several P450 enzymes (Ceppa et al., 1997; Nebbia et al., 2001). Witkamp et al. (1996) considered the formation of tiamulin metabolite inhibitory (MI) complexes with P450 enzymes to be the basis of the toxic interaction, similar to that reported with macrolide antibiotics (see review by Anadon and Reeve-Johnson, 1999). However, Szücs et al. (2004) reported no evidence of tiamulin MI complexes and that tiamulin directly inhibited CYP3A and two other enzymes, CYP1A2 and CYP2E1, involved in monensin-o-demethylation. Whether similar alterations in ionophore metabolism occur with other drugs are not clear but is an active area of research.

The incidence of ionophore toxicity in all species appears to be low (Novilla and Folkerts, 1986). This is based on periodic reviews of product complaints submitted to the US FDA, as well as from a perusal of the literature. For instance, from 1976 to June 30, 1992, Elanco Animal Health received information about 168 complaints of cattle mortality involving 2045 head where Rumensin was being fed and suspected as a cause of death. Other causes of death were ultimately found for all but 1532 head. Of the 1532 head, most deaths were believed to have been caused by mixing errors. Approximately one-half of the deaths occurred when there were mixing errors of greater than five times the intended dose. When compared to approximately 334 million head of beef cattle that received Rumensin during this time period, the prevalence rate of toxicity would be less than 0.0005% (Novilla and Laudert, 2009). This is remarkable considering the widespread use of ionophore products. In the United States, more than 90% of broiler chickens and about 75% of cattle marketed yearly have consumed ionophores at least part of their lifetime. More information and reports of adverse reactions are available on monensin than for the other ionophores because of monensin's long-standing and widespread use in food animals. However, all the other ionophores can produce a similar toxic syndrome following overdosage, misuse and drug interaction.

Over the years, several acute toxicity (LD_{50}) studies have been conducted in laboratory and domestic animals with monensin, lasalocid, salinomycin and narasin. Due to a change in FDA regulations, there are limited or no LD_{50} data for the other marketed ionophores. Available data for most species are shown in Table 78.2.

The LD_{50} of monensin varies from 214 mg/kg in broiler chickens to 1.4 mg/kg in horses, the most sensitive domestic animal species to ionophore toxicoses. In ionophore toxicoses, there is a progression of events from ingestion of a particular product. Dose and time factors influence the outcome. The greatest risk of intoxication is upon initial

TABLE 78.2 Acute Oral Toxicity of Ionophores in Various Animals[a]

Animal Species	Sex	Monensin[b]	Narasin[c]	Salinomycin[d]	Lasalocid[e]	Laidlomycin[f]
Chicken	C	214[100]	67	40	71.5	N.R.
Turkey	C	253[90]	N.D.	N.R.	N.R.	N.R.
Cattle	MF	26.4[12.6]	N.D.	N.R.	<10> 50[10]	N.R.
Horse	MF	1.38 ± 0.2[0.675]	0.8	N.R.	21.5	N.R.
Swine	MF	16.7 ± 3.6[4]	8.9	N.R.	N.R.	N.R.
Dog	M	[>20]	[>10]	N.R.	N.R.	N.R.
	F	[>10]	(MF)			
Rabbit	MF	41.7 ± 3.6[25.2]	[>10.75]	N.R.	40	N.R.
Rat	M	40.1 ± 0.4	22	48.9	122	63
	F	28.6 ± 3.8	24	47.6	(MF)	(MF)
Mouse	M	70 ± 9	15.8 ± 2.6	57.4	N.R.	N.R.
	F	96 ± 12	16.7 ± 2.1	(MF)		
Sheep	MF	11.9 ± 1.2[3]	N.D.	N.R.	N.R.	N.R.
Goat	MF	26.4 ± 4[4]	N.D.	N.R.	N.R.	N.R.
Trout	MF	>1000	N.D.	N.R.	N.R.	N.R.

C, combined LD_{50} values; *F*, female; *M*, male; *MF*, males and females represented; *N.D.*, not done; *N.R.*, no record.
[a]*LD_{50}: amount of drug (mg/kg) required to kill 50% of the group of animals (LD_0: no deaths) within 7 or 14 days after a single oral dose. No data available for maduramicin and semduramicin.*
[b]*Updated from Todd et al. (1984).*
[c]*From Novilla et al. (1994).*
[d]*Salinomycin sodium. Freedom of Information Summary. FDA NADA #D128686.*
[e]*From Galitzer et al. (1984); Lasalocid. Freedom of Information Summary. FDA NADA #96-298 V.*
[f]*Laidlomycin propionate potassium. Freedom of Information Summary. FDA NADA #1410025.*

exposure, since animals will not consume highly contaminated feed. After an overdose, repeated daily intake of high levels of ionophores is not possible when anorexia occurs (Potter et al., 1984; Matsuoka et al., 1996).

Laboratory and field studies have shown that there is a threshold dose for individual ionophores below which no adverse effects are observed. Safety studies have shown that consumption by horses of complete feed containing the maximum approved level of monensin for cattle is harmless. This is probably true for lasalocid and laidlomycin as well since there are no confirmed reports of ionophore toxicoses in horses used in cattle feedlots.

Results of acute toxicity studies with ionophores in domestic animals indicate that the horse is the most sensitive species; the chicken least sensitive; and cattle intermediate. From studies in ponies given toxic doses of monensin, Amend et al. (1981) found that the death pattern from single, high toxic doses by gavage varied from peracute death in less than 24 h; acute death in 24–96 h; subacute death in 4–14 days; and chronic death after 14 days. The latter is not a chronic toxicity by definition, but delayed death secondary to congestive heart failure (CHF), a recognized consequence of ionophore toxicoses. Death from CHF may occur in some animals that survive the acute toxic episode depending on the affected area in the heart and the cardiac reserve. In cattle, peracute death from monensin toxicity has not occurred. In fact, no deaths have been recorded earlier than 3 days even after high-level (LD_{50}) toxic exposure (Potter et al., 1984).

Blood-level studies suggest that horses, compared to cattle, are not able to clear monensin rapidly from the blood (Donoho, 1984). This was probably related to the oxidative efficiency of P450 demethylating enzymes in the liver. Working with liver microsomes from horses, pigs, broiler chicks, rats and cattle, Nebbia and associates (2001) found that horses had the lowest catalytic efficiency, which may explain the greater susceptibility of horses to the ionophore-induced toxicosis, relative to the other species. However, not all levels of monensin are toxic to horses (Matsuoka et al., 1996). In a subchronic feeding study in horses, all three horses provided a complete ration containing 330 ppm monensin (or 300 g/ton, 10 times the maximum cleared level of monensin in complete feeds for feedlot cattle) and one out of three horses given 121 ppm monensin died during the 1-month feeding period. However, three horses provided 33 ppm monensin maintained typical levels of feed intake and suffered no ill effects attributable to treatment (Table 78.3).

After evaluating the effects of monensin in either supplements or blocks in pasture horses, Matsuoka and coworkers (1996) made the following conclusions that may apply to other marketed ionophores as well: (1) horses on pasture may consume, at initial exposure, enough supplement containing high levels of monensin to be toxic and/or lethal; (2) following an initial high-level monensin exposure, consumption of treated feed, supplement or block is negligible; and (3) horses can consume certain levels of monensin without suffering any ill effect indicative of toxicity.

Clinical Signs

Physical signs reported for ionophore toxicoses across several animal species are as follows: anorexia, diarrhea, depression, hypoactivity/reluctance to move, dyspnea, leg weakness, ataxia, and recumbency. Most of these clinical signs occur in all animals studied but variations in their occurrence have been observed. For instance, diarrhea is commonly observed with monensin toxicity in cattle and poultry but has not been reported in either horses or dogs. The most consistent clinical sign in animals that have ingested toxic levels of ionophores is partial to complete anorexia (Novilla, 1992).

TABLE 78.3 Effect of Feeding Monensin in Complete Feed to Horses for 28 Days

Monensin Level	Effect
33 ppm (cattle use level)	Transient anorexia[a]
121 ppm (broiler use level)	May be toxic
330 ppm (10 × cattle use level)	Lethal

[a]*Occurred in week 2 and 3 of the study.*
Source: From Matsuoka, T., Novilla, M.N., Thomson, T.D., Donoho, A. L., 1996. Review of monensin toxicosis in horses. J. Equine Vet. Sci. 16, 8–15.

In chickens, anorexia is associated with diarrhea, drowsiness, extreme weakness, and sternal recumbency with legs extended posteriorly. In target animal safety and toxicity studies, depression of growth and feed conversion as well as higher mortality occur in broilers fed five times the recommended level of monensin for 8 weeks (Novilla, 2004). Broiler breeders exposed to high levels of ionophores manifest severe drops in egg production, anorexia, depression, paralysis, and death in sternal recumbency. Similar signs were reported in turkeys with toxicity induced by monensin, salinomycin, and narasin (Salyi et al., 1988). Mortality was variable but high death losses (up to 96.7%) were recorded with salinomycin (Halvorson et al., 1982).

In cattle, clinical signs of monensin toxicosis include anorexia, diarrhea, ataxia, recumbency, depression and non-responsiveness to visual stimuli (Van Vleet et al., 1983c; Potter et al., 1984). There is a definite correlation between onset of clinical signs and amount of monensin consumed. All intoxicated cattle manifest partial to complete anorexia. Severely intoxicated animals develop anorexia within 24 h. Animals exposed to lower levels may take up to 48 h to develop anorexia. Diarrhea usually is evident in 24–48 h in animals receiving high doses of monensin. Exposure to low doses may result in a delay of up to 5 days in the onset of diarrhea. Onset of depression follows a similar pattern, being observed by day 3 in animals receiving excessive monensin overdoses while being observed after 1 week in animals receiving less than excessive overdoses. Rapid breathing and ataxia may be present only in animals that have consumed extremely high levels. In cattle, death occurs without any manifestations of struggle.

Galitzer and coworkers (1982) found that lasalocid-intoxicated cattle manifested early signs of forced watery diarrhea, muscle tremors and greater cardiac and respiratory rates followed by or concurrent with anorexia. Delayed signs of cardiac insufficiency were evident 7–10 days after administration of the toxic dose. The temporal occurrence of clinical signs and mortality from ionophore toxicity was clearly documented by Potter et al. (1984) in a multiple bolus dosing trial with monensin in cattle (Table 78.4).

TABLE 78.4 Clinical Signs in Beef Cattle Gavaged With Multiple Doses (7 Days) of Monensin

Monensin (mg/kg/day)	Day First Observed					
	Anorexia	Diarrhea	Depression	Dyspnea	Ataxia	Death
0	–[a]	–	–	–	–	–
1.5	2	5	7	–	–	–
2.3	1	4	6	–	–	–
3.8	1	3	4	–	–	–
7.6	1	2	4	5	5	5
15.5	1	2	3	5	4	4

[a]*Not observed.*

TABLE 78.5 Clinical Signs of Ionophore Toxicoses in the Horse

Sign	Monensin	Lasalocid	Salinomycin	Narasin	Laidlomycin
Anorexia	X[a]	X	X	X	X
Diarrhea	–[b]	–	X	X	–
Depression	X	X	–	X	X
Dyspnea	X	–	X	X	X
Ataxia	X	X	X	X	X
Colic[c]	X	–	X	X	–
Leg weakness	X	X	X	X	X
Muscle tremors	X	–	–	X	X
Sweating	X	–	X	X	X
Recumbent	X	X	X	X	X

[a]*Observed.*
[b]*Not observed.*
[c]*Pain manifested by uneasiness, abnormal (wide) leg stance, pawing.*

The onset and severity of toxic effects induced by monensin were dose related. In the study, anorexia was the most consistent clinical sign of toxicity and no deaths occurred earlier than 4 days after exposure to high toxic doses of monensin. However, multiple bolus dosing does not simulate actual field conditions since repeated exposure to toxic levels is not possible when anorexia occurs. Further, the onset and severity of toxicity from bolus dosing is different than that via feed (Buck et al., 1976).

Sheep and goats have clinical signs similar to cattle (anorexia, diarrhea, ataxia) but affected lambs frequently exhibit labored breathing, frothing at the mouth and kicking at the abdomen (Agaoglu et al., 2002). Dogs with ionophore toxicoses become weak and develop a rapid onset of paresis progressing to flaccid paralysis of the anterior and posterior limbs, tongue laxity and dyspnea (Safran et al., 1993; Condon and McKenzie, 2002; Segev et al., 2004). In pigs, anorexia, diarrhea, lethargy, dyspnea, ataxia, knuckling at the fetlock and myoglobinuria were present prior to lateral recumbency and death from ionophore toxicoses (Van Vleet et al., 1983a,b; Plumlee et al., 1995).

As in cattle and other species, anorexia is the first and most consistent clinical sign finding in the horse with ionophore toxicosis (Table 78.5).

Diarrhea has not been observed with either monensin or lasalocid but was reported with salinomycin and narasin (Whitlock et al., 1978; Matsuoka et al., 1996). Profuse sweating was also observed with monensin, salinomycin, narasin and laidlomycin but not with lasalocid toxicity. Horses with leg weakness and ataxia generally progress to recumbency. Once recumbent, horses frequently attempt to rise with thrashing of the limbs until death supervenes. This is in contrast to cattle that die without signs of struggling.

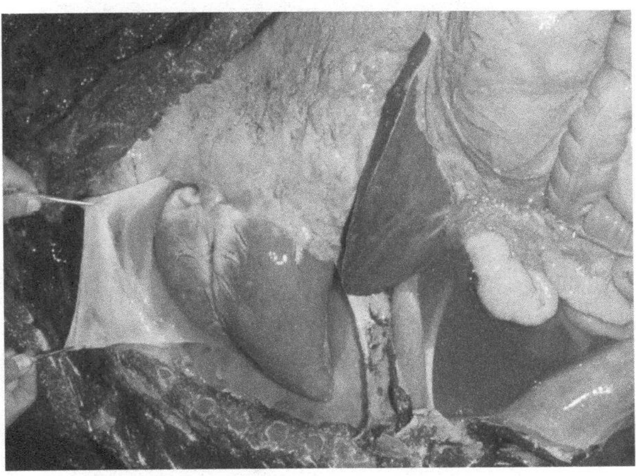

FIGURE 78.5 Thoracic and abdominal viscera from a mare that died 7 days following a single gavage dose of 1.65 mg monensin/kg body weight. Note the fluid accumulation in the body cavities and the pale areas and epicardial hemorrhages on the heart.

Postmortem Findings

Necropsy findings in animals with ionophore toxicoses include hemorrhages and pale areas in the heart, pale areas in some limb muscles, pulmonary edema, hydrothorax, ascites and inflammation of the stomach and intestines (Van Vleet et al., 1983a,b,c; Galitzer et al., 1986a,b; Novilla, 1992). Animals that die soon after exposure often will have no lesions, since they had not had time to develop or they may be masked by postmortem changes. Those with lethal doses surviving longer than a week may have hydropericardium, pulmonary edema, hydrothorax, ascites, reddish-mottled liver, and subcutaneous edema of the abdomen and limbs (Figs. 78.5 and 78.6).

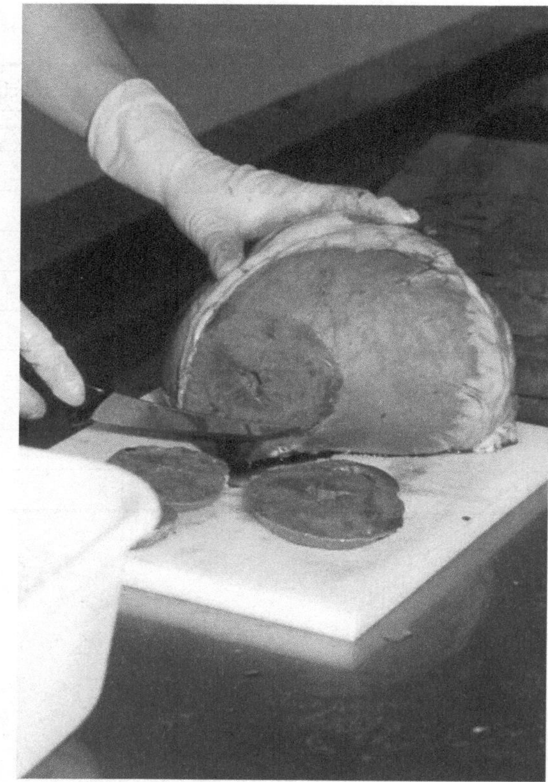

FIGURE 78.6 Diffuse pallor in cross-sections of the heart from the same mare described in Fig. 78.5 legend.

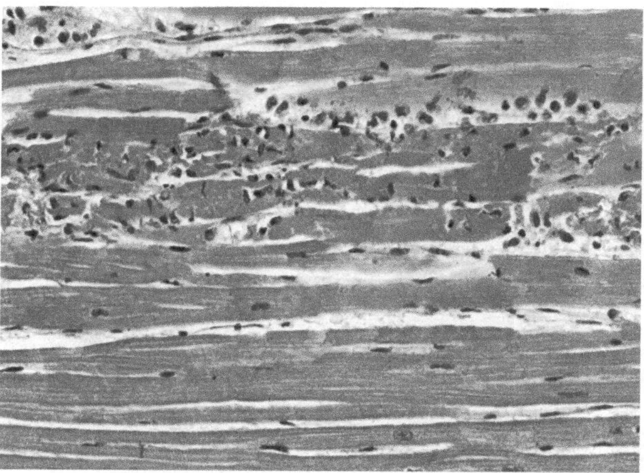

FIGURE 78.7 Early necrotic focus in the left ventricle of a gelding that died 20 h following gavage with 2.5 mg monensin/kg body weight. Necrotic muscle fibers have sparse infiltration of neutrophils and lymphocytes. H&E. Original magnification ×64.

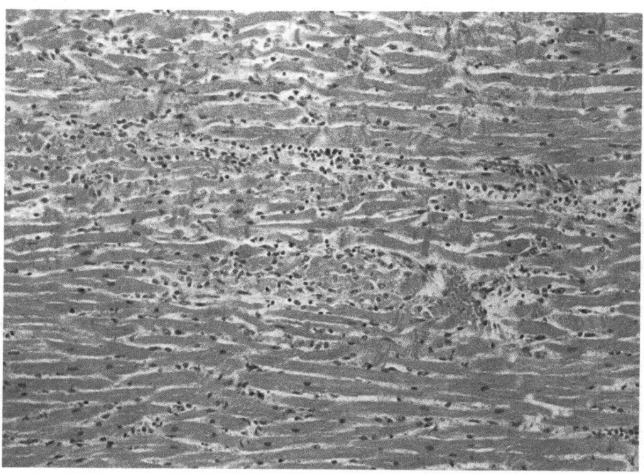

FIGURE 78.8 Larger foci of myofiber necrosis with contraction bands in the interventricular septum from a horse euthanized 72 h following a single oral dose of 1.65 mg monensin/kg body weight given by gavage. More cellular infiltrates with lymphocytes, macrophages, and few eosinophils are present. H&E. Original magnification ×10.

At necropsy, cutting the ventricular and thigh muscles transversely often shows the diffuse pallor of myonecrosis induced by toxic levels of ionophores. Skeletal muscle lesions may be quite severe in sheep, pigs and dogs, moderate in cattle and minimal to slight in horses. For this reason, myoglobinuria, evidenced by red urine, has been observed in pigs, sheep and dogs but not in cattle or horses.

Histopathologic Findings

Target organs damaged by toxic doses of monensin and other ionophores were identified to include the heart and skeletal muscles in all species studied (Todd et al., 1984; Van Vleet et al., 1991; Dowling, 1992; Novilla, 2004). In addition, neurotoxic effects have been reported for lasalocid (Shlosberg et al., 1985; Safran et al., 1993), narasin (Novilla et al., 1994) and salinomycin (Van der Linde-Sipman, 1999). The development of muscle lesions varies among species. The heart is primarily affected in horses, skeletal muscle in pigs and dogs, and there is about equal tissue predilection in rats, chickens and cattle. Morphologic effects include degeneration, necrosis and repair of cardiac and skeletal muscle fibers with a variable inflammatory component and secondary lesions of CHF. Neuropathic changes occurred in peripheral nerves and the spinal cord. Focal swelling, fragmentation, loss of axons and formation of digestion chambers filled with macrophages were observed in both sensory and motor nerves, and there was vacuolation with swelling, degeneration and fragmentation of myelin sheaths and axons in the spinal cord.

The most important change is a toxic myopathy characterized by focal areas of degeneration, necrosis and repair in cardiac and skeletal muscles with a variable inflammatory component (Novilla, 1992; Van Vleet et al., 1991). Muscle lesions are similar to those described for compound A204, the first polyether antibiotic tested at Lilly Research Laboratories (Todd et al., 1984). Doses and time factors influence the severity and distribution of lesions in ionophore toxicosis (Figs. 78.7 and 78.8).

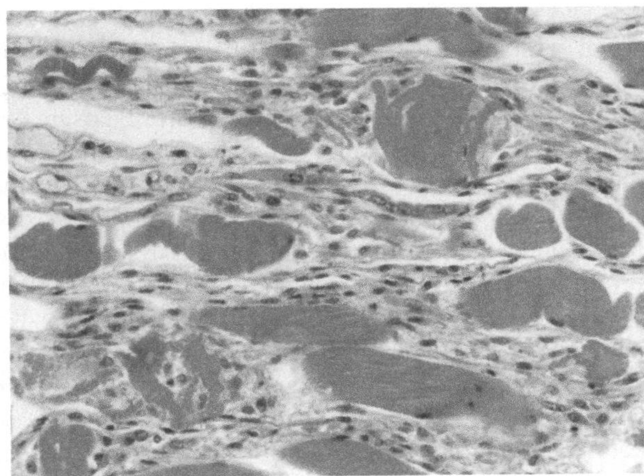

FIGURE 78.9 Skeletal muscle from a steer that died 6 days after a gavage dose of 39.8 mg monensin/kg body weight. Notice the fragmented and regenerating fibers. H&E. Original magnification ×80.

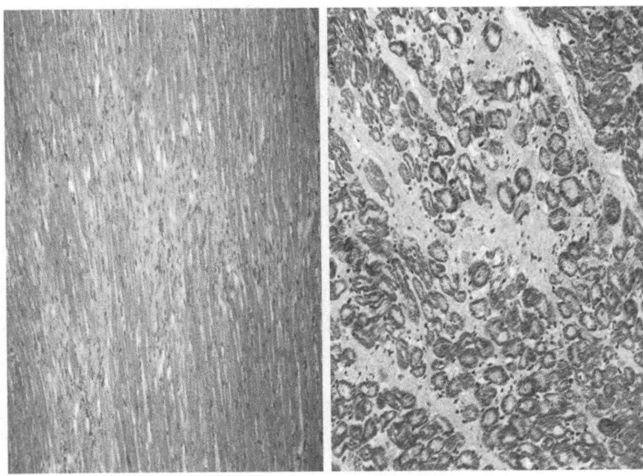

FIGURE 78.10 Hearts from animals that survived acute ionophore toxicity. (Left panel) Section of left ventricle with focal interstitial fibrosis from another steer, cohort of that described in Fig. 78.9 legend, euthanized 28 days after a gavage dose of 39.8 mg monensin/kg body weight. H&E. Original magnification ×20. (Right panel) Interstitial fibrosis in the left ventricle from a gelding that survived a gavage dose of 2 mg monensin/kg body weight for 4 months. Masson's trichrome. Original magnification ×32.

Generally, no significant lesions are seen by light microscopy in animals that die immediately, and animals that die after an acute course may have only a few scattered degenerated fibers in the heart and highly active muscles, such as the diaphragm. Lesions are most pronounced within 7–14 days following ingestion of a toxic dose and are accompanied by profound attempts at repair. Skeletal muscle fibers regenerate rapidly, and lesions are completely healed in about a month. Heart muscle fibers do not regenerate, but repair takes place by replacement fibrosis. Secondary lesions of CHF, including heart dilatation and hydropericardium, lung edema, liver necrosis and fluid accumulation in the thoracic and abdominal cavities, may be present, depending upon the severity of heart damage and the potential cardiac reserve (Figs. 78.9 and 78.10).

Observations to date indicate that in horses the heart suffers the greatest damage from monensin toxicoses with little or no involvement of skeletal muscles. This finding is in contrast to dogs and pigs in which the lesions are most pronounced in skeletal muscles. Chickens, cattle and rodents have about equal predilection for cardiac and skeletal muscle lesions.

Other Laboratory Findings

Mitochondrial swelling, myelin figures and lipid vesicles were observed ultrastructurally in cardiac and skeletal muscles of ponies given monensin at 4 mg/kg and observed for 79 h (Mollenhauer et al., 1981). Early degenerative changes of sarcoplasmic vacuolation from swollen mitochondria and accumulation of lipid were described in cattle and pigs with monensin toxicosis (Van Vleet et al., 1991). Severely injured mitochondria had marked swelling, disrupted cristae and dense matrical granules. Scattered myelin figures were present in muscle cells with numerous disrupted mitochondria. Subsequently necrosis occurred in degenerated myocytes and was characterized by dense fibers with intact sarcomeres or disrupted fibers with hypercontraction bands. Necrosis was followed rapidly by extensive macrophage infiltration with lysis of disrupted organelles and contractile material. Similar ultrastructural findings were observed in hearts and skeletal muscles of sheep given monensin and in skeletal muscles of broilers simultaneously given triacetyloleandomycin in the drinking water and monensin in the feed (Dowling, 1992). Regeneration as evidenced by myoblast proliferation was observed as early as 4 days posttreatment in pigs and sheep.

Hematologic parameters are not significantly affected by ionophore toxicosis (Van Vleet et al., 1983a,b,c; Condon and McKenzie, 2002; Segev et al., 2004). Elevation of serum enzymes, notably creatine phosphokinase (CPK), lactate dehydrogenase (LDH) and aspartate transaminase (AST), may indicate damage to cardiac and skeletal muscles (Amend et al., 1981; Van Vleet et al., 1983b,c; Galitzer et al., 1986b; Wilson et al., 1990). Alkaline phosphatase (ALP), inorganic phosphorus and total bilirubin (TB) levels are also higher, while serum levels of calcium and potassium are lower (Table 78.6).

The progressive hypokalemia and attendant cardiac conduction disturbances demonstrated in ponies were considered the life threatening events in early acute monensin toxicosis in equines (Amend et al., 1981). Consequent to muscle damage, significant increases in enzymes of muscle origin occur

TABLE 78.6 Some Biomarkers of Ionophore Toxicity

Elevated	Decreased	No Change
Aspartate transaminase	Calcium	Sodium
Creatine kinase	Potassium	
Lactic dehydrogenase		
Alkaline phosphatase		
Blood urea nitrogen		
Total bilirubin		
Cardiac troponin 1		

(Amend et al., 1981; Van Vleet et al., 1983a,b,c). AST, CPK, LDH, ALP, blood urea nitrogen, and TB are elevated, calcium (Ca) and potassium (K) transiently decrease while sodium (Na) levels are within normal limits. Cardiac troponins (both cTnI and cTnT) were reported to be highly sensitive and specific biomarker of myocardial injury in humans (O'Brien, 2008).The level of cardiac troponin I (cTnI), the preferred biomarker for cardiotoxicity in laboratory animals, ranged from 0.0 to 0.06 ng/mL while values of 0.08–3.68 ng/mL were found in six horses gavaged with a single dose of 1.0–1.5 mg monensin/kg body weight (Divers et al., 2009; Kraus et al., 2010). Since these monensin doses are close to the LD_{50} of 1.38 mg/kg body weight, it was not surprising that the biomarker picked up the presence of the myocardial injury caused by toxic doses of monensin, as it would for any significant injury to heart muscle.

Diagnosis and Differential Diagnosis

Since all ionophores in the market place are likely to produce a similar toxic syndrome in overdosage and misuse situations, six important criteria must be considered before a diagnosis of toxicity is given (Novilla, 2004). These include (1) history of feed-related problem, usually affecting a group of animals; (2) ionophore laboratory assays; (3) clinical signs manifested during the toxicity episode; (4) gross postmortem lesions; (5) microscopic pathology; and (6) exclusion of nutritional, infectious and other toxic factors.

History assumes great significance when the problem is connected to the introduction of newly formulated feed or supplement to the herd or flock. Since clinical signs and lesions are not pathognomonic, feed analysis for the amount and type of ionophore in the ration is necessary for diagnosis. With the availability of seven ionophores in the market place, the use of an efficient and highly selective laboratory assay is indicated. Newer methods have been developed to determine one or more ionophores in feeds and tissues (Bertini et al., 2003; Ebel et al., 2004). Several samples of the feed should be submitted for analysis, including residual material from the feeder, trough, auger, or feed bin. Feed assays may prove exposure to a particular product but significantly higher than the recommended levels must be found for a confirmatory diagnosis. Otherwise, concurrent use of an incompatible drug must be documented. Absent proof of a gross feed mixing error, a wide list of differential diagnoses need to be excluded in order to return a presumptive diagnosis.

Initially, ionophore toxicosis may be suspected when there is a history of a feed-related problem in a group of animals; clinical signs of anorexia, diarrhea, labored breathing, depression, locomotory disorder, recumbency and death; lesions affecting heart and skeletal muscles; or CHF. The clinical signs and lesions induced by toxic levels of ionophores are not pathognomonic. However, recent introduction of newly formulated feed or supplement to a flock or herd in which signs and lesions are present may cause one to suspect that acute intoxication has occurred. Dose and time factors influence the severity and distribution of lesions. Animals that die soon after exposure may not have muscle lesions discernible by light microscopy. Lesions are likely to be found in animals that survived longer than a week. The most active skeletal muscles may be involved when the heart is not affected or is only slightly affected. Since changes can be missed because of their focal distribution, more intense tissue sampling to include one section each of the atria, ventricles, and interventricular septum of the heart, the diaphragm, and muscles of the abdomen and thigh is desirable. Some animals with substantive heart damage from very high levels of monensin and other ionophores may later develop CHF.

Although a presumptive diagnosis of ionophore toxicosis can be made based on history, clinical signs, lesions, and considerations of differential diagnosis, specific assays are needed for confirmatory diagnosis. With seven ionophores currently in use, the need for confirmatory laboratory assays cannot be overemphasized. In monensin toxicosis, values greater than five times the recommended use level in the feed provided affected animals are usually confirmatory. Assays on stomach contents from per acute and acute cases of toxicity can prove exposure but values obtained have been low. Only minimal residues of monensin have been detected in target tissues of cattle and chickens given monensin (Donoho, 1984; Atef et al., 1993). Further, blood levels of monensin are low or undetectable even in intoxicated animals and accumulation in target tissues does not occur.

Ionophore toxicosis may be confused with acute infectious diseases, deficiencies and other intoxications (Van Vleet et al., 1983a,b,c; Dowling, 1992; Novilla, 2004). In the differential diagnosis of monensin toxicosis, myopathic conditions should be considered first. In cattle, these would include (1) ionophore toxicoses, (2) vitamin E and selenium deficiencies, (3) poisonous plant ingestion, e.g., senna, coyotillo, white snakeroot, vetch, and (4) the common, yet puzzling, sudden death syndrome with myocardial necrosis. Ionophore toxicosis usually involves an accompanying history of feed supplementation or feed change and usually involves many animals. Clinical signs are anorexia, diarrhea, lethargy, ataxia, and the suggestion of damage to striated muscles. Vitamin E and selenium deficiency occurs sporadically and produces prominent degeneration and necrosis with calcification of cardiac and skeletal muscles. Plant poisonings are usually localized to areas where the toxic plants are indigenous. For instance, coffee senna (*Cassia occidentalis*) poisoning occurs in the southeastern United States. It may cause anorexia, diarrhea, and the production of dark urine but generally causes more pronounced lesions in skeletal muscles than in the heart. The coyotillo plant (*Karwinskia huntholdtiana*) in southwest Texas and Mexico produces limberleg in sheep and goats characterized by progressive weakness of the legs, muscular incoordination, recumbency, respiratory distress, and death. Lesions are observed both in cardiac and skeletal muscles as well as peripheral nerves and the liver. White snakeroot (*Eupatorium rugosum*), a plant indigenous to much of eastern Canada and the United States, causes "trembles" in goats, sheep, cattle, horses, and swine. Cardiac and skeletal muscle lesions may be present in animals that ingested this plant. However, with trembles there is constipation, blood in feces, an odor of acetone in the breath and severe fatty degeneration in the liver and kidney that are not seen in ionophore toxicities. Hairy vetch (*Vicia villosa*) also produces myocardial necrosis but, unlike monensin toxicosis, it produces dermatitis, conjunctivitis and abortion as well as lesions in the kidneys, adrenal glands, lymph nodes, and thyroid gland. The syndrome of sudden death with myocardial necrosis in cattle, especially calves, is common but sporadic in occurrence and is associated with lesions in cardiac but not skeletal muscle (Bradley et al., 1981). Hence, clinical history and detailed pathologic studies will help distinguish among ionophore toxicosis, acute infectious diseases, deficiencies, and other intoxications.

From a clinical standpoint, respiratory diseases, particularly infectious bovine rhinotracheitis and the shipping fever complex, are initially considered in the differential diagnosis for cattle because of the respiratory difficulties that occur with ionophore toxicosis. At necropsy, however, pneumonic lesions are consistent with these diseases. Animals with acute bovine pulmonary edema and emphysema or fog fever, nitrogen dioxide intoxication, or rape, turnip, or kale poisoning also exhibit respiratory difficulties. But in these conditions gross lesions will include severe interstitial and interlobular emphysema or pneumonia or both rather than edema. The incoordination, stiff wobbly gait, and loss of visual reflexes may lead one to suspect polioencephalomalacia and thromboembolic meningoencephalitis. But in these conditions histologic lesions present in the brain are confirmatory. Unequivocal central nervous system lesions have not been found in cases of monensin toxicity in any species. However, lesions in the spinal cord and peripheral nerves occurred with lasalocid toxicosis in chickens (Shlosberg et al., 1985). Peripheral neuropathic changes have also been reported in cats exposed to salinomycin-contaminated feed (Van der Linde-Sipman et al., 1999) and in dogs given narasin (Novilla et al., 1994). Salt poisoning will cause nervous signs, paralysis, and diarrhea, but knowledge that insufficient amounts of water were available to the animals will also point to this problem. Eosinophilic meningoencephalitis is pathognomonic for salt poisoning in pigs, but this lesion does not occur in other species. Laboratory procedures used to confirm a diagnosis include assays of serum, cerebrospinal fluid and brain tissue for sodium concentrations (Buck et al., 1976). In cattle, urea toxicosis must be considered when sudden collapse, bloat, violent convulsions, terminal tetanic spasms, and high death losses occur within 10 min to 4 h from exposure to newly formulated feed. Deaths occurring earlier than 72 h have not been reported in cattle gavaged with high doses of monensin (Potter et al., 1984).

In poultry, differential diagnoses should include nutritional (focal) myopathy, coffee senna toxicity, botulism, sodium chloride (salt) toxicity, mycotoxicosis by cyclopiazonic acid and other myopathic mycotoxins, round heart disease and, in the turkey, the knockdown (downer) syndrome. Although no striated muscle lesions are produced in botulism and sodium chloride toxicity, clinical signs of limber neck and lesions of "water belly" may be confused with ionophore toxicoses. On the other hand, birds affected with salt poisoning may have enlarged hearts or have enlarged pale kidneys from urate nephrosis. Monensin per se does not produce "barebacks" in broiler chickens, and downers among replacement birds may be suffering from viral arthritis. Therefore, this common reovirus infection must be excluded as a cause of the problem in chicken flocks. In commercial turkeys reared in confinement, focal myopathy has been attributed to deficiencies in vitamin E or selenium associated with rapid growth (Wilson et al., 1990). Nutritional myopathy may mimic skeletal muscle lesions induced by ionophore toxicoses; but unlike those of nutritional myopathy, ionophore-induced lesions are monophasic and polyfocal with little or no mineralization. Muscle lesions also occur in deep pectoral myopathy, coffee senna toxicity and toxicoses from the mold toxins, cyclopiazonic acid and moniliformin. Their clinical presentation and presence of other lesions will help distinguish these conditions.

Round heart disease, also known as round heart-edema-ascites syndrome or spontaneous cardiomyopathy, occurs sporadically in turkeys and other fowl (Czarnecki, 1984). Clinical signs indicate the presence of heart failure but the exact cause has not been determined. A genetic predisposition has been suggested because it is more common in certain lines of turkeys, particularly those having a rapid rate of early muscle development. Some of the predisposing factors include low levels of oxygen and high levels of carbon dioxide in the incubator, poor brooder house ventilation and overcrowding during transport. Exposure to these factors may occur days or weeks prior to onset of illness. In contrast, monensin toxicity occurs as a sudden outbreak in a flock of birds accidentally provided toxic levels due to a feed mixing error. Among birds that survive the acute toxic episode, a few, depending upon the extent and location of heart damage and the potential cardiac reserve, may subsequently develop dilatation of the heart and secondary signs of CHF.

Another condition that needs to be distinguished from monensin toxicity is the turkey knockdown syndrome. Turkey knockdown has been defined as any condition affecting the neuromuscular system to the extent that a bird is unable to stand or walk (Wages, 1993). A necrotizing myopathy, particularly of the rear limbs, has been reported in turkeys with the knockdown syndrome (Cardona et al., 1993). Unfortunately, striated muscles have limited responses to injury (Van Vleet et al., 1991) and lesions induced by any ionophore, including monensin, are not pathognomonic (Novilla, 1992). Although monensin feed inclusion rates in knockdown cases are within or slightly above the maximum recommended level of 99 ppm (Wages, 1993; Cardona et al., 1993) monensin has been implicated as a causative factor because the clinical and pathologic findings are similar to those induced by monensin toxicity. However, unlike monensin toxicity, the turkey knockdown syndrome is characterized by: (1) low incidence and fatality rates; (2) acute onset of paresis/paralysis; (3) no anorexia, birds will eat if able to reach feeders; (4) no diarrhea; (5) affected birds are alert; (6) unable to vocalize; (7) presence of widespread skeletal muscle lesions that are subacute to chronic in character, generally no heart lesions; and (8) rapid recovery following change of feed. These observations were confirmed in an epidemiological, case controlled study of knockdown cases in the Shenandoah Valley of Virginia that evaluated various factors, including management, environment, health, feed, water, pathology and clinical pathology analytes (Evans et al., 2000). Serum vitamin E levels were significantly lower in affected birds (Meldrum et al., 2000). Feed and/or water intake alterations were highly correlated with the incidence of turkey knockdown and modification of practices affecting feed/water intake reduced the incidence of knockdown in one farm from 6 in 1999 to 0 in 2000.

In pigs, vitamin E and selenium deficiency, gossypol poisoning and porcine stress syndrome (PSS) should be considered in the differential diagnosis since skeletal or cardiac lesions may be found in these conditions (Van Vleet et al., 1983b, 1986). In monensin toxicosis, the striated muscle lesions appear more frequently and are more severe in skeletal muscle than in cardiac muscle. Myoglobinuria may also be present. Widespread cardiac and skeletal muscle lesions, vascular damage, dietetic hepatosis, and gastric ulceration may be found in vitamin E and selenium deficiency. With PSS, cardiac, and skeletal muscle lesions may or may not be observed following a history of stress.

For horses, the exertional myopathies, such as equine rhabdomyolysis (Monday morning disease) and hyperkalemic periodic paralysis, plant poisoning from coffee senna and white snakeroot, should be excluded along with blister beetle intoxication, colic, and laminitis (Whitlock et al., 1978; Amend et al., 1981; Novilla, 1992; Matsuoka et al., 1996). Complete herd history, clinical examination, successful supportive treatment and necropsy may help differentiate these conditions from ionophore toxicoses.

TREATMENT

When ionophore toxicity is suspected, a feed change to a nonionophore medicated ration must be made immediately and the affected group(s) of animals maintained on this ration until all diagnostic procedures are completed. In cattle presumably diagnosed with monensin toxicity, it is advisable to replace the suspected culprit feed with feed known to contain the approved concentration of monensin. This allows the rumen microbes of unaffected cattle to remain adapted to monensin and will promote overall herd performance (Novilla and Laudert, 2009). At the present time, there is no known antidote or treatment for ionophore toxicity. Although previous antidotal trials failed, the search continues (Mitema et al., 1988). Nonetheless, it may be difficult to find a drug that can block up to four pathogenic mechanisms, acting singly or in concert, that are involved in the toxicoses. Therapeutic interventions have been largely supportive. For horses, Amend et al. (1981) recommended supportive treatment with mineral oil, activated charcoal and aggressive fluid and electrolyte replacement with potassium and phosphorus supplementation, including means to reduce cardiac work. However, supportive therapy may not be practical on a herd or flock basis.

Van Vleet (1986), Van Vleet et al. (1983a, 1987) obtained protection against the development of clinical monensin toxicity in pigs treated with selenium and vitamin E (selenium as selenite at 0.25 mg/kg and vitamin E as α-tocopherol acetate at 17 IU/kg) prior to a single oral dose of 50 mg monensin/kg (LD_{50} 16.7 ± 3.57 mg/kg). A similar regimen in cattle administered toxic doses of monensin provided only partial protection but clinical signs in pigs with tiamulin-induced salinomycin toxicity were ameliorated following administration of vitamin E. The protection against the toxicoses was theorized to be produced by stabilization of cellular membranes since selenium and vitamin E are known to prevent and control peroxidation-mediated cellular injury (Tappel, 1981; Van Vleet, 1986). Similarly, the antioxidant property of zinc prevented adverse effects of salinomycin in chickens (Kamashi et al., 2004). Monensin, like all polyether carboxylic ionophores, is lipophilic and may produce dose-dependent membrane perturbations and increased lipid peroxidation, which could lead to degradative processes. Further studies are needed to determine whether antioxidants, such as vitamin E and selenium, or zinc administration may have important roles in the prevention and treatment of ionophore toxicoses.

Until proper and effective therapy is available, prevention of ionophore toxicoses by (1) proper use from the implementation of good feed manufacturing and feeding practices at the feed mill and farm level; (2) avoidance of overdosing of feeds for approved species, which may carry over to feeds for nontarget species; and (3) adherence to species restrictions will help prevent the adverse effects associated with this class of compounds.

CONCLUDING REMARKS AND FUTURE DIRECTIONS

Seven ionophores—monensin, lasalocid, salinomycin, narasin, maduramicin, laidlomycin and semduramicin—are marketed globally for use as anticoccidial drugs for poultry and/or growth promotants in ruminants. Off-label usage of ionophore products is known to occur since other uses continue to be investigated and applied in many countries. It is likely that basic and applied research on these versatile compounds could lead in the future to product line extensions to other target species and potential development of novel therapeutics for unmet needs in veterinary and human medicine.

Generally, these feed additives have been found to be safe and effective in target animal species, but toxic syndromes have resulted from overdosage, misuse, and drug interaction. Among the domestic species, horses are the most sensitive to ionophore toxicoses, poultry the least sensitive, and cattle intermediate. However, even for the horse, there is a threshold level of exposure below which no adverse effects are observed. Consumption of complete feed containing the maximum approved use levels of monensin, lasalocid, or laidlomycin is harmless. Dose and time factors influence the severity and outcome of the toxic exposure. Results of controlled studies and confirmed field reports of toxicity indicate that the greatest risk of intoxication is upon initial exposure to ionophore-containing feed or supplement. Following sublethal exposure, consumption of culprit feed or supplement is negligible because of anorexia. Animals that die acutely after high levels of exposure often will have few or no lesions. Those that die later have profound striated (cardiac and/or skeletal) muscle lesions and changes secondary to CHF in some animals that survive the acute toxic episode.

Confirmatory diagnosis requires efficient laboratory assays to determine the identity and amounts of the ionophore involved and a thorough consideration of differential diagnosis. These cannot be overemphasized. There is no known antidote or specific treatment for ionophore toxicoses and treatment is largely supportive. Judicious use, avoidance of overdosing, and adherence to species recommendation will enhance livestock production and help prevent the occurrence of adverse effects associated with this class of compounds.

REFERENCES

Adovelande, J.B., Schrevel, J., 1996. Carboxylic ionophores in malaria chemotherapy: the effects of monensin and nigericin on *Plasmodium falciparum in vitro* and *Plasmodium vinckelpetteri in vivo*. Pharmacol. Lett. 59, 309–315.

Agaoglu, Z.T., Akgul, Y., Keles, I., et al., 2002. Accidental salinomycin intoxication of Angora goats in Turkey. Small Ruminant Res. 45, 159–161.

Amend, J.F., Mallon, F.M., Wren, W.B., Ramos, A.S., 1981. Equine monensin toxicosis: some experimental clinicopathologic observations, Comp. Cont. Ed., 11. pp. S173–S183.

Anadon, A., Reeve-Johnson, L., 1999. Macrolide antibiotics, drug interactions and microsomal enzymes: implications for veterinary medicine. Res. Vet. Sci. 66, 197–203.

Atef, M., Ramadan, A., Abo El-Sooud, K., 1993. Pharmacokinetic profile and tissue distribution of monensin in broiler chickens. Br. Poult. Sci. 34, 195–203.

Becker, J.A., Speare, D.J., Daley, J., Dick, P., 2002. Effects of dose and treatment time on xenoma reduction in microsporidial gill disease in rainbow trout, *Onchorynchus mykiss* (Walbaum). J. Fish Dis. 25, 673–680.

Bergen, W.G., Bates, D.B., 1984. Ionophores: their effect on production efficiency and mode of action. J. Anim. Sci. 58, 1465–1483.

Bertini, S., Feirrero, S., Berny, P., 2003. A new improved high performance thin layer chromatography (HPTLC) method for the detection of ionophore antibiotics in feeds and animal tissues. J. Liq. Chrom. Rel. Technol. 26, 147–156.

Bradley, R., Markson, L.M., Bailey, J., 1981. Sudden death and myocardial necrosis in cattle. J. Pathol. 135, 19–38.

Brumbaugh, G.W., Simpson, R.B., Edwards, J.F., et al., 2004. Susceptibility of *Mycobacterium avium* sbsp *paratuberculosis* to monensin sodium or tilmicosin phosphate in vitro and resulting infectivity in a murine model. Can. J. Vet. Res. 88, 175–181.

Buck, W.B., Osweiller, G.D., Van Odder, C.A., 1976. Clinical and Diagnostic Veterinary Toxicology second ed. Kendall/Hunt Publishing Co, Dubuque, IA.

Buxton, D., Blewett, D.A., Trees, A.J., et al., 1988. Further studies in the use of monensin in the control of experimental ovine toxoplasmosis. J. Comp. Pathol. 98, 225–235.

Caldeira, C., Neves, W.S., Cury, P.M., et al., 2001. Rhabdomyolysis, acute renal failure, and death after monensin ingestion. Am. J. Kidney Dis. 38, 1108–1112.

Calo, M., Locascio, P., Licata, P., et al., 2002. Effects of monensin on Na+/K(+)-ATPase and Ca(++)-ATPase activities in chick skeletal muscle and myocardium after subacute treatment. Eur. J. Histochem. 46, 309–315.

Calo, M., Martini, D., Locascio Naccari, F., 2003. Effects of monensin on nitric oxide synthases in chick cardiac muscle. J. Vet. Pharmacol. Ther. 26 (Suppl. 1), 82–87.

Cardona, C.J., Galey, F.D., Bickford, A.A., et al., 1993. A syndrome in commercial turkeys in California and Oregon characterized by a rear-limb necrotizing myopathy. Avian Dis. 36, 1092–1101.

Carpenter, J.W., Novilla, M.N., 1992. Safety and physiologic effects of the anticoccidial drugs monensin and clasuril in sandhill cranes (*Grus canadensis*). J. Zoo Wild. Med. 23, 214–221.

Ceppa, L., Nachtman, C., Dacasto, M., et al., 1997. The effect of hepatic microsomal cytochrome P450 monooxygenases on monensin-sulfadimidine interaction in broilers. J. Vet. Pharmacol. Ther. 24, 73–76.

Condon, F.P., McKenzie, R.A., 2002. Fatal monensin toxicity in a dog after chewing a bovine intraruminal slow-release device. Aust. Vet. Pract. 32, 179–180.

Coyle, D., Walker, A., 2005 A study to determine the residues of monensin in edible tissues of growing cattle following treatment at 0.9 mg monensin/kg body weight for 28 days. Submitted to the European Medicines Agency CVMP by Elanco Animal Health, Division of Eli Lilly and Company, Indianapolis, IN.

Czarnecki, C.M., 1984. Cardiomyopathy in turkeys. Comp. Biochem. Physiol. 77, 591–598.

Davison, K.L., 1984. Monensin absorption and metabolism in calves and chickens. J. Agric. Food Chem. 32, 1273–1277.

Divers, T.J., Kraus, M.S., Jesty, S.A., et al., 2009. Clinical findings and serum cardiac troponin I concentrations in horses after intragastric administration of sodium monensin. J. Vet. Diagn. Invest. 21, 338–343.

Donoho, A.L., 1984. Biochemical studies on the fate of monensin in animals and in the environment. J. Anim. Sci. 58, 1528–1539.

Dowling, L., 1992. Ionophore toxicity in chickens: a review of pathology and diagnosis. Avian Pathol. 30, 358–368.

Duffield, T., Bagg, R., DesCoteaux, L., et al., 2002. Prepartum monensin for the reduction of energy associated disease in postpartum cows. J. Dairy Sci. 85, 397–405.

Ebel, J.G., Wachs, T., Henion, J.D., 2004. Rapid forensic selected reaction monitoring liquid chromatography/mass spectrometry determination of ionophore antibiotics found at toxic levels in animal feeds. J. Assoc. Off. Anal. Chem. 87, 25–30.

Evans, R.D., Edson, R.K., Watkins, K.L., et al., 2000. Turkey knockdown in successive flocks. Avian Dis. 44, 730–736.

Fajer-Avila, E.J., Covarrubias, M.S.M., Abad-Rosales, S., et al., 2005. Effectiveness of oral Elancoban™ and Avimix-ST™ against *Nematopsis* (Apicomplexa:Porosporidae) gametocyts infecting the shrimp *Litopenaeus vannamei*. Aquaculture 244, 11–18.

Frigg, M., Broz, J., Weber, G., 1983. Compatibility studies of ionophore anticoccidials with various antibiotics and chemotherapeutics in broiler chicks. Arch. Geflugelkunde 47, 213–220.

Galitzer, S.J., Bartley, F.F., Oehme, F.W., 1982. Preliminary studies on lasalocid toxicosis in cattle. Vet. Hum. Toxicol. 24, 406–409.

Galitzer, S.J., Kruckenburg, S.M., Kidd, J.R., 1986a. Pathologic changes associated with experimental lasalocid and monensin toxicosis in cattle. Am. J. Vet. Res. 47, 2624–2626.

Galitzer, S.J., Oehme, F.W., Bartley, E.E., Dayton, A.D., 1986b. Lasalocid toxicity in cattle: acute clinicopathological changes. J. Anim. Sci. 62, 1308–1316.

Greenstein, R.J., Su, L., Whitlock, R.H., Brown, S.T., 2009. Monensin causes dose dependent inhibition of *M. avium* subspecies *paratuberculosis* in radiometric culture. Gut Pathog. 1, 4.

Griffin, T., Ryback, M.E., Recht, L., et al., 1993. Potentiation of anti-tumor immunotoxins by liposomal monensin. J. Natl. Cancer Inst. 85, 292–298.

Gumila, C., Ancelin, M.L., Delort, A.M., et al., 1997. Characterization of the potent in vitro and in vivo antimalarial activities of ionophore compounds. Antimicrob. Agents Chemother. 41, 523–529.

Halvorson, D.A., Van Dijk, C., Brown, P., 1982. Ionophore toxicity in turkey breeders. Avian Dis. 26, 634–639.

Hamidinia, S.A., Shimelis, O.I., Tan, B., et al., 2002. Monensin mediates a rapid and selective transport of Pb(2+) Possible application of monensin for the treatment of Pb(2+) intoxication. J. Biol. Chem. 277, 3811–38120.

Hanley, H.G., Slack, J.D., 1982. Pharmacology of lasalocid. In: Westley, J.W. (Ed.), Polyether Antibiotics. Marcel Dekker, New York, NY, pp. 341–395.

Heuer, C., Schuken, Y.H., Jonker, L.J., et al., 2001. Effect of monensin on blood ketones bodies, incidence and recurrence of disease and fertility in dairy cows. J. Dairy Sci. 84, 1085–1097.

Holland, D.R., 1978 Cardiovascular and respiratory effects of sodium monensin, I.V. and P.O., in conscious dogs. Lilly Research Laboratories. Submitted to the European Medicines Agency CVMP by Elanco Animal Health, Division of Eli Lilly and Company, Indianapolis, IN.

Huczynski, A., 2012. Salinomycin-a new cancer drug candidate. Chem. Biol. Drugs Design. 79, 235–238, Perspective[a] 2011 John Wiley & Sons A/S http://dx.doi.org/10.1111/j.1747-0285.2011.01287.x.235.

Jones, T.C., Overstreet, R.M., Lotz, J.M., Frelier, F.P., 1994. *Paraphidioidina scolecoides* n. sp., a new aseptate gregarine from cultured Pacific white shrimp *Pennaeus vannamei*. Dis. Aquat. Org. 19, 67–75.

Kamashi, K., Reddy, A.G., Reddy, K.S., Reddy, V.R., 2004. Evaluation of zinc against salinomycin toxicity in broilers. Ind. J. Physiol. Pharmacol. 48, 89–95.

Kennington, A.S., Darby, J.M., Ehrenfried, K.M., et al., 1995. [14C] Monensin milk and tissue residues/metabolism in dairy cows. Submitted to the European Medicines Agency CVMP by Elanco Animal Health, Division of Eli Lilly and Company, Indianapolis, IN.

Kouyoumdjian, J.A., Morita, M.D., Sato, A.K., Pissolatti, A.F., 2001. Fatal rhabdomyolysis after acute sodium monensin (Rumensin) toxicity: case report. Arq. Neuropsiquiatr. 59, 596–598.

Kraus, M.S., Jesty, S.A., Gelzer, A.R., et al., 2010. Measurement of cardiac troponin 1 concentration by use of a point-of-care analyzer in clinically normal horses and horses with experimentally induced cardiac disease. Am. J. Vet. Res. 71, 55–59.

Kyriakis, S.C., Vlemmas, J.C., Mavromatis, J.C., et al., 1993. The effect of monensin in the control of transmissible gastroenteritis (TGE) of pigs. Swine Health Prod. 1, 15–18.

Long, P., Jeffers, T.K., 1982. Studies on the stage of action of ionophorous antibiotics against *Eimeria*. J. Parasitol. 68, 363–371.

Matsuoka, T., Novilla, M.N., Thomson, T.D., Donoho, A.L., 1996. Review of monensin toxicosis in horses. J. Equine Vet. Sci. 16, 8–15.

Mehlhorn, H., Pooch, H., Raether, W., 1983. The action of polyether ionophorous antibiotics (monensin, salinomycin, lasalocid) on developmental stages of *Eimeria tenella* (Coccidia, Sprozoa) in vivo and in vitro: study by light and electron microscopy. Z. Parasitenkd. 69, 457–471.

Meingassner, J.G., Schmook, F.P., Czok, R., Mieth, H., 1979. Enhancement of the anticoccidial activity of polyether antibiotics in chickens by tiamulin. Poult. Sci. 58, 308–313.

Meldrum, J.B., Evans, R.D., Robertson, J.L., et al., 2000. Alterations in levels of various antioxidant factors in turkey knockdown syndrome. Avian Dis. 44, 891–895.

Mitema, E.S., Sangiah, S., Martin, T., 1988. Effects of some calcium modulators on monensin toxicity. Vet. Hum. Toxicol. 30, 409–413.

Mollenhauer, H.H., Rowe, L.D., Cysewski, S.J., Witzel, D.A., 1981. Ultrastructural observations in ponies after treatment with monensin. Am. J. Vet. Res. 42, 35–40.

Mollenhauer, H.H., Morre, D.J., Rowe, R.D., 1990. Alteration of intracellular traffic by monensin: mechanism, specificity and relationship to toxicity. Biochim. Biophys. Acta 1031, 225–246.

Nebbia, C., Ceppa, L., Dacasto, M., et al., 2001. Oxidative monensin metabolism and cytochrome P450 3A content and functions in liver microsomes from horses, pigs, broiler chicks, cattle and rats. J. Vet. Pharmacol. Ther. 24, 399–403.

Nocerini, M.R., Honeyfield, D.C., Carlson, J.R., Breeze, R.G., 1985. Reduction in 3-methylindole production and prevention of acute bovine pulmonary edema and emphysema with lasalocid. J. Anim. Sci. 60, 232–238.

Novilla, M.N., 1992. The veterinary importance of the toxic syndrome induced by ionophores. Vet. Hum. Toxicol. 34, 66–70.

Novilla, M.N., 2004. Expert report on the safety file for monensin sodium. Submitted to the European Medicines Agency CVMP by Elanco Animal Health, Division of Eli Lilly and Company, Indianapolis, IN.

Novilla, M.N., Folkerts, T.M., 1986. Ionophores: monensin, lasalocid, salinomycin, narasin. In: Howard, J.L. (Ed.), Current Veterinary Therapy-Food Animal Practice. Academic Press, New York, NY, pp. 359–363.

Novilla, M.N., Laudert, S.B., 2009. Monensin Toxicity in Cattle. TechTalk Scientific Update from Elanco Animal Health, A Division of Eli Lilly and Company, Greenfield, IN.

Novilla, M.N., Todd, G.C., 1991. Cardiotoxicity of the ionophores – rat. In: Jones, T.C., Mohr, U., Hunt, R.D. (Eds.), Monographs on Pathology of Laboratory Animals Cardiovascular and Musculoskeletal Systems. Springer Verlag, Berlin.

Novilla, M.N., Owen, N.V., Todd, G.C., 1994. The comparative toxicology of narasin in laboratory animals. Vet. Hum. Toxicol. 36, 318–323.

O'Brien, P.J., 2008. Cardiac troponin is the most effective translational safety biomarker for myocardial injury in cardiotoxicity. Toxicology 245, 206–218.

Parker, R.J., Jones, G.W., Ellis, K.J., Heater, K.M., Schroter, K.L., Tyler, R., et al., 1986. Post-weaning coccidiosis in beef calves in the dry tropics: experimental control with continuous monensin supplementation via intraruminal devices and concurrent epidemiological observations. Trop. Anim. Health Prod. 18, 198–208.

Plumlee, K.H., Johnson, B., Galey, F.D., 1995. Acute salinomycin toxicosis of pigs. J. Vet. Diagn. Invest. 7, 419–420.

Potter, E.L., Van Duyn, R.L., Cooley, C.O., 1984. Monensin toxicity in cattle. J. Anim. Sci. 58, 1499–1511.

Pressman, B.C., 1976. Biological applications of ionophores. Annu. Rev. Biochem. 45, 501–530.

Pressman, B.C., Fahim, N.I., 1982. Pharmacology and toxicology of the monovalent carboxylic ionophores. Annu. Rev. Pharmacol. Toxicol. 22, 465–490.

Pressman, B.C., Fahim, N.I., 1983. Cardiovascular toxicity of ionophores used as feed additives. Adv. Exp. Med. Biol. 161, 543–561.

Reed, P.W., 1982. Biochemical and biological effects of carboxylic acid ionophores. In: Westley, J.W. (Ed.), Polyether Antibiotics. Marcel Dekker, New York, NY, pp. 185–302.

Reichenback, D.D., Benditt, E.P., 1982. Catecholamines and cardiomyopathy: the pathogenesis and potential importance of myofibrilar degeneration. Human Pathol. 1, 125–150.

Russell, J.B., Strobel, H.J., 1989. Mini-review: effect of ionophores on ruminal fermentation. Appl. Environ. Microbiol. 55, 1–6.

Safran, N., Aisenberg, I., Bark, H., 1993. Paralytic syndrome attributed to lasalocid residues in a commercial ration fed to dogs. J. Am. Vet. Med. Assoc. 202, 1273–1275.

Salyi, G., Szabo, E., Bago, G., et al., 1988. Narasin poisoning in turkeys. Acta Vet. Hung. 36, 107–114.

Sandercock, D.A., Mitchell, M.A., 2004. The role of sodium ions in the pathogenesis of skeletal muscle damage in broiler chickens. Poult. Sci. 83, 701–706.

Segev, G., Baneth, G., Levitin, B., et al., 2004. Accidental poisoning of 17 dogs with lasalocid. Vet. Rec. 135, 174–176.

Shaik, M.S., Ikediobi, O., Turnage, V.D., et al., 2001. Long-circulating monensin nanoparticles for the potentiation of immunotoxin and anticancer drugs. J. Pharm. Pharmacol. 53, 617–627.

Shier, W.T., DuBourdieu, D.J., 1992. Sodium- and calcium-dependent steps in the mechanism of neonatal rat cardiac myocyte killing by ionophores. Toxicol. Appl. Pharmacol. 116, 38–46.

Shlosberg, A., Weisman, Y., Klopper, U., Perl, S., 1985. Neurotoxic action of lasalocid at high doses. Vet. Rec. 117, 394.

Smith, C.K., Galloway, R.G., 1983. Influence of monensin on cation influx and glycolysis of *Eimeria tenella* sporozoites in vitro. J. Parasitol. 69, 666–670.

Smith, C.K., Galloway, R.B., White, S.L., 1981. Effect of ionophores on survival, penetration, and development of *Eimeria tenella* sporozoites *in vitro*. J. Parasitol. 67, 511–516.

Szücs, G., Tamasi, V., Laczay, P., Monostory, K., 2004. Biochemical background of toxic interaction between tiamulin and monensin. Chem. Biol. Interact. 147, 151–161.

Tappel, A.L., 1981. Vitamin E and selenium protection from in vitro lipid peroxidation. Ann. N.Y. Acad. Sci. 355, 18–31.

Taylor, R.W., Kauffman, R.F., Pfeifer, D.R., 1982. Cation complexation and transport by carboxylic acid ionophores. In: Westley, J.W. (Ed.), Polyether Antibiotics. Marcel Dekker, New York, NY, pp. 103–184.

Thomas, E.E., Smith, C.K., McGuffey, R.F., Quin, M.E., 1985. Monensin Provides Coccidiosis Control: Site and Mode of Action. Tech Talk Scientific Update from Elanco Animal Health, Division of Eli Lilly and Company, Indianapolis, IN.

Todd, O.C., Novilla, M.N., Howard, L.C., 1984. Comparative toxicology of monensin sodium in laboratory animals. J. Anim. Sci. 58, 1512–1517.

Van der Linde-Sipman, J.S., Van den Ingh, T.S.G.A.M., Van Es, J.J., et al., 1999. Salinomycin-induced polyneuropathy in cats: morphologic and epidemiologic data. Vet. Pathol. 36, 152–156.

Van Vleet, J.F., 1986. Interactions of nutritional status and ionophore feed additives in animals. In: Proc. 6th International Conference on Production Diseases in Farm Animals. Belfast, Northern Ireland, pp. 268–276.

Van Vleet, J.F., Amstutz, H.E., Weirich, W.E., Rebar, A.H., Ferrans, V. J., 1983a. Acute monensin toxicosis in swine: effect of graded doses of monensin and protection of swine by pretreatment with selenium-vitamin E. Am. J. Vet. Res. 44, 1460–1468.

Van Vleet, J.F., Amstutz, H.E., Weirich, W.E., et al., 1983b. Clinical clinicopathological and pathologic alterations of acute monensin toxicosis in swine. Am. J. Vet. Res. 44, 1469–1475.

Van Vleet, J.F., Amstutz, H.E., Weirich, W.E., et al., 1983c. Clinical, clinicopathologic and pathologic alterations in acute monensin toxicosis in cattle, Am. J. Vet. Res., 44. pp. 2133–2144.

Van Vleet, J.F., Runnels, L.J., Cook, J.R., Scheidt, A.B., 1987. Monensin toxicosis in swine: potentiation by tiamulin administration and ameliorative effect of treatment with selenium and/or vitamin E. Am. J. Vet. Res. 48, 1520–1523.

Van Vleet, J.F., Ferrans, V.J., Herman, E., 1991. Cardiovascular and skeletal muscle system. In: Hascheck, W.M., Rousseaux, C.G. (Eds.), Handbook of Toxicologic Pathology. Academic Press, San Diego, CA, pp. 539–624.

Wages, D.P., 1993. Turkey knockdown is a multi-faceted puzzle. Turkey World 69, 24–25.

Weisman, J., Herz, A., Jegana, J., et al., 1983. The effect of tiamulin administered by different routes and at different ages in turkeys receiving monensin in their feed. Vet. Res. Commun. 6, 189–198.

Whitlock, R.H., White, N.A., Rowland, G.N., Plue, R., 1978. Monensin toxicosis in horses; clinical manifestations. Proc. Am. Assoc. Equine Pract. 24, 473–486.

Wilson, B.W., Nieberg, P.S., Buhr, R.J., et al., 1990. Turkey muscle growth and focal myopathy. Poult. Sci. 69, 1553–1562.

Witkamp, R.P., Nijmeijer, S.M., Van Miert, A.S.J.P.A.M., 1996. Cytochrome P450 complex formation in rat liver by the antibiotic tiamulin. Antimicrob. Agents Chemother. 40, 50–54.

FURTHER READING

Food and Drug Adminstration, CFR Parts 556 and 558, 2004. Approval of supplemental NADA for the use of monensin Type A medicated articles to formulate Type and Type C medicated feeds for increased milk production efficiency in dairy cows. Fed. Reg. 69, 68783–68784.

Novilla, M.N., Muller, R.D., 2003. Ionophore Diagnostic Manual. Elanco Animal Health, A Division of Eli Lilly and Company, Greenfield, IN.

Chapter 79

Nonprotein Nitrogen (Urea) and Hyperammonemia

Rhian B. Cope

INTRODUCTION AND BACKGROUND

Nonprotein nitrogen (NPN) intoxication is a common occurrence in ruminants. It has been long recognized that ruminal microbes of cattle and sheep can utilize NPN to synthesize protein that can replace a portion of their host's total dietary protein requirements (Davis and Roberts, 1959; Dinning et al., 1948; Haliburton and Morgan, 1989; Hatch, 1977; Lloyd, 1981; Loosli and McDonald, 1968; Osweiler et al., 1985; Word et al., 1960). Given that feeding NPN is typically less expensive than feeding true protein, the practice of adding NPN to ruminant diets remains common. This practice is safe and beneficial if carefully managed. Feed-grade urea is usually the cheapest and most available nitrogen source for NPN supplementation. Other NPN compounds, which may be less readily available and more expensive, can be used as well (Table 79.1; Loosli and McDonald, 1968). Addition of NPN sources into the diet requires careful dietary nutritional examination and evaluation of the animal's circumstances if toxicity is to be avoided. Urea and other NPN sources are commonly combined with molasses, which acts as a readily available soluble carbohydrate source and provides the dietary energy needed by the rumen microflora to convert NPN sources to microbial protein. Many of these supplements are solids and can be directly mixed into mineral or grain supplements. Ammoniated beet pulp, citrus pulp, straw, silage, molasses and rice hulls have also been used to supplement the protein content of a ruminant's diet. Ruminants can also suffer NPN poisoning through accidental consumption of fertilizers containing >40% urea.

CHEMISTRY

The terms "ammonia" and "ammonium" are commonly not used according to their strictly chemical definitions in the veterinary literature. For clarity, in this chapter the following strict chemical definitions are used (NCBI):

Ammonia = Azane (IUPAC name) = NH_3; A gas

Ammonium = Ammonium cation = Azanium (IUPAC name); A water soluble cation

The important basic chemical relationships between ammonia (NH_3) and the ammonium cation (NH_4^+) are as follows (Lower and Fraser, 2016). In the presence of proton donors (i.e., Brønsted acids), ammonia (NH_3) undergoes protonation to the ammonium cation (NH_4^+):

$$H^+ + NH_3 \rightarrow NH_4^+$$

The ammonium cation (NH_4^+) is a weak acid ($pK_a = 9.26$) and in the presence of a OH^- donor (i.e., a Brønsted base) it undergoes hydroxylation to the uncharged ammonia molecule:

$$OH^- + NH_4^+ \rightarrow NH_3$$

Thus, in an aqueous environment the following equilibrium is established:

$$H_2O + NH_3 \leftrightarrow OH^- + NH_4^+$$

The balance of this equilibrium depends on the pH of the aqueous solution (Fig. 79.1).

In a low pH (approximately less than pH 8), more acid aqueous environment, the dominant reaction is the protonation of ammonia (NH_3) to the ammonium cation (NH_4^+),

Veterinary Toxicology. DOI: http://dx.doi.org/10.1016/B978-0-12-811410-0.00079-9

TABLE 79.1 Common Nonprotein Nitrogen Sources for Ruminants

	Formula	Nitrogen Content (%)	Protein Equivalent[a]
Ammonium acetate	$CH_3CO_2NH_4$	18	≈112
Ammonium bicarbonate	NH_4HCO_3	18	≈112
Ammonium carbonate	$NH_2CO_2NH_4$	36	≈225
Ammonium lactate	$CH_3CHOHCO_2NH_4$	13	≈81
Biuret	$NH_2CONHCONH_2H_2O$	35	≈219
Dicyanodiamide	$NH_2(:NH)NHCN$	67	≈419
Glutamine	$NH_2CO(CH_2)_2CHNH_2CO_2H$	19	≈119
Glycine	$NH_2CH_2CO_2H$	19	≈119
Urea (pure)	$(NH_2)_2CO$	46.7	≈292
Urea (feed grade)[b]		42–45	≈262–281
Common oil seed meals[c] (for comparison)	–	5.8–8.0	36–50

[a]*Nitrogen content (%) × 6.25.*
[b]*Diluted with various anticaking agents to prevent concentrated lumps forming.*
[c]*Includes cottonseed, soybean, linseed, coconut and similar oil extracted seed meals.*

i.e., the fractional composition (α) of the material almost completely consists (i.e., $\alpha \approx 1$) of the hydrophilic (i.e., less systemically bioavailable) ammonium cation (NH_4^+) form at pH $\leq \approx 8$ (the *red line* in Fig. 79.1).

In a high pH (approximately greater than pH 11), more alkaline aqueous environment, the dominant reaction is the hydroxylation of the ammonium cation (NH_4^+) to ammonia (NH_3), i.e., the fractional composition (α) of the material almost completely consists (i.e., $\alpha \approx 1$) of the more lipophilic (i.e., more systemically bioavailable) ammonia (NH_3) form at pH $\geq \approx 11$ (the *black line* in Fig. 79.1).

If the rumen pH equals the pK_a of the ammonium cation (NH_4^+; p$K_a = 9.26$), then 50% of the material will be in the ammonia form and 50% will be in the ammonium cation form.

NONPROTEIN NITROGEN UTILIZATION UNDER NORMAL CONDITIONS (RUMEN pH 6.5–7.0)

Following ingestion, NPN sources are rapidly converted to ammonia (NH_3) by microbial metabolism (typically hydrolyzed by bacterial urease in the case of urea; Loosli and McDonald, 1968). Ammonia (NH_3) is subsequently used by the rumen microflora for the synthesis of amino acids and proteins that are required for their growth. These processes are closely associated with the utilization of cellulose, other carbohydrates, and short chain fatty acids, etc., as energy sources by the rumen microflora. In particular, soluble readily available dietary carbohydrates (e.g., molasses) facilitate these microbial processes. The rate of ammonia production from NPN sources is about the same as for water soluble dietary proteins (e.g., casein). Since ruminant diets typically contain a high proportion of insoluble proteins, which are not utilized by the rumen microflora (i.e., bypass the forestomach with subsequent digestion and absorption in the stomach and small intestine), the rate of rumen ammonia production from NPN sources is usually much higher than that associated with normal foraging.

At normal rumen pH (i.e., pH 6.5–7.0), virtually all free ammonia (NH_3) that is not utilized for microbial protein synthesis and which is released into the rumen fluid, will be very rapidly protonated to ammonium cations (NH_4^+). Because ammonium cations (NH_4^+) are charged, they are poorly lipophilic and thus poorly absorbed across the rumen wall, i.e., toxicity is less likely under these conditions. The extremely small fraction of the material that remains in the more lipophilic ammonia (NH_3) form under these conditions can be systemically absorbed across the rumen wall and subsequently metabolized to urea (CH_4N_2O) in the liver. A portion of the urea produced is then excreted in the urine, i.e., lost to the animal (Loosli and McDonald, 1968).

In ruminants and camelids, a significant amount of systemically absorbed ammonia (NH_3) is recycled to the digestive tract in the form of urea in saliva or as urea transported from the blood across the rumen wall (fraction

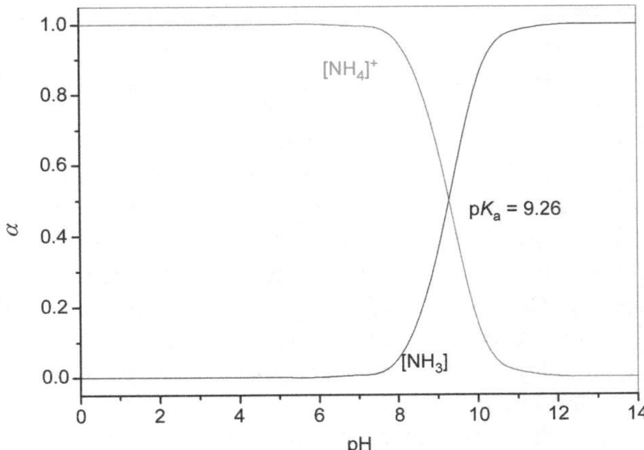

FIGURE 79.1 Acid–base fractional composition ($\alpha = 0 = 0\%$ fractional composition; $\alpha = 1 = 100\%$ fractional composition) as a function of pH for ammonia (NH_3) and ammonium ions (NH_4^+) (Fractional composition (α) for a simple monoprotic acid–base relationships can be calculated using the following equations:

$$\alpha_0 = \frac{[H^+]}{[H^+] + K_a} = \frac{[HA]}{[A^-] + [HA]}; \alpha_1 = \frac{K_a}{[H^+] + K_a} = \frac{[A^-]}{[A^-] + [HA]}).$$

ranges from 10% to 40% of nitrogen consumed in feed depending on species and conditions, water intake and the nature of the feed available also affect the response). Urea can also be directly absorbed through the rumen wall and can also be recycled to the digestive tract. Camelids, in comparison with ruminants, are much more efficient at conserving nitrogen under conditions of low protein nutritional stress. Under these conditions, this species excretes only 1%–2% of systemically available nitrogen, with the remainder being recycled into the rumen.

THE BIOLOGICAL VALUE OF RUMEN MICROFLORA PROTEIN

When NPN is used as the only source of dietary nitrogen, the rumen microflora can produce all the amino acids that are essential for growth, wool production, and milk production provided other dietary requirements are adequate, i.e., effective conversion of dietary NPN to tissue, wool and milk proteins occurs in ruminants (Loosli and McDonald, 1968). Irrespective of the dietary nitrogen source, the resultant microbial protein tends to have a biological value of 60%–70% (biological value measures the proportion of absorbed dietary protein from a food that is subsequently incorporated into the organism's proteins, i.e., it is a measure of how readily digested dietary protein can be used in protein synthesis in the cells of the organism). Insoluble rumen bypass dietary protein is still of value in particular circumstances (e.g., the rapid growth phases of pregnancy and postpartum periods of high milk production in highly productive animals).

TOXICITY

Depending on dose, all mammalian species are potentially susceptible to NPN poisoning via the consumption of ammonia-containing feeds (Hintz et al., 1970). However, NPN poisoning is most commonly observed in ruminants. In ruminants, if NPN is consumed at a rate that exceeds the capacity of the rumen microflora to convert it into microbial protein, then free NPN (typically free ammonia or free ammonium, depending on pH) will remain in the rumen fluid. At normal rumen pH (pH 6.5–7.0), free ammonia (NH_3) will be rapidly protonated to ammonium (NH_4^+) with the coproduction of hydroxyl ions (OH^-). This results in an increase in rumen pH (Lower and Fraser, 2016). When rumen pH rises above approximately pH 8, the ammonia–ammonium equilibrium reaction strongly favors the formation of free ammonia (NH_3; *black line* in Fig. 79.1). Since the free ammonia (NH_3) form is unionized and more lipophilic, these conditions also favor systemic absorption through the rumen wall. Once the systemic absorption of ammonia (NH_3) exceeds the animal's capacity to excrete it or metabolise it, hyperammonemia and toxicity develop. In non-NPN–adapted ruminants, these reactions can occur relatively quickly (e.g., within 30 min to hours in animals that are not adapted to NPN sources and/or after feed mixing errors).

Hyperammonemia inhibits the citric acid cycle (Hatch, 1977), resulting in metabolic lactic acidosis, interference with cerebral energy metabolism and failure of Na^+-/K^+-ATPase pumps with resultant hyperkalemia. Factors that potentially predispose ruminants to dietary ammonia poisoning include low energy diets, high rumen pH (e.g., rumen impaction), elevated body temperature (increases rumen microflora urease activity), and dehydration, stress, concurrent disease, alterations in rumen microflora, insufficient rumen microflora adaptation time and hepatic insufficiency. A lack of readily available soluble dietary carbohydrates markedly affects the rumen bacteria's ability to utilize the ammonia for protein synthesis.

Most NPN poisonings in ruminants occur as a result of inadequate implementation of an adaptation period, improper mixing of the supplement into the diet (including hot spots of NPN concentration), and unlimited/unrestricted access to palatable liquid NPN supplements. Adaptation of the rumen microflora to dietary NPN sources takes several days. The use of anticaking agents to prevent the formation of areas of high urea concentration in the ration is an important preventative strategy in solid preparations. NPN poisoning in monogastric animals is uncommon.

Toxic and lethal doses are difficult to establish in ruminants due to all the predisposing factors that can enhance or decrease their sensitivity to these compounds. The oral lethal dose for urea in horses is about 4.0 g/kg body weight and the oral lethal dose for ammonia salts is about 1.5 g/kg body weight (Hintz et al., 1970). A reported oral toxic dose for urea in nonacclimated cattle is 0.44 g/kg body weight (Word et al., 1960), whereas a lethal dose is in the 1.0–1.5 g/kg body weight range (Osweiler et al., 1985). Urea is recommended in ruminant rations at a rate of approximately 3% of a grain ration or 1% of the total ration. Well-adapted cattle can tolerate much higher levels in their diets. Biuret is considered one of the safest NPN compounds, and the reported lethal dose in cattle is 8.0 g/kg body weight (Haliburton and Morgan, 1989). A single dose of 116 g of urea caused clinical signs of toxicity in cattle, whereas a dose of 57 g did not (Dinning et al., 1948). Davis and Roberts (1959) reported that 0.3 g/kg body weight urea was toxic to nonacclimated cattle.

CLINICAL SIGNS

The onset of clinical signs following introduction of a NPN source into a nonadapted ruminant's diet can be extremely quick, commonly within 30 min of consumption. A delay in the onset of clinical signs may result from a wide variety of factors, including dose, method of introduction and, most importantly, degree of rumen microbial adaptation. Many cases of NPN poisoning in ruminants involve a history of some type of "recent feed change." Commonly reported clinical signs include uneasiness and ataxia, muscle tremors, excessive salivation, weakness, labored breathing, abdominal pain and bloat. The progression of clinical signs is usually rapid and recumbency, convulsions and death typically ensues within 4 h of the onset of the toxidrome. Hyperthermia, marked jugular pulse, cardiac arrhythmias, vomiting/regurgitation, and cyanosis have also been reported (Haliburton and Morgan, 1989). Affected animals rarely survive once clinical signs start without some type of rapid treatment.

DIAGNOSTIC CRITERIA

The diagnosis of NPN intoxication rests mainly on a compatible history of exposure to an NPN source, a clinical history that documents relevant risk factors, compatible clinical signs with rapid progression to death and clinical diagnostic laboratory data. Definitive postmortem changes are rare. Common findings at necropsy include generalized congestion of visceral organs, evidence of bloat and mild to moderate pulmonary edema. Subepicardial and myocardial hemorrhages have also been reported. There are several diagnostic aids that can assist the veterinarian in confirming NPN poisoning.

Assessing the rumen pH either antemortem or shortly after death is a potentially useful diagnostic tool. In animals that have recently succumbed to NPN intoxication, rumen pH is typically >8–10 (i.e., in the pH range that strongly favors the formation of ammonium cations [NH_4^+]). An elevated rumen pH postmortem will gradually revert to normal over time due to continued microbial activity. Other causes of excessive rumen pH can include rumen impactions or other problems leading to a "dead" (nonmotile) rumen or excessive salivary secretions (increased rumen pH).

Elevated ammonia concentrations in various biological specimens (e.g., serum, plasma, ocular fluid, and abomasal or rumen fluid) can be analytically confirmed by various methods. Ocular fluids are often considered to be the most reliable postmortem sample. All samples should be collected in well-sealed containers and frozen immediately for delivery to the diagnostic laboratory, to prevent loss of the volatile ammonia gas. Samples collected postmortem should be retrieved shortly after death because decomposition of tissues can cause spuriously high or low results. Ammonia concentrations typically >1.0 mg/dL in serum or plasma and/or >than 80 mg/dL in rumen or abomasum contents are generally diagnostically significant.

Lastly, ammonia, nitrogen, or urea levels can be assessed in the "suspect" feed source. These analyses should be quantitative, and the sampling technique used should assist the veterinarian in determining whether a mixing error or the presence of "hot spots" was responsible for the clinical problem.

TREATMENT

Very rapid intervention is necessary in order for affected animals to survive. This is rarely possible except in experimental settings. Poisonings generally occur on a large scale (rarely a single animal problem) and in a setting (e.g., feedlots, pastures typically located in more rural settings) where it usually nearly impossible to implement appropriate rapid therapies. Treatments are generally thought to be effective if aggressively initiated within 20 min after the onset of clinical signs; however, the prognosis is usually poor for recumbent animals. A triage decision to prioritize the treatment of animals that are still standing may be justifiable.

The immediate treatment objective is to lower the rumen pH to below pH 8 (i.e., shift the $NH_3 \leftrightarrow NH_4^+$ equilibrium in favor of the formation of the less bioavailable ammonium cation [$NH_4{}^+$] form). Five percent acetic acid (i.e., vinegar) should be administered by intrarumen intubation (2–6 L in cattle and 0.5–1.0 L in sheep and goats;

Lloyd, 1981) until the rumen fluid pH is <8 (i.e., rumen fluid pH should be clearly acidic on testing). Ideally, the rumen fluid pH should be periodically checked using pH papers during acetic acid administration in order to evaluate the effectiveness of this treatment.

The next treatment objective is to decrease the reaction rate of rumen microflora urease by reducing the temperature of the rumen contents. Following rumen acidification, a large volume (5–10 gallons) of cold water should be administered by intrarumen intubation.

Animals that respond to treatment often relapse and repeat treatment (usually using about half the amounts of acetic acid and cold water used in the first treatment) is typically required (can be aided by periodic monitoring of rumen pH after initial treatment). Recumbent and convulsing animals generally respond poorly to treatment.

Other nonspecific, supportive therapies may include anticonvulsant therapy (e.g., phenobarbital, pentobarbital) and intravenous fluid therapy to correct fluid deficits and any elemental or electrolyte abnormalities.

Animals that recover usually do not appear to suffer any recognizable long-term adverse effects, although abortions can occur in pregnant animals.

AMMONIA (NH_3) GAS

NPN poisonings resulting in hyperammonemia should not be confused with ammonia poisoning (covered in detail in the chapter on toxic gases). Synonyms include ammonia gas, anhydrous ammonia and liquid ammonia. Livestock can be poisoned by ammonia, either through inhalation or ingestion, through its use as a fertilizer. As described previously, ammonia (NH_3) readily dissolves in water to form the ammonium cation (NH_4^+) and hydroxyl ions (OH^-). This results in typical alkali burns (i.e., dissolution of tissue proteins). Anhydrous ammonia is colorless, highly irritating, and causes corrosive injury to the mucous membranes of the eyes, lungs, and skin. Inhalation of ammonia can lead to severe bronchiolar and alveolar edema, and airway destruction that can result in respiratory failure and death. Dermal contact or oral exposures lead to corrosive skin lesions and corrosive damage to the mucosal lining of the oral cavity, esophagus, and stomach.

CONCLUDING REMARKS AND FUTURE DIRECTIONS

All mammalian species are susceptible to urea/ammonia poisoning, although poisoning most commonly occurs in ruminants undergoing dietary supplementation with NPN. Diagnosis is based on clinical signs and analysis of the body tissues/fluids and feed for urea and ammonia levels. Treatment includes oral administration of acetic acid (vinegar) and symptomatic and supportive therapies.

REFERENCES

Davis, G.K., Roberts, H.F., 1959. Urea Toxicity in Cattle. Agricultural Experiment Station, Bulletin 611, Gainesville, FL.

Dinning, J.S., Briggs, H.M., Gallup, W.D., Orr, H.W., Butler, R., 1948. Effect of orally administered urea on the ammonia and urea concentration in the blood of cattle and sheep, with observations on blood ammonia levels associated with symptoms of alkalosis. Am. J. Physiol. 153, 41–46.

Haliburton, J.C., Morgan, S.E., 1989. Nonprotein nitrogen-induced ammonia toxicosis and ammoniated feed toxicity syndrome. Vet. Clin. North Am. Food Anim. Pract. 5 (2), 237–249.

Hatch, R.C., 1977. Veterinary toxicology. In: Jones, L.M., Booth, L.F. (Eds.), Veterinary Pharmacology and Therapeutics. The Iowa State University Press, Ames, IA, pp. 1253–1259.

Hintz, H.F., Lowe, J.E., Clifford, A.J., Visek, W.J., 1970. Ammonia intoxication resulting from urea poisoning by ponies. J. Am. Vet. Med. Assoc. 157, 963–966.

Lloyd, W.E., 1981. Urea and other nonprotein nitrogen sources. In: Howard, J.L. (Ed.), Current Veterinary Therapy. Food Animal Practice. W.B. Saunders, Philadelphia, PA, pp. 393–396.

Loosli, J.K., McDonald, I.W., 1968. Nonprotein Nitrogen in the Nutrition of Ruminants. FAO Agricultural Studies No. 73. Food and Agriculture Organization of the United Nations, Rome.

Lower, S., Fraser, S., 2016. All about acids and bases; and Acid-base equilibria and calculations (Chapters 9 and 21 (respectively)). In: Chem1 Virtual Textbook a reference text for General Chemistry. Ed. Lower S, Fraser S. Simon. <http://www.chem1.com/acad/webtext/virtualtextbook.html> (accessed 31.10.16.).

Osweiler, G.D., Carson, T.L., Buck, W.B., Van Gelder, G.A., 1985. Urea and nonprotein nitrogen. Clinical and Diagnostic Veterinary Toxicology. Kendall/Hunt Publishing Company, Dubuque, IA, pp. 160–166.

Word, J.D., Martin, L.C., Williams, D.L., et al., 1960. Urea toxicity studies in the bovine. J. Anim. Sci. 29, 786–791.

FURTHER READING

NCBI. (National Center for Biotechnology Information). PubChem Compound Database; CID 222. <https://pubchem.ncbi.nlm.nih.gov/compound/ammonia>. CID 223. <https://pubchem.ncbi.nlm.nih.gov/compound/ammonium> (accessed 31.10.16.).

Chapter 80

Water Quality and Contaminants

Michael P. Carlson

INTRODUCTION

Water is essential for all forms of life. The availability of adequate quantities and quality of water dictates the types of life and numbers of individuals that a locale can sustain. Competition for water among various users may limit water available for animal production and available water may be of poorer quality if water supplies become limited. Large-scale animal production practices and emphasis on animal performance may increase the demands on water delivery systems and increase concern about water quality.

Water quality generally refers to the suitability of water for some purpose and it may be assessed for any of several reasons, including: to determine if the available water is suitable for a particular production system, to determine if there has been a change in water quality, or to determine if adverse health effects that are occurring may be attributable to contaminated water. Assessment is usually made based on the amount of various chemicals found in the water compared to water quality standards.

What chemicals should be included in water quality assessment? What standards should be used to assess water quality?

The intent for this chapter is to provide the reader with information to aid in the assessment of drinking water quality for companion and production animals. Some of the more readily accessible water quality standards applicable to drinking water for animals will be highlighted. Information about the daily amounts of water required by animals is also provided to help assess cases of possible exposure of animals to water-borne poisons. Lastly, standards for cyanotoxins in water are discussed.

WHAT CHEMICALS SHOULD BE INCLUDED IN LIVESTOCK DRINKING WATER QUALITY ASSESSMENT?

There is no consensus about what chemicals should be included in a drinking water quality assessment for livestock. Various chemicals are included in livestock water quality monographs readily available on line, a sampling of which appears in Table 80.1. Those eight monographs are written by university experts and published by the university cooperative extension service (Faries et al., 1991; German et al., 2008; Higgins et al., not specified; Mukhtar, 1998; Raisbeck et al., not specified; Sallenave, 2016) or a governmental agency (Olkowski, 2009).

Faries et al. (1991), say that the most common water quality problems affecting livestock production are high mineral content, high nitrate or nitrite content, bacterial contamination, blue-green algae contamination, and accidental contamination from spills of agrichemicals or petroleum products. Practically, the chemicals included should be based on circumstances, which might include chemicals known to be present in local water at high concentrations or chemicals that might be etiological agents for adverse health effects being seen in the herd or animal group.

WATER QUALITY ANALYTICAL SERVICES

Water quality analytical services are available from academic, governmental, and commercial laboratories. Services at governmental laboratories may be limited to regulatory monitoring programs or to specimens related to water quality regulation violations and therefore may not be readily available to the general public.

Services offered may include water quality panels, anion panels, mineral panels, microbial culture and identification, and à la carte services.

Water quality panels commonly include some but not all of the following analytes: pH, total dissolved solids (TDSs), ammonia, chloride, phosphorus, nitrate, nitrite, and sulfate. Some include coliform counts. Panels may also include some metal cations, such as calcium, magnesium, potassium, and sodium, but often metal cation analytical services are offered separately. Analytes included in a panel depend upon the intended use of the water, e.g., irrigation, human consumption, or livestock consumption. A panel specifically for water intended for livestock consumption is preferable.

Veterinary Toxicology. DOI: http://dx.doi.org/10.1016/B978-0-12-811410-0.00080-5

TABLE 80.1 Chemicals Listed in Each of a Sampling of Livestock Water Quality Monographs

Chemical	Monograph							
	Faires	German	Higgins	Mukhtar	Olkowski	Pfost	Raisbeck	Sellenave
Al			X		X	X		
As	X		X	X	X	X	X	X
B	X							
Ba	X		X	X	X	X	X	X
Be					X			
Ca					X			
Cd	X		X	X	X	X		X
Cl	X							
Cr	X		X	X	X	X		X
Co	X		X		X			
Cu	X		X	X	X	X		X
F	X		X	X	X	X	X	X
Hardness		X	X			X		
Fe	X							
Pb	X		X	X	X			X
Mg								
Mn	X		X				X	
Mo	X		X	X	X	X		
Hg	X				X			X
NO_3^-	X	X	X	X			X	X
$NO_3^- + NO_2^-$					X	X		
NO_2^-	X			X	X	X		
Ni	X						X	
pH		X	X					
Phosphate						X		
Salinity	X	X	X	X		X	X	X
Se	X		X		X	X		X
Ag	X							
Na		X					X	
Sulfate	X	X			X	X	X	X
TDS	X				X	X	X	
V	X		X		X	X		
Zn	X		X	X	X	X		X

Water anion panels may include some or all of the following anions: nitrate, nitrite, chloride, phosphate, and sulfate.

Water mineral panels commonly include arsenic, cadmium, calcium, iron, lead, magnesium, manganese, phosphorus, potassium, selenium, sodium, and zinc, but other metals may also be included.

À la carte analytical services for individual analytes may be offered instead of or in addition to panels. Panels usually cost less than will a la carte services for all analytes included in the panels, even if only some of the analytes included in the panel are of interest.

Cost comparisons of analytical services offered by various laboratories can be challenging because of the varying analytical technology that is used to provide the services and varying number of analytes included in panels.

WHAT STANDARDS SHOULD BE USED TO ASSESS WATER QUALITY?

The assessment of water quality data requires standards against which to compare the results. Reports of water quality data may include graphical comparisons of the results to water quality standards, making results that fall outside of the standard limits easily identifiable. But what standards should be used to assess water intended for consumption by animals?

Water quality standards may be established by national, state or provincial, or local governments. Sometimes standards recommended by an international body such as the World Health Organization may be used. Governmental standards are usually applicable to water used for a particular purpose, e.g., human consumption, livestock consumption, or irrigation, or in a particular circumstance, e.g., agriculture land runoff water.

Generally, quality standards for water intended for human consumption are regulated with a rigor not applicable to water intended for animal consumption. Some regulations for water for use by humans are actionable, meaning the water quality regulating body can legally require that potable water be made available to replace water deemed unfit for human consumption. The scope of the regulating authority may be limited, e.g., regulations may apply to municipal water supplies but not to private supplies.

Regulations for drinking water for use by animals are generally not actionable and may be referred to as recommendations.

Standards for human drinking water may be realistically applied to water for companion animals because those animals often consume the same water as do their owners. But human drinking water standards are not necessarily what should be used to assess the quality of water for livestock. For example, the US human drinking water standard for nitrate + nitrite is 10 mg $NO_3^- - N + NO_2^- - N/L$ (US EPA, (a), (b)), whereas the livestock standard for nitrate + nitrite established by Canadian Council of Ministers of the Environment is 100 mg $NO_3^- - N + NO_2^- - N/L$ (Canadian Council of Ministers of the Environment (CCME), (a), (b)). That 10-fold difference can have a significant impact on water quality assessment. Animal owners may take unnecessary and costly actions to get water quality to meet the human standard.

What standards should be used to assess drinking water intended for animals? Raisbeck et al., (not specified) list several factors that need to be considered when assessing water quality for livestock or wildlife if the following question is posed by an animal owner or manager: "Will ⟨chemical name⟩ present in the water at ⟨concentration⟩ harm my animals?"

1. Many chemicals in water interact additively with the same chemicals in feedstuffs. In such circumstances, it is not the water concentration that is singly important but the total dietary content for those chemicals. For example, the nitrate is present in forages, so total nitrate exposure is the combination of nitrate in ingested feeds and water.
2. Water quality analytical methods do not necessarily measure the specific form of the chemical present in the water. For example, selenium is usually reported as total selenium and not as the actual chemical form present in the water, such as selenite or selenate. The toxicities of chemicals can differ significantly depending of the chemical form present.
3. Reports of water quality do not usually differentiate between animal species. The toxicity of chemicals can differ significantly between species. For example, the toxicity of nitrate is much higher for ruminants than it is for nonruminants.
4. Many chemical substances in the diet interact with each other. Those chemicals may be either nutrients or potential toxicants. For example, the absorption of copper depends upon the amounts of dietary molybdenum and sulfur-containing compounds.
5. Rate of exposure influences the rate at which adverse health effects may become evident. For example, the ingestion of nitrate-fertilizer-contaminated water usually produces adverse effects much more rapidly than does ingestion of high-nitrate-containing fresh forage.

DRINKING WATER QUALITY STANDARDS FOR ANIMALS

The authors of the monographs included in Table 80.1 include concentration limits for various chemicals, but the references from which those limits are taken are not always easily identified. Some cite primary and other secondary sources. Most of the standards included in the monographs written by US scientists seem to be based on the 1974 NAS recommendations (NAS Subcommittee on Nutrient and Toxic Elements in Water, 1974). The standards included in the monograph written by Olkwoski, a Canadian, are those established by Canadian governmental bodies (Canadian Council of Ministers of the Environment (CCME), (a), (b)).

Livestock water quality recommendations have been published by the US EPA (1973), the National Academy of Sciences (NAS) in 1974 (NAS Subcommittee on Nutrient and Toxic Elements in Water, 1974), and Canada (Canadian Council of Ministers of the Environment (CCME), (a), (b)). Table 80.2 lists water quality recommendations for selected chemicals for livestock taken from each of those sources

Those publications include recommendations for water use by animals other than livestock. Recommendations for other animals are listed in Table 80.3. Readers may find them to be more applicable than the livestock recommendations in certain circumstances.

US EPA Water Quality Criteria for Animals

The US EPA published proposed water quality standards for irrigation, livestock, aquatic life, wildlife, public freshwater, marine aquatic life, and recreational water in 1973 (US EPA, 1973). The criteria were formulated and published by the US EPA pursuant to the Federal Water Pollution Control Act Amendments of 1972 and the Water Quality Act of 1965. The report states: "Almost all of the criteria are taken from the recommendations of the National Academy of Science's report on Water Quality Criteria (in press) developed under contract to the Environmental Protection Agency." Those recommendations do not appear to have been revised since their publication.

National Academy of Sciences Recommended Limits in Drinking Water for Livestock and Poultry

The NAS report published in 1974 summarizes what was known at the time of publication about effects of nutrient and toxic substances that were found in water consumed by domesticated animals (NAS Subcommittee on Nutrient and Toxic Elements in Water, 1974). It also contains information about water requirements and the percentages of recommended intake of various substances provided by normal daily water consumption, and toxic concentrations for various species. The publication includes a table summarizing the effects of toxic concentrations of various chemicals in water for various domestic and laboratories animals. The information included in those tables is too extensive to reproduce in this chapter. Readers are urged to consult them as needed.

An ad hoc committee of the National Research Council's Committee on Animal Nutrition reviewed the scientific literature related to minerals and toxic substances in the diets and water for animals. Its findings and recommendations were published as a second revision of mineral tolerances of animals (Committee on Mineral and Toxic Substances in Diets and Water for Animals, 2005) Drinking water standards cited in that revision still refer to the 1974 NAS publication (NAS Subcommittee on Nutrient and Toxic Elements in Water, 1974).

Canadian Environmental Quality Guidelines

Canadian water quality standards for agricultural use, including livestock, were first published in a document titled *Canadian Water Quality Guidelines* in 1987 by the Canadian Council of Resource and Environment Ministers (CCREM). That organization was later renamed the Canadian Council of Ministers of the Environment (CCME). In April 1996, CCME began work that consolidated national environmental quality guidelines for water, soil, sediment, tissue residues and air into one document, which was published as *Canadian Environmental Quality Guidelines* by CCME. The guidelines are continually reviewed and updated as deemed necessary.

Water quality standards have continued to be revised and current information is readily available on the CCME Canadian Environmental Guidelines Summary Table websites (Canadian Council of Ministers of the Environment (CCME), (a), (b); Health Canada, 2012). The sites are designed to produce a listing of the chemicals and the guidelines of interest to the user.

Organic Contaminants

There are numerous organic chemicals, including many used in modern agricultural production, that are also included in various water quality tables. Such chemicals do not seem to be at issue for the quality of water for animals.

Organic Livestock Production

Drinking water quality pertaining to organic livestock production is not defined in the U.S. Code of Federal Regulations. Access to clean drinking water is mandated, as indicated in this extract (bold-faced font added), but "clean water" is not defined: "Year-round access for all animals to the outdoors, shade, shelter, exercise areas, fresh air, **clean water for drinking**, and direct sunlight, suitable to the species, its stage of life, the climate, and

TABLE 80.2 Water Quality Recommendations for Selected Chemicals for Livestock

Chemical	Toxic Effects[a]	Upper Concentration Limit (mg/L)		
		US EPA	NAS	Canadian
Arsenic	Mice @ 5 mg/L: nontoxic through three generations, tissue accumulation	0.2	0.2	0.025 (interim)
	Guinea pigs @ 1 mg/L: increased thyroid colloid			
Cadmium	Mice @ 5, 10 mg/L: reduced longevity at lower dose, 2-day generation did not survive at higher dose	0.050	0.05	0.08
	Rats @ 5 mg/L: reduced longevity			
	Rabbits @ 0.1 mg/L: swollen kidney epithelium @ 6 month			
	Dos @ 0–5 mg/L: tissue concentration proportional to intake			
Calcium	–	–	–	1000
Chloride	–	–	–	–
Chromium	Rats, rabbits @ 500 mg/L, 25 mg Cr^{6+}/L: first concentration is maximum nontoxic level based on growth, second concentration decreased water intake and tissue content 9X that when Cr^{3+} was substituted	1.0	1.0	0.050 (Cr^{III}, Cr^{VI}) (interim)
Copper	Steers @ 12 g $CuSO_4 \cdot 5H_2O$/day as drench: body weight decrease, fatal in 65 days	0.5	0.5	1.0 (cattle)
				5.0 (swine, poultry)
	Turkeys @ 625 mg/L: decreased feed & water intake, fatal			0.5 (sheep)
Fluoride	Calves and cattle @ 100, 11.8 mg/L: first concentration decreased feed intake, growth and Ca absorption, bones decalcified; second concentration mottled teeth	2.0	2.0	2.0
				1.0 (if also in feed)
	Sheep @ 5–20 mg/L: severe mottled teeth, decreased wool production, decreased health			
	Hogs @ 6–10 mg/L: severe mottling of teeth			
	Mice @ 10 mg/L: no innate toxicity			
Hardness	–	–	–	–
Iron	Cattle @ 17 mg/L: pasture irrigation water produced scouring, decreased body weight and milk production	No limit	–	–
Lead	Calves @ 100 mg/L: died after 4 months of drinking $Pb(NO_3)_2$	0.1	0.1	0.1
	Rats and mice @ 5, 25 mg/L: lower concentration reproduction ceased in second generation, higher concentration hypertension and higher death rates due to infections			
Mercury (inorganic)	Humans @ 30 μg/L, 75–30 mg/L: lower concentration readily absorbed into tissues, higher concentrations fatal	1.0	0.010	0.003

(Continued)

TABLE 80.2 (Continued)

Chemical	Toxic Effects[a]	Upper Concentration Limit (mg/L)		
		US EPA	NAS	Canadian
Nitrate (as N)	Studies cited, too numerous to list here, involved concentrations from 90 to 4158 mg nitrate–nitrogen/L in sheep, pigs, cattle, chickens, turkeys, and guinea pigs	23 ($NO_3^- + NO_2^-$)	100 ($NO_3^- + NO_2^-$)	100 ($NO_3^- + NO_2^-$)
(as NO_3^-)		100 ($NO_3^- + NO_2^-$)	440	
Nitrite (as N)	Studies cited, too numerous to list here, involved concentrations from 20 to 240 mg nitrite–nitrogen/L in pigs, cockerels, poults, chicks, laying hens, turkeys, rats, and guinea pigs	3.0	10	10
(as NO_2^-)		10	33	
Selenium	Rats and mice @ 2–3 mg Se^{4+}/L, 2–3 mg Se^{6+}/L: first concentrations decreased growth and caused early deaths in males; later concentrations caused no effects on growth or longevity, but tumorigenic, third generation failed to survive	0.05	–	0.05
Sulfate	Cattle @ 100, 3590 mg/L: first concentrations decreased water and feed intake, and creatinine excretion	–	–	1000
	Laying hens @ 2700 mg Na_2SO_4/L: reduced egg production			
Total dissolved solids	–	–	–	3,000
Zinc	Humans @ 5 mg/L: emetic	25	25.0	50
	Rats @ 5 mg/L: increased mortality with 11 ppm Se in diet			
	Hens @ 2320 mg/L: decreased water consumption; egg production stopped after 3 days; body weight decreased			
Microorganisms	–	5000 coliforms/dL (average of ≥2 samples/month), 20,000/dL (individual sample)	–	–
Fecal coliforms	–	1000/dL (average of ≥2 samples/month), 4000/dL (individual sample)	–	–

[a]*Summary of effects reported in Table 80.11 of NAS for the listed animals and at listed concentration or dosage.*

the environment: Except, that, animals may be temporarily denied access to the outdoors in accordance with §§205.239(b) and (c)" (National Organic Program, 2000).

No mention of drinking water appears in Article 14: "Livestock production rules" in the European Union's organic production regulation ("on Organic Production and Labelling (Sic) of Organic Products and Repealing Regulation (EEC) no 2092/91", 2007), but water is mentioned in Article 15 "Production rules for aquaculture animals," Paragraph 1.(b)ii (bold-faced font added): "husbandry practices, including feeding, design of installations, stocking densities, and **water quality** shall ensure that the developmental, physiological, and behavioural needs of animals are met" ("on Organic Production and Labelling (Sic) of Organic Products and Repealing Regulation (EEC) no 2092/91", 2007).

DRINKING WATER QUALITY STANDARDS FOR HUMANS

Drinking water quality standards for selected chemicals are listed in Table 80.4 that are published by the

TABLE 80.3 Water Quality Recommendations for Selected Chemicals for Aquatic Water Systems

Water System	Upper Concentration Limit (mg/L)				
	Freshwater Aquatic Life		Freshwater Wildlife	Marine Aquatic Life	
Agency	Canadian	US EPA	US EPA	Canadian	US EPA[a]
Chemical					
Arsenic	0.005	–	–	0.0125 (interim)	0.01 × 96-h LC_{50}; 0.5
Cadmium	0.000017 (interim)	0.03 in hard water, 0.004 in soft water	–	0.00012	0.01 × 96-h LC_{50}; 0.01 mg/L
Calcium	–	–	–	–	–
Chloride	–	–	–	–	–
Chromium	Cr^{III}: 0.0089 (interim)	0.03	–	Cr^{III}: 0.056 (interim)	0.01 × 96-h LC_{50}; 0.1 mg/L
	Cr^{VI}: 0.001			Cr^{VI}: 0.0015	
Copper	0.002 @ [$CaCO_3$] = 0–120 mg/L	0.1 is 96-h LC_{50}	–	–	0.01 × 96-h LC_{50}; 0.5 mg/L
	0.003 @ [$CaCO_3$] = 120–180 mg/L				
	0.004@ [$CaCO_3$] = >180 mg/L				
Fluoride	–			–	0.1 × 96-h LC_{50}; 1.5 mg/L
Hardness	–	–	–	–	–
Iron	0.300	–	–	–	0.3
Lead	0.001 @ [$CaCO_3$] = 0–60 mg/L	0.03	–	–	0.02 × 96-h LC_{50}; 0.1 LD_{50}
	0.002 @ [$CaCO_3$] = 60–120 mg/L				
	0.004 @ [$CaCO_3$] = 120–180 mg/L				
	0.007 @ [$CaCO_3$] = >180 mg/L,				
Mercury (inorganic)	Inorganic: 0.000026	0.0002 (total)	0.5 mg/kg in fish	Inorganic: 0.000016 (interim)	0.01 × 96-h LC_{50}; 0.1 mg/L
	MethylHg: 0.000004 (interim).	0.00005 (average)		MethylHg: no recommendation	
	May not protect against bioaccumulation	0.05 mg/kg (total body burden)			
Nitrate (as N)		–	–		–
(as NO_3^-)	13 (interim)			16 (interim)	
Nitrite (as N)		–	–	–	–
(as NO_2^-)	0.06				
Total dissolved solids	–	–	–	–	–

(Continued)

TABLE 80.3 (Continued)

Water System	Upper Concentration Limit (mg/L)				
	Freshwater Aquatic Life		Freshwater Wildlife	Marine Aquatic Life	
Agency	Canadian	US EPA	US EPA	Canadian	US EPA[a]
Chemical					
Selenium	0.001	–	–	–	0.01 × 96-h LC_{50}, 0.01 mg/L
Sulfate	–	–	–	–	–
Zinc	0.030			–	
Microorganisms	–	–	2000/dL	–	–
Fecal coliforms	–	–	2000/dL	–	–

[a]*Recommended concentration limits are expressed as the fraction of either lethal concentration- 50 (LC_{50}) or lethal dose-50 (LD_{50}). The concentration listed thereafter is the maximum concentration considered acceptable.*

United States (US EPA, (a), (b)), Canada (Health Canada, 2012) and the World Health Organization (World Health Organization, 2011). They are included in this chapter to allow readers to compare standards for animals and humans. The adverse health effects listed in US EPA documents for each chemical are also listed in the table.

In the United States, legal limits called maximum contaminant levels (MCLs) have been established for about 90 contaminants. If contaminant concentrations in public water supplies and certain private supplies are found to be above applicable MCLs, then the water supplier must take action to bring the contaminant concentration down below the MCL. Meanwhile, an alternate source of water that meets the standards must be provided.

In the United States, there are primary and secondary water standards for human drinking (US EPA, (a), (b)). Primary drinking water standards are legally enforceable, and water providers cannot provide water that contains contaminants higher than their respective MCLs. Secondary standards are nonenforceable guidelines for contaminants that may cause cosmetic effects, such as skin or tooth discoloration, or unacceptable aesthetic effects, such as unacceptable taste of, odor from or discoloration of the water.

Primary standards are established considering the adverse health effect caused by the contaminant and the dose at which such effects occur. A reference dose (RFD or RfD) is estimated based upon the amount of the contaminant to which a person may be exposed on a daily basis that is not anticipated to cause the adverse health effect over a person's life time. Consequently, the standards may not reflect the risk of adverse health effects in animals, and care should be use applying them to water intended for consumption by animals.

WATER CONSUMPTION TABLES

The dose of a water-borne contaminate may have to be estimated in cases of suspected toxicoses and may be calculated if the contaminant's concentration in the water and the amount of water consumed by the victims are known. Contaminant concentration in the water may be determined by analysis, but water consumption by the victims is rarely known with certainty.

Water consumption varies by species, weather condition, diet, and state of health. All of those factors and their interactions make the determination or estimation of minimal water requirements difficult if not impossible. Additionally, daily water requirements are not necessarily met solely by drinking water consumption.

Use water consumption data to calculate doses of water-borne poisons, if such data are available. If not, use the data in Table 80.5, which was taken from the NAS publication (NAS Subcommittee on Nutrient and Toxic Elements in Water, 1974), to estimate water consumption. Those data should be modified for situations falling outside of the defining parameters listed in the title.

RATIONALE FOR LIVESTOCK RECOMMENDATIONS

The rationales for the chemicals included in Table 80.2 livestock recommendations are included in the US EPA Proposed Criteria for Water Quality Volume (US EPA, 1973) 1 are summarized below. Information listed was what was known at the time the recommendations were formulated and may not reflect current knowledge of the effects of the chemicals. Our addenda are so noted.

TABLE 80.4 Water Quality Recommendations for Human Drinking Water: Selected Contaminants

Body Establishing Guidelines	Maximum Acceptable Concentration (mg/L)			Potential Health Effects From Exposure Above Maximum Acceptable Concentration (US EPA)
	US EPA	Canadian	WHO	
Chemical				
Arsenic	0.010	0.025	0.01 (provisional)	Skin damage or problems with circulatory system; may have increased risk of cancer
Cadmium	0.005	0.005	0.003	Kidney damage
Calcium	–	–	–	–
Chloride	250 (secondary)	≤250 (aesthetic objective)	No health concerns at usual concentrations	–
Chromium	0.1	0.05	0.05 (provisional)	Allergic dermatitis
Copper	1.3	≤1.0 (aesthetic objective)	2	Short-term exposure: gastrointestinal distress
				Long-term exposure: liver or kidney damage; in cases of Wilson's Disease consult physician about max. acceptable concentration
Fluoride	4.0	1.5 (adjust to 0.8–1.0, optimal for control of dental caries)	1.5	Pain and tenderness of the bones; mottled teeth in children
Hardness	–	–	–	–
Iron	0.3 (secondary)	≤0.3 (aesthetic objective)	No health concerns at usual concentrations	–
Lead	0.015	0.010	0.01	Infants and children: physical or mental development delays, slight attention span deficits and learning disabilities
				Adults: kidney problems, hypertension
Mercury	0.002 (inorganic)	0.001	0.001 (total)	Kidney damage
Nitrate (as N)	10		–	Infants <6 months old: blue-baby syndrome
(as NO_3^-)	–	45	50 (short term)	
Nitrite (as N)	1		–	Infants <6 months old: blue-baby syndrome
(as NO_2^-)	–	<3.2, where nitrite is measured in addition to nitrate	3 (short term)	
			0.2 (long term, provisional)	
Selenium	0.05	0.01	0.01	Hair or fingernail loss; numbness in extremities; circulatory problems
Sulfate	250 (secondary)	≤500 (aesthetic objective)	No health concerns at usual concentrations	–

(*Continued*)

TABLE 80.4 (Continued)

Body Establishing Guidelines	Maximum Acceptable Concentration (mg/L)			Potential Health Effects From Exposure Above Maximum Acceptable Concentration (US EPA)
	US EPA	Canadian	WHO	
Chemical				
Total dissolved solids	–	–	No health concerns at usual concentrations	–
Zinc	5 (secondary)	≤5.0 (aesthetic objective)	No health concerns at usual concentrations	–
Microbes	**US EPA**	**Canadian**	**WHO**	
Total coliforms	–	None in consecutive samples from same site; present in ≤10% of samples from distribution system in calendar month		
Fecal coliforms	–			
E. coli		None		

TABLE 80.5 Anticipated Water Consumption of Various Adult Animals of Medium Weight in Temperate Climates

Animal	Expected Consumption (L/day)
Beef cattle	26–66
Dairy cattle	38–110
Horses	30–45
Swine	11–19
Sheep, goats	4–15
Chickens	0.2–0.4
Turkeys	0.4–0.6

Source: Data are from NAS.

The EPA writes in its introduction to the document:

Acceptable limits specified in the recommendations were derived by the application of scientific judgment to lethal dose or lethal concentration data in a manner that provides a margin of safety to test organisms. For those substances whose effects are more aptly described as undesirable such as impairing aquatic habitats, causing taste and odor problems in water supplies, or reducing the aesthetic or recreational quality of a water body, limits which minimize these effects were established on the basis of field and laboratory investigations. Acceptable levels of toxic materials for which specific numerical maximum acceptable concentrations are not prescribed are determined by applying an application factor to locally derived LC_{50} data .... By basing criteria on effects on the most sensitive important species, a desirable degree of regional and local variation is introduced, allowing water quality standards to depend on local conditions.

An 'important species' in the criteria is defined as an organism that is: a) commercially or recreationally valuable; b) is rare or endangered; c) affects the well-being of some species within a) and b); or d) is critical to the structure and function of the ecological system. A 'rare or endangered' species is any species so officially designated by the U.S. Fish and Wildlife Service.

Arsenic

Toxicity of arsenic depends upon its chemical form, relating primarily to rate of excretion. Inorganic oxides are generally more toxic than are organic forms of arsenic. Acute toxicities for farm animals were given in Table 80.6.

Arsenic acid fed to lactating cows at up to 1.25 mg/kg body weight for eight weeks, equivalent to an intake of 60 L of water containing 5.5 mg arsenic/L daily by a

TABLE 80.6 Acute Toxicity of Inorganic Arsenic by Species

Species	Toxicity (g/Animal)
Poultry	0.05–0.10
Swine	0.15–1.0
Sheep and goats	10.0–15.0
Horses	10.0–15.0
Cattle	15.0–30.0

Wadsworth 1952 as cited by US EPA.

TABLE 80.7 Effects of Cadmium in Various Species

Species	Amount and Source	Effect
Human	15 mg/L in popsicles	Sickening
Male rats	4.5 mg Cd/kg bw	Permanent sterility
Rats or mice	5 mg/L in drinking water	Reduced longevity
Pregnant hamsters	2 mg/kg bw of $CdSO_4$ by i.v. injection	Dose on day 8 of gestation caused fetal malformations

Source: Data are from US EPA.

500 kg animal was absorbed and rapidly excreted in the urine with no increase of arsenic content of milk. No toxicity was observed.

Cadmium

Effects of cadmium in various species are listed in Table 80.7.

A small fraction of cadmium was absorbed in ruminants, with most of what was absorbed going to the kidneys and liver. The cow was "found to be very efficient in keeping cadmium out of its milk." Most major animal products, including beef and milk, seem "quite well protected against cadmium accumulation."

Chromium

Chromium is not readily absorbed by animals. Most of what is ingested is excreted in the feces. It does not appear to concentrate in mammalian tissue or its concentration to increase with age. It was concluded that up to 5 mg/L of chromium II or VI in drinking water should not be harmful to livestock. That level may be unnecessarily high and the 1.0 mg/L level was recommended to provide a "suitable margin of safety."

Copper

Copper is an essential trace element so some is required in the diet to maintain good health. Swine appear to be more tolerant of copper with dietary concentrations of 250 mg/kg or higher improving live weight gains and feed efficiency. Copper does not appear to accumulate in tissues. Sheep are very susceptible to copper toxicosis.

A diet containing 25 mg/kg fed to sheep is considered toxic. About 9 mg per animal per day is considered safe.

Fluorine

Author's addendum The terms "fluorine" and "fluoride" seem to be used synonymously in water quality literature, but they are very different chemicals. The chemical usually found dissolved in water is fluoride not fluorine. "Consumption of drinking water with 2.0 mg/L may produce some tooth mottling, but it is not excessive with respect to animal health or deposition in meat, milk or eggs. Chronic fluorosis of livestock has occurred with water content of 10–15 mg fluoride/L. Total ration content of 30–50 mg fluoride/L (sic) for dairy cattle is considered a safe upper limit. Transfer to milk occurs to a very small extent and to a greater degree in eggs. Fluoride at 1.0 mg/L in drinking water did not harm livestock.

Hardness (Author's Addendum)

Hard water does not appear to have a deleterious effect on animals, but it often is reported as part of water quality analysis. Hardness is a measure of the calcium and magnesium ions present in the drinking water. Water with high TDS or salinity may or may not be hard water. Hardness of water may be measured as grains/ gallon or in ppm. One grain per gallon is equivalent to 17 mg calcium and magnesium per liter. Water is classified according to calcium and magnesium salt content as follows: soft water ranges from 0 to 60 ppm, hard water varies from 120 to 180 ppm and very hard water is greater than 180 ppm.

Iron

Iron is essential to animal life and is not considered toxic. Dietary iron concentrations of at least 4000 mg/kg were found to cause phosphorus deficiency and to be toxic to weanling pigs. Concentrations fewer than 3000 mg/kg apparently were not toxic. "While iron occurs in natural water as very soluble ferrous salts, on contact with air they are oxidized and precipitated as ferric oxide,

TABLE 80.8 Effects of Nitrate and Nitrite Administered to Nonruminants

Species	Concentration, Dosage or Dose	Observed Effect(s)
Gilts from weaning through two farrowing seasons	330 mg/L (nitrate)	No adverse effects
Growing pigs	330 mg/L (nitrate)	No adverse effects
Chick and laying hens	Up to 300 mg/L (nitrite)	No effects on growth or production
Chicks and laying hens	Up to 200 mg/L (nitrite)	No effects on growth or production
Turkey pullets	200 mg/L (nitrite)	Decreased growth
Turkeys, laying hens and turkeys	200 mg/L (nitrite)	Reduced liver vitamin A stores
	50 mg/L (nitrite)	No adverse effects observed

Source: Data are from US EPA.

rendering them essentially harmless to animal live. It is therefore not considered necessary to set a limit for this element." Elevated dietary iron may antagonize copper, manganese and sulfur in lactating dairy cattle.

Lead

The toxicity of lead had not been clearly established quantitatively. Daily intake of 6–7 mg/kg body weight had been suggested as a threshold dosage in cattle, but that is difficult to establish. A concentration of 0.5 mg/L in drinking water is considered safe. Drinking water containing 5 mg/L consumed by rats and mice over the course of their lifetimes produced toxic effects. Death rates of older animals increased, especially in males. Death was not caused by overt lead toxicosis, but was due to an increased susceptibility to "spontaneous infections."

Mercury

Mercury content in surface water was found to usually be <5 μg/L, but methylation of mercury in bottom sediments bordering mercury deposits resulted in the continuous presence of mercury in solution. The relative stability of methylmercury and its high absorption from the gut contributes to its oral toxicity. It had been suggested that livestock blood and tissue lead content be kept below 0.1 and 0.5 mg/kg, respectively, to protect humans who might consume those tissues. The safe contamination level for fish consumed by humans had been set at 0.5 mg/kg by the US FDA. However, that did not take into consideration other possible sources of dietary mercury. "In view of these facts the limits prescribed herein are reduced by a factor of 10 to reduce the significance of levels from meat products in comparison with those of fish."

Nitrate and Nitrite

Nitrite is more toxic to livestock than is nitrate. Usually nitrite is produced by the reduction of nitrate to nitrite, which occurs in the rumen; in moistened feeds, such as freshly chopped green forage; or water containing sufficient organic matter to sustain microbes. Natural waters may contain "high levels" of nitrate, but they usually contain very low concentrations of nitrite. Nitrate in cattle feed did not seem to pose a hazard to humans consuming dairy products or meat produced from cattle eating the nitrate-containing feed.

"Animals fed nitrate continuously develop some degree of adaptation (sic) to it." "Assuming maximum water consumption by dairy cattle of three to four times the dry matter intake, the concentration of nitrate to be tolerated in water should be about one fourth of that tolerated in the feed. This would amount to about 300 mg/L of nitrate."

Effects of nitrate and nitrite at various concentrations given to nonruminants are summarized in Table 80.8.

It appeared that ingestion of water containing up to 300 mg/L nitrate or 100 mg/L nitrite was well tolerated by all classes of livestock and poultry studied under controlled experimental conditions.

Authors' addendum: Crowley and coworkers (1974) conducted a 35-month study in Wisconsin comparing reproductive efficiency and lactational performance for a 54-cow Holstein herd that consumed drinking water containing either 19 or 374 ppm nitrate. During the last 15 months of the study, cattle drinking the elevated nitrate-containing water had the highest services per conception and lowest first service conception rates. The average milk yield was not significantly different between the two groups but the total milk yield for the entire 35-month study was lower in the elevated water nitrate group. This small difference in milk yield in the elevated nitrate-containing drinking water was thought to be due to an increased dry period due to lower conception rates.

We have never encountered a case of acute nitrate or nitrite toxicoses due to the consumption of drinking water, unless the water had been hauled to the animals in a fertilizer tank. Such cases have always involved cattle and occur when the availability of drinking water is disrupted and drinking water must be hauled to the animals from someplace else. Such circumstances may occur when water freezes during stretches of very cold weather or the water pump fails and cannot be rapidly repaired. Deaths often occur relatively rapidly; owners often report finding dead victims within a few meters of the contaminated water tank. Ocular fluid collected from dead victims usually contains nitrate in excess of 100 μg nitrate/mL and nitrite in excess of 2 μg nitrite/mL. Ocular fluid collected from dead victims of forage nitrate toxicosis usually contains less nitrate than ocular fluid from dead victims of water nitrate toxicosis. If the fertilizer tank contained ammonium nitrate, then death may be the result of either excessive ammonia or nitrate exposure, and the determination of the exact cause of death is mostly academic. Under *no* circumstances do we recommend that a tank that has contained fertilizer be used to haul drinking water to animals, even if it has been "thoroughly washed out." Theoretically, a fertilizer tank may be cleaned sufficiently to haul drinking water, but not practically.

Total Dissolved Solids

"Total dissolved solids" is defined in the NAS publication (NAS Subcommittee on Nutrient and Toxic Elements in Water, 1974) as the concentration of all dissolved constituents in water. "Salinity" is often used synonymously with "total dissolved solids," although that assumes that all of the dissolved solids are saline. Salinity is more than a measurement of the total amount of sodium and chloride present in water. Salinity also includes anions, such as carbonates expressed as oxides, bromide and iodine expressed as chlorine, and cations such as calcium, magnesium, bicarbonate, and sulfate but does not include organic matter.

The US EPA does not include recommendations for TDS, but the NAS provides criteria for classification of water based upon TDS content established for the US Geological Society. Criteria for two classification systems are listed in Table 80.9. Note the differences in the classification and the use of brine in both, but with different criteria for inclusion in that classification. It has been our experience that those classifications contribute little to the assessment of water quality for animals, as we have never encountered an instance where those water classifications have been used to describe the TDS content. Nevertheless, they are included here.

More useful information about the use of saline waters for livestock is provided under the section titled "A Guide to the Use of Saline Waters for Livestock" in the NAS publication, starting on p. 48 (NAS Subcommittee on Nutrient and Toxic Elements in Water, 1974).

> *Several factors need to be considered in assessing the suitability of saline water for livestock use, including kind, age and sex of the animals; pregnancy or lactation status; physical exertion; climatic conditions; diet and its moisture and mineral content; production expectations; water salt content; access to other water sources; and the adaptation to available water sources. Weight given to those factors is largely a matter of judgment, but TDS is the single most reliable factor that can be determined.*

The NAS did not recommend the use of highly saline water for livestock but acknowledged that circumstances may arise such that saline water may be all that is readily available. Table 80.10 lists the guidelines for use of saline

TABLE 80.9 Water Classifications Based Upon Total Dissolved Solid Content

DeWiest Classification (1966)		Robinove et al., Classification (1958)	
Water Classification	**TDS Content (mg/L)**	**Water Classification**	**TDS Content (mg/L)**
Freshwater	<1000		
Brackish water	1000–10,000	Slightly saline	1000–3000
		Moderately saline	3000–10,000
Salty water	10,000–100,000	Very saline	10,000–35,000
		Brine	>35,000
Brine	>100,000		

Source: Data are from US EPA.

TABLE 80.10 Guide to Use of Saline Waters for Livestock and Poultry

Water TDS Content (mg/L)	Expected Health or Performance Effects
<1000	None expected for any livestock class
1000–2999	None expected for any livestock class. May cause temporary diarrhea or watery droppings in animals unaccustomed to the water
3000–4999	Should be none. May cause temporary diarrhea or be refused at first by animals unaccustomed to the water. Poor water for poultry, often causing watery droppings, increased mortality and decreased growth, especially in turkeys
5000–6999	Reasonably safe for dairy and beef cattle, sheep, swine and horses. Avoid use of water approaching the higher limit for pregnant or lactating animals. Unacceptable for poultry; use for poultry will almost always be accompanied by some type of problem, especially near the upper limit, such as reduced growth or production
7000–10,000	Unfit for poultry and probably swine. Considerable risk may exist for pregnant or lactating cows, horses, sheep and the young of those species. Considerable risk for animals subject to heavy heat stress or water loss. Generally use of such water should be avoided, although older ruminants, horses and even poultry and swine may subsist on it for long periods of low stress
>10,000	Unacceptable risks for any livestock class

Source: Taken from NAS[10].

water for livestock and poultry. If high-TDS water is to be used, the following points should be considered, too:

1. Alkalinities and nitrate should be considered whenever water contained >3000 mg TDS/L is to be used. Alkalinities of 2000 mg $CaCO_3$ detract from the suitability of water. Hydroxide is more harmful that carbonate, which is more harmful than bicarbonate.
2. If offered the choice between two water sources, one highly saline and one less saline, they will choose the less saline source.
3. Animals can tolerate high saline water for a few days if they are then given low saline water.
4. Water intake usually increases with soluble salt content, except in cases of extremely high saline content, which animals may refuse to drink.
5. Abrupt changes from a low to high saline water will likely cause more problems than a gradual change.
6. Decreased water intake is very likely accompanied by decreased feed intake. So, animals with high production expectations may not produce as well showing "deleterious effects from waters of lower salts content than animals on a maintenance regimen."
7. Highly saline water may furnish enough minerals to be considered in dietary mineral formulations. And salt content of the diet may contribute to the toxicity of saline water, particularly if salt is added to control feed intake. Generally, water should not normally be relied upon as a source on essential inorganic minerals.

Selenium

At the time that the US EPA formulated its recommendations, no substantiated case of livestock poisoning by selenium in waters had been found. However, selenium toxicosis was found in wildlife exposed to high-selenium–containing irrigation runoff water. Agricultural drainage water entering Kesterson Reservoir in California ranged from 0.140 to1.40 mg/L (140–1400 ppb) during 1983–85.

Sulfate

No recommendation for sulfate was made by the US EPA probably because the association between sulfate exposure and polioencephalomalicia in ruminants had not yet been discovered. The Canadian recommendation is 1000 mg/L. Exposure to elevated sulfates in drinking water can result in a transient diarrhea. Animals usually acclimate to an elevated level of drinking water sulfate in 3–7 days and no longer exhibit diarrhea. Methemoglobin was increased 450% in cattle consuming drinking water containing sulfates at 3493 ppm.

Zinc

Zinc is relatively nontoxic. The findings cited in the EPA document are summarized in Table 80.11. Increased zinc intake increased the zinc content of body tissue, but its accumulation was not great and tissue content fell rapidly after zinc intake was reduced.

TABLE 80.11 Zinc Toxicity in Diets for Various Animals

Dietary per Water Zn Content	Species and Effect(s)
1000 mg/kg in diet	Swine tolerated it
≥2000	Swine: toxic
2320 mg/L in water	Chickens: reduced water consumption, egg production, body weight
>500 mg/kg in diet, as oxide	Ruminants: toxic

Source: Data are from US EPA.

TABLE 80.12 Cyanotoxins on the US EPA Contaminant Candidate List (CCL)

Cyanotoxin	Number of Known Variants or Analogues	Most Common Cyanobacteria Producing the Toxin[a]
Microcystin-LR	80–90	*Microxystis*
		Anabaena
		Planktothrix
		Anabaenopsis
		Aphanizomenon
Cylindrospermopsin	3	*Cylindrospermopsis*
		Aphanizomenon
		Anabaena
		Lyngbya
		Rhaphidiopsis
		Umezakia
Anatoxin-a group[b]	2–6	*Anabaena*
		Planktothrix
		Aphanizomenon
		Cylindrospermopsis
		Oscillatoria

[a]*Not all species in the listed genera produce toxin and not all of those listed are equally important toxin producers.*
[b]*Anatoxin-a group does not include anatoxin-a(S), a cholinesterase-inhibiting organophosphate. In the United States, anatoxin-a(S) is not that common.*

CYANOTOXINS FROM WATER

Cyanotoxins are toxins produced by cyanobacteria; the organisms were previously called blue-green algae. Information about the toxicology of cyanotoxins may be found in the chapter on cyanobacterial (blue-green algae) toxins elsewhere in this book.

Currently cyanotoxins included on the US EPA Contaminant Candidate List (CCL) (US EPA, 2014) are listed in Table 80.12. Those included are believed to most commonly occur in US waters.

Many countries have developed regulations or guidelines for microcystin contamination of drinking water and those are mostly based on the World Health Organization provisional concentration for drinking water of 1.0 μg/L microcystin-LR (0.001 mg/L) (US EPA, 2014), but not necessarily so. For example, Canada has established a cyanobacterial toxin maximum acceptable concentration of 1.5 μg/L microcystin-LR (0.0015 mg/L) (Health Canada, 2012).

Standards for drinking water for animals have not been established.

TABLE 80.13 Critical Control Points for Assessing the Safety of Drinking Water

Control Point	Remarks
Water source	Groundwater less risky than surface waters. Water sources contaminated by surface runoff pose higher risks
Presence of cyanobacteria; tendency of bloom formation	Bloom formation less likely during periods of high flow or deep vertical mixing, and are more likely during periods of low flow or stagnation
	Historical evidence of algal blooms increases risk; blooms may be cyclic
	Nutrient input, especially nitrogen and phosphorus, increases risk
	Absence of cyanobacteria reduces risk
Cell lysis	Most cyanotoxins are cell-bound and may be removed with the cells. Lysis may occur naturally as the bloom dies, or artificially by treatment, pumping or transport
Water treatment systems	Cyanotoxins may be removed by filtration through activated charcoal or by oxidation, but effectiveness of treatment should be monitored

Source: Adapted from Table 5.1 in Falconer, Bartram, Chorus, et al.

Availability of analytical services for the detection of cyanotoxins in water is limited but growing. Cyanotoxins are not commonly part of water quality panels and must be purchased a la carte.

Safe Practices To Minimize Cyanotoxin Contamination of Drinking Water

Draw drinking water from sources that do not harbor cyanobacteria, such as groundwater or surface water not supporting cyanobacterial growth.

Cyanobacterial-contaminated water may be used for drinking water if the cyanobacterial cells are removed without lysing them because most cyanotoxins are cell bound. Removal of released cyanotoxins from the water may be possible, but it may also be difficult and expensive. Risk of cyanotoxicosis should be considered high after algae-infested water is treated with copper sulfate. Critical control points for assessing the safety of drinking water based on Falconer, et al., are listed in Table 80.13 (Falconer et al., 1999).

Algal blooms are usually regarded as more of a nuisance than a toxic hazard. They are often associated with unpleasant odors and offensive appearances. They may be regarded as normal in areas where they occur frequently or regularly, and their toxic potential may be unknown or disregarded. The presence of any algal bloom, regardless of its color, location, or time of occurrence should be considered to pose a high risk of cyanotoxicosis and all animals should be denied access to such areas, whether it is in the water or on the shore.

All animals should be denied access to bodies of water containing visible discoloration that cannot be attributed to some other source other than algae or cyanobacteria. Areas in which scum has formed should be considered very high risk for acute cyanotoxicosis, regardless of the color of the scum. Identification of the microbial components of the scum may help with the risk assessment.

REFERENCES

On Organic Production and Labelling (Sic) of Organic Products and Repealing Regulation (EEC) no 2092/91, Council Regulation (EC) No 834/2007 (2007).

Canadian Council of Ministers of the Environment (CCME). (a). Canadian Water Quality Guidelines for the Protection of Agriculture Water Uses: Summary Table. Retrieved February 15, 2017, from: <http://st-ts.ccme.ca/en/index.html>.

Canadian Council of Ministers of the Environment (CCME). (b). Canadian Water Quality Guidelines for the Protection of Aquatic Life: Summary Table. Retrieved February 15, 2017, from <http://st-ts.ccme.ca/en/index.html>.

Committee on Mineral and Toxic Substances in Diets and Water for Animals, 2005. Mineral Tolerance of Animals, second revised ed. National Research Council of the National Academies, Washington, DC.

Crowley, J., Jorgensen, N., Kahler, L., et al., 1974. Effect of Nitrate in Drinking Water on Reproductive and Productive Efficiency of Dairy Cattle. Wisconsin Water Resources Center, Madison, WI.

Falconer, I., Bartram, H., Chorus, I., et al., 1999. Safe levels and safe practices. In: Djhorus, I., Bartram, J. (Eds.), Toxic Cyanobacterial in Water: A Guide to Their Public Health Consequences, Monitoring and Management. E&FN Spon, London (pp. Chapter 5).

Faries, F., Sweeten, J., Reagor, J., 1991. Water Quality: Its Relationship to Livestock. Texas Agricultural Extension Service, College Station, TX.

German, D., Thiex, N., Wright, C., 2008. Interpretation of Water Analysis for Livestock Suitability. South Dakota State University, Brookings, SD.

Health Canada, (2012. Guidelines for Canadian Recreational Water Quality – third edition. Retrieved February 16, 2017, from: <https://www.canada.ca/en/health-canada/services/publications/healthy-living/guidelines-canadian-recreational-water-quality-third-edition.html>.

Higgins, S., Agouridis, C., Gumbert, A., not specified. Drinking Water Quality Guidelines for Cattle. Univ of Kentucky Cooperative Extension Service.

Mukhtar, S., 1998. Water Quality Guide for Livestock and Poultry. Texas Agricultural Extension Service, College Station, TX.

NAS Subcommittee on Nutrient and Toxic Elements in Water, 1974. Nutrients and Toxic Substances in Water for Livestock and Poultry. National Academy of Sciences, Washington, DC.

National Organic Program, 7 CFR Section 205.239, 2000.

Olkowski, A., 2009. Livestock Water Quality: A Field Guide for Cattle, Horses, Poultry, and Swine. Agriculture and Agri-Food Canada.

Raisbeck, M., Riker, B., Tate, C., et al., not specified. Water Quality for Wyoming Livestock & Wildlife. University of Wyoming Extension.

Sallenave, R., 2016. Water Quality for Livestock and Poultry. NM State University Cooperative Extension Service.

US EPA. (a). National Primary Drinking Water Regulation Table. Retrieved February 16, 2017, from: <https://www.epa.gov/ground-water-and-drinking-water/table-regulated-drinking-water-contaminants>.

US EPA. (b). National Secondary Drinking Water Regulation Table. Retrieved February 16, 2017, from: <https://www.epa.gov/dwstandardsregulations/secondary-drinking-water-standards-guidance-nuisance-chemicals>.

US EPA, 1973. Proposed Criteria for Water Quality. US EPA, Washington, DC.

US EPA, 2014. Cyanobacteria and Cyanotoxins: Information for Drinkings Water Systems. Retrieved February 27, 2017, from: <https://www.epa.gov/sites/production/files/2014-08/documents/cyanobacteria_factsheet.pdf>.

World Health Organization, 2011. Guidelines for Drinking-Water Quality, fourth ed. Retrieved February 27, 2017, from: <http://apps.who.int/iris/bitstream/10665/44584/1/9789241548151_eng.pdf>.

Section XVII

Analytical Toxicology

Chapter 81

Analytical Toxicology and Sample Submission Requirements

Michael Filigenzi

INTRODUCTION

Veterinary diagnostic toxicology combines the disciplines of veterinary toxicology and analytical chemistry to answer a deceptively simple question: Did a chemical make an animal sick or kill it, and if so, which chemical? This seemingly simple question may be extremely challenging to answer. Even in situations in which the diagnosis seems obvious, chemical testing is often required to confirm that diagnosis. Although laboratories sometimes receive requests for a "poison screen," there is in fact no such test. The biological systems involved, the toxicants, and the nature of analytical chemistry combine to provide a situation far too complex for any single test. Analysis may be required for pesticides, toxic metals, plant toxins, mycotoxins, algal toxins, drugs, industrial chemicals, and virtually any other chemical that might adversely affect the health of any of a wide variety of species. The types of samples that may require testing are nearly unlimited and include any type of animal tissue or bodily fluid, anything that an animal might ingest, and environmental samples. There are no standard analytical methods for many compounds and sample types, so the development and modification of analytical methods is a commonplace occurrence. At times, this method development occurs on an emergency basis due to the potential exposure of large numbers of animals to a particular chemical or due to the potential for a toxicant to enter the human food supply. Fortunately, the field of analytical chemistry is in a rapidly evolving state, with the constant introduction of new techniques and instrumentation that provide faster, more efficient analyses for broadening arrays of chemicals with ever increasing levels of sensitivity. In this chapter, we'll look at some of the techniques and instruments currently used in veterinary toxicology labs, how they are used, and what is involved in submitting samples for testing.

THE STRUCTURE OF A TOXICOLOGY LAB

Veterinary toxicology labs are usually headed by a veterinary toxicologist who is a Diplomate of the American Board of Veterinary Toxicology. It is the toxicologist's job to consult with those submitting samples to the lab, to direct the testing on samples, to review and interpret testing results, and report diagnoses. The toxicologist may also perform testing in the laboratory. The lab is staffed with specialized analytical chemists, who analyze the samples and report the results to the toxicologist. These labs vary in size and staff, ranging from two or three people up to a dozen or more.

Analytical procedures typically require some type of sample preparation (which can be quite complex) prior to the actual analysis. Therefore, the laboratory must have the required equipment and facilities for both of these steps. The laboratory must also have a means of maintaining records of sample receipts and of reporting the results of the analyses. These chores are typically handled by a computer systems known as Laboratory Information Management Systems, commonly abbreviated as "LIMS" systems.

ELEMENTAL AND INORGANIC CHEMICAL ANALYSIS

Elemental Analysis

Various types of elemental analysis comprise a valuable service offered by veterinary toxicology laboratories. These analyses are commonly used to help diagnose poisonings due to excessive levels of toxic elements such as heavy metals but are also used to diagnose deficiencies of trace level essential elements and to monitor animal health. Most labs offer tests that include panels of toxic heavy

Veterinary Toxicology. DOI: http://dx.doi.org/10.1016/B978-0-12-811410-0.00081-7

metals and/or trace elements at relatively low prices. These tests are commonly performed on serum, plasma, blood, or liver tissue (including liver biopsy samples) but are also run on many other types of samples, from feed to feathers. Both the sample preparation and analysis steps are usually done quickly and efficiently, resulting in short turnaround times. The techniques that are commonly used for the analysis of elemental species are as follow.

Atomic Absorption Spectroscopy (abbreviated as AAS or AA)

AA is based on the principle that many elements will absorb light at a specific wavelength when they are atomized. An AA spectrometer atomizes a sample in a flame or in a small carbon tube inside of a furnace that can be rapidly heated. The basic constituents of the instrument are the atomization source (either flame or furnace), a lamp producing light at a specific wavelength, a monochromator that allows only light of a specific wavelength to pass through it, and a detector (Fig. 81.1). The wavelength of the light from the lamp is matched to the specific element being tested for. When the sample is atomized in the furnace or flame, this light is passed through it with the monochromator set such that only light of that wavelength will strike the detector. Any decrease in light intensity reaching the detector as the sample is atomized is directly proportional to the concentration of the tested element in the sample. These instruments are relatively inexpensive and easy to use and may be used to test for most metallic elements. Detection limits are very low for some elements when using the furnace technique. The primary disadvantage of AA is that the lamp must be replaced whenever the element being tested needs to be changed. Since most labs provide analyses that include a number of metals or trace elements, this results in a significant efficiency problem. ICP and ICP-MS have largely replaced AA for the majority of elemental analyses due to their superior efficiency and sensitivity. Furnace AA is still a valuable technique for a fast low-level analysis of certain single elements.

Inductively Coupled Plasma Coupled Optical Emission Spectrometry (ICP-OES, or just ICP)

This technique is similar to AA in that it also involves atomization of the sample, but in the case of ICP, it's the emission of light that's measured rather than the absorbance. In ICP, thermal energy excites the atoms to a higher energy state. When the atoms relax to a lower state, they emit light at a frequency specific to the element. The thermal energy is supplied by a torch in which argon is subjected to radiofrequency energy to form a plasma, the temperature of which may be as high as nearly 10,000°C. The prepared sample is introduced into this torch, the elements absorb the thermal energy from the torch, and the light that is subsequently emitted at the various frequencies for the different elements is measured (Fig. 81.2). The fact that many frequencies may be differentiated allows for the simultaneous detection of many different elements in a single analysis. ICP-OES is a fast, selective, and sensitive technique that has been the mainstay of elemental analysis in veterinary toxicology for many years. It's important to note, however, that there can be interferences for some elements under some conditions. Analysts must be aware of these interferences and interpret data accordingly in order to produce accurate results. Although still widely used, ICP-OES is beginning to be superceded ICP-mass spectrometry for elemental analysis.

ICP-Mass Spectrometry (ICP-MS)

In addition to being excited to higher energy states, elements introduced into an ICP torch will also ionize; that is, they will form a charged species, e.g., Pb^+. This makes the ICP torch an excellent ion source for mass spectrometry. Mass spectrometers separate ions based on their atomic or molecular weight, which provides a high degree of selectivity in detection. (See below for a

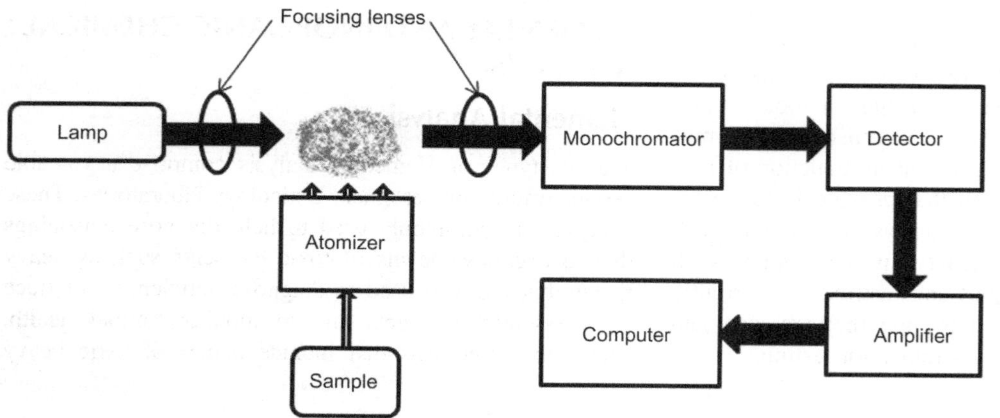

FIGURE 81.1 A diagram of an atomic absorption spectrophotometer.

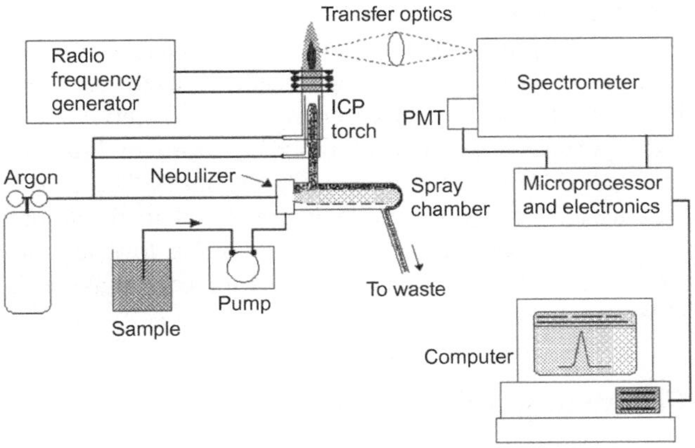

FIGURE 81.2 A diagram of an ICP-OES system.

detailed discussion of mass spectrometry.) Since the introduction of commercial ICP-mass spectrometer (ICP-MS) systems, they have become increasingly popular. Although ICP-MS systems are costlier and more complex than ICP-OES systems, they allow for the analysis of a wider array of elements with greater sensitivity without requiring any increased time for the analysis. There are fewer problems with interferences in ICP-MS, making data interpretation less complicated than with ICP-OES.

Sample Preparation for Elemental Analysis by AA, ICP, and ICP-MS

Sample preparation for elemental analysis typically involves digestion of the sample into its elemental constituents under strongly acidic conditions. All organic bonds are chemically destroyed by the acid, and the elemental components of those molecules are released into the solution. The resulting acidic digest is then diluted and analyzed.

Block Digestion

In this technique, a sample (a piece of liver tissue or a serum sample, for instance) is placed in a glass tube. A strong acid such as nitric acid is added to the tube and the tube is placed in a heating block. Heating the tube for several hours (or overnight) results in the sample being digested to its elemental constituents. The acid solution is then diluted and analyzed by AA, ICP, or ICP-MS. This is a simple and reliable technique that does not rely on complex equipment.

Microwave Digestion

In this technique, the sample is placed in an acid resistant vessel with a strong acid. The vessel is sealed and exposed to microwave irradiation, in a device similar to a microwave oven. This causes heat and pressure to build up within the vessel, digesting the sample. Once the sample is digested, pressure is released from the vessel and the solution is transferred out of the vessel, diluted, and analyzed.

Other Inorganic Analyses

Ion Chromatography

This technique is similar to other types of high-performance liquid chromatography (see below). In an ion chromatography column, separation of small ionic species occurs based on the strength of the attraction between the analytes and the stationary phase. Detection is based on conductivity or UV absorbance. Analyses for ions such as chloride, bromide, nitrate, sulfate, and fluoride are often performed using this method.

Nitrate/Nitrite

Nitrate and nitrite are commonly measured using convenient and inexpensive test strips, similar to pH paper. These give quantitative measurements of nitrate and nitrite in a variety of matrices including serum, feed, forage, and ocular fluid. A collaborative study of a method for nitrate analysis in forage samples using test strips was found to give good quantitative results (Jain et al., 1999). If necessary, results of screening using test strips may be confirmed by ion chromatography.

Cyanide

The cyanide concentration in a sample may be accurately quantified by distillation. The sample is mixed with water and acid and the liberated cyanide is distilled off. This solution is then mixed with a reagent that complexes with the cyanide to produce a colored derivative. The color intensity of the solution may then be accurately measured using a spectrophotometer, and this result may be used to provide the concentration of cyanide in the sample.

Cyanide may also be measured using test strips similar to those used for nitrate. The sample is mixed with water, and then a small amount of a strong acid is added to release any cyanide present. The test strip is dipped into the sample and the container is sealed while it incubates. The paper will change color if cyanide is present. The detection limit for this type of analysis is generally in the low part-per-million range, but the method does not provide an accurate measurement of cyanide concentration. It is, however, a fast and inexpensive screening method that may be followed up with the distillation method if necessary.

ORGANICS ANALYSIS

Introduction

Organic chemical analysis for veterinary diagnostics is a complicated proposition. Organic toxicants span a broad array of structural and chemical characteristics, and they must be identified and sometimes quantified in the presence of other chemicals that may be quite similar in their properties and present in far greater concentrations. In some cases, very low limits of detection—in the low part-per-billion range or even less—may be required to provide adequate diagnostic information. The field of organics analysis is currently dominated by techniques involving chromatography and mass spectrometry with some other techniques also in use.

ELISA

There are a variety of different types of analysis that involve the use of antibodies to bind to specific compounds within a sample. ELISA, which stands for "Enzyme Linked Immunosorbent Assay," is one such technique that is used in veterinary toxicology. A common type of ELISA test uses a multiwell plate, with each well containing immobilized antibodies specific for a given analyte. When a sample or sample extract is introduced to the well, any analyte that is present becomes immobilized by binding to the antibody. The remaining sample is rinsed out and a second solution is introduced. This solution contains another antibody specific to the analyte that is bound to an enzyme. A third solution containing the enzyme's substrate is added, and the reaction between enzyme and substrate produces a signal, usually in the form of a color change. A plate reader, which measures the intensity of the color change in each of the wells in the plate, may be used to quantify the concentrations of the analyte in the samples. ELISA tests require minimal equipment, are inexpensive to run, and they can be extremely sensitive. There is usually some potential for cross-reactivity of the antibodies with compounds other than the analytes, which can cause problems with false positive identifications. Therefore, ELISA may be used as a screening technique, with more selective techniques used to confirm positive identifications. Its use in veterinary toxicology is limited due to the lack of commercially produced test kits for many toxicants and sample types. ELISA kits are available for mycotoxin analysis in a variety of matrices as well as proteinaceous toxins, such as ricin and botulinum toxin.

Measurement of Acetylcholinesterase Activity

The activity of the enzyme acetylcholinesterase (AChE) is reduced by exposure to substances such as carbamate and organophosphate pesticides. Many labs use tests of AChE activity to check for the possibility of poisoning by such substances. These tests are typically run on blood or brain samples using a procedure known as the Ellman method (Ellman et al., 1961). This is an enzyme kinetic assay in which the substrate acetylthiocholine is hydrolyzed by AChE in the sample. The hydrolyzed acetylthiocholine immediately reacts with another reagent, providing a product with a yellow color. The rate of color change is measured with a spectrophotometer. The result is cholinesterase activity in micromoles of acetylthiocholine hydrolyzed per mL of blood or gram of brain per minute (μM/mL per min or μM/g per min). The activity measured in a given sample is compared to the normal activity level for that species. If the level is low, then followup analysis for organophosphate or carbamate pesticides may be done.

Chromatography

Introduction

Chromatography is a process of separation in which a mobile phase is passed through a stationary phase. Different constituents of the mobile phase will pass through the stationary phase at differing rates due to interactions with the stationary phase, resulting in their separation. While many different chromatographic techniques have been developed, only a few are commonly used in veterinary toxicology. These are discussed below. (Note that the use of mass spectrometers as detectors for chromatographic systems will be discussed in a separate section below.)

Thin Layer Chromatography (TLC)

In this technique, the stationary phase consists of a thin layer of a sorbent which is coated onto a flat plate (typically glass, but other materials may be used). Once the coating is dry, a few drops of the sample (or an extract of the sample) are carefully spotted onto a single point on the plate and the spot is allowed to dry. The plate is then set on edge into a container filled with enough solvent to cover a short portion of the plate's bottom edge. Capillary action causes the solvent to migrate up the sorbent coating. As solvent contacts the sample spot, the various components of that sample will migrate upward with it at different rates, causing them to separate. After a set period of time, the plate may be rotated 90 degrees and placed back into the solvent to provide a second dimension of separation. After a set period of time, the plate is removed and allowed to dry. Colored components may be identified visually, but many more compounds may be detected by illumination under UV light or by the application of various chemicals. In one method (Brazelton and Johnson, 2003), a variety of compounds were visualized on TLC plates by UV illumination and application of a sulfuric acid mixture that caused some components to turn black. TLC was once highly utilized and is very inexpensive, with no requirement for complex instrumentation. The use of TLC has waned in recent years, though, due to its limited separation capability and poor sensitivity as compared to instrumental techniques, such as gas chromatography and high-performance liquid chromatography. It can still be useful for some purposes, however. For instance, plants may be identified via comparison of TLC plates developed from unknown plant samples with those obtained from known plants. In such cases, it is not necessary to know the identity of each of the components, but only to match the patterns of components on the plates.

Gas Chromatography (GC)

In gas chromatography, the mobile phase consists of a gas, termed the carrier gas, which is passed through a tubular column containing the stationary phase coated on its internal surface. Sample extracts are introduced into the system by injection into a heated injector block that volatilizes the sample and introduces it into the stream of carrier gas and through the column. Separation of the chemical components occurs due to the different manners in which they interact with that stationary phase, resulting in different travel times through the column for the different components. At the end of the column, a detector responds to the different components as they elute (Fig. 81.3). The length of time it takes a compound to pass through the column, called the retention time, is a primary characteristic used to identify an analyte. As compounds elute from the column during the course of analysis, the detector response comes in the form of peaks (Fig. 81.4). The height and area of the peak are related to the concentration of the compound in the sample and are used to quantify its concentration. The width of the peak is a function of the separation power of the chromatographic system, with narrower peaks indicative of higher separation capability.

GC is an appropriate technique for analytes that are at least somewhat volatile, thermally stable, and are not significantly polar. Compounds such as chlorinated pesticides, organophosphate pesticides, PCBs, some plant alkaloids, some solvents, some drugs, gasoline, polynuclear aromatic hydrocarbons, and many others may be successfully analyzed using GC. Examples of compounds that are too polar for GC analysis include compounds with carboxylic acid, primary amine, or multiple hydroxyl moieties, although these may be analyzed with specialized columns or other specialized techniques.

The three primary components of a GC system are the injector, the column, which is housed in a precisely controlled oven, and a detector. The injector consists of a heated chamber with an inlet for carrier gas and an outlet to which the column is connected. The carrier gas is usually helium, although hydrogen, nitrogen, or other gases can be used. Most systems also include an autosampler, which automatically injects samples in a predetermined sequence, allowing for unattended operation of the instrument. Each of these components varies depending on analytical needs.

GC Columns

The column is the heart of the chromatographic system. Most GC columns in use today consist of a thin, hollow, silica capillary that can be internally coated with a wide variety of stationary phases. These columns provide extremely high separation capabilities with many options in terms of length, diameter, stationary phase, etc. Typical GC columns used in veterinary diagnostics are 15–30 m in length with internal diameters of 0.25–0.32 mm (Fig. 81.5). The choice of a GC column is based on the analyte(s) and the matrix in question. The column must be able to separate an analyte from as many other sample components as possible and the peak shape should be symmetrical and narrow. The retention time of the analyte must be consistent and repeatable irrespective of the concentration of other components in the mixture. The

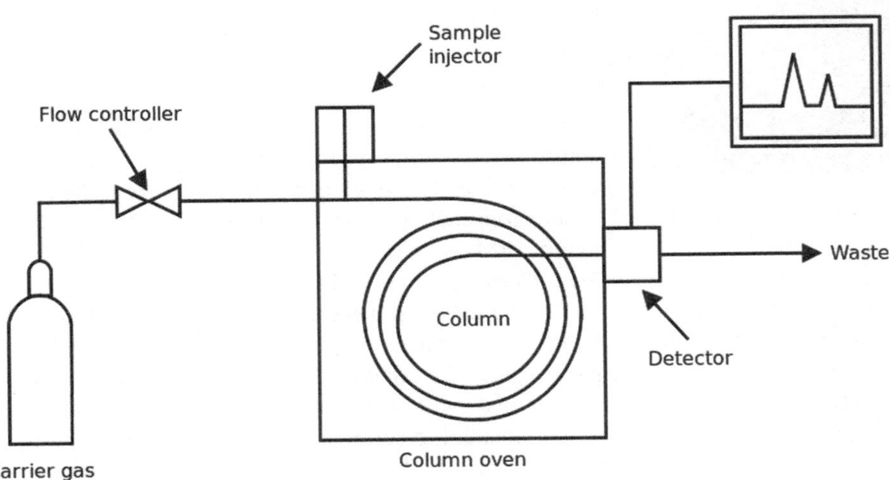

FIGURE 81.3 A diagram of a gas chromatograph.

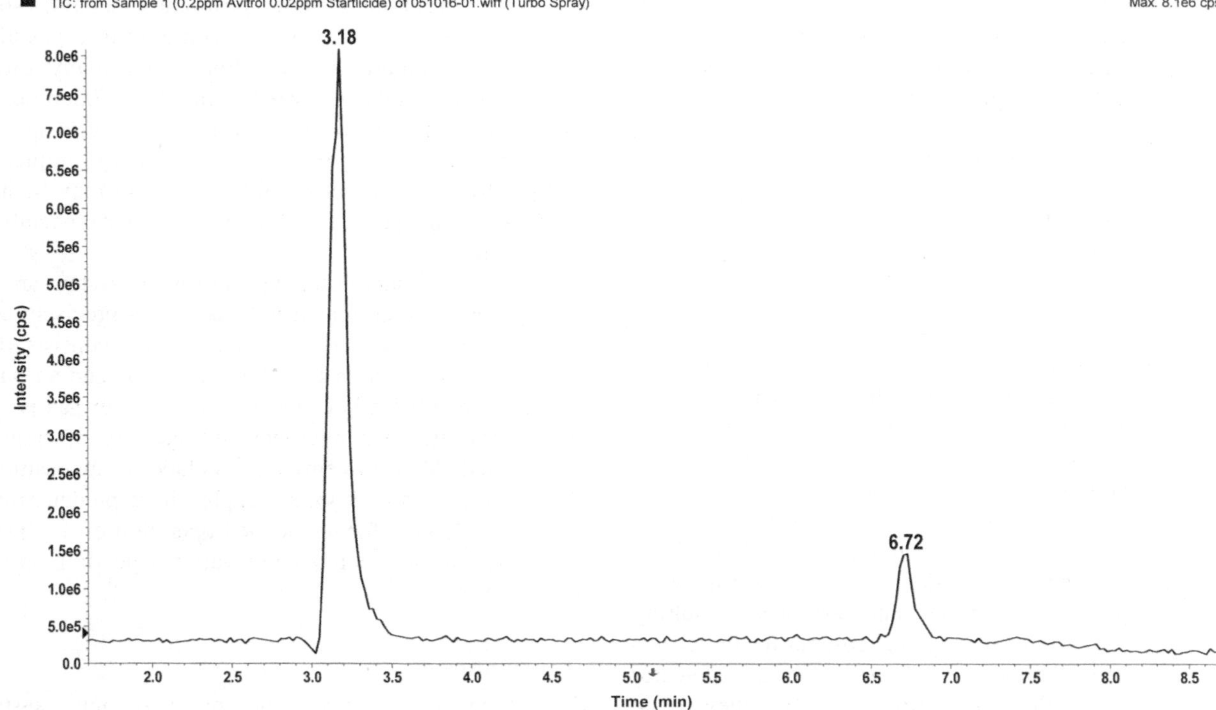

FIGURE 81.4 An example of a GC chromatogram. The *x*-axis is time, with the injection at time 0. The *y*-axis is the intensity of the detector response, normalized to the largest peak in the chromatogram. The two peaks shown each represent a different chemical eluting from the column into the detector and are labeled with their retention times.

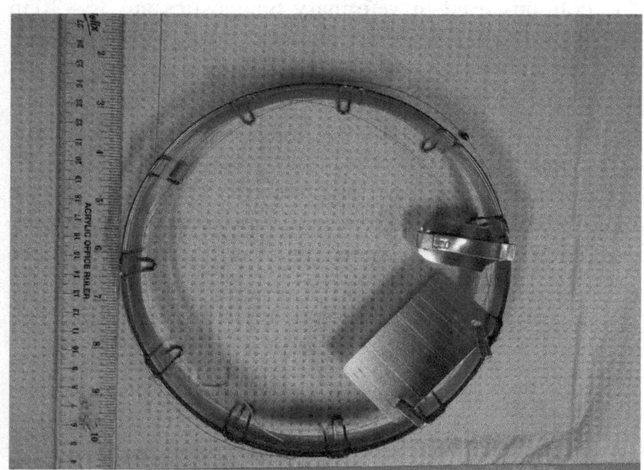

FIGURE 81.5 A typical GC column. This column is 15 m long and 0.25 mm in outer diameter.

retention time of a compound will depend on how it interacts with the column coating, the flow rate of the carrier gas, and the temperature of the GC oven. A higher oven temperature will provide for shorter retention times (and shorter analysis times) and vice versa. GC ovens are capable of heating to very consistent and accurate temperatures, which is necessary to insure repeatable retention times. They are also capable of temperature programming, a technique in which the temperature is increased at a specified rate during the course of analysis. This allows the analyst to essentially tune the analysis to help isolate the analyte from interfering compounds. It also allows for more rapid analysis without compromising separation, particularly when only a few analytes are involved. Increasing numbers of analytes usually results in slower temperature programs and longer analysis times.

GC Detectors

A wide array of detectors has been developed for GC analysis. They range from general-purpose detectors that respond to nearly any component eluting from the column to detectors that only respond to narrow classes of compounds. (Mass spectrometers will be considered separately from other types of GC detectors.)

Among the most generic used in veterinary diagnostics is the flame ionization detector (FID). In an FID, the gases exiting the column are mixed with hydrogen and air and burned within a small chamber. Combustion of carbon-containing compounds from the column creates an electrical current that changes as the different compounds elute. The change in current as a compound elutes is measured and detected as a chromatographic peak. FIDs are inexpensive, rugged, and sensitive, particularly to compounds containing mainly carbon and hydrogen. Their primary disadvantage for veterinary diagnostics involves the complex matrices typically analyzed. In order to be detected, the analyte must be present at a concentration high enough for it to stand out among the many other carbon-containing compounds in a sample. This problem may be mitigated to some extent with extraction and cleanup procedures that minimize the presence of interfering matrix components and/or with well-designed chromatographic separation. Nonetheless, FIDs have largely been replaced by detectors that allow for more specific modes of detection and, especially, by mass spectrometers.

The flame photometric detector (FPD) is an example of one that offers significantly more selectivity than the FID. In an FPD, the compounds eluted from the column are burned in a hydrogen rich atmosphere in similar fashion to the FID. The FPD takes advantage of the fact that compounds containing certain elements will emit light of specific wavelengths when combusted. A photomultiplier tube is used to measure the light produced as compounds elute from the column and are burned. A filter placed in between the end of the column and the photomultiplier tube is used to allow only light of a specific wavelength to be detected. Filters typically used are specific for the characteristic wavelengths of sulfur or phosphorus. Thus, as compounds elute from the column, only those containing the element that matches the filter will produce a response from the detector. A common application of these detectors in veterinary diagnostics is for analysis of organophosphate pesticides. These compounds may be detected at very low levels in extremely complex matrices because of the detectors ability to screen out any compounds that do not contain a phosphorus atom.

Another example of a highly selective detector is the electron capture detector (ECD). In an ECD, a beta-emitting radioactive source (typically ^{63}Ni foil) is placed such that the electrons are emitted into the column eluent. These electrons ionize the carrier gas resulting in an abundance of free electrons. These electrons are collected by an anode, which results in an electrical current that is constantly monitored. In the absence of electronegative species, this current remains constant. Electronegative species that elute from the column will capture electrons resulting in a change in the electrical current, which is then recorded as a chromatographic peak. Halogens are an example of a class of electronegative elements, and the ECD is extremely sensitive to organohalides. Common uses for the ECD in veterinary diagnostics include tests for organochlorine pesticides and for some pyrethroids. As with the FPD, the ability of the detector to respond selectively to a specific class of compounds results in highly sensitive assays in complex matrices. Low part-per-billion detection limits are commonly achieved in matrices, such as liver and adipose tissue with ECDs.

High-Performance Liquid Chromatography (HPLC)

Another type of chromatography commonly used in veterinary diagnostics is high-performance liquid chromatography (HPLC). In HPLC, the mobile phase is a stream of liquid and the stationary phase consists of fine particles coated with a sorbent. The particles are packed into a metal tube, typically 1–4.6 mm in diameter and 50–250 mm in length (Fig. 81.6). The sample extract is injected directly into the flowing mobile phase, which is pumped through the column under high pressure (typically in the range of 500–14,000 psi). Separation occurs based on the affinities of the different components in the sample for the adsorbent. Compounds that only adsorb weakly will quickly elute from the column while those that are more strongly adsorbed will take longer to elute. Different types of detectors are used to produce a response as compounds elute from the column. As with GC, compounds are identified by their characteristic retention times and detector response is in the form of peaks. Peak height and area correlate with the concentration of the compound in the sample and peaks should be as narrow and symmetrical as can be achieved.

HPLC is a complementary technique to GC. Injection and separation are performed at ambient temperature, which allows for the analysis of thermally labile compounds. The use of polar mobile phases, such as water, allow for the analysis of highly polar compounds that are typically not amenable to GC. Examples of compounds commonly analyzed by HPLC include carbamate

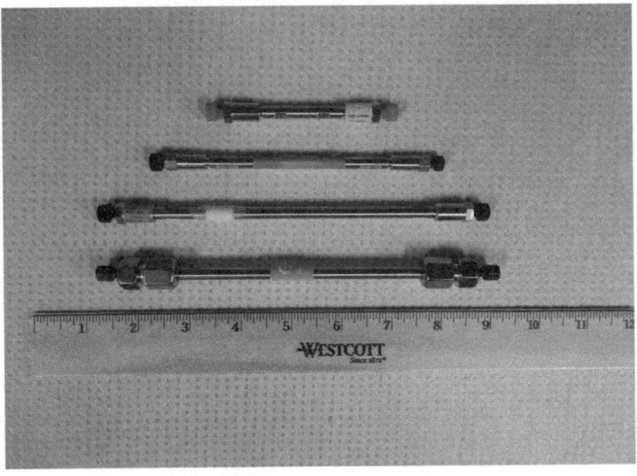

FIGURE 81.6 Several examples of typical HPLC columns. Those shown range in length from 50 to 150 mm in length and are 2.1 mm in diameter.

pesticides, drugs of abuse, pesticide and drug metabolites, mycotoxins, and marine toxins, such as domoic acid and microcystins. HPLC is also used for the separation of high molecular weight compounds such as proteins, although this type of analysis is not yet common in veterinary diagnostics.

In its most basic form, an analytical HPLC system consists of a high pressure pump, a mobile phase, an injector, a column, a detector, and the tubing that connects these components. Modern commercially produced systems typically include several other components. A degasser is used to remove dissolved gases such as nitrogen and oxygen from the mobile phase as the presence of these gases will result in inconsistent pressure in the system. An autosampler is used to automatically inject samples and a temperature controlled column compartment is provided in order to provide a consistent column temperature. Of these different components, it is the column, the mobile phase, and the detector that vary most depending on the required analysis.

HPLC Columns

As with GC, a wide variety of commercially produced HPLC columns allow for the analysis of many different classes of analytes in different matrices. The sorbent in the column (the "column packing") typically provides separation based on the polarity of the analytes, although factors such as the pK_a of the analyte may also be used to provide separation. The length and diameter of the column are also parameters that will affect the column's separation capabilities.

HPLC Mobile Phases

Mobile phases are chosen based on the separation needed, the type of column being used, and the detector. Typically, solvents such as water, methanol, and acetonitrile, are used. They often contain low concentrations of modifiers, such as acetic or formic acid or buffers that contain phosphate or acetate. These modifiers can greatly improve the peak shape and width for analytes and they may be crucial in providing good separation capabilities. Some of these modifiers, particularly phosphate buffers, are not compatible with the use of a mass spectrometer as the detector.

HPLC Detectors

Ultraviolet Light Detectors Ultraviolet spectrophotometric (UV) detectors are commonly used in veterinary diagnostics. These detectors measure light absorbed by the mobile phase at different wavelengths. As compounds that absorb light at a specific wavelength elute, the absorbance at that wavelength changes resulting in detection of the compound. For single wavelength detectors, the wavelength of light must be selected as part of the analysis, and only compounds that absorb light at that wavelength will be detected. Variable wavelength detectors allow for several different wavelengths or ranges of wavelengths to be used. Diode array detectors offer the capability to scan across a wide range of wavelengths, producing a UV spectrum, which can be used in addition to the retention time to support the identification of an analyte (Fig. 81.7).

Fluorescence Detectors Another type of HPLC detector commonly used in veterinary diagnostics is the fluorescence detector. These detectors use high intensity light of a specific wavelength to excite an analyte molecule to a higher energy state. The analyte quickly relaxes back to a lower energy state, emitting light at a specific wavelength as it does so. It is the emitted light that is detected and which provides the detector response. In order for this process to work, the analyte must contain a functional group, known as a fluorophore, which fluoresces. Aromatic ring structures and carbonyl groups are among those that offer

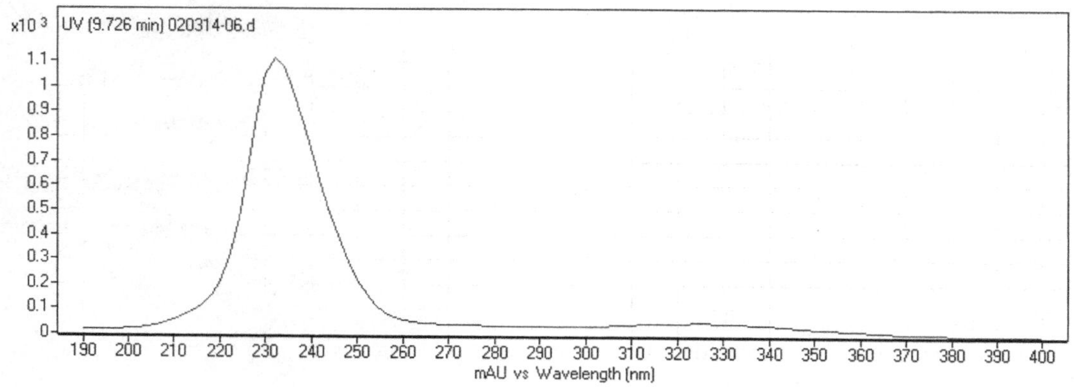

FIGURE 81.7 An example of a spectrum taken from an ultraviolet light absorption detector. The *x*-axis is wavelength in nanometers and the *y*-axis is intensity of detector response. The two distinctive features of this spectrum are the large peak at ~235 nm and the broad, low intensity peak centered at ~325 nm.

strong fluorescence activity. Molecules that do not contain fluorophores may be chemically modified by addition of an aromatic structure in order to analyze them by fluorescence. Fluorescence analysis is extremely sensitive and selective for those compounds containing fluorophores, making it a good choice for trace analysis in difficult matrices. Vitamin A, vitamin E, and some anticoagulant rodenticides are examples of chemicals that may be analyzed by HPLC with fluorescence detection.

Mass Spectrometry

Mass spectrometers are instruments that measure the mass (m) to charge (z) ratios of ions. (In most veterinary toxicological analyses, the charge on the molecule will be 1, and thus the m/z will be equivalent to the mass or molecular weight of the ion.) This simple concept is the basis of one of the most powerful techniques in analytical chemistry. Recall that a molecule's mass is calculated by adding the atomic weight of each of the atoms in the molecule. Thus, the molecular weight is directly related to a compound's atomic composition. Mass spectrometry also can provide information regarding the way these atoms are put together, i.e., the structure of the molecule.

A mass spectrum consists of a plot of a detector signal with m/z on the x-axis and signal intensity on the y-axis. Fig. 81.8 is the mass spectrum of caffeine obtained on a gas chromatograph-mass spectrometer. Note that there are signals obtained at various m/z values, each derived from a different fragment of the caffeine molecule. Also note the relative intensities of the different signals. These are characteristic for the caffeine molecule. (Somewhat confusingly, the signals at the different m/z ratios are called "peaks," just as the signals obtained at different retention times in a chromatographic analysis are also called "peaks.")

Most mass spectrometers used for organic analysis in veterinary diagnostics are interfaced to a chromatographic system. The selectivity of combined chromatography-mass spectrometry analysis is due to the fact that these techniques combine two orthogonal separations. The chromatographic portion of the analysis separates molecules based on properties, such as vapor pressure or polarity, providing retention time information. After this separation occurs, the molecules are further differentiated by their m/z ratios. The combination of both retention time and m/z data provides for a very selective analysis. This high selectivity is the reason these techniques are often considered the "gold standards" for providing high confidence in compound identification and quantitation.

Mass spectrometers are also combined with ICP systems, which allows for the identification of elements by

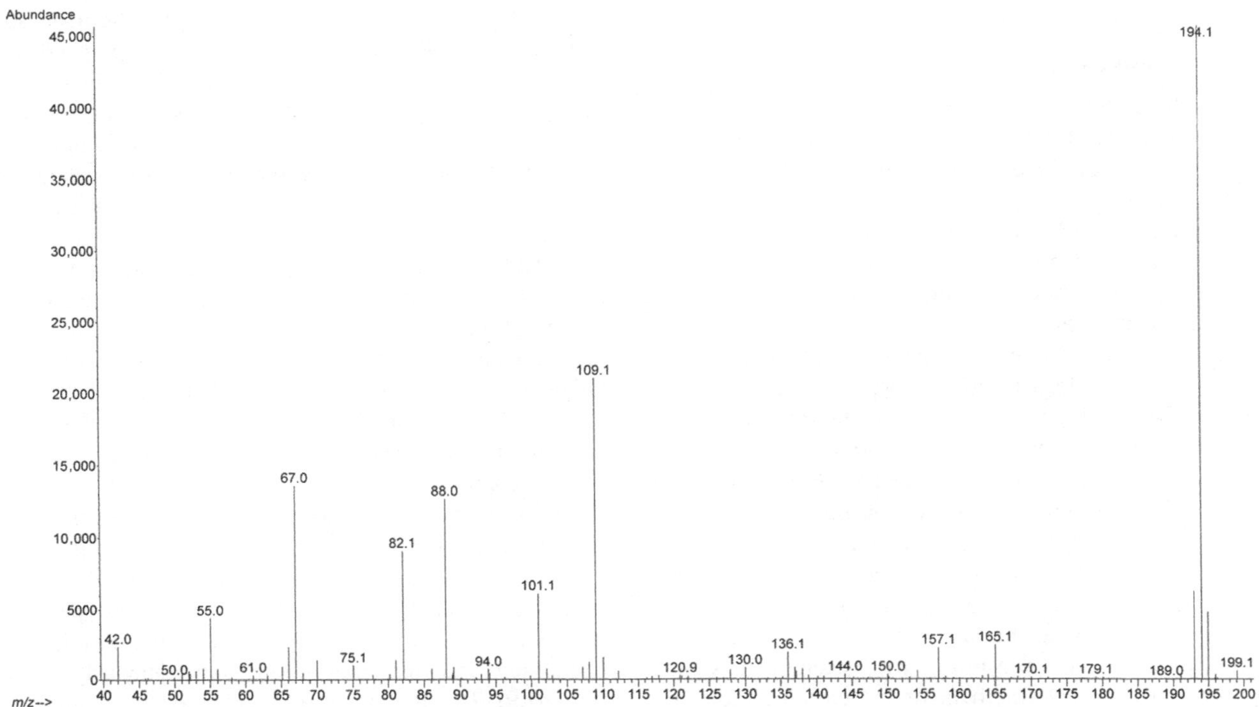

FIGURE 81.8 A mass spectrum of caffeine obtained by electron ionization. The x-axis is the mass-to-charge ratio (m/z, in this case equivalent to molecular weight) and the y-axis is intensity of response. The peak at m/z 194 is derived from intact caffeine while the other major peaks in the spectrum are derived from fragments of the caffeine molecule.

their atomic mass. Again, this provides for a very selective (as well as a very sensitive) method of analysis.

A mass spectrometer consists of three essential components: an ion source, a mass analyzer, and a detector. The mass analyzer and detector (and in some cases, the ion source) are maintained under high vacuum, so a vacuum system of some kind is also important. While a wide variety of ion sources and mass analyzers have been developed, only a few of these are commonly used in veterinary diagnostics. These are described below.

Ion Sources

For a compound to be analyzed by mass spectrometry, it must be present in the form of an ion; i.e., it must have a positive or negative charge on it. The vast majority of compounds of interest in veterinary diagnostics are not naturally present as ions. Therefore, some method of ionizing them must be used in order for them to be analyzed by MS. Common ionization methods used in veterinary diagnostics include ICP for elements, electron ionization (EI) for GC-MS, and electrospray for LC-MS.

ICP

In ICP-MS, the ICP torch functions as the ion source for the instrument. The ionized elements are then directed to the mass analyzer where they are detected based on their *m/z* ratios.

Electron Ionization (EI)

This is the technique commonly used in GC-MS. In EI, the ion source is housed in the vacuum chamber of the mass spectrometer. An electrical current is applied to a filament consisting of a thin wire. The current is set such that electrons are emitted from the filament with an energy of 70 eV. The end of the GC column is placed such that compounds elute from the column directly into the stream of electrons emitted from the filament (Fig. 81.8). A compound impacted by these electrons will emit an electron of its own, resulting in a positive charge on the compound. Additionally, the high energy level of these filament electrons will cause many compounds to break apart, with some of the fragments being ionized while others remain neutral. The resulting ions (intact molecules and/or their fragments) are then directed into the mass analyzer, which differentiates them based on *m/z*. The output of this process is what is typically recognized as a mass spectral "fingerprint," showing the *m/z* and relative abundance of each of the ions. Note that in Fig. 81.8, each of the signals represents a different fragment of the caffeine molecule. Keeping the electron energy precisely set at 70 eV ensures that the fragmentation of a given compound will happen consistently, always providing the same fragment ions with the same relative abundance levels. The standardization of the electron energy at 70 eV for all instruments provides consistency in mass spectra among instruments from different manufacturers and different laboratories. Therefore, a compound analyzed in one laboratory will provide the same spectrum when it's analyzed in any other laboratory. This has allowed for the development of mass spectral libraries, containing spectra for hundreds of thousands of different chemicals. Instrument software is provided with most GC-MS systems, which allows the analyst to search an obtained mass spectrum against all of those contained within the library. This library searching software provides an excellent means of identifying both targeted compounds suspected to be present and nontargeted ones that are not expected to be present in a sample at the time of analysis.

Electrospray Ionization (ESI)

Electrospray is the ionization method typically used in HPLC-MS. The coupling of GC with MS was a relatively easy undertaking as compared to coupling HPLC to MS. This is primarily due to the fact that mass analyzers must operate in a vacuum. Ions formed in an ion source must be physically moved to the mass analyzer, and this cannot occur if there are significant numbers of other molecules such as atmospheric nitrogen, oxygen, or water that get in the way. A typical GC system will introduce somewhere around 1 cc of carrier gas per minute into the mass spectrometer, and this amount of gas is easily pumped away using common types of vacuum pumps. A liquid chromatograph eluting directly into a mass spectrometer would introduce somewhere between 0.1 and 0.5 mL/min of solvent into the MS. This volume of solvent expands tremendously when vaporized, to the point that only extremely complex and expensive vacuum systems could pump it away and maintain vacuum. Various techniques were used to try to get around this issue, but none were seen as practical until the development of electrospray ionization. This technique involves directing the LC flow through a fine diameter needle. Voltage is applied to the needle as the solvent flows through it, resulting in a fine spray of charged droplets. (This is somewhat similar to how an electric paint sprayer works.) The droplets are directed at the front of the mass spectrometer. The electric charge helps to ionize molecules within the droplets while solvent from the HPLC mobile phase evaporates from the droplets as they pass between the needle and the mass spectrometer. In this manner, the bulk of the liquid is eliminated while any analytes present are simultaneously ionized (Fig. 81.9). This ionization mechanism differs significantly from EI, providing intact molecular ions without the fragmentation of EI. So instead of a somewhat unique molecular fingerprint, ESI usually produces ions of a single *m/z*

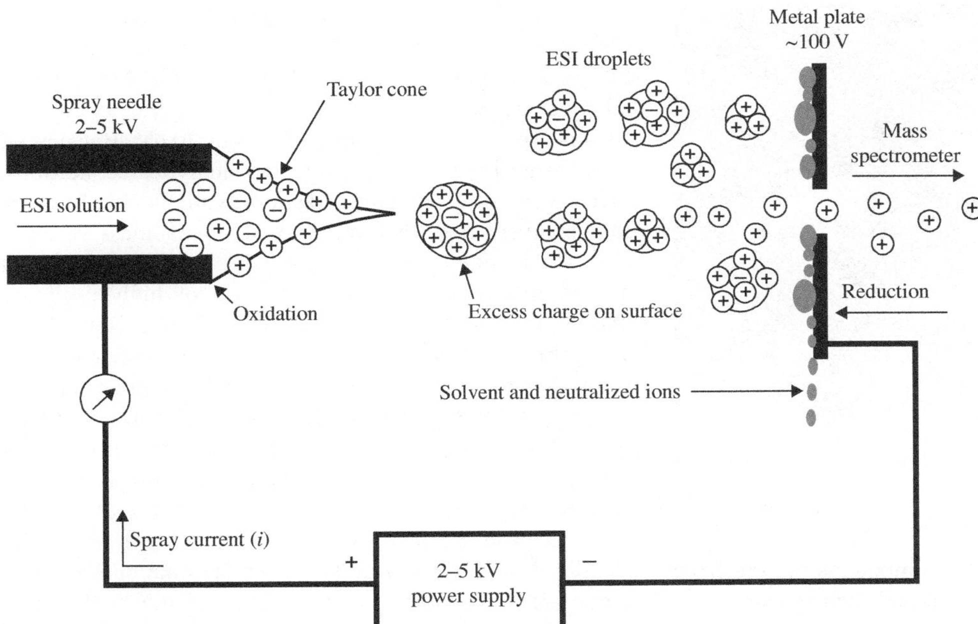

FIGURE 81.9 A simple electrospray ionization source. On the left is the electrically charged capillary tube connected to the exit of the HPLC column. Liquid from the column exits the capillary in the form of electrically charged droplets. As solvent molecules evaporate from the droplets, they become smaller and smaller until only gas phase ions are left. These are drawn into the mass spectrometer, on the right. The "Taylor Cone" refers to the characteristic shape of liquid exiting a capillary under high voltage conditions.

for a particular molecule. Typically, this is the protonated molecular ion $[M+H]^+$ for positive ions or the deprotonated $[M-H]^-$ for negative ions. Because only ions of a single *m/z* are formed, ESI is not very selective in and of itself; most molecules with the same molecular weight will give the same ion. The upshot of this is that the mass analyzer must do more than just provide the nominal *m/z* for the ion in order to achieve a selective analysis. Triple stage quadrupole instruments (see below, under Mass Analyzers) are commonly used to provide high selectivity with ESI. It's also important to note that only some types of molecules will ionize by this method. There must be a site on the molecule that is basic enough to accept a proton or acidic enough to lose one. Compounds containing nitrogen typically ionize well by accepting protons while compounds containing solely carbon and hydrogen do not. Compounds containing other atoms, such as oxygen, sulfur, and phosphorus, ionize to greater or lesser extents depending on their molecular structures.

While electrospray ionization is currently the method of choice for the vast majority of LC-MS analyses, it is not without issues, particularly when it comes to quantitative measurements. The detector response for a given concentration of a chemical in a standard solution is usually very different from that of the same concentration of that chemical in a sample extract. Typically, the response will be suppressed in the more complex sample matrix although enhancement of response also occurs. Quantitation relies on the comparison of response in a sample to the response in a standard, which can make it difficult to provide accurate data for concentrations of toxicants in matrices, such as tissue, body fluids, or feed. There are methods that can account for this variability in response and allow for accurate quantitation in such matrices, but they typically add time and cost to LC-MS analyses. This is in contrast to GC-MS analyses, in which such problems are much less common. Another issue with LC-MS analysis is that it typically does not allow for screening against a mass spectral library, as is common with GC-MS. The reason for this is explained in the section on triple stage quadrupole instruments.

Mass Analyzers

A bewildering array of mass analyzers have been developed over the years, ranging from extremely simple ones suitable for detecting explosives at airports to extremely complex instruments costing millions of dollars and requiring multiple PhD level scientists just to keep them running. Only one—the quadrupole analyzer—has commonly been used in veterinary toxicology.

The quadrupole analyzer is the most widely produced of the mass analyzers. It is relatively simple and the design and operation of these systems has matured greatly over the last forty years or so. A quadrupole analyzer consists of four round parallel metal rods arrayed in a square configuration (Fig. 81.10). Ions from the ion source are directed through the space between the four rods at one end and a detector is placed at the other end. Voltages on the rods can be manipulated such that only ions of a specific *m/z* will pass through from the ion source to the detector, making the analyzer an effective mass filter. These voltages can be rapidly changed, allowing ions of increasing *m/z* to sequentially pass through the analyzer. This results in a scan of a selected mass range over the course of a second or less. When the mass spectrometer is

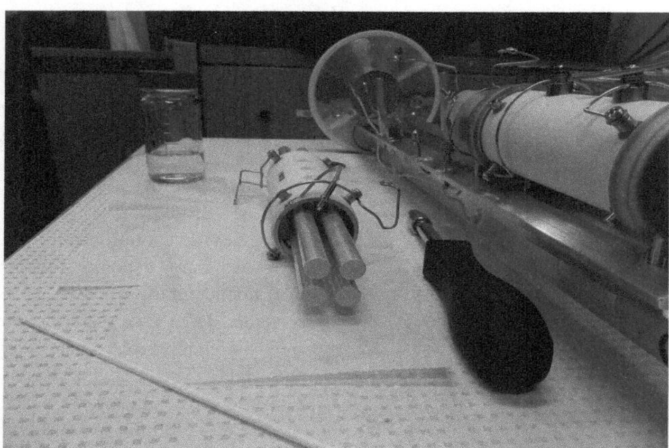

FIGURE 81.10 A photograph of a set of quadrupoles from the mass analyzer of an LC-MS instrument.

attached to a chromatograph the compounds eluting from the chromatograph may be ionized and then scanned on a second-to-second basis, providing spectra for compounds as they elute (Fig. 81.11). Quadrupole analyzers are commonly found in LC-MS, GC-MS, and ICP-MS systems.

Quadrupole analyzers are considered to be nominal mass analyzers; i.e., they separate ions on a whole number basis. An ion with an *m/z* of 100 can be distinguished from one with an *m/z* of 99 or 101 but not one of 99.5 or 100.3. This is not a problem in GC-MS analysis as the "mass spectral fingerprint" is a good identifier. This does present a problem in selectivity for ions generated using electrospray ionization, as there is no fragmentation provided and there may be thousands of compounds that provide the same single ion. The most common solution to this problem is to use triple stage quadrupole systems. These systems consist of three separate quadrupole analyzers in series. The first quadrupole (Q1) is set to select a single ion formed in the ion source—e.g., one of *m/z* of 300—and send only those ions to the second quadrupole. The second quadrupole (q2) is not used to select ions; rather, it is used to contain nitrogen or argon gas and to transmit ions to Q3. The ions selected in Q1 are accelerated into q2 where they collide with the gas molecules and break into fragments in a process somewhat analogous to the fragmentation process of EI. These fragments are then directed into Q3, which provides mass analysis of the fragments and the resulting "MS fingerprint" (Fig. 81.12). This process is referred to as MS/MS and with an HPLC, LC-MS/MS. Such systems provide a high level of selectivity and very high confidence in identifications when an assay is properly run. They can be extremely sensitive, detecting compounds down to the femtogram or even attogram level. They are also very complex and expensive instruments, and it is challenging for veterinary toxicology labs to obtain the funding required to purchase and operate them.

While GC-MS screening against a mass spectral library is a common type of analysis, there is no comparable analysis possible with LC-MS/MS. GC-MS systems all give the same mass spectrum for a given compound because of the standardization of EI at 70 eV. Because of differences in instrumentation and analytical conditions, there is no similar standardization available for LC-MS/MS analysis and therefore no standard mass spectral libraries available for this technique. It is possible to get around this problem through the use of high-resolution mass spectrometers, including time of flight and orbitraps. The primary difference between these and other analyzers is their ability to provide extremely high precision and accuracy in mass measurement. While a quadrupole analyzer is capable of distinguishing between ions of (for example) *m/z* 300 and 301, a high-resolution instrument may reliably differentiate ions of, e.g., *m/z* 300.001 and 300.002. The number of compounds with a molecular weight of 300.002 will be far fewer than the number with a nominal molecular weight of 300, and this is the basis for the selectivity of this mass spectrometer. This technique is termed "high-resolution, accurate mass spectrometry," or HRAMS. It allows for high selectivity without a requirement for fragmentation and may be used as an alternative to a triple stage quadrupole for most LC-MS analyses and it allows for nontargeted analysis like that of GC-MS screening. With a triple stage quadrupole instrument, ions of a single *m/z* must be selected in the first quadrupole in order for them to be fragmented and analyzed in the second and third quadrupoles. The instrument must be programmed to specifically allow only the selected ions through the first quadrupole and detect their fragment ions. Detection of nontargeted analytes is therefore not possible. In the HRAMS, data is gathered for all of the ions produced in the ion source within a specified mass range, with the selectivity coming from the precision and accuracy of the mass measurements rather than measurement of fragment ions. Instead of a mass spectral library, a database consisting of many compounds and their corresponding accurate mass ions is used for screening. While HRAMS use is currently rare in veterinary diagnostics, it is possible that more labs will purchase these instruments in the future. These systems are generally slightly less sensitive than the best triple stage quadrupoles, but the advantage of providing nontargeted analysis can be significant and the costs of the two types of systems are comparable.

Sample Preparation for Organics Analysis

The complicated nature of organics analysis is reflected in the broad array of techniques used for sample preparation. Generally speaking, the goal of sample preparation in veterinary toxicology is to extract the compounds(s) of

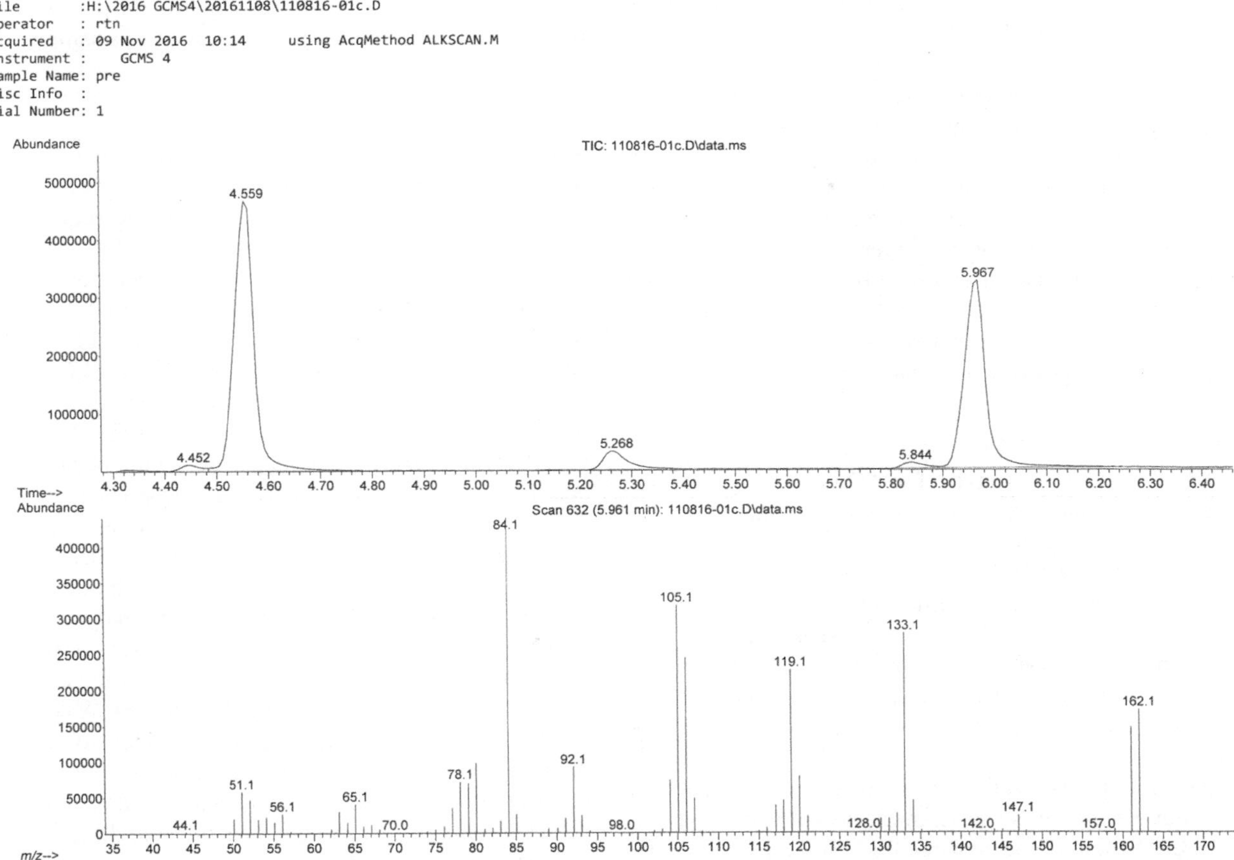

FIGURE 81.11 A segment from a GC-MS analysis. The chromatogram is above. Below is the mass spectrum obtained from the compound eluting at a retention time of 5.967 min.

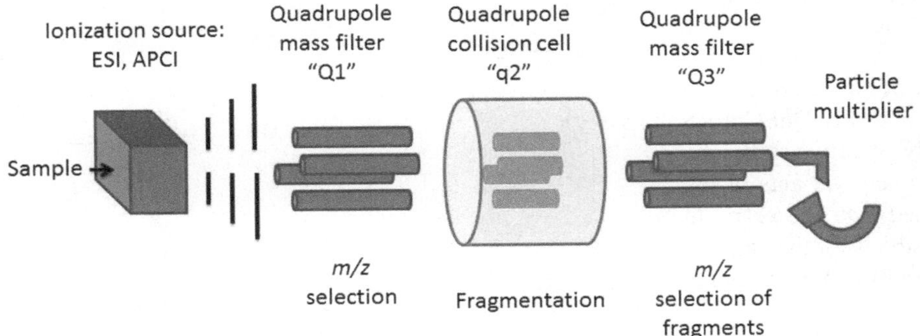

FIGURE 81.12 A diagram of a triple stage quadrupole instrument. Ions of a single *m/z* ratio are selected in Q1. Those ions are fragmented in the collision cell (q2) and the fragments are analyzed in Q3. The particle multiplier detects the fragment ions as they exit Q3.

interest from the sample into a solvent that is appropriate for the analytical technique. The first step of this extraction process for nonliquid samples usually involves homogenization into a solvent, such as water, methanol, or some other organic solvent. Once this has been accomplished, the analytes can be extracted from the liquid phase. The resulting extract may be subjected to cleanup procedures designed to remove potentially interfering compounds and it may be concentrated in order to provide lower detection limits. A few of the more common extraction methods follow.

Homogenization

This step involves the blending of nonliquid samples, such as feed or tissue with an organic solvent. The solvent is chosen based on the nature of the analyte(s) and the matrix. Typical extraction solvents include ethyl acetate, acetonitrile, hexane, and methylene chloride.

Liquid–Liquid Extraction (LLE)

In this technique, a donor phase is shaken with a nonmiscible acceptor phase. The donor phase may consist of a liquid sample, such as urine or serum, or it may be a homogenate of a nonliquid sample. When the acceptor phase is properly chosen, the analytes will partition into it. Organochlorine pesticides are a good example. Most are not very polar compounds, so if they are contained in an aqueous solution and that solution is shaken up with methylene chloride (which is not miscible with water), the organochlorines will partition into the less polar methylene chloride phase. The methylene chloride will settle out from the water and it can then be removed, subjected to further cleanup procedures, concentrated, or analyzed directly. LLE is a very effective technique for extracting many different types of compounds out of a sample

QuEChERS Extraction

QuEChERS is an acronym for "Quick, Easy, Cheap, Effective, Reliable, Safe." It describes a variant of LLE combined with a cleanup step that removes some potential interfering compounds. The technique was developed by Anastassiades and Lehotay for the analysis of a broad range of pesticides in food products (Anastassiades et al., 2003). The extraction is a type of "salting out" LLE, in which a high concentration of salt, usually sodium chloride or magnesium sulfate, is added to an aqueous phase (the sample or its homogenate). Acetonitrile serves as the acceptor phase. Normally, acetonitrile is miscible with water, but the high ionic strength of the salt water solution causes the acetonitrile to separate from the water. This high ionic strength will also cause many organic chemicals to partition into the acetonitrile phase, which is then removed from the water. Some of the potentially interfering sample components, such as pigments and fatty acids, may then be removed by adding a powdered sorbent to the solution. The interferences adsorb onto the sorbent, which is then removed from the solution. This type of cleanup is known as "dispersive solid phase extraction" or dSPE. QuEChERS has turned out to be an exceptionally effective, efficient, and versatile extraction method and many variants of the original procedure have been published over the years. In veterinary toxicology, QuEChERS methods for the analysis of anticoagulant rodenticides and for an LC-MS screening procedure have been published.

Solid Phase Extraction

Solid phase extraction (SPE) is a variant of liquid chromatography. A SPE cartridge consists of a small, open-ended container (often a syringe barrel) filled with particles coated with a sorbent. Some of these sorbents are the same types used in HPLC columns. The liquefied sample is passed through the sorbent, with different components adsorbing depending on their affinity for the sorbent. Adsorbed components may be eluted from the sorbent by passing a different solvent through it. Different mixtures of solvents may be used to first elute off potentially interfering compounds before eluting the analytes. In this way, SPE may provide both extraction and cleanup of a sample.

Derivatization Methods

There are some poisons that are not amenable to detection by any of the above methods. An example of such a compound is ethylene glycol. Its low molecular weight and high polarity make it unsuitable for GC analysis. It lacks a distinctive UV spectrum and does not contain a fluorophore, making it unsuitable for HPLC with UV or fluorescence detection. And it lacks any acidic or basic sites on the molecule making it unsuitable for LC-MS. In a case like this, the compound may be chemically altered into a derivative that is suitable for one of the above methods. Ethylene glycol can be reacted with phenylboronic acid to produce a derivative that is nonpolar and thermally stable, which can then be analyzed by GC with an FID or by GC-MS (Fig. 81.13). In some cases, the derivatization step can be automated. Ionophore antibiotics are an example of a class of compounds often analyzed using a post-column derivatization system. In these systems, the ionophores are mixed with reagents as they elute from the HPLC column, prior to entering the detector. A compound containing a fluorophore chemically binds to the ionophore molecule and the derivatized ionophore, which is now suitable for fluorescence analysis, then enters the detector. This results in high sensitivity and selectivity as well as good quantitative performance (Table 81.1).

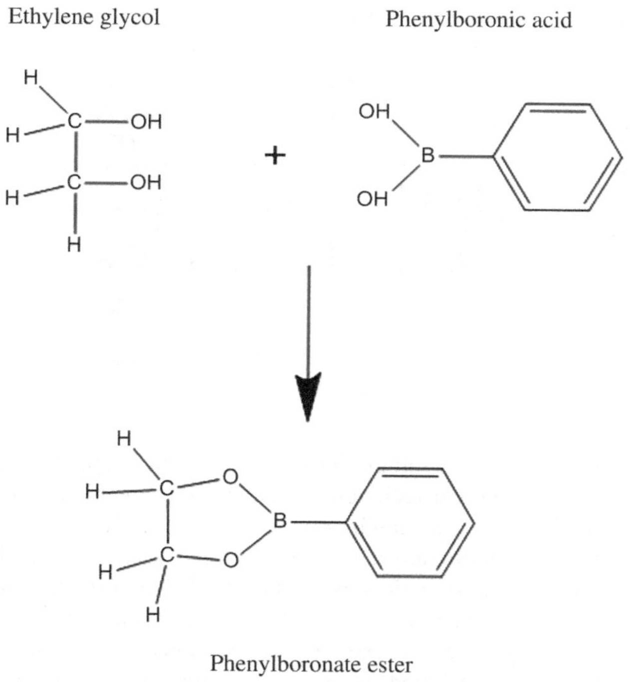

Ethylene glycol + Phenylboronic acid

Phenylboronate ester

FIGURE 81.13 The conversion of ethylene glycol into its borohydrate derivative. Ethylene glycol is too polar for gas chromatographic analysis, but the derivative is amenable to it.

TABLE 81.1 A Table of Various Analytical Techniques With Their Advantages, Disadvantages, and Some Common Uses

Technique	Advantages	Disadvantages	Appropriate Types of Analytes	Typical Analyses
Atomic absorption spectrophotometry	Quick setup. Relatively simple inexpensive instrument	Can only analyze for one element at a time	Most elements in the periodic table	Lead
ICP-OES	Fast multielement detection	Less sensitive than ICP-MS	Most elements in the periodic table	Various multielement tests
ICP-MS	Fast multielement detection, very sensitive	Instrument is more expensive and complex than ICP-OES	Most elements in the periodic table	Various multielement tests
Ion chromatography	Relatively simple, inexpensive instrumentation. Adequate sensitivity for most uses	Low level analysis in complex matrices may be difficult due to lack of selectivity	Small ionic atoms and molecules	Nitrate, halogens such as chloride and bromide
GC with ECD	Relatively simple, inexpensive instruments. Very sensitive for halogenated compounds. Provides accurate quantitation	Not as selective as mass spectrometry. May require second analysis for high confidence in identification	Halogenated organic chemicals which are nonpolar, volatile or semivolatile, and not thermally labile	Organochlorine pesticides, PCBs, some pyrethroids
GC with FPD	Relatively simple, inexpensive instrument. Very sensitive for compounds containing phosphorus or nitrogen. Provides accurate quantitation	Not as selective as mass spectrometry. May require second analysis for high confidence in identification	Organic chemicals containing phosphorus or nitrogen which are nonpolar, volatile or semivolatile, and not thermally labile	Organophosphate pesticides
HPLC with UV and/or fluorescence	Simple, relatively inexpensive equipment. Good sensitivity for some compounds. Provides accurate quantitation	Selectivity is dependant on the structure of the analyte. Sensitivity varies. May require second analysis for confirmation. May require complex sample preparation including cleanup steps	Most organic chemicals	Mycotoxins, anticoagulant rodenticides, vitamins, ionophore antibiotics (with post column derivatization)
GC–MS	Mature technology. Excellent selectivity. Can be quite sensitive depending on the analysis. No confirmation analysis is usually required. Provides accurate quantitation. Nontargeted analysis is possible	Works poorly for polar, nonvolatile, and thermally labile compounds. Fairly expensive instruments. Data interpretation for nontargeted screening can be complex and time consuming	Organic chemicals which are fairly nonpolar, volatile or semivolatile, and not thermally labile	Strychnine, metaldehyde, various types of pesticides, alkaloids, some types of drugs, ethylene glycol (after derivatization), nontargeted GC–MS screens
LC–MS/MS	Extremely sensitive and selective. Useful for a very broad range of compounds. No confirmation analysis is usually required. Can provide accurate quantitation	Complex, very expensive equipment. Requires specialized training to use the instrumentation and to properly interpret data. Analysis must be targeted for specific analytes. Quantitative analysis is often complicated	Organic chemicals which are sufficiently acidic or basic to attract a proton or to lose one	Pesticides, alkaloids, anticoagulant rodenticides, algal toxins, mycotoxins, drugs of abuse, antibiotics, amanitin, cardiotoxic glycosides, metabolites of drugs and toxicants

METHOD DEVELOPMENT IN VETERINARY ANALYTICAL TOXICOLOGY

It is not uncommon for laboratories to get requests for analyses for which they have no analytical method in place. Depending on the nature of the situation (the number of animals involved, the potential for a problem in the human food supply, etc.), the laboratory may need to develop a new method. These development projects may be fairly simple, involving the addition of a new analyte into an existing method or replicating a method from the scientific literature. These projects may also be quite complex, involving multiple trials to optimize the extraction and analysis conditions and even collaborative method validation among multiple laboratories. Good communication between the laboratory and their client is essential for the laboratory personnel to understand the client's needs and for the client to understand the process the laboratory will have to follow to meet those needs. Issues involving costs, turnaround times, detection limit requirements, and quantitative precision should be determined prior to the initiation of the development process. Laboratory personnel must make an honest determination of their ability to meet the client's needs and of the resources, which will be required for the successful development of the method.

Some questions to consider prior to the start of a method development project:

- What are the analytes and the sample types?
- What amount of sample is available? Is there enough that the lab will be able to provide relevant results?
- How much time is available for method development?
- How many samples will ultimately be analyzed using the new method?
- Will there be specific turnaround time requirements for sample analysis once the method is in place?
- What are the required detection limits?
- Will the method need to provide quantitative data or strictly qualitative (detected/not detected) results
- What is the end-use of the data? Will it be used for regulatory actions, legal proceedings, research, or other uses?
- Are there other specific data quality requirements? (For instance, does the lab need to follow FDA method validation guidelines?)
- What is the cost estimate for the development process?
- Once the method is in place, what is the cost estimate for sample analysis?

The development process will establish several aspects of the method. These include availability of analytical standards, selectivity, sensitivity, and the detection/quantitation/reporting limits. It's important that needs and expectations for these method parameters are established and that there is frequent communication between the laboratory and the client as development proceeds. Even the most experienced toxicologist or chemist can't foresee all of the possible problems that may arise during the development of a new method.

Analytical Standards

Most analytical methods rely on the comparison between the analysis of a sample and the analysis of a chemical standard. One of the first questions that must be resolved prior to method development is whether a chemical standard is commercially available. The standard usually consists of the pure analyte, purchased from a supply house that provides documentation of the identity and purity of the compound. The standard is analyzed to determine method parameters, such as the chromatographic retention time or mass spectrum, and to document that the instrument is functioning properly for the analysis. For quantitative methods, a standard is used to determine the response of the detector to a specific amount of the chemical in order to measure the concentration in a sample. Standards are also "spiked" into control samples prior to analysis in order to provide quality control (QC) information. The availability of pure analytical standards is critical to the performance of most testing in a toxicology lab.

Another type of standard is known as a "standard reference material" or SRM. An SRM consists of a sample such as feed or tissue in which the analyte is known to be present. The SRM is analyzed by a number of different labs in order to establish a reference concentration of the analyte. Labs may then purchase the reference material and analyze it in order to demonstrate the accuracy of the analytical process. SRMs are mostly used in elemental analysis, as they are rarely available for the types of organic tests performed in veterinary toxicology.

Selectivity

Selectivity describes the ability of a technique to reliably differentiate an analyte from the many other chemical components in a sample. A technique with a high degree of selectivity will be less prone to false positive detections than a technique with a lower degree of selectivity. A high degree of selectivity in a method gives a high degree of confidence in the identification of analytes. A method with a relatively low level of selectivity may require a second confirmatory test in order to confidently report a result. Method development generally involves analysis of samples known to be free of the analyte in order to ensure that the method can discriminate the analyte from other constituents in the matrix.

Sensitivity

Sensitivity describes the ability of a technique to detect low levels of an analyte. This varies significantly between analytes, techniques, and sample types. The need for sensitivity also varies. For instance, for postmortem diagnosis of oleander poisoning, it is necessary to be able to detect oleandrin at low part-per-billion levels in liver tissue while it is only necessary to detect low part-per-million levels in stomach or rumen content.

Detection/Reporting/Quantitation Limits

The detection limit is the lowest concentration of an analyte that can be detected in a sample. It may also be termed the "limit of detection" or "method detection limit." The detection limit for a given compound in an analysis is usually determined when the method is developed or initially set up in the lab. In reality, the absolute lowest detectible concentration of an analyte will vary somewhat from day to day (because of differences in the condition of the instrument) and from sample to sample (because of variability in sample matrices and differences in technique between analysts). Still, the detection limit as originally established is a good indicator of the sensitivity of the method and its applicability to a diagnostic investigation.

The reporting limit is the lowest concentration of an analyte that the laboratory is confident that it can detect in a specific sample or set of samples. This is typically verified with each set of samples by analyzing a control sample with the analyte added to it at the reporting limit concentration. Detection of the analyte in the fortified control sample provides evidence that the reporting limit is valid. The reporting limit will usually be higher than the detection limit, which means that it is possible to detect concentrations of the analyte that are between the reporting limit and the detection limit. Laboratories have different ways of reporting analytes that fall into this concentration range, such as stating that a compound is detected at a "trace" level. Whatever terminology is used should be explained in the laboratory's report.

The quantitation limit is the lowest concentration of an analyte that can be accurately measured in a sample. This concentration will be higher than the detection limit, but it may be greater than or equal to the reporting limit. As with the reporting limit, laboratories may have different practices for reporting concentrations that fall between the detection limit and quantitation limit.

Precision and Accuracy

In a quantitative method (i.e., one that provides a measure of the concentration of the analyte in the sample rather than just presence or absence of the analyte) the method's levels of precision and accuracy should be established. Precision reflects the repeatability of the measurement while accuracy reflects how close the measured value is to a true value. There are a number of ways of determining these parameters that will vary depending on the client's needs and the end-use of the data. The requirements for precision and accuracy will also vary. For instance, analyses used for regulatory purposes, such as those that measure levels of antibiotics in milk, must be as precise and accurate as is possible due to the fact that a measured level of an antibiotic above the established tolerance level will likely cause a significant economic loss for the milk producer. Again, it is important to establish the precision and accuracy requirements prior to initiation of the development process.

QUALITY ASSURANCE AND QUALITY CONTROL IN THE VETERINARY TOXICOLOGY LAB

Quality assurance (QA) and QC procedures are essential in providing reliable analytical data. QA refers to a structured program that spells out the various policies and procedures used to ensure that the data produced by a lab meets predetermined standards for quality. QA programs include written documentation for different elements, such as personnel training, data review, client confidentiality, records review, and many others. QC refers to specific procedures applied to testing to ensure that the data produced by that test continually meet standards for accuracy, precision, and other parameters. QC in veterinary toxicology labs typically involves the analysis of controls included with each batch of samples analyzed by a given test. These may include analytical standards, standard reference materials, negative control samples, and positive control samples. The goal is to demonstrate that the analysis will not produce false positive or false negative results and that any quantitative measurements fall within acceptable ranges of precision and accuracy.

Veterinary toxicology labs are typically accredited by the American Association of Veterinary Laboratory Diagnosticians (AAVLD). The AAVLD has set standards for QA programs that labs must meet in order to receive accreditation. Prior to receiving accreditation, labs must submit documentation demonstrating that their QA program meets these standards. A site visit is also conducted by AAVLD auditors in order to ensure that the QA program is being followed by all laboratory personnel. Renewal of accreditation, with QA program review and a site visit by auditors, occurs on a periodic basis. Labs that fail to meet AAVLD standards on an ongoing basis are subject to loss of accreditation.

Accreditation provides a laboratory's clients with confidence that the data provided meets accepted standards and that it can be defended against challenges in court or in other forums. It is important to note, however, that no level of QA, QC, or accreditation can substitute for well-trained, experienced analysts. This is particularly true in veterinary analytical toxicology due to the wide range of analytes and matrices and the complexity of some analyses.

SAMPLE SUBMISSION REQUIREMENTS

One of the first considerations prior to sending samples to a toxicology lab for analysis is not the actual samples but the circumstances surrounding the possible poisoning. A detailed clinical history is highly valuable in determining which chemicals might be responsible for the incident and what samples will provide the most relevant information. Any available information from postmortem examination, histopathology findings, etc. can be very helpful as well. Laboratories typically require that clients complete a submission form that is to be sent in with the samples. All of the relevant information surrounding the suspected poisoning should be included on the submission form or attached to it. A discussion with the laboratory's toxicologist prior to sample submission will also help significantly in narrowing down the possible samples and tests needed for the diagnosis.

When submitting samples for toxicological analysis, it is essential to submit the appropriate sample type for the test. A serum sample that is appropriate for one analysis may not be useful for another. It is also important to submit the amount of sample that the laboratory needs to perform the test. A test that is typically run on 1 g of liver tissue may still be run on 0.1 g of tissue, but the reporting limit will likely increase by a factor of 10. If this raises the reporting limit to a level well above that which would be associated with toxicity, then the test may have little diagnostic relevance. Laboratories typically list submission requirements on their websites, making this an easy way to determine whether a sample is appropriate for testing. At times, it may not be possible to submit the amount the lab requests, for instance, when tissue is being taken from small birds or other small animals. In such cases, the laboratory's toxicologist should be consulted prior to submission in order to determine whether it's worth testing or not. (It should be noted that one of the more common frustrations for laboratory personnel involves receiving a very small amount of a sample from a very large animal, such as a cow or horse.) It's also important to note that toxicology testing generally requires fresh tissue rather than fixed tissue, although there are cases in which fixed tissue may be suitable. Consult with the laboratory if only fixed tissue is available for testing.

Sampling of Feed and Forage

Sampling from large amounts of feed, hay, or forage presents a difficult problem in ensuring that the sample taken is representative of the entire amount of feed, bale (or bales) of hay, or pasture of forage. The distribution of toxic plants or chemicals may be very uneven. For instance, sampling for mycotoxins in grain and feed is notoriously difficult due to the potential for "hot spots" with very high concentrations of mycotoxins in otherwise uncontaminated grain. A number of subsamples should be taken from the pasture, stack, or bale and combined in order to provide the best possible representative sample. If sampling wet hay for nitrate, bear in mind that the nitrate is water-soluble and will migrate down through the hay with the water. The highest levels of nitrate are likely to be found at the water line. This part of the hay should be sampled and frozen prior to shipment. Other parts of the bale or stack should also be sampled (Arnold, 2012).

Sample Shipment

In the United States, packaging and shipping of diagnostic specimens is subject to federal government regulations published in the Code of Federal Regulations (CFR) Part 49, sections 100–185. These regulations are available on the Internet at http://www.ecfr.gov (accessed 17.02.17) and there are numerous other internet resources providing information on meeting them. It's important to note that the shipper (and not the transport company!) is responsible for the condition of the package until it reaches its destination. There are fines and other penalties that may be assessed for violation of these regulations, so it's important that samples are packaged correctly prior to shipment.

Apart from the shipping regulations, all samples must be packaged carefully in order to ensure that they remain intact during transit. Lids for blood and serum tubes must be secured. Other liquid samples should be shipped in screw cap tubes or vials with the lids secured with parafilm or tape. Tissue samples, feces, rumen content, pesticide bait, or similar samples should be carefully wrapped in aluminum foil and then placed in a sealable plastic bag. Handle each sample individually, taking care to avoid any potential for cross-contamination. Use a waterproof, permanent marker to label sample containers. These primary containers should be packed into a watertight secondary container with enough absorbent material to contain the entire contents of the package. The secondary container should, in turn, be placed inside of an outer container of sufficient strength to prevent damage during shipping.

REFERENCES

Anastassiades, M., Lehotay, S.J., Stajnbaher, D., Schenck, F.J., 2003. Fast and easy multiresidue method employing acetonitrile extraction/partitioning and "dispersive solid phase extraction" for the determination of pesticide residues in produce. J. AOAC Int. 86 (2), 412–431.

Arnold, B.S., 2012. Sample submission for toxicological analysis. In: Gupta, R. (Ed.), Veterinary Toxicology, Basic and Clinical Principles, second ed. Academic Press, London

Brazelton, W.E., Johnson, M., 2003. Thin layer chromatography convulsant screen extended by gas chromatography-mass spectrometry. J. Vet. Lab. Invest. 15 (1), 42–45.

Ellman, G.L., Courtney, D.K., Andres, V., Featherstone, R.M., 1961. A new and rapid colorimetric determination of acetylcholinesterase activity. Biochem. Pharmacol. 7, 88–95.

Jain, A.V., Ross, P.F., Carlson, M.P., 1999. Screening nitrate in forages with a strip test. Collaborative study. J. AOAC Int. 82 (1), 1–7.

Section XVIII

Prevention and Treatment

Chapter 82

Prevention and Treatment of Poisoning

Camille DeClementi

PREVENTION OF POISONING

Prevention of poisoning in household pets consists of controlling the animals' environment to decrease exposure to potentially dangerous substances. This requires animal caretakers to be diligent and knowledgeable of potential risks. While much of the advice offered to prevent poisoning will seem like common sense to many veterinarians, these guidelines are often unfamiliar to animal caretakers. Veterinarians are therefore encouraged to share this information with their clients.

Clients should be reminded to keep all veterinary and human medications, both prescription and over-the-counter (OTC), out of the reach of animals. Since some pets are able to climb onto high surfaces and open cabinets, medications are not adequately "out of reach" in those places. Owners should be instructed not to give their pets any medication, including their own, unless directed by their veterinarian. Clients may not realize that giving an OTC medication that they consider safe, like acetaminophen, could cause a life-threatening illness in their pet. Just one 500 mg acetaminophen tablet could cause life-threatening methemoglobinemia is an average-sized cat. Another example is the treatment of alopecia in cats with topical minoxidil solution. This has led to pleural effusion, pulmonary edema, and death (DeClementi et al., 2004). Clients should also store all other potentially hazardous products, including cleaning products, auto-care products, pesticides, and insecticides, out of the reach of their animals. Garbage cans should be sealed with tamper-proof lids.

Animal caretakers should be urged to read all label information before using a product on an animal or in the animal's environment and to follow the label instructions exactly. Veterinarians should mention that it is often not safe to use a product on an animal species for which it is not intended. For example, using a concentrated permethrin flea product labeled for dogs could prove deadly if used on a cat (Richardson, 2000a).

Since many plants are poisonous, clients will want to be aware of the plants in an animal's environment, including those in outside areas. Additionally, they should be alert to any fluids leaking from vehicles and clean up leaks immediately. If a rodenticide or other bait is necessary in the home or yard, the product should be placed in an area that is completely inaccessible to nontarget animals. The bait should be removed as soon as it is no longer needed. An animal's enclosure should be routinely checked, and unfamiliar or questionable items removed. Companion animals should be supervised, when possible, if they are outdoors, and a securely gated, confined area should be provided when animals are left unattended.

The guidelines for keeping household pets safe from poisoning are very similar to those for children, especially toddlers. Some pets may even be more at risk than children because, unlike children, they are commonly left unattended. They are also likely to chew open some containers, including those considered child-safe. The ASPCA website has additional information regarding poison prevention (http://www.aspca.org/pet-care/animal-poison-control).

Decreasing the risk of exposure to toxicants is also important in large animals. Caretakers should be urged to purchase hay and feed from reputable suppliers to examine the feed for recognizable contamination and to verify cleanliness and high quality. Feed should be stored in a clean, insect-free area at the appropriate moisture level to prevent damage and lessen the risk of contamination or mycotoxin growth (Osweiler, 2001).

Learning to identify poisonous plants and their potential effects is critical for large animal clients. Once poisonous plants have been recognized in an area, many strategies can be employed to limit exposure. The most effective strategy is to remove animals from poisonous plant-infested areas either by herding or fencing off those areas. If this is impossible, attempts should be made to reduce the poisonous plant populations via mechanical (burning or pulling), chemical (herbicides), biological

Veterinary Toxicology. DOI: http://dx.doi.org/10.1016/B978-0-12-811410-0.00082-9

(such as using the larvae of the cinnabar moth to control tansy ragwort), or other control methods. Since treatment with herbicides may increase palatability or toxicity in some plants, animals should not be allowed access to herbicide-treated areas until all treated plant material is dead and removed. Once the plant populations are controlled, good grazing management can be used to maintain the area in a condition that limits regrowth of the plants (Cheeke, 1998).

Large animal enclosures and barns should also be kept free of other potential toxicants, including insecticides, pesticides, petroleum products, and medicated feeds. Following label instructions is just as important for large animals as household pets. Medicated feeds, medications, and insecticides should be used only on the labeled species. If a pour-on amitraz product intended for cattle is instead used on horses, fatal ileus may result (Gwaltney-Brant, 2004).

STABILIZATION AND MONITORING

Toxicant exposures often require immediate or urgent attention. Television and movies have led the public to believe that every toxicant has an antidote; consequently animal caretakers may expect their veterinarian to provide one. Unfortunately, this expectation is far from reality. There are very few antidotes and when they do exist, they may be cost prohibitive or difficult to obtain. Therefore, it is critical for the clinician to concentrate on treating the patient and not the poison. Poisoning cases should be managed following the same principles of triage and patient stabilization as other emergencies. Decontamination and antidote administration, if available, should follow initial stabilization.

A detailed history should be taken after the patient is stabilized, but the following questions should be asked on presentation. To what toxicant was the animal exposed? What amount? When did the exposure occur? Has the patient shown any effects? Have any treatments been performed (e.g., dilution, emesis or bathing)? Have other animals also been exposed?

As in any emergency case, initial evaluation and stabilization of the patient should address the basic ABCs (airway, breathing, bleeding, cardiovascular, circulation and level of consciousness). The clinician must assure that the patient has an adequate airway and is not having difficulty breathing. If needed, an endotracheal tube should be placed or a tracheostomy performed to establish a patent airway. If the patient is dyspneic, 100% oxygen should be delivered via oxygen cage, mask or nasal cannula (Mathews, 2006). Oxygen supplementation is contraindicated in a paraquat exposure (Oehme and Mannala, 2006). Stress and handling should be minimized in a dyspneic patient.

The patient should be checked for bruising and for signs of active bleeding from the nose, mouth, anus and vulva or penis. The mucous membrane color and capillary refill time should be evaluated. Pulse rate, rhythm, and strength should be assessed. Electrocardiogram (ECG) and blood pressure monitoring should also be performed. If needed, an intravenous (IV) catheter should be placed and fluid therapy initiated. Attempts should be made to control life-threatening arrhythmias (Mathews, 2006).

The patient's level of consciousness should be determined. If the patient is actively seizing, diazepam, given as an IV bolus at a dosage of 0.5–1 mg/kg, is often the initial drug used for dogs and cats (Plumb, 2015). If this is not effective, other medications including phenobarbital, pentobarbital, and propofol may be useful. Inhalant anesthesia may also be used to control the seizure activity (Mathews, 2006). The reader is referred to a formulary or reference on emergency seizure control for recommendations on doses and drug choices for the species being treated. Since some diagnostic tests, including that for ethylene glycol, may give false results once injectable medications are administered, the clinician should obtain blood samples prior to administering these medications. Body temperature should be checked and thermoregulation initiated if needed.

Once the patient has been stabilized, a more thorough clinical evaluation can be completed including complete history, physical examination and appropriate diagnostic testing (Cantilena, 2001), and a treatment plan developed. The signalment and health history of the patient is important in developing a treatment plan. If the patient is a nursing or pregnant female, e.g., precautions will need to be taken to prevent exposure to the fetus or young. Or if the patient is taking a highly protein-bound medication, it is more at risk from an overdose of another protein-bound drug. If there is no known exposure to a toxicant but poisoning is suspected based on presentation and clinical findings, the questions in Table 82.1 may be helpful to reveal a cause.

Next, a complete treatment plan should be developed. It should include what method, if any, will be used to prevent further toxin absorption and if an antidotal therapy will be used. The plan should address any clinical signs not addressed in the initial stabilization. It should list what additional findings may yet develop and a plan of action for each. The plan should define how often the patient will be monitored and what indices will be evaluated. And it should determine what diagnostic tests are appropriate for the situation. The treatment plan may need to be updated as the case progresses.

Diagnostic testing will be governed by clinical findings, history and, in a known exposure, expected effects. The clinician should perform baseline testing and repeat as required throughout the course of the treatment.

TABLE 82.1 History Gathering Questions

- When was the patient last normal?
- How long have the signs been present?
- Were there any initial signs that are no longer present?
- Was the onset of the signs gradual or sudden?
- Are there other pets in the area? Are they affected?
- What was the location of the animal in the last few hours prior to development of signs? Was the animal supervised?
- Is the animal indoors or outdoors mostly?
- If the animal is outdoors, is it confined or does it roam?
- To what areas of the home or garage does the animal have access?
- Have any new foods or treats been introduced to the animal's diet?
- Any access to sugar-free products?
- Has there been any recent access to garbage?
- Has the animal chewed or destroyed anything recently?
- Are there any medications in the house (human, veterinary, prescription, OTC)?
- Could the animal have been exposed to illicit drugs?
- Are there children or teenagers in the household?
- Have there been any recent visitors who may have dropped medication?
- Are there any rodenticides or other baits being used in the home or yard?
- Could the animal have ingested any plants (indoors or outdoors)?
- Have any medications, herbal products or insecticides been administered to this or any other animals in the household recently?
- Are there any mushrooms growing in the yard?
- Is there a compost pile in the yard?
- Have any yard treatments been applied recently?
- Are there any livestock in the animal's environment?
- Have any livestock been recently euthanized or buried on the property?

Appropriate testing may include a packed cell volume and total solids to identify dehydration or blood loss in cases of anticoagulant exposure or agents that may cause gastrointestinal (GI) ulceration. A complete blood count (CBC) may be needed to check for inflammation or secondary infections in cases where GI ulceration and perforation are possible, such as in exposures to cationic detergents, corrosive materials or nonsteroidal antiinflammatory drugs (NSAIDs). Monitoring the CBC is also indicated in exposures that may cause bone marrow suppression such as estrogen overdoses.

A full chemistry panel is often appropriate. Blood glucose should be monitored closely with exposures to sulfonylurea hypoglycemic agents and in exposures to the sugar-free sweetener xylitol in dogs. Monitoring the renal values, blood urea nitrogen and serum creatinine is important in many exposures to identify dehydration and renal alterations if the patient was exposed to potential renal toxicants, such as lilies in cats, grapes and raisins in dogs, NSAIDs and ethylene glycol. In these cases, urinalysis is also indicated. Electrolytes should be monitored in cases where IV fluid therapy is required and in cases where the toxicant may lead to electrolyte abnormalities. For example, hypokalemia is a common effect in dogs that puncture albuterol inhalers (Vite and Gfeller, 1994).

Monitoring of acid–base status is important in some cases, such as exposures to aspirin and ethylene glycol. The cardiovascular system will need to be monitored, via ECG and evaluating blood pressure in exposures to certain agents, such as pseudoephedrine and the methylxanthines in chocolate. Other general testing including pulse oximetry, radiographs, and ultrasound may be required depending on the toxicant. Specific tests, such as an ethylene glycol test or serum iron panel, may also be suitable depending on the situation.

In addition to these physiological parameters, the patient's clinical signs, vitals, behavior, and mentation should be monitored frequently for the duration of the treatment and abnormalities addressed. The frequency and degree of monitoring will depend on the situation. The patient's attitude should be noted regularly. Respiratory and cardiovascular status should also be checked at regular intervals, especially in cases where these systems may be affected by the toxicant. Capillary refill time and mucous membrane color can be used to assess peripheral perfusion. Body temperature should be monitored if the toxicant, clinical findings, or treatments may cause abnormalities. Appetite, hydration status, bowel movements, and urinary output should also be noted.

DECONTAMINATION

Once the patient has been stabilized, decontamination should be considered to prevent additional exposure to the toxicant. Although the basics of decontamination are similar among species, the specific method of decontamination that is chosen in each case must be guided by the exposure circumstances and the species exposed. For all decontamination methods, consider sedation or anesthesia if the procedure will be very stressful for the patient, but only if the health of the patient will allow. The handler should wear appropriate protective clothing including gloves, and mask and eye gear to prevent personal exposure. Most exposures to toxicants can be broken down into ocular, dermal, and oral exposures. The following are methods of decontamination for each of these exposure types.

Ocular Exposure

Ocular exposures may cause effects ranging from mild irritation to corrosive injury and blindness depending on the substance, the concentration, the exposure time, and the sensitivity of the patient. With any ocular exposure, the eyes should be flushed repeatedly with tepid tap water or saline solution for a minimum of 20–30 min (Rosendale, 2002). An eyedropper can be used for smaller patients like birds or reptiles. With a larger patient, fill a plastic cup and slowly pour the contents over the ocular area. Patients can be given a mild sedative prior to flushing if needed and if the health of the patient will allow. If not sedated, the patient should be allowed to rest at regular intervals during the flushing to minimize stress. Fluorescein staining should be performed after flushing and again at 12–24 h postexposure to check for corneal ulceration. Additional treatment with ophthalmic and systemic medications may be necessary.

Dermal Exposure

Dermal exposure to a large variety of substances, including petroleum products, pesticides, and insecticides, corrosive or irritating materials and substances that are sticky (tar, asphalt, sap, and glue), may occur. Removal of such substances may be less stressful for the patient and safer for the handler if sedation is used. Sedatives should only be used if the health of the patient will allow. If not sedated, the patient should be allowed to rest at regular intervals to minimize stress.

In birds, dermal substances can be removed by using a water bottle to spritz the bird lightly with room temperature water. This procedure should be done in a warm environment to prevent chilling. The bird should be misted until the feathers no longer smell or feel of the product. If misting alone does not remove the product, and soap is needed, a liquid dishwashing detergent (e.g., Dawn) may be diluted in the bottle and applied. After removal of the substance, the bird should be rinsed via misting with plain water until all soap is removed. In cases of heavy exposure, birds may be bathed with liquid dishwashing detergent and rinsed well. After misting or bathing, the bird should be wiped with a dry towel and kept in a warm environment away from drafts until completely dry. The procedure for reptiles is similar.

For dermal exposures in mammals, bathing in a mild liquid dishwashing detergent and warm water is recommended. Baths may be repeated in order to remove the toxicant completely (Rosendale, 2002). The animal should then be rinsed well with warm water and towel dried, then kept in a warm environment until completely dry. For smaller patients, like cats, that resent being sprayed with water, the bucket technique may be helpful. Fill a bucket with warm soapy water and, while supporting the hind legs, immerse the patient up to the neck. Remove the patient and continue washing. Use a fresh bucket with plain warm water to rinse well.

If the patient has a sticky substance on its fur, feathers or skin, do not use solvents to remove it since these may be irritating or corrosive to the patient. Instead, to remove sticky substances from mammals, remove as much of the substance as possible by trimming the fur. Then work a small amount of vegetable oil, mineral oil, mayonnaise or peanut butter through the rest of the substance until it breaks down into "gummy balls." Afterward, wash with liquid dishwashing detergent as described above (Rosendale, 2002). For birds, do not trim the feathers, just use vegetable oil, mineral oil, mayonnaise or peanut butter and then mist as described above.

Oral Exposure

When a patient is exposed to a potentially dangerous substance by ingestion, the clinician has many options for decontamination including dilution, induction of emesis, lavage, removal via endoscopy or gastrostomy, use of adsorbents, cathartics and administration of enemas. Often, the best treatment plan will include more than one of these methods.

Dilution

Dilution with a small amount of milk or water is recommended in cases where irritants or corrosive materials have been ingested. A suggested dose is 2–6 mL/kg (Mathews, 2006), which would be approximately only one to two teaspoons in an average-sized cat. It is important to use only a small amount of liquid for dilution. Using excessive amounts could lead to vomiting and reexposure of the esophagus to the damaging material. For birds and reptiles, juicy fruits, and vegetables can be fed to accomplish dilution. Dilution is not recommended in patients who are at an increased risk for aspiration, including those who are obtunded (Rosendale, 2002) or actively seizing. Additionally, milk, yogurt and cottage cheese have been useful as demulcents in cases of oral irritation following ingestion of plants containing insoluble calcium oxalate crystals (*Philodendron* species, for example) (Means, 2004b).

Emetics

Emetics are usually most effective if used within 2–3 h postingestion (Rosendale, 2002) but in some instances emesis may be effective even after that time frame. For instance, if a timed-released medication was ingested or if the substance ingested could coalesce to form a bezoar in the stomach, emesis may be effective later than 3 h after the ingestion. Chocolate (Albretsen, 2004) and chewable medications may form bezoars. If the patient has not eaten in the previous 2 h, feeding a small moist meal before inducing vomiting can increase chances of an adequate emesis. Emetics generally empty 40%–60% of the stomach contents (Beasley and Dorman, 1990).

Dogs, cats, ferrets, and potbelly pigs are examples of domestic animals that are able to vomit safely. Emetics should not be used in rodents, rabbits, birds, horses and ruminants. Rodents are unable to vomit (Plumb, 2015) and rabbits have a thin-walled stomach putting them at risk for gastric rupture if they vomit (Donnelly, 2004). It is not safe to induce emesis in birds, horses or cattle.

Induction of emesis is contraindicated with ingestion of alkalis, acids or other corrosive agents. When one of these products is swallowed, the protective epithelial lining of the esophagus may be damaged. This damage can leave the muscular layer of the esophagus exposed and at risk for ulceration, perforation and scarring if vomiting does occur (Beasley and Dorman, 1990). Emesis is not recommended after ingestion of petroleum distillates due to the risk of aspiration. Preexisting conditions of the patient that can cause vomiting to be hazardous, such as severe cardiac disease or seizure disorder, must also be taken into account by the clinician when deciding whether to induce emesis. In all instances, the attending veterinarian must weigh the benefits of emesis against the risks. Emesis should not be attempted if the animal has already vomited or is exhibiting clinical signs, such as coma, seizures or recumbency, which make emesis hazardous. Additionally, if the patient has ingested a central nervous system (CNS) stimulant and is already agitated, the additional stimulation of vomiting could elicit seizures (Rosendale, 2002).

Hydrogen peroxide, apomorphine hydrochloride, and xylazine hydrochloride are commonly used emetics in the veterinary clinical setting. Data obtained from the ASPCA Animal Poison Control's toxicology database indicate that hydrogen peroxide and apomorphine are effective emetics in dogs. Emesis was successful in 92% of dogs when administered either 3% hydrogen peroxide or apomorphine. No significant adverse effects were reported in dogs after emetic use. Apomorphine was poorly effective as an emetic in cats. Xylazine was an effective emetic in 57% of cats. When emesis was successfully induced, 68% of patients vomited some portion of the ingested toxicant (Khan et al., 2009).

Hydrogen peroxide, at a 3% concentration, is a useful emetic when given orally. It is an ideal emetic for household use because the 3% concentration is used in many households for cuts and scrapes. Additionally, it is inexpensive and easy to administer. Hydrogen peroxide is thought to induce emesis via gastric irritation (Peterson, 2006). The dosage is 1–2 mL/kg (Beasley and Dorman, 1990) generally not to exceed 50 mL for dogs and potbelly pigs and 10 mL for cats and ferrets (Peterson, 2006). The dose can be administered with a syringe or turkey baster or can be mixed with a small amount of milk or ice cream to entice voluntary ingestion. Vomiting usually occurs within 10–15 min and the dose can be repeated once more if emesis is not initially successful. Walking or other gentle movement may be beneficial in initiating emesis.

Apomorphine hydrochloride is often used in the clinical setting to induce emesis in dogs. Use of apomorphine is considered controversial in cats (Plumb, 2015) and it is not very effective (Khan et al., 2009). Apomorphine hydrochloride is a synthetic opiate that stimulates the dopamine receptors in the chemoreceptor trigger zone to cause emesis. The dosage is 0.03 mg/kg, IV or 0.04 mg/kg, IM. Emesis is expected rapidly following IV administration, but may take 5 min with IM administration. Apomorphine can also be used conjunctivally by crushing and dissolving a portion of a tablet in a few drops of water. The solution is then administered into the conjunctival sac (Plumb, 2015). This route may be preferred since the eye can be rinsed after emesis has occurred to prevent additional systemic absorption and decrease the likelihood of adverse events. At doses used to induce emesis, adverse effects may include CNS depression and protracted vomiting. CNS stimulation and respiratory and cardiac depression may be seen with excessive doses (Plumb, 2015). The opiate antagonist naloxone can be used to reverse the CNS and respiratory effects, but will not block the emetic effect (Rosendale, 2002).

Xylazine hydrochloride is a potent α_2-adrenergic agonist used in the veterinary clinic setting primarily as a sedative. It has also been used, with some success, as an emetic in cats. Xylazine does not produce predictable emesis in dogs (Beasley and Dorman, 1990; Khan et al., 2009; Plumb, 2015). The recommended emetic dose in cats is 0.44 mg/kg IM. This is lower than the dose used for sedation in cats. Emesis is expected within 5 min of administration. Possible adverse effects include CNS and respiratory depression, hypotension, and bradycardia. These effects, as well as the emetic effects (Beasley and Dorman, 1990), can be reversed by giving an α_2-adrenergic antagonist, either yohimbine at a dosage of 0.1 mg/kg IV or atipamezole at a dosage of 25–50 μg/kg IM or slow IV (Plumb, 2015).

Lavage

Lavage is sometimes used in cases where emesis is contraindicated, not possible or has been unsuccessful. If the patient is agitated, seizing or recumbent or has other health concerns, such as recent abdominal surgery, that increase the risks associated with induction of emesis, lavage is an option. Lavage should also be considered in species, like rabbits and rodents, which are unable to vomit safely. Lavage is unlikely to remove as much ingested toxicant as emesis (Beasley and Dorman, 1990) and is associated with significant potential risks. For these reasons, it should not be chosen haphazardly as a decontamination method over emesis. Lavage should also not be used to remove caustic substances or volatile hydrocarbons for the same reasons emesis is contraindicated in such cases (Rosendale, 2002).

Gastric lavage can be used in mammals to remove recently ingested toxicants. If the patient is a species with cheek pouches, the cheek pouches should be emptied gently with a finger or swab prior to the lavage. In all instances, a cuffed endotracheal tube should be in place to prevent aspiration; therefore, general anesthesia must be performed unless the patient is comatose. Body temperature water (5–10 mL/kg) should be instilled via a large bore gastric tube with a fenestrated end, inserted to a length equal to the distance from the nose to the xiphoid cartilage (Beasley and Dorman, 1990). The head of the patient should be kept lower than the chest throughout the procedure. Gravity should be used to instill the water by holding the tube higher than the patient and then drained by moving the tube lower than the patient. The flushing process should be repeated multiple times (15–40) until the lavage fluid runs clear. With each flush, approximately the same amount of fluid instilled should be removed. The free end of the tube should be occluded before removal to prevent aspiration (Rosendale, 2002). The initial washings should be saved for toxicological testing if needed (Peterson, 2006).

In humans, hypernatremia following lavage with normal saline and hyponatremia following lavage with water have been reported. Additionally, one human study showed that as much as 25% of the fluid used for lavage passed into the small intestine. Thus, there is a concern that lavage may actually propel a toxicant into the small intestine where the absorptive surface area is greater. These risks should be limited by allowing the entire amount of fluid to drain out after each flush and by using only gravity to instill the water. Other risks associated with gastric lavage include esophageal or stomach damage or perforation, hypothermia and the accidental placement of the tube in the trachea and the instillation of fluid into the lungs (Rosendale, 2002).

A lavage technique can also be used in birds to remove recently ingested toxicants from the crop. To prevent injury to the patient and handlers, anxious and fractious birds should be anesthetized prior to the procedure. If the patient is under general anesthesia, an endotracheal tube should be placed to protect the airway (Richardson et al., 2001). The patient should be held with the head up and the mouth held open. The bird's head and neck should be extended to minimize esophageal damage. An appropriately sized feeding tube (soft plastic or rubber) is then passed into the crop. The crop should be palpated to assure correct placement. Then 10–20 mL/kg of warm saline is infused into the crop, the crop is massaged gently and the liquid is aspirated. The first washing can be kept for toxicological evaluation if needed. The cycle is repeated three or four times (Echols, 2005).

Adsorbents

Adsorbents may be utilized in addition to, or instead of emesis or lavage, to prevent further systemic absorption of a toxicant. These agents act by adsorbing to a chemical or toxicant in the upper gastrointestinal tract (GIT) and facilitating its excretion via the feces. The most commonly used adsorbent is activated charcoal. In the past, kaolin–pectin (Kaopectate) had also been recommended as an adsorbent and demulcent in some instances. However, Kaopectate, and most generic kaolin–pectin combinations, now contain bismuth subsalicylate as the active ingredient instead of kaolin and pectin. Some commercial-activated charcoal products also contain kaolin (Vet-A-Mix, Toxiban).

Activated charcoal is composed of large porous particles that are able to adsorb and therefore trap a wide range of organic compounds within the GIT. The surface binding area of these products is quite large, in the range of 900–1500 m^2/g (Rosendale, 2002). Charcoal tablets and capsules, found in pharmacies and used to control flatulence and bloating, are not likely to be as effective as the commercially prepared products (Buck and Bratich, 1986), as the concentration of the charcoal is often low and may have a smaller binding area.

The recommended dose of activated charcoal for all species of animals is 1–3 g/kg (or 1–3 mg/g) body weight (Buck and Bratich, 1986). There are many products on the market, including both liquid and powder forms. If using the powder formulation in dogs and cats, the total calculated dose of activated charcoal is mixed with 50–200 mL of warm tap water to make a slurry (Rosendale, 2002). In horses and ruminants, each gram of activated charcoal powder is mixed with 5 mL of water (Plumb, 2015). In symptomatic small animal patients and large animals, the activated charcoal liquid or prepared slurry is administered via stomach tube (Bailey and Garland, 1992). Small animals receiving activated charcoal via stomach tube should be sedated and have a cuffed endotracheal tube in place to prevent aspiration. In small animal patients where no clinical effects are present, activated charcoal can be given orally with a large syringe or can be mixed with a small amount of canned food or chicken broth and offered to the patient (Rosendale, 2002). Some patients, especially dogs, will voluntarily ingest the mixture. Many birds will regurgitate a portion of the activated charcoal dose given, and some dogs and cats will vomit after administration.

Repeated doses of activated charcoal may be indicated in some instances, such as cases where toxicants undergo enterohepatic recirculation. The first step in this process involves the toxicant being carried to the liver by either the portal vein after absorption from the GIT or via the systemic circulation. Once in the liver, the toxicant then enters the bile and is excreted into the GIT where it is again available for absorption. Many toxicants are known to undergo this type of recycling, including ibuprofen, marijuana and digoxin.

When repeated doses are indicated, half the original dose should be given at 4–8 h intervals, often for 2–3 days (Peterson, 2006). It is important to mention that with medications that are excreted in the bile, activated charcoal can be of benefit regardless of the route the medication was administered. Thus, if a patient received an overdose of injectable ivermectin subcutaneously, activated charcoal will still be a very valuable decontamination option. The ivermectin molecules will be carried to the GIT by the bile.

The use of activated charcoal does carry some risks and it does not bind all compounds equally. Some chemicals that are not effectively adsorbed include: ethanol, methanol, fertilizer, fluoride, petroleum distillates, most heavy metals, iodides, nitrates, nitrites, sodium chloride and chlorate. Activated charcoal should not be given to animals that have ingested caustic materials since it is unlikely to bind them, it can be additionally irritating to the mucosal surfaces and make visualization of oral and esophageal burns difficult (Buck and Bratich, 1986). If ethylene glycol testing will be performed, activated charcoal should be administered after blood is collected, since propylene glycol found in many formulations can cause a false positive on some of these tests. Additionally, the timing of the activated charcoal administration should be taken into account when deciding on dosing of other oral medications since the charcoal can also bind them.

Administration of activated charcoal carries a significant risk of aspiration. If the patient does aspirate the charcoal, the prognosis is poor. Hence proper placement of the stomach tube and a protected airway is a must in symptomatic patients. The patient may also experience constipation and black bowel movements, making it difficult to determine if melena is present. If the activated charcoal sits within the GIT for a significant period of time, it may release the compound it has adsorbed, leading to systemic absorption and recurrence of the clinical signs. It is for this reason that activated charcoal is frequently administered with a cathartic. In fact, many commercially available preparations do contain a cathartic, such as sorbitol.

Another possible adverse effect of activated charcoal administration is the development of hypernatremia. In humans, hypernatremia has been reported primarily in children when multiple doses of a charcoal–sorbitol mixture were administered. The hypernatremia is attributed to a water shift from the intracellular and extracellular spaces into the GIT as a result of the osmotic pull of the sorbitol cathartic (Allerton and Strom, 1991). The ASPCA Animal Poison Control Center (APCC) has also received reports of elevated serum sodium following activated charcoal administration in dogs. Hypernatremia seems to be more often reported in small dogs receiving multiple doses of activated charcoal, but it has also been reported in large dogs and in cases receiving only a single dose. Furthermore, unlike the human reports, hypernatremia has also been noted in cases where no cathartic was present in the charcoal product given (Ball, 2014). Perhaps one of the other components of the product is also osmotically active. In these cases, the APCC has found that administration of a warm water enema is very effective at lowering the serum sodium and easing the resultant central nervous system effects (Ball, 2014).

Cathartics

Cathartics enhance elimination of substances, including activated charcoal, by promoting their movement through the GIT. Since activated charcoal only binds to toxicants by weak chemical forces, without cathartics, the bound toxicant can eventually be released and reabsorbed (Rosendale, 2002). When used with activated charcoal, the cathartic should be given immediately following or mixed with the charcoal. Cathartics are contraindicated if the animal has diarrhea, is dehydrated, if ileus is present, or if intestinal obstruction or perforation are possible (Peterson, 2006).

There are bulk, osmotic, and lubricant cathartics. The most commonly used bulk cathartic is psyllium hydrophilic mucilloid (e.g., Metamucil). Psyllium is found in the ripe seed coatings of *Plantago* species. It absorbs water and swells in the intestine increasing bulk to induce peristalsis and decrease gastrointestinal transit time. The dose in dogs is 0.32–4.9 g/kg/day, and the dose in cats is one to four teaspoons per meal (Plumb, 2015). Psyllium can also be used in birds by mixing one-half teaspoon with 60 mL of baby food to form a gruel, then administering by a dosing syringe or eyedropper (Richardson et al., 2001).

Another bulking cathartic that can be used in dogs and cats is unspiced canned pumpkin. Dilute peanut butter, fruit, or vegetables can also be used as bulking cathartic agents in birds and reptiles. Timothy hay can be utilized in rabbits. Bulking cathartics are also used to assist the passage of physical agents through the GIT (Beasley and Dorman, 1990). Examples include small pieces of plastic, coins, button batteries, and sand in horses.

Osmotic cathartics have limited absorption from the GIT so they are able to pull electrolyte-free water into the GIT, thereby increasing the fluid volume and stimulating motility to hasten expulsion in the feces. There are saline and saccharide osmotic cathartics. Sorbitol is the most commonly used saccharide osmotic cathartic; it is the cathartic of choice and is frequently combined with activated charcoal in commercially prepared charcoal products. The dose is 1–2 mL/kg of a 70% solution (Peterson, 2006). Sorbitol can be utilized in mammals, birds, and reptiles.

The saline cathartics include sodium sulfate (Glauber's salts) and magnesium sulfate (Epsom salts). The recommended dose is 250 mg/kg. The use of magnesium sulfate has led to hypermagnesemia in some cases, which presents as depression of the central nervous and cardiovascular systems (Rosendale, 2002). Saline cathartics should not be used in patients with renal insufficiency or in birds or reptiles.

Of the lubricant cathartics, mineral oil is the most often used. Heavy mineral oil is preferred to light mineral oil since it is thought to carry less of a chance of systemic absorption and aspiration following oral administration. Mineral oil lubricates fecal material and the intestinal mucosa easing elimination and reduces absorption of water from the GIT, increasing fecal bulk and cutting transit time (Plumb, 2015). Mineral oil is not recommended as a cathartic following activated charcoal administration, as the mineral oil may render the charcoal less adsorptive (Buck and Bratich, 1986; Galey, 1992). Mineral oil has been recommended to bind lipid-soluble toxicants including metaldehyde, nitrate, and cantharidin (Stair and Plumlee, 2004; Plumb, 2015), and it is used to treat impaction in horses (Buck and Bratich, 1986). The recommended dose in horses is 2–4 L per 500 kg body weight (Brown and Bertone, 2001). Possible adverse effects include diarrhea and aspiration of the oil leading to lipid pneumonitis. Ensuring proper placement of the stomach tube and slow administration lessen the risk of aspiration (Plumb, 2015).

As mentioned earlier, hypernatremia attributed to sorbitol administration has been reported in humans. Because all cathartics alter the water balance in the GIT, electrolyte abnormalities, especially hypernatremia, are a potential risk to their use. A patient's hydration status should be monitored frequently and fluids administered, intravenously or via an enema, as needed.

Enemas

Enemas are also appropriate when elimination of toxicants from the lower GIT is desired (Beasley and Dorman, 1990). Many extended-release or controlled-release medications are absorbed from the entire GIT, including significant absorption from the colon (Buckley et al., 1995). Enemas can be used to move those medications quickly through the colon and lessen additional systemic effects. The general technique is to use plain warm water or warm soapy water. Commercial phosphate enema solutions should be avoided due to the risk of electrolyte and acid–base disturbances (Beasley and Dorman, 1990). Enemas are not recommended for birds since they already have a rapid gastrointestinal transit time. In reptiles, enemas may be useful since ingested materials often lag for prolonged periods in the colon.

Endoscopy/Gastrostomy

In some cases, endoscopy or gastrostomy may be indicated to prevent further clinical effects. Endoscopy can be used to remove small objects, such as pennies, lead paint chips and small batteries. These objects can also be removed via gastrostomy if endoscopy is not available. Gastrostomy is also used to prevent obstruction from expanding foreign objects. Expandable isocyanate-containing glues (i.e., Gorilla Glue) can swell once ingested to fill the entire volume of the stomach. A gastrostomy is needed in these cases to remove the mass (Horstman et al., 2003).

ANTIDOTAL THERAPIES

If an antidote to the toxicant a patient has been exposed to exists, the appropriate time to administer it will depend on the situation. In some instances, the antidote will be crucial in stabilizing the patient. For example, atropine should be used immediately in cases of organophosphate (OP) toxicosis in which the patient has life-threatening bradycardia and bronchial secretions (Gwaltney-Brant and Rumbeiha, 2002). On the other hand, in some cases, administration of the antidote is best done later. This is true for vitamin K_1 being used in anticoagulant rodenticide exposures. In a recent exposure, decontamination first would be the most appropriate course of action. In an anticoagulant patient is symptomatic, supportive measures like a blood transfusion should be started first since the vitamin K_1 will not be immediately life-saving (Merola, 2002).

Unfortunately, few antidotes exist. There is little economic incentive for pharmaceutical companies to seek approval for antidotal medications with only a small projected market (Post and Keller, 1999). Additionally, organizing clinical trials for antidotal medications is uniquely problematic. The US Food and Drug Administration has offered incentives to develop antidotal therapies through the Orphan Drug Act. As a result, at least one antidotal therapy was released for veterinary patients: fomepizole was approved for use in treating ethylene glycol intoxication (Cantilena, 2001). In situations where an antidote does exist, its use may be limited by its expense or availability.

Antidotes are generally divided into three groups, based on the mechanism by which they are protective. The groups are chemical antidotes, pharmacological antidotes and functional antidotes. Chemical antidotes act directly on the toxicant. They may decrease the toxicity of the agent or increase its excretion. Pralidoxime chloride, e.g., does both; it binds to OP insecticide molecules making them unable to bind to their target, and the pralidoxime–insecticide complex is then readily excreted (Mowry et al., 1994).

Pharmacological antidotes antagonize the poison at the target site. Flumazenil, e.g., has a high affinity for benzodiazepine receptors, thus it competes with benzodiazepines to reverse their depressive effects (Gwaltney-Brant and Rumbeiha, 2002). Functional antidotes act to lessen the symptoms of the poisoning. They have no interaction with the toxicant. An example of a functional antidote is the use of methocarbamol to control fasciculations and tremors associated with tremorgenic mycotoxins (Schell, 2000). Below are some examples of antidotal therapies available for use in veterinary medicine.

Antidotes for Amitraz: Atipamezole and Yohimbine

Amitraz, a synthetic formamidine pesticide, is used topically to control ticks, mites, and lice on cattle, pigs and dogs as well as to treat demodectic mange in dogs (Grossman, 1993). It is also available in a topical spot-on solution and collar form for tick control in dogs (Plumb, 2015). The acaricide action of amitraz is not well understood, but it may have effects on the CNS of susceptible organisms. It also exhibits significant alpha-2 adrenergic activity (Plumb, 2015). This activity is believed to be responsible for the clinical signs associated with amitraz toxicosis including ataxia, CNS depression, hypotension, hyperglycemia, mydriasis, hypothermia, gastrointestinal stasis and bradycardia. In dogs, toxicosis can occasionally result from exposure to a topical product but is more commonly due to ingestion of an amitraz-containing collar (Grossman, 1993; Gwaltney-Brant, 2004).

Atipamezole (Antisedan) is alpha-2 adrenergic antagonist labeled for use as a reversal agent for the sedative medetomidine. It has been used successfully in the treatment of amitraz toxicosis to reverse the CNS, bradycardia, gastrointestinal stasis, and hyperglycemia (Grossman, 1993; Gwaltney-Brant, 2004). The recommended dose in dogs is 50 μg/kg IM. The drug has a good margin of safety; dogs injected with 10 times the therapeutic dose did not have significant effects. Potential adverse effects of atipamezole administration include vomiting, diarrhea, hypersalivation, and trembling (Plumb, 2015). In cases where an amitraz collar was ingested and has not been retrieved from the GIT, the atipamezole dose may need to be repeated each time signs recur until the collar is passed through the GIT.

Yohimbine is another alpha-2 adrenergic antagonist that has been used to counter the toxic effects of amitraz. The recommended dose in dogs is 0.11 mg/kg IV. Yohimbine has a short half-life (1.5–2 h in dogs); consequently, the dose may need to be repeated. Potential adverse effects include temporary apprehension or CNS excitation, tremors, hypersalivation, elevated respiratory rate, and hyperemic mucous membranes. Careful dosing is recommended, because tremors and seizures have been reported in dogs receiving five times the therapeutic dose (Plumb, 2015).

Antidotes for Anticholinesterase Agents: Atropine and Pralidoxime

Atropine is used to counter the muscarinic effects of anticholinesterase agents. Acetylcholine (ACh) is a neurotransmitter that transmits impulses at cholinergic nerve synapses and neuromuscular junctions. The enzyme acetylcholinesterase (AChE) is responsible for the hydrolysis of ACh. Anticholinesterase agents, which include the carbamate and OP insecticides, produce their effects by binding with AChE to disrupt the breakdown of ACh. The ACh accumulates within the synapse leading to overstimulation of the end organ (Meerdink, 2004). There are two basic cholinergic receptor types: muscarinic and nicotinic. The muscarinic are the postganglionic parasympathetic receptors in smooth muscle, the heart, and endocrine glands. Overstimulation of these receptors leads to a complex of signs, often described as SLUDDE, which includes *s*alivation, *l*acrimation, *u*rinary incontinence, increased peristalsis and *d*iarrhea, increased bronchial secretions and *d*yspnea, miosis, nausea, *e*mesis, and abdominal discomfort. Excessive stimulation of the nicotinic receptors, which are found in the skeletal muscles and autonomic ganglia, leads to tremors, and possibly seizures, potentially followed by muscle fatigue, weakness and paralysis (Meerdink, 1989; Gupta and Milatovic, 2012; Gupta et al., 2015).

Atropine competes with the accumulated ACh in the synapse to block only the muscarinic effects. Atropine does not block the nicotinic effects. The dosage used to counter anticholinesterase agents is: dogs and cats 0.2–2 mg/kg; cattle 0.5 mg/kg; and horses 0.2 mg/kg. In all of those species, one-quarter of the dose is given IV and the remainder intramuscularly (IM) or subcutaneously (SC) (Plumb, 2015). In some cases, administration of atropine may need to be repeated, but great care should be exercised to prevent over-atropinization. Auscultation should be performed to monitor the patient for bradycardia and continued bronchial secretions, since these are the most life threatening of the muscarinic signs. Additional atropine should only be given if these signs are present. The patient will not die from miosis or hypersalivation. Horses are quite susceptible to ileus caused by atropine administration, and a total dose of no more than 65 mg is recommended for a horse of average weight (Meerdink, 2004).

Atropine is not an effective antidote for other types of insecticides including pyrethroids. When presented with a suspected case of anticholinesterase exposure, the clinician can use a test dose of atropine to assist in making a preliminary diagnosis. The patient should be given the preanesthetic dose of atropine (0.02 mg/kg) IV. If this dose is able to produce typical anticholinergic signs such as mydriasis and tachycardia, then the patient has likely *not* been poisoned by an anticholinesterase agent (Fikes, 1990). If the patient truly had been poisoned by an anticholinesterase agent, the dose of atropine required to produce those effects would be at least 10 times higher (0.2 mg/kg).

Pralidoxime chloride (2-PAM) is used with atropine in the treatment of OP poisoning to relieve nicotinic signs, such as tremors and muscle fasciculations (Fikes, 1990). 2-PAM reactivates the AChE enzyme that has been inactivated by the OP. Normally, acetylcholine (ACh) binds to the enzyme at the anionic binding site. OPs and carbamates bind nearby on the esteric site, thus physically blocking the anionic site from ACh and inactivating the enzyme. 2-PAM is able to squeeze in via nucleophilic attack and bind to the anionic binding site. It then attaches to the OP forming a pralidoxime–OP complex. This complex detaches from the enzyme reactivating it and is then excreted in the urine (Fikes, 1990; Mowry et al., 1994; Plumb, 2015).

Administration of 2-PAM is most effective if given within 24 h of exposure (Plumb, 2015). If the OP remains attached to the AChE much longer, aging of the bond may occur so that it can no longer be broken by 2-PAM (Meerdink, 1989; Mowry et al., 1994; Marrs and Vale, 2006; Gupta and Milatovic, 2012). There are instances when later administration is warranted. For example, in large OP exposures, pralidoxime may still be of some benefit if given within 36–48 h (Plumb, 2015). And 2-PAM may still be indicated even later if clinical signs have been present for an extended period of time (Fikes, 1992). Please see Table 82.2 for dosing information.

Treatment with 2-PAM should continue until the animal is asymptomatic. If no improvement is seen after 24–36 h following initiation of treatment, 2-PAM should be discontinued (Fikes, 1990). In acute feline chlorpyrifos toxicosis, cats with persistent tremors can be maintained on 1–2 times daily treatment for up to 4 weeks. The typical presentation in these cats differs from the classical signs expected from other OPs. The onset may be delayed 1–5 days and the cats have neurological signs, including tremors, especially of the muscles of the back, neck and top of head, ataxia and seizures in addition to nonspecific

TABLE 82.2 Pralidoxime Dosing in OP Treatment

Species	Dosing Instructions
Dogs and cats	Pralidoxime works best when combined with atropine
	Pralidoxime at 20 mg/kg, 2–3 times a day
	Initial dose may be given either IM or slow IV
	Subsequent doses may be given IM or SQ
Cattle	30 mg/kg IM q 8 h
Horses	20 mg/kg (may require up to 35 mg/kg) slow IV and repeat every 4–6 h

depression and anorexia, which can persist for 2–4 weeks (Fikes, 1992).

As indicated in Table 82.2, when given IV, administration of 2-PAM should be slow. Rapid IV administration can cause tachycardia, muscle rigidity, transient neuromuscular blockade, and laryngospasm. At therapeutic doses, 2-PAM is generally safe and has no significant adverse effects. However, careful dosing is recommended. At high doses, 2-PAM may exhibit anticholinesterase activity including muscle weakness, ataxia, vomiting, hyperventilation, seizures, respiratory arrest, and death. The LD_{50} in dogs is 190 mg/kg (Plumb, 2015).

Patients receiving 2-PAM should be monitored for hypersensitivity reactions. 2-PAM is generally not recommended for carbamate toxicosis because AChE inhibition due to carbamates is rapidly reversible (Plumb, 2015), and 2-PAM has less affinity for carbamates than OPs (Meerdink, 2004). In addition, there is evidence that 2-PAM can reduce the protective effects of atropine in the treatment of one carbamate, carbaryl (Fikes, 1990). Since the drug is excreted by the kidneys, patients with underlying renal impairment should receive a decreased dose and be monitored closely for signs of toxicity (Plumb, 2015).

Cyproheptadine HCl

Cyproheptadine HCl has been successful in treating serotonin syndrome in dogs and people (Gwaltney-Brant and Rumbeiha, 2002). Cyproheptadine is an antihistamine that is most commonly utilized in veterinary practice as an appetite stimulant for cats. It also is a potent serotonin antagonist (Plumb, 2015).

Serotonin is a neurotransmitter in the CNS. It also acts to promote platelet aggregation and as a stimulant on the smooth muscle of the respiratory, gastrointestinal and cardiovascular systems. The term serotonin syndrome is used to describe the characteristic signs that develop from excessive serotonin including autonomic, neuromuscular, behavioral and cognitive abnormalities (Gwaltney-Brant et al., 2000). Excess serotonin may result from use or accidental overdose of medications that increase brain serotonin levels. These medications include selective serotonin reuptake inhibitors, like venlafaxine (Effexor), paroxetine HCl (Paxil), and fluoxetine HCl (Prozac) as well as 5-hydroxytryptophan, which is a serotonin precursor sold OTC as a dietary supplement (Gwaltney-Brant and Rumbeiha, 2002). See Table 82.3 for a list of medications that carry a high potential of increasing brain serotonin levels.

Dogs with serotonin syndrome typically have hyperthermia, central nervous abnormalities including tremors, seizures, ataxia, excitation or depression and hyperesthesia, and gastrointestinal effects of vomiting, diarrhea, and abdominal discomfort (Gwaltney-Brant and Rumbeiha, 2002). Death is possible if the signs are not controlled quickly. When used as a serotonin antagonist, the recommended dose of cyproheptadine in dogs is 1.1 mg/kg q 4–6 h until signs do not recur (Plumb, 2015). The dose can be given orally if the patient is alert, not vomiting and activated charcoal was not given within 2 h. In those instances, the dose can be crushed, mixed with a small amount of saline and given per rectum. The drug should be discontinued after the first two doses if little or no improvement is noted (Gwaltney-Brant et al., 2000). A similar dose of cyproheptadine has also been of some benefit in controlling vocalization and disorientation in some cases of baclofen toxicosis (Wismer, 2004).

TABLE 82.3 Drugs With High Serotonergic Potential

Amitriptyline (e.g., Elavil)	Lithium
Amphetamines (e.g., Adderall)	Meperidine (e.g., Demerol)
Clomipramine (e.g., Clomicalm)	Moclobemide
Dexfenfluramine	Paroxetine (e.g., Paxil)
Fenfluramine (e.g., Ponderal)	Phenelzine
Fluoxetine (e.g., Prozac)	Selegiline (e.g., Anipryl)
Hydroxytryptophan	Sertraline (e.g., Zoloft)
Imipramine (Tofranil)	Tranylcypromine
Isocarboxazid	Tryptophan
	Venlafaxine (e.g., Effexor)

Digoxin Immune Fab

Digoxin immune Fab fragments (e.g., Digibind from GlaxoSmithKline) are a promising treatment for life-threatening digoxin toxicosis. The Fab fragments are used as a specific antidote for digoxin since they inactivate the drug by directly binding to it. The fragments are produced by first immunizing sheep with digoxin–human albumin complexes. In response, the sheep produce antibodies that are collected, purified, and cleaved with papain into Fab fragments and Fc portions (Kittleson and Kienle, 1998). Digoxin immune Fab fragments are quite expensive, so their use may be cost prohibitive and they may be difficult to obtain. A local human hospital pharmacy may be willing to sell the product to the veterinary clinic if needed.

Digoxin and other digitalis glycosides are thought to cause their effects by inhibition of the sodium–potassium ATPase pump (Na^+/K^+-ATPase) through competition with potassium for binding sites (Kittleson and Kienle, 1998). Fab fragments can actually remove a digoxin molecule that is bound to the ATPase since their affinity for digoxin is much stronger than the affinity of digoxin for the Na^+/K^+-ATPase target (Gwaltney-Brant and Rumbeiha, 2002). Fab fragments may also be used as an effective antidote for digitoxin toxicosis since they bind to it, though with less affinity than for digoxin. Moreover, sufficient cross-reactivity exists with cardiac glycosides derived from *Bufo* toads and a wide variety of plants; consequently, Fab fragments may be effective at controlling toxicoses from these agents as well (Clark et al., 1991; Gwaltney-Brant and Rumbeiha, 2002). See Table 82.4 for a list of plants containing cardiac glycosides that Fab fragments may be effective against.

The antidotal use of Fab fragments is indicated for treatment of potentially life-threatening cardiac glycoside toxicoses. Fab fragments should be considered when the patient has developed cardiac arrhythmias that are unresponsive to other antiarrhythmic therapy. Ideally, the appropriate dose of Fab fragments is determined by using the patient's serum digoxin level. In some cases, the laboratory at a local human hospital may be willing to perform serum levels for the veterinarian. If a serum level can be obtained, the following formula is used to calculate the number of vials (Gwaltney-Brant and Rumbeiha, 2002). This formula assumes each vial will bind 0.5 mg of digoxin:

$$\text{Dose (number of vials)} = \frac{\text{Serum digoxin concentration (ng/mL)} \times \text{Body weight (kg)}}{100}$$

In cases where the cost of the calculated number of vials is prohibitive, if digoxin levels cannot be measured, or if the Fab fragments are being used to treat another

TABLE 82.4 Plants Containing Cardiac Glycosides

Plant Species	Common Name
Acokanthera oblongifolia	
Adonis microcarpa	Pheasant's eye
Asclepias physocarpa	Balloon cotton bush
Bryophyllum tubiflorum	Mother of millions
Calotropis procera	King's crown
Carissa laxiflora	
Cerbera manghas	Sea mango
Convallaria majalis	Lily of the valley
Cryptostegia grandiflora Helleboros.	Rubber vine
Nerium oleander	Oleander
Thevetia neriifolia	Yellow oleander

cardiac glycoside, treatment can be initiated with one to two vials and the patient observed for improvement. The reconstituted Fab fragments are administered intravenously over approximately 30 min. If the clinician feels the patient's clinical signs are immediately life-threatening, the product can instead be given as a bolus. Fab fragments act quickly and dramatically. The patient's cardiac status is expected to begin improving within 20–90 min of administration and complete resolution of the clinical effects is usually seen within 4 h (Gwaltney-Brant and Rumbeiha, 2002). If significant improvement does not occur, additional vials may need to be given.

While monitoring the patient, it is important to note that the total serum digoxin concentration will be markedly increased with most commercial assays after Fab fragment administration. This occurs because previously tissue-bound digoxin binds to the Fab fragments, and the Fab–digoxin complexes then move into the blood to be excreted by the kidneys (Ward et al., 1999). Since these patients have a compromised cardiovascular system as a result of the toxicosis, it is likely that renal perfusion is also compromised. These animals should be monitored carefully because decreased renal clearance of Fab–digoxin complexes may allow for dissociation of the toxin and recurrence of signs (Gwaltney-Brant and Rumbeiha, 2002).

The patient should also be monitored for hypokalemia. Elevated serum potassium is expected with cardiac glycoside toxicosis due to interference with the Na^+/K^+-ATPase pumps. After administration of the Fab fragments, potassium moves quickly back into the cells leading to a significant drop in serum potassium levels. Serum potassium levels should be checked frequently within the first few hours and hypokalemia treated if needed (Gwaltney-Brant and Rumbeiha, 2002). The patient should also be monitored for anaphylaxis, fever, and hypersensitivity reactions (Ward et al., 1999).

Antidotes for Ethylene Glycol: Ethanol and Fomepizole

Ethanol can be used as an antidote for ethylene glycol poisoning. Ethylene glycol is found in many products at many concentrations. Most animal intoxications occur from ingestion of antifreeze since these products may have concentrations of ethylene glycol exceeding 90%. With intoxication, the gastrointestinal, central nervous, cardiopulmonary and renal systems can be affected. Death is usually due to acute renal failure. The ethylene glycol itself does not cause the life-threatening clinical findings. It must be converted, primarily in the liver, to its more toxic metabolites including glycolic, glycoxalic, and oxalic acids (Dalefield, 2004). The first step in the metabolism is conversion of the parent ethylene glycol molecule to glycoaldehyde via the enzyme alcohol dehydrogenase (ADH). Ethanol is also metabolized by ADH, therefore it competes for the enzyme, allowing time for ethylene glycol to be excreted unchanged in the urine (Mathews, 2006). Early intervention is very important to prevent the conversion to toxic metabolites. If a toxic dose was ingested and treatment is not initiated within a few hours of exposure, the patient's prognosis is grave.

The dosing recommendations for ethanol vary among authors. Intermittent dosing is possible, but a continuous rate infusion (CRI) is preferred to avoid high blood concentrations of the ethanol, which can exacerbate the potential clinical effects (Mathews, 2006). See Table 82.5 for examples of intermittent and CRI dosing recommendations for dogs and cats.

Ethanol is easy to obtain and is inexpensive. However, significant adverse effects will likely develop at the high doses required for treatment of ethylene glycol toxicosis, including severe respiratory and CNS depression and metabolic acidosis. Since the signs of ethylene glycol intoxication mirror those effects, gauging patient progress can be challenging (Plumb, 2015).

Fomepizole, also called 4-methylpyrazole (4MP), is an antidote for ethylene glycol toxicosis in dogs. 4MP was once sold as Antizol-Vet, which is no longer on the market, so it now must be compounded. Studies have found that 4MP can also be used in cats but must be used at higher doses to be effective (Connally et al., 2002). 4MP is a synthetic ADH inhibitor that works similarly to ethanol to prevent the conversion of ethylene glycol to its toxic metabolites. However, while ethanol acts by competing for the enzyme, 4MP forms a complex with ADH and its coenzyme (Connally et al., 1996). Fomepizole is significantly more expensive than ethanol, but has a therapeutic advantage because it causes fewer serious side effects (Gaddy, 2001). Dose-related CNS depression is the only adverse effect expected and tends to be mild if it develops. Cats are more at risk, because they require higher doses. Since 4MP has few serious risks, treatment is recommended in cases where exposure to ethylene glycol is suspected but not confirmed (Gwaltney-Brant and Rumbeiha, 2002).

4MP is excreted in the urine and accumulates over time depending on the dosage amount and frequency of administration. Since the drug accumulates, lower doses are given following the initial dose (Gaddy, 2001). In dogs, an initial dose of 20 mg/kg of the 5% reconstituted solution is given IV. At 12 and 24 h after the first dose, additional doses of 15 mg/kg are given. Finally, at 36 h after the first dose, a dose of 5 mg/kg is given. In cases where the patient has not fully recovered following the above doses, additional dosing of 3 mg/kg every 12 h is recommended (Gwaltney-Brant and Rumbeiha, 2002).

The dosing schedule in cats is an initial dose of 125 mg/kg IV, then subsequent doses at 12, 24 and 36 h with 31.25 mg/kg (Plumb, 2015). Treatment in cats with either 4MP or ethanol must begin within 3 h postingestion of ethylene glycol or prognosis is grave. In dogs, fomepizole is most effective if given within 3–6 h of ethylene glycol ingestion; however, some benefit was seen as late as 36 h postingestion. A late dose may prevent additional injury to the kidneys (Gwaltney-Brant and Rumbeiha, 2002).

Flumazenil

Flumazenil, 1,4-imidazobenzodiazepine, is a benzodiazepine antagonist (Plumb, 2015). It is derived from the antibiotic anthramycin (Gwaltney-Brant and Rumbeiha, 2002) and blocks benzodiazepines by competition for the benzodiazepine receptor in the CNS (Plumb, 2015). Flumazenil has a higher affinity for the receptor than that of the benzodiazepines; as a result, it displaces receptor-bound benzodiazepines to reverse their depressive effects (Gwaltney-Brant and Rumbeiha, 2002).

Flumazenil has been used as a successful therapy for benzodiazepine toxicosis in dogs and cats (Wismer, 2002). It is also used to improve neurological signs in dogs with severe hepatic encephalopathy (Plumb, 2015).

TABLE 82.5 Ethanol Dosing in EG Treatment

	Intermittent Dosing	CRI
Dogs	Start with a 20% solution	Start with a 5% solution
	Give 5.5 mL/kg IV q 4 h for 5 treatments	Give at CRI rate of 5.5 mL/kg/h
	Then give 5.5 mL/kg IV q 6 h for 4 additional treatments	
Cats	Start with a 20% solution	Start with a 5% solution
	Give 5 mL/kg IV q 6 h for 5 treatments	Give at CRI rate of 5 mL/kg/h
	Then give 5 mL/kg IV q 8 h for 4 additional treatments	

Flumazenil has been used in humans, with some success, to reverse ethanol and tegretol-induced CNS depression. Consequently, it is reasonable to assume flumazenil also could be effective in small animal patients in such cases (Gwaltney-Brant and Rumbeiha, 2002).

The recommended flumazenil dose in dogs and cats is 0.01 mg/kg administered by IV injection (Plumb, 2015). The medication rapidly crosses the blood–brain barrier and a swift reversal of benzodiazepine-induced sedation is expected within 1–2 min (Gwaltney-Brant and Rumbeiha, 2002). The dose may need to be repeated multiple times, since flumazenil's half-life is shorter than most of the benzodiazepines. The half-life of flumazenil is only 1 h in humans (Plumb, 2015), but the half-life of diazepam in the dog is 6 h. The patient should be monitored carefully for recurrence of signs and additional doses of flumazenil given as needed. Repeat doses should not be given in asymptomatic patients. Flumazenil may act as a benzodiazepine agonist if administered at high doses despite its antagonist action at therapeutic doses (Gwaltney-Brant and Rumbeiha, 2002).

Flumazenil is a costly medication and carries the risk of significant adverse effects. It should be reserved for cases where the patient has life-threatening benzodiazepine-induced clinical signs. The drug should be given through a patent IV catheter, because extravascular leakage can cause extensive local tissue irritation and necrosis (Gwaltney-Brant and Rumbeiha, 2002). In humans, vomiting, cutaneous vasodilation, vertigo, ataxia and blurred vision have been reported following flumazenil administration (Plumb, 2015). Seizures and death are also rarely reported in humans after treatment with flumazenil (ASHSP, 2003).

Flumazenil may lower the seizure threshold and is contraindicated in cases when seizures are anticipated. It also may increase intracranial pressure and should not be used in patients with head trauma (Gwaltney-Brant and Rumbeiha, 2002). Additionally, flumazenil is contraindicated in patients with life-threatening tricyclic antidepressant toxicosis and should be used only after careful consideration in cases of multiple drug overdosage (Plumb, 2015). Most human deaths and seizures associated with flumazenil followed use in cases of tricyclic antidepressant toxicosis (ASHSP, 2003).

Lipid Emulsion

Intravenous infusion of a lipid emulsion (ILE) has been used successfully in humans to treat intoxication with local anesthetic medications and the antidepressant buproprion (Crandell and Weinberg, 2009; O'Brien et al., 2010). Research studies in dogs, rats, and rabbits have shown ILE to be effective in managing bupivacaine, verapamil, propranolol and clomipramine toxicosis. ILE use in the treatment of companion animal intoxications has also been reported: lidocaine intoxication in a cat and moxidectin toxicosis in a puppy (Crandell and Weinberg, 2009; O'Brien et al., 2010).

Lipid emulsions are made from purified soybean oil in water, are commonly used in medicine to provide intravenous (parenteral) nutrition and are the delivery mechanism for certain hydrophobic drugs like propofol. The mechanism by which ILE is effective at treating toxicoses is not yet fully understood. However, the fact that ILE seems to be most effective in treating overdosage of lipid-soluble medications suggests that the infusion expands the amount of plasma lipid that acts as a sink in which the offending drug can gather reducing free drug concentrations. In theory, the drug is trapped in the plasma lipid so it is not available to act on other tissues (Crandell and Weinberg, 2009; O'Brien et al., 2010).

The APCC uses the following dosing protocol. Using a 20% product, give an initial bolus of 1.5 mL/kg slowly then start a continuous rate infusion (CRI) of 0.25 mL/kg/min for 30–60 min. Four hours after the CRI is finished, check the serum for hyperlipidemia and to see if the serum is orange or yellow. If the serum looks normal, repeat the initial bolus and CRI again. If hyperlipidemia or a color change is present, check the serum for resolution every 2 h. Repeat the initial bolus and CRI once the hyperlipidemia or color change resolves. If a third dose is needed, follow the above directions beginning 4 h after the second CRI finishes. Do not give more than three doses if there has been no significant response.

ILE may be effective in treating intoxications with many lipid-soluble medications including local anesthetics (lidocaine, bupivacaine, ropivicaine), macrocyclic lactones (ivermectin, moxidectin), calcium channel blockers (diltiazem, verapamil, amlodipine), beta-blockers (propranolol), antidepressants (buproprion, clomipramine, doxepin, sertraline), and muscle relaxants (baclofen, cyclobenzaprine) (Plumb, 2015). Possible side effects of administering ILE include induction of pancreatitis, creation of a fat embolism, immunosuppression, phlebitis, thrombosis, hypertriglyceridemia, and hepatic lipidosis (Crandell and Weinberg, 2009; O'Brien et al., 2010).

Methocarbamol

The skeletal muscle relaxant methocarbamol has proved to be very useful in the management of severe muscle fasciculations, tremors and seizures associated with a variety of toxicologic agents. The exact mechanism by which methocarbamol works is unknown, but it is thought to act centrally to block nerve impulses in the brain stem, spinal cord and subcortical levels of the brain (Gwaltney-Brant and Rumbeiha, 2002).

Methocarbamol has been used successfully in veterinary medicine to treat the following types of toxicoses: permethrin in cats (Richardson, 2000a), metaldehyde (Richardson et al., 2003), strychnine (Gwaltney-Brant and Rumbeiha, 2002; Plumb, 2015) and tremorgenic mycotoxins (Schell, 2000). It is able to reduce the severity of tremors without causing the severe CNS depression often encountered when using a barbiturate medication (Gwaltney-Brant and Rumbeiha, 2002).

The dosage for dogs and cats is 55–220 mg/kg administered slowly IV at a rate of no more than 2 mL/min (Schell, 2000). Methocarbamol administration should be repeated if the signs recur; however, the total dose should not exceed 330 mg/kg in a 24-h period to avoid CNS and respiratory depression (Gwaltney-Brant and Rumbeiha, 2002; Richardson et al., 2003). The dosage for horses is 4.4–55 mg/kg by slow infusion (Plumb, 2015). The drug should not be given SQ, and extravasation of methocarbamol should be avoided, as the solution can be irritating (Plumb, 2015).

In dogs and cats, adverse effects may include sedation, salivation, emesis, lethargy, weakness, and ataxia. Slow administration of the drug can help to avoid salivation and emesis. Sedation and ataxia can be seen in horses following methocarbamol administration. This medication is contraindicated in animals intended for food purposes and in patients hypersensitive to it. The manufacturer lists known or suspected renal insufficiency as a contraindication to injectable methocarbamol therapy since the injectable product contains polyethylene glycol 300, which has been found to increase acidosis and urea retention in renal-impaired humans (Plumb, 2015). For this reason, veterinary patients treated with injectable methocarbamol should receive IV fluid support and have kidney values monitored if renal impairment is suspected or is a possible outcome of their clinical signs. For example, patients with prolonged tremors or seizures can release muscular myoglobin. The myoglobin is excreted by the kidneys and can lead to renal damage (Volmer, 2004).

Naloxone HCl

Naloxone HCl (Narcan) is an injectable opiate antagonist used to reverse the effects of opiate medications. It is able to reverse opioid agonist/antagonists, such as butorphanol as well. This drug is also being investigated for treatment of other conditions like septic, hypovolemic and cardiogenic shock (Plumb, 2015).

Naloxone is a pure opiate antagonist, and it has no analgesic activity or other agonist effects. Although the exact mechanism for its activity is not fully understood, it is thought the drug acts as a competitive antagonist by binding to multiple opioid receptor sites. The drug apparently has its highest affinity for the *mu* receptor, which makes it an ideal antagonist since most of the clinically useful opioids work by binding to the *mu* receptor (Plumb, 2015; Volmer, 2006).

Naloxone reverses most of the effects of opioids including analgesia and respiratory and CNS depression (Plumb, 2015). It does not reverse the emetic actions of apomorphine in dogs (Volmer, 2006). At high doses, naloxone increases dopamine levels and acts as a GABA antagonist (Plumb, 2015).

Because orally administered naloxone is only minimally absorbed and the drug is destroyed rapidly in the digestive tract, an injectable formulation is preferred. The onset of action is normally within 1–2 min when given IV and within 5 min when given IM. The duration of action is usually 45–90 min but may be as long as 3 h. Since the duration of action of naloxone may be shorter than the medication being reversed, additional doses may be required (Plumb, 2015).

The recommended dosage for dogs and cats is 0.01–0.04 mg/kg IV, IM or SC; and for horses, 0.01–0.05 mg/kg IV (Plumb, 2015). In patients that have been intentionally given an opioid to treat a painful condition, abrupt reversal can lead to tachycardia, vasoconstriction and hypertension. In these cases, the unwanted CNS and respiratory depression can be reversed without reversing the analgesia. To achieve this, dilute 0.04–0.1 mg of naloxone in 5–10 mL of normal saline and give slowly to effect by dosing 0.5–1 mL per minute (Mathews, 2006).

Naloxone is considered quite safe at therapeutic doses. Very high doses have been associated with seizures in a few patients perhaps due to GABA inhibition. It is contraindicated in patients that are hypersensitive to it and should be used with caution in animals with preexisting cardiac abnormalities due to the potential cardiovascular adverse effects (Plumb, 2015).

N-Acetylcysteine

N-Acetylcysteine (NAC) is used to prevent methemoglobinemia and hepatic necrosis in acetaminophen (APAP) toxicosis. APAP is metabolized in the liver primarily via glucuronidation and sulfation to nontoxic metabolites. However, other pathways of metabolism exist that yield the toxic metabolites *N*-acetyl-para-benzoquinoneimine (NAPQI) and para-aminophenol (PAP) (Aronson and Drobatz, 1996; McConkey et al., 2009). In a significant APAP exposure, the glucuronidation and sulfation pathways become saturated, leading to increased production of NAPQI and PAP. NAPQI is produced through the P450 mixed function oxidase system and is normally inactivated through conjugation with glutathione (Richardson, 2000b). PAP is produced by deacetylation and is removed both through conjugation with glutathione and by *N*-acetylation. Dogs and cats are deficient in the enzymes needed for *N*-acetylation (McConkey et al., 2009).

Initially the excess NAPQI and PAP will be detoxified through conjugation with glutathione. However, once glutathione stores are depleted, the NAPQI metabolite can lead to liver necrosis and the PAP metabolite can lead to methemoglobinemia. NAPQI binds to hepatic cell membranes causing oxidative injury to the bi-lipid layer and potential cellular death and necrosis (Richardson, 2000b). PAP causes redox cycling in the red blood cells (RBCs) leading to oxidation of the hemoglobin to methemoglobin, which is unable to carry oxygen (McConkey et al., 2009). While all species can develop both hepatic and RBC effects, dogs more commonly develop hepatic necrosis, whereas cats more commonly develop methemoglobinemia and Heinz body anemia (Taylor and Dhupa, 2000).

There are at least two mechanisms by which NAC prevents methemoglobinemia and hepatic necrosis from APAP. NAC binds directly with NAPQI rendering it inactive and therefore nontoxic. NAC is a precursor for glutathione production. It restores and maintains glutathione levels by increasing synthesis (Richardson, 2000b). NAC administration may also lead to increased serum sulfate, which could reestablish the sulfation pathway to nontoxic metabolites (Aronson and Drobatz, 1996) (Fig. 82.1).

The therapeutic dose of NAC for dogs and cats is a loading dose of 140 mg/kg PO or IV (as a 5% solution), then 70 mg/kg PO or IV every 6 h for seven treatments. The number of additional treatments varies between authors; some recommend up to 17 treatments (Plumb, 2015). Presently, both an injectable form and oral solution are on the market. When given orally, NAC can cause gastrointestinal irritation so proper dilution is important.

Pamidronate Disodium

Pamidronate disodium (Aredia) is a biphosphonate used in the treatment of hypercalcemia associated with malignancy and vitamin D_3 toxicity in dogs and cats (Plumb, 2015). Vitamin D_3, also called cholecalciferol, is found in some rodenticides. Calcipotriene, which is an analog of cholecalciferol, is found in some human prescription topical antipsoriasis medications (e.g., Dovonex) (Pesillo et al., 2002). Since vitamin D_3 plays an important role in calcium and phosphorus homeostasis, oral exposure to these rodenticides or topical medications can lead to significant elevations in serum calcium and phosphorus levels. Vitamin D_3 enhances calcium and phosphorus absorption from the GI tract. In addition, it works with parathyroid hormone to promote calcium reabsorption in the kidney and mobilization of calcium from the bone via osteoclastic-mediated bone resorption (Rumbeiha et al., 2000; Morrow, 2001).

Calcium maintains cell membrane stability and is a second messenger in several cellular responses (Pesillo et al., 2002). Therefore, increasing serum calcium can cause many cellular effects including altered cell

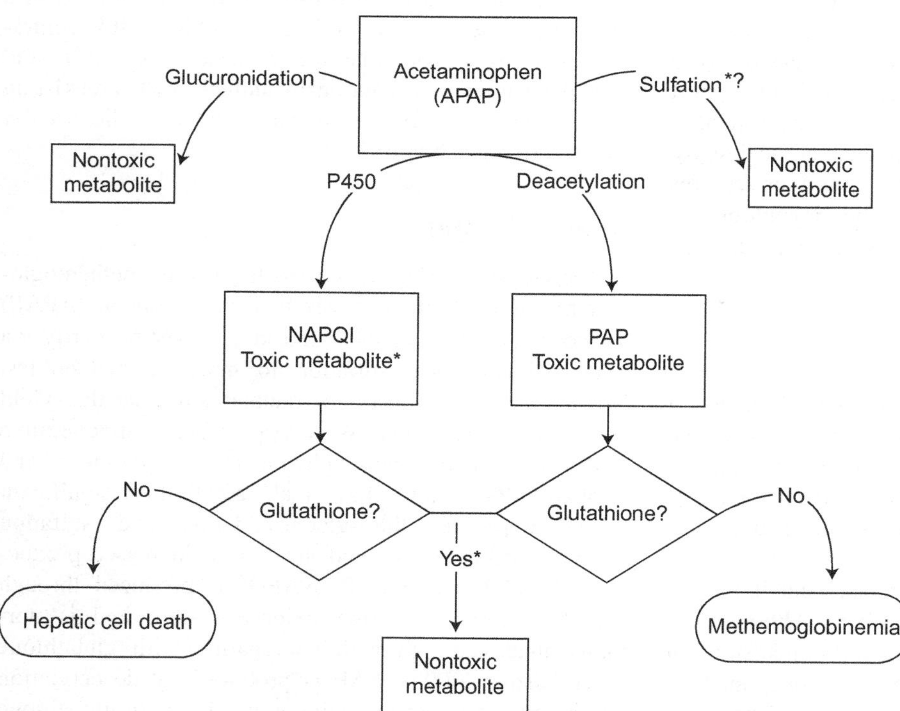

FIGURE 82.1 The metabolism of acetaminophen (APAP). Areas of *N*-acetylcysteine (NAC) action are indicated with an *.

membrane permeability, a decrease in cellular energy production and cellular necrosis (Morrow, 2001). Patients poisoned by vitamin D_3 and its analogs often present with polyuria, polydipsia, vomiting, anorexia, lethargy, hypercalcemia and hyperphosphatemia (Pesillo et al., 2002). If elevations in serum calcium and phosphorus concentrations go unchecked, the plasma calcium phosphorus product ($Ca \times P$) can rise above 60, leading to soft tissue mineralization (Morrow, 2001). Mineralization of the kidneys and heart can lead to a life-threatening decrease in function of these organs.

Pamidronate acts to decrease serum calcium levels by binding to hydroxyapatite crystals in the bone to prevent their dissolution and bone resorption. It also interrupts osteoclast activity and induces osteoclast apoptosis (Plumb, 2015). Some authors suggest pamidronate may decrease intestinal absorption of calcium as well (Pesillo et al., 2002).

The recommended dose of pamidronate is 1.3–2 mg/kg given as a slow IV infusion over several hours (Plumb, 2015). Pamidronate must be given in saline and should not mix with any IV fluid containing calcium (e.g., Ringer's). In most cases, a single dose will be effective in lowering calcium levels back to normal (Gwaltney-Brant and Rumbeiha, 2002). However, some patients may require an additional dose 5–7 days after the initial treatment (Morrow, 2001). Calcium levels should be monitored once daily for at least 10 days after they have returned to normal. Pamidronate is most effective if given within 24–36 h of the exposure, prior to development of soft tissue mineralization (Gwaltney-Brant and Rumbeiha, 2002).

Anemia, thrombocytopenia and granulocytosis have been reported in humans following pamidronate administration. In dogs, hypersensitivity reactions, electrolyte abnormalities including hypomagnesemia and hypocalcemia, arrhythmias and renal toxicity are possible (Plumb, 2015). Slow infusion of the drug over at least 2 h may help in avoiding renal effects. Use of pamidronate in dogs with impaired renal function is controversial since it may confound renal injury (Gwaltney-Brant and Rumbeiha, 2002).

Pamidronate now comes in a generic form and its use may be more cost effective than using salmon calcitonin in vitamin D_3 toxicosis. Pamidronate lowers plasma calcium concentrations within 24–48 h of a single IV dose. Calcitonin requires dosing several times daily due to its short half-life. Additionally, with calcitonin therapy, saline diuresis, and treatment with diuretics and corticosteroids must also be performed, requiring many days, sometimes multiple weeks, of hospitalization. In most cases treated with pamidronate, treatment can be performed on an out-patient basis once the calcium has returned to the normal range (Morrow, 2001; Pesillo et al., 2002). Pamidronate is also preferred to calcitonin since patients may become refractory to calcitonin treatment after 10 days of therapy (Rumbeiha et al., 2000; Morrow, 2001).

Phytonadione (Vitamin K_1)

Phytonadione, a naphthoquinone derivative identical to naturally occurring vitamin K_1, is used in the treatment of anticoagulant toxicosis resulting from anticoagulant rodenticides, the medication warfarin or moldy sweet clover (Plumb, 2015). All household pets, including pocket pets, may be exposed to anticoagulant rodenticides and the medication warfarin. Livestock and horses are more likely to be poisoned by the dicoumarol in moldy sweet clover, but they can also be exposed to rodenticides (Knight, 2004).

Anticoagulants block clotting factor activation. Vitamin K_1 is involved in the activation of precursor clotting factors into functional factors. During the activation, vitamin K_1 is converted to inactive vitamin K_1 epoxide. Normally, vitamin K_1 epoxide is reactivated by vitamin K_1 epoxide reductase. Anticoagulants work by inhibiting this enzyme and halting the recycling of vitamin K_1 (Merola, 2002). As a result, the number of active clotting factors decreases.

The vitamin K_1-dependent clotting factors are II, VII, IX, and X. These factors are involved in all three pathways of the coagulation system: the extrinsic, intrinsic, and common (Means, 2004a). Active bleeding is not expected for 3–7 days after the ingestion because the body has a reserve of active clotting factors. When these degrade naturally or are consumed, clinical signs are possible. If an external source of vitamin K_1 is provided, the factors will be activated normally (Merola, 2002).

Bleeding can occur anywhere within the body and the presenting clinical signs will relate to where the bleeding has occurred. The signs may be vague and nonspecific. In dogs, dyspnea, coughing, lethargy, and hemoptysis are commonly reported due to bleeding into the chest cavity (Merola, 2002). With moldy sweet clover poisoning in livestock, prolonged bleeding in some members following routine surgical procedures, like castration or dehorning, is often the first indication of a problem within the herd (Knight, 2004).

The dose for vitamin K_1 in household pets is 1.5–2.5 mg/kg orally twice daily. Pocket pets and other small patients can be given the injectable formulation orally if a suitable tablet size is not available. Small patients should be dosed at the high end of the range and larger patients (e.g., large breed dogs) should be started at the low end (Means, 2004a). Vitamin K_1 should be given with a fatty meal to enhance absorption. In dogs, giving the medication with canned food caused a four- to five-fold increase in bioavailability (Plumb, 2015).

Oral administration is preferred since the vitamin K_1 will be carried, via the portal circulation, directly to the liver where the activation of clotting factors occurs (Merola, 2002). Additionally, vitamin K_1 injections have been associated with anaphylactic reactions and hematoma formation (Plumb, 2015). However, IM administration is recommended by many authors for livestock, perhaps for ease of administration. The recommended dose for cattle, horses, swine, sheep, and goats is 0.5–2.5 mg/kg IM (Knight, 2004; Plumb, 2015).

The length of vitamin K_1 administration depends on the toxicant. Warfarin exposures generally require a 14-day course. Second generation anticoagulant rodenticides should be treated for 30 days, except for bromadiolone, which should be treated for 21 days (Means, 2004a). Moldy sweet clover poisoning should be treated for 1–2 weeks (Knight, 2004). In all cases, a prothrombin time should be checked 48–72 h after the course of vitamin K_1 is complete. If this test is abnormal, resume vitamin K_1 therapy for an additional 7 days (Merola, 2002).

Blood transfusions may be required in severely symptomatic patients, since it may take 6–12 h for the liver to produce active clotting factors following initiation of vitamin K_1 therapy (Plumb, 2015). Exercise restriction is indicated in all patients during this lag time to prevent active bleeding (Merola, 2002). Substituting vitamin K_3 (menadione) for vitamin K_1 is not recommended, as it is not as effective and is nephrotoxic in horses (Merola, 2002; Knight, 2004).

CONCLUDING REMARKS AND FUTURE DIRECTIONS

Proper client education is crucial to poison prevention. However, when poisonings do occur, the clinician should concentrate on treating the patient and not the poison. The same principles of history collection, physical examination, and patient monitoring that are used in other cases should be applied when managing a poisoning patient. Appropriate decontamination and antidotal therapies should be decided on after initial patient stabilization.

REFERENCES

Albretsen, J.C., 2004. Methylxanthines. In: Plumlee, K.H. (Ed.), Clinical Veterinary Toxicology. Mosby, St. Louis, MO, pp. 322–326.

Allerton, J.P., Strom, J.A., 1991. Hypernatremia due to repeated doses of charcoal-sorbitol. Am. J. Kidney Dis. 17, 581–584.

American Society of Health System Pharmacists, 2003. American Hospital Formulary Service Drug Information. American Hospital Formulary Service, Bethesda, pp. 2421–2423.

Aronson, L.R., Drobatz, K., 1996. Acetaminophen toxicosis in 17 cats. J. Vet. Emerg. Crit. Care. 6, 65–69.

Bailey Jr, E.M., Garland, T., 1992. Management of toxicoses. In: Robinson, N.E. (Ed.), Current Therapy in Equine Medicine 3. W. B. Saunders Company, Philadelphia, pp. 346–353.

Ball, A., 2014. Managing hypernatremia after activated charcoal administration. Vet. Med. 109, 128–130.

Beasley, V.R., Dorman, D.C., 1990. Management of toxicoses. Vet. Clin. North Am. Small Anim. Pract. 20, 307–337.

Brown, C.M., Bertone, J., 2001. The 5-Minute Veterinary Consult Equine. Lippincott Williams & Wilkins, Philadelphia, PA, pp. 816–817.

Buck, W.B., Bratich, P.M., 1986. Activated charcoal: preventing unnecessary death by poisoning. Vet. Med. 81, 73–77.

Buckley, N.A., Dawson, A.H., Reith, D.A., 1995. Controlled release drugs in overdose, clinical considerations. Drug Safety 12, 73–84.

Cantilena Jr, L.R., 2001. Clinical toxicology. In: Klaassen, C.D. (Ed.), Casarett and Doull's Toxicology: The Basic Science of Poisons, sixth ed. McGraw-Hill, New York, NY, pp. 1109–1122.

Cheeke, P.R., 1998. Natural Toxicants in Feeds, Forages, and Poisonous Plants. Interstate Publishers, Inc, Danville, CA.

Clark, R., Curry, S., Selden, B., 1991. Digoxin-specific Fab fragments in the treatment of oleander toxicity in the canine model. Ann. Emerg. Med. 20, 1073–1077.

Connally, H.E., Forney, S.D., Grauer, G.F., et al., 1996. Safety and efficacy of 4-methylpyrazole treatment of suspected or confirmed ethylene glycol intoxication in dogs: 107 cases (1983–1995). J. Am. Vet. Med. Assoc. 209, 1880–1883.

Connally, H.E., Hamar, D.W., Thrall, M.A., 2002. Resident Forum Abstract from 8th IVECCS San Antonio, Texas. Safety and efficacy of high dose fomepizole as therapy for ethylene glycol intoxication in cats. J. Vet. Emerg. Crit. Care 12, 191.

Crandell, D.E., Weinberg, M.D., 2009. Moxidectin toxicosis in a puppy successfully treated with intravenous lipids. J. Vet. Emerg. Crit. Care 19, 181–186.

Dalefield, R., 2004. Ethylene glycol. In: Plumlee, K.H. (Ed.), Clinical Veterinary Toxicology. Mosby, St. Louis, MO, pp. 150–154.

DeClementi, C., Bailey, K.L., Goldstein, S.C., Orser, M.S., 2004. Suspected toxicosis after topical administration of minoxidil in 2 cats. J. Vet. Emerg. Crit. Care 14, 287–292.

Donnelly, T.M., 2004. Rabbits. Basic anatomy, physiology, and husbandry. In: Quesenberry, K.E., Carpenter, J.W. (Eds.), Ferrets, Rabbits, and Rodents Clinical Medicine and Surgery, second ed. Saunders, St. Louis, MO, pp. 136–139.

Echols, S., 2005. Collecting diagnostic samples in avian patients. In: Rupley, A.E. (Ed.), The Clinics Collection Veterinary Clinics of North America Exotic Animal Practice. W.B. Saunders Company, Philadelphia, PA, pp. 60–63.

Fikes, J.D., 1990. Organophosphorus and carbamate insecticides. Vet. Clin. North Am. Small Anim. Pract. 20, 353–367.

Fikes, J.D., 1992. Feline chlorpyrifos toxicosis. In: Kirk, R.W., Bonagura, J.D. (Eds.), Current Veterinary Therapy XI. W.B. Saunders Company, Philadelphia, PA, pp. 188–191.

Gaddy, J., 2001. Pharm profile fomepizole. Comp. Cont. Educ. Pract. Vet. X, 1073–1074.

Galey, F.D., 1992. Diagnostic toxicology. In: Robinson, N.E. (Ed.), Current Therapy in Equine Medicine 3. W.B. Saunders Company, Philadelphia, PA, pp. 337–340.

Grossman, M.R., 1993. Amitraz toxicosis associated with ingestion of an acaricide collar in a dog. J. Am. Vet. Med. Assoc. 203, 55–57.

Gupta, R.C., Milatovic, D., 2012. Toxicity of organophosphates and carbamates. In: Marrs, T.C. (Ed.), Mammalian Toxicology of Insecticides. Royal Society of Chemistry Publ, Cambridge, pp. 104–136.

Gupta, R.C., Zaja-Milatovic, S., Dettbarn, W.-D., Malik, J.K., 2015. Skeletal muscle. In: Gupta, R.C. (Ed.), Handbook of Toxicology of Chemical Warfare Agents. Academic Press/Elsevier, Amsterdam, pp. 577–597.

Gwaltney-Brant, S., 2004. Amitraz. In: Plumlee, K.H. (Ed.), Clinical Veterinary Toxicology. Mosby, St. Louis, MO, pp. 177–178.

Gwaltney-Brant, S.M., Rumbeiha, W.K., 2002. Newer antidotal therapies. Vet. Clin. North Am. Small Anim. Pract. 32, 323–339.

Gwaltney-Brant, S.M., Albretsen, J.C., Khan, S.A., 2000. 5-Hydroxytryptophan toxicosis in dogs: 21 cases (1989–1999). J. Am. Vet. Med. Assoc. 216, 1937–1940.

Horstman, C.L., Cornell, K.K., Eubig, P.A., et al., 2003. Gastric outflow obstruction after ingestion of wood glue in a dog. J. Am. Anim. Hosp. Assoc. 39, 47–51.

Khan, S., McLean, M.K., Hansen, S., et al., 2009. ASPCA Animal Poison Control Center uses its databases to study the efficacy and safety of three different emetics in dogs and cats utilizing 3R principles. In: Poster Presented at 7th World Congress on Alternatives and Animal Use in the Life Sciences. Rome, Italy.

Kittleson, M.D., Kienle, R.D., 1998. Small Animal Cardiovascular Medicine. Mosby, St. Louis, MO, pp. 159–166.

Knight, A.P., 2004. Coumarin glycosides. In: Plumlee, K.H. (Ed.), Clinical Veterinary Toxicology. Mosby, St. Louis, MO, pp. 388–390.

Marrs, T.C., Vale, J.A., 2006. Management of organophosphorus pesticide poisoning. In: Gupta, R.C. (Ed.), Toxicology of Organophosphate and Carbamate Compounds. Academic Press/Elsevier, Amsterdam, pp. 715–733.

Mathews, K.A., 2006. Veterinary Emergency and Critical Care Manual. Lifelearn Inc., Guelph, ON, pp. 4–8, 12–17, 85, 630–640, 655–659.

McConkey, S.E., Grant, D.M., Cribb, A.E., 2009. The role of para-aminophenol in acetaminophen-induced methemoglobinemia in dogs and cats. J. Vet. Pharmacol. Ther. 32, 585–595.

Means, C., 2004a. Anticoagulant rodenticides. In: Plumlee, K.H. (Ed.), Clinical Veterinary Toxicology. Mosby, St. Louis, MO, pp. 444–446.

Means, C., 2004b. Insoluble calcium oxalates. In: Plumlee, K.H. (Ed.), Clinical Veterinary Toxicology. Mosby, St. Louis, MO, pp. 340–341.

Meerdink, G.L., 1989. Organophosphorus and carbamate insecticide poisoning in large animals. Vet. Clin. North Am. Food Anim. Pract. 5, 375–389.

Meerdink, G.L., 2004. Anticholinesterase insecticides. In: Plumlee, K.H. (Ed.), Clinical Veterinary Toxicology. Mosby, St. Louis, MO, pp. 178–180.

Merola, V., 2002. Anticoagulant rodenticides: deadly for pests, dangerous for pets. Vet. Med. 97, 716–722.

Morrow, C., 2001. Cholecalciferol poisoning. Vet. Med. 96, 905–911.

Mowry, J.B., Chylea, P.A., Furbee, R.B., 1994. Organophosphate insecticides. In: Chernow, B. (Ed.), Essentials of Critical Care Pharmacology, second ed. Williams & Wilkins, Baltimore, MA, pp. 522–524.

O'Brien, T.Q., Clark-Price, S.C., Evans, E.E., et al., 2010. Infusion of a lipid emulsion to treat lidocaine intoxication in a cat. J. Am. Vet. Med. Assoc. 237, 1455–1458.

Oehme, F.W., Mannala, S., 2006. Paraquat. In: Peterson, M.E., Talcott, P.A. (Eds.), Small Animal Toxicology, second ed. Elsevier Inc, St. Louis, MO, pp. 964–977.

Osweiler, G.D., 2001. Mycotoxins. Vet. Clin. North Am. Equine Pract. 17, 547–566.

Pesillo, S.A., Khan, S.A., Rozanski, E.A., Rush, J.E., 2002. Calcipotriene toxicosis in a dog successfully treated with pamidronate disodium. J. Vet. Emerg. Crit. Care 12, 177–181.

Peterson, M.E., 2006. Toxicological decontamination. In: Peterson, M. E., Talcott, P.A. (Eds.), Small Animal Toxicology, second ed. Elsevier Inc, St. Louis, MO, pp. 127–141.

Plumb, D.C., 2015. Plumb's Veterinary Drug Handbook. eighth ed. PharmaVet Inc., Stockholm, pp. 11–13, 77–78, 88–89, 93–96, 202–203, 273–274, 312–315, 409–411, 420–422, 454–455, 471–472, 697–698, 728–730, 757–759, 811–812, 857–858, 877–879, 913–914, 1099–1103,1104–1105, 1239–1241.

Post, L.O., Keller, W.C., 1999. An update of antidote availability in veterinary medicine. Vet. Human Toxicol. 41, 258–261.

Richardson, J.A., 2000a. Permethrin spot-on toxicoses in cats. J. Vet. Emerg. Crit. Care. 10, 103–106.

Richardson, J.A., 2000b. Management of acetaminophen and ibuprofen toxicosis in dogs and cats. J. Vet. Emerg. Crit. Care. 10, 285–291.

Richardson, J.A., Khan, S.A., Means, C., Murphy, L.A., 2001. Managing pet bird toxicoses. Exotic DVM. 3.1, 23–27.

Richardson, J.A., Gwaltney-Brant, S.M., Huffman, J.D., et al., 2003. Metaldehyde toxicoses in dogs. Comp. Cont. Educ. Pract. Vet. 25, 376–379.

Rosendale, M.E., 2002. Decontamination strategies. Vet. Clin. North Am. Small Anim. Pract. 32, 311–321.

Rumbeiha, W.K., Braselton, W.E., Fitzgerald, S.D., et al., 2000. Use of pamidronate disodium to reduce cholecalciferol-induced toxicosis in dogs. Am. J. Vet. Res. 60, 9–13.

Schell, M.M., 2000. Tremorgenic mycotoxin intoxication. Vet. Med. 95, 283–286.

Stair, E.L., Plumlee, K.H., 2004. Blister beetles. In: Plumlee, K.H. (Ed.), Clinical Veterinary Toxicology. Mosby, St. Louis, MO, pp. 101–103.

Taylor, N.S., Dhupa, N., 2000. Acetaminophen toxicity in cats and dogs. Comp. Cont. Educ. Pract. Vet. 22, 160–170.

Vite, C.H., Gfeller, R.W., 1994. Suspected albuterol intoxication in a dog. J. Vet. Emerg. Crit. Care. 4, 7–12.

Volmer, P.A., 2004. Pyrethrins and pyrethroids. In: Plumlee, K.H. (Ed.), Clinical Veterinary Toxicology. Mosby, St. Louis, MO, pp. 188–190.

Volmer, P.A., 2006. "Recreational" drugs. In: Peterson, M.E., Talcott, P.A. (Eds.), Small Animal Toxicology, second ed. Elsevier Inc, St. Louis, MO, pp. 273–311.

Ward, D.M., DeFrancesco, T.C., Forrester, S.D., Troy, G.C., 1999. Treatment of severe chronic digoxin toxicosis in a dog with cardiac disease, using ovine digoxin-specific immunoglobulin G Fab fragments. J. Am. Vet. Med. Assoc. 215, 1808–1812.

Wismer, T., 2004. Baclofen overdose in dogs. Vet. Med. 99, 406–410.

Wismer, T.A., 2002. Accidental ingestion of alprazolam in 415 dogs. Vet. Human Toxicol. 44, 22–23.

Index

Note: Page numbers followed by "*f*" and "*t*" refer to figures and tables, respectively.

B

C

D

E

F

G

H

I

J

K

L

M

N

O

P

Q

R

T

U